Anesthesia Review

Anesthesia Review

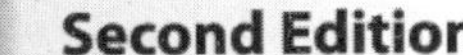

Second Edition

Kaushik Jothinath
MBBS DNB FIACTA FCA
Consultant Pediatric Cardiac Anesthesiologist
G Kuppuswamy Naidu Memorial Hospital
Coimbatore, Tamil Nadu, India

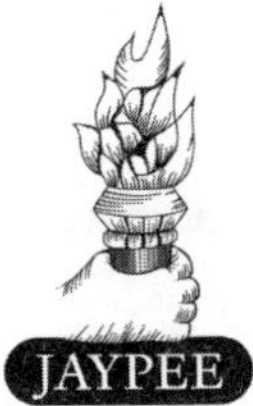

JAYPEE BROTHERS MEDICAL PUBLISHERS
The Health Sciences Publisher
New Delhi | London

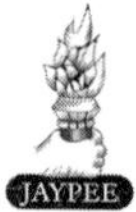

Jaypee Brothers Medical Publishers (P) Ltd

Headquarters
EMCA House
23/23-B, Ansari Road, Daryaganj
New Delhi 110 002, India
Landline: +91-11-23272143, +91-11-23272703
+91-11-23282021, +91-11-23245672
E-mail: jaypee@jaypeebrothers.com

Corporate Office
Jaypee Brothers Medical Publishers (P) Ltd.
4838/24, Ansari Road, Daryaganj
New Delhi 110 002, India
Phone: +91-11-43574357
Fax: +91-11-43574314
E-mail: jaypee@jaypeebrothers.com

Overseas Office
JP Medical Ltd.
83, Victoria Street, London
SW1H 0HW (UK)
Phone: +44-20 3170 8910
E-mail: info@jpmedpub.com

EU GPSR Authorised Representative
Logos Europe, 9 rue Nicolas Poussin
17000, La Rochelle, France
Phone: +33 (0) 6 67 93 73 78
E-mail: Contact@logoseurope.eu

Website: www.jaypeebrothers.com
Website: www.jaypeedigital.com

Inquiries for bulk sales may be solicited at: jaypee@jaypeebrothers.com

Anesthesia Review

First Edition: 2016

Second Edition: **2021** Reprint : 2024, 2025, 2026

ISBN 978-93-90020-75-1

Printed at K.K. Printers, Kundli, Haryana-131 028.

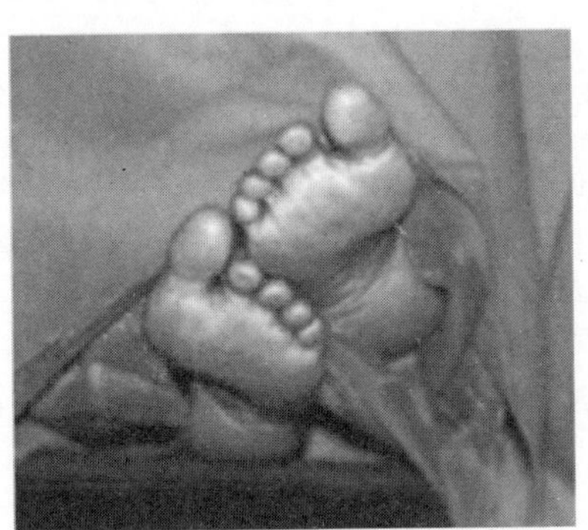

AT THY LOTUS FEET

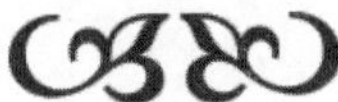

Preface

It was during my postgraduate years that I realized that the subject of anesthesiology does not have a comprehensive and examination-oriented book. The pursuit of DNB as a postgraduation degree itself is an arduous task, owing to the difficult work schedule, and high expectations from the students at the time of examinations. This problem is compounded manifold for the subject of anesthesiology, as it is a discipline in which the students have to have a wide base of knowledge.

Most of the textbooks available today are not student-friendly as there is a lot of information in them, from which the examinee has to pick and retain in memory only those details which are necessary. As a result, there is a whole lot of unwanted information to which he is subjected, which may be confusing at the time of examinations. Secondly, there is no single textbook which gives all the details in an examination-oriented format. As a result, the student is forced to study from several different textbooks spanning multiple subjects. Also, owing to the importance of knowledge of various clinical guidelines, it becomes mandatory for the anesthesiology examinee to be familiar with the latest guidelines across a wide variety of disciplines. I have attempted to address these problems by compiling a book, which is student-friendly, well researched and is based on the most recent clinical practice guidelines.

This book has been written to cater to the DNB anesthesiology board examinations in a comprehensive and point-based system. Also, most of the references are from standard textbooks in order to prevent confusion arising due to numerous research papers published in the recent past.

Therefore, the information has been provided in a highly concise, crisp and readable manner to help you crack the anesthesiology boards.

Hope you enjoy reading it and wishing you all the best to crack your boards!!

Kaushik Jothinath

Acknowledgments

My humble gratitude to my teacher, father figure and guiding spirit, Dr Krishnadasan, without whom this book would not have materialized. Your encouragement and motivation have been vital in bringing forth this second edition.

I am also indebted to Dr Sathya Swaroop Patnaik for his help during those difficult years when life looked uncertain. He was an invaluable guide and helping hand, who showed me the way during this arduous journey. Bhishma sir, the man who lives up to his name, will always be remembered for the exceptional moral support he gave, during those years.

I sincerely acknowledge all my anesthesiology professors Dr Debadas Bagchi, Dr Pandey, Dr Anand, Dr Hemadri, Dr Kolli S Challam, Dr Prabhakar, Dr Jayashree Simha, Dr Iyer, Dr Vasanth Nayak, Dr Prabhakar, Dr Parameshwar, Dr Suma, Dr Murthy, Dr Rehana, Dr Jalaja, Dr Ramachandra, Dr Sowmini, Dr Kumaresan, Dr Manjunath, Dr Niranjan, Dr Vaishali and Dr Anita for their enormous help and guidance during the formative years of this book. I am also immensely thankful to my mentors Dr Vindhya Kumar, Dr Shivananda N.V and Dr Nagaraj. I have been immensely lucky to have learnt the art of anesthesia from you all.

My humble gratitude to the CEO of GKNM hospital Dr. Raghupathy Veluswamy for the immense support given to me for the second edition of this book. I would also like to thank my teachers in the department of Anesthesiology, GKNM hospital, Dr Rajani Sundar, Dr Soundaravalli Balakrishnan, Dr Sai Gopalakrishnan, Dr Anandhi Arul and Dr Palaniappan for being the sturdy, unrelenting backbone behind the entire process of giving shape to the second edition.

I am also thankful to my colleagues Dr Karthik Babu, Dr Manikandan and Dr Naresh Kumar from GKNM Hospitals for their valuable guidance and support.

I sincerely acknowledge Dr S Muralidharan, Dr P Chandrashekhar, Dr Sundar Ramanathan, Dr Madhav Rao and Dr Shobha Menon from GKNM Hospitals for their valuable inputs into this book.

My acknowledgement would be incomplete if I do not mention my colleague and friend Dr Vijayakumar Raju who inspires everyone around with his sheer hard work and will power as a congenital heart surgeon.

I will be indebted to my closest friend Mahesh T. Venkataramani, whose constant inputs and feedback at various stages made this book what it is

My biggest source of strength has been my group of friends, Dr Satya Swaroop Patnaik, Dr Anoop Pothen John, Dr Gokulakrishnan, Dr Aamir Farooq Siddique, Dr Abhinay Indrakumar Reddy and Dr Sandeepan.

I also appreciate the continuous moral support given by my parents and wife during this process. Thank you for your patience.

I am also thankful to all my colleagues and staff at Sri Sathya Sai Institute of Higher Medical Sciences, Manipal Hospital and GKNM hospital for rendering a helping hand.

I appreciate Shri Jitendar P Vij (Group Chairman) and Mr Ankit Vij (Managing Director), M/S Jaypee Brothers Medical Publishers (P) Ltd, for their patience, encouragement and punctuality for publishing this book.

I would also like to thank Ms Chetna Malhotra Vohra (Associate Director–Content and Strategy), Ms Saima Rashid (Publishing Manager) and Mr Santosh Kumar (Commissioning Editor) from Jaypee Brothers for their thoughtful insights into making this second edition a more user friendly version.

Finally I would like to thank all my students for making the first edition of this book an enormous success story.

I owe this book to everyone who contributed directly or indirectly. Any oversight is purely unintentional.

Contents

1 CHAPTER

Anesthetic Pharmacology

DRUG INTERACTIONS

Classification

- Pharmaceutical interactions
- Pharmacokinetic interactions:
  - Absorption
  - Distribution
  - Cardiac output alterations
  - Ion trapping
  - Protein binding
  - Metabolism
  - Hepatic biotransformation
  - Elimination
- Pharmacodynamic interactions:
  - Affecting hemodynamics
  - Affecting analgesia/hypnosis

Problems Due to Drug Interactions

- One drug may antagonize action of other
- Toxicity due to drug interaction
- Reduced therapeutic window of warfarin/digoxin/theophylline
- Unable to identify the drug producing clinical effect
- Increased idiosyncratic reactions: MAO inhibitors with meperidine

Pharmaceutical Interaction

Introduction

Chemical/physical interaction which occurs before a drug is administered/absorbed systemically.

Types

- Incompatibility between two drugs in solution:
  - Thiopentone precipitates when given with succinylcholine
  - Sodium bicarbonate reduces solubility of bupivacaine and precipitates it
  - Sodium bicarbonate inactivates catecholamines
- Drugs forming toxic compounds:
  - Halogenated agents + Baralyme → CO + heat
  - Sevoflurane + Baralyme → Sevo-olefin
  - $NO + O_2 \rightarrow NO_2$ (toxic at > 10 ppm concentration)

Pharmacokinetic Interactions

I. Absorption

- Altered mechanism of absorption:
  - Oral tetracycline inactivated with $Mg^{2+}/Ca^{2+}/Al^{3+}$ antacids
  - Oral anti-diarrheals (kaolin/pectin) absorb digoxin
  - Bile acid binding residue cholestyramine binds to warfarin and reduces absorption
- Reduced regional perfusion:
  - Reduced local anesthetic absorption when adrenaline added

II. Distribution

- Cardiac output altering distribution:
  - Thiopentone/propofol/remifentanyl causes reduced cardiac output
  - Volatile anesthetics reduce cardiac output and have increased CNS effect
- Ion trapping:
  - Drug induced changes in pH causing altered distribution
  - Antacids/H_2 blockers/proton pump inhibitors reduce absorption of acidic drugs
  - Altered urinary pH affects renal clearance of drugs
- Plasma protein binding:
  - Displacement of bilirubin by sulphonamides causing *kernicterus*
  - Displacement of warfarin by phenylbutazone/phenytoin

III. Metabolism

- Acetylcholine esterases/nonspecific esterases:
  - Neostigmine/pyridostigmine increases succinylcholine effects

- Neostigmine increases action of ester local anesthetics:
  - Procaine
  - Cocaine
  - Tetracaine

❖ MAO inhibitors interaction:
- They increase action of indirect acting sympathomimetics:
  - Ephedrine
  - Amphetamine
- They may cause hypertensive crises due to tyramine present in aged cottage cheese: ***Wine and cheese reaction***
- They increase action of direct acting sympathomimetics to a lesser extent:
  - Epinephrine,
  - Norepinephrine
- When given with meperidine it causes ***serotonin syndrome***:
  - Excitation and hyperpyrexia
  - HTN, diaphoresis, rigidity
  - Seizures, coma and death

IV. Hepatic Biotransformation

❖ Drugs with high extraction ratio (ER $\geq$ 0.7):
- Examples of drugs with high ER:
  - Lidocaine
  - Propranolol
- Blood flow to liver is rate limiting as metabolism is at maximum
- Lidocaine concentration increases due to:
  - Reduced hepatic blood flow due to reduced cardiac output
  - Vasopressors: Isoproterenol and noradrenaline

❖ Drugs with low extraction ratio (ER $\leq$ 0.3):
- Examples of drugs with low ER:
  - Diazepam
  - Mepivacaine
  - Alfentanyl
- Activity of hepatic enzymes is rate limiting as enzyme induction can increase metabolism
- Midazolam and fentanyl are competitive inhibitors of CYP3A4
- Propofol inhibits CYP3A4 and reduces clearance of midazolam by 37%
- Erythromycin increases effect of alfentanyl
- Cimetidine inhibits metabolism of warfarin, diazepam, phenytoin and morphine
- Ketoconazole inhibits clearance of midazolam, theophylline, warfarin and digoxin
- Etomidate inhibits cytochrome P450 dependant 17 α hydroxylase and 11 β hydroxylase
- This causes reduced synthesis of cortisol and aldosterone

❖ Enzyme inducers:
- Phenobarbitone
- Phenytoin
- Rifampicin
- Carbamezipine
- Ethanol

❖ Enzyme inhibitors:
- Cimetidine
- Ketoconazole
- Erythromycin
- Disulfiram
- Ritonavir

V. Elimination

❖ Ion trapping: Phenobarbital (weak acid) excretion is increased in acidic urine

❖ Ion secretion:
- Probenecid inhibits secretion of penicillin
- Quinidine reduces V_d and clearance of digoxin

Pharmacodynamic Interactions

I. Additive Interactions

❖ Occurs when drugs with similar mechanism of action are combined

❖ Rocuronium + vecuronium: Additive effect

❖ 2 volatile anesthetics or N_2O + VA: Additive effect

II. Antagonistic Interaction

❖ SCH + NDMR

❖ Neostigmine + NDMR

❖ Flumazenil + Benzodiazepines

❖ Naloxone + opioid

❖ Butorphanol + midazolam: increased sedation but less anterograde amnesia than midazolam alone

III. Synergistic Interaction

❖ Small doses of 2 drugs producing larger effects

❖ Opioid potentiation by NSAIDs

❖ NDMR potentiation by volatile anesthetics

❖ Aminosteriod + benzylisoquinoline NDMR

IV. Pharmacodynamic Interactions Affecting Hemodynamics

❖ Tricyclic antidepressants can increase effects of direct/indirect acting agonists

❖ β_2 agonists may cause tachycardia and ectopic rhythms

V. Interactions Affecting Analgesia/Hypnosis

- Opioid – hypnotic:
  - Fentanyl reduces barbiturate need
  - Opioids potentiate propofol
- Opioid – Benzodiazepine:
  - Fentanyl potentiates midazolam
- Opioid – volatile anesthetic:
  - Fentanyl at 1.67 ng/mL blood concentration reduces isoflurane MAC by 50%
  - Butorphanol and nalbuphine also reduces MAC
- Benzodiazepine – hypnotic
  - Thiopentone potentiates midazolam
  - Propofol hypnosis increased with midazolam
- α_2 agonist interaction:
  - Dexmedetomidine potentiates opioids and benzodiazepines (BZDs)
  - Dexmedetomidine reduces halothane MAC by almost 100%
- Three way interactions:
  - Propofol dose reduces by 86% in combination with midazolam and alfentanyl
  - Enflurane MAC reduces with dexmedetomidine and fentanyl

THIOPENTONE

Introduction

- Introduced by Waters and Lundy in 1934
- Thio-barbiturate which is commonly used as a hypnotic inducing agent

Chemistry

- Derivative of barbituric acid formed by condensation of urea and malonic acid
- Oxygen in barbituric acid replaced by:
  - Sulphur at urea derived carbon position 2
  - Branched chain group at carbon position 5
- This gives the drug short duration of action
- S (–) isomers of thiopental are more potent than R (+) isomers
- Commercial preparations are racemic mixtures

Presentation

- Hygroscopic yellow powder
- Clinically used as 2.5% solution
- Contains thiopentone with 6% anhydrous Na_2CO_3 stored under atmosphere of nitrogen
- Nitrogen prevents precipitation of insoluble acid formed by atmospheric carbon dioxide
- Solution has highly alkaline bacteriostatic properties with pH of 10.8 and pKa of 7.6
- Reconstitution:
  - Should not be reconstituted with Lactated Ringers or acidic solutions
  - This will cause a reduction in alkalinity of the solution
  - Thus, barbiturates will precipitate as free acids
  - Once reconstituted, it can be used for 1 week if refrigerated

Mechanism of Action

- Two principle mechanisms of action:
  - Enhancement of synaptic actions of inhibitory neurotransmitters: GABA receptors
  - Blockade of synaptic actions of excitatory neurotransmitters:
    - Inhibits synaptic transmission of glutamate, adenosine receptors
    - This blocks excitatory CNS transmission
- At $GABA_A$ receptors:
  - Positive allosteric modulation:
    - Thiopentone binds to $GABA_A$ receptor
    - This increases channel opening time of Cl^- channels
    - Thus chloride conductance through the ion channel increases
    - This causes hyperpolarization of the cell membrane
    - Thus, threshold of excitability of postsynaptic neuron is increased
  - Reduces dissociation of GABA from receptors:
    - Occurs at lower concentrations
    - Rate of dissociation of GABA from $GABA_A$ receptor is reduced
    - This causes sustained inhibition of RAS
    - This may be responsible for hypnotic action of thiopentone
  - Mimics GABA action by directly stimulating $GABA_A$ receptors

Pharmacodynamics

- Central nervous system: Cerebro-protective effect:
  - Sedation
  - Rapid induction of anesthesia
  - *Antalgesic in lower doses:* Reduces pain threshold
  - Anti-convulsant
  - Depresses respiratory center
  - Depresses vasomotor center
  - *Retrograde amnesia: Midazolam causes anterograde amnesia*

- Reduced cerebral blood flow, cerebral vasoconstriction
- Reduces ICP, depresses cerebral metabolism
- Reduces intra-ocular pressure

❖ Respiratory system:
- Depresses respiratory center:
  - Causes transient apnea
  - This is followed by a more prolonged period of respiratory depression
- Preserves laryngeal reflexes
- Coughing, laryngeal spasm, bronchoconstriction especially in asthmatics
- Reduces ventilatory response to hypercarbia

❖ Cardiovascular system:
- Hypotension and tachycardia
- Negative inotropism
- Reduces cardiac output by about 20%
- Reduces peripheral vascular resistance

❖ Genitourinary system:
- Reduces renal plasma flow
- Increases ADH secretion
- Reduces urine output
- Uterine tone is unaffected
- Crosses blood-placental barrier
- Fetal plasma concentration is lower and more delayed

❖ Autonomic nervous system:
- Reduces intestinal activity
- Constriction of splanchnic vasculature
- Inhibits vasomotor center
- Constriction of pupil followed by dilatation
- Loss of pupillary and eyelash reflexes

❖ Metabolic: Transient reduction in K^+ levels

Dosage

❖ Intravenous: given as 2.5% solution (25 mg/mL) in a dose of 3–5 mg/kg

❖ Can be given rectally as 5–10% solution in a dose of 50 mg/kg body weight

Pharmacokinetics

❖ Onset of action: within *one brain arm circulation time (30 seconds)*

❖ Duration of action: 5–10 minutes

❖ Absorption: Absorbed when given orally/rectally

❖ Distribution:
- 72–86% protein bound, mostly to albumin
- Volume of distribution 2.5 L/kg
- Lipid soluble, un-ionized form of the drug crosses BBB
- Rapid onset of action as:
  - High blood flow to brain
  - Lipophilicity of drug
  - Low degree of ionization

❖ Redistribution:
- Initial high uptake of drug by the brain causes plasma concentration to decrease
- This results in reversal of the concentration gradient
- This causes movement of the drug back into blood subsequently
- Accounts for the brief duration of anesthesia following bolus dose of thiopentone

❖ Metabolism:
- Hepatic metabolism with extraction ratio of 0.15 (low)
- Indicates that approximately 15% of the drug presented to the liver is extracted
- Oxidation results in formation of active metabolite pentobarbital
- Initially after bolus dose, decay follows first order kinetics
- With longer infusions and higher doses hepatic metabolic capacity is exceeded
- This results in zero order kinetics
- Thiopentone causes hepatic enzyme induction

❖ Excretion:
- Predominantly in urine
- Excreted as inactive metabolic
- Less than 1% is directly eliminated unchanged in urine

Implications of Pharmacokinetics

❖ Dose should be reduced in CRF and liver failure patients as serum albumin will be low: More amount of free drug in circulation

❖ Concurrent administration of warfarin and aspirin may displace thiopentone from proteins resulting in toxicity

❖ Dose should be reduced in hypovolemia as blood flow to skeletal muscle is reduced while brain and heart perfusion is maintained

Clinical Uses

❖ Induction of anesthesia:
- 3–5 mg/kg IV is induction dose
- Loss of consciousness (LOC) occurs in one brain-arm circulation time (30 seconds)
- LOC lasts for around 5–15 minutes

❖ Treatment of raised ICT:
- Produces cerebral vasoconstriction and reduces cerebral blood flow

- 37.5 mg/kg thiopentone required to produce iso-electric EEG
- Hemodynamic instability may complicate high dose thiopentone
- Thiopentone is preferred to isoflurane for raised ICT
- Isoflurane requires 2 MAC to produce equivalent EEG suppression

❖ Cerebral protection:
- Useful in focal ischemia, but not global cerebral ischemia like in cardiac arrest
- Reduces incidence of neuropsychiatric complications following cardiopulmonary bypass
- Cerebral protection occurs due to:
  - Reduction in $CMRO_2$
  - Reverse steal phenomenon ***(Robin Hood effect)*** on CBF
  - Free radical scavenging
  - Stabilization of lysosomal membranes
  - Excitatory amino acid receptor blockade

❖ To verify wet epidural tap:

❖ Used to verify if the fluid coming out of the epidural catheter is CSF or LA

❖ Local anesthetic (LA) solutions are highly acidic preparations

❖ If fluid coming out of catheter is LA solution, thiopentone being highly alkaline will precipitate on being added

Side Effects

❖ Cardiovascular:
- Myocardial depression especially when given in high doses
- Hypotension due to peripheral venodilatation
- Histamine release: Hypotension
- Heat loss and hypothermia due to vasodilation

❖ Respiratory:
- Transient apnea
- Bronchospasm/laryngospasm during intubation if inadequate depression of laryngeal reflexes by barbiturates

❖ Liver: Modest reduction in hepatic blood flow

❖ Kidney: Modest reduction in renal blood flow and GFR

❖ Tolerance

❖ Venous thrombosis:
- Due to deposition of barbiturate crystals in the vein
- Occurs frequently when vecuronium is given after thiopentone injection
- Diluting thiopentone injection to 2.5% reduces this incidence

❖ Intra-arterial injection:
- Clinical features:
  - Immediate intense pain
  - Vasoconstriction with blanching of extremity
  - This can result in cyanosis and gangrene
- Mechanism of action:
  - Endothelial damage causes inflammatory response
  - This leads to arteritis and micro-embolization causing occlusion of artery
- Treatment and prevention:
  - Use only 2.5% solution thiopentone
  - Let angio-catheter remain in place
  - If angio-catheter has been removed:
    - Inject vasodilator into more proximal location in artery
    - Injected more proximally because affected artery will be in spasm
  - Inject saline into angio-catheter to dilute the drug
  - Lidocaine, apaverine and phenoxybenzamine used to produce vasodilation
  - Heparin/urokinase is considered if thrombosis occurs
  - Sympathetic blockade: stellate ganglion/brachial plexus block may be used

❖ Allergic reaction:
- May occur even without prior exposure to thiopentone
- Aggressive and early therapy with epinephrine, fluids and steroids
- Unusually high mortality rate

❖ Immuno-suppression:
- Bone marrow suppression and leucopenia occurs
- Also inhibits neutrophil function
- Occurs with long term and high dose administration
- Results in increased incidence of nosocomial infections

Contraindications

❖ Porphyria:
- Thiopentone causes hepatic enzyme induction
- Thus, it may stimulate the enzyme δ- aminolevulinic acid synthetase
- This is the enzyme responsible for production of porphyrins
- Thus, acute worsening of porphyria may result

❖ Status asthmaticus

❖ Shock, pericardial tamponade

❖ Uncompensated myocardial disease

PROPOFOL

Introduction

Propofol is a substituted isopropylphenol which is commonly used as an induction agent in anesthesia.

Chemistry

- Chemically 2–6 disopropylphenol
- Propofol unlike ketamine and thiopentone is a non-chiral compound

Presentation

- Propofol is an oily compound which is insoluble in water
- Therefore, it requires a lipid vehicle for emulsification
- Commercial preparations contain propofol molecule, a carrier and preservative compound
- Preservatives are used because the lipid carrier acts as a potent medium for bacterial growth

Preparations

- There are various preparations for propofol depending on:
  - Carrier molecule
  - Propofol concentration
  - Preservative compound
- The various preparations are:
  - Generic propofol:
    - Contents:
      - 1% propofol
      - 2.25% glycerol
      - 10% soyabean oil
      - 1.2% egg phosphatide
    - Preservative used: sodium metabisulfite
    - pH: 4.5–6.5
  - Cremophor EL:
    - Earlier used as the carrier
    - Withdrawn due to anaphylaxis
  - Diprivan:
    - Contents:
      - 1% propofol
      - 2.25% glycerol
      - 10% soyabean oil
      - 1.2% egg phosphatide
    - Preservatives: NaOH, disodium edetate (EDTA)
    - pH: 7–8.5
  - Ampofol low-lipid emulsion
    - Contents:
      - 1% propofol
      - 0.6% egg lecithin
      - 0.5% soyabean oil
    - Preservatives: None because of low lipids
    - Equipotent to diprivan but causes more pain or injection
    - Less bacterial growth
  - Aquavan:
    - Alternative to lipid emulsion formulations
    - It is water soluble
    - Contains pro-drug *fospropofol* (phosphorylated pro-drug)
    - Propofol is liberated after hydrolysis by alkaline phosphatases
    - Prevents lipid associated side effects like:
      - Pain, hypertriglyceridemia
      - Pulmonary embolism
    - Properties:
      - Larger V_d
      - Higher potency
      - Longer time to peak effect
      - Prolonged pharmacological action
  - Non-lipid formulations with cyclodextrin carrier:
    - Structurally sugar molecules
    - Forms guest-host complexes which migrate between hydrophilic center of the cyclodextrin molecular and the water soluble phase
    - After injection, propofol migrates out of the cydodextrin into blood
  - 2% formulations:
    - Contains 2% propofol and medium to long chain fatty acids
    - Decreased incidence of pain on injection due to long chain and medium chains
    - Mixing of propofol with any drug is not recommended
    - May be mixed with lignocaine to reduce pain on injection
    - This may result in coalescence of oil droplets causing pulmonary embolism

Mechanism of Action

- $GABA_A$ receptor:
  - Propofol binds to β subunit of $GABA_A$ receptor
  - α and γ_2 subunits also contribute to modulatory effects of propofol on $GABA_A$
  - Prevents dissociation of GABA from the receptor
  - This causes prolonged activation of the receptor
  - Chloride influx occurs as a result causing hyperpolarization and inhibition of post-synaptic neurons
- Inhibits ACH release in hippocampus through $GABA_A$ action
- Inhibits NMDA receptor

Pharmacodynamics

- Central nervous system:
  - Rapid smooth induction
  - Rapid and clear headed recovery
  - Cerebroprotective:
    - Antioxidant properties
    - Reduces intra-cranial pressure, $CMRO_2$ and cerebral perfusion pressure
  - Cerebrovascular autoregulation and reaction to changes in $PaCO_2$ not affected
  - Produces burst suppression on EEG: Anti-convulsant
  - Produces same degree of memory impairment as midazolam
  - Seizures and abnormal motor activity may sometimes occur
  - Tolerance occurs to repeated dosing
  - Increases dopamine in *nucleus accumbens*: Results in drug abuse
- Cardiovascular system:
  - Decrease in:
    - Arterial blood pressure:
      - Reduction in systolic, diastolic and mean pressures
      - Effects exaggerated in old patients, hypovolemia and LV dysfunction due to CAD
      - Inhibits baroreceptor reflex to hypotension
    - PVR: Due to more impotent inhibition of sympathetic nervous tone
    - Cardiac output, stroke volume index and cardiac index:
      - Occurs due to reduced intracellular Ca^{2+} availability
      - This is secondary to inhibition of trans-sarcolemmal Ca^{2+} influx
  - Heart rate:
    - May increase, decrease or remain unchanged
    - Response depends on hypotension and baroreceptor suppression
    - Causes bradycardia and asystole sometimes
    - Heart rate response to atropine is attenuated
    - Bradycardia is reversed by isoprenaline
  - Does not alter SA node or AV node function: safe in WPW syndrome and ablative procedures
  - Suppresses supra-ventricular tachycardia
  - Potentiates oculocardiac reflex
- Respiratory system:
  - Produces short duration apnea (30–60 sec) after induction in 25–30% patients
  - Decreases tidal volume and frequency of breathing
  - Response to CO_2 and hypoxemia is reduced by direct action on carotid body receptors
  - Produces bronchodilation and reduces intraoperative wheezing
  - Hypoxic pulmonary vasoconstriction is intact but attenuated
  - *Laryngeal reflexes are lost*
- Hepatic and renal functions:
  - Prolonged infusion:
    - Causes hepatocellular injury resulting in acidosis
    - Increases phenols in urine:
      - This causes phenol urea resulting in green color urine
      - However, it does not alter renal function
  - Urinary uric acid excretion increases resulting in turbid urine
  - Decreases hepatic blood flow
- Intraocular pressure:
  - Decreases intraocular pressure following intubation
  - Potentiates oculo-cardiac reflex
- Coagulation: Does not alter coagulation profile

Pharmacokinetics

- Distribution:
  - Volume of distribution 3.5–4.5 L/kg
  - 97% is plasma protein bound
  - Onset of action: 30–45 seconds (one brain-arm circulation time)
  - Duration of unconsciousness produced is around 10 minutes
- Metabolism: Undergoes hepatic and extra-hepatic metabolism:
  - Hepatic metabolism:
    - Rapid metabolism
    - Conjugation to soluble, inactive compounds with glucuronide and sulfate
    - Cytochrome P_{450} actions:
      - Ring hydroxylation occurs forming 4-hydroxypropofol
      - This has one-third the hypnotic activity of propofol
  - ***Extrahepatic metabolism***:
    - Lungs:
      - Are responsible for 30% uptake and first pass elimination after bolus dose
      - Propofol is metabolized to 2-disopropyl-quinol
    - Kidney and brain: Contains UDP-glucuronyl transferase
- Excretion:
  - Less than 0.3% excreted unchanged in kidneys
  - Metabolites are also excreted in kidney
  - 2% is eliminated in feces

- No influence of renal dysfunction on renal clearance
- Hepatic dysfunction also does not affect elimination

❖ Fospropofol
- Endothelial cell alkaline phosphatase hydrolyses it to release propofol
- Each mg of fospropofol liberates 0.54 mg of propofol

Clinical Uses

❖ Induction of anesthesia:
- Results in rapid induction with rapid and smooth recovery
- Induction dose: 1.5–2.5 mg/kg IV in adults
- Higher doses in children due to higher central compartment volume and clearance rate
- Complete awakening results without residual CNS effects

❖ Intravenous sedation:
- 25–100 µg/kg/min IV infusion
- Prompt recovery occurs following stoppage of infusion
- Low incidence of postoperative nausea and vomiting

❖ Maintenance of anesthesia:
- 100–300 µg/kg/min IV infusion
- Used only for short procedures
- Longer procedures (72 hours): propofol not preferred due to higher cost

❖ Non-hypnotic therapeutic applications:
- Antiemetic effects:
  - Due to:
    - Reduced release of glutamate and aspartate in olfactory cortex
    - Inhibits CTZ and vagal nuclei
    - Has anti-dopaminergic properties
    - Also reduces serotonin levels in *area postrema*
  - 10–15 mg given IV (sub-hypnotic doses)
- Effective for PONV especially if non-vagal in nature and chemotherapy induced vomiting

❖ Antipruritc actions:
- 10 mg propofol given IV
- Due to ability to depress spinal cord activity
- Used for:
  - Pruritis due to intrathecal opioids
  - Cholestatic jaundice associated pruritis

❖ Anticonvulsant: 1 mg/kg IV reduces seizure duration in patients undergoing ECT

❖ Chronic intractable headache: 20–30 mg IV given every 3–4 minutes (maximum 400 mg)

❖ Also used for laryngospasm and for cerebroprotection

Immediate Side Effects

❖ Hypotension and bradycardia: augmented by concomitant opioids

❖ Pain on injection:
- *Most common* side effect
- Occurs especially on injection into smaller veins
- Preventive measures:
  - Inject into larger veins
  - Avoid veins on dorsum of hand
  - Pretreatment with opioids/NSAIDs
  - Prior administration of 1% lidocaine
  - Change carrier composition to long and medium chain fatty acids

❖ Allergic reactions:
- Was more with cremaphor-EL which was withdrawn from production
- Occurs due to isopropyl side chain and phenol nucleus

❖ Proconvulsant action:
- Spontaneous excitatory activity due to increased subcortical activity
- Caution in administration of propofol with poorly controlled epileptic patients
- Myoclonus associated with meningismus occurs in some cases

Side Effects on Prolonged Administration

❖ Bacterial growth:
- Lipid carrier is a potent culture medium
- Supports the growth of E. coli and pseudomonas
- Preventive measures:
  - Aseptic technique: Disinfect neck of ampule with 70% isopropyl alcohol
  - Withdraw drug with sterile syringe
  - Discard unused contests within 6 hours
  - Flush IV cannula after administration of drug

❖ Abuse potential:
- Due to dopamine accumulation in *nucleus accumbens*
- Causes intense dreaming, amorous behavior and sexual fantasies
- Hallucinations occur on recovery from effects of propofol

❖ *Propofol infusion syndrome*

❖ Pancreatitis: Due to prolonged administration of preparations with lipid carriers

❖ Thrombophlebitis in rare cases

❖ Hypertriglyceridemia

❖ Immunosuppression:
- Inhibits phagocytosis and killing of bacteria
- Reduces proliferative lymphocyte activity

PROPOFOL INFUSION SYNDROME

Introduction

Features which occurs in patients receiving propofol infusions for long duration (> 48 hrs).

Incidence

- More common in children
- More common if used for sedation in TBI
- Can occur with prolonged infusion (> 48 hrs)

Risk Factors

- Pediatric age group
- Cumulative dose:
  - > 75 μg/kg/min
  - > 4 mg/kg/hr
- Duration of infusion > 48 hrs
- Severe inciting illness
  - CNS origin (TBI)
  - Sepsis
  - Respiratory origin
  - Pancreatitis
- Catecholamines/corticosteroid supplementation
- Inadequate delivery of carbohydrates
- Subclinical mitochondrial disease

Pathophysiology

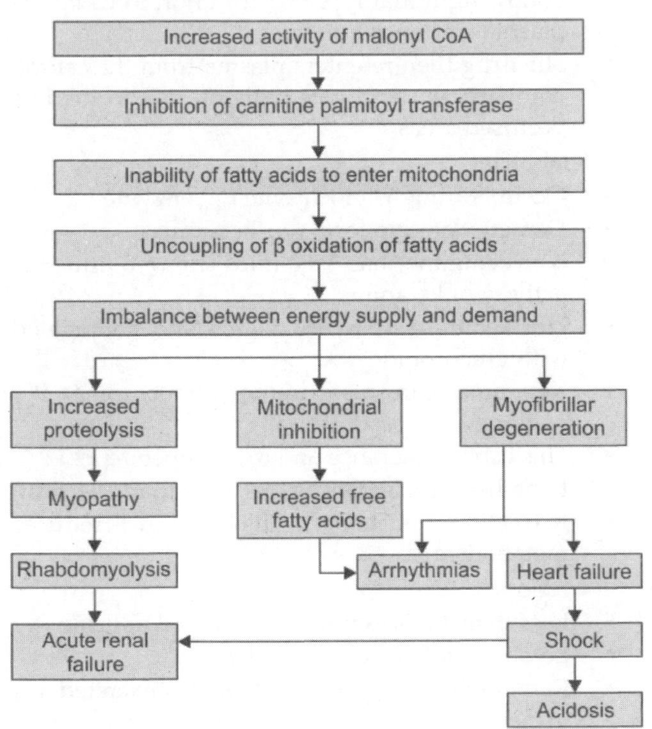

Clinical Features

- Profound metabolic acidosis (base deficit > 10 mmol/l)
- Lactic acidosis
- Hyperkalemia
- Hyperlipidemia hypertriglyceridemia
- Acute refractory bradycardia, sinus arrest, asystole
- Cardiomyopathy, cardiac failure, hypotension
- Fatty liver, hepatomegaly
- Skeletal myopathy, rhabdomyolysis
- Acute renal failure

Early Markers

- Unexplained metabolic acidosis
- Elevated serum lactate
- Elevated creatinine kinase
- Elevated myoglobin levels
- Hyperlipidemia
- ECG changes (ST segment elevation in V1 to V3)

Investigations

- ABG for metabolic acidosis
- Triglycerides
- Lactate
- Creatinine kinase
- Myoglobin

Prevention

- Avoid high dose propofol
- Minimize duration of infusion
- Avoid infusion in:
  - Children
  - Mitochondrial disease
- Early and adequate carbohydrate intake
- Avoid lipid overload
- High index of suspicion – serum triglycerides after 2 days of continuous infusion

Treatment

- Mainly supportive
- Stop propofol infusion
- Start alternative sedation
- Hemodynamic maintenance:
  - IV crystalloids/colloids
  - Vasopressors/inotropes
  - Transvenous pacing
- Nutritional support:
  - Avoid additional lipids
  - Add dextrose to IV fluids (4–8 mg/kg/hr glucose)

- Renal support:
  - Dialysis
  - Continuous renal replacement therapy
- Maintain oxygenation
- **ECMO** has been tried

KETAMINE

Introduction

This is a phencyclidine derivative widely used for induction of anesthesia.

Chemistry

- Phencyclidine derivative
- Two optical isomers:
  - S (+) and R (–) ketamine
  - Racemic mixture of the two is usually used commercially
  - Isomers are pharmacodynamically and pharmacokinetically different

No.	Property	S (+) Isomer	R (–) Isomer
1.	Action	More intense	Less intense
2.	Potency	Analgesia is four time more potent	Less potent
3.	Metabolism	Rapid hepatic biotransformation	Slower biotransformation
4.	Recovery	More rapid	Slower
5.	Emergence reaction	Lower incidence	Higher incidence
6.	Salivation	Less	More
7.	EEG suppression	More potent	Less potent
8.	Apoptosis	More anti-apoptotic	Less
9.	Therapeutic index	More	Less
10.	Affinity	More receptor affinity	Less

Preparation

- Available in 1%, 5% and 10% concentrations
- It is partially water soluble, 5 to 19 times as lipid soluble as thiopentone
- Preparation has a pKa of 7.5
- Preservative:
  - *Benzethonium chloride used as preservative which is neurotoxic*
  - S (+) isomer preparations do not have preservative (less neurotoxic)
  - Only these preservative free preparations are used for intrathecal administration

Mechanism of Action

- NMDA receptor:
  - Causes non-competitive inhibition of NMDA receptor
  - Decreases presynaptic glutamate release
  - Potentiates GABA effect
- Opioid receptors: Interacts with μ, κ and δ receptors
- Monoaminergic receptor: Interacts and thus interferes with pain pathway
- Muscarinic receptors:
  - Acts as an antagonist at muscarinic receptors
  - This causes the bronchodilator and delirious effects of ketamine
- Sodium channels: Attributes mild local anesthetic like properties
- Cytokines:
  - Suppresses neutrophil production of cytokines
  - Also, directly inhibits cytokines in circulation causing analgesic properties

Pharmacokinetics

- Distribution:
  - Less plasma protein bound
  - Large volume of distribution (V_d = 3 L/kg)
  - Rapid onset of action as:
    - Highly lipid soluble (5–10 times that of thiopentone)
    - Ketamine induced vasodilatation:
      - Causes increased cerebral blood flow
      - This causes increased drug delivery
  - Onset of action 30–60 seconds
- Redistribution:
  - Following initial rapid distribution to CNS, the plasma concentration falls
  - The drug then re-enters plasma from the central compartment and gets redistributed to the less perfused areas
- Metabolism:
  - Occurs through cytochrome P_{450} enzyme
  - Demethylated to form nor-ketamine
  - Nor-ketamine has one-third to one-fifth the activity of ketamine
  - Nor-ketamine is hydroxylated and conjugated with glucuronide
  - Ketamine can also induce cytochrome P_{450} enzyme
  - This causes tolerance and drug dependence
  - High hepatic clearance rate (more than 1 L/min)
  - Reduction in hepatic blood flow reduces metabolism
- Excretion:
  - Less than 4% is excreted unchanged in urine
  - Less than 5% is excreted in feces
  - Remaining conjugated metabolites excreted via urine

Pharmacodynamics

- Central nervous system:
  - Analgesia:
    - Greater for somatic non-visceral pain
    - Reduces spinal cord sensitization by blocking NMDA receptors in dorsal horn
    - Also reduces transmission of impulses in medullary RAS: Important for affective component of pain
  - Anesthesia: Called ***Dissociative Anesthesia***:
    - Definition: Cataleptic state where profound analgesia and amnesia occurs even though patient appears conscious and maintains protective reflexes
    - Mechanism:
      - Causes dissociation between thalamo-cortical tract and limbic system
      - Inhibition of thalamo-cortical tract occurs with stimulation of limbic system
      - This causes functional disorganization of nonspecific pathways in midbrain and thalamus
    - Characteristics:
      - It is a *cataleptic state*
      - Open eyes with slow and nystagmic gaze
      - Appears awake but non-communicative
      - Various degrees of hypertonus and purposeless skeletal muscle movements
      - Amnesia: No recall of surgery/anesthesia
      - Cough, swallowing and corneal reflexes are present
      - Reflexes should not be assumed to be protective
      - Profound analgesia present
  - Intracranial pressure:
    - Potent vasodilator
    - Increases cerebral blood flow by 60%
    - Increases ICP in normo-capneic patients
    - May cause reduction in ICP in ventilated patients
    - Cerebrovascular response to CO_2 is preserved
  - Neuro-protection:
    - Antagonist of NMDA receptors
    - This causes neuro-protection in cerebral ischemic states
  - EEG:
    - Abolishes α-rhythm
    - β-rhythm slowly progresses to δ-rhythm, which coincides with loss of consciousness
    - High doses cause burst suppression pattern
    - Has anti-convulsant activity though myoclonus may present occasionally
- Autonomic nervous system:
  - Pupillary dilation, nystagmus
  - Increased salivation and lacrimation
- Cardiovascular system:
  - Blood pressure:
    - Increases blood pressure
    - SBP increases by 20–40 mm Hg, DBP by smaller amount
    - Rise in BP occurs progressively during first 3–5 minutes
    - This is followed by a fall over next 20–30 minutes
  - Critically ill patients:
    - In these patients catecholamine stores are exhausted
    - Direct negative inotropic effect of ketamine may manifest in critically ill patients
    - Administration on ketamine may therefore cause cardiovascular collapse
  - Also increases heart rate, cardiac output, cardiac work, myocardial oxygen demand
  - Enhances arrhythmogenicity of adrenaline
  - Mechanisms of cardiovascular effect:
    - Direct stimulation of CNS resulting in increased central sympathetic flow
    - Inhibition of baroreceptor reflex through NMDA receptors in nucleus tractus solitarius
    - Inhibition of nor-epinephrine reuptake in post-ganglionic sympathetic nervous system: results in increased plasma catecholamine concentration
- Respiratory system:
  - Ventilation:
    - No significant depression of ventilation occurs
    - Has no effect on central respiratory drive
    - Ventilatory response to CO_2 is preserved
    - Breathing frequency reduced for 2–3 minutes after administration
    - Apneacan occur with large dose/with concomitant benzodiazepines
  - Upper airway reflexes:
    - Airway reflexes are preserved
    - However airway is not completely protected as silent aspiration may occur
  - Salivary and tracheo-bronchial secretions:
    - Ketamine increases trachea-bronchial and salivary secretion
    - Secretions are especially problematic in children as it causes laryngospasm
    - Pretreatment with anti-sialogogues mandatory

- Bronchodilation:
  - May be useful in asthmatics
  - Bronchodilation occurs due to:
    - Reduced uptake of catecholamines
    - Increasedlevels of circulating catecholamines
    - Muscarinic antagonism
    - Inhibition of Ca^{2+} channel
- Coagulation: Inhibits platelet aggregation by reducing formation of inositol 1, 4, 5 – triphosphate
- Hepatic and renal function: Not significantly altered

Clinical Uses

- Analgesia:
  - 0.2–5 mg/kg IV analgesic dose of ketamine
  - Indications:
    - Cancer pain
    - Chronic central and peripheral neuropathic pain
    - Fibromyalgia, migraine
    - Phantom limb and ischemic limb pain
    - Complex regional pain syndrome
- Neuraxial analgesia:
  - 0.5–1 mg/kg neuraxial dose of ketamine
  - Mechanism of action:
    - Due to systemic and spinal effects
    - Spinal effects:
      - Action on spinal opioid receptors
      - LA action through sodium channels
  - Affinity of ketamine is 10,000 times weaker than morphine
  - S (+) isomer preparations with no preservative is used
  - Preservative in the racemic mixture formulation is neurotoxic
- Induction of anesthesia:
  - Induction doses:
    - 1–2 mg/kg IV dose
    - 4–8 mg/kg IM dose
  - Consciousness is lost in 30–60 seconds after IV administration
  - Loss of consciousness occurs 2–4 minutes after IM administration
  - Return of consciousness occurs after 10–20 minutes
  - Full orientation attained 60–90 minutes after last dose
  - No retrograde amnesia present
  - Preferred agent in:
    - Children
    - Skin grafting/debridement/burn dressing
    - Hypovolemic shock
    - Known asthmatics/bronchospasm
    - Congenital heart disease especially with right to left shunts
    - Septic shock, provided catecholamine stores are intact
- Sedation:
  - 2 mg/kg/hr IV effusion used for postoperative sedation
  - Especially useful in pediatric patients for:
    - Cardiac catheterization
    - Radiotherapy/radiological studies
    - Dressing change
    - Dental work
- Adjunct to regional anesthesia:
  - 0.5 mg/kg IV given along with 0.03 mg/kg midazolam
  - Used during application of painful blocks
- Reversal of opioid tolerance:
  - Useful in reversing opioid tolerance
  - Acts through interactions between NMDA, nitric oxide pathway, and μ-opioid receptors
- Improvement of mental depression:
  - Postoperative depression unproved in patients with mental depression
  - Improves depression apart from providing analgesia in chronic pain syndrome
- ***Restless legs syndrome***: Inhibits neuro-inflammation in spinal cord

Contraindications

- Raised ICP, head trauma
- Open ocular injury: As ketamine increases IOP
- Ocular examination/operations: As ketamine causes nystagmus
- Schizophrenia, delirium tremens
- Coronary artery disease
- Pulmonary hypertension, right heart failure
- Systemic hypertension
- Vascular aneurysmal surgery

Side Effects

- Central nervous system:
  - Raised intracranial pressure, myoclonus
  - Nystagmus, raised intraocular pressure
- Central nervous system: Raised systemic BP, tachycardia
- Respiratory:
  - Transient apnea in rare cases
  - Sialorrhea and laryngospasm especially in children

- Allergic reactions: very rare
- Tolerance and drug abuse
- Increased bleeding tendency
- *Emergence reaction:*
  - Description: Emergence from ketamine anesthesia is associated with visual, auditory and proprioceptive illusions which may progress to delirium
  - Clinical features:
    - Transient cortical blindness, altered short term memory
    - Vivid and brightly colored dreams with morbid content and nightmares
    - Hallucinations:
      - May occur upto 24 hours after administration of ketamine
      - Usually disappear within a few hours
    - *Extra-corporeal experiences*:
      - Patient feels a sensation of floating out of body
      - This is due to lack of appreciation of gravity
      - Occurs due to reduced somatic and proprioceptive sensation
  - Incidence: Increased incidence in:
    - Females
    - Age more than 15 years: As children are unable to communicate the dreams occurance
    - Dosage more than 2 mg/kg IV
    - History of personality problems/frequent dreaming
  - Mechanisms:
    - Due to depression of inferior colliculus and medical geniculate body
    - This causes mis-interpretation of auditory and visual stimuli resulting in illusions
    - Extra-corporeal experiences due to κ-receptor stimulation
  - Prevention:
    - Pretreatment with benzodiazepines: Midazolam best
    - Co-administration of thiopental, inhaled anesthetics or propofol
    - Benzodiazepines given 5 minutes IV before ketamine usage
    - Prospective discussion with patients about side effects

Drug Interactions

- Hemodynamic depression rather than stimulation when used with:
  - Inhaled agents
  - Diazepam/midazolam
  - Verapamil
- Enhances neuromuscular blocking actions of non-depolarizing drugs
- Pancuronium enhances cardiac stimulating properties
- Succinylcholine apnea may be prolonged
- Seizures when aminophylline is given along with ketamine
- When used with tricyclic antidepressants (TCAs):
  - TCAs and ketamine prevent nor-epinephrine reuptake
  - This results in severe hypotension, cardiac failure and myocardial ischemia

ETOMIDATE

Introduction

- Initially developed as an anti-fungal agent
- Hypnotic activity discovered later during animal testing
- First introduced as an induction agent to clinical practice in 1972
- Unique properties of hemodynamic stability with minimal respiratory depression

Chemistry

- Carboxylated imidazole
- Structurally unrelated to other anesthetic agents
- Structurally R- (+) -pentylethyl-1H-imidazole-% carboxylate sulphate

Presentation

- Imidazole ring causes lipid solubility at physiological pH
- At acidic pH however, it becomes water soluble
- Thus, it is formulated as a 0.2% solution with 35% propylene glycol for injection
- This may be responsible for pain on injection

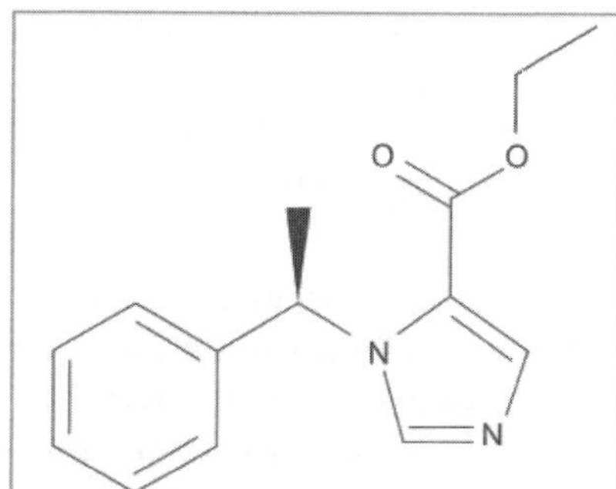

Fig. 1: Etomidate.

Mechanism of Action

- *Positive modulation* of GABA receptor:
  - Occurs at clinical doses
  - R+ isomer of etomidate binds to $GABA_A$ receptor
  - This increases the receptors affinity for GABA
  - Thus lower concentration of GABA is required to activate the $GABA_A$ receptor
- *Allosteric agonism*:
  - Occurs at high, supraclinical doses
  - Etomidate directly activates $GABA_A$ receptor
- *Disinhibitory effects*:
  - May have disinhibitory effect extrapyramidal pathways
  - Myoclonus seen in 30–60% of patients on induction with etomidate

Pharmacodynamics

- Central nervous system:
  - Decreases $CMRO_2$ (45%), cerebral blood flow (34%)
  - Produces a decline in intracranial pressure (50%)
  - Cerebral perfusion pressure increased or maintained
  - PONV more common than propofol or barbiturate
  - Lacks analgesic properties
  - Associated with grand mal seizures
  - EEG activity increases in epileptogenic foci
- Cardiovascular system:
  - Minimal effects on cardiovascular system- makes it a unique drug
  - Hemodynamic stability due to lack of effect on sympathetic nervous system
  - Causes mild reduction in peripheral vascular resistance, mean arterial pressure
  - Myocardial contractility and cardiac output are usually unchanged
  - Maintains myocardial oxygen demand-supply ratio
  - Useful in patients with valvular heart disease, IHD with poor cardiac function
- Respiratory system:
  - Less effects on respiratory system
  - Induction usually does not cause apnea unless opioids have been administered
  - May be associated with brief period of hyperventilation following induction
  - Does not induce histamine release
- Endocrine system:
  - Transiently inhibit enzymes involved in cortisol and aldosterone synthesis
  - Results in decreased cortisol synthesis and adrenocortical suppression
  - Dose-dependant reversible inhibition of 11β-hydroxylase
  - Adrenal suppression may last upto 72 hours following induction
  - Adrenal suppression action of etomidate more potent compared to sedation

Pharmacokinetics

- Onset of action:
  - Very rapid onset of action due to high lipid solubility
  - Large unionized fraction at physiological pH contributes to rapid onset
  - Hypnosis achieved in one brain-arm circulation time
- Duration of action:
  - Provides hypnosis for 5–10 minutes
  - Awakening occurs predominantly due to redistribution
- Absorption:
  - Oral transmucosal administration has been used in the past
  - Rectal administration has also been attempted
  - Available currently only for intravenous injection
- Distribution:
  - Highly protein bound (75% plasma protein bound)
  - Large peripheral V_d of 74.9 L/kg
- Metabolism:
  - By hepatic microsomal enzymes and plasma esterases
  - High hepatic extraction ratio 0.5 + 0.9
  - Rapidly hydrolyzed to carboxylic acid and an ethanol leaving group
- Excretion:
  - Elimination $T_{1/2}$ of 2.9–5.3 hours
  - Primarily excreted in urine
  - Renal excretion: 2% excreted unchanged, 85% as metabolites
  - Biliary elimination: 13% as metabolites

Clinical Uses

- Induction of anesthesia:
  - Especially useful in those with poor cardiovascular reserve
  - Reasonable choice during neurosurgical procedures
  - Useful in trauma patients with questionable intravascular volume status
- Short term sedation:
  - Useful in hemodynamically unstable patients
  - Useful for cardioversion, primary percutaneous intervention
- Maintenance of anesthesia: not used now due to adrenal suppression
- Treatment of Cushings syndrome
- Intraoperative mapping of seizure foci:
  - Useful to map foci prior surgical ablation
  - This is due to property of enhancing EEG activity in epileptogenic foci

Dosage

- Can be used in doses of 0.2–0.6 mg/kg IV for induction
- Usual induction dose is 0.3 mg/kg IV
- 0.04–0.05 mg/kg/hr infusion in refractory cases of Cushings

Adverse Effects

- Emergence delirium
- Pain on injection:
  - More with aqueous preparations compared with propylene glycol
  - Reduced with cyclodextrin and medium chain FA formulations
  - Reduced by IV xylocard 20–40 mg immediately prior to etomidate injection
- Nausea and vomiting
- Myoclonus:
  - Reduced by premedication with midazolam
  - Split dose induction has been useful in some studies
  - Thiopentone and dexmedetomidine have also been useful
  - Magnesium sulphate 60–90 seconds prior to injection reduces myoclonic activity

Validation

- *CORTICUS* trial:
  - Corticosteroid Therapy of Septic Shock trial
  - Enrolled 500 septic shock patients, 20% of whom received etomidate
  - Observed that patients receiving etomidate had higher 28-day mortality
  - Steroid supplementation provided no benefits in these patients
  - Other studies have reported conflicting results
  - Larger well designed trials are required to define the impact of single dose etomidate in critically ill patients

MIDAZOLAM

Introduction

This is a commonly used short acting benzodiazepine.

Chemistry

- Water soluble compound
- Imidazole ring present which accounts for:
  - Water solubility
  - Short duration of action
  - Rapid metabolism
- Non-chiral in nature: no isomers

Preparation

- Clear, colorless solution
- 1/2/5 mg/mL of solution for IV injection
- Midazolam syrup preparation has 2 mg/mL
- Acidic pH of 3.5
- Compatible with lactated Ringers solution
- Characterized by *pH dependant ring opening phenomenon:*
  - At pH less than 4, ring remains open and thus it is water soluble
  - At pH more than 4 (physiological pH), ring closes and it becomes a highly lipid soluble drug

Mechanism of Action

- Acts mainly through BZD receptors:
  - Found at synapses concentrated in cortex and mid-brain
  - These are closely related to $GABA_A$ receptors
  - BZD receptors facilitate $GABA_A$ receptor opening
  - This opens up chloride channels: Causes hyperpolarization of the synaptic membrane
- Kappa opioid agonist activity which explains spinal analgesia

Routes of Administration

- Oral administration: 0.25 mg/kg given as 2 mg/mL syrup
- Intramuscular administration: 0.07–0.08 mg/kg
- Intravenous administration: 0.02–0.03 mg/kg
- Intrathecal administration: 0.3–2 mg given usually
- Epidural administration: 0.03–0.05 mg/kg

Pharmacodynamics

- Central nervous system:
  - Hypnosis, sedation, anxiolysis
  - *Anterograde amnesia* which is more potent and longer lasting than sedative effect
  - Reduces cerebral metabolic oxygen requirements which has a ceiling effect
  - Reduces cerebral blood flow, especially in regions associated with arousal, attention and memory
  - Little or no change in intra-cranial pressure
  - Potent anticonvulsant, no cerebroprotective effects
  - When administered intrathecally or epidurally, it has anti-nociceptive effect
  - Muscle relaxant through actions on spinal internuncial gamma neurons
- Cardiovascular system:
  - Reduces systolic BP by 5% and diastolic BP by 10%
  - No effect on cardiac output: most useful in congestive cardiac failure
  - Reduces peripheral vascular resistance
  - Increases heart rate
- Respiratory system:
  - Reduction in tidal volume but increase in respiratory rate
  - Dose dependant reduction in ventilation with 0.15 mg/kg IV
  - Transient apnea with doses more than 0.15 mg/kg
  - Impaired ventilatory response to hypercapnea
  - Better avoided in COPD patients
  - Ventilatory depression more when 0.05 mg/kg IV used for induction
- Others:
  - Reduces hepatic and renal blood flow
  - Reduces adrenergic but not cortisol response to stress
  - Inhibits phagocytosis and leucocyte bactericidal activity

Pharmacokinetics

- Absorption:
  - Absorbed well and very quickly when given orally
  - Oral bioavailability 50%
  - IM bioavailability 80–100%
- Distribution:
  - V_d of 1–1.5 L/kg may increase to 3 L/kg in critically ill patients
  - 96% plasma protein bound
  - Short duration of action due to:
    - High lipid solubility
    - Rapid redistribution
    - Short context sensitive half time: can be used for continuous infusion
- Metabolism:
  - By hepatic and small intestinal by cytochrome P_{450}
  - Converted to 1 and 4 hydroxy-midazolam
  - 1-hydroxy-midazolam has half the activity of midazolam
  - This may be responsible for prolonged sedation in renal insufficiency
  - Metabolism is slowed in the presence of cytochrome P_{450} inhibitors:
    - Cimetidine, erythromycin
    - Calcium channel blockers, antifungal drugs
  - Hepatic clearance is also reduced by concomitant fentanyl administration
  - Finally 1 and 4 OH-midazolamare conjugated with glucuronide
- Excretion:
  - In urine as glucuronide conjugates
  - Renal impairment has little effect
  - Elimination half life of 1.5–3.5 hours
- Onset of action within 30–60 seconds
- Peak effect within 3–5 minutes
- Duration of action 15–80 minutes

Uses

- Preoperative medication:
  - Most commonly used premedication in children for conscious sedation
  - Oral midazolam syrup 2 mg/mL in dose of 0.25 mg/kg
  - Administered at least 20 minutes prior to surgery
- Intravenous sedation:
  - 0.03–0.05 mg/kg given IV
  - Continuous IV infusion can be used at 4 μg/kg/min
  - Useful for:
    - Endoscopy and procedures performed under local anesthesia
    - Monitored anesthesia care
  - Used with caution in patients with COPD and old age
- Induction of anesthesia:
  - 0.1–0.2 mg/kg IV
  - Causes slower onset of unconsciousness compared with thiopental
  - Onset can be quickened by prior administration of opioids
  - Fentanyl 50 or 100 μg IV can be given preceding midazolam by 1–3 minutes

- Maintenance of anesthesia:
  - 0.25 to 1 mg/kg/hour
  - Used as supplement to opioids and propofol
  - Reduces MAC of volatile agents by around 15%
  - Produces gradual awakening which is rarely associated with nausea or emergence reactions
- Post-operative sedation: 1–7 mg/hr IV in intubated patients
- ***Paradoxical vocal cord motion:***
  - Causes non-organic upper airway obstruction and stridor
  - Midazolam 0.5–1 mg IV can be used effectively
- Chronic pain including de-afferentiation syndrome

Side Effects

- Occasional discomfort at site of injection
- Ventilatory depression and apnea especially with doses > 0.15 mg/kg
- Withdrawal phenomenon like irritation and insomnia in prolonged infusions
- Transient apnea in geriatric patients and those with COPD
- May accelerate cognitive decline in elderly patients with long term use
- May inhibit platelet aggregation by causing conformational change in platelet membranes

Drug Interactions

- Antacids and food reduce absorption from GIT
- Cimetidine, erythromycin, calcium channel blockers inhibit metabolism of midazolam
- Metabolism of midazolam is also inhibited by fentanyl
- Alcohol, inhaled anesthetics, opioids and α_2 agonist exert synergistic sedative effects
- Analgesic actions of opioids are reduced by BZDs
- Depressant actions of opioids are potentiated by BZDs
- Flumazenil:
  - Is specific antagonist at BZD receptor
  - Reverses all effects except respiratory depression

DIAZEPAM

Chemistry

- Lipid soluble benzodiazepine
- Non chiral compound with no isomers

Presentation

- Available as tablets containing 2/5/10 mg
- Syrup contains 0.4 mg/1 mg/mL
- 10 mg suppository or 2/4 mg/mL solution available for rectal administration
- Clear yellow solution with 5 mg/mL for IM/IV injection
- Insoluble in water and thus dissolved in organic solvent like propylene glycol
- Slightly acidic with pH of 6.6–6.9
- Also available as soyabean formulation for IV injection

Mechanism of Action

- Acts mainly through BZD receptors:
  - Found at synapses concentrated in cortex and mid-brain
  - These are closely related to $GABA_A$ receptors
  - BZD receptors facilitate $GABA_A$ receptor opening
  - This opens up chloride channels: causes hyperpolarization of the synaptic membrane
- Kappa opioid agonist activity which explains spinal analgesia

Routes of Administration

- Oral dose of up to 60 mg/day in divided doses in adults
- Intravenous dose: 5–20 mg, increasing according to clinical effect
- Rectally used in children with febrile seizures

Pharmacodynamics

- Central nervous system:
  - Anxiolytic and decreases aggression
  - Paradoxical excitement may occur
  - Sedation, hypnosis, *anterograde amnesia*
  - Anticonvulsant activity:
    - Act by selectively inhibiting limbic system especially hippocampus
    - This is different from bartiturates
    - Barbiturates inhibit seizures by non-selective CNS depression
  - Analgesic: Especially with spinal analgesia
  - Muscular relaxation through actions on spinal gamma internuncial neurons
- Cardiovascular system:
  - Transient reduction in BP and systemic vascular resistance
  - Reduction in cardiac output
  - Reduction in myocardial oxygen consumption
  - Coronary blood flow increases secondary to coronary vasodilation
- Respiratory system:
  - Ventilatory depression causing reduced tidal volume

- Large doses may produce apnea
- Ventilatory depression reversed by surgical stimulation but not by naloxone
- Depressant action exaggerated in:
  - Patients with COPD
  - Concomitant administration of other CNS depressants (alcohol, opioids)

Pharmacokinetics

- Absorption:
  - Rapidly absorbed after oral and rectal administration
  - Bioavailability of 86–100%
  - Absorption after intramuscular administration is slow and erratic
- Distribution:
  - Volume of distribution:
    - V_d of 1–1.5 L/kg
    - Increase in fat content of body, as with old age and female gender, increases the V_d
  - Plasma protein binding:
    - 96–98% plasma protein bound, mainly to albumin
    - Reduced levels of plasma proteins:
      - Occurs in cirrhosis and CRF
      - Reduction in plasma levels of albumin occurs
      - This causes a reduction in plasma protein binding
      - Increased propensity of side effects of diazepam occurs
  - Diazepam rapidly crosses placenta
- Metabolism:
  - Metabolized by hepatic microsomal enzymes by N-demethylation (oxidation)
  - Desmethyl-diazepam, oxazepam and temazepam are the active metabolites formed
  - Contribute to return of drowsiness which occurs 6–8 hours after administration of diazepam
  - Metabolites are then conjugated with glucuronide
  - Metabolism is inhibited by cytochrome P_{450} enzyme inhibitors
  - Enterohepatic circulation present
- Elimination:
  - Excreted in urine as glucuronide derivative
  - Less than 1%is excreted unchanged
  - Elimination half-life of 20–40 hours
  - This is prolonged in cirrhosis due to reduced protein binding of drugs
  - Elimination half life also prolonged in elderly due to fat content causing increased V_d
  - Context sensitive half time longer than midazolam

Uses

- Short term treatment of anxiety
- Premedication in adults
- Status epilepticus, febrile seizures in children
- Delirium tremens and alcohol withdrawal (second drug of choice to chlordiazepoxide)
- Treatment of local anesthetic induced seizures 0.1 mg/kg IV
- Tetanus, lumbardisc prolapse and other spastic conditions for muscle relaxation

Side Effects

- Drowsiness, ataxia, headache
- Tolerance, dependence
- Withdrawal symptoms: insomnia, anxiety, confusion, psychosis, perceptual disturbances
- Gastrointestinal: Nausea, vomiting, abdominal pain
- Allergic reactions and rashes
- Thrombophlebitis:
  - Highly irritant to veins
  - Soyabean oil preparation is less irritant and may be preferred
- CNS intoxication when plasma concentration is 1000 ng/mL
- Ventilatory depression especially in COPD and old patients

Drug Interactions

- Reduces MAC value of inhaled anesthetic
- Diazepam potentiates non-depolarizing muscle relaxants
- Cimetidine reduces clearance of diazepam by inhibiting cytochrome P_{450}
- Drug cannot be removed by hemodialysis due to the high protein binding
- Synergistic CNS depression on administration with opioids and alcohol

REMIMAZOLAM

Introduction

- Ultra short acting imidazo-benzodiazepine
- Similar to midazolam but with the pharmacokinetic properties of remifentanyl

Chemistry

- Chemically (methyl 3-[(4S) -8-bromo-1-methyl-6-(2-pyridinyl) -4H-imidazo [1,4] benzodiazepine-4-yl] propanoate)

- Carboxylic ester moiety incorporated into benzodiazepine core
- Molecular formula $C_{21}H_{19}BrN_4O_2$
- Average mass 439.305 Da
- Water soluble compound

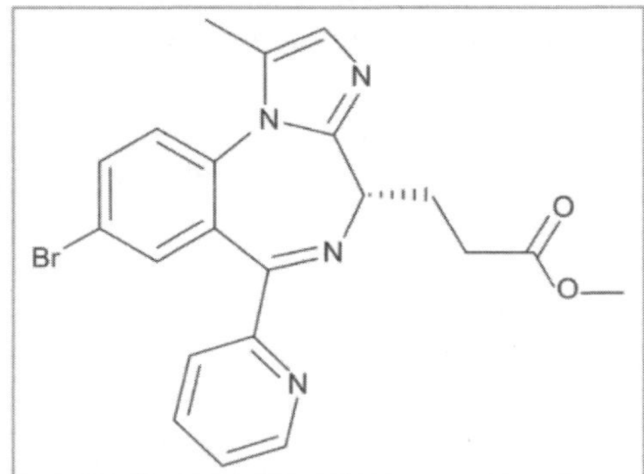

Mechanism of Action

- Remizolam is a high affinity, selective ligand for BZD site on $GABA_A$ receptors
- Binding to receptor site opens up GABA-activated chloride channels
- This initiates cell membrane hyperpolarization by increasing chloride ion influx
- Thus, neuronal transmission is inhibited
- Action on GABA receptors is dose-dependent:
  - Lower doses produce anxiolysis
  - Higher doses produce sedation and hypnosis

Pharmacodynamics

- Central nervous system:
  - Sedative, hypnotic, amnesia, muscle relaxant, anticonvulsant properties
  - Sedation, amnesia and anticonvulsant property mediated by α_1 subunit of $GABA_A$ receptor
  - Anxiolysis and muscle relaxation mediated by α_2 subunit of $GABA_A$ receptor
  - Reduces cerebral oxygen consumption and $CMRO_2$
- Respiratory system:
  - Less depression of respiratory drive compared to midazolam
  - Minimal risk of apnea
- Cardiovascular system: minimal effects on cardiovascular system

Pharmacokinetics

- Onset of action: 1–3 minutes
- Peak action: 4 minutes
- Duration of action: 10 minutes
- Context sensitive half time:
  - Follows first order kinetics even with prolonged infusions
  - Context sensitive $T_{1/2}$ of 7–8 minutes after 2 hour infusion
  - Thus, no accumulation occurs on prolonged infusions
- Distribution:
  - Volume of distribution 34.8 + 9.5 litres
- Metabolism:
  - Dose-independent ester hydrolysis by tissue esterases
  - Hydrolysed to inactive metabolite CNS 7054
  - This ester hydrolysis is responsible for short duration of action of remimazolam
- Clearance:
  - Clearance rate of 70.3 + 13.9 L/hr
  - Elimination $T_{1/2}$ of 24 minutes

Indications

- Premedication
- Procedural sedation
- In combination with opioids for TIVA
- ICU sedation

Dosage

- Premedication: 0.075 mg/kg
- Induction dose: 0.1–0.3 mg/kg
- Maintenance of general anesthesia: 0.72–3 mg/kg/hr
- Maintenance of sedation: 0.72–3 mg/kg/hr

Adverse Effects

- Headache
- Somnolence

Advantages

- Fast onset of action (faster compared to midazolam)
- Ultra short acting
- Short context sensitive half time
- Organ-independent metabolism like remifentanil
- Can be safely used in those with hepatic or renal impairment
- Lesser propensity to cause apnea
- Weaker circulatory suppression compared to propofol
- No injection site pain as with propofol
- Action is reversible with flumazenil (better safety profile)

Validation

- Lower incidence of cardiac arrest, compared with propofol sedation
- Not yet been approved for clinical use
- Undergoing phase II-III licensing trials in Europe, Japan and United States

REMIFENTANYL

Introduction

Ultra short-acting synthetic opioid with ester side chain, susceptible to metabolism by blood and tissue esterases.

Mechanism of Action

- 4-anilido-piperidine compound
- Pure μ-receptor agonist
- μ-receptor stimulation causes intracellular calcium accumulation
- This increases K^+ conductance causing hyper-polarization of excitable cell membranes
- This reduces membrane excitability causing pre and post-synaptic effects

Pharmacodynamics

- Central nervous system:
  - Minimal sedative/hypnotic activity
  - Dose dependant analgesic effects
  - Peak effect occurs between 1–3 minutes
  - Concentration dependant slowing of EEG
  - Muscle rigidity with bolus doses
  - Drug is injected over 60 seconds to avoid muscle rigidity
  - Lesser suppression of motor evoked potentials (compared with other opioids)
  - Preserves cerebral auto-regulation (if < 0.5 μg/kg/min)
  - Miosis from stimulation of Edinger-Westphal nucleus
  - MEAC = 0.75 ng/mL
- Respiratory system:
  - Dose dependent ventilatory depression (maximum with 2 μg/kg IV)
  - Reduces tidal volume and respiratory rate
  - Reduces ventilatory response to hypoxia and hypercarbia
  - No bronchospasm as it does not cause histamine release
  - Respiratory parameters recover more rapidly than other opioids
- Cardiovascular system:
  - Brief increase in systolic BP and heart rate if bolus dose > 1 μg/kg is given
  - Dose dependent reduction in SBP and heart rate otherwise (causes 20% reduction in MAP)
  - Greater hemodynamic changes in CAD patients
  - May also reduce contractility and cardiac output
- Gastrointestinal:
  - Dose dependant nausea and vomiting
  - Delays gastric emptying and biliary drainage
  - Effects resolve more quickly

Pharmacokinetics

- Ultra short acting opioid
- Termination of action by:
  - Redistribution of drug from effect site
  - Hydrolysis by blood and tissue non-specific esterases
- Absorption:
  - Not effective orally
  - Volume of distribution: 0.3–0.5 L/kg
  - 70% plasma protein bound
- Metabolism: by blood and tissue non-specific esterases
- Excretion:
  - Clearance = 3–5 L/min
  - Elimination half-life = 10 minutes
  - Context sensitive half-life = 4 minutes after 4 hour infusion

Uses in Anesthesia

- Induction and maintenance of anesthesia
- Conscious sedation in ESWL and colonoscopy
- Component of TIVA
- *Fast-track cardiac anesthesia*
- Postoperative analgesia
- Reduces MAC of isoflurane by 65%
- Reduces MAC-BAR by 60%
- Obstetric analgesia

Dosage and Administration

- Induction of general anesthesia:
  - Opioid induction: 2–5 μg/kg bolus
  - Balanced anesthesia: 1 μg/kg over 60 seconds followed by 0.25–0.5 μg/kg/min
- Maintenance of anesthesia:
  - Balanced anesthesia: 0.2–0.25 μg/kg/min
  - High dose opioid maintenance: 1–3 μg/kg/min

- Nitrous-narcotic technique: 0.6 μg/kg/min
- Cardiac surgery: 1–3 μg/kg/min and reduced during hypothermia

❖ TIVA: 0.25–0.5 μg/kg/min

❖ Conscious sedation:
- 12.5–25 μg boluses intermittently
- 0.01–0.2 μg/kg/min infusion
- 0.2–0.25 μg/kg/min for colonoscopy/ESWL
- 0.05–0.1 μg/kg/min as an adjunct to LA or RA

❖ Post op pain: 0.05–0.15 μg/kg/min

❖ Monitored anesthesia care:
- 0.1 μg/kg/min given 5 minutes prior to stimulus
- Wean to 0.05 μg/kg/min as tolerated
- Adjust, increase/decrease in increments of 0.025 μg/kg/min
- Reduce dose accordingly at the time of administration of midazolam/propofol
- Avoid administration of bolus doses

❖ Labor analgesia:
- May have maternal, fetal and neonatal side effects
- 0.2–1 μg/kg boluses with lock out intervals of 1–5 minutes
- 0.1 μg/kg/min infusion may be used

Dose Adjustments

❖ Pediatric patients may require twice as much remifentanyl (0.15 μg/kg/min)

❖ 50% reduction in dose required in old age

❖ No dosage adjustments required in CRF

Side Effects

❖ Respiratory depression

❖ Muscle rigidity

❖ Transient hypertension and tachycardia, bradycardia

❖ Postoperative shivering and pruritus

❖ Subjective side effects: Dry mouth, itching, flushing, sweating

❖ Impaired performance of psychomotor tests

Disadvantages

❖ Rapid loss of analgesia with development of opioid induced hyperalgesia postoperatively

❖ Opioid tolerance

❖ Intraoperative awareness as it has minimal hypnotic properties

Contraindications: Not used in spinal/epidural as additive as the preparation has glycine

CLONIDINE

Introduction

Selective partial α_2 agonist which is an aniline derivative.

Mechanism of Action: Primarily sympatholytic action:

Acute Use

❖ Direct action:
- Direct sympatholytic action on spinal preganglionic sympathetic neurons
- This reduces sympathetic tone and increases vagal tone

❖ Indirect action:
- Stimulates prejunctional α_2 receptors as it is structurally similar to norepinephrine
- This opens up K^+ channels and pre-synaptic Ca^{2+} channels
- This causes inhibition of adenylyl cyclase resulting in reduced neurotransmitter release
- Therefore, post-synaptic transmission reduces from pontine locus ceruleus
- This results in sedation and analgesia
- Also, reduced post-synaptic transmission causes reduced central sympathetic outflow
- This results in hypotension and bradycardia

Chronic Use

Acts by reducing responsiveness of blood vessels to vasoactive substances and sympathetic stimulation

Pharmacokinetics

❖ Absorption:
- Rapidly absorbed orally
- Oral bioavailability around 70–90%

❖ Distribution:
- 20–40% plasma protein bound
- Volume of distribution 2L/kg
- Peak plasma levels in 60–90 minutes

❖ Metabolism and excretion:
- Half life = 12–24 hours
- 50% metabolized in liver to glucronide conjugates
- 50% excreted unchanged in urine
- Elimination half-life = 9–12 hours

❖ Duration of action:
- Hypotension after single dose for 8 hours
- Transdermal administration requires around 48 hours to achieve therapeutic levels

Pharmacodynamics

❖ Receptor-wise action:
- α_{2a}: Sedation, analgesia, anxiolysis
- α_{2b}: Reduces shivering and vasoconstriction
- α_{2c}: Startle response
- α_2: α_1 = 220: 1 for clonidine

- Central nervous system:
  - Supraspinal (*locus ceruleus*), spinal (*substantia gelatinosa*) and peripheral analgesia
  - Sedative and anxiolytic
  - Reduces shivering and cerebral blood flow
  - Reduces IOP
- Cardiovascular:
  - Cardio-protective properties
  - Hypotension (due to reduces central and peripheral sympathetic outflow)
  - Reduction in SBP more than reduction in DBP
  - Transient HTN may occur immediately after injection due toα_1 action
  - No effect on baroreceptor reflexes
  - Bradycardia, well maintained cardiac output
- Respiratory:
  - Does not induce profound respiratory depression
  - Mildly potentiates opioid induced respiratory depression
- Gastrointestinal: Reduces gastric motility, anti-sialogogue
- Genitourinary: Maintains GFR and renal blood flow
- Endocrines: Reduces catecholamine, renin levels and insulin secretion

Indications

- Anesthetic indications:
  - Premedication:
    - Oral 2.5–4.5 µg/kg preoperatively reduces anxiety
    - Transdermal patch:
      - 0.2 µg/day patch is applied on the night before surgery
      - This is continued for 72 hours postoperatively
  - Protection against perioperative MI:
    - 300 µg clonidine P.O 90 minutes before surgery
    - This is continued for 72 hours at 200 µg/day
  - Induced hypotension
  - Reduce intubation response
  - Analgesia:
    - Epidural clonidine for reflex sympathetic dystrophy, intraop and postop pain
    - 1–1.5 µg/kg IV bolus (upto 2 µg/kg)
    - 1–2 µg/kg/hour IV infusion
  - As an additive to prolong neuraxial blockade
  - Postoperative shivering:
    - 75 µg bolus can be given IV
    - 1 µg/kg as it reduces vasoconstriction
  - Postoperative nausea and vomiting
  - PICU sedation: 1 µg/kg/hour with midazolam 350 µg/kg/hour
  - Clonidine can be used with lidocaine for IVRA
- Non-anesthetic uses:
  - Severe hypertension, rennin dependant HTN: 0.2–0.3 mg/day
  - Pheochromocytoma:
    - Aids in diagnosis of pheochromocytoma
    - 300 µg clonidine is administered orally
    - This reduces catecholamine concentration in normal patients
    - Catecholamines remain raised in the presence of pheochromocytoma
  - Treatment of opioid withdrawal, panic disorder
  - Treatment of cancer chemotherapy associated emesis and diabetic diarrhea
  - Treatment of spasticity, attention deficit hyperkinetic disorder, schizophrenia

Dose

- 1–2 µg/kg: IV, IM, caudal, spinal and epidural routes
- 2–4 µg/kg: Rectal and nasal routes
- 4–5 µg/kg: Oral dose
- 0.2 mg/day via transdermal route

Anesthetic Advantages

- General anesthesia:
  - Reduced anesthetic requirements:
    - Volatile anesthetics:
      - Reduced by 40–60% if acute clonidine use
      - Reduced by 10–20% if on chronic clonidine therapy
    - Also has opioid sparing and MAC sparing properties
  - Hemodynamics:
    - More stable cardiovascular course
    - Reduced stress response
    - Reduces laryngoscopic and intubation response
    - Obtunds tourniquet induced hypertension
  - Postoperative:
    - Better pain relief especially postoperatively
    - Reduces postoperative agitation in children
    - Reduces postoperative shivering, nausea and vomiting
    - Reduces postoperative oxygen consumption
  - Others:
    - Reduced dose of cardioactive anesthetics
    - Blocks narcotic induced muscle rigidity
    - Reduces propofol requirement for LMA insertion

- Regional anesthesia:
  - Prolongs duration of analgesia (50% prolongation of bupivacaine)
  - Reduces peak plasma concentration of local anesthetics
  - Slight sedation provided for 1–3 hours postoperatively
  - Does not cause urinary retention after neuraxial block
  - Reduces duration of motor block

Side Effects

- Drowsiness, dry mouth, constipation, impotence
- Bradycardia and hypotension (especially if intrathecal dose ≥ 150 µg)
- Orthostatic hypotension (rare)
- Rashes (rare) and fluid retention
- Glucose intolerance
- Rebound hypertension:
  - Occurs in patients taking more than 1.2 mg/day
  - Occurs 18 hours after sudden discontinuation of clonidine
  - Lasts for around 72 hours
  - Characterized by:
    - Hypertension and tachycardia
    - Insomnia, flushing, headache, apprehension, and sweating
  - Treatment:
    - Hydralazine, SNP
    - Restart clonidine (transdermally if patient has vomiting)

Drug Interactions

- Co-administration of TCAs, phenothiazines and butyrophenones can precipitate hypertensive crisis
- Reduces anesthetic requirements

Contraindications

- Avoid in first 6 months of life as respiratory depression can occur due to reduced clearance in neonates
- Reduce dose if GFR is less than 10 mL/min and in liver disease

DEXMEDETOMIDINE

Introduction

Selective and complete α-agonist introduced in 1999 which is more selective for α_2 receptors than clonidine.

Chemistry

- D-enantiomer of medetomidine
- High ratio of specificity for α_2 receptors (α_2: α_1 = 1600: 1)
- Belongs to imidazole subclass of α_2 agonists
- Freely soluble in water

Pharmacokinetics

- Distribution:
  - 94% plasma protein bound
  - Volume of distribution 2–3 L/kg
  - Rapid onset of action within 5 minutes
  - Peak effect within 15 minutes
  - Context sensitive half-life:
    - 4 minutes after 10minute infusion
    - 250 minutes after 18 hours infusion
- Metabolism: metabolized in liver:
  - N-methylation and hydroxylation reactions
  - This is followed by conjugation with glucuronide
- Elimination:
  - Via kidney and feces
  - Elimination half-life 2–3 hours
  - Clearance of 10–30 mL/kg/min

Mechanism of Action

- Dexmedetomidine selectively activates α_2 receptors (G-protein coupled receptors)
- 3 types of α_2 receptors exist:
  - α_{2a} receptors:
    - Present in peripheral tissues
    - *Postsynaptic* α_{2a} stimulation causes vasoconstriction
    - *Presynaptic* α_{2a} stimulation inhibits norepinephrine release
    - This inhibits vasoconstriction
  - α_{2b} and α_{2c} receptors:
    - Present in brain and spinal cord
    - α_{2b} and α_{2c} stimulation causes sympatholysis, sedation and analgesia
- α_2 activation by dexmedetomidine causes the following changes:
  - Reduction in activity of adenylyl cyclase
  - Increase in K^+ channel activity
  - Inhibition of opening of voltage gated Ca^{2+} channels

Pharmacodynamics

- Central nervous system:
  - Causes arousable sedation
  - Sedation: Hypnosis (α_2 stimulation in locus ceruleus)
  - Analgesia:
    - Supraspinal analgesia: Locus ceruleus
    - Spinal analgesia: Substantia gelatinosa

- Anxiolysis, dose dependant amnesia
- Preserves cerebral oxygen supply-demand ratio
- Reduces cerebral blood flow by α_2 mediated vasoconstriction
- Reduces cerebral metabolic rate

❖ Respiratory system:
- Reduces minute volume
- Maintains ventilatory response to carbon dioxide
- Demonstrates hypercarbic arousal phenomenon like natural sleep

❖ Cardiovascular system:
- Reduces heart rate, SVR, myocardial contractility and cardiac output
- Hypotension and bradycardia for 5 minutes after loading dose
- Limiting bolus dose to 0.4 μg/kg reduces incidence of hypotension
- Reduces incidence of perioperative MI
- Increases sweating threshold, reduces vasoconstriction and shivering threshold

Side Effects

❖ Systemic hypotension with rapid IV boluses (give less than 0.4 μg/kg over 20 minutes)

❖ Bradycardia, AV dissociation, sinus arrest/cardiac arrest

❖ Dryness of mouth, transient hypertension

Uses

❖ ICU sedation:
- FDA approved for sedation less than 24 hours duration in adults
- Loading dose of 0.5–1 μg/kg followed by 0.1–1 μg/kg/hr infusion
- Has opioid sparing properties with more stable hemodynamics
- Useful for conducting daily wake-up tests in mechanically ventilated patients
- Reduced incidence of delirium and coma

❖ Off-label indications:
- Premedication:
  - 0.33–0.66 μg/kg IV given 15 minutes before surgery
  - 1 μg/kg given transmucosal
  - 3–4 μg/kg given orally
  - 2.5 μg/kg IM given 45–90 minutes before surgery
  - Advantages of dexmedetomidine premedication:
    - Reduces thiopentone requirement by 30%
    - Reduces volatile anesthetic requirement by 25%
- Maintenance of anesthesia:
  - 0.5–0.8 μg/kg IV bolus
  - Followed by 0.4 μg/kg/hr infusion
  - Advantages:
    - Opioid sparing properties
    - Reduces narcotic requirement in OSAS patients
    - Low postoperative pain scores
- TIVA: Useful when:
  - Spontaneous ventilation has to be maintained
  - Access to airway difficult
  - Rapid awakening is required
- Monitored anesthesia care:
  - Dose: 0.7 μg/kg/min IV infusion
  - Indications:
    - Patients receiving LA/RA
    - Pediatric patients undergoing MRI
    - Awakes craniotomies requiring patient cooperation
    - Awake carotid end-arterectomy
    - Cardiac catheterization studies in children
    - Awake fibreoptic intubation:
      - 1 μg/kg loading dose IV over 10 minutes
      - 0.2–0.7 μg/kg/hr maintenance dose
- IVRA: 0.5 μg/kg added to lidocaine improves quality of anesthesia and postoperative analgesia
- Treatment of narcotic, benzodiazepine, alcohol and recreational drugs withdrawal

Advantages

❖ Excellent sedation

❖ Potentiates benzodiazepine induced hypnosis and opioid induced analgesia

❖ Potent MAC sparing and opioid sparing properties

❖ Reduces BP, heart rate and plasma catecholamine levels

❖ Little respiratory depression while weaning off mechanical ventilation

❖ Improved cardiac outcome in non-cardiac patients

❖ Reduces emergence delirium associated with ketamine

Drug Interactions

❖ Sedation antagonized with ***atipamezole*** 50 μg/kg (α_2 antagonist)

❖ Reduces volatile anesthetic requirements (by 25%)

❖ Reduces opioid requirements

❖ Potentiates benzodiazepine mediated hypnosis and opioid analgesia

❖ INH and other cytochrome inhibitors may increase dexmedetomidine levels

MAGNESIUM SULPHATE

Introduction

- Mg^{2+} is the second most prevalent intracellular cation after K^+
- Therapeutic range = 4–6 mEq/L

Presentation

- Clear, colorless solution
- Contains 2.03 mmol/L of ionic Mg^{2+}

Physiology

- Is a *natural physiological antagonist of calcium*
- Upto one half of total body magnesium is present in bones (50%)
- 20% is present in skeletal muscle
- 1% is present in ECF, 30% is plasma protein bound
- Activates upto 300 enzyme systems
- ATP becomes fully functional only after chelation to magnesium
- Regulates calcium access into cells and action of calcium within cells
- Presynaptic release of ACH depends on action of magnesium

Mechanism of Action

- Anticonvulsant action:
  - Mechanism is unclear
  - CNS depressant action
  - Reduces CNS irritability
  - Secondary action through cerebral vasodilation which reverses cerebral vasospasm
- Muscle relaxation:
  - Reduces NMJ irritability
  - Reduces pre-synaptic release of ACH
  - Reduces sensitivity to ACH
  - Reduces uptake and binding of intracellular Ca^{2+}
- Antihypertensive actions:
  - Vasodilatation by direct action on blood vessels
  - Reduces sympathetic tone by sympathetic blockade
  - Reduces catecholamine release

Pharmacodynamics

- Central nervous system:
  - CNS depressant, reduces CNS irritability
  - Anticonvulsant
  - Possible analgesic effect by antagonism at NMDA receptors
- Cardiovascular system:
  - Cardioprotective action
  - Vasodilation, reduces SVR, hypotension
  - Slows SAN impulse formation and prolongs SA conduction time
  - Prolongs PR interval and AV nodal effective refractory period: bradycardia
  - Attenuates arrhythmogenic and vasoconstrictive action by adrenaline
  - Reduces reperfusion injury with minimal myocardial depression
- Respiratory system:
  - Effective bronchodilator due to smooth muscle relaxation
  - Attenuates hypoxic pulmonary vasoconstriction
  - Maintains intact respiratory drive
- Gastrointestinal:
  - Osmotic laxative if given orally
  - Antacid properties
- Genitourinary:
  - Renal vasodilatation, diuresis
  - Uterine tocolytic, increased placental perfusion
- Others:
  - Inhibits platelet function
  - Prolongs clotting time
  - Reduces thromboxane A_2 synthesis
  - Inhibits thrombin induced platelet aggregation

Pharmacokinetics

- Absorption: 25–65% of ingested magnesium is absorbed
- Distribution: 30% plasma protein bound
- Excretion: More than 50% of magnesium dose is excreted in kidney

Clinical Uses

- Central nervous system:
  - Subarachnoid hemorrhage:
    - Reduces newischemic deficits and improves outcome
    - To be started within 4 days of subarachnoid hemorrhage
  - Postoperative shivering: 30 mg/kg IV
  - Cerebral edema
- Cardiovascular system:
  - Anti-arrhythmic:
    - 1–2 gm IV over 5–10 minutes
    - Followed by 1–2 gm/hour IV
    - Alternatively, 25–50 mg/kg IV over 10–20 minutes

- For treatment of:
  - Torsades-de-pointes, QT_c prolongation
  - Intractable VT, VF, multifocal atrial tachycardia
  - Dysrhythmias associated with:
    - Alcoholism
    - Hypokalemia
    - Digitalis toxicity
    - MI, catecholamine release
    - Post cardiac surgery
- In supraventricular tachycardias:
  - 2–2.5 g IV bolus followed by 1.75 g/hr infusion
  - Rarely used now: only used for rate control in SVT
- As a component of cardioplegia: to reduce effects of calcium
- To treat autonomic hyper-reflexia secondary to spinal cord injury

❖ Respiratory system:
- Suppression of intubation response
- To reduce fasciculation after succinylcholine administration
- Management of intractable bronchospasm
- Spasms occurring with tetanus

❖ Gastrointestinal system:
- As a component of total parental nutrition
- Anti-aspiration prophylaxis: antacid properties of MgO useful

❖ Genitourinary:
- Severe PIH:
- *Drug of choice* for seizure control and prevention
- IV regimen:
  - 4 g in 20% solution IV given over 10 minutes
  - This is followed by 1 gm/hour infusion
  - Alternatively, 40–60 mg/kg IV bolus followed by 15–30 mg/kg/hr
- IM regimen:
  - 5 g (10 mL of 50% solution) IM in both buttocks
  - This is followed by 5 g Q4H in alternate buttocks
  - Continued till 24 hours post-partum
- Preterm labor:
  - 4 g IV over 15 minutes loading dose
  - This is followed by 1–4 gm/hr infusion
- Antepartum hemorrhage

❖ Dyselectrolytemias:
- Hypomagnesemia
- Refractory hypokalemia
- Refractory hypocalcemia

❖ Others:
- Thrombophlebitis
- Malignant hyperthermia therapy
- Patients undergoing pheochromocytoma resection
- Patients undergoing surgeries involving aortic cross-clamping
- Barium poisoning

Interactions

❖ Neuromuscular blocking agents:
- Prolongs action of NMBAs (by reducing ACH release and sensitivity to ACH)
- 30–50% of normal dose of NMBAs used in the presence of $MgSO_4$
- More interaction seen with vecuromium.

❖ Succinylcholine:
- Prevents K^+ release and reduces fasciculations
- Reduces incidence and severity of muscle pain
- May prolong phase-II block

❖ Opioids: Enhances sedative action of opioids

Side Effects

❖ Minor side effects: warmth, flushing, nausea, headache, dizziness

❖ May cause fetal and neonatal hypermagnesemia when used in PIH

❖ Pain on IM injection of $MgSO_4$

❖ Reduced DTR is useful sign to predict magnesium toxicity

Serum level	Clinical features
2.5–5 mg/dL	Reduced cardiac conduction, nausea
	Wide QRS
	Increased PR interval
5–7 mg/dL	Sedation and hypoventilation
	Reduced deep tendon reflexes
	Muscle weakness
7–12 mg/dL	Hypotension
	Bradycardia
	Diffuse venous dilation
	Loss of DTR
More than 12 mg/dL	Areflexia
	Respiratory paralysis
	Coma
	Cardiac arrest, complete heart block

SUGAMMADEX

Introduction

- Novel selective reversal binding agent
- Also called ORG 25963

Structure

- Modified γ-cyclodextrin
- Lipophilic core and hydrophilic periphery
- Modification of the γ-cyclodextrin extended the cavity size
- This allowed greater encapsulation of rocuronium molecule

Mechanism of Action

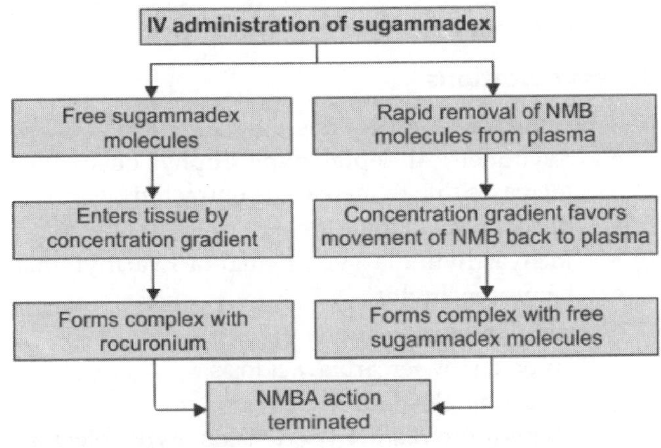

Pharmacokinetics

- Volume of distribution = 12–15L
- Plasma half-life = 2.2 hours
- Nometabolism occurs
- Clearance = 90 mL/min

Key Features

- Unique mode of action
- Rapid reversal from any depth of NM blockade
- Faster speed of reversal than neostigmine
- Usually well tolerated
- Low risk of residual blockade
- Dosing for multiple situations: immediate, moderate and deep block reversal

Advantages

- Useful in conditions where succinylcholine is contraindicated:
  - Ocular surgeries
  - Hyperkalemia
  - Burns
- Avoids side effects of SCH
- Useful for RSI with rocuronium
- Avoids need and side effects of cholinesterase inhibitors
- 9–12 times faster than neostigmine
- Immediate reversal of NMBA (3 minutes after rocuronium dose)
- Re-curarization is rare and occurs only insufficient sugammadex doses
- Same efficacy for vecuronium and rocuronium but as vecuronium is 7 times more potent, blockade is less

Dosage

- Routine reversal:
  - 2 mg/kg given IV
  - Used if some amount of spontaneous recovery has occurred
  - Upto occurence of T_2 following NMB
- Profound blockade:
  - 4 mg/kg given IV
  - Used if 1–2 post-tetanic convulsions have occurred
- Immediate reversal:
  - 16 mg/kg given IV
  - Used within 3 minutes after rocuronium administration

Side Effects

- Interacts with remifentanyl
- Anaphylaxes
- Caution in patients with renal dysfunction
- Impairment of taste (bitter metallic taste)

Present Status

- Still undergoing trials
- Has no effect on succinylcholine/mivacurium/atracurium
- Not used regularly due to concern over rare allergic reactions

EPHEDRINE

Introduction

Sympathomimetic amine used as a stimulant, appetite suppressant, concentration aid, decongestant and to treat hypotension associated with anesthesia.

Chemistry

- Alkaloid derived from ephedra vulgaris
- Four stereo-isomers are present: D (+) ephedrine and L (–) ephedrine

- It is a substituted amphetamine and structural methamphetamine analogue
- Enantiomers with opposite stereochemistry around chiral centre is called ephedrine while those with same stereochemistry is called pseudoephedrine

Mechanism of Action

- Sympathomimetic amine
- Indirect stimulation of adrenergic receptors by increasing the activity of norepinephrine on post-synaptic α_1, α_2 and β_1 receptors
- Direct α receptor activation: Controversial
- Also crosses blood brain barrier: Weak CNS activation

Pharmacokinetics

- $T_{½}$ of 3–6 hours
- Onset of action 5 minutes
- Duration of action 1 hour
- Biotransformation in liver
- Excreted mostly unchanged in urine

Indications

- Treatment of anesthesia induced hypotension:
  - Especially following spinal anesthesia
  - 750 µg/kg IV in titrated doses
- Treatment of bronchitis:
  - Due to bronchodilator action
  - Pseudoephedrine has less bronchodilator action
- ECA stack:
  - Component of thermogenic weight loss pills
  - Contains ephedrine, caffeine and aspirin
  - Speeds up metabolism and causes faster burning of food
  - Taken by body builders before work-outs to increase concentration, alertness and energy levels
- ***Coast guard cocktail***:
  - Along with promethazine (25 mg), ephedrine 25 mg forms part of coastguard cocktail
  - Used to combat sea sickness
  - Promethazine prevents vomiting
  - Ephedrine fights drowsiness due to promethazine

Adverse Reactions

- Neurological:
  - Restlessness, insomnia
  - Hallucination (rare), hostility
  - Confusion, mania, delusion, paranoia
- Cardiovascular:
  - Tachycardia, arrhythmias
  - Angina, hypertension
- Respiratory: Dyspnea, pulmonary edema
- Gastrointestinal: Anorexia, nausea
- Genitourinary:
  - Diuresis due to increased renal blood flow
  - Difficult micturition due to internal urethral sphincter constriction (rare)
- Dermatological: Flushing, diaphoresis, acne vulgaris
- Miscellaneous:
  - Dizziness, headache
  - Tremors, hyperglycemia

Dosage

- Intramuscular/subcutaneous: 25–50 mg repeated as per BP response
- Intravenous: 750 µg/kg or 25 mg/cm^2 of body surface area

Contraindications

- Absolute contraindications:
  - Asymmetrical septal hypertrophy: obstruction-increases due to increased contractility
  - Pheochromocytoma
  - Tachyarrhythmias: ventricular tachyarrhythmias
  - Hypersensitivity
- Relative contraindications:
  - Hypoxia, hypercarbia, acidosis
  - Closed angle glaucoma
  - Hyperthyroidism, hypertension, hypovolemia
  - Diabetes insipidus, impaired adrenal function
  - Prostatic hypertrophy, pregnancy (category C drug)
- Abuse potential:
  - Ephedrine increases concentration more than caffeine: Used by students and athletes
  - Used to synthesize methamphetamine by Birch reduction (using ammonia and Li^{2+})

Drug Interactions

- Not to be used with SSRIs (serotonin and norepinephrine reuptake inhibitors)
- Not to be used with bupropion: Increases norepinephrine levels
- Not to be used with MAO inhibitors
- Caution with concomitant use of halothane: sensitizes to arrhythmias

PHENYLEPHRINE

Introduction

Synthetic sympathomimetic agent which acts as a vasoconstrictor.

Chemistry

- Chemically m-hydroxy-α [(methyl-amino) methyl] benzyl alcohol hydrochloride
- Molecular formula: $C_9H_{13}NO_2$

Clinical Pharmacology

- Predominantly α_1 adrenergic agonist
- No direct stimulating effects on CNS
- Peripheral vasoconstrictor and causes reflex bradycardia
- Onset of action:
  - 10–15 minutes following IM/subcutaneous
  - Onset is immediate following IV administration
- Duration of action:
  - 1–2 hours for IM/subcutaneous administration
  - 20 minutes for IV administration

Pharmacokinetics

- Metabolized in liver by MAO enzyme
- Route of elimination of metabolites not identified

Indications

- Hypotensive states
  - Circulatory failure
  - Central neuraxial block
  - Following labor analgesia (preferred to ephedrine)
  - Drug induced hypotension.

Dosage

- In adults:
  - IM or subcutaneous administration: 2_5 mg with further 1–10 mg supplements
  - Intravenous administration:
    - 100–500 µg at rate of 180 µg/min
    - Taper to 30–60 µg/min according to response
- In children: 100 mg/kg IM or subcutaneous

Contraindications

- Patients on MAO inhibitors or within 14 days of ceasing such therapy
- Severe hypertension, hyperthyroidism
- Ischemic heart disease
- Occlusive vascular disease: Atherosclerosis, hypertension, aneurysm
- Arrhythmias, diabetes mellitus, closed angle glaucoma

Adverse Effects

- Extravasation may cause tissue necrosis
- Hypertension: Headache, vomiting, cerebral hemorrhage, pulmonary edema
- Reflex bradycardia, arrhythmias, angina, palpitation, cardiac arrest, dizziness, flushing
- Urinary retention, difficulty in micturition
- Altered glucose metabolism
- Transient tingling sensation, cooling of skin

Drug Interactions

- May cause VF if used with halothane/cyclopropane
- May increase risk of arrhythmias if given along with cardiac glycosides, quinidine/TCA
- Reverses action of antihypertensives

Overdose

- Headache, vomiting, hypertension, reflex bradycardia, cardiac arrhythmias, acidosis
- Treat symptomatically with supportive measures
- Counter hypertension with α-blocker like phentolamine 5–60 mg IV over 10–30 minutes and repeat as necessary

DOPAMINE

Introduction

Endogenous catecholamine which is immediate precursor to nor-epinephrine.

Chemistry and Presentation

- Naturally occurring catecholamine
- It is a non-chiral compound
- Presented as a clear, colorless solution
- Contains 40/160 mg per mL of dopamine hydrochloride
- 200 mg of dopamine present per ampoule

Mechanism of Action

- Direct action is by action on receptor
- Indirect action occurs by releasing nor-epinephrine
- 25% of IV dose is converted to nor-epinephrine
- Dose wise difference in the site of action
- Site of action:
  - At dose of 0.5 µg/kg/min: on D_1 and D_2 receptors
  - At dose of 5–10 µg/kg/min: on β_1 and β_2 receptors
  - At dose of more than 10 µg/kg/min: α_1 action predominates

Dosage

- Given only as continuous infusion as it is rapidly metabolized
- Diluted in D5/normal saline as alkaline solutions inactivate dopamine
- Central vein is preferred for infusion

- Lowest dose should be used to maintain the desired BP
- Usually used in doses of 5–15 µg/kg/min

Pharmacodynamics

- Central nervous system:
  - Nausea and vomiting by stimulation of CTZ
  - Raised intraocular pressure
- Autonomic nervous system:
  - Vasodilatation of splanchnic circulation
  - Reduces gastrointestinal motility
- Cardiovascular system: Dose dependant action:
  - At dose of 0.5 µg/kg/min:
    - Causes vasodilatation
    - Decreases diastolic BP
  - At dose of 5–10 µg/kg/min:
    - Positive inotropic effect
    - Increased chronotropism
    - Venoconstriction: Causes reduction in preload
    - Systemic vasodilatation: Causes reduction in afterload
    - Modest increase in systemic BP
    - Predisposes to arrhythmias due to norepinephrine release
  - At dose of more than 10 µg/kg/min:
    - Raised systolic BP but no increase in cardiac output
    - Causes non-epinephrine release
    - Coronary vasoconstriction
- Respiratory system:
  - Reduces ventilatory response to hypoxia
  - Increases intrapulmonary shunting
- Genitourinary:
  - Reduces renal vascular resistance
  - Increases renal blood flow and causes diuresis
  - Creatinine clearance is unaltered
- Endocrine:
  - Aggravates partial hypopituitarism
  - Reduces growth hormone secretion in critically ill patients
  - Aggravates sick euthyroid syndrome
  - Inhibits insulin secretion: Hyperglycemia
  - Inhibits aldosterone secretion causing diuresis

Pharmacokinetics

- Absorption:
  - Not effective orally
  - Volume of distribution 1.8–2.5 L/kg
- Metabolism:
  - 75% of administered dose:
    - Rapidly metabolized in plasma, liver and kidneys
    - Metabolized by MAO and COMT
    - Metabolized to homovanillic acid and 3,4 dihydroxyphenyl acetic acid
  - 25% of administered dose: Converted to norepinephrine in adrenergic nerve terminals
- Excretion:
  - Excreted in urine as homovanillic acid
  - Small fraction is excreted unchanged
  - Elimination half life of 2 minutes
- Onset of action within 5 minutes
- Duration of action 10 minutes

Side Effects

- Pain on extravasation:
  - Most common due to intense vasoconstriction
  - Treated by local infilteration of phentolamine
- Cardiovascular:
  - Tachycardia, arrhythmias
  - Angina and hypertension
  - Palpitation
- Others:
  - Mesenteric ischemia
  - Hyperglycemia
  - Potentiates development of MODS
  - Raised intraocular pressure
  - Nausea and vomiting due to stimulation of CTZ
  - Gangrene of extremities when used in occlusive vascular diseases and DM

Uses

- Low cardiac output states
- Septic shock
- Following cardiopulmonary bypass
- To maintain blood pressure in post surgery patients

Contraindications

- Right heart failure
- Pulmonary hypertension
- Pheochromocytoma
- Tachyarrhythimias

Drug Interactions

- Concurrent use of volatile anesthetics predisposes to arrhythmias
- Inactivated by alkaline solutions like $NaHCO_3$
- Dopamine action is blocked by phenothiazines (metoclopramide and droperidol)
- Phosphodiesterase inhibitors may accentuate action of dopamine

Renal Dose Dopamine

- Refers to continuous small dose infusion (0.5 μg/kg/min)
- Causes improvement in urine output when used in low doses
- This is thought to be due:
  - An overall improvement in cardiac output with dopamine
  - This causes an increased renal blood flow and inhibits aldosterone secretion
  - This results in improved urine output
- Diuresis is not due to any specific action of dopamine
- No studies to prove reduction in incidence of ARF when dopamine is administered to patients at risk for developing ARF
- No evidence of improved creatinine clearance or reduced need for dialysis with dopamine administration
- May increase risk for MODS by causing GI mucosal ischemia and translocation of bacterial toxins

DOBUTAMINE

Chemistry

- Is a synthetic isoprenaline derivative
- Has two isomers, levo (L–) and dextro R (+)

Presentation

- 12.5/50 mg/mL of dobutamine hydrochloride
- Presented as a clear colorless solution
- 250 mg of dobutamine per ampoule

Mechanism of Action

- Mainly β_1 agonist:
  - Stimulates adenalyl cyclase
  - This causes an increase in c-AMP levels
  - This increases cell membrane permeability to calcium
- Also acts as a weak β_2 agonist
- At doses above 5 μg/kg/min levo-dobutamine also exerts weak α_1 action

Route of Administration

- Ineffective when administered orally
- Used with 5% dextrose/normal saline to avoid inactivation by alkaline solution
- Usually in doses of 5–15 μg/kg/min (> 20 μg/kg/min causes tachyarrhythmias)

Pharmacodynamics

- Central nervous system: Stimulation at highest doses
- Cardiovascular system:
  - Positive inotropic effect
  - Increases SA node automaticity: tachycardia
  - Increases AV nodal conduction velocity
  - Increases myocardial perfusion
  - Causes coronary vasodilation
  - Improves cardiac index
  - Reduces left ventricular end diastolic pressure
  - Reduces systemic vascular resistance
  - Reduces pulmonary arterial occlusion pressure
- Genitourinary:
  - Increased urine output due to increase in cardiac output
  - Has no renal vasodilator effect
- Others:
  - Reduces blood glucose
  - Increases natural-killer cell activity
  - Increases cutaneous heat loss due to cutaneous vasodilatation

Pharmacokinetics

- Absorption: Not effective orally
- Distribution: Volume of distribution = 0.2 L/kg
- Metabolism:
  - Mainly by COMT methylation
  - Converted to 3-O-methyl-dobutamine and conjugated with glucuronide
- Excretion:
  - In urine as conjugated products
  - 20% excreted in feces
  - Elimination half life of 2 minutes
- Onset of action within 1–2 minutes
- Duration of action 10 minutes

Uses for Inotropic Support in

- Myocardial infarction
- Cardiomyopathy
- Low output cardiac failure
- Cardiogenic shock
- Septic shock
- Post-cardiac surgery
- For cardiac stress testing in those in whom exercise testing cannot be done

Side Effects

- Arrhythmias, tachycardia, hypertension, angina
- Fatigue, nervousness, headache, paresthesias, tremors

- Allergy, tachyphylaxis
- Increased heat loss
- Dyspnea, nausea

Contraindications

- Cardiac tamponade
- *Aortic stenosis*
- Mitral stenosis
- Allergy

MILRINONE

Introduction

- Synthetic, non-catecholamine inotropic agent with vasodilator properties (inodilator)
- Action is distinct from catecholamines and digoxin

Chemistry

- Bipyridine derivative of amrinone
- Inotropic potency 20–30 times that of amrinone
- Structurally related to theophylline and caffeine
- Chemically 1, 6- dihydro-2-methyl-6-oxo [3, 4`-bipyridine]-5-carbonitrile lactate
- Structural formula- $C_{12}H_9N_3O$
- Molecular weight 211.224 g/mol

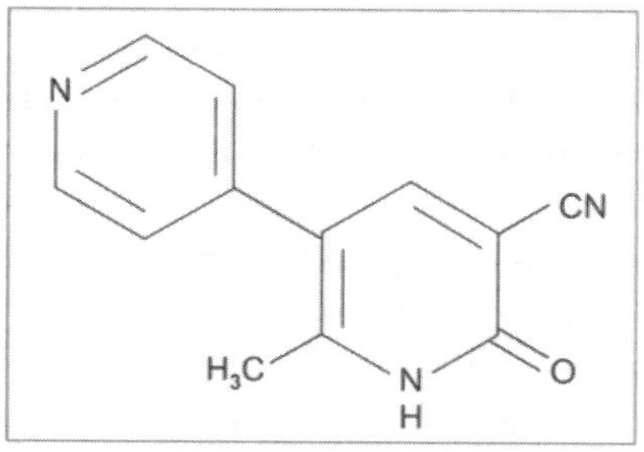

Preparation

- Stable as a lactate salt
- Colorless to pale yellow in color
- Available as a sterile aqueous solution to be diluted prior to use
- Stored at controlled room temperature between 15–30 °C
- Diluents 1/2NS, NS or D5W
- Diluted solutions may be stored for upto 72 hours

Mechanism of Action

- Selective inhibitor of cAMP phosphodiesterase III isoenzyme
- This inhibition decreases hydrolysis of cAMP
- This leads to accumulation of cAMP in myocardium and vascular smooth muscle
- This stimulates protein kinases within myocardial cells
- Ultimately, storage and release of calcium from sarcoplasmic reticulum is potentiated
- This increase in intracellular ionized calcium results in positive inotropism
- Milrinone also enhances effects of catecholamines
- This increases intracellular cAMP levels through β-receptors

Pharmacokinetics

- Onset of action: 5–15 minutes
- Peak action: 2 minutes
- Duration of action: 3–5 hours
- Therapeutic range: 100–300 ng/mL
- Absorption:
  - Rapidly and almost completely absorbed after oral administration
  - Bioavailability of 92%
- Distribution:
  - Volume of distribution of 0.38 L/kg when given as bolus dose
  - Volume of distribution 0.45 L/kg when given as an infusion
  - 70% plasma protein bound
- Metabolism:
  - Hepatic metabolism (12%)
  - Glucuronidation is main pathway of metabolism
  - Milrinone-O-glucuronide forms major metabolite
- Elimination:
  - Primarily urinary clearance
  - Clearance rate of 2.3 mL/kg/min
  - 83% drug excreted unchanged in urine, 12% as O-glucuronide metabolite
  - Terminal elimination $T_{1/2}$ of 2.3 hours
  - No evidence of tachyphylaxis for upto 48–72 hours

Pharmacodynamics

- Positive inotropic action:
  - Produces a prompt and dose related increase in cardiac output
  - Increases cardiac index, reduces LVEDP and PCWP
  - No increase in myocardial oxygen consumption
  - Improves diastolic function
  - Useful in right heart failure: increases contractility, reduces PVR

- Vasodilatation:
  - Produces vascular smooth muscle relaxation
  - Reduces arterial and venous pressures
  - This reduces afterload in heart failure patients
- Positive chronotropic action:
  - Mild- moderate increase in heart rate
  - Less tachycardia compared with dobutamine
  - Enhances AV nodal conduction
  - This can cause increase in ventricular response rate in those with AF

Indications

- For short term intravenous treatment of acute decompensated heart failure
- For treatment of cerebral vasospasm after aneurysmal subarachnoid hemorrhage

Dosage

- Cardiac failure:
  - 50 µg/kg IV given slowly over 10 minutes
  - 5–17% fall in mean arterial pressure may be seen with loading dose
  - Followed by a continuous infusion of 0.375–0.75 µg/kg/min
- Cerebral vasospasm:
  - Intra-arterial injection 4 mg over 30 minutes to main artery in vasospastic territory
  - Upto 15 mg repeat dose can be given in same territory
  - This is followed by an IV infusion for upto 14 days

Contraindications

- Uncorrected LVOTO, RVOTO, HOCM:
  - Inotropic activity exacerbates outflow tract obstruction
  - These lesions require surgical correction prior to inotropic support
- Renal impairment:
  - Terminal elimination $T_{1/2}$ may be prolonged in the presence of renal failure
  - Dose has to be reduced in those with creatinine clearance < 50 mL/min
- Acute myocardial infarction:
  - Effects of milrinone following acute MI are unknown
  - Milrinone is avoided in these circumstances
- Atrial fibrillation/flutter with fast ventricular rates
- Pregnancy, breast feeding mothers:
  - FDA pregnancy risk category C
  - Should be used during pregnancy only if benefits outweigh risks
  - Safety and effectiveness in pediatric population not established

Side Effects

- Severe:
  - Arrhythmias:
    - High incidence of ventricular arrhythmias (12%)
    - Non-sustained VT (2.8%), sustained VT (1%), VF (0.2%)
    - Torsades de pointes
    - *Atrial fibrillation: Use of milrinone is independent risk factor for AF*
    - Arrhythmias more common in:
      - Those with preexisting arrhythmias
      - Hypokalemia
      - Digitalis toxicity
  - Bronchospasm
  - Anaphylactic shock
- Moderate:
  - Premature ventricular ectopics (8.5%)
  - Supraventricular tachycardia (2.8%)
  - Hypotension, angina
  - Hypokalemia (0.6%)
  - Thrombocytopenia (0.4%)
  - Elevated liver enzymes
- Mild:
  - Headache (2.9%)
  - Tremors (0.4%)
  - Nausea and vomiting
  - Rashes, injection site reaction

VASOPRESSIN

Introduction

Hormone secreted by posterior pituitary gland.

Chemistry and Preparation

- Nanopeptide, containing 8-L-arginine vasopressin
- Molecular formula $C_{46}H_{65}N_{15}O_{12}S_2$
- 1 mL ampoules with 40/20 IU of vasopressin
- Molecular weight 1084.23

Physiology

- Synthesized as prohormone in *magnocellular neuron cell bodies* of *supraoptic and paraventricular nuclei* of posterior hypothalamus
- Bound to a neurohypophysin and transported to axonal terminals
- Synthesis transport and storage takes 1–2 hrs

Stimuli for Release of Vasopressin

Increased plasma osmolarity
Hypercapnea
Pain
Nausea
Chemical mediators:
ACH
Histamine
Angiotensin

Severe hypovolemia
Hypoxia
Stress
Pharyngeal stimuli

Dopamine
Prostaglandins
Catecholamine

Mechanism of Action

No.	Receptor	Location	Mode of action	Actions
1.	V1	Renal coronary	G protein receptors	Direct vasoconstrictor
		Systemic circulation	Activate phospholipase C	Pulmonary vasodilator (NO)
		Myometrium		
		Platelets		
2.	V2	Distal tubule	G protein receptors	Antidiuretic action
		Collecting ducts	Activate adenalyl cyclase	Induces factor VIII release
			Increase cAMP	Induces vWF release
			Mobilize aquaporin channel	
			Aquaporin channels inserted	
			Into apical membrane of renal collecting duct cells	
3.	V3	Pituitary gland	G protein receptor	Neurotransmitter in memory
			Increases intracellular Ca^{2+}	Consolidation
			Mediated by NO	Regulates body temperature
				Stimulates ACTH release

Pharmacodynamics

I. Cardiovascular

- Potent splanchnic portal cerebral pulmonary coronary vasoconstrictor
- Contracts especially capillaries small arterioles and venules
- Platelet aggregation and thrombus formation through endothelial vWF

II. Central Nervous System

- Stimulates ACTH release from anterior pituitary
- Neurotransmitter for memory, body temperature and BP

III. Renals

- Antidiuresis by increasing water resorption by renal tubules
- Contraction of bladder uterus GIT

Pharmacokinetics

- Administered IV/IM/SC
- Duration of action 2–8 hrs
- NOT PROTEIN BOUND
- V_d = 140 mL/kg
- Plasma T1/2 = 10–35 mins
- Normal plasma concentration < 4 pg/mL
- Metabolized in liver
- Excreted by kidneys (65%) and metabolism by vasopressinase (35%)

Indications

I. Cardiopulmonary resuscitation

- VF/PEA/Asystole
- As alternative to epinephrine
- Causes sustained increase in MAP as opposed to epinephrine
- 40 mg IV repeated every 3–5 mins regardless of initial rhythm
- Pediatric CPR: Dilute 1 IU/kg in 50 mL NS and infuse @ 1 mL/hr (0.33 IU/kg/min)

II. Shock

- SEPTIC: 0.01–0.04 IU/min
- ANAPHYLACTIC: 2–10 IU bolus followed by 2–6 IU/hr
- HEMORRHAGIC: 2–10 IU bolus followed by 0.8IU/kg/min titrated to BP
- VASODILATORY: 2–6 IU/hr in post cardiotomy patients

III. Abdomen

- Abdominal distention:
  5 IU IM increased to 10 IU IM and repeated at 3–4 hr intervals
- Variceal Bleed:
  20 IU in 100 mL 5% D over 15 mins bolus
  Given IV or rarely intra arterial infusion
  Reduces Portal blood flow and variceal pressure

IV. Central Diabetes Insipidus

- Given IV/intranasally on cotton pledgets/sprays
- 5–10 IU IM or SC TID/BD
- 2.5–10 IU IM/SC TID or QID for children

V. Bleeding Anomalies

- In von Willibrands disease and mild hemophilia
- Impaired platelet function due to NSAIDs/renal failure

VI. Other Vasodilatory States

- Hypotension with SAB/epidural
- Triple H therapy with phenylephrine
- Hormone replacement in brain death
- Periop refractory hypotension in patients on ACE inhibitors
- Shock after pheochromocytoma excision resistant to catecholamines
- Carcinoid crisis as sympathomimetics are contraindicated

Side Effects

- Local/systemic allergic reactions
- Abdominal cramps
- Nausea vomiting flatus
- GIT ischemia
- Tremors, vertigo, severe headache
- Bronchospasm, sweating, urticaria
- Cutaneous gangrene on extravasation
- Thrombophlebitis
- Water intoxication: Hyponatremia drowsiness headache coma

Contraindications

- Anaphylaxis
- Hyperbilirubinemia
- Chronic renal failure
- Peripheral vascular disease
- A/c bowel ischemia/MI
- Caution in
- Migraine
- Asthma
- Epilepsy
- Heart failure

Pregnancy: Category C

Drug Interactions

I. Potentiation of ADH Action By

- Carbamezepine
- Clofibrate
- Fludrocortisone
- Chlorpropamide
- Tricyclic antidepressants

II. Potentiation of Pressor Action By

- Ganglion blocking agents

III. Negate ADH Action

- Demeclocycline
- Lithium
- Alcohol
- Heparin
- Norepinephrine

MECHANISM OF ACTION OF LOCAL ANESTHETICS

Pharmacokinetics

- Only 1–2% of local anesthetic volume injected eventually reaches the nerve fibre
- The action is exerted on the nerve fiber in three phases:
  - Delivery phase:
    - Drug diffuses through many layers before it reaches the axons
    - Two main types of movement of drugs occurs:
      - Mass movement (due to injection)
      - Diffusion along concentration gradient
    - Factors affecting drug delivery:
      - Amount of fat and fibrous tissue surrounding the nerve
      - Absorption into vascular and lymphatic channels
    - Example:
      - More amount of fat and fibrous tissue is present in sciatic nerve
      - Spinal nerve roots on the other hand, are almost naked in CSF
      - LA gets absorbed into blood vessels around peripheral nerves
      - Thus, lesser amount of local anesthetic is available for delivery to the sciatic nerve
      - Addition of vasoconstrictor thereby increases drug delivery
      - Drugs like bupivacaine are extensively bound to plasma proteins
      - Thus, less amounts of free drug is available for vascular absorption
      - Therefore, adding epinephrine to bupivacaine does not increase its duration of action
  - Induction phase:
    - Refers to diffusion of local anesthetic from nerves outer surface towards center

- Thus, axons at the outer layer of nerve (mantle fibers) supplying proximal part of limb are blocked earlier than those in the inner layer (core fibers), supplying distal part of limb
- Implications:
  - In IVRA, local anesthetics are present in veins of axon
  - These are more densely packed in core region
  - Local anesthetic molecules diffuse from core to mantle
  - Hence, the block progresses from distal to proximal
  - In supraclavicular blocks, paresis precedes analgesia
  - This is because motor fibers of shoulder girdle area are present in mantle position of nerve fibers
- Recovery phase:
  - During recovery phase, the diffusion gradient is reversed
  - Nerve core contains higher concentration of LA
  - Therefore, it loses drug for more time (as more drug has to diffuse out)
  - Thus, proximal limb area recovers faster than distal areas

Molecular Basis of Action

- Locus of action:
  - Voltage gated sodium channels:
    - LA acts on inactivated and activated channels more than resting state channels
    - This is according to ***Modulated receptor hypothesis***
    - Thus binding of LA stabilizes the channels in a non-conducting state
  - Voltage gated K^+ channels
  - L-type Ca^{2+} channels
  - NMDA receptors
  - Nicotinic ACHR
- Active species:
  - Local anesthetics have a pKa of 7.5–9.5
  - Thus they are more often electrically charged molecules
  - The neutral form of LA is necessary to pass through axonal membrane
  - But, protonated form is necessary to block Na^+ channels
- Types of blockade:
  - Phasic blockade/use dependent blockade:
    - Refers to potentiation of anesthetic block by repetitive depolarization
    - Greater number of Na^+ channels are blocked at same drug concentration by repetitive stimulation
    - This is because more channels are in open state
    - This results in potentiation by repetitive depolarization
  - Tonic blockade:
    - Refers to degree of inhibition of single impulses measured without preceding stimulus
    - Indicates reduction in number of Na^+ channels in open state for a given drug concentration
    - Use dependant blockade is explained by modulated receptor hypothesis
  - Other drugs with local anesthetic action:
    - Ketamine, inhaled anesthetics
    - Pethidine, tricyclic antidepressants

Neurophysiological Implications

- Myelination of nerve fibers:
  - LA have to diffuse through lesser tissue to reach axons in small diameter fibers
  - Thus, smaller diameter fibers are more sensitive to LA action
  - Also, myelin stores LA at induction but draws them away from axon during drug diffusion
  - Thus myelinated fibres are blocked by LA slowly
  - Type B autonomic preganglionic and type C fibers are therefore more sensitive
- *Minimum blocking concentration (C_m):*
  - Lowest concentration of LA in vitro which will block given nerve within reasonable time (usually 10 minutes) is called C_m
  - This is similar to MAC value of inhaled anesthetics
  - Factors affecting C_m:
    - Dilution by tissue fluid
    - Fibrous tissue barriers
    - Drug absorption and metabolism
    - Elimination and distribution of LA
- *Differential nerve blockade*:
  - Refers to complete blockade of 1 nerve modality (sympathetic) with partial blockade of other modalities (sensory and motor)
  - Occurs due to 3 reasons:
    - Impulse in smaller fibres (B and C) blocked before larger fibers (Aδ and Aγ)

- Some fibres are more susceptible due to lack of myelin (C fibers)
- Axons per se may be differentially sensitive to block as some may have K^+ channels while some do not

- Increasing concentration of LA ensures C_m of larger fibers is attained
- This negates differential blockade occurring commonly
- Orderly progression of block from first to last:
  - Temperature
  - Proprioception
  - Motor
  - Sharp pain
  - Light touch

❖ *Threshold block phenomenon/**Wedensky block:***
- Phenomenon where, when C_m of a nerve fibre has been reached, it no longer conducts a single impulse but allows 2nd/3rd member of a train of impulses to breach the block
- Occurs as the conducted impulse briefly lowers the firing threshold of the nerve
- Another nerve impulse arriving during this phase will induce just enough depolarization to trigger an action potential
- This phenomenon is more pronounced in thinner axons
- Noxious stimuli trigger impulses in high frequency barrages through thin axons
- Thus, patient may not feel pain to a pin prick but may react to a high intensity stimulus like a surgical incision
- As anesthetic concentration progressively rises above the Cm, fewer impulses in a train are conducted as blockade becomes more profound

❖ *Decremental conduction*:
- Sufficient volume of LA is required to suppress conduction across a critical length of nerve fiber
- As membrane depolarization from an action potential spreads passively across a nerve fiber a critical length of fibre should be blocked to prevent passive firing of AP from adjacent membrane/Nodes of Ranvier
- Too short an exposure length allows impulse to skip over membranes and bigger APs
- Concentration of LA, which blocks 84% of sodium channel conductance at 3 successive Nodes of Ranvier, prevents any impulse propogation

Cardiac Action of Local Anesthetics

❖ Local anesthetics can be both proarrhythrogenic and is also used to Rx arrhythemias.

❖ Use of lidocaine in arrhythmias:
- Mainly used in ventricular tachy-arrhythmias
- Lidocaine targets open cardiac Na^+ channels
- It limits the rate of firing in ventricular tissue by increasing AP threshold in a phasic manner
- Thus, due to faster firing rates in VT, more number of Na^+ channels are open and also remain open for longer times
- Thus, use dependant blockade helps to reduce rate of ectopic ventricular firing while not affecting normal impulses
- This occurs due to 2 main differences between heart and peripheral nerves:
  - At RMP, few channels are in open state while in peripheral nerve, 30% may be in active state
  - Cardiac action potential produces depolarization which lasts several 100 milli seconds while neuronal impulse is only 1 msec
- Lidocaine thereby acts by delaying rate of spontaneous phase 4 depolarization by preventing or diminishing the gradual decrease in K^+ permeability that occurs
- In higher doses, lidocaine reduces conduction in AV node and Purkinje fibers

❖ Bupivacaine toxicity:
- Bupivacaine differs from lidocaine (mainly bradycardiogenic) in being arrhythmogenic
- It effects the storage and release of cytoplasmic Ca^{2+} thus affecting membrane excitability

LOCAL ANESTHETIC TOXICITY

Introduction

Adverse reactions with local anesthetics include systemic toxicity, localized neural and skeletal muscle toxicity and drug specific side effects.

Mechanism of La Toxicity

❖ Local anesthetics inhibit carnitine acyl carnitine translocase

❖ This prevents transfer of acyl COA across mitochondrial membrane

❖ This reduces fatty acid metabolism and reduces available energy at the cellular level

❖ This results in cardiac arrest

Systemic Toxicity

❖ Most toxic reactions involve CNS

❖ CVS depression is rare but is more serious and difficult to manage

- Neurotoxicity:
  - Factors affecting CNS toxicity:
    - Rate of drug injection also influences toxicity
    - Anesthetic potency:
      - Convulsions occur at:
        - Dose of 5 mg/kg of bupivacaine
        - Dose of 20 mg/kg of lidocaine
      - Thus, CNS toxicity relationship of lidocaine: bupivacaine is 4: 1
  - Phases of toxicity:
    - Initial phase of excitation: Due to selective blockade of inhibitory pathways
    - Later, CNS depression due to inhibition of both inhibitory and facilitatory pathways
  - Respiratory acidosis, hypercarbia and acidosis decrease toxic threshold as:
    - Hypercarbia increases cerebral blood flow: more LA delivery to brain
    - Acidosis reduces plasma protein binding: decreased V_d and more free drug for diffusion
    - Decreased intracellular pH causes:
      - Increased conversion to cationic form which is responsible for LA action
      - Conversion to poorly diffusible cationic form: Increases intracellular LA concentration
  - ***Cauda equina syndrome***:
    - 5% lidocaine and 0.5% tetracaine on repeated doses pool around cauda equina
    - Neurotoxic potential: from most toxic to least toxic:
      - Lidocaine = tetracaine
      - Bupivacaine
      - Ropivacaine
    - Sodium metabisulphate and low pH propentiate development of cauda equina
  - ***Transient neurological symptoms***:
    - 5% lidocaine, lithotomy position, obesity and outpatient status are risk factors for TNS
    - Occurs due to:
      - Local nerve root irritation in lithotomy position
      - More common with continuous injection of lidocaine via intrathecal catheters
      - This causes chromatolysis and vacuolysis of spinal neurons in ***Obersteiner-Redleich*** zone
- Cardiovascular toxicity:
  - Local anesthetics cause increased conduction time and myocardial depression
  - This results in:
    - Prolonged PR interval, QRS duration
    - SA node depression, sinus bradycardia and sinus arrest
    - AV nodal dissociation and idioventricular rhythm
  - Dose dependent negative inotropism: more intense with more potent LA
  - CC/CNS ratio:
    - Refers to ratio of dose required for causing cardiac to that required for neurotoxicity
    - CC/CNS ratio is 7 for lidocaine
    - This means 7 times as much lidocaine is required for cardiovascularcollapse as for convulsions
    - CC/CNS ratio is 3.5 for bupivacaine
  - Cocaine causes HTN and VPCs which are treated with CCBs and adrenergics
  - Bupivacaine more cardiotoxic due to:
    - Molecular structure per se
    - Also due to higher lipid solubility and protein binding
- Peripheral vascular toxicity:
  - Has biphasic action on smooth muscles of blood vessels
  - Vasoconstriction occurs, followed by vasodilatation
  - Cocaine is an exception which produces only vasoconstriction by inhibiting norepinephrine uptake
  - Increased heart rate, BP and cardiac output
  - This is followed by profound cardiovascular depression and circulatory collapse
- Other system toxicity:
  - Membrane stabilizing property results in:
    - Neuromuscular blockade
    - Ganglion blockade
    - Anticholinergic activity
  - Hematological: Lidocaine inhibits coagulation by:
    - Inhibiting thrombosis
    - Inhibiting platelet aggregation
    - Enhanced fibrinolysis

Local Tissue Toxicity

- Localized skeletal muscle damage:
  - Mostly commonly by bupivacaine and etidocaine
  - Muscle damage is reversible
  - Occurs due to hypercontraction which causes lytic degeneration and necrosis
  - Rapidly reversed within 3–4 weeks of injection
- Local ischemia or neurotoxicity may occur

Drug Specific Toxicity

- Methemoglobinemia:

- Following large doses (> 600 mg) of prilocaine
- Due to formation of O-toluideine in liver which:
- Oxidizes hemoglobin to meth-hemoglobin
- Spontaneously reversible
- Treated with IV methylene blue

❖ Drug allergy:
- More to amino esters like procaine
- Rare with amino-amides
- Due to drugs being derivatives of PABA
- Allergy also to preservatives sodium metabisulphite/methyl paraben

Treatment

❖ Stop local anesthetic injection

❖ Instruct patient to hyperventilate if conscious

❖ Minor reactions may be allowed to resolve spontaneously

❖ Protect airway: Intubate if necessary

❖ Provide supplemental oxygen if seizures present

❖ Anticonvulsants:
- Thiopentone 50–75 mg or diazepam 2.5–10 mg IV
- Midazolam 2 mg, propofol 1 mg/kg IV

❖ Cardiac arrest:
- Transvenous/transarterial pacing
- ACLS protocol based resuscitation
- Use amiodarone/bretylium instead of lidocaine for ventricular arrhythmias
- Vasopressors like epinephrine, vasopressin and norepinephrine
- Massive doses of atropine/adrenaline required for bupivacaine cardiotoxicity
- ***IV lipid emulsion (Intralipid)*** in refractory cases
- Cardiopulmonary bypass

❖ Local ischemic or neurotoxicity due to vascular compromise:
- Warm compresses
- IV phentolamine
- Nitroglycerine cream

❖ Treat meth-hemoglobinemia
- If methemoglobin > 30% methylene blue IV at 1–2 mg/kg
- Upto 50 mg/kg can be given in adults
- Given as 1% solution in 5 minutes and repeated in1 hour
- Ascorbic acid 200–500 mg orally
- N acetylcysteine can also be used
- Exchange transfusion recommended in severe cases

❖ Drug scavenging nano particles:
- Structure:
  - Contain yellow oil hydrophobic core with soluble hydrophilic cover
  - Also contains a nonionic polymer made of ethylene oxide and polypropylene oxide
- Mechanism of action:
  - Nanoparticles have large surface area to volume ratios
  - This aids in the treatment of LA toxicity
  - Nanoparticles are made of polyacrylic acid spheres
  - These can soak up drug molecules in the body like a sponge
  - Thus, they sequester bupivacaine from the acqueous phase of human blood
- Advantages:
  - Can penetrate deep into tissues through fine capillaries due to small size
  - Enter cells to evade detection by RES

PREVENTION OF LAST

Procedural

❖ Use ultrasound guided nerve blocks

❖ Avoidance of multiple simultaneous nerve blocks

❖ Use low dose while giving blocks with high LA absorption

❖ (Intercostal > epidural > brachial)

❖ Use of adrenaline as marker for intravenous injection

❖ Aspiration before injection of LA

❖ Injection in graded aliquots

❖ Use of continuous catheter techniques as:
- Allows use of less toxic drugs (lidocaine rather than bupivacaine)
- Avoids rapid injection of high doses
- Allows sufficient time interval between doses

Drugs

❖ Use of less toxic drugs (lidocaine, prilocaine > ropivacaine, levobupivacaine > bupivacaine)

❖ Restrict total anesthetic dosage to lowest effective dose

❖ When large doses are required fractionate doses

❖ Allow sufficient time interval before subsequent drug dosages

❖ Avoid rapid epidural injections

❖ Avoid combination of LA as toxic doses of combinations not known

❖ Use adjuvants to reduce dosage of LA

❖ Avoid excessive sedation to allow early LAST detection

Patient Factors

- Reduced LA dose in those with:
  - Obesity
  - Pregnancy
  - Old age
  - Cardiac failure
  - Liver failure
  - Renal failure

LIPID EMULSION THERAPY FOR LA TOXICITY

Introduction

- First clinical application by ***Rosenblatt and Litz***
- It is used only when more conventional methods of treatment have failed

Pharmacological Basis

- Lipid emulsion on administration creates a lipid bank
- Wayward local anesthetic molecules are deposited into this bank
- Thus, concentration of LA molecules into this bank prevents progression of toxicity
- This prevents progression of CNS to CVS toxicity
- This is advantageous as there are a number of options to revert CNS toxicity, but CVS toxicity is refractory to most resuscitative techniques

Mechanism of Action of Lipid Emulsions

- Prevents LA induced inhibition of carnitine acyl carnitine translocase
- Lipid droplets also segregate the unbound bupivacaine
- Provides instant energy source as it contains fat molecules
- Acts on nitric oxide pathway and reverses inhibitory effects of bupivacaine

Indications

- Toxicity of any lipid soluble drug:
  - Sertraline, quetiapine, bupropion
  - Lamotrigine, clomipramine
  - Verapamil, bupivacaine, ropivacaine
- Intralipid forms a component of parenteral nutrition formulations
- Some propofol and etomidate preparations use propofol as carrier

Composition of Intralipid

- Available in 10, 20 and 30% concentrations
- Contains emulsion of soya bean, egg phospholipids and glycerine (Lytic cocktail)
- Provides omega 6 essential fatty acids, linoleic acid and linolenic acid

Dosage: *Weinberg regimen:*

- Intralipid used as 20% solution, 1 mL/kg given over 1 minute
- Dose can be repeated every 3–5 minutes upto a dose of 3 mL/kg
- This is followed by an infusion of 0.25 mL/kg/min which is continued till hemodynamic stability is achieved
- Rate is increased to 0.5 mL/kg/min if hypotension occurs
- A total maximum dose of 8 mL/kg is recommended

Side Effects

- Altered reticulo-endothelial system function and inflammatory responses
- Increased risk of infections and thrombophlebitis
- Allergy and anaphylaxis, especially if soya bean is present
- Pulmonary, splenic and cerebral fat emboli
- Pulmonary hypertension
- May cause raised ICP after traumatic brain injury
- May induce weakness and seizures in children

Drug Interactions

- Causes warfarin resistance by facilitating its binding to albumin
- May interfere with ECMO circuit

HEPARIN

Introduction

- Discovered in 1916
- One of the strongest acids found in nature (negatively charged anion)
- Anticoagulant which delays clotting by direct and indirect actions on coagulation system

Chemistry

- Negatively charged anion
- Extracted from bovine lung/porcine intestinal mucosa
- Also present in basophils, mast cells, liver, lymph nodes and thymus
- Is a glycosaminoglycan formed by altering residues of D-glucosamine and L-iduronic acid
- Mixture of highly sulfated glycosaminoglycans which are acid mucopolysaccharides
- Molecular weight of 3000–60000 Da (with mean of 15,000 Da: UFH) Presentation

- Packed in two formulations:
  - Heparin sodium containing 1000/5000/25000 IU/mL
  - Heparin calcium containing 25000 IU/mL
- 1 IU of heparin is defined as that volume of heparin containing solution which will prevent 1 mL of citrated sheep blood from clotting for 1 hour after addition of 0.2 mL of 1: 100 calcium chloride
- Heparin must contain at least 120 USP (United States Pharmacopeia) units per mL
- 1 mg of heparin = 100 IU

Mechanism of Action

- Anticoagulant action:
  - Indirect action:
    - Pentasaccharide sequence of heparin binds to scaffolding present on antithrombin
    - This increases antithrombotic activity of AT by 1000 times
    - AT then inactivates factors V, VII, IX, X, XI and XII
    - Arginine center of AT binds to these serine proteases and inhibits them
    - Factor IIa is 10 times more sensitive than Xa to inhibition by UFH
    - Principal action is inhibition of thrombin induced activation of factors V and VII
    - Anti-thrombin is therefore also called ***Heparin cofactor***
  - Direct action:
    - Also directly binds to several serine proteins (IX, X, XI, XII)
    - This facilitates their action on AT
- Antithrombotic action: Inhibits platelet function by:
  - Inhibiting platelet aggregation
  - Inhibiting vWF and collagen cross linking

Routes of Administration

- Poorly absorbed from GIT as it is less lipid soluble: oral dose is ineffective
- Subcutaneous and intravenous administration preferred
- IM dose avoided as increases risk of hematoma formation

Pharmacokinetics

- Absorption:
  - Poorly absorbed orally
  - Bioavailability is the same (40%) for IV/subcutaneous administration
  - Onset of action:
    - IV administration is immediate
    - S/C administration is delayed by 1–2 hours
- Distribution:
  - One-third of dose binds to antithrombin III
  - Remaining two-third of dose binds to:
    - Albumin, fibrinogen
    - Proteases, platelet factor 4
    - Histidine rich glycoprotein, fibronectin, vitronectin and vWF
  - Volume of distribution 40–100 mL/kg
  - Highly plasma protein bound
- Metabolism: Desulfated and depolymerized in liver, kidney and RES by heparinases
- Excretion:
  - Mainly by depolymerization in endothelium and macrophages (JPME)
  - Small amounts excreted unchanged in kidney
  - Clearance: 0.5–2 mL/kg/min
  - Elimination half-life: 2.5 hours
  - Elimination and thus duration of action is prolonged in:
    - High dose (thus, dose response curves are not linear)
    - Hepatic and renal dysfunction
    - Hypothermia< 37 C (as during CPB)
  - Does not cross placenta unlike warfarin: not teratogenic

Pharmacodynamics

- Anticoagulant: Inhibits factors V,VII, IX, X, XI, XII, XIII
- Anti-thrombotic: Inhibits platelet aggregation
- Lipolysis:
  - Is precursor of lipoprotein lipase
  - Also increases other lipase activity in plasma
  - This reduces plasma free fatty acid concentration
- Anti-inflammatory action: Through mast cells
- Angiogenesis: Inhibits vascular smooth muscle proliferation
- Osteolytic:
  - Suppresses osteoblast formation
  - Stimulates osteoclasts and causes bone loss
- Increases blood vessel permeability

Lab Evaluation

- ***Lee-Whites whole blood clotting time***
- aPTT: Kept at 1.5–2.5 times the normal value (30–35 seconds)

- ACT:
  - Kept at more than 480 seconds for CPB
  - 180–480 seconds: Questionable anticoagulant effect
  - If less than 180 seconds: Inadequate anticoagulant effect
- Thrombin time: More than 16 seconds preferred (normal is 14–16 seconds)
- BART (Blood activated recalcification time): normal 65–125 seconds
- No need of monitoring for LMWH due to its higher bioavailability and half life

Clinical Uses

- Venous thromboembolism prophylaxis: 3500 IU S/C Q8H, started 2 hours before surgery
- Fat embolism: increased lipase action and clears FFA from blood
- Treatment of pulmonary embolism
- Disseminated intravascular coagulation: 50–100 IU/kg bolus followed by 10–15 IU/kg/hr
- Priming of cardiopulmonary bypass and hemodialysis circuits: 300–500 IU/kg
- Maintaining patency of indwelling catheters (IBP, CVP): 3–4 IU half hourly
- Coronary Artery disease:
  - Unstable angina, Non-Q-wave STEMI
  - 5000 IUIV followed by 32000 IU/24 hour infusion
- Atrial fibrillation with embolic complication while on standard dose warfarin and in pregnant patientswith prosthetic valves: long term heparin therapy

Contraindications

- Absolute contraindications:
  - Bleeding diathesis, thrombocytopenia
  - Intraocular surgeries
  - Intracranial surgeries
  - History of allergy to heparin
  - Threatened abortion
- Relative contraindications:
  - Patients undergoing neuraxial blockade
  - For tests which involve complement and Ig osmotic fragility
  - Severe hypertension, endocarditis
  - Hemorrhoids, GIT ulcers, large malignancies, tuberculosis
  - Chronic alcoholics, hepatic and renal dysfunction

Side Effects

- Hemorrhage:
  - *Most common* side effect
  - Risk increases with:
    - Pre-existing coagulation defects
    - Concurrent use of other drugs which inhibit coagulation
    - Chronic alcoholism
    - Other serious concurrent illness
- Allergy: as heparin is derived from animal tissues
- Cardiovascular changes:
  - Reduces MAP, pulmonary arterial pressure and SVR on rapid infusion
  - This is due to direct relaxant effect on vascular smooth muscle
- Osteoporosis:
  - Occurs if high dose heparin given for more than 5 months
  - This is because heparin inhibits osteoblasts and stimulates osteoclasts
- Aldosterone suppression
- Altered cellular morphology:
  - Heparin alters cellular morphology of stored blood
  - Heparinized blood is hence not used for tests which involve osmotic fragility
- Increased thrombotic tendency:
  - Heparin may reduce anti-thrombin activity to one-third of normal
  - It may therefore paradoxically increase thrombotic tendency
- Heparin resistance:
  - Occurs due to anti-thrombin deficiency
  - This may necessitate high doses of heparin together
  - Administration of FFP may restore AT III levels to normal
  - This is seen in inflammatory disorders due to raised plasma protein concentration
  - This reduces the amount of free drug available for action
- Heparin induced thrombocytopenia

Drug Interactions

- Nitroglycerine increases heparin requirement
- Increased concentration of free propranolol and diazepam when administered with heparin as heparin displaces these drugs from protein binding sites
- OCPs (estrogen containing): Reduce levels of AT and thus may cause heparin resistance
- Increased bleeding tendencies when used with aspirin and clopidogrel
- Alcohol increases risk of heparin induced bleeding

Heparin Reversal

- Protamine
- Platelet factor 4:
  - Heparin binding protein which is present in α-granules of platelets
  - It is released during platelet aggregation and reverses heparin anticoagulation
  - Recombinant PF_4 can be used in protamine allergy
- Heparinase I: Heparin degrading enzyme which lyses heparin at its α-glycoside linkages
- Histidine rich glycoprotein, vitronectin: Physiologically present

HEPARIN INDUCED THROMBOCYTOPENIA

Introduction

Life threatening prothrombotic complication of heparin administration.

Incidence

- 2.6% incidence with UFH, 0.2% incidence with LMWH
- 8% patients have antibodies to heparin
- 3% of these patients develop thrombocytopenia
- Only 1% patients undergo thrombotic complications

Mechanism

- Mechanism of HIT I:
  - Non-immune mediated mechanism
  - Occurs due to drug binding to platelets
  - This inhibits platelet aggregation
- Mechanism of HIT II:
  - Immune mediated mechanism
  - Heparin complexes with PF4 and forms the antigen
  - IgG antibodies develop against this antigen and bind to heparin-PF4 complexes
  - This causes endothelial injury, complement activation and heparin neutralization
  - This results in platelet aggregation and platelet (white) clots

Risk Factors

- Can occur with any dose of heparin, any route of administration
- Highest incidence with full dose UFH
- Bovine UFH> porcine UFH > LMWH > danaparoid
- Surgical patients > medical patients

Clinical Features

- Onset on day 5–10 after heparin exposure
- Triad of signs in heparin induced thrombocytopenia:
  - Thrombocytopenia
  - Tachyphylaxis to heparin and heparin resistance
  - Thrombotic complication
- Thrombocytopenia:
  - May begin within hours in patients previously exposed
  - Can even occur with catheter flush doses
- Tachyphylaxis: Antibodies disappear within 3 months of discontinuation
- Thrombotic complications:
  - Can cause venous/arterial thrombii in iliac arteries and aorta
  - Manifestations:
    - DVT, pulmonary embolism
    - DIC, stroke, MI, splanchnic ischemia
    - Gangrene of legs and arms
  - Risk of thrombosis persists upto 30 days after cessation of heparin
  - Highest risk within first 10 days of diagnosis

Types

Feature	HIT I	HIT II
Synonym	Heparin associated thrombocytopenia	Heparin induced platelet activation
Incidence	More common	Less common
Severity	Mild	Severe, life threatening
Incidence	30–40% of heparinized patients	0.5–6% patients
Type	Non-immunological	Immunological
Mechanism	Drug induced platelet aggregation	Due to heparin interaction with PF_4
Antiplatelet antibodies	Absent	Present
Platelet count	Less than 1,00,000/ mm^3	Less than 50,000/ mm^3
Onset	Less than 3 days of therapy	6–10 days of heparin therapy
Resolution	Spontaneous	Not spontaneous
Complications	Benign	Severe with end organ damage
Thrombosis	Not seen	Causes stroke and amputation
Diagnosis	Solely clinical	Enzyme assays
Therapy	No specific therapy	Specific therapy indicated

Determination of Risk

- *Warkentins criteria*
- To determine probability of heparin induced thrombocytopenia:

Criteria	2 Points	1 Point	0 Point
Thrombocytopenia	> 50% fall	30–50% fall	< 30% fall
Onset	Onset on day 5–10	Onset after day 10	Platelet count fall too early
	< 1 day if heparin in past 3 months		No recent heparin exposure
Sequelae	New thrombosis	Progressive thrombosis	None
	Skin necrosis	Erythematous skin lesion	
	Post-heparin acute reaction		
Other causes	No other cause	Other cause possible	Definite other cause
Pretest probability score			
6–8	High probability		
4–5	Intermediate probability		
0–3	Low probability		

Diagnosis

- Platelet aggregation studies: Simple and cost effective
- Antibody assays:
  - Functional assays:
    - PF_4-Ig assay
    - Serotonin release assay: Gold standard
  - ELIZA: easy and rapid
- Mainly clinical diagnosis: Suspect HIT if:
  - Declining platelet count to less than 50% 0f baseline value
  - Occurs within 5–10 days of heparin therapy
  - Other causes of thrombocytopenia have been excluded
  - Condition resolves after cessation of therapy

Prevention of Hit

- Immediate evaluation if heparin resistance/tachyphylaxis
- Minimize dose and duration of heparin
- Use LMWH/porcine heparin
- No heparin bonded vascular catheters
- Heparin less catheter flush solution
- Avoid platelet transfusion: helps in formation and extension of thrombus
- Add heparin to list of drug allergies in patients medical chart

Treatment

- HIT I requires no specific treatment
- HIT II:
  - Discontinue heparin immediately
  - Anticoagulation for CPB with HIT:
  - Give antithrombotic drugs which do not produce immune mediated thrombocytopenia Alternatives:
    - Warfarin, anerod
    - Orgaran, danaparoid
  - Platelet transfusion if platelet count is low
  - LMWH have a high incidence of cross reaction with heparin dependant antibodies and is not useful

Anticoagulation in HIT

Anticoagulation in active HIT: Avoid heparin in any route:

Procedure	Agent	Dose	Monitor
CPB	Lepirudin	0.25 mg/kg bolus	ECT
		0.5 mg/kg infusion	
	Argatroban	0.1 mg/kg bolus	ACT
		5–10 µg/kg/min infusion	
PCI	Argatroban	350 µg/kg bolus	ACT
		25 µg/kg/min infusion	
	Danaparoid	2250 IU bolus	
		200 IU/hr infusion	

Anticoagulation in subacute HIT: Avoid heparin in any route:

Drug	Dose	Monitor
Lepirudin IV	0.4 mg/kg	aPTT
	0.15 mg/kg/hr	
Argatroban IV	2 µg/kg/hr	aPTT
Danaparoid S/C	1500–2250 IU Q12H	Anti-Xa levels

Anticoagulation in Patients with History of HIT

- Heparin re-exposure considered for short term anticoagulation (CPB)
- Alternative anticoagulants to be used for long term indication

Anticoagulation in Pregnancy with History of Hit

- No heparin use in active/subacute HIT
- Danaparoid can be used
- Not known if fondaparunix/DTI crosses placenta.

Differential Diagnosis

- Aplastic anemia, septicemia
- Leukemia, DIC

- Alcoholism
- Drugs: drug induced thrombocytopenia:
  - Quinidine, cytotoxic drugs
  - Gold, rifampicin
  - Sulfa drugs, valproate

Feature	HIT	DIT
Platelet count	50,000/mm³	Less than 10000/mm³
Mechanism	F_{cr} activation	F_{ab} mediated
Thrombosis	Yes	No
Bleeding	Rarely	Yes

LOW MOLECULAR WEIGHT HEPARIN

Introduction

They are produced from unfractionated heparin by chemical and enzymatic depolymerization.

Chemistry

- Mean molecular weight 4000–6500 Da
- Ranges from 2000–10,000 Da
- Fragments are one-third the size of heparin
- Chain length of 13–22 sugars

Types

- Nadroparin: By N_2O depolymerization
- Enoxaparin: Benzylation followed by alkaline depolymerization
- Dalteparin: N_2O depolymerization
- Ardeparin: Peroxidative depolymerization
- Tinzaparin: Enzymatic depolymerization with heparinase
- Reviparin: N_2O depolymerization
- Danaparoid: Prepared from animal gut mucosa

Mechanism of Action

- Smaller size molecule and thus retains full anti-Xa activity with less anti-IIa activity
- Anti Xa: Anti IIa = 4: 1
- Also binds directly to factor VII and reduces production of prothrombinase

Pharmacokinetics

- Route of administration: subcutaneous
- Absorption: Absorbed completely, 90% bioavailability
- Distribution:
  - Less protein bound (only 10%)
  - Half-life is 2–4 times longer than UFH
- Metabolism: Partially by desulfonation and depolymerization
- Excretion:
  - Not depolymerized by endothelial cells which occurs rapidly
  - Excreted only through renal route
  - Thus the duration of action is prolonged

Monitoring

- Monitoring is generally not required as anticoagulant effect is predictable
- LMWH also reduces risk of bleeding
- aPTT is a relatively insensitive indicator
- Anti-Xa levels are measured to monitor LMWH (should be kept at 0.5–0.8 IU/mL)
- PT and INR also used

Uses

- Prevention of VTE:
  - Enoxaparin 20–40 mg S/C given 6 hours preoperatively
  - LMWH continued once daily thereafter
- Treatment of VTE
- Treatment of unstable angina and NQWMI: 1 mg/kg enoxaparin Q12H

Reversal: Reversal of low molecular weight heparin:

- 1 mg protamine given for every 100 anti-Xa units (for enoxaparin)
- Protamine is given within first 8 hours of administering LMWH
- If bleeding continues, 0.5 mg protamine/100 anti-Xa units can be administered
- Smaller doses needed beyond 8 hours after LMWH administration
- Protamine neutralizes 65% of anti-Xa activity and 90% of anti-IIa activity

Advantages over UFH

- Protects against VTE better
- Greater efficacy: Safety ratio
- Once daily dose possible due to long DOA
- No monitoring required
- Less hemorrhage, osteoporosis, HIT

Classification of Anticoagulants

- Used in-vitro:
  - Heparin
  - Sodium citrate: 1.65 gm/350 mL of blood
  - Sodium oxalate
  - Sodium edetate

- Used in-vivo:
  - Parenteral agents:
    - Heparin (UFH, LMWN)
    - Heparinoids:
    - Heparan sulfate
    - Ancrod
    - Dextran sulfate
  - Oral anticoagulants:
    - Coumarin derivatives:
      - Warfarin, acenocoumarin
      - Dicoumarol, ethyl bicoumacetate
    - Inandione: phenindione

HEPARIN ALTERNATIVES

Classification

- Direct thrombin inhibitors:
  - Lepirudin, bivalirudin
  - Debigatran etixilate
  - Argatroban, ximelagatran
- Anti-Xa agents:
  - Danaparoid, rivaroxaban
  - Fondaparinux
- Warfarin
- Defibrinogenating agents: ancrod

Direct Thrombin Inhibitors

Introduction

In contrast to the indirect inhibition of thrombin caused by heparin, DTIs require no preceding interaction prior to their effect on thrombosis (factor IIa).

Properties

- More specific
- Do not cross-react with HIT antibodies
- Acts on both soluble and thrombus bound thrombin
- Anti-inflammatory property
- Suppresses platelet function
- Used to treat arterial/venous thrombotic disorders

Lepirudin/Desirudin

- Chemistry:
  - Recombinant hirudin derivative
  - Is present in saliva of ***hirudomedicinalis***
  - Derived from yeast cells
- Kinetics:
  - Half-life of 1.3 hours with peak effect in about 4 hours
  - Eliminated through renal clearance and effect is therefore prolonged in renal failure
- Indications:
  - Anticoagulation with renal replacement therapy
  - CPB in heparin induced thrombocytopenia
- Dose:
  - 0.4mg/kg bolus followed by 0.15 mg/kg/hr infusion
  - When INR reaches 2, reducelepirudin rate by 50%
  - Stop infusion when INR reaches 2.5
  - aPTT titrated to 1.5–2.5 times baseline
- Monitoring:
  - ECT (Ecarin clotting time)
  - aPTT, ACT
  - PT, INR, TEG
- Contraindications:
  - Patients with recent biopsy
  - Stroke, major surgery
  - Major bleeding, uncontrolled hypertension
- Benefits:
  - Rapid onset of action
  - Short half-life
  - Does notcross react with HIT antibodies
  - Risk of bleeding is not increased
- Reversal:
  - No antidote, factor VIIa may be tried for reversal
  - Emergency reversal can be done with plasmapheresis, hemofilteration and peritoneal dialysis

Argatroban

- Small (molecular weight of 500 Da) arginine derivative
- Promotes nitric oxide release
- Half-life of 40–50 minutes
- Undergoes hepatic metabolism and excretion and is therefore useful in CRF
- FDA approved for use in PCI
- Dose: 2 µg/kg/min infusion
- Monitor ACT and aPTT
- Maintain aPTT at 1.5–3 times baseline
- Contraindicated when there is active bleeding

Bivalirudin

- Direct thrombin inhibitor
- Dose: 0.75 mg/kg followed by 1.75 mg/kg/hr infusion

Ximelagatran

- Oral prodrug of DTI melagatran
- Converts to melagatran which binds to clot bound and free thrombin

- Elimination half-life of 3 hours, cleared by kidneys
- Monitoring of coagulation is not necessary during therapy
- Does not increase incidence of bleeding
- Withdrawn from market due to hepatotoxicity: transiently increases transaminase levels

Dabigatran Etexilate

- New oral prodrug of DTI dabigatran used for DVT prophylaxis
- Has low molecular weight
- Dosage: 200 mg OD 1–4 hours after surgery
- Epidural avoided for 36 hours after a dose and 12 hours before next dose

Anti-Xa Agents

Danaparoid

- Derived from porcine intestinal mucosa
- Composed of heparin, dermatan and chondroitin sulphate
- Is a univalent DTI and anti Xa agent
- Anti-Xa: Antithrombin activity = 28: 1
- Molecular weight of 527 Da
- Half life of 40–50 minutes with elimination by renal clearance
- In heparin induced thrombocytopenia, 25 μg/kg/min to 350 μg/kg
- Monitoring:
  - ACT maintained at 250–300 seconds
  - Anti-Xa assay (0.5–0.8 U/mL is normal)
- Has low risk of bleeding
- Emergency clearance can be done by plasmapheresis

Fondaparinux

- Synthetic anticoagulant
- Contains 5 saccharide units
- These bind to antithrombin and inhibit factor Xa directly and indirectly
- 100% oral bioavailability
- Rapid onset of action (25 minutes after subcutaneous injection)
- Peak action 1–2 hours
- Elimination half-life 15 hours
- Elimination unchanged by kidneys and is therefore prolonged in CRF
- Useful to prevent DVT and pulmonary embolism
- Given 2.5 mg subcutaneously once daily

Rivaroxaban

- Potent, selective *oral* Xa inhibitor
- 10 mg Q6-8H after surgery
- Remove epidural at least 20 hours after initial dose
- Next dose of epidural is delayed 4 hours after catheter removal

Defibrinogenating Agents: Ancrod

- Defibrinogenating agent
- It is derived from Malayan pit viper venom
- Multiple mechanisms of action:
  - Cleaves fibrinogen to prevent clot formation
  - Reduces blood viscosity causing improved blood flow: Reperfusing agent
  - Thrombus modification
  - Altered hemostasis
- It also limits brain damage in stroke
- Half-life of 3–5 hours, mainly eliminated via renal clearance
- Given subcutaneously or via IV infusion
- Contraindications:
  - Bleeding disorders, platelet counts < 1,00,000/mm^3 (except HIT)
  - Planned surgery
  - Active GIT ulcers, renal stones
  - Uncontrolled hypertension

FONDAPARINUX

Introduction

Fondaparinux is a synthetic glycopyranoside antithrombotic agent.

Chemistry

- Fondaparinux is a synthetic pentasaccharide
- Molecular formula is $C_{31}H_{43}N_3Na_{10}O_{49}S_8$
- Molecular weight of fondaparinux is 1728 Da

Mechanism of Action

- Fondaparinux binds specifically to anti-thrombin III (AT III)
- This in turn potentiates the neutralization of factor Xa by AT III by 300 times
- Neutralization of factor X_a interrupts the conversion of prothrombin to thrombin
- This inhibits fibrinogen conversion to fibrin and clot propagation

- Fondaparinux however, does not have an effect on:
  - Platelet function
  - Inactivation of thrombin (Factor II)
  - Fibrinolysis
  - Bleeding time
- Fondaparinux does not have an antidote to reverse its action
- Monitoring of anticoagulation is usually not required with fondaparinux

Measurement of Action

- PT, INR and aPTT are relatively insensitive measures of the factor X_a activity
- Monitoring of anticoagulation is usually not required with fondaparinux
- Monitoring therapy may however be indicated in high risk populations such as:
  - Renal impairment
  - Pregnant women
- Monitoring pharmacodynamics can be done using fondaparinux plasma concentrations
- Plasma concentrations are quantified via anti-factor Xa activity
- Activity of fondaparinux is expressed as milligrams of fondaparinux calibrator
- The anti-Xa activity increases with increasing drug concentrations

Pharmacokinetics

- Peak action: Occurs 3 hours after subcutaneous injection
- Peak plasma concentration: 0.34–0.50 mg/L
- Duration of action:
  - Effects persist for 2–4 days (3–5 half lives) in those with normal renal function
  - Effects may last longer in those with renal impairment
- Absorption:
  - Absorption is rapid and complete following subcutaneous injection
  - Absolute bioavailability is 100% on subcutaneous injection
- Distribution:
  - Distributes minimally in the extravascular fluid compartment
  - Binds specifically to antithrombin III and is highly specific (almost 94%)
  - Thus, it binds minimally to other plasma proteins and RBCs
  - Volume of distribution V_d of 7–11 liters
- Metabolism:
  - At present, there is no evidence of metabolism
  - Majority of a dose is eliminated unchanged by the kidneys
- Elimination:
  - Eliminated unchanged by the kidneys
  - Up to 77% of a S/C or IV dose is eliminated unchanged by kidneys
  - Elimination $T_{1/2}$ is 17–21 hours
- Renal impairment:
  - Fondaparinux elimination is prolonged in those with renal impairment
  - This is because elimination is mainly via urinary excretion of unchanged drug
- Hepatic impairment: Pharmacokinetics has not been studied in patients with hepatic impairment
- Pregnancy:
  - Pregnancy category B
  - Drug should be used during pregnancy only if clearly needed

Dosage

- First dose is administered 6–8 hrs post surgery to reduce risk of major bleeding
- Dose of 2.5 mg once daily S/C for DVT prophylaxis in patients > 50 kg weight
- Dose for treatment of DVT and pulmonary embolism:
  - 5 mg subcutaneously OD for patients < 50 kg weight
  - 7.5 mg subcutaneously OD for patients 50 -100 kg weight
  - 10 mg subcutaneously OD for patients > 100 kg weight

Indications

- Prophylaxis of DVT in patients undergoing:
  - Surgery for hip fractures for minimum 14 days post surgery (up to 1 month)
  - Hip replacement surgery for minimum 14 days post surgery (up to 1 month)
  - Knee replacement surgery for minimum 14 days post surgery (up to 1 month)
  - Abdominal surgery for up to 10 days post surgery
- DVT prophylaxis in those with heparin induced thrombocytopenia
- Treatment of DVT, administered in conjunction with warfarin
- Treatment of acute pulmonary embolism, in conjunction with warfarin
- Management of unstable angina, NSTEMI, STEMI

Contraindications

- Severe renal impairment, with creatinine clearance < 30 mL/min
- As prophylactic therapy in patients weighing less than 50 kg in those undergoing:
  - Surgery for hip fractures
  - Hip and knee replacement
- Patients with active major bleeding
- Thrombocytopenia
- Patients at increased risk of bleeding:
  - Congenital or acquired bleeding disorders
  - Active angioplastic GI disease
  - Hemorrhagic stroke
  - Use of concomitant platelet inhibitor therapy
- Bacterial endocarditis
- Hypersensitivity to fondaparinux

Adverse Effects

- Hepatotoxicity: Therapy can be associated with increase in aminotransferase levels
- Major bleeding, especially in:
  - Those receiving therapeutic doses of fondaparinux
  - Patients weighing less than 50 kg
  - Renal impairment
- Spinal and epidural hematomas when used with neuraxial anesthesia
- Thrombocytopenia with thrombosis, similar to HIT
- Serious allergic reactions

PROTAMINE

Introduction

- Protamines are nucleoproteins found in the sperm cells of fish
- These were developed in the 1930s as a heparin reversal agent
- Till date, it is the only FDA approved agent available for heparin neutralization

Chemistry

- Protamine is a basic polypeptide occurring in combination with a nucleic acid
- It was originally derived from sperm of salmon, in the form of salmine
- Salmine molecular structure is $ARG_{51}ALA_4VAL_4ILE_1PRO_7SER_6$
- Molecular weight of salmine is close to 6000 Da
- Thus, it is a simple protein with the following properties:
  - Low molecular weight
  - Rich in arginine
  - Strongly basic (pH between 6.8–7.1
- Other types of protamine:
  - Sturine from sturgeon
  - Clupeine from herring sperm
- It is currently produced using recombinant techniques
- Available in glass ampoules of 5 mL, each containing 50 mg, with a shelf life of 2 years
- Should be stored between 15–30 °C, taking care to prevent freezing
- Diluted solutions should be discarded as it does not contain any preservative

Mechanism of Action

- Neutralization of unfractionated heparin:
  - Protamine is cationic at a pH of 6.8–7.1 while heparin is anionic at a pH of 5–7.5
  - Protamine binds covalently with heparin to form a stable ionic complex
  - This results from a polyanionic-polycationic interaction
  - This ionic complex is free of anticoagulant activity
  - The complex is eventually removed by the reticulo-endothelial system
  - Thus, protamine neutralizes the anticoagulant effect of unfractionated heparin
- Neutralization of low molecular weight heparin:
  - The ability of protamine to neutralize heparin varies with the heparin chain length
  - Thus, short chain fragments cannot be neutralized with protamine
  - This results in incomplete neutralization of anti-Xa activity and thus, LMWH
- Direct anticoagulant effect of protamine:
  - Protamine has a direct anticoagulant effect when administered:
    - In the absence of heparin
    - In doses larger than those required to neutralize heparin
  - This anticoagulant effect is due to protamine's anti-thromboplastin activity
  - This results in the inhibition of thrombin generation and anticoagulant effect

Pharmacokinetics

- Onset of action:
  - Onset of action occurs within 30–60 seconds of IV administration

- Heparin neutralization occurs within 5 minutes of IV administration

❖ Peak action: Not known
❖ Duration of action: 2 hours, depending on body temperature
❖ Absorption:
  - Protamine can only be administered intravenously
  - Protamine administered in any other way does not neutralize heparin

❖ Distribution: Volume of distribution V_d 12.3 liters
❖ Metabolism:
  - Protamine-heparin complexes may be partially metabolized by fibrinolysin
  - This in turn frees up heparin from protamine

❖ Elimination:
  - Mechanism of elimination has not yet been discovered
  - Clearance of 2.2 L/min
  - Elimination $T_{1/2}$ of 7.4 minutes
  - Protamine is cleared from blood at a rate much faster than heparin
  - Also, S/C or IM heparin administration may cause prolonged anticoagulation
  - Therefore further doses may be required in these scenarios to neutralize heparin
  - This is based on ACT measurements, usually taken 5–15 mins after protamine

❖ Pregnancy category C: should be given to a pregnant woman only if clearly needed
❖ No dosage adjustment is required in those with renal or liver dysfunction

Indications and Dosage

❖ Heparin neutralization:
  - 1.5 mg protamine is administered per 100 units of heparin
  - Dose is monitored with aPTT 5–15 minutes after dose and again after 2–8 hours
  - Dosage according to time elapsed since heparin dose:
    - Less than 30 minutes: 1–1.5 mg/100 units heparin
    - 30–120 minutes: 0.5–0.75 mg/100 units of heparin
    - 120 minutes: 0.25–0.375 mg/100 units of heparin

❖ Dalteparin/tinzaparin neutralization:
  - 1 mg protamine per 100 units of dalteparin or tinzaparine
  - aPTT is measured 4 hours after protamine administration
  - If aPTT remains elevated 0.5 mg protamine per 100 units dalteparin/tinzaparin

❖ Enoxaparine neutralization:
  - 1 mg protamine/mg enoxaparine if dose has been administered within last 8 hrs
  - 0.5 mg protamine/mg enoxaparine if dose was administered beyond last 8 hrs

Contraindications

❖ Fish allergy
❖ Previously vascetomized patients
❖ Hypersensitivity

Adverse Effects

❖ Hypotension:
  - Slow IV administration is recommended
  - Rate of administration should be < 50 mg every 10 minutes
  - Rapid IV infusion causes hypotension
  - Risk factor for hypotension with protamine use:
    - High dose
    - Rapid rate of administration
    - Repeated doses
    - Previous administration of protamine or protamine containing drugs like:
      - NPH insulin
      - Protamine zinc insulin
    - Previous vasectomy
    - Allergy to fish

❖ Protamine reaction:
  - Characteristics of protamine reactions:
    - Sudden onset
    - Severe bronchospasm with extreme difficulty in ventilation
    - Hyperinflation of lungs
    - Pulmonary hypertension with normal LA pressures
    - Progression to fulminant non-cardiogenic pulmonary edema
    - Significant mortality
  - Risk factors for protamine reactions:
    - Preexisting pulmonary HTN secondary to valvular heart disease
    - Prior protamine exposure from insulin use
    - Post vasectomy patients
    - Allergy to vertebrate fish

- Types of reactions:
  - Type I reactions:
    - Brief hypotension
    - Most likely secondary to histamine release
  - Type II reactions:
    - Type II reactions are mainly allergic
    - Classified further into:
      - Type II A: True anaphylactic reaction
      - Type II B: Early anaphylactoid reaction
      - Type II C: Delayed anaphylactoid reaction
  - Type III reactions:
    - Acute pulmonary hypertension is classified as type III reaction
    - RV failure and cardiovascular collapse can be precipitated
    - Biventricular failure can occur rarely
    - Thought to be mediated by both immune and non-immune factors
    - It is an extremely rare complication
- Management:
  - Administration of supportive therapy:
    - Epinephrine, dopamine
    - Vasopressors- norepinephrine
    - Inodilators: Milrinone
    - Steroids
    - Methylene blue
  - Heparin administration:
    - This can reverse heparin-protamine complexes
    - Thromboxane release from macrophages may thus be stopped
    - This may theoretically help control severity of protamine reactions
  - Potassium replacement
  - Nitric oxide therapy
  - Inhaled prostacyclin (PGI_2)

- Anaphylaxis
- Flushing
- Pulmonary hypertension
- Circulatory collapse
- Nausea and vomiting

Protamine Alternatives

- Hexadimethrine bromide:
  - Also called polybrene
  - Used earlier, but no longer available for clinical use
- rPF4: most promising agent
- If risks of adverse reactions to protamine outweigh risk of bleeding, spontaneous reversal of heparin preferred

EPSILON AMINO CAPROIC ACID

Introduction

6-amino-hexanoic acid which acts as an inhibitor of fibrinolysis.

Chemistry

- Chemically, it is 6-amino-hexanoic acid
- Molecular formula: $C_6H_3NO_2$
- Packed as 250 mg/mL of EACA with 0.9% benzyl alcohol as preservative

Pharmacokinetics

- Volume of distribution: 30 ± 8litres
- Distributes throughout extravascular and intravascular compartments
- Penetrates RBCs and other tissue cells
- Eliminated renally with clearance = 116 mL/min
- Elimination half-life of approximately 2 hours

Indications: Excessive bleeding due to:

- Systemic fibrinolysis: Pathological condition associated with:
  - Cardiac surgery, porto-caval shunt
  - Hematological disorders like aplastic anemia
  - Abruptio, liver cirrhosis
  - Carcinoma of prostrate, lung, stomach
- Urinary fibrinolysis: Normal physiological phenomenon associated with:
  - Complications following severe trauma
  - Following anoxia and shock

Dosage

- Priming dose of 5 g oral/IV (through slow infusion)
- Followed by 1–1.25 g doses at hourly intervals
- This is continued for 8 hours or until bleeding stops
- Dose more than 30 grams in 24 hour period is not recommended

Contraindications

- When there is evidence of active intravascular clotting process
- In presence of DIC without using concomitant heparin
- Hematuria of upper urinary tract origin:
  - EACA can cause intra-renal obstruction
  - Form clots in renal pelvis and ureters causing obstruction
- Early pregnancy unless benefits out-weighs the risks as teratogenicity not established

- Not recommended in children and neonates:
  - Preservative benzyl alcohol can cause ***Gasping syndrome***
  - Syndrome consists of:
    - Gasping respiration
    - Hypotension, bradycardia
    - Cardiovascular collapse

Adverse Effects

- General:
  - Edema, headache, malaise
  - Hypersensitivity, anaphylaxis
- Local: Injection site reaction, pain, necrosis
- Neurological:
  - Confusion, dizziness
  - Convulsion, hallucinations
  - Delirium, intracranial hypertension
  - Stroke, syncope
- Cardiovascular:
  - Bradycardia
  - Hypotension (especially if rapid IV boluses)
  - Peripheral ischemia
  - Thrombosis
- Respiratory:
  - Dyspnea
  - Nasal congestion
  - Pulmonary embolism
- Genitourinary: Raised blood urea nitrogen, renal failure
- Dermatological: Pruritis, rashes
- Musculoskeletal:
  - Raised CPK levels, myalgia
  - Muscle weakness, myopathy
  - Myositis, rhabdomyolysis
- Hematological:
  - Agranulocytosis
  - Leukopenia
  - Coagulation disorders, thrombocytopenia

Overdose: Causes transient hypotension, ARF and death

NITROUS OXIDE

Introduction

Prepared by ***Joseph Priestly*** in 1776.

Properties

- Colorless, odourless, inorganic gas
- Non explosive and non-inflammable but supports combustion
- Gas at room temperature, becomes liquid under pressure
- Manufactured by heating ammonium nitrate in a controlled process
- Low blood gas partition coefficient (BGPC 0.47%)
- High MAC value (105%)
- Poor solubility but more soluble than oxygen
- More soluble than nitrogen (35 times)
- 1.5 times heavier than air

Pharmacodynamics

I. Central Nervous System

- Weak anesthetic
- Powerful analgesic
- Mild evaluation of ICP as it increases CBF and CBV
- Increases cerebral O_2 consumption
- Maximum analgesic effect at 35% concentration

II. Neuromuscular

- No muscle relaxation
- Skeletal muscle rigidity at high concentration

III. Respiratory System

- Increased respiratory rate, reduces tidal volume
- Reduces ventilatory response to hypoxia and hypercarbia
- ***Diffusion hypoxia*** on emergence

IV. Cardiovascular System

- Slight direct myocardial depression
- Offset by sympathetic stimulation
- Opioids can block sympathomimetic effects
- Increases pulmonary vascular resistance

V. Hepatic and GIT

- Reduces hepatic blood flow
- May cause PONV by stimulating CTZ and vomiting centre in medulla

VI. Renals

- Increases renal vascular resistance
- Reduces renal blood flow: Reduced GFR and urine output

Pharmacokinetics

- Mainly eliminated unchanged through lungs
- < 0.01% undergoes reductive metabolism by anerobic bacteria in GIT
- Small amounts diffuse through skin

Mechanisms of Action

- Analgesic action through stimulation of opioid receptors
- Anxiolytic action through stimulation of GABA receptors

Anesthetic Uses

- As a supplement to anesthesia
- As carrier gas for inhalational agents
- As analgesic agent in: *As entonox*
    - Obstetrics for labor analgesia
    - Burn dressing
    - Dental pain
    - Acute trauma and fracture reduction

Contraindications

Absolute

- Neurosurgery
- Middle ear surgeries
- Congenital heart diseases with pulmonary HTN
- Significant respiratory compromise
- Laparoscopic surgeries
- Pneumothorax/air embolism/bowel obstruction

Relative

- History of stroke/hypotension
- Vitamin B_{12}/folate deficiency
- Pregnancy

Effects on Closed Gas Spaces

Highly Compliant Spaces

- Spaces normally contain nitrogen which:
    - Has low solubility
    - BGPC of nitrogen is 0.015
    - BGPC of N_2O is 0.47
- Therefore, entrance of N_2O into the space is not countered by an equal loss of N_2
- This increases the volume of the space
- Expansion occurs in cases of:
    - Pneumothorax, pneumoperitoneum
    - Air embolus
    - ETT cuff and cuff of inflatable balloons (Swann Ganz catheter)
- 75% N_2O in pneumothorax doubles the volume in 10 min and triples it by 30 mins
- 4 hrs of N_2O at 100% increases ETT cuff volume by 300–350%

Poorly Complaint Spaces

- Increased IOP after intravitreal SF_6 for retinal detachment surgery
- Middle ear pressure: Tympanic membrane rupture and displacement of TM graft during tympanoplasty
- Increased ICP during neurosurgery

Toxicity

Bone Marrow Toxicity

- Can cause bone marrow depression: Megaloblastic anemia and pernicious anemia
- Irreversibly oxidizes cobalt atom in vitamin B_{12}
- This inhibits vitamin B_{12} dependent enzymes
    - Methionine synthetase: Myelin formation
    - Thymidylate synthetase: DNA synthesis
- Complete bone marrow failure after several days of exposure
- More than 12 hrs exposure causes mild and > 24 hrs causes marked changes

Neurotoxicity

- Neurodeficits on prolonged exposure:
    - Peripheral neuropathy
    - Subacute degeneration of cord after several months
- Prevented by pretreating patients with large doses of folinic acid
- This gets converted to 5,10 methylene THF and causes thymidine synthesis

Reproductive Toxicity

- No significant effect on sperms
- Reduced fertility and increased spontaneous abortion rates on chronic exposure
- Teratogenic effects

Immunological Toxicity

- Alters chemotaxis
- Alters neutrophil mobility

Environmental toxicity: *NIOSH recommendation*
Theatre pollution: Recommended maximum level of N_2O < 25 ppm parts of air

Desirable Properties

- Inexpensive
- Poor solubility: Ensures quick induction and recovery
- ***Second gas effect***: Accelerates anesthetic effect

- Lessens respiratory irritation produced by isoflurane/sevoflurane
- Weak anesthetic but powerful analgesic
- Has little effect on respiration
- Has little effect on BP and heart rate

Undesirable Properties

- Limited potency, MAC of 105
- Cannot produce anesthesia alone
- MAC_{awake} for N_2O suppresses awareness but not recall
- Reduces delivered O_2 concentration and thus increases risk of hypoxia
- Diffusion hypoxia at emergence
- Impaired pulmonary function: Increased risk of hypoxia
- Can expand bowel gas, pneumothorax, air embolism, ETT cuff volume
- Can increase ICP, IOP and middle ear pressure
- Increases $CMRO_2$, CBF, ICP
- Increases pulmonary vascular resistance
- Does not provide ischemic preconditioning like volatile anesthetics
- Increases muscle tone and rigidity when used alone
- Can cause bone marrow depression and neurotoxicity
- Supports combustion

Current Status: Due to increased number of undesirable properties, it is proposed that eliminating N_2O use leads to safer anesthetic delivery devices.

NITRIC OXIDE

Introduction

- Vasoactive gas naturally produced from L-arginine, primarily in endothelial cells which is an important messenger molecule
- Formerly called endothelium derived relaxation factor (EDRF)

Chemistry

- Colourless, colorless, corrosive
- Only slightly soluble in water
- Unstable in air, undergoes spontaneous oxidation and forms NO_2

Presentation

- Stored in aluminium or stainless steel cylinders
- Typically have 40 L capacity at high pressures (2000 PSIG)
- Stored as 100/1000/2000 ppm of NO in nitrogen

Sites at Which Nitric Oxide is Biological Mediator

- Vascular endothelium
- Platelets
- Marcrophages
- Brain tissue

Diseases Associated with Abnormal Nitric Oxide Production

- Ageing, smoking
- HTN, obesity, Type I and II DM, atherosclerosis
- Dyslipidemias:
  - Hypercholesterolemia
  - Hypertriglyceridemia
- Heart failure
- Multiple sclerosis
- Ulcerative colitis
- Arthritis

Administration

- Injected into patient limb of inspiratory circuit of ventilator
- To be stored prediluted in nitrogen
- Not injected between patient and ventilator to avoid over-dosage
- Not allowed to contact air/oxygen until it is used (to prevent NO_2 formation)
- Use of sodalime in inspiratory limb to absorb the formed $NO_2$is advocated
- Delivered safely via face mask/nasal cannula/ET tube

Mechanism of Action

- Nitric oxide diffuses out from endothelial cells and enters vascular smooth muscle
- It then stimulates guanylate cyclase and increases c-GMP levels causing vasodilation
- NO also causes vasodilation by reducing cytosolic calcium

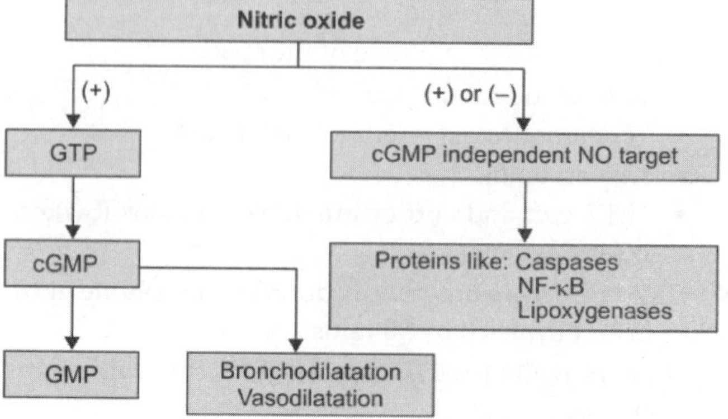

Pharmacokinetics

- Absorption:
  - Highly lipid soluble
  - Freely diffuses across cell membranes
- Metabolism:
  - Rapidly converted to nitrates and nitrites in presence of oxygen
  - Reacts with oxidized hemoglobin to form methemoglobin
  - Half-life less than 5 seconds

Pharmacodynamics

- Central nervous system:
  - Acts as neurotransmitter in CNS
  - Important role in modulation of:
    - State of arousal
    - Pain perception
    - Apoptosis
    - Long term neuronal depression and excitation
  - Peripheral neurons with NO control regional blood flow in corpus cavernosum
- Cardiovascular:
  - Direct vasodilatation
  - Indirect vasodilatation by inhibiting AT-II medicated vasoconstriction
  - Antithrombotic effect by inhibiting platelet aggregation
  - Anti-proliferative action by inhibiting smooth muscle hyperplasia
  - Anti-inflammatory by inhibiting leukocyte adhesion to vascular endothelium
  - Anti-apoptotic
- Respiratory:
  - Selective pulmonary vasodilator when inhaled
  - Preferentially increases blood flow to well ventilated areas
  - Selective to pulmonary blood vessels as it rapidly binds to hemoglobin with high affinity and gets inactivated before reaching systemic circulation
  - Improves ventilation-perfusion relationship
  - Bronchodilatation
  - Anti-inflammatory
- Gastrointestinal:
  - Determinant of GI motility
  - Modulates morphine induced constipation
- Genitourinary:
  - Role in regulation of renin production
  - Role in Na^+ homeostasis in kidney
  - Physiological mediator of penile erection
- Immunological:
  - Toxic to pathogens, important in host-defense mechanisms
  - Inhibits leucocyte adhesion to vascular endothelium
  - Scavenges superoxide anion
- Hematological:
  - Reduces platelet aggregation
  - Prolongs bleeding time by inhibiting platelet function

Advantages

- Selective pulmonary vasodilator
- Devoid of systemic action
- Dilates blood vessels in those lung regions which are well ventilated
- Favorably affects ventilation-perfusion relationship
- Low toxicity if safety precautions followed

Disadvantages

- Stringent safety precautions required
- NO_2 induced pulmonary edema
- Methemoglobinemia
- Ciliary depletion in terminal bronchioles on chronic use
- Corrosive to metal
- Requires monitoring

Uses

- Pulmonary hypertension:
  - For persistent pulmonary HTN secondary to:
    - Meconium aspiration
    - Pneumonia, sepsis
    - Hyaline membrane disease
    - Congenital diaphragmatic hernia
    - Pulmonary hypoplasia
  - Inhalational NO called INO_{max}
  - Recommended dose: 0.5–20 ppm (upto 80 ppm)
  - Lowest effective dose to be used
  - Onset time for reducing PVR and RV-SWI: 1–2 minutes
  - Should be maintained upto 14 days or until underlying oxygen desaturation has resolved
- ARDS:
  - Effect on outcome not demonstrated conclusively
  - Mechanism of action in ARDS:
    - Selective pulmonary vasodilatation
    - Reduces pulmonary capillary pressure
    - Reduces pulmonary transvascular albumin flux
    - Improves oxygenation

- Intraoperative:
  - Used for lung and cardiac transplants
  - Reduces the incidence of fatal pulmonary HTN post-transplant
  - Pulmonary vasoreactivity testing in catheterization laboratory
  - To treat pulmonary HTN following CABG: 20–40 ppm
  - Pulmonary hypertensive crises following congenital heart disease repair: 10 ppm
  - Insertion of LVAD: To reduce PVR after LVAD insertion
- Pulmonary diseases:
  - Reduces rate of bronchopulmonary dysplasia but additional studies needed
  - COPD patients and bronchospasm:
  - Improves oxygenation when used with 1 L/min O_2 via facemask
  - If used alone, it may reduce oxygenation
- Indirect effects:
  - Drugs like NTG (releasing NO) for angina
  - Drugs altering NO activity protects brain in stroke, Alzheimer and Parkinsons

Monitoring no Levels

- Chemiluminescent reaction:
  - $NO + O_3 \quad NO_2 + O_2$ + light
  - Light is detected by photodetector
- Electrochemical analysis

Toxic Effects

- Meth-hemoglobinemia:
  - Neonates at greater risk as they have reduced levels of methemoglobin reductase
  - If inhaled concentration around 500–2000 ppm
  - Occurs 8 hours after inhalation
- Pulmonary edema if NO_2 levels more than 10 ppm
- Acute lung injury and pneumonitis:
  - Due to elevated NO_2 levels which gets converted to HNO_3 in presence of water
  - This results in the formation of ***Acid Rain***
  - Occurs if environmental levels ≥ 25 ppm for more than 8 hours
- Chronic use/sustained elevation:
  - Direct tissue toxicity
  - Results in ciliary depletion and epithelial hyperplasia of terminal bronchioles
  - Cardiovascular collapse associated with septic shock
- Abrupt discontinuation:
  - Worsens PaO_2 and oxygenation
  - Increase in pulmonary artery pressures
- Headache in hospital staff
- Others:
  - Alveolar hemorrhage, sepsis
  - Atelectasis, hyperglycemia
  - Stridor, cellulitis
  - Hematuria
- Raised LV filling pressure due to direct negative inotropic actions
- Caution in patients with severe LV dysfunction

Contraindications: In neonates dependant on right-left shunt

XENON

Properties

- Colorless, odourless, non-explosive
- Density is 3.2 times that of air
- Viscosity is 1.7 times that of air
- BGPC = 0.15, MAC value = 63%
- Boiling point = 108.1 C
- Molecular weight = 54 kDa

Ideal Anesthetic Agent

- Smooth induction, rapid emergence
- Environmentally safe, no occupational hazards
- Non-toxic, non-allergic
- No carcinogenic potential
- No fetoxicity
- Very low chances of diffusion hypoxia
- Produces anesthesia, analgesia and some degree of muscle relaxation
- Does not cause respiratory depression to the point of apnea
- Cardiac stable, not metabolized in body and eliminated completely by lungs

Mechanism of Action

- Inhibits NMDA receptors: Anesthetic and analgesic actions
- Serotonin inhibitor: Used in management of PONV
- Central and peripheral nociception

Stages of xenon anesthesia: 4 stages of anesthesia with 70% xenon and 30% oxygen

- Stage 1: Whole body paresthesia and hypoalgesia
- Stage 2: Euphoria, increased psychomotor activity
- Stage 3: Analgesia, partial amnesia (after 3–4 minutes)
- Stage 4: Surgical anesthesia with degree of muscle relaxation

Pharmacodynamics

- Central nervous system:
  - Neuroprotective as:
    - NMDA antagonist
    - Anti-apoptotic effects
    - Activation of K^+ channels
  - Some degree of muscle relaxation
  - Increases ICP and CBF in traumatic brain injury patients
  - Produces anesthesia and amnesia
- Cardiovascular:
  - Mild sympatholytic effect
  - Negative inotropic effects
  - Ischemic preconditioning: protects from brief periods of ischemia
  - No significant change in blood pressure
- Respiratory:
  - Increases airway resistance
  - Increases turbulence and work of breathing due to increase in density and viscosity
  - Very low BGPC (0.115): Low chances of diffusion hypoxia

Use in Anesthesia

- Xe^{133} isotope is most commonly used
- MAC value of 63%
- MAC_{AWAKE} of 33%
- 50% xenon causes increase in pain threshold and reduces consciousness
- 80% xenon produces profound analgesia
- Delivered via ***Physioflex*** machine with rotating meters to measure gas flow

Other Uses

- Induction agent
- Nuclear medicine to diagnose ventilation-perfusion mismatch
- To find out functional capacity of lung parenchyma
- CT scans of brain and lungs to:
  - Diagnose early infarct and vasospasm
  - Evaluation of head trauma
  - Confirmation of brain death
  - Locate seizure foci

Disadvantages: High cost and low availability

HALOTHANE HEPATITIS

Definition: Jaundice occurring in a patient who is previously exposed to halothane within 3 weeks with fever, rashes and lab evidence of raised liver enzymes like SGOT, SGPT and antibodies

Incidence

- Male: Female: 1: 2
- Type I halothane hepatitis: 25–30%
- Type II halothane hepatitis: 1: 6000–35000
- In children: 1: 1,00,000–2,00,000 (rare)

Classification

- Type I halothane hepatitis:
  - Mild form
  - Benign features
  - Self limiting disease
  - Mild rise in serum transaminase and glutathione-S-transferase
- Type II halothane hepatitis:
  - Severe form
  - Causes massive centrilobular necrosis
  - Results in fulminant liver failure

Clinical Features

- High grade fever lasting for 3–14 days
- Jaundice: onset within 1–2 days after fever
- Nausea, vomiting anorexia
- Chills, myalgia, rash
- Moderate liver enlargement with tenderness

Lab Findings

- Raised serum bilirubin
- Raised serum ALT, AST and alkaline phosphatase
- Increased prothrombin time
- Increased GST > 2 is specific index

Metabolism and Mechanism

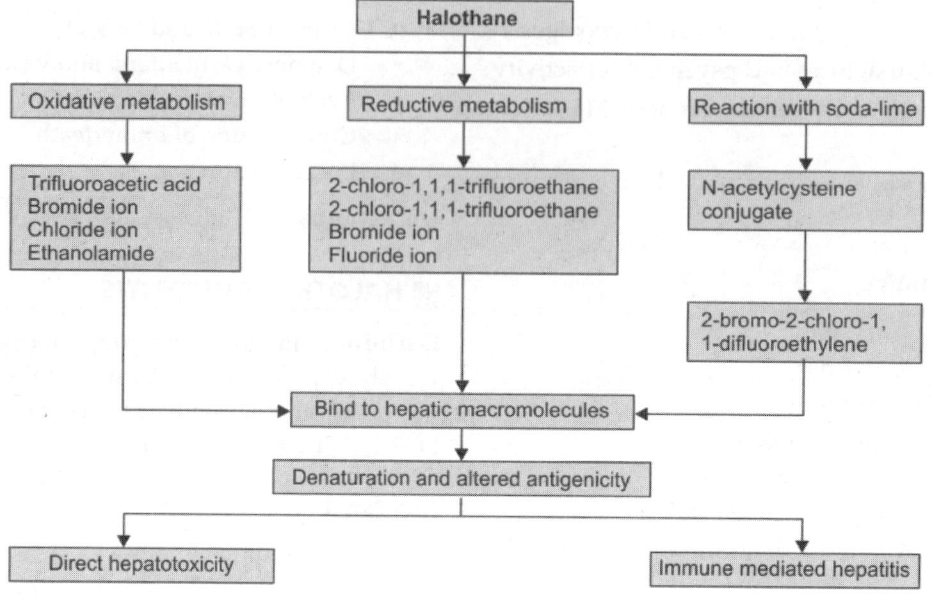

Risk Factors

- Multiple exposures at intervals < 6 weeks
- Prior history of post anesthetic fever/jaundice
- Duration: Prolonged exposure, major surgeries
- Obesity, middle age, pregnancy
- Male: Female ratio: 1: 2
- Enzyme induction (alcohol/barbiturates)
- Drug allergy, recent viral hepatitis

Predisposing Factors

- Pregnancy
- Viral hepatitis
- Burns
- Hypoxia, hypercarbia

Guidelines for safe use: Avoid halothane if:

- Age more than 70 years
- Obese females
- Preexisting liver disease/biliary surgery
- If family history of unexplained jaundice after halothane
- Recent halothane exposure within 6 weeks

Prognosis

- If fulminant liver failure occurs, 50% deaths
- Hepatic encephalopathy also results in 50% deaths

NEPHROTOXICITY OF FLUORINATED AGENTS

Mechanisms of Nephrotoxicity

- Reduced renal blood flow
- Inorganic fluoride production is directly nephrotoxic
- Vinyl halide production
- BCDFE induced nephrotoxicity

Fluoride Induced Nephrotoxicity

Mechanism

- Fluoride inhibition of adenylate cyclase:
  - Prevents normal action of ADH on DCT
  - Therefore unable to concentrate urine
- Fluoride induced intrarenal vasodilation:
  - Shunting of blood from cortex to medullary area
  - This interferes with counter current multiplier mechanisms

Toxic Levels

No.	Fluoride levels	Manifestations
1.	< 50 μmol/L	No evidence of toxicity
2.	50–80 μmol/L	Moderate injury
3.	80–120 μmol/L	Severe injury
4.	> 120 μmol/L	Most often fatal

Clinical Features

- Polyuria (inability to concentrate urine)
- Hyperosmolarity
- Hypernatremia
- Increased plasma creatinine

Factors Affecting Toxicity

Individual Agents

- Methoxyflurane *most nephrotoxic* and causes high output renal failure

- Enflurane: Only transient reduction in renal concentrating ability
- Isoflurane:
  - Resistant to defluorination
  - No significant increased in fluoride concentration on prolonged administration
- Sevoflurane:
  - Due to low blood solubility, even though fluoride concentration increases, it falls very rapidly after surgery and toxicity is very rare
  - Not nephrotoxic
- Desflurane:
  - No evidence of nephrotoxicity
  - No biotransformation
- Halothane: Not nephrotoxic

Metabolism

- Intrarenal metabolism causes more nephrotoxicity than metabolism in liver
- Methoxyflurane and enflurane undergo more intrarenal metabolism to fluoride
- Therefore they are more nephrotoxic
- Sevoflurane undergoes more hepatic metabolism
- Thus sevoflurane is less nephrotoxic even though fluoride concentration is more

Vinyl Halide Nephrotoxicity

Mechanism: Reaction of fluorinated volatile anesthetic agents with CO_2 absorbent produces trifluromethyl vinyl ether (*Sevo-olefin/compound A*)

β Lyase Pathway

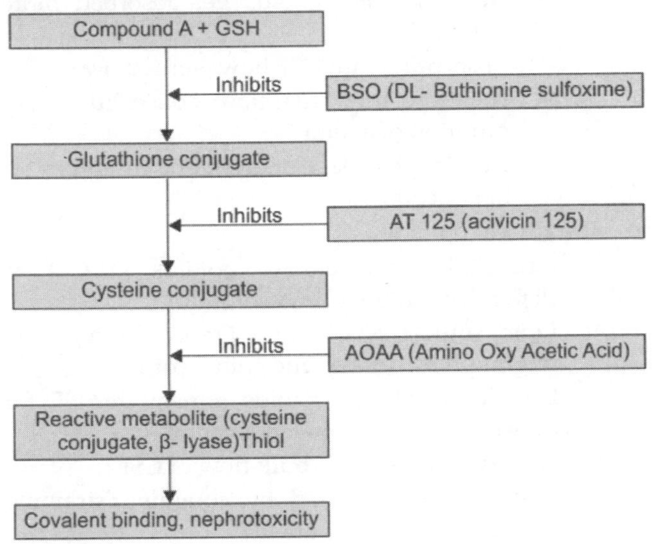

Factors Affecting Toxic Levels

- Total exposure rather than absolute concentration is more important determinant of toxicity
- 150–300 ppm-hours of compound A exposure (i.e., 50 ppm for 3 hrs)
- Compound A production more with baralyme than sodalime
- More production occurs with increased temperature of absorbent
- Hyperventilation causes increased temperature increasing compound A levels

Recommendations to Reduce Nehrotoxicity

- Use fresh gas flow of at least 2 L/min while using sevoflurane to prevent accumulation of metabolites in breathing circuit
- Most important factor determining blood levels is inspired FGF rate
- Renal changes with prolonged sevoflurane exposure is usually transient
- Patients with preexisting renal disease not to be exposed to sevoflurane
- Lower threshold for renal toxicity is 150 ppm – hrs of compound A

BCDFE Induced Nephrotoxicity

- Produced due to reaction of halothane with CO_2 absorbent
- 75% less nephrotoxic than compound A
- BCDFE is ***bromochlorodifluoro ethane***
- Chance of BCDFE causing nephrotoxicity when halothane is used as sole anesthetic is negligible

Methods of Studying Nephrotoxicity

- Creatinine clearance
- Maximal urinary osmolality
- Urinary N-acetyl β macroglobulin
- Urinary excretion of alanine amino peptidase

HERBAL TOXICITY

No.	Drug	Common use	Toxicity
1.	Ephedra	Weight loss	Halothane arrhythmias
		Antitussive	MAO-I: increased sympathetic effect
		Bacteriostatic	Oxytocin: HTN
			Stroke, HTN, cardiac arrest
2.	Garlic	Lipid lowering	Potentiates warfarin
		Antiplatelet	Reduces platelet aggregation
		Antihypertensive	
		Antioxidant	

Contd...

Contd...

No.	Drug	Common use	Toxicity
3.	Echinacea	Common cold prevention	Hepatotoxic
			Inhibits CYP1A2
			Induces CYP 3A
4.	Ginger	Nausea	Inhibits thromboxane A2 synthetase
		Antispasmodic	
5.	Gingko	Circulatory stimulant	Inhibits Platelet Activating Factor
			Increases bleeding
6.	Kava	Anxiolytic	Hepatotoxic
			Potentiates BZDs
			Potentiates barbiturates
7.	Licorice	Gastric ulcer	Hypokalemia
		Gastritis	Hypertension
		Cough, bronchitis	Edema
8.	Vitamin E	Anti-ageing	Increased bleeding
		Reduce stroke	Hypertension
		Reduce atherosclerosis	Reduces platelet aggregation
		Improve wound healing	
9.	St. Johns wort	Depression	Reduces digoxin efficacy
			Reduces warfarin efficacy
			Reduces anticonvulsant efficacy
			Prolongs emergence
			Cardiovascular toxicity
			CYP3A induction
10.	Valerian	Sedative	Potentiates barbiturates
		Anxiolytic	

INTRATHECAL/EPIDURAL OPIOIDS

Introduction

Analgesia provided by intrathecal administration of opioids is not associated with sympathetic denervation, skeletal muscle weakness or loss of proprioception.

Mechanism of Action

- Analgesia following epidural placement of opioids is by diffusion across dura mater
- They act on the μ receptors present in substantia gelatinosa of the spinal cord
- Lipophilic opioids rely mainly on systemic absorption from epidural space to act on systemic opioid receptors
- Epidural administration of these drugs (fentanyl/sufentanyl) may therefore offer no clinical advantages over IV administration
- Analgesia is specific for visceral rather than somatic pain

Pharmacokinetics

- Epidural opioids:
  - Movement of opioids from epidural space depends on their lipid solubility
  - Lipid soluble opioids:
    - Have a quick onset and short duration of action
    - Opioids can get absorbed into epidural fat and CSF
    - They also get absorbed into systemic circulation via ***Batsons plexus***
    - Time for peak CSF concentration after epidural administration:
      - Fentanyl: 20 minutes
      - Sufentany l: 6 minutes
      - Morphine: 1–4 hours
    - Time for peak blood concentration after epidural administration:
      - Fentanyl: 5–10 minutes
      - Morphine: 10–15 minutes
    - Only 3% of epidural morphine reaches CSF
    - Addition of epinephrine to epidural opioids reduces systemic absorption
    - Lipophilic drugs get absorbed more into systemic circulation than CSF
    - They also depend more on systemic opioid receptors on epidural administration
  - Water soluble opioids:
    - Water soluble opioids get absorbed more into CSF
    - Absorption into CSF however is slower
    - Therefore, they have slower onset but longer duration of action
    - They depend less on systemic receptors for their action
- Intrathecal opioids:
  - Cephalad movement of opioids in CSF is dependant on their lipid solubility
  - Lipid soluble opioids are limited in cephalad migration by uptake into spinal cord
  - Less lipid soluble opioids remain in CSF for transfer to more cephalad location
  - The cause of ascent is bulk flow of CSF
  - This can be increased by coughing/straining (but not position of patient)

- They can reach upto cisterna magna, 3rd, 4th and lateral ventricles (within 3–6 hours) through bulk flow

Dosages: (Epidural close = 5–10 times SA dose)

- Fentanyl:
  - Intrathecal: 5–25 μg
  - Epidural: 50–100 μg
  - Onset of action: 5–10 minutes (faster)
  - Duration of action: 2–4 hours (shorter)
- Morphine:
  - Intrathecal: 0.1–0.3 mg
  - Epidural: 1–5 mg
  - Onset of action: 30–60 minutes (delayed)
  - Duration of action: 6–24 hours (longer)
- Alfentanyl: epidural: 0.5–1 mg
- Sufentanyl:
  - Intrathecal: 2–10 μg
  - Epidural: 10–50 μg
- Hydromorphone: Epidural: 0.5–1 mg
- Diamorphone:
  - Intrathecal: 1–2 mg
  - Epidural: 4–6 mg
- Meperidine/Pethidine:
  - Intrathecal: 10–30 mg
  - Epidural: 20–60 mg
- Methodone: epidural: 4–8 mg
- Butorphanol:
  - Intrathecal: 5–25 μg/kg
  - Epidural: 1–4 mg

Advantages of Neuraxial Opioids

- Longer duration of analgesia: better post-operative pain control
- No associated sympathetic denervation
- No associated muscle weakness
- No loss of proprioception

Side Effects of Neuraxial Opioids

- Side effects are less common in those chronically exposed to opioids
- Pruritis:
  - *Most common* side effect of neuraxial opioids: 1% incidence
  - More common in obstetric patients due to interaction with estrogen receptors
  - May be localized to face, neck, thorax or generalized
  - Due to cephalad migration and interaction with μ receptors in trigeminal nucleus
  - Treatment:
    - Anti-histaminics and naloxone
    - Naltrexone and nalbuphine also can be used
- Urinary retention:
  - More common in young males
  - Occurs due to interaction with μ receptors in sacral spinal cord
  - This causes inhibition of sacral parasympathetic outflow: Increased bladder capacity
  - Epidural morphine also causes detrusor relaxation within 15 mins, lasting up to 16 hrs
  - Treatment: low dose naloxone (0.5–1 μg/kg)
- Ventilatory depression:
  - May be early or late ventilatory depression
  - Incidence of 1% and is equal to incidence following IV administration of opioids
  - Early depression: Within 2 hours of injection:
    - More with lipophilic opioids, unlikely with morphine
    - Occurs due to systemic absorption of LA
    - Cephalad migration of opioids in CSF might also be responsible
  - Delayed depression: After 72 hours of injection:
    - More common with hydrophilic opioids
    - Occurs due to cephalad migration of LA
    - LA subsequently interact with opioid receptors in ventral medulla
    - Characteristically occurs 6–12 hours after epidural or intrathecal morphine
    - Usually does not occur after 24 hours of administration
  - Factors increasing risk:
    - Concomitant IV sedative administration
    - Coughing, straining
    - Advanced age, raised intrathoracic pressure
  - Obstetric patients are at low risk due to ventilatory stimulation by progesterone
  - Treatment:
    - Naloxone 0.5–1 μg/kg upto 1–2 μg/kg
    - Infusion: 0.5–5 μg/kg/hr
- Nausea and vomiting:
  - Due to spread to area postrema in medulla oblongata
  - More common with hydrophilic opioids
  - Treatment:
    - Metaclopramide (0.2 mg/kg), ondansetron 4 mg IV
    - Droperidol 25–50 μg/kg, transdermal scopolamine patch (1.25 mg)
    - Naloxone 0.5–1 μg/kg

- ❖ Sedation:
  - More often with sufentanyl
  - May be due to depression of ventilation causing carbon dioxide narcosis
  - Paranoid psychosis, catatonia, hallucinations which are naloxone reversible also occur
- ❖ CNS excitation:
  - Tonic rigidity similar to seizures occurs rare
  - Myoclonus progressing to grand-mal seizures
  - May be due to cephalad migration and interaction with non-opioid receptors in brainstem and basal ganglion
  - This causes blockade of glycine/GABA mediated inhibition
- ❖ Viral reactivation:
  - Reactivation of herpes simplex virus
  - Occurs commonly 2–5 days after epidural morphine in obstetric patients
  - Occurs due to cephalad migration and interaction with trigeminal nucleus
- ❖ Neonatal morbidity:
  - May cause increased blood levels in neonates: respiratory depression
  - Negligible concentration in breast milk (fenta/sufenta)
- ❖ Miscellaneous:
  - Sexual dysfunction: sustained erection, inability to ejaculate
  - Ocular: miosis, nystagmus, vertigo (naloxone reversible)
  - Delayed gastric emptying
  - Peripheral edema due to:
    - Oliguria
    - Water retention due to release of vasopressin (from cephalad migration)
  - Spinal cord damage due to preservatives: spasms, paresis, paralysis

STEROID THERAPY IN PERIOPERATIVE PERIOD

Introduction

Increasingly used in peri-operative period.

Indications

- ❖ Peri-operative steroid replacement therapy
- ❖ Postoperative nausea and vomiting (PONV)
- ❖ Day – care surgery
- ❖ Anaphylaxis
- ❖ Septic shock
- ❖ Anti – inflammatory uses
- ❖ Hyper reactive airway
- ❖ Analgesic adjunct
- ❖ Cerebral edema
- ❖ Spinal cord injuries
- ❖ Specific surgeries

Comparison of Steroids

Compound	Anti-inflammatory potency	Na retention potency	DOA	Equivalent dose
Cortisol	1	1	8–12 h	20
Cortisone	0.8	0.8	8–12 h	25
Dexamethasone	25	0	36–72 h	0.75
Prednisone	4	0.8	12–36 h	5
Prednisolone	4	0.8	12–36 h	5
Triamcinolone	5	0	12–36 h	4
Betamethasone	25	0	36–72 h	0.75

I. Steroid Replacement Therapy

Indications:

- ❖ Adrenal suppression
- ❖ Axis separation due to steroid intake – > 5 mg prednisone for at least one month in past 6 months
  - Rhematoid arthritis
  - Ulcerative colitis
  - Bronchial asthma

Dosage:

For patient currently on steroids:

<10 mg/day prednisolone	Assume normal HPA axis	Additional cover not required
>10 mg/day prednisolone	Minor surgery	25 mg hydrocortisone @ induction
	Moderate surgery	Usual preoperative steroid
		25 mg hydrocortisone at induction
		100 mg/day for 24 hrs
	Major surgery	Usual preoperative steroid
		25 mg hydrocortisone at induction
		100 mg/day for 48–72 hrs
High dose immu-nosuppression		Usual immunosuppressive dose at induction

For patients stopped taking steroids:

< 3 months	treat as if on steroids
> 3 months	no peri-operative steroids necessary

Advantages:

- ❖ Prevents stress induced hypotension and shock
- ❖ Prevents secondary adrenal insufficiency
- ❖ Prevents hypothalmo pituitary axis suppression

Disadvantages:

- ❖ Catabolic effects
- ❖ Affects wound healing
- ❖ Impairs glucose metabolism

II. Anti-inflammatory Uses

Indications:
- ❖ Anaphylactic reactions –
  - Blood transfusions
  - Drug allergies
- ❖ Solid organ transplant
- ❖ Spinal cord injuries (within 8 hrs of injury)
- ❖ Autoimmune disorders

Mechanism of action:
- ❖ Inhibit production of interleukins, cytokines, chemotactic agents
- ❖ Reduced secretion of proteolytic enzymes
- ❖ Decreased leucocyte margination
- ❖ Diminished inflammatory response

III. Hyper–Reactive Airways

Indications:
- ❖ History of asthma
- ❖ Recent upper respiratory tract infection
- ❖ Difficult airway
- ❖ Multiple intubation attempts
- ❖ Aspiration
- ❖ Airway surgeries
- ❖ COPD
- ❖ Foreign body bronchus

Mechanism of action:
- ❖ Anti – inflammatory
  - Decreased mucosal edema
  - Prevents bronchoconstrictor release
- ❖ Enhance efficacy of bronchodilators

IV. Postoperative Nausea and Vomiting

Optimal dose 10 mg IV
Most effective if given before induction

Mechanism of action:
- ❖ Decreased production of inflammatory mediators
- ❖ Improves blood brain barrier function
- ❖ Synergistic effect with 5-HT3 antagonists

V. Day Care Surgery

12 mg betamethasone IM 30 minutes prior to surgery

Mechanism of action:
- ❖ Decreased incidence of PONV
- ❖ Decreased postoperative pain
- ❖ Establishes early oral intake
- ❖ Elevates level of endorphins

VI. Anaphylaxis

100 mg hydrocortisone IV after initial therapy with epinephrine 0.5 mL of 1: 1000 IM or SC
IV. methyprednisolone 125 mg Q6H in very severe cases

VII. Cerebral Edema

Loading dose dexamethasone 8–32 mg IV

Mechanism of action:
- ❖ Reduces vasogenic edema
- ❖ Stabilizes cerebral endothelium
- ❖ Increases cerebral glucose utilization
- ❖ Electrolyte shifts favoring trancapillary efflux of fluid
- ❖ Inhibits release of free radicals
- ❖ Increased lysosomal activity of cerebral capillaries

VIII. Spinal Cord Injury

Methyprednisolone 30 mg/kg IV loading dose
5.4 mg/kg/hr infusion for 23 hrs
To be used within 8 hrs of cord injury

IX. Specific Surgeries

250 mg methylprednisolone prior to and for 2 days post esophageal resection

ICU SEDATION

Aims

- ❖ Improve patient comfort
- ❖ Analgesia
- ❖ Reduce incidence of ICU delirium
- ❖ Facilitate mechanical ventilation
- ❖ Facilitate therapeutic interventions

Drugs Used

Induction Agents

- ❖ Propofol: < 75 µg/kg/min for < 48 hrs to avoid PRIS
- ❖ Thiopentone: To treat refractory raised ICP
- ❖ Ketamine

Benzodiazepines

- ❖ Midazolam: Accumulation of metabolites (hydroxymidazolam) in ARF
- ❖ Lorazepam: Causes increased incidence of ICU delirium

Opioids

- ❖ Morphine: Accumulates on prolonged usage
- ❖ Fentanyl, alfentanyl, sufentanil: Long context sensitive T1/2
- ❖ Remifentanil: Useful adjunct, 0.1–0.15 µg/kg/min

Inhalational: AnaConDa for isoflurane use

α_2 **Agonist:**
- Dexmedetomidine 0.1–1 µg/kg/hr infusion for duration < 24 hrs
- Clonidine 4 µg/kg/hr in NICU sedation protocols

Antipsychotics
- Olanzipine
- Quetiapine
- Haloperidol

Types
- Hypnotic based sedation
- Analgosedation with remifentanyl

Recommendations
- Ideally should be protocol based sedation
- Titrated to sedation scores
- Should resemble normal sleep wake cycle
- Avoid over/under sedation
- Avoid neuromuscular blocking agents
- ***Sedation holiday***

ICU Sedation Protocols

Patient Targeted Sedation Protocols:
- Once in 4 hrs assessment of pain and distress
- Bolus doses given by nurse
- Continuous infusion started if increased frequency of boluses

Daily Interruption of Continuous Sedation
- Continuous infusion
- Interrupted daily
- Assess distress and pain
- Restart at half the previous dose if increased distress

Sedation Assessment

Ramsays sedation scale:

Score	Description
1	Confused, irritable
2	Comfortable, oriented
3	Responds to vocal commands
4	Brisk response to auditory stimulus/ glabellar tap
5	Sluggish response to auditory stimulus/ glabellar tap
6	No response

Advantages
- Better patient comfort
- Pain free
- Reduced anxiety and ICU delirium
- Reduced post traumatic stress syndrome
- Facilitates mechanical ventilation and therapeutic interventions

Disadvantages

Oversedation
- ICU sedation itself is risk factor for delirium
- Respiratory depression
- Hypoxia, hypercarbia in extubated patients
- Hemodynamic instability
- Delayed weaning
- Long ICU stay, long hospital stay

Undersedation
- Pain, delirium, anxiety
- Self extubation
- Ventilator asynchrony
- Raised airway pressure
- HTN, arrhythmias, MI

ROLE OF NEUROMUSCULAR BLOCKERS IN ICU

Indications for NMB in ICU
- To facilitate mechanical ventilation:
  - To facilitate endotracheal intubation
  - Enable patients to tolerate ventilation
  - High pulmonary inflation pressure: ARDS
  - Prone ventilation
- Facilitate permissive hypercapnea
- Hyperventilation for raised ICP
- Facilitate therapeutic/diagnostic procedures
- To reduce oxygen consumption:
  - Abolish shivering
  - Reduce work of breathing
- Treatment of tetanus and status epilepticus

Complications of Muscle Paralysis in ICU
- Short term use:
  - Specific drug side effects
  - Inadequate ventilation if ventilator failure/ disconnection
  - ICU awareness: Inadequate sedation/analgesia

- Long term use:
  - Complications of immobility:
    - DVT, pulmonary embolism
    - Peripheral nerve injuries
    - Decubitus ulcers
  - Inability to cough: retention of secretions, pneumonia
- Dysregulation of nACH receptors
- Residual paralysis:
  - Persistent neuromuscular blockade
  - *Critical illness myopathy*
  - *Critical illness neuropathy*
  - Use of vecuronium in renal failure patients
  - High dose steroids in asthmatics
- Unrecognized effects of drugs/metabolites:
  - Succinylcholine, 3-desacetylvecuronium, laudanosine
  - Metabolic acidosis
  - Hypovolemia
  - Cerebral excitation

Risk Factors for Development of Neuromuscular Dysfunction

- Female sex, steroid administration
- Hypercapnea, increased duration of mechanical ventilation
- Sepsis
- Dysfunction of more than 2 organ systems

Recommendations for Neuromuscular Blockade in ICU

- Avoid use of neuromuscular blockers:
  - Maximize use of analgesics and sedatives
  - Manipulate ventilator modes and parameters
- Minimize use of succinylcholine as:
  - Up-regulation of ACHRs occurs due to immobilization
  - This causes high incidence of cardiac arrest due to hyperkalemia
  - Contraindicated in patients with total body immobilization for more than 24 hours
- Minimize dosage of neuromuscular blocking agents:
  - Use only in patients who cannot be managed otherwise
  - Administer only when required and to achieve a well defined goal
  - Administer as bolus doses rather than continuous infusions
  - Use peripheral nerve stimulator with TOF monitoring
  - Continuously allow recovery from paralysis
  - Do not administer NMBAs for more than 2 days continuously
  - Drug requirement increases with time due to receptor up-regulation
  - Avoid combining non-depolarizing agents with steroids
- Choice of non-depolarizing muscle relaxants:
  - Steroid based relaxants like vecuronium/pancuronium have prolonged action
  - These drugs may cause residual palsy
  - Atracurium causes residual palsy in 70% cases if NM blockade exceeds 2 days
  - Cisatracurium is better as lesser chances of residual palsy
  - Laudanosine accumulation is less with cisatracuriumcompared with atracurium
- Consider alternative therapy:
  - Avoid vecuronium in females with renal failure
  - Use isoflurane in place of muscle relaxants for treatment of status asthmaticus
  - Reduce dose of steroids in asthma patients

LEVOSIMENDAN

Introduction

Inodilator with a unique non-catecholamine action.

Mechanism of Action

- Cardiac troponin C:
  - Binds to cardiac troponin C in a calcium-dependant manner
  - This stabilizes troponin C and the kinetics of actin-myosin cross-bridges
  - Increased actin-myosin cross bridge formation results
  - This occurs without an accompanying increase in myocardial ATP consumption
  - This results in the positive inotropic effect of levosimendan
- ATP-sensitive K^+ channels:
  - Opens ATP-sensitive K+ channels in the vascular smooth muscle
  - Causes vasodilatation of systemic and coronary resistance vessels
  - Causes vasodilatation of systemic capacitance vessels
  - Thus, it reduces systemic vascular resistance
- Luteotropic action:
  - During diastole, there is a fall in intracellular Ca^{2+} concentration

- Levosimendan mediated myofilament responsiveness depends on intracellular Ca^{2+} levels
- Thus, diastolic relaxation is not hampered by levosimendan
- Thus, force of contraction is increased without impairing ventricular relaxation

Pharmacokinetics

- Linear pharmacokinetics
- Distribution:
  - Volume of distribution V_d 0.2 L/kg
  - 97–98% plasma protein bound, primarily to albumin
- Metabolism:
  - Primarily metabolized by conjugation to cyclic or N-acetyled cysteinyl glycine
  - 5% is metabolized in the intestine to aminophenylpyridazinone (OR-1855)
  - OR-1855 is metabolized by N-acetyl transferase to active metabolite OR-1896
  - OR-1855 and OR-1896 are active metabolites
- Elimination and excretion:
  - Peak plasma concentration is achieved 2 days after termination of the infusion
  - Clearance is 3 mL/min/kg
  - $T_{1/2}$ of levosimendan is 1 hour
  - $T_{1/2}$ of the active metabolites is 75–80 hours
  - This accounts for the prolonged hemodynamic effects of the drug
  - Effects last for 7–9 days after discontinuation of a 24-hour infusion
  - 54% is excreted in urine and 44% in feces
  - > 95% of the dose is excreted within 1 week

Indications

- Acutely decompensated chronic heart failure
- Post cardiac surgery
- Following PTCA

Contraindications

- Hypersensitivity to levosimendan or any of its excipients
- Severe hypotension and tachycardia
- Severe left ventricular outflow tract obstruction, HOCM
- Severe renal impairment (creatinine clearance <30 mL/min)
- Severe hepatic impairment
- History of Torsades-de-Pointes

Dosage

- 3 µg/kg to 24 µg/kg bolus given over 10 minutes
- Followed by a 0.05–0.2 µg/kg/min for 24 hours
- Dose individualized as per the patients clinical condition and response
- Not recommended in pregnant patients unless benefits to mother outweigh risks to fetus
- Avoided in lactating women
- Not recommended for use in children <18 years age due to limited clinical experience

Adverse Effects

- Hypokalemia
- Headache, dizziness, insomnia
- Hypotension
- Atrial fibrillation, ventricular extrasystoles
- Ventricular tachycardia
- Diarrhea, vomiting, nausea, constipation

Drug Interactions

- Increased risk of hypotension when used concomitantly with vasodilators or inodilators

DIGOXIN

Introduction

- Cardiac glycoside derived from digitalis purpurea; the foxglove plant
- Therapeutic benefits of digitalis first described by William Withering in 1785

Chemistry

- Belongs to the group of drugs cardiac glycosides
- The glycosides are composed of 2 portions: A sugar and a cardenolide
- Consists of 3 sugars and the aglycone digoxigenin
- Molecular formula is $C_{41}H_{64}O_{14}$
- Molecular weight is 780.95

Composition

- Exists as odourless white crystal, insoluble in water
- Solution contains a vehicle 40% propylene glycol and 10% alcohol
- Injection is buffered to a pH of 6.8–7.2
- This is done with 0.17% sodium phosphate and 0.08% anhydrous citric acid

Mechanism of Action

- Inhibits membrane protein Na^+-K^+ ATPase
- This causes intracellular Na^+ accumulation

- This in turn stimulates the Na^+-Ca^{2+} exchanger
- Thus, excess intracellular Na^+ is pumped out in exchange for extracellular Ca^{2+}
- This causes an increased intracellular Ca^{2+} levels
- This in turn promotes calcium release from the sarcoplasmic reticulum
- Thus, more calcium is available to bind to troponin C
- Ultimately results in increased myocardial contractility

Pharmacodynamics

- Cardiovascular system:
  - Increases contractility: *Positive inotropic effect*
  - Reduces SA firing rate: *Negative chronotropic effect*
  - Reduces conduction velocity through AV node: *negative dromotropic effect*
  - This prolongs refractory period of AV node
  - Increased rate of phase 4 depolarization (increased ventricular automaticity)
  - Decreased refractory period in atria and ventricles
  - *Neurohormonal deactivating effect:*
    - Digoxin causes baroreceptor sensitization through its indirect effects
    - This results in increased afferent inhibitory activity
    - This causes reduced activity of the sympathetic system
    - Renin angiotensin system is also suppressed
  - High doses:
    - High doses of digoxin may increase sympathetic outflow from the CNS
    - This may be responsible for features of digoxin toxicity

Pharmacokinetics

- Onset of action:
  - 30–120 minutes following PO dose
  - 5–30 minutes following IV dose
- Peak action:
  - 2–6 hours following PO dose
  - 1–4 hours following IV dose
- Duration of action: 2–4 days following PO or IV dose
- Absorption:
  - Following oral administration, 60–80% is absorbed from tablets
  - 80% absorbed following intramuscular injection
  - IM injection avoided due to severe pain/irritation
- Distribution:
  - 25% plasma protein bound
  - Has a large apparent V_d
  - Crosses both the blood-brain barrier and placenta
- Metabolism:
  - Only a small percentage of digoxin dose is metabolized (16%)
  - Hepatic metabolism via hydrolysis, oxidation and conjugation
  - Metabolites include 3-β-digoxigenin and 3-keto-digoxigenin
  - These are conjugated with glucuronide and sulfate
- Elimination:
  - Undergoes renal elimination
  - Elimination follows first-order kinetics
  - 50–70% of digoxin dose is excreted unchanged by the kidneys
  - Elimination $T_{1/2}$ is 40 hours
  - Elimination $T_{1/2}$ is prolonged to 84–120 hours in anuric patients
  - Long $T_{1/2}$ which makes it difficult to titrate dosage

Serum Digoxin Levels

- Therapeutic level is approximately 0.5–2.5 ng/mL
- Serum levels may be drawn 6–8 hours after administration of a dose
- Values more than 3 ng/mL indicative of toxicity
- Conditions refractory to toxicity:
  - Children
  - Hyperkalemia
  - Atrial arrhythmias

Indications

- Supraventricular tachyarrhythmias for control of ventricular response rate
- Mild-moderate heart failure

Contraindications

- Hypersensitivity
- WPW syndrome:
  - Digoxin slows AV nodal conduction
  - This may encourage antegrade conduction across accessory pathways
  - Thus, SVT may be precipitated
- Uncontrolled ventricular arrhythmias
- Sinoatrial block, AV block: May worsen

- Idiopathic hypertrophic subaortic stenosis as inotropic effect may increase LVOTO
- Acute myocardial infarction as in increases myocardial oxygen demand
- Hypokalemia, hypercalcemia, hypomagnesemia: predisposes to digitalis toxicity
- Renal impairment (reduced dose warranted)

Dosage

- Rapid digitalizing regimen (loading dose):
  - Intravenous:
    - 8–12 µg/kg total loading dose
    - 50% of the calculated dose is administered initially
    - One fourth of the remaining dose is given Q6–8H
    - The remaining one-fourth can be given Q6-8H based on clinical response
  - Oral:
    - 10–15 µg/kg total loading dose
    - 50% of the calculated dose is administered initially
    - One fourth of the remaining dose is given Q6-8H
    - The remaining one-fourth can be given Q6-8H based on clinical response
- Maintenance dose:
  - Oral:
    - 0.125–0.5 mg/day as maintenance dose based on clinical effect
    - Dose increased every 2 weeks based on response and serum drug levels
  - Intravenous: 0.1–0.4 mg per day
- Dose adjustment required in geriatric age as therapeutic threshold is further reduced
- Use only if benefits to mother outweigh risk to fetus in pregnancy and lactation

Adverse Effects

- Central nervous system: Fatigue, headache, weakness, blurring of vision, yellow vision
- Gastrointestinal: Anorexia, nausea, vomiting, diarrhea
- Hematology: Thrombocytopenia, maculopapular rashes
- Others: Gynecomastia following prolonged use
- Digoxin toxicity:
  - Has an extremely low therapeutic index
  - 20% of patients show toxicity at some point of time
  - Cardiac manifestations are the most frequent and serious sign of toxicity
  - Peak cardiac effects occur 3–6 hours following overdosage
  - These effects may last for 24 hours or longer
  - Precipitating factors:
    - Hypokalemia, hypomagnesemia, hypercalcemia
    - Alkalosis, acidosis, renal insufficiency, hypothyroidism
  - Presentation:
    - Can produce virtually any type of arrhythmia
    - Usually toxicity results in increased automaticity and conduction block
    - Multiple rhythm disturbances in the same patient are common
    - Can result in:
      - Premature atrial contraction
      - Premature ventricular depolarization
      - AV block
      - Accelerated junctional tachycardia
      - VT or VF refractory to countershock
      - Asystole or VF is usually fatal
  - Therapy:
    - Discontinue digoxin therapy
    - Increase serum potassium levels to upper limit of normal (4–5.5 mEq/L)
    - Treat ventricular arrhythmias with phenytoin, lidocaine or amiodarone
    - Treat atrial arrhythmias with phenytoin or amiodarone
    - Beta blockers may be used
    - Atropine or ventricular pacing may be required if AV block develops
    - Cardioversion may be used, but arrhythmias are usually refractory
    - ***DIGIBIND:***
      - Resistant arrhythmias treated with digoxin immune Fab (*Digibind*)
      - This binds to digitalis glycoside molecule in the blood
      - The complex is then excreted by the kidneys
      - Used as plasma level may take several days to fall to safe limits
      - This is due to the prolonged $T_{1/2}$ of digoxin
- Validation ***RADIANCE trial:***
  - 12 week, double blind placebo controlled study
  - Enrolled 178 patients with NYHA class II-III heart failure
  - Showed better preservation of exercise capacity in those treated with digoxin

- Continued treatment reduced the risk of developing worsening heart failure
- Similar conclusions were reached in the PROVED trial and DIG trial

❖ *AFFIRM trial:*
- Included 4060 patients with AF considered at high risk for stroke
- Patients were randomized to rate control vs rhythm control over a 4 year period
- Concluded that digoxin increased all-cause mortality in patients with AF

AMIODARONE

Introduction

❖ Potent class III anti-arrhythmic agent

❖ Unique drug as it has actions of all four anti-arrhythmic drug classes

Chemistry

❖ It is a benzofuran derivative

❖ Iodine containing compound with 2 iodine molecules

❖ Contains 37.3% iodine by weight

❖ Structurally similar to thyroxine

❖ Structural formula is $C_{25}H_{29}I_2NO_3.HCl$

❖ Molecular weight of 681.8 daltons

Mechanism of Action

❖ Unique drug with actions of all four antiarrhythmic drug classes

❖ Blocks Na^+ channels- Class I action

❖ Anti-adrenergic action- Class II action

❖ Ca^{2+} channel blockade- Class IV action

❖ Prolongs QT interval

❖ Delays AV nodal conduction

❖ Prolongs action potential duration

❖ Increases refractoriness of all cardiac tissue

❖ Primarily exerts its actions via 2 major actions:
- Prolongation of myocardial cell action potential duration and refractory period
- Non-competitive antagonism of α and β adreno-ceptors

Pharmacodynamics

❖ Electrophysiological effects:
- Acts on all parts of the action potential
- Decreases sinus rate by 15–20%
- Prolongs PR and QT intervals
- Slows heart rate and AV nodal conduction (Ca^{2+} channel, β-receptor blockade)
- Slows intracardiac conduction (sodium channel blockade)
- Prolongs refractoriness (via potassium and sodium channel blockade)

❖ Other actions:
- Relaxes vascular smooth muscle, reduces peripheral vascular resistance
- Mild negative inotropic effect following intravenous dose

Pharmacokinetics

❖ Onset of action:
- 2 days- 3 weeks required for initial response following oral dose
- 30 minutes following IV dose

❖ Peak action: 1 week- 3 weeks following oral dose

❖ Duration of action:
- Upto 50 days following discontinuation of therapy
- Antiarrhythmic actions persist for weeks-months after discontinuation of therapy

❖ Absorption:
- Slow and variable absorption following oral dose
- Low bioavailability (22–95%)
- Absorption is enhanced when taken with food

❖ Distribution:
- Highly protein bound (96% protein bound)
- Highly lipid soluble and stored in high concentrations in fat and muscle
- Volume of distribution 66 L/kg
- Crosses blood-brain barrier and placenta

❖ Metabolism:
- Undergoes hepatic metabolism via CYP2C8 and CYP3A3/4
- Produces active metabolite N-desethylamiodar-one (DEA)
- Undergoes enterohepatic recirculation

❖ Elimination:
- Elimination $T_{1/2}$ of parent drug is 26–107 days
- Elimination $T_{1/2}$ of DEA metabolite is 14–75 days
- Eliminated via feces (major) and urine (minor)

Dosage

❖ Intravenous dose:
- 150 mg bolus over 10 minutes
- This dose can be repeated if necessary in 10–30 minutes
- This is followed by an infusion of 1 mg/min for

6 hours
- This is followed by an infusion of 0.5 mg/min for 18 hours

- Oral dose:
  - 800–1600 mg/day for those who have received IV amiodarone for < 1 week
  - 600–800 mg/day for those who have received IV amiodarone for 1–3 weeks
  - 400 mg/day for those who have received IV amiodarone for > 3 weeks

Indications

- Long term therapy:
  - Secondary prevention of life threatening ventricular arrhythmias
  - Atrial fibrillation
- Acute therapy:
  - Ventricular tachyarrhythmias
  - Hemodynamically stable wide complex tachyarrhythmias
  - Atrial fibrillation

Contraindications

- Known hypersensitivity to amiodarone or ***iodine***
- Cardiogenic shock
- Severe sinus node dysfunction
- Second or third degree AV block

Adverse Effects

- Therapeutic range: 0.8–2.8 µg/mL
- Toxicity range: More than 2–2.5 µg/mL
- Short term effects:
  - Anaphylaxis
  - Cardiovascular:
    - Potent vasodilation and negative inotropism may be associated
    - Torsades de Pointes:
      - Amiodarone blocks potassium channels and prolongs QT interval
      - This may predispose to Torsades de Pointes
    - Sinus bradycardia, heart block:
      - Occurs due to β receptor blockade
      - May require supplemental pacing
- Long term effects:
  - Pulmonary:
    - Subacute pulmonary fibrosis
    - Eosinophilic pneumonia
    - Bronchiolitis obliterans
  - Gastrointestinal:
    - Hepatitis, cirrhosis
    - Pancreatitis
  - CNS:
    - Photosensitivity, corneal microdeposits, optic neuropathy
    - Pseudotumor cerebri
    - Parkinsonism
  - Endocrine:
    - Hypothyroidism, hyperthyroidism
    - SIADH
  - Hematology:
    - Hemolytic anemia
    - Aplastic anemia, pancytopenia
    - Thrombocytopenia

CISATRACURIUM

Introduction

- Intermediate-onset, intermediate-duration non-depolarizing muscle relaxant
- It is a diastereoisomer of atracurium

Chemistry

- Benzyl-isoquinolinium compound
- Contains isoquinoline molecule to which benzyl group is attached
- It is the 1R *cis* -1'R *cis* isomer of atracurium
- Chemical formula $C_{53}H_{72}N_2O_{12}$
- Average molecular weight 929.161 g/mol

Presentation

- 5 mg in 2.5 mL ampoule
- Refrigerated at 2–8 °C
- Requires proper temperature maintenance
- This is because it undergoes organ-independent, temperature-dependant degradation

Mechanism of Action

- Competitive acetylcholine receptor antagonist
- Binds to nicotinic acetylcholine receptors at motor endplate
- This blocks acetylcholine's access to its receptors
- Thus, competitive blockade of neuromuscular transmission results

Pharmacokinetics

- Onset of action: 2–3 minutes
- Peak action: 3–5 minutes
- Duration of action: 55–65 minutes

- Context sensitive half time:
  - Rate of recovery after infusion is independent of duration of infusion
  - Recovery following infusion is thus, comparable to that following bolus doses
- Absorption:
  - Following IV administration, absorption is essentially complete
  - Absorption is poor following oral administration
- Distribution:
  - Rapidly distributes into ECF
  - Volume of distribution is limited by large molecular weight and high polarity
  - Volume of distribution Vd 161 mL/kg
  - Binding to plasma proteins not successfully studied
  - This is due to rapid degradation at physiological pH
- Metabolism:
  - Largelyindependentofhepaticbiotransformation
  - Lacks the ester hydrolysis, which occurs with atracurium
  - Undergoes Hofmanns elimination (77%):
    - Is *a organ-independent, pH and temperature-dependant* chemical process
    - Loses positive charges by molecular fragmentation to form:
    - Laudanosine (tertiary amine):
      - Is an inactive metabolite
      - Potentiates seizure activity as it is a CNS stimulant
      - Laudanosine is metabolized to des-methyl metabolites
      - These are conjugated with glucuronic acid and excreted in urine
      - Cisatracurium is 5 times as potent compared to atracurium
      - Thus, it produces 5 times lesser laudanosine
    - Monoquaternary acrylate:
      - Is an inactive metabolite
      - This undergoes hydrolysis by non-specific esterases
      - Monoquaternary alcohol metabolite is formed
      - This metabolite also undergoes Hofmanns elimination
- Elimination:
  - Renal elimination is 16% of total dose
  - Plasma clearance 5.2 mL/kg/min
  - Elimination $T_{1/2}$ of cisatracurium is 23.5 minutes
  - Elimination $T_{1/2}$ of laudanosine is 3.1 hours

Indications

- To facilitate endotracheal intubation
- To provide skeletal muscle relaxation during surgery
- To facilitate mechanical ventilation in ICU

Dosage

- 0.15- 0.2 mg/kg IV intubation dose
- 0.02 mg/kg IV supplemental dose (given 40–50 minutes after initial dose)
- 1–2 µg/kg/min continuous infusion dose
- Maximum bolus dose up to 0.4 mg/kg IV
- No dosage adjustments required in those with renal/hepatic dysfunction

Contraindications

- Known hypersensitivity to cisatracurium, atracurium or benzenesulfonic acid
- Has not been studied in neonatal population
- Preterm neonates:
  - Commercial preparations contain benzyl alcohol
  - This is potentially toxic to neural tissue
  - Rare reports of death in preterm infants

Adverse Effects

- Bronchospasm
- Bradycardia
- Flushing
- Pruritus
- Myositis ossificans
- Anaphylaxis

Interactions

- Action potentiated by:
  - Volatile anesthetics, ketamine
  - Aminoglycosides, tetracycline, lincomycin, clindamycin
  - Propranolol, calcium channel blockers, lignocaine
  - Furosemide, thiazide, mannitol
- Decreased action with chronic phenytoin, carbamazepine therapy

VECURONIUM

Introduction

- It is an intermediate acting, aminosteroid, nondepolarizing, competitive NMBA

- It was the first non-depolarizing NMBA with shorter duration of action to be introduced
- It the standard of comparison of other NMBAs due to:
  - Intermediate duration of action
  - Lack of cardiovascular side effects

Chemistry

- It is the 2-desmethyl derivative of pancuronium, making it a mono-quarternary analogue
- Chemically it is a bis-quaternary aminosteroid
- Chemical formula is $C_{34}H_{57}BrN_2O_4$
- It has a molecular weight of 637.74 Da

Presentation

- As a lyophilized powder containing:
  - Citric acid monohydrate 20.75 mg
  - Disodium hydrogen phosphate dihydride 16.25 mg
  - Mannitol 170 mg
  - Sodium hydroxide or phosphoric acid
- On dilution, a clear, colorless isotonic solution is obtained
- Mannitol is added to alter the tonicity
- The sodium hydroxide or phosphoric acid adjusts the pH to 4
- After reconstitution, the solution remains stable for 24 hours

Mechanism of Action

- Vecuronium binds competitively to nicotinic acetylcholine receptors (n-ACHR)
- Thus, it competes with acetylcholine for binding sites on nicotinic N_2 receptors
- By doing so, it blocks impulse transmission from motor nerve ending to striated muscle
- Following IV administration of 0.08–0.10 μg/kg vecuronium:
  - Excellent intubating conditions is produced within 90–120 minutes
  - Muscle paralysis adequate for surgical dissection is produced within 3–4 minutes

Pharmacodynamics

- Cardiovascular system:
  - Minimal cardiovascular effects
  - With large doses following changes are seen:
    - Slight decrease (12%) in SVR
    - Slight increase (9%) in cardiac output
    - Bradycardia due to unchecked action of fentanyl and propofol
- Respiratory system:
  - Neuromuscular blockade produces apnea
  - Histamine release and bronchospasm may be seen rarely
- Central nervous system:
  - Vecuronium has no effect on ICP or IOP
  - Prolonged infusions (> 6 days) may be associated with myopathy
- ANS: LES sphincter tone is unaltered after administration of vecuronium
- Metabolic: May decrease PT and aPTT

Pharmacokinetics

- Onset of action:
  - Within 90–120 seconds following intubating dose
  - Onset time can be prolonged in patients with increased volume of distribution
  - It is also prolonged in conditions with increased circulation time such as:
    - Old age
    - Cardiovascular disease
    - Edematous states
- Peak action: within 3–5 minutes of IV administration
- Duration of action:
  - 25–40 minutes under balanced anesthesia
  - May be prolonged in renal and hepatic dysfunction
- Distribution:
  - 60–80% plasma protein bound
  - V_d in adult patient 0.3–0.4 L/kg
  - Distribution $T_{1/2}$ of 2.2 + 1.4 minutes
  - Mainly distributed in extracellular compartment
  - It does not cross the blood- brain barrier
  - Clinically insignificant doses may cross the placenta
- Metabolism:
  - Extent of metabolism is relatively low
  - Metabolized in liver by deacetylation to active metabolite:
    - 3- desacetyl vecuronium (3- OH vecuronium)
    - 17- desacetyl vecuronium (17-OH vecuronium)
    - 3,17 desacetyl vecuronium

- These metabolites have approximately 50% NM blocking potency of vecuronium
- In the absence of renal and hepatic dysfunction, plasma concentration of the metabolite is very low

❖ Elimination:
- Biliary excretion is the main route of elimination
- 40–75% is excreted in the feces
- 25–30% is excreted in urine as unchanged drug
- Within 24 hours of IV administration, 40–80% of the dose is excreted in bile
- Plasma clearance is 3–6.4 mL/kg/min
- Elimination $T_{1/2}$ averages 71 + 20 minutes
- Recovery is 95% complete 45–65 minutes after administration of IV dose

Indications

❖ As an adjunct to general anesthesia to facilitate endotracheal intubation

❖ To facilitate skeletal muscle relaxation during surgery

❖ To facilitate mechanical ventilation in ICU

❖ To treat shivering due to therapeutic hypothermia following cardiac arrest

Dosage

❖ ED_{90} of vecuronium is approximately 0.057 mg/kg

❖ Intubating dose: 0.08–0.10 mg/kg IV

❖ Maintenance dose: 0.02–0.03 mg/kg IV

❖ As an infusion, dose is 0.8–1.2 μg/kg/min

❖ The drug is non-cumulative with repeated administration

❖ Dosage to maintain paralysis following succinylcholine administration:
- 0.03–0.05 mg/kg IV
- Vecuronium has to be given only after recovery of paralysis from succinylcholine

❖ Dosage adjustments may be required in the following scenarios:
- Severe obesity:
  - Dose is calculated taking into account lean body mass
  - This results in administration of lesser doses, compared to dose calculated by total body mass
- Renal, hepatic failure:
  - Elimination may be delayed in these patients
  - Therefore, doses have to be more widely spaced
  - Thus, the dose administered during a procedure is eventually reduced
  - This effectively reduces the total dose administered during a procedure

Contraindications

❖ Hypersensitivity to vecuronium bromide

Adverse Effects

❖ Hypersensitivity reactions

❖ Histamine release and histaminoid (anaphylactoid) reactions

❖ Bradycardia, hypotension

❖ Myopathy with prolonged infusions (> 6 days)

Drug Interactions

❖ Increased effect of vecuronium:
- Volatile anesthetic agents
- High doses of ketamine, etomidate and propofol
- Aminoglycoside antibiotics
- Polypeptide antibiotics
- Diuretics
- Thiamine
- MAO inhibitors
- Protamine
- Magnesium salts
- Coadministration of other NMBAs

❖ Variable effect of vecuronium seen during coadministration of depolarizing muscle relaxants like succinylcholine

Physiological Interactions

❖ Conditions which antagonize vecuronium NMB:
- Respiratory alkalosis
- Hypercalcemia
- Demyelinating lesions
- Peripheral neuropathies
- Denervation
- Muscle trauma

❖ Conditions which potentiate vecuronium NMB:
- Dyselectrolytemias:
  - Severe hypocalcemia
  - Hypokalemia
  - Hypermagnesemia
- Metabolic and respiratory acidosis
- Eaton-Lambert syndrome
- Myasthenia gravis

THIOPENTONE VS PROPOFOL

Property	Thiopentone	Propofol
Chemistry	Thio-barbituric acid	2,6-di-isopropyl phenol
	S (+) and R (–) isomers present	Non-chiral compound: no isomers
Presentation	Hygroscopic yellow powder	Oily emulsion
	Water soluble	Fat soluble
	6% Na_2CO_3 preservative	Sodium metabisulphite preservative
	Used as 2.5% solution	Used as 1% solution
	Alkaline pH 10.8	Acidic pH 4.5–6.5
	Bacteriostatic due to alkalinity	Promotes bacterial growth due to lipid carrier
Mechanism of action	Direct and indirect action on $GABA_A$	No direct $GABA_A$ action
	Also on n-ACHR and glutamate receptors	Acts on NMDA receptors
Pharmacodynamics		
Central nervous system	Residual effects: hangover	Clear headed recovery
	Anticonvulsant	Causes myoclonus
	Antalgesic	Analgesic
Cardiovascular	Tachycardia	Rarely bradycardia and asystole
Respiratory	Bronchospasm, laryngospasm	Bronchodilatation
	Preserved laryngeal reflexes	Laryngeal reflexes are blunted
Hepatic	Reduces hepatic blood flow	Hepatocellular injury on long term infusions
Renal	Reduces urine output	Phenoluria: green color urine
Pharmacokinetics	Absorbed rectally	Not absorbed
	Vd 2.5 L/kg	Vd 3.5–4.5 L/kg
	72–86% plasma protein bound	97% plasma protein bound
	Hepatic oxidative metabolism	Hepatic metabolism by hydroxylation
	No extra-hepatic metabolism	Extrahepatic metabolism in lungs and kidney
	Excreted in urine	Excreted in urine and feces
	Enzyme inducer	No enzyme induction
Uses	Induction agent 3–5 mg/kg	Induction agent 1.5–2 mg/kg
	Raised ICP	Anticonvulsant
	Cerebroprotection	Antiemetic 10–15 mg IV
	Checking wet epidural tap	Antipruritic 10 mg IV
Side effects	Hypotension, tachycardia	Asystole, bradycardia
	Allergy due to histamine release	Allergy due to cremaphor-EL
	Arterial thrombi	Not common
	No increased risk	Increased risk of pancreatitis
	Rare	Pain on injection common
	Not common	Liver damage on prolonged infusion (PRIS)
Contraindications	Porphyria	Drug allergy
	Status asthmaticus	
	Cardiac tamponade, shock	

DOPAMINE VS DOBUTAMINE

Property	Dopamine	Dobutamine
Chemistry	Natural endogenous catecholamine	Synthetic derivative
	Non-chiral compound	Two isomers present: L (–) and R (+)
Presentation	40 mg/mL of dopamine	50 mg/mL of dobutamine
	200 mg/ampoule of dopamine	250 mg/ampoule of dobutamine
Mechanism of action	α_1, β_1, β_2, D_1, D_2 receptors	β_1, weak β_2 and α_1 actions
	Dosewise variation in action:	Less than 5 µg/kg/min: β_1 action
	0–5 µg/kg/min: D_1 and D_2 action	More than 5 µg/kg/min: α_1 action
	5–10 µg/kg/min: β_1 and β_2 action	No indirect action
	More than 10 µg/kg/min: α_1 action	
Pharmacodynamics		
Cardiovascular		
Cardiac output	Increased	Increased
Heart rate	Increased	Increased (less likely)
Arrhythmias	Stimulates	Stimulates
Coronary vasculature	Vasoconstriction	Vasodilatation
Myocardial O_2 demand	Increased	Not increased
Systemic vascular resistance	Increased	Decreased
	Vasodilatation in brain and kidney	Vasodilatation in skin and skeletal muscle
	Increases pulmonary artery pressure	Decreases pulmonary artery pressure
Renal blood flow	Increased	Increased (less prominent effect)
Pharmacokinetics	V_d = 1.8–2.5 L/kg	V_d = 0.2 L/kg
	Onset of action within 5 minutes	Onset of action within 1–2 minutes
	Eliminated in urine	In urine and feces
Uses	Post surgery cases	Low cardiac output states
	Not used commonly	Stress testing
	Septic shock	Not used commonly
	Not used	Cor-pulmonale, right heart failure
	Mainly in cardiac surgical ICU	Mainly in cardiac CCU
Side effects	Nausea and vomiting prominent	Rare
	Rare	Allergy present
	Raised IOP	No increase in IOP
	Hyperglycemia	Reduces blood glucose
	Potentiates development of MODS	Does not potentiate
Contraindications	Pulmonary HTN, cor pulmonale	Used in these patients
	Used in these patients	Aortic stenosis, mitral stenosis
	Allergies are rare	Allergies

MIDAZOLAM VS PROPOFOL

Property	Midazolam	Propofol
Chemistry	Benzodiazepine, imidazole ring	2,6-diisopropyl phenol
	Water soluble	Lipid solubel
Presentation	Syrup with 2 mg/mL	No oral preparation
	IV preparation with 1/2/5 mg/mL	1% solution
	pH of 3.5	pH of 4.5–6.5
	pH dependant ring opening phenomenon	Not present
	No preservative	EDTA or sodium metabisulphite
	Mixed with lactated ringers	Not recommended
Mechanism of action	Agonist at BZD receptor	$GABA_A$ stimulant
	κ-opioid agonist	Inhibits ACH release from hippocampus
	No action on NMDA receptor	NMDA inhibition
Routes of administration	Oral, IV, IM, epidural, intrathecal	Only IV administration
Dose	1.5–2 IV	1.5–2 mg/kg IV
Pharmacodynamics		
Central nervous system	Anterograde amnesia	Absent
	Muscle relaxant	No muscle relaxation
	Not cerebroprotective properties	Cerebroprotective
	Not present	Myoclonus, abnormal motor activity
	Cannot produce isoelectric EEG	Can produce isoelectric EEG
Cardiovascular system	No reduction in cardiac output	Reduced cardiac output
	Not present	Bradycardia and asystole
Respiratory system	Intact laryngeal reflexes	Laryngeal reflexes lost
Others	Absent	Phenoluria possible
	No hepatocellular injury	Hepatocellular injury on long infusion
Pharmacokinetics	V_d of 1–1.5 L/kg	V_d of 3.5–4.5 L/kg
	96–98% plasma protein bound	97% plasma protein bound
	Onset of action 30–60 seconds	Onset of action 30-45 seconds
	Duration of action 15–80 minutes	Duration of action 10 minutes
	Only hepatic metabolism	Extra-hepatic metabolism present
	Excreted in urine	Excreted in urine and feces
	Elimination $T_{1/2}$ 1.5–3 hours	Elimination $T_{1/2}$ 10–70 minutes
Uses	Mainly as premedication	Mainly as induction agent
	Also useful as anticonvulsant	Also used for cerebroprotection
	Used in paradoxical vocal cord motion	Used as antiemetic and antipruritic
Side effects	Rare	Pain on injection
	Ventilatory depression	Transient apnea
	Withdrawal phenomenon on long term use	Dependence and abuse potential common

MIDAZOLAM VS DIAZEPAM

Property	Midazolam	Diazepam
Chemistry	Water soluble BZD	Lipid soluble BZD
Preservative	Syrup: 2 mg/mL	Syrup: 0.4 mg/1 mg/mL
	IV presentation: 1/2/5 mg/mL	5 mg/mL solution
	Not available	Available as rectal suppository
	No solvent required	Propylene glycol as solvent
	Water soluble	Fat soluble
	pH 3.5	pH 6.6–6.9
	pH dependant ring opening phenomenon	No such phenomenon
	Not available	Soyabean formulation to reduce pain
Route of administration	Oral/IV/IM/epidural/spinal	Oral/IV/IM/rectal
Pharmacokinetics	50% oral bioavailability	86–100% oral bioavailability
	80–100% IM bioavailability	IM absorption slow and erratic
	V_d 1–1.5 L/kg	V_d 1–1.5 L/kg
	96–98% plasma protein bound	96–98% plasma protein bound
	Duration of action 15–80 minutes	Longer duration of action
	Onset of action 30–60 seconds	Onset of action late
	Short context sensitive half life	Very long context sensitive half life
	Metabolized by hepatic hydroxylation	
	1 hydroxy-midazolam active metabolite	Desmethyl-diazepam active metabolite
	Hepatic clearance 10 times faster	Hepatic clearance slow
	Renal elimination	Renal elimination
	Elimination $T_{1/2}$ 1.5–3 hours	Elimination $T_{1/2}$ 20–40 hours
	Absent	Enterohepatic circulation present
	No effect	Produces coronary vasodilatation
Uses	Mainly premedication in children	Rarely used in children
	Used for IV sedation and induction	Used in alcohol withdrawal, delirium
	Can be used as infusion for ICU sedation	Not used as infusion
Side effects	Inhibits platelet aggregation	Does not inhibit aggregation
	No pain	Pain on injection common
	Less common	Allergic reactions
	Less common	Nausea and vomiting

UFH VS LMWH

Property	UFH	LMWH
Mean molecular weight	15,000 Da	4000 Da
Anti-Xa: IIa activity	1: 1	4: 1
Inhibition of platelets	Yes	No
Bioavailability	40%	90%
Protein binding	More	Less (10%)
Excretion and metabolism	Endothelial cells and kidney	Only kidney
Elimination $T_{½}$:	Shorter	Longer
$T_{1/2}$ IV administration	1 hour	2 hours
$T_{1/2}$ S/C administration	2 hours	4 hours
Monitoring	Required	Not essential
VTE prevention	Lesser	Better
Thrombocytopenia	High (2–6%)	Low (0.2%)
Hemorrhage	High	Low
Osterporosis	High	Low
Protamine neutralization	Full	Anti-Xa 65%, anti-IIa 90% reversed
Anticoagulant effect	Inconsistent	Consistent

CLONIDINE VS DEXMEDETOMIDINE

Clonidine	Dexmedetomidine
α2: α1 = 220: 1	α2: α1 = 1600: 1
Aniline derivative	Imidazole derivative
Primarily analgesic adjuvant	Primary sedative
Anti-hypertensive	Analgesic
Vd = 2L/kg	Vd = 2–3 L/kg
T ½ = 12-24 hours	T ½ = 2 hours
20-40% protein bound	94% protein bound
Elimination T ½ = 9-12 hours	Elimination T ½ = 2-3 hours
PO, IV, transdermal, epidural routes of administration	IV, IM, PO, transmucosal
Doses: 4–5 μg/kg oral, 1–2 μg/kg IV	0.5–1 μg/kgIV, 2-4 μg/kg PO, 1–2 μg/kg nasal
Uses: antihypertensive, PMI prophylaxis	Mainly ICU sedation and MAC

REMIMAZOLAM VS PROPOFOL

No.	Characteristic	Remimazolam	Propofol
1.	Chemistry	Benzodiazepine	Alkyl phenol
2.	Solubility	Water soluble	Fat soluble
3.	Preparation	Aqueous solution	Needs lipid carrier
4.	Metabolism	Ester hydrolysis	
5.	Pain on injection	Absent	Present
6.	Circulatory depression	Less common	More common
7.	Apnea	Less common	More common
8.	Onset of action	1–3 minutes (longer)	
9.	Context sensitive $T_{1/2}$	Shorter	Longer
10.	Organ damage	Nil	Propofol infusion syndrome
11.	Reversibility	Flumazenil antagonism	Not reversible

SUGGESTED READING

1. Aitkenhead, A.K., Thompson, K., Rowbotham, D.J., Moppett, I. (2013). *Smith and Aitkenheads Textbook of Anesthesia.* 6th ed. Philadelphia: Churchill Livingstone Elsevier.
2. ASHP. (2010). AHFS Drug Information. *American Society of Health System Pharmacists.* 1507.
3. Barash, P.G. (2017). *Clinical Anesthesia.* 8th ed. China: Wolters Kluwer.
4. Butterworth, J., Mackey, D., Wasnik, J. (2018). *Morgan and Mikhails Clinical Anesthesiology.* 6th ed.New York: McGraw-Hill Education/Medical.
5. Davis, P.J., Cladis, F. (2017). *Smiths anesthesia for infants and children.* 9th ed. Philadelphia: Elsevier.
6. FDA. (n.d.). *FDA pharmacology classes.* [online]Available from www.accessdata.fda.gov: <https://www.accessdata.fda.gov/spl/data/70dfc0ee-1ced-425d-b1b4-60935c2413d4/70dfc0ee-1ced-425d-b1b4-60935c2413d4.xml>
7. Flood, P. (2015). *Stoeltings Pharmacology and Physiology in Anesthetic Practice.* 5th ed. China: Wolters Kluwer.
8. Granick, S. (2012). Induction of the synthesis of d-aminolevulinic acid synthetase in liver parenchyma cells in culture by chemicals that induce porphyria. *The Journal of Biological Chemistry.* 2247-9.
9. Gropper, M., Eriksson, L., Fleisher, L., Wiener-Kronish, J., Cohen, N., Leslie, K. (2020). *Millers Anesthesia.* 9th ed. Philadelphia: Elsevier Saunders.
10. Judge, S.E. (1983). Effect of general anesthetics on synaptic ion channels. *British Journal of Anaesthesia.* 191-200.
11. Kaplan, J.A. (2017). *Kaplans Cardiac Anesthesia.* 7th ed. Philadelphia: Elsevier.
12. Miller, R.D., Eriksson, *L., Fleisher, L,* Wiener-Kronish, J., Cohen,N., Young, W. (2014). *Millers Anesthesia.* 8th ed. New York: Elsevier Health.
13. Murray, M.J. (2015). *Fausts Anesthesiology Review.* 4th ed. Philadelphia: Elsevier.
14. Ratuapli, S.K., Bobba, B., Zafar, H. (2010). Heparin induced thrombocytopenia in a patient treated with fondaparinux. *Clinical Advances in Hematology and Oncology.* 61-5.

2 CHAPTER

Neuroanesthesia

PHYSIOLOGY OF INTRACRANIAL PRESSURE

Introduction

Intracranial pressure (ICP) is the pressure within the intracranial space relative to the atmospheric pressure.

Properties

- Total skull volume = 1400–1700 mL
- Total brain volume = 1120–1360 mL
- CSF volume = 140–170 mL
- Blood volume = 140–170 mL

Normal Intracranial Pressures

- 7–15 mm Hg in adults and young children
- 3–7 mm Hg for young children
- 1.5–6 mm Hg for term neonates
- > 20 mm Hg = Raised ICP

Factors Determining ICP

- *Monroe–Kellie doctrine*:
  - States that the contents of the cranium are in a state of constant volume
  - Cranium consists of 3 principle components:
    - Brain tissue
    - Cerebrospinal fluid (CSF)
    - Intracranial blood
  - The cranial vault is an indistensible structure
  - Thus, the volume of its components must be in equilibrium
  - An increase in volume of 1 component causes a reduction in the volume of the other component
- Normally, a small increase in volume is compensated by:
  - Elastance of intracranial components
  - Translocation of CSF from the intracranial cavity into thecal sac
  - Extrusion of venous blood into extracranial veins
- *Intracranial compliance* refers to the degree of increase in ICP in response to an increase in volume of intracranial contents

Intracranial Pressure–Volume Curve

- Relationship between intracranial pressure and volume follows a sigmoidal curve
- Volume expansion of up to 30 mL results in insignificant changes in ICP
- This is because of extrusion of CSF volume and venous blood from the cranium
- When these compensatory mechanisms have exhausted, ICP rises rapidly
- ICP rises until it equilibrates with the cerebral arteriolar pressures
- Thereafter, rise in ICP is halted as cerebral arterioles begin to collapse
- This cessates the cerebral blood flow completely.

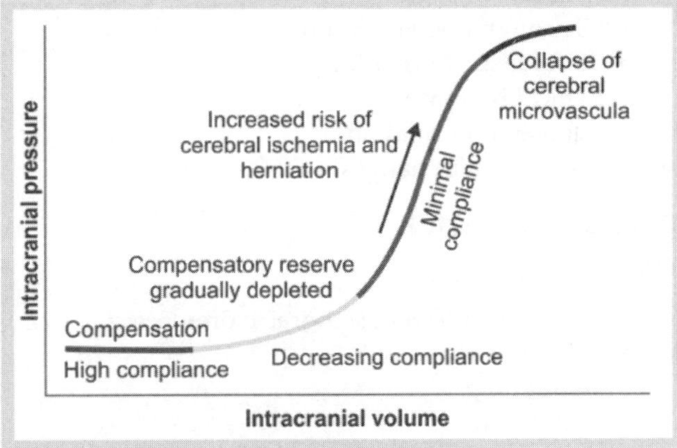

Fig. 1: Intracranial pressure volume curve.

Factors Affecting ICP

- Factors affecting brain tissue:
  - Cerebral swelling:
    - Traumatic brain injury
    - Acute liver failure
    - Hypercarbia
  - Mass effect:
    - Tumors
    - Contusion
    - Subdural hematoma
    - Epidural hematoma
    - Abscess
- Factors affecting CSF flow:
  - Obstruction to CSF flow:
    - Hydrocephalus
    - Meningeal disease
    - Infections
  - Increased CSF production: Choroid plexus tumors:
    - Papilloma
    - Carcinoma
- Factors affecting intracranial blood volume:
  - Increased cerebral blood flow:
    - Aneurysms
    - Hypercarbia
  - Increased venous pressure:
    - Venous sinus thrombosis
    - Heart failure
  - Metabolic disorders:
    - Hypoosmolality
    - Hyponatremia
    - Uremic encephalopathy
    - Hepatic encephalopathy

Effects of Raised ICP

- Cerebral ischemia due to a reduction in Cerebral Perfusion Pressure (CPP)
- Impaired autoregulation—lower limit of autoregulation is raised with increasing ICP
- Herniation of brain:
  - Through open cranium
  - Subfalcine herniation
  - Uncal herniation
  - Tonsillar herniation
- Hemodynamic changes—*Cushings reflex*

Causes of Raised ICP

Physiological Causes

- Increase in abdominal/thoracic pressure:
  - Valsalva maneuver
  - Coughing
  - Intubation
- Increased metabolic demands:
  - Fever
  - Seizures
- Hypervolemia:
  - Fluid overload
  - Head down tilt
- Hypoperfusion:
  - Anemia
  - Cerebral ischemia
- Relative hypoventilation:
  - Sleep
  - Sedation
  - Hypercarbia
  - Hypoxemia

Pathological Causes

- Acute causes:
  - Intraparenchymal hemorrhage:
    - Hemorrhagic stroke
    - Aneurysmal rupture
    - Postoperative intracranial hemorrhage
  - Traumatic hemorrhage:
    - Epidural hematoma
    - Acute subdural hematoma
  - Acute cerebral edema:
    - Acute hyponatremia
    - Hepatic coma
    - Uremic encephalopathy
    - Reyes syndrome
    - *Traumatic Brain Injury* (TBI) causing cerebral contusion
    - Severe hypertension
- Chronic causes:
  - Slow growing lesions:
    - Primary brain tumors
    - Metastatic tumors
    - Abscess
  - Disturbance in CSF absorption, production or flow:
    - Hydrocephalus
    - Meningeal disease
    - Idiopathic intracranial hypertension
    - Chronic subdural hematoma
  - Congenital anomalies:
    - Arnold–Chiari malformation
    - Stenosis of aqueduct of Sylvius

Pathophysiology

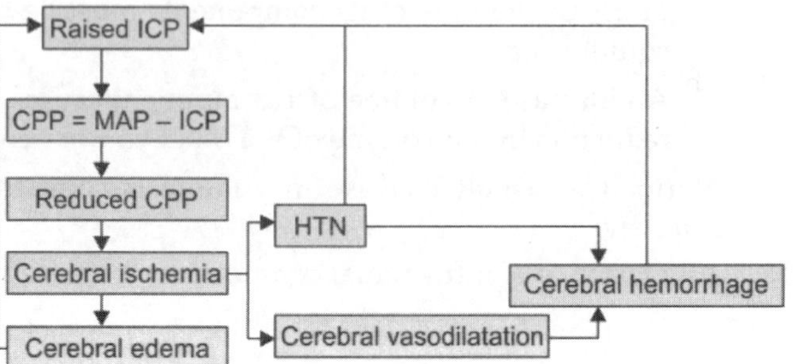

Anesthetic Drugs and ICP

No.	Drug	Effect on ICP	Mechanism
1.	Induction agents		
	Thiopentone	Reduces CBF, CBV and ICP	Cerebral vasoconstriction
			Reduced $CMRO_2$
	Propofol	Reduces CBF, CBV and ICP	Cerebral vasoconstriction
			Reduced $CMRO_2$
	Ketamine	Increases CBF, CBV and ICP	
2.	Opioids	Increases CBF, CMR	Cerebral vasodilatation
		Maintains ICP	Systemic hypotension
3.	Nitrous oxide	Increases ICP	Cerebral vasodilatation
			Reversed with IV anesthetic
4.	Volatile agents	Reduce ICP at <1 MAC	Vasoconstriction and reduced CBF
		Increase ICP at > 1 MAC	Vasodilatation and increased CBF
5.	Succinylcholine	Increases CVP, ICP	Muscle fasciculations
6.	NDMR	Maintains ICP	No effect

CEREBRAL BLOOD FLOW

Introduction

- CNS receives 15% of cardiac output, though it represents only 2% of the body weight
- This is due to the high cerebral metabolic rate

Normal Values

Parameter	Normal
CBF	45–55 mL/100 g/min
CBF to gray matter	75–80 mL/100 g/min
CBF to white matter	20 mL/100 g/min
$CMRO_2$	3–3.5 mL/100 g/min
Cerebral vascular resistance	1.5–2.1 mm Hg/100 g/min/mL
Cerebral venous PO_2	32–44 mm Hg
Cerebral venous SO_2	55–70%
ICP (supine)	8–12 mm Hg

Factors Affecting CBF

- Chemical/metabolic/humoral:
  - PaO_2
  - $PaCO_2$
  - $CMRO_2$:
    - Arousal/pain
    - Temperature
    - Seizures
    - Anesthetics
  - Vasoactive agents:
    - Anesthetics
    - Vasodilators
    - Vasopressors
- Myogenic:
  - Autoregulation
  - Mean arterial pressure
- Rheological: Blood viscosity
- Neurogenic pathways:
  - Extracranial sympathetic and parasympathetic pathway
  - Intraaxial pathways

Factors Affecting CBF

Metabolism

- Increase in $CMRO_2$ increases CBF
- CBF increases with seizures, pain, anxiety, acidosis
- CBF decreases with coma, hypothermia, alkalosis, anesthetic agents
- The proportional increase in CBF with $CMRO_2$ is called ***Flow-Metabolism coupling***
- When $CMRO_2$ increases, local byproducts of metabolism increase:
  - K^+ ions
  - H^+ ions
  - Lactate, adenosine
  - ATP
- This increase in local byproducts is thought to mediate flow-metabolism coupling

$PaCO_2$

- Hypocapnea causes cerebral vasoconstriction and a reduction in cerebral blood flow
- Changes in CBF caused by $PaCO_2$ are dependent on pH alterations in brain ECF
- Changes are more in gray than in white matter due to increased vascular density
- Hypercapnea on the other hand produces cerebral vasodilatation
- CO_2 dissolves with H_2O in CSF and forms H_2CO_3
- The H^+ ions generated cause vasodilation of CBV
- 1 mm Hg rise in $PaCO_2$ causes increase in CBF of 1–2 mL/100 g/min
- Though the changes in CBF with $PaCO_2$ levels occur rapidly, they are not sustained
- CBF returns to normal over a period of 6–8 hours after normalization of pH
- This, in a patient with sustained hypoventilation, rapid normalization of $PaCO_2$ should be avoided

- At $PaCO_2 \geq 90$ mm Hg, narcosis occurs
- At $PaCO_2 \leq 20$ mm Hg, cerebral ischemia with left shift of Hb dissociation curve occurs

PaO_2

- Not an important determinant of CBF
- Changes in PaO_2 from 60 mm Hg to > 300 mm Hg have little influence on the CBF
- Effect of PaO_2 on CBF is mediated through:
  - Peripheral and neuraxial chemoreceptors
  - Lactic acid and other local metabolic products of acidosis
- CBF begins to increase when:
  - PaO_2 falls below 60 mm Hg
  - Cerebral venous PO_2 reduces from 35 to 30 mm Hg

Temperature

- Hypothermia decreases $CMRO_2$ by 6–7% for every °C
- Complete suppression of EEG occurs at 18–20°C
- Hyperthermia increases CBF and $CMRO_2$
- Between 37–42°C, both CBF and $CMRO_2$ increase
- However, above 42°C, a dramatic reduction in $CMRO_2$ occurs

Viscosity

- Not a target of manipulation for those at risk of cerebral ischemia, unless HCT > 55%
- Only modest alterations of CBF occurs when HCT is between 33–45%
- CBF will increase with reduction in HCT below 30%
- This may be due to:
  - Reduction in blood viscosity with reduced hematocrit
  - Compensatory response to reduced oxygen delivery
- In focal cerebral infarcts, a HCT of 30–34% will cause optimal delivery of O_2
- However, manipulation of viscosity provides no additional benefit in reducing the extent of injury in acute ischemic stroke

Anesthetic Agents

No.	Agent	Effect
1.	Inhalational agents	Reduce CBF at < 1 MAC (reduces $CMRO_2$)
	Halothane = enflurane > desflurane>	Increase CBF at > 1 MAC (vasodilation)
	Isoflurane > sevoflurane	***Luxury Perfusion*** occurs at >1 MAC when CBF increases but $CMRO_2$ decreases
2.	Nitrous oxide	Increases CBF by cerebral vasodilation
3.	Intravenous anesthetics:	
	Ketamine	Increases CBF
	Thiopentone	Decreases CBF
	Propofol	Decreases CBF
	Etomidate	Decreases CBF
	Benzodiazepines	Decrease CBF
4.	Opioids	
	Morphine	Increases CBF due to histamine release
	Fentanyl and others	Modest reduction in CBF and $CMRO_2$
		May increase CBF if system is hypotension
5.	Nondepolarizing muscle relaxants	Increase CBF at high doses due to histamine release
6.	Succinylcholine	Increases CBV due to fasciculation induced increase in CVP
7.	Lidocaine	1.5–2 mg/kg boluses
		Effective in controlling acute rise in ICP
8.	Droperidol	Reduces CBF without significant change In $CMRO_2$
9.	Dopamine, adrenaline	Increase CBF

Monitoring CBF

Quantitative Global and Regional CBF

- ***Kety–Schmidt technique***:
  - Considers nitrous oxide (N_2O) to be a freely diffusible intravascular tracer
  - N_2O is administered by inhalation and is measured from IJV
  - Cannulation of jugular bulb is necessary and thus is invasive
  - Measures global hemispheric blood flow and derives $CMRO_2$
- ***Radioactive Xenon washout***:
  - Xe^{133} administered by IV/inhalation (less common)
  - Multiple detectors next to head measure CBF
  - However, accuracy is impaired in low flow conditions
  - Also, areas with no flow cannot be detected (***look through phenomenon***)
- ***Stable Xenon CT***:
  - Stable non-radioactive xenon is inhaled and routine CT scan taken
  - Kety–Schmidt equation is used to derive the CBF

- This process can be repeated at 20 minute intervals after a drug challenge
- Repeat CT scan can be used to test vessel reactivity and cerebrovascular reserve
- This procedure requires xenon inhalation at 26–33%
- Thus, it may be impractical in patients requiring high FiO_2
- Also, xenon is expensive and at 30% causes significant cerebral vasodilation
- This provides a static, non-continuous value of CBF
- Currently used for research purposes only

❖ *CT perfusion scan*:
- CT scans taken after contrast injection helps identify vascular abnormalities
- Computer examines transit time of contrast and derives regional CBF
- Measures intracranial blood flow and shows areas of abnormal CBF
- Uses include:
  - Diagnosis of acute infarction
  - Vasospasm
  - Autoregulation
  - Cerebral vascular reserve

❖ ***Position Emission Tomography***:
- Measures accumulation of positron emitting radioisotopes within an object
- Radioisotopes distribute to different compartments based on pharmacokinetic properties
- The radioisotope (^{15}O) uptake is then measured with a cyclotron
- Measures regional CBF, CBV, $CMRO_2$ and glucose consumption
- Provides the only true measure of CBF adequacy, the oxygen extraction fraction (OEF)
- Expensive, available only in few centers

❖ ***Perfusion weighted MRI***:
- Protons in arterial blood en route to brain are labelled with an inversion pulse
- This is then compared with a control image without an inversion pulse
- This creates an intra-arterial contrast with the intracranial contents
- This provides a quantifiable data set which is used to calculate CBF
- However, it may prove challenging and time consuming in unstable patients

Semiquantitative/Qualitative CBF

❖ Single photon emission computed tomography (SPECT):
- Relies on the emission of gamma-emitting tracers that emit a single photon
- Uses ^{99m}Tc-hexamethylpropyleneamine oxide (HMPAO)
- This radioisotope crosses the BBB and is distributed in proportion to CBF
- The radioisotope is injected intravenously to map the CBF
- Noninvasive, involves less radiation than a CT scan
- Regional distribution of blood can be quantified but not absolute CBF
- The study cannot be repeated to assess efficacy of therapeutic interventions
- Clinical applications include:
  - Assessment of acute stroke
  - Cerebral vasospasm
  - Occlusive vascular disease
- Relatively simple, widely available and inexpensive

Bedside Methods

❖ Thermal diffusion flowmetry (TDF):
- Based on thermal conductivity of brain tissue to measure quantitative CBF
- TD probes are placed on the brain surface during surgery
- Probes are placed subdurally on the cortex to measure superficial CBF
- Alternatively, probes can be placed through a burr hole and secured with a bolt
- It provides only a single CBF measurement from a small volume of tissue
- Thus, this method does not measure global CBF
- Also, it is an invasive method thus, predisposing to bleeding and infection
- Normal values are between 40–70 mL/100 gm/min

❖ Laser Doppler flowmetry (LDF):
- Provides continuous, qualitative measurements of microvascular perfusion
- A small fibreoptic laser probe is applied on the brain surface during surgery
- This illuminates a tissue volume of 1 mm^3 with monochromatic laser light
- The photons are then scattered by moving red blood cells
- The fraction of shifted and nonshifted photons gives an estimate of CBF
- However, this technique has the same limitations as TDF

- Jugular venous oximetry ($SjvO_2$):
  - An oximetric sensor is placed in the jugular bulb to assess global oxygenation
  - This sensor measures the oxygen saturation of jugular venous blood ($SjvO_2$)
  - Jugular bulb is the final common pathway for venous blood from the brain
  - Thus, $SjvO_2$ reflects the balance between global cerebral O_2 demand and supply
  - Therefore $SjvO_2$ does not provide regional CBF measurements
  - $SjvO_2$ is measured intermittently or continuously using fibreoptic catheters
  - Normal $SjvO_2$ is between 55–75%
- Direct brain tissue oxygen monitoring ($PbtO_2$):
  - These are the most commonly used monitors to assess cerebral oxygenation
  - Two commonly used systems are Licox and Neurotrend
  - This technique uses a modified Clark electrode to measure the O_2 content
  - $PbtO_2$ is displayed in mm Hg and the normal value is above 20 mm Hg
  - Values less than 20 mm Hg should be treated
  - $PbtO_2$ less than 15 mm Hg indicates brain hypoxia or ischemia
  - $PbtO_2$ values less than 10 mm Hg indicates severe brain hypoxia
  - Values less than 5 mm Hg are associated with cell death and a poor outcome
  - However, changes in PaO_2 can cause alterations in $PbtO_2$
  - Thus, $PbtO_2$ is not specific for changes in cerebral blood flow
- Near infrared spectroscopy:
  - Technique which measures regional cerebral oxygen saturation (rSO_2)
  - Provides noninvasive bedside measurements of cerebral oxygenation
  - Bilateral electrodes are placed on the frontotemporal region
  - Technique is based on reflectance oximetry
  - Normal values range between 60–80%
  - However, NIRS is affected by the arterial oxygen content
  - Therefore, it is not specific for changes in CBF
  - It is useful for neonates as the thin skull permits transillumination
  - However, in adults a reflectance mode is used due to thickness of the skull
  - Thus, it is prone for contamination by reflectance from extracranial vessels
- Cerebral microdialysis (MD):
  - Used as a bedside monitor to analyze brain tissue biochemistry
  - Microdialysis catheter is placed in at-risk tissue
  - Technique collects low molecular weight substances from the interstitial space
  - These are then analyzed to assess abnormalities in brain metabolism
  - Thus, since it measures changes in metabolism, it is not specific for CBF
  - Changes in MD values precede changes in other physiological variables
  - Thus, it is possible to treat adverse events before they cause irreversible injury
  - Analytes measured are:
    - Lactate-pyruvate ratio (LPR): value > 40 indicates hypoxia
    - Lactate–glucose ratio
    - Glycerol levels: 4–8 fold rise is seen in severe ischemia
- Transcranial Doppler USG:
  - Low frequency (2 mHz) pulsed wave probe is used
  - Insonation of basal cerebral vessel is done through acoustic cranial window
  - Reflected ultrasound from cerebral arteries determines the blood flow velocity
  - The resistive index is then used to calculate turbulent blood flow
  - This is a noninvasive technique which can be used in the ICU
  - However, it may not be possible to obtain acoustic windows in 5–10% patients
  - Also, reproducibility of readings is operator dependent.

CEREBRAL AUTOREGULATION

Introduction

- Physiological response whereby CBF remains constant despite a change in CPP due to alterations in cerebrovascular resistance
- CBF closely autoregulated between MAP 70–150 mm Hg
- Above and below this range, the CBF is pressure dependent (pressure passive)

Mechanism

- Neurogenic hypothesis:
  - This mechanism occurs through the extensive nerve supply to cerebral vessels

- However, autonomic influence on the normal cerebrovascular tone is limited
- In this way, cerebral circulation differs from systemic circulation
- At lower limits of autoregulation however, sympathetic activity modifies CBF
- Thus during shock, sympathetic activity shifts the autoregulatory curve to the right

❖ Myogenic hypothesis (***Bayliss Effect***):
- Smooth muscles in resistance arteries respond directly to CPP alterations
- Thus, changes in CPP cause direct change in tone of vascular smooth muscle
- This maybe due to endogenous nitric oxide release
- Also due to autonomic innervations of cerebral blood vessels

❖ Metabolic coupling:
- This mechanism modifies CBF in proportion to changes in $CMRO_2$
- Reduction in CBF stimulates vasoactive substance release from the brain
- This in turn stimulates cerebral vessel dilatation
- Occurs when metabolic demands of tissues exceeds cerebral blood flow
- This is primarily due to *Flow-Metabolism Coupling*
- Principal mediators include:
  - Nitric oxide
  - Vasoactive peptides
  - Prostaglandins (PGE_2, PGI_2, PGF_2)
  - Endothelin.

Factors Affecting Autoregulation

❖ Hypertension:
- In patients with chronic HTN, autoregulation curve shifts to right
- Lower limit of autoregulation is therefore higher
- Thus, BP which may be adequate in a normal patient may cause ischemia in a hypertensive patient
- Shift of autoregulation curve is modified by anti-hypertensive therapy

❖ Hypotension:
- Autoregulation is impaired during hypotension
- Autoregulation is better preserved with pharmacological hypotension
- In case of hypovolemic hypotension, autoregulation is poorly preserved

❖ Chemical sympathectomy:
- Used along with sodium nitroprusside/trimethophan
- Cerebral autoregulation curve is shifted to the left
- Similar changes occur during sympathetic blockade
- May extend lower limit of tolerable hypotension

Autoregulation impaired in

❖ Areas of relative ischemia
❖ Surrounding mass lesions
❖ After grand mal seizures
❖ After head injury

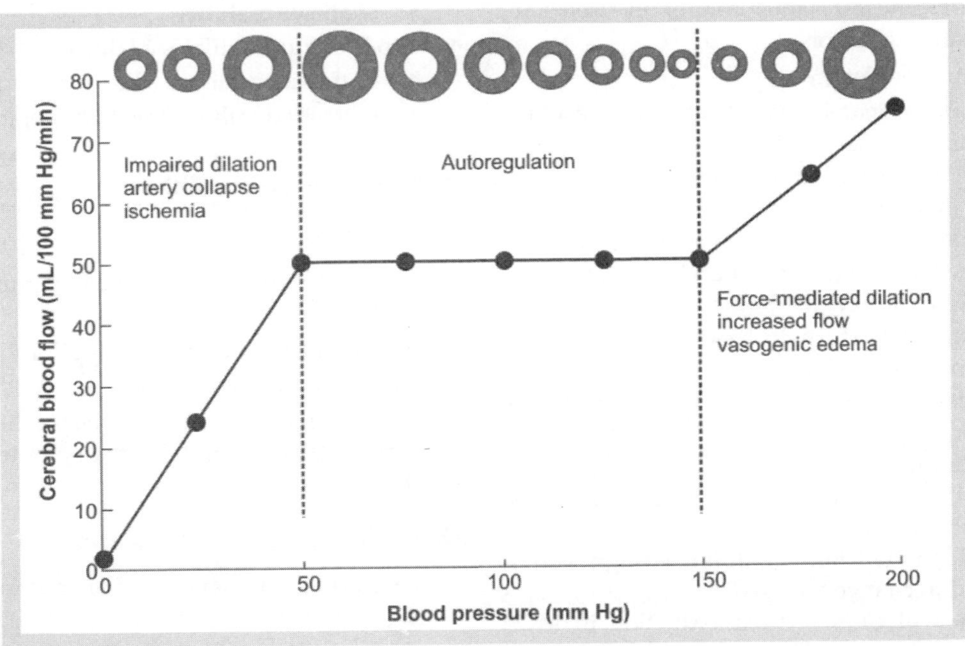

Fig. 2: Cerebral autoregulation curve.

- During episodes of hypoxia/hypercarbia
- Volatile anesthetics (except sevoflurane)
- Brain tissue acidosis:
  - Hypoxia
  - Hypercarbia
  - In areas surrounding infarcts

Types of Autoregulation

- *Static autoregulation*: Response to slow changes in arterial BP/CPP
- *Dynamic autoregulation*: Response to rapid changes in arterial BP/CPP

Tests of Autoregulation

- Static autoregulation
  - Older method which used Kety-Schmidt technique or ^{133}Xe uptake technique
  - Changes in MAP are produced by mechanical methods like head up tilt
  - Measurements of MAP and CBF are taken at baseline and after the maneuver
  - These are used to assess the intactness of autoregulation
  - Drugs which change the MAP with no effect on metabolism are used now
  - This yields 2 values of CBF at two different levels of MAP
  - Any difference in CBF is thereby indicative of cerebral autoregulation
  - Phenylephrine test is most commonly used static test of autoregulation
- Dynamic autoregulation
  - Determines dynamic changes of CBF in response to dynamic changes in MAP
  - After a change in MAP, CBF will first react to the change in MAP
  - Thereafter, CBF will return to the baseline value
  - The time taken to return to baseline is a measure of degree of autoregulation
  - The faster the return to baseline, better is the degree of autoregulation
  - These tests are carried out with transcranial Doppler
  - Thigh cuff test:
    - A BP cuff is tied around the thigh and inflated to above SBP for 2–3 mins
    - Sudden deflation of inflated thigh cuff is used to change the MAP
    - This will cause a brief reduction in MCA flow velocity on TCD
    - Thereafter, flow velocity returns to baseline
    - Cerebral autoregulation is defined by the slope of CVR (CPP/CBF) recovery
    - Steeper the slope of CVR, better is the autoregulation
  - Carotid compression test:
    - Observes changes in CBF with ipsilateral carotid artery compression
    - Measures TCD changes in middle cerebral artery flow velocity
    - Brief compression (< 5 seconds) of I/L common carotid artery is performed
    - Intact autoregulation results in vasodilatation during this period
    - Releasing the compression causes a transient hyperemic overshoot
    - If autoregulation is impaired, this response is absent.

Autoregulatory Failure

- Refers to the disturbance in cerebral autoregulation in disease states
- The final pathway of autoregulatory dysfunction is termed *vasomotor paralysis*
- Autoregulatory failure may occur due to:
  - Acute ischemia
  - Mass lesions
  - Trauma
  - Inflammation
  - Prematurity
  - Neonatal asphyxia
  - Diabetes mellitus
- Types of autoregulatory failure:
  - Right sided failure (due to hyperperfusion)
  - Left sided failure (due to hypoperfusion)

THERMOREGULATION

Introduction

- Mean core temperature in healthy humans is 36.5°C–37.3°C
- Peripheral temperature is typically 2°C–4°C lower than the core temperature
- Thermoregulation refers to the mechanism by which hypothalamus maintains the body temperature at a stable level

Physiology of Thermoregulation

- Thermoregulation is based on multiple signals coming from different tissues
- The processing of thermal information occurs in three phases:

- Afferent input
- Central regulation
- Efferent responses

❖ Thermoregulatory efferent response involves control of:
  - Basal metabolic rate
  - Muscular activity
  - Sympathetic activity
  - Vascular tone
  - Hormonal activity

❖ There is an orderly progression of responses in proportion to the need

❖ Threshold temperature is the temperature at which an efferent response is triggered

❖ Inter-threshold range:
  - Range over which autonomic responses are not activated
  - It is bound by:
    - Sweating threshold at the upper end
    - Vasoconstriction threshold at lower end
  - No autonomic thermoregulatory response occurs in this range
  - Normally this range is only a few tenths of a degree centigrade (0.2°C)
  - This interthreshold range increases under general anesthesia
  - Thus, under anesthesia, thermoregulatory responses will be blunted

Pathways of Thermoregulation

Afferent Sensing Pathway

❖ Thermo-sensitive cells (receptors) are found in most parts of the body like:
  - Hypothalamus and other parts of brain
  - Spinal cord: Deep abdomen
  - Deep thorax: Skin surface (each 20% input)

❖ Receptors for perception of cold are different from those for heat perception

❖ Cold receptors are triggered when the core temperature falls below a set threshold

❖ Impulses are then conducted to the thermoregulatory center in the hypothalamus

❖ This pathway represents the afferent sensing pathway for thermoregulation

❖ Heat receptor generated impulses are transmitted through the unmyelinated C fibers

❖ The same fibers are responsible for conduction of pain sensation

❖ Thus, patients are often unable to distinguish between extreme pain and heat or cold

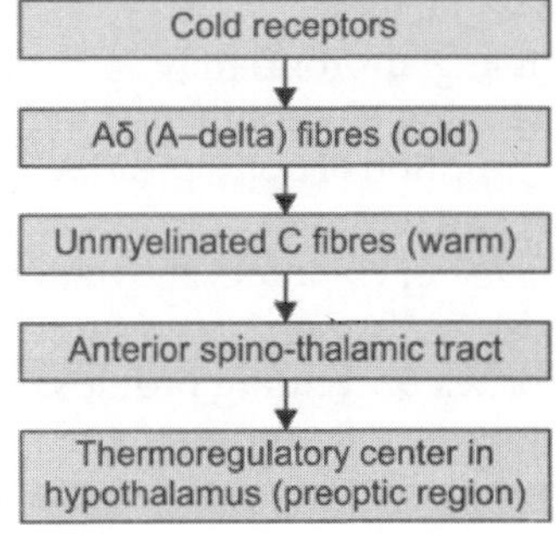

Central Regulation

❖ Hypothalamus integrates the afferent input and coordinates various efferent outputs

❖ Input received from the skin surface and deep tissues is compared by hypothalamus

❖ Input is compared with threshold temperature for each thermoregulatory response

❖ Hypothalamus then stimulates appropriate efferent pathways to produce a response

❖ Threshold temperature for vasoconstriction is 36.5°C

❖ Threshold temperature for shivering is 36°C

❖ Mediators involved in establishing thresholds include:
  - Norepinephrine
  - Dopamine
  - Serotonin
  - Acetylcholine
  - Prostaglandin E_1
  - Neuropeptides

Efferent Responses

❖ Behavioural responses:
  - These are the most effective responses for thermoregulation

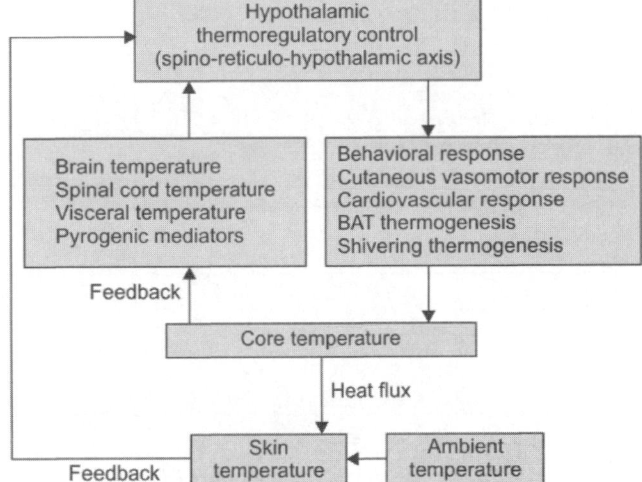

Fig. 3: Threshold range.

- Responses include:
  - Dressing appropriately
  - Modifying environmental temperature
  - Assumption of body positions which oppose skin surfaces
  - Increasing voluntary movements to generate heat
- ❖ Other responses preventing heat loss include:
  - *Vasoconstriction*: Reduces cutaneous heat loss
  - *Nonshivering thermogenesis*: Especially in newborn
  - Shivering:
    - Increases heat production by 100–200%
    - Occurs after vasoconstriction
    - Does not occur in newborn
    - It is ineffective in children up to several years old.

Thermoregulation during General Anesthesia

- ❖ Under GA, behavioral regulation is not relevant as patients are unconscious
- ❖ Thus thermoregulatory responses under anesthesia include:
  - Autonomic responses
  - External thermal management
- ❖ Autonomic responses are also markedly blunted under anesthesia
- ❖ Therefore under GA, alterations in autonomic thresholds include:
  - Increase in warm response threhold
  - Decrease in cold response threshold
- ❖ Thus, interthreshold range increases almost 10-fold (from 0.2°C to 2°C–4°C)
- ❖ Altered efferent responses during general anesthesia include:

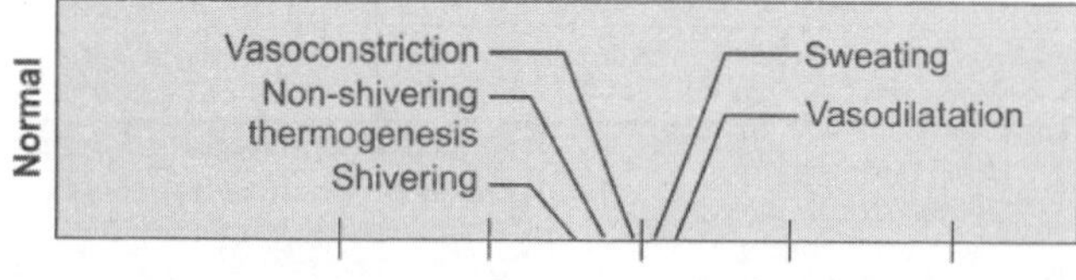

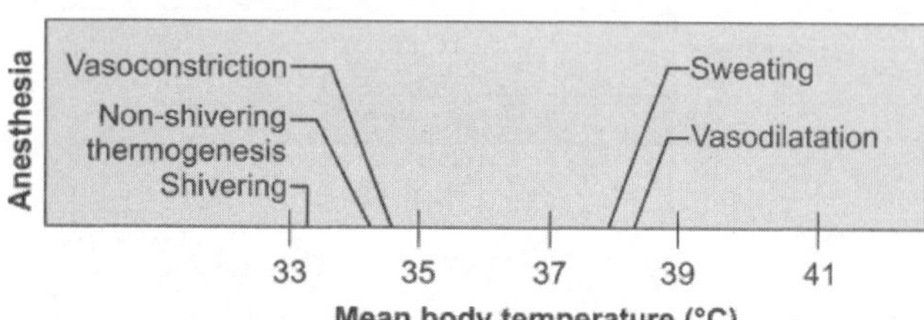

Fig. 4: Interthreshold range under anesthesia.

- Increase in interthreshold range 2–4° C
- Irrelevant behavioral regulation
- Nonshivering thermogenesis not significant in adult
- Impaired shivering response due to muscle paralysis

Effect of General Anesthetics on Thermoregulation

No.	Agent	Sweating threshold	Cold threshold
1.	Propofol	Increase	Linear decrease
2.	Opioids	Increase	Linear decrease
3.	Dexmedetomidine	Increase	Linear decrease
4.	Clonidine	Slight increase	Decrease
5.	Volatile agents	Slight increase	Nonlinear decrease
6.	Fentanyl + N_2O	Slight increase	Nonlinear decrease

Thermoregulation Under Regional Anesthesia

- ❖ Hypothermia during regional anesthesia is as severe as during GA
- ❖ Under regional anesthesia, behavioural regulation is impaired
- ❖ This is because behavioural regulation is largely determined by skin temperature
- ❖ Thus, though core temperature reduces, skin temperature increases due to vasodilation
- ❖ Patient therefore does not feel cold in spite of having a reduced core temperature
- ❖ Also, regional anesthesia blocks all thermal input from anesthetized regions
- ❖ Thus, RA inhibits tonic cold signals from legs to thermoregulatory center
- ❖ The hypothalamus wrongly interprets this as warming of legs
- ❖ Thus, it reduces the vasoconstriction and shivering threshold by up to 0.6°C
- ❖ Peripheral vasoconstriction and shivering is inhibited in blocked areas
- ❖ However, these reflexes are preserved in muscle mass proximal to these areas
- ❖ Supplementation with sedatives further impairs thermoregulation
- ❖ Also, regional anesthesia itself impairs the thermoregulatory center.

Thermoregulation in Combined General-Regional Anesthesia

- ❖ Core temperature does not plateau in combined GA-RA
- ❖ Thus, it continues to decrease throughout surgery
- ❖ Core temperature management and monitoring is very important in these cases

Phases of Hypothermia Under General Anesthesia

- Phase I: ***Redistribution phase:***
  - Occurs during the first hour of GA
  - Causes the largest drop in core temperature (0.5–1.5°C)
  - At the same time, peripheral temperature increases from 33°C to 35°C
  - Accounts for 81% of temperature reduction
  - Redistribution is caused by vasodilatation induced by general anesthetics
  - This causes redistribution of heat from the core to periphery
  - This redistribution occurs along temperature gradient
- Phase II: ***Linear phase:***
  - Occurs for next 2–4 hours after GA
  - During this phase linear reduction in core temperature occurs
  - This is mainly due to heat loss exceeding heat production under GA
  - Heat loss occurs by radiation > convection > evaporation> conduction
- Phase III: ***Plateau phase:***
  - Occurs after 3–4 hours of GA
  - Core temperature stops reducing and stabilizes
  - Represents normal steady state when heat loss equals heat production
  - Usually occurs once thermoregulatory vasoconstriction sets in
  - Reduces heat lost from body
  - However, this phase is absent in peripheral/ autonomic neuropathy

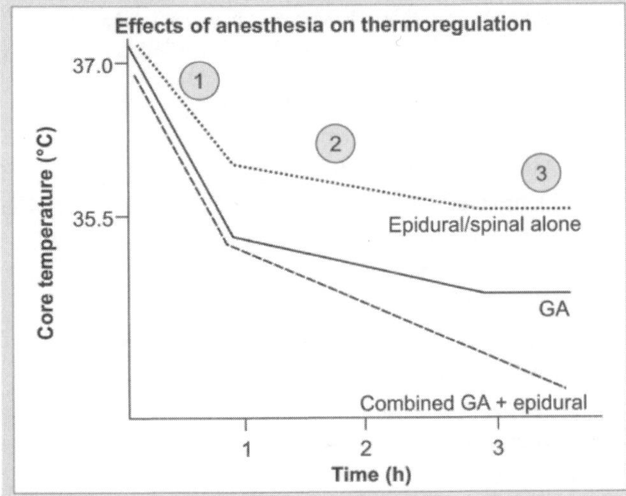

Fig. 5: Thermoregulatory curves under anesthesia.

Phases of Hypothermia During Regional Anesthesia

- Phase I: ***Redistribution phase***:
  - Core temperature reduces during first hour after RA due to vasodilatation
  - At the same time, peripheral temperature increases due to redistribution
  - This accounts for the largest drop in core temperature during RA
- Phase II: ***Linear phase:***
  - Occurs during the next 2–4 hours after RA
  - Mainly due to heat loss exceeding heat production
- Phase III: ***Plateau phase***:
  - *Plateau phase is absent under RA*
  - This is because RA blocks nerve supply to blood vessels in the legs
  - This prevents any thermoregulatory vasoconstriction

Thermoregulation in Newborn

- No shivering/effective vasoconstriction occurs
- Have a larger surface area to weight ratio which increases heat loss
- Newborns also have lesser subcutaneous fat for insulation
- *Nonshivering thermogenesis* is however very effective
- No thermoregulatory sweating occurs in newborns

SHIVERING

Introduction

- Spontaneous, oscillatory, asynchronous muscular activity which augments heat production as a thermoregulatory response to hypothermia
- It is defined as the fasciculations of the face, jaw, head or muscle hyperactivity lasting longer than 15 seconds

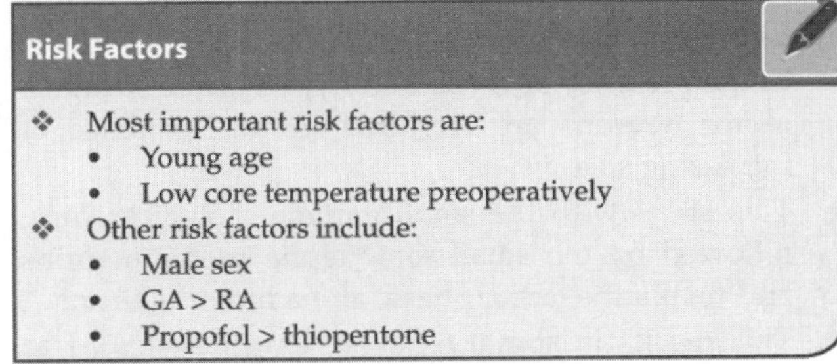

Risk Factors

- Most important risk factors are:
  - Young age
  - Low core temperature preoperatively
- Other risk factors include:
  - Male sex
  - GA > RA
  - Propofol > thiopentone

Etiology

- Increased heat loss due to:
  - Evaporation during skin preparation
  - Radiation and convection from skin

- Low ambient temperature (< 21°C)
- Cold IV fluids and irrigation fluids
- Humidification of gases

❖ Redistribution due to:
- Peripheral vasodilatation:
  - Regional anesthesia
  - Volatile anesthetics
- Reduced thermoregulatory threshold
- Sepsis induced vasodilatation
- Allergy

❖ Altered thermoregulation due to:
- Paralysis and anesthesia impaired shivering and behavioural regulation
- Impaired thermoregulatory vasoconstriction
- Absent nonshivering thermogenesis in anesthetized adults
- Volatile anesthetics interfere with hypothalamic thermostat
- Reduced basal metabolic rate (0.83 kcal/kg/hr)

Incidence

❖ Up to 40% following all anesthetics
❖ 65% after general anesthesia
❖ 33% after regional anesthesia

Pathogenesis

❖ Elicited when preoptic region of hypothalamus is cooled
❖ Stimulation of κ-opioid, NMDA and 5-HT receptors occurs
❖ Efferent signals from hypothalamus descend via medial forebrain bundle
❖ Mesencephalic reticular formation and medullary reticular formation exert descending influence on spinal cord which increases muscle tone
❖ Spinal α motor neurons are the final common pathway for shivering
❖ A typical cold tremor has a specific rhythm in the form of grouped discharges
❖ In the presence of continued hypothermic stimulus motor neurons are recruited in the sequence of increasing size
❖ This starts with the small gamma motor neurons, followed by the small tonic alpha motor neurons and finally the larger phasic alpha motor neurons
❖ This results in spinal reflexes being manifested as clonic activity
❖ This in turn increases heat production by up to 600%
❖ This is a last resort defence which is activated only when other responses are insufficient to maintain core temperature

Pathophysiology

❖ The fundamental tremor frequency on electromyogram is 200 Hz
❖ This is modulated by a slow 4–8 cycles/min waxing and waning pattern
❖ EMG demonstrates two distinct shivering patterns:
- Tonic pattern:
  - Resembles normal shivering
  - Normal thermoregulatory responses to hypothermia
- Clonic pattern:
  - Resembles pathological clonus
  - Not a normal component of thermoregulatory shivering
  - Occurs specifically on recovery from volatile anesthetics

Factors Potentiating Shivering

❖ Pain
❖ Adrenal suppression
❖ Uninhibited spinal reflexes
❖ Pyrogens
❖ Decreased sympathetic activity
❖ Respiratory alkalosis

Shivering Assessment

Bedside Shivering Assessment Scale:

Score	Type of shivering	Location
0	None	No shivering on palpation of masseter/neck/chest muscles
1	Mild	Shivering localized to neck and thorax only
		May be seen only as artifact on ECG
2	Moderate	1+ Shivering involving gross movement of upper extremities
3	Severe	Involving gross movements of trunk, upper and lower extremities

Effects of Hypothermia and Shivering

❖ Central nervous system:
- Altered mental status
- Decreased MAC (5–7% per 1°C cooling)
- Increased residual sedation
- Increased residual paralysis
- Delayed awakening
- Slow EEG with increased SSEP latency
- Protects against cerebral ischemia
- Increased IOP and ICP
- Decreases $CMRO_2$ by 8%

❖ Cardiovascular:
- Increased release of norepinephrine and epinephrine

- Increases peripheral and pulmonary vascular resistance
- Decreases venous capacitance and cardiac output
- Increases heart rate and blood pressure
- Increases chances of MI
- Increased troponin I levels
- Dysrhythmias (VF, if < 28°C)

❖ Altered coagulation due to:
- Platelet sequestration
- Decreased platelet function
- Decreased clotting factor function
- Increased blood loss and blood transfusion

❖ Impaired wound healing due to:
- Increased postoperative infection
- Impaired phagocytosis and oxidative killing
- Impaired chemotaxis
- Moderate hyperglycemia

❖ Oxygenation:
- Shift of oxyhemoglobin dissociation curve to left
- Increased oxygen consumption (100–200%) and CO_2 production
- Increased tissue hypoxia and metabolic acidosis
- Jeopardized marginal tissue grafts

❖ Others:
- Impairs renal function
- May interfere with planned procedure done under monitored anesthesia:
  - ESWL
  - Colonoscopy
- Decreases reliability of pulse oximetry, ECG and IBP monitoring
- Incidental trauma
- Wound pain by stretching incision site
- Decreased drug metabolism—interferes with recovery from anesthesia

Prevention

❖ Maintain OT temperature between 21–23°C
❖ Maintain intraoperative normothermia
❖ Adequate prewarming for 30 minute prior to regional anesthesia
❖ Ketamine 0.5 mg/kg IV before GA/RA
❖ Ondansetron 8 mg IV given during induction of anesthesia prevents PAS
❖ Correct underlying problems:
- Sepsis
- Hypothermia

❖ Warming IV fluids and irrigating solutions:
- 1 unit of blood or 1 litre crystalloid at room temperature reduces mean body temperature by 0.25°C
- Withhold reversal of intraoperative muscle relaxation in intubated patients

Treatment

I. Rewarming

❖ Active rewarming:
- Attempt at restoring body temperature above shivering threshold
- Mechanism of action:
  - Increasing body heat content
  - Limiting heat redistribution from core to periphery
  - Decreasing radiant heat loss
- Usually not very effective as:
  - Skin surface contributes only 20% to control of shivering
  - Available warmers increase mean skin temperature only few degrees
- These measures are usually ineffective when core temperature falls < 35°C
- Available alternatives include:
  - Circulating water mattresses:
    - Not very effective
    - Increased risk of burns due to combination of:
      - Active warming of the back
      - Reduced perfusion to the back
  - Forced air warmers at 40–43°C—*most effective*
  - Radiant infrared lamps

❖ Passive rewarming:
- These measures are of limited benefit
- Maintain OT temperature at 21–23°C
- Insulators used to cover head and body surface such as:
  - Cotton blankets
  - Surgical drapes
  - Plastic sheets
  - Reflective composites
- Single layer of each reduces heat loss by 30%
- Using multiple layers or prewarming insulators not very useful
- Cover head of infants with blankets/aluminium foil

II. Humidification

❖ Limited role as only 10% of heat produced is lost via respiratory tract
❖ Respiratory loss remains almost constant during anesthesia
❖ Thus, fraction of heat lost during major surgeries reduces drastically
❖ HME is breathing circuits (infants and children)

III. Supplemental Oxygen

IV. Drugs

- *Opioids*:
  - Due to activation of central μ and κ receptors
  - Meperidine:
    - 0.35–0.4 mg/kg (12.5–25 mg IV)
    - Central κ opioid action
    - ***Most effective*** opioid for shivering
  - Tramadol: 25–50 mg or 1–2 mg/kg IV
  - Butorphanol: 1–2 mg IV
  - Fentanyl
  - Alfentanil 250 μg IV
- *5–HT Antagonists*:
  - Action based on ***monoamine theory of thermoregulation***
  - States that balance between 5–HT and norepinephrine in the hypothalamus controls hypothalamic thermostat
  - 5-HT causes shivering and vasoconstriction
  - Thus, 5-HT antagonists may be used to prevent shivering
  - Ketanserin 10 mg IV
  - Ondansetron may also be used for prevention of shivering
- α_2 *Agonists*:
  - Clonidine 1.5 μg/kg or 75 μg IV
  - Dexmedetomidine 0.5 μg/kg/hr
  - Decreases vasoconstriction and shivering threshold
  - However, use for sole purpose of preventing PAS is not recommended
- *Anticholinergics*:
  - Physostigmine 0.04 mg/kg IV
  - Chlorpromazine 10–25 mg IV
- *NMDA Antagonists:*
  - Ketamine –0.5 mg/kg IV
  - Magnesium sulphate:
    - 50 mg/kg IV bolus
    - Followed by 15 mg/kg/hr continuous infusion
- *Analeptics*:
  - Doxapram 100 mg or 1.5 mg/kg IV
  - Methylphenidate
- *Others*:
  - Propofol 10–50 μg/kg/min
  - Nefopam 0.15 mg/kg IV
  - If uncontrolled, IV vecuronium 0.1 mg/kg IV followed by mechanical ventilation
- *Shivering associated with sepsis*:
  - PG synthetase inhibitors [Acetaminophen (PR), aspirin]
  - Glucocorticoids

Columbia Antishivering Protocol for Therapeutic Hypothermia

BSAS Score	Step	Intervention	Dose
0	Baseline	Acetaminophen	650–1000 mg Q4–6H
		Buspirone	30 mg Q8H
		Magnesium sulphate	0.5–1 gm/hr IV
		Skin counterwarming	43°C
1	Mild sedation	Dexmedetomidine	0.2–1.5 μg/kg/hr
		OR	
		Meperidine	50–100 mg IM or IV
2	Moderate sedation	Dexmedetomidine	0.2–1.5 μg/kg/hr
		AND	
		Meperidine	50–100 mg IM or IV
3	Deep sedation	Propofol	50–75 μg/kg/min
	Paralysis	Vecuronium	0.1 mg/kg

NONSHIVERING THERMOGENESIS

Introduction

- Defined as hypothermia induced increase in metabolic heat production which is not associated with muscle activity
- Also called *chemical thermogenesis*

Physiology

- NST occurs from few hours after birth up to 2 years of age
- Occurs predominantly in brown fat or Brown Adipose Tissue (BAT)
- Other sites of NST:
  - Liver
  - Skeletal muscle
  - Brain
  - White fat
- Norepinephrine, glucocorticoids and thyroxine are chief mediators for NST
- NST can be inhibited by:
  - Surgical sympathectomy
  - Pharmacological agents:
    - Ganglionic blockers
    - Beta blockers
    - Volatile anesthetics
    - Fentanyl
    - Propofol

Mechanism of NST

- NST represents the primary mechanism in newborns to respond to heat loss

- NST increases the metabolic heat production by up to 200%
- Mitochondria present in brown adipose tissue are unique
- This is because they can uncouple oxidative phosphorylation
- This results in heat production instead of generation of ATP
- This is mediated by the presence of uncoupling protein 1 (UCP–1 or thermogenin)
- Activation of brown fat metabolism results in a redirection of cardiac output
- Higher proportion of cardiac output is diverted through brown fat
- This proportion may reach as high as 25% of the cardiac output
- This in turn facilitates direct warming of the blood

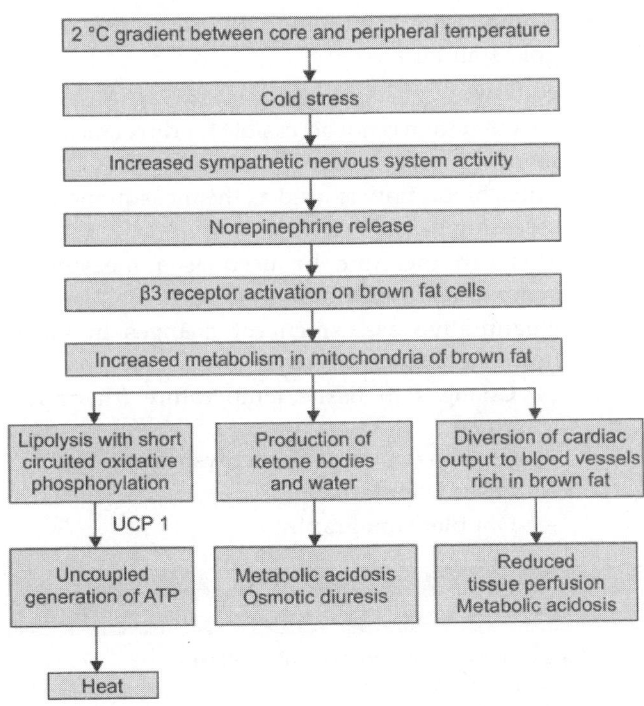

Brown Fat

- Brown fat is adipose tissue with high vascularity
- Ample source of blood vessels is partly responsible for the brown color of tissue
- Abundant mitochondria in its multinucleated cells also contributes to the color
- These mitochondria are densely packed with cristae
- They also have an increased content of respiratory chain components
- Constitutes 2–6% of infants total body weight
- Also richly innervated by sympathetic nervous system
- Six main sites with brown fat:
  - Between scapulae
  - In small masses around blood vessels of the neck
  - Large deposits in axilla
  - Medium sized masses in the mediastinum
  - Around kidneys, adrenals
  - Around major blood vessels of thorax like internal mammary artery
- Causes of insufficient BAT:
  - Preterm infants
  - Intrauterine Growth Retardation (IUGR)
- Regeneration of brown adipose tissue in adults may occur due to:
  - Sustained sympathetic stimulation
  - Chagas disease
  - Hibernoma (benign brown fat tumor)
  - Marked cold acclimatization

Efficacy

- Increases heat production by up to 200% in infants
- However, it does not compensate for the decreased ability of newborns to:
  - Reduce heat loss through cutaneous vasoconstriction
  - Increase heat production through shivering
- NST is not functional or relevant in adults
- Shivering is primary mechanism of heat production in adults
- Heat production increased only slightly in non-anesthetized adults

Prevention of Hypothermia in Neonates

- Important as it causes increased hypoxia and metabolic acidosis
- Maintain neutral thermal environment
- Skin surface warming:
  - Hot water warmers
  - Infrared radiant heaters
  - Convection heaters
  - Use plastic wrap/covers/hats to reduce heat loss from head and other areas
  - Use of head caps useful in infants in contrast to adults
- Prevent heat losses
  - Transport newborn in incubator and not bed with overhead heaters
  - Increase OT temperature to maximum levels (around 26°C if tolerable)
  - Air humidification

- Place patient on forced air warming blanket to reduce conductive heat loss
- Use of warm IV fluids—place fluid warmer close to IV access site.

TESTS OF AUTONOMIC NERVOUS SYSTEM

Introduction

- ANS is responsible for the regulation and integration of internal organ function
- However, clinical symptoms of ANS disorders are non-characteristic
- Thus, in order to identify ANS disorders, detailed assessment of its function is required
- Tests of the ANS system therefore are vital in diagnosing these disorders

Indications

- Syncope
- Central autonomic degeneration (e.g. Parkinsonism)
- Pure autonomic failure
- Postural tachycardia syndrome
- Autonomic and small fiber peripheral neuropathies
- Diabetic neuropathy
- Hereditary neuropathy
- Sympathetically mediated pain
- Evaluating response to therapy

Patient Preparation

- Refrain from heavy meals, coffee and nicotine for 3–4 hours before testing
- Alcohol should be withheld for 8 hours prior to testing
- Withhold anticholinergic medication for 48 hours before test
- Withhold sympathomimetic medications for 24–48 hrs before test
- Patients are instructed to wear loose fitting clothes
- Patients should be housed in a quiet room with neutral temperature and humidity
- Before testing patients should be lying down or seated for 30 minutes

Biosignals Used During ANS Tests

- Heart rate recording:
  - Continuous ECG monitoring allows precise evaluation of heart rate response
  - Heart rate response is a major indicator of parasympathetic function
  - 3-lead ECG is connected with electrodes on anterior chest wall
  - Reference electrode is placed in the midaxillary line at T_4 level
  - Tests of heart rate variability (HRV) is measured in the form of R–R interval
  - Computer aided HRV calculations are most specific and accurate
  - The ECG signal is digitized at a sampling frequency of 256 Hz
  - The RR interval duration is then displayed over the interval number producing the tachogram
- Blood pressure recording:
  - Blood pressure is an indicator of vascular tone
  - Regulation of vascular tone is primarily carried out by the sympathetic NS
  - Thus, BP variation is used as a measure of sympathetic NS activity
  - Continuous or intermittent recording can be done
  - Brachial/wrist/finger blood pressure cuffs may be used
  - Noninvasive continuous BP recording is the gold standard
- Blood flow:
  - Vascular tone is not accessible for direct measurement
  - Thus, blood flow is used as the measurement for assessing vascular tone
  - This can therefore be used as a measure of sympathetic vasomotor system
  - Quantitative assessment of changes in blood flow can be measured by:
    - Changes in tissue temperature (thermometry)
    - Changes in volume (plethysmography)
    - Laser Doppler
    - Doppler sonography

Types of Tests for Autonomic Nervous System

- Tests of autonomic cardiovascular reflexes:
  - Valsalva maneuver
  - Respiratory sinus arrhythmia
  - Orthostatic test (active standing)
  - Pressor functional tests:
    - Isometric handgrip test
    - Cold pressor test
    - Mental arithmetic
  - Head up tilt
  - Baroreflex sensitivity test
- Analysis of heart rate variability
- Microneurography
- Tests of sudomotor function:
  - Thermoregulatory sweat test
  - Sympathetic skin response
  - Quantitative sudomotor axon reflex test

Tests of Autonomic Cardiovascular Reflexes

I. Valsalva Maneuver

- Physiology:
  - Valsalva maneuver evaluates function of the baroreceptor reflex
  - It refers to a voluntary forced expiration against a resistance
  - The maneuver consists of four phases:
    - Phase I:
      - Characterized by brief increase in intrathoracic pressure
      - This causes mechanical compression of the aorta
      - This causes a transient increase in blood pressure (1–2 sec)
      - This activates baroreceptors simultaneously
      - Therefore slight bradycardia occurs
    - Phase II:
      - Increased intrathoracic pressure persists
      - This reduces the venous return and preload to the heart
      - Therefore there is a drop in stroke volume and blood pressure
      - There is a reflex peripheral arterial vasoconstriction
      - This results in concomitant compensatory tachycardia
    - Phase III:
      - Expiration is stopped during this phase
      - This results in short lasting pulmonary vascular expansion
      - As a result, blood pressure falls further during this phase
      - This causes a compensatory tachycardia
    - Phase IV:
      - This marks the completion of rise in intrathoracic pressure
      - Thus, venous return and stroke volume increases
      - This causes an abrupt rise in blood pressure
      - However, the arterial vascular bed is still vasoconstricted
      - Baroreceptor activation occurs during this phase
      - This results in bradycardia
- Procedure:
  - Maneuver is performed with the subject seated after 15 mins rest
  - Baseline BP and heart rate are measured 3 minutes before the test
  - Patient is asked to blow into a special tube connected to a pressure transducer
  - The pressure transducer is used to measure expiratory pressure
  - Patient takes deep inhalation, complete exhalation followed by deep inhalation again
  - Patient then exhales deeply into the mouth piece of this tube for 15 seconds
  - Expiratory pressure is maintained at 40 mm Hg for these 15 seconds
  - BP and heart rate are measured throughout the maneuver
  - Measurement is continued for 60 seconds after the maneuver
  - The maneuver is repeated thrice and mean values are taken
- Interpretation:
  - Valsalva ratio:
    - It is the most important index of parasympathetic NS function
    - Valsalva Ratio = $\dfrac{\text{Longest RR interval in phase IV}}{\text{Shortest RR interval in phase II}}$
    - Normal ratio > 1.21
    - Value less than 1.21 indicates parasympathetic NS dysfunction
  - Blood pressure variation:
    - This is an index of sympathetic NS dysfunction
    - Fall in BP at the beginning of phase II should be less than 21 mm Hg
    - BP should return to baseline value by the end of phase II or in phase III
- Contraindications:
  - Geriatric patients
  - Respiratory disease
  - H/o recent retinal detachment surgery
- Sources of error:
  - Faulty breathing through mouth piece resulting in inadequate seal
  - Hypovolemia
  - Medical deconditioning
  - Hypothyroidism
- *Summary*:

Stimulus	Expiratory pressure of 40 mm Hg for 15 seconds
Afferent	Baroreceptors, glossopharyngeal and vagus nerves
Central	Nucleus tractus solitarius
Efferent	Vagus and sympathetic nervous system
Response	Maximum: Minimum heart rate > 1.21

II. Respiratory Sinus Arrhythmia

- Physiology:
  - Physiologically, inhalation causes an increase in heart rate
  - On the other hand, exhalation causes a decrease in heart rate
  - This is mainly due to changing parasympathetic activity
  - Dependence of HR on respiration is called respiratory sinus arrhythmia (RSA)
  - During metronomic breathing, heart rate reaches both extremes
  - Thus, the ratio of 2 extremes is used to assess parasympathetic NS function
- Procedure:
  - Done with patient supine
  - Patient is instructed to breathe deeply and evenly
  - Breathing is done at rate of 6 breaths/minute, each breath lasting 5 seconds
  - This provides maximum heart rate variability
  - One or two trials of this metronomic breathing is recorded
  - This deep breathing pattern potentiates sinus arrhythmia
  - In patients with ANS disease, reduced HRV is seen with respiration
  - Test duration should be limited to 2 minutes
  - This is in order to prevent errors due to respiratory alkalosis
- Results:
  - I:E ratio:
    - Calculated as I:E ratio = $\frac{\text{Longest R-R interval}}{\text{Shortest R-R interval}}$
    - Normal value should be more than 1.2
  - E:I difference:
    - Calculated as: {(RR interval during expiration) – (RR interval during inspiration)}
    - Normal value should be more than 15 beats per minute
    - Values are considered pathological if less than 10 bpm
- Sources of error:
  - Poor respiratory effort
  - Hypocapnea
  - Salicylates
  - Positioning
  - Obesity

- *Summary*:

Stimulus	Metronomic breathing (6 breaths/min)
Afferent	Pulmonary receptors, cardiac mechanoreceptors
	Vagus nerve, Glossopharyngeal nerve
	Respiratory center
Central	Nucleus Tractus Solitarius
Efferent	Vagus nerve
Response	HR increase during inspiration
	HR decreases during expiration

III. Active Orthostatic Maneuver: ***(Schellong test)***

- Physiology:
  - During transition from lying to standing, redistribution of blood occurs
  - Blood gets redistributed to the veins of the lower limbs (400–600 mL)
  - This leads to a short term reduction in venous return to the heart
  - Thus, stroke volume and blood pressure reduces
  - In the presence of a healthy ANS, blood pressure changes only slightly
  - However a profound changes in BP occur in patients with ANS disorders
  - The initial response is a drop in systolic and diastolic BP during first 30 sec
  - This triggers a compensatory response causing tachycardia
  - This is followd by a phase of early stabilization lasting 1–2 min
  - The third phase occurs on prolonged orthostasis lasting more than 5 min
- Procedure:
  - Baseline heart rate is measured in supine position
  - Patient is then asked to stand up quickly
  - Heart rate variability is measured for at least 1 minute of active standing
  - BP measurements are done every 2.5 minutes for a 5–10 minute interval
  - Difference between baseline supine and minimal BP after standing is measured
  - This is the best test to diagnose idiopathic orthostatic hypotension
  - Heart rate changes indicate parasympathetic nervous system function
  - BP changes indicate sympathetic nervous system function
- Interpretation:
  - ***Ewing ratio*** (30:15 ratio):
    - 30:15 ratio = $\frac{\text{HR at 15 seconds of standing (maximal)}}{\text{HR at 30 seconds of standing (minimal)}}$
    - Normal ratio > 1.04

- Orthostatic BP difference:
  - Orthostatic BP difference = (supine BP) – (minimal standing BP)
  - A drop in BP within 3 minutes of standing indicates orthostatic hypotension
  - Less than 20 mm Hg is normal for systolic BP
  - Less than 10 mm Hg is normal for diastolic BP

❖ Sources of error:
- Hypovolemia
- Medical deconditioning
- Hypothyroidism

❖ *Summary*:

Stimulus	Decreased central blood volume
Afferent	Baroreceptors, ergoreceptors
	Vagus nerve, glossopharyngeal nerve
Central	Nucleus tractus solitarius
	rostral ventrolateral medulla
Efferent	Vagus nerve
Response	Heart rate increases at 15 seconds
	Heart rate decreases at 30 seconds

IV. Pressor Functional Tests

❖ Physiology:
- Pressor stimuli are applied in these tests
- This results in the stimulation of peripheral receptors and cerebral activation
- Thus sympathetic afferents are stimulated independant of baroreceptor afferents
- This leads to an increase in the heart rate and blood pressure

❖ Procedure:
- Isometric handgrip test:
  - Sustained hand grip is obtained using a hand dynamometer
  - The BP changes in the other arm is measured over a 3 minute period
  - Blood pressure is measured every minute for 3 minutes
  - Initial DBP is subtracted from DBP just before release of hand grip
- Cold pressor test:
  - One hand is immersed in cold water (4°C) for 60–90 seconds
  - This leads to activation of peripheral cold receptors
  - This in turn causes sympathetic activation
  - Rise in diastolic BP is used to evaluate the ANS
- Mental arithmetic test:
  - Patient is asked to solve an arithmetic problem during a 2 minute interval
  - This usually involves serial subtraction (100 minus 7)
  - This aims at activating the central sympathetic outflow
  - The difference in blood pressure is then calculated

❖ Interpretation:
- Isometric hand grip test normal value: rise in DBP should exceed 16 mm Hg
- Cold pressor test normal value: rise in diastolic BP should exceed 15 mm Hg
- Mental arithmetic test normal value: rise in SBP should exceed 10 mm Hg

❖ Sources of error:
- Valsalva maneuver during the test (especially handgrip test)
- Hyperventilation during cold pressor test

V. Tilt Table Test

❖ Physiology:
- This test is similar to orthostatic test in the physiological challenges it provides
- However there is an important difference in that this test is passive
- Active standing involves contraction of calf muscles
- This in turn increases the venous return to the heart
- This pumping action may mask ANS disorders
- In the tilt table test, calf muscle contraction is avoided
- Therefore this test is more sensitive for ANS dysfunction

❖ Procedure:
- The test is carried out early in the morning, after midnight starvation
- Patient lies supine on an automated tilt table for around 15 minutes
- This is followed by a 30–40 minute period of tilting to 60–80°
- Patient is instructed to report any symptoms during the upright tilt
- BP and heart rate are measured throughout the test
- Baseline BP is recorded followed by measurements for at least 3 minutes
- Patient is then returned to the horizontal supine position
- HR and BP are monitored till they return to baseline

❖ Interpretation:
- Sensitivity of this test exceeds that of orthostatic hypotension
- Normal values:
  - No symptoms
  - Decrease in systolic BP < 20 mm Hg
  - Decrease in diastolic BP < 10 mm Hg

- Postural tachycardia syndrome:
  - Tilt test time is extended to 90 minutes and heart rate changes recorded
  - An increase by 30 bpm would confirm orthostatic tachycardia
- Variations:
  - Splanchnic vasodilatation: Test carried out after food intake
  - Muscular vasodilatation: Test carried out after physical activity
  - ***Lower body negative pressure test***: Test carried out after application of negative pressure
- *Summary*:

Stimulus	Decreased central blood volume
Afferent	Baroreceptors
	Vagus nerve, glossopharyngeal nerve
Central	Nucleus tractus solitarius
	Rostral ventrolateral medulla
	Hypothalamus
Efferent	Sympathetic vasomotor
Response	Fall in SBP with tilting
	Fall in DBP with tilting

VI. Baroreceptor Sensitivity Testing

- Baroreceptor stimulation is accomplished by the administration of IV phenylephrine
- The subsequent rise in BP causes bradycardia
- Changes in SBP and RR intervals are presented in the form of a graph
- Baroreceptor sensitivity is calculated as the slope of linear regression between beat-to-beat SBP values and values of RR interval
- Normal value should be above 10 ms/mm Hg
- This test can also be performed by baroreceptor decompression using SNP/NTG

Analysis of Heart Rate Variability

- Physiology:
  - This method has become one of the most popular methods of ANS evaluation
  - This method is based on the fact that even at rest RR interval changes constantly
  - These fluctuations are based on interactions between sympathetic and parasympathetic systems
  - Variations due to parasympathetic activity are quick and transient
  - Those due to sympathetic activity are slow and long lasting
- Procedure:
  - HRV is measured from time domain or frequency domain analysis
  - This analysis is doneover a full 24-hour ECG recording
- Interpretation:
  - Values used to measure HRV include:
  - Standard deviation of Normal-to-Normal (NN) intervals (SDNN)
    - Standard deviation of average NN interval (SDANN)
  - Square root of mean squared differences of successive NN intervals (rMSDD)
  - Proportion of differences in consecutive NN intervals longer than 50 ms (pNN50)

Microneurography

- Tungsten electrodes are inserted selectively into muscle or skin fascicles
- Thus, sympathetic activity from large superficial nerves is directly recorded
- This technique allows two separate recordings of sympathetic activity:
  - Activity of vessels of muscle (MSNA)
  - Activity of vessels of skin (SSNA)

Sudomotor Function Tests

I. Thermoregulatory Sweat Test

- Sweat secretion is measured after raising body temperature by 1–1.4°C
- Indicators like alizarin red which change color on exposure to moisture are used
- The patient is placed in a sweat chamber with:
  - Air temperature at 45–50°C
  - Humidity at 35–50%
- The dye is scattered on the complete ventral skin surface
- Eyes, ears and perioral regions are omitted
- Peak response of sweat glands occurs after 35–45 minutes
- Normal subjects demonstrate generalized perspiration
- Digital images of the sweating patterns are taken
- The anhidrotic skin area is divided by the total skin area
- This value is expressed as a percentage
- Since it marks anhidrotic areas topographically, it can be used to diagnose:
  - Neuropathies
  - Ganglionopathies
  - Generalized autonomic failure

II. Sympathetic Skin Response (SSR)

- Physiology:
  - The electrical resistance of skin changes in response to sweat secretion

- This test is based on this change in the electrical resistance of skin
- Electrical potentials are measured using electrodes placed on the skin
- The change in potentials reflects sympathetic cholinergic activity of sweat glands

❖ Procedure:
- Standard EMG instrument is used
- Sweep speed of 10 sec and band pass filter of 1–2000 Hz is used
- Small recording electrode is attached to palms of hand and soles of feet
- Stable baseline is recorded before administering the stimulus
- Stimuli used can be:
  - Electrical stimuli: peripheral nerve stimulation of:
    - Median nerve
    - Tibial/peroneal nerve
    - Supraorbital nerve
  - Physiological stimuli:
    - Loud noise
    - Flash
    - Touch
    - Inspiratory gasps
- Sympathetic sudomotor skin response is noted
- Recordings can be obtained simultaneously from hands and feet
- 3–4 trials are obtained

❖ Interpretation:
- Normal response: monophasic/biphasic deflection which habituates with time
- Abnormal response: absent SSR

III. Quantitative Sudomotor Axon Reflex Test (QSART)

❖ This test assesses sudomotor nerve fibers by direct activation using acetylcholine

❖ This stimulates the cutaneous axon reflex and local sweat production

❖ A sudorometer which measures the sweat volume is used for the test

❖ Multicompartment sweat capsules attached to the skin at 4 different sites are required

❖ Sweat glands are stimulated using acetylcholine iontophoresis in one compartment

❖ The other compartment is used to measure the skin humidity

❖ The change in skin humidity over time allows us to measure the sudomotor function

IV. Sudoscan

❖ Recent technique utilizing reverse iontophoresis and chronoamperometry

❖ This test assesses chloride content of the skin as a measure of sudomotor output

❖ Application of electrical current induces shift of Cl^- ions from sweat glands to skin surface

❖ This results in a current between the anode and a reference electrode

❖ The amplitude of the current is proportional to the cutaneous chloride concentration

GLASGOW COMA SCALE

Introduction

❖ Neurological scale which describes the extent of impaired consciousness in acute medical patients

❖ Published in 1974 by two neurosurgeons ***Bryan Jennett and Graham Teasday***

Components

❖ The scale assesses patients according to three aspects of responsiveness:
- Best eye opening response
- Best motor response
- Best verbal response

❖ The score is expressed as the sum of the individual elements

❖ The scale can be applied to all adults and children above 2 years of age

Sl No.	Components	Score
I.	**Eye opening**	
	No eye opening	1
	Opens eyes to painful stimuli	2
	Opens eye to speech/command	3
	Opens eyes spontaneously	4
II.	**Motor response**	
	No response	1
	Abnormal extension to pain (decortications)	2
	Abnormal flexion to pain (decerebration)	3
	Withdrawal from pain	4
	Localizes pain	5
	Obeys commands	6
III.	**Verbal Response**	
	No verbal response	1
	Incomprehensible sounds	2
	Inappropriate words	3
	Confused	4
	Oriented	5

Glasgow Coma Scale in Intubated Patients

- In intubated patients, the verbal response represents a non-testable aspect
- In these patients therefore, a combined score is not used
- The GCS score is noted only with its individual testable components
- Thus only motor and eye opening scores are reported individually
- The suffix NT is added to their score to indicate non-testability

Glasgow Coma Scale in Preverbal Children

Sl No.	Components	Score
I.	**Eye opening**	
	No eye opening	1
	Opens eyes to painful stimuli	2
	Opens eye to speech/command	3
	Opens eyes spontaneously	4
II.	**Motor response**	
	No response	1
	Abnormal extension to pain (decortications)	2
	Abnormal flexion to pain (decerebration)	3
	Withdrawal from pain	4
	Localizes pain	5
	Obeys commands	6
III.	**Verbal response in children 0 to 2 yrs**	
	No response	1
	Moans in response to pain	2
	Cries in response to pain	3
	Irritable/cries	4
	Coos and babbles	5

Procedure

- Painful stimuli used:
  - Supraorbital pressure
  - Earlobe pinch
  - Trapezius squeeze
  - Sternal rub (avoided due to risk of bruising and difficulty in interpretation)
  - Nailbed pressure
- Decorticate/extensor response:
  - Abducted arm
  - Internal rotation of shoulder
  - Pronation of forearm
  - Wrist extension
- Flexor/decerebrate response:
  - Adducted arm
  - Internal rotation of shoulder
  - Pronation of forearm
  - Wrist flexion

Factors Interfering with Assessment

- Preexisting factors:
  - Language barriers
  - Intellectual deficit
  - Hearing loss/speech impediment
- Effects of current treatment:
  - Intubation/tracheostomy
  - Sedation/paralysis
- Effects of other injuries:
  - Orbital/cranial fracture
  - Spinal cord damage
  - Nerve injuries

Uses

- Risk stratification and guidance of therapy in patients with TBI:
  - Patients with low GCS score need emergent management such as securing the airway
  - Patients with high scores can be evaluated further with neuroimaging
- Allows continuous assessment of prognosis of the patient
- Key component for prediction of neurological outcomes
- As part of other ICU scoring systems and guidelines:
  - ATLS guidelines
  - BTF guidelines
  - APACHE II score
  - SOFA score

Prognostication

No.	Prognosis	Score	Description
I.	Mild disability	13–15	
II.	Moderate disability	9–12	Loss of consciousness > 30 mins Physical/cognitive impairment May/may not resolve Benefit from rehabilitation
III.	Severe disability	3–8	Comatose Unconscious state No meaningful response No voluntary activities
IV.	Vegetative state	3	Sleep –wake cycles Arousable but no interaction No localized response to pain
V.	Persistent vegetative state	3	Vegetative state > 1 month
VI.	Brain death	3	No brain function

Disadvantages

- Response cannot be elicited in
  - Severe facial injury/orbital injury (eye opening response)
  - Injury to limb (motor response)
  - Intubated patients (vocal response)
  - Drugs:
    - Alcohol intoxication
    - Sedatives
    - Neuromuscular blocking agents
  - Nerve injuries
  - Spinal cord injuries
  - Dysphasia
- Limited application in children below 36 months
- Long term prognosis cannot be predicted on this alone
- Does not check memory of patient

Glasgow Coma Scale Pupils Score

- Aims at combining the 2 key indicators of severity of TBI into a single index
- Obtained by subtracting Pupil Reactivity Score (PRS) from Glasgow Coma Scale (GCS)
- Thus, GCS – P = GCS – PRS
- Pupil Reactivity Score:
  - Both pupils unreactive to light –2
  - One pupil unreactive to light –1
  - Both pupils reactive to light –0
- GCS–P score may range from 1 to 15
- Shown to be useful or prediction of outcomes after TBI

Modifications

- Abbreviated GCS/*AVPU SCALE*
  - Simplified scale useful in risk stratification and triaging of patients
  - However, it cannot be used to establish a baseline to detect subsequent changes
  - Score consists of 4 components:
    - A = alert
    - V = responds to vocal stimuli
    - P = responds to painful stimuli
    - U = unresponsive
- Full Outline of Unresponsiveness Score (*FOUR score*):
  - Similar to the GCS score but includes brainstem examination
  - It may have a greater utility than the GCS core in coma diagnosis
  - Has a similar sensitivity and specificity compared with GCS score in predicting coma outcome
  - However, it is more difficult to perform

No.	Components	Score
1.	**Eye response**	
	Eyelids remain closed with pain	0
	Eyelids closed, but open to pain	1
	Eyelids closed, but open to loud voice	2
	Eyelids open but not tracking	3
	Eyelids opened or blinks to command	4
2.	**Motor response**	
	No response to pain/generalized myoclonus state	0
	Extensor response to pain	1
	Flexor response to pain	2
	Localizes pain	3
	Thumbs up, fist or peace sign	4
3.	**Brainstem reflexes**	
	Absent pupil, corneal and cough reflex	0
	Absent pupil AND corneal reflex	1
	Absent pupil OR corneal reflex	2
	One pupil wide and fixed	3
	Pupil and corneal reflex present	4
4.	**Respiration**	
	Breathes at ventilator rate/apnea	0
	Breathes above ventilator rate	1
	Not intubated, irregular breathing	2
	Not intubated, Cheyne–Stokes breathing pattern	3
	Not intubated, regular breathing pattern	4

HORNER'S SYNDROME

Introduction

- Neurological syndrome whose symptoms include ptosis, miosis and anhidrosis
- Can be produced by a lesion anywhere along the sympathetic pathway supplying head, eye and neck
- Also called:
  - ***Claude Bernard Horner syndrome***
  - ***Oculosympathetic palsy***
- Called ***Von Passow syndrome*** when associated with heterochromia iridis
- Apical bronchogenic carcinoma is the most common cause of Horner's syndrome

Anatomy

- Sympathetic pathway is a three neuron pathway which consists of:
  - Ist order neurons:
    - Extends from hypothalamus to the first synapse
    - Synapse is located in lateral grey matter in cervical spinal cord (C_8–T_2)
    - This is also called the ***ciliospinal center of Budge***

- IInd order neurons:
  - Consists of preganglionic neurons from spinal cord
  - These travel through brachial plexus over the lung apex
  - The neurons then ascend to the superior cervical ganglion
  - This is located near the angle of mandible
- IIIrd order neurons:
  - Consists of postganglionic neurons from superior cervical ganglion
  - These neurons ascend within the adventitia of internal carotid artery
  - It ascends through the cavernous sinus, in close relation to CN VI
  - Oculosympathetic pathway then joins the ophthalmic division of trigeminal nerve
  - They then supply the pupils and blood vessels of eye

❖ Oculomotor nerve supplies the elevator of eyelid (***Mueller muscle***)

❖ Nasociliary nerve supplies the blood vessels

❖ Long ciliary nerve innervates the pupils

❖ Site of lesion is on the ipsilateral side of symptoms

Etiology

❖ Lesions of first order neurons (central):
- Hemispherical lesions:
  - Lateral medullary syndrome (Wallenberg syndrome)
  - Demyelinating diseases (multiple sclerosis)
  - Cavernous sinus thrombosis
  - Arnold Chiari malformation
- Brainstem lesions:
  - Stroke
  - Vasculitis
  - Encephalitis
  - Basal meningitis
  - Demyelination
  - Tumors: pontine glioma
- Cervical cord lesions:
  - Trauma
  - Myelitis
  - Syringomyelia
  - Demyelination
  - Intramedullary tumors:
    - Gliomas
    - Ependymomas
  - Arteriovenous malformations
  - Infarctions

❖ Lesions of second order neurons (preganglionic):
- Pulmonary apical lesions:
  - Subclavian artery aneurysm
  - Pancoast tumor (tumor in apex of lung)
  - Mediastinal tumors
  - Cervical rib
  - *Klumpkes palsy*: Avulsion of lower brachial plexus
- Thyroid malignancies

❖ Lesions of third order neurons (postganglionic):
- Superior cervical ganglion:
  - Trauma
  - Jugular venous ectasia
  - During surgical neck dissection
- Internal carotid artery:
  - Dissection
  - Aneurysm
  - Trauma
  - Arteritis
  - Thrombosis
  - Tumor
- Skull base lesions
  - Nasopharyngeal carcinoma
  - Lymphoma
- Cavernous sinus lesions:
  - Tumors
  - Invasive pituitary tumors
  - Inflammation
  - Thrombosis
  - Carotid aneurysm

❖ Miscellaneous:
- Congenital
- Cluster headache
- Orbital lesions
- Otitis media

❖ Procedural:
- During nerve blocks:
  - Cervical plexus block
  - Stellate ganglion block
  - Interscalene block
- During carotid artery stenting/endarterectomy
- During tube thoracostomy
- During thoracic surgery

Components

❖ Ptosis

❖ Miosis

❖ Anhidrosis (ipsilateral)

❖ Enophthalmos

❖ Loss of ciliospinal reflex

❖ Conjunctival redness

Classification of Horner's Syndrome

- First order syndrome:
  - Hemisensory loss
  - Dysarthria, dysphagia
  - Ataxia
  - Vertigo, nystagmus
- Second order syndrome:
  - Pain in face, neck, axilla, shoulder or arm
  - Associated with cough, hemoptysis
- Third order syndrome:
  - Diplopia due to CN VI palsy
  - Numbness in distribution of first or second division of trigeminal nerve

Clinical Features

- In all patients:
  - Ptosis:
    - Ptosis is usually minor (less than 2 mm) and is thus partial
    - Occurs due to loss of innervation to Muellers muscle
    - This causes paralysis of the lower and upper eyelid
    - This results in the so called *upside-down ptosis*
    - Levator palpebrae superioisis is however unaffected
  - Miosis
  - Ipsilateral anhidrosis:
    - Refers to the inability to sweat on the same side of the face
    - Present in first or second order syndromes
    - Involves entire side of face if lesion is present in common carotid artery (CCA) area
    - Involves only medial side of forehead and side of nose if lesion is distal to CCA bifurcation
  - Enophthalmos:
    - True enophthalmos refers to posterior displacement of the eyeball within the orbit
    - This is usually due to changes in the volume of the orbital contents
    - True enophthalmos however is uncommon in Horner's syndrome
    - Apparent enophthalmos which is seen in Horner's is due to ptosis
    - This causes a narrowing of the palpebral fissure
    - This gives an illusion of enophthalmos
  - Loss of ciliospinal reflex
    - Also called the pupillary-skin reflex
    - Afferent pathway for this reflex is via cervical pain fibers
    - Efferent pathway is via sympathetic fibers from lower cervical cord
    - Therefore, this reflex is lost in Horner's syndrome
    - Ipsilateral pupils fail to dilate when back of the neck is pinched
    - Inconsistent sign and is difficult to elicit
- In some patients:
  - ***Anisocoria***:
    - Condition where the affected pupil dilates slower than normal pupil
    - The degree of anisocoria is more marked in the dark, than in the light
    - Dilation lag:
      - This occurs when the light source is moved away from the eye
      - An asymmetry in pupil redilation is seen between the 2 eyes
      - The Horner pupil redilates more slowly by 15–20 seconds
  - ***Heterochromia iridis***:
    - Seen in congenital Horner's syndrome
    - Refers to the difference in color between the two irises
    - The affected iris is lighter in color
    - This is because formation of iris pigment is under sympathetic control
    - In congenital Horner's syndrome, sympathetic chain is disrupted early
    - Thus, formation of iris pigment (melanin) is hampered
    - However, this is apparent only if natural color is relatively dark
  - ***Hortons headache***: Refers to association of Horner's syndrome with cluster headache
  - ***Harlequin sign***:
    - Refers to asymmetrical facial flushing
    - Seen in infants and children
    - Occurs due to impaired sympathetic vasodilatation
    - Ipsilateral side of the face is associated with:
      - Impaired flushing
      - Decreased skin temperature
    - This may be associated with:
      - Conjunctival injection
      - Nasal stuffiness
      - Increased near point of accomodation

Variants

- ***Raeder paratrigeminal syndrome:***
  - Term used for patients who have Horner's syndrome with ipsilateral headache
  - Thus, it refers to a triad of:
    - Episodic retrobulbar/orbital pain

- Miosis
- Ptosis
- Types of Raeder's syndrome:
  - Type I Raeder's syndrome:
    - Seen in mass lesions of the middle cranial fossa
    - Triad of symptoms is associated with lesions of CN III–VI
  - Type II Raeder's syndrome:
    - Considered to be a migraine variant
    - Relatively benign form
    - Not associated with any cranial nerve findings

Investigations

- Pharmacological tests:
  - Pharmacological tests are useful to:
    - Confirm the diagnosis of Horner's syndrome
    - Localize the lesion
  - Cocaine drop test:
    - Cocaine cause pupillary dilatation in normal patients
    - 2–4% cocaine is instilled into each eye
    - The response is evaluated 1 hour after cocaine administration
    - Mydriatic failure is seen in Horner's syndrome
    - Anisocoria more than 1 mm confirms Horner's syndrome
    - This is due to sympathetic denervation seen in Horner's syndrome
    - This occurs regardless of the level of sympathetic interruption
    - Therefore, this test is not useful for localization of lesions
  - Apraclonidine test:
    - *Test of choice* currently for diagnosis of Horner's syndrome
    - Uses 0.5–1% apraclonidine for the test
    - Apraclonidine is a weak α_1 agonist and strong α_2 agonist
    - In the normal eye, apraclonidine instillation has no effect
    - However, in Horner's syndrome, upregulation of α_1 receptors occurs
    - This causes ipsilateral denervation supersensitivity of α_1 receptors
    - This results in ipsilateral pupillary dilatation and lid elevation
    - Thus, in Horner's syndrome, apraclonidine instillation causes:
      - Ipsilateral pupillary dilatation by 2 mm due to α_1 action
      - Pupillary constriction in the normal eye due to α_2 action
    - However upregulation of receptors takes 6–8 days
    - This can result in false negative results
  - Hydroxyamphetamine (HA) test:
    - Topical hydroxyamphetamine aids localization of the lesion
    - HA stimulates the release of stored endogenous norepinephrine into the neuromuscular junction at the dilator iris muscle
    - This causes dilatation of the pupil
    - This test differentiates 3rd order lesions from 1st and 2nd order lesions
    - Two drops of 1% hydroxyamphetamine are instilled into each eye
    - The response to HA helps localizing the lesion
    - This is done by comparing the response with the normal eye:
    - 1st and 2nd order lesions dilate the affected pupil to a greater extent
    - 3rd order lesions do not dilate the affected pupil to that extent
- Nonpharmacological tests:
  - Complete blood count
  - *Urine analysis*: Vanillylmandelic acid (VMA) in children for neuroblastoma
  - *X-ray chest*: Apical bronchogenic carcinoma
  - CT scan brain for stroke
  - MRI (head neck and chest)
  - MR angiography for carotid artery dissection in case of painful Horner's syndrome

Treatment: Treat the cause.

GUEDEL'S STAGES OF ANESTHESIA

Introduction

- Described by ***Arthur E Guedel*** in 1920 with ether
- Regarded obsolete now due to use of rapid acting IV induction agents and muscle relaxants
- Depth estimated with BIS/entropy
- With thiopentone induction patient directly enters Stage III, Plane II

Prerequisites

- For use with sole inhalational anesthetic ether
- Premedicated with atropine
- IV anesthetic agents/morphine/muscle relaxants not used

Stages

Plane	Extent	Description
Stage I: Stage of Analgesia and Amnesia		
Plane	*Extent*	*Description*
	Beginning of induction to LOC	Loss of memory intellect perception of time, space Sensation of pain present Altered reaction to pain Used for minor surgeries IInd stage labour analgesia/dental procedures
Divided into 3 planes by *Joseph F Artusio*		
I.		Patient does not experience amnesia/analgesia
II.		Complete amnesia, but only partial analgesia
III.		Complete analgesia and amnesia
Stage II: Stage of delirium/excitement		
	LOC to onset of regular breathing (RB)	Loss of eyelash reflex Other reflexes intact Struggling coughing vomiting possible Irregular respiration with breath-holding Patient should not be stimulated Reaction to stimulus maybe violent and injurious
Stage III: Stage of surgical anesthesia		
Plane	*Extent*	*Description*
	Onset of RB to respiratory paralysis (RP)	
Divided into 4 Stages:		
I.	Onset of RB to cessation of eye movement	Loss of eyelid and conjuctival reflex Loss of swallowing reflex Marked eyeball movement possible
II.	Cessation of eyeball movement to commencement of intercostals palsy	Loss of corneal and laryngeal reflexes Pupil centrally fixed mid-dilated reactive to light Increased secretion of tears Automatic and regular respiration Loss of movement to skin stimulation
III.	Commencement to completion of intercostal palsy	Loss of light reflex Pupils dilated Persistence of diaphragmatic respiration Progressive intercostals palsy ***Desired plane for surgery***
IV.	Intercostal palsy to diaphragmatic palsy	
Stage IV: Stage of medullary paralysis		
	Stoppage of respiration till death	Medullary paralysis Respiratory arrest and vasomotor collapse Pupils widely dilated, muscles relaxed

MALIGNANT HYPERTHERMIA

Introduction

- Autosomal dominant life-threatening disorder which manifests as a hypermetabolic crisis causing rapidly increasing body temperature and extreme acidosis
- Usually occurs when the susceptible individual is exposed to a volatile anesthetic or succinylcholine
- Identified as a separate clinical entity by ***Denborough*** in 1960

Incidence

- Depends on the prevalence of MH susceptibility
- Varies from 1:10000 to 1:50000
- Occurs more commonly in males than females
- Most common in children under 19 years age
- Mortality in the absence of dantrolene approaches 70%

Etiology

- Autosomal dominant with reduced penetrance
- Occurs due to multiple mutations in:
  - Ryanodine receptor type 1:
    - Also called RYR1 receptor or dihydropyridine receptors (DHP)
    - Situated on chromosome 19
    - Occurs in 50% of patients with MH
    - Accounts for MHS1 variant of MH
    - Encodes skeletal muscle isoform of calcium release channel of sarcoplasmic reticulum
  - Calcium voltage gated channel subunit alpha 1S gene:
    - Also called CACNA 1S gene
    - Occurs in less than 1% cases of MH
    - Accounts for MHS5 variant of MH
    - Encodes α-subunit of L-type calcium channel isoform of sarcolemma
  - CACNA2D1 gene

Pathophysiology

- Occurs due to abnormal functioning of calcium release units (CRU)
- CRU is a macromolecular assembly of interacting proteins
- These units participate in excitation–contraction coupling
- The ryanodine receptor (RYR1) is a central part of CRU
- In MH, RYR1 gene undergoes mutation causing increased sensitivity to VAs

- This causes unregulated expulsion of calcium from the sarcoplasmic reticulum
- Calcium enters the intracellular space causing sustained muscular contraction
- This muscular contraction generates more amount of heat than the body can dissipate
- Initially aerobic metabolism sustains the muscular hyperactivity for sometime
- This however results in increasing cellular acidosis and CO_2 production
- Over a period of time metabolism slowly changes to anerobic metabolism
- Once all energy stores are depleted, rhabdomyolysis results
- MH occurs due to exposure to trigerring factors such as:
  - Volatile anesthetics
  - Succinylcholine
  - Caffeine
  - Ryanodine
  - 4 chloro-m-cresol
  - K^+ depolarization

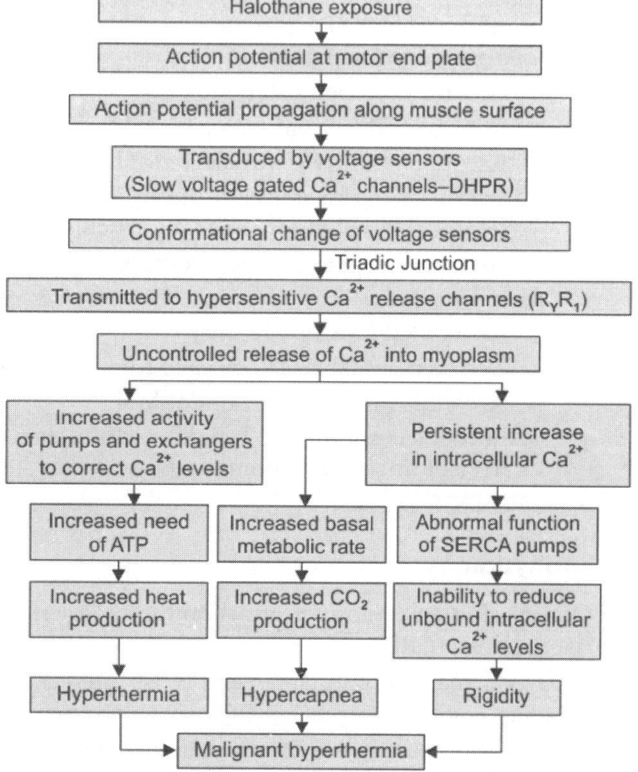

Risk Factors for Malignant Hyperthermia

- Neuromuscular disorders:
  - Strabismus, ptosis
  - Meningomyelocele
  - Hypoplastic mandible, poor dental enamel, cleft palate
  - Myotonic dystrophy, muscular dystrophy
  - Pectus carinatum
  - Kyphoscoliosis
  - Osteogenesis imperfecta
  - Clubfoot
- Syndromes:
  - ***Duchenne's*** muscular dystrophy
  - ***Becker's*** dystrophy
  - ***King-Denborough*** syndrome
  - Short stature
  - Mental retardation
  - Cryptorchidism
  - Kyphoscoliosis
  - Pectus deformity
  - Slanted eyes
  - Low set ears
  - Webbed neck
  - Winged scapulae
  - Arthrogryposis multiplexa congenita
  - Periodic paralysis
- Surgeries:
  - Tonsilectomy, adenoidectomy, dental surgery
  - Orthopaedic surgery (joint dislocation)
  - Ophthalmic surgery (squints)
  - Head and neck surgery
- Body habitus:
  - Short, stocky stature (Marfanoid features too)
  - Bulky muscles, rounded belly
  - Muscle hypertrophy, atrophied muscle groups, muscle cramps
  - Intolerance to caffeine

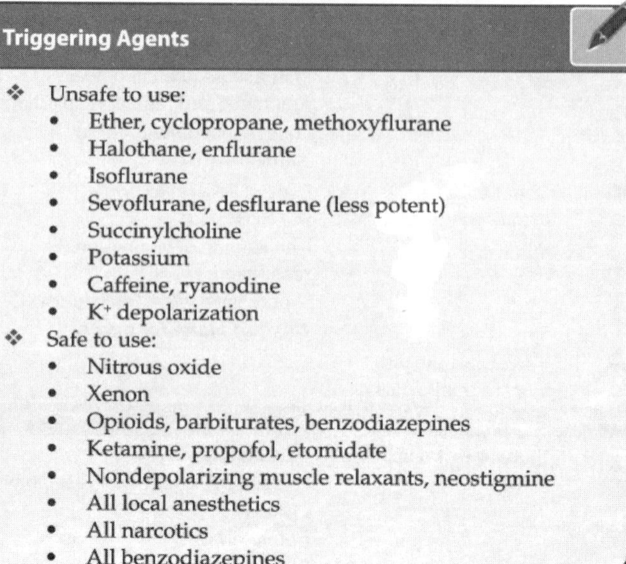
Triggering Agents

- Unsafe to use:
  - Ether, cyclopropane, methoxyflurane
  - Halothane, enflurane
  - Isoflurane
  - Sevoflurane, desflurane (less potent)
  - Succinylcholine
  - Potassium
  - Caffeine, ryanodine
  - K^+ depolarization
- Safe to use:
  - Nitrous oxide
  - Xenon
  - Opioids, barbiturates, benzodiazepines
  - Ketamine, propofol, etomidate
  - Nondepolarizing muscle relaxants, neostigmine
  - All local anesthetics
  - All narcotics
  - All benzodiazepines

Clinical Features

- Onset of syndrome:
  - Acute onset of symptoms
  - If succinylcholine is used fulminant MH can occur within 5–10 minutes
  - Can be delayed up to 4 hours postoperatively
  - Earliest signs of MH under anesthesia include:
    - Tachycardia *(earliest sign)*
    - Hypercarbia
    - Muscle rigidity
- Features of hypermetabolism:
  - Tachypnea, cyanosis, mottling of skin
  - Hypercarbia with adequate ventilation is the *most sensitive* sign
  - E_TCO_2 may be more than 100 mm Hg
  - Increased O_2 consumption with decreased SpO_2
  - Unexpected metabolic acidosis (pH may be < 7)
  - Reduced mixed venous oxygen saturation
- Features of hyperthermia:
  - Fever:
    - Inconsistent and *late* presenting sign
    - Can increase by more than 1°C rise every five minutes
    - Core temperature may exceed 43°C
  - Sweating
  - Hyperthermia may not be prominent if:
    - Heat loss exceeds production
    - Cardiac output decreases early
- Increased sympathetic activity:
  - Tachycardia: *Cardinal and earliest* sign
  - Hypertension
  - Arrhythmias:
    - Ventricular ectopy
    - Ventricular tachycardia
    - Ventricular fibrillation
- Muscle damage/rigidity:
  - Masseteric spasm presents early
  - Generalized rigidity in the presence of neuromuscular blockade *(specific sign)*
  - Presence of muscle rigidity is pathognomonic of MH
  - Increase creatinine kinase:
    - Peak levels seen 12–18 hours after anesthesia
    - Usually exceeds 20,000 IU/L
  - Myoglobinemia, myoglobinuria
  - Hyperkalemia, hypernatremia, hyperphosphatemia
- Complications:
  - Acute renal failure
  - DIC
  - Cardiac failure: Pulmonary edema
  - Cerebral edema, coma, paralysis
  - Hepatic failure

Variations in Presentation

- MH associated with less rigidity
- MH associated with less hyperthermia
- Masseteric spasm/rigidity (MMR)

Factors Affecting Severity

- Depends on 4 variables:
  - Genetic predisposition
  - Absence of inhibiting factors
  - Persistence of anesthetic/non-anesthetic triggers
  - Presence of potentiating environmental factors
- Factors delaying onset of MH:
  - Preoperative hypothermia
  - Preadministration of:
    - Barbiturates
    - Propofol
    - Nondepolarizing muscle relaxants

Intraoperative Diagnosis

- Usually occurs within minutes of using succinylcholine/volatile agents
- Occurs in the immediate postoperative period
- Rarely seen beyond 4 hours postoperatively
- Diagnostic indicators include:
  - Unexpected increase in E_TCO_2
  - Unexplained tachycardia, arrhythmias
  - Unstable BP
  - Tachypnea, cyanosis, if spontaneous ventilation
  - Increased temperature, sweating, mottling of skin
  - Muscle rigidity in the presence of adequate neuromuscular blockade
  - Combined metabolic and respiratory acidosis
  - CO_2 absorbent becomes warm to touch as the reaction with CO_2 is exothermic

Investigations

- Combined metabolic and respiratory acidosis
- Dyselectrolytemias:
  - Hyperkalemia:
    - Occurs due to elevated potassium from muscle breakdown
    - May occur early in muscular patients
  - Increased ionized calcium
  - Hyperphosphatemia
  - Hypernatremia
  - Hypermagnesemia

- Decreased MvO_2
- Elevated creatinine kinase:
  - Creatinine kinase levels are usually above 20,000 IU/L
  - Levels may exceed 1,00,000 IU/L
  - These levels peak approximately 14 hours after acute MH
  - Should be monitored every 6 hrs for the first 24 hours
- Other investigations:
  - Increased myoglobin levels
  - Presence of urinary myoglobin
  - Increased pyruvate, LDH, aldolase levels

Larach's Clinical Grading Scale

- Muscle rigidity:
  - Generalized rigidity 15
  - Masseteric rigidity 15
- Myonecrosis:
  - CK >20000 (with succinylcholine) 15
  - CK >10000 (without succinylcholine) 15
  - Cola colored urine 10
  - Myoglobin is urine > 60 μg/L 5
  - Serum $K^+ > 6$ mEq/L 3
- Respiratory acidosis:
  - $E_TCO_2 > 55$ with controlled ventilation 15
  - $PaCO_2 > 60$ with controlled ventilation 15
  - $E_TCO_2 > 60$ with spontaneous ventilation 15
  - Inappropriate hypercarbia 15
  - Inappropriate tachypnea 10
- Temperature:
  - Rapid increase in temperature 15
  - Inappropriate temperature > 38.8°C 10
- Cardiac involvement:
  - Inappropriate tachycardia 3
  - VT or VF 3

Score range	MH Rank	Likelihood of MH
0	1	Almost never
3–9	2	Unlikely
10–19	3	Somewhat less than likely
20–34	4	Somewhat greater than likely
35–49	5	Very likely
More than 50	6	Almost certain

Diffferential Diagnosis

- Pheochromocytoma:
  - Severe HTN usually present (pheochromocytoma > thyrotoxicosis > MH)
  - Not associated with muscle rigidity and acidosis
- Thyrotoxicosis:
  - Severe HTN seen in thyrotoxicosis, compared with MH
  - Not associated with muscle rigidity and acidosis
- Sepsis:
  - Persistent rigidity is rare in sepsis
  - However, rigors associated with fever may be present
  - This can be treated effectively with:
    - NSAIDs
    - Antibiotics
    - Cardiovascular support
  - MH does not respond to such treatment
- Mitochondrial myopathies
- Rhabdomyolysis
- Muscular dystrophy
- Neuroleptic malignant syndrome
- Contrast dye/drug anaphylaxis
- Drug abuse/toxic overdose
- Heat stroke
- Diabetic coma, hypokalemic periodic paralysis
- Serotonin syndrome—drug induced hyperthermia
- Hypoxic Encephalopathy (Brainstem/hypothalamic injury)

Screening for Malignant Hyperthermia

- Plasma CK values: (more than 20000 IU/L)
  - If increased in close relatives of patients with MH, considered to have MH (without contracture testing)
  - If normal on several occasions it has no predictive value and contracture studies are necessary
  - Nonspecific test
- *Caffeine Halothane Contracture Test (CHCT)*:
  - Most sensitive test
  - Considered to be the definitive test to rule out MH
  - Negative result in this test therefore rules out MH
  - It is an in vitro bioassay using the patients skeletal muscle
  - Skeletal muscle biopsy is (3–4 inch) taken from vastus lateralis muscle
  - Muscle is divided into strips measuring:
    - 15–30 mm × 2–3 mm width
    - 2–3 mm thickness
  - These strips are mounted in a muscle bath apparatus
  - Strips are then stimulated at 0.1–0.2 Hz to check for muscle viability

- Halothane and caffeine are added to the muscles strips
- Patients susceptible to MH show high levels of contractile force
- This usually occurs at much lower agonist concentration
- This test has a sensitivity of 97% and specificity 78%
- Other variants of this test includes In Vitro Contracture Test (IVCT)

❖ Genetic tests:
- Tests for most common RYR1 mutations on chromosome 19
- This uses B-lymphocytes present in the blood
- These tests usually have a low sensitivity (25–30%) and high specificity

❖ Intralymphocytic calcium assay:
- Intracellular calcium assays using B lymphocytes indicate MH susceptibility
- Increased intracellular Ca^{2+} response to caffeine indicate MH susceptibility
- This test is still in experimental stages

❖ Nuclear magnetic resonance spectroscopy (using forearm ischemia):
- Evaluates ATP depletion during graded exercise
- MH patients have greater breakdown of ATP and creatine phosphate

❖ In vivo microdialysis:
- Small quantity of caffeine/halothane is injected through microdialysis catheter into the thigh muscle
- Samples of local CO_2 and lactate levels taken

Treatment

❖ Call for help:
- Additional personnel to be mobilized as MH management is labor-intensive
- Notify the surgeon to stop the surgical procedure as soon as possible

❖ Discontinue trigger:
- Discontinue all anesthetic agents
- Insert charcoal filters into inspiratory and expiratory limb of anesthesia circuit
- Secure another anesthesia machine with ambu bag support
- This machine may be used if clinical picture worsens in spite of charcoal filters
- E cylinder of oxygen is kept ready
- Change anesthesia circuit and soda lime
- General anesthesia can then be maintained with propofol infusion
- Hyperventilate with
  - 100% FiO_2
  - Target a minute ventilation more than 10 L/min
  - O_2 flow rates should be increased to 10 L/min

❖ Monitor:
- Pulse oximeter: IBP
- E_TCO_2
- Urine output
- ECG
- CVP (individualized)
- Temperature: ABG/electrolytes
- Coagulation parameters for DIC:
  - PT, INR
  - Platelet count
  - FDP, fibrinogen
- Muscle tone

❖ Optimize ventilation:
- Increase inspired oxygen to 100%
- Increase ventilation rate and tidal volume to maximize ventilation
- Secure airway with ETT in case of spontaneously breathing patient
- Non-depolarizing muscle relaxants may be used for intubation

❖ Secure additional intravascular access:
- Wide bore IV cannula for resuscitation
- Arterial line/CVP
- Foleys catheter (as every 20 mg dantrolene has 3 g mannitol)
- Nasogastric tube

❖ Dantrolene:
- Mechanism of action:
  - Dantrolene is a hydantoin derivative
  - It interferes directly with muscle contraction
  - It binds to RYR1 receptor and inhibits calcium ion release
  - This prevents the sudden surge in myoplasmic calcium concentration
  - Available in 2 preparations (Revonto and Ryanodex)
- Timing of administration:
  - Dantrolene is administered as soon as possible after diagnosis of MH
  - A 20 minute delay in administration increases complications by 30%
- Loading dose:
  - IV 2.5 mg/kg is given rapidly through large bore IV cannula
  - This is usually sufficient to achieve therapeutic levels
  - Dantrolene preparations have a high pH
  - Thus, large bore IV cannula is preferred to avoid venous irritation

- Repeat doses:
  - Definitive guidelines on redosing do not exist
  - Need to redose should be individualized based on patient response
  - 1 mg/kg is repeated every 5–10 mins until signs of MH subside
  - This is indicated by:
    - Decrease in E_TCO_2
    - Decrease in muscle rigidity
    - Decrease in heart rate
  - Up to 10 mg/kg IV may be given, especially in muscular individuals
- Maintenance dose:
  - IV 1 mg/kg is given Q4–6H for 24 hrs after last observed sign of MH
  - This is in order to prevent relapse which occurs in 20% patients
  - Relapse usually occurs around 12–13 hours after the initial reaction
  - Additional boluses of dantrolene may be required in case of relapses
  - Dantrolene is discontinued when all the following criteria are met:
    - Metabolic stability for more than 24 hour
    - Absence of muscle rigidity
    - Core temperature less than 38°C
    - No evidence of myoglobinuria
    - Decreasing creatinine kinase trends

❖ Control hyperthermia:
- Indications:
  - Cooling is initiated when core temperature is above 39°C
  - Cooling is stopped at 38°C to prevent hypothermia
- Treatment options:
  - Refrigerated IV fluids (20 mL/kg)
  - Body surface cooling:
    - Circulating water mattress
    - Cooling blanket packed with ice
  - Ice packs on groin and axilla
  - Gastric, rectal, wound and peritoneal lavage with iced saline.
  - In case of intractable hyperthermia:
    - Cold peritoneal dialysis
    - Cardiopulmonary bypass/ECMO

❖ Symptomatic therapy:
- Acidosis:
  - Sodium bicarbonate 1–2 mEq/kg IV when base deficit > 8 mEq/L
  - Maximum dose 50 mEq
- Cardiovascular support:
  - Cardiac glycosides and inotropes
  - Antiarrhythmics: IV lidocaine is useful for ventricular arrhythmias
  - Calcium channel blockers:
    - Coadministration with dantrolene is *contraindicated*
    - This is because it may worsen hyperkalemia and hypotension
    - Thus, CCBs should not be used to treat hypertension
- Hyperkalemia:
  - Treated when:
    - Abnormal ECG waveforms:
    - Peaked T waves
    - Ventricular ectopics
    - Ventricular arrhythmias
    - Serum K^+ more than 6 mEq/L in the absence of ECG changes
  - Treatment options:
    - Calcium gluconate 10% 10 mL over 10 minutes
    - Insulin 0.15 IU/kg IV
    - Glucose: 1 mL/kg 50% dextrose
    - Dantrolene is best to reverse hyperkalemia

❖ Monitor urine output:
- Maintain urine output of 1–2 mL/kg/hour
- Mannitol 0.5 g/kg or furosemide 1 mg/kg IV may be used
- Urine dipstick for heme may be used to check for myoglobinuria

❖ Postoperative care:
- Monitor:
  - Cardiovascular and respiratory stability
  - Urine output
  - Coagulation profile
  - Acid base and electrolytes
- Maintain body temperature below 38°C
- Administer dantrolene 1 mg/kg IV Q4–6H
- Maintain urine output 1–2 mL/kg/hour
- Symptomatic treatment of muscle pain
- Sodium bicarbonate administered to maintain alkaline urine

ANESTHESIA FOR MH SUSCEPTIBLE PATIENTS

Choice of Anesthetic Technique

❖ Administration of *trigger–free* anesthesia is the primary goal in these patients

❖ Regional anesthesia is safe and is the preferred technique

❖ Epidural anesthesia is the *safest technique* for Caesarean section

- If GA is used, non-triggering anesthetic technique should be employed
- TIVA is a safe alternative

Technique of General Anesthesia

Preoperative Preparation

- Adequate reassurance and counselling
- Ensure availability of adequate quantity of dantrolene
- Adequate premedication to ensure low normal heart rate
- Premedication with opioids, benzodiazepines, barbiturates
- Anticholinergics and antihistaminics are safe
- Phenothiazines can be avoided
- Routine dantrolene prophylaxis is not recommended as:
  - Oral absorption does not ensure adequate plasma dantrolene levels
  - May cause severe respiratory depression especially in neuromuscular diseases

OT Preparation

- Ventilator preparation
- Equipment for rapid ABG and electrolyte measurement
- Cooling aids
  - Hypothermic blanket
  - Crushed ice
  - Cold saline
- Monitors:
  - Pulse oximeter
  - ECG
  - Capnogram
  - NIBP
  - Temperature monitor
  - Exhaled gas analyzer:
    - Used to confirm absence of volatile gases
    - This is because plastic components of the machine absorb VAs
    - Thus, previously absorbed gases may be emitted during anesthesia
    - Exhaled gas analyzers ensure absence of these gases

Machine Preparation

- Vapor free anesthesia machine should be ensured prior to induction
- Alterations in the machine include:
  - Removal/sealing of vapourizers to avoid accidental administration
  - Replacement of the used soda lime
  - Replacement of fresh gas flow hose, reservoir bag
  - Fresh circuit should be used
  - Charcoal filters:
    - Attached to both inspiratory and expiratory limbs of the circuit
    - Done to absorb any residual traces of VA
    - Prior to insertion of the filter:
      - Circuit is flushed with FGF > 10 L/min for 90 seconds
      - This reduces sevoflurane concentration to 5 ppm within 10 min
- Clean the breathing circuit of traces of volatile anesthetics:
  - Unused breathing bag is attached to the Y–piece of the circle system
  - The ventilator is set to inflate the bag periodically
  - The machine is flushed with high flows (10 L/min) for at least 20 minutes
  - Manufacture recommendations regarding duration have to be followed

Malignant Hyperthermia Cart

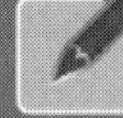

- Drugs:
  - Dantrolene:
    - At least 36 vials of Revonto preparation should be available
    - This is the maximum dose (10 mg/kg) for a 72 kg patient
    - At least 3 vials of the Ryanodex preparation should be available
  - Sterile water for injection
  - 8.4% sodium bicarbonate 50 mL 5 ampuoles
  - 50% dextrose 50 mL 2 ampuoles
  - 10% calcium chloride 10 mL 2 ampuoles
  - 2% lidocaine 20 mL 2 vials
- Refrigerated solutions:
  - 0.9% normal saline 1000 mL 4 bags
  - Cold packs 8 numbers
- Other equipment:
  - 50 mL syringes 5 numbers
  - Large bore IV catheters (different sizes)
  - Nasogastric tubes (different sizes)
  - Irrigation syringes 60 mL
  - Airway equipment
- Nursing supplies:
  - Irrigation tray with piston
  - Large plastic bags for ice
  - Test strips for hemoglobin and glucose
- Monitoring equipment:
  - CVP kits (different sizes)
  - Transducer kits for arterial and central venous pressure
  - Core temperature probes

Induction

- Safe induction agents include:
  - Thiopentone
  - Propofol
  - Ketamine
  - Etomidate
- IV fentanyl 2 μg/kg with thiopentone 3–4 mg/kg or propofol 1–2 mg/kg
- Ketamine or etomidate may be used safely in unstable patients
- Intermediate acting nondepolarizing MR can be used for muscle relaxation
- Ventilation with 100% FiO_2
- Topical anesthesia of vocal cords with LA during intubation reduces the response

Maintenance

- Safe gaseous agents include:
  - Nitrous oxide gas
  - Xenon
- O_2 + air + fentanyl 1 μg/kg boluses + NDMR
- MH is unlikely if no signs of MH occur during the first hour of anesthesia

Postoperative

- Vigilant monitoring
- Extubate in calm environment
- Minimum PACU stay of 2 hours recommended
- Adequate IVF and oral intake reduces chances of fever due to dehydration

TREATMENT OF RAISED ICP

Introduction

- Normal ICP values:
  - 7–15 mm Hg in adults and young children
  - 3–7 mm Hg for young children
  - 1.5–6 mm Hg for term neonates
  - 20 mm Hg = Raised ICP
- Goal of treating ICP is to maintain a cerebral perfusion pressure (CPP) of 50–70 mm Hg

Management Goals

Airway: Early tracheal intubation if GCS < 8 or unable to meet respiratory goals

Respiratory

- Avoid hypoxia, maintain SpO_2 > 97%, PaO_2 > 80 mm Hg
- Maintain $PaCO_2$ between 35 to 37 mm Hg
- Hyperventilation with $PaCO_2$ between 30 to 35 mm Hg only if indicated

Cardiovascular

- Avoid hypotension, maintain MAP ≥ 100 mm Hg
- Replace intravascular volume
- Avoid hypotonic and glucose containing solutions
- Use blood as necessary, reverse existing coagulopathy
- Vasopressors, as necessary to maintain cerebral perfusion pressure

Central Nervous System

- Monitor ICP, avoid ICP > 20 mm Hg
- Maintain CPP between 60–70 mm Hg
- Adequate sedation and analgesia
- Hyperosmolar therapy
- Maintain serum sodium < 155 mEq/L, P_{osm} < 320 mOsm/L
- CSF drainage
- Treat seizures

Metabolic

- Monitor blood glucose
- Aim for blood glucose below 200 mg/dL
- Avoid hyperthermia
- DVT thromboprophylaxis

GENERAL MEASURES (BTF 2016 Guidelines)

I. Treatment of Cause

- Treatment of the cause of raised ICP is the best therapy
- This includes:
  - Evacuation of blood clot
  - Resection of tumor
  - CSF diversion (shunts)
  - Treatment of metabolic disorder

II. Airway

- Intubation if altered consciousness to:
  - Reduce risk of aspiration
  - Maintain oxygenation and ventilation
- Minimize further elevations in ICP during intubation:
  - Careful positioning
  - Appropriate choice of induction and paralytic agents
  - Adequate sedation
  - Administration of lidocaine prior to intubation
- PEEP:
  - PEEP values less than *10 cm H_2O* is recommended
  - ICP and CVP monitoring is used if higher PEEP required

- PEEP may increase ICP as it causes:
  - Increase in intrathoracic pressure
  - Reduction in cerebral venous outflow

III. Sedation

- Adequate sedation reduces ICP by:
  - Reducing metabolic demand
  - Reducing venous congestion
  - Alteration of cerebral vascular tone
  - Reducing ventilator asynchrony
- Barbiturates:
  - Usually the preferred agents if hemodynamically stable
  - Administration of high doses to induce burst suppression is not recommended
  - High dose therapy is used to control raised ICP refractory to standard therapy
- Propofol:
  - It is an useful alternative but only for short term sedation
  - Caution is required while using high dose therapy
  - Propofol infusion syndrome (PRIS) occurs on long term therapy
  - Short half life allows frequent neurological assessment
  - Propofol sedation does not improve mortality or long term outcomes
- Inhalational agents such as isoflurane dose < 1 MAC have been used

IV. Fluid Therapy

- Patients with elevated ICP do not require fluid restriction
- Goal of fluid therapy should be to maintain:
  - Euvolemia
  - Normosmolarity or hyperosmolarity
- Maintain serum osmolality more than 280 mOsm/L
- Avoid hypotonic fluids:
  - 5% dextrose
  - 0.45% normal saline
- Use isotonic fluids:
  - Normal saline
  - Lactated ringers
- Role of colloids in raised ICP is controversial

V. Anticonvulsants

- Anticonvulsant therapy is instituted on suspicion of seizures
- Prophylactic anticonvulsant therapy:
  - Refers to the administration of anticonvulsants to prevent seizure occurrence
  - Indications for prophylactic anticonvulsant therapy:
    - Supratentorial cortical lesions
    - Subdural hemorrhage
    - Subarachnoid hemorrhage
- Phenytoin:
  - *Drug of choice* at present
  - Dose of 15 mg/kg IV bolus administered at a rate of less than 50 mg/min
- Insufficient evidence to recommend levetiracetam over phenytoin at present
- But due to safe clinical profile of levetiracetam, it can be considered as first choice

SPECIFIC MEASURES (BTF 2016 Guidelines)

I. Hyperosmolar Therapy to Reduce Brain Water

- Mechanism of action:
  - Establishes osmotic gradient across blood brain barrier to reduce brain ECF
  - Reduces brain water content and CSF pressure in 20 mins
  - Compensatory cerebral vasoconstriction in response to an increase in cerebral blood flow
  - Rise in BP causes autoregulatory cerebral vasoconstriction and reduction in cerebral blood volume
- Mannitol:
  - This is the most commonly used agent for hyperosmolar therapy
  - IV mannitol (20%) 0.25–1 gm/kg can be given over 10–15 minutes
  - Repeat dosing can be given at 0.25–0.5 gm/kg
  - Up to 2 gm/kg can be tried if serum osmolarity is above 320 mOsm/kg
  - Hypotension (SBP less than 90 mm Hg) should be avoided
  - Sudden exposure to high osmolarity can cause vasodilation and increase CBF
- Hypertonic saline:
  - Appears to have a greater efficacy in managing elevated ICP
  - Dose:
    - 3% saline is infused at 20–40 mL/hour
    - It is titrated to maintain serum sodium levels 145–155 mEq/L
    - 30 mL supplement of 23.4% saline is used for acute ICP elevations

- Advantages:
  - No electrolyte disturbance (as seen with mannitol)
  - Brisk diuresis (seen with mannitol) is absent
- Can cause:
  - Osmotic demyelination
  - Rebound increase in ICP
  - Coagulopathies
  - Volume overload
  - Electrolyte abnormalities and renal failure
- Administration:
  - Hypertonic saline should be given via central line
  - This is due to the high risk of extravasation when using peripheral lines
  - It is tapered off slowly to prevent rebound hyponatremia
- In the presence of hyperchloremic acidosis use a mixture of:
  - Sodium chloride
  - Sodium acetate

❖ Mannitol with 0.5–1 mg/kg frusemide may be more effective than mannitol alone

❖ Other alternatives: Urea, glycerol, sorbitol, HS–dextran

❖ Current evidence:
- Insufficient evidence about effects of hyperosmolar therapy on clinical outcomes
- Insufficient evidence to support the use of any specific hyperosmolar agent

II. CSF Drainage

❖ External ventricular drain, ventriculostomy

❖ Subarachnoid catheter/screw

❖ Lumbar drain

❖ Maybe difficulty if ventricular collapse associated with edema

❖ Trauma and infection may occur

❖ Shunt procedures

III. Reduce Cerebral Blood Volume

❖ Position:
- Patients are positioned to maximize cerebral venous outflow
- Neutral head position is important
- Avoid flexing/turning the head sideways to avoid IJV obstruction
- 15–30° elevation of head end is recommended to increase venous drainage
- Avoid restrictive neck taping
- Minimize stimuli causing Valsalva responses (endotracheal suctioning)
- Abdominal decompression as increased IAP reduces venous outflow from lumbar veins

Hyperventilation

❖ Indications:
- Brief periods of hyperventilation ($PaCO_2 < 35$) for:
  - Acute neurological deterioration
  - Tonsillar herniation
- Prolonged hyperventilation not recommended
- Short periods to improve surgical field Guidelines:
- Limit reduction in $PaCO_2$ to 25 mm Hg as:
  - Below 25 mm Hg, very little additional benefit
  - Increased chances of cerebral ischemia due to vasoconstriction
- In craniotomy patients, $PaCO_2$ to be increased after retractors are removed to minimize residual pneumotocele

❖ Disadvantages:
- Hyperventilation causes cerebral vasoconstriction
- This reduces CBF when $CMRO_2$ is high
- Therefore increased chances of cerebral ischemia
- CBF and ICP return to normal in 8–12 hours due to reduction in CSF bicarbonate levels by altered function of carbonic anhydrase

IV. Increase MAP

❖ Adequate IV resuscitation to maintain euvolemia

❖ Phenylephrine,dopamine and norepinephrine used to ensure CPP between 60–70 mm Hg

❖ Intraoperative BP maintained within 10% of awake values

V. Excise Mass Lesions

❖ Tumor/hematoma excision

❖ This is most definitive treatment

Other Measures

I. Steroids

❖ 4 mg dexamethasone QID

❖ Not recommended in head injury management protocols routinely

❖ Restores blood brain barrier and reduces edema

❖ Improves viscoelastic property

❖ Takes 48–72 hrs to act

❖ Administer 48 hrs before surgery for action to be apparent

II. Hypothermia

❖ Head injured patients with mild hypothermia (< 35°C) had better outcomes

❖ Not routinely recommended

❖ Increases risk of pneumonia, wound infections, and coagulopathies

III. Cerebral Vasoconstrictors

❖ Dihydroergotamine is precapillary vasoconstrictor
❖ Used in refractory intracranial hypertension in patients with TBI
❖ Limited experience

Refractory Intracranial Hypertension

❖ High dose barbiturate (***Pentobarb coma***).
❖ Thiopentone 10–15 mg/kg IV
❖ Aggressive hyperventilation
❖ Surgical options:
  • Hemicraniectomy
  • Frontal/temporal lobectomy
  • Decompressive craniectomy
  • Decompressure exploratory laparotomy

ANESTHESIA FOR RAISED ICP

Anesthetic Considerations

❖ Maintain CPP around 60–70 mm Hg
❖ Avoid increase in CBF and ICP
❖ *Loose brain* which facilitates access to lesion
❖ IPPV to control $PaCO_2$ and good oxygenation

Preoperative Evaluation

Clinical Features

❖ Early:
  • Headache
  • Focal neuro deficits
  • Vomiting
  • Papilledema, blurred vision
  • Seizures
❖ Headache which is postural and awakens patient at nightlate:
  • Hypertension, bradycardia, Cheyne Stokes breathing ***(Cushing's triad)***
  • Agitation, drowsiness, coma
  • Apnea
  • Ipsilateral followed by bilateral pupillary dilation
  • Decorticate followed by decerebrate posturing
  • Obtain history of medication to reduce ICP

Investigations

❖ Routine blood: Complete blood count, coagulation profile, blood group and type
❖ RFTS and LFTS
❖ *X-ray skull*: ***Silver beaten appearance***
❖ *CT/MRI*:
  • Midline shift, obliteration of sulci
  • Ventricular effacement/enlargement, edema

Preoperative Preparation

❖ Dehydration and dyselectolytemia due to vomiting and diuresis corrected
❖ Continue steroid therapy if patient is on chronic steroid therapy
❖ Loading dose of phenytoin 15 mg/kg IV
❖ Loss of conscious and any focal neuro deficits documented
❖ Avoid sedation in drowsy patients
❖ In awake patients, benzodiazepines on night before and morning of surgery
❖ IV fluids at <30 mL/kg/day if cerebral edema present

Induction

❖ Thiopentone 3–5 mg/kg or propofol 1.5 mg/kg + fentanyl 2–3 µg/kg + vecuronium 0.15 mg/kg
❖ Rapid inhalational induction in children
❖ *Rapid sequence induction* with cricoid pressure and scholine if difficult airway
❖ Smooth unhurried induction to avoid increase in ICP
❖ Avoid coughing and straining
❖ IV lidocaine 1–1.5 mg/kg to avoid raised ICP at intubation
❖ Avoid obstructing neck with ETT ties to avoid increasing venous pressure

Monitoring

❖ *Pulse oximetry*: Foleys catheter
❖ E_TCO_2
❖ Temperature
❖ ECG
❖ Neuromuscular monitoring
❖ *NIBP/IBP*: Central Venous Pressure
❖ ICP monitoring

Ventilation

❖ Controlled mandatory ventilation
❖ Normocapnia/mild hypocapnea (30–35 mm Hg)
❖ Avoid PEEP
❖ If used, PEEP < 10 mm Hg recommended

Position

❖ 15 –30° head up tilt to improve venous drainage
❖ Head in neutral position
❖ Avoid undue flexion/turning of head to avoid IJV compression
❖ Avoid undue abdominal pressure to avoid increasing IAP

Maintenance

- O_2 + air + isoflurane/seroflurane (0.5 –1 MAC) + fentanyl boluses + NDMR
- Avoid nitrous oxide as it increases ICP
- TIVA is a good alternative which allows good ICP control
- Enflurane contraindicated in neurosurgery as it causes seizures especially with hypocapnea
- Mannitol can be used before craniotomy—facilitates brain retraction without causing contusion in deep seated tissues

Hemodynamics

- Aim for CPP around 60–70 mm Hg
- Maintain MAP > 80 mm Hg
- Failure of cerebral autoregulation occurs if CPP < 50 mm Hg
- Thus, patient is more susceptible to cerebral ischemia during hypotension
- Maintain BP around 10% of preoperative values
- Hypotonic solutions avoided to prevent fluid flux across blood brain barrier—***RL avoided***
- Maintain high plasma osmolality
- Control BP with fluids and vasopressors
- Moderate hypothermia (around 35°C) beneficial

Extubation

- Fully reverse neuromuscular blockade
- Assess neurological status before extubation
- Extubate fully awake
- Hypertension at extubation increases risk of postoperative hematoma

Postoperative

Monitoring

- Pulse oximetry
- Temperature
- NIBP/IBP
- ECG
- Urine output

Care

- Continue to maintain patients airway
- Adequate sedation and analgesia
- Assess and document size and reactivity of pupils
- Deep vein thrombosis prophylaxis

Complications

- *Delayed awakening*: Shivering
- *Seizures*: PONV
- *HTN/hypotension*: Cerebral edema
- *Pain*: Postoperative hematoma

PERIOPERATIVE CEREBRAL PROTECTION

Introduction

- Neuro protection is defined as the treatment initiated before the onset of ischemia, intended to modify cellular and vascular biological responses to deprivation of energy supply so as to increase tolerance of neural tissue to ischemia
- Protection means prevention of a foreseeable insult highly likely to occur given the circumstances

Physiological Basis

- Cerebral metabolism is unique as energy is mainly spent in:
  - Neuronal excitation to generate action potentials
  - Conduction of these impulses
- Cerebral metabolism has 2 components:
  - Functional component:
    - Accounts for 60% of the total neuronal energy utilization
    - This component is important for generating action potentials
    - The functional component maybe assessed using EEG
    - Anesthetic agents reduce this functional component
    - These anesthetic agents are:
      - Thiopentone
      - Propofol
      - Etomidate
      - Volatile anesthetics
    - Thus ideal anesthetic technique produces at the most a 60% reduction in O_2 use
  - Cellular integrity component:
    - This accounts for the remaining 40% of neuronal energy utilization
    - This component maintains neuronal integrity and homeostasis
    - Only hypothermia reduces the functional and integrity component
    - Anesthetic agents have no effect on the integrity component

Categories of Cerebral Ischemia

	Focal	Global
Transient	Embolus with reperfusion	Cardiac arrest with reperfusion
Permanent	End vessel occlusion	Brain death

Types of Ischemic Events

- Anticipated events:
  - Cerebral aneurysm clipping
  - Carotid endarterectomy
  - Cardiopulmonary bypass
- Unanticipated events:
  - Cardiac arrest
  - Spontaneous stroke

Physiological Neuroprotective Interventions

1. *Hypothermia*

- Types of hypothermia:
  - Prophylactic: When applied early after injury, prior to increase in ICP
  - Therapeutic hypothermia: When applied as treatment for refractory raised ICP
- Mechanisms of protection:
  - Reduces cerebral metabolism
  - Membrane stabilizing action
  - Increases blood brain barrier stability
  - Preserves ATP and reduces calcium influx
  - Maintenance of ion homeostasis
  - Reduces levels of excitatory amino acids
  - Reduces free radicals
  - Suppresses cytokine production
- Guidelines for use:
  - Mild hypothermia is recommended for routine neurosurgery
  - No such effect is seen following focal ischemia
  - Beneficial temperature threshold is 33–35°C
  - Deep hypothermia < 20°C if prolonged cardiac arrest
  - Early institution of hypothermia is more beneficial following the neural insult
- Disadvantages:
  - Reduced metabolism of drugs
  - Coagulopathy
  - Arrhythmias
  - Immunosuppression

2. *Cerebral Perfusion Pressure*

- CPP is a surrogate measure for the delivery of nutrients to the brain
- Since MAP and ICP determine CPP, it is important to maintain normotension
- However, CPP values above 70 mm Hg was associated with poorer outcomes
- Recommended target CPP values for a favorable outcome is between 60–70 mm Hg

3. *Arterial CO_2 Levels*

- Normocapnea with $PaCO_2$ between 35–45 mm Hg is the goal
- Under normal circumstances, $PaCO_2$ is the most powerful determinant of CBF
- CBF at all times should be appropriate to the cerebral metabolic rate
- Low $PaCO_2$ results in low CBF and causes cerebral ischemia
- High $PaCO_2$ on the other hand may result in cerebral hyperemia and high ICP
- Since cerebral metabolic rate is not routinely measured, normocapnia is recommended
- Hyperventilation is recommended only in the presence of cerebral herniation
- Prolonged prophylactic hyperventilation with $PaCO_2$ < 25 mm Hg is not advised

4. *Glycemic Control*

- Serum glucose levels increase during situations of severe stress such as surgical stress
- Controlling this response with insulin leads to significant improvement in outcomes
- However, "tight glucose control strategies" may have deleterious CNS effects
- Strict glycemic control has not shown to improve mortality/outcomes
- Thus, at present no recommendations have been made regarding glycemic control
- However, glycemic intervention is advised if plasma glucose exceeds 250 mg/dL
- Glycemic control should aim at plasma sugars less than 200 mg/dL

5. *Seizure Prophylaxis*

- Refers to the practise of administering anticonvulsants to prevent the occurrence of seizures
- Acute irritation of the cortical surface during surgery may cause seizures
- Advantages of preventing seizures using anticonvulsants include:
  - Limiting the derangement in acute physiology
  - Preventing the development of chronic epilepsy
  - Preventing brain herniation
- At present, routine prophylactic use of phenytoin or valproate is not recommended
- However, other anticonvulsants such as levetiracetam have minimal side effects
- These may be administered prophylactically for:
  - Supratentorial craniotomies
  - Patients who have sustained recent TBI or SAH

6. *Arterial Blood Pressure*

- Acceptable arterial blood pressure must be discussed prior to the surgery
- Intraoperative hypotension has been shown to correlate with diffuse cerebral edema
- Recommended targets for systolic blood pressure:
  - More than 100 mm Hg for patients 50–69 years old
  - More than 110 mm Hg for patients 15–49 years old and above 70 years
- Safe target would be to maintain the systolic pressures within 10% of awake values

Pharmacological Interventions

1. *Barbiturates*

- Considered ***gold standard*** of brain protective anesthetics during focal ischemia
- Hypothermia is for global ichemia and barbiturates for focal ischemia
- Mechanism of action:
  - Metabolic suppression and oxygen consumption
  - Improved metabolic coupling
  - Membrane stabilization
  - Free radical scavenging
  - Altered ion homeostasis
  - Reduced glutamate activity
  - Reduced intracellular calcium
  - Increased GABA activity and NMDA antagonism
- Barbiturate therapy to reduce ICP requires high doses which results in a fall in BP
- The hypotensive effect will therefore offset any ICP lowering action on the CPP
- Thus, high doses which produce EEG burst suppression are not recommended
- High doses may however be considered in those refractory to conventional therapy

2. *Propofol*

- Reduces the cerebral metabolism and oxygen consumption
- Mechanism of action:
  - Increased GABA activity
  - Free radical scavenging
  - Limits lipid peroxidation
- Propofol may be used for short term control of ICP
- However, it is not associated with improvement in mortality or 6–month outcomes
- High dose therapy is avoided as it can produce significant mortality

3. *Volatile Anesthetics*

- All volatile anesthetic agents are dose dependent cerebral vasodilators
- The CBF differences between iso, sevo and desflurane is not clinically significant
- The net CBF effect of volatile anesthetics depends on:
  - Concentration of the volatile anesthetic
  - Extent of previous cerebral metabolic rate depression
  - Simultaneous blood pressure changes
  - Simultaneous changes in $PaCO_2$
- Volatile anesthetic administration may be effective when:
  - Applied during ischemic insult
  - Used as preconditioning therapy
- No trial data exists at present to guide clinical practice

4. *Steroids*

- Administration of steroids helps in limiting the formation of edema
- Neurological benefits of steroid therapy include:
  - Restoration of altered vascular permeability in brain edema
  - Reduction in CSF production
  - Attenuation of free radical production
- When therapy is begun 48 hours prior to surgery, it improves the clinical condition
- Reduction in ICP however, occurs 48–72 hours after initiation of steroid therapy
- However, currently steroids are recommended only in patients with refractory ICP
- This is because high dose steroid therapy was associated with increased mortality

5. *Osmotherapy*

- Hyperosmolar agents are used to reduce the brains ICF and ECF volume
- Both osmotic and loop diuretics have been used, though osmotic agents are widely used
- Mannitol:
  - Reduces ICP via:
    - Simple brain tissue dehydration
    - Reduction of blood viscosity
  - Most commonly used dose is 1 gm/kg given over 10–15 minutes
  - It is the most commonly used agent for ICP management
  - But the eventual diuresis produced may be undesirable in hypotensive patients

- Hypertonic saline (HS):
  - Useful as repeated administration of mannitol may result in unwanted diuresis
  - In addition HS may be effective in patients who are refractory to mannitol
  - However, at present there is insufficient evidence to support any specific osmolar agent

MYASTHENIA GRAVIS

Introduction

- Myasthenia gravis is a chronic acquired autoimmune disorder of neuromuscular junction characterized by weakness and fatigueability of voluntary muscles with improvement following rest
- It is a type II hypersensitivity immune response
- It is the most common disorder of neuromuscular transmission

Incidence

- Prevalence ranges from 7–20 per 1,00,0000
- More common in females than males with a 3:2 ratio
- Peaks of incidence:
  - 3rd decade in females
  - 6th –7th decade for men
- Mean age of onset:
  - 28 years in females
  - 42 years in males
- Current in hospital mortality rate is around 2.2%
- Old age and respiratory failure are strong predictors of mortality

Associated Autoimmune Disorders

- Rheumatoid arthritis
- SLE
- Neuromyelitis optica
- Autoimmune thyroid disease
- SIADH
- Cushing's syndrome
- Hypogammaglobulinemia
- RBC Aplasia

Etiopathogenesis

- Autoimmune disorder
- Types of autoantibodies are:
  - Antibodies (Abs) to n–ACh receptors:
    - 90% patients have antibodies to n–ACh receptors
    - Antibodies bind to the ACh receptor
    - This causes AChR dysfunction by:
      - Blocking ACh binding to its receptor
      - Internalizing AChR
      - Activating complement mediated destruction of AChR
    - Usually associated with thymic pathology
  - Muscle specific kinase antibodies (MuSK):
    - Directed against muscle specific receptor tyrosine kinase
    - Usually present in those who are seronegative for n-AChR Abs
    - MuSK is a protein that mediates NMJ formation during development
    - Usually not associated with thymic pathology
    - Usually causes 2 types of myasthenia:
      - Oculobulbar form: diplopia, ptosis and dysarthria
      - Myopathic form: respiratory and proximal muscle weakness
- Seronegative myasthenia gravis:
  - Subset of patients who do not have anti-AChR or MuSK antibodies
  - Also called double seronegative myasthenia gravis
  - Occurs in 6–12% of patients with myasthenia gravis
  - Clinical findings are similar to sero positive myasthenia gravis
- Role of thymus:
  - Majority of patients with AChR–Ab positive MG have thymic abnormalities:
    - Hyperplasia in 60–70%
    - Thymoma in 10–12%
  - The thymus contains myoid cells which express AChR on their surface
  - The autoimmune T cells attack the AChR units on the myoid cells
  - Thus, germinal centers are created in the thymus which contain:
    - Myoid cells
    - Complement
    - Autoantibodies
  - Autoantibodies in the germinal center mature to recognize muscle AChR
  - Thus, the thymus plays an important part in the generation of auto–antibodies

Clinical Classification

I. Myasthenia Gravis in Pediatric Age

- Neonatal transient myasthenia gravis:
  - Occurs in babies born to mothers with myasthenia gravis

- Seen in 15–20% babies born to myasthenic mothers
- Circulating anti-AChR antibodies are passively transferred
- Presents within 12–48 hours of birth and lasts for 2–4 weeks
- Characterized by:
  - Feeble cry
  - Poor feeding effort
  - Respiratory difficulty
  - Ptosis and facial weakness

❖ Neonatal persistent myasthenia gravis:
- Very rare in occurrence
- Usually has no detectable antibodies to AChR
- Onset occurs within 2–3 months of age

❖ Juvenile myasthenia: Similar to adult myasthenia gravis

II. Myasthenia Gravis in Adults: Osserman and Genkins Classification

Class	Name	Description
I.	Ocular myasthesia	• Involves ocular muscles only • Ptosis and diplopia • Electrophysiologic tests of other muscles is negative
II. Generalized myasthenia		
IIa.	Mild	• Slow onset • Usually ocular • Spreading to bulbar and skeletal muscles • Good response to drug therapy • No respiratory muscle involvement • Low mortality rate
IIb.	Moderate	• Slow onset • Ocular with more severe involvement of peripheral muscles • Dysarthria, dysphagia, etc • Fair response to drug therapy • No respiratory muscle involvement • Patients activities limited • Low mortality rate
III.	Acute Fulminating Myasthenia	• Rapid onset • Progresses within 6 months • Severe bulbar and skeletal muscle involvement • Poor response to treatment • Involves respiratory muscles • Patients activities limited • Low mortality rate
IV.	Late severe myasthenia	• Develops 2 years after onset of group I or II symptoms • Progression may be gradual or rapid • Severe bulbar and skeletal involvement • Poor response to treatment • Involves respiratory muscles • Patients activities limited • High mortality

Clinical Features

❖ Muscle weakness:
- Fluctuating muscle weakness is the *cardinal feature*
- Often associated with true muscle fatigue
- Fatigue manifests as worsening contractile force of the muscle (not tiredness)
- Weakness worsens with exertion and improves on rest
- Fatigue is absent upon awakening in the morning early in the disease course
- Weakness worsens as the day progresses
- As the disease progresses, the fatigue free intervals are lost
- Symptoms will then be continuously present with fluctuating severity
- Ocular weakness:
  - Occurs as first manifestation in more than 50% patients
  - Presents with ptosis and diplopia
  - More than 50% of these patients develop generalized weakness in 2 yrs
  - Ptosis:
    - Occurs due to weakness of eyelid muscles
    - Can be:
      - Symmetrical/asymmetric
      - Unilateral/bilateral
    - Degree of ptosis varies throughout the day
    - Ptosis typically alternates between eyes
    - It may become so severe as to occlude vision
    - Varying severity between eyes may result in unilateral ptosis
  - Extraocular muscle involvement:
    - Varies from single muscle involvement to total ophthalmoplegia
    - Typically produces binocular diplopia
    - Diplopia disappears on closing or occluding one eye
    - Diplopia may be horizontal or vertical
    - Muscle fatigue can also cause nystagmus
  - Pupil usually spared
  - Progress to more generalized weakness in 80–85% patients
  - If it remains ocular for 2 yrs, chances of generalizing are rare

❖ Bulbar muscles:
- Bulbar muscle involvement results in:
  - Dysarthria
  - Dysphagia
  - Resultant weight loss

- This typically produces weakness on prolonged chewing *(fatiguable chewing)*
- Involvement of palatal muscles produces:
  - Nasal regurgitation
  - Nasal twang in voice
  - Hypophonic voice
- Involvement of facial muscles:
  - Involves elevators of angles of mouth
  - This results in an *expressionless face*
  - Typically involves:
    - Levator angulii oris
    - Levator labii superioris
    - Orbicularis oris
  - This produces the ***Myasthenic snarl*** on attempting to smile
  - Mid–lip rises but outer corners of mouth fail to move

❖ Limb muscles:
- Occurs in 15–20% patients with myasthenia gravis
- Proximal muscles are more involved resulting in:
  - Difficulty in climbing stairs
  - Difficulty in lifting hands
- Upper limbs are affected more than the lower limbs
- Weakness of neck extensors:
  - Involves rectus capitis posterior major and minor
  - This results in the weight of head overcoming the extensor power
  - Thus, patient is unable to maintain the head upright
  - This worsens later in the day producing the *dropped–head syndrome*
- Weakness may also involve:
  - Wrist and finger extensors
  - Foot dorsiflexors
- Respiratory muscle involvement:
  - Produces the most serious symptoms in myasthenia gravis
  - Causes dyspnea, especially in supine position
  - This may lead to impending respiratory failure and myasthenic crisis
  - Myasthenic crisis may be precipitated by:
    - Surgery
    - Infections
    - Medications
    - Tapering of immunosuppression
- Diaphragmatic involvement:
  - Produces reduced forcefulness of cough
  - Patients are usually unable to project their voice

❖ Mass effect:
- Cough, dyspnea
- SVC syndrome

❖ Cardiovascular:
- Focal myocarditis
- LV diastolic dysfunction
- Atrial fibrillation
- AV conduction delay

Phases of Myasthenia Gravis

❖ Active phase:
- This has the most severe symptoms and most fluctuations
- Occurs 5–7 years after the onset of the disease
- Myasthenic crisis occurs most frequently during this period

❖ Plateau phase:
- During this phase symptoms persist but stabilize
- Symptoms may worsen due to:
  - Medication error
  - Infections
  - Tapering of medications

❖ Remission phase:
- Remission may occur in some patients
- Patients may be free of symptoms and off medications entirely

Factors Aggravating Myasthenic Crisis

❖ Physical and emotional stress
❖ Infections—especially pulmonary and viral
❖ Pregnancy
❖ Surgery
❖ Heat and exposure to bright sunlight
❖ Drugs
- Cardiovascular drugs:
  - Beta blockers, lidocaine
  - Quinidine, procainamide
  - Penicillamine, verapamil
- Antibiotics:
  - Aminoglycosides, erythromycin
  - Clindamycin, ciprofloxacin
  - Ampicillin, streptomycin
- Other drugs:
  - Phenytoin, lithium
  - Corticosteroids, interferon α
  - Magnesium, NMBAs

Diagnosis

❖ Clinical examination:
- Monitor prolonged upward gaze
- Holding outstretched hand in abduction
- Determine vital capacity

- Edrophonium/Tensilon test:
  - Not used commonly (drug is rarely available)
  - Edrophonium is an acetylcholinesterase inhibitor with:
    - Rapid onset of action (30–45 seconds)
    - Short duration of action (5–10 minutes)
  - Edrophonium thus prolongs the presence of acetylcholine in the NMJ
  - This results in an immediate improvement in the muscle strength
  - The test requires obvious ptosis or ophthalmoplegia for correct diagnosis
  - Patients show improvement in ptosis after edrophonium administration
  - This effect lasts for the duration of action of the drug (10 minutes)
  - Procedure:
    - IV edrophonium 2 mg is given initially
    - This is followed by 2 mg every 60 seconds up to a total dose of 10 mg
    - Incremental administration avoids precipitating muscarinic side effects
    - Thus, the test is avoided in patients with:
      - Cardiac disease
      - Bronchial asthma
  - Sensitivity of the edrophonium test is between 80–90%
  - Positive test can also occur in:
    - Motor neuron disease
    - Brainstem tumors
    - Compressive cranial neuropathies
- Curare test: (rarely used nowadays)
  - Regional test:
    - Tourniquet is applied to both arms
    - 0.2 mg of d-tubocurarine (diluted to 20 mL) is given in one arm
    - 20 mL normal saline is given in the other arm
    - Reduced twitch response is seen in the d-TC arm within 6 minutes
    - This is suggestive of myasthenia gravis
  - Systemic test:
    - 0.5–1 mg increments of d-tubocurarine is given
    - Up to a maximum dose of 0.03 mg/kg IV can be given
    - Increased chances of respiratory failure during the test—not preferred
- Ice pack test:
  - Can be used in patients with ptosis
  - Test relies on the fact that NM transmission improves at lower temperature
  - Icepacks are placed over the patients eyelids for 2 minutes
  - This causes direct cooling of the eyelid muscles
  - The icepacks are then removed and extent of ptosis is immediately assessed
  - Test is positive when improvement of ptosis occurs
  - Sensitivity is as high as 80% in patients with prominent ptosis
  - This test is not helpful in patients with extraocular muscle weakness
- Serological tests:
  - Anti–AChR antibodies:
    - Found in 85% patients with generalized myasthenia
    - Found in 50% patients with only ocular myasthenia
    - Test is not useful for assessment of severity of disease
    - Should be conducted prior to initiation of modulating therapy
  - MuSK antibodies (muscle specific kinase):
    - Seen in 8% patients
    - Commonly seen only in AChR antibody negative patients (38–50%)
    - Usually not associated with thymomas (unlike AChR antibodies)
  - LRP4 antibodies:
    - Seen in approximately 1% of patients
    - Usually seen in younger females with mild disease
    - Not commonly associated with thymic pathology
  - Seronegative MG:
    - Seen in 6–12% of patients
    - More likely to have pure ocular myasthenia gravis
- Electrophysiological tests:
  - Repetitive nerve stimulation:
    - Most frequently used electrodiagnostic test
    - The recording electrode is placed over motor endplate
    - Motor nerve supplying the muscle is stimulated repetitively (2–3 Hz)
    - The compound muscle action potential (CMAP) is recorded
    - In normal muscle physiology, there is no change in the CMAP
    - In myasthenia, there is a progressive decline in CMAP amplitude
    - This is called the decremental response
    - A decline of more than 10% is considered positive for myasthenia
  - Single fiber electromyography:
    - Most sensitive electrodiagnostic test for myasthenia

- Allows simultaneous recording of APs of 2 muscle fibers innervated by the same axon
- Usually studies a limb and a facial muscle
- Time interval between the 2 APs is called jitter
- Has a sensitivity as high as 98%
- However specificity is low as it can be positive in:
  - Motor neuron disease
  - Lambert-Eaton syndrome
  - Polymyositis
- Nystagraphy
- Stapedius reflexometry

Differential Diagnosis

- Ocular myasthenia:
  - Thyroid ophthalmopathy
  - Myotonic dystrophy
  - Chronic progressive external ophthalmoplegia
- Generalized myasthenia:
  - Amyotrophic lateral sclerosis
  - Lambert–Eaton myasthenic syndrome
  - Guillaine Barre syndrome

Treatment

- Anticholinesterases:
  - Prolong the duration of action of ACH at post–synaptic membranes
  - This is the initial therapy for patients with mild–moderate MG
  - Most patients with MuSK antibodies show poor response to pyridostigmine
  - Pyridostigmine is usually given 30–120 mg per day PO in 3–6 divided doses
  - Maximum dose is 120 mg given 4th hourly
  - Glycopyrrolate 1 mg may be added with each dose to reduce cholinergic effect
  - ACHE inhibitors provide only symptomatic relief
  - Side effects:
    - Cholinergic crisis
    - Occurs due to excessive ACH at NMJ
    - Weakness occurs due to persistent depolarization of muscle membranes
- Corticosteroids:
  - Initiated in patients who respond poorly to pyridostigmine
  - Corticosteroids reduce the amount of ACHR antibodies
  - Also reduces anti-ACHR reactivity of peripheral blood lymphocytes
  - 1 mg/kg or 40–60 mg prednisolone PO is given on alternate days
- Immunosuppressants:
  - Azathioprine and cyclosporine are used most commonly
  - 50–100 mg/day PO azathioprine
  - Slowly increased till WBC count is 3000–4000 cells/cc
  - Many months may be required before maximal therapeutic effect
  - Cyclosporine takes only 1–2 months to show maximal therapeutic effect
  - Causes nephrotoxicity and hepatotoxicity
  - Cyclophosphamide, tacrolimus, rituximab and mycophenolate mofetil also used
- Plasmapheresis:
  - Mechanism:
    - Also called therapeutic plasma exchange
    - Directly removes circulating antibodies from plasma
    - However, blood cells are returned back to circulation
    - This requires a large bore venous access (central venous catheter)
  - Beneficial effects:
    - Patients condition improves rapidly and is seen within days
    - However, the beneficial effect is short lived and lasts 3–6 weeks
    - Associated with antibody rebound in absence of concurrent immunotherapy
  - This technique is used along with IV immunoglobulins for myasthenic crisis
  - Course of treatment:
    - 5 exchanges are done on alternate days over 7–14 days
    - 3–5 Liters of plasma is processed per exchange
    - Replacement fluid used is albumin
  - Plasmapheresis reduces pseudocholinesterase levels
  - This in turn increases the duration of action of succinylcholine
- Intravenous immunoglobulins:
  - This consists of pooled immunoglobulin from donors
  - Beneficial effects:
    - Seen in less than 1 week
    - Action lasts for 3–6 weeks
  - Total dose is 2 g/kg given over 2–5 days
  - 400 mg/day for 5 days given IV
  - Commonly used for treatment of myasthenic crisis
  - May be associated with acute nephrotoxicity due to high sucrose content

- Role of thymectomy:
  - Approaches:
    - Sternal splitting
    - Transcervical
    - Video assisted thoracoscopy (VATS)
    - Robotic surgery
  - Patients with thymoma:
    - 10–15% patients with myasthenia gravis have thymoma
    - In these patients thymectomy is indicated when surgically feasible
    - Radiotherapy and chemotherapy is given in unresectable disease
    - Less than 25% undergo resolution of symptoms after thymectomy
  - Patients without thymoma:
    - Thymectomy in these patients is recommended in:
      - Age less than 60 years
      - Generalized myasthenia gravis
      - Presence of AChR antibodies
    - Thymectomy in these patients is associated with:
      - Reduced need for immunosuppressive therapy
      - Minimal clinical manifestations
      - May be associated with remission
  - Contraindications:
    - Prepubertal children
    - Those patients with only ocular symptoms.

Anesthetic Management of Myasthenia Gravis Patient: Preoperative Assessment

History

- Muscles involved
- Duration and severity of disease
- Total daily requirement of pyridostigmine
- Evaluate severity of myasthenia
- Assess involvement of respiratory and bulbar muscles

Lab Investigations

- Complete blood count: Especially if patients have been on cyclosporine therapy
- Thyroid function tests
- Serum electrolytes as hypokalemia increases muscle weakness
- Blood glucose levels as these patients will be on long term steroid therapy
- LFTs and RFTs: Especially if cyclosporine has been administered
- ECG as pyridostigmine may cause bradycardia
- Chest X-ray for aspiration pneumonia
- Preoperative ABG and PFTs:
  - Used as a baseline to help extubation
  - Serial FVC measurements are used for respiratory reserve
  - Flow volume loops:
    - Mediastinal extension of thymoma may cause airway obstruction
    - Maximal inspiratory and expiratory flow volume loops obtained
    - Separate loops obtained in supine and upright positions
    - This measures the nature of obstruction (fixed/dynamic)
- CT/MRI of thymus
- Serological tests for:
  - Lupus erythematosus
  - Antinuclear antibodies
  - Rheumatoid factor
- Bone densitometry in older patients

Predictors of Postoperative Myasthenic Crisis

- Duration of myasthenia gravis more than 6 years
- History of concomitant COPD
- History of myasthenic crisis
- Preoperative bulbar symptoms
- Dose of pyridostigmine > 750 mg/day
- Vital capacity less than 2–2.9 L
- Serum AChR antibody titers > 100 nmol/mL
- Intraoperative blood loss more than 1000 mL

Preoperative Preparation and Premedication

- Patients should be admitted while in remission 24 hours before surgery
- Preoperative physiotherapy and incentive spirometry are important
- Discuss need for postoperative ventilation and obtain consent
- *To be scheduled as first case of the day in OT*
- Anticholinesterase therapy: *Controversial*
  - Continue the anticholinesterase therapy up to the morning of surgery
  - However this may alter the effect of depolarizing and non-depolarizing NMBAs
  - Also, the response to NMBA reversal agents may be unpredictable
  - Pyridostigmine is the most commonly used drug:
    - Onset of action: 15–30 minutes
    - Peak action: 2 hours

- Duration of action: 3–4 hours
- In case of IV supplementation, IV dose is 1/30th the oral dose
- 1 mg pyridostigmine IV is equivalent to 30 mg pyridostigmine PO

❖ Steroid therapy:
- Usual morning dose of steroids have to be continued
- Indications of stress dose steroids (IV supplementation):
  - Moderate surgical stress:
    - Lower extremity revascularization
    - Total joint replacement
  - Major surgical stress:
    - Cardiac surgery
    - Esophagogastrectomy
    - Proctocolectomy
  - Patients who have taken more than 5 mg prednisolone:
    - For more than 3 weeks within 6 months of surgery
    - With Cushingoid features

❖ Immunotherapy has to be withheld on the morning of surgery

❖ Antiaspiration prophylaxis if bulbar muscles are involved

❖ IM glycopyrrolate/atropine to reduce secretions from anticholinesterase therapy

❖ Premedication:
- Smallest effective dose of benzodiazepines may be given
- This is achieved by administering incremental 0.5 mg doses of IV midazolam
- Continuous monitoring for bulbar weakness is essential
- Avoid opioids as respiratory depression is possible

❖ Preoperative plasmapheresis in poorly controlled patients

Anesthetic Considerations

❖ To be scheduled as first case in the day

❖ Regional anesthesia:
- Use regional anesthesia/local anesthetic techniques where possible
- Midthoracic or higher levels can paralyze accessory muscles of breathing
- Thus, high neuraxial blocks should be avoided
- Care while administration of supraclavicular/interscalene block as:
  - Phrenic nerve may be inadvertently blocked
  - This may result in ipsilateral diaphragmatic palsy
  - In poorly controlled patients this may precipitate myasthenic crisis

❖ Increased risk of aspiration if bulbar muscles are involved

❖ Reduced dosage of ester local anesthetics which inhibit plasma cholinesterase

❖ Use short acting anesthetic agents to minimize respiratory depression on emergence

❖ Consider reversal with sugammadex rather than neostigmine

❖ Patients have reduced respiratory reserve:
- Avoid premedication with opioids
- Postoperative ventilation maybe required

Considerations for Neuromuscular Blockade

Succinylcholine

❖ Variable response to succinylcholine occurs in patients with myasthenia

❖ This may be due to the reduced number of ACH receptors

❖ In patients not receiving anticholinesterase therapy:
- Succinylcholine resistance occurs
- This is due to the reduced number of functional AChR at the NMJ
- ED_{95} in these patients is 2.6 times that of normal patients
- Thus, dose can be increased to 2 mg/kg in these patients

❖ In patients receiving anticholinesterase therapy:
- Plasma cholinesterase activity is inhibited
- Succinylcholine metabolism is thereby reduced
- Thus, more succinylcholine is available at the motor end plate
- In effect, the duration of action of succinylcholine increases

❖ In patients who have received plasmapheresis also:
- Plasma cholinesterase levels reduce
- Duration of action of succinylcholine is prolonged

❖ Formation of phase II block occurs with repeat doses of succinylcholine

Nondepolarizing Muscle Relaxants

❖ As a rule, NMBAs are avoided unless absolutely necessary

❖ Patients are extremely sensitive to NDMR as AChRs are reduced by 70%

- Administration of NMBAs and reversal agents have an unpredictable response as:
  - Patients are extremely sensitive to NDMR
  - Patients are resistant to DMR
  - Treatment with anticholinesterases affects the degree of relaxation
- Profound weakness occurs in response to precurarizing dose of muscle relaxants
- Long acting NDMRs like pancuronium are avoided
- Safe NMBAs include:
  - Atracurium
  - Vecuronium
  - Cisatracurium
  - Rocuronium
- When used, these agents are reversed with sugammadex
- Role of mivacurium:
  - Not used as it is metabolized by pseudo cholinesterase
  - Thus, use of pyridostigmine inhibits metabolism of mivacurium
  - Thus, concomitant therapy with pyridostigmine may prolong its action
- Cisatracurium is preferable as:
  - Short $T_{½}$
  - Small V_d
  - Lack of cumulative effect
  - High clearance
  - Spontaneous reversal
- Initial doses of NDMR reduced to 10–20% of normal dose
- Dosage should ideally be titrated with train-of-four response with nerve stimulator
- Corticosteriods may block effects of steroidal relaxants like vecuronium

Monitoring

- *Pulse oximetry*: Temperature
- E_TCO_2
- CVP if significant fluid shifts
- BP-IBP if cardiovascular instability
- Baseline ABG
- Urine output
- Frequent blood sugars
- Neuromuscular monitoring with:
  - Mechanomyogram
  - Twitch monitor
  - Integrated electromyographic monitor
  - Accelograph monitor
- Response to orbicularis oculi is reduced more than adductor pollicis due to ocular involvement

Induction

- Neuromuscular blockade avoided as much as possible
- Propofol (2 mg/kg) + remifentanyl (4–5 μg/kg) + O_2 + N_2O may be used for induction
- Good intubating conditions may be achieved at 2.5 minutes with this technique
- Volatile agents like isoflurane/sevoflurane provide muscle relaxation for intubation
- This effect is however dose dependent
- Thus, NDMRs are used if cardiovascular depressant effects of VA are pronounced
- Initial dose of NDMR is reduced to 10–20% of the normal dose
- LA sprayed on vocal cords to reduce intubation response (4% lidocaine)
- In case of rapid sequence induction, 2 mg/kg SCH can be used safely
- Insert orogastric tube if early return to oral intake not predicted

Maintenance

- Maintanance with O_2 + N_2O + isoflurane + remifentanyl infusion
- Role of NMBAs:
  - Cisatracurium preferred in reduced doses
  - 10–25% of ED_{95} of intermediate acting MRs sufficient for most cases
  - If SCH is used, other MRs are avoided till muscle function has returned
- Controlled ventilation to ensure adequate gas exchange
- TIVA with remifentanyl and propofol infusions can be a safe alternative technique
- Role of dexmedetomidine:
  - Dexmedetomidine for transternal thymectomy is associated with asystole
  - Dexmedetomidine accentuates pyridostigmine associated vagal activity

Extubation

- Reversal should be accomplished with sugammadex rather than neostigmine
- Patient should be extubated in fully awake planes
- Extubation criteria:
  - Ability to maintain normocapnea and adequate oxygenation
  - Train of four ratio > 0.9
  - Ability to generate negative inspiratory pressure >–20 cm H_2O
  - Peak occlusion pressure > 30 cm H_2O
  - FVC > 15 mL/kg with sustained head lift > 5 seconds

- Mechanical ventilation continued till spontaneous recovery of NM function occurs
- Thorough pulmonary toilet is essential prior to extubation
- Use of sugammadex:
    - IV sugammadex 2–4 mg/kg can be used
    - Usually reverses deep NDMR within 4–5 minutes in myasthenia
    - Sugammadex reversal is not affected by anticholinesterase therapy
    - Shown to safely and predictably reverse NMB by steroidal NDMR
- Use of anticholinesterase reversal agents:
    - Patient may be reversed if preoperative symptom control is good
    - Avoid reversal otherwise, as it increases the risk of cholinergic crisis
    - Thus, the dose of neostigmine should be titrated in incremental doses

Postoperative Management

Monitoring

- Pulse oximetry
- Neuromuscular monitoring
- ECG
- Urine output
- BP
- Temperature
- CVP
- ABG and Glucose

Analgesia

- Adequate pain control is necessary
- Use lower doses of opioids to avoid respiratory depression
- Epidural opioids decreases systemic opioid requirements
- Regional anesthesia supplementation should be used where possible
- NSAIDs are useful for their opioid sparing properties
- Multimodal analgesia is key to prevent precipitation of myasthenic crisis

Ventilation

Leventhal Orkin and Hirsh Scoring

No.	Category	Points
1.	Duration of more than 6 years	12
2.	History of COPD	10
3.	Pyridostigmine dose > 750 mg/day	8
4.	Vital capacity < 2.9 L	4

- Score >12 points indicates need for postoperative ventilation
- Not a very specific score
- Even patients with <12 score may require ventilation for:
    - Transternal thymectomy
    - Upper abdominal surgery

Management

- Physiotherapy and incentive spirometry are essential
- Pyridostigmine therapy is resumed as soon as possible post surgery
- Repeated PEFR and FVC measurement to monitor impending respiratory failure
- ABG changes occur very late
- Anticholinesterase therapy:
    - Dosage of neostigmine should be titrated with neuromuscular monitoring
    - Dose titration:
        - 2.5–5 mg IV boluses are given initially
        - 1 mg boluses are then given every 2–3 minutes
        - Dose increased up to the maximal equivalent dose of pyridostigmine
        - 1 mg neostigmine = 30 mg pyridostigmine
        - Oral anticholinesterase therapy is resumed as soon as possible

Complications

- Cholinergic crisis:
    - Occurs due to overdosage of anticholinesterase reversal agents
    - Associated with paradoxical weakness
    - Weakness is seen along with signs of cholinergic excess:
        - Salivation, lacrimation
        - Defecation, emesis
        - Bradycardia
        - Respiratory secretions
        - Bronchospasm
    - ACH induced pupillary contriction (miosis) occurs
    - No improvement/worsening of symptoms with 10 mg tensilon
    - Treatment includes:
        - IV atropine 0.4–2 mg
        - IV glycopyrrollate 0.2–1 mg
        - Profound bradycardia may necessitate electrical pacing Myasthenic crisis:
    - Defined as delayed extubation for more than 24 hours post surgery

- Occurs in postoperative period due to:
  - Underdosage of anticholinesterase reversal agents
  - Residual anesthetic action
  - Stress of surgery
  - Stress associated with infections
  - Administration of drugs known to exacerbate neuromuscular weakness
- Usually causes respiratory and bulbar muscle weakness
- This results in:
  - Dysphagia, change in phonation
  - Weak cough
  - Difficulty in handling secretions
  - Tachypnea with shallow tidal volume breaths
  - Use of accessory muscles of respiration
- ABG shows:
  - Hypocapnia in the initial stages due to hyperventilation
  - Hypercarbia in later stages due to impending respiratory failure
  - Pupillary dilatation may be seen due to hypercarbia
- Tensilon test can be used for diagnosis of myasthenic crisis
- Rapid improvement in symptoms occurs with 10 mg tensilon
- Urgent rapid therapy with plasma exchange or IVIg may be required
- Profound bradycardia may necessitate electrical pacing

EATON-LAMBERT/MYASTHENIC SYNDROME

No.	Feature	Myasthenia Gravis	Lambert-Eaton syndrome
1.	Gender	Female > Male	Male > Female
2.	Age at onset	20–40 yrs	50–70 yrs
3.	Presentation	Weakness of ocular, bulbar, facial	Weakness of proximal muscles
		Fatigue with activity	Increased strength on activity
		Muscle pain uncommon	Muscle pain common
		Normal deep tendon reflexes	Reduced or absent deep tendon reflexes
4.	Pathology	15–20% patients have thymoma	Small cell carcinoma of lung
5.	Electromyography	Voltage decreases to repeated stimulus	Voltage increases to repeated stimulus
6.	Response to MR	Increased sensitivity to NDMR	Increased sensitivity to NDMR
		Resistance to scholine	Increased sensitivity to NDMR
7.	Antibodies	Anti ACHR	Ca^{2+} channel associated synaptogamin
		MUSK antibodies	
8.	Dysautonomia	Absent	Present
9.	Treatment	Anticholinesterase	3,4 diaminopyridine
		Plasmapheresis	Less responsive plasmapheresis
		IV immunoglobulins	
10.	Response to ACHE	Good response	Poor response

HYPERTHERMIA AND NEUROLEPTIC MALIGNANT SYNDROME

Introduction

- Hyperthermia is an elevation in body temperature above 40°C or 104 °F characterized by an unchanged setting of thermoregulatory center
- Fever is an elevation of body temperature which occurs in conjunction with an increase in hypothalamic set point
- Normal body temperature = 36.8°C ± 0.4°C

Etiology

- Heat stroke:
  - Exertional heat stroke
  - Non-exertional:
    - Anticholinergics
    - Antihistaminics
    - Antiparkinsonian
    - Diuretics
    - Phenothiazines
- Drug induced:
  - Amphetamine, cocaine, phencyclidine
  - MDMA (ecstasy), LSD
  - Salicylates, lithium, anticholinergics
  - Sympathomimetics
- Neuroleptic malignant syndrome:
  - Phenothiazines, butyrophenones, metaclopramide, domperidone

- Fluoxetine, loxapine, thiothixene, molindone
- Withdrawal of dopaminergic agents

❖ Serotonin syndrome:
- Selective serotonin reuptake inhibitors
- MAO inhibitors
- Tricyclic antidepressants

❖ Malignant hyperthermia:
- Volatile anesthetics
- Succinylcholine

❖ Endocrinopathy:
- Thyrotoxicosis
- Pheochromocytoma
- Diabetic ketoacidosis

❖ CNS disorders:
- Cerebral hemorrhage
- Status epilepticus
- Hypothalamic injury
- Meningitis, encephalitis, brain abscess

❖ Generalized infection:
- Sepsis
- Malaria
- Typhoid
- Tetanus

Complications of Hyperthermia

No.	System	Initial	Delayed
1.	Vital signs	Hypotension	
		Hyperthermic rebound	
		Hypothermic overshoot	
2.	Muscular	Shivering	
		Rhabdomyolysis	
3.	Neurological	Delirium	Cerebral edema
		Seizures	
		Coma	
4.	Cardiac	Heart failure	
5.	Pulmonary	Pulmonary edema	ARDS
6.	Renal	Oliguria	Renal failure
7.	Gastrointestinal	Diarrhoea	Hepatocellular necrosis
			Mucosal GI hemorrhage
8.	Metabolic	Hypokalemia	Hyperkalemia
		Hypernatremia	Hypocalcemia
			Hyperuricemia

NEUROLEPTIC MALIGNANT SYNDROME

Introduction

❖ Life-threatening neurological emergency associated with the use of neuroleptic (antipsychotic) medications resulting in a classical tetrad of:
- Hyperthermia
- Rigidity
- Autonomic dysfunction
- Change in mental status

Incidence

❖ Ranges from 0.02–3% among patients taking antipsychotic medications

❖ Mostly occurs in young adults although age is not a risk factor

❖ Can occur across all age groups

❖ Occurs more commonly in males

❖ Mortality rate of 10–20%

Etiology

❖ Most commonly seen with high potency first generation antipsychotic agents

❖ However, the syndrome can occur with every class of antipsychotic medication

❖ Symptoms usually develop within 2 weeks of initiating antipsychotic therapy

❖ It is an idiosyncratic reaction and is not dose dependent

❖ Risk factors include:
- Higher doses
- Recent and rapid dose escalation
- Switch of antipsychotic agents
- Parenteral administration
- Concomitant use of lithium/psychotropic drugs
- Withdrawal of L–dopa in Parkinsons patients

❖ Medications associated with NMS include:
- Antipsychotic medications:
  - Aripiprazole, chlorpromazine
  - Clozapine, olanzapine
  - Fluphenazine, paliperidone
  - Haloperidol, quetiapine
  - Perphenazine, risperidone
  - Thioridazine, ziprasidone
  - Amisulpride, zotepine
- Antiemetic agents:
  - Domperidone, metaclopramide
  - Droperidol, prochlorperazine
  - Promethazine

Pathophysiology

❖ Dopamine receptor blockade theory:
- NMS occurs due to dopamine D_2 receptor antagonism
- D_2 receptor blockade in hypothalamus causes an elevated temperature setpoint

- This causes impairment of heat dissipating mechanisms and hyperthermia
- D_2 blockade in nigrostriatal pathways results in Parkinsonism like symptoms

❖ Muscle mitochondrial dysfunction theory:
- Toxic effects of the drug causes changes in mitochondrial function
- This results in increased calcium release from sarcoplasmic reticulum
- This causes hyperthermia, rigidity and increased muscle breakdown

Clinical Features

❖ Classical tetrad of symptoms:
- Hyperthermia
- Rigidity
- Autonomic instability
- Changes in mental status

❖ Tetrad of symptoms slowly evolve over 1–3 days

❖ Muscular rigidity:
- Rigidity is generalized and severe
- Increased tone is characterized by lead pipe rigidity
- Superimposed tremors cause cogwheel phenomenon
- Other motor abnormalities include:
  - Dystonia, opisthotonus
  - Trismus, chorea

❖ Mental status change:
- Initial manifestation in up to 82% patients
- However due to underlying psychiatric illness it may not be appreciated
- Presents as confusion, psychomotor agitation and delirium
- Evolves to profound encephalopathy with stupor and eventual coma

❖ Hyperthermia:
- Temperatures above 38°C is seen in 87% patients
- Temperature above 40°C is seen in 40% patients
- Less common in NMS associated with second generation antipsychotics

❖ Autonomic instability:
- Associated with tachycardia and dysrhythmias
- Results in profuse diaphoresis and labile blood pressure

Investigations

❖ Serum creatinine kinase levels:
- CK values are usually elevated
- More severe rigidity leads to higher CK values
- Typically range between 1000–1,00,000 IU/L
- CK values may be normal early in the disease, before rigidity develops
- CK values above 1000 IU/L correlate well with disease severity and prognosis

❖ Mild elevation in LDH, AST, ALT, alkaline phosphatase levels

❖ Leucocytosis (10,000–40,000 cells/mm^3), thrombocytosis

❖ Hyperuricemia, hyperphosphatemia, myoglobinemia

❖ Dyselectrolytemias:
- Hypocalcemia
- Hypomagnesemia
- Hypo and hypernatremia
- Hyperkalemia
- Metabolic acidosis

❖ Myoglobinuric AKI due to rhabdomyolysis

Diagnostic Criteria

American Psychiatric Association

❖ Major criteria:
- Fever
- Muscle rigidity

❖ Minor criteria:
- Diaphoresis
- Dysphagia
- Tremor
- Incontinence
- Altered mental status
- Mutism
- Tachycardia
- Labile blood pressure
- Leucocytosis
- Elevated CK levels

❖ Diagnostic requirement: Both major and at least 2 minor criteria must be present

Differential Diagnosis

❖ Serotonin syndrome

❖ Malignant hyperthermia

❖ Malignant catatonia

❖ Central anticholinergic syndrome

❖ Meningitis, encephalitis

Treatment

❖ Discontinue causative agent:
- Antipsychotic medications are stopped immediately
- Psychotropic drugs potentiate the syndrome and should be stopped:
  - Lithium
  - Anticholinergic therapy
  - Serotonergic agents

- If L–dopa therapy has been stopped in Parkinsons patients, it has to be restarted

❖ Supportive measures:
- Cardiorespiratory support with:
  - Mechanical ventilation
  - Antiarrhythmic drugs
  - Pacemakers
  - Antihypertensives can be used for HTN:
    - Clonidine is a very effective agent
    - SNP is advantageous as:
      - It facilitates cooling through cutaneous vasodilatation
      - Reduces blood pressure by vasodilatation
- Maintain euvolemia:
  - IV fluids are used to maintain hydration
  - Insensible losses due to fever and diaphoresis should be accounted for
  - Urine is alkalanized to prevent ATN due to rhabdomyolysis
- Cooling and supportive measures:
  - Cooling blankets used to lower core temperature
  - More aggressive methods may be required in extreme hyperthermia:
    - Iced water gastric lavage
    - Ice packs in axilla
    - Administration of acetaminophen

❖ Specific therapy:
- Recommendations for specific treatment are unclear and disputed
- Dantrolene:
  - It is a direct acting muscle relaxant
  - Less well defined role in NMS as compared to MH
  - Reduction of rigidity and hyperthermia can be seen within minutes
  - Initial dose of 1–2.5 mg/kg IV
  - Repeated every 10 minutes up to maximum dose of 10 mg/kg/day
  - Dantrolene is continued for 10 days and then tapered to prevent relapses
- Bromocriptine:
  - Believed to restore the lost dopaminergic tone
  - For treatment of muscular rigidity
  - 2.5 mg is given PO Q6H
  - The dose is titrated to a maximum of 40 mg/day
  - Bromocriptine is continued for 10 days and then tapered to prevent relapses
- Amanditine:
  - Has dopaminergic and anticholinergic effects
  - Used as an alternative to bromocriptine
  - Initial dose is 100 mg given PO or via Ryles tube
  - Titrated to a maximum dose of 200 mg Q12H
- Other medications reported as useful include:
  - Levodopa
  - Apomorphine
  - Carbamazepine
  - Bupropion

❖ Electroconvulsive therapy:
- Used in refractory NMS
- However, it is associated with multiple side effects such as:
  - Status epilepticus
  - Aspiration pneumonia
  - Ventricular arrhythmias

❖ Resumption of antipsychotics:
- Waiting period of 2 weeks following complete resolution for oral medication
- Waiting period of 6 weeks is recommended for parenteral therapy
- Consider resumption with different neuroleptic than the offending agent

HYDROCEPHALUS

Introduction

❖ Congenital/acquired disease causing excessive amount of CSF accumulation within the ventricles or subarachnoid space resulting in:
- Raised ICP
- Ventricular dilatation

Incidence

❖ Incidence of congenital hydrocephalus is 0.6–1.2 cases per 1000 children

❖ Incidence of acquired hydrocephalus is not known

❖ Incidence is increasing due to better survival of preterm infants with intraventricular hemorrhage

❖ Death usually arises due to tonsillar herniation secondary to raised ICP

Etiology

❖ Excessive CSF production:
- Choroid plexus papilloma
- Choroid plexus carcinoma

- Obstruction of CSF pathways:
  - Within ventricular system
    - Lateral ventricle (atrium/body/foramen of ***Monroe)***
    - Third ventricle
    - Acqueductal stenosis
    - Fourth ventricle ***(Dandy–Walker)***
  - Within subarachnoid space
    - Basal cisterns (Chiari, post infectious)
    - Convexity
- Decreased absorption:
  - Obstruction at arachnoid villi:
    - Plugging by tumor cells
    - Protein
    - Blood
    - Bacteria
  - Obstruction of dural venous sinuses:
    - Thrombus
    - Haematological malignancies
    - Infections
  - Obstruction of extracranial venous sinuses:
    - Achondroplasia

Classification

- Communicating hydrocephalus:
  - CSF escapes from ventricular system but not absorbed by arachnoid villi
  - This occurs due to:
    - Obstruction of CSF absorption in subarachnoid space
    - Excessive CSF production
  - Radiographic hallmark is the dilatation of entire ventricular system
  - Causes:
    - Obstruction of absorption:
      - Post-infectious etiology
      - Blood in CSF due to SAH/intraventricular hemorrhage
      - Proteins
      - Tumor cells—choroid plexus papilloma
    - Excessive production:
      - Functional choroid plexus papilloma
      - Choroid plexus carcinoma
- Non-communicating hydrocephalus
  - Also called obstructive hydrocephalus
  - This is the most common cause of hydrocephalus in children
  - Occurs due to structural obstruction of CSF flow within the ventricular system
  - Obstruction to CSF flow can occur at the level of:
    - Foramen of Monroe
    - Aqueduct of Sylvius
    - Fourth ventricle
  - Dilatation of the ventricles occurs proximal to the obstruction
  - Causes include:
    - Infections:
      - Abscess
      - Meningitis –TB/pyogenic
      - Encephalitis
      - Post infectious adhesions
    - Neoplastic:
      - Astrocytoma
      - Ependymoma
      - Choroid plexus papilloma
      - Oligodendroglioma
      - Medulloblastoma
      - Meningioma
    - Vascular:
      - Cerebellar hematomas
      - AV malformation
      - Aneurysm
- Congenital hydrocephalus:
  - Arachnoid cyst
  - Colloid cyst
  - Chiari malformation
  - ***Dandy–Walker*** malformation
  - Atresia of outlet formen

Clinical Features

- Factors determining presentation:
  - Time of onset:
    - Fusion of cranial suture lines prevents increases in intracranial volume
    - Signs of raised ICP will therefore be absent if hydrocephalus develops prior to fusion of sutures
    - In these children, enlarging head circumference is the predominant feature
  - Rate of rise of ICP:
    - Slow accumulation of CSF allows physiological adjustments to occur
    - Thus, symptoms may develop late in these cases
  - Associated structural abnormalities:
    - Hydrocephalus caused by space occupying lesions present early
    - These children may have focal neurodeficits along with hydrocephalus

- In infants:
  - Symptoms:
    - Headache:
      - Occurs due to distortion of meninges and blood vessels
      - Occurs early in the morning on awakening
      - Associated with nausea and vomiting due to raised ICP in posterior fossa
    - Behavioral changes:
      - Characterized by head banging and aggressive behavior
      - Irritability and apathy may be seen
      - This occurs due to raised ICP
    - Developmental delay:
      - Psychomotor delay and gait disturbances seen in older children
      - With progression, brainstem dysfunction causes lethargy
  - Signs:
    - Cranium:
      - Thin and shiny skin
      - Dilated scalp veins
      - Abnormal skull percussion sound (cracked pot/Macewen sign)
      - Bulging anterior fontanelle
      - *Frontal bossing*: Abnormally prominent forehead
      - Cranial enlargement/deformity:
        - Measured between:
          - » Frontal area of head 1–2 cm above glabella
          - » Most prominent part of occiput posteriorly
  - Serial measurements are made to track the disease progress
    - Neurological:
      - Spastic palsy of lower limbs due to stretching of motor fibers
      - Diplopia due to compression of CN III or CN VI
      - ***Sunset Sign***:
        - Occurs due to impairment of upward gaze
        - This results in inferiorly deviated eyes
        - Thus, sclera above the cornea becomes visible
        - Occurs due to pressure on the midbrain
    - Ocular:
      - Strabismus, ptosis
      - Papilledema with absent pulsations in retinal blood vessels
      - Loss of corneal reflex
    - Cardiovascular:
      - ***Cushing's triad*** comprising of:
        - Hypertension
        - Bradycardia
        - Altered respiratory rate
      - Occurs due to distortion of the brain stem

Variations

- Normal pressure hydrocephalus:
  - Cerebral ventricles are pathologically enlarged with normal ICP
  - Most commonly seen in older adults (above 60 years)
  - Believed to occur due to chronic periventricular ischemia
  - This causes increased compliance of ventricular wall and enlargement
  - Associated with classical triad of:
    - Abnormal gait
    - Dementia
    - Urinary incontinence
- Hydrocephalus ex–vacuo:
  - Ventricular dilatation with normal ICP is seen
  - Usually seen in association with atrophy of brain tissue
  - Occurs due to reduced volume of brain causing enlarged ventricles
  - Thus, enlargement of ventricles is not associated with raised ICP
  - There may be focal distortion of the normal anatomy

Differential Diagnosis

- Megalencephaly:
  - ***Hurler's syndrome, Tay Sachs disease***
  - No increase in ICP or ventricular size
- Chronic subdural hematoma
  - Large head
  - Located in parietal region
  - No sunset sign/scalp vein prominence
- Hydrencephaly
- Rickets, achondroplasia
- Hemolytic anemia

Diagnosis

- Serial head circumference measurement
  - Increase of more than 2 cm every month during first 3 months of life

- Normal head circumference measurements:
  - At birth –35 cm
  - 3 months –41 cm
  - 6 months –43 cm
  - 2 year –49 cm
- ❖ Skull radiographs:
  - Persistent widening of sagittal and coronal suture > 0.5 cm after 2 weeks of life
  - CT Scan/MRI for confirmation and etiology
  - Cranial USG for ventricular size
  - Shunt scan for site of malfunction if preexisting shunt present

Surgical Management

- ❖ Surgical excision of obstructive lesion
- ❖ Extracranial shunts:
  - Ventriculoperitoneal shunt (*most common*)
  - Ventriculoatrial shunt
  - Ventriculopleural shunt
  - Lumboperitoneal shunt
- ❖ External ventricular drain (EVD)
- ❖ Endoscopic ventriculostomy

Ventriculoperitoneal Shunt

- ❖ A catheter is inserted via a burrhole into the frontal horn of lateral ventricle
- ❖ The burrhole is created in the occipitoparietal or frontal region
- ❖ The catheter is always inserted on the non-dominant side (right side)
- ❖ A valve system is present which:
  - Allows CSF drainage once ICP exceeds a certain value
  - Prevents CSF draining too rapidly with changes in posture
- ❖ The valve system is placed subcutaneously beneath the postauricular area
- ❖ The distal end of the valve system is connected to a catheter
- ❖ This catheter is passed through a subcutaneous tunnel to a point near epigastrum
- ❖ It is then inserted into peritoneal space through small laparotomy
- ❖ Inadvertent gastrotomy can occur if stomach is inflated during insertion
- ❖ A flushing device is present in the burrhole to keep the system clear
- ❖ Complications include:
  - Shunt malfunction
  - Infections
  - Overdrainage

Lumboperitoneal Shunt

- ❖ Done in lateral position
- ❖ Catheter positioned is lumbar CSF space via Tuohy needle
- ❖ Catheter tunnelled subcutaneously to anterior abdominal wall
- ❖ Inserted into peritoneal space via small laparotomy

Endoscopic Ventriculostomy

- ❖ Rationale:
  - Creates a hole in floor of third ventricle
  - This allows CSF to flow into the prepontine cistern and subarachnoid space
  - May be used for treatment of obstructive hydrocephalus
  - It is not useful for patients with communicating hydrocephalus
- ❖ Procedure:
  - Burrhole is created in the skull
  - Percutaneous flexible neurendoscope is passed through burrhole
  - Ventriculostomy created in the floor of third ventricle
  - This bypasses the obstruction which is causing the hydrocephalus
- ❖ Advantages:
  - Minimally invasive as it is done through a burrhole
  - Absence of any indwelling catheter (foreign body)
- ❖ Disadvantages:
  - Can damage structures in the floor of third ventricle
  - Damage to basilar artery/branches and nerve injury is possible
  - Associated with bradycardia, asystole and arrhythmias

External Ventricular Drain

- ❖ Done as an emergency procedure for acute hydrocephalus
- ❖ This is used as a temporizing maneuver until a permanent shunt can be placed
- ❖ This system consists of a small catheter inserted into the lateral ventricle
- ❖ The catheter is connected to a closed collecting device for CSF collection
- ❖ EVD should be clamped during transfer of patient
- ❖ Also height of the drainage bag should be kept constant with respect to the patient
- ❖ This is because sudden, rapid CSF drainage causes rupture of cortical veins and SDH

Anesthetic Considerations 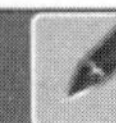

- Difficult IV access if multiple prior surgeries
- Difficult airway due to macrocephaly
- Risk of aspiration due to:
  - Altered sensorium
  - Increased propensity for vomiting
- Maintain normal blood pressure to maintain cerebral perfusion
- Maintain normothermia
- Dyselectrolytemia may be present due to vomiting/hormonal alterations
- Avoid factors causing an increase in ICP:
  - Hypoxia
  - Hypercapnea
  - Succinylcholine
  - Ketamine
- Presence of pre-existing EVD:
  - Risk of dislodgement during transfer of the patient
  - Risk of rapid CSF drainage (due to non-clamping) and SDH
  - Avoid changing height of the drainage bag with respect to the head
- Risk of venous air embolism (especially ventriculo–atrial shunts)
- Risk of latex allergy especially in those with associated meningomyelocele

Preanesthetic Assessment

History

- Vomiting: Suggests increase ICP and delayed gastric emptying
- Drug history:
  - Steroids: Glucose intolerance
  - Anticonvulsants: Enzyme induction
- Immunization history for congenital rubella

Examination

- Airway assessment: Difficult airway due to enlarged head
- Pulmonary compliance and renal function assessed
- Neurological status and gag reflex to assess ability to protect airway
- Level of consciousness which is an indicator of raised ICP

Investigations

- Complete blood count
- Electrolytes
- ECG
- Blood glucose
- Renal Function Tests
- Arterial blood gas
- Liver Function Test
- Skull X-ray
- CT scan
- *Ultrasonography*: For size site and vascularity of lesions

Preoperative Optimization and Premedication

- NPO orders:
  - 6 hrs solids, milk
  - 4 hrs breast milk
  - 2 hrs water, clear fluids
- Informed consent
- Secure or evaluate existing intravenous access as it may be required for:
  - Acute interventions
  - Rapid sequence induction
- Correct dehydration/electrolyte imbalance occurring due to vomiting and diuretics
- Restrict IV fluids to 30 mL/kg/day if cerebral edema is present
- Avoid glucose containing IV fluids as:
  - It decreases osmolality
  - Increases cerebral edema
  - Also has poor postoperative neurological outcome
- *Avoid routine use of premedication* as raised ICP alters the level of consciousness
- Avoid atropine and if sympathetic nervous system is immature
- Prophylactic phenytoin is usually required:
  - 15 mg/kg IV loading dose
  - This is followed by single daily dose of 3–4 mg/kg
- Antibiotic prophylaxis as per hospital protocol
- Emotional preparation in older children
- Compression stocking for DVT prophylaxis
- In the presence of a pre-existing EVD:
  - Close the EVD prior to transport to avoid excess CSF drainage
  - Determine the maximum permissible time for clamping the EVD
  - The safe time interval for clamping the EVD is usually 15 minutes
  - The height of the bag with respect to the head should not be changed
  - In the presence of an open EVD, lowering the bag may drain CSF quickly
  - This may lead to collapse of the ventricles and rupture of cortical bridging veins
  - This ultimately results in subdural hematoma
  - Care must be taken while shifting to prevent dislodgement of the EVD catheter

Monitoring

- ECG
- Pulse oximetry
- E_TCO_2
- Urine output
- NIBP/IBP if hemodynamically unstable

- Core temperature as the procedure entails exposure of large surface area of body
- Fontanelle palpation for online trend monitoring of ICP

Induction

- Inhalational induction:
  - Used when IV access unavailable
  - Technique is avoided when child is stuporus
  - Sevoflurane is the *agent of choice* as:
    - Minimal effect on cerebral hemodynamics
    - Cardiac stability
    - Absence of airway irritation
- Intravenous induction:
  - *Rapid sequence induction* is the preferred technique
  - This is due to increased chances of vomiting and aspiration as a result of:
    - Raised ICP
    - Delayed gastric emptying time
  - Succinylcholine 1–1.5 mg/kg, fentanyl 2–3 µg/kg, thiopentone 3–4 mg/kg
  - Succinylcholine can marginally raise the ICP
  - However, this effect can be offset by:
    - Hyperventilation
    - Adequate dose of intravenous anesthetic agents
  - Hyperventilation with low inspiratory pressures is preferred
  - Deep planes at intubation to avoid coughing which increases ICP
  - *IV lidocaine avoided as it may cause sudden cardiac arrest*
  - RAE tube may be used as airway is remote

Position

- Supine with the head turned to opposite direction
- Patients with raised ICP are placed in 30° head up position
- Minimal neck rotation/flexion should be ensured after positioning
- This improves cerebral venous drainage
- Patients with posteriorly placed shunt tubing are placed in lateral position
- All extremities should be adequately padded and axillary roll should be placed

Maintenance

- Isoflurane/sevoflurane and fentanyl boluses are used to maintain anesthesia
- Minimal doses of volatile agents should be used as it increases CBF and ICP
- Remifentanyl infusion 0.5 µg/kg/min ensures adequate analgesia
- Vecuronium or atracurium can be used for muscle paralysis
- Nitrous oxide is avoided as it:
  - Increases cerebral blood flow
  - Increases cerebral blood volume
  - Causes gastric distension (may cause inadvertent gastrostomy during laparotomy)
  - Postoperative nausea and vomiting causing raised ICP
- Additional muscle relaxation provided before laparotomy
- Opioid boluses are usually required during burrowing of the subcutaneous tunnel

Ventilation

- Spontaneous ventilation not preferred as it:
  - Increases the risk of venous air embolism (ventriculoatrial shunts)
  - Increases chances of pneumothorax (ventriculopleural shunts)
- Spontaneous ventilation is avoided at the time of opening the cranial vault
- Normocapnea is the goal if ICP is normal
- Hyperventilation with $PaCO_2$ between 25–30 mm Hg in patients with raised ICP

Hemodynamics

- No significant blood loss/third space loss occurs during surgery
- Blood loss may occur from burrhole if dural veins are enlarged
- Avoid hypothermia from cooling and evaporation:
  - Overhead warmer
  - Drape the limbs properly
  - Use warm IV solutions
- Sudden hypotension occurs during cannulation of the ventricle due to fall in ICP
- Bradycardia/arrhythmias may occur due to shift in intracranial content

Emergence

- Adequate reversal of neuromuscular blockade should be ensured prior to extubation
- Extubate fully awake after full recovery of protective reflexes
- Avoid coughing/straining during extubation
- Gastric contents should be suctioned out prior to extubation

- Postoperative ventilation is preferred in the presence of preoperative apnea/bradycardia due to intracranial abnormalities

Postoperative Management

Pain

- Usually associated with only minor postoperative discomfort
- Analgesic options include:
  - Paracetamol
  - Low dose morphine during the first 24 hours
  - LA infilteration over abdominal incision at end of surgery

Management

- Continue IV fluids until the resumption of adequate oral intake
- Maintain normothermia
- If focal neurological signs appear, urgent CT scan to rule out intracranial hematoma

Monitoring

- Pulse oximetry
- Urine output
- Blood pressure
- CNS status
- ECG
- Temperature

Complications

- Nausea, vomiting
- Seizures
- Shunt infection/obstruction—acute hydrocephalus
- Pneumothorax/hemothorax if subcutaneous trocar penetrates pleura
- *Venous air embolism* (common in ventriculoatrial shunt)
- Blood loss if dural veins are breached
- Subdural hemorrhage if CSF is drained too rapidly due to rupture of bridging veins
- Inadvertent tunnelling of VP shunt into chest cavity

MENINGOMYELOCELE

Introduction

- Meningomyelocele is NTD causing hernial protrusion of a part of meninges and spinal cord through a cleft in the vertebral column with a corresponding defect in the skin
- It is the *most common* primary neural tube defect
- It is also called:
  - Spina bifida
  - Open spinal dysraphism (as the neural tissue is exposed)
- Neural tube defects or myelodysplasia refers to abnormality in fusion of embryological neural groove that normally closes in first month of gestation

Anatomy

- The defect results from failure of neural tube closure within 28 days of conception
- At the superior margin of the lesion in the midline is a small opening
- This in the opening into the central canal of the closed spinal cord
- CSF from the central canal oozes out from this opening if the sac has not ruptured
- The embryonic ventral sulcus runs caudally in the midline
- On either side of the sulcus are the motor plates
- The motor nerves exit from the ventral surface of these plates
- The outer lateral plates are the sensory plates
- Sensory nerves enter at the lateral edge of these plates
- At the lateral edge, the defect is attached to the dysplastic meninges and skin

Incidence

- Ranges from 1–7 per 1000 live births
- Highest rates seen in China, Ireland, Great Britain and India
- Girls are more commonly affected

Clinical Features

- Usually obvious at birth due to the grossly visible lesion
- Appears as red fleshy plaque seen through a defect in vertebral column (spina bifida)

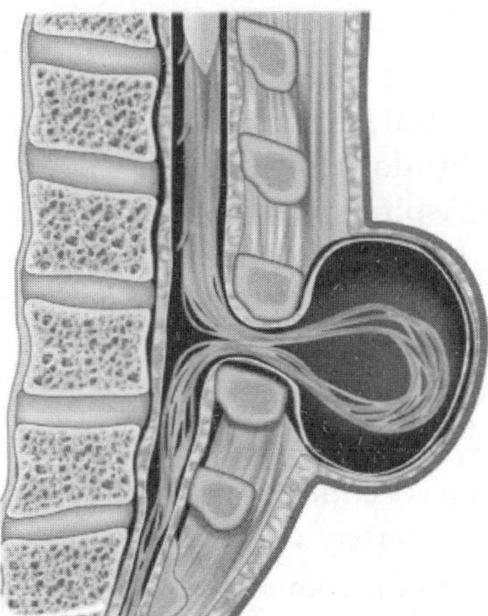

Fig. 6: Meningomyelocele.

- A protruding membranous sac containing meninges, CSF and nerve roots may be seen
- The exposed neural tissue may be flat or elevated by the CSF sac below
- Seen in lumbosacral or sacral region in up to 80% of cases
- However, any segment of the vertebral column may be involved
- Neurological problems:
  - Isolated meningocele patients are usually born without CNS deficits
  - Motor deficits occur if spinal cord is tethered caudally by sacral roots
  - Characterized by:
    - Flaccid/spastic paraplegia
    - Absence of sensations
  - Chiari II malformation is commonly seen with meningomyelocele
  - Components of Chiari II malformation:
    - Downward displacement of cerebellar tonsils and medulla
    - Meningomyelocele
  - Varying degrees of brainstem dysfunction occur due to Chiari malformation
  - Hydrocephalus:
    - Seen in 90% of patients with spina bifida
    - Commonly seen in children with higher vertebral lesions
    - Leads to multiple hospitalizations for shunt revisions
    - Thus, it is a major cause of morbidity and mortality
  - Brainstem dysfunction:
    - Occurs in 20% patients
    - Vocal cord and other cranial nerve palsy due to:
      - Pressure on brainstem
      - Focal infarcts of brainstem
    - Clinical features:
      - Stridor, apnea
      - Aspiration pneumonia
      - Lack of coordination and spasticity
      - Bradycardia, hypertension
- Orthopedic problems:
  - Congenital skeletal deformities of feet, knees, hips and spine
  - Scoliosis occurs in most children with lesion above L_2 vertebra
  - Other lesions commonly seen are:
    - Kyphosis
    - Clubfoot
    - Rocker bottom foot
    - Ankle valgus
    - Hip deformities such as contractures, subluxation and dislocation
- Bowel and bladder problems:
  - Innervation of the bowel and bladder are affected in almost all patients
  - This results in the loss of anal urethral and bladder sphincter tone
  - Bowel disturbances include:
    - Bowel incontinence in 60–70% of patients
    - Decreased bowel motility, constipation and fecal impaction
  - Bladder disturbances seen include:
    - Neurogenic bladder
    - Recurrent UTI complicated by gram negative sepsis
    - Severe dilatation of upper urinary tract
    - Bladder exstrophy and prolapsed uterus
- Associated abnormalities:
  - Latex allergy:
    - Due to:
      - Impaired immune system
      - Repeated exposure to latex products from frequent hospitalization
      - Daily bladder catherization for those with neurogenic bladder
    - Limit latex exposure especially
    - ***Latex free surgical environment***
  - Other associated conditions:
    - ***Klippel Feil syndrome***
    - Congenital cardiac defects
    - Clubfoot
    - Dislocation of hips
    - Scoliosis

Timing of Intervention

- Meningomyelocele exposes neural tissue and places the patient at risk for infections
- Delay in the surgical repair results in:
  - Increased risk of infections
  - Progressive neurological dysfunction
  - Decreased motor function
- Infection occurs in less than 7% patients if repaired within 48 hours of birth
- Thus, meningomyelocele is a neurological emergency
- It is repaired preferably within first 48 hours of birth
- If infected surgery is done only when three 24 hour CSF cultures are sterile

Investigations

- General investigations:
  - Complete blood count, electrolytes, blood glucose, RFTS
  - Blood for grouping and cross matching
  - Ultrasonography of head, menigomyelocele sac and kidney if possible
  - Chest X-ray, X-ray spine
  - Cultures from lesion and draining CSF
- Diagnostic investigations:
  - Prenatal ultrasound—pick up rate of 100%
  - Elevated maternal serum α feto protein: 50 –90% pick up
  - Amniotic fluid α feto protein is more reliable and done between 14–16 wks gestation
  - Amniotic fluid acetylcholine esterase
  - CT and MRI confirms anomaly, Neural tube defects and spinal cord anomalies

Management

- Surgery not done if Lorber's selection criteria are met:
  - Severe paraplegia at or below L_3
  - Severe kyphosis/scoliosis
  - Gross hydrocephalus
  - Other associated gross congenital anomalies
  - Major intracerebral birth injury
- Most centers close defect and place shunt for hydrocephalus at same time
- Repaired within 24–48 hours of birth
- Surgical steps include:
  - Release of neural placode
  - Closure of dura in a watertight fashion
  - Mobilization of adjacent soft tissue flaps
  - Layered closure of soft tissue flap

Preoperative Assessment

- History:
  - Drug history
  - Folic acid supplementation during pregnancy
  - Recurrent UTI
  - History of itching/rashes/wheezing on exposure to latex
- Examination:
  - Neurological examination:
    - Lesions above level of T4 result in paraplegia
    - Lesions below S1 usually allow ambulation
  - Vocal cord mobility
  - Ventilatory response to hypoxia and hypercarbia
  - Gastro-esophageal reflux and aspiration
  - Other life-threatening congenital anomalies

Anesthetic Considerations

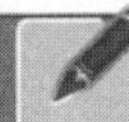

- Care during intraoperative positioning to avoid cyst rupture:
  - Use of circular gel pad/doughnut in supine position
  - Prone position can be used as alternative
- Preoperative nursing in prone position to avoid cyst rupture
- Difficult airway if large meningomyelocele present at cervical level
- High incidence of hypothermia due to:
  - Exposure of large surface area
  - High third space loss
  - Loss of autonomic control below the level of the lesion
- Considerations in fluid management:
  - High third space loss due to exposure of large surface area
  - Potential for intraoperative blood loss during dissection of skin flaps to cover defect
- Anesthetic considerations arising from associated defects:
  - Arnold Chiari malformation
  - Congenital heart disease
  - Prematurity
- Latex allergy: Latex free surgical environment to be ensured
- Considerations due to brainstem dysfunction:
  - Absent/reduced response to hypoxia and hypercarbia
  - Impaired swallowing and gag reflex predisposing to postoperative aspiration
- Avoid high oxygen concentrations to prevent *retinopathy of prematurity*
- Prevent infection: Antibiotics in preoperative period

Preoperative Preparation and Premedication

- NPO guidelines
- Informed consent
- Nurse in prone position
- Cover placode with saline soaked Telfa pads/sterile sponges to prevent dessication
- Antibiotic therapy in preoperative period according to hospital protocol
- Fluid therapy to correct deficits as intraoperative third space loss is substantial

Anesthetic Management

Done in latex free surgical environment.

Monitor

- Pulse oximetry
- $E_T CO_2$
- NIBP
- ECG
- Precordial stethoscope
- Invasive blood pressure monitoring if:
  - Large size defects

- Multilevel meningomyelocele where significant mobilization of skin is needed
- Encephalocele requiring craniotomy

❖ Central venous line in repairs of nasal encephalocele done in semi–sitting position

❖ Blood loss as it may be large volume but insidious

❖ Electromyography to identify functional nerve roots

Induction

❖ *Inhalational induction*:
- Done if no intravenous access
- Sevoflurane is the *agent of choice*

❖ *Intravenous induction*:
- Adequate preoxygenation
- Propofol 1–2 mg/kg + NDMR + fentanyl 1–2 μg/kg
- RAE tube may be used
- *Rapid sequence induction* in the presence of:
  - Large hydrocephalus
  - Large cervical meningomyelocele
- If large cervical meningomyelocele awake intubation in lateral/supine position
- Patients with nasal encephalocele may have airway obstruction

Position

❖ During induction:
- Supine position
- Defect rests in *doughnut* to minimize trauma
- Lateral position may be tried if defect is large

❖ During surgery:
- Prone position
- Rolls placed under chest and hips to free the abdomen
- Abdomen and chest to be free to avoid pressure on epidural veins
- This helps in reducing intraoperative blood loss
- Prevent injury to exposed neural tissue
- Extremities in relaxed position and adequately padded
- Avoid excess rotation of neck

Maintenance

❖ O_2 + isoflurane + titrated fentanyl boluses

❖ High O_2 concentrations avoided to prevent *retinopathy of prematurity*

❖ Avoid NMBAs as nerve stimulator is used for identification of neural structures

❖ Opioid doses are limited to prevent postoperative apnea

Hemodynamics

❖ Large third space losses occur and are to be replaced with normal saline

❖ Possibility of underestimating fluid and blood loss from deficit is high

❖ Increased blood loss when large amount of skin is required to cover defect

❖ Excessive blood loss may warrant transfusion

❖ Rupture of cyst with CSF leakage can occur

❖ This is replaced with full strength balanced salt solution

❖ Avoid hypothermia using radiant heat warmers

❖ Drying/thermal injury to neural tissues from radiant heat warmers has to be prevented

Extubation

❖ Adequate reversal of neuromuscular blockade has to be ensured

❖ Fully awake extubation preferred for:
- Neonates at risk for postoperative apnea
- Severe central neurodeficits
- Craniotomy for encephalocele

❖ Criteria for extubation:
- Intact cough and gag reflex
- Negative inspiratory force of 15–30 cmH_2O
- Forced vital capacity breath in excess of 10 mL/kg
- Air leak around ETT with peak airway pressure below 25 cmH_2O
- Acceptable oxygenation and ventilation on minimal ventilatory support

❖ Residual airway obstruction due to blood may occur in surgery for nasal encephalocele

Postoperative Management

Management

❖ Nurse in prone position

❖ Prevent hypothermia

❖ Humidified gases to be used

❖ Monitoring:
- ECG
- NIBP
- Pulse oximetry
- Urine output
- Temperature
- Neurological status for hydrocephalus especially in the absence of VP shunts

Analgesia

❖ NSAIDs

❖ Low dose morphine

❖ Use of narcotics is limited postoperatively

- This is because these children are susceptible to respiratory depression
- LA infilteration around wound site
- *Multimodal analgesia*

Complications

- *Respiratory*: Especially in those with brainstem abnormalities
  - Stridor and laryngospasm
  - Post extubation apnea
  - Bronchospasm
  - Prolonged breath holding
- Cardiovascular complications:
  - Bradycardia
  - Hypotension
  - Tachycardia
  - Arrhythmias (especially in association with Chiari malformation)
- Cranial nerve palsy causing inspiratory stridor
- Brainstem herniation
- Hydrocephalus

Regional Anesthesia

- Spinal anesthesia with hyperbaric 0.5% tetracaine has been used
- 2 out of 14 infants had adverse postoperative respiratory events
- This was seen when subarachnoid block was supplemented with midazolam sedation
- No evidence of anesthesia induced CNS depression was seen

Prevention of Neural Tube Defects

Folate Supplementation

- Decreases risk of neural tube defects by 70%
- 0.4 mg/day of folic acid for primary prevention
- If previously delivered child with NTD, 5 mg/day for subsequent prevention
- Prophylaxis is given for 2 months before and 3 months after conception

POSTERIOR FOSSA SURGERY

Introduction

- Posterior fossa is the deepest cranial fossa
- The important contents of the posterior fossa require special considerations by surgeons and anesthesiologists

Anatomy

- Components:
  - Neuronal components:
    - Cerebellum
    - Pons
    - Medulla
    - Fourth ventricle
    - Lower cranial nerves
  - Vascular components:
    - Vertebral arteries
    - Basilar arteries
    - Superior petrosal sinus
    - Transverse sinus
    - Sigmoid sinus
- Boundaries
  - *Superiorly*: Dural layer of tentorium cerebelli
  - *Floor*: Occipital bone
  - *Laterally*: Petrosal and mastoid components of temporal bone
  - *Anteriorly*: Clivus of occipital bone
- Importance
  - Vital neuronal and vascular structures are contained within the space
  - Relatively small masses in this restrictive compartment can cause brain herniation
  - Pons and medulla contain major sensory and motor pathways:
    - Cardiovascular and respiratory centres
    - Lower cranial nerve nuclei
    - Reticular activating system (RAS)
    - Networks for protective reflexes like gag, cough, eye blink
  - CSF flows out from third ventricle to fourth ventricle and out on surface of brain through ***foramen of Magendie and Luschka*** Any obstruction at the foramen will cause hydrocephalus.

Posterior Fossa Lesions

- Tumors:
  - Axial tumors:
    - Medulloblastoma (commonest)
    - Cerebellar astrocytoma
    - Brainstem glioma
    - Ependymoma
    - Choroid plexus papilloma
    - Dermoid tumors
    - Hemangioblastoma
    - Metastatic tumors

- Cerebellopontine angle tumors:
  - Schwannoma
  - Meningioma
  - Acoustic neuroma
  - Glomus jugular tumor
- ❖ Cranial nerve lesions:
  - Trigeminal neuralgia (CN V)
  - Hemifacial spasm (CN VII)
  - Glossopharyngeal neuralgia (CN IX)
- ❖ Vascular lesions:
  - Aneurysm of:
    - Superior cerebellar artery
    - Posterior inferior cerebellar artery
    - Vertebral artery
    - Basillar artery
  - AV malformation
  - Cerebellar hematomas: Spontaneous and traumatic
  - Cerebellar infarction
  - Hemangiomas
- ❖ Craniocervical abnormalities:
  - Atlanto–occipital instability:
    - Congenital
    - Acquired
  - Atlanto–axial instability:
    - Congenital
    - Acquired
- ❖ Others:
  - Cysts:
    - Epidermoid cyst
    - Arachnoid cyst
- ❖ Abscesses
- ❖ Arnold–Chiari malformation

Posterior Fossa Surgeries

- ❖ Tumor excision/debulking
- ❖ Foramen magnum decompression
- ❖ Vascular procedures
- ❖ Decompression of cranial nerve V (***Tic Douloureaux***):
  - Dissection along intracranial portion of nerves
  - Identification of offending blood vessel which encroaches on nerve
  - Placement of insulating Teflon pad between blood vessel and nerve
- ❖ Decompression of CN VII (Hemifacial spasm) and CN IX (Glossopharyngeal Neuralgia)
- ❖ Balloon compression of trigeminal ganglion:
  - Rapid inflation of Fogarty type balloon within ***Meckel's cave***
  - Balloon is introduced percutaneously through cheek and beneath maxilla
  - General anesthesia is preferred as it is a very painful procedure
  - Profound bradycardia is sign of adequate compression of the ganglion

Surgical Approaches to Posterior Fossa

- ❖ Suboccipital approach
- ❖ Supracerebellar intratentorial approach
- ❖ Transtemporal approach
- ❖ Transoral approach

Complications of Posterior Fossa Surgery

- ❖ Venous air embolism (VAE):
  - VAE occurs in almost 76% patients undergoing posterior fossa surgery
  - This is commonly seen in sitting position as:
    - Operative site is 20 cm above the heart
    - This creates a subatmospheric pressure in the dural venous sinuses
    - Also, the venous sinuses are kept open by the dura and bone in the fossa
    - This provides an excellent portal for air entry in hypovolemic patients
    - Aspiration of air into the venous sinuses is the end result
  - Factors modifying severity of VAE:
    - Position of the patient
    - Volume and rate of air entering venous sinuses
    - Central venous pressure
    - Type of ventilation
  - Clinical feature depends on the rate of air entry:
    - Single large bolus:
      - Causes air lock in right heart
      - This results in:
        - Acute right ventricular failure
        - Arrhythmias
        - Myocardial ischemia
        - Frank cardiovascular collapse
    - Slow entrainment of large volume of air:
      - The entrained air enters into pulmonary circulation
      - This impairs blood flow distal to the pulmonary artery
      - This causes a progressive increase in CVP and PA pressure
      - This ultimately leads to:
        - Ventilation perfusion mismatch
        - Pulmonary edema
        - Bronchoconstriction
  - The lethal dose of air in humans is:
    - 3–5 mL/kg
    - 200–300 mL bolus

- Pneumocephalus:
  - Complication of surgery in the sitting position
  - Techniques used to reduce brain volume during surgery encourage intracranial air entry
  - This can raise the ICP once cranium is closed
  - Sufficient air entry into epidural or dural spaces causes a mass effect
  - Nitrous oxide aggravates pneumocephalus and, is avoided
  - Clinical features:
    - Delayed recovery
    - Neurological deficits
    - Headache, confusion, agitation
    - Convulsions
    - Herniation and cardiac arrest
  - Treatment:
    - High flow oxygen therapy
    - Burr hole and aspiration of air
- Quadriplegia:
  - Caused by prolonged focal pressure on the spinal cord
  - Occurs secondary to acute flexion of the head during prolonged surgery
  - Particularly common in sitting position
  - Episodes of significant hypotension during surgery may aggravate the insult
- Airway obstruction due to:
  - Macroglossia:
    - Occurs due to obstruction to venous and lymphatic drainage of tongue
    - Potentiating factors:
      - Prolonged surgery
      - Increased neck flexion
      - Use of oropharyngeal airways
  - Partial damage to vagus nerve
  - Increased flexion of cervical spine
- Brain stem damage:
  - Due to postoperative posterior fossa swelling
  - This can sometimes occur few hours after a good initial recovery
  - Detected by deterioration in CNS status after surgery
  - Posterior fossa swelling due to:
    - Tendency of cerebellum to swell after prolonged retraction
    - Bleeding and hematoma
    - Reduced respiration may result from and also may increase swelling
- Cranial nerve injuries:
  - Can occur during dissection on floor of fourth ventricle
  - CN IX, X and XII, VII and VIII may get injured
  - This results in:
    - Loss of patency of upper airway
    - Decreased gag reflex
- Other complications:
  - Postoperative nausea and vomiting especially after CP angle surgeries
  - CSF leak (most common complication)
  - Meningitis
  - Wound infection
  - Hydrocephalus
  - Hematomas
- Hemodynamic perturbations especially in the presence of autonomic neuropathy

Anesthetic Goals

- Facilitate surgical access:
  - Decrease brain volume
  - Control ICP
- Minimize nervous tissue trauma
- Maintain respiratory stability
- Maintain cardiovascular stability
- Facilitate rapid awakening

Anesthetic Considerations

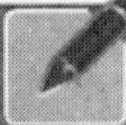

- Facilitate optimal brain relaxation for surgical exposure
- Maintain cerebral perfusion pressure
- Considerations for sitting position:
  - Hemodynamic alterations: Hypotension
  - Venous air embolism, paradoxical air embolism
  - Macroglossia and airway obstruction
  - Pneumocephalus
- Brain stem and cranial nerve manipulation:
  - Hemodynamic alterations
  - Vital centre dysfunction
  - Cranial nerve injury causing poor gag reflex postoperatively
  - Vocal cord palsy and stridor
  - Delayed awakening: Reticular activating system
  - Poor preoperative nutrition and dehydration due to dysphagia
  - Facilitate rapid and smooth emergence

Preoperative Considerations and Premedication

- History:
  - Nausea, vomiting
  - Aspiration
  - Hoarseness, dysphagia
- Examination:
  - Assess intracranial pressure status:
    - Hydrocephalus is common in posterior fossa lesions

- Assess for:
  - Level of consciousness
  - Headache
  - Histroy of vomiting
- Assess ICP response to steroids
- If hydrocephalus is present, EVD may be required prior to surgery
- Assess cranial nerve dysfunction:
  - Lower cranial nerve dysfunction causes loss of gag reflex
  - This predisposes to aspiration pneumonia
  - In the presence of bulbar dysfunction, prepare for:
    - Postoperative ventilation
    - Tracheostomy
- Assess the hydration status:
  - These patients are prone to dehydration as a result of:
    - Reduced oral intake from altered sensorium
    - Administration of diuretics
    - Presence of diabetes insipidus
    - Use of IV contrast agents for imaging
  - Preoperative fluid administration may be required in these cases
- Cardiovascular system:
  - Tolerance of sitting and prone position
  - Echo for paten foramen ovale (predisposes to PAE in sitting position)
  - Preoperative uncontrolled HTN predisposes the patient for hypotension
- Respiratory system:
  - Indirect laryngoscopy for vocal cord palsy and Mallampatti grade
  - Have reduced levels of consciousness and impaired airway reflexes
  - Increased chances of silent aspiration if bulbar palsy

❖ Special investigations:
- Coagulation status
- Echocardiography: Bubble contrast for detection of PFO
- Pulmonary function tests
- Auditory function for schwanomma surgery
- Scans should be examined for:
  - Size of lesions
  - Degree of edema
  - Presence of hydrocephalus
- Blood glucose in patients on chronic steroids
- Premedication:
  - Ensure availability of adequate cross matched blood
  - Premedication is usually witheld in patients with abnormal intracranial elastance
  - Preoperative steroid therapy is continued
  - Preoperative fluid therapy to correct electrolyte imbalance

Positions used for Posterior Fossa Surgery

❖ Prone position:
- Procedure:
  - Head is secured with three-point fixation in adults
  - Mayfield horseshoe rest can be used for head fixation in children
  - Neck is flexed to allow optimal surgical access
  - Avoid abdominal compression while positioning
  - This increases cerebral venous pressure and bleeding
  - Ensure adequate padding of:
    - Elbows, knees
    - Genitals
    - Superficial peripheral nerves (ulnar, tibial)
  - Breasts should be tucked inwards to avoid pressure on nipples
  - Chest and pelvis should be adequately supported
  - Fibreoptic confirmation of ETT after positioning is recommended
  - This is to rule out distal migration of the ETT following neck flexion
  - Check for patency of intravascular catheters after final positioning
- Advantages:
  - Allows good access to midline structures
  - Incidence of venous air embolism is lesser compared with sitting position
- Disadvantages:
  - Malposition of endotracheal tube occurs frequently
  - Increased bleeding is seen in prone position
  - Associated with complications such as:
    - Neuropathies
    - Facial and airway edema
    - Blindness due to:
      - Retinal artery thrombosis
      - Ischemic optic neuropathy

❖ Lateral position:
- Used for unilateral procedures in upper posterior fossa
- Provides access to:
  - Cerebellopontine angle

- Cerebellum
- Infracerebellar region
- Procedure:
  - Lower arm is placed next to the body
  - Upper arm is flexed and supported with pillows
  - Neck is flexed and head is rotated towards floor
  - Avoid nerve damage by ensuring adequate padding of:
    - Dependent shoulder
    - Greater trochanter
    - Common peroneal nerve at fibular head
    - Infra-axillary roll placed to avoid pressure on axillary neurovascular bundle
    - A pillow should be placed between slightly flexed legs
    - Avoid jugular vein compression due to excess flexion/rotation of neck.
- Advantages:
  - Better access to ETT compared to prone position
- Disadvantages: Damage to eyes possible
  - Significant bleeding from superior petrosal sinus during dissection
  - Nondependent shoulder may be in surgeons way

❖ Supine position:

- Procedure:
  - Patient placed supine with neck rotated laterally
  - Roll is placed under ipsilateral shoulder to avoid stretching brachial plexus
  - Adequate padding of pressure points is important
- Useful for:
  - Surgery at the cerebellopontine angle, particularly for small tumors
  - Trigeminal neuralgia
  - Acoustic neuroma
  - Advantages: Circumvents the problem of field invasion by nondependent shoulder seen in lateral position
- Disadvantages: Extreme neck rotation may result in brachial plexus injuries

❖ Sitting position:

- Use of sitting posture for surgery is declining
- Provides optimal access for:
  - Midline posterior fossa lesions
  - Upper cervical lesions
  - Fourth ventricular tumors
  - Tumors of CP angle
- Procedure:
  - Using standard OT table, remove head portion
  - Place back vertically to 60°
  - Legs slightly flexed to ensure buttocks are firm against vertical portion
  - Head is held by Mayfield pin fixator mounted on frame across table
  - Minimum of 2 finger gap between chin and suprasternal notch
  - Maintain head up tilt: prevents venous congestion
  - Forehead rests on horshoe ring mounted on frame
  - Padding of elbows, ischial spines, heels, forehead
  - All catheters and endotracheal tube secured well
- Advantages: (advantages are mostly surgical)
  - Better spatial orientation and surgical exposure
  - Better preservation of cranial nerve function
  - Lesser surgical blood loss
  - Better gravitational venous and CSF drainage
  - Reduces ICT
  - Easier ventilation in obese patients
  - Easier facial nerve monitoring as the face is visible
- Disadvantages: (disadvantages are all anesthetic)
  - Hemodynamic instability especially in patients with higher ASA grade due to:
    - Peripheral pooling of blood
    - Positive pressure ventilation
    - Anesthetic agents
  - Venous air embolism, paradoxical air embolism
  - Pneumocephalus, quadriplegia
  - Peripheral brachial neuropathies
  - Exaggerated neck flexion can result in:
    - Jugular compression
    - Tongue swelling, tongue necrosis
    - Cervical cord ischemia
- Contraindications:
  - Absolute contraindications:
    - Ventriculoatrial shunts
    - Right–left cardiac shunts
  - Relative contraindications:
    - Patent foramen ovale
    - Extremes of age
    - Uncontrolled hypertension
    - COPD
    - Severe autonomic neuropathy

Anesthethic Technique

Induction

- Adequate preoxygenation
- Thiopentone 3–5 mg/kg + vecuronium 0.15 mg/kg + fentanyl 1–2 µg/kg bolus
- Propofol 1–2 mg/kg can be used as an alternative
- Induction agents are given slowly to avoid hypotension and reduction in CPP
- Lidocaine 1.5 mg/kg or labetolol 5 mg increments to reduce BP response to intubation
- Armoured endotracheal tube used to prevent kinking
- NGT inserted if patient is at increased risk for postoperative bulbar dysfunction
- Protect eyes

Monitoring

- Pulse oximetry
- E_TCO_2
- ECG
- Temperature
- Urine output
- Invasive BP monitoring
- Neuromuscular monitoring
- Central venous pressure especially in sitting posture surgeries
- Precordial stethoscope
- Electrophysiological monitoring:
  - SSEP, spontaneous/evoked electromyographic activity
  - Brainstem/auditory evoked potential
  - Cranial nerve function through electromyography:
    - CN VII for acoustic neuroma: As it is stretched across capsule of tumor
    - From tongue for hypoglossal nerve
    - From glottis through electrodes in specialized ETT to monitor CN X
- Coagulation studies:
  - Used for extremely vascular tumors (meningiomas)
  - This is because intraoperative coagulopathy can occur
- Monitor for venous air embolism: Transesophageal echocardiography

Maintenance

- O_2 + isoflurane/sevoflurane (0.5–1 MAC) ensures balanced anesthesia
- Fentanyl 4–6 µg/kg provides intraoperative analgesia
- NMBAs should be used to ensure immobility in the pin holder
- Advantages of neuromuscular blockade include:
  - Ensuring an immobile field
  - Reduction of airway pressure
  - Facilitation of hyperventilation
  - Maintenance of lighter anesthetic planes
  - Reduction of injury due to patient movement
- NMBAs may be avoided in select cases to allow assessment of cranial nerve function
- Propofol infusion at 50–100 µg/kg/min may provide better surgical access
- Desflurane avoided as it promotes coughing at extubation
- Vasopressors may be required to maintain hemodynamics in chronic HTN patients
- Reverification of ETT position after final positioning of patient is important
- Alternatively, TCI with propofol 3–6 µg/mL + remifentanyl 0.15–0.25µg/kg/min can be used
- Avoid nitrous oxide as it:
  - Increases cerebral metabolic rate and worsens outcome of VAE
  - Increases chances of postoperative pneumocephalus
- Lumbar CSF drainage done sometimes as it:
  - Improves surgical conditions
  - Reduces incidence of postoperative CSF leaks
- Measures to reduce tumor edema:
  - 3% saline better than mannitol especially if anuric renal failure is present
  - Loop and osmotic diuretics are avoided (especially in sitting position) as:
    - They predispose patients to hypovolemia
    - This may aggravate hypotension
    - This may also aggravate pre-existing dyselectrolytemias
    - Also, the size of pneumocephalus may increase
- At the time of application of Mayfield fixator:
  - Marked hypertensive response may occur
  - Infilteration of pin sites of *Mayfield* with local anesthetic reduces this response
  - Additional remifentanyl 0.5 µg/kg or propofol 0.5 mg/kg bolus may help
  - Short acting β-blockers and direct acting vasodilators may be used
- Intermittent pneumatic compression devices should be applied to calves and feet
- IV morphine during skull closure for postoperative analgesia when remifentanyl is used

Ventilation

- Traditionally spontaneous ventilation was used
- This was to allow detection of change in respiratory patterns
- These changes would indicate surgical manipulation of the respiratory centre
- This technique is not used nowadays
- This is because proximity of cardiovascular and respiratory centers permits cardiovascular signs to serve as an indicator of injury to respiratory centre
- Advantages of controlled ventilation include:
  - Maintenance of lighter planes of anesthesia which allows:
    - Better cardiovascular stability
    - Early extubation
  - Allows hyperventilation to optimize surgical exposure
- Controlled ventilation with mild hypocapnia (30 to 35 mm Hg) is preferred

Hemodynamics

- Intraoperative hemodynamic manipulations:
  - Modest hypotension is preferred as it facilitates surgical exposure
  - BP brought close to normal prior to closure to assess adequacy of hemostasis
  - Surgical intervention/retraction of brainstem may alter vitals
  - In case of drastic changes, inform surgeon to retract or dissect more gently
  - Sudden changes in BP increases chances of damage to respiratory centre
- Preserve cardiovascular responses to brainstem manipulation by:
  - Avoiding atropine
  - Avoiding long acting β–blockers
- Maintain normothermia
- Fluid management:
  - Glucose containing fluids are avoided due to detrimental effects hyperglycemia
  - Normal saline used as maintenance fluid
  - Blood/colloid is used to replace active blood loss
  - FFP and platelets given if intraoperative coagulopathy develops
- Intraoperative cardiovascular responses may include:
  - Bradycardia and hypotension
  - Tachycardia and hypertension
  - Bradycardia and hypertension
  - Ventricular arrhythmia

Effects of Surgical Brainstem Manipulation

Area	Signs	Changes in monitor
CN V	Hypertension, bradycardia	IBP, ECG
CN VII	Facial muscle involvement	EMG
CN X	Hypotension, bradycardia	IBP, ECG
Pons, medulla	Arrhythmias	ECG
	Hypotension/hypertension	IBP
	Tachycardia/bradycardia	ECG
	Irregular breathing pattern	$ETCO_2$

Extubation

- Anesthetic goals at extubation:
  - Prevent abrupt rise in blood pressure
  - Allow rapid awakening
  - Allow rapid return of motor strength
  - Minimize coughing and straining on ETT
- Feasibility of extubation depends on:
  - Patients preoperative neurological condition
  - Duration of surgery and anesthesia
  - Nature of surgery (extensive brainstem manipulation causing edema)
- Prerequisites at extubation:
  - Adequate neuromuscular reversal
  - Fully awake planes
  - Obey commands
  - Return of protective airway reflexes
- Airway obstruction due to airway edema and macroglossia possible post extubation

Postoperative Management

Management

- Postoperative nausea and vomiting:
  - PONV can increase the ICP and risk of postoperative bleeding
  - Thus, aggressive management of PONV is required
  - Dexamethasone and ondansetron may be used to prevent PONV
- Elective postoperative ventilation preferred if:
  - Poor preoperative neurological status
  - Extensive manipulation of medullary structures
  - Occurrence of adverse intraoperative event such as brainstem injury
  - Prolonged surgery with significant tissue retraction
  - Significant intraoperative blood loss
  - Lesions more than 30 mm diameter with mass effect
  - Postoperative cerebral edema

Monitor

- Pulse oximetry
- Urine output
- NIBP/IBP
- Temperature
- ECG
- Neurological status

Pain

- NSAIDs avoided
- Low dose morphine given only in the absence of respiratory depression
- Multimodal analgesia

Complications

- Venous air embolism
- Pneumocephalus
- Quadriplegia
- Postoperative nausea and vomiting especially after CP angle surgeries
- Hemodynamic perturbations
- Postoperative airway obstruction
- Brainstem damage
- Cranial nerve damage
- Other complications:
    - Postoperative nausea and vomiting especially after CP angle surgeries
    - CSF leak (most common complication)
    - Meningitis
    - Wound infection
    - Hydrocephalus
    - Hematomas

CIRCLE OF WILLIS

Introduction

- This represents a free anastomosis between blood vessels supplying the brain
- Equalizes pressure in arteries of the two sides: also called ***circulus arteriosus***

Situation

Located in interpeduncular subarachnoid cistern

Formation

- *Anteriorly*: Anterior communicating artery
- *Posteriorly*: Basilar artery as it divides into right and left posterior cerebral artery
- Each side:
    - Anterior cerebral artery
    - Internal carotid artery
    - Posterior communicating artery
    - Posterior cerebral arteryB

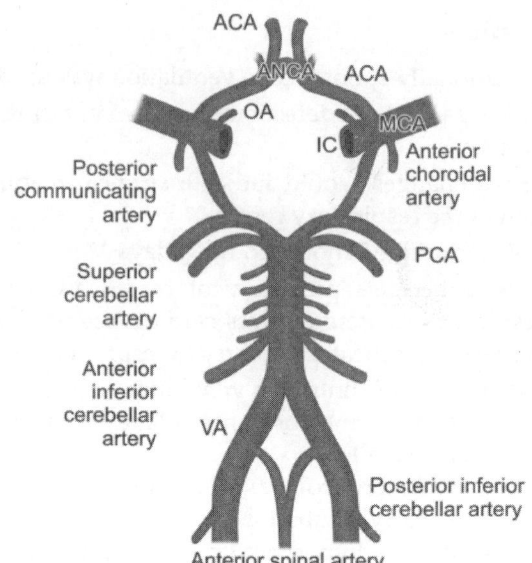

Fig. 7: Circle of Willis.

Branches of Internal Carotid Artery

- Ophthalmic artery
- *Anterior cerebral artery*: Larger branches
- Middle cerebral artery
- *Posterior communicating artery*: Smaller branches
- Anterior choroidal artery

Branches of Cranial Part of Vertebral Artery

- Meningeal artery
- Anterior spiral artery
- Posterior spinal artery
- Posterior inferior cerebellar artery
- Medullary artery

Branches of Basilar Artery

- Pontine artery
- Labyrinthine artery
- Anterior inferior cerebellar artery
- Superior cerebellar artery
- Posterior cerebral artery

CAROTID ENDARTERECTOMY

Introduction

- Prophylactic revascularization surgery done in patients with carotid atherosclerotic lesions to prevent stroke
- This surgery carries a risk of high morbidity and mortality
- Thus, risk–benefit analysis is important for patient selection

Incidence

- Stroke is third leading cause of death
- 10–15% of patients with carotid territory strokes and TIAs have > 50% carotid stenosis
- Risk of recurrent stroke is highest in first few days after the initial event

Etiology

- Atheromatous plaque most common at bifurcation of common carotid artery
- Clot embolism into distal cerebral blood vessels may cause reduced blood flow
- Cerebrovascular sequelae occur due to:
  - Embolization of thrombus
  - Atheromatous debris
  - Hypoperfusion secondary to stenosis

Physiological Effects

Occurs due to temporary blood flow obstruction:

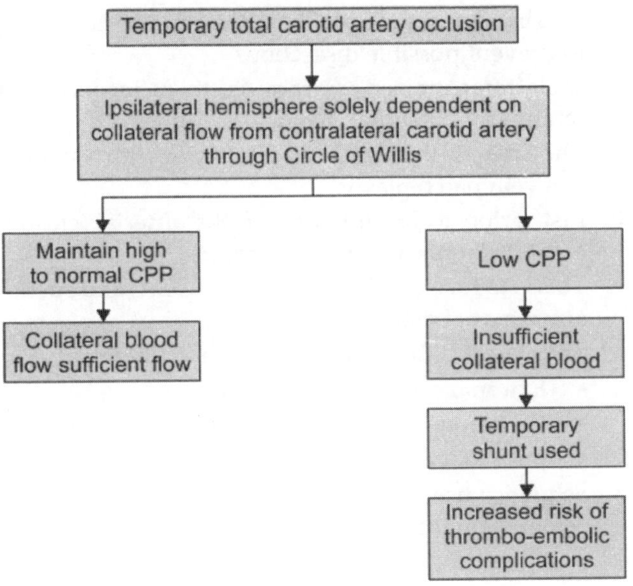

Presentation

- Wide range of presentation based on severity
- Incidental: Asymptomatic finding during investigation of arterial disease
- Asymptomatic bruit
- *Amaurosis fugax*:
  - Transient attacks of monocular blindness
  - Due to embolus into ophthalmic artery
- *Transient ischemic attacks:*
  - Last less than 24 hours
  - Paresthesias, clumsiness, speech impediment
- *Reversible ischemic neuro-deficit (RIND):*
  - Lasts less than 3 weeks
  - Stroke/CVA
  - 30% one-year mortality rate

Treatment

- Medical therapy:
  - Only approved therapy is with recombinant TPA
  - To be given within 3 hours of onset of symptoms
  - Risk factor control: HTN, diabetes, hyperlipidemia, cardiac disease
- Carotid end arterectomy:
  - Controversial role
  - Currently it is the *gold standard*
- Extra–intracranial bypass surgery:
  - Less commonly used
  - Branch of superficial temporal artery is anastomosed to cortical branch of MCA
  - The surgery is done via burr hole and is useful in distal carotid or MCA lesions
- Endovascular therapy:
  - Carotid angioplasty and stenting (CAS) used as alternative to CEA
  - CAS avoids the risks associated with open surgery
  - Perioperative morbidity may be lesser than that of CEA
  - However, the risk of perioperative stroke is higher than that of CEA
  - It has been approved as an acceptable alternative to CEA by the FDA
  - However in many European countries CEA is still regarded as the safer option
  - Currently CAS can be recommended for patients with:
    - Surgically inaccessible lesions
    - Past neck irradiation
  - Major morbidity from CAS may arise due to:
    - Dislodged atherothrombotic debris
    - Arterial wall dissection
    - Arterial rupture
    - Stent restenosis

Indications of CEA NASCET Trial

- Symptomatic carotid atherosclerosis:
  - Effective in reducing the risk of ischemic stroke provided:
    - Stenosis severity should be 70–99%
    - A minimum life expectancy should be at least 5 years
    - All of the following should be present along with the above criteria:

- Surgically accessible carotid lesion
- Absence of clinically significant systemic disease:
  - Cardiac disease
  - Pulmonary disease
- No ipsilateral endarterectomy

❖ Asymptomatic carotid atherosclerosis:
- CEA is beneficial for selected patients when stenosis severity is 60–99%
- The benefits may be greater for men than for women
- The degree of benefit is not as high as for symptomatic patients
- The benefits of CEA for asymptomatic carotid stenosis is delayed
- This is because of the high incidence of perioperative morbidity
- Thus, significant benefit accrues only after 2 years of CEA

Contraindications of CEA

❖ Absolute contraindication: Asymptomatic complete carotid occlusion

❖ Relative contraindications:
- Prior neck irradiation
- Concurrent tracheostomy
- Prior radical neck dissection with or without radiation
- Contralateral vocal cord paralysis from prior endarterectomy
- Surgically inaccessible atypical lesion location
- Severe recurrent carotid restenosis

Timing of Surgery

❖ The benefit of CEA is highest when performed within 2 weeks of the ischemic event

❖ Also, the benefits from surgery declines more rapidly in women than in men

Procedure

❖ Incision is made along the anterior border of SCM

❖ Alternatively, a transverse incision is made at the level of carotid bulb: high approach

❖ Platysma and subcutaneous tissues are divided

❖ Carotid sheath is exposed and internal carotid artery is identified

❖ Heparin 5000 IU after exposure of common carotid artery bifurcation

❖ ACT is preferably maintained between 200–250 seconds

❖ Routine monitoring of ACT is not required as the duration of surgery is short

❖ Carotid stump pressures can be obtained after clamping the proximal CCA and ECA

❖ Mean pressures above 30–50 mm Hg imply adequate collateralization

❖ Cross clamp is applied sequentially to:
- Internal carotid artery (ICA): Clamped first to prevent embolization
- Common carotid artery (CCA)
- External carotid artery (ECA)

❖ A longitudinal arteriotomy is performed below the level of the bifurcation

❖ This incision is extended proximally and distally

❖ A carotid shunt is inserted (from CCA to ICA) based on:
- Surgical preference
- Anesthetic technique (general anesthesia)
- Carotid stump pressures (< 30–50 mm Hg)

❖ The carotid plaque is then freed and removed through dissection

❖ Tacking sutures are placed at the end of arterectomy to prevent possible dissection

❖ Endarterectomized surface is then inspected to remove any residual plaque

❖ The artery is then repaired directly or with a saphenous vein patch plasty

❖ Just prior to completion of the arterial closure, carotid clamps are briefly released

❖ This is to forward flush the vessel (CCA) and suction any residual debris

❖ The clamp is then removed sequentially from:
- External carotid artery (ECA)
- Common carotid artery (CCA)
- Internal carotid artery (ICA)

❖ Sequence used to prevent any debris from entering cerebral circulation

❖ Problems of shunting:
- Air embolism
- Kinking of shunt
- Shunt occlusion against side of blood vessel wall
- Injury/disruption of distal ICA
- May impair surgical access to artery: increases cross–clamp time

Preoperative Assessment

❖ Goals of preoperative assessment:
- Risk stratification
- Evaluation of benefits of revascularization
- Optimization of pre–existing disease

- Identification of occult cardiac disease requiring immediate management
- Formulation of anesthetic plan

❖ History:
- 60% patients have asymptomatic CAD
- Asses severity of preoperative symptoms of CVA
- Age and female sex: increased incidence of CVS and CNS complications
- HTN: SBP 180 mm Hg increases risk of stroke and postoperative death
- History to rule out peripheral vascular disease, COPD

❖ Investigations:
- Hb, hematocrit, urinalysis, BUN, serum creatinine
- ECG: Arrhythmias, MI, LVH
- Chest X-ray: Cardiomegaly, pulmonary edema, COPD
- Doppler angiography and oculoplethysmography
- MR angiography

❖ Examination:
- Head and neck for potential airway problems
- Evidence of any positional ischemia
- Blood pressure:
  - Determine BP and HR from time of preoperative clinic to perioperative period
  - Helps determine range of patients acceptable values of BP
  - Intraoperatively, maintain hemodynamics within this range

Preoperative Risk Stratification

❖ Medical risk factors:
- Angina
- Myocardial infarction within 6 months
- Congestive cardiac failure
- Severe HTN (>180/110 mm Hg)
- Chronic obstructive lung disease
- Age more than 70 years
- Severe obesity

❖ Neurological risk factors:
- Progressing neurological deficits
- New neurological deficit (< 24 hours)
- Frequent daily TIAs
- Multiple cerebral infarcts

❖ Angiographic risk factors:
- Contralateral carotid artery occlusion
- Internal carotid artery siphon stenosis
- Proximal or distal plaque extension
- High carotid bifurcation

Risk Group	Characteristics	Morbidity (%)
1.	Neurologically stable No major medical risk factors No major angiographic risk factors	1%
2.	Neurologically stable No major medical risk Significant angiographic risk	2%
3.	Neurologically stable Major medical risk Major angiographic risk	7%
4.	Neurologically unstable Major medical risk Major angiographic risk	10%

Anesthetic Technique for CEA

❖ General anesthesia:
- More commonly used for carotid end arterectomy
- Advantages:
  - Reduces cerebral oxygen consumption the most
  - Reduces stress response to surgery
  - Ensures a secure airway
  - Reduces patient discomfort
  - Easier control of blood pressure
  - May be indicated when:
    - Extreme preoperative anxiety
    - Patient preference
    - Inability to communicate/cooperate
    - Neurocognitive dysfunction
    - Patient is unable to lie down supine (e.g., CCF, severe COPD)
- Disadvantages:
  - Volatile anesthetics impair cerebral autoregulation
  - Requires special cerebral function monitors
  - More labile BP: BP fluctuations common
  - Increased incidence of MI
  - Increased requirement of vasoactive drugs

❖ Regional anesthesia:
- More commonly used for carotid artery stenting (CAS)
- Advantages:
  - Provides awake patient: *Gold standard* of cerebral function monitoring
  - Allows monitoring of cerebral function continuously
  - Eliminates the need for expensive monitoring techniques
  - BP and cerebral perfusion unaltered: more stable BP

- Lower incidence of hypotension during and after the procedure
- Better postoperative recovery
- Reduced incidence of MI
- Reduced requirement of vasoactive drugs
- Reduces hospital costs
• Disadvantages:
  - Patient has to lie still with neck turned for more than 90 minutes
  - Requires high level of patient cooperation
  - Volatile anesthetic induced neuroprotection is absent
  - Patient and surgeon cooperation is required
  - Discomfort during surgery: May require additional IV sedation
  - Increases perioperative blood pressure
  - Loss of control of airway if intraoperative seizures or sudden LOC
  - Remote airway: Difficult to control airway in emergency
  - Awake patient may panic and become combative: Loss of control of surgical field

❖ Combined GA with LA:
  • Superficial cervical plexus block with light GA
  • Dexmedetomidine used for sedation
  • Reduced need of shunt and no stroke
  • Clonidine 1 μg/kg/hr better
  • Clonidine also gives more hemodynamic stability postoperaitvely
❖ Evidence: ***GALA trial***:
  • Largest multicentric randomized trial for GA vs LA in CEA
  • Primary outcomes studied included:
    - Stroke at 30 days post surgery
    - Myocardial infarction at 30 days post surgery
    - Death at 30 days post surgery
  • 3526 patients were studied
  • There was no difference between the 2 techniques regarding primary outcome
  • Also, the 2 groups did not differ in terms of:
    - Quality of life
    - Length of hospital stay
  • However, regional anesthesia was associated with:
    - Lesser operative cost
    - Lesser incidence of early neurocognitive decline
  • Concluded that both GA and LA appear to be equally safe

Anesthetic Goals 

❖ Maintain adequate cerebral blood flow
❖ Maintain normal BP, PaO_2 and $PaCO_2$ throughout the procedure
❖ Avoid myocardial ischemia and infarction
❖ Ablation of surgical pain and stress responses
❖ To have awake patient at the end of surgery for CNS examination

Preoperative Preparation and Premedication

❖ Informed consent
❖ NPO orders
❖ Surgical duration is short, typically lasting less than 90 minutes
❖ Therefore, long acting agents like lorazepam are avoided
❖ Short acting benzodiazepines preferred: IV midazolam 0.05 mg/kg
❖ Aspirin and clopidogrel are continued in the perioperative period
❖ Discontinuing aspirin therapy may cause increased risk of MI and TIA
❖ Antianginal, statins and antihypertensives are continued on the day of surgery

Regional Anesthesia

❖ Techniques: C_2 to C_4 segment blockade by:
  • Superficial cervical block
  • Deep cervical block
  • Combined deep and superficial cervical block
  • Cervical epidural block
❖ Superficial cervical plexus block:
  • This is the most common regional technique used for CEA
  • Midpoint of posterior border of SCM is used as the point of entry
  • EJV usually crosses the SCM at this point
  • 10–15 mL of LA is infilterated along posterior border of SCM
  • Usually, this is done in the cranial–caudal fashion
  • Additional LA may be required on entering the carotid sheath
  • This may be provided by local infilteration by the surgeon
❖ Deep cervical plexus block:
  • This is a paravertebral block of the C_2–C_4 nerve roots

- Procedure:
  - Head is turned away and the neck is extended
  - Palpate for:
    - C_2 transverse process below mastoid process
    - C_6 at the level of cricoid cartilage
  - C_3 and C_4 are at 2 cm intervals along a line joining C_2 to C_6
  - The needle is inserted deep at the desired level
  - Penetration in continued until contact is made with lateral edge of transverse process
  - Needle is then walked off the transverse process in a caudal direction
  - The tip of the needle now lies above the spinal nerve root within the sulcus of the transverse process
  - 5–8 mL LA is then injected at each of C_2, C_3 and C_4
  - Alternate approach consists of a single injection at the level of C_3
  - Additional LA may be required on entering the carotid sheath
  - This may be provided by local infilteration by the surgeon
- Complications:
  - Phrenic nerve block
  - Vertebral artery injection
  - Injection into CSF
  - Laryngeal nerve palsy: Respiratory distress
- Contraindicated in anticoagulated patients
- Clinical use:
  - Addition of deep cervical plexus provides more rapid onset of action
  - However, its use for CEA is restricted as:
    - Quality of anesthesia is similar to superficial plexus block
    - Associated with life-threatening complications

❖ Cervical epidural:
- Not routinely used
- Provides good operating conditions
- Major complications:
- Dural puncture
  - Total spinal
  - Puncture
  - Respiratory paralysis

General Anesthesia

Induction

❖ Adequate preoxygenation

❖ Insertion of 1 medium bore IV catheter is sufficient as major blood loss is rare

❖ Central venous access is usually not required

❖ Propofol/etomidate + fentanyl 2–5 μg/kg IV is the preferred combination

❖ Etomidate is useful in patients with low cardiac reserve

❖ Other opioid alternatives include:
- Sufentanil 0.5–1 μg/kg
- Remifentanyl 0.2–0.5 μg/kg bolus

❖ Vecuronium/rocuronium can be used to facilitate intubation

❖ Succinylcholine is contraindicated in patients with a recent paretic cerebral infarct

❖ Both hypotension and HTN are detrimental and avoided at the time of induction

❖ Laryngoscopy and intubation responses are blunted with:
- Lidocaine 1–1.5 mg/kg
- Additional opioid supplements
- Supplemental hypnotic agents
- Increasing dose of volatile anesthetic agents
- IV esmolol 0.5 mg/kg boluses
- IV NTG 5–25 μg boluses

❖ Flexometallic ETT:
- May be used, although not absolutely essential
- Its flexibility facilitates positioning without encroaching the surgical field

❖ Phenylephrine 50–100 μg IV can be used for hypotension at induction

Position

❖ Reverse Trendelenburg with head up and feet up to reduce venous pooling

❖ Head turned away from operating side

❖ Shoulders raised with support placed between shoulder blades

❖ Head kept in position with head ring

❖ Drapes heaped up like tent away from patients face to prevent claustrophobia

Monitors

❖ Non-specific monitors:
- ECG, pulse oximetry
- NIBP in both arms as PVD causes differences between the two arms
- E_TCO_2, VA concentration
- Esophageal stethoscope
- Airway pressure, FiO_2
- Arterial line for IBP and blood gasses
- PA catheter/CVP via subclavian/femoral vein only if decompensated CCF
- TEE in high-risk patients

- Cerebral function monitors:
  - Awake patient:
    - *Gold standard* of monitoring cerebral function during LA
    - Patient is given a squeaky toy in the contralateral hand
    - The patient squeezes this toy in response to oral command
    - Contralateral hand grip is assessed in response to command
    - Observe for loss of consciousness and speech assessment
    - Abnormal response warrants insertion of a carotid artery shunt
    - Absence of new neurodeficits after a test clamp of 1 minute indicates adequate collateral flow
    - Orientation in time and place, mental tasks like counting to 100 can be done
  - Carotid artery stump pressure:
    - Stump pressure and waveform are measured following cross–clamping
    - Technique measures pressure in ICA once CCA and ECA are clamped
    - A needle connected to a transducer is used to measure the waveforms
    - This needle is inserted into the ICA distal to the carotid cross clamp
    - The waveform generated resembles perfusion pressure in Circle of Willis
    - Stump pressure less than 30–50 mm Hg associated with hypoperfusion
    - Not reliable as it is a single, one-time measurement
    - This method is no longer widely used
  - Transcranial Doppler:
    - Probe is placed on the petrous temporal bone
    - Measures blood flow velocity in the MCA
    - May be technically impossible to perform in 10–13% of patients
    - A reduction in flow velocity of > 60% at the time of clamping indicates cerebral hypoperfusion
    - Detects and quantifies embolic signals
  - Somatosensory evoked potentials:
    - Can be used to monitor brain function during CEA
    - Also evaluates deep brain structures
    - Stimulation of median nerve activates areas of cerebral cortex supplied by:
      - MCA
      - Boundary zone of ACA and MCA
    - Advantages:
      - Allows us to selectively monitor specific vascular territories
      - Monitors subcortical pathways not captured on EEG
      - Sensitivity to ischemia is equivalent to EEG
    - However, volatile agents can reduce amplitude of SSEP
  - EEG/processed EEG:
    - Most commonly used technique for monitoring brain function
    - Both raw and processed EEG (like BIS) have been used
    - Does not monitor deep brain structures
    - Only frontal cerebral cortex is monitored
    - Changes in EEG however are not ischemia specific
    - It is affected by:
      - Changes in temperature
      - Changes in $PaCO_2$
      - Depth of anesthesia
      - Noise in OT
    - *Gold standard* in anesthetized patients
    - Consider shunt placement if EEG changes occurs
    - Maybe false negative in patients with preexisting neurodeficits
    - Deterioration in EEG begins when CBF falls below 15 mL/100 g/min
    - Cellular metabolic failure occurs when CBF drops < 12 mL/100 g/min
    - Most common EEG changes of ischemia:
      - Ipsilateral attenuation
      - Ipsilateral attenuation with slowing
      - Ipsilateral slowing without attenuation
      - Difficult to interpret and requires skill and experience

Cerebral Protection

- Thiopentone/propofol used along with volatile anesthetics
- Mild hypocarbia beneficial
- Maintain mild hypothermia

Maintenance

- Procedure duration is typically short (around 90 minutes)
- Maintain light planes of anesthesia:
  - Permits EEG monitoring
  - Maintains BP in high normal range

- Air + O_2 + isoflurane/sevoflurane 1 MAC used to maintain balanced anesthesia
- TIVA with remifentanyl and propofol are other options
- Nitrous oxide is avoided as:
  - It increases CBF and $CMRO_2$
  - Causes postoperative nausea and vomiting–wound hematoma
- Intermediate action NDMR used to avoid high dose of VA
- Small doses of opioids used to avoid postoperative respiratory depression:
  - Fentanyl 3 µg/kg
  - Sufentanil 0.5–1 µg/kg
  - Remifentanyl 0.05–0.2 µg/kg/min infusion
- Spray trachea with 100 mg lidocaine to reduce ETT stimulation during surgery
- Heparin 75–100 IU/kg IV is given before carotid cross clamping
- ACT monitoring is not required as the procedure itself is relatively short

Ventilation

- Normocarbia/moderate hypocarbia (30–35 mm Hg) is preferred
- Hypercarbia is usually avoided
- This is because hypercarbia also dilates blood vessels in normal areas
- This results in the ***cerebral steal phenomenon***

Hemodynamics

- Patients who are HTNsive pre–induction have hypotension post–induction
- Vasoactive agents like ephedrine/adrenaline used to increase BP during induction
- Hemodynamic responses at various phases of surgery:
  - Bradycardia and hypotension:
    - Rarely asystole can occur
    - Common during traction on carotid artery during dissection
    - Traction on carotid artery is misinterpreted as HTN
    - This stimulates the parasympathetic output from baroreceptor reflex
    - This results in bradycardia with hypotension
    - Treatment:
      - Treat with anticholinergics
      - Ask surgeon to stop manipulation
      - 1% lidocaine infilteration around carotid sheath
      - This prevents further episodes of bradycardia
      - Fluid boluses
      - Administration of vasopressors such as:
        - Phenylephrine
        - Ephedrine
        - Hypertension:
    - Arises during:
      - Traction on the carotid artery at the time of dissection
      - Following application of carotid cross clamp
    - Mild increases in BP up to 20% are acceptable
    - However, excessive increases should be treated
    - 1% lidocaine infilteration around carotid sheath obtunds this response
    - Antihypertensives which may be used in refractory HTN include:
      - NTG
      - Esmolol
- Hemodynamic management during cross clamping:
  - Cross clamping interrupts blood flow through the ipsilateral carotid artery
  - However, perfusion may occur through the collateral blood vessels
  - These include:
    - Circle of Willis
    - Facial artery
    - Ophthalmic artery
    - Leptomeningeal collaterals
  - This requires a 10–20% rise in MAP at the time of clamping to preserve CPP
  - The agents used to achieve this include:
    - Phenylephrine
    - Ephedrine
- Use non-glucose containing IV fluids: Lactated Ringers is ideal
- Total IV fluids 5 mL/kg/hour as fluid overload may cause postoperative HTN
- Isovolemic hemodilution with dextran/hestarch to reduce viscosity
- Hyperglycemia increases ischemic injury: Maintain blood sugar less than 200 mg%
- Warming equipment for OT, IV fluids and hot air blanket for patient

Extubation

- Confirm neurological integrity before extubation
- Extubate in deep planes to limit hypertensive response
- Tight hemodynamic control at emergence
- Patient to be wide awake after extubation to allow CNS examination
- Heparin is usually not reversed following arteriotomy closure
- If however, hemostasis is inadequate small dose protamine can be given IV (2 mg/kg)

POSTOPERATIVE CARE

Management

- Supplemental oxygen mandatory as the ventilatory response to PaO_2 is reduced in case of bilateral loss of carotid body function
- Blood pressure:
  - BP is maintained within the range of patient's preoperative value
  - If HTN persists, IV 5 mg labetolol increments given
  - Usually HTN peaks 2–3 hours postoperatively and persists for 24 hours
  - Rule out other causes of HTN:
    - Pain
    - Bladder distension
    - Hypoxia
    - Hypercarbia
- Postoperative ICU detention is warranted if more than 4 of following are present:
  - Stroke
  - CCF
  - HTN
  - MI
  - Arrhythmias
  - Chronic kidney disease

Monitors

- ECG
- Pulse oximetry
- IBP
- Temperature
- Urine output
- CNS status

Analgesia

- Reduced incidence of postoperative pain as CEA is only superficial surgery
- Minimal opioids are required usually
- Paracetamol with LA block is usually effective

Complications

- Perioperative stroke/neurodeficits:
  - 5–6% incidence
  - Predictors of stroke:
    - Emboli during wound closure
    - Reduction CBF at cross clamping
    - Inadequate collateral circulation
  - Prevention of periprocedural stroke:
    - Antiplatelet therapy:
      - Aspirin is started prior to the procedure
      - It is continued indefinitely after the procedure
      - There is insufficient evidence for DAP in CEA
    - Anticoagulation:
      - Heparin is administered prior to clamping the carotid artery
      - Target ACT is around 200–250 seconds
      - However routine monitoring of ACT is not required
    - Carotid shunting during surgery:
      - Shunting maintains blood flow when the ICA is clamped
      - However, it can dislodge thrombi into the distal circulation
      - Not found to be associated with reduced risk of perioperative stroke
- Cerebral hyperperfusion syndrome (CHS):
  - Occurs in approximately 3% patients following CEA
  - Usually occurs within a few hours of revascularization
  - However, can be seen up to 28 days later
  - This occurs because autoregulation is impaired in hypoperfused areas
  - On revascularization these vessels fail to constrict in response to increased perfusion
  - This results in an increase in cerebral perfusion by at least 100% causing CHS
  - Usually presents with:
    - Headache, seizures
    - Focal neurodeficits
    - Cerebral haemorrhage
- Cranial nerve damage:
  - Vagus nerve
  - Hypoglossal nerve
  - Marginal mandibular nerve
  - Posterior auricular nerve
- Myocardial infarction
- Altered BP regulation: HTN/hypotension (HTN more common)
- Carotid body dysfunction:
  - This abolishes cardiorespiratory response to hypoxemia
  - Respiratory regulation becomes totally dependent on changes in $PaCO_2$
- Impaired baroreceptor function
- Respiratory insufficient due to:
  - RLN/hypoglossal nerve injury
  - Neck hematoma
  - Deficient carotid body function
- Wound hematoma
- Tracheal compression and deviation

INTRACRANIAL ANEURYSMS

Introduction

- Intracranial aneurysms result from progressive degeneration of the blood vessel wall
- Despite improvements in the treatment the morbidity and morality remains high

Incidence

- More common in women
- Incidence increases with age
- 0.2 to 9.9% in general population
- SAH resulting from ruptured aneurysms is responsible for 5% of all strokes
- 30–day mortality rate following aneurysmal SAH is 45%
- Only 1/3 of patients treated for ruptured intracranial aneurysms have good outcomes

Anatomy

- 85% of intracranial aneurysms are seen in anterior cerebral circulation
- Remaining 15% of aneurysms are seen in the posterior cerebral circulation
- ***Most common*** in Anterior communicating artery complex (ACOM)
- Usually occurs at the junctions of blood vessels in the Circle of Willis
- Multiple aneurysms can occur in 20% cases
- Common sites of occurrence in anterior circulation include:
  - Junction of anterior communicating artery with anterior cerebral artery
  - Junction of posterior communicating artery with internal carotid artery
  - Bifurcation of middle cerebral artery
- Common sites of occurrence in the posterior circulation include:
  - Top of basilar artery
  - Junction of basilar artery and anterior inferior cerebellar artery
  - Junction of vertebral artery and posterior inferior cerebellar artery
- Small aneurysms (<10 mm diameter) have rupture rate = 0.05% per year
- Large aneurysms (>10 mm diameter) have rupture rate = 0.5% per year

Risk Factors

- Genetic factors:
  - Hereditary syndromes:

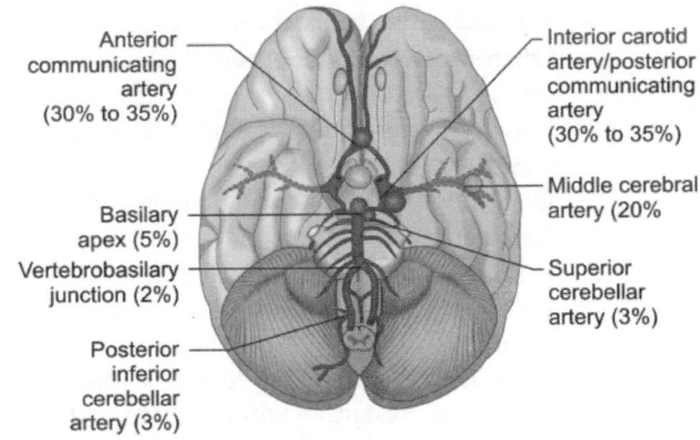

Fig. 8: Intracranial aneurysms.

    - Ehlers Danlos syndrome
    - Pseudoxanthoma elasticum
    - Autosomal dominant polycystic kidney disease
    - Familial aldosteronism type I
    - Moyamoya syndrome
  - Familial aneurysms:
    - Family members of patients with aneurysms are at increased risk
    - Family history of aneurysm confers an almost 3.6 times greater risk
    - Mode of inheritance is variable:
      - Autosomal dominant
      - Autosomal recessive
      - Multifactorial transmission
- Other factors:
  - Cigarette smoking
  - Hypertension
  - Alcohol consumption
  - Estrogen deficiency during menopause
  - Coarctation of aorta

Clinical Features

- Unruptured aneurysms:
  - Mostly asymptomatic in the absence of rupture
  - Symptoms, when present, includes:
    - Headache
    - Loss of visual acuity
    - Cranial neuropathies (particularly CN III palsy)
    - Pyramidal tract dysfunction
    - Facial pain
- Ruptured aneurysms:
  - Headache:
    - Sudden onset, severe headache
    - Location of the headache is not specific

- Headache may be localized or generalized
- Often described as the *worst headache of my life*
- Usually peaks within one hour (instantaneous peaking)
- Often referred to as ***thunderclap headache***
- ***Sentinel headache***:
  - Present in some patients with SAH
  - Occurs weeks prior to the aneurysm rupture
  - History of sudden and severe headache
  - May represent a minor hemorrrhage (warning leak)

- Associated symptoms:
  - Brief loss of consciousness
  - Vomiting
  - Neck pain
  - Neck stiffness
  - ***Terson syndrome:***
    - Refers to pre–retinal hemorrhages
    - Implies a poor prognosis
    - Usually seen in patients with higher grades of SAH
    - May indicate a more abrupt increase in ICP

❖ Aneurysmal rupture occurs most often during non-strenuous activity, rest or sleep

❖ However, onset of symptoms during Valsalva maneuver or exertion suggests SAH

❖ Aneurysmal rupture during pregnancy occurs:
- Most commonly between 30–40 weeks of gestation
- In the immediate postpartum period
- Rarely at time of labor

Grading of Severity of SAH

❖ Grading systems were designed to allow better assessment of surgical risk

❖ Clinical grading systems include the WFNS and Hunt–Hess scales

❖ Fisher grading system is used to report CT findings

❖ Patients with higher clinical grades are more likely to develop:
- Vasospasm
- Elevated ICP
- Impaired autoregulation
- Cardiac arrhythmias
- Myocardial dysfunction World Federation of Neuro Surgeons grades (*WFNS grade*)

Grade	GCS Score	Motor deficit
I	15	Absent
II	14–13	Absent
III	14–13	Present
IV	12–7	Present/absent
V	6–3	Present/absent

Modified Hunt-Hess clinical Grades for SAH

Grade	Description
0	Unruptured aneurysm
I	Asymptomatic
	Minimal headache
	Slight nuchal rigidity
II	Moderate –severe headache
	Nuchal rigidity
	Cranial nerve palsies
	No other neurological deficits
III	Drowsiness, confusion
	Mild focal neurological deficits
IV	Stupor
	Mild or severe hemiparesis
	Possible early decerebrate rigidity
	Vegetative disturbances
V	Deep coma
	Decerebrate rigidity
	Moribund appearance

Surgical mortality and morbidity of SAH according to clinical grades:

Hunt–Hess grade	Mortality (%)	Morbidity (%)
0	0–2%	0–2%
I	2–5%	0–2%
II	5–10%	7%
III	5–10%	25%
IV	20–30%	25%
V	30–40%	35–40%

Investigations

❖ Routine blood chemistry and hematology

❖ Blood grouping, typing and screening

❖ Platelet count and coagulation profile

❖ ECG changes
- Morphological changes:
  - ST elevation/depression
  - T wave flattening/inversion: ***Canyon T waves***
  - Appearance of U waves
  - Rarely appearance of Q waves
  - Prolonged QT interval (> 55 msec)
- Rhythm disturbances:
  - Include:
    - Sinus bradycardia
    - Sinus tachycardia

        - AV dissociation
        - Ventricular tachycardia
        - Ventricular fibrillation
    - Usually resolve within 10 days following SAH
    - Susceptible to Torsades de pointes due to increased QT_c
- *Echocardiography*: Higher grades of SAH are associated with LV dysfunction
- CT brain shows high density (white) blood clot in basal subarachnoid cisterns

Treatment (ACC/AHA 2012 Guidelines)

- Surgical management:
    - Comprises of placement of a clip across the neck of the aneurysm
    - Can be used in patients with ruptured and unruptured aneurysms
    - May involve inducing transient cardiac arrest with adenosine boluses
    - This is done in patients with a large aneurysm with a broad base
    - This reduces the risk of intraoperative aneurysmal rupture
    - Incidental aneurysms >6 mm in anterior circulation should be treated
    - Intraoperative angiography can be used to facilitate accurate clip placement
    - *Disadvantages*: New neurodeficits may occur due to:
        - Brain retraction
        - Temporary artery occlusion
        - Intraoperative hemorrhage
- Endovascular therapy:
    - Coil embolism:
        - Platinum coils are inserted into the lumen of aneurysm
        - A local thrombus forms around the coils
        - This obliterates the aneurysmal sac
        - The procedure is often performed under general anesthesia
        - Complications:
            - Intraprocedural aneurysmal rupture
            - Thromboembolism
    - Newer techniques:
        - Stent assisted coiling
        - Balloon assisted coiling
        - Flow diverters

Timing of Surgery

- Timing of surgical intervention is controversial
- Early surgery: Within 24–72 hours of SAH
    - Indications:
        - Patients with unstable hemodynamics
        - Seizures/mass effect from thrombus
        - Large bleed
        - Evidence of active bleeding
        - Aneurysmal growth
    - Advantages:
        - Reduced incidence of rebleeding which is prime cause of death
        - Subsequent vasospasm can be aggressively treated
        - Reduced hospital stay
        - Reduced medical complications (DVT, pneumonia, atelectasis)
    - Disadvantages:
        - Technically difficult as brain is edematous and clot is friable
        - Increased risk of intraoperative aneurysmal rupture
- Delayed surgery: 11–14 days after SAH
    - Traditionally preferred to allow:
        - Resolution of cerebral edema
        - Reabsorption of subarachnoid haemorrhage
        - Stabilization of aneurysmal clot
    - Highest morbidity and mortality when surgery is done between days 7–10
    - This is because the incidence of cerebral vasospasm peaks at this time
    - At present, surgery is delayed only if:
        - Hemodynamics are stable
        - Advanced age

Preoperative Evaluation and Preparation

- Evaluate and optimize associated medical conditions:
    - ECG and ECHO are essential as cardiopulmonary dysfunction maybe present
    - Cardiac abnormalities include:
        - Ischemia
        - LV dysfunction
        - Pulmonary edema
- Evaluate neurological status:
    - Assess for intracranial hypertension and hydrocephalus
    - Counceling required for grade I and II patients who are anxious
    - WFNS grading is done before and after surgery to assess progress after surgery
- Evaluate dyselectrolytemias and anemia:
    - Hyponatremia is common following SAH due to development of SIADH
    - Anemia is corrected to maintain hemoglobin levels between 8–11.5 g/dL

- Premedication:
  - Premedication is *best avoided* as it may reduce consciousness levels
  - Use of premedication is restricted to:
    - Extremely anxious patients
    - Good clinical grade
  - Choice of drugs:
    - Small doses of short acting benzodiazepines or opioids are titrated
    - Narcotics are preferred to benzodiazepines
    - Dosages:
      - IV fentanyl 50–150 µg
      - IV morphine 1–5 mg
      - IV midazolam 1–2 mg
  - Respiration should be monitored following premedication
  - This is because hypoventilation may increase $PaCO_2$
  - This may in turn increase the ICP and aggravate intracranial HTN
- Other medications to be continued prior to surgery include:
  - Anticoagulants
  - Calcium channel blockers
  - Steroids
- Fluid resuscitation required in the presence of cerebral salt wasting syndrome
- Fluid restriction is required in the presence of SIADH

Anesthetic Considerations

- Avoid acute HTN at intubation with attendent risk of aneurysmal rupture
- Maintain adequate perfusion to the brain
- Minimize transmural aneurysmal pressure during dissection and clipping
- Maintain high normal MAP to prevent critical reduction of cerebral blood flow
- Preparedness to perform precise manipulations of MAP during clipping/hemostasis
- Provide adequate brain relaxation to:
  - Optimize brain access
  - Minimize retraction
- Account for enzyme induction in those patients on anticonvulsants preoperatively
- Hyperventilation:
  - Should be avoided in patients with good clinical grade
  - Should be used in patients with poor clinical grade
- Provide therapeutic adjuncts as required:
  - Induced hypothermia
  - Metabolic suppression
  - Induced hypotension
  - Adenosine induced transient cardiac standstill

Monitoring

- Pulse oximetry
- E_TCO_2
- ECG
- IBP is mandatory and inserted prior to induction if possible
- Core temperature
- Central venous access secured if:
  - Prophylactic fluid loading is used to treat vasospasm
  - Preexisting hypovolemia is present
  - Large intraoperative fluis shift is expected using osmotic/loop diuretics
  - Myocardial dysfunction is present preoperatively
  - Need to administer vasoactive medication perioperatively
- Urine output
- Neurocritical care monitors:
  - Jugular saturation catheter
  - Brain tissue oxygen intraparenchymal probe
  - Ventricular catheters
  - Transcranial Doppler
- Neurophysiological monitors:
  - EEG and SSEP may be used
  - Useful to monitor:
    - Cerebral perfusion during induced hypotension
    - Perfusion during aneurysmal clip application

Induction

- Adequate preoxygenation
- 2 large bore intravascular catheters (including a 16 G catheter) are usually sufficient
- IV thiopentone 3–5 mg/kg + fentanyl 2–3 µg/kg + vecuronium 0.1 mg/kg
- Other induction agents which can be used are:
  - IV propofol 1.5–2 mg/kg
  - IV etomidate 0.3–0.4 mg/kg
  - IV midazolam 0.1–0.2 mg/kg
- IV sufentanil (0.3–0.5 µg/kg) and remifentanyl are useful alternatives
- Any anesthetic technique which allows good hemodynamic control can be used
- Careful and slow induction is key to minimize changes in transmural pressure
- Rupture during induction occurs in 1% patients with 75% mortality
- Deep planes should be maintained especially during:
  - Intubation

- Insertion of Mayfield pins
- Scalp incision
- Turning bone flap
- Opening dura

❖ Mechanisms of blunting the sympathetic response at intubation:
- High dose narcotics:
  - Fentanyl 5–10 g/kg
  - Sufentanil 0.5–1 g/kg
  - Remifentanil 1–1.5 g/kg
- IV lidocaine 1.5–2 mg/kg
- β-adrenergic agonists such as:
  - IV esmolol 0.5 mg/kg
  - IV labetalol 10–20 mg given in 5 mg increments
- Deepening the plane using high dose isoflurane/sevoflurane:
  - Useful in patients with good clinical grade
  - Avoided in patients with raised ICP

❖ Lumbar CSF drain may be required

❖ IV Mannitol 0.5–1 gm/kg just before opening dura mater

❖ Mannitol is repeated 15 minutes after opening dura

Position

❖ Anterior circulation aneurysms:
- Usually approached through the frontotemporal incision (pterional incision)
- Patient is positioned supine and head slightly turned

❖ Basilar tip aneurysms:
- Approached through a subtemporal incision
- Patient therefore lies in the lateral position

❖ Aneurysm in vertebral system:
- Approached through a suboccipital craniotomy
- Patient remains in seated or park bench position

❖ After final positioning always ensure:
- Padding of pressure points
- All extremities are supported
- Head and neck position remains neutral to rest of the body
- Position of the ETT remains unchanged

Ventilation

❖ ETT with IPPV is the preferred technique

❖ Hyperventilation:
- May be used to alter the brain relaxation:
  - Should be avoided in patients with good clinical grade
  - Should be used in patients with poor clinical grade
- Mild hypocapnia (30–35 mm Hg) is used before the dura is opened
- Moderate hypocapnia (25–30 mm Hg) is used after dura is open
- Relative normocapnia is used when induced hypotension is being employed
- Normocapnia should be maintained once the aneurysm is clipped

Maintenance

❖ Any technique which allows adequate brain relaxation may be used

❖ Balanced anesthesia with isoflurane/sevoflurane (<1 MAC) is commonly used

❖ Desflurane may be avoided as it causes sympathetic stimulation in higher doses

❖ Opioid infusion may be used to maintain analgesia:
- Fentanyl 1–2 µg/kg/hour
- Sufentanil 0.1–0.2 µg/kg/min
- Remifentanil 0.1–0.3 µg/kg/min

❖ Atracurium/vecuronium boluses may be used for muscle relaxation

❖ Nitrous oxide avoided as it reduces intracranial compliance

❖ TIVA with propofol and remifentanil is an alternative technique

❖ Continuous infusion of propofol (even for balanced anesthesia) is used to control BP

❖ Infusions up to 150–200 µg/kg/min may be used to provide brain relaxation

❖ $T_{1/2}$ of NDMR may be reduced in patients on anticonvulsants

❖ Thiopentone 3–5 mg/kg may be given before temporary aneurysm clipping

❖ If temporary occlusion lasts > 10 mins recirculation established

❖ Additional thiopentone administered before applying temporary clip

❖ Fentanyl and sufentanil infusion is stopped 1 hour before applying the surgical dressing

❖ Remifentanyl infusion can be continued until 5 minutes before dressing application

❖ Total narcotic dosage should not exceed:
- 10 µg/kg of fentanyl
- 2 µg/kg of sufentanil

Brain Relaxation

❖ Various maneuvers may be used to ensure brain relaxation:
- Reverse Trendelenburg positioning
- Mannitol:

- IV mannitol 0.5–2 g/kg given over 30 minutes
- Action begins in 4–5 minutes
- Action peaks in 30–45 minutes
- Acute reduction in PVR may result when mannitol is given rapidly

- 3% hypertonic saline:
  - May be used as an alternative to mannitol
  - Avoids the volume shifts seen with mannitol
- Lumbar CSF drain:
  - Usually kept closed till surgeon is just about to open the dura mater
  - 20–30 mL of CSF is drained at this point
  - Drainage rate should not exceed 5 mL/min
  - Sudden aspiration of CSF fluid may cause reflex HTN
  - Drain is left open until the dura is closed at the end of procedure
  - This allows CSF to accumulate following dural closure
  - This is important to reduce the size of postoperative pneumocephalus
  - Use of lumbar CSF drains is declining
- Hyperventilation
- Propofol:
  - IV bolus 100–200 mg
  - Followed by infusion of 150–200 g/kg/min

Hemodynamics

- Normotension:
  - Maintain normotension prior to clipping to maximize cerebral perfusion
  - In the presence of significant vasospasm, higher BP has to be maintained
  - Important during temporary occlusion to maximize collateral circulation
- Normovolemia:
  - Maintain normovolemia to maximize cerebral perfusion
  - After securing aneurysmal clipping, CVP is raised to 10–12 mm Hg
  - This is done with boluses of crystalloid/colloid/blood
  - Postoperative hematocrit of 30–35% is desirable
  - Hemodilution reduces risk of vasospasm and improves perfusion
- Deliberate hypotension:
  - Usually avoided
  - Used in the presence of active bleeding preventing surgical visualization
  - MAP of 40–50 mm Hg is required if active arterial bleeding
- Contraindicated in patients with:
  - Cardiovascular disease
  - Cerebrovascular disease
  - Intracerebral hematoma
  - Fever/anemia/renal disease
- Largely replaced by temporary clipping of feeding blood vessels
- Induced hypertension:
  - Maybe required during temporary clipping to maintain collateral circulation
  - SBP is increased to 20% above baseline with IV phenylephrine boluses
- Fluids:
  - Potential for massive sudden blood loss exists
  - Thus, adequate blood should be readily available
  - Crystalloid isotonic solutions without glucose are used before aneurysmal clipping
  - Ringer's lactate is not used as it is relatively hypo–osmolar
  - Other fluids which may be beneficial are:
    - Plasmalyte A
    - Normosol
    - Normal saline
  - Aim to maintain:
    - Normovolemia prior to aneurysm clipping
    - Mild hypervolemia after aneurysm clipping

Interventions during Temporary Clipping

- Vascular clips may be applied temporarily to the parent artery
- This improves surgical visualization for application of permanent clip to the aneurysm
- Temporary clipping < 2 minutes: no intervention
- Temporary clipping > 2 minutes:
  - Increase FiO_2 to 100%
  - Increase concentration of volatile anesthetic
  - Consider phenylephrine to maintain the MAP
- Temporary clipping > 10 minutes:
  - Consider augmenting blood pressure
  - This may preserve perfusion via collaterals
  - Increased concentration of volatile agent to induce burst suppression

Cardiac Standstill Using Adenosine

- Usually implemented in patients with large aneurysms and a wide base
- A dose response is first established with 2–3 incremental boluses of adenosine

- A duration of approximately 30 seconds of asystole is then induced
- This is usually achieved with an average dose of 30–36 mg adenosine
- Recovery of cardiac rhythm is usually spontaneous
- The standstill may be followed by rebound tachycardia and HTN
- This technique is avoided in patients with:
  - Preexisting conduction abnormalities
  - Severe bronchial asthma

Extubation

- Anesthetic goals at extubation:
  - Prevent abrupt rise in blood pressure
  - Allow rapid awakening to facilitate neurological assessment
  - Allow rapid return of motor strength
  - Minimize coughing and straining on ETT
- Feasibility of extubation depends on:
  - Patients preoperative neurological condition
  - Duration of surgery and anesthesia
- Prerequisites at extubation:
  - Adequate neuromuscular reversal
  - Mild cerebral edema during surgery
  - Short period of temporary clipping
  - Fully awake planes
  - Obey commands
  - Return of protective airway reflexes
- Prevent HTN at extubation using:
  - IV labetalol boluses
  - IV esmolol boluses
  - IV hydralazine boluses
  - IV SNP infusions
- Postoperative ventilation is preferred in:
  - Patients with intraoperative complications
  - Poor preoperative clinical grade

Intraoperative Aneurysmal Rupture

- Occurs most commonly as neck of aneurysm is dissected
- Temporary clip is used to stop hemorrhage from main blood vessel
- *Uncontrolled bleeding*: Deliberate hypotension is used to allow surgical access
- Deliberate hypotension can be achieved with:
  - Fentanyl boluses
  - Thiopentone 3–5 mg/kg boluses
  - Labetolol 5–10 mg increments
  - Sodium nitroprusside incremental boluses
- Normotension restored following control of bleeding

POSTOPERATIVE MANAGEMENT

Management

- Hypertension can occur due to:
  - Pain
  - Hypercarbia
  - Pre–existing hypertension
- Treated by treating cause/using antihypertensives
- Hypotension avoided by using intravascular volume resuscitation

Pain

- NSAIDs are avoided
- Low dose opioids may be used depending on neurological status
- *Multimodal analgesia*

Complications

1. Vasospasm
   - Angiographic vasospasm occurs in 40–60% patients after SAH
   - However, clinically significant vasospasm has a lower incidence (20–30%)
   - Angiographic vasospasm is seen 72 hours after SAH
   - Peak incidence between 7–10 days after initial SAH
   - Causes delayed cerebral ischemia

Etiology

- Exact mechanism of vasospasm has not yet been established
- One or more vasoactive substances present in the blood incite an inflammatory reaction on extravasation
- Oxyhemoglobin and its metabolites play an important role
- Thought to occur due to presence of BOXES (bilirubin oxidation products)
- These accumulate around blood vessels following metabolism of oxyhemoglobin
- This incites an inflammatory response including:
  - Free radicals
  - Cytokines
  - Cell–adhesion molecules
  - Haptoglobin

Diagnosis

- Presents as focal and fluctuant neurodeficits
- Cerebral angiography is the ***gold standard***
- Transcervical Doppler USG showing flow velocity >120 cm/sec in MCA suggests vasospasm

Treatment

- Calcium Channel Blockers:
  - Patients with SAH coming to OT must receive nimodipine
  - Nicardipine is IV alternative
  - Minimal effects on hemodynamics during anesthetic induction
  - No reduction in vasospasm on angiography but reduction in morbidity
  - Reduces incidence of cerebral infarction by 34%
  - Reduces incidence of poor outcome post SAH by 40%
- Triple H therapy:
  - Hypertension, hypervolemia and hemodilution to optimize cerebral perfusion
  - Induced HTN with dopamine/phenylephrine
  - Raise MAP to 20–30 mm Hg above baseline systolic BP
  - Hypovolemia to reduce HCT to low 30s
  - Complications:
    - Pulmonary edema
    - Cardiac failure
    - Myocardial infarction
    - Hypertensive intracranial hemorrhage
- Angioplasty:
  - Reduces severity of vasospasm
  - Increases risk of blood vessel dissection and rupture
- Endovascular infusion of vasodilators:
  - Papaverine, verapamil and nicardipine used
  - Papaverine being neurotoxic is less favored
  - Intraarterial verapamil is better alternative
- Intracisternal fibrinolytic therapy:
  - Urokinase/r–TPA used to remove vasospastic agents from subarachnoid space
  - Removal of subarachnoid blood done at the same time following exposure of the brain
- Endothelin an antagonist:
  - *Clazosentan* undergoing phase III trials
  - Magnesium and simvastatin too undergoing trials

2. Rebleeding
   - Most often within first 48 hours following initial SAH
   - Chance of rebleeding in first 24 hours is 4%
   - Chance of rebleeding after 1 year is 11%
   - Mortality rate in rebleeds is 42%
3. Intracranial HTN
   - Usually requires no treatment as ICP becomes normal by end of first week
   - Emergency ventriculostomy if:
     - Severe intracranial HTN
     - Intracerebral/Intraventricular hemorrhage
     - Vasospasm
     - Hydrocephalus
4. Hyperemic complications
   - Comprise cerebral edema/haemorrhage occurring during endovascular embolization/surgical resection
   - Theories to explain it:
     - *Normal Perfusion Pressure Breakthrough theory (NPPB)*
     - *Occlusive hyperemia theory*
   - SPECT imaging identifies patients at risk of developing NPPB
   - NIRS (near infrared spectroscopy) detects hyperemic status after AVM resection by measuring cortical O_2 saturation.
5. SIADH
6. Cerebral Salt Wasting Syndrome
   - Triad of:
     - Hyponatremia
     - Volume contraction
     - High urinary sodium > 50 mmol/L
7. SAH associated myocardial dysfunction
   - Reversible stunning like injury
   - Associated with high troponin levels
   - ECG changes as described in investigations

ANESTHESIA FOR PARKINSON'S DISEASE

Introduction

- First described by ***James Parkinson*** in 1817
- *Most common* movement disorder
- *Second most common* neurodegenerative disorder (after Alzheimer's disease)
- Parkinson's disease (PD) is the most common cause of Parkinsonism
- Parkinsonism is the name given to the clinical syndrome with:
  - Impairment of voluntary movement (bradykinesia)
  - Rigidity
  - Tremors
  - Postural instability

- PD is caused by the degenerative loss of dopaminergic neurons in the brain
- Also called "***shaking palsy***" or "***the happy disease***"

Risk Factors

- Idiopathic: Accounts for almost 75% cases
- Positive family history: *PARK 1* and *PARK 13* genes
- Genetic factors:
  - Autosomal dominant inheritance with poor penetrance
  - Mutations in α–synuclein gene (SNCA)
- Male gender
- Living in rural areas
- Farming and agricultural work
- Infections: Postencephalitic Parkinson's disease, AIDS
- Environmental factors:
  - MPTP–induced Parkinsons
  - Herbicides and insecticides may increase risk of Parkinsons disease
  - High consumption of dairy products increases risk of PD
- History of:
  - Depression
  - Traumatic brain injury
  - Low levels of sunlight derived vitamin D

Factors Associated with Reduced Risk of Parkinsons

- Coffee and caffeine intake
- Cigarette smoking
- Aerobic exercise
- Ibuprofen
- Statins

Pathogenesis

- Characterized by death of dopaminergic neurons in substantia nigra of basal ganglia
- Mechanisms of cell death:
  - Mitochondrial dysfunction
  - Oxidative stress
  - Excess nitric oxide formation
  - Deficient neurotrophic support
  - Immune mechanisms
- Cell death in substantia nigra causes a decrease in dopamine production
- Dopamine deficiency causes increased activity of inhibitory nuclei in basal ganglia
- This causes inhibition of thalamic nuclei receiving outflow from basal ganglia
- Excessive thalamic inhibition causes suppression of cortical motor system
- This causes akinesia, rigidity and tremors
- Inhibition of brainstem locomotor areas cause abnormalities of posture and gait

Parkinson's Syndrome

- Caused by conditions which affect brainstem/disrupt dopaminergic pathway
- Clinical features are that of Parkinsons disease but etiology is different
- Causes:
  - Cerebrovascular disease: Atherosclerosis, multi–infarct disease
  - Repeated head trauma
  - Intracranial neoplasms
  - Toxins:
    - ***Wilsons disease***
    - Carbon monoxide poisoning
    - Heavy metal poisoning
  - Drugs
    - Phenothiazines
    - Butyrophenones
    - Metoclopramide
    - Reserpine
    - *Chronic trichloroethylene exposure*

Parkinson Plus Syndromes

- Refers to neurodegenerative conditions associated with features of Parkinsons
- These are associated with more extensive pathologies in brain and brainstem
- They have multiple clinical features in addition to Parkinsonian features
- Therefore, they are called Parkinson plus syndromes
- Causes:
  - Progressive supra–nuclear palsy
  - Cortico–basal degeneration
  - Multiple system atrophy
  - Striatonigral degeneration
  - ***Shy–Drager syndrome***
  - Diffuse Lewy body disease

Clinical Features

- Classical triad:
  - Tremors
  - Muscle rigidity
  - Bradykinesia
- Severity of motor symptoms is an independent predictor of mortality

- Tremors:
  - Presenting symptom in 70–80% of patients with PD
  - *Resting tremors* oscillating at 4–5 Hz
  - Characteristic ***pill rolling*** quality
  - Most noticeable when the tremulous body part is at rest
  - Ceases at the onset of movement
  - Thus, it is the least disabling of all the manifestations
- Muscle rigidity:
  - Refers to increased resistance to passive movement about a joint
  - Occurs in 75–90% PD patients
  - Rigidity begins unilaterally and typically on the same side as the tremor
  - Rigidity eventually progresses to the contralateral side
  - Rigidity along with tremors causes ***cog wheeling*** nature of rigidity
- Bradykinesia:
  - Refers to the paucity and slowness of movements
  - It is the major cause of disability in PD
  - Usually starts with a reduction in amplitude of finger excursions
  - This results in the reduced manual dexterity of fingers
  - This may lead to a difficulty in simple tasks like:
    - Buttoning clothes
    - Tying shoelaces
  - Bradykinesia of the lower limbs may result in shuffling gait
  - Severe bradykinesia results in disturbed sleep patterns
  - Handwriting becomes micrographic
- Posture and gait:
  - Slightly flexed posture
  - Loss of postural reflexes is a commonly associated feature
  - Retropulsion (several steps backwards) or propulsion (several steps forward) on losing balance
  - Lack of arm swing, with small rapid steps causes ***festinant gait***
  - Gait initiation failure, gait hypokinesia and ***freezing gait*** at later stages
- Others:
  - Expressionless facial features: ***mask like facies*** *(hypomimia)*
  - Primitive reflexes like glabellar tap sign can be elicited
  - Decreased eye blink rate
- Autonomic dysfunction:
  - Orthostatic hypotension
  - Seborrhea, sialorrhea
  - Urinary and bowel disturbances
  - Sleep disorders, depression, anxiety

Investigations

- Predominantly clinical diagnosis
- MRI:
  - Usually normal
  - Can detect cerebrovascular etiology or neurodegenerative etiology
- Sphincter electromyography:
  - Reflects degeneration of ***Onuf's*** nucleus
  - Useful to distinguish Parkinsons disease from multiple system atrophy

ANESTHETIC CONSIDERATIONS

- Central nervous system:
  - Muscle rigidity
  - Tremors:
    - Difficult ECG interpretation
    - Inaccurate NIBP recordings
    - Difficult IV access
  - Postoperative delirium:
    - 8-fold increase in incidence of postoperative delirium in PD patients
    - Most commonly due to multiple drug interactions
- Autonomic nervous system:
  - Orthostatic hypotension: Gradual change in posture recommended
  - Defective temperature regulation: Prone for hypothermia
- Respiratory system:
  - Upper airway dysfunction:
    - *Difficult airway* on account of:
      - Flexion deformity of neck
      - Risk of aspiration due to upper airway muscle dysfunction
    - Excessive salivation: antisialogogue is mandatory
    - Pharyngeal dysfunction:
      - Causes dysphagia in patients with PD
      - This makes them prone for aspiration pneumonia
    - Intrinsic laryngeal muscle dysfunction: Prone for postoperative laryngospasm
    - Sleep apnea: In postencephalitic Parkinsons

- Lower airway dysfunction:
  - Obstructive airway disease:
    - Seen in 35% of PD patients
    - Abnormal function of upper airway is seen in PD
    - This causes obstructive ventilatory pattern
  - Muscle rigidity may impair ventilation
- Cardiovascular system:
  - Intraoperative cardiac arrhythmias common
  - Hypertension: Intubation response should be blunted
  - Hypovolemia
- Gastrointestinal system:
  - Poor nutrition: Dyselectrolytemia
  - Susceptible to reflux: Post extubation aspiration possible
  - Abnormal glucose metabolism
- *Urological*: Difficulty in micturition
- Pharmacological considerations:
  - Avoid drugs precipitating PD:
    - Phenothiazines: Metoclopramide (due to anti-dopaminergic action)
    - Butyrophenones: Droperidol (due to anti–dopaminergic action)
  - Anesthetic agents:
    - Halothane avoided as it sensitizes heart to catecholamines
    - Ketamine avoided as it causes exaggerated sympathetic response
    - Fentanyl (even at normal doses) may exacerbate muscle rigidity
    - Alfentanil may cause dystonic reactions
    - Succinylcholine may cause hyperkalemia
  - Drug interactions:
    - Avoid meperidine with selegiline: Causes ***Serotonin syndrome***

Potential Drug Interactions in Parkinson's Disease

- Induction agents:
  - Propofol:
    - Avoid for stereotactic procedures
    - May abolish tremors
  - Etomidate: Probably safe
  - Thiopental: Probably safe
- Analgesics:
  - Fentanyl: Possible muscle rigidity
  - Morphine: Possible muscle rigidity
- Neuromuscular blocking agents:
  - Succinylcholine: Possible hyperkalemia
  - Nondepolarizing agents: Probably safe
- Volatile agents:
  - Isoflurane: Probably safe
  - Sevoflurane: Probably safe
- Metaclopramide: Exacerbates Parkinsonism

PREOPERATIVE ASSESSMENT

History and Examination

- Drug history:
  - Dose of medicines
  - Timing of medication
  - Control of symptoms with medications
- Note down side effects of anti–PD drugs that the patient is taking
- Assess for systemic features associated with PD:
  - Pharyngeal muscle dysfunction:
    - Dysphagia
    - Sialorrhea
  - Respiratory impairment
  - Orthostatic hypotension, hypertension
  - Difficulty in micturition, bowel disturbances
  - Akinesia, tremors, muscle rigidity
  - Confusion, hallucinations
  - Speech impairment

Investigations

- *Complete blood count*: Respiratory infections
- *Blood glucose estimation*: Altered glucose metabolism
- Renal function tests
- *Serum albumin/transferring*: For nutritional status
- *Electrocardiography*: Pre-existing arrhythmias (usually VPCs)
- *Chest X–ray*: Aspiration pneumonia
- *Pulmonary function tests*: Obstructive ventilatory pattern
- Arterial blood gas
- MRI

Choice of Anesthetic Technique

- Regional anesthesia is preferred over general anesthesia
- However, regional anesthesia can be technically difficult as:
  - Tremors
  - Rigidity can make positioning difficult
  - Twitches from peripheral nerve stimulator hard to discern
  - Poor cooperation if patient has dementia
- Advantages of regional anesthesia:
  - Patient remains conscious
  - Avoids effects of general anesthesia and muscle relaxants which mask tremors
  - Reduced risk of postoperative respiratory complications
  - Prevents PONV-can resume anti-PD medications in immediate postoperative period

Preoperative Preparation

- NPO orders:
  - 6 hours for solids
  - 2 hours for clear liquids
- Informed consent
- Assess and discuss need for possible postoperative ICU/HDU stay
- Anti-aspiration prophylaxis:
  - IV ranitidine 1 mg/Kg
  - 30 mL sodium citrate given preoperatively
- It is *imperative to continue PD medications* up to the time of surgery
- Oral PD medication can be given 20 minutes prior to surgery in prolonged surgeries
- Securing IV access may be difficult in patients with persistent tremors
- IV glycopyrrolate 0.2 mg as an anti-sialogogue
- IV midazolam 0.03 mg/kg for anxiolysis and sedation

Monitors

- Pulse oximetry
- ECG—may show artefacts due to tremors
- NIBP
- Unreliable due to tremors
- Capnography
- Temperature
- Urine output
- Neuromuscular monitoring
- Invasive hemodynamic monitoring for those with severe PD or cardiac comorbidities

Induction

- Adequate preoxygenation
- Thiopentone is *avoided* as it decreases dopamine release from striatal neurons
- Ketamine is avoided as it may lead to an exaggerated sympathetic response
- Propofol is the induction agent of choice as it reduces tremors
- Propofol 1–2 mg/kg + fentanyl 2 μg/kg + vecuronium 0.1 mg/kg IV
- Rapid sequence induction for severe PD with risk of aspiration pneumonia
- High dose opioids avoided as it may cause *wooden chest*
- Nasogastric tube inserted after intubation
- Foleys catheter may be inserted in severe PD to prevent postoperative urine retention

Maintenance

- O_2 + air + isoflurane (1 MAC) + fentanyl boluses
- *Halothane avoided* as it sensitizes the heart to catecholamines
- Isoflurane and sevoflurane are less arrhythmogenic
- Levodopa may be administered via NG tube in case of prolonged surgeries
- This is because abrupt withdrawal of levodopa can cause skeletal muscle rigidity
- This may lead to difficulty in intraoperative ventilation

Positioning

- Difficult positioning due to muscle rigidity
- Gradual change of position due to autonomic instability
- Adequate padding at pressure points essential

Hemodynamics

- Adequate fluid resuscitation perioperatively is important
- This is due to dehydration caused by vomiting associated with anti–PD drugs
- Autonomic insufficiency further alters the response to hypovolemia
- Precipitous hypotension may occur at induction due to:
  - Relative hypovolemia
  - Catecholamine depletion
  - Autonomic instability
  - Sensitization to catecholamines
  - Coadministration of bromocriptine/selegeline
- Directly acting vasopressors should be used to treat hypotension such as:
  - Phenylephrine
  - Epinephrine

Extubation

- Fully reversed, awake extubation
- Adequacy of ventilation and recovery from NMDR established before extubation
- Assess:
  - Spontaneous breathing pattern
  - Presence of gag reflex
  - Ability of patient to focus
  - Presence of 4 twitches/sustained tetanus
- Adequate suction to remove excessive secretions before extubation

POSTOPERATIVE

Management

- Anti–PD drugs to be started as soon as possible after surgery

- This is because the elimination $T_{1/2}$ of levodopa is brief
- Interruption of these drugs for more than 6 hours results in loss of therapeutic effect
- L–Dopa can be administered via nasogastric tube if required
- Good physiotherapy and early ambulation to aid postoperative recovery
- Breathing exercises and spirometry to prevent chest infections
- Diphenhydramine 25 mg IV can be used to reduce postoperative tremors
- Avoid using phenothiazines and haloperidol

Pain

- Opioids may be used but have to be replaced with NSAIDs as soon as possible
- PCA may be difficult to operate
- NSAIDs (ketorolac) useful as they do not interfere with respiratory function
- Local anesthetic infilteration useful
- Multimodal analgesia best

Complications

- Pathological reflexes at emergence:
  - Babinski's reflex
  - Hyperreactive stretch reflexes
  - Ankle clonus
  - Decerebrate posturing
- Aggravated rigidity
- Postoperative laryngospasm, respiratory failure
- Aspiration pneumonia: *Most common*
- PONV: Domperidone *antiemetic of choice*
- Postoperative confusion, hallucinations

ANESTHESIA FOR DEEP BRAIN STIMULATION

Introduction

- Deep brain stimulation (DBS) was first used in the 1970s for treating chronic pain
- It is a well tolerated surgical treatment predominantly used for movement disorders
- DBS is now the most commonly used surgical procedure for treating advanced PD
- Currently it has become an effective treatment for patients with movement disorders

Indications

- FDA approved indications:
  - Parkinson's disease
  - Essential tremors

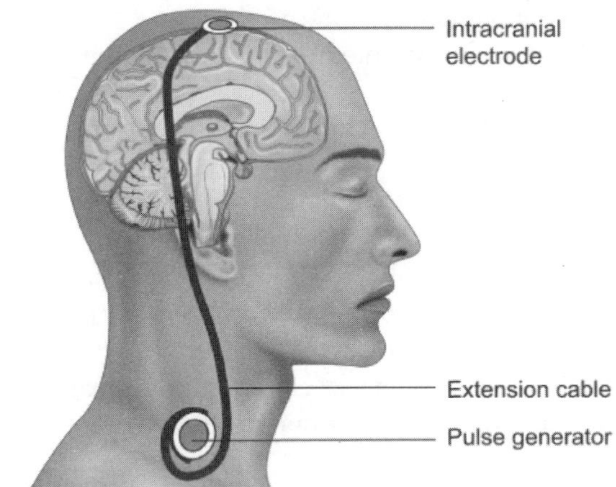

Fig. 9: Deep brain stimulation.

  - Dystonia
  - Obsessive compulsive disorder
- Off label indications include:
  - Epilepsy
  - Depression
  - Tourette's syndrome
  - Alzheimers disease
  - Anorexia

Indications for DBS in PD 

- Levodopa dosing required more than four times daily
- Inconsistent response to medical treatment
- Severe motor fluctuations despite optimal oral levodopa therapy
- Motor fluctuations causing disability/reduced quality of life
- Severe refractory tremor

Efficacy

- Currently FDA approved for used in:
  - PD of at least 4 years duration and 4 months of motor complications
  - Essential tremors
  - Dystonia
  - Obsessive compulsive disorder
- When used in PD, it has shown to improve symptoms due to:
  - Tremors
  - Rigidity
  - Bradykinesia
  - Drug induced dyskinesias

Therapeutic Targets for DBS

- Most common therapeutic targets for movement disorders are:
  - Subthalamic nucleus (STN)

- Globus pallidus interna (GPi)
- Ventralis intermedius nucleus of the thalamus (Vim)

- Therapeutic targets for obsessive compulsive disorders:
  - Subcallosal cingulate gyrus
  - Anterior limb of internal capsule
  - Nucleus accumbens
- Stimulating the STN and GPi are both effective in improving PD symptoms
- DBS to the STN is associated with a greater reduction in anti–PD medication doses

Mechanism of Action

- Currently the mechanism of action of DBS is not clear
- Mechanism of action may differ depending on the site of stimulation
- Stimulation of STN:
  - Results in hyperpolarization or *neuronal jamming*
  - This results in the inhibition of its activity
- Stimulation of GPi:
  - Results in activation of GABAergic neurons
  - This in turn inhibits GPi neurons
- Stimulation of the Vim:
  - Activates output to neurons in the reticular nucleus
  - This results in inhibitory signals being sent to thalamic nuclei
  - This results in the improvement in symptoms

Predictors of Efficacy of DBS

- Preoperative levodopa responsiveness:
  - Most important determinant of DBS outcomes
  - Outcome of DBS will be as good as the best preoperative levodopa response
  - Symptoms unresponsive to levodopa are unlikely to respond to DBS
- Other predictors of good outcome:
  - Young age
  - Mild cognitive impairment
  - Absence of/well controlled psychiatric illness

Device Used

- The device consists of three components:
  - Intracranial electrode
  - Extension cable
  - Implanted pulse generator
- The electrode is a coiled wire insulated in polyurethane
- It has 4 iridium electrodes for implantation in the target tissue
- The lead is connected by an extension cable to the implanted pulse generator
- PG is a programmable single or dual channel internal pulse generator
- This sends electrical impulses at the pre-programmed levels to stimulate the target site
- The PG is placed subcutaneously below the clavicle or in the abdomen.

Surgical Technique

- Performed best by a surgical team experienced in stereotactic neurosurgery
- Typically, surgery involves 2 procedures:
  - Placement of electrodes into the target area of the brain
  - Internalization of the lead and implantation of pulse generator
- The procedure may be completed on the same day or as a two–stage procedure
- Internalization of the PG may be done 3 days–2 weeks after the procedure
- Advantages of a two–staged procedure:
  - Useful in prolonged procedures and uncooperative patients
  - *Microlesion effect*:
    - Caused by the edema around the implanted electrode
    - This causes improvement in patients symptoms without any stimulus
    - This impairs the ability to check for stimulation induced benefits
- Surgery begins with the placement of a rigid head frame to the patients skull
- MRI is then done to visualize intracranial structures and establish reference points
- Commonly used head frames include:
  - ***Cosman–Roberts–Wells frame***
  - ***Leksell frame***
- After imaging, patient is transferred to the operating room
- Patient is positioned in the supine/semi sitting position with the frame fixed to bed
- Method of localizing the specific target for electrode placement includes:
  - Micro Electrode Recordings (MERs)
  - Macro–stimulation testing of awake patient
- MERs are obtained to detect and amplify activity of individual neurons
- The electrode is then inserted 10–15 mm above the target site
- It is advanced 0.5–1 mm along its trajectory towards the target nuclei
- Continuous spontaneous neuronal discharges are simultaneously recorded

- Localization of the specific target area is done using:
  - Variations in the spontaneous firing rate
  - Movement related changes in firing rates
- The electrode is secured and wound is closed after radiological confirmation
- In bilateral DBS, a second incision is made on the other side and procedure is repeated
- Electrodes are tunnelled subcutaneously on the side of the neck
- The electrodes are then connected to the pulse generator
- The pulse generator is usually placed in the infraclavicular area or abdomen

Goals of Anesthesia

- Providing optimal surgical conditions
- Optimizing patient comfort
- Facilitating intraoperative monitoring
- Facilitating target localization
- Rapid diagnosis and treatement of complications

Anesthetic Considerations

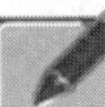

- Procedure related considerations:
  - Long procedure: Fatigue and discomfort
  - Preoperative polypharmacy
  - Altered pharmacokinetics due to preoperative medications
  - Selective continuation of preoperative medications: Requires discussion with surgical team
  - Mutiple locations for procedure and transport due to intraoperative MRI
  - Stereotactic frame application causing remote airway problems
  - Surgery in sitting/semi-sitting position
  - Intraoperative stimulation testing of patient requiring alert and conscious patient
  - Microelectrode recordings: May be altered by anesthetic agents
- Disease related considerations:
  - Parkinsons disease:
    - Pharyngeal dysfunction: Increased incidence of aspiration pneumonia
    - Laryngeal dysfunction: Increased incidence of laryngospasm
    - Autonomic dysfunction causing:
      - Hemodynamic instability
      - Rapid development of hypothermia
    - Difficult airway
    - Postoperative delirium
  - Psychiatric patients:
    - Severe preoperative anxiety
    - Drug interactions with preoperative medications
  - Chronic pain:
    - Opioid resistance
    - Opioid sparing anesthetic technique
  - Alzheimers disease:
    - Difficult intraoperative communication
    - Postoperative delirium

Effects of Anesthetic Agents on MER

Agent	Effects
Local anesthetics	Nil
Benzodiazepines	Amelioration of tremors
	Interference with MER
Opioids	Rigidity
	Suppression of tremors
Propofol	Dyskinetic effects
	Abolishes tremors
	Attenuates MER signals
Dexmedetomidine	High dose abolishes MER
	Hypotension, bradycardia

Choice of Anesthetic Technique

- Local anesthesia with monitored anesthesia care:
  - Local anesthesia is injected at the sites of pin insertion and incision for burr hole
  - Long acting agents are preferred:
    - 0.5% bupivacaine
    - 0.5% levobupivacaine
    - 0.75% ropivacaine
  - Monitored anesthesia care is provided to keep the patient comfortable
  - Proper positioning is important to maximize patient comfort
  - Supplemental oxygen may be delivered via face mask or nasal prongs
  - Other noteable factors while providing MAC include:
    - Restriction of fluid therapy to prevent intraoperative bladder distention
    - Patients are encouraged to void just before surgery for the same reason
    - Appropriate methods to prevent intraoperative hypothermia
  - Additional infilteration may be required for closure in prolonged procedures
  - Neurological medications should be withheld 15 minutes prior to MER
  - In case sedation is required during the procedure, short acting agents are used
  - Agents used include:
    - Propofol
    - Remifentanyl
    - Dexmedetomidine
  - In case sedative agents are being used, they are stopped 15 min before MER
- Scalp block with monitored anesthesia care:
  - Scalp block is achieved by blocking individual nerves including:
    - Supraorbital nerve

- Supratrochlear nerve
- Auriculotemporal nerve
- Zygomaticotemporal nerve
- Greater occipital nerve
- Lesser occipital nerve
- This technique is less painful compared with local anesthetic infilteration
- Complications include:
  - Transient facial palsy can occur during drug injection
  - This interferes with the assessment of intraoperative nerve injury
  - Intraarterial injection
- Scalp block is usually avoided in patients with coagulopathy
- In case sedation is required during the procedure, short acting agents are used
- Agents used include:
  - Propofol
  - Remifentanyl
  - Dexmedetomidine

❖ Conscious sedation with asleep–awake–asleep (AAA) technique:
- Aims to have:
  - A comfortably sedated patient
  - Minimally depressed consciousness at certain times during surgery
  - Ability to maintain airway patency
  - Ability to respond to verbal stimulation
- Frequently used drugs include short acting agents such as:
  - Propofol
  - Remifentanyl
  - Dexmedetomidine
- Benzodiazepines are avoided as the alter the threshold for stimulation
- Adjuncts to maintain airway patency include:
  - Oral/nasopharyngeal airway
  - Cuffed oropharyngeal airway
  - Laryngeal mask airway
- LMA is the preferred technique
- Conscious sedation is initiated once the patient arrives in the OR after MRI
- When the surgeon is ready to begin mapping, anesthetic plane is lightened
- The patient is allowed to emerge from anesthesia and airway is removed
- Smooth emergence is essential and disastrous complications can occur due to:
  - Valsalva maneuver
  - Coughing
  - Vomiting
  - Patient movement
- Thus, this is the most crucial part of surgery
- Once mapping is completed, sedation is resumed till the end of surgery
- This constitutes the asleep–awake–asleep technique of conscious sedation

❖ General anesthesia:
- Indicated in patients with:
  - Excess anxiety
  - Chronic pain syndromes with opioid tolerance
  - Severe movements due to off drug state
  - Severe dystonia or choreoathetosis
  - Pediatric patients
  - Critically ill patients
- Advantages:
  - Provides a secure airway
  - Securing airway access may be difficult in the presence of stereotactic frame
  - Provides more patient comfort
- Disadvantages:
  - Anesthetic agents may interefere with MERs
  - Thus, intraoperative mapping and stimulation testing will be difficult

ANESTHETIC MANAGEMENT FOR GENERAL ANESTHESIA

Preoperative Evaluation and Premedication

❖ Assessment should include:
- Severity of Parkinsons disease
- Prior responsiveness to levodopa therapy
- Prior history of obstructive sleep apnea
- Thorough airway assessment
- Assessment for intraoperative positioning:
  - History of orthostatic hypotension
  - History of limitation of joint mobility
- Need for invasive vascular access based on severity of disease

❖ Assessment should also be done for chronic pain and psychiatric illnesses

❖ Ability to cooperate during the procedure should be assessed

❖ This is important as:
- Most of the times surgical duration is prolonged
- Intraoperative anxiety increases BP and leads to intracranial hemorrhage

❖ Drug and procedural history:
- History should be obtained regarding previous medications
- Most patients will have multiple prior medications

- History should also be obtained regarding implanted ferrous metals and pacemakers
- This is because DBS usually involves intraoperative MRI
- Discuss with the surgical team about continuation of preoperative neurological drugs
- This is because some patients may require a "drug–off" state to facilitate mapping
- In case of severe symptoms, reduced dose of regular medication may be given
- Sedative premedications are avoided (including opioids and benzodiazepines)

Monitors

- Pulse oximetry
- ECG
- Noninvasive BP
- E_TCO_2
- Invasive blood pressure monitoring indicated in the presence of:
  - Labile blood pressure
  - Patients with severe comorbidities
- Urine output
- Bispectral index
- Neuromuscular monitoring

Induction

- Adequate preoxygenation
- Propofol is commonly used for intravenous induction
- Propofol 1–2 mg/kg + fentanyl 1–2 µg/kg + rocuronium 1 mg/kg IV
- Alternatives for induction include etomidate and ketamine
- Rapid sequence induction used for severe PD with risk of aspiration pneumonia
- LMA may be used in case intraoperative emergence is planned
- In all other cases ETT is used to secure the airway
- Foleys catheter may be inserted in severe PD to prevent postoperative urine retention
- Stereotactic head frame is placed following endotracheal intubation
- Patient is then shifted to the MRI suite to obtain the coordinates for the target nuclei
- Following MRI, patient is shifted back to the OR and positioned

Maintenance

- O_2 + air + sevoflurane (0.8–1 MAC) + fentanyl boluses
- Short acting volatile agents like sevoflurane and desflurane are preferred
- This is to facilitate emergence in case patient needs to be awakened intraoperatively
- NMBAs are avoided if movement related neuronal discharges are elicited
- Alternatively, TIVA may be used with:
  - Remifentanil 0.02–0.1 µg/kg/min
  - Propofol 75–200 µg/kg/min
- If MER is planned during surgery use:
  - Low dose inhalational anesthetic (0.5 MAC)
  - Low dose opioid (0.02–0.1 µg/kg/min)
  - Low dose propofol (75 µg/kg/min)
- Analgesic supplementation is required during tunnelling of the electrode cable
- This part of the procedure is extremely painful
- Postoperative MRI may be performed to rule out surgical complications
- Following this, the stereotactic frame is removed

Positioning

- Difficult positioning due to muscle rigidity
- Gradual change of position due to autonomic instability
- Adequate padding at pressure points essential
- Proper positioning is important to minimize perioperative complications
- Use of clear plastic drapes is preferred to allow constant monitoring of position
- Flexion of lower cervical spine and extension of atlanto–occipital joint is ensured
- This makes the airway patent and aids airway access in case of emergencies
- Legs should be flexed and supported under the knees
- This is in order to maintain stability when the patient is elevated to sitting position

Hemodynamics

- Vasodilatation associated with anesthetic induction may cause severe hypotension
- Autonomic insufficiency alters response to hypovolemia and worsen hypotension
- Precipitous hypotension may therefore occur at induction due to:
  - Relative hypovolemia
  - Catecholamine depletion
  - Autonomic instability
  - Sensitization to catecholamines
  - Coadministration of bromocriptine/selegeline

- Directly acting vasopressors should be used to treat hypotension such as:
  - Phenylephrine
  - Epinephrine

Extubation

- Fully reversed, awake extubation
- Adequacy of ventilation and recovery from NMDR established before extubation
- Assess:
  - Spontaneous breathing pattern
  - Presence of gag reflex
  - Ability of patient to focus
  - Presence of 4 twitches/sustained tetanus
- Adequate suction to remove excessive secretions before extubation

Postoperative Management

- Monitors
  - Pulse oximetry
  - Noninvasive blood pressure
  - Electrocardiography
- Management
  - Head up nursing is preferred
  - Anti-PD drugs to be started as soon as possible after surgery
  - This is because the elimination $T_{1/2}$ of levodopa is brief
  - Interruption of these drugs for more than 6 hours results in loss of therapeutic effect
  - L-Dopa can be administered via nasogastric tube if required
  - Good physiotherapy and early ambulation to aid postoperative recovery
  - Breathing exercises and spirometry to prevent chest infections
  - Diphenhydramine 25 mg IV can be used to reduce postoperative tremors
  - Avoid using phenothiazines and haloperidol
- Pain
  - Opioids may be used but have to be replaced with NSAIDs as soon as possible
  - PCA may be difficult to operate
  - NSAIDs (ketorolac) useful as they do not interfere with respiratory function
  - Local anesthetic infilteration useful
  - Multimodal analgesia best
- Complications
  - Under MAC:
    - Coughing, sneezing
    - Aspiration
    - Pulmonary edema
    - Combative behavior, agitation
    - Bronchospasm
    - Intracranial hemorrhage
    - Seizures
- Under GA:
  - Hypertension Venous air embolism
  - Arrhythmias
  - Focal neurodeficits

Anesthetic Considerations in Patients with Pre-Existing DBS

- Preoperative assessment:
  - Identification of specific device type
  - Severity of symptoms once device is turned off
  - Note down anatomical course of the DBS extension cable
  - Oral medications are resumed if severe symptoms appear after switching off device
- DBS systems may produce artifacts and interfere with ECG recordings
- Interaction with electrocautery:
  - Intraoperative electrocautery may burn neural tissue around electrodes
  - Electrocautery may also reprogram the device spontaneously
  - Thus, the device should be turned off for procedures requiring electrocautery
  - Bipolar cautery is safer compared to unipolar cautery
  - If unipolar cautery is used:
    - The grounding pad should be placed far away from the PG
    - Lowest possible source of energy should be used for cautery
    - Cautery should be used in short irregular pulses
- Interaction with defibrillators:
  - Safety of cardiac defibrillators has not been established in patients with DBS
  - If defibrillators have to be used:
    - Paddles must be positioned as far as possible from the DBS-PG
    - Lowest possible source of energy must be used for cardioversion
    - Function of the DBS-PG should be re-checked after using defibrillator

ANESTHESIA FOR GUILLAIN-BARRE SYNDROME

Introduction

Guillain-Barre syndrome is an acute demyelinating polyneuropathy characterized by an ascending motor weakness, sensory and autonomic dysfunction following a prodromal illness.

Etiology

Precipitating Events

- Triggering infection:
  - Campylobacter jejuni
  - Cytomegalovirus
  - Epstein Barr virus
  - Mycoplasma pneumonia
- Immunizations:
  - Rabies vaccine
  - Swine flu
- Lymphomas/Hodgkins disease
- Traumatic events
- Surgery

Pathogenesis

- Precipitating events trigger autoimmune response
- Auto-antibodies formed against glycolipids and gangliosides
- This causes multifocal demyelination and secondary axonal degeneration
- Demyelination causes conduction blockade resulting in motor paralysis

Clinical Features

Symptoms

Motor Weakness

- Rapidly evolving progressive ascending motor paralysis
- Starts in lower limbs and ascends cranially
- Weakness may involve respiratory muscles and cause respiratory failure
- Deep aching pain in muscles and back
- Lower cranial nerve involvement: Difficulty in swallowing, maintaining airway
- Bulbar weakness: Facial nerve palsy
- Ophthalmoplegia

Sensory Disturbances

- Pain: Severe lower back pain
- Numbness and paraesthesias: Starts distally and ascends upwards
- Sensory ataxia and dysarthria

Signs

- Flaccid areflexic paralysis: Diminishes DTR with absent proprioception
- Muscle wasting within 2 weeks of onset of symptoms
- Autonomic dysfunction:
  - Labile blood pressure
  - Orthostatic hypotension
  - Resting tachycardia
  - Arrhythmias
  - Urinary retention
  - Paralytic ileus
  - Hyperhydrosis
- Metabolic derangements: Hyponatremia due to SIADH

Types

Acute Inflammatory Demyelinating Polyradiculoneuropathy (AIDP)

- *Most common* form
- Due to inflammation of myelin sheaths of peripheral nerve axons
- Causes slowing and blockage of conduction through peripheral nerves
- Secondary axonal damage occurs in severe cases
- Symmetrical ascending motor weakness: Hypo/areflexia

Acute Motor Axonal Neuropathy (AMAN)

- Associated with precedent Campylobacter jejuni infection
- Selective motor nerve and axonal involvement
- Antibodies bind to ganglioside antigens on axonal cell membrane
- Macrophage invasion, inflammation and axonal damage follows
- Clinical features similar to AIDP but tendon reflexes preserved

Acute Motor and Sensory Axonal Neuropathy (AMSAN)

- Both motor and sensory fibers involved
- Antibody mediated motor and sensory axonal damage
- Clinical features similar to AMAN but involves sensory symptoms
- More severe and associated with prolonged/partial recovery

Miller-Fisher Syndrome

- Antiganglioside antibodies to GQ1b causes ophthalmoplegia

- Causes demyelination of nerve roots
- Ataxia, areflexia and ophthalmoplegia characteristic
- 25% patients develop limb weakness

Chronic Inflammatory Demyelinating Polyradiculoneuropathy

- Slowly progressive with relapsing course
- Clinical features similar to AIDP

Investigations

Diagnostic

- Raised ESR, CRP
- Anti–GM1, anti–GD1a, anti–GQ1b antibodies
- Serology:
  - Campylobacter jejuni
  - Mycoplasma pneumonia
  - Cytomegalovirus
  - Epstein–Barr virus
- Stool culture: Campylobacter jejuni
- CT scan: To rule out other causes, raised ICP
- MRI: Excludes cervical nerve involvement
- Lumbar puncture: Raised protein with normal cell count and glucose
- Nerve conduction studies: Demyelinating pattern with axonal loss

To Rule Out Complications

- Complete blood count
- Liver function tests: Raised ALT and AST, gamma GT, creatine kinase
- Renal function tests
- Chest X-ray: Aspiration pneumonia
- Features of SIADH
- Autonomic function tests
- PFTs: Reduced vital capacity, maximal inspiratory and expiratory pressures
- Arterial blood gases: Progressive respiratory failure

Differential Diagnosis

Neurological

- Myasthenia gravis
- Eaton-Lambert syndrome
- Multiple sclerosis
- Transverse myelitis

Metabolic

- Hypokalemic periodic paralysis
- Hypermagnesemia
- Hypophosphatemia
- Acute intermittent porphyria

Infective

- Post diphtheria neuropathy
- Polio
- Botulism
- Tick paralysis

Toxins

- Heavy metal poisoning: Lead
- Biological toxins: Snake, scorpion
- Drugs: Nitrofurantoin, aminoglycosides

Others

- Acute polymyositis
- Critical illness myopathy

Diagnostic Criteria

Essential Criteria

- Progressive weakness of more than one limb
- Areflexia
- Duration of progression < 4 weeks

Supportive Criteria

- Relative symmetry
- Mild sensory signs/symptoms
- Cranial nerve involvement, especially bilateral CN VII involvement
- Recovery beginning 2–4 weeks after progression ceases
- Autonomic dysfunction
- Absence of fever at onset
- Typical CSF, EMG and nerve conduction studies

Management

Monitor

- Pulse oximetry: Desaturation is late sign
- Blood pressure: Invasive monitoring as autonomic instability
- ECG
- Arterial blood gases: Evidence of respiratory failure
- Others:
  - Head lift
  - Upper limb weakness
  - Respiratory rate
  - Vital capacity measured thrice daily
  - Maximal inspiratory and expiratory pressures

Airway

- 30% patients require ventilation
- Indications for intubation:
  - Vital capacity < 15 mL/kg or < 1L

- Maximum inspiratory pressure < 30 cm H_2O
- Maximum expiratory pressure < 40 cm H_2O
- Bulbar involvement with weak cough and dysphagia
- Evidence of respiratory failure
- Autonomic instability

❖ Tracheostomy if prolonged respiratory support needed

Deep Vein Thromboprophylaxis

❖ Subcutaneous low molecular weight heparin
❖ Pneumatic compression devices
❖ Early physiotherapy and ambulation

Nutrition

❖ Early resumption of enteral nutrition via nasogastric tube
❖ Paralytic ileus common: Treat with metaclopramide/domperidone
❖ Total parenteral nutrition when enteral measures are inadequate

Immunomodulatory

❖ Intravenous immunoglobulins:
- Most effective if administered within 2 weeks of onset
- 400 mg/kg IV for 5 days
- Indications:
  - Muscle weakness
  - Respiratory depression
- Contraindications:
  - Previous anaphylaxis to IVIg
  - IgA deficiency
- Side effects:
  - Nausea, headache
  - Erythroderma
  - Fluid overload
  - Acute renal failure

❖ Plasma exchange:
- Best if commenced within one week of onset of symptoms
- Beneficial up to 30 days after onset of symptoms
- Involves passage of blood through cell separator
- Plasma fraction is removed and replaced with FFP or human albumin
- Thus, antibodies associated with auto–immune response are removed
- 40–50 mL/kg plasma exchange for 4–5 days
- Indications:
  - Muscle weakness
  - Respiratory weakness
- Contraindications:
  - Coagulopathy
  - Sepsis
  - Hemodynamic instability
- Side effects:
  - Nausea, vomiting
  - Coagulopathy
  - Immunosupression
  - Hypocalcemia

Others

❖ Frequent turning to avoid pressure sores
❖ Prompt correction of dyselectrolytemias
❖ Physiotherapy: For clearance of secretions, prevention of sequelae of limb disuse
❖ Suction clearance of secretions

Corticosteroids

❖ Of historical significance to suppress immune response
❖ No longer used as no evidence of improving long term prognosis

Anesthetic Considerations

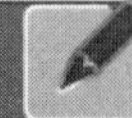

Neurological

❖ Careful limb positioning: Compression nerve palsies common
❖ Neuropathic pain common in postoperative period
❖ Higher incidence of postoperative cognitive decline and depression

Respiratory

❖ Cranial nerve involvement: Upper airway obstruction causing postoperative respiratory failure
❖ Susceptible to aspiration pneumonia due to:
- Bulbar palsy causing difficulty in swallowing
- Laryngeal paralysis

❖ Perioperative respiratory dysfunction: Intercostal and diaphragmatic weakness
❖ Possibility of prolonged postoperative ventilation

Cardiovascular

❖ Arrhythmias common:
- Atrial fibrillation
- Paroxysmal atrial tachycardia
- Ventricular tachyarrhythmias
- Prolonged QT interval
- Atrioventricular blocks
- Asystole

❖ Autonomic dysfunction:
- Labile blood pressure, orthostatic hypotension
- Avoid drugs with negative impact on cardiovascular function

Contd...

Contd...

- Exaggerated response to endotracheal intubation, surgical incision
- Arrhythmias common during endotracheal suction
- Gradual change of posture to avoid hemodynamic disturbances
- Treat hypotension with:
  - Volume expansion
  - Direct acting adrenergic agents
  - Sensitive to vasoactive drugs due to denervation supersensitivity
- Deep vein thrombosis: High risk due to immobility

Gastrointestinal

- Poor oral intake due to bulbar weakness: Dyselectrolytemias
- Early institution of enteral/parenteral feeding
- Susceptible to paralytic ileus in postop period: Treat with prokinetic agents

Pharmacological

- Succinyl choline absolute contraindication as it causes:
  - Severe hyperkalemia
  - Life-threatening arrhythmias
  - Sudden hyperkalemic cardiac arrest
  - Rhabdomyolysis
- More sensitive to non-depolarizing muscle relaxants: avoid NMBAs
- Use intermediate acting NMBAs with neuromuscular monitoring when indicated
- Avoid drugs which prolong action of NMBAs:
  - Aminoglycosides
  - Calcium channel blockers
  - Ranitidine
  - Anticonvulsants
- Use short acting anesthetic agents: To prevent postop respiratory failure
- Sensitive to local anesthetics: Profound hypotension and bradycardia possible

Preoperative Assessment and Preoperative Preparation

- Assess airway, mouth, dentition and neck
- Assess bulbar function to prevent aspiration during induction
- Assess respiratory muscle function: Vital capacity, mouth occlusion pressures, cough
- Assess autonomic function: ECG, postural hypotension, excessive sweating
- Correct electrolyte imbalance/hyponatremia
- NPO orders:
  - 6 hrs solids
  - 2 hrs clear fluids
- Informed consent
- Anti-aspiration prophylaxis
  - Metaclopramide 10 mg IV
  - 30 mL of non-particulate 0.3 M sodium citrate

Monitor

- Pulse oximetry
- Blood pressure
- *ECG*
- $ETCO_2$
- Temperature
- Urine output
- Neuromuscular monitoring mandatory
- Invasive pressure monitoring: For autonomic instability, blood loss anticipated

Position

- Careful positioning to avoid compression palsy
- Gradual change of posture to avoid hypotension

Induction

- Rapid sequence induction
- Propofol 2 mg/kg + fentanyl 1–2 µg/kg + rocuronium 0.1 mg/kg
- Profound hypotension with induction of anesthesia
- Prevent intubation response: IV xylocard 1.5–2 mg/kg 90 seconds before intubation
- Ryles tube inserted

Maintenance

- O_2 + air + isoflurane + fentanyl boluses + vecuronium boluses
- Reduced requirement of NDMRs: Reduce dosage
- Pneumatic compression devices applied

Ventilation

- Controlled ventilation preferred
- Profound hypotension may occur at the initiation of positive pressure ventilation

Hemodynamics

- Profound hypotension during:
  - Induction of anesthesia
  - Change in posture
  - Blood loss
- Exaggerated HTN with intubation/surgical incision
- Treat hypotension with:
  - Volume expansion
  - Direct acting adrenergic agents
  - Exaggerated response to direct acting adrenergic agents
- Normal temperature maintained to prevent hypothermia induced delayed awakening

Extubation

Fully reversed and extubated when fully awake.

Indications for postoperative ventilation:

- Vital capacity < 15 mL/kg or < 1L
- Maximum inspiratory pressure < 30 cm H_2O
- Maximum expiratory pressure < 40 cm H_2O
- Bulbar involvement with weak cough and dysphagia
- Evidence of respiratory failure
- Autonomic instability

Postoperative Management

Management

- Care of skin, bladder and bowel
- Vigorous chest physiotherapy to prevent hospital acquired pneumonia
- DVT prophylaxis instituted as soon as possible after surgery

Monitors

- Pulse oximetry
- Blood pressure
- ECG
- Temperature
- Arterial blood gas
- *Muscle strength*: Head lift, vital capacity

Analgesia

- Multimodal analgesia useful
- Analgesic adjuncts: Useful for opioid sparing properties
  - Anticonvulsants: Gabapentin better than cabamezepine
  - Tricyclic antidepressants

ANESTHESIA FOR EPILEPSY PATIENTS

Introduction

- Seizures are episodes of transient neurological change due to hypersynchronous and hyperexcited neuronal activity
- Epilepsy is defined as a disorder of the brain characterized by a predisposition to epileptic seizures
- For practical purposes, epilepsy is defined by the presence of any of the following:
  - At least 2 unprovoked seizures occurring > 24 hours apart
  - One unprovoked seizure and a probability of further seizures:
    - Similar to the general recurrence risk of at least 60%
    - Occurring over the next 10 years
  - Diagnosis of epilepsy syndrome
- Epilepsy is considered resolved for patients who have remained:
  - Seizure free for the last 10 years
  - Off anti–seizure medications for last 5 years

Incidence

- Epilepsy is the second most frequent neurological disease
- It affects approximately 1% of the worlds population
- The incidence of epilepsy increases linearly with age
- Acute symptomatic seizures are more common in older patients
- Incidence of seizures in patients older than 60 years is 0.55–1 per 1000
- The prevalence of epilepsy in older adults is 3–4 times higher than in young adults
- Age is therefore an independent risk factor for the development of epilepsy

Classification

- *Level 1 diagnosis*: Seizure type
  - Generalized onset seizures:
    - Motor seizures
    - Absence seizures
  - Focal onset seizures:
    - Motor seizures
    - Absence seizures
  - Unknown onset seizures
  - Unclassified seizures
- *Level 2 diagnosis*: Epilepsy based on seizure type
  - Generalized epilepsy
  - Focal epilepsy
  - Generalized and focal epilepsy
  - Unclassified types
- *Level 3 diagnosis*: Epilepsy syndromes
  - Dravet syndrome
  - West syndrome
  - Lennox–Gastaut syndrome
- *Level 4 diagnosis*: Epilepsy with etiology

Etiology

- Genetic syndromes:
  - Epilepsy syndromes

- Juvenile myoclonic epilepsy
- Benign rolandic epilepsy

❖ Trauma:
- Depressed skull fractures
- Intracranial hemorrhages

❖ Tumors: *More common* with anterior hemisphere tumors

❖ Infections:
- Meningitis
- Encephalitis

❖ Cerebrovascular disease:
- Hemorrhage
- Infarction

❖ Cerebral degenerative disease:
- Alzheimers disease
- Multi–infarct dementia
- Multiple sclerosis

❖ Metabolic disorders:
- Hypo/hypercalcemia
- Hypoglycemia
- Hypo/hypernatremia
- Hypomagnesemia

Differential Diagnosis

❖ Syncope:
- Micturition syncope
- Cough syncope
- Cardiac syncope
- Carotid sinus syncope

❖ Transient ischemic attack (TIA)

❖ Basilar migraine

❖ Hyperventilation syndromes

❖ Narcolepsy and cataplexy

Effect of Antiepileptic Drugs (AEDs) on Anesthesia

❖ AEDs have pharmacokinetic and pharmacodynamic interactions with anesthetic agents

❖ This can affect:
- The efficacy of both AEDs and anesthetic agents
- The risk of perioperative seizures

❖ Induction of cytochrome P450 enzymes:
- Enzyme induction reduces the concentration of co–administered drugs
- This may lead to a reduced plasma concentration and efficacy of these drugs
- Drugs with a reduction in plasma concentration include:
  - Immunosuppressants
  - Antibiotics
  - Amiodarone
  - β-blockers
  - Calcium channel antagonists
- AEDs causing enzyme induction include:
  - Carbamazepine
  - Phenytoin
  - Phenobarbital
  - Primidone

❖ Inhibition of cytochrome P450 enzymes:
- Sodium valproate is an AED causing enzyme inhibition
- This reduced the clearance of concurrently administered medications
- This action may in turn contribute to drug toxicity of concurrent drugs

❖ Drugs which do not have any action on cytochrome P450 enzymes:
- Gabapentin
- Lamotrigine
- Levetiracetam
- Tiagabine
- Vigabatrin

❖ Drugs which produce sedation:
- Oxcarbazepine
- Lamotrigine

❖ Changes in hematopoietic system:
- Carbamezepine: Hematopoietic depression
- Sodium valproate: Thrombocytopenia, platelet dysfunction

❖ Metabolic changes:
- Topiramate is associated with asymptomatic non-anion gap metabolic acidosis
- This can lead to intraoperative metabolic acidosis

Effect of Anesthetic Drugs on Epilepsy

❖ Inhalational anesthetics:
- Proconvulsant actions:
  - Nitrous oxide (in animal models)
  - Sevoflurane (when used in high concentrations with hypocapnia)
  - Enflurane
- Anticonvulsant actions:
  - Isoflurane
  - Desflurane

❖ Opioids:
- Proconvulsant actions:
  - After IV administration: Meperidine

- After intrathecal administration:
  - Fentanyl
  - Alfentanil
  - Sufentanil
  - Morphine
- Opioids enhancing EEG activity in patients with focal epilepsy:
  - Remifentanil
  - Alfentanil
- Anticonvulsant actions: None of the opioids have anticonvulsant properties
- Neutral effect: When used intravenously:
  - Fentanyl
  - Morphine

❖ IV anesthetic agents:
- All agents produce excitatory activity on induction of anesthesia
- However, at higher doses, all agents act as anticonvulsants
- Anticonvulsant actions (at high doses):
  - Thiopentone
  - Methohexital
  - Pentobarbital
  - Propofol
  - Ketamine
- Proconvulsant actions (in order of highest incidence):
  - Etomidate
  - Thiopentone
  - Methohexital
  - Propofol

❖ Benzodiazepines:
- All benzodiazepines are anticonvulsants
- Examples include:
  - Midazolam
  - Diazepam
  - Lorazepam

❖ Neuromuscular blocking agents:
- Do not have any pro-convulsant or anti-convulsant actions
- Drugs causing EEG activation include:
  - Atracurium metabolite laudanosine:
    - Produces clinical evidence of seizures in animals
    - Has not been replicated in human beings
    - However, caution using atracurium in hepatic failure patients
    - Half life of laudanosine in these patients is prolonged
    - This can predispose them to seizures
  - Succinylcholine:
    - Produces EEG activation related to an increase in CBF
    - Not associated with any seizure activity however

❖ Local anesthetics: Can cause seizures due to:
- Accidental IV administration
- Rapid systemic absorption from a highly vascular area

Anesthetic Goals

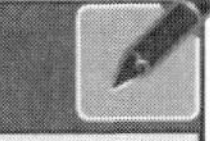

❖ To maintain hemodynamic stability
❖ Avoid any increase in ICP
❖ Minimize impact on electrocorticographic monitoring
❖ Provide neuro-protection
❖ Avoid secondary systemic insults
❖ Facilitate rapid and smooth emergence

Anesthetic Considerations

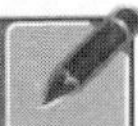

❖ Anesthetic requirements are reduced with use of AEDs which produce sedation:
- Oxcarbazepine
- Lamotrigine

❖ Ensure rapid recovery for postoperative neurological assessment
❖ Management of perioperative refractory status epilepticus
❖ Anesthetic considerations arising from drug interactions:
- Avoid anesthetic drugs potentiating seizure activity:
  - Enflurane
  - Sevoflurane (especially > 1 MAC)
  - Methohexital
  - Etomidate
  - Alfentanil, meperidine, tramadol
- Enzyme induction causing reduced drug efficacy:
  - Carbamezepine
  - Phenytoin
  - Phenobarbital
  - Primidone
- Enzyme inhibition causing drug toxicity: Sodium valproate

❖ Considerations due to concomitant medical problems:
- Psychiatric disorders
- Tuberous sclerosis
- Neurofibromatosis

Choice of Anesthetic Technique

❖ Regional anesthesia is the safest technique
❖ Factors known to precipitate seizures have to be avoided
❖ Sedation and anxiolysis is mandatory to prevent hyperventilation
❖ This in turn reduces the seizure threshold
❖ Local anesthetic agents may cause convulsions are lower than normal concentrations
❖ Thus, the safe maximal dose should be reduced in these patients

Preoperative Assessment

- History:
  - Epilepsy:
    - Etiology of seizures
    - Type and pattern of seizures
    - Frequency and control of seizures
    - Epilepsy free interval
    - Triggers for seizures:
      - Fasting
      - Stress
      - Sleep deprivation
      - Alcohol, drugs
  - Antiepileptic therapy:
    - Type of drugs
    - Duration of therapy
    - Recent change in therapy: Escalation/de-escalation of therapy
- Examination:
  - Risk factors for aspiration and airway obstruction
  - Difficult airway:
    - Craniosynostosis in case of maternal AED therapy
    - Gingival overgrowth from AED therapy
  - Complications of antiepileptic therapy:
    - Acidosis
    - Renal, liver damage
    - Coagulopathies
- Investigations:
  - Complete blood count
  - LFTs: Especially in those on ethosuximide, valproate, carbamezepine
  - Coagulation abnormalities
  - ECG and echocardiography: Especially if tuberous sclerosis/murmurs
  - Plasma levels of antiepileptic therapy for poorly controlled epilepsy
  - EEG
  - CT scan: For detecting structural abnormalities
  - MRI: For detecting small brain lesions
  - SPECT: Single photon emission tomography for cerebral blood flow
  - PET: For cerebral blood flow and glucose metabolism

Preoperative Preparation and Premedication

- Neurologist review if recent change in nature of seizures
- Informed consent to be taken
- NPO orders:
  - 6 hours for solids
  - 2 hours for clear fluids
- Avoid prolonged preoperative starvation to prevent metabolic disturbances
- Perioperative management of AEDs:
  - Continue antiepileptic therapy on the morning of surgery
  - Re–establish antiepileptic medication as soon as practical after surgery
  - When multiple doses are likely to be missed, start parenteral AED supplementation
  - Alternative AEDs have to be started in case parenteral formulation of the routine AED is not available
- Need for possible prolonged postoperative ventilation to be explained
- Use anti–emetics with low likelihood of producing dystonias, when indicated
- Thus, in these patients, ondansetron is the preferred antiemetic
- Sedation is beneficial as hyperventilation reduces seizure threshold
- BZDs are *premedicants of choice* for their anxiolytic and anticonvulsant properties
  - Midazolam 0.03 mg/kg IV is commonly used
  - Long acting benzodiazepines may be useful such as:
    - Diazepam 10 mg PO
    - Lorazepam 2–4 mg PO

Monitoring

- Monitors chosen depending on the type of surgery
- Pulse oximetry
- Electrocardiography
- Noninvasive blood pressure
- E_TCO_2
- Neuromuscular monitoring
- Urine output
- Temperature
- Invasive hemodynamic monitoring in ASA III, IV patients
- Repeated ABG, blood glucose estimation if prolonged surgery

Induction

- Adequate preoxygenation
- Thiopentone 4–5 mg/kg + fentanyl 2 µg/kg + vecuronium 0.1 mg/kg IV
- However, enzyme induction can lead to rapid metabolism of vecuronium
- However, NMBAs such as cisatracurium provide stable pharmacokinetics

- Rapid sequence induction for status epilepticus/ prolonged seizures
- Avoid:
  - Propofol, ketamine and etomidate for induction
  - High induction dose (>0.5 mg/kg) or prolonged infusion of atracurium
  - Succinylcholine for RSI
  - Rocuronium is preferred for RSI

Maintenance

- O_2 + air + isoflurane (1 MAC) + fentanyl boluses used
- Isoflurane is *volatile anesthetic of choice*
- Desflurane also may be used
- Nitrous oxide use is controversial
- Fentanyl and cisatracurium or vecuronium boluses may be titrated
- Increased requirements of opioids and NMBAs due to enzyme induction by AEDs
- Avoid:
  - Halothane (risk of halothane hepatitis)
  - Enflurane (any concentration)
  - Sevoflurane (> 1.5 MAC) contraindicated
  - Alfentanil and pethidine

Ventilation

- Controlled ventilation is preferred
- Avoid hypoxia
- Maintain normocapnea
- Avoid hyperventilation as hypocapnea reduces seizure threshold

Hemodynamics

- Maintain normovolemia during all stages of surgery
- Avoid hypotension, maintain MAP to around 20% of preoperative values
- Avoid hypoglycemia, hyponatremia during prolonged surgery
- Normal saline is the fluid of choice due to slightly higher osmolality
- Avoid fluids which contribute to metabolic acidosis:
  - Lactated ringers
  - Fluids containing glucose

Extubation

- Early emergence is a priority in epileptic patients
- Early awakening facilitates a rapid and complete neurological assessment
- Plane of extubation is determined by the type of surgery
- Emergence response may be blunted with lignocaine, esmolol or labetolol

Postoperative Management

- Management
- Restart AED therapy as soon as possible after surgery:
  - If NPO for 12–24 hours postoperatively:
    - Estabilsh regular oral feeds
    - Restart oral AEDs once oral feeding established
  - If NPO for > 24 hours postoperatively:
    - Replace oral AEDs by parenteral AEDs 2–3 times a day
    - Restart oral AEDs once oral feeding is established
- Monitoring
  - Pulse oximetry
  - Electrocardiogram
  - Blood pressure
  - Urine output
  - Plasma levels of AEDs for 48 hours postoperatively
- Pain
  - Avoid pethidine and tramadol for postoperative analgesia
  - Regional blocks safe
  - Multimodal analgesia preferred
- Complications
  - Status epilepticus
  - *Infections*: Neutropenia, aplastic anemia due to AED
  - Halothane hepatitis

STATUS EPILEPTICUS

Introduction

- Generalized convulsive status epilepticus (GCSE):
  - Defined as continuous seizure activity lasting > 5 minutes duration
  - Risk of long-term complications increases when duration exceeds 30 minutes
- Focal status epilepticus (complex partial status epilepticus):
  - Defined as seizure activity lasting > 10 minutes with impaired consciousness
  - Risk of long–term complications increases when duration exceeds 60 minutes
- Absence status epilepticus:
  - Defined as continuous seizure activity lasting >15 minutes duration
  - Duration which determines the risk of long–term complications is not defined for absence seizures

Incidence

- Incidence (all types of status epilepticus) ranges from 7–41 per 1,00,000 patients
- Incidence of generalised convulsive status epilepticus is 7 per 1,00,000
- Incidence of status epilepticus is highest at extremes of age
- Up to 10% of adults with epilepsy will have one or more episodes of status in their life

Classification

- Generalized convulsive status epilepticus (GCSE)
- Subtle status epilepticus
- Non-convulsive status epilepticus:
  - Absence SE
  - Complex partial SE
- Simple partial status epilepticus

Etiology

- Stuctural brain injury:
  - Stroke
  - Hypoxic injury
  - Tumors
  - Subarachnoid hemorrhage
  - Head injury
- Infections:
  - Meningitis
  - Brain abscess
  - Encephalitis
- Drugs:
  - Antiseizure drug withdrawal
  - Overdose of drugs which reduce seizure threshold:
    - Imipenem
    - Lithium
    - Cocaine
    - Theophylline
    - Isoniazid
    - Bupivacaine, lidocaine
  - Withdrawal of:
    - Barbiturate
    - Benzodiazepines
    - Alcohol
- Metabolic derangements:
  - Hypoglycemia
  - Hyponatremia
  - Hypocalcemia
  - Hypomagnesemia
  - Hepatic encephalopathy
  - Uremic encephalopathy

Clinical Features

- Generalized convulsive status epilepticus:
  - *Impaired consciousness is always seen* in GCSE
  - Bilateral tonic stiffening of the body is seen
  - This is followed by rhythmic symmetric jerking of the limbs
  - Associated with serious side effects
  - This followed by/associated with urinary incontinence
  - Tongue biting is a common complication
- Subtle status epilepticus:
  - Consists of electrical seizure activity with an absent motor response
  - It is considered as an advanced stage of GCSE
  - *Associated with impaired consciousness*
  - Associated with worse prognosis
- Absence status epilepticus:
  - Present with an apparent state of low alertness
  - *Depressed level of consciousness* associated with:
    - Decreased spontaneity
    - Slow speech
  - EEG demonstrates generalized spike and wave discharges
- Complex partial status epilepticus:
  - Rarely seen
  - Arise mainly in the limbic cortex (mesial temporal lobe)
  - Present with features such as:
    - Staring, unresponsiveness
    - Automatisms, atypical anxiety
    - Déjà vu, profound stupor
- Simple partial status epilepticus:
  - Rarely seen
  - Seizures are localized to discrete areas of the cortex
  - *Alterations in the level of consciousness is not seen*
  - Associated with progression of focal jerking activity of the limb
  - This is called the *Jacksonian march*
  - May be associated with impairment of consciousness

Differential Diagnosis

- Myoclonic jerks
- Septic rigors
- Dystonia
- Pseudostatus epilepticus

Management

- *Stage 1*: Active seizures (within 0–5 minutes):
  - General measures:

- Secure IV access
- Monitors (ECG, pulse oximetry)
- Check airway and breathing
- Maintain airway, oxygenation
- Check point of care blood glucose levels
- Provide IV glucose if indicated
- Provide adequate patient protection

❖ *Stage* 2: Established status epilepticus (more than 5 minutes):
- Treatment goal within 5–10 minutes
- General measures:
  - Oxygen supplementation
  - Consider intubation
  - Treat medical complications
  - Investigations:
    - Random blood glucose
    - LFT, RFT, electrolytes
    - Toxicology screening
    - Serum magnesium, phosphorous
    - CSF analysis once stabilized
    - CT/MRI brain once stabilized
- Benzodiazepines are first line drugs: Use one of:
  - IV lorazepam 2 mg up to maximum of 0.1 mg/kg
  - IV diazepam 10–20 mg
- At least 1 parenteral AED is added along with benzodiazepines:
  - IV fosphenytoin 20 phenytoin equivalents/kg at 150 mg/min
  - IV phenytoin 20 mg/kg at 50 mg/min
  - IV levetiracetam 2000–4000 mg

❖ *Stage* 3: Refractory status epilepticus:
- Treatment goal less than 30 minutes
- General measures:
  - Intubate the patient
  - Shift to neuro ICU for admission
  - Continuous EEG monitoring
  - Consider treating acidosis if present
- Drug therapy: One of the following is used for refractory SE:
  - IV midazolam:
    - 0.2 mg/kg bolus dose
    - This is followed by an infusion of 0.05–0.2 mg/kg/hour
  - IV propofol 1 mg/kg followed by 1–10 mg/kg/hour infusion
  - Phenobarbital 20 mg/kg at 50–75 mg/min

Complications

❖ Central nervous system:
- Cerebral hypoxia
- Cerebral edema
- Cerebral hemorrhage
- Cerebral venous thrombosis

❖ Cardiovascular system:
- Myocardial infarction
- Hyper/hypotension
- Arrhythmias
- Cardiac arrest
- Cardiogenic shock

❖ Respiratory system:
- Apnea
- Respiratory failure
- Pneumonia
- Pulmonary edema

❖ Metabolic:
- Hyponatremia
- Hypoglycemia
- Hyperkalemia
- Metabolic acidosis
- Acute tubular necrosis
- Acute hepatic necrosis
- Acute pancreatitis

❖ Miscellaneous:
- Disseminated intravascular coagulation
- Rhabdomyolysis
- Fractures

CAUSES OF PERIOPERATIVE SEIZURES

I. Central Nervous System

❖ Preexisting epilepsy
❖ Previous history of traumatic brain injury (TBI)
❖ ***Breakthrough seizures***: Due to missed dose of anti–convulsants
❖ Trauma
❖ Intracranial hemorrhage
❖ Cerebral venous thrombosis
❖ Intracranial space occupying lesions (ICSOL):
- Tumors
- Abscesses

II. Metabolic Disturbances

❖ Hypoxia
❖ Hypercarbia/Hypocarbia
❖ Hyponatremia
❖ Hypocalcemia
❖ Hypomagnesemia
❖ Hypoglycemia: ***Neuroglycopenia***
❖ Hypothermia

III. Infections

- Febrile seizures
- Toxemias:
  - Encephalitis
  - Meningitis
  - Parasitemias: Schistosomiasis/tapeworm
  - Sepsis

IV. Peripartum

- Ecclampsia
- Amniotic fluid embolism
- Magnesium sulphate toxicity

V. Drugs

Proconvulsant Drugs

- Dopaminergic antagonists: Metaclopramide
- Tricyclic antidepressants
- Antipsychotics: Clozapine, olanzapine
- Antiepileptics: Phenytoin/carbamazepine at supra–therapeutic range
- Methylxanthines: Theophylline/aminophylline
- Prostaglandins
- Beta blocker toxicity
- Beta lactam antibiotics: Infants/history of meningitis/supra–tentorial craniotomy

Anesthetic Agents

- Volatile anesthetics:
  - Enflurane: Especially at > 2 MAC
  - Sevoflurane: Proconvulsant at > 1.5 MAC when associated with hyperventilation
- Induction agents:
  - Etomidate:
    - Has a dose dependent action
    - Proconvulsant action at smaller induction doses
    - Burst suppression seen at higher doses
  - Methohexitone
  - Ketamine: Proconvulsant with subcortical electrical activation
  - Propofol:
    - Dose dependent action
    - Proconvulsant action at smaller induction doses
    - Burst suppression at higher doses
- Atracurium/cisatracurium:
  - Occurs due to laudanosine formation
  - Accumulation at high doses/repeated prolonged dosing
  - Laudanosine levels > 17 μg/mL is epileptogenic
- Meperidine: in renal failure/at high doses
- Tramadol in renal failure patients
- Pentazocine

Medication Errors

- Local anesthetic systemic toxicity (LAST)
- Intrathecal tranexemic acid/repeat doses of tetracaine

Drug Withdrawal

- Alcohol withdrawal
- Sedative drug withdrawal: Diazepam withdrawal
- Antiepileptic withdrawal: Phenobarbital, carbamezepine

ANESTHESIA FOR AWAKE CRANIOTOMY

Introduction

- Awake craniotomy refers to surgery that is performed on the brain while the patient is in a state of awareness
- This allows for functional testing of the cortex during the procedure

Indications

- Eloquent cortex refers to the areas of the brain which control:
  - Motor function
  - Sensory function
  - Language function
- Awake craniotomy allows functional mapping of lesions close to the eloquent cortex
- Anatomical indications:
  - Resection of tumors in eloquent cortex:
    - Frontal lobe:
      - Motor area
      - ***Brocas*** speech area
    - Temporal lobe: ***Wernickes*** speech area
  - Lesions resected usually include:
    - Seizure foci
    - Arteriovenous malformations
    - Aneurysms
    - Tumors
- Functional indications:
  - Deep brain stimulation:
    - Parkinsons disease
    - Dystonias
  - Stereotactic brain biopsies

Contraindications

- Absolute contraindications:
  - Uncooperative patient
  - Extreme anxiety
  - Patients with impaired communication:
    - Inability to speak
    - Difficulty in hearing
- Relative contraindications:
  - Obstructive sleep apnea
  - Morbidly obese
  - Difficult airway
  - Vascular tumors
  - Tumor with dural involvement: painful
  - Low occipital tumors: prone position
  - Inexperienced surgeon

Steps of Surgery

- Cortical mapping:
  - The surgeon stimulates cortical areas of interest
  - This is done using monopolar or bipolar stimulator probes
  - The patients response to stimulation is monitored
  - Different types of mapping may be done:
    - Motor mapping:
      - Patient is observed for involuntary movements in contralateral limb
      - Movement disturbances help in mapping motor areas
    - Sensory mapping: Patient reports abnormal sensations such as paresthesias
    - Language mapping:
      - Tests may involve:
        - Naming objects
        - Counting numbers
        - Reading single words
        - Repeating complex sentences
      - Patient is monitored during stimulation for:
        - Speech arrest
        - Expressive/receptive aphasia
    - Visual mapping:
      - Involves monitoring for abnormal visual phenomena
      - Responses monitored include:
        - Visual hallucinations
        - Visual field cuts
- Electrocorticographic (ECoG) recordings:
  - ECoG recordings are performed for localization of epileptogenic focus
  - Electrodes are placed on the surface of the brain adjacent to epileptogenic foci
  - The electrodes are used to stimulate these foci as ECoG recordings are made
  - Quality of ECoG recordings is affected by the anesthetic agents administered
  - Epileptogenic foci may require stimulation by the administration of:
    - Methohexital 10–50 mg
    - Thiopentone 25–50 mg
    - Propofol 10–20 mg
    - Etomidate 2–4 mg

Anesthetic Goals

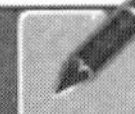

- Preoperative goals:
  - Establish rapport with the patient
  - The requirement for awake surgery should be reinforced
  - Detailed explanation about the procedure to allay patient anxiety
  - Individualize premedication based on:
    - Procedural demand (ECoG)
    - Anxiety levels
- Intraoperative considerations:
  - To facilitate excision of maximum amount of the lesion
  - Modify anesthetic technique to minimize interference with ECoG recordings
  - To maximize patient cooperation:
    - Optimal analgesia
    - Adequate sedation and anxiolysis
    - Comfortable positioning
    - Prevent nausea, vomiting and seizures
  - Smooth transition between anesthesia and consciousness:
    - *Asleep*: Sufficient depth of anesthesia during opening and closing of skull flap
    - *Awake*: Maintain full consciousness during brain mapping
  - Maintain homeostasis:
    - Safe airway and adequate ventilation
    - Hemodynamic stability
    - Normal ICP
    - Appropriate cerebral blood flow and perfusion
  - Facilitate rapid emergence for postoperative neurological evaluation
- Postoperative considerations:
  - Vigilant postoperative monitoring for neurological status and complications
  - Aggressive seizure control

Preoperative Assessment

- Evaluate seizure history:
  - Type and pattern of seizures
  - Frequency of seizures
  - Previous and current anticonvulsant therapy
  - Complications of anticonvulsant therapy
  - Plasma concentrations of drugs

- Airway assessment:
  - Ease of mask ventilation
  - Mallampatti score, predictors of difficult laryngoscopy
  - *Obstructive apnea risk*: Obesity, sleep apnea, retrognathia
  - Important as anesthetist should be prepared for emergency intubation, in lateral position
- Evaluate nausea and vomiting risk:
  - Past anesthesia exposure
  - Kinetosis
- Evaluate hemorrhagic risk:
  - Type of lesion
  - Antiplatelet therapy
  - Medical history
- Evaluate intracranial pressure:
  - Type of lesion
  - Radiological and clinical signs
- Evaluate patient cooperation:
  - Anxiety
  - Pain tolerance
  - Neurological deficits
  - Psychological status

Preoperative Preparation

- Informed consent
- NPO orders:
  - 6 hours for solids
  - 2 hours for clear fluids
- Psychological preparation of patient for awake surgery:
  - Patient should be given a clear outline regarding:
    - Details of the procedure
    - Position adopted during the procedure
    - Varying states of sedation and awareness
    - ECoG testing process (motor vs verbal)
  - Reassure that procedure will be entirely painless
  - Possibility of nausea on traction of temporal lobe explained
- Anti–epileptic medications are continued on the day of surgery
- Good IV line is secured, arterial line maybe inserted under LA
- Preoperative antibiotics administered as per hospital protocol
- Antiemetic prophylaxis: ondansetron 4–8 mg IV
- For procedures involving ECoG:
  - Benzodiazepines are avoided in patients undergoing ECoG as:
    - BZDs suppress seizure foci
    - This may interfere with ECoG recordings
  - Clonidine 2–3 μg/kg PO maybe given one hour before surgery
- For procedures not involving ECoG:
  - Premedication is individualized based upon:
    - Baseline neurological status
    - Patients level of anxiety
    - Comorbidities
    - Plan of anesthetic technique
  - Short acting benzodiazepines such as midazolam may be useful
- IV dexamethasone 8 mg before surgery:
  - Reduces ICP
  - Reduces incidence of PONV

OT Preparation

- Suction apparatus (S)
- Oxygenation: Airway devices (O)
- Anesthetic drugs: Local anesthetics, sedatives (A)
- Pharmacy: Other medications (antiemetics, vasopressors, anticonvulsants) (P)
- Monitors (M)
- Emergency drugs: Atropine, adrenaline (E)
- OT temperature to be suitable
- Surgical table covered with soft, thick dressing
- Position all instruments in order to minimize movement of objects and personnel
- Audio–video recorder system to record patient responses during cortical mapping

Monitors

- Pulse oximetry
- ECG
- NIBP
- E_TCO_2
- Respiratory rate
- Temperature
- Continuous IBP: For recording BP and periodic ABGs
- Urine output: Foleys catheter inserted if:
  - Expected duration of surgery more than 4 hours
  - Intraoperative mannitol administration
- BIS monitoring:
  - Facilitates regulation of anesthetic dose
  - Allows rapid awakening for intraoperative language testing
  - However, placement of leads may not be possible for frontal craniotomies
- Central venous catheter placement if large blood loss anticipated
- Ramsay sedation score/VAS score for adequacy of sedation/analgesia

Position

- Positioning during awake craniotomy should ensure:
  - Patient comfort
  - Access to the patient during surgery
- Supine, lateral or semi-lateral position is used, depending on surgical requirements
- The patients head is held in skull pins with a May-field apparatus
- Once the pins are applied, repositioning is usually not feasible
- Extreme flexion and rotation of the head is avoided to minimize airway obstruction
- Adequate padding is provided and pressure points are checked
- Draping should allow:
  - Constant, unimpeded access to airway
  - Visualization of the patient to allow intra-operative assessment
- Drapes are tented upwards from the patient on the side of the anesthesia team
- Tenting, along with the use of clear transparent drapes prevents claustrophobia

Anesthetic Techniques

I. Local Anesthesia

- Scalp can be anesthetized for awake craniotomies using:
  - Scalp block
  - Regional field block with LA infiltration around incision and pin sites
- Scalp block:
  - Requires bilateral injection of six cranial nerves
  - Approxiamtely 40 mL of local anesthetic solution is required
  - Local anesthetics used include:
    - 0.25% bupivacaine
    - 0.2% ropivacaine
    - 0.25% levobupivacaine
  - Epinephrine 1:2,00,000 is co-administered to minimize systemic absorption
  - The six nerves that are blocked with scalp block include:
    - i. Supraorbital nerve
    - ii. Supratrochlear nerve
    - iii. Zygomatico–temporal nerve
    - iv. Auriculotemporal nerve
    - v. Lesser occipital nerve
    - vi. Greater occipital nerve
- Local anesthetic infilteration of trigeminal nerve trunk is used for analgesia of dura
- Precautions to avoid LAST:
  - Limit scalp infiltration to < 2.5 mg/kg lean body weight for bupivacaine
  - In case of redosing:
    - One fourth the initial dose can be given within 2–4 hours of initial dose
    - One–half the initial dose can be given within 4–8 hours of initial dose
    - Full dose can be repeated after 8 hours of the initial dose
- IV sedation required until the dura is opened as the patient might be distressed

II. Conscious Sedation

- Introduction:
  - Comprises sedation and analgesia, carefully titrated to different surgical planes
  - Used in conjunction with LA infilteration
  - Requires good regional anesthesia of scalp with carefully titrated anesthetics
- Goals of conscious sedation:
  - Adequate analgesia
  - Patient should respond to verbal/tactile stimulation
  - Airway should be maintained without intervention
  - Ventilation should be adequate
  - Hemodynamics should be stable without support
- Drugs used:
  - Fentanyl + droperidol in incremental doses: ***neuroleptanalgesia*** (used earlier)
  - Propofol infusion + fentanyl boluses
  - Propofol + remifentanyl infusion as Target Controlled Infusion
  - Dexmedetomidine infusion
- Technique:
  - Radial arterial line is inserted under LA
  - Indications for Foleys catheter:
    - Expected surgical duration more than 4 hours
    - Intraoperative administration of mannitol
  - Patients position is adjusted on surgical table to be comfortable
  - Scalp block is performed with ropivacaine/levo-bupivacaine
  - This is reinforced with infilteration of pin–sites and surgical incision line
  - Analgesia and sedation co–administered with short acting agents:
    - Propofol 50–150 μg/kg/min IV
    - Remifentanyl 0.05 μg/kg/min is added 5 mins before pin placement

- Remifentanyl is reduced to 0.01 μg/kg/min after placement of pins
- Ramsay score of 3–4 is targeted during pin–fixation and craniotomy
- Dexmedetomidine is an effective alternative
- It can be used alone or in conjunction with:
  - Propofol
  - Opioids
- Benzodiazepines are avoided in patients requiring ECoG
- Nasal airway can be used with supplemental oxygen to maintain the airway
- IV mannitol 0.25 gm/kg can be administered at the time of skull opening
- Hemodynamic management:
  - IV labetolol 5–10 mg when SBP > 150 mm Hg with HR > 50 bpm
  - IV hydralazine 5 mg when SBP > 150 mm Hg with HR < 50 bpm
- Sedation is terminated 20 minutes prior to intra–operative monitoring
- Patient is maintained fully awake till end of brain mapping/tumor removal
- In case of pain arising during resection/dural opening:
  - Paracetamol 1 g IV
  - Remifentanyl increased to 0.025–0.05 μg/kg/min
- Sedation recommenced at the end of tumor resection when dural closure initiated:
  - Propofol 15 μg/kg/min IV and titrated to sedative effect
  - Remifentanyl 0.01 μg/kg/min IV
  - Ramsay score of 2–4 maintained until removal of Mayfield fixators
- IM diclofenac 1 mg/kg is given half hour before end of surgery
- Repetition of scalp block can be done for postoperative analgesia

❖ Advantages:
- Full cooperation of patient if successful
- Does not require ETT/LMA insertion
- Facilitates accurate monitoring of brain function

❖ Disadvantages:
- Maintaining optimal sedation with adequate control of airway is difficult
- Over–sedation causes respiratory depression
- Under–sedation makes the patient uncooperative
- Emergency airway intervention is risky at the time of intraoperative seizures
- Accidental fire:
  - Oxygen is administered using an unsecured airway during surgery
  - This increases the risk of fire with the use of electrocautery

III. Asleep-Awake-Asleep (AAA) Technique

❖ *Introduction*: Technique involves general anesthesia with intraoperative wake up

❖ Components:
- General anesthesia is induced at the beginning of surgery
- Airway is secured with either ETT/LMA
- Anesthetic planes are maintained till the time of dural opening
- Once the dura is opened, the patient is awakened and extubated
- This allows the patient participation during cortical mapping

❖ Phases:
- *Phase 1*: Induction of GA with ETT/LMA until brain is exposed
- *Phase 2*: Patient is gradually awakened and extubated to allow brain mapping
- *Phase 3*: GA is induced after resection of tumor and ETT/LMA reinserted

❖ Technique:
- Phase 1:
  - First part of procedure is done under general anesthesia
  - TIVA with propofol and remifentanyl infusion is the *technique of choice*
  - BIS monitoring is used to guide target-controlled infusions
  - ProSeal LMA is preferred during the first phase for airway control
  - Advantages of supraglottic airway devices:
    - Allow controlled ventilation
    - Avoid airway obstruction
    - Facilitate smoother intraoperative transition to awake state
  - Benzodiazepines are avoided in patients requiring ECoG
  - IV mannitol 0.25 gm/kg is administered at the time of skull opening
  - Hemodynamic management:
    - IV labetolol 5–10 mg (SBP >150 mm Hg with HR > 50 bpm)
    - IV hydralazine 5 mg (SBP >150 mm Hg with HR < 50 bpm)
- Phase 2:
  - Dose of remifentanyl reduced after dural opening

  - This allows the patient to breathe spontaneously
  - Propofol infusion rate is then reduced and stopped to awaken patient
  - LMA/ETT is then removed when patient is fully awake
  - Patient is maintained awake till completion of resection
- Phase 3:
  - After resection of lesion, propofol and remifentanyl are restarted
  - LMA may be reinserted to secure the airway
  - This technique carries minimal risk of coughing, straining and vomiting
  - Securing the airway with ETT may not be possible during this stage

❖ Alternate techniques:
- Alternatively, LMA is kept in-situ during awake phase
- This can cause coughing and straining when the patient awakens
- ETT with catheter attached spirally to ETT is used as alternative to LMA
- Local anesthetic is injected into catheter to provide for airway anesthesia during awake phase
- This allows tube tolerance during the awake phase with ETT in-situ

❖ Advantages:
- Allows titratable levels of anesthesia
- Guarantees patient immobility and maximum patient comfort
- Allows adequate oxygenation and ventilation
- Fast and reliable wake-up
- Patient feels less psychological stress and discomfort

❖ Disadvantages:
- Physical stress associated with intubation
- Awake phase may cause airway irritation, coughing and raised ICP
- Patient movement possible during awake phase with rigid Mayfield head fixation
- Reinsertion of airway devices maybe difficult at end of surgery
- Residual anesthetic effect during awake phase affects evaluation of cortical function
- Longer hospital stays

IV. Asleep–Awake (AA) Technique

❖ Done in two phases:
- Phase 1: Patient is induced and ETT/LMA is inserted
- Phase 2:
  - After exposure of brain, patient is awakened
  - ETT/LMA is then removed
  - Patient is left awake or lightly sedated thereafter till the end of surgery

❖ Advantages:
- Avoids re–induction of GA at the end of surgery
- Avoids problems relating to reinsertion of airway device

❖ Disadvantages:
- Awake phase may cause airway irritation, coughing and raised ICP
- Patient movement possible during awake phase with rigid Mayfield fixation
- Last part of surgery involves administering sedation without securing airway

Postoperative Management

❖ Monitors
- Pulse oximetry
- ECG
- Invasive blood pressure

❖ Analgesia
- Opioids increase risk of sedation, PONV
- NSAIDs may cause postoperative intracranial hemorrhage
- Scalp infilteration along with paracetamol effective and reduces need for opioids

❖ Complications
- Anesthesia related:
  - Airway obstruction
  - Desaturation/hypoxia
  - Raised ICP
  - Hypertension/hypotension
  - Tachycardia/bradycardia
  - Nausea/vomit
  - Shivering
  - LA systemic toxicity
  - Pain
  - Poor cooperation–conversion to general anesthesia

❖ Surgery related:
- Focal seizures
- Generalized seizures
- Aphasia
- Bleeding
- Raised ICP
- Venous air embolism

TRANSPHENOIDAL HYPOPHYSECTOMY

Introduction

- Hypophysectomy refers to the excision/destruction of pituitary gland
- The most widely used approach is the endonasal endoscopic approach
- Anesthetic management is challenging as it involves:
  - Neurosurgical management
  - Principles of endocrine management

Anatomy

- Pituitary gland lies within pituitary fossa (***sella turcica***) of skull base
- Boundaries of the fossa are:
  - Floor: Roof of sphenoid sinus
  - Lateral walls: Cavernous sinus (with carotid artery and CN III, IV and VI)
  - Roof: Diaphragm sella with pituitary stalk
- Hormones secreted:
  - Anterior lobe (adenohypophyses)
    - Luteinizing hormone (LH)
    - Follicle stimulating hormone (FSH)
    - Growth hormone (GH)
    - ACTH
    - Thyroid stimulating hormone (TSH)
    - Prolactin
    - Melanocyte stimulating hormone
  - Posterior lobe:
    - Oxytocin: Formed in hypothalamus
    - Vasopressin

Pathology

- Pituitary tumors are classified into two types:
  1. Functional tumors which secrete hormones, causing distinct syndromes
  2. Non-functional/non-secretory tumors
- Pituitary tumors can also be classified according to their size:
  - Macroadenomas (more than 10 mm)
  - Microadenomas (less than 10 mm)
- Most of the pituitary tumors are benign
- Location of the tumor:
  - Anterior pituitary gland is the most common site of adenomas
  - Most commonly seen adenomas are prolactinoma and nonsecreting adenomas
  - Craniopharyngiomas and *Rathkes pouch cysts* are found in the intermediate lobe
  - Lesions of the posterior pituitary gland are rare
- Hyposecretion of hormones:
  - Due to:
    - Tumor compression
    - Necrosis after postpartum hemorrhagic shock (***Sheehans syndrome)***
    - Head injury
    - Radiation/surgical/chemical hypophysectomy
  - Order in which endocrine function lost (GnRH >GH > ACTH > TSH)
- Hypersecretion of hormones:

Location	Hormone	Type	Clinical presentation
Ant pituitary	Prolactin	Prolactinoma	Galactorrhea Amenorrhea Infertility, hypogonadism
	ACTH	Basophilic adenoma	Cushing's syndrome Centripetal obesity Diabetes mellitus HTN Difficult airway
Suprasellar	Non secretory	Craniopharyngioma Rathkes cleft cyst Suprasellar extension of pituitary lesion	SIADH Panhypopituitarism Visual symptoms Hydrocephalus

Clinical Presentation

- Due to hypersecretion of pituitary hormones:
  - Growth hormone:
    - Gigantism in prepubertal age
    - Acromegaly in adults
  - *ACTH*: Cushing's syndrome
  - Prolactin: Galactorhea, infertility, secondary amenorrhea
- Mass effect if large (> 1 cm diameter) tumor:
  - Headache
  - Hydrocephalus (rare): If suprasellar extension
  - Visual field defects due to optic chiasm compression
  - ***Bitemporal hemianopia** classical*
  - Hypopituitarism if hemorrhage into tumor
  - Cranial nerve palsies: CN III, IV, VI

Surgical Procedure

- Three transsphenoidal approaches are used commonly:
  - Sublabial
  - Nasal aperture
  - Posterior nasopharynx
- Precise navigation to the sella is critical
- This is because the sella is bounded by the carotid arteries and optic nerve

- Techniques used to guide navigation are:
  - Intraoperative fluoroscopy
  - Neuronavigation devices
- Intraoperative visualization is using wither:
  - Operating microscope
  - Endoscope
- The pituitary fossa is entered by removing the bony floor
- After incising dura, tumor is removed using trans-sphenoidal curettes and suction
- After tumor removal, sella is reconstructed with subcutaneous abdominal fat
- Nasal packs are inserted before the end of the procedure

Advantages of Transnasal Approach

- Relatively non-invasive as it utilizes the nasal passages and sinuses to reach the sella
- Shorter operative times
- Lower estimated blood loss
- Less pain
- Lesser incidence of postoperative diabetes insipidus
- Shorter hospital stay

Disadvantages of Transnasal Approach

- Surgical access to the pituitary is limited
- May be difficult to completely excise large tumors
- Rapid blood loss from cavernous sinus due to fracture of the sella turcica floor

Anesthetic Goals

- Provide a relaxed brain for surgical exposure
- Maintain normal intracranial pressure
- Provide perioperative hemodynamic stability
- Maintain adequate cerebral blood flow and oxygen supply
- Maintain metabolic homeostasis
- Provide adequate renal protection
- Facilitate rapid and smooth recovery from anesthesia
- Rapid treatment of any intraoperative complication

Preoperative Anesthetic Considerations

General

- Remote airway
- Raised ICP
- Oropharyngeal packing
- Use of submucosal epinephrine to decrease bleeding

Acromegaly

- OSAS
- Hypertension
- Diabetes mellitus and glucose intolerance
- Increase ventilation perfusion mismatch
- Peripheral neuropathy
- Skeletal muscle weakness
- Osteoporosis
- Poor ulnar collateral blood flow
- Difficult airway due to:
  - Dental malocclusion
  - Enlarged tongue and epiglottis
  - Thich pharyngeal and laryngeal soft tissues
  - Enlarged jaw
  - Thick vocal cords
  - Subglottic narrowing
  - Thyroid enlargement
  - Rarely RLN palsy

Cushings

- HTN
- Fragile skin
- OSAS
- Perioperative steroid cover
- DM
- Osteoporosis
- Obesity and GERD
- Raised intravascular volume state
- Increased infection
- Muscle weakness
- Electrolyte imbalance
- Prolactin secreting tumors
- No anesthetically important endocrinopathy

TSH

Correct hypothyroidism preoperatively.

Preoperative Preparation

- NPO orders
- Informed consent
- Make note of visual disturbances and cranial nerve palsies preoperatively
- Counsel and train the patient to breathe via the mouth preoperatively
- Prepare nasal mucosa to minimize intraoperative bleeding:
  - Traditionally cocaine was used for nasal infiltration
  - Xylometazoline nasal drops administered 10–15 minutes before induction
  - Lignocaine with adrenaline may be infilterated just prior to surgical incision

- IV access is placed in upper extremity on the side opposite to the surgeon
- Bruising may occur on IV access
- IV cefuroxime 1.5 g for surgical antibiotic prophylaxis
- Sedative premedication is avoided if:
  - Difficult airway is anticipated
  - History of obstructive sleep apnea seen with:
    - Acromegaly
    - Cushing's disease
- If premedication is necessary:
  - Short acting benzodiazepines like midazolam are preferred
  - Sedatives are administered in small doses and titrated to effect
  - Sedative and opioid antagonist should be available prior to premedication
- Antiaspiration prophylaxis:
  - IV metaclopramide 10 mg
  - IV ranitidine 1 mg/kg
- Perioperative glucocorticoids:
  - Use of glucocorticoids preoperatively is done in conjunction with the surgeon
  - This is because dexamethasone inhibits the HPA axis for over 24 hours
  - This may result in false diagnosis of pituitary insufficiency postoperatively
  - When used, IV dexamethasone 4–10 mg can be administered

Induction

- Adequate preoxygenation especially when difficult airway is anticipated
- Any IV agent can be used for induction depending on patient factors
- Thiopentone 3–5 mg/kg or propofol 1–2 mg/kg used for induction
- Fentanyl 1–2 µg/kg and vecuronium 0.1 mg/kg can be used to facilitate intubation
- Smaller size RAE tube used to minimize chances of airway trauma
- ETT is secured to lower jaw at corner of mouth opposite to surgeons dominant hand
- Small esophageal stethoscope and temperature probe can lie with ETT
- Entire bundle of ETT, stethoscope and temperature probe is covered with a towel
- This is then clipped below the lower lip to protect it from preparation solutions
- Appropriate size of ETT should be used as undersizing the ETT can cause airway fire
- Fibreoptic intubation is used to secure the airway if difficult airway anticipated
- Throat pack is placed after intubation to prevent blood accumulation in:
  - Stomach leading to postoperative retching and vomiting
  - Glottis causing coughing at extubation
- Proper eye cover as exophthalmos increases chances of corneal abrasion

Lumbar Drains

- Lumbar CSF drains may be inserted after induction of anesthesia
- This is especially useful in patients at a high risk of postoperative CSF leak
- Lumbar drains are preferably inserted in the lateral position
- This is to avoid the risk of rapid loss of CSF during drain insertion
- Uses of lumbar CSF drain:
  - Removal of CSF and reduction of CSF pressure
  - To improve surgical exposure by injection of saline
- Lumbar drains are not allowed to drain continuously
- The volume and timing of CSF should be discussed with the surgeon
- Placement of lumbar drain is associated with a high incidence of PDPH

Monitoring

- SpO_2
- Nerve stimulator at lower extremity
- E_TCO_2
- Temperature
- ECG
- *Urine output*: Foleys catheter is indicated if:
  - Diabetes insipidus
  - Expected duration of surgery is more than 4 hours
- NIBP
- Invasive blood pressure monitoring:
  - Indicated when multiple blood samples have to be taken such as:
    - Invasive tumors
    - Diabetes mellitus
    - Diabetes insipidus
    - Syndrome of Inappropriate Antidiuretic Hormone secretion
  - Small percentage of acromegaly patients have poor ulnar arterial flow
  - Thus, status of collateral circulation has to be checked using Allens test

- Femoral or brachial arteries may be used for patients with positive Allens test
- Intraoperative visual evolved potential in surgeries near visual pathway

Position

- Supine position with neck extended
- After intubation, the table is turned 90° with respect to the anesthesia machine
- Head may be secured with Mayfield pins or supported on a headrest
- Slight head up tilt is provided to avoid venous engorgement and venous air embolism
- Arm on the surgeons side is usually tucked along the patients side
- Anesthesiologist usually has access to the opposite side upper and lower extremities
- Joints and pressure points should be carefully padded

Maintenance

- O_2 + air + isoflurane + remifentanyl 0.05–2 µg/kg/min
- Mucosal surface of nose infilterated with LA + epinephrine prior to incision
- Deep planes are preferred during:
  - Incision, made under lower lip
  - Drilling of sphenoid bone
- Cisatracurium/vecuronium is used to maintain muscle relaxation
- Transphenoidal surgery ends quickly following reconstruction of skull base defect
- Thus, NMBAs have to be titrated depending on the patient needs
- If suprasellar extension is present:
  - 10–40 mL saline/air is injected via the lumbar drain
  - This is done to increase intraventricular pressure
  - This causes prolapse of suprasellar part of tumor into surgical field
- Deliberate hypotension during surgery facilitates repair
- Valsalva maneuver is used after tumor resection to check for CSF leak

Ventilation

- IPPV with ETT
- If no suprasellar extension:
  - Modest hyperventilation to maintain $PaCO_2$ 30–35 mm Hg
  - This helps in decreasing the brain volume
  - Also minimizes the extent to which arachnoid mater bulges into sella
- If suprasellar extension present:
  - Normocapnea/hypercarbia which helps to deliver lesion into sella for excision

Hemodynamics

- Hypotensive anesthesia is preferred to facilitate surgical exposure
- Upper limits of hemodynamic goals during surgery:
  - Normotension for patients without HTN
  - In patients with HTN, BP is maintained within 20% of baseline
- Blood loss is limited unless carotid artery/cavernous sinus ruptures
- If intraoperative diabetes insipidus occurs:
  - Fluid management should be altered
  - Hourly maintenance fluid plus 2/3rd of previous hour urine output used
  - *1/2 normal saline or 5% dextrose is the fluid of choice*
- If hourly fluid requirement > 350–400 mL, use desmopressin

Extubation

- Fully awake extubation after full reversal
- Remove throat pack and thorough suctioning
- Extubate after return of spontaneous respiration and airway reflexes
- Smooth emergence is important to prevent increases in venous pressure
- Harmful effects of retching:
  - Can cause epistaxis
  - Also cause disruption of the surgical wound
  - May result in upward displacement of nasal flora
  - This inturn predisposes the patient to meningitis
- Measures to prevent coughing during extubation:
  - IV lignocaine 1–1.5 mg/kg
  - Continuation of remifentanil infusion at 0.05–0.1 µg/kg/min until extubation
  - ***Bailey maneuver***:
    - Involves substitution of ETT by LMA in deep planes
    - This is useful for patients in whom coughing is particularly detrimental

Postoperative Management

- Management
  - CSF drainage via lumbar drain for 24–48 hours if CSF leak occurs during surgery
  - IV fluid maintenance

- Prophylaxis against PONV:
  - Important as vomiting can:
    - Increase venous pressure
    - Cause epistaxis
    - Disrupt the surgical wound
  - Drugs used:
    - IV ondansetron 4 mg
    - IV dexamethasone 4–10 mg

❖ Monitor
- SpO_2, NIBP, ECG, temperature
- Foleys catheter and urine output
- Electrolytes and serum osmolarity

❖ Analgesia
- Morphine 0.1–0.2 mg/kg is *analgesic of choice*
- Avoid high dose opioids—sedation causes airway obstruction

❖ Complications
- Hemorrhage from cavernous sinus/carotid artery
- Postoperative hematoma:
  - Tight surgical packing of sella causes backward pressure on the optic nerve
  - Thus, it presents as postoperative visual defects/changes in mental status
- Diabetes insipidus:
  - If damage occurs to posterior lobe of pituitary
  - Usually occurs within 4–12 hours postoperatively and is transient
  - Suspect if > 1 L dilute urine (specific gravity <1.005) within 12 hours
  - Associated with:
    - Plasma sodium concentration >143 mEq/L
    - Plasma osmolarity >295 mOsm/kg
    - Urine osmolarity < 300 mOsm/kg
    - High urine output > 2 mL/kg/hour
- Venous air embolism
- Cranial nerve palsies
- Aiway obstruction:
  - Especially common if preoperative OSAS
  - Occurs due to nasal pack which usually stays for 24–48 hours
  - Obligate oral breathing is required in these patients postoperatively
  - This may not be adequate if patient has upper airway obstruction due to:
    - Large tongue
    - Increased pharynageal soft tissue
- SIADH, hypopituitarism
- CSF leak, meningitis, headache, PONV

ANESTHESIA FOR MRI

Introduction

MRI is a diagnostic technique which uses electromagnetic fields to perform noninvasive imaging.

Principle

❖ Based on principle that atomic nuclei with odd number of protons or neutrons have potential to act as magnetic dipoles

❖ Since biological tissues have high water content, H^1 detection is the basis of MRI

❖ Patients are placed within strong magnetic field

❖ Pulses of radiofrequency (RF) energy are applied

❖ This results in intermittent release of RF energy from H^1 nuclei

❖ This energy is detected by a series of close fitting receiving antennae known as coils

❖ The RF signals are collected and interpreted by computer to produces images

❖ Strength of magnetic field during MRI measured in Tesla

❖ One Tesla is equal to 10,000 Gauss(G)

❖ The magnetic field of earth is ≃ 0.5–1.5 G

❖ Most common strength of scanners is 0.5 and 1.5T

❖ Increased strength is associated better spatial resolution

Uses of MRI

❖ Central nervous system:
- Posterior fossa tumors
- Head trauma
- Cerebral infracts
- Dementia
- Intracranial infections

❖ Others:
- Spinal cord
- Cardiac chambers
- Musculoskeletal system—tendon/muscle/ligament injuries
- Intrathoracic disorders
- Intraabdominal disorders

Advantages of MRI

❖ Noninvasive

❖ Obtains images in multiple planes simultaneously:
- Transverse

- Sagittal
- Coronal/oblique

- Excellent spatial resolution and soft tissue contrast
- Not affected by bony artefacts
- Does not employ ionizing radiation
- Requires little patient preparation
- May provide intravascular contrast without IV contrast media
- Does not in itself produce biologically deleterious effects

Problems of MRI

- Remoteness of location
- Lack of trained personnel to assist in the event of emergency
  - Minimum consideration given to anesthetic requirements in design of area like: Lack of pipeline gases and suction
  - Lack of waste gas exhaust capabilities
- Limitations from the magnetic field of imager

Safety Issues

- Implanted ferromagnetic objects:
  - Includes:
    - Intraocular foreign bodies
    - Scissors
    - Oxygen cylinders
    - Laryngoscopes and stylets
  - These may move in the magnetic field and can become dangerous projectiles
  - Some objects may become inactivated/dislodged such as:
    - Implanted pacemakers
    - AEDs
    - Cochlear implants
    - Cerebrovascular clips
  - These may cause hemorrhage/motile injury to adjacent structures
- Metal objects/electronic monitors:
  - May produce RF waves which interfere with images generated by MRI
  - This can result in the generation of degraded and distorted images
  - Alternate, specially adapted monitors and equipment are required
  - These should be positioned as far away from the magnet as possible
- Thermal injury:
  - RF energy may be absorbed by tissues/other objects
  - This results in localized heating
  - Unlikely that body temperature increases by more than 1°C
  - Thermal effects may not be great enough to cause tissue damage
- Noise pollution:
  - Noise generated by the scanner can be as high as 125 dB
  - This may cause temporary/permanent hearing loss
  - Difficult to monitor heart sounds via esophageal/precordial stethoscope
  - Ear is protected with ear plugs
- Pregnancy: Pregnant patients in first trimester should not enter scanner

Zones of MR Suite

ZONE I	Public free access
ZONE II	Interface between public zone and MR suite
	All movement by non-MRI personnel supervised
ZONE III	Area where introduction of ferromagnetic objects forms a hazard
	Separated from zone II by physical restriction (locked doors)
ZONE IV	Scanner room
	Marked lighted signs

Indications for Anesthesia in MRI

- Trauma and shock
- Children
- Ventilated/other ITU patients
- Intraoperative MRI for stereotactic neurosurgery
- Mental illness
- Patients with severe movement disorders
- Patients whose position is limited by pain
- Patients with learning difficulties
- Claustrophobic patients

Anesthetic Goals

- Maintain patient safety and comfort throughout MRI
- Absolute immobility to obtain best possible images
- Not painful: Hypnosis, amnesia and immobility are aims
- Rapid recovery
- Equipment used should be
  - MRI safe: can be used with no additional risk to patient
  - MRI compatible:
    - As well as being MR safe, it does not degrade images produced
    - Its function is not altered by the scanner

Anesthetic Considerations

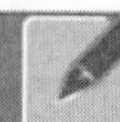

- Remote location of MR suite
- Remote airway with limited patient access and visibility
- Need to exclude ferromagnetic components
- Interference/malfunctioning of monitoring equipment due to magnetic field
- Potential degradation of images by RF currents from leads/monitoring equipment
- Necessity to not move anesthetic/monitoring equipment once examination has started to prevent degradation of magnetic field homogeneity
- Limited access to MR suite for emergency personnel

Preoperative Assessment

- All female patients to have pregnancy test
- Assess all implanted devices:
  - Type of orthopedic implant
  - Pacemaker and internal defibrillators—*MRI contraindicated*
  - Aneurysms clips, cochlear implants, prosthetic heart valves, may get dislodged/heat up/cause induction of electric currents
  - Metal workers may have intraocular foreign bodies–screen by plain radiography before MRI
- Tattoos may heat up in magnetic field due to presence of FeO

Contraindication of MRI

- Obese patients may not fit into bore of magnet
- Cardiac pacemakers and ICDS as the following may occur:
  - Heating of leads
  - Inhibiting of pacemaker output of rapid pacing
  - *Reed* switch malfunction
  - ICD malfunction
  - Torque on pacemaker pack
- Pregnancy in first trimester
- Suspected ferromagnetic intraocular foreign bodies
- Ferromagnetic vascular clip patients
- Titanium clips are an exception as they are non-ferromagnetic
- Hemodynamically unstable patients on infusion pumps as pumps cannot be taken inside

Monitoring in MRI Suite

- General principles:
  - Must conform to ASA standards
  - Important as direct patient visualization in the MRI suite is difficult
  - MR compatible monitors are used and are placed 6–8 feet from the magnet bore
  - If monitors are non-MR compatible, they are placed outside the scan room
  - Long cables are passed through specially shielded holes in walls
  - MR–compatible anesthesia machine with piped anesthetic gases to be available
  - Non-MR compatible machines kept outside 50 G line and bolted onto floor
  - All gas cylinders to be MR compatible
- Specific monitors:
  - Pulse oximeters should have fibreoptic cables to avoid burns
  - Capnograph—delay in obtaining signal as sampling tube will be longer
  - NIBP is safe provided the connections of the cuff and hose are plastic
  - Precordial and esophageal stethoscopes are useless
  - Temperature monitoring is difficult unless probes with RF filters are used
  - ECG:
    - Cables to be shielded and use specific electrodes
    - May have ST–T changes similar to pericarditis due to magnetic field
    - ECG may be completely distorted due to the static magnetic field
  - Padding to be placed between patients skin and monitor cables to prevent burns

Anesthetic Management

Choice of Anesthesia

- GA with ETT/LMA commonly used
- Children between 3–7 years may require sedation
- Older children are often compliant without sedation
- Younger children sleep deeply enough after feeds

Site of Induction

- Best induced outside MRI room, where effects of magnet on laryngoscope and equipment is not a problem
- Patient transferred to docking table and shifted on non-ferromagnetic trolley

Airway Management

- Remote airway as access under the magnet is limited
- LMA is the most commonly used airway adjunct
- MR compatible LMAs are available
- Pilot balloon is taped away from scan site as spring inside may cause artefact
- Patients with poor gag reflex/pregnant patients require intubation

- Preformed ETT is used with pilot balloon taped away from scan site
- Flexometallic tube not used as they degrade images
- Plastic laryngoscope with lithium battery and aluminium spares are used
- Airway to be clear as partial airway obstruction may cause increased respiratory movement and image artefact

Maintenance

- Easier with sevoflurane, as this avoids need for MR compatible infusion pumps
- TIVA with propofol and remifentanyl infusion is alternative
- Circuits have to be very long to go into chamber
- Use long extension lines for IV lines
- Contrast used is Gadolium DTPA which has very low incidence of anaphylaxis

Awakening

Patient is awakened once shifted back to induction area where conventional monitoring can be resumed.

Sedation in MRI

Adults

- Oral benzodiazepines most commonly used
- IV sedation bolus midazolam/low dose propofol with remifentanyl infusion
- Monitor pulse oximetry, E_TCO_2 if possible
- Short MR sequences improves patient compliance

Children

- Children < 3 years sleep deeply after feed
- Children >7 years are often compliant without sedation
- Chloral hydrate, benzodiazepines and low dose propofol infusions used
- Conscious sedation does not ensure compliance due to noise
- Supplemental O_2 and adequate monitoring mandatory

BRAIN DEATH

Introduction

- Brain death is the absence of clinical brain function when the proximate cause is known and demonstrably irreversible
- Death is irreversible loss of capacity for consciousness, combined with irreversible loss of capacity to breathe
- Cerebral death/persistent vegetative state is cessation of function of cerebral cortice's Brainstem function controlling respiratory centres ANS and endocrine and immune systems are preserved with a flat cortical EEG
- Brainstem death:
  - Concept first developed in UK
  - Involvement of bilateral cerebral cortices not required
  - Does not require EEG for confirmation
  - Based on rationale that brain stem and not cortices control respiration,ciculation homeostasis and reticular formation for consciousness

Mechanism of Brain death

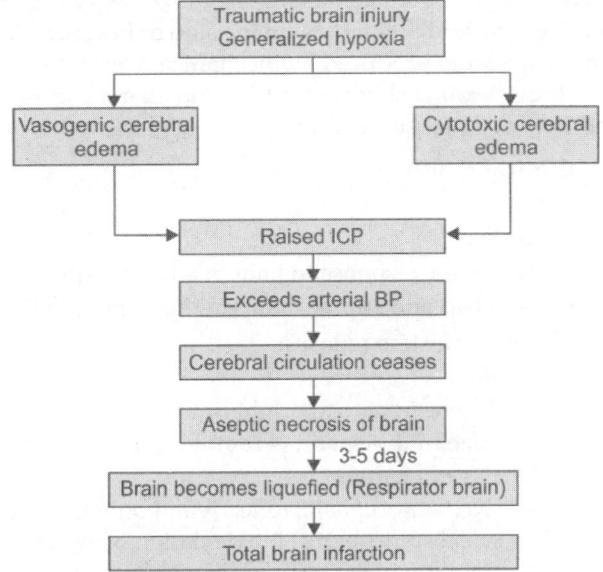

Areas of Brain Involved

- Ascending Reticular Activating System (ARAS)
- Primary respiratory center in reticular core of medulla
- Circulatory center (nucleus tractus solitarius)
- Thermoregulatory centers in hypothalamus
- Pituitary gland
- CNS control over immune system:
  - Increased cytokines (IL–1β, TNFα) seen
  - Increased ICAM and VCAM
- Brain death does not include lower portion of spinal cord caudal to C_2

Diagnostic Criteria

American Academy of Neurology 1995

- Two examinations required, separated by at least 6 hours

- Diagnosis done by 2 or 3 physicians who are independent of transplant team
- At least one physician should be a specialist in neurology/neurosurgery/anesthesia

1. **Prerequisites**

- Clinical/neuroimaging evidence of acute CNS catastrophe
- Exclusion of complicating causes:
  - Severe electrolyte imbalance
  - Acid base disorders
  - Endocrine disturbance
- No dug intoxication/poisoning
- Core temperature >32°C (90°F)

Lazarus sign: Spontaneous/reflex movements due to intact spinal cord at time of skin incision or in synchrony with respiration produced by mechanical ventilation.

Arm flexion, shoulder adduction, hands crossed and opposed just below chin.

2. **Clinical Findings**

- Coma:
  - GCS 3
  - No motor response to pain in all extremities
  - Nail bed and supraorbital pressure included
- Absent brainstem reflexes:
  - Pupils
    - No responses to bright light
    - Size mid position (4 mm) to dilated (9 mm)
  - Ocular movement:
    - No oculocephalic reflex (valid only if no cervical spine injury) No deviation of eyes to irrigation of ear with 50 mL cold water
  - Facial senses and facial motor responses:
    - No corneal reflex with throat swab
    - No jaw reflex
    - No grimacing on nailbed/TM joint/supraorbital ridge pressure
  - Pharyngeal/tracheal reflexes:
    - No response to stimulation of posterior pharynx
    - No cough response to bronchial suctioning
- *Apnea testing*: Most important and mandatory
  - Prerequisites:
    - Core temperature >36.5°C or 97°F
    - Systolic BP >90 mm Hg
    - Euvolemia/positive fluid balance in last 6 hrs
    - $PaCO_2$ normal/$PaCO_2$ = 40 mm Hg
    - Preoxygenate to make PaO_2 >200
  - Connect pulse oximeter and disconnect ventilator
  - Deliver 100% O_2 at 6 L/min into trachea
  - Look for respiratory movements (abdomen/chest excursions)
  - Measure PaO_2, $PaCO_2$ and pH 8 minutes after and reconnect ventilator
  - Absent respiratory movements with $PaCO_2$ > 60 mm Hg or 20 mm Hg increase over baseline $PaCO_2$ levels indicate brain death
  - If respiratory movements present: Not brain death, repeat test for confirmation
  - After connecting ventilator draw ABG if:
    - SBP < 90 mm Hg
    - Pulse oximeter shows desaturation
    - Cardiac arrhythmias present
    - If $PaCO_2$ > 60 mm Hg or > 20 mm Hg increase over baseline $PaCO_2$ it indicates brain death

Brain Death Guidelines in Children

Differences from adult guidelines:

- 3 separate longer observation periods required
- 2 corroborating EEGS and 1 EEG with radionucleide angiography required

1. History

- Determine cause of coma
- Exclude remediable/reversible causes

2. Clinical Examination

- Coma and apnea
- Absent brainstem function
  - Midposition/fully dilated pupils
  - Absent spontaneous eye movements
  - Absent bulbar muscle movements
  - Absent corneal, gag, cough, rooting and sucking reflexes
  - Absent respiratory movements on apnea test
- Patient not hypothermic/hypotensive for age
- Flaccid tone
- Absent spontaneous/induced movements excluding spinal cord events

3. Observation Period

- 7 days to 2 months: 2 examination and EEG separated by > 48 hrs
- 2 months to 1 year: 2 examinations and EEG separated by > 24 hrs
- Older than 1 year: At least 12 hour observation

4. Laboratory Testing

- EEG: Through 30 minute period
- Angiography: Lack of visualization of cerebral circulation

- Other techniques:
  - Xenon CT
  - Digital subtraction angiography (DSA)
  - Transcranial Doppler
  - Evoked potentials

Confirmatory Tests

- Mandatory in children <1 year
- Strongly recommended in children
- Not mandatory in adults

1. Cerebral Angiography

- Contrast injected under high pressure in anterior/posterior circulation
- No intracerebral filling to be detected at level of entry of carotid artery/vertebral artery into skull
- External carotid artery should be patent
- Filling of superior longitudinal sinus may be delayed

2. EEG

- Minimum of 8 scalp electroles to be used
- Interelectrode impedance to be between 100–10000 ohms
- Distance between electrodes to be at least 10 cm
- Sensitivity should be increased to at least 2 μv for 30 minutes
- EEG should show lack of reactivity to intense somatosensory/audiovisual stimuli

3. Transcranial Doppler USG

- Probe at temporal bone above zygomatic arch
- Alternative is suboccipital transcranial window for vertebrobasilar artery
- Should show lack of diastolic/reverberatic flow and small systolic peaks in early systole

4. Cerebral Scintigraphy

- $Tc^{99}m$ used
- Isotope to be injected within 30 minutes after reconstitution
- Static images immediately at 30 min, 60 min and 2 hrs later

5. Evoked Potentials

- BAEP and SSEP of median nerve used
- Loss of waves II, III, IV and V regarded as brain-death
- Bilateral absence of N20–P22 responses with median nerve stimulation is confirmatory

6. CT Angiography

- Noninvasive
- Average global flow <5 mL/dL/min confirms brain-death

7. MRI

8. PET Scan

ANESTHESIA FOR ECT

Introduction

- Consists of programmed electrical stimulation of CNS to initiate seizure activity
- Introduced by ***Cerlitti and Bini*** in 1938

Mechanism of Action

- Changes in blood–brain barrier permeability
- Regional cerebral blood flow changes and electrolyte changes
- Changes in neuro–endocrine activity
- Acute discharge of neuro–endocrine units (ACTH, prolactin)
- Changes in ion transport, neurotransmitters and biogenic amines

Indications

- Acute life-threatening severe endogenous depression:
  - Drug resistance: 2 medications at adequate dose for adequate period of time
  - Associated with suicidal tendencies
  - Very poor fluid intake
- Acute catatonia
- Mania resistant to treatment
- Mania where treatment is limited by side effects
- Bipolar mood disorders
- Schizophrenia with affective component
- Catatonia

Contraindications

- Absolute contraindications:
  - Myocardial infarction in last 3 months
  - Cerebrovascular accident in last 3 months
  - Raised ICP, pheochromocytoma
- Relative contraindications:
  - Recent intracranial surgery, intracranial mass lesion
  - Untreated cerebral aneurysm

- Retinal detachment, glaucoma
- Cochlear implants, cardiac conduction defects
- Aortic aneurysm, uncontrolled angina
- Major bone fractures, severe osteoporosis
- DVT (not anticoagulated), high risk pregnancy

Physics

- Electric current applied transcutaneously
- Two electrodes are positioned unilaterally/bilaterally
- Phases of GTCS induced:
  - Latent phase: for 2–3 seconds
  - Tonic phase: for 10–12 seconds
  - Clonic phase: for 30–50 seconds
- Bilateral ECT more commonly performed
- Unilateral ECT performed on non-dominant hemisphere and has advantage of reducing cognitive side effects

Technique

- Usually performed at dedicated ECT suites or offsite locations such as PACU
- Two scalp electrodes are usually placed with psychiatrist guidance
- Typical electrode positions include:
  - Bilateral or bitemporal scalp electrodes
  - Right unilateral electrodes: ***d'Elia positioning***:
    - One electrode is placed on the right temple
    - Other electrode is placed to the right of the vertex of the skull
  - Bifrontal electrodes: Placed above the outer canthus of each eye
- Dose of stimulus:
  - Dose of the stimulus is described in multiples of the *seizure threshold* (ST)
  - ST is determined by initially setting the device to a small amount of charge
  - If this dose does not produce a seizure, the device is reset to a higher dose
  - The dose is incrementally increased to induce a seizure
  - This dose is the seizure threshold for the particular patient
  - The usual dose for bitemporal leads is 1.5–2 times the seizure threshold
  - Typical setting during ECT:
    - Pulse 60 Hz
    - Duration 0.75 msec
    - Total stimulus duration 1.25 seconds
- Optimal seizure duration more than 15 seconds and less than 120 seconds
- If seizure lasts more than 120 seconds, it should be pharmacologically terminated
- Done 3 times a week for 6–12 treatment sittings
- This is followed by weekly/monthly maintenance therapy
- ECT is done till improvement is seen or treatment is deemed unsuccessful

Physiological Changes

- Cardiovascular system:
  - Initial parasympathetic response (lasts 10–15 seconds):
    - Bradycardia, hypotension
    - Rarely asystole
    - Premature atrial/ventricular complexes, VT
  - Late sustained sympathetic response:
    - Usually peaks at 3–5 minutes
    - 20% increase in heart rate
    - 30–40% increase in systolic BP
    - Increased myocardial O_2 consumption
    - Reduced myocardial oxygen supply
    - Oxygen demand–supply imbalance
    - LV systolic and diastolic dysfunction
    - Cardiac arrhythmias:
      - Sinus tachycardia
      - PVCs, bigeminy, trigeminy, VT
  - ECG changes:
    - ST depression, T wave inversion
    - No changes in myocardial enzyme levels
- Central nervous system:
  - Increased cerebral oxygen consumption and glucose utilization
  - Increased cerebral blood flow (1.5–7 times baseline)
  - Increased intracranial pressure
  - Increased blood brain barrier permeability
  - Transient ischemic deficits, intracranial hemorrhage
  - Prolonged seizures, status epilepticus
  - Cognitive adverse effects, permanent memory loss
- Other changes:
  - Increased intraocular pressure
  - Increased intragastric pressure
  - Reflux esophagitis
  - Nausea, myalgia, feeling of general unease
  - Damage to crewnism bridges, or other dental supports

Complications

- **Neurological:**
  - Short term memory loss, headache
  - Cerebrovascular accidents
  - Status epilepticus
  - Emergence agitation
  - Drowsiness, confusion, disorientation
  - Attention deficit
- **Cardiovascular:**
  - MI, CCF
  - Sudden death
  - Pulmonary edema
  - Transient arrhythmias
- **Others:**
  - Myalgia, weakness
  - Nausea, anorexia
  - Fractures, dislocation
  - Amenorrhea, pulmonary aspiration

Anesthetic Goals

- Rapid and smooth induction
- Adequate amnesia
- Adequate muscle relaxation
- Airway protection
- Control of hemodynamics
- Prevention of complications and bodily injuries
- Rapid and smooth emergence

Anesthetic Considerations

- Difficult history taking
- Drug interactions
- Short duration of procedure
- Antiaspiration prophylaxis
- Hemodynamic alterations
- Use anesthetic drugs which do not alter seizure activity
- Peri-procedural complications
- Associated medical conditions which increase perioperative risk:
  - Unstable or severe cardiovascular disease
  - Space occupying intracranial lesion
  - Recent cerebral hemorrhage
  - Unstable vascular aneurysm
  - Severe pulmonary disease

Anesthetic Considerations of Psychotropic Drugs

- Selective serotonin reuptake inhibitors (SSRI):
  - Cholinesterase inhibition:
    - Mainly occurs with:
      - Fluoxetine
      - Sertraline
    - This prolongs the duration of action of succinylcholine
  - Development of serotonin syndrome:
    - Occurs if other drugs with serotonergic potential are co-administered
    - Drugs causing serotonin syndrome when administered with SSRIs are:
      - Metaclopramide
      - Ondansetron
      - Fentanyl
- Tricyclic antidepressants (TCAs):
  - Interaction with other vasopressor agents:
    - TCAs inhibit uptake of norepinephrine and serotonin at the synaptic cleft
    - This potentiates vasopressor effects of indirect sympathomimetic agents like:
      - Ephedrine
      - Metaraminol
  - Anticholinergic effect may be accentuated by coadministration of other anticholinergic agents
  - TCAs may cause disturbances on ECG:
    - Prolongation of QTc interval
    - Widening of QRS complex
    - Conduction delay
- MAO inhibitors:
  - Interaction with vasopressors:
    - Use of indirect sympathomimetic agents is contraindicated
    - Thus, ephedrine and metaraminol should not be used in these patients
    - Concomitant use of these agents causes exaggerated vasopressor effect
  - Interaction with other drugs:
    - Coadmininstration of meperidine is contraindicated
    - This can precipitate a serotoninergic reaction
- Lithium:
  - Can aggravate cognitive dysfunction following ECT
  - Lithium can also prolong the duration of action of succinylcholine and NDMRs
- Anticonvulsant mood stabilizers:
  - Adversely alter the seizure induction and duration during ECT
  - Enzyme induction by carbamazepine increases anesthetic requirements
- Antipsychotics:
  - Enhance the effects of CNS depressants and thus lower anesthetic requirements
  - Associated with an increased risk of extrapyramidal syndromes:
    - Akathisia
    - Tardive dyskinesia
    - Parkinsonian tremors

- May be associated with neuroleptic malignant syndrome
- ❖ Benzodiazepines:
  - Increase the seizure threshold and reduce the seizure duration
  - Also reduce the anesthetic requirements during the procedure

Preoperative Evaluation

- ❖ History and examination:
  - Difficult history taking, maybe unreliable
  - Evaluate coexisting CNS, CVS disease, osteoporosis and fragile bones
  - Rule out contraindications for ECT
  - Consider other cardiac, respiratory and musculoskeletal medications
- ❖ *Investigations*: Routine blood investigations, ECG, CXR, RFT
- ❖ Preoperative psychotropic drug administration:
  - To be continued:
    - Selective serotonin reuptake inhibitors:
      - Paroxetine
      - Sertraline
      - Fluoxetine
    - Selective norepinephrine reuptake inhibitors:
      - Venlafaxine
      - Des-venlafaxine
      - Duloxetine
    - Tricyclic antidepressants:
      - Amitriptyline
      - Nortriptyline
      - Imipramine
      - Desipramine
    - Monoamine oxidase inhibitors: are continued preoperatively only if:
      - Anesthesiologist is familiar with MAO safe technique
      - Withdrawal of drug will exacerbate the depressive syndrome
    - Antipsychotics:
      - Chlorpromazine
      - Clozapine
      - Quetiapine
      - Olanzapine
      - Risperidone
      - Thioridazine
  - To be withheld:
    - Lithium: 1–2 doses are withheld preoperatively
    - Anticonvulsant mood stabilizers:
      - Carbamezepine
      - Valproate
      - These are withheld on the night before the planned procedure
    - Benzodiazepines: Tapered and discontinued prior to planned ECT
- ❖ MAO inhibitors: Timing of discontinuation:
  - Moclobemide stopped 24 hours preoperatively
  - Stopped 2 weeks prior to surgery:
    - Tranylcypromine
    - Phenelzine
    - Isocarboxacid

Premedication

- ❖ NPO for 6–8 hours
- ❖ Informed consent
- ❖ Anticholinergic premedication:
  - Severe bradycardia and hypotension may occur during the first episode of ECT
  - This occurs due to delivery of subconvulsive stimulus
  - This leads to excessive parasympathetic discharge causing bradycardia and salivation
  - However, anticholinergic medications are *not routinely indicated* in ECT
  - This is due to the undesirable effects associated with tachycardia
  - Used only for patients with prior history of:
    - Severe bradycardia during ECT
    - Excessive salivation during ECT
  - Drugs used:
    - IV glycopyrollate 0.2 mg IV
    - IV atropine 0.2–0.4 mg
- ❖ Sedatives (especially benzodiazepines) are avoided due to risk of:
  - Delayed emergence
  - Increased seizure threshold
  - This would make seizure induction more difficult
- ❖ Anti–aspiration prophylaxis:
  - 0.3 M sodium citrate 15 mL
  - H_2 antagonist: ranitidine 1 mg/kg IV
  - Metoclopramide 10 mg IV
- ❖ Headache prophylaxis:
  - Headache is most common adverse effect of ECT
  - Acetaminophen or ibuprofen may be administered prophylactically
  - IV ketorolac 30 mg is given for patients refractory to conventional NSAIDs
- ❖ Blunting sympathetic response (not routinely used):
  - Atenolol 25–50 mg PO
  - Sublingual nifedipine 10 mg

OT Preparation

- Skilled assistant
- Emergency drugs:
  - β blockers: atenolol/labetolol/esmolol
  - Nicardipine IV
  - IV NTG/hydralazine
- Airway equipment:
  - Ambu bag, airways, face mask
  - Laryngoscope, ETT, stylet, LMA
- Defibrillator

Choice of Drugs

Induction Agents

Drug	Dose	Advantage	Disadvantage
Methohexital	0.75–1 mg/kg	*Drug of choice*	Reduced availability
		Minimal anti-convulsant effect	Myoclonus
		Rapid onset, short duration	Reduces seizure duration
Etomidate	0.15–3 mg/kg	Reduces seizures threshold	Hyperdynamic response
		Prolongs seizure duration	Causes pain on injection
			Longer emergence time
			Increases muscle tone, PONV
Propofol	0.75 mg/kg	Better cardiovascular stability	Pain on injection
		Reduced PONV	Short acting
		Faster emergence	Reduces seizure duration
		As good as methohexital	Significant anticonvulsant action
Thiopentone	2–5 mg/kg	Resistant cases	Reduced cardiovascular stability
		Longer DOA compared to propofol	Causes raised ICT
			Emergence agitation
Ketamine	Not used due to adverse cardiovascular actions		

Muscle Relaxants

Drug	Dose	Advantage	Disadvantage
Succinylcholine	0.5–1 mg/kg	*Drug of choice*	Raises ICP, IOP, IGP
		Partial block reduces ECT seizures	
Mivacurium	0.15 mg/kg		May need reversal

Other Agents

- Remifentanyl:
  - Used in patients in whom seizures are difficult to elicit
  - Advantages of remifentanil:
    - Reduces the dose of ECT required to induce seizures
    - Increases seizure duration
    - Attenuates hypertensive response to seizures
- Caffeine/theophylline:
  - Reduces seizure threshold
  - Prolongs seizures
  - Used for seizure augmentation

Monitors

- ECG, NIBP
- Pulse oximetry
- Visual observation of limb for duration of seizure
- EEG for central seizure
- EMG for peripheral seizure

Procedure

- Preoxygenation:
  - Done with supplemental oxygen via nasal cannula or face mask
  - Aims at maintaining oxygen saturation close to 100%
- Induction:
  - Anesthesia is usually induced with IV propofol in the absence of methohexital
  - This ensures appropriate level of anesthesia for 8–10 minutes
- Neuromuscular blockade:
  - Plan of anesthesia is ensured prior to administration of NMBA
  - Neuromuscular blockade minimizes risk of physical trauma
  - This usually arises due to uncontrolled tetanic muscle contractions
  - IV succinylcholine 1 mg/kg is the NMBA of choice
- Airway management:
  - Patient ventilated with oral airway, face mask and self inflating bag
  - Ventilation is usually done with 100% oxygen
  - ETT intubation is usually not required as the procedure duration is short
  - LMA may be useful in patients with difficult mask ventilation
- Airway is secured with ETT only in the presence of increased risk of aspiration:
  - Pregnancy

- GERD
- Hiatus hernia
- Bite block:
  - Inserted post induction in order to prevent dental and soft tissue injury
  - Bite block should be made of flexible material
  - Maximal cushioning should be provided in the molar area
  - Final position of bite block:
    - Tongue should be pushed inferiorly and posteriorly in the mouth
    - Chin is held firmly against the bite block
- Ventilation and oxygenation:
  - Ventilation with 100% oxygen ensures hyperoxia
  - Hyperventilation is used prior to delivery of the electrical stimulus
  - This induces moderate hypocarbia with $ETCO_2$ of 30 mm Hg
  - Hyperoxia along with hypocarbia increases seizure duration and intensity
  - This optimizes the ECT stimulus efficiency and minimizes postictal side effects
- Electrical stimulation:
  - Stimulus is applied through two electrodes placed on the patients scalp
  - If seizure lasts more than 120 seconds, it is terminated with IV diazepam 5 mg
- Hemodynamic management:
  - Parasympathetic response:
    - ECT stimulation may result in bradycardia or asystole
    - This is due to electrical stimulation of:
      - Motor nucleus of vagus nerve
      - Nucleus ambiguous of medulla oblongata
    - This increases the parasympathetic discharge to SA node suddenly
    - However, the resultant bradycardia and asystole are self limited
    - If persistent, atropine may be used to treat bradycardia
  - Sympathetic response:
    - Sympathetic responses seen during electrical stimulation include:
      - Increase in heart rate by 20%
      - Increase in systolic blood pressure by 30–40%
      - Increase in cardiac output by 80%
    - These responses last for 5–10 minutes postictally
    - Drugs used to counter these responses include:
      - IV esmolol 0.5–1 mg/kg repeated every 3–5 minutes
      - IV metaprolol 1–5 mg followed by 5–15 mg Q6H
      - IV labetolol 5 mg repeated every 10 minutes up to 300 mg
      - Other alternatives include:
  - SNP 0.1–3 μg/kg/min infusion
  - GTN 0.1–3 μg/kg/min infusion
  - Calcium channel blockers:
    - IV nicardipine 100–500 μg followed by 5–15 mg/hour
    - IV clevidipine 1–2 mg/hour infusion
  - Fenoldopam 0.1–1.6 μg/kg/min

Postictal Care

- Oxygen supplementation till fully awake
- IV midazolam 0.05 mg/kg to reduce emergence agitation
- A detailed record of the anesthetic technique and NMBAs used should be made
- This is because the treatment is repeated over weeks
- Consistent patient condition must be provided during each ECT therapy session
- Complications:
  - Postictal confusion, agitation
  - Aggression: Treated with midazolam
  - Headache: Most common adverse effect
  - Reversible memory loss and cognitive impairment
  - Nausea, fractures and dislocation
  - Dental and oral injury
  - Laryngospasm, exacerbation of IHD

SUGGESTED READING

1. [No Authors](1988). Data from Report of World Federation of Neurological Surgeons Committee on a universal subarachnoid hemorrhage grading scale. *Journal of Neurosurgery*, 68(6), 985–6.
2. Adityanjee. (1991). The myth of elevated serum creatine phosphokinase levels and neuroleptic malignant syndrome. *British Journal of Psychiatry*, 158, 706–7.
3. Aitkenhead, A. R., Thompson, J., Rowbotham, D. and Moppett I. (2013). *Smith and Aitkenheads Textbook of Anesthesia*. 6th edition. Netherlands: Churchill Livingstone Elsevier.
4. Alharbi, S., Harsh, G. and Ajlan, A. (2018). Perioperative lumbar drain utilization in transphenoidal pituitary resection. Neurosciences, 23(1), 46–51.
5. Allen, G. C., Larach, M. G. and Kunselman, A. R. (1998). The sensitivity and specificity of the caffeine halothane contracture test: a report from the North American Malignant Hyperthermia Registry. The North American Malignant Hyperthermia Registry of MHAUS. *Anesthesiology*, 88(3), 579–88.
6. American Psychiatric Association. Task Force on Electro convulsive Therapy. (2001). *The practise of ECT: recommendations for treatment, training and privileging: a task force report of the APA*. Washington. 6(2), 85–120.

7. Andrade, C., Sundar, S., Arumugham, and Thirthalli, J. (2016). Adverse effects of electroconvulsive therapy. *Psychiatric Clinics of North America*, 39(3), 513–30.
8. Armstead, W. M. (2017). Cerebral blood flow autoregulation and dysregulation. *Anesthesiology Clinics*, 34(3), 465–77.
9. Bajwa, S. S. and Bajwa, S. K. (2011). Anesthesia and intensive care implications for pituitary surgery: recent trends and advancements. *Indian Journal of Endocrinology and Metabolism*, 15(7), S224–32.
10. Baraka, A. (1992). Suxamethonium block in the myasthenic patient. *Anaesthesia*, 47(3), 217–9.
11. Barry, E. and Hauser, W. A. (1993). Status epilepticus: the interaction of epilepsy and acute brain disease. *Neurology*, 43(8), 1473–8.
12. Benatar, M. (2006). A systematic review of diagnostic studies in myasthenia gravis. *Neuromuscular Disorders*, 16(7), 459–67.
13. Bhagat, H. and Dash, H. H. (2006). Anestehsiologist's role in the management of an epileptic patient. *Indian Journal of Anesthesia*, 50(1), 20–6.
14. Billman, G. E. (2011). Heart rate variability—a historical perspective. *Frontiers in Physiology*, 2:86.
15. Bilotta, F., Gelb, A. W., Stazi, E., Titi, L., Paoloni, F. P. and Rosa, G. (2013). Pharmacological perioperative brain neuro protection: a qualitative review of RCTs. *British Journal of Anesthesiology*, 110(Suppl 1), i113–20.
16. Bindu, B., Bindra, A. and Rath, G. (2017). Temperature management under general anesthesia: compulsion or option. *Journal of Anesthesiology and Clinical Pharmacology*, 33(3), 306–16.
17. Bini, L. (1938). Experimental researches on epileptic attacks induced by the electrical current. *American Journal of Psychiatry*, 16, 136–8.
18. Blencowe, H., Kancherla, V., Moorthie, S., Darlison, M. W. and Modell, B. (2018). Estimates of global and regional prevalence of neural tube defects for 2015: a systematic analysis. *Annals of the New York Academy of Sciences*, 1414(1), 31–46.
19. Borgialli, D. A. et al., (2016). Performance of the pediatric Glasgow Coma Scale score in the evaluation of children with blunt head trauma. *Academic Emergency Medicine*, 23(8), 878–84.
20. Brambrink, A. M. and Kirsch, J. R. (2012). *Essentials of neurosurgical anesthesia and critical care*. New York: Springer.
21. Brennan, P. M., Murray, G. D. and Teasdale, G. M. (2018). Simplifying the use of prognostic information in TBI: the GCS-Pupils score: an extended index of clinical severity. *Journal of Neurosurgery*, 128(6), 1612–20.
22. Brilstra, E. H., Algra, A., Rinkel, G. J. E., Tulleken, C. A. F. and van Gijn, J. (2002). Effectiveness of neurosurgical clip application in patients with aneurysmal SAH. *Journal of Neurosurgery*, 97(5), 1036–41.
23. Brott, T. G., Halperin, J. L. and Abbara, S. (2011). ASA/ACCF/AHA/AANN/AANS/ACR/ASNR/CNS/SAIP/SCAI/SIR/SNIS/SVM/SVS guideline on the management of patients with extracranial carotid and vertebral artery disease. *Stroke*, 42, 464–540.
24. Bryson, E. O., Aloysi, A.S., Farber, K. G. and Kellner, C. H. (2017). Individualized anesthetic management for patients undergoing ECT: a review of current practise. *Anesthesia Analgesia*, 124(6), 1943–56.
25. Butterworth, J. F., Mackey, D. C. and Wasnick, J. D. (2013). *Morgan and Mikhails Clinical Anesthesiology*. 6th edition. New York: McGraw Hill Education. Retrieved 2018. [Viewed 26th May 2020] https://accessmedicine.mhmedical.com/book.aspx?bookID=2444.
26. Carey, C. M., Tullous, M. W. and Walker, M. L. (1994). *Pediatric Neurosurgery*. 3rd edition. Philadelphia: Saunders.
27. Carney, N. et al., (2017). Guidelines for the management of severe traumatic brain injury, 4th edition. *Neurosurgery*, 80(1), 6–15.
28. Caroff, S. N. and Mann, S. C. (1993). Neuroleptic malignant syndrome. *Medical Clinics of North America*, 77(1), 185–202.
29. Chakrabarti, R., Ghazanwy, M. and Tewari, A. (2014). Anesthetic challenges for DBS: a systematic approach. *North American Journal of Medical Sciences*, 6(8), 359–69.
30. Chin, R. F., Neville, B. G. R. and Scott, R. C. (2004). A systematic review of the epidemiology of status epilepticus. *European Journal of Neurology*, 11(12), 800–10.
31. Choi, H., Pack, A., Elkind, M. S. V., Longstreth, Jr., W. T., Ton, T. G. N. and Onchiri, F. (2017). Predictors of incident epilepsy in older adults: The Cardiovascular Health Study. *Neurology*, 88(9), 870–7.
32. Choi, H. A. et al. (2011). Prevention of shivering during therapeutic temperature modulation: The Columbia Antishivering Protocol. *Neurocritical Care*, 14(3), 389–94.
33. Choukalas, C. G. et al., (2010). Mask ventilation, hypocapnia and seizure duration in electroconvulsive therapy. *Journal of Clinical Anesthesiology*, 22(6), 415–9.
34. Connolly, Jr., E. S. et al., (2012). AHA/ASA guidelines for the management of aneurysmal subarachnoid hemorrhage: a guideline for healthcare professionals. *Stroke*, 43(6), 1711–37.
35. Cottrell, J. E. and Patel, P. (2017). *Cottrell and Patels Neuroanesthesia*. 6th edition. Philadelphia: Elsevier.
36. Crossley, A. W. (1992). Perioperative shivering. *Anesthesia*, 47, 193–5.
37. Crossley, A. W. (1992). Six months of shivering in a district general hospital. *Anesthesia*, 47(10), 845–8.
38. Danks, R.A., Aglio, L. S., Gugino, L. D. and Black, P. M. (2000). Craniotomy under local anesthesia and monitored conscious sedation for the resection of tumors involving eloquent cortex. *Journal of Neurooncology*, 49(2), 131–9.
39. Davis, P. J. and Cladis, F. P. (2017). *Smiths Anesthesia for Infants and Children*. 9th edition. Philadelphia: Elsevier.
40. Demirel, S., Attigah, N., Bruijnen, H., Hakimi, M., Macek, L. and Böckler, D. (2012). Eversion carotid endarterectomy is associated with impaired postoperative hemodynamic stability compared with conventional technique. *Annals of Vascular Surgery*, 26(6), 755–65.
41. Duffy, C. and Matta, B. F. (2000). *Anesthesia for Posterior Fossa Surgery*. London: Greenwich Medical Media.
42. Edwards, P. et al., (2005). Final results of the MRC CRASH trial: a randomized placebo-controlled trial of intravenous corticosteroid in adults with head injury—outcomes at 6 months. *Lancet*, 365(9475), 1957–9.
43. Erickson, K. M. and Cole, D. (2012). Anesthetic considerations for awake craniotomy for epilepsy and functional neurosurgery. *Anesthesiology Clinics*, 30(2), 241–68.

44. Espay, A. J. et al. (2017). Deconstructing normal pressure hydrocephalus: ventriculomegaly as early sign of neurodegeneration. *Annals of Neurology*, 82(4), 503–13.
45. European Malignant Hyperthermia Group. (2018). *European Malignant Hyperthermia Group Recommendations*: Perioperative management of malignant hyperthermia suspected or susceptible patients. [Viewed 26th May 2020] https://www.emhg.org/recommendations-1/2018/2/27/perioperative-management-of-mh-suspected-or-susceptible-patients.
46. Fantini, S., Sassaroli, A., Tgavalekos, K. T. and Kornbluth, J. (2016). Cerebral blood flow and autoregulation: current measurement techniques and prospects for noninvasive optical methods. *Neurophotonics*, 3(3), 031411.
47. Fasano, A., Daniele, A. and Albanese, A. (2012). Treatment of motor and non-motor features of Parkinson's Disease with deep brain stimulation. *Lancet Neurology*, 11(5), 429–42.
48. Fisher, R. S. et al., (2014). ILAE official report: a practical clinical definition of epilepsy. *Epilepsia*, 55(4), 475–82.
49. Fuhrman, B. P. and Zimmerman, J. (2017). *Fuhrman and Zimmerman's Pediatric Critical Care*. 5th edition. Philadelphia: Elsevier.
50. GALA Trial Collaborative Group, et al., (2008). General anaesthesia versus local anaesthesia for carotid surgery (GALA): a multicentric randomized controlled trial. *Lancet*, 372(9656), 2132–42.
51. Gennarelli, T. A. Champion, H. R., Copes, W. S. and Saccoand, W. J.. (1994). Comparison of mortality, morbidity and severity of 59,713 head injured patients with 114,447 patients with extracranial injuries. *Journal of Trauma*, 37(6), 962–8.
52. Gill, M., Steele, R., Windemuth, R. and Green, S. M. (2006). A comparison of 5 simplified scales to the out-of-hospital Glasgow Coma Scale for the prediction of TBI outcomes. *Academic Emergency Medicine*, 13(9), 968–73.
53. Gregory, G. A. and Andropoulos, D. B. (2012). *Gregory's Pediatric Anesthesia*. 5th edition. West Sussex, United Kingdom: Wiley-Blackwell.
54. Grob, D., Brunner, N., Namba, T. and Pagala, M. (2008). Lifetime course of myasthenia gravis. *Muscle Nerve*, 37(2), 141–9.
55. Grotta, J. C. et al. (2016). *Stroke: Pathophysiology, Diagnosis and Management*. 6th edition. Philadelphia: Elsevier.
56. Guilfoyle, M. R., Helmy, A., Duane, D. and Hutchinson, P. J. A. (2013). Regional scalp block for post-craniotomy analgesia: a systematic review and meta-analysis. *Anesthesia Analgesia*, 116(5), 1093–102.
57. Halliday, A. et al., (2004). Prevention of disabling and fatal strokes by successful carotid endarterectomy in patients without recent neurological symptoms: randomized controlled trial. *Lancet*, 363(9420), 1491–502.
58. Hermesh, H., Aizenberg, D., Weizman, A., Lapidot, M., Mayor, C. and Munitz, H. (1992). Risk for definite neuroleptic malignant syndrome: a prospective study in 223 consecutive in-patients. *British Journal of Psychiatry*, 161, 254–7.
59. Hilz, M. L. and Dütsch, M. (2006). Quantitative studies of autonomic function. *Muscle Nerve*, 33(1), 6–20.
60. Hye, R. J. et al., (2016). Anesthetic type and risk of myocardial infarction after carotid endarterectomy in the Carotid Revascularization Endarterectomy Versus Stenting Trial (CREST). *Journal of Vascular Surgery*, 64(1), 3–8.e1.
61. Jagannathan, S. and Krovvidi, H. (2014). Anesthetic considerations for posterior fossa surgery. *Continuing Education in Anesthesia Critical Care and Pain*, 14 (5), 202–6.
62. Jaradeh, S. S. and Prieto, T. E. (2003). Evaluation of the autonomic nervous system. *Physical Medicine and Rehabilitation Clinics of North America*, 14(2), 287–305.
63. Kanosue, K., Zhang, Y. H., Yanase-Fujiwara, M. and Hosono, T. (1994). Hypothalamic network for thermoregulatory shivering. *American Journal of Physiology*, 267 (1 Pt 2), R275–82.
64. Kim, T. W. and Nemergut, M. E. (2011). Preparation of modern anesthesia workstations for malignant hyperthermia susceptible patients: a review of past and present practise. *Anesthesiology*, 114(1), 205–12.
65. Kofke, W. A.. (2010). Anesthetic management of the patient with epilepsy or prior seizures. *Current Opinion in Anesthesiology*, 23(3), 391–9.
66. Lacomis, D. (2005). Myasthenic crisis. *Neurocritical Care*, 3(3), 189–94.
67. Larach, M. G, Brandom, B. W., Allen, G. C., Gronert, G. A. and Lehman, E. B. (2008). Cardiac arrests and deaths associated with malignant hyperthermia in north america from 1987 to 2006. *Anesthesiology*, 108(4), 603–11.
68. Larach, M. G. et al. (1994). A clinical grading scale to predict malignant hyperthermia susceptibility. *Anesthesiology*, 80(4), 771–9.
69. Leng, L. Z., Greenfield, J. P., Souweidane, M. M., Anand, V. K. and Schwartz, T. H. (2012). Endoscopic endonasal resection of craniopharyngiomas: analysis of outcome including extent of resection, cerebrospinal fluid leak, return to preoperative productivity and body mass index. *Neurosurgery*, 70(1), 110–23.
70. Leventhal, S. R, Orkin, F. K. and Hirsh, R. A. (1980). Prediction of the need for postoperative mechanical ventilation in myasthenia gravis. *Anesthesiology*, 53(1), 26–30.
71. Longnecker, D. E., Brown, D. L., Newman, M. F. and Zapol, W. (2012). *Longneckers Anesthesiology*. 2nd edition. New York: McGraw-Hill Professional.
72. Longnecker, D. E., Newman, M., Zapol, W., Sandberg, W. and Mackey, S. (2017). *Longneckers Anesthesiology*. 3rd edition. New York: McGraw-Hill Education.
73. Lopez, M. B. (2018). Postanesthetic shivering- from pathophysiology to prevention. *Romanian Journal of Anesthesia and Intensive Care*, 25(1), 73–81.
74. Low, P. A. (2003). Testing the autonomic nervous system. *Seminars in Neurology*, 23(4), 407–21.
75. MacLennan, D. H. (1992). The genetic basis of malignant hyperthermia. *Trends in Pharmacological Sciences*, 13(8), 330–4.
76. Makikallio, T. H., Tapanainen, J. M., Tulppo, M. P. and Huikuri, H. V. (2002). Clinical application of heart rate variability analysis by methods based on nonlinear dynamics. *Electrophysiology Review*, 6(3), 250–5.
77. Maltete, D. et al., (2004). Subthalamic stimulation in Parkinson disease: with or without anesthesia? *Archives of Neurology*, 61(3), 390–2.

78. Marcucci, G. et al., (2012). High-risk patients for carotid endarterectomy: turned down cases are rare. *Journal of Cardiovascular Surgery*, 53(3), 333–43.
79. Martignago, S., Fanin, M., Albertini, E., Pegoraro, E. and Angelini, C. (2009). Muscle histopathology in myasthenia gravis with antibodies against MuSK & AChR. *Neuropathology & Applied Neurobiology*, 35(1), 103–10.
80. Mathias, C. (2003). Autonomic diseases: clinical features and laboratory evaluation. *Journal of Neurology, Neurosurgery and Psychiatry*, 31–41.
81. Matsuda, M., Watanabe, K., Saito, A., Matsumura, K. I. and Ichikawa, M. (2007). Circumstances, activities and events precipitating aneurysmal subarachnoid hemorrhage. *Journal of Stroke and Cerebrovascular Diseases*, 16(1), 25–9.
82. Matsukawa, T., Sessler, D. I. and Sessler, A. M. (1995). Heat flow and distribution during induction of general anesthesia. *Anesthesiology*, 82, 662–73.
83. McQuillan, P. M., Allman, K. G. and Wilson, I. H. (2007). *Oxford American Handbook of Anesthesiology*. 2nd edition. Oxford: Oxford Medical Publications.
84. Meredith, W., Rutledge, R., Fakhry, S. M., Emery, S. and Kromhout-Schiro, S. (1998). The conundrum of the Glasgow Coma Scale in intubated patients: a linear regression prediction of the Glsgow verbal score from the Glasgow eye and motor scores. *Journal of Trauma*, 44(5), 839–45.
85. Miller, R. D., Cohen, N. H. and Eriksson, L. I. (2015). *Miller's Anesthesia*. 8th edition. Philadelphia: Elsevier Saunders.
86. Mokri, B. (2001). The Monroe Kellie hypothesis: application in CSF volume depletion. *Neurology*, 56(12), 1746–8.
87. Morrison, D. A., Bibby, K. and Woodruff, G. (1997). The harlequin sign and congenital Horner's syndrome. *Journal of Neurology Neurosurgery and Psychiatry*, 62(6), 626–8.
88. Mughal, M. and Longmuir R. (2009). Current pharmacological testing for Horner's syndrome. *Current Neurology and Neuroscience Reports*, 9, 384–9.
89. National Institute for Health and Care Excellence. (2018). *NICE Guidelines for Depression in Adults: Recognition and Management*. Retrieved from National Institute for Health and Care Excellence. -[Viewed 26th May, 2020]. https://www.nice.org.uk/guidance/CG90.
90. NE, G. (2016). Myasthenia gravis. *New England Journal of Medicine*, 375(26), 2570–81.
91. Nemergut, E.C., Dumont, A. S., Barry, U. T. and Laws, E. R. (2005). Perioperative management of patients undergoing transphenoidal pituitary surgery. *Anesthesia Analgesia*, 101(4), 1170–81.
92. Nemergut, E. C. and Zuo Z. (2006). Airway management in patients with pituitary disease: a review of 746 patients. *Journal of Neurosurgical Anesthesiology*, 18(1), 73–7.
93. North American Symptomatic Carotid Endarterectomy Trial Collaborators, et al., (1991). Beneficial effects of carotid endarterectomy in symptomatic patients with high-grade carotid stenosis. *New England Journal of Medicine*, 325(7), 445–53.
94. Noyce, A. J., Bestwick, J. P., Silveira-Moriyama, L., Hawkes, C. H. and Giovannoni, G. (2012). Meta-analysis of early nonmotor features and risk factors for Parkinsons disease. *Annals of Neurology*, 72, 893–901.
95. Odekerken, V. J. J. et al., (2013). Subthalamic nucleus versus globus pallidus bilateral deep brain stimulation for advanced Parkinson's disease (NSTAPS) study: a randomized controlled trial. *Lancet Neurology*, 12(1), 37–44.
96. Osborn, I. and Sebeo, J. (2010). Scalp block during craniotomy: a classic technique revisited. *Journal of Neurosurgical Anesthesiology*, 22(3), 187–94.
97. Oya, A., Asakura, H., Koshino, T. and Araki, T. (1997). Thermographic demonstration of nonshivering thermogenesis in human newborns after birth: its relation to umbilical gases. *Journal of Perinatal Medicine*, 25, 447–54.
98. Ozaki, M. et al., (1994). Thermoregulatory thresholds during epidural and spinal anesthesia. *Anesthesiology*, 81(2), 282–8.
99. Perks, A., Cheema, S. and Mohanraj, R. (2012). Anesthesia and epilepsy. *British Journal of Anesthesia*, 108,(4), 562–71.
100. Perlmuter, L. C., Sarda, G., Casavant, V. and Mosnaim, A. D. (2013). A review of the etiology, associated comorbidities and the treatment of orthostatic hypotension. *American Journal of Therapeutics*, 20(3), 279–91.
101. Petrides, G. et al., (2009). Seizure threshold in a large sample implications for stimulus dosing strategies in bilateral electroconvulsive therapy: a report from CORE. *The Journal of electroconvulsive therapy*, 25(4), 232–7.
102. Pilley, S. F. and Thompson, H. S. (1975). Pupillary dilatation lag in Horner's syndrome. *British Journal of Ophthalmology*, 59(12), 731–5.
103. Potters, J. W. and Klimek, M. (2015). Awake craniotomy: improving the patient's experience. *Current Opinions in Anesthesiology*, 28(5), 511–6.
104. Prabhakar, H., Singhal, V. and Gupta, N. (2019). *Co-existing Diseases and Neuroanesthesia*. 1st edition. Singapore: Springer Nature Singapore Pte Ltd.
105. Rath, G. P., Bithal, P. K., Chaturvedi, A. and Dash, H. H. (2007). Complications related to positioning in posterior fossa craniectomy. *Journal of Clinical Neurosciences*, 14(6), 520–5.
106. Riazi, S., Larach, M. G., Hu, C., Wijeysundera, D., Massey, C. and Kraeva, N. (2014). Malignant hyperthermia in Canada: characteristics of index anesthetics in 129 malignant hyperthermia susceptible probands. *Anesthesia and Analgesia*, 118(2), 381–7.
107. Rintoul, N. E. et al., (2002). A new look at myelomeningoceles: functional level, vertebral level, shunting and the implications for fetal intervention. Pediatrics, 109(3), 409–13. Hines, R. L. and Marschall, K. E. (2017). *Stoeltings Anesthesia and Co-existing Disease*. 7th edition. Philadelphia: Elsevier.
108. Roberts, I. and Sydenham, E.(2012). Barbiturates for acute TBI. *Cochrane Database of Systematic Reviews*, 12, CD000033.
109. Rosner, M. J., Rosner, S. D. and Johnson, A. H. (1995). Cerebral perfusion pressure: management protocol and clinical results. *Journal of Neurosurgery*, 83, 949–62.
110. Ruskin, K. J., Rosenbaum, S. H. and Rampil, I. J. (2014). *Fundamentals of Neuroanesthesia—A Physiological Approach to Clinical Practice*. 1st edition. Oxford: Oxford University Press.
111. Sarang, A. and Dinsmore, J. (2003). Anesthesia for awake craniotomy: evolution of a technique that facilitates awake neurological testing. *British Journal of Anesthesia*, 90(2), 161–5.
112. Sawaya, R., Bindal, R. K., Lang, F. F. and Abi-Said, D. Metastatic brain tumors. In: Kaye, A. H. and Laws E. R. (eds). (2001). *Brain tumors: an encyclopedic approach*. 2nd edition. New York: Churchill Livingstone.

113. Scheffer, I. E. et al., (2017). ILAE classification of the epilepsies: position paper of the ILAE commission for classification and terminology. *Epilepsia*, 58(4), 512–21.
114. Schievink, W. I. (1997). Intracranial aneurysms. *New England Journal of Medicine*, 336(1), 28–40.
115. Schmoker, J. D., Shackford, S. R., Wald, S. L. and Pietropaoli, J. A. (1992). An analysis of the relationship between fluid and sodium administration and intracranial pressure after head injury. *Journal of Trauma and acute Care Surgery*, 33(3), 476–81.
116. Selvarajah, D. et al., (2015). Sudoscan: a simple, rapid and objective method with potential or screening for diabetic peripheral neuropathy. *PLoS One*, 10:e0138224.
117. Sessler, D. I., Rubinstein, E. H. and Moayeri, A. (1991). Physiological responses to mild perianesthetic hypothermia in humans. *Anesthesiology*, 75, 594–610.
118. Sivasankar, C., Schlichter, R. A., Baranov, D. and Kofke, W.A. (2016). Awake craniotomy: a new airway approach. *Anesthesia Analgesia*, 122(2), 509–11.
119. Sorrentino, E. et al., (2012). Critical thresholds for cerebrovascular reactivity after traumatic brain injury. *Neurocritical Care*, 16, 258–66.
120. Steiner, L. A. and Andrews, P. J. D. (2006). Montioring the injured brain: ICP amd CBF. *British Journal of Anesthesia*, 97(1), 26–38.
121. St George, R. J., Nutt, J. G., Burchiel, K. J. and Horak, F. B. (2010). A meta-regression of the long-term effects of deep brain stimulation on balance and gait in PD. *Neurology*, 75(14), 1292–9.
122. Sundt, T. M., Sandok, B. A. and Whisnant, J. P. (1975). Carotid endarterectomy. Complications and perioperative assessment of risk. *Mayo Clinic Proceedings*, 50(6), 301–6.
123. Tameem, A. and Krovvidi, H. (2013). Cerebral physiology. *Continuing Education in Anesthesia Critical Care and Pain*, 13(4), 113–8.
124. Taylor, M. D. and Bernstein, M. (1999). Awake craniotomy with brain mapping as the routine surgical approach to treating patients with supratentorial intra-axial tumors: a prospective trial of 200 cases. *Journal of Neurosurgery*, 90(1), 35–41.
125. Teasdale, G. et al., (1974). Assessment of coma and impaired consciousness. A practical scale. *Lancet*, 2(7872), 81–4.
126. Teunissen, L. L., Rinkel, G. J., Algra, A. and van Gijn, J. (1996). Risk factors for subarachnoid hemorrhage: a systematic review. *Stroke*, 27(3), 544–9.
127. The Committee on Standards and Practice Parameters, et al., (2013). Practice Guidelines for Postanesthetic Care: An Updated Report by the American Society of Anesthesiologists Task Force on Postanesthetic Care. *Anesthesiology*, 118, 291–307.
128. Tintinalli, J., Stapczynski, J. and John Ma, O. (2015). *Tintinallis Emergency Medicine: A Comprehensive Study Guide*. 8th edition. New York: McGraw-Hill Education.
129. Tintinalli, J. E. et al., (2016). *Tintinallis Emergency Medicine*. 8th edition. New York: McGraw-Hill Education.
130. Treiman, D. M. (1994). *Current Diagnosis in Neurology*. St. Loius: Mosby.
131. Trinka, E. et al., (2015). A definition and classification of status epilepticus—a report of the ILAE task force on classification of status epilepticus. *Epilepsia*, 56(10), 1515–23.
132. Unic-Stojanovic, D., Babic, S. and Neskovic, V. (2012). General versus regional anesthesia for carotid endarterectomy. *Journal of Cardiothoracic and Vascular Anesthesia*, 29(1), 178–84.
133. Venkatraghavan, L., Rakhman, E., Krishna, V., Sammartino, F., Manninen, P. and Hutchison, W. (2016). The effect of general anesthesia on the microelectrode recordings from pallidal neurons in patients with dystonia. *Journal of Neurosurgical Anesthesiology*, 28(3), 256–61.
134. Vetrugno, R., Liguori, R., Cortelli, P. and Montagna, P. (2003). Sympathetic skin response. *Clinical Autonomic Research*, 13(4), 256–70.
135. Viscomi, C. M, Abajian, J. C. and Wald, S. L. (1995). Spinal anesthesia for repair of meningomyelocele in neonates. *Anesthesia and Analgesia*, 81, 492–5.
136. Vymazal, T., Krecmerova, M., Bicek, V. and Lischke, R. (2015). Feasibility of full and rapid neuromuscular blockade recovery with sugammadex in myasthenia gravis patients undergoing surgery: a series of 117 cases. *Therapeutics and Clinical Risk Management*, 11, 1593–6.
137. Wappler, F. (2010). Anesthesia for patients with a history of malignant hyperthermia. *Current Opinion in Anesthesiology*, 23(3), 417–22.
138. Wells, D. G. and Davies, G. G. (1987). Hemodynamic changes associated with electroconvulsive therapy. *Anesthesia Analgesia*, 66(11), 1193–5.
139. Welter, M. L. et al., (2002). Clinical predictive factors of subthalamic stimulation in Parkinson's disease. *Brain*, 125(Pt 3), 575–83.
140. Wijdicks, E. F., Bamlet, W. R., Maramattom, B. V., Manno, E. M. and McClelland, R. L. (2005). Validation of a new coma scale: the FOUR score. *Annals of Neurology*, 58(4), 585–93.
141. Williams, D. R., Evans, A. H., Fung, V. S. C., Hayes, M., Iansek, R. and Kimber, T. (2017). Practical approaches to commencing device assisted therapies for Parkinson's disease in Australia. *Internal Medicine Journal*, 47(10), 1107–13.
142. Yeoh, T. Y., Manninen, P., Kalia, S. K. and Venkatraghavan, L. (2017). Anesthesia considerations for patients with an implanted deep brain stimulator undergoing surgery: a review and update. *Canadian Journal of Anesthesia*, 64(3), 308–19.
143. Yi, J. S., Guptill, J. T., Stathopoulos, P., Nowak, R. J. and O'Connor, K. C. (2018). B cells in the pathophysiology of myasthenia gravis. *Muscle Nerve*, 57(2), 172–84.
144. Zaza, A. and Lombardi, F.. (2001). Autonomic indexes based on the analysis of heart rate variability: a view from the sinus node. *Cardiovascular Research*, 50(3), 434–52.
145. Zuercher, M., Ummenhofer, W., Baltussen, A. and Walder, B. (2009). The use of Glasgow Coma Scale in injury assessment: a critical review. *Brain Injury*, 23(5), 371–84.
146. Zygmunt, A. and Stanczyk, J. (2010). Methods of evaluation of autonomic nervous system function. *Archives of Medical Sciences*, 6(1), 11–8.
147. Zöllei, E., Paprika, D. and Rudas, L. (2003). Measures of cardiovascular autonomic regulation derived from spontaneous methods and the valsalva maneuvre. *Autonomic Neuroscience*, 103(1–2), 100–5.

3 CHAPTER

Cardiac Anesthesia

PHYSIOLOGY OF FETAL CIRCULATION

Introduction

- Fetal pulmonary and systemic circulation are essentially in parallel instead of in series
- In adults, pulmonary and systemic circulation are in series
- Several changes occur at the time of birth, to ensure conversion to adult circulation

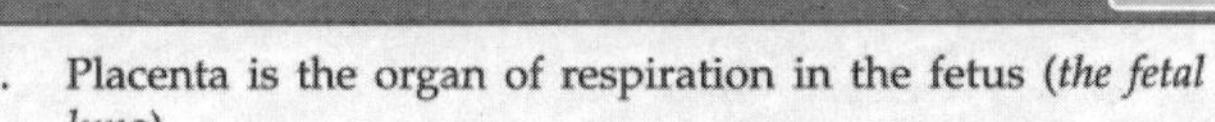

Differences between Fetal and Adult Circulation

1. Placenta is the organ of respiration in the fetus (*the fetal lung*)
2. Gas exchange does not occur in the collapsed lungs
3. Pulmonary and systemic circulations occur in parallel

Contd...

Contd...

4. Presence of three shunts:
    - Ductus arteriosus
    - Foramen ovale
    - Ductus venosus
5. Pulmonary circulation is a high resistance circuit (high PVR)
6. Systemic circulation is low resistance (low SVR)
7. Fetal heart is RV dominant

Fetal Circulation

- Fetal blood volume during the 3rd trimester is 120–160 mL/kg body weight
- Total blood volume of the term neonate is approximately 500 mL

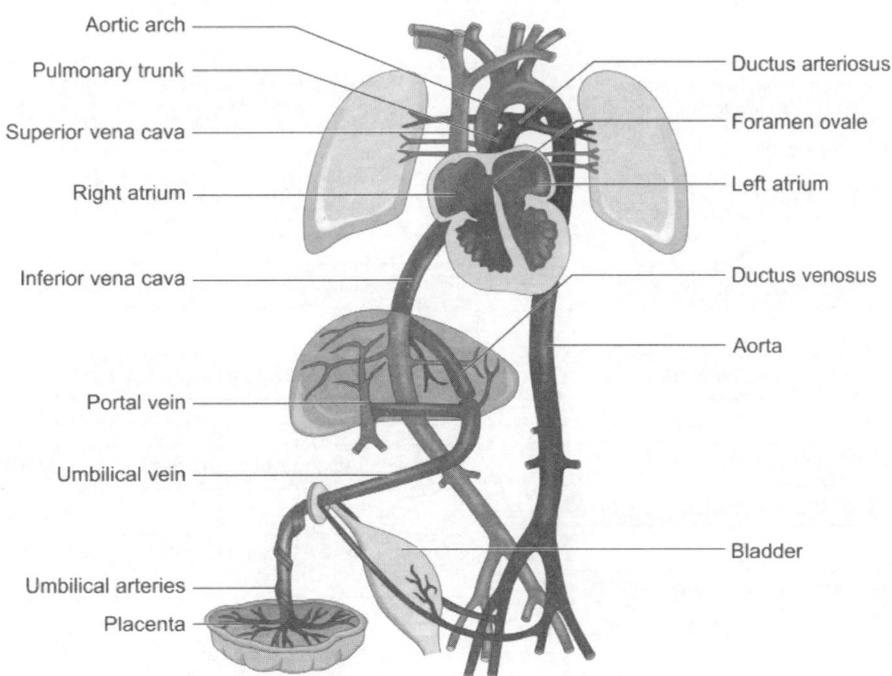

Fig. 1: Fetal circulation.

- Fetal pulmonary circulation is essentially a high resistance circuit
- This is due to collapsed nature of the lungs in utero
- Pulmonary capillaries are formed only after 24–25 weeks of gestation
- These later come to lie close to an immature alveolar epithelium

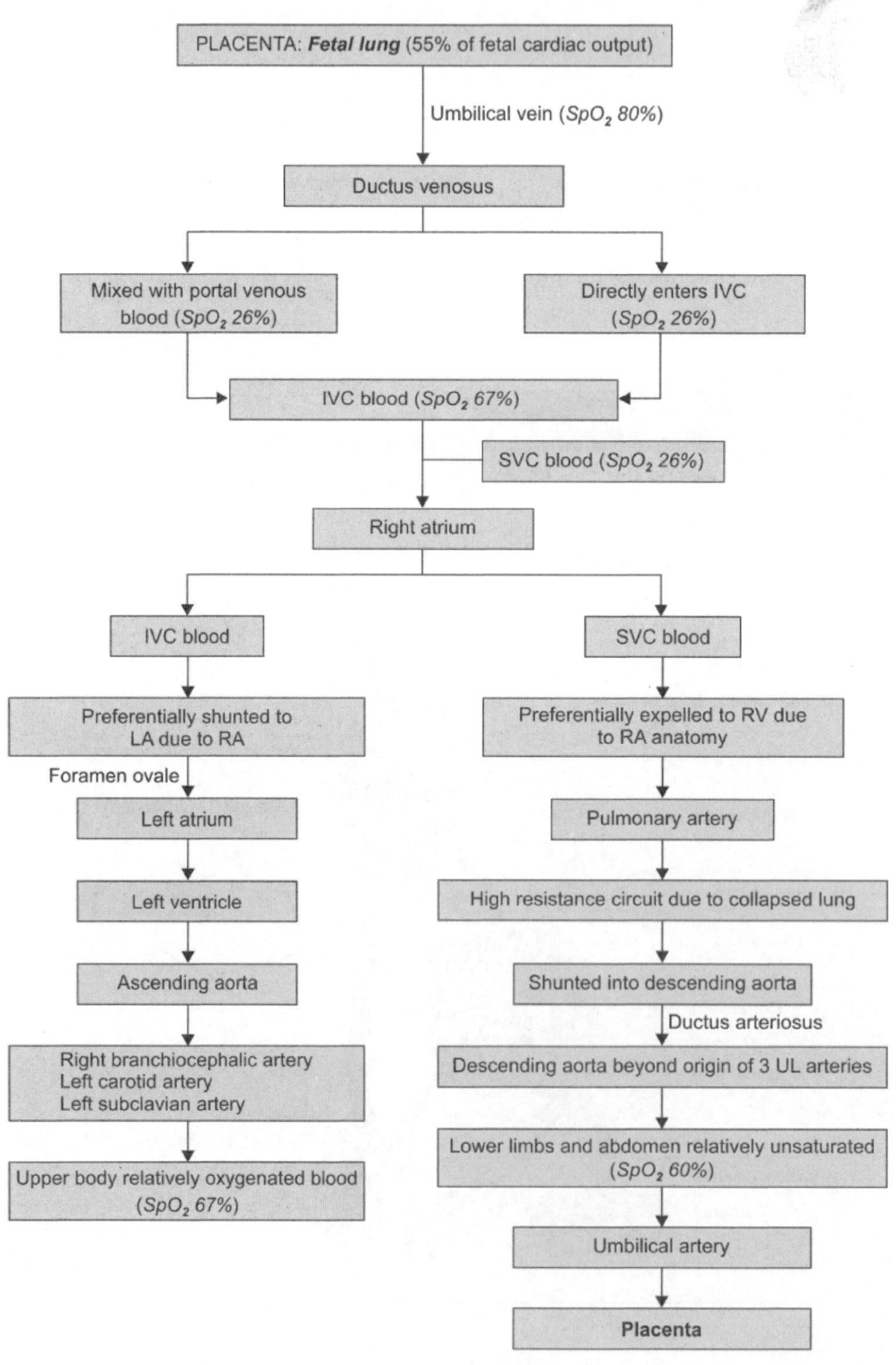

Changes Occurring at Birth

- The major cardiopulmonary adaptations at birth are:
  - Recovery from birth asphyxia
  - Reflex initiation of breathing and expansion of lungs
  - Establishment and maintenance of adequate spontaneous ventilation
  - Conversion of fetal parallel circulation into series adult circulation
- Closure of ductus arteriosus:
  - At birth, there is an increase in SVR with the clamping of umbilical cord
  - Along with this, there is a reduction in PVR, with lung expansion and first breath
  - This causes SVR to rise above PVR, causing a reversal of shunt across the DA
  - Thus, shunting is predominantly left-right across the ductus arteriosus
  - This results in highly oxygenated blood traversing the DA, stimulating its closure
  - Chemical mediators which aid in DA closure:
    - Prostaglandins
    - Bradykinin
    - Acetylcholine
  - Physiological closure occurs at 10–15 hrs of life
  - Anatomical closure occurs at 2–4 weeks of life
  - Factors causing reduction in PVR at birth:
    - Clamping of umbilical cord:
      - This separates the fetus from the placenta, its source of oxygen
      - Thus, source of oxygenated blood is removed
      - This causes fetus to become increasingly asphyxic
      - Finally, the newborn is forced to take its first breath
      - With the first breath, several factors cause a reduction in PVR:
        - Expansion of the lung
        - Increase in alveolar oxygen content
        - Increase in pH
        - Nitric oxide relaxation of pulmonary vasculature
      - Respiratory efforts are usually initiated within 30 seconds
      - Respiratory efforts become sustained within 90 seconds
    - ***Vaginal squeeze***:
      - Fetal thorax passes through the narrow vaginal vault
      - Outward recoil of chest occurs as it passes through the vagina
      - This makes intrapleural pressure negative (–30 to –50 mm Hg)
      - This causes expansion of lung
      - Vaginal squeeze is absent in cesarean section causing TTN
- Closure of foramen ovale:
  - At birth, SVR increases, while PVR decreases
  - This causes LA pressure to rise above RA pressure
  - Eventually, this results in closure of the flap valve, the foramen ovale
  - Functional closure of foramen ovale occurs soon after birth
  - Anatomical closure occurs between 3 months and 1 year of life
  - Factors causing raised SVR at birth:
    - Clamping of cord:
      - Causes increased umbilical artery pressure which raises SVR
      - Pushes around 100 mL of blood from placental circulation into systemic circulation (*placental transfusion*)
    - Increased LA pressure:
      - Increased pulmonary blood flow occurs due to reduction in PVR
      - This increases pulmonary venous return into left heart
      - Thus LA pressure increases, closing foramen ovale
    - Vaginal squeeze:
      - Around 20–30 mL/kg of ultrafilterate is present in fetal lungs
      - At birth, chest wall is squeezed as it passes through vaginal vault
      - Thus, ultrafilterate gets pushed into systemic circulation (90 mL)
- Fate of ductus venosus (DV):
  - Once the umbilical cord is clamped, flow through the umbilical vein (UV) ceases
  - Thus, the low resistance shunting of UV blood to the IVC through the DV stops
  - Thus all blood entering the liver has to pass through the hepatic sinusoids
  - The ductus venosus atrophies over a period of time
  - The atrophied ductus venosus forms the *ligamentum venosum* of the liver
- Thus the two sites of right to left shunting are closed at birth
- This converts fetal parallel circulation into adult circulation in series

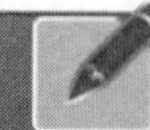

Fate of Fetal Anatomical Shunts

- Umbilical artery forms the medial umbilical ligament
- Left umbilical vein forms the ligamentum teres of the liver
- Ductus venosus forms the ligamentum venosum of the liver
- Ductus arteriosus forms the ligamentum arteriosum
- Foramen ovale closes and forms the fossa ovalis

CLASSIFICATION OF CONGENITAL HEART DISEASE

Lesions Causing Outflow Tract Obstruction

- Left ventricular outflow tract (LVOT) obstruction:
  - Parachute mitral valve
  - Congenital mitral stenosis
  - Coarctation of aorta
  - Aortic stenosis
- Right ventricular outflow tract (RVOT) obstruction: pulmonary valve stenosis

Lesions Causing Left-Right Shunting

- Ventricular septal defects (VSD)
- Atrial septal defects (ASD)
- Patent ductus arteriosus (PDA)
- Endocardial cushion defects
- Partial anomalous pulmonary venous return (PAPVR)

Lesions Causing Right-Left Shunting

- With decreased pulmonary blood flow:
  - Tetralogy of Fallot (TOF)
  - Pulmonary atresia
  - Tricuspid atresia
  - Ebsteins anomaly
  - Pulmonary AV fistula
- With increased pulmonary blood flow:
  - Transposition of great arteries (TGA)
  - Truncus arteriosus (TA)
  - Total anomalous pulmonary venous return (TAPVR)
  - Double outlet right ventricle (DORV)
  - Hypoplastic left heart syndrome (HLHS)

CORONARY CIRCULATION

Introduction

- The coronary arteries encircle the heart like a crown on its epicardial surface
- Hence it is called coronary circulation
- Coronary circulation averages around 250 mL/min at rest
- This amounts to around 5% of the cardiac output

Components

- Main components of coronary circulation are:
  - Right coronary artery
  - Left main coronary artery
- Origin of coronary arteries:
  - Originate from the coronary sinuses present on the proximal aorta
  - Arise from just beyond the cusps of aortic semilunar valves
  - Coronary arteries are the first branches of proximal aorta
- Right coronary artery (RCA):
  - Smaller than the left coronary artery
  - Arises from the anterior or right coronary sinus
  - Emerges from the surface of heart between the pulmonary trunk and right auricle
  - Winds around inferior border of the heart to reach diaphragmatic surface of heart
  - Traverses along the posterior interventricular groove
  - Terminates by anastomosing with the left coronary artery
  - Branches of right coronary artery:
    - Large branches:
      - Right marginal artery
      - Posterior descending artery (PDA)
      - Posterior left ventricular artery (PLV)
    - Small branches:
      - Right atrial branch
      - Infundibular artery
      - Sinoatrial nodal artery
      - AV nodal artery
      - Terminal branches
  - Areas of distribution:
    - Right atrium
    - Ventricles:
      - Most of RV, except areas along anterior interventricular groove
      - Small part of LV adjoining posterior interventricular groove
    - Posterior part of the interventricular septum
    - Whole conducting system of heart except:
      - Part of left branch of AV bundle
      - Sinoatrial node in 40% cases

❖ Left main coronary artery (LMCA):
  - Called ***widow artery*** as occlusion of this artery commonly results in sudden death
  - Larger than right coronary artery
  - Arises from posterior or left coronary sinus
  - Emerges from the surface of the heart between pulmonary trunk and left auricle
  - Soon after its emergence on the surface, the LMCA gives rise to its branches
  - Branches of left coronary artery:
    - Large branches:
      - Left circumflex (LCX) artery—gives rise to obtuse marginals (OM)
      - Left anterior descending (LAD) artery—gives rise to:
        - Diagonal branches
        - Septal perforators
    - Small branches:
      - Left atrial branches
      - Branches supplying pulmonary artery
      - Terminal branches
  - LCX is the continuation of LMCA and runs along the left anterior coronary sulcus
  - It winds around the left border of the heart to reach the posterior surface
  - It terminates in the posterior interventricular groove by anastomosing with RCA
  - Areas of distribution:
    - Left atrium
    - Ventricles:
      - Most of LV, except for area along posterior interventricular groove
      - Small part of RV adjoining anterior interventricular groove
    - Anterior part of interventricular septum
    - Part of left branch of AV bundle

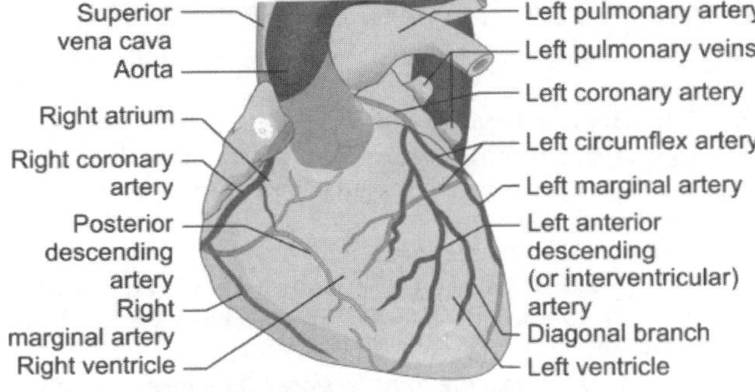

Fig. 2: Coronary circulation.

Anatomical Distribution of Blood Flow

Coronary artery	Part of myocardium supplied	Part of conduction system supplied
Right coronary artery		
Posterior descending artery	Right atrium	Sinoatrial node (60%)
Right marginal artery	Right ventricle	Atrioventricular node (85–90%)
	Inferior LV surface (85%)	Proximal part of bundle of His
	Posterior LV surface (85%)	Part of posterior fascicle of LBB
Left coronary artery		
Left anterior descending artery	Anterior surface of LV	Most of RBB
	Part of lateral surface of LV	Anterior fascicle of LBB
	Most of interventricular septum	Part of posterior fascicle of LBB
Left circumflex artery	Left atrium	Sinoatrial node (40%)
	Part of lateral surface of LV	Atrioventricular node (10–15%)
	Inferior surface of LV (15%)	
	Posterior surface of LV (15%)	

Anatomical region of heart	Coronary artery
Inferior wall	Right coronary artery
Anteroseptal wall	Left anterior descending artery
Anteroapical wall	Distal left anterior descending artery
Anterolateral wall	Circumflex artery
Posterior wall	Right coronary artery

Cardiac Dominance

❖ The artery giving rise to posterior descending artery is called the dominant artery

❖ Most often, PDA arises from right coronary artery

❖ Therefore, most often coronary circulation is *right dominant coronary circulation*

❖ In about 10% of hearts, RCA is small and does not give rise to PDA

❖ In these cases, LCX continues as PDA

❖ Such cases are called *left dominant coronary circulation*

❖ In rare instances, PDA is supplied by both the RCA and LCX

❖ The coronary circulation is then called *co-dominant coronary circulation*

Microvascular Network

- Epicardial coronary vessels distribute blood to different regions of the heart
- This is through the complex coronary microvascular network
- Epicardial arteries give rise to smaller arterioles comprising the microvascular network
- Branches of these penetrate the myocardium and supply the subendocardium with blood
- The diameter of these feeder branches is narrower and these are essentially end arteries
- These arterioles form the primary sites of vascular resistance and regulation of blood flow
- The arterioles further branch into capillaries, which lie adjacent to the cardiac myocytes
- This results in a high capillary-myocyte ratio and short blood diffusion distances
- This ensures adequate oxygen delivery and waste product removal from the myocytes
- The capillaries eventually form venules, which join and give rise to coronary veins

Coronary Veins

- Coronary veins travel alongside the corresponding epicardial coronary arteries
- Venous drainage of the heart is by three means:
  - Coronary sinus
  - Anterior cardiac veins
  - ***Venae cordis minimae or Thebesian veins***
- Coronary sinus:
  - This is largest vein draining the heart
  - Receives 85% of coronary blood flow

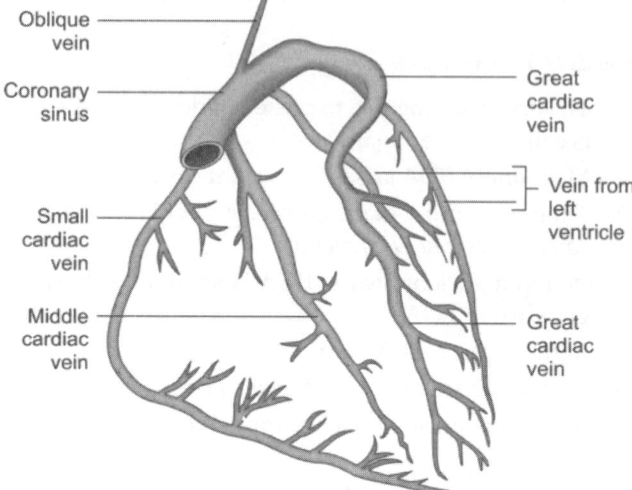

Fig. 3: Coronary veins.

  - Lies in the left posterior coronary sulcus, on posterior surface of the heart
  - It is about 30 mm long and ends by opening into posterior wall of right atrium
  - Veins draining into coronary sinus:
    - Great cardiac vein:
      - Lies along anterior interventricular groove
      - Joins left end of coronary sinus
    - Small cardiac vein:
      - Lies along RCA
      - Joins right end of coronary sinus
    - Middle cardiac vein:
      - Lies along posterior interventricular groove
      - Joins right end of coronary sinus
    - Posterior vein of left ventricle:
      - Runs on diaphragmatic surface of left ventricle
      - Joins the middle portion of coronary sinus
    - Oblique vein of left atrium:
      - Also called ***vein of Marshall***
      - Develops from the left common cardinal vein
      - Runs on posterior surface of left atrium
      - Joins the left end of coronary sinus
    - Right marginal vein: accompanies marginal branch of RCA
- Anterior cardiac veins:
  - 3–4 small veins running on anterior wall of right ventricle
  - Drain directly into the right atrium
  - These along with Thebesian vein receive remaining 15% of coronary venous blood
- Thebesian veins:
  - Numerous small veins present in all the 4 chambers of the heart
  - These veins open directly into the cavities

Peculiarities of Coronary Circulation

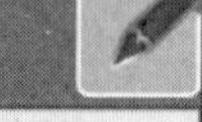

- *Phasic flow*: blood flow occurs predominantly during diastole
- Coronary arteries are *end arteries*
- *High oxygen extraction* occurs from the coronary circulation
- Regulation of coronary circulation is determined by its own metabolism
- Transmural flow redistribution:
  - A gradient exists for CBF across the wall of the heart
  - Subendocardial myocardium receives lesser blood flow
  - This is due to more compression of the subendocardium
  - Thus, subendocardium is more prone to ischemia

PHYSIOLOGY OF CORONARY CIRCULATION

Introduction

- Unique as it is intermittent rather than continuous as in other organs
- During systole, intramyocardial pressure in LV approaches systemic arterial pressure
- This almost completely occludes the intramyocardial part of coronary artery
- This produces the ***Throttling effect*** on coronary vessels
- Therefore, coronary blood flow almost ceases during isovolumetric contraction phase
- Therefore, coronary perfusion occurs predominantly during diastole
- Maximal coronary flow occurs during isovolumetric relaxation

Peculiarities of Coronary Circulation

- *Phasic flow*: blood flow occurs predominantly during diastole
- Coronary arteries are *end arteries*
- *High oxygen extraction* occurs from the coronary circulation
- Regulation of coronary circulation is determined by its own metabolism
- Transmural flow redistribution:
  - A gradient exists for CBF across the wall of the heart
  - Subendocardial myocardium receives lesser blood flow
  - This is due to more compression of the subendocardium
  - Thus, subendocardium is more prone to ischemia

Coronary Perfusion Patterns

- Normal coronary flow is approximately 250 mL/min at rest
- Left ventricle is perfused only during diastole
- This is because the left ventricle generates almost 120 mm Hg pressure during systole
- Thus, due to throttling effect, CBF to LV ceases during systole
- In contrast, right ventricle is perfused during systole and diastole
- This is because right ventricular systolic pressure is normally only around 30 mm Hg
- This constitutes the phasic nature of coronary blood flow

Determinants of Coronary Blood Flow

- Physical factors:
  - Patency of coronary vessels
  - Coronary steal
  - Coronary perfusion pressure
- Chemical factors:
  - Coronary perfusion time (heart rate)
  - Myocardial metabolism
  - Autoregulation
- Neural factors: autonomic innervation
- Hormonal factors
- Cardiac reflexes

Patency Of Coronary Vessels

- Coronary vessel luminal diameter can be reduced by:
  - Deposits of lipids
  - Smooth muscle proliferation
  - Endothelial dysfunction
- Critical stenosis occurs when CBF is unable to meet increases in metabolic demand
- This typically occurs when the luminal diameter is reduced by 50%
- Resting CBF is affected when the luminal diameter is reduced by 80%

Coronary Steal

- Phenomenon where physiological or pharmacological vasodilatation of a myocardial segments vasculature is associated with steal of blood from another myocardial segment
- This occurs when there is a significant stenosis in a large epicardial artery
- Blood flow to this diseased segment remains normal at rest as the distal vascular bed is already maximally vasodilated
- In this scenario, any vasodilatory stimulus such as exercise or vasodilatory drugs would reduce the vascular resistance of neighboring non-ischemic regions
- The vascular resistance of the diseased region is minimally affected as the vascular bed in this region is already maximally dilated
- Thus, CBF increases to the non-ischemic regions, furthering the ischemic process in the diseased regions thereby resulting in coronary steal

Coronary Perfusion Pressure

- Coronary perfusion pressure (CPP) = (Arterial diastolic BP or DBP) – (LVEDP)

- Thus, CPP can reduce due to either:
  - Decrease in arterial diastolic blood pressure (DBP)
  - Increase in left ventricular end diastolic pressure (LVEDP)
- Diastolic blood pressure:
  - Arterial diastolic pressure is more important determinant of CBF than MAP
  - When arterial diastolic pressure is decreased, coronary blood flow decreases
  - Factors causing reduced diastolic blood pressure:
    - Aortic regurgitation
    - Large PDAs
- Left ventricular end diastolic pressure (LVEDP):
  - Increase in LVEDP occurs with diastolic dysfunction
  - Mechanisms causing raised LVEDP:
    - Abnormal detachment of actin-myosin cross bridges
    - Delayed removal of cytosolic calcium
  - Raised LVEDP can be due to various factors like:
    - Abnormal left ventricular diastolic distensibility
    - Impaired left ventricular filling
    - Chamber stiffness
    - Delayed relaxation

Coronary Perfusion Time

- Heart rate is a very important factor regulating CBF
- Maximal coronary flow occurs during isovolumetric relaxation phase due to:
  - Dilated coronary vessels
  - High aortic diastolic pressure
- Changes in heart rate affect diastolic time more than the systolic time
- Thus, tachycardia shortens the diastolic time and reduces coronary perfusion time
- Extreme tachycardia can produce ischemia in normal hearts
- ***Diastolic Pressure Time Index (DPTI):***
  - It is a useful measure of how tachycardia affects coronary blood supply
  - DPTI = (CPP) x (Diastolic time)
  - DPTI represents the time spent in diastole at a certain perfusion pressure
  - It reflects the time during which diastolic pressure fills the coronary arteries
  - Thus, tachycardia reduces diastolic time and thereby decreases DPTI

Myocardial Metabolism

- Normal basal cardiac oxygen consumption is 8–10 mL O_2/min/100 g myocardium
- Flow-metabolism coupling:
  - Refers to the link between myocardial metabolism and blood flow
  - Represents the negative feedback control system of coronary circulation
  - This is important as the myocardium has a very high basal oxygen consumption
  - The myocardium extracts 70–80% of oxygen delivered to it by the coronaries
  - This compares to only 25% oxygen extraction in other tissues
  - Oxygen consumption for various myocardial activities:
    - Basal requirements 20%
    - Electrical activity 1%
    - Volume work 15%
    - Pressure work 64%
  - Therefore, myocardium cannot compensate for reduction in blood flow by extracting more oxygen from blood
  - Any increase in metabolic demand must be met by an increase in CBF
  - This phenomenon is called *Flow-Metabolism coupling*
  - Factors which cause coupling:
    - Oxygen
    - Carbon dioxide
    - Nitric oxide
    - Adenosine (*most important*)
    - K_{ATP} channels
    - Reactive oxygen species (H_2O_2)
  - ***Berne hypothesis***:
    - Used to describe role of adenosine in flow-metabolism coupling
    - Increased myocardial metabolism causes adenosine nucleotide degradation
    - This produces increased extracellular levels of adenosine
    - Adenosine reaches precapillary sphincters of coronary system
    - This causes a strong vasodilatory response
    - Thus, CBF increases in response to an increase in metabolic demand

Autoregulation

- Refers to the ability of an organ to maintain constant blood flow despite changes in arterial perfusion pressure

- In response to increased myocardial metabolism, coronary arterial tone reduces
- This essentially constitutes coronary autoregulation
- Characteristically occurs between MAP of 50–120 mm Hg
- Beyond this range, blood flow becomes increasingly pressure dependent
- Autoregulation occurs by metabolic coupling in blood vessels less than 150 µm
- Critical mediator for autoregulation is hypoxia, acting directly, or via adenosine
- Mechanisms of autoregulation:
  - Myogenic response:
    - Responsible for fast regulation of CBF
    - Increase in passive stretch due to increased perfusion pressure causes active smooth muscle contraction
    - Decrease in passive stretch due to decrease in perfusion pressure causes active relaxation of smooth muscle
  - Metabolic response:
    - Responsible for slow regulation of CBF
    - Effective autoregulation is coupled to coronary venous PO_2
    - Autoregulation is observed when coronary venous PO_2 is below 32 mm Hg
    - Decreased perfusion pressure leads to hypoxia
    - Hypoxia produces increased adenosine levels
    - This causes vasodilatation and leads to increase in CBF

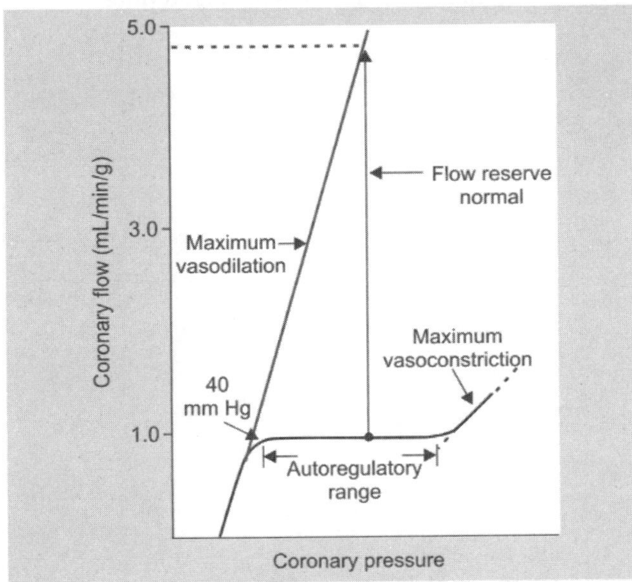

Fig. 4: Coronary autoregulation curve.

Neural Control

- Autonomic influences in coronary blood flow are generally weak
- α_1 receptors:
  - Are primarily present in the epicardial coronary arteries
  - These receptors cause vasoconstriction
  - May be responsible for producing an *anti-steal effect* in ischemic regions
  - By producing vasoconstriction in normal vessels, these receptors increase CBF in vessels with stenosis
  - This constitutes the anti-steal effect
- β_2 receptors:
  - Are primarily present in the intramyocardial and subendocardial vessels
  - Stimulation of these receptors causes vasodilatation
- Sympathetic innervation:
  - From superior, middle and inferior cervical ganglia: mainly stellate ganglion
  - Also from first four thoracic ganglia
  - Sympathetic stimulation mainly causes β_2 activation and vasodilatation
- Parasympathetic innervation:
  - Predominantly by vagus nerve
  - Parasympathetic effets on coronary circulation are usually minor and weak
  - Stimulation causes weak vasodilatation

Hormonal Control

- Peptide hormones controlling coronary blood flow include:
  - Antidiuretic hormone:
    - Has little effect in physiological concentrations
    - Causes intense vasoconstriction in stressful conditions
  - Angiotensin II:
    - Causes vasoconstriction independent of synmpathetic innervations
    - It also causes intense vasoconstriction through indirect mechanisms:
      - Enhanced calcium influx
      - Release of endothelin
  - Atrial natriuretic peptide
  - Vasoactive intestinal peptide
  - Calcitonin gene-related peptide:
    - Along with substance P, it releases EDRF
    - This causes maximal coronary vasodilatation

Cardiac Reflexes

- ***Anrep's reflex:***
  - Increased venous return causes increased right atrial pressures
  - This leads to reflex increase in CBF
  - Typically occurs during exercise
- ***Gastro-coronary reflex***:
  - Distention of stomach with a heavy meal causes reflex coronary vasoconstriction
  - This reduces the CBF and predisposes to ischemia

Effects of Anesthetic Agents

- Most volatile agents are coronary dilators through:
  - Action on ATP sensitive K^+ channels
  - Stimulation of adenosine A_1 receptors
- Halothane > isoflurane > desflurane > sevoflurane (negligible)
- Volatile agents protect against reperfusion injury
- They also reduce myocardial O_2 requirements during ischemia and infarction

CARDIAC ACTION POTENTIAL

Introduction

- Action potential (AP) for skeletal muscle is due to abrupt opening of fast Na^+ channels
- For cardiac muscle, AP is generated by opening of:
  - Fast sodium channels causing a spike
  - Slower L-type calcium channels causing the plateau

Characteristics of Cardiac Action Potential

- Action potential recorded in ventricular muscle fiber averages 105 millivolts
- Thus, intracellular potential rises from –85 mV to +20 mV every beat
- After the initial spike, the membrane remains depolarized for about 0.2 seconds
- This phase is called the plateau of cardiac action potential
- This increases the duration of cardiac AP to 15 times that of skeletal muscle AP
- This is followed by an abrupt repolarization to resting membrane potential (RMP)

Types of Cardiac Action Potential

- Fast-response action potentials:
  - Seen in ordinary cardiac muscle cells
  - Characterized by:
    - Rapid depolarization with substantial overshoot
    - Rapid reversal of overshoot potential
    - Long plateau phase
    - Rapid repolarization phase to stable high resting membrane potential
- Slow-response action potentials:
  - Seen in pacemaker cells (SA node and AV node)
  - Characterized by:
    - Slower initial depolarization phase
    - Lower amplitude overshoot
    - Shorter and less stable plateau phase

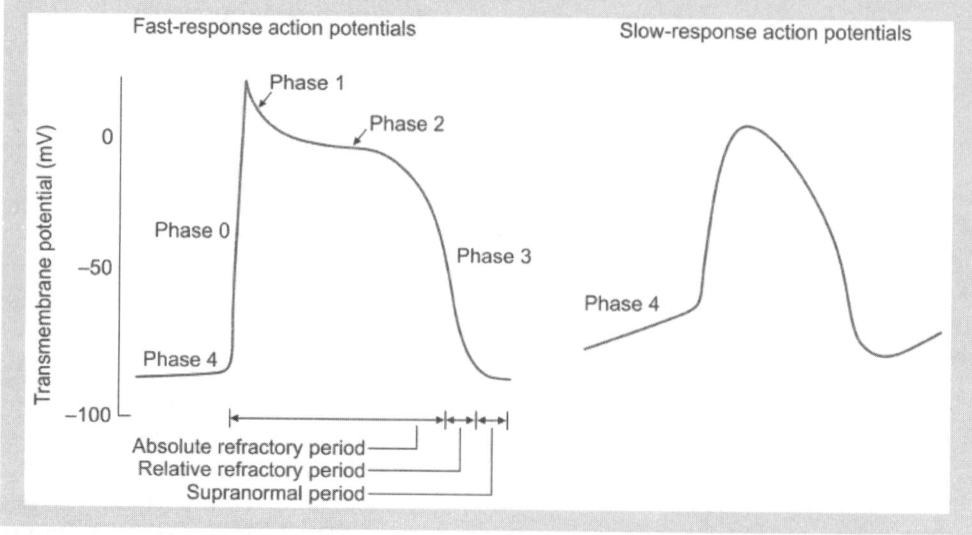

Fig. 5: Types of cardiac action potential.

- Repolarization to unstable, slowly depolarizing RMP
- This unstable RMP is also called:
  - Phase 4 depolarization
  - Diastolic depolarization
  - Pacemaker potential

Differences from Skeletal Muscle AP

- Sodium and calcium channels:
  - Skeletal muscles:
    - Skeletal muscle AP is generated solely by fast sodium channels
    - These remain open for only few thousandths of a second
    - This causes rapid entry of Na^+ into cells and depolarization
    - Following this, abrupt closure of the channels occur causing repolarization
  - Cardiac muscles: AP is caused by opening of 2 types of channels:
    - Fast sodium channels:
      - Cause rapid entry of Na^+ into cardiac myocytes and depolarization
      - Results in the generation of the spike of cardiac AP
    - L-type slow calcium channels:
      - Also called calcium-sodium channels
      - They are slower to open and remain open for longer duration
      - This results in influx of large amounts of Na^+ and Ca^{2+}
      - The channel remains open for longer duration of time
      - This results in formation of a plateau
      - Ca^{2+} ions which enter during this phase trigger contractile process
- Permeability of potassium ions:
  - Following onset of AP, membrane permeability for K^+ reduces in cardiac myocyte
  - This is not seen in skeletal muscle fibers
  - Decreased outflow of K^+ ions during AP prevents early return of AP to baseline
  - This contributes to the formation of plateau on cardiac myocyte AP

Phases of Normal Action Potential

Phase	Name	Event	Ion flux	Changes
0.	Upstroke/depolarization	Fast Na^+ channels open	Na^+ influx	MP becomes +ve
1.	Early rapid repolarization	Fast Na^+ channels close	K^+ efflux	Repolarization
2.	Plateau phase	Slow Ca^{2+} channels open	Ca^{2+} influx	Plateau formation
		Fast K^+ channels close	Reduced K^+ efflux	
3.	Final repolarization	Slow Ca^{2+} channels close	K^+ efflux	Return of MP to baseline
		Slow K^+ channels open		
4.	Resting potential	Normal permeability restored	K^+ efflux	MP becomes –90 mV
			Na^+ and Ca^{2+} influx	

Characteristics of Pacemaker Cells

- Pacemaker cells are characterized by slow depolarization during diastolic interval
- This results in an unstable RMP in pacemaker cells
- This is also called pacemaker potential
- This occurs due to:
  - Decreased permeability to K^+ during resting phase:
    - This prevents influx of K^+ ions during resting phase
    - Thus, RMP moves away from K^+ equilibrium potential (– 90 mV)
  - Increased permeability to Na^+ during resting phase:
    - This results in slow influx of Na^+ ions
    - Thus, RMP becomes progressively more positive
  - Increase in Ca^{2+} permeability during diastole:
    - Results in progressive influx of Ca^{2+} ions late in diastole
    - This contributes to diastolic depolarization

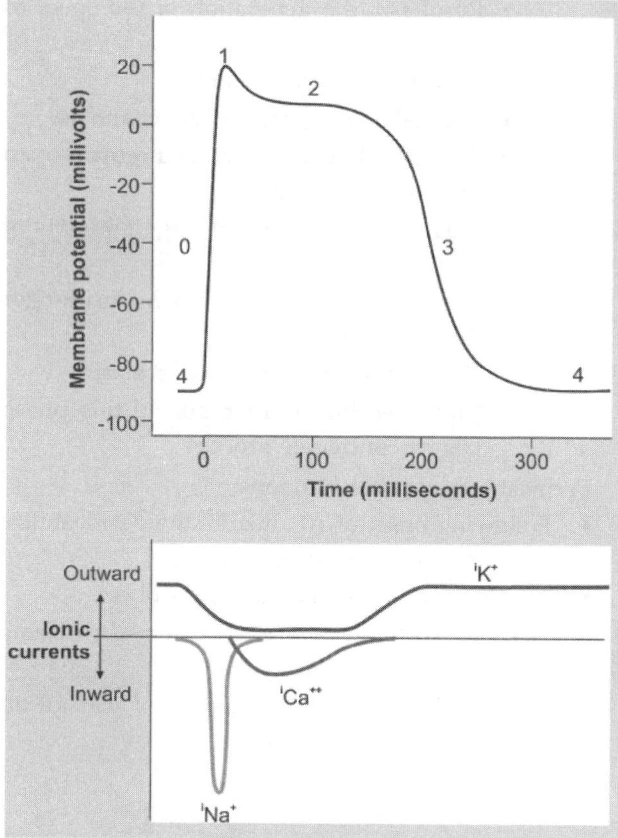

Fig. 6: Phases of cardiac action potential.

Channels Involved in Generation of Cardiac AP

No.	Channel	Gating mechanism	Function
1.	K^+ channel (K_{ir})	Voltage gated	Maintains high K^+ permeability during phase 4
	Inward rectifier		Its decay contributes to diastolic depolarization
			Its suppression contributes to plateau phase
2.	Fast Na^+ channel	Voltage gated	Accounts for phase 0 of AP
	(Nav 1.5)		Inactivation contributes to phase 1 of AP
3.	K^+ channel (K_{to})	Voltage gated	Contributes to phase 1 of AP
	Transient outward		
4.	L- Ca^{2+} channel	Both	Contributes to phase 2 of AP
	Slow inward		Inactivation contributes to phase 3 of AP
	Cav 1.2		Enhanced by sympathetic stimulation
5.	K^+ channels	Voltage gated	Causes phase 3 of AP
	Delayed rectifier		Enhanced by increased intracellular Ca^{2+}
	K_s, K_t, K_{ur}		
6.	K^+ channel	Ligand gated	Increases K^+ permeability when ATP is low
	ATP-sensitive		
7.	K^+ channel	Ligand gated	Responsible for effects of vagal stimulation
	ACH activated		Decreases diastolic depolarization
			Hyperpolarizes RMP
			Shortens phase 2 of AP

Events in Action Potential

Myocardial Cells

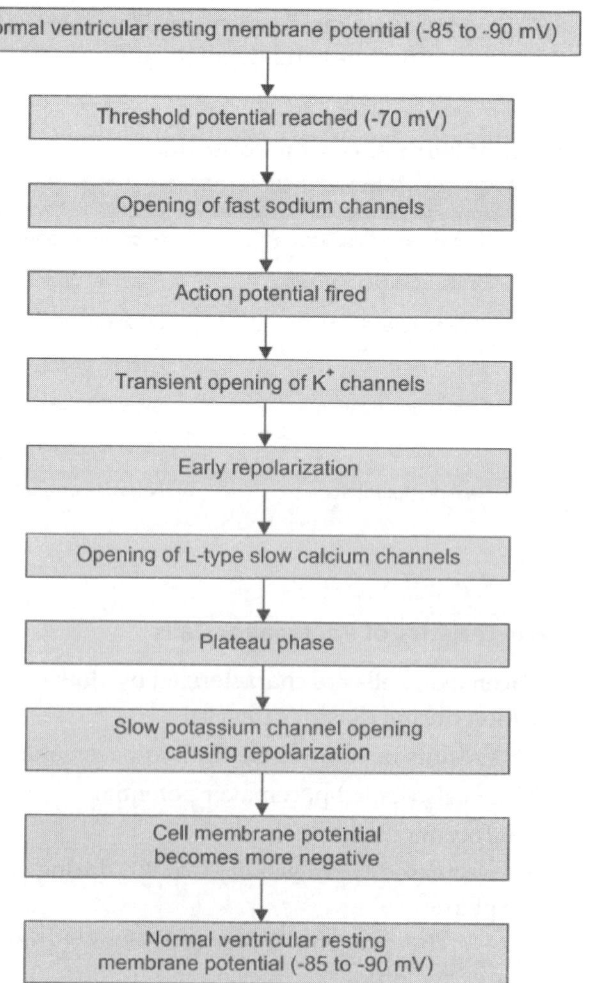

Pacemaker Cells

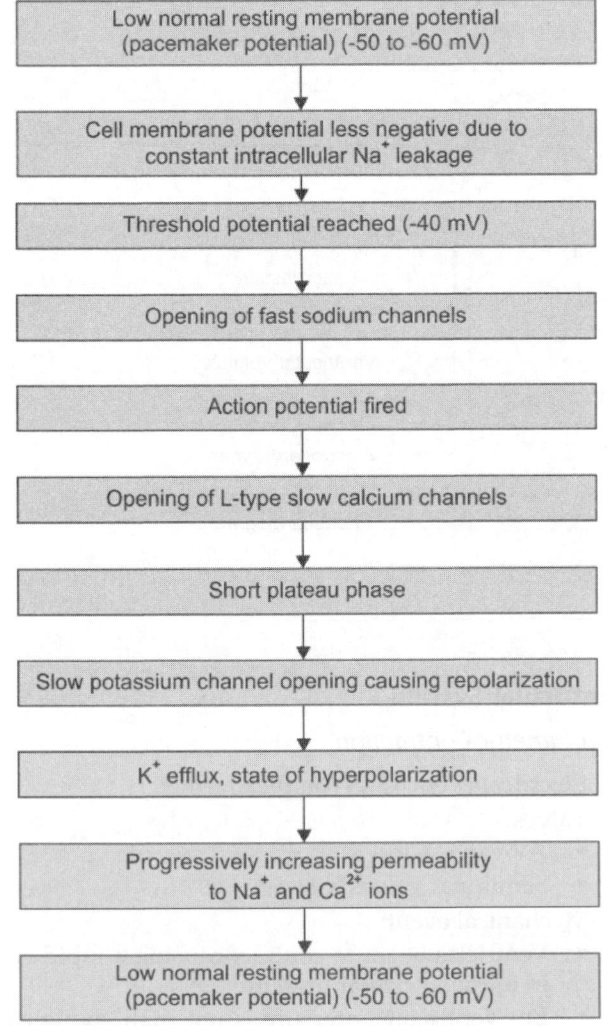

Physiological and Pathological Changes in AP

- Catecholamines:
  - Catecholamines cause an increase in the size of plateau current
  - This leads to higher influx of Ca^{2+} ions during plateau phase
  - This results in increased contractility of cardiac myocyte
  - Thus, contractility of cardiac myocyte is proportional to size of plateau current
  - CCBs block the L-type calcium channels and cause negative inotropism
- Acute ischemia:
  - Acute myocardial ischemia and hypoxia results in shortening of plateau phase
  - This occurs due to activation of ligand gated K_{ATP} channels
  - Normal intracellular ATP levels is approximately 5 mM
  - Reduction in ATP levels triggers opening of K_{ATP} channels
  - This results in early onset of repolarization and shortening of depolarization
- Chronic heart failure (HF):
  - Chronic HF causes ventricular hypertrophy
  - This causes reduced expression of transient outward K^+ channels
  - This leads to:
    - Delayed repolarization
    - Prolonged plateau phase causing calcium overload
    - Increased propensity for arrhythmias due to after-depolarization

CARDIAC CYCLE

Introduction

- Sequence of electrical and mechanical events occurring during course of a single heart beat
- The cardiac cycle integrates various changes during systole and diastole:
  - Pressure changes
  - Volume changes
  - Valvular dynamics
  - Electrocardiographic events
- The normal duration of cardiac cycle is approximately 0.83 seconds

Phases of Cardiac Cycle

- Atrial systole (100 msec)
- Ventricular systole (350 msec):
  - Isovolumetric contraction (30–50 msec)
  - Ejection phase (300 msec)
- Ventricular diastole (450 msec):
  - Isovolumetric relaxation (60–80 msec)
  - First rapid filling phase (150 msec)
  - Diastasis/slow filling phase (120 msec)
  - Second rapid filling phase (100 msec).

Events in Cardiac Cycle

Atrial Systole

- Electrical event:
  - Electrical activation of atria
  - P wave, PR interval

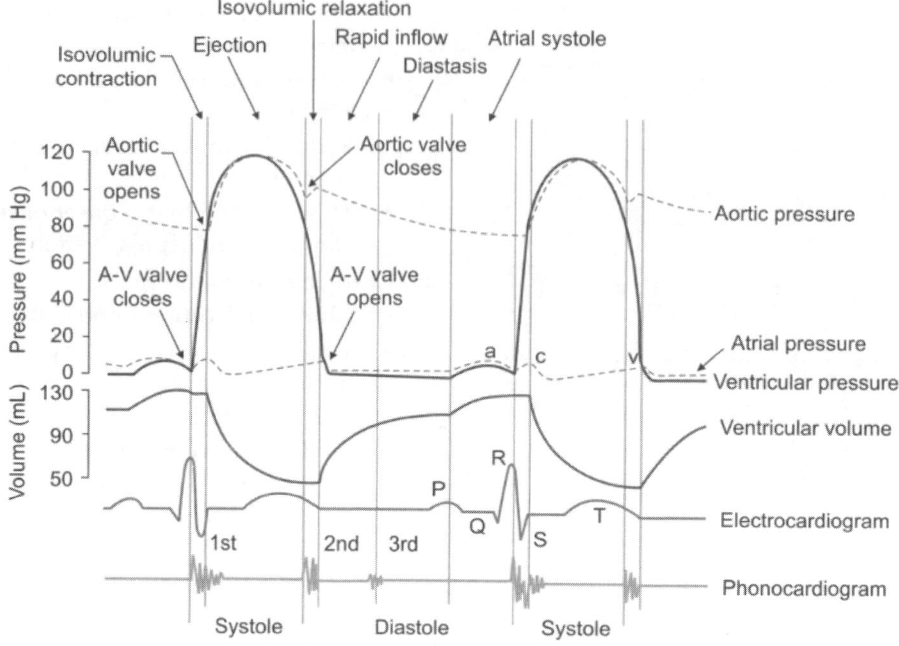

Fig. 7: Cardiac cycle.

- Valves:
  - AV valve: open
  - Semilunar valves: closed
- Mechanical event:
  - Atrial systole/atrial kick
  - Atrial muscles contract from superior portion of atria towards AV septum
  - Pressure within the atrial rises and blood in ejected across the open AV valve
  - 25–30% cardiac output is produced by atrial kick in normal individuals
  - Fully completed before ventricle begins to contract
  - Atrial systole lasts for approximately 100 msec
- Pressure-volume event:
  - *a* waves in JVP
  - Atrial pressure increases
- Heart sound event:
  - Fourth heart sound S_4 is produced by atrial contraction
  - Fourth heart sound is not heard normally
  - Causes of abnormal audible S_4:
    - Massive pulmonary embolism
    - Cor pulmonale
    - Hypertrophic obstructive cardiomyopathy
    - Tricuspid regurgitation

Ventricular Systole

Isovolumetric Contraction

- Electrical event: QRS complex formed
- Valves:
  - AV valve: Closed
  - Semilunar valves: Closed
- Mechanical event:
  - Ventricles begin to contract causing a rapid rise in intraventricular pressure
  - But ventricular pressure is not high enough to open the semilunar valves
  - However, ventricular pressure at this stage exceeds atrial pressure
  - This forces the atrio-ventricular valves to close
  - Since blood is not ejected from the ventricles, ventricular volume is constant
  - Thus, this stage is called isovolumetric contraction
- Pressure volume event:
  - Responsible for *c* wave in JVP
  - Contraction is isovolumetric, while intraventricular pressure increases
  - Rapid rise in intraventricular pressure occurs during this phase
  - Maximum rate of rise of pressure (dP/dt_{max}) is used as an index of contractility
- Heart sound event: S_1 produced due to closure of atrio-ventricular valves

Ejection Phase

- Electrical event: falls on QT segment
- Valves:
  - AV valves: Closed
  - Semilunar valves: Open
- Mechanical event:
  - Ventricular pressure rises to a level higher than the aortic and pulmonary pressures
  - Thus, semilunar valves are forced open at the beginning of this phase
  - This produces ejection of blood across the semilunar valves
  - During initial one-third of this phase, 70% of ventricular emptying occurs
  - This is called the *rapid ejection phase*
  - During the latter two-third of this phase, remaining 30% of emptying occurs
  - This is called the *slow ejection phase*
- Pressure volume event:
  - Opens up semilunar valve
  - Ejects blood, causing a sudden reduction in ventricular pressure
  - Only 2/3rd of the EDV is ejected during systole called stroke volume (70–80 mL)
  - The residual volume in the ventricle is called end-systolic volume (40–50 mL)
  - Proportion of EDV ejected during systole is called ejection fraction (50–70%)
- Heart sound event: No event

Ventricular Diastole

Isovolumetric Relaxation

- Electrical event: T wave due to repolarization
- Valves:
  - AV valve: closed
  - Semilunar valves: closed
- Mechanical event:
  - Ventricular relaxation begins during this phase and pressure rapidly falls
  - When ventricular pressure falls below aortic pressure, semilunar valves close
  - Atrio-ventricular valves are closed, with closed semilunar valves
  - No ventricular volume change occurs as both AV and semilunar valves are closed
  - Therefore, this phase is called isovolumetric relaxation phase
- Pressure volume event:
  - Atrial pressure increases, as blood collects passively
  - v waves occur in JVP
  - Ventricular pressure continues to fall
  - Ventricular volume is minimal
- Heart sound event:
  - S_2 occurs when semilunar valves close
  - S_2 is usually split as aortic valve opens before pulmonary valve

Rapid Filling Phase

- Electrical event: No events
- Valves:
  - AV valves: Open
  - Semilunar valves: Closed
- Mechanical event:
  - Ventricular pressure continues to drop during ventricular diastole
  - However, atrial filling during this stage causes atrial pressure to rise
  - Eventually, atrial pressure increases above the ventricular pressure
  - This forces atrio-ventricular valves to open, causing rapid ventricular filling
- Pressure volume event:
  - Blood from atria enters ventricles
  - Ventricular volume increases rapidly
- Heart sound event:
  - S_3 produced due to rapid passive filling of blood
  - S_3 is usually not audible in adults
  - Causes of audible S_3 gallop:
    - Myocardial infarction
    - Congestive cardiac failure
    - Hypertension

Diastasis

- Electrical event: No events
- Valves:
  - AV valve: Open
  - Semilunar valve: Closed
- Mechanical event:
  - At the end of rapid filling phase, atrio-ventricular pressure gradient reduces
  - Rest of blood which has accumulated slowly in the atria flows into ventricles
  - Ventricle reaches its natural, inherent relaxed volume
  - Thus, the rate of filling slows down (diastasis)
- Pressure volume event: Ventricular volume increases more slowly
- Heart sound event: No events

Second Rapid Filling Phase

- Electrical event: P wave, PR interval
- Valves:
  - AV valve: Open
  - Semilunar valve: Closed
- Mechanical event:
  - Occurs due to atrial systole/atrial kick
  - Volume of blood in ventricle at end of this phase is end-diastolic volume (EDV)
  - EDV is typically 120–150 mL
  - The pressure corresponding to this volume is the end-diastolic pressure (EDP)
  - EDP is typically 4–9 mm Hg
- Pressure-volume event:
  - *a* waves in JVP
  - Atrial pressure increases
- Heart sound event: S_4 produced

CONDUCTION SYSTEM OF HEART

Sinoatrial Node

- Location:
  - On the RA wall at SVC-RA junction
  - 10–20 mm long, 2–3 mm wide, 2–3 mm thick
  - Located 1 mm below epicardial surface
  - ***Crista terminalis***
  - 50% cells have pacemaker activity
  - Densely innervated with postganglionic adrenergic and cholinergic nerve terminals
  - SA nodal discharge is modulated by adrenergic and muscarinic receptors
  - Density of receptors in the SA node is three-times that of adjacent atrial tissue
- Blood supply:
  - 60% RCA via SA nodal artery
  - 40% LCA
- Function:
  - Primary pacemaker of heart as it has fastest heart rate
  - Conduction to RA, interatrial septum, LA
- Intrinsic pacemaker activity:
  - 60–100 bpm
  - Called *sinus rhythm*

Internodal Pathways

- Three pathways exist:
  - ***Bachmann's*** anterior bundle
  - ***Wenckebach's*** middle bundle
  - ***Thorel's*** posterior bundle
- Function: Conducts impulses between SA node and AV node

Atrioventricular Node

- Location:
  - In the floor of RA
  - Situated just behind septal leaflet of tricuspid valve
  - Present near opening of coronary sinus
  - Located in ***Triangle of Koch*** formed by:
    - Tendon of Todaro superiorly
    - Attachement of septal leaflet of tricuspid valve inferiorly
    - Mouth of coronary sinus at the base
- Anatomy:
  - Fibers are smaller with lesser gap junctions: permits for AV nodal delay
  - Three functional regions:
    - Atrionodal region
    - Nodal region
    - Nodal-His regions
  - AV delay occurs at Atrionodal and Nodal regions
- Blood supply:
  - In 85–90% patients branch of the RCA
  - In 10–15% patients branch of left circumflex artery
- Function:
  - Receives impulses from SA node
  - Delays relay allowing atria to empty before ventricles contract
  - Fibers in lower part of AV node may exhibit automatic impulse formation
  - This may be responsible for junctional rhythm
- Intrinsic pacemaker activity:
  - 40–60 bpm
  - Called *junctional rhythm*

Bundle of His

- Location: Upper part of interventricular septum
- Anatomy:
  - Divides into right and left Bundle of His
  - Right BOH has 3 fascicles
  - Left BOH has 3 fascicles:
    - Anterior fasciculus
    - Septal fasciculus
    - Posterior fasciculus
- Blood supply:
  - Dual blood supply to left posterior fasciculus via LAD and PDA

- Therefore, the BOH is relatively resistant to ischemic damage

❖ Function:
- Receives impulses from AV node
- Conducts them to Purkinje fibers

❖ Intrinsic pacemaker activity: 40–60 bpm

Purkinje Fibers

❖ Location:
- In ventricular myocardium
- Penetrates only inner one-third of ventricular endocardium
- Form interweaving network on the endocardial surface of both ventricles

❖ Function:
- Fastest speed of conduction
- Receives impulses from Bundle of His
- Conducts them to ventricular myocardium

❖ Intrinsic pacemaker activity: 20–40 bpm

Variations

Prexcitation syndromes:

❖ Terms used to describe rhythm that originate from above the ventricles but in which impulse travels via a pathway other than AVN and BOH

❖ Types:
- ***Wolff-Parkinson-White syndrome*** via ***bundle of Kent***
- ***Lown-Ganong-Levine syndrome*** via ***James bundle***
- ***Mahaim fibers***

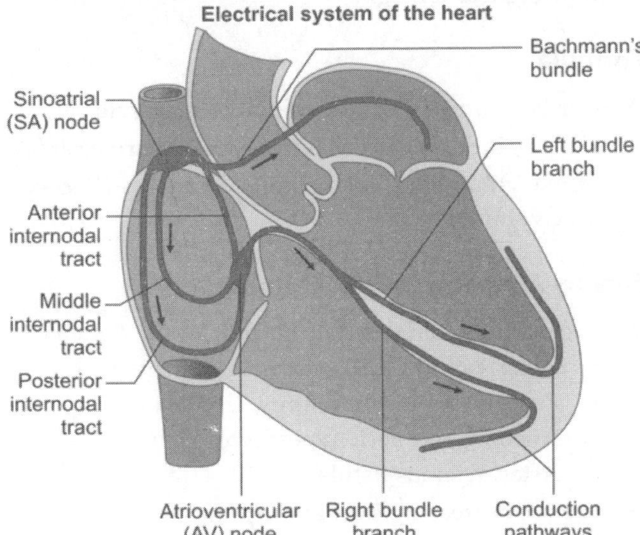

Fig. 8: Conduction system of heart.

PREEXCITATION SYNDROME

Introduction

Preexcitation is a term used to describe rhythms that originate from above the ventricle but in which the impulse travels via a pathway other than the AV node and BOH.

Embryology

❖ During fetal life, strands of myocardial tissue form connection between the atria and ventricles, outside the normal conduction system

❖ These strands normally become nonfunctional soon after birth

❖ In patients with preexcitation syndrome these connections persist

❖ These strands form congenital malformations of working myocardial tissue

Types of Malformations

❖ Accessory pathways: bypass part or whole of the normal conduction system

❖ Bypass tracts: when one of the accessory pathway is attached to normal conductive tissue.

Examples

There are 3 major forms of preexcitation syndromes:

❖ ***Wolff-Parkinson-White (WPW) syndrome***:
- The accessory pathway is called *Bundle of Kent*
- This connects atria directly to ventricles, by passing the normal conduction system
- Thus, the AV node is bypassed
- Hence AV nodal delay does not occur

❖ ***Lown–Ganong–Levine syndrome***:
- The accessory pathway is called *James bundle*
- This connects atria directly to lower part of AV junction
- Thus it partially bypasses AV node

❖ ***Mahaim fibers***:
- These cause an unnamed preexcitation syndrome
- Fibers originate below AV node and insert into ventricular wall
- This bypasses the ventricular conducting system

Incidence

❖ 1.5–3.1 per 1000 individuals

❖ More commonly occurs in men

❖ WPW syndrome is *most common* type of preexcitation syndrome

Description

- WPW syndrome
  - Delta waves
  - Short PR interval
  - Wide QRS duration (> 0.12 seconds)
- LGL syndrome:
  - No delta waves
  - Short PR interval
  - Normal QRS duration
- Mahaim fibers
  - Delta wave present
  - Normal PR interval
  - Widened QRS complexes

Pathophysiology

- Patients with WPW are predisposed to tachyarrhythmias because of:
  - Accessory pathway bypassing the AV nodal delay
  - Pathway also provides a mechanism of reentry
- Two types of reentry are seen in WPW syndrome:
  - Antidromic conduction:
    - Rare variety
    - Occurs in an impulse generated from SAN
    - This travels via to ventricles via accessory pathway
    - Bypasses AV node on the way to ventricles
    - Impulse reenters atria via AV node
  - Orthodromic conduction:
    - More common
    - Occurs in an impulse generated from SAN
    - This enters ventricles via AV node
    - Impulse reenters atria via accessory pathway of Kent

Clinical Features

- Palpitations, anxiety
- Light headedness, dizziness, weakness
- Chest discomfort, dyspnea, signs of shock
- Complications: Three main types of dysrhythmias:
  - AV nodal reentrant tachycardia: *most common*
  - Atrial fibrillation
  - Atrial flutter: least common

Treatment

- Stable, symptomatic patient with orthodromic AVRT (narrow QRS):
  - Oxygen administration, IV access secured
  - Vagal maneuvers to convert rhythm
  - IV adenosine: May transiently increase risk of atrial fibrillation
  - IV calcium channel blockers/β blockers: Cause transient AV block
  - Avoid digoxin and verapamil as:
    - Conduction through AVN is slowed
    - This may speed up conduction through accessory pathway
- Stable, symptomatic patient with antidromic AVRT (wide QRS):
  - Oxygen administration
  - IV access secured
  - IV procainamide/amiodarone
  - Amiodarone preferred in CHF patients
- Unstable patients: synchronized cardioversion

CARDIAC OUTPUT

Definition

Volume of blood ejected per minute from LV to aorta to support the metabolic demands of peripheral tissues.

Normal Values

- Males: 5–6 L/min
- Females: 10–20% less than males
- Children:
  - 350–400 mL/kg/min at birth
  - 150–200 mL/kg/min after first week of life
- Cardiac index: 3.2 L/min/m^2 (2.5–4.2 L/min/m^2)
- Body surface area calculated from nomogram based on weight and height

Formula

- Cardiac output = stroke volume x heart rate
- Cardiac index = cardiac output/body surface area
- Stroke volume = (End diastolic volume) – (End systolic volume)

Factors Affecting Cardiac Output

- Factors increasing cardiac output:
  - Fever, raised BMR, exercise, pregnancy
  - Posture: supine, lithotomy, Trendelenburg
  - Anemia, beri-beri, hyperthyroidism
  - Arteriovenous fistula
- Factors decreasing cardiac output:
  - Sleep, heart rate more than 120 bpm
  - *Posture*: standing up, sitting

- Reduced ventricular compliance due to:
  - Myocardial infarction
  - Valvular heart disease
  - Cardiac tamponade
  - Left ventricular hypertrophy
- Reduced venous return due to:
  - Hemorrhage
  - Acute venodilatation, spinal anesthesia
  - Venous obstruction
  - Intermittent positive pressure ventilation

Factors Affecting Stroke Volume

Preload

Definition:

- Represents filling of heart chamber with blood during diastole
- Represents the muscle length prior to contraction or end diastolic fiber length
- Venous return is the amount of blood flowing from veins into RA each minute

Formula:

- $\text{Venous return} = \frac{(\text{Arterial pressure}) - (\text{RA pressure})}{\text{Total peripheral resistance}}$
- 55% to 60% of blood in body is in systemic veins
- Equivalent of EDV of LV in intact heart (normal around 120 mL)

Determinants of preload:

- Determinants of ventricular filling:
  - Venous return, blood volume
  - Rhythm (artrial contraction)
  - Heart rate
  - Distribution of blood volume:
    - Posture
    - Intrathoracic pressure
    - Pericardial pressure
    - Venous tone (major determinant)
- Determinants of ventricular compliance:
  - Hypertrophy, asynchrony
  - Ischemia, fibrosis
  - Pericardial disease
  - Overdistension of contralateral ventricle
  - Increased pleural/airway pressure
  - Tumors, surgical compression

Measurement of preload:

- Pulmonary artery pressure, PCWP
- CVP: is poorest estimate of LV preload
- LVEDV via echocardiography
- LVEDP via cardiac catheterization

Afterload

Definition:

- Force which the heart must pump against, in ejecting blood from the heart
- SVR accounts for 95% of resistance to ejection

Formula:

$$\text{SVR} = \frac{(\text{MAP} - \text{RAP})}{\text{CO}} \times 80$$

$$\text{PVR} = \frac{(\text{PAP} - \text{LAP})}{\text{CO}} \times 80$$

- Normal SVR = 900–1500 dynes seconds/cm^{-5}
- Normal PVR = 150–250 dyne sec/cm^{-5}
- SVR represents ratio of pressure to cardiac output

Factors affecting aferload:

- Viscosity and density of blood
- Aortic pressure, SVR
- Aortic valve area, vascular distensibility
- Volume and thickness of LV
- Systolic intraventricular pressure

Contractility

Definition:

- Myocardiums intrinsic ability to generate work from a given end diastolic fiber length
- Intrinsic force of myocardial contraction in inotropic state

Factors affecting:

- Increased by:
  - Sympathetic activity
  - Calcium
  - Noradrenaline
  - Digoxin
- Decreased by:
  - Parasympathetic activity:
  - Increased K^+ levels
  - Magnesium ions
  - Acidosis, hypoxia
  - β blockers, calcium channel blockers

Measurement of contractility:

- Ejection fraction
- Isovolumetric contraction phase indices (d_p/d_t)
- Load dependent indices (slope of end systolic – pressure volume relation)
- Preload recruitable stroke work
- LV systolic wall thickening

Heart Rate

Normal: 60–80 bpm

Formula:

- Maximum heart rate = (220 - age in years)
- Normal intrinsic heart rate = 118 bpm – (0.57 × age)

  Factors increasing heart rate: exercise, fever, stress, high BMR

  Factors decreasing heart rate: sleep, hypothermia, low BMR

  CO decreases progressively when heart rate ≥120 bpm, as diastolic filling time reduces

Frank Starlings Law

Introduction

- Force of contraction of muscle is directly proportional to initial length of muscle fiber
- Represents the ability of heart to change its force of contraction and therefore stroke volume in response to changes in venous return

Uses

- Illustrates relationship between CO and LVEDV
- Illustrates relationship between SV and RAP

MYOCARDIAL OXYGEN SUPPLY DEMAND BALANCE

Introduction

- Normal cardiac oxygen consumption = 80–100 mL O_2/100 g myocardium
- Normal oxygen supply = 250 mL/min
- Myocardium usually extracts 75–80% oxygen in arterial blood, compared with 25% in most other tissues
- Thus, it cannot compensate for a decrease in blood flow by extraction of more oxygen from hemoglobin
- This must be met with, by an increase in CBF

Factors Affecting Supply

- Coronary blood vessel diameter
- Autonomic innervation
- Autoregulation
- Coronary steal
- Coronary perfusion pressure:
  - Aortic diastolic blood pressure
  - LVEDP/RVEDP
- Arterial oxygen content:
  - Arterial oxygen tension
  - Hemoglobin concentration
- Heart rate: diastolic time
- Exogenous substances:
  - Oxygen, carbon dioxide
  - Nitric oxide
  - Adenosine
  - K^+, Ca^{2+}
  - pH, osmolarity

Factors Affecting Demand

- Basal requirements (20%)
- Heart rate (most important)
- Wall tension:
  - Preload (ventricular radius)
  - Afterload
- Contractility

VENTRICULAR PRESSURE-VOLUME LOOPS

Introduction

- Cardiac function is characterized by ventricular pressure-volume loops
- Aids to visualize changes in ventricular function in response to changes in preload, afterload and inotropy

Method

The LV pressure is plotted against LV volume at multiple time points in cardiac cycle

Phases of Pressure Volume Loop 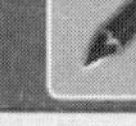

- Phase I: Ventricular filling:
  - From point a- point b
  - Point b represents the EDV and EDP
- Phase II: Isovolumetric contraction (point b- point c)
- Phase III: Ejection phase:
  - From point c- point d
  - Point d represents the ESV and ESP
- Phase IV: Isovolumetric relaxation phase (point d- point a)

Events during the Pressure Volume Loop

- PHASE 1: *ventricular filling in diastole:*
  - At the beginning of this phase:
    - Ventricular volume is 50 mL (ESV of previous heart beat)
    - Ventricular pressure 2–3 mm Hg
  - Phase begins with opening of the mitral valve
  - This initiates ventricular filling
  - Initially, ventricular pressure remains constant

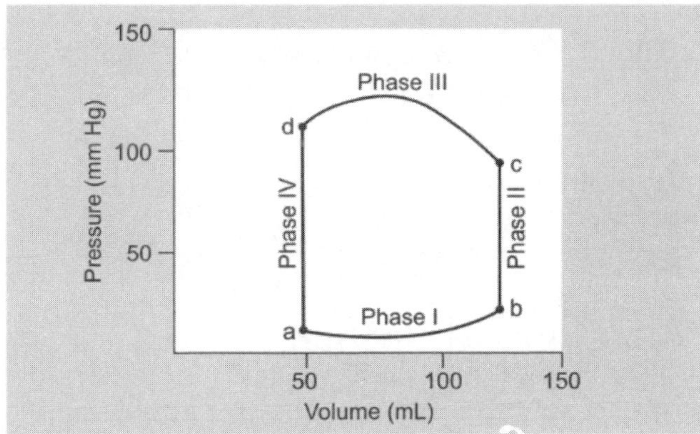

Fig. 9: Phases of pressure volume loop.

- Over time, as the ventricular volume increases, the preload increases
- Thus, there is a simultaneous increase in intraventricular pressure
- This results in a horizontal line as ventricular volume constantly changes
- At the end of this phase:
  - Ventricular volume: 120 mL (EDV)
  - Ventricular pressure: 5–7 mm Hg (EDP)

❖ PHASE II: *isovolumetric contraction*:
- At the beginning of this phase:
  - Ventricular volume: 120 mL
  - Ventricular pressure: 5–7 mm Hg
- Phase begins with the closure of mitral valve, at the onset of systole
- Ventricle has begun to contract but volume remains constant
- This is because sufficient pressure has not developed to exceed pressure in aorta
- This results in a vertical line as volume remains constant
- Greater the afterload, more pressure is required to overcome it
- At the end of this phase:
  - Ventricular volume: 120 mL
  - Ventricular pressure: 80 mm Hg

❖ PHASE III: *ejection period*:
- At the beginning of this phase:
  - Ventricular volume: 120 mL
  - Ventricular pressure: 80 mm Hg
- Phase begins with opening of aortic valve
- This occurs when intraventricular pressure exceeds aortic pressure
- Blood is continually ejected from the ventricle
- This occurs until pressure in aorta exceeds intraventricular pressure
- At this point aortic valve closes
- This again results in a horizontal line as the ventricular volume changes
- At the end of this phase:
  - Ventricular volume: 50 mL (ESV)
  - Ventricular pressure: 100 mm Hg

❖ PHASE IV: *isovolumetric relaxation*:
- At the beginning of this phase:
  - Ventricular volume: 50 mL
  - Ventricular pressure: 100 mm Hg
- Phase begins immediately after closure of aortic valve
- At this point, intraventricular pressure is lesser than aortic pressure
- However, intraventricular pressure exceeds the atrial pressure
- Thus, ventricle begins relaxing with a closed AV valve and semilunar valve
- This maintains a constant ventricular volume
- At the end of phase IV, atrial pressure begins to exceed ventricular pressure
- This causes AV valve to open
- This allows resumption of ventricular filling and increased ventricular volume
- Intraventricular pressure constantly reduces resulting in a vertical line
- At the end of this phase:
  - Ventricular volume: 50 mL
  - Ventricular pressure: 2–3 mm Hg

Pressure Volume Loop in Mitral Stenosis

❖ Mitral stenosis prevents diastolic filling of the left ventricle
❖ Thus, MS diminishes the LV preload reserve
❖ This results in reduced LV volumes during both systole and diastole
❖ Thus, LVEDV and LVEDP are reduced with an accompanying decline in stroke volume
❖ This results in a reduced width of curve (i.e., stroke volume) and low LVEDV
❖ The universal reduction in LV volumes causes a leftward shift in the PV loop

Pressure Volume Loop in Mitral Regurgitation

❖ Mitral regurgitation is characterized by systolic regurgitation of blood into LA
❖ The regurgitation begins early in the cycle of ventricular systole

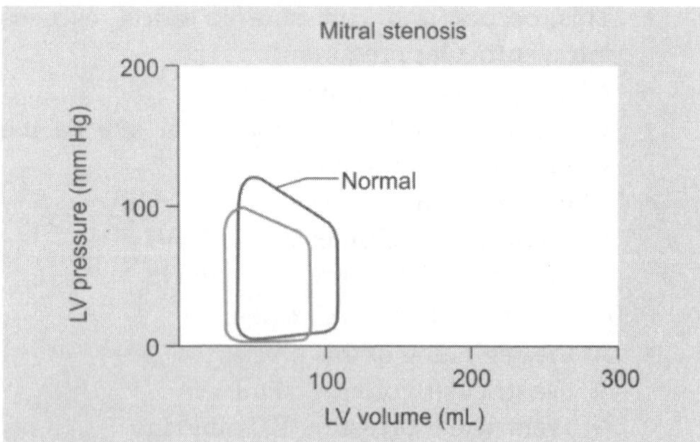

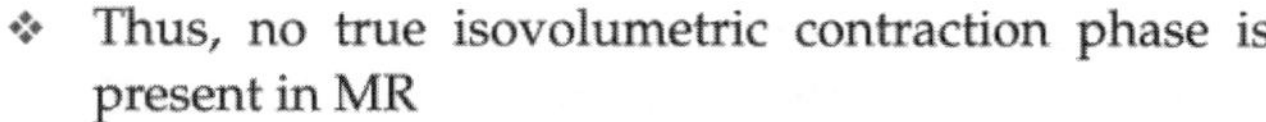
Fig. 10: Pressure volume loop in mitral stenosis.

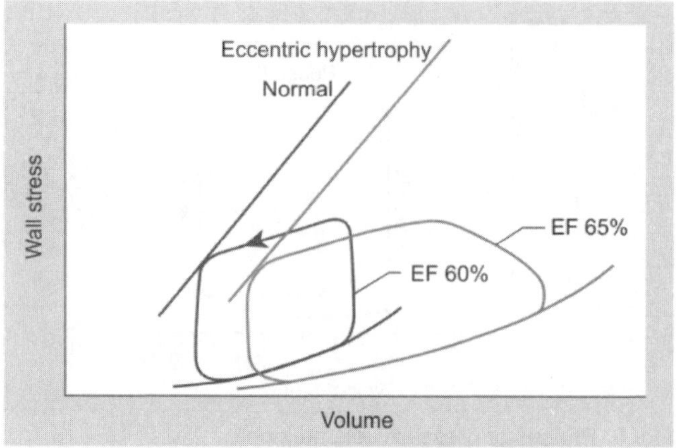

Fig. 11: Pressure volume loop in mitral regurgitation.

- Thus, no true isovolumetric contraction phase is present in MR
- This is because blood flows back into LA during this phase
- Since the LV volume is constantly decreasing, phase II is represented by an oblique line
- Phase III and IV are predominantly normal
- However, during ventricular filling, LV receives both:
  - Pulmonary blood from pulmonary veins
  - Regurgitant blood volume due to mitral regurgitation
- Thus, volume of LV at the end of ventricular filling is higher than normal
- Thus, LVEDP and LVEDV (represented by *point b)* are higher
- The universal increase in ventricular volumes results in rightward shift of PV curve
- Also, width of PV loop is increased causing an increase in stroke volume
- This is because blood is ejected into aorta and also back into LA during systole

Pressure Volume Loop in Aortic Stenosis

- The diastolic compliance of hypertrophied LV wall is reduced
- Thus, the diastolic slope of phase I is steeper
- This is because small changes in ventricular volume produce large changes in pressure
- Thus, EDP is higher (*point b*) compared with an unchanged EDV
- Also, the aortic valve opens at a much higher LV pressure
- Thus, *point c* is shifted higher in the curve

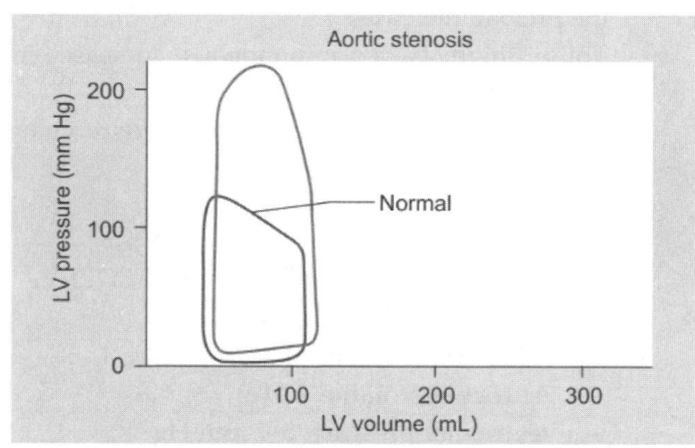

Fig. 12: Pressure volume loop in aortic stenosis.

- The peak pressure generated at end of systole (*point d*) is also much higher
- Both these changes are due to the high transvalvular pressure gradient
- LV emptying is impaired causing a reduced stroke volume (small width of loop)

Pressure Volume Loop in Aortic Regurgitation

- Phase I is characterized by ventricular filling by antegrade flow from mitral valve
- This is followed by isovolumetric contraction phase
- This phase is very brief due to the low aortic diastolic pressure
- Phase III is characterized by ventricular ejection into the aorta
- This is followed by isovolumetric relaxation
- However, there is no true isovolumetric relaxation phase in AR

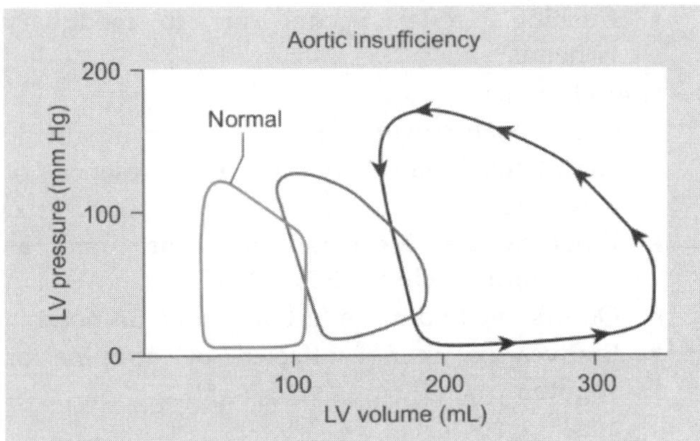

Fig. 13: Pressure volume loop in aortic regurgitation.

- This is because the ventricle fills continuously from AR during diastole
- Thus, ventricular volume constantly increases during isovolumetric relaxation
- Thus, *point a* at end of phase IV is placed more distal than *point d*
- The PV curve itself is grossly shifted to the right
- This is due to a massive increase in LVEDV with minimal change in filling pressure
- This is because of high ventricular diastolic compliance
- This occurs due to a phenomenon called ***creep***
- Creep refers to time-dependent increase in LV dimension due to volume related stress
- Over time, LV adapts to the chronic volume overload related stress
- Thus, LV filling pressure is low and is relatively insensitive to changes in volume status
- Also, the ventricle ejects more volume of blood with every contraction
- This is because of the increased volume of blood within LV from:
  - Antegrade flow via mitral valve
  - Retrograde flow via incompetent AV
- Thus, the area under curve (stroke volume) is increased

ASSESSMENT OF VENTRICULAR FUNCTION

Assessment of Systolic Function

- Initial rate of rise of arterial pressure tracing
- Change in ventricular pressure overtime during systole (d_p/d_t)
- Ejection fraction
- Ventricular pressure-volume loops
- Preload recruitable stroke work
- LV systolic wall thickening

Assessment of Diastolic Function

Using Doppler ECHO via TTE/TEE

Ejection Fraction

Introduction

- Fraction of end diastolic volume which is ejected from the ventricle
- This measures systolic function of heart

Calculation

$$\text{Ejection fraction} = \frac{\text{Stroke volume}}{\text{End diastolic volume}} = \frac{\text{(EDV-ESV)}}{\text{EDV}}$$

Normal value: 0.67 ± 0.08

Measurement

- Transthoracic ECHO
- Transesophageal ECHO
- Cardiac catheterization
- Radionucleotide studies

Grading of LV Dysfunction

Ejection fraction	Grade
40–50	Mild dysfunction
25–40	Moderate dysfunction
Less than 25	Severe dysfunction

Factors Reducing Ejection Fraction

- MI/ischemia
- HOCM/DCM
- Myocarditis, amyloid infilterates
- Chronic pressure/volume overload
- HTN, LVF/CCF
- Congenital and valvular heart diseases
- Anemia
- Hypo/hyperthyroidism/pheochromocytoma

Assessment of Diastolic Function

- Flow velocities across mitral valve measure during diastole
- Three patterns of diastolic dysfunction based on isovolumetric relaxation time, which is the ratio of peak early diastolic flow (E) to peak atrial systolic flow (A)
- Deceleration time (DT) of E (DT_E) also measured and used to categorize diastolic dysfunction

CAUSES OF INTRAOPERATIVE BRADYCARDIA

Introduction

- Bradycardia is one of the most common arrhythmias that occur during anesthesia
- It may be hemodynamically significant particularly in patients with heart disease

Causes

Intrinsic

- Systemic causes:
  - Hypoxia
  - Hypercarbia
  - Hypothermia < 34°C
  - *Raised ICT*: ***Cushing's reflex***
  - Drugs:
    - Opioids, volatile anesthetics, succinylcholine, vecuronium
    - Beta blockers, calcium channel blockers
    - Anticholinesterase inhibitors (neostigmine)
- Cardiac causes:
  - Sick sinus syndrome, sinus bradycardia
  - Junctional rhythm
  - AV nodal blocks
  - Myocardial infarction

Vagal Response

- Traction on:
  - Extraocular muscles: ***oculocardiac reflex***
  - Oropharynx (laryngoscopy and intubation, extubation)
  - Bronchus, peritoneum, bowel, rectum
- Right atrial distension
- Bladder distension

Direct Effect

- Narcotics
- Volatile anesthesia
- Regional anesthesia
- High spinal/spinal shock

Intrinsic Causes

- Hypoxemia:
  - *Most common* cause
  - Causes cardiovascular and respiratory depression: bradycardia, hypotension, decreased minute ventilation
- Raised ICT: causes Cushing's reflex:
  - Consists of hypertension, bradycardia, irregular respiration
  - Cushing's reflex occurs due to medullary ischemia
- Hypothermia:
  - Causes tachycardia initially due to sympathetic stimulation especially in the presence of shivering
  - Proportionate reduction in heart rate as temperature reduces below 34°C
  - Occurs due to direct effect of cold on SA node
  - Bradycardia is not affected by atropine or vagotomy

Vagal Response

- Occurs due to stimulation of:
  - Oropharynx
  - Bronchus
  - Rectum
  - Peritoneum
- Stimulation causes bronchospasm, bradycardia and hypotension in lightly anesthetized patient
- Prevented by:
  - Using atropine IV
  - Topical anesthesia with local anesthetics
  - Adrenergic blocking agents
  - Deep anesthetic planes
  - Vasodilating agents

Direct Anesthetic Effect

- Volatile anesthetics:
  - Mostly occurs with enflurane, isoflurane, halothane
  - Volatile agents directly depress SA node
  - Occurs after slope of phase II depolarization by affecting calcium flux across membrane
- Regional block: Mild bradycardia on release of tourniquet may be seen
- IV local anesthetic:
  - Fetal bradycardia seen when IV local anesthetic is given to mother
  - Paracervical block associated with 20–30% chance of bradycardia
- Succinylcholine:
  - Bradycardia seen after first dose of SCH in children
  - In adults 80% cases present with bradycardia after second dose of SCH if given within 5 minute after first dose
  - This is due to:
    - Choline molecule from breakdown of SCH may sensitize patient to subsequent SCH

- SCH may directly stimulate peripheral sensory receptors to produce bradycardia
- SCH stimulation of parasympathetic NS

❖ Vecuronium: Lacks vagolytic effect and thus may cause bradycardia

❖ Spinal anesthesia: Bradycardia following SA is mediated by 3 reflexes:
- ***Atrial/Bainbridge reflex***:
  - Reduction in venous return occurs following SAB
  - This causes reduced efferent output to cardioaccelerator fibers from the atria
  - This causes bradycardia
- ***SA node stretch reflex***:
  - Stretch receptors not stimulated in SAN due to reduced venous return following SAB
  - This causes bradycardia
- ***Bezold Jarisch reflex***:
  - Reduced venous return causes increased contractilility of ventricle
  - This causes stretching of baroreceptors present in inferoposterior wall of left ventricle
  - This in turn increases vagal output from vasomotor center causing bradycardia

DIAGNOSIS AND MANAGEMENT OF PERIOPERATIVE ARRHYTHMIAS

Introduction

Arrhythmias are the most common perioperative cardiac abnormality in patients undergoing both cardiac and non-cardiac surgery.

Etiology

Patient Related Factors

❖ Geriatric age: *old age* increases chances of *atrial fibrillation*

❖ Thrombosis: coronary/pulmonary

❖ History of coronary artery disease/recent cardiac ischemia

❖ Subarachnoid hemorrhage

❖ Toxins: digoxin toxicity

❖ Trauma:
- Cardiac tamponade
- Tension pneumothorax

Anesthesia Related Factors

❖ Light anesthetic plane/pain

❖ Drugs:
- Halothane Enflurane
- Catecholamines Aminophylline

❖ Central neuraxial block: Causes pharmacological sympathetectomy

❖ Electrolyte imbalance:
- Hypo/hyperkalemia
- Hypo/hypermagnesemia: *torsades de pointes*

❖ Mechanical irritation:
- Central venous lines
- Pulmonary artery catheter
- Chest tubes
- Tracheal intubation/extubation

Surgery related Factors

❖ Non-cardiac surgery:
- Traction on intestines
- Carotid surgery – direct pressure on carotid body
- Oculocardiac reflex
- Neurosurgical causes

❖ Cardiac surgery:
- Cardiac compression on beating heart
- Pericardial traction
- Atrial sutures
- Venous cannulation
- Following release of aortic cross clamp

Miscellaneous Factors

❖ Hypovolemia

❖ Hypoxia

❖ Hypercapnea

❖ Hypoglycemia

❖ Hypothermia/Fever

❖ Acidosis

❖ Thyrotoxic crisis

Classification

Bradyarrhythmias

❖ Sinus bradycardia

❖ Heart block:
- First degree
- Second degree
- Complete heart block

Tachyarrhythmias

❖ Narrow QRS (SVT) tachyarrhythmias:
- Sinus tachycardia
- Atrial premature complexes
- Unifocal/multifocal atrial tachycardia
- Atrial flutter
- Atrial fibrillation
- Paroxysmal supraventricular tachycardia (PSVT)
- AV reciprocating tachycardia (AVRT)
- AV nodal reentrant tachycardia (AVNRT)

- Wide QRS tachyarrhythmias:
  - Ventricular premature extrasystole
  - Ventricular tachycardia
  - Ventricular fibrillation
  - Torsades de pointes

Mechanisms

Automaticity Enhanced

- Normal: Sinus tachycardia
- Abnormal:
  - Unifocal atrial tachycardia
  - Accelerated idioventricular rhythms
  - VT post myocardial infarction

Triggerred Activity

- Early after depolarization: Torsades de pointes
- Late after depolarization:
  - Some VT
  - Digitalis induced arrhythmias

Reentry: Sodium Channel Dependent

- Long excitable gap:
  - Atrial flutter
  - Circus movement tachycardia in WPW syndrome
  - Monomorphic VT
- Short excitable gap:
  - Atrial flutter
  - Atrial fibrillation
  - Circus movement tachycardia in WPW syndrome
  - Polymorphic VT
  - Monomorphic VT
  - Bundle branch reentry
  - Ventricular fibrillation

Reentry: Calcium Channel Dependent

- AV nodal reentrant tachycardia (AVNRT)
- Circus movement tachycardia in WPW
- Ventricular tachycardia

Diagnosis

Tachyarrhythmias

- Sinus tachycardia:
  - Rhythm – Regular
  - Rate –100 - 180 bpm
  - QRS duration – normal
  - P wave – visible before each QRS complex
  - PR interval – normal

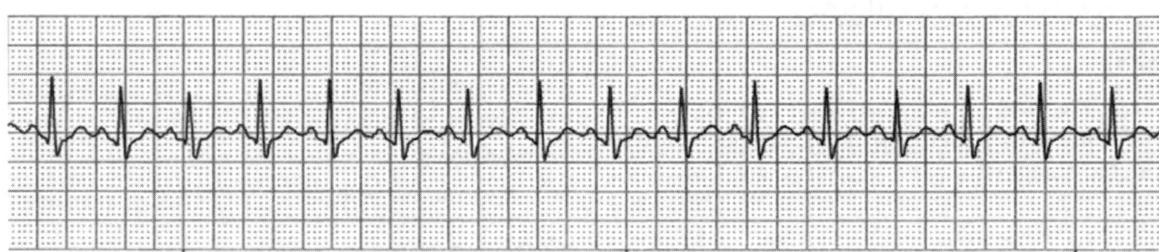

- Unifocal atrial tachycardia:
  - Rhythm – regular
  - Rate – 75–200 bpm (ventricular), 120–250 bpm (atrial)
  - QRS duration – normal
  - P wave –P wave with consistently abnormal morphology
  - PR interval – usually normal
- Multifocal atrial tachycardia:
  - Rhythm – irregular
  - Rate – 75–200 bpm (ventricular), 120–250 bpm (atrial)
  - QRS duration – normal
  - P wave – P waves of atleast 3 different morphologies
  - PR interval – variable

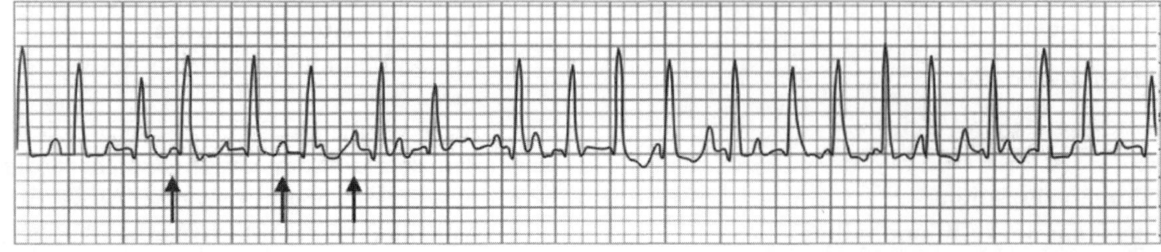

- Atrial fibrillation:
  - Rhythm – irregularly irregular
  - Rate – 100–160 bpm (ventricular), 400–600 bpm (atrial)
  - QRS duration – usually normal
  - P wave – indistinguishable, ***fibrillatory*** waves
  - PR interval – not measurable

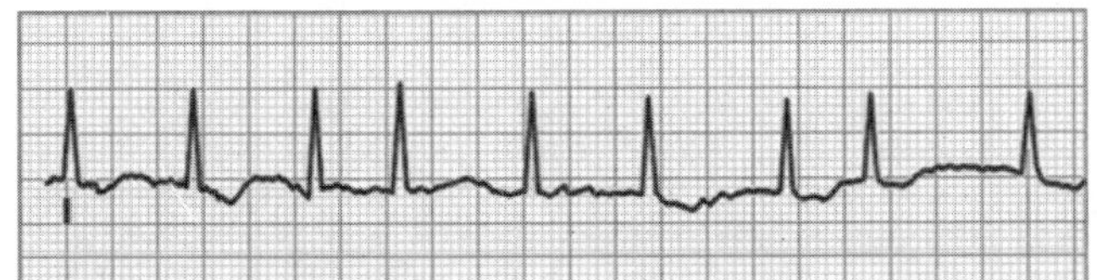

- Atrial flutter:
  - Rhythm – regular
  - Rate—around 110 bpm (ventricular), 250–350 bpm (atrial)
  - QRS duration – usually normal
  - P wave—replaced with multiple ***saw-tooth flutter waves***
  - P wave rate—300 bpm, flutter wave: QRS complexes = 2:1
  - PR interval—not measurable

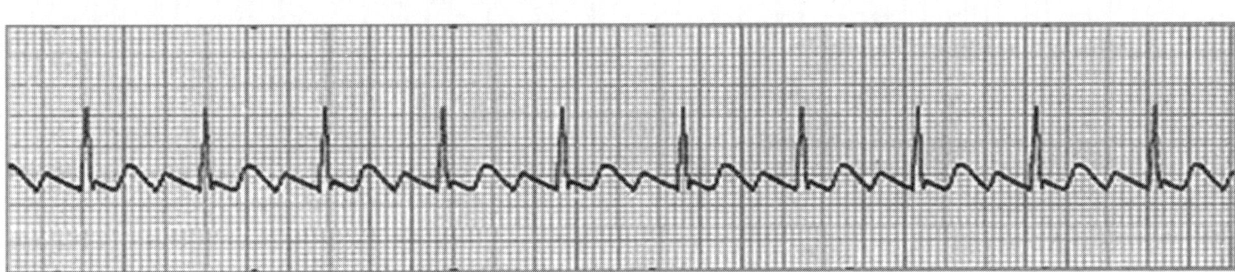

- AV nodal reentrant tachycardia:
  - Rhythm – regular
  - Rate – 180–250 bpm
  - QRS duration – normal, <120 msec
  - P wave – absent (buried within QRS complex) or occurs immediately after QRS complex
  - PR interval – unmeasurable

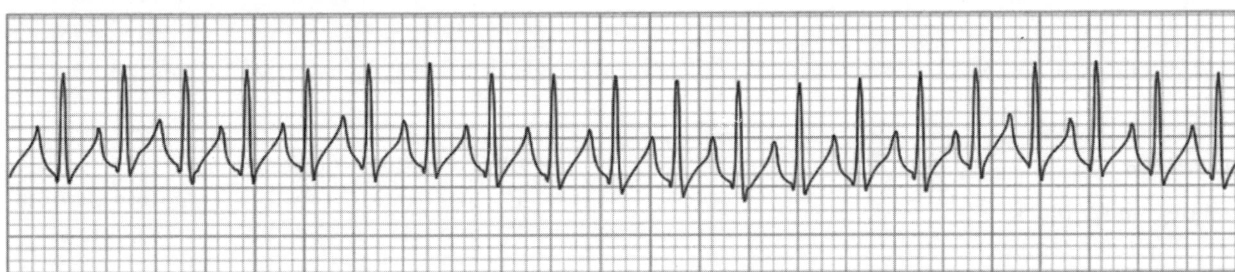

- AV reciprocating tachycardia:
  - Rhythm – regular
  - Rate – 150–250 bpm
  - QRS duration – normal in orthodromic, wider in antidromic with ***delta*** waves
  - P wave – follows each narrow QRS complex in orthodromic AVRT
  - PR interval – usually normal
  - Orthodromic AVRT: P wave follows each narrow regular QRS complex
  - Antidromic AVRT: wider QRS complexes with ***delta*** waves

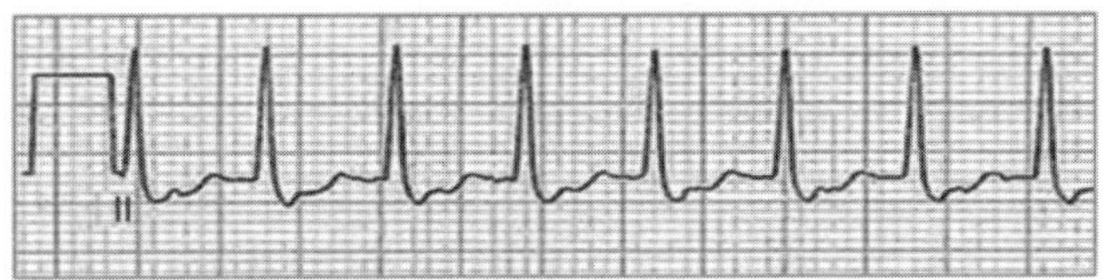

- AV junctional tachycardia:
  - Rhythm – regular
  - Rate – 70–130 bpm (ventricular), 60–100 bpm (atrial)
  - QRS duration – usually normal or widened with aberrant ventricular conduction

- P wave—inverted/abnormal morphology, irregular relationship with QRS complexes
- PR interval – <120 msec if present

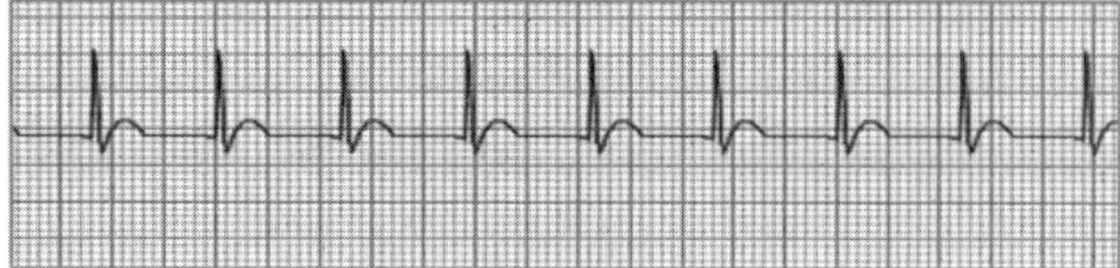

- Ventricular tachycardia
  - Rhythm – regular
  - Rate – 180–190 bpm
  - QRS duration – prolonged
  - P wave – not seen
  - PR interval – no measurable

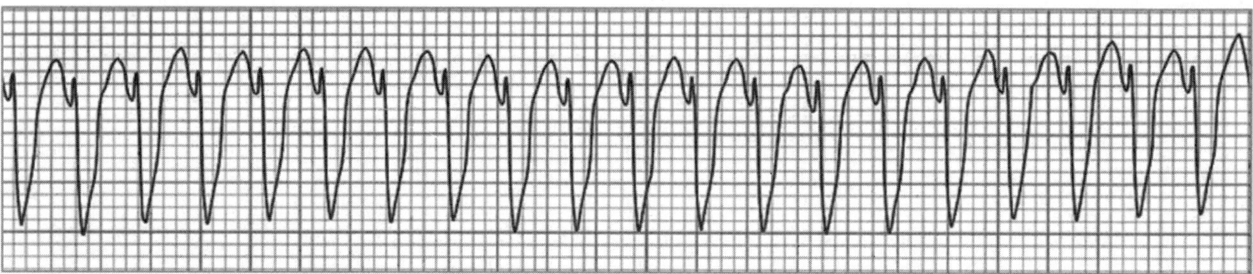

- Ventricular fibrillation:
  - Rhythm – irregular
  - Rate – >300, disorganized
  - QRS duration – not recognizable
  - P wave – not seen
  - PR interval – not measurable

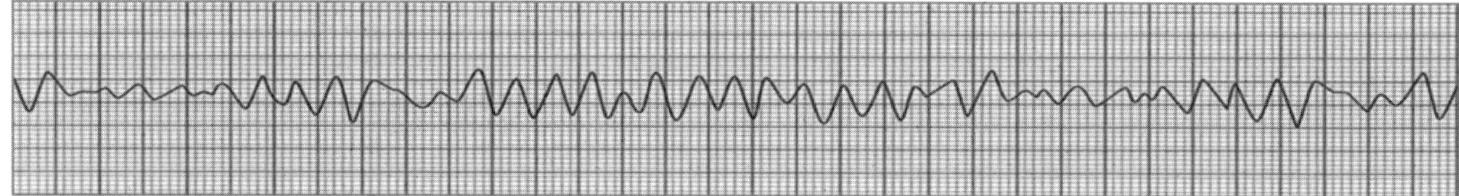

Bradycardia

- Ist degree AV block
  - Rhythm – regular
  - Rate – normal
  - QRS duration – normal
  - P wave – ratio 1:1
  - PR interval – prolonged > 20 msec

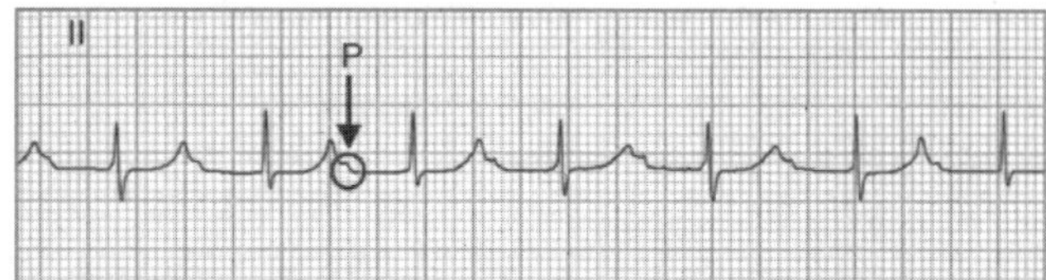

- IInd degree AV block Type I (Wenckebach)
  - Rhythm – regularly irregular
  - Rate – normal or slow
  - QRS duration – normal
  - P wave – ratio 1:1 for 2–4 cycles and then 1:0
  - P wave rate – normal but faster QRS rate
  - PR interval – progressive lengthening of PR interval until a QRS complex is dropped

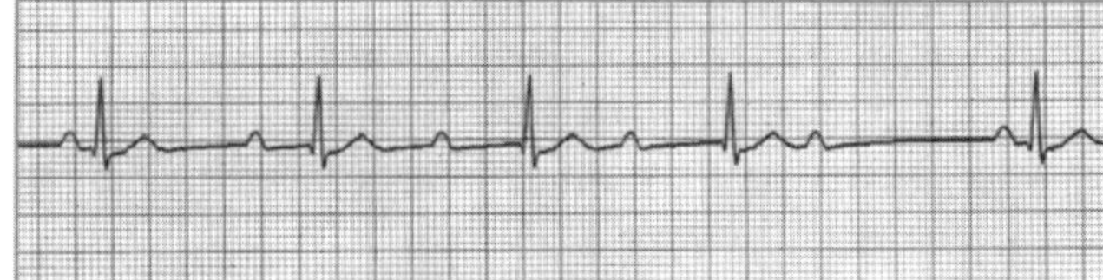

- IInd degree AV block Type II (Mobitz)
  - Rhythm – regular
  - Rate – normal or slow
  - QRS duration – prolonged
  - P wave – ratio 2:1, 3:1
  - PR interval – normal or prolonged but constant

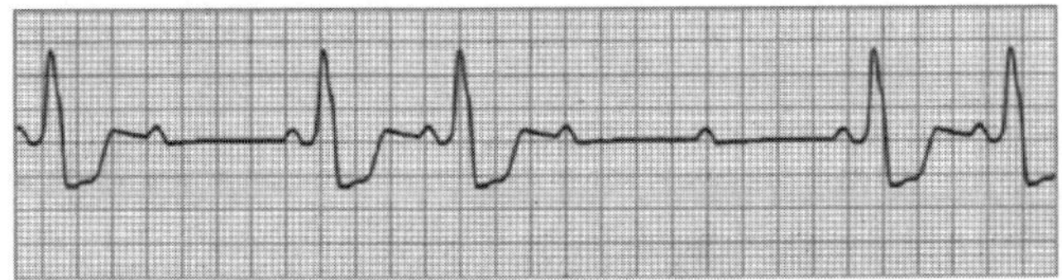

- IIIrd degree AV block
  - Rhythm – regular
  - Rate – slow
  - QRS duration – prolonged
  - P wave – unrelated
  - P wave rate – normal but faster than QRS rate
  - PR interval – variation

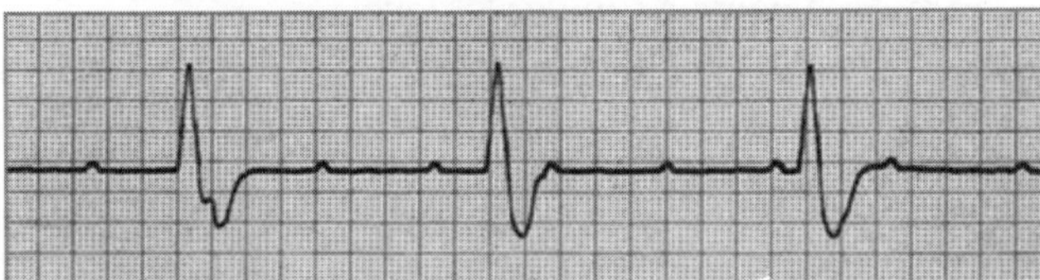

Management

General

- Ensure adequate oxygenation and ventilation
- Deepen plane of anesthesia
- Ensure optimum PaO_2, $PaCO_2$
- Correct acid base imbalance and dyselectrolytemias
- Reevaluate for cardiac pathology
- Prepare:
  - Anti-arrhythmic drugs
  - Anti-ischemic drugs
  - Pacing equipment
  - Defibrillator
- Vagal maneuvers:
  - Carotid massage
  - Ocular massage
  - Valsalva maneuver

Specific Arrhythmia Treatment

Supraventricular tachycardia:

- Adenosine – ***drug of choice*** – 0.1 mg/kg bolus followed by 0.2 mg/kg after 2 minutes if refractory
- Verapamil – ***second drug of choice*** – 0.1–0.2 mg/kg at 1 mg/min
- Diltiazem – 0.25 mg/kg at 2.5 mg/min followed by 0.35 mg/kg if refractory
- Metoprolol – 0.1 mg/kg given every 5 mins to a maximum of 0.3 mg/kg
- Rapid overdrive pacing
- Radiofrequency ablation:
  - For AVNRT, focal atrial tachycardia, atrial flutter, atrial fibrillation
  - Ablation around pulmonary veins, coronary sinus, right atrium, SVC
  - Reduces frequency of recurrent atrial fibrillation in 60% patients

Atrial fibrillation:

- Rate control:
  - Diltiazem: (***rule of 15*** in adults)
    - 0.25 mg/kg at 2.5 mg/min
    - Repeat the dose after 15 min if refractory
    - Infusion at 2.5 mg/kg/hr titrated to control ventricular rate
  - Verapamil:
    - 0.1 mg/kg at 1 mg/min
    - Repeated in 30 mins
    - Watch for prolonged hypotension
  - Beta blockers:
    - Esmolol 0.25–0.5 mg/kg followed by 0.05 mg/kg/min titrated to a maximum of 0.2 mg/kg/min
    - Propranolol 0.15 mg/kg given over 2 mins
  - Digoxin:
    - 5–10 µg/kg IV rapid digitalizing dose
    - Half the total calculated dose administered first
    - Remaining dose administered in fractions at 6–8 hour intervals
- Anticoagulation:
  - Unfractionated heparin 80 IU/kg followed by 18 IU/kg infusion
  - Maintain aPTT 1.5 to 2 times reference value
  - Gradually shift to warfarin therapy
  - Maintain INR of 2–3 to prevent thromboembolic sequelae
- Restore sinus rhythm:
  - DC cardioversion:
    - 200 J with monophasic defibrillator
    - 120–200 J with biphasic defibrillator
    - 0.5–1 J/kg increased to 2 J/kg if ineffective
  - Chemical cardioversion:
    - Procainamide
      - 10–15 mg/kg over 30–60 min until one of the four situations arise:
        - Arrhythmia suppression
        - Hypotension develops
        - QRS prolongation > 50% from baseline
        - Maximum of 17–20 mg/kg has been administered
      - Maintenance dose 1–4 mg/min

- Ibutilide:
  - < 60 kg 0.01 mg/kg over 10 min
  - >60 kg 1 mg over 10 min
- Dofetilide:
  - Dose adjusted according to creatinine clearance
  - 250–500 mics PO Q12H
- Propafenone:
  - 150–300 mg PO Q8H immediate release
  - 225–325 mg PO Q12H extended release
- Amiodarone:
  - 5 mg/kg bolus dose over 20 mins
  - 1 mg/min infusion for 6 hrs
  - 0.5 mg/min maintenance for 18 hrs

Ventricular tachycardia/ventricular fibrillation:

- Unsynchronized DC defibrillation
  - 200 J unsynchronized defibrillation with biphasic defibrillator
  - 360 J unsynchronized defibrillation with monophasic defrillator
  - In children:
    - First shock 2J/kg, second shock 4 J/kg
    - Subsequent shocks > 4 J/kg up to maximum of 10 J/kg
- Resistant VT/VF:
  - Lidocaine:
    - 50–100 mg IV over 5 mins
    - Followed by 2–4 mg/min infusion
  - Amiodarone
    - 5 mg/kg bolus dose over 20 mins
    - May repeat twice for refractory cases
  - Bretilium:
    - 5–10 mg/min over 2–5 min
    - Followed by 1–2 mg/min

MYOCARDIAL PROTECTION

Introduction

Myocardial protection refers to the set of pharmacological and physiological strategies aimed at attenuating the intensity of myocardial ischemia-reperfusion injury during cardiac surgery and its consequences on myocardial function.

History

- Early efforts with topical hypothermia:
  - Caused postoperative myocardial depression
  - Also lead to myocardial contracture ***"stone heart"***
- This later led to potassium cardioplegia introduced by ***Melrose*** in 1958:
  - 2 mL of 25% solution of tri-potassium citrate and 18 mL warm blood
  - 9: 1 blood: potassium ratio was used
  - Such high levels of potassium caused refractory ventricular fibrillation
  - This predisposed the heart to permanent myocardial damage
  - Therefore, this technique was abandoned
- Techniques like intermittent cross clamping with hypothermia were used till the 1970s
- In 1973, Gay and Ebert reintroduced hyperkalemic cardioplegia using lower K^+ levels
- K^+ levels used were less than 20 mmol/L
- This prevented the permanent myocardial damage seen earlier with hyperkalemic cardioplegia

Goals of Myocardial Protection

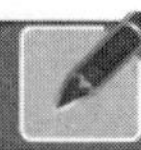

- To provide a quiet bloodless field
- To avoid iatrogenic injury as a result of:
  - Extracorporeal circulation
  - Cross clamping
  - Revascularization of ischemic segment of myocardium
  - Release of cross clamp
- Terminate clinical ischemia secondary to coronary occlusion or severe hypotension
- Limitation of myocardial damage by reduction of:
  - Intracellular acidosis
  - Edema
  - Depletion of high energy phosphate stores (ATP)
- Preservation of coronary endothelial function
- Prevent or reduce reperfusion injury

Determinants of Myocardial Oxygen Supply

- Oxygen content of blood
- Aortic root pressure
- Autonomic innervation
- Ventricular pressure
- Local vascular resistance, autoregulation, coronary steal
- Diastolic perfusion time (Heart rate)
- Exogenous drugs

Determinants of Oxygen Consumption: MvO_2

- Myocardial contractility (inotropy) = velocity of pressure development (d_p/d_t)
- Wall tension = $\frac{\text{Pressure} \times \text{Radius}}{2 \times \text{Wall thickness}}$
- Heart rate

- ❖ Basal oxygen consumption
- ❖ Work = Area within systolic pressure – volume loop

Mechanisms of Myocardial Ischemia-Reperfusion Injury

- ❖ Direct myocellular injury from ischemia
- ❖ Myocellular edema from ischemia-reperfusion injury
- ❖ Depletion of high energy phosphates (ATP)
- ❖ Intracellular acidosis due to anerobic metabolism
- ❖ Altered intracellular calcium homeostasis causing intracellular calcium overload
- ❖ Oxygen derived free radical generation during reperfusion
- ❖ Complement activation associated with inflammation occurring with ischemic injury

Phases of Myocardial Injury

- ❖ 15 minutes of coronary occlusion results in 6 hours of LV depression
- ❖ Myocardial injury sustained in the surgical setting is divided into 3 phases
  - Antecedent ischemia:
    - Also called ***Unprotected ischemia***
    - Occurs prior to institution of CPB or delivery of cardioplegia solution.
  - Protected ischemia: Occurs during electively initiated chemical cardioplegia
  - Reperfusion injury: Occurs:
    - During intermittent infusion of cardioplegia solution
    - After removal of cross clamping
    - After discontinuing CPB

Etiology of Ischemia and Reperfusion Injury

- ❖ Antecedent ischemia:
  - Prolonged hypotension
  - Arrhythmias
- ❖ Protected ischemia:
  - Reperfusion injury at initiation of CPB:
    - At initiation of CPB, oxygen demand of myocardium reduces by 50%
    - But extracorporeal oxygenation results in high oxygen content of blood
    - The myocardium is perfused with this highly oxygenated blood
    - Therefore, there is an abrupt withdrawal of antecedent ischemic conditions
    - This can lead to reperfusion injury at the onset of CPB itself
  - Maldistribution of cardioplegia:
    - Maldistribution of cardioplegia occurs distal to coronary occlusion
    - This can lead to ischemic injury to myocardium
  - Delay between intermittent infusions of cardioplegia solutions
  - During interruption of continuous cardioplegia strategies
  - Inadequate delivery of retrograde cardioplegia:
    - To areas of right heart directly emptying into Thebesian veins
    - Malposition of retrograde cardioplegia cannula
  - Excessive infusion pressure of cardioplegia solution causing microvascular injury
  - Low oncocity of cardioplegia solutions causing extravasation and edema
- ❖ Reperfusion injury:
  - Kinked grafts
  - Tight anastomoses
  - Air emboli
  - Ventricular fibrillation at low perfusion pressures
  - Once converted to post- CPB:
    - Hypotension
    - Persistent arrhythmias

Phases of Myocardial Protection

- ❖ Pretreatment therapy:
  - Includes measures taken against antecedent ischemia
  - Includes ischemic and pharmacological preconditioning
  - Exert protection at cellular and mitochondrial levels
  - Aims to:
    - Reduce myocardial oxygen demand
    - Optimize myocardial oxygen supply
    - Maintain adequate perfusion pressures
- ❖ Induction phase:
  - Includes protection strategies employed at the time of initiation of CPB
  - Aims to:
    - Arrest the heart
    - Induce hypothermia
    - Resuscitates the heart that is energy depleted or failing
- ❖ Maintenance phase:
  - Involves strategies to maintain myocardial protection on CPB

- Includes strategies like:
  - Intermittent cardioplegia administration
  - Maintenance of hypothermia
- Aims to:
  - Reoxygenate the heart
  - Restore nutrient supply to the heart
  - Wash out metabolic waste products
  - Restore ionic balance to the heart

❖ Reperfusion and reanimation phase:
- Involves strategies employed at the time of declamping and thereafter
- Aims to:
  - Repolarize the heart after hyperkalemic arrest
  - Establish ionic homeostasis
  - Increase aerobic metabolic capacity after suppression by hypothermia
  - Remove gradient between cold myocardium and warm systemic blood
  - Deliver drugs which work specifically at reperfusion

Methods of Myocardial Protection

I. Measures against Antecedent Ischemia

❖ Emergent revascularization

❖ Minimize ischemic injury during ongoing ischemia:
- Anticoagulation
- Antiplatelets
- Nitroglycerin
- IABP

❖ Continue all preoperative cardiovascular drugs:
- Antiarrhythmics
- β-blockers
- Calcium channel blockers
- Nitrates, aspirin
- Digoxin
- α_2 agonists like clonidine and mivazerol
- Statins

❖ Premedication: sedation for CABG patients

❖ Conversation to reduce level of anxiety

❖ Nutritional repletion with GIK infusion

❖ Intubation response suppression:
- Lignocaine: 1.5–2 mg/kg IV 90 seconds before intubation
- $MgSO_4$: 20–60 mg/kg IV
- Nitroglycerin drip: 0.5–10 µg/kg/min
- Labetolol/esmolol: 20 mg IV or 300 µg/kg IV respectively
- Deepen planes of anesthesia: Inhalational or fentanyl 1 µg/kg
- Brief duration of laryngoscopy: < 10 seconds

❖ Control of heart rate to <80 bpm in patients with coronary artery disease

❖ Adequate hydration to enable heart to tolerate hypotension prior to initiation of CPB

❖ Anesthetic preconditioning with volatile anesthetics

❖ Avoidance of cross clamping:
- Preference of OPCAB
- Normothermic CPB without application of cross clamp
- Normothermic or hypothermic fibrillatory arrest

II. Measures against Protected Ischemia

These measures are taken during the period of CPB:

❖ Asystole with cardioplegia:
- Warm or cold cardioplegia
- Antegrade or retrograde cardioplegia
- Crystalloid or blood cardioplegia

❖ Hypothermia

❖ Hypocalcemia

❖ Buffering

❖ Intermittent cross clamping with brief periods of reperfusion

❖ Hypothermic ventricular fibrillation

❖ Left ventricular venting

III. Measures against Reperfusion Injury

❖ Prompt deairing

❖ Controlled reperfusion

❖ Prompt DC version of arrhythmias

❖ Postconditioning

❖ Substrate washout- hot-shot warm blood cardioplegia

❖ Oxygen free radical scavenging

❖ IV sedation with propofol

❖ Anti-ischemic agents:
- ATP sensitive potassium channel openers:
  - Cromokalim
  - Pinacidil
  - Nicorandil
- Agents which increase intravascular adenosine:
  - 5-amino-4-imidazole carboxyamide riboside deaminase inhibitors
  - Transport inhibitors

- Monoclonal antibodies directed against neutrophil/endothelial components of adhesive glycoprotein complexes

Asystole and Cardioplegia

Rationale of Use

- Continued electromechanical activity after cross clamping increases the rate of high energy phosphate depletion
- This causes a more rapid fall in ATP reserves before anoxic arrest ensues
- Intentional chemical induction of diastolic arrest avoids depletion of ATPs
- This conserves myocardial energy reserves
- Reserves can be used during ischemia to maintain ionic and metabolic homeostasis
- Total electro-mechanical silence reduces oxygen demand by about 80–90% of which:
  - 30–40% of this reduction is contributed by ventricular decompression
  - The remainder is contributed by asystole accomplished by chemical cardioplegia

Methods of Inducing Rapid Asystole

- Hyperkalemia
- Hypermagnesemia
- Hypocalcemia
- Calcium channel blockers
- Infusion of local anesthetic agents

Hyperkalemic Asystole

- Potassium rich solutions used as cardioplegia to ensure diastolic arrest
- Usual concentration of potassium in cardioplegia solutions is 8–10 mEq/L
- Blood may be added to cardioplegia solution in a 4:1 ratio of cardioplegia: blood
- Final hematocrit of cardioplegia solution is 16–20%
- Antegrade cardioplegia:
  - Delivered to the myocardium via coronary arteries
  - Initial dose of cardioplegia is usually 15–20 mL/kg, up to 1000 mL
  - Cardioplegia delivery:
    - Flow is started at a rate of 150 mL/min/m^2
    - Adjusted to obtain appropriate aortic root pressure
    - Delivered at a perfusion pressure not exceeding 70–100 mm Hg
- Retrograde cardioplegia:
  - Delivered usually as an adjunct to antegrade cardioplegia
  - Initial dose and target of delivery is the same as antegrade cardioplegia
  - However, perfusion pressures are maintained at less than 40 mm Hg

Hypothermia

Benefits

- Hypothermia reduces myocardial oxygen demand
- At 22°C, myocardial O_2 demand reduces from 80 to 0.3 mL/100 g /min
- Hypothermia below 22°C does not significantly reduce myocardial oxygen demand
- Thus, temperatures below 22°C fail to improve myocardial protection unless imposed for 4–6 hours
- Most often moderate hypothermia (24–28°C) is used to obtain beneficial effects of hypothermia while avoiding deleterious effects of profound hypothermia

Rationale

- Major methods of myocardial protection by hypothermia is:
  - Reduction in myocardial metabolic rate
  - Reduction in oxygen demand of myocardium
- ***Vant Hoffs law/Q_{10} effect***:
  - MVO_2 reduces by 50% for every 10°C reduction in temperature.
  - Greatest reduction in MVO_2 occurs between 37°C and 25°C
  - At 28°C, a reduction in metabolic rate by 50% occurs
  - Q_{10} is the ratio of metabolic rates at two different temperatures
  - Normally, Q_{10} = 2 to 2.2
- Greatest protection at 24–28°C with little additional protection at temperature < 24°C.
- Hypothermia is achieved on CPB by two methods:
  - Passive cooling: patients core temperature is allowed to equalize with ambient temperature
  - Active cooling:
    - Using heat exchanger
    - Using topical ice slush
    - Ice jacket
    - Cold cardioplegia at 4–10°C, maintain myocardial temperature at 15–20°C

Advantages of Hypothermia

S. No.	Advantages
1.	Reduces myocardial metabolism
2.	Reduces oxygen requirement
3.	Reduced rate of degradative reactions
4.	Reduced progression of ischemic injury
5.	Reduced tolerable period of ischemia
6.	Reduced potassium needed to accomplish arrest
7.	Prolongs cardiac arrest
8.	Inhibits intracellular Ca^{2+} gain
9.	Reduces excitatory neurotransmitters

Disadvantages of Hypothermia

S. No.	Disadvantages
1.	Reduces rate of reparative process
2.	Increased myocellular swelling
3.	Increases inotropic state and MVO_2 per beat
4.	Induces fibrillation
5.	Impairs oxygen dissociation
6.	Impairs autoregulation
7.	Poses threat of phrenic nerve ***freeze injury*** on local application of ice
8.	Increases rouleaux formation in RBCs

Hypocalcemia

- Calcium plays a central role in excitation – contraction coupling
- Calcium is needed to transduce electrical signals into a mechanical event
- However, during ischemia, intra- and extracellular calcium homeostasis becomes altered
- Ca^{2+} accumulation occurs during ischemia and myocardium becomes Ca^{2+} overloaded
- Intracellular calcium overload also occurs as sarcoplasmic reticulum releases Ca^{2+}
- Calcium concentration may be so high as to cause contractures
- Therefore, reduction of extracellular calcium is important for myocardial protection
- Reduction of extracellular calcium can be done by using:
  - Direct chelation with citrate phosphate dextrose (CPD) in cardioplegia solution
  - Reducing the amount of calcium added in crystalloid cardioplegia solutions
  - Adding magnesium to cardioplegia, which acts as a calcium channel blocker
  - K_{ATP} channel openers such as:
    - Cromokalim
    - Aprikalim
    - Diazoxide
- ***Calcium paradox:***
  - Refers to sudden influx of Ca^{2+} which occurs on perfusing a tissue with perfusates containing Ca^{2+} after a period of profound hypocalcemia
  - This occurs when calcium is completely absent from cardioplegia solutions
  - Therefore, intracellular calcium is completely depleted
  - During reperfusion, massive amount of calcium reenters the cell
  - This causes severe myocardial damage and calcium paradox
  - Therefore, calcium should be present in small amounts in cardioplegia solutions

Intermittent Cross Clamping

- In this technique, aortic cross clamp is applied and the heart is fibrillated using a fibrillator
- Distal coronary anastomosis is performed on a cross clamped, fibrillating heart
- The clamp is removed for reperfusion and reapplied for the next distal anastomosis
- To be successful, each duration of fibrillation should be short
- Energy consumption:
  - Fibrillating heart is lesser than a beating cross clamped heart
  - However, asystolic heart has the least energy consumption
- Avoided in cases of:
  - Left ventricular hypertrophy
  - Aortic regurgitation

LV Venting

- Ventricular distension is detrimental to ventricular function during CPB and reperfusion
- Therefore, LV venting plays an important role in myocardial protection
- Causes of dysfunction due to LV distension:
  - Increased wall stress, which increases myocardial oxygen demand
  - Direct myocardial damage due to excessive stretch
  - Reduced subendocardial perfusion
  - Increased LA pressure causing pulmonary edema
  - Interference with surgical exposure—prolongs CPB time

- Causes of LV distension:
  - On cardiopulmonary bypass:
    - Aortic cross clamping
    - Antegrade cardioplegia administration
    - Aortic regurgitation
    - Patent ductus arteriosus
    - Major Aorto-Pulmonary Collateral Arteries (MAPCAS)
  - At the time of reperfusion:
    - Ventricular fibrillation
    - Cardiac arrest
    - Cross clamp release
- Sources of blood to the LV after application of aortic cross clamp:
  - Non-coronary collateral flow (bronchial veins 100 mL/min)
  - Aortic regurgitation
  - Major Aorto-Pulmonary Collateral Arteries
  - Large PDA
  - ASD
  - VSD
- Importance:
  - Distension of LV causes mechanical damage to muscle from excessive stretching
  - Venting improves preservation by reducing myocardial oxygen demand
  - Venting also reduces wall tension due to a reduction in radius of ventricle
  - It facilitates subendocardial perfusion by reducing wall tension
  - It prevents pulmonary venous hypertension with pulmonary edema
- Sites of LV vent application:
  - Indirect LV vent via right superior pulmonary vein (RSPV):
    - Advantages:
      - Tackles all sources of blood to LV
      - Optimal decompression
      - Best method in the presence of aortic regurgitation
      - Avoids direct LV incision
    - Disadvantages:
      - Useless in the presence of mitral regurgitation
      - Dislodges clots present in LA
      - Can cause damage to RSPV
      - Difficult to insert
      - Can cause air entry into LV
      - Contraindicated in the presence of mitral prosthesis
  - Direct LV vent via LV apex:
    - Advantages:
      - Tackles all sources of blood to LV
      - Optimal decompression
      - Tackles aortic regurgitation
      - Easy to insert
    - Disadvantages:
      - Can cause LV aneurysm
      - Vent can get occluded by myocardial tissue
      - Dislodges LV thrombus and risks systemic embolism
      - Can result in coronary disruption
      - LV dysfunction
      - Can cause bundle branch block
      - Causes air entry into LV
      - Postoperative bleeding
  - Indirect LV venting via LA appendage:
    - Advantage: easy to insert
    - Disadvantages:
      - Does not tackle aortic regurgitation
      - Dislodges clot in LA appendage
      - Can cause air entry into LV
  - Ascending aorta:
    - Advantages:
      - Easy of insertion
      - Can be used to vent even after LV starts ejecting
    - Disadvantages:
      - Not useful in the presence of aortic regurgitation
      - Can cause air in the aortic root and systemic embolization
      - Not useful at the time of administration of cardioplegia
  - Pulmonary artery:
    - Advantages:
      - Easy to insert
      - Reduces air entry into the left heart
    - Disadvantages:
      - Not useful in the presence of aortic regurgitation
      - Does not handle all the sources of blood into LV
      - Can cause distortion of PA anatomy and PA damage
- Uses of LV venting:
  - Prevents myocardial distension
  - Reduces myocardial rewarming
  - Prevents ejection of air: used to aspirate air from heart during de-airing procedure
  - Facilitates surgical exposure eg. when working on aortic valve

- Complications of LV venting:
  - Damage to the corresponding structure
  - Air entry into left heart and embolization
  - Dislodgement of thrombi
  - Mitral valve incompetence

Substrate Washout

- Warm hyperkalemic cardioplegia administered at the end of the surgical repair
- This called hot-shot or terminal warm blood cardioplegia
- This allows maintenance of asystole with replenishment of metabolic substrates

Controlled Reperfusion

- Pressure generated during reperfusion is important to limit myocardial damage
- After cross clamp removal, perfusion pressure is limited to 10 mm Hg during first 1–2 min
- This is done by reducing pump flows appropriately
- Pump flows are then increased to maintain a mean pressure of 70 mm Hg
- Restriction of MAP during first 1–2 min of reperfusion is called controlled reperfusion

Oxygen Radical Scavenging

- Hydrogen peroxide is an important transitional molecule in the oxygen radical cascade
- It is involved in ischemic reperfusion injury
- Infusion of cardioplegia is also a form of reperfusion during which injury can occur
- Scavengers which inhibit free radicals can be administered as a pretreatment therapy
- Free radical scavengers which can be used:
  - Glutathione
  - Mannitol
  - Allopurinol

Anesthetic Preconditioning

- Involves myocardial exposure to volatile agents to reduce ischemia-reperfusion injury
- Characteristics of anesthetic preconditioning:
  - Effect depends on:
    - Duration of administration
    - Concentration of the drug
  - Maximal effect is attained with 1.5–2 MAC of volatile anesthetic
  - Does not depend on ischemic preconditioning
  - Does not require preemptive ischemic episodes
  - Has only slightly protective effect on the heart
- Mechanisms involved in anesthetic preconditioning:
  - Extracellular signaling pathways acting via G-protein coupled receptors
  - Mitogen activated protein kinase
  - Adenosine receptor activation
- Volatile anesthetics reduce MvO_2 due to:
  - Direct negative inotropic, lusitropic and chronotropic effects
  - Reduction in LV afterload (reduces SVR)
  - Reduce oxygen free radicals
  - Cause coronary vasodilatation
- Examples of volatile anesthetic preconditioning:
  - Halothane:
    - Attenuates ST segment changes caused by brief coronary artery occlusion
    - Reduces ST elevation more than sodium nitroprusside and propranolol
  - Isoflurane and sevoflurane:
    - Reduce myocardial reperfusion injury
    - Improve functional recovery after global ischemia
- Procedure:
  - To be initiated at > 1 MAC for 15–30 minutes prior to aortic cross clamping
  - Initiated again several minutes before release of aortic cross clamp
  - This is done via oxygen-air supply line of extracorporeal circuit
  - Volatile agents are continued for at least 2–5 minutes after reperfusion
- Stages of preconditioning:
  - Preconditioning occurs in 2 stages
  - Shows that protective effects outlast drug elimination time
    - Early preconditioning: lasting for 1–2 hours after exposure
    - Late preconditioning: reappears after 24 hours and lasts up to 72 hours
- Other agents used in anesthetic preconditioning:
  - Xenon
  - Adenosine
  - Nicorandil
  - Norepinephrine
  - Morphine via δ receptors

Propofol

- Propofol exhibits myocardial protection like isoflurane in patients undergoing CABG
- However, the degree of protection offered is lesser than preconditioning with isoflurane

- Propofol is similar in structure to phenol based free radical scavengers like vitamin E
- Thus, propofol acts as a strong free radical scavenger and antioxidant
- Infusion of propofol results in significant reduction in myocardial oxygen consumption.
- High dose propofol (100 μg/kg/min) administered for CABG or OPCAB showed:
  - Improved troponin levels
  - Reduced inotropic requirements
  - Better hemodynamic function

Recent Advances

- Esmolol:
  - Recent interest in use of high dose esmolol to induce profound bradycardia
  - Esmolol used to induce hypocontractile state during continuous perfusion on CPB
  - Hyperkalemic arrest of the heart is not employed to provide myocardial protection
  - Strategy used as an alternative to prevent hyperkalemic cardioplegic arrest
  - Studies shoed that esmolol treated patients had:
    - Lesser myocardial edema
    - Lesser morphological changes in the left ventricle
    - Lesser lactate release
    - Comparable cardiac function
    - Decreased inotropic support
- Mitochondrial transition pore inhibition:
  - Inhibition of opening of mPTP protects against reperfusion injury
  - Agents used include:
    - Cyclosporine A
    - Sanglifehrin A
    - NIM 811
- Statin therapy:
  - Statins have myocardial protective properties unrelated to LDL cholesterol lowering effect
  - Vascular endothelium is protected by statin therapy and associated NO release
  - Treatment with statins before ischemia or at reperfusion reduces infarct size
  - Better outcomes are reported in CABG patients on preoperative statin therapy

CARDIOPLEGIA

Introduction

- Cardioplegia is the solution used to produce intentional, temporary cessation of the heart for cardiac surgery, in which cardiac standstill is usually achieved using high potassium concentrations
- Cardioplegia solutions usually contain 20–30 mEq/L of potassium
- Solutions containing > 40–50 mEq/L of K^+ are avoided as they cause endothelial damage

Mechanism of Action of Cardioplegia

- Potassium present in the cardioplegia solution arrests the heart in diastole
- This reduces myocardial oxygen demand by > 80% and allows longer ischemic times
- When a cardioplegia solution containing 10 mEq/L of potassium is administered, transmembrane potential (TMP) is reduced from –85 mV to –65 mV
- This renders the myocardium unexcitable and in a state of depolarized arrest
- At this TMP, voltage-dependant fast Na^+ channels are blocked
- Thus, there is no phase 0 of the action potential
- Wash out of hyperkalemic cardioplegia solution by non-coronary collateral flow causes resumption of electrical and mechanical activity
- This is countered by intermittent (every 20–30 min) replenishment of cardioplegia solution

Mechanisms of Myocardial Protection

- Produces immediate asystole
- Reduces oxygen demand to less than 10% of that of the working heart
- Initiates hypothermia and maintains low myocardial temperature
- Provides intermittent oxygenation when used as multidose regimens
- Improves anerobic metabolism
- Prevents reperfusion injury and calcium paradox
- Causes less activation of lymphocytes
- Upregulates protective heat shock proteins

Goals

- To provide a quiet and bloodless field
- Limitation of myocardial damage by reduction of:
  - Intracellular acidosis
  - Edema
  - Depletion of ATP stores
- Preservation of coronary endothelial function and myocardial flow
- Reduce reperfusion injury

Types

I. Based on Temperature

- Warm cardioplegia
  - Delivered at 37°C
  - Mechanical activity of the heart is suspended
  - However, since myocardium continues to be warm, basal metabolism continues
  - Thus, oxygen consumption is constantly higher than when myocardium is cool
  - Therefore, prolonged ischemia is not advisable when using warm cardioplegia
  - Thus, warm cardioplegia is usually administered continuously
  - Also, metabolic requirement of the warm myocardium is higher
  - Crystalloid based cardioplegia is usually unable to meet this energy requirement
  - Thus, blood is an essential component of warm cardioplegia
  - Single hot shot warm cardioplegia used for initiation and termination of arrest
- Tepid cardioplegia:
  - Delivered at 29° C
  - Provides benefits of warm cardioplegia and minimizes myocardial hypothermia
- Cold cardioplegia:
  - Delivered at 4–10° C
  - This cools the myocardium to 15–16° C
  - Mechanical activity of the heart is suspended
  - Also, administration at low temperature minimizes basal oxygen consumption
  - Thus, cardioplegia can be administered intermittently

II. Based on Contents

- Crystalloid cardioplegia:
  - Using uncommonly nowadays
  - Does not contain hemoglobin and thus has low oxygen carrying capacity
  - Thus, crystalloid cardioplegia depends on dissolved oxygen for oxygen delivery
  - Therefore, crystalloid cardioplegia is effective only in the presence of myocardial hypothermia
- Blood cardioplegia:
  - Produced by mixing crystalloid cardioplegia with blood in a defined ratio
  - Usually done using 4:1 concentration of cardioplegia: blood
  - Final hematocrit of blood cardioplegia is usually 16–20%
  - Advantages of blood cardioplegia:
    - Improves systolic function recovery
    - Decreases ischemic injury
    - Decreases myocardial anerobic metabolism
  - Blood useful as:
    - Acts as source of oxygen to heart as blood has higher O_2 carrying capacity
    - Blood is a rich source of buffering agents
    - Also provides free radical scavengers and colloids
    - Preferred in anemic and pediatric patients
- Microplegia:
  - Uses blood minimally diluted with crystalloid cardioplegia
  - Contains bare minimal elements which are necessary for producing asystole
  - Usually delivered continuously and at tepid temperatures
  - Therefore, aerobic metabolism is maintained throughout the duration of arrest
  - Avoids myocardial edema associated with the low hematocrit of cardioplegia
  - Thus, myocardial recovery and ventricular function may be better
  - Clinical studies with microplegia are limited

Methods of Delivery

- Anterograde cardioplegia:
  - Delivered into coronary arteries via the aortic root
  - Delivered with a cannula placed between aortic cross clamp and aortic valve
  - Can be delivered via the grafts in CABG once distal anastomoses has been made
  - Administration into grafts allows the surgeon to check the patency of each graft
  - Most physiological method of cardioplegia delivery
  - Targets of delivery:
    - Typical initial dose is 10–15 mL/kg, up to 1000 mL
    - Flow is started at a rate of 150 mL/min/m^2
    - It is adjusted to maintain optimal aortic root perfusion pressure
    - Perfusion pressure should not exceed 70–100 mm Hg
  - Cannot be used in the presence of aortic regurgitation as:
    - Difficult to obtain aortic root pressure in the presence of AR
    - Regurgitant blood causes LV distension and increases wall tension
    - Significant portion of CP fails to perfuse coronaries due to AR

- Suboptimal protection can occur in the presence of coronary disease as:
  - Uneven distribution of cardioplegia occurs due to occluded coronaries
  - Combined administration via retrograde route beneficial in these cases

❖ Retrograde cardioplegia:
- Delivered into coronary veins via coronary sinus
- Usually administered through a balloon tipped cannula placed in coronary sinus
- Targets of delivery are similar to antegrade cardioplegia
- However, perfusion pressure is kept below 40 mm Hg at the time of administration
- Better distribution of cardioplegia in:
  - Significant coronary artery disease
  - Aortic regurgitation
  - Aortic valve surgeries
- Provides suboptimal protection to:
  - Right ventricular myocardium
  - Posterior one-third of interventricular septum

❖ Combined cardioplegia:
- Uses antegrade and retrograde routes of administration simultaneously
- Thought to be superior to either of the above

Timing of Delivery

❖ Intermittent cardioplegia:
- Initially 1–1.5 L of *high potassium* cardioplegia (CP) delivered
- Then 200–500 mL of *low potassium* CP infused at periodic intervals of 20–40 minutes
- High potassium CP solution contains 20–30 mEq/L of potassium
- Low potassium CP solution contains 10–20 mEq/L of potassium

❖ Continuous cardioplegia:
- Delivered at low flows
- Continuous warm cardioplegia advocated for long surgeries
- Concern about protection of right ventricle and posterior septum in this method

Common Additives to Cardioplegia

❖ *Potassium*: produces and maintains diastolic arrest

❖ *Magnesium*: mitigates effects of calcium ions

❖ *Citrate Phosphate Dextrose (CPD)*: lowers free calcium concentration

❖ Buffers:
- Bicarbonate prevents increased build up of acid metabolites
- *Alternate buffers*: histidine, THAM (tromethamine)

❖ Mannitol:
- High osmolarity of mannitol controls myocardial edema
- Acts as free radical scavenger

❖ Membrane stabilizing agents:
- Procaine
- Lidocaine
- Glucocorticoids

❖ Energy substrates:
- Glucose
- Glutamate
- Aspartate
- Blood/crystalloid

Composition of Common Cardioplegia Solutions

❖ ***St. Thomas cardioplegia***:
- Clinically validated in 1989
- Sold commercially as Plegisol
- Provides short periods of aystole (20 minutes)
- Components:
  - Na^+ – 110 mmol/L
  - K^+ – 16 mmol/L
  - Mg^{2+} – 16 mmol/L
  - Ca^{2+} – 1.2 mmol/L
  - HCO_3^- – 10 mmol/L

❖ ***Del Nido cardioplegia***:
- Developed by Dr Pedro del Nido and patented for use in 1995
- Initially developed for use in immature hearts (pediatrics)
- Use has been extended for other surgeries
- Base of the solution is Plamalyte A with a composition similar to plasma
- Provides longer periods of myocardial quiescence (40 minutes)
- Salient features of this fluid are:
  - Low calcium content (provided by blood)
  - Hyperkalemia (24 mEq/L)
  - Mannitol for scavenging and osmotic properties
  - Sodium bicarbonate as buffering agent
  - Lidocaine to stabilize cell membrane and reduce arrhythmias

- Components:
  - Mannitol 16.3 mL of 20% solution, 3.26 g
  - Magnesium sulfate 4 mL of 50% w/v solution, 2 g
  - Sodium bicarbonate 13 mL of 8.4% solution, 13 mEq
  - Lidocaine 13 mL of 1% solution, 130 mg
  - Potassium chloride 13 mL of 2 mEq/mL solution, 26 mEq

❖ *Custodial*:
- Also called Bretschneider or HTK (histidine-tryptophan-ketoglutarate) solution
- Solution was developed in Germany
- Currently mainly used for perfusing and flushing organs from organ donors
- Also used for preservation of organs for transplant
- Components:
  - Sodium chloride 15 mmol/L
  - Potassium chloride 9 mmol/L
  - Magnesium chloride 4 mmol/L
  - Histidine hydrochloride 18 mmol/L
  - Histidine 180 mmol/L
  - Tryptophan 2 mmol/L
  - Mannitol 30 mmol/L
  - Calcium chloride 0.015 mmol/L
  - Potassium hydrogen ketoglutarate 1 mmol/L

Strategies to Reduce Ischemic Injury with Cardioplegia

No.	Principle	Mechanism	Component
1.	Reduce O_2 demand	Hypothermia	Blood/crystalloid
			Ice slush/lavage/ice jacket
		Asystole	Potassium chloride
			Hyperpolarizing agents
2.	Substrate supply and use	Oxygen	Blood, PFC
		Glucose	Blood, glucose, citrate-phosphate-dextrose
		Amino acids	Glutamate, aspartate
		Buffers	Blood, bicarbonate, phosphate, THAM, histidine
3.	Control calcium influx	Hypocalcemia	Citrate, magnesium
			Calcium channel blockers
			Potassium channel openers
4.	Reduce edema	Hyperosmolar solutions	Glucose
			Potassium chloride
			Mannitol
		Moderate infusion pressure	Less than 50 mm Hg

Adverse Effects of Cardioplegia

❖ Excessive cardioplegia:
- Absence of electrical activity
- AV conduction block

❖ Poorly contractile heart at termination of bypass

❖ Persistent systemic hyperkalemia

Cardioplegia Circuits

Two types of circuits:

❖ Recirculating circuit:
- For asanguinous cardioplegia (crystalloid) delivery
- Crystalloid CP solution is kept running constantly in the circuit
- It is delivered to a patient on removing a clamp thus directing flow away from recirculation circuit and to patient

❖ Non-recirculating circuit:
- For sanguinous cardioplegia (blood containing) delivery
- Involves shunting of arterialized blood from oxygenator into the CP circuit
- Here it is mixed with a crystalloid base solution and delivered
- Makes only a single pass through heat exchanger

Recent Advances

❖ Adenosine enhanced cardioplegia:
- Studied in several clinical trials
- Used in concentration of 15–50 μmol/L
- Advantages of adenosine enriched cardioplegia:
  - Lesser inotropic requirements
  - Better ventricular function
- Further studies are warranted to justify routine use

❖ Arginine enhanced cardioplegia:
- L-arginine acts as a precursor for endogenous NO production
- This reduces neutrophil adherence to endothelium and endothelial damage
- Used in concentration of 15 g L-arginine per liter of cardioplegia
- Postoperative markers of myocardial injury like troponin T and I were reduced

❖ ***Adenocaine cardioplegia***:
- Refers to a combination of adenosine and lignocaine in cardioplegia
- This is used as an alternative to hyperkalemic cardioplegia

- Both adenosine and lignocaine have desirable properties like:
  - Cardioprotection
  - Vasodilatation
  - Anti-arrythmic properties
  - Anti-inflammatory properties
- Advantages of adenocaine cardioplegia:
  - Can be delivered at normal potassium concentrations
  - Can be used as warm or cold cardioplegia
  - Can be delivered intermittently or continuously
- Provides comparable ventricular functional recovery to hyperkalemic cardioplegia
- Requires further validation in large scale trials

REPERFUSION INJURY

Introduction

Injury characterized by myocardial, vascular or electrophysiological dysfunction that is induced by the restoration of blood flow to a previously ischemic tissue.

Pathophysiology: Factors causing reperfusion injury include:

- ❖ Microvascular occlusion:
  - Reperfusion occurs due to restoration of blood flow in epicardial arteries
  - However, distal flow may remain impaired due to microvascular occlusion
  - This may be due to:
    - Embolization of clot or plaque material
    - Formation of new thrombus
    - Direct cellular toxicity
    - Vasocontriction
- ❖ Myocyte hypercontracture:
  - Reperfusion can result in myocardial hypercontracture and band necrosis
  - Hypercontracture state occurs due to:
    - Increased intracellular calcium:
      - During ischemia, intracellular Ca^{2+} increases due to sarcolemmal damage
      - This process is exacerbated by reperfusion and restoration of normal extracellular pH
      - Restoration of pH reverses function of Na^{+}/Ca^{2+} channel
      - This produces further influx of calcium into the cell
    - Re-energization of myocyte:
      - Sudden return of circulation provides oxygen and energy substrate
      - This stimulates myofibrils in an environment of excess calcium
      - This produces uncontrolled and excessive contraction
- ❖ Reactive oxygen species:
  - Reperfusion results in the production of free radicals
  - Free radical generation continues for many hours after reperfusion
  - Free radicals generated include:
    - Superoxide anion
    - Hydrogen peroxide
    - Hypochlorous acid
    - Nitric oxide derived peroxynitrite
    - Hydroxyl radical
- ❖ Leukocyte aggregation:
  - Reperfusion of previously ischemic tissues triggers leukocyte aggregation
  - Multiple factors trigger leukocyte aggregation like:
    - Release of cytokines and complement from injured myocardium
    - Diminished release of nitric oxide
    - Expression of new adhesion molecules
- ❖ Platelet activation:
  - Circulating platelets become activated during reperfusion
  - Degree of activation is proportional to the duration of preceding ischemia
- ❖ Complement activation:
  - Complement activation is commonly seen in reperfusion injury
  - This injures the endothelium and makes it incabable of generating NO
  - This sets in motion a cycle of vasoconstriction and myocardial mecrosis
- ❖ Apoptosis:
  - Programmed cell death may play an important role in reperfusion injury
  - Apoptotic cells appear in the ischemic penumbra regions during reperfusion

Types of Reperfusion Injury

- ❖ Reversible injury:
  - Arrhythmias
  - Myocardial stunning
- ❖ Irreversible injury:
  - Myocyte necrosis
  - Apoptosis

Clinical Features of Reperfusion Injury

- Arrhythmias:
  - Clinical precipitants of reperfusion arrhythmias:
    - Thrombolytic therapy
    - Primary percutaneous coronary intervention
    - Post-cardiac surgery
  - *Most common* arrhythmia after reperfusion is accelerated idioventricular rhythm
  - Reperfusion arrhythmias may be caused by:
    - Mitochondrial dysfunction
    - Accumulation of intracellular calcium (Ca^{2+} dependent arrhythmias)
    - Oxygen derived free radicals
  - More commonly seen with reperfusion after short periods of ischemia
  - Prolonged ischemia results in irreversible injury and electrical silence
  - Other arrhythmias commonly associated with reperfusion:
    - Premature ventricular contractions
    - Ventricular tachycardia
    - Ventricular fibrillation
    - Complete heart block
- Myocardial stunning:
  - Refers to transient myocardial systolic dysfunction occurring after reperfusion
  - Results from intracellular calcium overload seen with reperfusion
  - Reperfusion causes loss of myocardial compliance and diastolic dysfunction
  - This together with systolic dysfunction reduces stroke volume and cardiac output
  - Stunning recovers over a period of time, with no obvious morphological injury
  - Short-term inotropic therapy augments vital organ perfusion during this period
- Myocardial necrosis:
  - Necrosis is myocellular injury occurring with edema and sarcolemmal dysfunction
  - This results in local hypercontracture and contraction bands
  - Subesequently, intracellular contents are released into the extracellular space
  - These include larger molecules like:
    - Creatinine kinase (CK-MB)
    - Troponin T and I
  - Manifests clinically as myocardial infarction
  - Reperfusion recruits regions of myocardium in the ischemic penumbra
  - This increases infarct size, especially with reperfusion after prolonged ischemia
  - Global necrosis causing contracture state results in ***stone heart***
- Apoptosis:
  - Cells targeted for apoptosis undergo DNA fragmentation in specific areas
  - This causes condensation of nuclear material
  - The cell eventually breaks apart into discrete cell membrane bound vesicles
  - These are then removed by the macrophages via phagocytosis
  - Apoptosis occurring post reperfusion causes myocardial dysfunction and stunning

Myocardial Blush Grade

- Used to evaluate the risk of reperfusion injury following percutaneous intervention
- Found to be an important predictor of successful intervention along with TIMI flow grade

Blush grade	Angiographic finding
0	Absence of myocardial blush or contrast density
1	Minimal myocardial blush or contrast density
2	Moderate myocardial, less than ipsilateral non-infarct related coronary
3	Normal myocardial blush, comparable with ipsilateral non-infarct related coronary

Potential Therapies

- No treatment directed at reperfusion injury has shown improved clinical outcomes
- This is because reperfusion injury is multifactorial
- This warrants simultaneous administration of multiple therapies
- This may not be possible owing to the hemodynamically instability seen with the injury
- Potential therapies include:
  - Ishemic preconditioning
  - Glycoprotein IIb-IIIa inhibitors:
    - Platelet activation is an important contributor to reperfusion injury
    - GP IIb-IIIa inhibitors are potent inhibitors of platelet activity
    - GP IIb-IIIa inhibitors help in preventing reperfusion injury
    - Multiple studies have shown good outcomes with GPIIb-IIIa inhibitors
    - Significant benefit is seen when GPIIb-IIIa inhibitors are given prior to onset of reperfusion

- Adenosine:
  - Has several beneficial properties like:
    - Vasodilatation
    - Platelet inhibition
    - Direct cardioprotective effect
  - Usually used as an adjunct during primary reperfusion for acute MI
  - Can be administered intravenously or intracoronary
  - Needs further large scale trials to establish clinical benefit
- Vasodilators:
  - Papaverine:
    - Improves angiographic TIMI flows
    - Associtated with ventricular arrhythmias on intracoronary administration
  - ACE inhibitors:
  - Beneficial effects:
    - Free radical scavenger
    - Vasodilatation of coronary bed
  - ACE inhibitors enhance coronary blood flow
  - But, they fail to improve regional ventricular function
- Ion channel modulation:
  - Ranolazine:
    - It is a late sodium channel inhibitor
    - This decreases sodium-dependent intracellular calcium overload
    - Thus, it may be effective in the prevention of reperfusion injury
  - K_{ATP} openers:
    - K_{ATP} channels are involved in microvascular dilatation
    - Nicorandil has shown benefit in small clinical trials
    - Better perfusion and ventricular function seen with K_{ATP} openers
- Antioxidant therapy:
  - Requires further investigations to establish clinical benefit
  - Agents used include:
    - Erythropoietin
    - Estrogen
    - Heme oxygenase
    - Cyclosporine
- Other experimental therapies include:
  - Intravenous sodium nitrite
  - Losmapimod (p38-MAPK inhibitor)
  - Delcasertib (protein kinase C inhibitor)
  - Endovascular cooling

MYOCARDIAL CONDITIONING

Introduction

- Myocardial ischemic preconditioning refers to the adaptive mechanism by which a brief period of reversible ischemia increases the heart's tolerance to subsequent longer periods of ischemia
- Anesthetic preconditioning refers to administration of volatile anesthetics before prolonged coronary artery occlusion in order to increase the ***critical ischemia time*** (CIT_{50})
- CIT_{50} is the duration of circulatory disruption, compatible with 50% tissue survival

Biochemical Mechanisms of Myocardial Conditioning

- Up-regulation and activation of mitochondrial and sarcolemmal K_{ATP} channel: acts by reducing coronary vascular tone
- G proteins and coupled receptor ligands:
  - Due to activation of δ_1 opioid receptors
  - These in turn activate G_i and G_s protein
- Protein kinases: PKC, PKG and $P_{13}K$ involved in cardioprotective signal transduction
- Reactive oxygen species:
  - Volatile anesthetics stimulate small bursts of reactive oxygen species (superoxide, H_2O_2 and peroxynitrite)
  - These paradoxically initiate downstream signaling and protect from subsequent ischemic injury
- Adenosine receptor (especially A_1 and A_3 subtypes)
- Tyrosine kinase
- Na^+: H^+ exchanger
- COX_2, NFKB and NO systems are implicated for delayed preconditioning

Beneficial Effects of Myocardial Conditioning

- CABG: Better ejection fraction and cardiac index after CABG
- OPCAB: Preconditioning less used now due to use of coronary shunts intraoperatively
- Heart transplant: Improves contractile function after global myocardial hypothermia, which occurs when donor heart is stored
- Cardiomyoplasty: Skeletal muscle preconditioning prior to cardiomyoplasty augments systolic function and limits diastolic dysfunction

Conditions which Benefit from Preconditioning

- Extreme CAD with poor collaterals
- Severe LVH with reduced subendocardial perfusion
- Anticipated prolonged ischemic time
- Senescent myocardium prone to tissue damage from calcium overload

Types of Myocardial Conditioning

- Based on mode of stimulus:
  - Ischemic conditioning:
    - Application of cycles of brief, intermittent ischemia
    - Rarely used clinically nowadays
  - Pharmacological conditioning:
    - Drugs used to mimic endogenous triggers
    - May be receptor or non-receptor mediated
  - Other stimuli:
    - Hyperthermia
    - Hypoxia
    - Trauma
- Based on site of application:
  - Local conditioning:
    - Stimulus applied to the circulation supplying the organ of interest
    - Used more commonly
  - Remote conditioning:
    - Stimulus applied to a circulation bed distal to the organ of interest
    - Used less frequently
- Based on timing of stimulus:
  - Preconditioning:
    - Used most commonly
    - Stimulus applied prior to the lethal ischemia-reperfusion injury
  - Perconditioning:
    - Stimulus applied during lethal ischemia-reperfusion injury
    - Not used frequently
  - Postconditioning:
    - Stimulus applied at the time of reperfusion
    - Requires further studies as it has not yet shown clinical benefit
- Based on the protective window period:
  - Acute or early conditioning:
    - Begins immediately after the preconditioning stimulus
    - Lasts for 2–4 hours after application of the stimulus
    - Provides intense myocardial protection against myocardial necrosis
    - But, protection is not provided against myocardial stunning
    - Also, myocardial protection conferred is of short duration
  - Chronic or delayed conditioning:
    - Begins after 12–24 hours of application of the stimulus
    - Myocardial protection lasts for 2–3 days after application of the stimulus
    - Provides strong protection against myocardial stunning
    - Less intense protection against myocardial necrosis
    - Myocardial protection lasts for longer duration of time

Stimuli Used for Conditioning

- Ischemia
- Volatile anesthetics:
  - Isoflurane
  - Halothane
  - Sevoflurane
  - Desflurane
- *Adenosine*: acts through A_1, A_2 and A_3 receptors
- Others:
  - Phenylephrine
  - Bradykinin
  - Nitric oxide
  - Acadesine
  - Acetylcholine
  - Opioids: acts through δ_1 and K receptors

Ischemic Preconditioning

- Experimental preconditioning with LAD occlusion:
  - Ischemic preconditioning was initially introduced by Murry in 1986 in *dogs*
  - Four 5-minute cycles of LAD occlusion preceded prolonged LAD occlusion
  - This reduced infarct size by almost 75%
- Preconditioning with intermittent aortic cross clamping:
  - First human preconditioning done in 1993
  - Aorta was clamped for two 3-minute intervals each
  - This was followed by 2 minutes of reperfusion
  - This was followed by 10-minute intervals of aortic cross clamping and induced VF
  - Preconditioned patients showed lower postoperative troponin I levels
  - Stimulus most commonly used now is intermittent aortic cross clamping

- ❖ Most studies show ischemic conditioning provides additional myocardial protection over cardioplegia alone
- ❖ Beneficial effects of preconditioning include reduction in:
  - Infarct size
  - Microvascular damage
  - Mitochondrial dysfunction
  - Endothelial injury
  - Apoptosis
  - Neutrophil accumulation
- ❖ Application of intermittent ischemia, however risks multiple complications like:
  - Arrhythmias
  - Embolic events due to repeated clamping of aorta
  - Damage to vascular endothelium
  - Prolonged surgical time

Ischemic Postconditioning

- ❖ Two main mechanisms involved in reperfusion injury include:
  - Rapid equalization of intracellular and extracellular pH
  - Intracellular calcium overload
- ❖ Postconditioning attenuates reperfusion injury arising through these two mechanisms
- ❖ Post conditioning allows maintenance of low intracellular pH during reperfusion
- ❖ This mitigates reperfusion injury occurring via the RISK and SAFE cytokine pathways
- ❖ Postconditioning stimulus consists of two 30 s cycles of clamping the aorta
- ❖ This was followed by a 30 s period of declamping prior to cessation of CPB
- ❖ Evaluated in a small trial in adults undergoing valve surgeries
- ❖ Postconditioned patients showed:
  - Reduced peak CKMB levels post surgery
  - Reduced inotropic requirements

Remote Ischemic Pre-conditioning (RIPC)

- ❖ First discovered by Przyklenk in dogs in 1993
- ❖ Brief ischemia applied to remote area of the body leads to myocardial protection
- ❖ Thus, conditioning of one organ (skeletal muscle) confers protection of a distal organ (heart)
- ❖ Remote areas which are used clinically for preconditioning stimulus now are:
  - Kidney
  - Skeletal muscle
- ❖ Stimulus maybe applied through the use of blood pressure cuff applied on the arm or leg
- ❖ Increased muscle mass of lower limbs makes it more effective at providing RIPC
- ❖ Procedure:
  - BP cuff is inflated for 2 cycles of 3-minutes each
  - This is followed by 2 minutes of reperfusion
  - Alternatively, cyclical inflation of BP cuff prior to cross clamping is used
- ❖ Advantages of RIPC:
  - Avoids complications of repeated cross clamping seen with local preconditioning
  - Remote conditioning can be applied before, during and at the onset of reperfusion
  - Thus, it can be used as a pre, per and post-conditioning stimulus
- ❖ Mechanisms of remote ischemic preconditioning:
  - Humoral factors
  - Neural pathways
  - Systemic response via transcription of anti-inflammatory gene

Inhibitors of Preconditioning

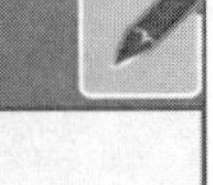

- ❖ Adenosine antagonists
- ❖ δ_1 opioids
- ❖ Glibenclamide:
  - As they close K_{ATP} channels
  - Discontinue glibenclamide 24–48 hours preoperatively
- ❖ Pertussis toxin
- ❖ Hyperglycemia

Anesthetic Preconditioning

- ❖ Involves myocardial exposure to volatile agents to reduce ischemia-reperfusion injury
- ❖ Characteristics of volatile anesthetic preconditioning:
  - Effect depends on:
    - Duration of administration
    - Concentration of the drug
  - Maximal effect is attained with 1.5–2 MAC of volatile anesthetic
  - Does not depend on ischemic preconditioning
  - Does not require preemptive ischemic episodes
  - Has only slightly protective effect on the heart

- Mechanisms involved in anesthetic preconditioning:
  - Extracellular signaling pathways acting via G-protein coupled receptors
  - Mitogen activated protein kinase
  - Adenosine type I (A_1) receptor activation
  - Reactive oxygen species
  - Altered neutrophil function
  - Mitochondrial and sarcolemmal K_{ATP} channels
- Volatile anesthetics reduce MvO_2 due to:
  - Direct negative inotropic, lusitropic and chronotropic effects
  - Reduction in LV afterload (reduces SVR)
  - Reduce oxygen free radicals
  - Cause coronary vasodilatation
- Beneficial effects of volatile anesthetic preconditioning:
  - Improves coronary perfusion
  - Reduces myocardial oxygen demand
  - Preserves energy dependant vital cellular processes
  - Negative inotropic effects
  - Negative chronotropic effects
  - Negative lusitropic effects
  - Reduces in LV afterload
- Examples of volatile anesthetic preconditioning:
  - Halothane:
    - Inhibits platelet thrombus formation by increasing platelet cAMP
    - Attenuates ST segment changes caused by brief coronary artery occlusion
    - Reduces ST elevation more than sodium nitroprusside and propranolol
    - Preserves contractile function and ultrastructural integrity at reperfusion
  - Isoflurane:
    - Reduces impact of reperfusion injury
    - Increases ratio of myocardial oxygen supply: demand
    - Beneficial to LV diastolic function during ischemia
    - Reduces troponin I and CK-MB levels after cardiac surgery
  - Sevoflurane:
    - Reduces impact of reperfusion injury
    - Improves functional recovery after period of global ischemia
    - Enhances endothelial nitric oxide release
    - Increases blood flow to collateral dependent myocardium
    - This action is via the calcium activated K^+ channels (BK_{ca})
  - Desflurane:
    - Beneficial to LV diastolic function during ischemia
    - Attenuates effects of free radicals on LV function
    - Reduces adhesion of neutrophils and platelets after myocardial reperfusion
- Procedure:
  - To be initiated at > 1 MAC for 15–30 minutes prior to aortic cross clamping
  - Initiated again several minutes before release of aortic cross clamp
  - This is done via oxygen-air supply line of extracorporeal circuit
  - Volatile agents are continued for at least 2–5 minutes after reperfusion
  - However, for maximal protection, administration throughout surgery is required
- Stages of preconditioning:
  - Preconditioning occurs in 2 stages
  - Shows that protective effects outlast drug elimination time
    - Early preconditioning: lasting for 2–4 hours after exposure
    - Late preconditioning:
      - Reappears after 24 hours and lasts up to 72 hours
      - May be species specific:
        - Occurs with sevoflurane
        - Absent when preconditioning is done with isoflurane
- Other agents used in anesthetic preconditioning:
  - Xenon
  - Adenosine
  - Nicorandil
  - Norepinephrine
  - Morphine via δ receptors

CARDIOPULMONARY BYPASS: BASIC CIRCUITRY

Introduction

- CPB is a form of extracorporeal circulation in which:
  Patients blood is rerouted outside the vascular system
  Functions of heart and lungs is temporarily assumed by surrogate technology
- Almost 25–30% of patients circulating volume is outside the body during CPB.

Goals

- To provide a quiet and bloodless field
- To limit myocardial damage by reduction of:
  - Intracellular acidosis
  - Edema
  - Depletion of ATP stores
- Preservation of coronary endothelial function and myocardial flow
- Reduce reperfusion injury

Types of Extracorporeal Circuitry

- Cardiopulmonary bypass (CPB)
- Left heart bypass
- Cardiopulmonary support
- Extracorporeal Membrane Oxygenation (ECMO)

Components

- Venous line
- Venous reservoir
- Arterial pump
- Heat exchanger
- Oxygenator
- Arterial line filter
- Arterial line
- Accessory pumps:
  - Cardiotomy suction
  - LV vent
  - Cardioplegia pump
- Accessory devices:
  - Ultrafilter
  - Volatile agent vaporizers
  - In line blood gas monitor
- Prime

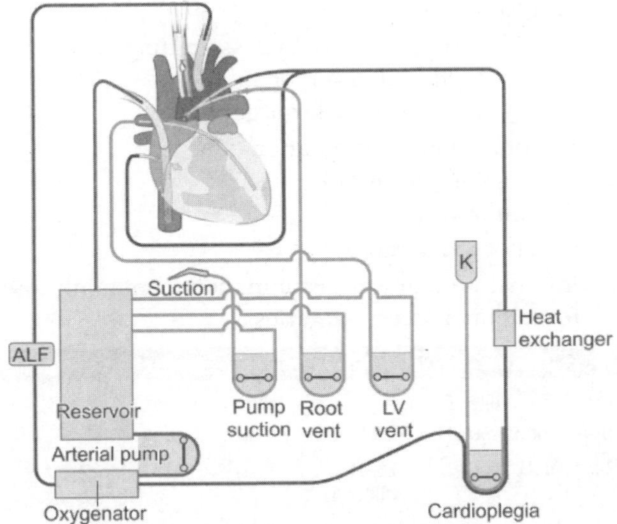

Fig. 14: Cardiopulmonary bypass circuitry.

VENOUS LINE AND CANNULAE

Description

- Venous tubing:
  - Connects the venous cannulae to the venous reservoir
  - Made of medical grade plasticizer such as DEHP
  - However, DEHP tubing may undergo spallation on long-term use
  - It has also been found to be carcinogenic
- Venous cannulae:
  - Aims to divert all blood from systemic venous circulation into CPB circuit
  - Made of medical grade polyvinyl chloride with surface coatings which:
    - Alter bioactivity of surface to reduce markers of subclinical coagulation
    - Attenuate cytokine and other inflammatory markers
  - Ends of cannulae are formed to permit easy vascular entry
  - Appropriate size cannula should be chosen to:
    - Maximize flow through the cannula
    - Minimize injury to blood vessel

Principles of Venous Drainage

- Venous return is accomplished by gravity siphonage
- Suction assisted venous return may be used to augment venous return
- Amount of venous drainage depends upon:
  - Patients blood volume
  - Height difference between patient and venous reservoir
  - Resistance in venous cannula and venous lines
  - Venous clamping
- For adequate venous drainage:
  - Venous reservoir must be adequately below level of patient
  - Venous line should be free of air bubbles as air lock removes gravitational siphon effect

Troubleshooting Venous Return

- Excessive venous drainage:
  - Occurs when rate of drainage is more than speed of return via arterial cannula
  - Causes collapse of venous wall around cannula if gravitational effect is high
  - This may manifest as chattering or fluttering of venous lines

- Treated by:
  - Partial occlusion of venous line by clamps
  - Addition of volume to venous reservoir
  - Administration of vasoconstrictive drug
- Reduced venous drainage:
  - Occurs when return from the venous cannula is reduced
  - Treated by:
    - Increasing height difference between patient and reservoir
    - Addition of volume to venous reservoir
    - Removal of air locks in venous line
    - Repositioning of venous cannula
    - Upsizing venous cannula

Types of Venous Cannula

- Standard tapered venous cannula
- Wire reinforced cannula
- Right angled tip cannula:
  - Tip is made of metal or hard plastic
  - This is to optimize ratio of internal to external diameter
  - Usually preferred for congenital heart surgeries

Types of Venous Cannulation

- Single atrial cannulation:
  - Cannula present in RA which drains blood from both RA and IVC
  - It is simpler, faster, less traumatic with one less incision
  - Interferes least with caval return when off bypass
  - Venous drainage is dependent on position of heart
  - Thus, it may be reduced in circumflex position during CABG
- Bicaval cannulation/single stage cannula:
  - Two separate cannulae are placed in SVC and IVC
  - Cannulae are snared to prevent systemic venous blood from entering the heart
  - Advantages:
    - Used anytime when right heart entry is anticipated
    - Provides best caval decompression when correctly positioned
  - Disadvantages:
    - Does not allow emptying of RA and RV once cannulae are snared
    - Causes greater interference with venous flow when not on CPB

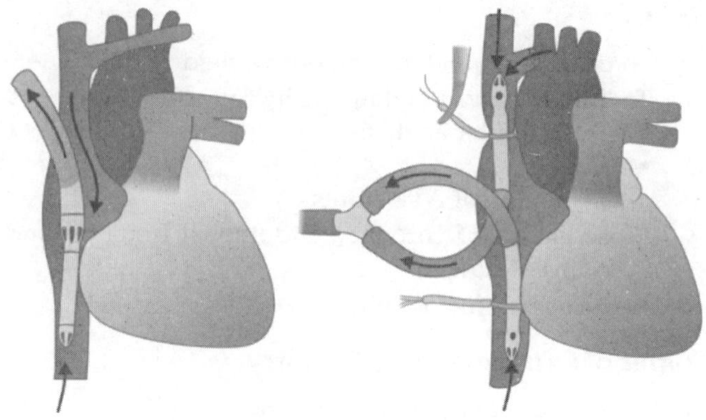

Fig. 15: Types of venous cannulation.

    - Presence of LSVC may require separate cannula for LSVC
  - Commonly used for:
    - Congenital heart surgeries (ASD, VSD)
    - Tricuspid valve surgeries
    - Mitral valve surgeries
- Cavo-atrial cannulation/dual stage cannulation:
  - Single cannula is inserted via the RA appendage
  - Cannula is designed such that:
    - Portion lying in RA is wide with additional holes
    - Portion lying in IVC (tip) is narrow
  - Cannula is positioned within the RA and extends into IVC
  - Provides superior decompression of right heart:
    - IVC and RA blood is emptied via the cannula tip
    - Cannula has additional set of holes to drain SVC
  - Commonly used for:
    - Coronary artery bypass grafting
    - Aortic valve surgeries
    - Ascending aorta surgery
- Femoral venous cannulation done in:
  - In emergent situation
  - Aortic surgery
  - Thoracic surgery
- Internal jugular vein cannulation: commonly used for minimal access surgeries

Feature	Bicaval	Atrial	Cavoatrial
Number of incisions	2	1	1
Speed of cannulation	Slowest	Fast	Fast
Technical difficulty	Most difficult	Easy	Moderately easy
Right heart exclusion	Complete	Absent	Absent

Contd...

Contd...

Feature	Bicaval	Atrial	Cavoatrial
Coronary sinus return	Excluded	Included	Included
Right heart decompression	None	Good	Best
Caval drainage	Best	Good (except IVC)	Good (except SVC)
Rewarming due to systemic return	Absent	Present	Present
Myocardial protection	Best	Suboptimal	Controversial

VENOUS RESERVOIR

Description

- Venous reservoirs for membrane oxygenators (MO):
  - Reservoir is positioned between venous line and systemic pump
  - Thus, it is the first component of ECC directly receiving the venous drainage
  - Blood from the reservoir passes through systemic pump and then through MO
  - Serves as a holding tank to buffer imbalances between:
    - Venous return
    - Arterial flow
  - Blood flows into the reservoir via gravitational drainage
  - Thus, if the venous reservoir is allowed to empty, air can enter arterial line
  - This may result in fatal air embolism
- Venous reservoirs for bubble oxygenators (BO):
  - Venous reservoirs for bubble oxygenators may be placed beyond the oxygenator
  - It is usually included as an integral part of the bubble oxygenator
  - In this case, venous return directly enters the oxygenation chamber of BO
  - Thus, venous reservoirs for BO is referred to as ***arterial reservoir***

Types of Venous Reservoirs

- Open system reservoirs:
  - Consist of polycarbonate hard-shell reservoirs
  - Usually equipped with integral cardiotomy reservoir
  - Thus, they have integral screen and depth filters for filtration of cardiotomy blood
  - Open system also has integrated positive and negative pressure release valves
  - These are necessary for application of vacuum to augment venous return
  - Venous return is improved by applying suction to the venous reservoir
  - This is called vacuum assisted venous drainage (VAVD)
  - In open systems, air escapes to atmosphere at the top of the reservoir
  - Open systems are preferred for:
    - Reduction in blood utilization
    - Improved safety profile
- Closed system reservoirs:
  - Consist of collapsible PVC bags
  - Do not have an integral cardiotomy reservoir
  - Thus, these systems require a separate cardiotomy reservoir
  - Have reduced contact surface of blood with air or plastic
  - Separate centrifugal pump may be used to increase venous return
  - This is called kinetic-assisted venous drainage (KAVD)
  - Buoyant air accumulates within the bag and must be actively aspirated

Clinical Uses

- Buffering of flow imbalances:
  - Reservoir acts as buffer for imbalances between venous return and arterial flow
  - It provides time for the perfusionist to act if venous drainage is reduced
  - This prevents pumping of air into systemic circulation causing air embolism
- Facilitates displacement of blood from circulation at strategic times during the operation
- Serves as gross trap for air which enters the venous line
- Serves as a site where blood, fluids and drugs can be added

ARTERIAL PUMPS

Types of Arterial Pumps

- Roller pumps
- Centrifugal pumps

Roller Pumps

- These are positive displacement pumps
- Structure:
  - Internal diameter of the ECC tubing ranges from 1/8 to 5/8 inch/minute

- Tubing which traverses the raceway is called pump header
- Pumping mechanism is also referred to as the pump head
- All roller pumps have manual cranks to allow manual pumping

❖ Functioning:
- Function by occluding a point in the tubing between:
  - Stationary raceway
  - Rotating roller
- The occlusive point of contact is then rolled along a length of the tubing
- This process forces an antegrade motion of blood within the tubing:
  - Forward flow of blood in front of the occlusion point
  - Aspiration of blood into the tubing behind the occlusive point
- Capacity for displacement of fluid depends upon:
  - Volume of tubing occluded by the roller (tubing stroke volume)
  - Number of revolutions per minute (rpm) of the roller

❖ Disadvantages:
- Air embolism:
  - Roller pumps generate extremely high positive and negative pressures
  - This can pump massive quantities of air into systemic circulation
  - Thus, risk of air embolism is high
- Under-occlusive pump roller may produce retrograde flow
- Over-occlusive pump roller:
  - May result in spallation of tubing
  - Excessive tube compression leads to microfragmentation
  - This leads to the formation of plastic microemboli
  - Spallation refers to the development of plastic microemboli

❖ Complications:
- Occlusion of pump inflow:
  - Causes development of negative pressure in ECC tubing
  - This can cause cavitation and air embolism
- Occlusion of pump outflow:
  - Increased pressure may develop proximal to occlusion
  - This causes tubing connection to separate or tube to burst

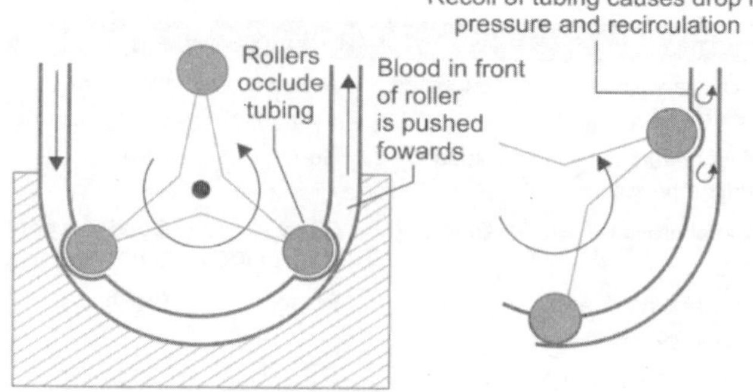

Fig. 16: Roller pumps for CPB.

- RBC hemolysis due to:
  - Over-occlusion of ECC tubing
  - Excessive revolutions per minute of roller pump

❖ Pulsatile CPB:
- Pulsatile flow is possible with some roller pumps
- Pulsations are produced by instant variations in rate of rotation of roller heads
- Advantages of pulsatile flow:
  - Increased tissue perfusion: increases renal and cerebral blood flow
  - Increased oxygen extraction
  - Reduces release of stress hormones
  - Reduces SVR during CPB

Centrifugal Pumps

❖ These are nonocclusive kinetic energy pumps

❖ Also called constrained vortex pumps

❖ They are used extensively for VADs and ECMO circuits (CentriMag) due to:
- Preload and afterload sensitivity
- Inherent safety features
- Low cost

❖ Functioning:
- Generate flow by magnetically coupling:
  - High speed revolution of a reusable motor and
  - Plastic plates, fins or channels inside a disposable cone
- This produces a constrained vortex which propels fluid forwards
- This produces antegrade motion of blood within the cone:
  - Forward flow of blood through opening on side of cone
  - Aspiration of blood into the point of the cone

- Blood flow is dependent upon:
  - Revolutions per minute (rpm) of the cones
  - Total circuit resistance

❖ Indications:
- VAD for left heart support up to 6 hours
- VAD for right heart support up to 30 days
- ECMO (CentriMag) for days-weeks
- Left heart bypass during repair of thoracic aortic aneurysms
- Veno-venous bypass during liver transplantation

❖ Advantages:
- Generation of high-volume output with moderate pressure development
- Reduced risk of RBC trauma and hemolysis as they are non-occlusive.
- Reduced risk of cavitation and massive air embolism
- Elimination of tubing wear off and spallation

❖ Disadvantages:
- Unable to generate extremely high/low pressures as they are non-occlusive
- In case of air embolism:
  - Air will remain within the cone
  - Pump will de-prime and not be able to generate forward flow
  - Thus, centrifugal pumps are unable to pump large volumes of air
  - Thus, risk of air-embolism is reduced
- Retrograde flow:
  - Centrifugal pumps lack a point of tubing occlusion
  - This allows retrograde flow from patients high pressure arterial system
  - This occurs when revolution of pump goes below a critical threshold
  - Causes of retrograde flow:
    - Power disruption
    - Pump failure
  - Flow can be directed retrogradely into:
    - Oxygenator
    - Venous reservoir
- Heating:
  - Downstream occlusion results in heating of fluid in the pump head
  - This occurs due to hydrodynamic processes in the magnetic coupling
  - Increase in temperature may lead to:
    - Blood trauma and hemolysis
    - Coagulation defects
- Cannot produce pulsatile flow

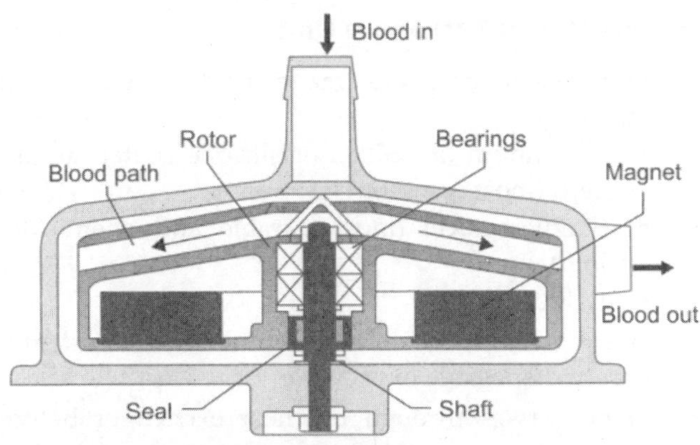

Fig. 17: Centrifugal pump for CPB.

Feature	Roller pumps	Centrifugal pumps
Property	Occlusive	Non-occlusive
Afterload dependence	Output independent of afterload	Output inversely proportional to afterload
Output quantification	Output = rpm × volume per revolution	Requires flow meter to determine output
Retrograde flow	Retrograde flow less frequent	Allows retrograde flow
Pulsatile flow	Better pulsatile flow capability	Poor pulsatile flow capability
Arterial line rupture	Arterial line bursts on clamping	Arterial line does not burst
Air embolism	Can pump massive air volumes	Does not pump massive air volumes
Spallation	Common	Less common
Hemolysis	Common	Less common
Platelet damage	More common	Less common
Cost	Cheaper	Expensive

HEAT EXCHANGER

Introduction

❖ Heat exchanger (HE) facilitates management of patients blood temperature on CPB

❖ Hypothermia is common on CPB as up to 25–30% of patients blood is outside the body

Components of Heat Exchange Unit

❖ Heat exchanger

❖ Source of hot and cold water

❖ Regulator or blender

❖ Temperature sensors

Design of Heat Exchanger Unit

- Heat exchangers are made from a variety of materials:
  - Aluminum (anodized or silicone coated anodized) (most common)
  - Stainless steel (most durable and chemically inert)
  - Polypropylene
- Heat exchangers are currently included as integral part of disposable oxygenator
- Blood passes through the heat exchanger before undergoing gas exchange
- This is in order to minimize risk of formation of gas microbubbles from the blood
- Bubbles are formed when blood saturated with gas is rewarmed quickly
- Heat exchangers consist of 2 phases:
  - Water from the heat exchanger passes through on one side
  - Patients blood passes on the other side
- Direction of blood flow is countercurrent to that of the water
- This helps in optimizing heat transfer across the heat exchanger
- They usually have an in-built filter to filter air bubbles formed during rewarming
- Separate heat exchangers are required for administration of cardioplegia solution

Functioning

- Temperature of water entering the HE is controlled by an external heater/cooler device
- Heat transfer occurs by conduction where thermal energy passes from water to blood
- Both cooling and warming of the patient can be achieved in the heat exchanger
- This is facilitated by altering the temperature of water flowing through HE (4–42°C)
- The blood is consequently warmed/cooled and maintained at the desired temperature
- Effectiveness of heat exchanger depends upon:
  - Total surface area
  - Thickness of conductor walls
  - Thermal conductivity
  - Residence time of blood within the device

Heater/Cooler Units

- Consist of a system providing thermoregulated water supply
- Can circulate water at a wide range of temperatures (4–42°C)
- Water is pulled from the cooler/heaters reservoir and reaches the HE unit
- Alternatively, water may be pumped from the reservoir into the HE unit
- Water reaches the heat exchanger unit in BGED through ½ inch internal diameter tubes

Disadvantages

- Heat exchanger malfunction occurs commonly during CPB
- Heater/cooler unit requires frequent maintenance:
  - Drainage of water supply
  - Sanitation of:
    - Internal pump
    - Conduit tubing
    - Internal surface of reservoir

Complications

- Air emboli:
  - Gas bubbles may be formed in the heat exchange unit
  - This occurs if rewarming is carried out rapidly after blood is saturated with gas
- Water leakage:
  - Water may leak into the blood compartment of the BGED rarely
  - This can result in hemolysis and hyperkalemia
- Aluminum toxicity:
  - Rare possibility of aluminum toxicity
  - Occurs when blood levels exceed 200 mg/L
  - Aluminum oxide concretions form with long-term use of ECC support devices (ECMO)
- *Mycobacterium* contamination of the water in heater/cooler units

BLOOD GAS EXCHANGE DEVICES

Introduction

- Devices which replace the function of lung in pulmonary gaseous exchange
- Performs gaseous exchange through a blood gas interface

Types of Blood Gas Exchange Devices (BGED)

- Membrane oxygenators
- Bubble oxygenators
- Film oxygenators

Membrane Oxygenators (MO)

- Most frequently used oxygenator currently
- Functioning:
  - MOs are made of 3 distinct compartments:
    - Blood space containing venous blood
    - Gas space containing fresh gas flow
    - Heat exchange space containing water (maintains temperature)
  - Venous blood entering MO is directed across the exterior surface of the fibers
  - Fresh gas is concurrently circulated through the inside of the fibers
  - Thus, blood and gas are separated with a limited or absent blood-gas interface
  - Separate gas inlet and outlet ports are present to refresh gas within the gas space
  - Gas exchange is determined by:
    - Surface area of membrane
    - Partial pressure of venous O_2 and CO_2
    - Blood flow
    - Ventilation flow (called sweep rate)
    - Gas flow and composition
  - PaO_2 is determined by FiO_2 of fresh gas
  - $PaCO_2$ is determined by sweep rate of ventilating gas
- Design:
  - Materials used in membranes:
    - Microporous polypropylene (PPL):
      - Excellent capacity for gas exchange
      - Good biocompatibility
      - It is extruded into thin straws with:
        - Outer diameter of 200–400 µm
        - Wall thickness of 20–50 µm
        - Total surface area of 2–4 m^2
        - Microscopic pores on the sides of fibers (0.5–1 µm)
    - Silicon:
      - Transfer gases directly by diffusion across the membrane
      - Do not have blood gas interface
      - More suitable for long-term perfusion (ECMO)
    - Microporous polymethyl pentene (PMP):
      - Designed as a non-porous true diffusion membrane
      - PMP membranes are more biocompatible compared with PPL
      - Suitable for long-term perfusion (ECMO)
      - Limits transfer of volatile agents
      - Thus it requires anesthetic supplementation
  - Usually positioned after the roller pumps
  - This is because of high resistance in most membrane oxygenators
  - This necessitates blood to be pumped through membrane oxygenators
  - Microporous membrane oxygenators:
    - Initially have a blood gas interface
    - On exposure to blood, a thin protein film is formed on the membrane
    - This acts as a diffusible barrier to gas exchange
    - Thus, blood-gas interface diminishes over time
- Advantages:
  - Can arterialize up to 7 L/min of venous blood
  - Allows independent control of PaO_2 and $PaCO_2$:
    - PaO_2 is determined by FiO_2 of fresh gas
    - $PaCO_2$ is determined by sweep rate of ventilating gas
- Disadvantages:
  - Gas emboli:
    - Microscopic pores (0.5–1 µm) are present on the side of the fibers
    - These pores are small enough to:
      - Prevent leakage of plasma and formed elements
      - Allow gaseous exchange
    - Thus, increase in driving pressure in the gas space may result in g E
  - Bio-membrane formation on prolonged use

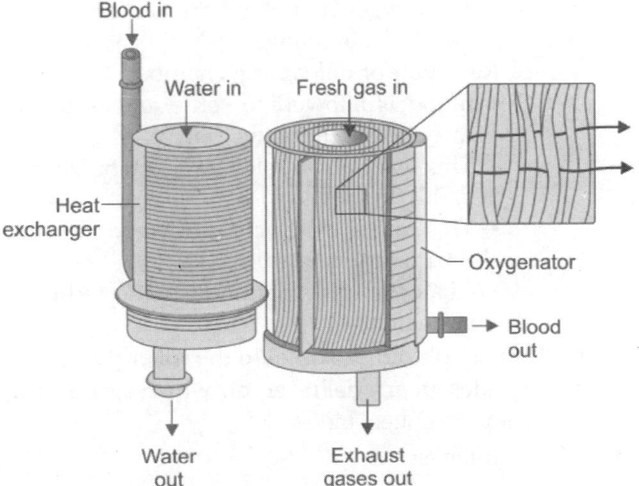

Fig. 18: Membrane oxygenator.

Bubble Oxygenators (BO)

- Not used commonly
- Functioning:
  - BOs use a direct blood: gas interface
  - Gas exchange occurs through direct blood: gas contact and dispersion of gas
  - Either 100% oxygen or mixture of CO_2 and O_2 (carbogen) is used
  - This gas is passes through a column of deoxygenated blood for gas exchange
  - Gas exchange is affected by:
    - Quantity of gas
    - Size of bubbles produced by gas sparger:
      - Small bubbles:
        - Effective for oxygen exchange
        - Poor for carbon dioxide exchange
      - Large bubbles:
        - Effective for carbon dioxide exchange
        - Poor for oxygen exchange
- Design:
  - Divided into two sections:
    - Mixing or oxygenating chamber:
      - Fresh gas flows through a perforated plate (gas sparger plate)
      - This results in the formation of gas bubbles
      - Diffusion takes place on the bubble surface
      - By using small bubbles a large surface area develops
      - Diffusion of gas occurs due to difference in:
        - Partial pressure of gases in bubbles
        - Partial pressure of dissolved gases in blood
      - The oxygenated blood then enters a reservoir/heat exchanger
    - Reservoir or defoaming chamber:
      - Blood is allowed to settle and is passed through a defoaming matrix
      - This causes bubbles to destabilize and break down
      - This causes destruction of blood elements if CPB time > 90 min
      - Coalescence of foam is also affected using surfactants
  - Usually placed proximal to the roller pump
  - Includes an arterial reservoir which serves as an atrium to collect blood
- Disadvantages:
  - Causes denaturation of plasma proteins
  - Increase RBC fragility and cause hemolysis
  - Causes platelet activation
  - Generates gaseous microemboli (GME)

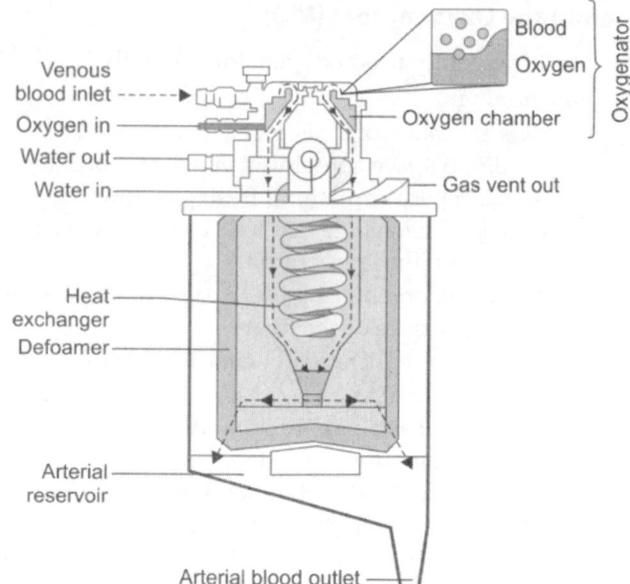

Fig. 19: Bubble oxygenator.

Circuit Design for Various BGED

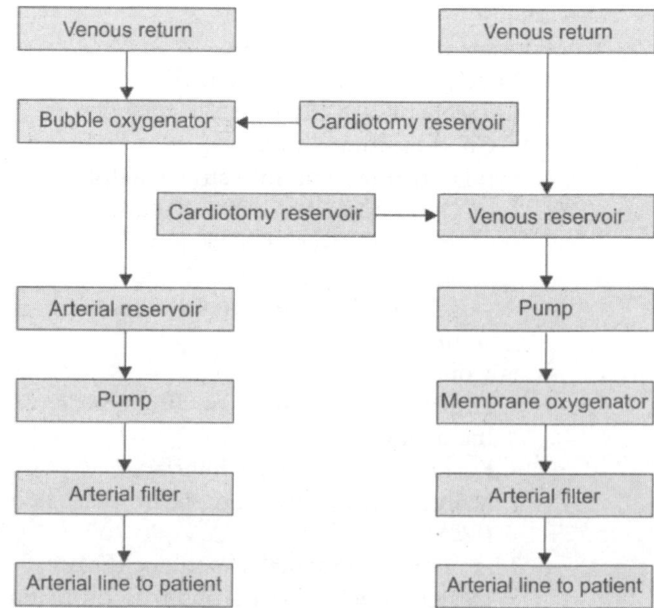

Film Oxygenators

- Used historically
- Utilizes a stationary 0.7 mm screen oxygenator
- Blood was distributed over the screen producing a film

- This increases the surface area of the blood in contact with oxygen
- Gas exchange occurs by diffusion

Gas Supply System for BGED

- Oxygenators require a gas supply system
- Typical gas supply system consists of:
  - Gas source supplying:
    - Oxygen
    - Air
    - Carbon dioxide (rarely)
  - Gas blender to blend oxygen-air and determine FiO_2
  - Flow regulator to determine sweep gas rate and $PaCO_2$
  - Flow meter
  - Oxygen analyzer
  - Volatile anesthetic vaporizer

ARTERIAL LINE FILTER

Introduction

- Arterial line filters are an integral part of CPB circuits
- They are important to reduce the load of gaseous and particulate emboli
- They have been shown to reduce the rate of post-CPB neurocognitive dysfunction

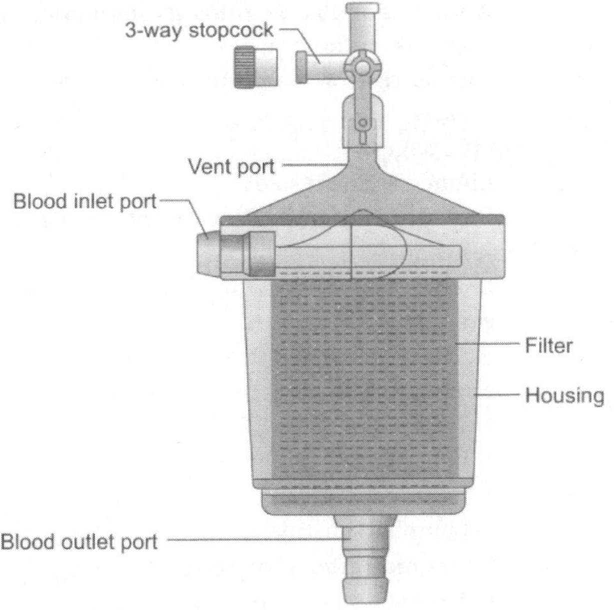

Fig. 20: Arterial line filter.

Design

- Placed in arterial line as the last component through which blood passes before it returns to patient
- Blood enters tangentially through the inlet port at the top of the arterial filter
- This encourages entrained air bubbles to rise to the top from where they are vented out
- This is done through a recirculation line connecting the filter to the venous reservoir
- The recirculation line may be used to measure ABG of post-oxygenator blood samples
- Blood then passes through the screen microfilter with pores to encourage further filtration
- Pore sizes can range from 20 to 40 µm which removes:
  - Gaseous microemboli
  - Particulate emboli:
    - Thrombi
    - Fat globules
    - Calcium
    - Tissue debris
- 20 µm filters are superior to 40 µm filters in reducing cerebral embolic counts
- Arterial line filters always have a bypass limb which is normally clamped
- This is unclamped in case it becomes clogged/develops high resistance

Types

- Microporous screen filters:
  - Used most commonly
  - Filter material is pleated within the housing unit to provide larger surface area
  - Trap emboli whose size is larger than their effective pore size
- Depth filters: consist of dense fiber material packed in polycarbonate housing

ARTERIAL LINE AND CANNULA

Introduction

- Arterial cannula closes the loop of the CPB circuit
- This is done by returning oxygenated blood to the systemic circulation
- Arterial cannulas are conventionally placed in the ascending aorta

Types of Cannula

- Metal tipped right angled cannula:
  - Tip of the cannula is made of metal
  - Reduces the ID-OD ratio
  - Plastic flange is included to secure its position on the aorta

- Plastic right angled cannula with molded flange:
  - Tip of the cannula is made of hard plastic (polycarbonate)
  - Reduces the ID-OD ratio
  - Plastic flange is molded to secure its position on the aorta
- Diffusion tipped angled cannula:
  - Inverted cone occludes the tip of the cannula
  - This disperses the arterial flow through the side ports
  - This design directs the systemic flow in four directions
  - Avoids jetting-effect seen with conventional single lumen cannulas
- Luer port incorporated cannulas:
  - Luer port is present proximal to the tip of the cannula
  - Luer port is incorporated to allow de-airing.

Sites of Cannulation

- Ascending aortic (AA) cannulation:
  - Most commonly used cannulation site
  - Readily accessible site for cannulation and is thus convenient to use
  - Produces antegrade perfusion through the arterial tree
  - Advantages:
    - Allows use of wide range of cannula sizes
    - Avoids local arterial access complications
    - Avoids limb ischemia seen with femoral cannulation
    - Low risk of dissection
  - Complications:
    - High risk of athero-embolism (Porcelain aorta)
    - Risk of malperfusion of aortic arch vessels
    - Aortic dissection (0.01–0.1%)
    - Complications due to incorrect cannulation:
      - Selective arterial perfusion:
        - Occurs especially in neonates
        - Length of insertion of cannula may be too long for patient
        - Thus, it may selectively enter innominate artery
        - This causes:
          - Hyperperfusion of right carotid artery
          - Hypoperfusion of left carotid artery
        - This may results in cerebral overperfusion and hemorrhage
      - Inappropriate size of arterial cannulas:
        - Small cannulas result in generation of high-velocity jets
        - This may result in a venturi effect and cause arterial steal
        - This causes selective hypoperfusion of aortic arch branches
  - *Contraindication*: Porcelain aorta
- Femoral artery cannulation:
  - Preferred site for when aortic cannulation is contraindicated (Porcelain aorta)
  - However, it requires a separate incision and arterial exposure for cannulation
  - Being a smaller artery, acceptable cannula sizes are limited
  - Produces retrograde perfusion through the arterial tree
  - Indications:
    - Aneurysm of ascending aorta extending up to arch
    - Antegrade aortic dissection extending up to arch
    - Surgery involving multiple procedures of ascending aorta
    - For peripheral cannulation under local anesthesia in unstable patients
    - Redo-sternotomies with limited retro-sternal space
    - Minimal access surgeries
  - Advantages:
    - Allows cannulation prior to sternotomy in high risk sternotomies
    - Avoids risk of malperfusion of aortic arch vessels
  - Disadvantages:
    - Limited cannula size
    - Provides retrograde flow (un-physiological)
  - Complications:
    - Limb ischemia especially when duration of cannulation > 6 hours
    - Aortic dissection in 0.2–1% patients
    - Local arterial access complications:
      - Tears, dissections
      - Late stenosis and thrombosis
      - Pseudoaneurysm
      - Lymphatic fistulas
    - Retrograde arterial dissections:
      - Most serious complication
      - Rare in occurrence (0.2–1.3%)

- May result in retroperitoneal hematoma formation
- Rarely results in retrograde dissection extending to aortic root
  - Wound infections possible
- Contraindications:
  - Peripheral vascular disease affecting femoral artery
  - Extensive atheromas of descending aorta

❖ Axillary/subclavian cannulation:
- Rarely used for arterial cannulation
- Requires a separate incision and arterial exposure
- Being a smaller artery, acceptable cannula sizes are limited
- Produces antegrade flow through the arterial tree
- Indications:
  - Aortic dissection extending to aortic arch
  - Porcelain aorta with severe peripheral vascular disease
  - Minimal access surgeries
- Advantages:
  - Less risk of atheroembolism compared with femoral and aortic cannulation
  - Better collateral flow reducing risk of limb ischemia
  - Avoids retrograde flow through the aorta (as in femoral cannulation)
  - Reduced risk of malperfusion during aortic dissection surgery
  - Allows selective antegrade cerebral perfusion
- Disadvantages:
  - Requires separate incision
  - Limited choice of cannula sizes
  - Risk of limb ischemia
  - Possible risk of malperfusion of aortic arch vessels
- Complications:
  - Local wound infections
  - Aortic dissection can occur in 0.75% patients
  - Brachial plexus injury
  - Axillary and subclavian arterial injury
- *Contraindication*: occlusive PVD of brachial vessels

❖ Other less commonly used access sites include:
- Innominate artery
- Brachial artery
- Common carotid artery
- Abdominal aorta

Hemodynamic Considerations during Cannulation

❖ Optimal arterial BP required during arterial cannulation as:
- If too high, increased chances of aortic dissection and tears
- If too low aorta may collapse

❖ Optimal pressure during arterial cannulation:
- Mean blood pressure of 60–65 mm Hg is preferred
- Systolic blood pressure of 90–100 mm Hg is preferred

Complications

❖ *Jetting effect*:
- Occurs due to high velocity flow through the tip of arterial cannula
- This damages the aortic wall and can lead to multiple adverse effects:
  - Dislodgement of atherosclerotic plaques (***sand-blasting effect***)
  - Hemolysis due to shear stress

❖ Arterial dissection due to poor hemodynamics during insertion/removal of cannula

Common Approaches to Cannulation

Procedure	Venous	Arterial	Cardioplegia	Vent
CABG	2-stage RA	AA	Root and/or coronary sinus	Aortic root
AVR	2-stage RA	AA	Root and/or coronary sinus	LV and aortic root
MVR	Bicaval	AA	Root and/or coronary sinus	LV and aortic root
Aortic root not including arch	2-stage RA	AA	Root and/or coronary sinus	LV and aortic root
Aortic arch	2-stage RA	Femoral artery	Root and/or coronary sinus	LV and aortic root
Redo surgeries	Femoral vein	Femoral artery	Root and/or coronary sinus	Aortic root
Intracardiac procedures	Bicaval	AA	Root and/or coronary sinus	LV and aortic root

CARDIOTOMY SUCTION AND RESERVOIR

❖ Cardiotomy suction:
- Aspirates blood from surgical field and returns it to main pump reservoir
- Use is initiated 3 minutes after heparin administration to ensure anticoagulation
- Use is terminated after reversal of heparin effect (half total dose of protamine)
- Excessive suction pressure may cause RBC trauma due to high negative pressure

- This occurs due to amount of air which is aspirated with blood
- The air-blood mixture causes turbulence and high shear stresses
- This can injure both RBCs and platelets
- This damage to RBCs precludes blood salvage from cardiotomy
- Disadvantages of cardiotomy suction:
  - Hemolysis
  - Particulate and gaseous microemboli
  - Fat globule formation
  - Platelet injury

❖ Cardiotomy reservoir:
- Receives blood that has been aspirated from surgical field through various vents
- It consists of 2 parts:
  - Defoaming chamber:
    - Consists of a plastic sponge material
    - Sponge is impregnated with anti-foam A to lower surface tension
  - Storage chamber:
    - Has markings on the outer shell to measure volume
    - Also has micro and macrofilters to remove debris

❖ Cell saver suction devices:
- Aspirates blood with controlled vacuum
- RBCs are automatically washed with saline and separated from fluid by centrifugation
- They are then returned to venous reservoir on extracorporeal circuit
- It removes microaggregates fat, air and tissue debris

LEFT VENTRICULAR VENT

❖ Ventricular distension is detrimental to ventricular function during CPB and reperfusion

❖ Therefore, LV venting plays an important role in myocardial protection

❖ Causes of dysfunction due to LV distension:
- Increased wall stress, which increases myocardial oxygen demand
- Direct myocardial damage due to excessive stretch
- Reduced subendocardial perfusion
- Increased LA pressure causing pulmonary edema
- Interference with surgical exposure—prolongs CPB time

❖ Causes of LV distension:
- On cardiopulmonary bypass:
  - Aortic cross clamping
  - Antegrade cardioplegia administration
  - Aortic regurgitation
  - Patent ductus arteriosus
  - Major Aorto-Pulmonary Collateral Arteries (MAPCAs)
- At the time of reperfusion:
  - Ventricular fibrillation
  - Cardiac arrest
  - Cross clamp release

❖ Sources of blood to the LV after application of aortic cross clamp:
- Non-coronary collateral flow (bronchial veins 100 mL/min)
- Aortic regurgitation
- Major Aorto-Pulmonary Collateral Arteries
- Large PDA
- ASD
- VSD

❖ Importance:
- Distension of LV causes mechanical damage to muscle from excessive stretching
- Venting improves preservation by reducing myocardial oxygen demand
- Venting also reduces wall tension due to a reduction in radius of ventricle
- It facilitates subendocardial perfusion by reducing wall tension
- It prevents pulmonary venous hypertension with pulmonary edema

❖ Sites of LV vent application:
- Indirect LV vent via right superior pulmonary vein (RSPV):
    - Advantages: Tackles all sources of blood to LV
    - Optimal decompression
    - Best method in the presence of aortic regurgitation
    - Avoids direct LV incision
  - Disadvantages:
    - Useless in the presence of mitral regurgitation
    - Dislodges clots present in LA
    - Can cause damage to RSPV
    - Difficult to insert
    - Can cause air entry into LV
    - Contraindicated in the presence of mitral prosthesis

- Direct LV vent via LV apex:
  - Advantages:
    - Tackles all sources of blood to LV
    - Optimal decompression
    - Tackles aortic regurgitation
    - Easy to insert
  - Disadvantages:
    - Can cause LV aneurysm
    - Vent can get occluded by myocardial tissue
    - Dislodges LV thrombus and risks systemic embolism
    - Can result in coronary disruption
    - LV dysfunction
    - Can cause bundle branch block
    - Causes air entry into LV
    - Postoperative bleeding
- Indirect LV venting via LA appendage:
  - Advantages: easy to insert
  - Disadvantages:
    - Does not tackle aortic regurgitation
    - Dislodges clot in LA appendage
    - Can cause air entry into LV
- Ascending aorta:
  - Advantages:
    - Ease of insertion
    - Can be used to vent even after LV starts ejecting
  - Disadvantages:
    - Not useful in the presence of aortic regurgitation
    - Can cause air in the aortic root and systemic embolization
    - Not useful at the time of administration of cardioplegia
- Pulmonary artery:
  - Advantages:
    - Easy to insert
    - Reduces air entry into the left heart
  - Disadvantages:
    - Not useful in the presence of aortic regurgitation
    - Does not handle all the sources of blood into LV
    - Can cause distortion of PA anatomy and PA damage

❖ Uses of LV venting:
- Prevents myocardial distension
- Reduces myocardial rewarming
- Prevents ejection of air: used to aspirate air from heart during de-airing procedure
- Facilitates surgical exposure, e.g., when working on aortic valve

❖ Complications of LV venting:
- Damage to the corresponding structure
- Air entry into left heart and embolization
- Dislodgement of thrombi
- Mitral valve incompetence

CARDIOPLEGIA PUMP

❖ Allows optimal control over infusion pressure, rate and temperature of cardioplegia

❖ Separate heat exchanger ensures accurate control of temperature of cardioplegia solution

❖ This solution may be infused from a cold IV fluid bag given under pressure or by gravity

ULTRAFILTER/HEMOFILTER/ HEMOCONCENTRATOR

❖ Used to increase patient's hematocrit during CPB without transfusion

❖ Contains hollow semipermeable fibers which can function as membrane

❖ Blood is passed through fibers either from arterial side/venous reservoir

❖ This is done using an accessory pump

❖ Hydrostatic pressure forces water and electrolytes across the fiber membrane

❖ This allows separation of aqueous phase of blood from cellular and proteinaceous elements

❖ Effluents of up to 40 mL/min can be removed

❖ Can be used post bypass to concentrate pump blood before it is given back to patient

❖ Conserves coagulation factors, platelets and albumin

IN LINE BLOOD GAS MONITORS

❖ Noninvasive flow-through devices to measure blood gases in arterial and venous lines

❖ Arterial monitor provides continuous assessment of arterial oxygenation

❖ Venous oximetry provides rapid assessment of balance of oxygen supply and demand

AUTOMATIC DATA COLLECTION SYSTEMS

❖ To assist preoperative calculation, processing and storing data during bypass

❖ This allows perfusionist to attend to more important tasks

CPB PRIMING SOLUTIONS

Introduction

- Fluid contained within CPB tubing prior to initiation of CPB is called prime
- This creates a fluid filled circuit to ensure continuity with the patient
- Fluid filled circuits are mandatory prior to initiation of CPB
- This is important to prevent air embolism during CPB

Types of Prime

- Sanguinous prime (SP):
  - Uses blood to fill the CPB circuit
  - This was used historically
  - SP ensures close matching of prime with patients own rheological characteristics
  - This required large volumes of blood (8–10 units of heparinized blood)
  - This was associated with massive histamine release
  - This resulted in a high incidence of ***capillary leak syndrome***
  - Thus, this practice was stopped due to:
    - Increased demand for blood
    - Scarcity of supply
    - Capillary leak syndrome
- Asanguinous prime:
  - Uses balanced salt solutions (BSS) to fill the CPB circuit
  - Initiation of CPB with asanguinous prime results in significant hemodilution
  - This reduces the oxygen carrying capacity of the CPB-perfusate
  - However, tissue oxygenation is maintained due to reduced viscosity of perfusate
  - Safe levels of hemodilution depends upon:
    - Patients metabolic rate
    - Cardiovascular reserve
    - Degree of atherosclerotic disease
    - Core temperature
  - Calculation of resultant hematocrit (HCT_r):

$$HCT = \frac{HCT_r = (BV_p \times HCT_p)}{(BV_p \times PV)}$$

Where:
HCT_r = resultant hematocrit
HCT_p = patient's initial hematocrit
BV_p = patient's blood volume
PV = prime volume of extracorporeal circuit

- Factors affecting hematocrit during CPB:
  - Preoperative anemia/polycythemia
  - Preoperative hypovolemia/hypervolemia
  - CPB circuit volume (miniature circuits produce less hemodilution)
  - CPB prime constitution
  - Pre-CPB blood loss
  - Crystalloid cardioplegia volume
  - Added crystalloids during CPB to maintain venous reservoir volume
- Minimal hematocrit of 20–24% is required to ensure tissue oxygenation

Components of Prime

- Asanguinous prime:
  - Crystalloid solutions:
    - BSS are preferred due to similar osmolarity and electrolyte composition
    - Most frequently used BSS are:
      - Ringers lactate
      - Plasmalyte
      - Normosol A
    - Glucose containing solutions are avoided
    - This is because high blood glucose is associated with CNS dynsfunction
    - Thus, blood sugars on CPB are restricted to below 180 g/dL
  - Colloid solutions:
    - Priming with crystalloids reduces colloid oncotic pressure of the perfusate
    - This promotes edema due to interstitial expansion with plasma water
    - Thus, colloids may be added to reduce this effect
    - A significant decline in plasma albumin occurs post-CPB
    - Thus, albumin is the most commonly used colloid in CPB-prime
    - However, the benefits of albumin addition is still controversial
  - Average prime volume is 1500–2500 mL
  - Minimal volume used is based on body weight/BSA
- Sanguinous prime:
  - Useful in patients with small circulating blood volumes
  - This is because CPB prime volume exceeds circulating blood volume
  - Thus, use of asanguinous prime may result in:
    - Severe anemia
    - Hypoproteinemia

- Thus, blood may be added to the CPB.prime in:
  - Children
  - Small adults
  - Patients with preoperative anemia to prevent dilutional anemia
- ❖ Other components which are added to make up prime:
  - Heparin for anticoagulation (2–2.5 IU per mL of prime)
  - Mannitol for diuresis 25–50 grams
  - Albumin to reduce postoperative edema
  - Calcium to prevent hypocalcemia due to citrate in transfused blood (200 mg/L)
  - Corticosteroids for anti-inflammatory action

Retrograde Autologous Priming

- ❖ This refers to the process of displacing prime solutions with patients own blood
- ❖ This reduces hemodilution occurring at the onset of CPB
- ❖ Initiated once the patient has been anticoagulated and cannula are in place
- ❖ The venous cannula is allowed to slowly drain the patients blood volume
- ❖ Trendelenburg position is necessary to improve RA filling pressure
- ❖ Circuit prime is slowly removed as the venous blood is drained to minimize hemodilution
- ❖ Hypotension may occur during venous emptying
- ❖ Phenylephrine may be administered to maintain systemic perfusion pressures
- ❖ Indications:
  - Limited blood availability
  - Rare blood group types
  - Jehovahs witness patients
- ❖ *Disadvantages*: may result in transient ST-changes and myocardial ischemia during drainage

PULSATILE CPB

Introduction

- ❖ Early mechanical pumps delivered non-pulsatile flow which is un-physiological
- ❖ Pulsatile CPB refers to intermittent delivery of high amplitude pressure and flow pulses during CPB

Rationale

- ❖ Pulsatile flow during CPB is more physiological
- ❖ This improves major organ perfusion and augments oxygen delivery at tissue level
- ❖ Improved tissue oxygenation occurs as a result of:
  - Motion of tissue fluid around cell membranes
  - Improvement in tissue microcirculation
  - Increased diffusion
  - Enhanced oxygen consumption

Mechanisms of Action

- ❖ Decreases systemic vascular resistance
- ❖ Increases capillary patency
- ❖ Reduces venous sludging
- ❖ Enhances lymphatic drainage, reducing edema
- ❖ Attenuated inflammatory response to CPB

Effects of Pulsatile Flow

- ❖ Effects on blood: reduced hemolysis compared to non-pulsatile flow
- ❖ Effects on hemodynamics and microcirculation:
  - Pulsatile flow decreases SVR due to:
    - Increased baroreceptor afferent activity
    - This inhibits vasomotor discharge and causes reduced SVR
    - Changes in catecholamine levels
    - Hydraulic energy of pulsatile flow maintaining microcirculatory patency
  - Pulsatile flow preserves microcirculation and improves tissue metabolism
- ❖ Effect on endocrine system:
  - Reduced circulating levels of catecholamines
  - Reduced renin activity
  - Decreased angiotensin II levels
  - Decreased anti-diuretic hormone levels
- ❖ Effects on renal function:
  - Better preservation of renal function
  - Increased urine output
  - Intrarenal redistribution of blood flow to preserve cortical perfusion
- ❖ Effects on cardiovascular system:
  - Improves myocardial oxygen extraction
  - Improves subendocardial perfusion
  - Decreases intramyocardial arteriovenous shunting
  - Increases flow through myocardial microcirculation
- ❖ Pulmonary effects:
  - Decreases PVR
  - Does not produce any change in gas exchange
- ❖ Effects on central nervous system:
  - Improve cerebral microcirculation
  - Preserves CBF when autoregulation is impaired

Blood Pumps Used for Pulsatile CPB

- Roller pumps:
  - First pulsatile roller pump made by Stockert company in 1970
  - Pulsatility of roller pumps is achieved through 2 modifications:
    - Modification of pump head design with low inertia
    - Incorporation of *stepping motor* mechanism
  - Pulsatility is produced by the *ripple-flow pattern*
  - Output produced by roller pumps cannot be described as physiologically pulsatile
  - Thus, roller pumps may not be the most effective way of producing pulsatile CPB
- Ventricular blood pumps:
  - Most physiological means of producing pulsatile CPB
  - Operate in a manner similar to the cardiac ventricles
  - Consists of a compressible sac with 2 one-way valves
  - Valves allow blood to flow into the sac in one direction only
  - These systems are driven using hydraulic mechanisms
  - The hydraulic mechanism uses distilled water as the drive medium
  - The distilled water is pumped into the sac present in the blood chamber
  - This displaces a volume of blood from the blood chamber producing forward flow
  - The output from the ventricular system depends upon:
    - Frequency of compression of the sac
    - Stroke volume of the sac
  - Widespread use of these pumps is hampered due to high cost
- Compression plate pumps:
  - Compression plate pumps function similar to ventricular pumps
  - A length of the CPB tubing is placed on the rigid backplate
  - This is compressed by the moving plate to produce forward pulsatile flow
  - Unidirectional flow is ensured by valves present on inlet and outlet of the tube
- Centrifugal pumps: cannot produce pulsatile flow as it requires very high rotational speeds
- Pulsatile assist devices:
  - Intermittent occlusive devices utilizing intra-aortic balloon pump apparatus
  - Pulse is generated by repeated inflation and deflation of the balloon within aorta
  - This can be used at the beginning and termination of CPB to produce pulsations

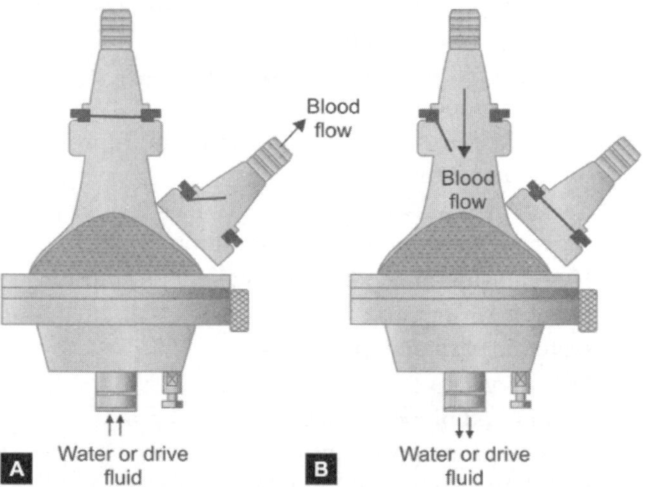

Figs. 21A and B: Ventricular blood pump for pulsatile CPB.

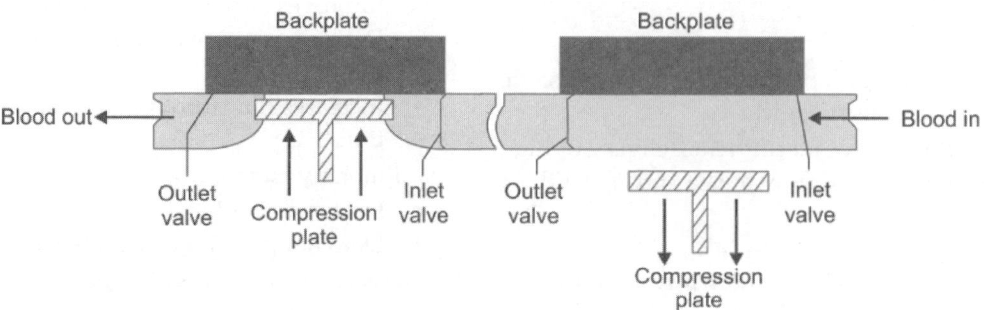

Fig. 22: Compression plate pump for pulsatile CPB.

Circuit Design

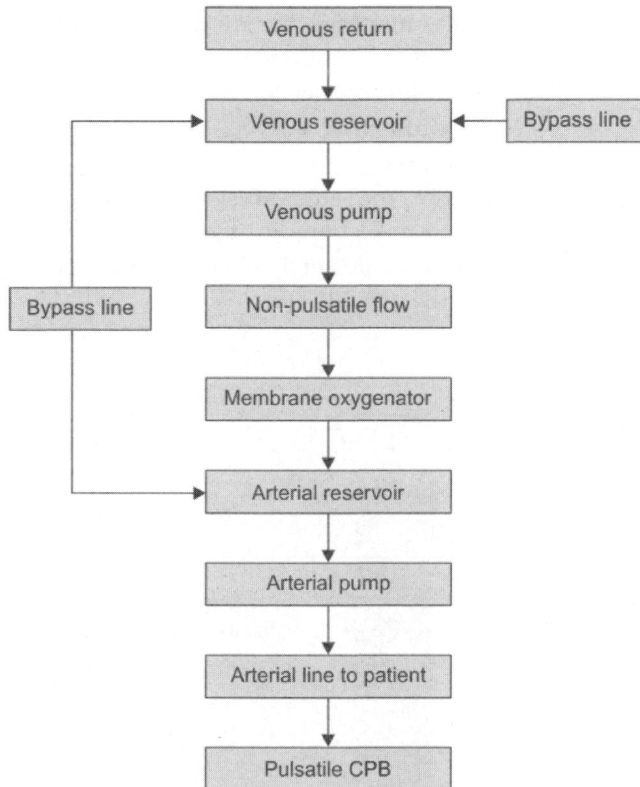

Factors Influencing Pulsatile CPB

- Hemodilution
- Drugs which alter systemic vascular resistance
- Degree of hypothermia
- Changes in perfusion flow rate
- Type of pump employed

Advantages

- Superior organ preservation
- Better postoperative cardiac, renal and pulmonary outcomes
- Increases regional CBF after DHCA
- Increases CBF when autoregulation is impaired
- Reduces neuronal cell loss following global cerebral ischemia
- Decreases need for inotropic support post-CPB
- Reduces hospital stay
- Better outcomes following pediatric open heart surgeries

Disadvantages

- Increases complexity of CPB
- Enhances destruction of RBCs and platelets

ULTRAFILTRATION

Introduction

- Utrafiltration (UF) refers to movement of water across a membrane due to hydrostatic pressure gradient
- Patients undergoing CPB develop fluid overload and electrolyte imbalances
- Exposure to foreign material increases capillary permeability
- This causes shifting on fluid into the extravascular space
- Ultrafiltration during CPB helps to attenuate these changes during CPB

Mechanism of Action

- UF is achieved through filtration of water across a semipermeable membrane
- The semipermeable membrane (SPM) permits water and small molecules to move across
- This is done using energy derived from hydrostatic pressure gradient
- Hydrostatic pressure gradient is created because:
  - Blood is rich in solutes
  - Ultrafiltrate side of the membrane does not have solutes
- Thus, small molecular solutes follow the concentration gradient across the membrane
- This results in the transfer of solutes from the blood into the ultrafiltrate
- This causes generation of a convection current or *solute drag*
- There also exists a pressure differential between:
  - Blood side of SPM
  - Ultrafiltrate side of SPM which is at atmospheric pressure
- This transmembrane pressure (TMP) results in the removal of plasma water from blood
- Thus, the ultrafiltrate becomes rich in water and small molecular solutes
- Typically solutes > 65,000 Da are not removed by ultrafiltration
- Cellular elements, plasma proteins and protein bound solutes are not removed by UF
- Thus, blood compartment loses water and undergoes hemoconcentration
- Rate of fluid removal depends upon:
  - Membrane permeability
  - Transmembrane pressure
  - Blood flow
  - Hematocrit

❖ Membrane permeability is determined by:
  - Pore size
  - Membrane material
  - Membrane thickness

Technical Considerations

❖ Ultrafiltrator design:
  - Ultrafilters are made of a microporous membrane extrudes into hollow fibers
  - Hollow fibers are 180–200 µm in diameter
  - Pores of the membrane are between 5 and 10 nm
  - Thousands of hollow fibers are configured in a bundle
  - These fibers are encased in a solid polycarbonate shell
  - Ultrafiltrators are designed to have high filtration rates (*high flux*)
  - Typical rate of UF varies from 2 to 50 mL/hour/mm Hg transmembrane pressure

❖ Ultrafiltration circuit:
  - Hemofilter is configured as a passive shunt parallel to the CPB circuit
  - It is configured as a passive shunt from a high-pressure level to low-pressure level
  - Thus, flow through UF is dependent on pressure differential between:
    - Inflow line
    - Outflow line
  - Inflow into the circuit is through a connection from the high-pressure arterial line
  - The inflow line is therefore placed distal to the arterial pump
  - The outflow line from the UF returns to a low-pressure port
  - The outflow line connection can be located in:
    - Venous reservoir
    - Venous line
  - Tubing from the effluent side of the UF is attached to a collection canister
  - The collection canister is usually placed 60–90 cm below the ultrafiltrator

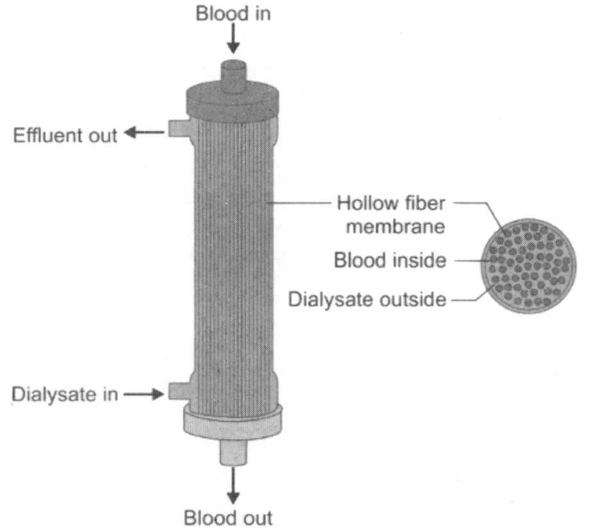

Fig. 23: Design of hollow fiber ultrafilter.

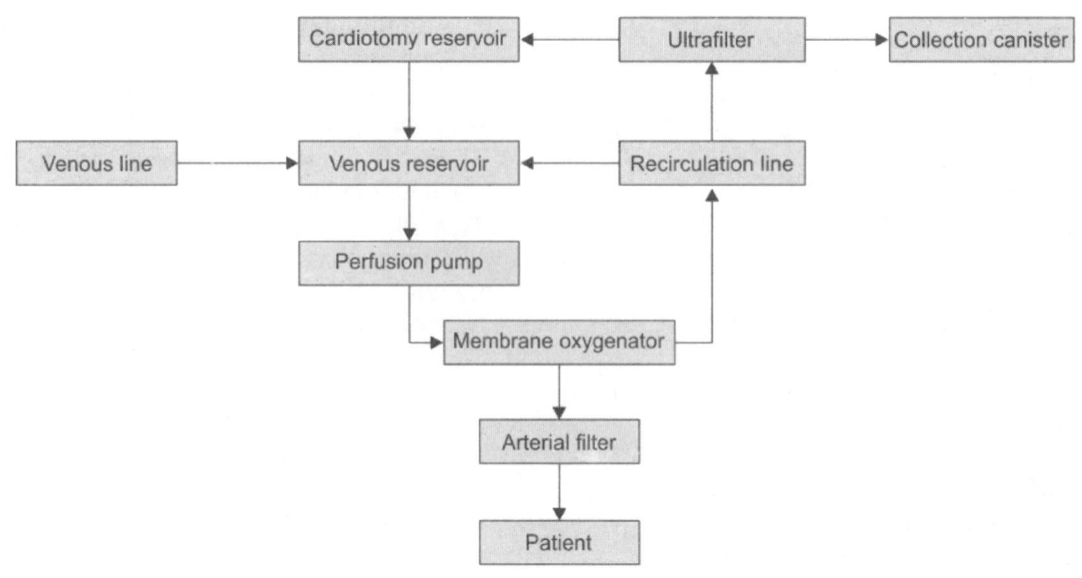

Indications

- Congestive cardiac failure
- Renal failure
- Neonatal cardiac surgeries

Uses of Ultrafiltration

- Hemoconcentration:
  - UF removes plasma water without causing any flux of cellular elements
  - Thus, it results in hemoconcentration
  - This prevents anemia and reduces the need for postoperative blood transfusion
- Reduction of tissue edema:
  - Solutes > 65,000 Da are not removed by ultrafiltration
  - Thus, plasma proteins concentration is increased during UF
  - This results in an increase in colloid oncotic pressure
  - Thus, tissue edema is prevented postoperatively
  - Optimization of electrolytes:
    - UF cause diffusion of electrolytes and other small solutes
    - This results in optimization of electrolytes and BUN in renal failure patients
- Inflammatory response:
  - Cytokine and complement factors are filtered during UF
  - Thus, UF greatly attenuates the inflammatory response

Advantages

- Decreases total body water
- Prevents anemia
- Reduces requirement for blood transfusion
- Prevents reduction in plasma protein levels
- Decreases myocardial edema
- Improves LV systolic function
- Decreases lung water
- Improves pulmonary compliance
- Reduces postoperative ventilatory support
- Optimizes intraoperative fluid balance
- Reduces inflammatory mediators and attenuates SIRS
- Improves perioperative hemostasis
- Decreases postoperative blood loss

Factors Influencing Outcomes of Ultrafiltration

- Ultrafiltration related variables:
  - Type of ultrafiltration
  - Duration of UF
  - Volume of ultrafiltrate obtained
- Patient related variables:
  - Young age
  - Presence of pulmonary arterial HTN
  - Complex surgery requiring long CPB time
- CPB related variables:
  - Prime volume
  - Use of sanguinous prime
  - Complex CPB techniques such as DHCA
  - Use of concomitant anti-inflammatory therapies such as steroids

Disadvantages of Ultrafiltration

- May result in hypovolemia and hemodynamic instability
- RBC trauma and increase in free plasma hemoglobin
- Anticoagulation:
  - Heparin being a large molecule is not filtered by UF
  - Thus, UF increases concentration of heparin in hemoconcentrated blood
- Increase in CPB time with MUF
- Adds to cost of surgery

Types of Ultrafiltration

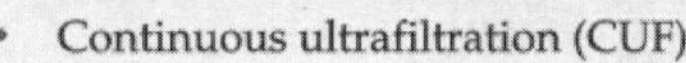

- Continuous ultrafiltration (CUF)
- Modified ultrafiltration (MUF)
- Zero-balanced ultrafiltration (ZBUF)
- Dilutional ultrafiltration (DUF)
- Prime ultrafiltration (PUF)

Continuous Ultrafiltration

- Performed during CPB from the time of rewarming to termination of CPB
- Aims primarily at removing excess plasma water and concentrate cellular elements
- Electrolytes and small solutes are also removed in equal concentration to plasma water
- Thus, plasma concentration of diffusible solutes remains unchanged
- Cytokine and complement levels reach their peak during rewarming
- Thus, CUF during this period greatly attenuates the inflammatory response

- However, continuous loss of volume may result in depletion of reservoir volume
- Thus, this technique of ultrafiltration is limited by the blood reservoir volume

Modified Ultrafiltration

Introduction

- In MUF, ultrafiltration is done following termination of CPB
- Residual contents of ECC are ultrafiltered and transfused back to the patient
- This is performed when the patient is still cannulated and attached to ECC
- Thus, this technique of UF is not limited by the reservoir volume

Technique

- Arteriovenous MUF:
  - Requires a separate roller pump
  - The cardioplegia pump system is usually preferred as:
    - It is already connected to the arterial side of ECC
    - Contains heat exchanger which prevents cooling of the patient
    - Enables pressure monitoring
  - The roller pump draws blood from the patient through the arterial line
  - Blood is then passed through the ultrafilter and concentrated
  - The return volume is pumped back into the patient through venous line into RA
  - This allows removal of excess water from the plasma and salvage of CPB blood
  - Once the venous reservoir is emptied, BSS is added to the reservoir
  - MUF is continued until all the residual blood is transfused to the patient
  - This leaves the CPB circuit primed with crystalloid
- Veno-venous MUF:
  - Blood is drawn from the right atrium and returned to the RA
  - Efficacy of MUF is limited due to recirculation

Advantages

- MUF is most effective in pediatric patients
- This is because of:
  - Use of large prime volumes relative to patients blood volume
  - Use of DHCA during surgery
- Advantages include:
  - Reduction in postoperative morbidity
  - Reduced blood loss and postoperative transfusion
  - Reduced inflammatory mediators
  - Improvement of myocardial systolic function
  - Improvement in cerebral oxygenation
- Additionally, MUF allows almost all the circuit contents to be concentrated and transfused without risk of hypervolemia
- MUF efficacy does not depend on the venous reservoir volume

Disadvantages

- Increases CPB time by 10–20 minutes
- Protamine administration has to be withheld during MUF

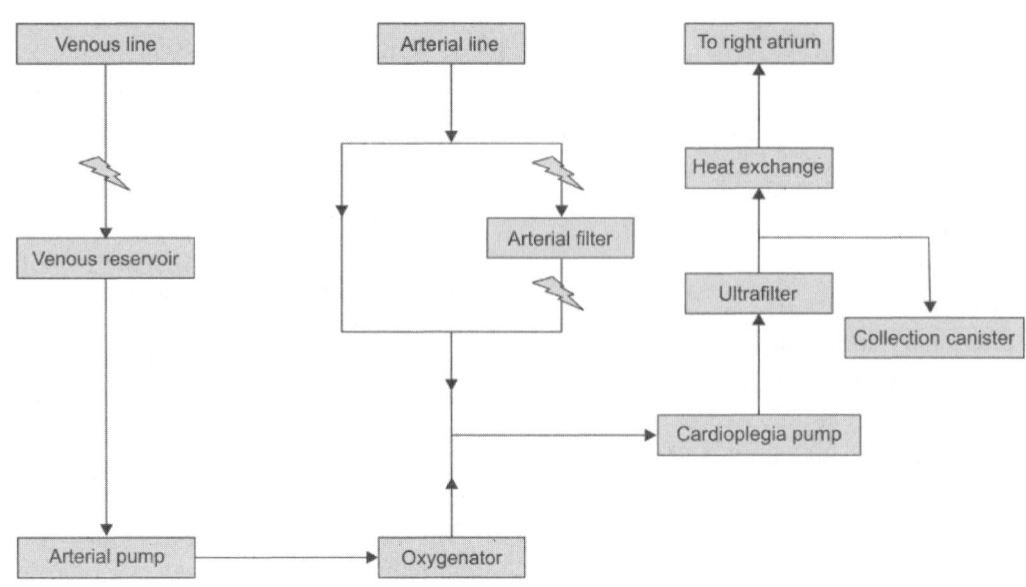

Complications

- Air embolism:
  - During MUF, blood is actively drawn from arterial line
  - This may result in entrainment of air from aortic cannulation site purse strings
  - Air can also be entrained due to development of negative pressure within circuit
  - This can occur due to kinking or clamping of aortic cannula/line
- Diastolic run-off:
  - High blood flows may be used to maintain flow through the MUF circuit
  - This may result in diastolic run-off and increase risk of intracranial steal
  - This can lead to reduced cerebral blood flow velocities and low cerebral MvO_2

Endpoints for MUF

- Hematocrit 40%
- Time based end-points: usually restricted to 10–20 minutes
- Completion of total salvage of circuit contents
- Filtrate volume-based end point

Zero-Balanced Ultrafiltration

- ZBUF is a modification of CUF
- It is also performed during rewarming phase of CPB
- ZBUF is a technique where filtered plasma water is replaced with equal volume of BSS
- Thus, plasma volume following ZBUF remains constant
- Therefore, ZBUF does not result in hemoconcentration and improved HCT
- BSS used commonly during ZBUF:
  - Hartmanns solution
  - Ringers lactate
  - Plasmalyte A
  - Normosol
- These solutions contain acetate or lactate which undergo conversion to bicarbonate
- This balances the bicarbonate lost during ZBUF filtration
- ZBUF may be used to treat hyperkalemia during CPB
- In these cases, BSS cannot be used as they contain potassium > 4 mEq/L
- Thus, normal saline may be used as the ZBUF replacement fluid
- ZBUF aims to remove inflammatory mediators primarily
- Also, since BSS is added to the venous reservoir, reservoir volume remains constant

Prime Ultrafiltration

- Banked PRBCs are used in pediatric patients to prime CPB circuit
- This may result in hyperkalemia and high lactate levels within the prime
- These have to be normalized prior to initiation of CPB to prevent cardiac arrest
- Ultrafiltration may be used in these cases prior to initiation of CPB to normalize prime
- The volume removed may be replaced with BSS to attain the necessary HCT
- This is called prime ultrafiltration
- Advantages:
  - Lowers plasma concentration of bradykinin and HMW kininogen
  - Reduces hyperkalemia and hyperlactatemia
  - Attenuates inflammatory response

Dilutional Ultrafiltration

- DUF is a modification of MUF
- Technically similar to ZBUF modification of CUF
- In this, BSS is added to the reservoir during MUF to maintain reservoir volume
- Ultrafiltration typically is performed at 40–70 mL/kg/hour
- Small aliquots of Plasmalyte A (< 20 mL/kg) is added during UF
- Volume of BSS is titrated to maintain safe reservoir volume

BLOOD GAS MANAGEMENT STRATEGIES ON CPB

Introduction

- Solubility of oxygen and carbon dioxide increases at low temperatures
- Thus, blood gas management strategies during hypothermia of CPB vary

Physiology

- Changes in $PaCO_2$ and PaO_2 with cooling:
  - According to Henrys law:
    - Amount of dissolved gas is proportional to its partial pressure above the liquid

$$H = C/P$$

- Where:
    - H = Henrys law constant
    - C = Concentration of gas in solution
    - P = Partial pressure of the gas
- Temperature affects the equilibrium constant (H) for the solvation process
- Thus, with cooling solubility of CO_2 and O_2 increases resulting in an increase in C
- This causes a reduction in the partial pressure of the gases (P)

❖ Changes in pH with cooling:
- Proton dissociation is an endothermic reaction where:

$$HA = H^+ + A^-$$

- Hypothermia promotes equilibration to the left with increased formation of HA
- Thus, concentration of protons in solution reduces
- This causes a linear reduction in pH with temperature causing alkalosis

Rationale

❖ During hypothermic CPB, solubility of CO_2 and O_2 increases

❖ This results in increased presence of gases in solution

❖ Thus, measured partial pressures of gases in blood samples will be low

❖ This causes reduced PaO_2 and $PaCO_2$ in vivo:
- $PaCO_2$ reduces by 5 mm Hg for each degree below 37°C
- $PaCO_2$ reduces by 2 mm Hg for each degree below 37°C

❖ Blood gas analyzers warm the blood to 37°C prior to measurement

❖ Thus, the results will show a higher PaO_2 and $PaCO_2$ and lower pH than actually present

❖ Modern blood gas machines can calculate pH values for the actual patient temperature

❖ This is calculated by application of ***Rosenthal correction factor*** to pH measured at 37°C

❖ Change in pH = 0.015 pH units per degree change in temperature

❖ Thus, two different strategies exist for management of ABGs at hypothermia:
- Alpha stat:
    - Here pH measured by the ABG machine is not temperature corrected
    - Blood samples are measured at 37°C, resulting in:
        - Higher PaO_2 levels
        - Higher $PaCO_2$ levels
        - Lower pH levels
    - Thus, patients actual $PaCO_2$ values are not known
    - In this strategy, ABGs are simply compared to normal results at 37°C
- pH-stat strategy:
    - Here, pH measured by the machine is corrected to patients temperature
    - This is done using Rosenthal factor
    - This results in higher pH levels (alkaline pH)
    - The alkaline pH is treated during CPB by addition of carbon dioxide

ALPHA-STAT STRATEGY

Introduction

❖ Refers to patient temperature-uncorrected method of measuring ABGs

❖ No CO_2 is added to the oxygenator gas to compensate for hypothermic pH variations

❖ This is a mechanism which prevails naturally in reptiles

Rationale

❖ Alpha is the degree of dissociation of ions

❖ Alpha refers to the ratio of:
- Protonated histidine-imidazole groups
- Total histidine-imidazole groups

❖ Alpha value of 0.55 is considered optimal for the function of intracellular enzymes

❖ Alpha value and total CO_2 levels remain constant during cooling

❖ Therefore, structure and function of intracellular enzymes remains unchanged

❖ Thus, in this strategy external CO_2 is not added to maintain pH

Changes Occurring during Alpha Stat Management

❖ Results in lower cerebral blood flows than during pH-stat management

❖ But, flow-metabolism coupling is maintained due to reduced metabolic requirements

❖ As pH is more alkaline, brain tissue pH is increased

❖ Shifts ODC to the left increasing affinity of hemoglobin to oxygen

Current Use

- Preferred in adult patients
- Strategy is used commonly during rewarming following DHC:
  - This is because embolic load is maximal during rewarming
  - Use of pH-stat during this phase by addition of CO_2 causes cerebral vasodilatation
  - This may increase chances of cerebral embolism
  - Thus, alpha-stat strategy is preferred during rewarming

Advantages

- Preserves cerebral autoregulation
- Maintains cerebral flow-metabolism coupling
- Optimizes intracellular enzyme activity
- Avoids cerebral vasodilatation
- Reduces cerebral embolic load
- Better cerebral protection due to intracellular alkaline pH

Disadvantages

- Causes less metabolic suppression during hypothermia
- Intracellular alkalosis during cooling
- Suboptimal cerebral oxygenation during rapid rewarming
- Shifts ODC to the left increasing affinity of oxygen to hemoglobin
- Requires higher hematocrit as ODC is shifted to left

PH-STAT STRATEGY

Introduction

- In this method, pH is maintained constant at the patients own temperature
- Thus, hypothermia induced alkalosis is corrected by addition of CO_2
- Aims at maintaining normal $PaCO_2$ and pH values in-vivo in hypothermic blood
- It is a mechanism which prevails naturally in hibernating animals

Rationale

- During hypothermia, pH becomes progressively alkaline
- With pH-stat strategy, this is corrected by addition of carbon-dioxide
- This results in the intracellular pH becoming more acidotic

Method

- Accomplished usually by reducing sweep speed of the air-oxygen mixture
- Rarely, CO_2 may be added to the inspired fresh gas flow delivered to the oxygenator
- Target values maintained using this strategy are:
  - pH of 7.40
  - $PaCO_2$ of 40 mm Hg

Changes Occurring during pH Stat Management

- Compared to alpha-stat, pH-stat leads to higher $PaCO_2$ levels
- This results in an increased cerebral blood flow
- Addition of CO_2 also causes respiratory and intracellular acidosis
- Intracellular acidosis also causes a shift in ODC to the right

Current Use

- Preferred in pediatric patients
- Used during cooling for DHCA as:
  - Addition of CO_2 results in cerebral vasodilatation
  - Thus, CBF is improved prior to institution of DHCA
  - Thus, cerebral cooling is enhanced and more uniform due to increased CBF

Advantages

- Causes sustained dilatation of cerebral blood vessels
- Increases cerebral blood flow
- Enhances cerebral oxygenation
- Causes quick and evenly distributed brain cooling
- Maintains normal intracellular pH during cooling
- Causes faster recovery of intracellular pH
- Shifts ODC to right causing increased availability of oxygen to the tissues
- Improves neurological outcomes in pediatric patients

Disadvantages

- Autoregulation of brain perfusion is lost
- CBF varies with perfusion pressure
- Increases embolic load to the brain
- Increases risk of regional ischemia through steal phenomenon in collaterals
- Increases risk of cognitive function when CPB time > 90 minutes
- Increases intracranial pressure and may cause cerebral edema

Differences between Alpha and pH Stat

No.	Feature	pH-stat	Alpha stat
1.	Aim	Constant pH	Constant OH^-/H^+
2.	Rationale	Temperature-corrected	Temperature-uncorrected
3.	Addition of carbon dioxide	Done	Not done
4.	Total carbon dioxide	Increased	Constant
5.	Intracellular state	Acidosis	Neutral
6.	Cerebral blood flow	Increased	Maintained
7.	Cerebral autoregulation	Lost	Maintained
8.	Cerebral embolic load	Increased	Decreased
9.	Intracerebral steal phenomenon	Present	Absent
10.	Cognitive dysfunction	Present	Rare
11.	Cerebral cooling	Uniform	Non-uniform
12.	ODC curve	Shifts to right	Shifts to left
13.	Patient preference	Pediatrics	Adults

Current Recommendations

- In adults, alpha-stat strategy during moderate hypothermia produces better outcomes
- No specific recommendations have been made for DHCA in adults
- In pediatric patients undergoing DHCA:
  - pH-stat strategy is used during cooling
  - Alpha-stat strategy is used during rewarming

PATHOPHYSIOLOGY OF CPB

Introduction

- Surgical procedures performed using CPB are unique
- This is because they produce physiological alterations not seen in other surgeries

Cardiovascular Changes during CPB

- Changes at the onset of CPB:
  - Hemodilution
  - Reduced systemic vascular resistance due to:
    - Hemodilution
    - Dilution of catecholamine
- Changes during CPB: slow rise in systemic vascular resistance due to:
  - Hypothermia
  - Rise in hematocrit
  - Stress response due to CPB
  - Closure of microvasculature
- Changes during rewarming:
  - Fall in systemic vascular resistance
  - Fall in mean arterial pressure
- Microcirculatory changes:
  - Precapillary arteriolar constriction
  - Interstitial edema
  - RBC deformability
  - Platelet and WBC aggregation
  - Reduced lymphatic drainage
  - Loss of pulsatile flow
- Ventricular dysfunction occurs following CPB due to:
  - Inadequate cardioplegia
  - Ventricular distension due to inadequate venting
  - Prolonged hypotension
  - Ischemia-reperfusion injury
  - Prolonged ventricular fibrillation
  - Microcirculatory changes

Pulmonary Changes during CPB

- Atelectasis due to:
  - Neuromuscular blockade during anesthesia
  - Cessation of ventilation
  - Resorption atelectasis due to perioperative use of high FiO_2
  - Surfactant depletion due to anesthesia and CPB
  - Use of low-tidal volume ventilation strategies
- Changes in lung mechanics due to:
  - Decreased vital capacity, FRC and lung compliance
  - Increased airway resistance
  - Opening of pleural cavity during surgery
- Acute lung injury (*pump-lung*) due to:
  - Capillary leak syndrome from histamine release
  - Pulmonary particulate emboli causing:
    - Complement activation
    - Neutrophil migration
    - Cytokine production
    - Arachidonic acid metabolites
  - Increased cytokine levels due to high perioperative FiO_2
- Altered pulmonary vascular resistance due to:
  - Pulmonary endothelin I
  - Reduced expression of nitric oxide by pulmonary endothelium
- Thus, pulmonary dysfunction following CPB can result from:
  - Intrapulmonary shunting and V/Q mismatch
  - Dead space ventilation
  - Hypoxic pulmonary vasoconstriction

- Vasoconstriction due to:
  - Circulating catecholamines
  - Sequestered neutrophils
- Damage to alveolar basement membrane due to:
  - Free radical injury
  - Complement activation
- Hydrostatic pulmonary edema due to inadequate LV venting
- Ischemia reperfusion injury
- Systemic inflammatory response
- Pulmonary emboli

❖ Treatment and prevention of CPB related pulmonary dysfunction:
- Atelectasis:
  - Use of CPAP immediately after separation from CPB
  - Use of recruitment maneuver post-CPB
  - *Open lung concept*:
    - It is an extrapolation of recruitment maneuver
    - Uses PCV to generate:
      - High airway pressure (40 cmH_2O)
      - Inverted I:E ratio (1:1)
- Acute lung injury:
  - Use of heparin coated circuits
  - Use of membrane oxygenators
  - Use of hemofiltration to reduce lung water
  - Use of leukocyte depletion filters
  - Perioperative use of protective lung ventilation strategy
  - Use of inhale nitric oxide

Changes in Neurological Function during CPB

❖ Factors affecting of neurological function during CPB:
- Temperature
- Mean arterial pressure
- Partial pressure of carbon dioxide
- Blood glucose levels
- Pulsatility of CPB
- Duration of CPB

❖ Etiology for adverse neurological outcomes following CPB:
- Cerebral embolism:
  - Air embolism (more common)
  - Particulate emboli from dislodgement of atherosclerotic plaques
- Hypoperfusion due to low MAP
- Hyper-perfusion as during inadvertent selective innominate A cannulation
- Inflammatory response

❖ Neurological complications following CPB:
- Type 1 neurological outcome:
  - Consists of:
    - Cerebral death
    - Non-fatal strokes
  - Risk factors for type 1 outcomes:
    - Aortic atherosclerosis
    - History of neurological disease
    - Older age
    - New transient ischemic attacks (TIAs)
- Type 2 neurological outcome (more common):
  - Consists of:
    - New intellectual deterioration at discharge
    - New onset seizures
  - Risk factors for type 2 outcomes:
    - Advanced age
    - Systolic HTN
    - Pulmonary disease
    - Alcoholism

Changes in Blood during CPB

❖ Changes in RBCs: Accelerated hemolysis due to:
- Exposure to foreign surface
- Presence of air-fluid interface
- Cardiotomy suction
- Excessive occlusion pressure of roller pump
- High flow rates on CPB

❖ Changes in WBCs:
- Activation of neutrophils and monocytes
- Sequestration in lung, heart and skeletal muscle during cooling
- Re-entry of sequestered WBCs into circulation during rewarming
- Release of immature WBCs from bone marrow causing neutrophilia

❖ Changes in platelets:
- Reduction in platelet count by 30–50% due to:
  - Hemodilution
  - ECC surface adhesion
  - Mechanical disruption from shear stress
  - Hypothermia
  - Sequestration in lungs and spleen
  - Consumptive coagulopathy
- Reduced platelet response to stimulation by ADP and thrombin
- Reduced adherence capacity of platelets due to low vWF levels
- Contact activation on exposure to circuit

- Changes in coagulation system:
  - Activation of contact system:
    - Also called kinin-kallikrein system
    - Consists of:
      - Factor XII
      - Factor XI
      - Prekallikrein
      - High-molecular weight kininogen (HMWK)
    - Contact with negatively charged surface of ECC activates factor XII
    - This causes activation of:
      - The contact system
      - Intrinsic coagulation cascade
  - Plasmatic coagulopathy following CPB due to:
    - Fibrinogen depletion
    - Consumptive coagulopathy
    - Residual heparinization
    - Hyperfibrinolysis due to release of tissue plasminogen activator
- Changes in plasma proteins:
  - Denaturation of proteins due to air-blood interface
  - Altered enzyme function causing coagulopathy
  - Aggregation of proteins causing microcirculatory occlusion

Changes in Kidney during CPB

- Depression of renal function due to:
  - Non-pulsatile flow
  - Renal microcirculatory changes
  - Redistribution of blood from cortex to outer medulla
  - Reduced blood flow during hypotension
  - Depressed tubular function due to hypothermia
- Acute tubular necrosis from hemoglobinuria due to hemolysis
- Risk factors for renal dysfunction:
  - Preoperative risk factors:
    - High serum creatinine
    - Elevated creatinine clearance (most important)
    - Advanced age > 63 years
    - Preoperative nephrotoxic agents such as:
      - Radiocontrast agents
      - ACE inhibitors
      - Aminoglycosides
      - NSAIDs do not increase risk of AKI if preoperative renal function is normal
  - Operative risk factors:
    - Prolonged CPB time > 130 minutes
    - Use of intra-aortic balloon pulsations
    - Development of systemic inflammatory response
    - Inappropriate hemodilution on CPB
- Prevention and treatment of AKI during CPB:
  - Judicious fluids to maintain euvolemia during surgery is key
  - Avoidance of large amounts to saline to prevent hyperchloremia
  - Avoidance of nephrotoxic colloids such as HES and albumin
  - Fenoldopam 0.05 μg/kg/min may be useful
  - Corticosteroids: routine use is not recommended to preserve renal function
  - Furosemide: routine use is not recommended
  - *Mannitol*: does not improve renal outcome
  - Renal-protective dose of dopamine: no longer used as:
  - No proven clinical benefit
  - Increased incidence of atrial fibrillation

Changes in Endocrine System

- Pituitary hormones:
  - Anterior pituitary hormones are not significantly altered during CPB
  - In patients with pituitary adenomas however, pituitary apoplexy may occur
  - Significant increase in ADH secreted by posterior pituitary can occur with CPB
- Thyroid hormones:
  - CPB results in the development of *sick-euthyroid syndrome*
  - This is characterized by:
    - Low serum T_3 levels
    - Normal or reduced T_4 levels
    - Reduced free thyroxine levels
    - Normal TSH levels
- Adrenal hormones:
  - Marked elevation of catecholamines is seen following CPB
  - Increased secretion of ACTH and cortisol can occur during CPB
  - Natriuretic hormones (ANP and BNP) are increased following CPB
- Hormones of RAA axis:
  - Levels of renin, angiotensin II and aldosterone increase after CPB
  - Conversely, ACE secretion by the lungs is depressed by CPB

- ❖ Glucose homeostasis is altered during CPB due to:
  - Reduced insulin production
  - Insulin resistance
  - Reduce glucose utilization due to hypothermia and reduced metabolism
  - Stress response resulting in:
    - Increased gluconeogenesis
    - Increased glycogenolysis
  - Increased renal reabsorption of glucose

Systemic Inflammatory Response after CPB (SIRAB)

- ❖ Initiation of the inflammatory response occurs due to:
  - Contact activation to circuit on repeated passage of blood through ECC
  - Contact activation to cardiotomy sucker
  - Ischemia-reperfusion injury
  - Endotoxemia
- ❖ Activation of immune response by:
  - Factor XII (principal event triggering inflammation)
  - Complement activation:
    - Anaphylo-toxins C3a, C5a
    - C1q, C3b
  - Other mediators such as:
    - Cytokines
    - Leukotrienes
    - Kallikrein-Bradykinin
    - Platelet activating factor
    - Nitric oxide
- ❖ Immune response consists of:
  - Cellular immune responses:
  - Neutrophils:
    - Neutrophil rolling
    - Neutrophil adhesion
    - Neutrophil migration to intestitium
    - Reduction in lymphocyte count
  - Endothelial response: damage due to:
    - Surgical damage
    - Turbulent flow during CPB
    - Shear stress
    - Ischemia-reperfusion injury
- ❖ Methods to prevent SIRAB:
  - Surgical strategies:
    - Preference for off-pump techniques (OPCAB)
    - Preoperative selective digestive decontamination
    - Reduce cardiotomy suction use
  - CPB strategies:
    - Use of cell saver to filter cardiotomy suction blood
    - Filter for cardiotomy suction blood
    - Miniaturization of CPB circuit
    - Use of heparin coated CPB circuit
    - Use of centrifugal pumps
    - Priming the CPB circuit with colloids
    - Use of pulsatile CPB
    - Use of ultrafiltration
  - Pharmacological adjuncts:
    - Corticosteroids: suboptimal results in multicentric trials
    - Pexelizumab (C5 complement inhibitor)
    - Protease inhibitors (aprotinin)
    - Cyclosporine

VENTRICULAR SEPTAL DEFECT

Introduction

- ❖ It refers to an abnormal communication between the two ventricles
- ❖ First identified by Dalrymple in the year 1847

Incidence

- ❖ VSDs are the most common congenital heart lesions in children
- ❖ They are the second most common congenital heart lesion in adults
- ❖ Isolated VSDs account for around 15–20% of all congenital heart defects
- ❖ Incidence of isolated VSDs is about 0.3% of newborns
- ❖ As many as 90% of them eventually close spontaneously
- ❖ Incidence is higher in premature infants and also slightly higher in males
- ❖ This does not include those seen as a part of cyanotic CHDs

Embryology

- ❖ Single ventricle divided into two by the union of:
  - Membranous portion of ventricular septum
  - Bulbus cordis
  - Endocardial cushions
- ❖ Formation of septum occurs in fifth week of intrauterine life
- ❖ Development of VSD due to:
  - Peri-membranous VSD: Defects in development of membranous septum

- Outlet VSD: failure of fusion of conus septum
- Inlet VSD: failure of fusion of endocardial cushion with muscular septum
- Muscular VSD: inadequate fusion of medial walls of right and left ventricles

Anatomy

- Ventricular septum is divided into:
  - Small membranous portion
  - Large muscular portion
- Membranous septum:
  - Is a small area immediately beneath the aortic valve
  - Membranous defects involving adjacent muscular septum are called peri-membranous defect
- Muscular septum:
  - It has three parts:
    - Inlet septum
    - Trabecular septum: also called muscular septum
    - Outlet septum: also called infundibular or conal septum
  - Trabecular septum is further divided into anterior, posterior, middle and apical portions
- Peri-membranous VSDs (PM-VSD):
  - Located in the membranous septum, inferior to crista supraventricularis
  - These are the most common type of VSD
  - 70% VSDs are peri-membranous VSDs
  - These defects are also called:
    - Membranous defects
    - Cono-ventricular/infra-cristal defects
    - Subaortic VSDs
  - Peri-membranous defects are situated:
    - Just beneath the aortic valve
    - Behind the septal leaflet of the tricuspid valve
  - Aneurysm of the ventricular septum:
    - PM-VSDs can undergo complete or partial closure by septal leaflet of TV
    - This forms a tricuspid valve pouch or aneurysm of the septum
  - Aortic cusp prolapse:
    - PM-VSDs may cause prolapse of the aortic cusp into the defect
    - Right aortic cusp is commonly involved causing aortic regurgitation
  - Bundle of His:
    - It is closely related to posteroinferior margin of PM-VSDs
    - Thus, heart block is a potential complication of corrective surgery
  - According to the accompanying defect in the muscular septum, PM-VSDs are classified as:
    - Peri-membranous inlet: AV canal type
    - Peri-membranous trabecular
    - Peri-membranous outlet: tetralogy type
- Outlet VSDs:
  - Also called:
    - Infundibular VSDs
    - Conal or conal-septal VSDs
    - Subpulmonic or subarterial VSDs
    - Subarterial double committed VSDs
  - Accounts for 5–7% of defects in Western countries
  - More common in the Asian population (up to 30% incidence)
  - Defect is located immediately beneath the pulmonary and aortic valve
  - Therefore, part of its rim is formed by the aortic and pulmonary annulus
  - May be associated with aortic regurgitation secondary to aortic cusp prolapse
  - These defects rarely undergo spontaneous closure
- Inlet VSDs:
  - Also called AV canal type VSDs
  - Accounts for 5–8% of all VSDs
  - Defect is located posterior and inferior to peri-membranous defect
  - These defects do not close spontaneously
  - Bundle of His is closely related to antero-superior quadrant of inlet VSDs
  - These defects are also closely related to septal leaflet of tricuspid valve
- Muscular VSDs:
  - Account for 5–20% of all VSDs
  - Frequently appear to be multiple
  - Depending on the location of the defect in the trabecular septum, they are classified as:
    - Anterior trabecular VSDs (anterior-muscular)
    - Mid-trabecular VSDs (mid-muscular)
    - Posterior trabecular VSDs (posterior-muscular)
    - Apical muscular VSDs
  - Mid-muscular VSD is located posterior to septal band
  - Apical muscular defect is located near cardiac apex: Difficult to visualize and repair
  - Anterior defects are usually multiple, small and tortuous

- Swiss cheese pattern:
  - Multiple muscular defects present
  - Involve all components of ventricular septum
  - Extremely difficult to close surgically

Classification

- Surgical classification:
  - Type 1: also called infundibular or outlet VSDs
  - Type 2: also called membranous VSDs
  - Type 3: also called inlet or atrioventricular canal type of VSDs
  - Type 4: also called muscular or trabecular VSDs
- Anatomical classification:
  - Peri-membranous VSD (70%):
    - Peri-membranous inlet extension (AV canal type)
    - Peri-membranous trabecular extension (typical type)
    - Peri-membranous outlet extension (Tetralogy type)
  - Muscular VSDs (25%):
    - Inlet VSDs
    - Trabecular VSDs:
      - Anterior trabecular VSDs (anterior-muscular)
      - Mid-trabecular VSDs (mid-muscular)
      - Posterior trabecular VSDs (posterior-muscular)
      - Apical muscular VSDs
    - Subarterial or outlet VSDs
    - Inlet VSDs

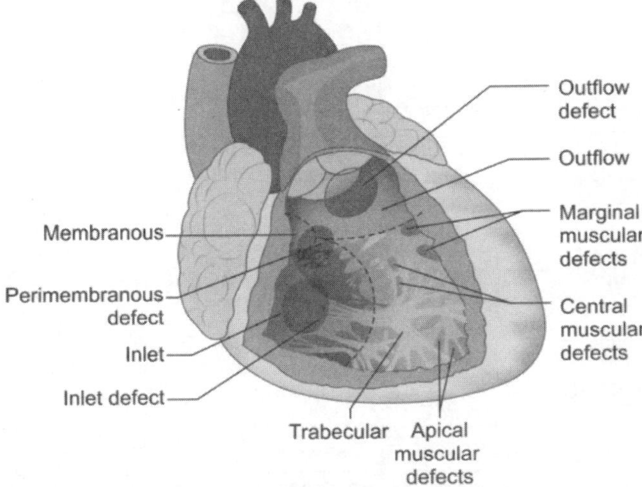

Fig. 24: Type's of VSD.

- Classification according to size of VSD:
  - Small VSD:
    - Left-right shunting occurs across the VSD
    - Only small amount of blood gets shunted into RV
    - RV pressure becomes 25–30% of LV pressure
    - This shunted volume enters PA, LA and then LV
    - But, owing to small volume of shunt, chamber enlargement does not occur
    - Degree of volume work on the LV is also too small to produce LVH
    - Clinical findings are:
      - Absent or minimal chamber enlargement
      - Shunt itself produces a regurgitant systolic murmur
      - P_2 is normal as the PA pressure is normal
      - X-ray and ECG are essentially normal
  - Moderate VSD:
    - Left-right shunting occurs across the VSD
    - Significantly larger quantity of blood is shunted across into the RV
    - The RV pressure becomes 30–50% of the LV pressure
    - Shunting is at ventricular level during systole
    - Since RV is also contracting, shunted blood directly goes into PA
    - Thus, shunted blood entering RV is directed immediately into PA, LA and LV
    - Thus, RV does not enlarge in moderate sized VSDs
    - However, enlargement of PA, LA and LV occurs
    - Also, pulmonary vascular markings become more prominent
    - Clinical findings are:
      - Shunt produces a regurgitant systolic murmur
      - Elevated PA pressure may produce slight increase in intensity of P_2
      - Relative mitral stenosis produces a mid-diastolic rumble at apex
    - ECG findings:
      - Volume overwork done by the LV is significant: LVH occurs
      - However, there are no signs of RV enlargement
    - X-ray shows hypertrophy of LA and LV with pulmonary plethora
  - Large VSD:
    - Left-right shunting occurs across the VSD
    - Large quantity of blood is shunted across into the RV

- The RV pressure becomes 60–80% of the LV pressure
- Shunting is at ventricular level during systole
- Since RV is also contracting, shunted blood directly goes into PA
- Owing to large size of VSD, LV pressure gets directly transmitted to RV
- This results in enlargement of RV, PA, LA and LV
- Clinical findings are:
  - Shunt produces a regurgitant murmur
  - Loud P_2 due to grossly elevated PA pressures
  - Relative mitral stenosis produces a mid-diastolic rumble at apex
- ECG shows biventricular hypertrophy with LA enlargement
- X-ray shows:
  - Biventricular hypertrophy
  - LA enlargement
  - Pulmonary plethora

- Large VSD with Eisenmangers syndrome:
  - Pulmonary vascular occlusive disease results
  - This produces irreversible changes in the pulmonary arterioles
  - PVR increases to reach systemic levels
  - Also, RV pressure becomes equal to LV pressure
  - This decreases magnitude of L-R shunt and results in a bidirectional shunt
  - Thus, volume overload on the LA and LV reduces
  - However, RV enlarges owing to raised PVR
  - This results in enlargement of RV, while LA and LV remain normal in size
  - Clinical signs are:
    - Cyanosis and clubbing occurs
    - Reduced intensity of shunt murmur due to reduced volume of shunt
    - Single and loud P_2 owing to elevated PA pressures
  - ECG show signs of RVH
  - Chest X-ray:
    - Shows RV enlargement with normal sized LA and LV
    - Main PA and hilar segment remains enlarged
    - Peripheral pulmonary oligemia occurs

Pathophysiology

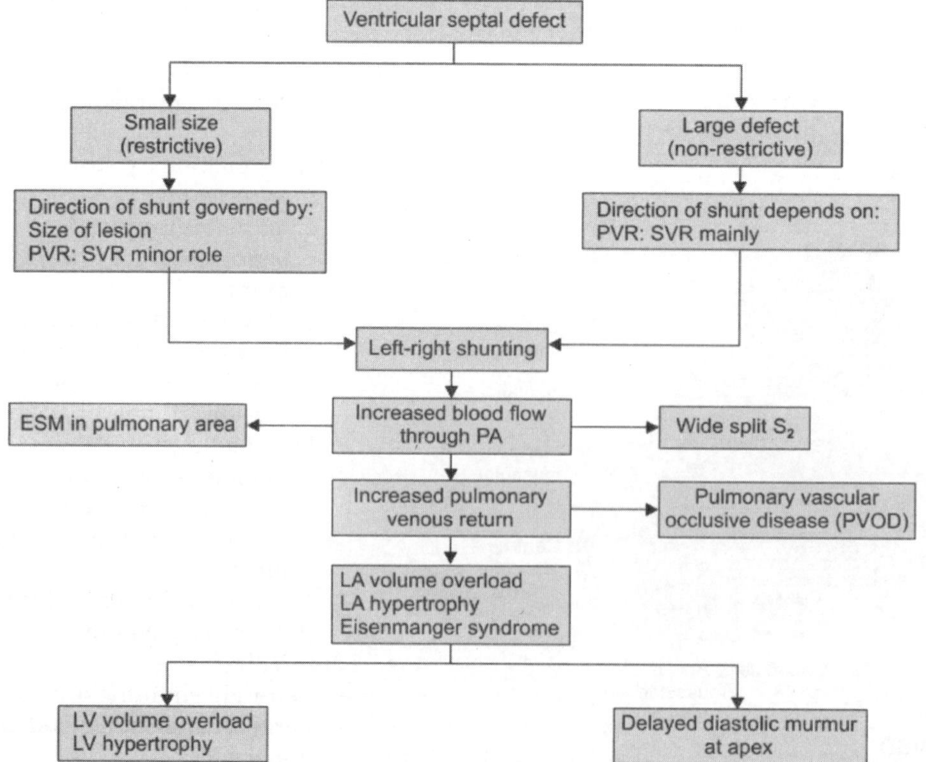

Clinical Features

- Small VSDs:
  - Symptoms:
    - Usually asymptomatic
    - Normal growth and development
  - Signs:
    - Well developed and acyanotic
    - Intensity of P_2 is normal
- Moderate VSD:
  - Symptoms:
    - Delayed growth and development
    - Decreased exercise tolerance
    - Repeated LRTIs
    - Congestive cardiac failure
  - Signs:
    - Systolic regurgitant murmur
    - Split S_2 with loud P_2
    - Mid-diastolic rumble of relative mitral stenosis
- Large VSDs:
  - Large VSD with CCF:
    - Symptoms:
      - Delayed growth and development
      - Decreased exercise tolerance
      - Repeated LRTIs
      - Congestive cardiac failure
    - Signs:
      - Palpation:
        - Precordial bulge and hyperactivity
        - Systolic thrill at lower left sternal border
        - LV type of apex
      - Auscultation:
        - Heart sounds:
          - S_1: masked by pansystolic murmur
          - S_2: widely split, increased intensity of P_2
          - S_3: in small left-right shunts
        - Murmurs:
          - Shunt murmur:
            - Grade 2–3/6 pansystolic murmur
            - Heard in left third/fourth ICS
          - Flow murmur:
            - Pulmonary ESM
            - Diastolic rumble due to relative MS
            - Diastolic decrescendo murmur of AR in infundibular VSDs
  - Eisenmangers syndrome:
    - Symptoms:
      - Dyspnea on exertion
      - Decreased level of activity
      - Chest pain, syncope, hemoptysis
      - Cyanosis
    - Signs:
      - Cyanosis, clubbing, polycythemia
      - S_2 is loud and single due to pulmonary HTN
      - Reduced intensity of shunt murmur

Assessment of Severity

- Small VSD:
  - Pansystolic murmur
  - S_2 normally split with normal P_2
  - No delayed diastolic murmur
  - X-ray and ECG are essentially normal
- Large VSD:
  - Pansystolic murmur becomes shorter, softer and appears like ESM
  - S_2 widely split, increased intensity of P_2
  - Delayed diastolic murmur present
  - ECG shows biventricular hypertrophy with P-mitrale

Investigations

- Complete blood count:
  - Polycythemia
  - Thrombocytopenia
- Baseline ABG:
  - For PaO_2 and electrolytes
  - Check K^+ levels if on digoxin therapy
  - Blood glucose for hypoglycemia
- Renal function tests
- Coagulation profiles:
  - Associated coagulopathy may be present
  - PT, INR, platelet count, APTT to be checked
- ECG:
  - Small VSD: normal ECG
  - Moderate VSD:
    - Occasional left atrial hypertrophy
    - Left ventricular hypertrophy
  - Large VSD:
    - Left atrial hypertrophy (P-mitrale) may or may not be present
    - Biventricular hypertrophy
  - Large VSD with Eisenmangers:
    - Absence of left atrial or ventricular hypertrophy
    - Only right ventricular hypertrophy present
- Chest X-ray:
  - Small VSD: normal X-ray
  - Moderate VSD:

- LA and LV enlargement
- Pulmonary plethora
- Large VSD:
  - Left atrial hypertrophy may or may not be present
  - Biventricular enlargement
  - Pulmonary plethora
- Large VSD with Eisenmangers:
  - Right ventricular hypertrophy on lateral view
  - Main PA and hilar branches are prominent
  - Peripheral pulmonary oligemia

❖ Echocardiography:
- Provides definite diagnosis
- Used to:
  - Study size, site and number of VSDs
  - Estimate PA pressure using modified Bernoullis equation
  - Identify associated defects
  - Estimate direction and magnitude of shunt
- Assessment of location of VSD: usually closely related to valves:
  - Membranous VSD is closely related to aortic valve
  - Inlet VSD is closely related to tricuspid valve
  - Infundibular VSD is closely related to semilunar valves
- Membranous VSDs:
  - Visualized in apical and subcostal five chamber views
  - Seen in LVOT just under aortic valve
  - In parasternal short axis view:
    - Seen at the level of aortic valve
    - Seen adjacent to tricuspid valve
- Inlet VSDs:
  - Best imaged in apical or subcostal four chamber view beneath AV valves
  - Can also be seen equally well in parasternal short axis view
  - Simple inlet VSD is seen beneath the AV valve
  - In AV canal type of VSD there may be straddling of AV valves
- Infundibular VSDs:
  - Lies inferior to semilunar valves
  - Those lying inferior to pulmonary valve:
    - Sub-pulmonary infundibular VSD
    - Supra-cristal infundibular VSD
  - Those lying inferior to aortic valve:
    - Subaortic infra-cristal VSD
    - Also called ***ToF type or cono-ventricular VSD***
- Trabecular VSDs:
  - Can lie anywhere from membranous septum to cardiac apex
  - Four types of VSDs are present:
    - Anterior
    - Mid-muscular
    - Apical
    - Posterior

❖ Cardiac catheterization: done to determine:
- Location and size of VSD
- Magnitude of shunt
- Q_p: Q_s ratio
- Pulmonary and systemic vascular resistance
- Ventricular function

Natural History

❖ Spontaneous closure of VSD:
- Occurs in 30–40% patients during first six months of life
- More common with:
  - Small sized VSDs which regress in size over time
  - Membranous and trabecular VSDs
- Spontaneous closure is rare with inlet and outlet type of VSDs

❖ Large VSDs:
- Congestive failure occurs at 6–8 weeks of age
- PVOD may start developing as early as 6–12 months of age
- Resulting right-left shunt usually does not occur till teenage years

❖ Infundibular stenosis:
- May develop rarely in large defects
- Results in right-left shunting rarely
- Effectively, left-right shunting reduces

Treatment (Indian Guidelines 2019)

❖ Medical management:
- Close follow-up
- Treat anemia and recurrent chest infections
- Congestive cardiac failure (CCF):
  - Trial for 3–4 months to see if growth failure can be improved
  - Diuretics: furosemide 1 mg/kg or 2–3 mg/kg IV or oral
  - Digoxin:
    - 20–50 µg/kg PO followed by 8–10 µg/kg maintenance dose
    - Reduce by 25% when giving IV therapy

- Afterload reduction:
  - Captopril used
  - May raise potassium levels: cautious use with spironolactone
- Feeding:
  - Frequent feeding with high calorie diet
  - Oral or nasogastric feeding may be used

- Anemia:
  - Maintenance of hematocrit is important
  - Anemia causes increase in left-right shunt, thereby worsening CCF
  - Oral iron therapy can be supplemented

❖ Timing of closure:
- Small VSDs:
  - Followed up annually till 10 years age
  - Closure is indicated on development of:
    - Infective endocarditis
    - Aortic cusp prolapse with AR
    - Significant RVOT obstruction
- Moderate VSDs:
  - Closure within 2–5 years age in asymptomatic patients
  - Closure within 1–2 years age in medically controlled symptomatic patients
  - Urgent closure in symptomatic patients refractory to medical therapy
- Large VSDs:
  - Closure within 6 months of age in medically controlled large VSDs
  - Urgent closure for:
    - VSDs refractory to medical therapy
    - VSD associated with AR

❖ Device closure:
- Pre-requisites:
  - Weight > 8 kg (5 kg for muscular VSDs)
  - Left-right shunt > 1.5:1
- Indications:
  - Class I indications:
    - Mid-muscular/apical VSDs which are difficult to close surgically
    - Post-surgical residual VSDs
  - Class IIb indications: PM-VSDs > 4 mm from aortic valve
- Contraindications:
  - VSD with irreversible PVOD
  - Inlet and subpulmonic VSDs
  - Pre-existing LBBB or conduction defects
  - Associated CHD lesions requiring surgery
- Done with:
  - Muscular septal occluder for muscular VSDs
  - Amplatzer duct occluder II (ADO II) for PM-VSDs
  - Konar-MF VSD occluder (associated with lower incidence of CHB)
- Associated with:
  - Heart block
  - Hemodynamic instability
  - Aortic regurgitation
  - Mitral and tricuspid regurgitation
  - Device embolization (rarely)
  - Vascular access site complications
  - Blood loss

❖ Surgical closure:
- Indications:
  - Inlet/subpulmonic VSD
  - VSD with associated defects
- Procedure:
  - Approaches to VSD:
    - Right atrial approach
    - Transpulmonary approach through pulmonary artery
    - Right ventricular approach using right ventriculotomy
    - Left ventricular approach (avoided)
  - Right atrial approach used for most membranous and inlet VSDs
  - Distortion of tricuspid valve occurs frequently with this approach
  - Approach through incision in main PA used for outlet VSD
  - Apical VSD requires right or left ventriculotomy
  - These approaches are however avoided
  - This is because ventricular dysfunction can occur postoperatively
  - Surgical closure done with dacron or pericardial patch repair
- Contraindications:
  - Development of PVOD with right-left shunt
  - PVR: SVR $\geq$ 0.50
  - If PVR $\leq$ one-third of SVR, progression of PVOD postoperatively is rare
- PA banding: (Class I)
  - Done very rarely as palliative surgery to reduce excess PA flow
  - Indications:
    - Multiple VSDs (***Swiss cheese*** appearance)
    - Surgically inaccessible VSDs
    - Contraindications to CPB such as sepsis

Anesthesia for VSD

Anesthetic Goals

- Rhythm: Sinus rhythm
- Rate: Maintain age appropriate rate
- Contractility: Maintain contractility
- Preload: Avoid fluid overload, especially if signs of CCF
- Afterload: Prevent reduction in afterload (increases R-L shunt)
- SVR: Maintain or prevent reduction in SVR
- PVR: Prevent increase in PVR
- Ventilation:
  - Avoid hypoxia
  - Avoid hypercarbia
  - Avoid hyperventilation and hyperoxemia
  - Avoid hyperinflation and atelectasis
- Temperature: Maintain, prevent hypothermia
- Hematocrit: Maintain, prevent anemia or polycythemia
- Most important factor which determines how the shunt behaves are SVR and PVR
- Other factors do not affect flow dynamics as much as SVR and PVR

Factors Causing Increased Left-Right Shunt

- Low hematocrit
- Increased SVR, reduced PVR
- Hyperoxemia
- Hyperventilation
- Negative airway pressure

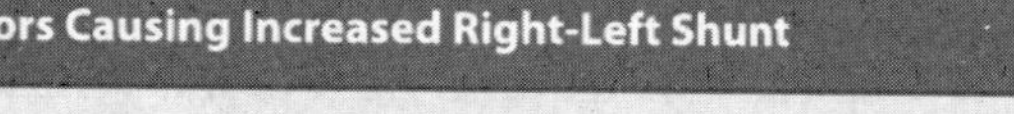

Factors Causing Increased Right-Left Shunt

- Polycythemia
- Reduced SVR, high PVR
- Hypoxia
- Hypoventilation, hypercarbia
- PEEP

Preoperative Preparation and Premedication

- Preoperative assessment includes:
  - History of:
    - Symptoms
    - Previous palliative surgery (PDA/COA)
    - Current medications
    - URTI, immunization
  - Examination should include airway for anticipated difficult intubation
  - Investigation including coagulation profile, ABG and electrolytes
- Fasting guidelines: Avoid hypoglycemia and dehydration
  - 6 hours for solids
  - 4 hours for breast milk
  - 2 hours for clear fluids and water
- Informed consent
- Treat preoperative URTI/LRTI adequately
- Premedication (in children ≥ 6 months age):
  - Oral: Midazolam 0.5 mg/kg with atropine 10 μg/kg
  - Intramuscular: Morphine 0.1 mg/kg with atropine 10 μg/kg
  - Avoid premedication in:
    - Children less than 6 months age
    - Those with right-left shunts
- Continue all medications except diuretics and anticoagulants
- Infective endocarditis prophylaxis as indicated

Regional Anesthesia

- Used in non-cardiac surgery where applicable
- Can be used safely provided sudden reduction in SVR is prevented
- Caudal anesthesia:
  - 2 mg/kg bupivacaine + 4 mg/kg lidocaine used
  - Care to prevent reduction in SVR at the time of induction
  - Reduction in SVR causes acute right-left shunting and rapid desaturation
- Contraindicated if coagulation abnormalities present

Monitors

- Pulse oximeter, E_TCO_2
- ECG, NIBP
- Airway pressure monitor
- IBP, CVP, PAC and PCWP as demanded by the procedure
- Left upper limb not to be used for NIBP/IBP in patients who underwent surgery for CoA
- Foleys catheter, urine output
- Transesophageal echocardiography
- ABG, electrolytes, blood glucose and hematocrit
- Temperature monitoring

Induction

- Adequate preoxygenation
- Patients with IV line in place:
  - Good LV function:
    - Thiopentone 3–4 mg/kg + vecuronium 0.1 mg/kg
    - Fentanyl 2 μg/kg can be used to ensure analgesia

- Poor LV function: ketamine 1–2 mg/kg + vecuronium 0.1 mg/kg

❖ Patients with no IV line:
- Inhalational induction with sevoflurane if good LV function
- IM ketamine 5 mg/kg if poor LV function

❖ 100% FiO_2 is avoided during mask ventilation to prevent increase in L-R shunting

❖ Induction agents are given slowly in incremental doses to prevent sudden drop in SVR

❖ IV induction is slow in patients with left-right shunt

❖ Avoid air bubbles in IV line:
- They cause paradoxical systemic air embolism
- Transient right-left shunt occurs during forceful injection
- This results in crossing over of air bubbles to left heart
- These air bubbles may travel towards the brain via:
  - Brachiocephalic artery
  - Left common carotid artery
- This results in paradoxical air embolism

Maintenance

❖ If good LV function:
- O_2 + air + 1% isoflurane
- Fentanyl 1 µg/kg and vecuronium 0.1 mg/kg intermittent boluses

❖ If poor LV function:
- O_2 + fentanyl 2 µg/kg/hour infusion
- Vecuronium 0.1 mg/kg and midazolam 0.05 mg/kg intermittent boluses

❖ Avoid nitrous oxide as it increases pulmonary HTN and size of air bubbles

Ventilation

❖ Use low FiO_2 as hyperoxemia increases left-right shunt

❖ Maintain $PaCO_2$ between 35 and 45 mm Hg

❖ Small PEEP is preferred as patients have increased pulmonary blood flow

❖ Avoid:
- Hyperventilation and hyperoxemia: increases left-right shunt
- Hypoxia, hypercarbia and acidosis: increases right-left shunt

Hemodynamics

❖ Judicious fluids as required if poor LV function

❖ Avoid anemia as left-right shunt increases (maintain hematocrit ≥ 10 g%)

❖ Maintain normothermia as hypothermia increases left-right shunt

❖ Measures to address bradycardia while coming off CPB:
- Epicardial pacing with pacemaker box
- Isoprenaline 0.01–0.05 µg/kg/min
- Prolonged pacemaker support if complete heart block post-VSD correction

❖ Inodilators are preferred in patients with severe PAH while coming off CPB:
- Milrinone 0.5–1 µg/kg/min
- Dobutamine 3–5 µg/kg/min

CPB Considerations

❖ Usually require short bypass runs

❖ Aorto-bicaval cannulation is preferred

❖ Tricaval cannulation required in the presence of LSVC

❖ Moderate hypothermia is used (28–32°C)

❖ Closure of VSD is done under cardioplegic myocardial protection

❖ LV vent is required and placed in LSPV

❖ Hematocrit is maintained > 24% on CPB

Extubation

❖ Postoperative ventilation required if:
- Poor preoperative cardiovascular reserve
- Congestive cardiac failure

❖ Reversal with neostigmine 0.05 mg/kg and glycopyrrolate 0.02 mg/kg

❖ Extubate when:
- Patient fully awake
- Hemodynamically stable
- Adequately rewarmed
- Normal acid base status and ABG

Postoperative Care

Management

❖ Adequate analgesia to prevent crying

❖ Avoid factors which precipitate pulmonary hypertension:
- Crying, stress
- Hypoxia, hypercarbia
- Acidosis

Analgesia

- Titrated opioids to avoid undue sedation
- Patient controlled analgesia
- Ketorolac 0.5 mg/kg or paracetamol 15 mg/kg IV as adjuvants
- Caudal/epidural analgesia where applicable
- Multimodal analgesia preferable

Monitors

- Pulse oximetry, E_TCO_2
- ECG, NIBP/IBP
- Temperature, urine output
- Echocardiography for LV function and residual VSDs
- CVP, PA pressure

Complications

- Arrhythmias:
  - Right bundle branch block
  - Right bundle branch block with left anterior hemiblock
  - Complete heart block
- TV regurgitation common, AR rarely
- RV/LV dysfunction which persists for years later
- Residual pulmonary HTN/VSD
- Rarely, cerebrovascular accidents and stroke
- Infective endocarditis

ATRIAL SEPTAL DEFECT

Introduction

It is an abnormal communication between the two atria.

Incidence

- Most common acyanotic congenital heart defect
- Fourth most common congenital heart defect
- Occurs as an isolated anomaly in 6–10% of all congenital heart defects
- Incidence of 1 in 1500 live births
- More common in females (male: female ratio of 1:2)
- Accounts for 30–40% of clinically important intra-cardiac adult shunts
- PFO is present in more than 20–25% of adults

Embryology

- Inter-atrial septum develops between 4th and 6th weeks of gestation
- A depression is formed in roof of common atrium, which enlarges as a crest
- This forms the *septum primum* (SP)
- SP extends downwards to meet the endocardial (EC) cushions formed in atrio-ventricular canal
- The opening between the atria formed before the SP meets EC is called ostium primum (OP)
- This is closed when the endocardial cushion fuses with septum primum
- As the septum primum extends downwards, fenestration appear superiorly which ultimately unite together and form the *ostium secundum* (OS)
- At the same time, a thin septum called the septum secundum develops to right of septum primum
- This grows and covers the OS in an incomplete fashion, resulting in the formation of foramen ovale
- After birth, with the increase in SVR and decrease in PVR, foramen ovale usually closes but may persist in 25% causing PFO

Classification

- Types:
  - Ostium primum ASD (15%)
  - Ostium secundum ASD (50–70%)
  - Sinus venosus ASD (10%)
  - Coronary sinus ASD (< 1%)
- Ostium primum ASD (OP-ASD):
  - Isolated OP-ASDs account for 15% of all ASDs
  - Occur due to failure of fusion of endocardial cushions
  - Thus, OP-ASDs exist within the spectrum of AV canal defects
  - Isolated OP-ASDs are also called partial or incomplete AV canal defect
  - Atrial communication occurs due to absence of AV canal portion of atrial septum
  - Common AV valve annulus is present with two AV valve orifices
  - AV valve tissue is adherent to the crest of IV septum (no ventricular level shunt)
  - Superior and inferior bridging leaflets of AV valve meet at the ventricular septum
  - This forms cleft of the mitral valve, through which AV valve regurgitation occurs

- Thus, OP-ASDs are associated with cleft AML and mitral regurgitation
- Margins of OP-ASD:
  - Superior margin: Septum primum
  - Anterior margin: Common AV valve annulus
  - Posterior margin: Septum primum
- As AV annulus forms one of the margins, device closure is not possible
- Associated defects:
  - Cleft mitral valve
  - Double orifice mitral valve
  - Subaortic stenosis
  - Coarctation of aorta
  - PDA
  - TOF

❖ Ostium secundum ASD (OS-ASD)
- OS-ASDs account for 50–70% of all ASDs
- Defects maybe multiple in 7.3% of patients with OS-ASD
- *Most common* type of true ASD
- Occurs as a result of true deficiency in septum primum tissue
- Defect is present at the site of fossa ovalis
- Range in size from few millimeters to larger than 30 mm in diameter
- Defects less than 5 mm in fossa ovalis area is considered as PFO
- Also, PFOs have a valve effect of septum primum opposition to septum secundum
- Allows left to right shunting from LA to RA
- Anomalous pulmonary venous return is present in 10% cases of OS-ASD
- Associated with mitral valve prolapse and mitral regurgitation
- Margins of OS-ASD defects:
  - Superior margin: Septum secundum
  - Anterior margin: AV canal septum
  - Posterior margin: Septum secundum
  - Inferior margin: septum primum, left venous valve of IVC

❖ Sinus venosus ASD (SV-ASD):
- Less common, compared to OS-ASDs and are not true ASDs
- SV-ASDs account for 10% of all ASDs
- SVC type:
  - More common variety of SV-ASD
  - Occurs due to absence of sinus venosus septum between SVC and RUPV
  - Commonly associated with anomalous drainage of RUPV into RA
  - RUPV may sometimes be connected to SVC, above level of RA
  - Patient will be mildly desaturated due to entry of SVC blood into LA
- IVC type:
  - Less common type of SV-ASD
  - Occurs due to absence of sinus venosus septum between IVC and RLPV
  - Commonly associated with anomalous drainage of RLPV into IVC
  - Also called ***scimitar syndrome***
- Usually, presence of SV-ASDs precludes device closure

❖ Coronary sinus ASD (CS-ASD):
- One of the less common forms of ASD and are not true ASDs
- Wall of the coronary sinus within the LA is deficient or completely absent
- LA blood shunts into the sinus and through the ostium into RA
- Produces clinical shunting similar to other ASDs
- Persistent LSVC associated with a CS-ASD is called ***Raghib syndrome***
- Device closure may be possible in some cases with partial CS unroofing

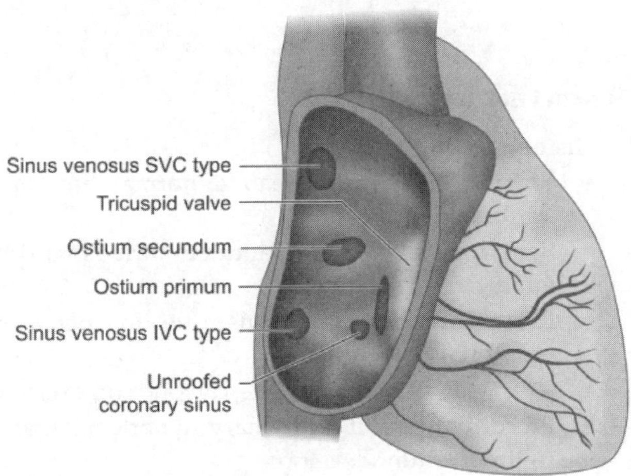

Fig. 25: Types of ASD.

Pathophysiology

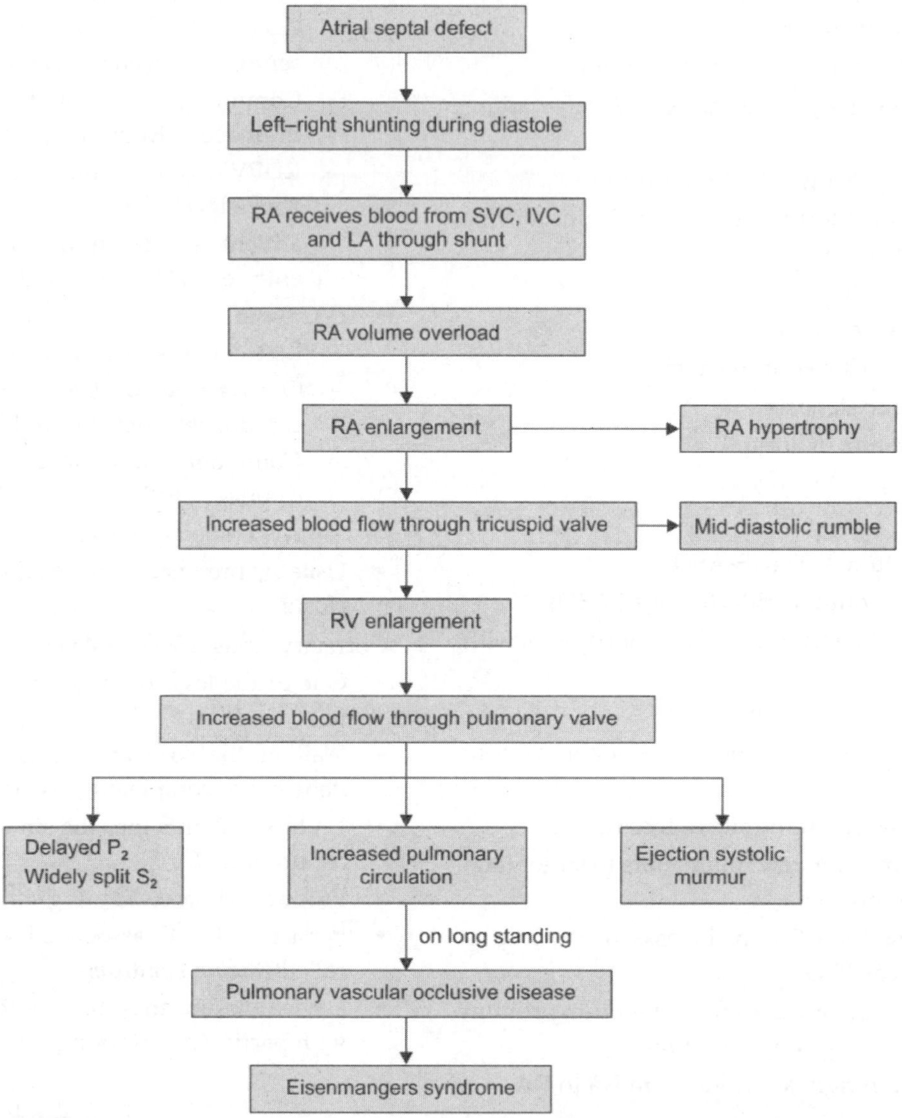

Clinical Features

- History:
  - Majority of patients lead a normal life until adulthood
  - Symptoms of CCF and failure to thrive in 3rd to 4th decades
  - Recurrent chest infections due to increased pulmonary blood flow
  - Cyanosis, clubbing, fatigue, dyspnea on exertion
  - Precordial pain if pulmonary hypertension and right-left shunt develops
  - Mild dyspnea, fatigue are most common early symptoms
- Examination:
  - Inspection:
    - Skeletal anomalies (***Holt-Oram syndrome***)
    - Facial anomalies (***Downs syndrome***)
    - Visceral anomalies (asplenia)
    - Prominent left costal cartilage from cardiomegaly
    - Gracile habitus: long bones with poorly developed skeletal muscles
  - Palpation:
    - Parasternal impulse
    - Systolic thrill in left second ICS
    - Palpable P_2

- Auscultation:
  - Findings present only in relatively large L-R shunts
  - Findings may be absent in poorly compliant RV (infants and toddlers)
  - Sounds:
    - S_1: loud, accentuated
    - S_2: wide and fixed split with increased P_2 intensity:
      - Widely split as:
        - Blood flow through pulmonary valve is more
        - This causes delayed pulmonary valve closure
        - Thus, S_2 is widely split
      - Fixed S_2 splitting as:
        - It does not vary with inspiration
        - RV is already fully loaded with shunted blood
        - Further inspiration cannot draw more blood into RV
        - This causes fixed splitting of S_2
    - S_3: Inconstant
  - Murmurs:
    - Shunt murmur absent
    - Flow murmur:
      - Results in mid-diastolic rumble
      - Occurs in large L-R shunts
      - Large volume of blood passes across tricuspid valve
      - This causes relative tricuspid stenosis and the flow murmur
      - Heard at left lower sternal edge
    - Delayed diastolic murmur of TR
    - Ejection systolic murmur of PV

Complications

- Usually in 3rd to 4th decade
- Congestive cardiac failure
- Eisenmanger syndrome
- Pulmonary vascular occlusive disease
- Arrhythmias:
  - Atrial flutter
  - Atrial fibrillation, PSVT
  - Atrioventricular conduction abnormalities

Assessment of Severity

If ASD is large:

- Cardiomegaly is more
- Increased intensity of ESM and delayed diastolic murmur

Investigations

- Complete blood count, renal function tests, coagulation profile
- Baseline ABG and blood glucose
- Chest X-ray:
  - Cardiomegaly with enlargement of RA and RV
  - RV enlargement seen in lateral X-ray as obliteration of retrosternal space
  - Pulmonary plethora when L-R shunt is significant
  - Prominent main PA segment
  - Localized dilation of SVC at the entrance of anomalous pulmonary veins
- Electrocardiogram:
  - Findings present only in relatively large L-R shunts ($Q_p : Q_s > 1.5$)
  - Right axis deviation of +90° to +180°
  - Right ventricular hypertrophy
  - RBBB with rsR` pattern in V_1
  - In about 50% patients with SV-ASDs, P-axis is less than 30°
- Echocardiogram:
  - Purpose: to show size and position of defect
  - Views:
    - Best seen in subcostal four chamber view
    - OS-ASD seen as a dropout in mid-atrial septum
    - OP-ASD seen as defect in lower atrial septum
    - SV-ASD seen as defect in posterosuperior atrial septum
  - Quantification of shunt:
    - Indirect sign of L-R shunt is RA, RV and PA enlargement
    - Pulsed wave Doppler shows maximum L-R shunting during diastole
    - RV volume overload is indicated by:
      - Paradoxical motion of interventricular septum
      - Increased RV dimensions
  - Transesophageal echocardiography done if:
    - Transthoracic echo is ambiguous
    - To determine adequacy of margins of the defect
    - To look for any atrial thrombus
- Catheterization:
  - Not routinely indicated
  - Used only if:
    - Inconsistency in clinical data
    - Significant PAH
    - Associated anomalies

Treatment (Indian Guidelines 2019)

- Medical treatment:
  - Consists of treatment of:
    - Recurrent chest infections
    - *Congestive cardiac failure*: diuretics and digoxin
    - Arrhythmias
  - Exercise restriction is usually unnecessary
  - IE prophylaxis indicated only if associated MVP or other defects
  - Spontaneous closure: occurs in more than 80% cases when:
    - ASD size 3–8 mm
    - Within 1.5 years of age
- *Age of intervention*:
  - Asymptomatic child:
    - May be delayed up to 4–5 years for SV-ASD (class IIa)
    - 2–4 years for all other types of ASDs (class I)
  - Symptomatic ASD in infancy:
    - Early closure is recommended (class I)
    - Rule out other associated lesions:
      - TAPVC
      - Left ventricular inflow obstruction
      - Aortopulmonary window
  - Delayed presentation beyond recommended age:
    - Elective closure irrespective of age at presentation (class I)
    - Symptomatic sequelae of paradoxical air embolism (class IIa)
    - PVR should be within operable range
- Surgical treatment:
  - Indications:
    - ASD with L-R shunt associated with RV volume overload
    - Q_p:Q_s > 1.5
    - No evidence of irreversible pulmonary vascular occlusive disease
    - OP-ASDs
    - SV- ASDs
    - Coronary sinus ASDs
  - Contraindications:
    - High PVR > 10 units/m^2
    - High PVR > 7 units/m^2 with vasodilators
    - Irreversible pulmonary vascular occlusive disease
  - Procedure:
    - Through midline sternotomy traditionally
    - Simple sutures are used for direct closure of small ASDs
    - Pericardial patch or Dacron patch can be used for larger ASDs
    - Minimally invasive techniques with smaller incisions becoming popular
  - SV-ASD with PAPVC:
    - Tunnel created between RUPV and ASD using pericardial or Teflon patch
    - Pericardial gusset may be placed in SVC to prevent SVC obstruction
  - Warden procedure:
    - Done when RUPV is directly connected to the SVC
    - SVC is divided above level of RUPV entry
    - Cardiac end of SVC is oversewn
    - Pericardial baffle is placed to drain RUPV blood into LA through the ASD
    - Proximal SVC is sewn to RA appendage
  - Coronary sinus ASD:
    - Ostium of coronary sinus is closed with pericardial patch
    - Care taken to avoid conduction tissues
    - This results in drainage of coronary sinus into LA

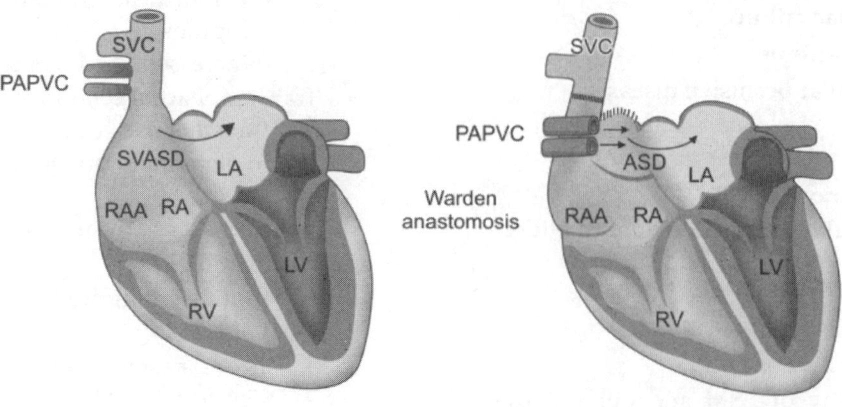

Fig. 26: Warden's procedure.

- Transcatheter closure:
  - Indications:
    - ASD with L-R shunt associated with RV volume overload
    - $Q_p:Q_s > 1.5$
    - < 38 mm diameter
    - No evidence of irreversible pulmonary vascular occlusive disease
  - Patient selection:
    - Device closure is reserved only for OS-ASDs
    - Adequate rim (> 5 mm) of tissue around defect should be present
    - Absence of other associated anomalies like PAPVC
  - Contraindications:
    - Deficit rims (especially IVC rim)
    - Weight < 15 kg
    - Defect size > 20 mm/m^2
  - Devices available:
    - Sideris buttoned device
    - Angel Wings device
    - CardioSEAL device
    - Amplatzer ASD occlusion device
    - *Amplatzer septal occluder (most commonly used)*
  - Advantages:
    - Avoidance of CPB
    - Avoidance of pain, surgical scar
    - Lesser duration of hospital stay
    - Rapid recovery
  - Disadvantages: Higher rate of residual leak compared to surgical closure
  - Complications:
    - Immediate complications:
      - Device embolization
      - Cardiac tamponade
    - Long-term complications:
      - Thrombus formation (more common with cardioSEAL)
      - Erosion of device with perforation of atria
      - Encroachment of device over mitral or aortic valve leaflets
      - Impaired return from pulmonary veins
      - Reactive or hemorrhagic pericarditis
      - Migration or dislodgement of device
  - Follow-up:
    - Aspirin prophylaxis:
      - Started 48 hours prior to procedure
      - Continued for 6 months post-procedure
    - Antibiotic prophylaxis for 6 months post procedure
    - Echo studies to check for:
      - Residual atrial shunt:
        - Reported in 7% patients immediately after device closure
        - These are usually not hemodynamically significant
        - 97% of shunts close completely in the long run
      - Unobstructed flow from pulmonary veins
      - Unobstructed flow from vena cavae and coronary sinus
      - Mitral and tricuspid valve function
  - Results:
    - Reversal of RV volume overload:
      - May occur < 3 weeks post-procedure in children
      - Occurs 9 months post-procedure in adults
    - Abnormal motion of IV septum normalizes shortly post-procedure
    - RBBB pattern:
      - Degree of RBBB diminishes in 61% patients
      - In 2.5% patients it becomes more prominent post-device closure

Natural History

- Spontaneous closure:
  - Occurs in 40% patients within first 4 years of life
  - 100% spontaneous closure seen in defects less than 3 mm size at 1.5 years of age
  - 80% spontaneous closure seen in defects between 3–8 mm size at 1.5 years of age
  - Defects more than 8 mm rarely close spontaneously

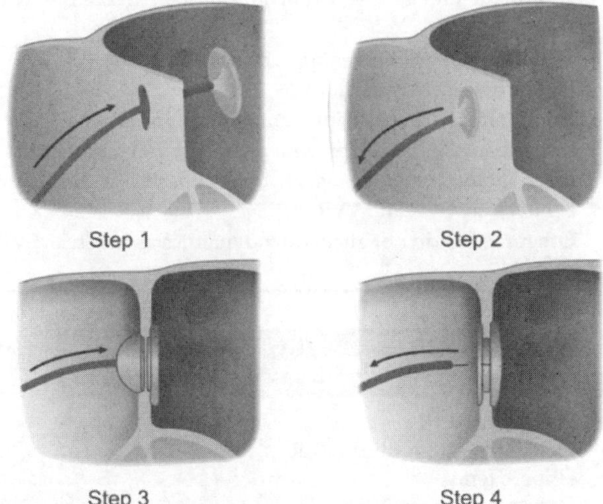

Fig. 27: Transcatheter closure of ASD.

- Congestive cardiac failure:
  - Occurs in large untreated ASDs
  - Usually develops in 3rd and 4th decade of life
  - Atrial arrhythmias (flutter and fibrillation may occur in adults)
  - Infective endocarditis usually is rare in patients with isolated ASDs
  - CVAs due to paradoxical embolism through the ASD is a rare complication

Anesthesia for ASD

Premedication

- Treat preoperative URTI/LRTI adequately
- Informed consent
- Fasting guidelines:
  - 6 hours: Solids
  - 2 hours: Clear fluids, water
- Large bore IV cannula to be secured for volume resuscitation
- IV cannula secured on left hand in the presence of LSVC
- Premedication: morphine 0.1 mg/kg and glycopyrrolate 20 µg/kg IV
- Continue all preoperative medication except diuretics
- Surgical antibiotic prophylaxis as indicated

Anesthetic Goals

- Rhythm: Sinus rhythm
- Rate: Maintain age appropriate rate
- Contractility: Maintain contractility
- Preload: Avoid fluid overload, especially if signs of CCF
- Afterload: Prevent reduction in afterload (increases R-L shunt)
- SVR: Maintain or prevent reduction in SVR
- PVR: Prevent increase in PVR
- Temperature: Maintain, prevent hypothermia
- Hematocrit: Maintain, prevent anemia or polycythemia
- Most important factor which determines how the shunt behaves are SVR and PVR
- Other factors do not affect flow dynamics as much as SVR and PVR

Factors Causing Left-Right Shunt

- Low hematocrit
- Increased SVR, reduced PVR
- Hyperoxemia
- Hyperventilation
- Negative airway pressure

Factors Causing Right-Left Shunt

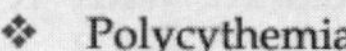

- Polycythemia
- Reduced SVR, high PVR
- Hypoxia
- Hypoventilation, hypercarbia
- PEEP

OT Preparation

- Anesthesia machine with circuit
- Airway equipment:
  - ETT, laryngoscope airways, suction apparatus
  - *DLT if minimally invasive surgery is planned*
- Other equipment:
  - TEE probe and machine
  - Defibrillator, temporary pacemaker
  - Equipment for thermal homeostasis
- Drugs:
  - Anesthetic drugs:
    - Thiopentone, propofol
    - Morphine, fentanyl
    - NDMR
  - Emergency drugs:
    - Atropine, adrenaline
    - Phenylephrine, ephedrine
    - Dopamine, dobutamine, NTG, isoprenaline

Monitors

- Pulse oximeter, E_TCO_2
- ECG, NIBP
- Airway pressure monitor
- IBP may be used for beat-beat BP monitoring
- CVP:
  - Can be used for administration of vasoactive agents
  - Also used as an auxiliary indicator of fluid status
  - CVP monitoring is especially important in SV-ASD repair
  - This is because surgery may cause iatrogenic narrowing of SVC-RA junction
  - Thus, continuous CVP monitoring allows early detection of SVC syndrome
- PA catheter is usually not required
- Foley's catheter, urine output
- Nasopharyngeal temperature
- Transesophageal echocardiography
- ABG, electrolytes, blood glucose and hematocrit

Induction

- Adequate preoxygenation
- Patients with IV line in place:
  - Good RV function:
    - Thiopentone 3–4 mg/kg + vecuronium 0.1 mg/kg
    - Fentanyl 2 μg/kg can be used to ensure analgesia
  - Poor RV function: Ketamine 1–2 mg/kg + vecuronium 0.1 mg/kg
- Patients with no IV line:
  - Inhalational induction with sevoflurane if good RV function
  - IM ketamine 5 mg/kg if poor RV function
- 100% FiO_2 is avoided during mask ventilation to prevent increase in L-R shunting
- Induction agents are given slowly in incremental doses to prevent sudden drop in SVR IV induction is slow in patients with left-right shunt
- Avoid air bubbles in IV line:
  - They cause paradoxical systemic air embolism
  - Transient right-left shunt occurs during forceful injection
  - This results in crossing over of air bubbles to left heart
  - These air bubbles may travel towards the brain via:
    - Brachiocephalic artery
    - Left common carotid artery
  - This results in paradoxical air embolism

Maintenance

- If good LV function:
  - O_2 + air + 1% isoflurane
  - Fentanyl 1 μg/kg and vecuronium 0.1 mg/kg intermittent boluses
- If poor LV function:
  - O_2 + fentanyl 2 μg/kg/hour infusion
  - Vecuronium 0.1 mg/kg and midazolam 0.05 mg/kg intermittent boluses
- Avoid nitrous oxide as it increases PVR and the size of injected air bubbles

Ventilation

- ET intubation and CMV preferred
- Use low FiO_2 as hyperoxia increases left-right shunt
- Maintain $PaCO_2$ between 30 and 40 mm Hg
- Avoid hyperventilation as it increases L-R shunting
- Small PEEP preferred as patients have increased pulmonary blood flow
- Avoid:
  - Hyperventilation and hyperoxemia: increases left-right shunt
  - Hypoxia, hypercarbia and acidosis: increases right-left shunt

Hemodynamics

- Judicious fluids as required if poor RV function
- Transient hypotension is best treated with phenylephrine boluses
- This is because phenylephrine causes increase in both SVR and PVR
- Avoid anemia as left-right shunt increases (maintain hematocrit ≥ 10 g%)
- Maintain normothermia as hypothermia increases left-right shunt
- Patients with ASD treated early usually do not require inotropic support
- Inotropes used for patients with pulmonary HTN during weaning of CPB:
  - Isoprenaline 0.01–0.05 μg/kg/min
  - Dobutamine 3–5 μg/kg/min
  - Milrinone 0.5–1 μg/kg/min
- Inhaled nitric oxide may be required for patients with severe PAH
- Pacemaker support may be required especially for ostium primum defects
- Rhythm disturbances are rare in OS-ASD and SV-ASD

CPB Considerations

- Usually require short bypass runs
- Aorto-bicaval cannulation is preferred
- Tricaval cannulation required in the presence of LSVC
- Moderate hypothermia is used (28–32°C)
- Closure of ASD is done under cardioplegic myocardial protection
- ETT may be used to cannulate the SVC in some centers
- Inflation of the ETT cuff is used to snare the SVC
- LV vent is required and placed in LSPV
- For surgical repair of SV-ASD, LV vent may be placed directly through the LA
- Hematocrit is maintained > 24% on CPB

Extubation

- Early extubation in OT or early postoperative period possible
- Neostigmine 0.05 mg/kg and glycopyrrolate 0.02 mg/kg used for reversal
- Extubate when:
  - Fully awake
  - Hemodynamically stable
  - Adequate rewarmed
  - Normal ABG

Postoperative Care

Analgesia

- Cautious use of opioids to avoid undue sedation
- Patient controlled analgesia
- Ketorolac 0.5 mg/kg or paracetamol 15 mg/kg IV as adjuvants
- Caudal/epidural analgesia used where applicable
- Multimodal analgesia

Monitors

- Pulse oximetry, E_TCO_2
- Urine output, NIBP/IBP
- CVP/PAC
- ECG, ABG
- Echocardiography
- Temperature

Complications

- Air embolism, cerebrovascular accidents
- SVC obstruction (due to SV-ASD closure)
- Arrhythmias:
  - Transient atrial arrhythmias (Atrial fibrillation and flutter) common
  - Complete heart block occurs in OP-ASD
- Severe brady/tachyarrhythmias rare
- Mitral regurgitation especially in ostium primum

PATENT DUCTUS ARTERIOSUS

Introduction

- The persistence of ductus arteriosus beyond 3 months after a full-term birth is called PDA
- It refers to a communication between descending aorta and pulmonary artery
- Also called ***Botallos duct***

Incidence

- 1 in 2000 live births
- Constitutes 5–10% of all congenital heart diseases
- More common in premature neonates:
  - Occurs in 45% neonates < 1750 grams birth weight
  - Occurs in 80% neonates < 1200 grams birth weight
- Incidence increases in congenital rubella syndrome

Embryology

- Aortic arch develops between 5 and 6 weeks of gestation
- This occurs from the truncus arteriosus as six paired arches
- Pulmonary artery arises from 6th arch
- When pulmonary vascularization is established:
  - Communication with right dorsal aorta regresses
  - Communication with left dorsal aorta persists
- This persistent communication forms the ductus arteriosus
- Thus, the ductus arteriosus is derived from the sixth aortic arch
- It develops during the sixth-week of intrauterine life from the distal part of left 6th arch
- Persistence of this communication beyond 3 months after birth causes PDA

Anatomy

- PDA is most commonly left sided
- It has diameter of 8–10 mm and length of 5–10 mm
- It arises close to the origin of LPA
- Inserted into lesser curvature of aorta, 5–10 mm distal to origin of left subclavian artery
- Relations of PDA:
  - Left main bronchus: posteriorly
  - Vagus nerve: anteriorly
  - Recurrent laryngeal nerve encircles ductus and ascends into neck
- In small children, wall of DA is thick and strong
- As age advances, wall becomes thin and friable especially in those with pulmonary HTN
- Anatomical types of PDA:
  - Tubular
  - Cylindrical
  - Window/funnel shaped
  - Elongated

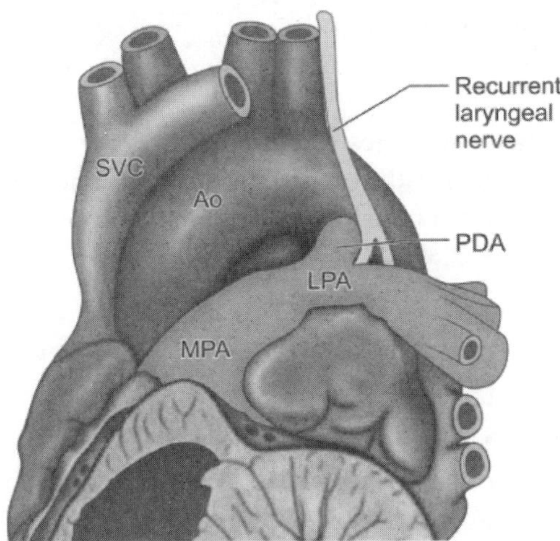

Fig. 28: Patent ductus arteriosus.

- Complex
- Aneurysmal which can be spontaneous/ acquired from:
  - Mycotic infections
  - Trauma
  - Hypertension

❖ Closure of ductus arteriosus:
- Functional closure of DA:
  - Begins within 12–15 hours after birth
  - Occurs due to:
    - Medial smooth muscle contraction
    - Protrusion of intimal cushions into PDA lumen
    - Usually completed by the second day of life
- Permanent anatomical closure:
  - Usually begins 2–3 weeks after birth
  - Occurs due to:
    - In-folding of endothelium
    - Necrosis and proliferation of sub-intimal layers
    - This leads to fibrosis and formation of ligamentum arteriosum
    - Usually completed within 1st 2 months of life

Pathophysiology

❖ Amount of blood flow through the PDA depends on:
- Size and shape of communication
- Difference between SVR and PVR

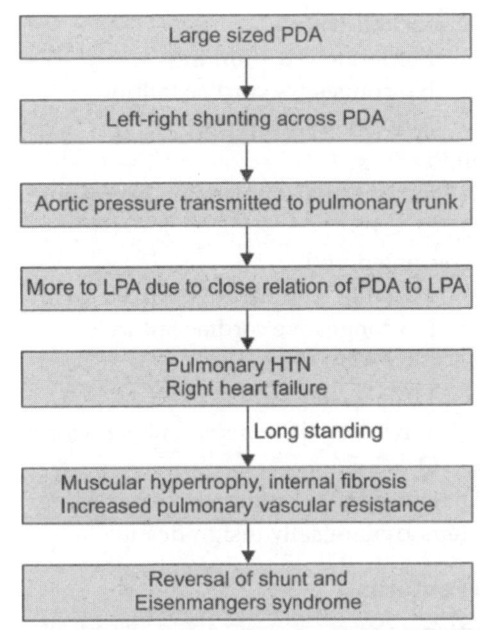

Ductus Dependent Cardiac Malformations

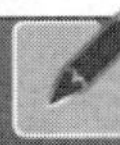

❖ Duct dependent pulmonary circulation:
- Pulmonary atresia/stenosis associated with:
  - VSD
  - ASD
  - TGA
- Critical pulmonary stenosis
- Tricuspid atresia associated with:
  - ASD
  - VSD

❖ Severe tetralogy of Fallot

❖ Duct dependent systemic circulation:
- Severe congenital aortic stenosis
- Coarctation of aorta
- Interrupted aortic arch
- Hypoplastic left heart syndrome

❖ Lesions with parallel circulation requiring intermixing of blood: TGA

Classification Of PDA

❖ Large PDA:
- > 5 mm internal diameter on lateral angiography
- Q_p: Q_s > 2.2
- Associated with:
  - Significant L-R shunting
  - Congestive cardiac failure
  - Severe PAH
  - Early onset PVOD

❖ Moderate PDA:
- 3–5 mm internal diameter on lateral angiography
- Q_p: Q_s 1.5–2.2

- Associated with:
  - Moderate L-R shunting
  - No congestive cardiac failure
  - Mild-moderate PAH
- Small PDA:
  - 1–3 mm internal diameter on lateral angiography
  - $Q_p : Q_s < 1.5$
  - Associated with:
    - Minimal left heart overload
    - No congestive cardiac failure
    - No PAH
- Silent PDA:
  - < 1 mm internal diameter on lateral angiography
  - $Q_p : Q_s < 1.5$
  - Diagnosed incidentally on echocardiography
  - Hemodynamically insignificant

Clinical Features

Presentation

- Usually asymptomatic when the duct is small
- Symptoms of congestive cardiac failure in older infants when the duct is large:
  - Recurrent LRTIs
  - Failure to thrive
  - Cough, dyspnea, tachypnea
  - Tachycardia
  - Hepatosplenomegaly
- Symptoms in preterm neonates:
  - Apnea and bradycardia in neonates who are not ventilated
  - Failure to wean from mechanical ventilation
- Clinical signs:
  - Wide pulse pressure with bounding peripheral pulse
  - Hyperdynamic precordium
  - Systolic and systolic-diastolic murmurs
  - *Hallmark: continuous machinery* murmur present in first/second left ICS
  - ***Graham-Steele*** murmur:
    - Seen in Eisenmanger syndrome
    - High pitched diastolic decrescendo murmur
    - Characteristic of pulmonary valvular insufficiency

Associated Anomalies

- Extra-cardiac anomalies:
  - Mental retardation
  - Eye defects
  - Deafness
  - Sternal deformities
  - Scoliosis
  - Clubfoot
- Cardiac anomalies:
  - Lesions with restricted pulmonary blood flow:
    - Pulmonary atresia/stenosis associated with:
      - VSD
      - ASD
      - TGA
    - Tricuspid atresia associated with:
      - ASD
      - VSD
  - Lesions with restricted systemic blood flow:
    - Mitral stenosis with ASD
    - Aortic stenosis with ASD/VSD
    - Preductal CoA
    - Interrupted aortic arch
    - Hypoplastic left heart syndrome
- Syndromes:
  - ***Charge syndrome***: iris coloboma, heart, choanal atresia, micrognathia, difficult airway
  - ***Edwards syndrome***: Trisomy 18, micrognathia, small mouth, difficult airway
  - ***Goldenhaar syndrome***: CoA, maxillary/mandibular hypoplasia, spine abnormalities
  - ***Vater syndrome***
  - ***Pataus syndrome***: Trisomy 13

Natural History

- Spontaneous closure rate in preterm neonates is between 35% and 75% within 1 year of life
- Rate of spontaneous closure post-infancy is 0.6% per year
- Small PDAs in full term neonates may close up to 3 months of age
- Large PDAs are unlikely to close spontaneously

Differential Diagnosis

- Venous hum: Disappears when the patient becomes supine
- VSD with aortic regurgitation: to- and -fro murmur rather than continuous murmur
- Systemic arterio-venous fistula:
  - Wide pulse pressure with bounding pulse similar to PDA
  - Continuous murmur is however localized to the site of AV- fistula
- Pulmonary arteriovenous fistula:
  - Continuous murmur present (over back rather than 2nd left ICS as in PDA)

- Presence of cyanosis and clubbing with no cardiomegaly
- Coronary arteriovenous fistula
  - Machinery murmur is also seen in coronary AV fistulas
  - However, they are located over precordium and not 2nd left ICS as in PDAs
- Ruptured sinus of Valsalva:
  - Characterized by sudden onset chest pain and CCF
  - Marfanoid features commonly present
  - Associated with to- and -fro murmur

Complications

- Congestive cardiac failure
- Infective endocarditis
- Pulmonary vascular occlusive disease (PVOD)
- PDA aneurysm

Investigations

- Complete blood count, electrolytes
- Coagulation profile including PT, APTT, platelet count
- Serum proteins, calcium levels
- Arterial blood gas, urine analysis, urine specific gravity
- X-ray chest:
  - Normal or ventricular hypertrophy in small PDAs
  - Large PDAs:
    Enlargement of LA, LV, ascending aorta and aortic arch
    Plethoric pulmonary vasculature
- ECG:
  - Usually normal in small PDAs
  - Signs of LVH:
    - Tall R-waves and peaked T-waves in II, III, aVF, V_5, V_6
    - Prominent Q-waves in V_5 and V_6
  - Signs of LA enlargement: broad notched P-waves in leads I and II
  - Right ventricular hypertrophy in PVOD
- Echocardiography:
  - Most important diagnostic modality
  - Transthoracic echo is used as PDAs are difficult to visualize on TEE
  - Useful for assessment of:
    - Size and anatomy
    - Left atrial and ventricular dimensions
    - Estimation of PA pressure
    - Suitability for device closure
- Cardiac catheterization:
  - Rarely required for establishing diagnosis
  - Currently indicated for:
    - Device closure of PDA
    - Ruling out irreversible PVOD

Medical Management

- Usually reserved for neonates with small PDAs with minimal symptoms
- They can be medically managed up to 6 months to allow spontaneous closure
- Patency at 6 months warrants some form of intervention to ensure closure
- For neonates in congestive cardiac failure stabilization may be attempted for 48 hours:
  - Fluid restriction
  - Furosemide:
    - May promote patency of DA
    - This is due to its effects on prostaglandin metabolism
  - Digoxin:
    - No benefit in children < 1250 g as it does not increase SVR
    - But it may reduce heart rate and thus decrease cardiac output

Methods of Maintaining PDA Patency in Duct-dependent Lesions

- Role of prostaglandins:
  - Prostaglandins which may be used to keep the ductus patent are:
    - PGE_1
    - $PGF_{2\alpha}$
    - PGI_2
  - Done in order to promote flow through pulmonary artery
  - Dose varies from 0.05–0.2 μg/kg/min and titrated to favorable effect
  - Side effects of prostaglandins:
    - Fever
    - Hypotension
    - Cutaneous flushing
    - Tachycardia
    - Apneic spells
    - Seizures
- PDA ductal stenting:
  - Done using a high-flexibility coronary stent
  - Can be used to maintain ductal patency for up to 6 months

- Used as palliation in patients with high surgical risk:
  - Hypoplastic left heart syndrome
  - TGA during first week of life

Indications for Closure of PDA (Indian Guidelines 2019)

- Early closure (within 3 months) recommended for large or moderate PDA with:
  - Congestive cardiac failure (Class I)
  - Severe failure to thrive (Class IIa)
  - Pulmonary arterial HTN (Class I)
- Delayed closure:
  - At 6 months–1 year for moderate PDA with number of signs of CCF/PAH (Class I)
  - At 12–18 months for small PDAs
- Patients presenting > 12 months with CCF should be evaluated for PVOD before closure
- Choice of interventional technique:
  - Device closure:
    - Is the preferred technique due to lesser morbidity
    - Avoided in preterm neonates due to high risk of complications
    - Preferred for PDAs < 10 mm diameter with favorable morphology
  - Surgical ligation is preferred for:
    - Preterm neonates
    - Progressively enlarging ductal aneurysm
    - PDA endarteritis
    - Aneurysmal PDA
    - Abnormally contoured PDA not amenable to device closure
  - Pharmacological closure:
    - Used mainly in preterm neonates prior to considering surgical closure
    - Not preferred for term neonates owing to high failure rates

Techniques of Closure of Ductus Arteriosus

- Pharmacological closure:
  - Indomethacin:
    - Reduces synthesis of prostaglandins by inhibiting cyclo-oxygenase
    - Dose:
      - Neonates < 48 hours old:
        - 0.2 mg/kg IV bolus
        - Followed by 2 doses of 0.1 mg/kg IV Q12H
      - Neonates 2–7 days: 0.2 mg/kg IV Q12H for 3 doses
      - Neonates > 7 days:
        - 0.2 mg/kg IV bolus
        - Followed by 2 doses of 0.25 mg/kg IV Q12H
    - Associated side effects like:
      - Increased bleeding time
      - Renal and hepatic insufficiency
      - Sepsis
      - Necrotizing enterocolitis
    - Contraindications:
      - High BUN > 25 mg/dL or creatinine > 1.8 mg/dL
      - Low platelet count < 80,000 cells/mm^3
      - Necrotizing enterocolitis (NEC)
      - Hyperbilirubinemia
  - Ibuprofen:
    - Useful as an alternative to indomethacin
    - Dose:
      - 10 mg/kg bolus
      - Two doses of 5 mg/kg Q24H
    - Advantages over indomethacin:
      - Lower incidence of oliguria
      - Less deleterious effects on CBF
- Transcatheter closure:
  - Small PDAs < 2.5 mm are closed by the ***Gianturco stainless coils***
  - Larger PDAs are closed by ***Amplatzer PDA device***
  - Amplatzer device can be used for PDAs up to 4–10 mm diameter
  - Multiple coils may be used to occlude PDAs up to 5 mm diameter
  - Complications of device closure:
    - Residual leaks
    - Coil embolization into pulmonary artery (most common)
    - Hemolysis
    - Left pulmonary artery stenosis
    - Aortic occlusion with Amplatzer device
    - Femoral vessel occlusion
- Surgical closure:
  - Reserved for those in whom non-surgical closure is not feasible
  - Either by division/ligation of PDA done through posterolateral thoracotomy
  - Duct is ligated with a braided ligature or using a surgical clip
  - CPB is not required for PDA ligation

- It is a safe technique with operative mortality is < 1%
- Thoracoscopic technique:
  - Associated with less pain
  - Reserved for infants > 3 kg weight
  - Thus, its use is limited
  - This is because surgery is usually done is low-weight neonates
  - Contraindicated in the presence of severe PAH

Effects of Various Drugs on Ductus Patency

- Drugs causing PDA contraction:
  - Increased PaO_2: hyperoxia
  - $PGF_{2\alpha}$, Indomethacin, aspirin
  - Acetylcholine, succinylcholine, histamine
  - NSAIDs
  - Norepinephrine
- Drugs causing PDA relaxation:
  - PGE_1, PGE_2
  - Hypoxemia, acidosis
  - High altitude
  - Hypothermia

Anesthetic Considerations

- Surgery is usually performed in preterm/low weight infants
- Neonates in severe failure may be ventilated preoperatively
- Avoid hypothermia: Causes PDA relaxation and increased left-right shunting
- Avoid hemodilution
- Cross matched blood must be available as PDA may be severed during ligation
- Postoperative ventilation may be required if heart failure is present
- Left lateral thoracotomy approach
- Avoid hypoxia/hyperoxia:
  - Tidal volume: Adjusted to keep peak inspiratory pressure between 15 and 25 cmH_2O
  - E_TCO_2: Maintain between 35 and 45 mm Hg
  - SpO_2: Maintained between 87% and 92%
  - PaO_2: Maintained between 50 and 70 mm Hg

Preoperative Evaluation

History

- Birth trauma
- Respiratory and cardiovascular status
- History of maternal drug intake
- Fluid status

Examination

- Airway examination
- Fluid status:
  - Skin turgor
  - Mucous membrane
  - Anterior fontanelle
- Cardiovascular and abdominal examination
- Preoperative cardiorespiratory support is noted:
  - Additional inotropic support
  - Ventilatory settings required

Investigations

- Complete blood count, arterial blood gas
- Electrolytes, coagulation profile
- Urine analysis, urine specific gravity
- X-ray chest and abdomen

Preoperative Medications

- Informed consent
- Orally hydrated till 2 hours before surgery
- If this is not possible, IV hydration to be started
- 2 large bore IV cannulae are usually sufficient
- Umbilical venous catheter may be used in newborns
- Judicious fluid administration to prevent overload
- Continue inotropic support if present
- Children under 6 months may not require any preoperative sedation
- Midazolam 0.5 mg/kg PO 30 minutes before surgery may be given

Monitoring

- ECG
- Pulse oximeter in right hand and lower limb to detect inadvertent aortic ligation
- Invasive BP monitoring in right hand or in lower limbs
- End tidal CO_2, inspiratory pressure gauge
- Urinary bag, precordial/esophageal stethoscope
- Esophageal/axillary temperature probe
- Doppler transducer, arterial blood gas monitoring
- Central line:
  - Routine monitoring of CVP is usually not required
  - Central venous access may be considered for administering inotropic infusions

Induction

- Adequate preoxygenation as apnea and bradycardia can occur

- Following changes are seen on induction:
  - Prolonged time for onset of action IV agents
  - No change is seen with onset of inhalational induction
- Patients with IV line in place:
  - Good LV function:
    - Thiopentone 3–4 mg/kg + vecuronium 0.1 mg/kg
    - Fentanyl 2 µg/kg can be used to ensure analgesia
  - Poor LV function: Ketamine 1–2 mg/kg + vecuronium 0.1 mg/kg
- Patients with no IV line:
  - Inhalational induction with sevoflurane if good LV function
  - Start IV line (largest possible)
  - Fentanyl 1 µg/kg + vecuronium 0.1 mg/kg + glycopyrrolate 20 µg/kg
  - IM ketamine 5 mg/kg if poor LV function
- Avoid succinylcholine as it causes contracture of ductus arteriosus

Position

Right lateral decubitus as left posterolateral thoracotomy has to be done

Maintenance

- Sevoflurane + NDMR + fentanyl 2 µg/kg or sufentanil 1.5 µg/kg
- N_2O not to be used if pulmonary hypertension is present

Hemodynamics

- Fluid therapy:
  - Maintenance with 5% dextrose in 1/4 th strength NS
  - Maintenance fluids at 4 mL/kg/hour
  - Restrictive fluid strategy is preferred
  - IV tubing to be bubble free to prevent embolization
  - Maintain hematocrit: Hemodilution associated with an increase in left-right shunt
  - Replace blood loss with PRBCs or 1:3 crystalloid if hematocrit > 30%
- Watch for:
  - Bradycardia while surgical manipulation of the ductus
  - Systolic hypotension at the time of ligation of the ductus
  - Abrupt increase in DBP and mean BP with interruption of DA
  - Increased DBP due to the elimination of low resistance pulmonary circulation

Ventilation

- IPPV with pediatric bellows
- Ventilatory goals:
  - Tidal volume adjusted to keep peak inspiratory pressure between 15 and 25 cmH_2O
  - FiO_2 adjusted to keep PaO_2 between 50 and 70 mm Hg
  - Maintain SpO_2 between 87% and 92%
  - High FiO_2 avoided to prevent retinopathy of prematurity
  - E_TCO_2 to be maintained between 35 and 45 cm H_2O
- Hypoventilation:
  - Causes hypoxic pulmonary vasoconstriction
  - Reverses shunt to right-left shunt
- Hyperventilation:
  - Reduces pulmonary vascular resistance
  - Causes an increase in left-right shunt
- Lung compliance is reduced by lung retraction and packing during the procedure
- Hand ventilation may be required with ***Jackson-Reese*** circuit to:
  - Compensate for changes in pulmonary compliance during thoracotomy
  - Allow adequate field exposure during surgery
  - Deairing pleural cavity before closure

Intraoperative Complications

- Tear/avulsion of ductus arteriosus with profuse bleeding
- Bradycardia while handling ductus arteriosus
- Inadvertent left pulmonary artery/aortic ligation
- Phrenic nerve/recurrent laryngeal nerve injury
- Trauma to thoracic duct
- Left lung injury from pressure and retraction of lung
- Systemic embolization from calcification of aorta
- Residual shunt with ligation

Extubation

- Fully awake extubation in lateral decubitus position
- Majority extubated on table/soon after surgery
- Only sick children require postoperative ventilation
- Done after full reversal with neostigmine and atropine

Postoperative

Management

- May be considered to have normal cardiovascular system postoperatively
- Do not require routine infective endocarditis prophylaxis for subsequent surgeries

Analgesia

- Local anesthetic infiltration
- Paravertebral block
- Intrapleural block
- Thoracic epidural
- Opioid analgesia
- Paracetamol rectal suppository

Complications

- Postoperative hypertension related to baroreceptor dysfunction
- Left recurrent laryngeal nerve injury
- Phrenic nerve injury
- Chylous leak
- Pneumothorax due to inadvertent lung injury (rare)
- Aneurysm formation
- Systemic thromboembolism
- Reduced systemic blood flow causing:
  - Renal dysfunction
  - Necrotizing enterocolitis due to gastrointestinal hypoperfusion

COARCTATION OF AORTA

Introduction

- Defined as a discrete narrowing of descending aorta located at site of insertion of PDA
- The narrowing is usually present between:
  - Left subclavian artery proximally
  - Ductus arteriosus distally
- Earlier classified as pre-ductal, juxta-ductal and post-ductal CoA
- This classification is obsolete as all CoAs are considered to be juxta-ductal
- First described by Morgagni in 1760
- First repair performed by ***Crafoord and Nylin*** in 1944

Prevalence

- Accounts for approximately 5–8% of all congenital heart defect
- Incidence of 3–4 per 10,000 live births
- Occurs as an isolated finding in 25% of cases
- Seen in association with other cardiac defects in 75% cases, most commonly VSDs
- It is also commonly associated with bicuspid aortic valve (up to 60%)
- Most common near ductus arteriosus but also occurs in lower thorax and abdominal aorta

Embryology

- Aortic arch normally arises from left 4th arch of primitive arches of truncus arteriosus between 5th and 7th weeks of gestation
- Aorta proximal to site of ductal insertion, arising from left 4th arch is the *most common* site of CoA (called preductal CoA)
- Anomalous development occurs from 6th primitive aortic arch to the point of fusion of the two dorsal aortae resulting in post ductal CoA
- Aortic luminal diameter maybe reduced to as little as 1–3 mm

Morphology

- Usually found in descending thoracic aorta just distal to origin of left subclavian artery
- Constriction consists of localized medial thickening with in-folding of tunica media
- This may result in narrowing of aorta via:
  - Formation of a shelf along posterior aortic wall within the lumen of aorta
  - Concentric narrowing of the lumen of aorta
- Constriction is more commonly discrete in nature
- A ductal sling of tissue usually encircles the aortic site of coarctation
- Untreated coarctation leads to the formation of significant collateral vessels
- These collaterals arise proximal to the coarctation and supply the lower part of the body
- Coarctation may be associated with various cardiac anomalies:
  - Hypoplasia of isthmus of aorta
  - Hypoplastic transverse arch
  - Hypoplastic left heart syndrome
  - VSDs, atrioventricular canal defect
  - Transposition of great arteries
  - Taussig Bing syndrome
  - Shones complex:
    - Parachute mitral valve
    - Supra-mitral ring
    - Subaortic stenosis
    - Coarctation of aorta/interrupted aortic arch

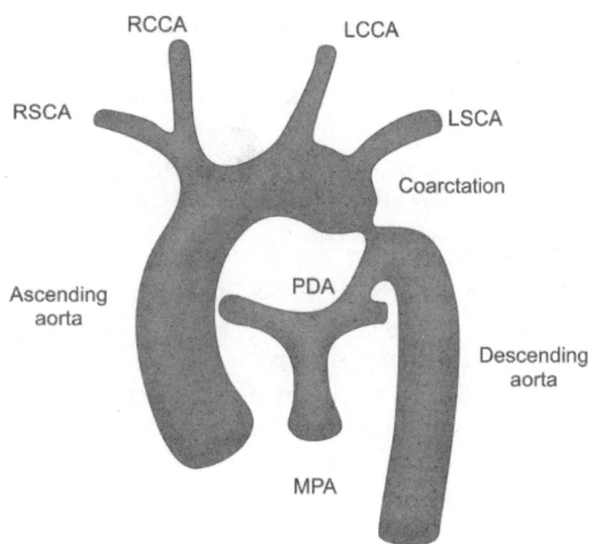

Fig. 29: Coarctation of aorta.

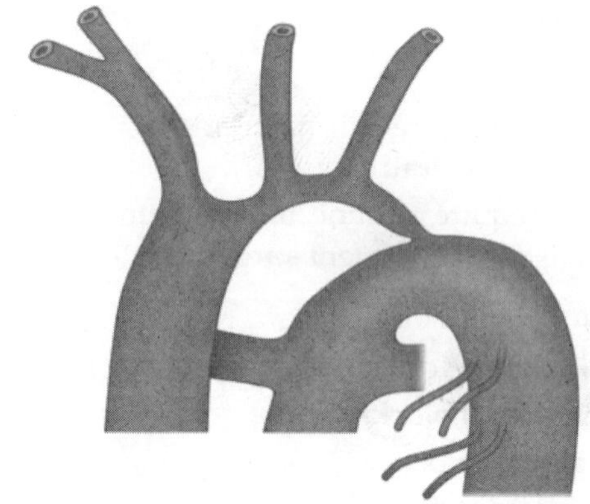

Fig. 30: Coarctation with hypoplasia of aortic arch.

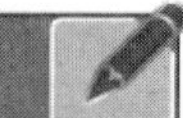

Classification

- Thoracic aortic CoA:
  - *Discrete coarctation*: localized shelf like lesion within aortic lumen
  - *Tubular coarctation*: uniform tube-like narrowing of part of aortic arch
- Coarctation associated with hypoplastic aortic arch:
  - Definition of hypoplastic arch is varied
  - *Moulaerts definition*: arch is hypoplastic when:
    - Diameter of proximal arch < 60% of diameter of ascending aorta
    - Diameter of distal arch < 50% of diameter of ascending aorta
    - Diameter of aortic ishmus < 40% of diameter of ascending aorta
  - Currently aortic arch z-scores are used to diagnose arch hypoplasia
- Lower thoracic CoA
- Abdominal aortic CoA

Etiology

- Genetic factors:
  - Strong familial association with autosomal dominant inheritance
  - Associated syndromes:
    - Turner syndrome
    - Noonan syndrome
    - Williams- Beuren syndrome
- Acquired coarctation of aorta:
  - Takayasus arteritis
  - Following cardiac surgery

Pathogenesis

- Ectopic ductal tissue theory:
  - Most coarctations are closely related to the site of PDA insertion (juxta-ductal)
  - In CoA, ectopic fibro-ductal tissue is present in the aorta beyond PDA
  - This abnormal extension of ductal tissue into aorta results in ectopic ductal tissue
  - PDA closure causes contraction of the ectopic ductal tissue
  - This results in the formation of the coarctation shelf and CoA
- Hemodynamic theory:
  - Reduced antegrade intrauterine blood flow in aorta alters endothelial development
  - This may lead to the development of localized intimal hyperplasia and CoA

Pathophysiology

- Patients with critical coarctation of aorta:
  - In neonates, closure of the DA causes severe obstruction to LV outflow
  - This results in:
    - Acute LV failure
    - Elevated LA pressures
    - Left-right shunting across PFO
  - In the presence of additional VSD, massive L-R shunting occurs
  - This may worsen LV failure and pulmonary edema
- Patients with non-critical coarctation of aorta:
  - Heart failure does not develop in these patients due to compensatory mechanisms:
    - Concentric myocardial hypertrophy
    - Increase in LV end-diastolic volume

- Increase in preload-recruitable cardiac output
- Increased sympathetic outflow resulting in increased inotropy
- Development of collateral circulation which helps to:
  - Decrease LV afterload
  - Maintain perfusion to lower body
- Failure to correct the CoA eventually leads to CCF with varying duration of onset

❖ Pressure gradients between 30 and 40 mm Hg develop which stimulates collateral circulation development

Collateral Circulation

❖ Intercostal artery
❖ Internal mammary artery
❖ Internal thoracic artery
❖ Subdivision of subclavian artery
❖ Superior epigastric artery
❖ Perhaps anterior spinal and vertebral artery
❖ Patients with collaterals are less likely to develop paraplegia following aortic cross clamping

Clinical Presentation

❖ Symptoms:
- Neonates:
  - Asymptomatic in the presence of PDA or minor CoA
  - Features of congestive cardiac failure:
    - Occurs in neonates with severe CoA
    - These neonates have a duct-dependent systemic circulation
    - Closure of PDA results in drastic increase in LV afterload
    - This results in:
      - CCF and pulmonary edema within 1–3 weeks of age
      - Tachycardia, tachypnea, dyspnea, poor feeding
      - Poorly perfused lower body resulting in:
        - Absent femoral pulses
        - Severe metabolic acidosis
        - Renal failure and oliguria
        - Cardiovascular collapse
- Older children:
  - Heart failure is rare beyond neonatal period
  - Presenting features include:
    - Chest pain, cold extremities
    - Limb claudication with physical exertion
    - Refractory HTN
- Adults:
  - Refractory HTN
  - Headache, epistaxis
  - Lower limb claudication on exertion
  - Rarely heart failure and aortic dissection

❖ Signs:
- Pulses in lower limb will is delayed/diminished/absent
- Pulse in upper limb is bounding
- BP decreased in lower limb
- Upper limb BP may exceed lower limb BP by > 20 mm Hg
- Localization of lesion:
  - CoA located at aortic isthmus, distal to let SCA when:
    - Pulse is present in right arm
    - Pulse is present in right carotid artery
    - Absent or weak in both lower limbs
  - CoA is proximal to left subclavian artery take off when:
    - Pulse is present in right arm
    - Pulse is absent in left arm and legs
    - Right arm BP is more than left arm BP
  - CoA is associated with aberrant right SCA:
    - Anomalous RSCA may have its origin distal to CoA segment
    - Pulse is palpable in left arm from LSCA
    - Pulse is absent in right upper arm due to anomalous RSCA
    - Pulse is absent in bilateral lower limbs
- Systolic thrill may be palpable in suprasternal notch area
- Auscultation:
  - S_3 gallop, diffuse ejection systolic murmur
  - Systolic ejection murmur:
    - Grade 2–3 radiating over right upper sternal border
    - Occasionally heard posteriorly in interscapular area left of midline
  - Ejection click of bicuspid aortic valve
  - Diastolic murmur of aortic regurgitation
- Metabolic acidosis and oliguria/anuria due to CCF

❖ Others:
- Differential cyanosis:
  - Occurs due to severe CoA with large PDA and an R-L shunt
  - R-L shunt into descending aorta causes lower limb cyanosis
  - Upper half receives oxygenated blood from blood vessels (bv) originating above CoA

- Lower half is perfused with deoxygenated blood from RV via PDA
- Thus, preductal saturation is higher than post-ductal saturation

❖ ***Suzmans sign:***
- Most prominent over scapula
- Continuous pulsations present in the back due to formation of scapular collaterals
- Best visualized with the patient bending forwards

Investigations

❖ ECG:
- Right ventricular hypertrophy with RBBB seen more commonly in neonates
- Left ventricular hypertrophy with left axis deviation in adults

❖ Chest X-ray:
- Heart size normal or slightly enlarged with or without ascending aortic dilation
- ***Figure of 3 sign:***
  - Seen in frontal chest X-ray
  - Occurs in one- third to one- half the patients with aortic coarctation
  - Refers to the contour formed by the coarctation segment of the aorta
  - Aortic segment affected by CoA forms a shape resembling the number 3
  - Upper arc is formed by pre-stenotic dilatation of left SCA and aortic arch
  - Indentation occurs at CoA site, between the 2 bulges, known as the *tuck*
  - Lower arc is formed by the post-stenotic dilatation of the descending aorta
  - May be associated with a prominent LV border
- Reverse 3 or E sign:
  - Seen in left anterior oblique view during barium esophagography
  - Occurs due to contour formed by the coarctation segment
  - Represents mirror image of pre and post-stenotic dilatation, seen on X-ray
  - Also called ***E- sign***
- Pulmonary edema and pulmonary venous congestion
- Inferior rib notching:
  - Also called ***Roeslers sign or Docks sign***
  - Etiology:
    - Occurs secondary to dilated intercostal collateral arteries (ICA)
    - Dilated ICAs bypass the CoA and supply the descending aorta (DA)
  - Description:
    - Intercostal vessels erode the inferior margins of the ribs
    - Uncommon in children below 5 years age
    - Seen in 75% of adults with coarctation
    - Commonly involves the 4th to 8th ribs
    - Occasionally involves the 3rd and 9th ribs
    - 1st and 2nd ribs are almost never involved
    - This is because:
      - 1st and 2nd ICA arise from the costo-cervical trunk
      - This is a branch of the subclavian artery
      - These ICAs do not communicate with the aorta
      - Thus, 1st and 2nd ICA are not involved in collateral formation
      - Therefore, 1st and 2nd ribs are not involved in rib notching
- Bilateral rib notching:
  - Coarctation lies distal to the origin of both SCA
  - Thus, collaterals arise from both the SCA and cause bilateral rib notching
- Unilateral right rib notching:
  - Coarctation lies between brachiocephalic trunk and origin of left SCA
  - Hence collaterals form between right SCA (brachiocephalic trunk) and DA
- Unilateral left rib notching:
  - Coarctation lies distal to origin of both SCA
  - This usually would result in bilateral rib notching
  - But, unilateral notching occurs when RSCA origin is aberrant
  - Aberrant right SCA usually arises distal to the coarctation segment
  - Thus collaterals form from the left SCA to the descending aorta
  - Collaterals do not form on the right as RSCA arises distal to coarctation
- Other causes of inferior rib notching:
  - Interrupted aortic arch
  - Subclavian artery occlusion
  - Arteriovenous malformation of the chest wall
  - Pulmonary arteriovenous malformation
  - Superior vena caval obstruction

❖ Echocardiography:
- Shelf like membrane in posterior descending aorta from suprasternal notch view
- Doppler evaluation across the CoA to determine severity of obstruction

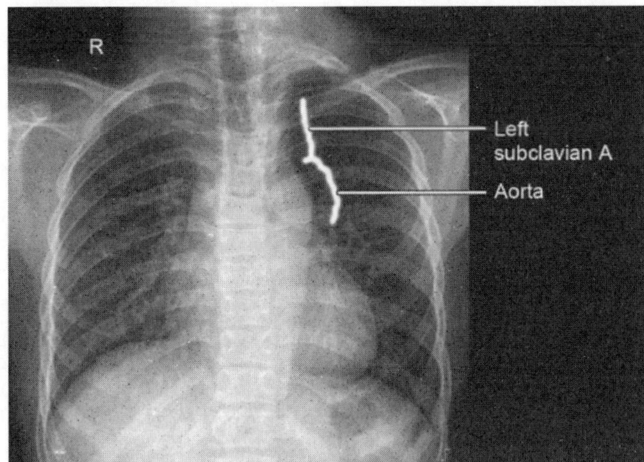

Fig. 31: Figure of 3 sign chest X-ray in coarctation of aorta.

- Left ventricular dysfunction
- Associated defects like hypoplastic arch, VSD, bicuspid aortic valve

❖ Computerized tomography: rarely required in the presence of diagnostic uncertainty

❖ Cardiac catheterization:
- Generally not required as a diagnostic tool
- Indicated when:
  - Information from ECHO is incomplete
  - Concern over collateral flow that may affect the surgical plan
- Studies pressure differential between ascending and decending aorta
- Confirms VSD, TGA, bicuspid aortic valve

Treatment

❖ Medical therapy:
- Oxygen therapy, digitalization, diuretics and inotropic support for children with CCF
- PGE_1 to maintain ductal patency if systemic perfusion depends on R-L shunt

❖ Indications for intervention:
- Patients with peak CoA gradient > 20 mm Hg (class I)
- Patients with peak CoA gradient < 20 mm Hg in the presence of:
  - LV dysfunction due to tight CoA (class I)
  - Severe LV hypertrophy (class IIa)
  - Upper limb HTN (class IIa)
  - Significant collateral formation (class IIa)
- > 50% narrowing at CoA site, relative to aortic diameter, irrespective of gradient

❖ Age at intervention:

LV dysfunction	CCF	Upper limb HTN	Gradient	Age
Severe	Severe	Severe	> or < 20 mm Hg	Immediate
Absent	Absent	Mild	> 20 mm Hg	Beyond 3–6 months age
Absent	Absent	Absent	> 20 mm Hg	1–2 years age
Absent	Absent	Absent	< 20 mm Hg	Regular follow-up

❖ Interventional therapies:
- Balloon angioplasty:
  - Causes damage to tunica intima and media
  - This can increase risk of aneurysm formation and dissection
  - Reserved for sick infants who cannot undergo surgery
  - Allows successful resuscitation prior to definitive surgical repair
  - Also can be considered as an option for early recurrence of CoA
  - Significant risk of aneurysm formation exists
- Stent placement:
  - Uses endovascular bare-metal stents (BMS) or covered stents (CS)
  - Adequate landing zone should be ensured prior to deployment of CS
  - This is in order to avoid occlusion of LSCA or LCCA
  - Use in children < 25 kg is controversial
  - Used most commonly for re-coarctation following surgical repair
  - Risk of aneurysm formation present although lesser than for angioplasty

❖ Surgical therapy:
- Resection and anastomosis:
  - *Surgery of choice* when feasible especially for neonates and infants
  - Involves extensive mobilization of tissues:
    - Site of coarctation
    - Descending aorta
  - Arch of aorta up to ascending aorta
  - Clamps are placed on the DA and arch
  - Coarctation segment and isthmus are excised
  - The two ends are then anastomosed together
  - Mortality rate is low in uncomplicated patients
  - Residual obstruction can occur in up to 34% patients at early follow-up
- Subclavian flap angioplasty:
  - Following application of clamps, left SCA is ligated distally
  - LSCA is laid open along its length with incision extending into the CoA

- The opened SCA is folded down and used as a flap to enlarge the CoA
- Less popular as:
  - High incidence of residual obstruction
  - High risk of aneurysm formation
  - Sacrifices LSCA (small risk of hemi-smallness of left arm)
- May be combined with end-to-end anastomosis for long-segment CoA

- Interposition grafts:
  - Done primarily in older patients
  - Substantial mobilization of tissue is required for end-end anastomosis
  - This may not be possible in older patients
  - Thus, interposition grafts are used to relieve obstruction
- Dacron patch aortoplasty:
  - Longitudinal incision is made across the area of CoA
  - The aortotomy is then repaired with a synthetic dacron patch
  - Seldom used
  - High risk of aneurysm formation along suture lines
  - May be used for patients with complex redo-arch reconstruction

Anesthetic Management

Preoperative Preparation and Premedication

- Evaluate:
  - Patients physical status
  - Associated cardiac and other medical problems
  - Whether patient has been optimally treated

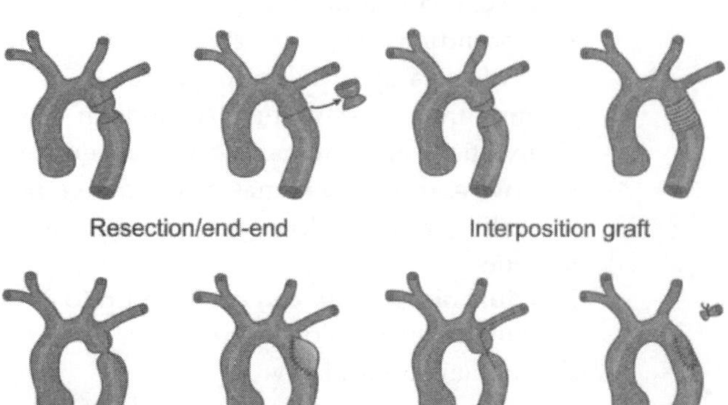

Fig. 32: Coarctation of aorta repair techniques.

- Discuss the plan of surgery with the surgical team:
  - Resection with end-end anastomosis: via thoracotomy
  - CoA repair + VSD closure: via sternotomy and CPB
  - Hypoplastic arch repair: via sternotomy and DHCA
- NPO orders
- Informed consent
- Large bore IV cannulation to enable volume resuscitation
- IV cannulas are placed on left hand in case thoracotomy is planned
- Sedation:
  - Not required for children < 6–9 months age
  - Sedation for other patients is individualized as per needs
  - 0.2–0.5 mg/kg midazolam orally within 15–30 minutes of induction
  - Better to give sedation in holding area of operating room
- Temperature:
  - Maintain thermally neutral environment during transfer of patient
  - Done to minimize stress on heart due to changes in SVR from vasoconstriction
  - Measures used include:
    - Passive measures such as clear plastic wrap
    - Active methods such as:
      - Warming blankets
      - IV fluid warmers
- Antisialogogue: anticholinergic premedication like glycopyrrollate useful
- Antibiotic chemoprophylaxis as per hospital protocol

Monitoring

- Pulse oximeter probe on right arm
- ECG lead placement to take into account right lateral decubitus position
- Invasive blood pressure:
  - Blood pressure is typically measured at 2 sites:
    - Preductal in the right radial artery
    - Post ductal in the femoral artery (either side)
  - Measurement at 2 sites enables continuous monitoring of CoA gradient
  - Left arm BP not used as LSCA may be clamped/used for surgical repair of CoA

- Right arm BP:
  - Provides information regarding cerebral circulation during clamping
  - This enables us to titrate preductal pressures during clamping such that:
    - HTN of cerebral circulation is avoided
    - Hypotension in vessels distal to the clamp is avoided
- ❖ Central venous pressure monitoring for fluid therapy and vasoactive medications
- ❖ Nasopharyngeal temperature, urine output
- ❖ BIS and neuromuscular monitoring as early extubation is preferred
- ❖ NIRS especially if DHCA and retrograde cerebral perfusion is planned
- ❖ Transesophageal echocardiography for CPB correction of associated defects

Induction and Intubation

- ❖ Adequate preoxygenation
- ❖ Techniques of induction:
  - In hemodynamically stable patients with good LV reserve:
    - Thiopentone 3–5 mg/kg with fentanyl 2 μg/kg
    - Propofol can be used alternatively
    - Induction agent given slowly to avoid myocardial depression
    - Neuromuscular paralysis with vecuronium 0.1 mg/kg
  - In patients with suspected/known reduction in LV function:
    - Etomidate 0.15–0.3 mg/kg and vecuronium 0.1 mg/kg
    - Ketamine may be used as an alternative
    - Fentanyl is given for analgesia once hemodynamically stable
    - Combined benzodiazepine with narcotic induction:
      - Midazolam 0.1–0.3 mg/kg and fentanyl 5–20 μg/kg
      - Neuromuscular paralysis with vecuronium 0.1 mg/kg
- ❖ In patients with no intravenous access inhalational induction with sevoflurane
- ❖ High FiO_2 is avoided in the presence of duct dependent physiology
- ❖ In these cases, lower body perfusion depends on R-L shunt through the PDA
- ❖ High FiO_2 reverses the shunt flow across PDA and lower body perfusion
- ❖ Debubbling is done scrupulously to avoid possibility of paradoxical embolization
- ❖ Ketamine and other agents which increase SVR to be avoided in patients with:
  - Bicuspid aortic valve
  - Significant AS/AR
- ❖ Left-to-right shunting may cause slight decrease in rate of IV induction
- ❖ Right-to-left shunting may increase rate of inhalational induction

Position

- ❖ Right lateral decubitus position if thoracotomy is planned
- ❖ Supine position for surgeries involving CPB

Maintenance

- ❖ Primarily narcotic based in patients with depressed myocardial function with:
  - Fentanyl 10–25 μg/kg or sufentanil 1–2.5 μg/kg total dose
  - Low dose inhalational agent used to maintain balanced anesthesia
- ❖ Avoid N_2O due to:
  - Potential for myocardial depression in those getting narcotics
  - Also causes enlargement of air bubbles
- ❖ Neuromuscular blockade with vecuronium/pancuronium
- ❖ $NaHCO_3$ (2 mEq/kg) is administered during release of aortic clamp in thoracotomy patients
- ❖ Precautions for DHCA:
  - Ice wrap around the head when temperature < 25°C is maintained
  - High dose methylprednisolone 30 mg/kg on CPB
  - Thiopentone 10 mg/kg administered on CPB

Ventilation

- ❖ Conventional ventilatory modes and settings are used with low FiO_2
- ❖ Low TV ventilation may be required to aid surgical exposure during thoracotomy
- ❖ Recruitment maneuver may be used just prior to chest closure to prevent atelectasis

Hemodynamics

- Maintenance fluids:
  - Isotonic crystalloids such as plasmalyte and lactated Ringers may be used
  - Dextrose containing fluids may be used in neonates
- Ductal manipulation may cause bradycardia:
  - Atropine should be immediately available
  - Manipulation of aorta should be suspended temporarily
- Avoid left-to-right shunting by preventing:
  - Respiratory alkalosis
  - Hyperoxia
  - Excessive reduction in hematocrit
  - Reduction in pulmonary vascular resistance
  - Increases in systemic vascular resistance
- During aortic clamping:
  - Maintain post-ductal MAP above age appropriate levels
  - This is to prevent lower body hypoperfusion and paraplegia
  - Vasodilators and β-blockers may be used to control pre-ductal BP during clamping
- Following release of aortic cross clamp:
  - There may be sudden, brief, severe hypotension immediately following release
  - Aggressive control of HTN is required thereafter
  - Pre-ductal and post-ductal gradients are checked to rule out residual CoA
- In patients with VSD:
  - Avoid hypervolemia to avoid increase in left-to-right shunting
  - Avoid increase in pulmonary artery pressure and pulmonary vascular congestion
  - Avoid sudden reduction in SVR
- Temperature:
  - Mild hypothermia (35°C) is preferred intraoperatively
  - This is because the risk of paraplegia post-procedure has been found to be lower
- Blood:
  - Blood loss is usually minimal during thoracotomy procedures
  - Given judiciously to avoid reduction in oxygen delivery
  - Administered at slow rates not likely to provoke cardiac failure
- Coagulation products generally not required in non-CPB cases

CPB Considerations

- CPB is used for hypoplastic arch repairs or CoA with associated defects
- Traditional CPB with cardioplegic myocardial protection used
- Single venous cannulation is usually used
- Bi-caval cannulation may be required in the presence of intracardiac defects
- Target temperature:
  - 24–28°C with very low flow CPB
  - Arch augmentation may require even lower temperature up to 18°C
- Minimal dilutional hematocrit of 25% is tolerated
- Pump flows are reduced during aortic clamp as only upper body is being perfused
- NIRS is constantly monitored and maintained within 20% of baseline values
- Higher pump flows may be required during cooling:
  - This is because lower body is under-perfused due to CoA
  - Thus, cooling of lower body may be slower
  - Higher pump flows during this phase may assist in cooling

Postoperative Management

Management

- Healthy older individuals can be extubated early in postoperative period
- Delayed weaning and extubation (12–24 hours) for:
  - Sicker patients with limited cardiopulmonary reserve
  - Preoperative heart failure
  - Complex arch repairs
- Prior to weaning, check:
  - Patient must be rewarmed to a normal body temperature
  - Fluid, electrolytes and coagulation status
  - Hemoglobin levels
  - Recovery of muscle strength and CNS status
- Hemodynamic management:
  - Inotropic support may be required in the presence of LV failure
  - Inotropes may be weaned following extubation
  - Strict control of blood pressure is important
  - Systolic BP is titrated to maintain strict control between 80 and 90 mm Hg

- Fluid therapy:
  - Fluid restriction is usually not required following surgery
  - Restrictive strategy may be used in surgeries done on CPB
  - Oral feeds are resumed slowly once:
    - Hemodynamically stable
    - Confirmation of bowel sounds
    - Normal abdominal examination

Early Complications

- Hypertension:
  - Most patients develop HTN in immediate postoperative period (within 24 hours)
  - Occurs due to:
    - Increased catecholamine levels, especially norepinephrine
    - Increased plasma renin activity
  - Strict control of BP is important during the 1st 24–48 hours to prevent:
    - Anastomotic leaks
    - Post-coartectomy syndrome
    - Minimize bleeding
  - Drugs used to control postoperative HTN include:
    - β-blockers
    - Nicardipine
    - Nitroglycerin and nitroprusside
    - ACE inhibitors once oral feeding is established
- Chylothorax: rare in infants, higher in adults
- Transient renal failure
- Paraplegia:
  - Incidence of 0.4%
  - Due to:
    - Ischemia of thoracic spinal cord from prolonged cross clamping
    - Spinal cord HTN below the level of aortic cross clamping causing cord infarction
    - Hyperthermia to 38–40°C during cross clamping
  - Maintain distal aortic press > 60 mm Hg to reduce incidence of neurological injury
  - Spinal cord infarction is rare if aortic cross clamp time is < 20 mins
  - If cross clamp time > 20 mins, consider placement of a temporary shunt
  - Hypothermia may offer cord protection by reducing spiral cord oxygen requirements and consumption
- Post-coartectomy syndrome:
  - Necrotizing mesenteric arteritis presenting with:
    - Ileus
    - Abdominal pain and distension
    - Melena, vomiting
    - Fecal incontinence and bowel necrosis
  - Thought to occur due to sudden reperfusion of mesenteric vessels following repair
  - Common in collapsed neonates with poor lower body perfusion
  - Less common now due to better control of postoperative HTN
- Injury to recurrent laryngeal nerve
- Injury to phrenic nerve causing diaphragmatic palsy.

Late Complications

- Recurrent coarctation:
  - Occurs in > 85% patients treated with catheter interventions
- Persistent HTN:
  - Rare if surgery is done below 5 years age
  - Incidence of almost 50% when surgery is conducted at later age

Natural History and Surgical Outcomes

- 50% mortality in first month of life
- ≥ 80% mortality in first 3 months of life
- Mortality reduces to 1–2% following surgery for isolated CoA
- Early surgery is associated with better long-term survival
- Fatality of >75% by age 46 years due to:
  - Rupture of aorta
  - Congestive cardiac failure
  - Bacterial endocarditis
  - Intracerebral bleed

TETRALOGY OF FALLOT

Introduction

- First described by Etienne-Louis Arthur Fallot in 1888
- Term tetralogy of Fallot was assigned in 1924 by Maude Abbot
- First palliative shunt done by Alfred Blalock and Helen Taussig in 1945
- First intracardiac repair done in 1954 by Lillehei using human controlled cross circulation
- First intracardiac repair using pump oxygenator was by Kirklin in 1955

Anatomical Components

- Anatomical components of tetralogy of Fallot includes:
  - Overriding of aorta
  - Non-restrictive large subaortic outlet VSD
  - Right ventricular outflow tract obstruction
  - Right ventricular hypertrophy
- Anatomical components of trilogy of Fallot includes:
  - Atrial septal defect
  - Pulmonary stenosis
  - Right ventricular hypertrophy
- Anatomical components of pentalogy of Fallot includes:
  - Large subaortic outlet VSD
  - Right ventricular out flow tract obstruction
  - Overriding of aorta
  - Right ventricular hypertrophy
  - Atrial septal defect

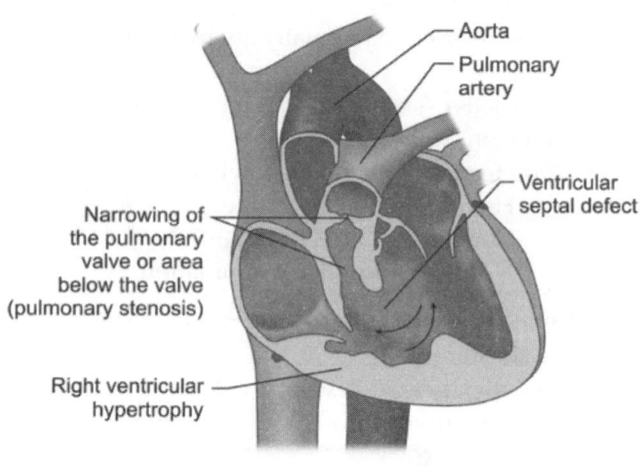

Fig. 33: Anatomy of TOF.

Incidence

- Most common cyanotic congenital heart disease
- Accounts for 5% of all congenital heart diseases
- 3.3 per 10,000 live births

Embryology

- TOF is characterized by underdevelopment of the subpulmonary infundibulum
- Anatomical findings are due to antero-cephalad displacement of the conal septum
- All the tenets of TOF can be explained by the singular deviation of outlet septum
- The conal septal deviation produces:
  - Overriding of aorta
  - Narrowing of RVOT
  - Large malalignment VSD
- Deviation of the spiral septum results in:
  - Anomalies of pulmonary valve:
    - Bicuspid pulmonary valve
    - Pulmonary valvular stenosis/atresia
  - Unusually large aortic root and ascending aorta
- Minor anomalies of the anterior leaflet of tricuspid valve also exist as this leaflet is formed by the coral septum

Anatomy

- VSD is large and unrestrictive and perimembranous
- RVOT obstruction can be at the level of:
  - Infundibulum of RV
  - Pulmonary valve/annulus
  - Main pulmonary artery
  - Peripheral pulmonary arteries
- Infundibular stenosis due to hypertrophy of subpulmonic muscle: ***crista ventricularis***

Associated Anomalies

- Patent foramen ovale: 50–60%
- Right aortic arch: 15–25%
- Left superior vena cava: 8–10%
- Additional VSDs (usually in muscular septum): 3–5%
- PDA: 4%
- Coronary artery abnormalities 3–5%:
  - LAD arising from RCA
  - RCA arising from left coronary artery
  - Large branch of RCA supplying conus region
  - Single right/left coronary artery
  - Coronary artery crossing RVOT
- Other syndromes:
  - DiGeorge syndrome 15%
  - VACTERL syndrome
  - CHARGE syndrome
  - Rare associations:
    - Downs syndrome
    - Pataus syndrome
    - Edwards syndrome

Pathophysiology

- Initial presentation of TOF patients depends on the degree of RVOTO
- Most commonly, cyanosis is mild at birth and progresses with age
- This is due to increasing hypertrophy of the RV infundibulum
- RVOT obstruction:
  - Usually results in dynamic obstruction at infundibulum

- Caused by:
  - Highly muscularized outlet septum on one side
  - Thickened septo-parietal band on the other side
- Can be increased by increases in heart rate and contractility
- Degree of RVOT obstruction determines the pathophysiological changes

❖ Mild-moderate RVOT obstruction
- Predominant shunt is left-right
- Clinical picture and presentation may be that of congestive cardiac failure:
  - Failure to thrive
  - Recurrent respiratory tract infections
- Patient is usually acyanotic (called ***pink tet***):
  - Patient with TOF with source for adequate PA blood flow from:
    - Antegrade flow across pulmonary valve
    - PDA
    - Major aorto-pulmonary collateral arteries: MAPCAs
    - Naturally occurring PA collaterals:
      - Intercostal artery
      - Bronchial arteries
  - Patient with TOF and insignificant RVOT obstruction
- Cyanosis increases with age (usually within first 6–12 months)

❖ Severe RVOT obstruction:
- Predominant shunt is right-left shunt
- Clinical picture and presentation is that of central cyanosis soon after birth
- RVOTO is nearly always due to hypoplastic pulmonary valve annulus
- Severe RV infundibular hyperplasia may or may not be present
- Cyanosis is constant in these patients due to fixed nature of RVOTO

❖ Acute increase in right-left shunt is due to:
- Reduced SVR: Hypotension
- Increased PVR: Hypoxia, hypercarbia, acidosis
- Increased RVOT obstruction: Tachycardia, increased contractility

❖ Congestive cardiac failure in cyanotic TOF:
- Since the VSD decompresses RV, CCF is rare in TOF
- CCF occurs only if cyanotic TOF is associated with:
  - Anemia
  - Infective endocarditis, myocarditis
  - Systemic HTN
  - Aortic regurgitation/pulmonary regurgitation

Classification of Tetralogy of Fallot

❖ TOF with pulmonary stenosis
❖ TOF with complete AV canal defect
❖ TOF with pulmonary atresia
❖ TOF with absent pulmonary valve syndrome

Clinical Features

❖ Symptoms:
- Time of presentation depends upon the degree of RVOTO
- Most neonates are acyanotic and become cyanosed gradually as RVOTO increases
- Cyanosis occurs in neonatal period when RVOTO is severe
- Clubbing in late presentations
- *Hypercyanotic tet spells*
- Pink TOF when RVOTO is less severe:
  - Failure to thrive, malnourishment
  - Recurrent respiratory tract infections
  - Exertional dyspnea in older children

❖ Signs:
- Central cyanosis
- Clubbing may be present beyond 3 months of life
- RV parasternal heave
- S_1 is normal
- Single audible S_2 due to:
  - Delayed closure of PV due to slow pressure drop in the stenotic RVOT
  - Valvular pulmonary stenosis
  - Overriding of aorta
- P_2 is faint as hardly any blood flow occurs through PA
- Single S_2 helps to differentiate TOF from isolated VSD or PS
- VSD murmur is not heard as it is unrestrictive
- Ejection systolic murmur:
  - Heard along mid and upper left sternal border radiating to the back
  - Intensity of murmur is inversely proportional to degree of RVOTO
  - Murmur disappears during cyanotic spells
- Continuous murmur occurs in the presence of:
  - PDA (heard below left clavicle)
  - VSD with pulmonary atresia:

    - Occurs extensively over anterior and posterior chest bilaterally
    - Due to major aortopulmonary collateral circulation (MAPCAs)
- Complications:
  - Paradoxical air embolism
  - Polycythemia
  - Coagulation defects
  - Pulmonary, renal/cerebral thrombosis: Especially if hematocrit > 65%
  - Cerebral abscess
  - Infective endocarditis
  - Cardiomyopathy, AR: Occur late and cause death
- Without surgical correction:
  - 25% die in 1st year of life
  - 40% die by 4 years
  - 70% die by 10 years
  - 90% die by 40 years
- Assessment of severity: more severe if:
  - Malnourished, inactive due to congestive cardiac failure
  - Cyanosis is severe due to increased right-left shunt
  - Shorter and less intense ESM: Implies PV is more tight

HYPERCYANOTIC TET SPELLS

Introduction

- Important manifestation of TOF with a dynamic and hypertrophic infundibulum
- Characterized by paroxysmal episodes in which cyanosis acutely worsens

Precipitating Factors

- Crying, fear, anxiety
- Feeding
- Defecation
- Exercise
- Concomitant illnesses such as dehydration and respiratory infections

Presentation

- Usually occurs in infants between 3 and 24 months of age
- Peak incidence occurs at 2–3 months age
- Cyanotic spells are less common beyond 2 years age
- Commonly occurs in acyanotic/mildly cyanotic patients
- Occur most commonly in morning and begins with irritability and crying
- Progressive increase in rate and depth of respiration follows
- Increasing cyanosis which terminates with syncope/seizures
- Each attack is potentially fatal
- Frequency varies from once in few days to numerous attacks per day

Mechanism

- Increasing dynamic right ventricular outflow tract obstruction:
  - Results in increasing cyanosis due to:
    - Reduced antegrade blood flow to the lungs
    - Increasing right-left shunt causing systemic desaturation
  - Precipitated by:
    - Increased heart rate
    - Increased contractility:
      - Surgical stimulus
      - Inotropes
    - Hypovolemia
- Decrease in SVR:
  - SBP < 60 mm Hg triggers episodes
  - Drugs:
    - Volatile anesthetics
    - Histamine releasers
    - Ganglionic blockade

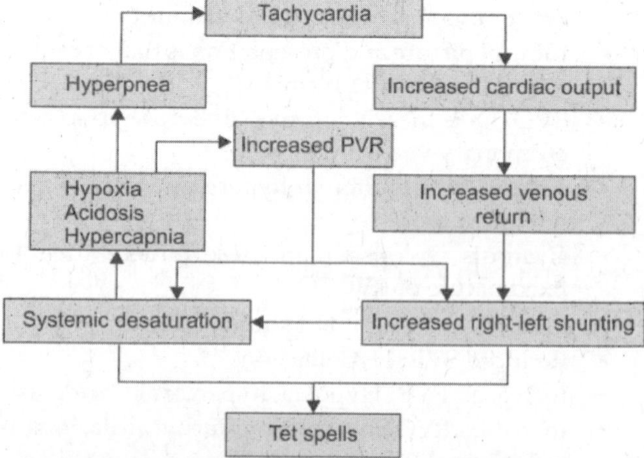

Theories of TET Spells

- Woods theory:
  - Postulates that hypoxic spells are due to RVOT spasm
  - This precipitates a cycle of progressively increasing right-left shunting

Contd...

Contd...

- This results in systemic desaturation and metabolic acidosis
- This theory does not explain cyanotic spells in TOF with pulmonary atresia

❖ Catecholamine release theory:
- Postulates that the precipitating event is catecholamine release
- This leads to increased myocardial contractility and RVOT spasm
- This theory does not explain cyanotic spells in TOF with pulmonary atresia

❖ Guntheroths theory:
- Precipitating event is hyperpnea causing increased venous return
- This leads to cyanosis through:
  - Increase in R-L shunting
  - Increased oxygen demand due to increase in work of breathing

❖ Kotharis theory:
- Discredits other theories associated with RVOT spasm
- Stimulation of right ventricular mechanoceptors precipitates tet spells

❖ Morgans theory:
- Postulates that hypoxic spells are due to vulnerable respiratory center
- Vulnerable respiratory center over-reacts to hypoxic stimuli like crying
- This causes an increase in cardiac output and heart rate
- This in turn increases the venous return causing increased R-L shunting
- Respiratory center again responds to the fall in PaO_2 and causes hyperpnea
- This results in a vicious cycle

❖ Youngs theory: Precipitated by atrial tachycardia

Other Conditions Causing TET Spells

- ❖ Tricuspid atresia
- ❖ Transposition of great arteries
- ❖ Single ventricle physiology with associated pulmonary stenosis

Treatment of TET Spells

❖ Reduce PVR:
- Hyperventilate with 100% oxygen (facemask 6 L/minute)
- Correct acidosis with IV 8.4% sodium bicarbonate:
  - 1 mL/kg can be given slow IV
  - This is diluted in equal quantity of sterile water
  - The resultant volume is given over 5–10 minutes
  - The dose may be repeated after 10 minutes

❖ Reduce RVOT obstruction:
- Deepen anesthetic plane:
  - Morphine:
    - 0.05–0.1 mg/kg slow IV over 5–10 minutes
    - 0.1–0.2 mg/kg IM
  - Ketamine 1–2 mg/kg IV
  - Fentanyl 1–2 μg/kg IV
- β-blockers:
  - Esmolol:
    - 0.5 mg/kg given over 1–2 minutes
    - This is followed by 50–300 μg/kg/min for up to 48 hours
  - Metaprolol:
    - 0.1 mg/kg given slow IV over 5 minutes
    - May be repeated every 5 minutes up to maximum of 3 doses
    - Can be followed by infusion of 1–2 μg/kg/minute
  - Propranolol:
    - 0.1–0.2 mg/kg IV
    - Can be repeated up to 3–4 times a day if required
- Volume administration:
  - Improves pulmonary arterial flow by increasing venous return
  - Reducing in blood viscosity favors pulmonary flow
  - 10–20 mL/kg ringers lactate/normal saline bolus is used

❖ Increase SVR:
- *Knee chest position*
- Correct anemia
- Phenylephrine:
  - 0.5–2 μg/kg slow IV bolus
  - Can be repeated every 10–15 minutes
  - Can be used as a continuous infusion 0.025–0.05 μg/kg/min
- Norepinephrine 0.01–0.02 μg/kg/min infusion
- Intubation and emergent surgery if unresponsive
- Abdominal aorta/ascending aortic compression

❖ Prophylaxis against further recurrence with PO propranolol 0.25–1 mg/kg Q6-8H

Investigations

❖ Complete blood count:
- Secondary polycythemia is commonly seen

- Thrombocytopenia:
  - Commonly seen in TOF patients
  - Megakaryocyte maturation occurs in the pulmonary circulation
  - R-L shunting decreases pulmonary blood flow in TOF patients
  - This causes shunting of megakaryocytes to systemic circulation
  - Other mechanisms causing thrombocytopenia include:
    - Decreased megakaryocyte production
    - Increased platelet destruction
    - Increased platelet activation

❖ ECG:
- Right atrial enlargement and right ventricular hypertrophy
- Characteristics on ECG include:
  - Right axis deviation
  - Prominent R-waves anteriorly
  - Prominent S-waves posteriorly
  - Upright T-wave in V1
  - qR pattern in right sided chest leads

❖ Chest X-ray:
- May be normal/slightly enlarged cardiac size
- Cardiomegaly in unusual and is seen in:
  - Pink tetralogy
  - TOF with associated AV canal defect
  - TOF with pulmonary atresia and MAPCAs
  - TOF with absent pulmonary valve
- *Boot shaped heart or* ***Coeur-en-sabot:***
  - Means clog-shaped heart in French
  - Seen in association with leftward rotation of cardiac axis
  - Characteristic components:
    - Upturned cardiac apex:
      - Cardiac apex forms acute angle with diaphragm
      - Occurs due to RV hypertrophy
    - Concavity of pulmonary conus:
      - Due to underdeveloped MPA and RV infundibulum
      - Results in absent MPA segment of left heart border
    - Oligemic pulmonary fields:
      - Due to diminished peripheral pulmonary vascularity
      - Oligemia is in proportion to degree of cyanosis
- Other features seen include:
  - Right sided aortic arch
  - Right atrial enlargement
  - Rib notching in the presence of MAPCAs

❖ Echocardiogram:
- Perimembranous VSD
- Aortic override
- Delineates VSD, atrioventricular valve anatomy
- Used to determine whether there is continuity between MPA and RPA/LPA
- Also diagnose PDA or LSVC
- Doppler ECHO:
  - To estimate gradient between RV and MPA
  - Also helps in estimating level of RVOT obstruction

❖ Cardiac catheterization studies:
- Provides information on:
  - Level of RVOT obstruction
  - Presence of MAPCAs

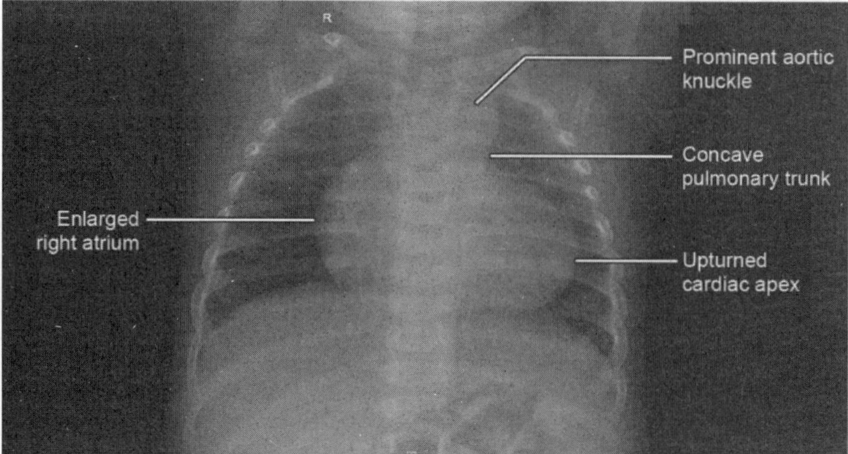

Fig. 34: Boot shaped heart on chest X-ray.

- Presence of additional VSDs
- Coronary artery anomalies
- May be useful for determining need for coiling of MAPCAs prior to surgery

❖ CT angiogram:
- To determine presence of MAPCAs
- To assess adequacy of PA anatomy for complete repair (***McGoon ratio)***

Management

Medical Management

❖ Treat hypercyanotic spells
❖ Prevent factors which precipitate spells like prolonged examination or venipunctures
❖ Patients with frequent spells are treated with propranolol 0.5–1 mg/kg Q6-8H PO
❖ Hemoglobin maintained > 14 g/dL using oral iron supplementation
❖ Repeated phlebectomies to maintain hematocrit < 60%
❖ Prostaglandin infusion in newborns with significant cyanosis
❖ Infective endocarditis prophylaxis is essential prior to surgical correction

Surgical Management

Types of Surgeries

❖ Palliative procedures:
- Balloon dilation of pulmonary valve
- Placement of RVOT stents
- PDA stenting
- Systemic-pulmonary shunts:
  - Classic BT shunt:
    - Involves end to side anastomosis
    - Right subclavian A (RSCA) to right pulmonary artery A (RPA)
  - Modified BT shunt:
    - Utilizes synthetic graft made of goretex material
    - Involves side to side anastomosis
    - Right subclavian to right pulmonary artery
  - Waterstons shunt: ascending aorta to right pulmonary artery
  - Potts shunt: descending aorta to left pulmonary artery

❖ Definite correction via intracardiac repair includes:
- VSD closure with dacron/pericardial patch via:
  - Transatrial approach via right atrium

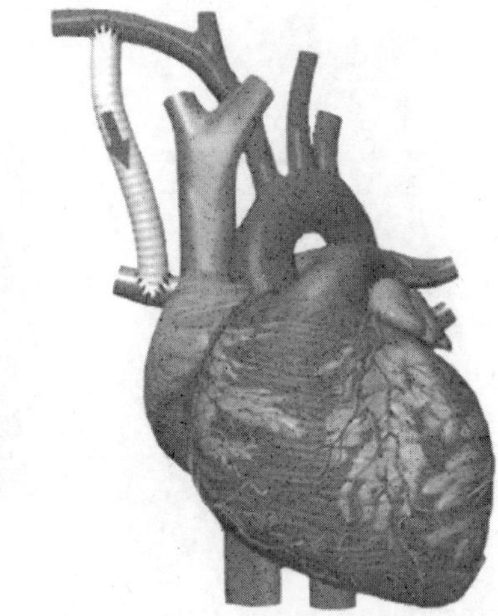

Fig. 35: Modified Blalock Taussig shunt.

  - Transpulmonary approach via pulmonary artery
  - Right ventriculotomy approach
- Excision of obstructing RVOT bundles
- Pulmonary valvotomy in case of fusion of pulmonary valve cusps
- Transannular patch (TAP) in case of narrow pulmonary annulus

❖ Rastellis procedure:
- External conduit placed from body of RV to PA beyond the stenosis
- This is done if a major coronary artery crosses the RVOT
- Ventriculotomy avoided in this region in such a situation
- This is the only contraindication to definitive correction after 2 months of age

Timing of Surgery

❖ Stable with minimal cyanosis total repair at 6–12 months age (Class I)
❖ Symptomatic patients with cyanosis or tet spells: (Class I)
- Palliation or ICR at < 6 months age
- RVOT/PDA stenting may be used as alternative to palliative surgery
- Choice of surgery depends upon PA anatomy

❖ TOF with anomalous coronary artery cross RVOT: (Class I)
- < 10 kg: palliative aorto-pulmonary shunt
- > 10 kg: total ICR using conduit (Rastellis procedure)

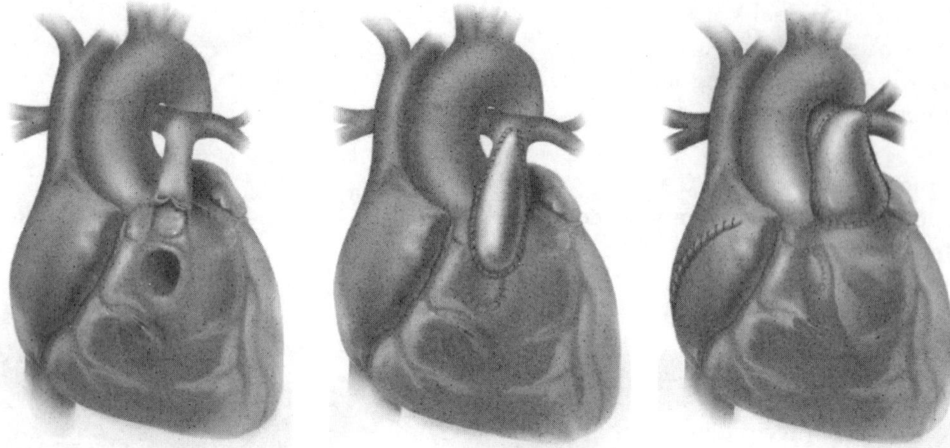

Fig. 36: Total intracardiac repair.

ANESTHETIC MANAGEMENT FOR DEFINITIVE CORRECTION

Preoperative Assessment

- History and clinical examination: check for:
  - Upper respiratory infections
  - Ear discharge
  - Loose teeth
  - Neurodeficits
- Evaluate frequency of cyanotic spells and prophylactic therapy
- Assess patency of veins as multiple phlebotomies may have been performed
- Investigations:
  - Serum electrolytes, hematocrit, platelet count
  - Coagulation profile, blood glucose, acid base status
  - Degree of RVOT obstruction and presence of LSVC noted

Preoperative Preparation and Premedication

- NPO guidelines:
  - 6 hours solids, 4 hours breast milk, 2 hours clear fluids
  - Maintain oral feeds/administer IV fluids to avoid dehydration
  - Scheduled as first case in the day to maintain intravascular volume status
- IV cannulation:
  - Large bore IV cannula is inserted for volume resuscitation
  - Two large bore IV cannulas are preferred
  - IV cannula may be inserted on left hand in the presence of LSVC
  - This enables saline contrast administration to confirm presence of LSVC
- Premedicate to avoid sympathetic stimulation:
  - Midazolam 0.5–1 mg/kg 20 minutes before surgery PO
  - Morphine 0.05–0.1 mg/kg slow IV
  - Sedation is avoided in infants < 6 months age
- Anticholinergic to avoid bradycardia associated with anesthetic induction:
  - Glycopyrrolate 10 μg/kg IV
  - Important as patient is already β blocked: profound bradycardia can occur
- Antibiotics:
  - Class IIa recommendations for infective endocarditis prophylaxis
  - Cefazoline 25 mg/kg IV
  - Vancomycin 20 mg/kg IV if penicillin allergy, given over 1 hour
- Continue propranolol up to and on day of surgery
- Continue PGE_1 infusion if already present to keep PDA patent

Monitoring

- Pulse oximetry
- Blood pressure:
  - NIBP and IBP used
  - Location of IBP:
    Arteries on the side affected by previous shunts are avoided
    Left radial artery or femoral artery (either side) may be cannulated
  - Allows continuous BP assessment and ABG sampling

- ECG, E_TCO_2
- Rectal and esophageal temperature probe
- Urine output
- Central venous catheter:
  - Right IJV/femoral vein
  - Left IJV may be cannulated if left sided SVC is present
  - Useful for inotropic administration postoperatively
- Transesophageal echocardiography:
  - For LV and RV function
  - Presence of residual VSD/intracardiac air post correction
- PA catheter:
  - Not necessary
  - Rarely used to assess PA and LA pressures

Anesthetic Goals

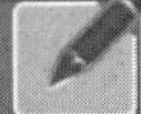

- Rhythm: Maintain sinus rhythm
- Heart rate: Maintain low-normal heart rate
- Contractility: Reduce contractility
- Preload: Maintain adequate preload
- Afterload: Prevent reduction in afterload
- SVR: Maintain SVR
- PVR: Minimize PVR

Anesthetic Considerations

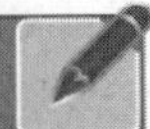

- Maintain adequate preoperative hydration and sedation
- Schedule as first case in the day to prevent hypovolemia
- Difficult IV access due to repeated phlebotomy
- Chances of excessive bleeding due to thrombocytopenia
- Deep planes of anesthesia preferable
- Avoid:
  - Histamine releasing agents as they reduce SVR:
    - Atracurium
    - Morphine
    - Pethidine
  - Excessive PEEP as it decreases preload
  - Air bubbles in IV line to prevent paradoxical air embolism

Induction

- Adequate preoxygenation for 5 minutes
- If IV line present: Induction with ketamine 2 mg/kg and vecuronium 0.1 mg/kg
- If IV line is not present:
  - Inhalational induction: with 100% oxygen and sevoflurane
  - IM induction:
    - With ketamine 5 mg/kg IM
    - Obtain IV access
    - Administer IV vecuronium 0.1 mg/kg
- IV fentanyl 2 µg/kg may be used to provide analgesia
- IV induction is faster than inhalational induction
- Intubate in deeper planes to prevent intubation response
- Leak above 22–25 cmH_2O preferred if uncuffed ET tube is used
- Baseline ABG is taken for postoperative comparison
- $ETCO_2$- $PaCO_2$ difference is noted as it may be high due to R-L shunting
- Acidosis if present, is corrected
- Cross matched blood to be readily available
- Avoid:
  - Air bubbles in tubing to prevent PAE
  - Histamine releasing drugs as it reduces SVR
  - Excitement/agitation at the time of induction

Maintenance

- 100% O_2 with isoflurane/sevoflurane
- Lower FiO_2 may be used if physiology-appropriate saturation is maintained
- N_2O is usually avoided
- If used, 50% N_2O with 50% oxygen preferred
- Fentanyl 5–10 µg/kg or sufentanyl 1–2 µg/kg is used to provide intraoperative analgesia
- Vecuronium or pancuronium boluses may be used to ensure neuromuscular blockade
- Tet spells are managed as mentioned earlier

Ventilation

- Avoid increased peak airway pressure
- Avoid excessive PEEP
- Mild hyperventilation: maintain $PaCO_2$ around 30 mm Hg
- N_2O does not cause much increase in PVR, but 100% O_2 preferred to avoid hypoxia
- A small PFO may be left behind post ICR in some patients
- This serves to:
  - Decompress the RV during RV dysfunction
  - Maintain LV preload during severe RV dysfunction
- This may result in mild desaturation following complete repair in TOF

Hemodynamics

- Hemodynamic goals to be maintained are:
  - Maintain SVR, and euvolemia
  - Avoid increases in PVR
  - Slow heart rate preferable
  - Provide mild myocardial depression
- Dissection around PDA and manipulation of PDA may result in profound bradycardia
- Postoperatively:
  - More volume may be required to prevent hypotension
  - This is due to hypertrophy causing a poorly compliant RV and diastolic dysfunction
  - Thus, higher CVP has to be maintained to ensure adequate RV forward output
  - Factors contributing to diastolic dysfunction include:
    - Right ventriculotomy
    - Myocardial edema following CPB
    - Inadequate myocardial protection of hypertrophied RV
    - Residual RVOT obstruction
    - Volume overload of RV due to residual VSD
    - Volume overload of RV due to pulmonary regurgitation
  - Excessive bleeding may occur postoperatively due to:
    - Thrombocytopenia
    - Coagulopathy
    - Accelerated fibrinolysis
  - Thus, plasma and platelets may be required in post-bypass period
  - Inotropes which are commonly used while coming-off CPB are:
    - Adrenaline 0.05–0.15 μg/kg/min
    - Milrinone 0.5–1 μg/kg/min
  - Arrhythmias:
    - Common owing to close proximity of conduction system to VSD patch
    - Complete heart block is commonly seen postoperatively
    - Epicardial pacing is used till edema around the VSD patch subsides
    - Atrioventricular pacing is the preferred mode of pacing

Considerations for CPB

- Bicaval cannulation is used as transatrial approach is used commonly
- Tricaval cannulation is used in the presence of LSVC
- After institution of CPB, administer:
  - Opioids, benzodiazepines and muscle relaxants
  - Repeat antibiotic on CPB
- Initiation of CPB causes hemodilution
- Slightly higher hematocrit 30–36% is preferred on CPB owing to preoperative cyanosis
- Pulmonary overperfusion is avoided by:
  - Clamping any preexisting shunt (systemic-pulmonary)
  - Clipping of PDA
  - Clipping of MAPCAs
- LV venting is important as left heart return may be high in the presence of MAPCAs
- Moderate hypothermia (28–32°C) is used for intracardiac repair on CPB
- Deep hypothermic arrest:
  - 18–20°C can be used for deep hypothermic arrest
  - Ice wraps for the head are important at low flows
  - pH-stat blood gas management is preferred
- Blood cardioplegia with Delnidos cardioplegia solution may be used for cardiac arrest
- Monitor:
  - Blood gases every 20–30 minutes to ensure adequate gas exchange and perfusion
  - Mixed venous O_2 saturation to assess tissue perfusion
  - ACT every 20–30 minutes to ensure adequate anticoagulation
  - ACT maintained 480 sec on CPB
  - Urine output: maintain urine output at 1–2 mL/kg/hour
- After heart is closed, Trendelenburg position is given for deairing to remove air bubbles
- Inotropic support with epinephrine/milrinone can be initiated after aortic unclamping
- Patients with thickened RV are sensitive to volume changes during weaning of CPB
- Weaning from CPB is initiated after:
  - Nasopharyngeal temperature reaches 36.5°C
  - Patient has stable rhythm and hemodynamics
- Heparin is reversed with protamine after coming of CPB

Extubation

- Usually mechanically ventilated post operatively, for 24–48 hours
- Once patient is fully awake, hemodynamically stable and peripherally warm, patient is extubated

Postoperative

Management

- Infants may be ventilated for 24–48 hours following surgery
- Epicardial pacing is continued postoperatively until sinus rhythm is established
- Requirement of epicardial pacing for > 10 days warrants permanent pacemaker implantation
- RV dysfunction is common postoperatively
- Junctional ectopic tachycardia:
  - Common in the postoperative period
  - Tachycardia is poorly tolerated as both systolic and diastolic dysfunction exist
  - Thus, diastolic filling time is important to maintain forward cardiac output
  - Treated with:
    - Magnesium sulphate
    - Amiodarone

Monitoring

- SpO_2, IBP, ECG
- CVP, ABG
- Urine output, blood glucose
- Peripheral temperature, airway pressure
- Echocardiography

Pain

- Adequate analgesia important
- Multimodal analgesia useful
- NSAIDs are avoided due to risk of bleeding
- Morphine 0.1 mg/kg IV or fentanyl 0.5 μg/kg IV boluses
- Erector spinae block may be useful for supplemental analgesia

Complications

- Immediate complications:
  - Arrhythmias:
    - Left anterior hemiblock/complete heart block/RBBB
    - Junctional ectopic tachycardia
  - Residual lesions:
    - VSD
    - Residual RVOT obstruction
    - Residual PS/RVOTO
  - Pulmonary regurgitation as valve is frequently excised
  - Low output state
  - Coagulopathies
  - Renal failure
  - Stroke
  - Infection
- Late complications:
  - RVOT obstruction
  - RVOT aneurysm
  - Residual VSD
  - Valvular insufficiency

ANESTHETIC MANAGEMENT FOR SHUNT PROCEDURES

Preoperative Assessment

- History and clinical examination: check for:
  - Upper respiratory infections
  - Ear discharge
- Evaluate frequency of cyanotic spells and prophylactic therapy
- Investigations:
  - Serum electrolytes, hematocrit, platelet count
  - Coagulation profile, blood glucose, acid base status
  - Degree of RVOT obstruction is noted

Preoperative Preparation and Premedication

- NPO guidelines:
  - 6 hours solids, 4 hours breast milk, 2 hours clear fluids
  - Maintain oral feeds/administer IV fluids to avoid dehydration
  - Scheduled as first case in the day to maintain intravascular volume status
- Large bore IV cannula is inserted for volume resuscitation
- Premedication:
  - Palliative procedures are usually done in infancy
  - Thus, sedative premedication is avoided
- Antibiotics:
  - Class IIa recommendations for infective endocarditis prophylaxis
  - Cefazoline 25 mg/kg IV
  - Vancomycin 20 mg/kg IV if penicillin allergy, given over 1 hour
- Continue propranolol up to and on day of surgery
- Continue PGE_1 infusion if already present to keep PDA patent

Monitoring

- Pulse oximetry:
  - Usually placed on hand opposite to the side of proposed shunt
  - Occasionally placed on both upper and lower extremity

- Blood pressure:
  - NIBP and IBP are used
  - NIBP cuff is used during induction
  - Arterial line is placed following induction
  - Site of IBP should avoid arteries affected by the planned procedure
  - Same side subclavian artery will be clamped, obliterating radial pulse
  - Thus, left radial artery or femoral artery (either side) may be cannulated
  - Arterial cannulation allows continuous BP assessment and ABG sampling
- ECG
- E_TCO_2:
  - Baseline E_TCO_2-$PaCO_2$ is gradient is noted
  - This is because PA is partially clamped during anastomosis
  - This reduces pulmonary blood flow and E_TCO_2
  - Thus, E_TCO_2-$PaCO_2$ gradient may be used to adjust ventilation
- Rectal temperature probe
- Urine output
- Central venous catheter:
  - Right IJV/femoral vein cannulated
  - Used for administration of inotropic support
  - Auxillary indicator of intravascular volume status

Anesthetic Goals

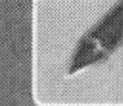

- Rhythm: Maintain sinus rhythm
- Heart rate: Maintain low-normal heart rate
- Contractility: Reduce contractility
- Preload: Maintain adequate preload
- Afterload: Prevent reduction in afterload
- SVR: Maintain SVR
- PVR: Minimize PVR

Anesthetic Considerations

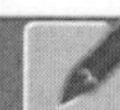

- May be done on CPB or without the use of CPB depending upon patient characteristics
- Maintain adequate preoperative hydration and sedation
- Schedule as first case in the day to prevent hypovolemia
- Chances of excessive bleeding due to thrombocytopenia
- Deep planes of anesthesia preferable
- Avoid:
  - Histamine releasing agents as they reduce SVR:
    - Atracurium
    - Morphine
    - Pethidine
  - Excessive PEEP as it decreases preload
  - Air bubbles in IV line to prevent paradoxical air embolism

Induction

- Adequate preoxygenation for 5 minutes
- *If IV line present*: induction with ketamine 2 mg/kg and vecuronium 0.1 mg/kg
- If IV line is not present:
  - Inhalational induction: with 100% oxygen and sevoflurane
  - IM induction:
    - With ketamine 5 mg/kg IM
    - Obtain IV access
    - Administer IV vecuronium 0.1 mg/kg
- IV fentanyl 2 μg/kg may be used to provide analgesia
- IV induction is faster than inhalational induction
- Intubate in deeper planes to prevent intubation response
- Leak above 22–25 cm H_2O preferred if uncuffed ET tube is used
- Baseline ABG is taken for postoperative comparison
- $ETCO_2$- $PaCO_2$ difference is noted as it may be high due to R-L shunting
- Acidosis if present, is corrected
- Cross matched blood to be kept readily available
- Avoid:
  - Air bubbles in tubing to prevent PAE
  - Histamine releasing drugs as it reduces SVR
  - Excitement/agitation at the time of induction

Position

- Lateral position: If thoracotomy
- Supine position: If midline sternotomy

Maintenance

- 100% O_2 with isoflurane/sevoflurane
- Lower FiO_2 may be used if physiology-appropriate saturation is maintained
- N_2O does not cause much increase in PVR, but 100% O_2 preferred to avoid hypoxia
- If used, 50% N_2O with 50% oxygen preferred
- Fentanyl 1 μg/kg/hour is used to provide intraoperative analgesia
- Vecuronium boluses may be used to ensure neuromuscular blockade
- Tet spells are managed as mentioned earlier
- Heparin 1 mg/kg may be administered prior to partial-clamping of RPA

Ventilation

- Avoid increased airway pressure
- Avoid excessive PEEP
- Mild hyperventilation: maintain $PaCO_2$ around 30 mm Hg
- Maintain mild alkalosis
- Reduction of tidal volume may be required to aid surgical exposure
- E_TCO_2-$PaCO_2$ gradient is used to titrate ventilation
- 100% O_2 preferred during anastomosis to avoid hypoxia as:
  - SpO_2 may decrease with lung compression during surgical manipulation
  - SpO_2 may further decrease with clamping of PA to facilitate anastomosis
- Post BT-shunt SpO_2 of > 80% is targeted
- FiO_2 is reduced appropriately to minimum tolerated levels

Hemodynamics

- Hemodynamic goals to be maintained are:
  - Maintain SVR, and euvolemia
  - Avoid increases in PVR
  - Slow heart rate preferable
  - Provide mild myocardial depression
- Blood loss may occur during anastomosis of the shunt
- Partial clamping of PA is important to prevent PA distortion
- This helps to maintain pulmonary blood flow during anastomosis
- Severe desaturation at the time of cross-clamp may necessitate institution of CPB
- Once shunt is completed and graft is in place, diastolic BP reduces due to runoff into PA
- Postoperatively:
  - More volume may be required to prevent hypotension
  - This is due to hypertrophy causing a poorly compliant RV and diastolic dysfunction
  - Thus, higher CVP has to be maintained to ensure adequate RV forward output
  - Excessive bleeding may occur postoperatively due to:
    - Thrombocytopenia
    - Coagulopathy
    - Accelerated fibrinolysis
  - Thus, plasma and platelets may be required in postoperative period
  - Inotropes which are commonly used in the postoperative period are:
    - Adrenaline 0.05–0.15 μg/kg/min
    - Dopamine 5–10 μg/kg/min
  - Dopamine is preferred as it also increases flow through the new shunt

Intraoperative Complications

- Hypercyanotic tet spells
- Bleeding
- Severe desaturation during chest closure due to:
  - Change in relation of intrathoracic contents
  - Distortion of PA
  - Kinking of the shunt

Extubation

- Patients are usually extubated soon after surgery
- Criteria for extubation:
  - Spontaneous ventilation
  - Normal ABG
  - Normothermia
  - Stable hemodynamics
  - Controlled bleeding

Postoperative

Management

- Prolonged intubation is not advised
- Postoperative period is characterized by the presence of systemic run-off into PA
- This occurs across a non-compliant artificial shunt
- Thus, alterations in SVR and PVR cause major fluctuations in systemic perfusion and PaO_2
- Therefore, sudden changes in SVR and PVR should be avoided
- Low dose heparin is initiated 1–2 hours after surgery to maintain shunt patency
- Heparin is usually initiated at 10 IU/kg/hour infusion
- Once enteral feeding is established, heparin may be transitioned to low-dose aspirin

Monitoring

- SpO_2, IBP, ECG
- CVP, ABG
- Urine output, blood glucose
- Peripheral temperature, airway pressure
- Echocardiography

Pain

- Adequate analgesia important
- Multimodal analgesia useful
- NSAIDs are avoided due to risk of bleeding
- Morphine 0.1 mg/kg IV or fentanyl 0.5 μg/kg IV boluses

Complications

- Desaturation due to:
  - Lung collapse
  - Shunt occlusion/kinking
- Bleeding
- Pneumothorax
- Pulmonary hyperperfusion and pulmonary edema
- Desaturation due to small shunt size
- Shunt thrombosis

ANESTHETIC MANAGEMENT OF TOF PATIENT WITH BRAIN ABSCESS

Introduction

- Brain abscess is commonly seen in cyanotic CHD (CCHD) due to:
  - Polycythemia-induced cerebral infarcts
  - Absence of pulmonary phagocytic clearance of pathogens due to R-L shunt
  - Poor host immunity
- Among all CCHD, TOF is most commonly associated with brain abscess (13–70%)

Surgical Considerations

- Brain abscesses are usually managed by aspiration followed by antibiotic therapy
- Antibiotic therapy is continued for 6–8 weeks following aspiration
- Craniotomy and surgical excision is reserved for:
  - Abscesses refractory to antibiotic therapy
  - Large and superficial abscesses
  - Abscesses in non-eloquent brain regions causing mass effect
  - Multiloculated abscesses

Anesthetic Considerations

- Unique as it requires titration of contrasting goals:
  - Hemodynamic goals of TOF
  - Intracranial hemodynamics for intracranial mass

Contd...

Contd...

- Considerations due to TOF:
  - Perioperative hemodynamic instability due to:
    - Congestive cardiac failure
    - Arrhythmias
    - Infective endocarditis
  - Increased perioperative incidence of cyanotic spells
  - Preoperative infective endocarditis prophylaxis
  - Polycythemia induced coagulation defects
  - Paradoxical air embolism
- Considerations due to brain abscess:
  - Raised intracranial pressure causing:
    - Fluid and acid base imbalances due to vomiting
    - Perioperative seizures
  - Maintenance of intracranial hemodynamics
  - Postoperative meningitis.

Anesthetic Techniques

- Scalp block:
  - May be used as the sole anesthetic technique in older patients
  - May be used to augment analgesia in younger patients receiving GA
  - 0.75% plain ropivacaine is used to administer scalp block
  - Addition of adrenaline is avoided as it may cause tachycardia
  - Advantages:
    - Reduces hemodynamic response to pin holder application
    - Decreases severity of postoperative pain
  - Disadvantages:
    - Absence of secure airway
    - This may necessitate airway instrumentation during the procedure
    - Poor control over oxygenation
- General anesthesia:
  - Advantages:
    - Controlled ventilation provides better oxygenation

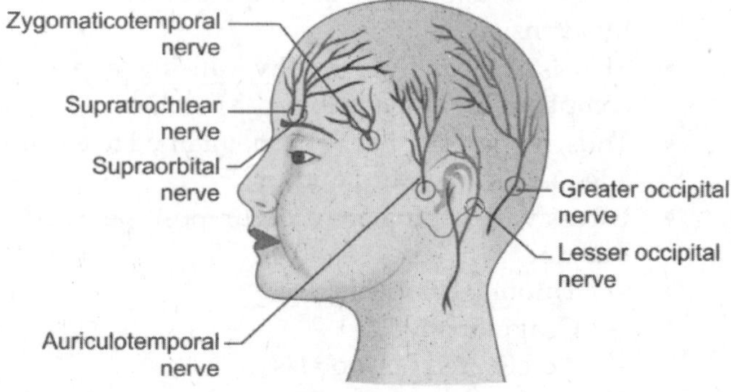

Fig. 37: Scalp block.

- Allows better control of ventilatory parameters
- Provides secure airway
- Disadvantages:
  - Risk of hemodynamic instability
  - PPV may cause compression of pulmonary blood vessels
  - This reduced pulmonary blood flow and gas exchange
- Useful in:
  - Small, uncooperative children
  - Patients with high ICP
  - Associated seizures, congestive cardiac failure
  - Hemodynamic instability
  - Frequent cyanotic spells

Anesthetic Goals

- Avoid hypoxemia
- Ensure adequate hydration
- Maintain SVR
- Minimize PVR
- Avoid sudden increases in systemic oxygen demand

Hemodynamic Goals

- Rhythm: Maintain sinus rhythm
- Heart rate: Maintain low-normal heart rate
- Contractility: Reduce contractility
- Preload: Maintain adequate preload
- Afterload: Prevent reduction in afterload
- SVR: Maintain SVR
- PVR: Minimize PVR

Preoperative Assessment and Preparation

- Thorough preoperative assessment documenting:
  - Current cardiac and neurological status
  - Associated conditions
  - History of prior abscess surgeries
  - History of previous shunt surgeries
  - Current medications
- Preoperative investigations should include:
  - Coagulation profile
  - Echocardiography
- Phlebotomy may be indicated in patients with hematocrit > 60%

Premedication

- NPO orders
- Prolonged preoperative fasting should be avoided
- Clear fluids should be given up to 2 hours before surgery
- Preoperative medications are continued on the morning of surgery:
  - Anti-seizure medications
  - Propranolol
- Aspirin for surgically palliated patients is withheld in view of closed space surgery
- Gentle separation from parents is necessary to avoid precipitation of tet spells
- Large bore IV access is secured to facilitate volume resuscitation

Monitors

- Pulse oximetry, E_TCO_2
- NIBP, nasopharyngeal temperature
- Invasive blood pressure monitoring:
  - Artery on the side opposite to previous palliative shunt is cannulated
  - Arterial line is useful as it allows:
    - Continuous beat-to-beat monitoring of IBP
    - Frequent ABG sampling
- Central vein is cannulated to allow:
  - Administration of vasoactive drugs
  - Estimation of fluid status of the patient

Induction

- Adequate preoxygenation
- *Ketamine is avoided* as the induction agent to avoid detrimental increase in ICP
- Incremental boluses of thiopentone/propofol may be used for induction
- Fentanyl 2 μg/kg ensures adequate analgesia
- Vecuronium is the preferred agent to facilitate neuromuscular paralysis
- Air filters in IV lines are essential to prevent air embolism
- Infective endocarditis prophylaxis is administered 30 minutes prior to surgical incision
- Deep anesthetic planes are preferred at intubation to:
  - Prevent sudden increase in ICP
  - Prevent precipitation of tet spells

Maintenance

- Balanced anesthesia with oxygen + air + sevoflurane
- Sevoflurane is the preferred agent as it prevents:
  - Cerebral vasodilatation
  - Excessive myocardial depression

- Nitrous oxide is usually avoided to prevent postoperative pneumocephalus
- These patients are prone to tet spells perioperatively
- Thus, these spells should be treated aggressively with:
  - 100% FiO_2
  - Phenylephrine
  - Beta blockers
  - Fluid boluses
  - Sodium bicarbonate
- High doses of opioids are avoided to:
  - Prevent delayed recovery
  - Enable early assessment of neurological status

Ventilation

- Prevent increase in intracranial pressure:
  - Avoid increased airway pressure
  - Avoid excessive PEEP
  - Mild hyperventilation: maintain $PaCO_2$ around 30 mm Hg
  - Maintain mild respiratory alkalosis
- Frequent ABGs are necessary as pulse oximeter may be unreliable in severe cyanosis

Hemodynamics

- Hemodynamic goals to be maintained are:
  - Slow heart rate preferable
  - Maintain SVR to minimize R-L shunting
  - Avoid increases in PVR to encourage antegrade flow across RVOT
  - Provide mild myocardial depression
- Hydration is important to prevent increased blood viscosity and thromboembolism
- Hypovolemia can also exacerbate RVOT obstruction
- Allowable blood loss is usually more owing to preoperative polycythemia
- Transfusion trigger is reserved for blood loss > 25% of total blood volume
- Brain relaxation:
  - Mannitol:
    - Useful as it decreases:
      - Intracranial pressure
      - Cerebral edema
      - Blood viscosity
    - However, it can precipitate tet spells by causing dehydration
    - Thus, mannitol should be used cautiously
  - Hyperventilation is useful as it also increases antegrade RVOT flow

Extubation

- Early extubation is preferred to:
  - Enable early assessment of neurological status
  - Prevent further reduction in pulmonary blood flow due to PPV
- Once patient is fully awake, hemodynamically stable and peripherally warm, patient is extubated

Postoperative

Management

- Propped up nursing
- Judicious fluid administration to prevent sudden increase in ICP
- Administration of 100% oxygen following extubation
- Early resumption of oral feeds post-extubation

Monitoring

- SpO_2, IBP, ECG
- CVP, ABG
- Urine output, blood glucose

Pain

- Adequate analgesia important to prevent precipitation of tet spells
- Multimodal analgesia useful
- NSAIDs are avoided due to risk of bleeding
- Morphine is administered cautiously post-extubation to prevent respiratory depression
- Scalp block may be useful for postoperative analgesia

Complications

- Tet spells are more common during surgery for brain abscess
- Cerebral edema
- Brainstem herniation
- Seizures

MITRAL REGURGITATION

Introduction

- Mitral regurgitation permits systolic blood flow from LV to flow back into left atrium
- Mitral valve apparatus consists of six components:
  - LA wall
  - Mitral valve annulus
  - Mitral leaflets
  - Chordae tendineae

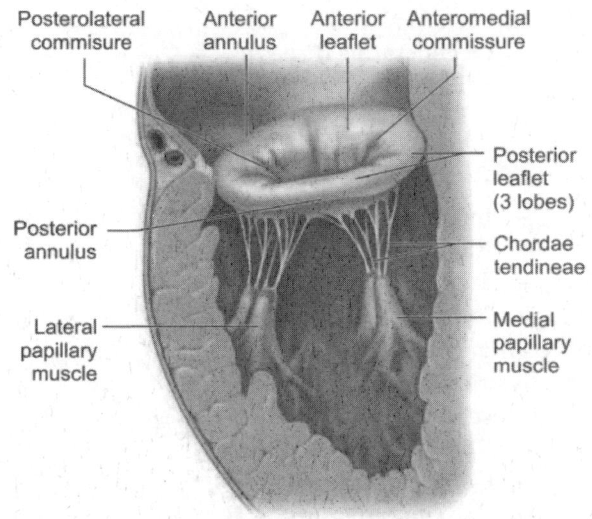

Fig. 38: Mitral valve apparatus.

- Papillary muscles
- Wall of left ventricle

❖ Abnormalities of any component may result in mitral regurgitation

Causes

No.	Cause	Characterictics	Location
Functional/secondary mitral regurgitation			
1.	Annular dilatation	Dilated cardiomyopathy	Annulus
2.	LV ischemia	Ischemic heart disease	Tensor apparatus
Organic/primary mitral regurgitation			
Chronic Mitral Regurgitation			
1.	Congenital	Cleft mitral valve	Leaflet
		Double orifice mitral valve	
2.	Mitral prolapse	Myxomatous degeneration	Leaflet
		Redundant tissue	
		Ruptured chordae	
3.	Rheumatic	Thickened leaflets	Leaflet
		Calcified leaflets	
		Commissural fusion	
4.	Miscellaneous	Fenfluramine	Leaflet
		Infective endocarditis	Leaflet
		Mitral annular calcification	Leaflet
		Ehler-Danlos disease	Leaflet
		Marfan syndrome	Leaflet
Acute Mitral Regurgitation			
1.	Endocarditis	Perforated leaflets	Leaflet
		Vegetations	
2.	Post MI	Papillary muscle rupture	Tensor apparatus
3.	Post chest trauma	Papillary muscle rupture	Tensor apparatus

Causes of Acute and Chronic Mitral Regurgitation

❖ Acute mitral regurgitation:
- Disorders of mitral annulus:
  - Infective endocarditis (abscess)
  - Inadvertent trauma during open heart surgery
  - Paravalvular leak caused by suture interruption
- Disorders of mitral leaflet:
  - Infective endocarditis:
    - Leaflet perforation
    - Vegetation interfering with valve closure
  - Trauma during PBMV
  - Tumors
  - Myxomatous degeneration
  - Libman Sacks endocarditis
- Rupture of chordae tendineae:
  - Idiopathic (spontaneous)
  - Myxomatous degeneration:
    - Mitral valve prolapse
    - Marfan syndrome
    - Ehler-Danlos syndrome
  - Infective endocarditis
  - Acute rheumatic fever
- Papillary muscle disorders:
  - Coronary artery disease causing papillary muscle rupture
  - Acute global LV dysfunction
  - Infiltrative disease (amyloidosis, sarcoidosis)
  - Trauma

❖ Chronic mitral regurgitation:
- Inflammatory causes:
  - Rheumatic heart disease
  - Systemic lupus erythematosus
  - Scleroderma
- Degenerative causes:
  - Myxomatous degeneration (Barlow click-murmur syndrome)
  - Marfan syndrome
  - Ehler-Danlos syndrome
  - Pseudoxanthoma elasticum
  - Mitral valve annular calcification
- Infective endocarditis
- Structural causes:
  - Ruptured chordae tendineae:
    - Spontaneous rupture
    - Secondary to myocardial infarction
    - Endocarditis

- Rupture or dysfunction of papillary muscle due to myocardial infarction
- Dilatation of mitral valve annulus:
  - Congestive cardiomyopathies
  - Aneurysmal dilation of left ventricle
- Hypertrophic cardiomyopathy

- Congenital causes:
  - Mitral valve clefts: partial, complete AV canal defects
  - Parachute mitral valve

Pathophysiological Causes of Mitral Regurgitation

- Type I:
  - Normal leaflet motion
  - Occurs due to:
    - Mitral annular dilatation
    - Mitral valve clefts
    - Mitral valve perforation
  - Causes:
    - Ischemic cardiomyopathy
    - Dilated cardiomyopathy
    - Valve perforation due to infective endocarditis
    - Congenital mitral valve clefts
- Type II:
  - Increased mitral leaflet motion
  - Occurs due to:
    - Billowing of mitral valve
    - Prolapse of mitral valve
    - Flail mitral valve
  - Causes:
    - Degenerative disease:
      - Fibroelastic deficiency
      - Marfan syndrome
      - Barlow disease
      - Ehler-Danlos syndrome
    - Infective endocarditis
    - Rheumatic heart disease
    - Trauma
    - Ischemic cardiomyopathy
- Type IIIa:
  - Restricted mitral leaflet opening
  - Causes:
    - Rheumatic heart disease
    - Carcinoid disease
    - Radiation therapy
    - Lupus erythematosus
    - Mucopolysaccharidosis
- Type IIIb:
  - Restricted mitral leaflet closure
  - Causes:
    - Ischemia cardiomyopathy
    - Dilated cardiomyopathy

Pathophysiology

- Chronic mitral regurgitation:
  - Regurgitation of blood into LA occurs during systole
  - On long standing, the LA dilates, making it more compliant

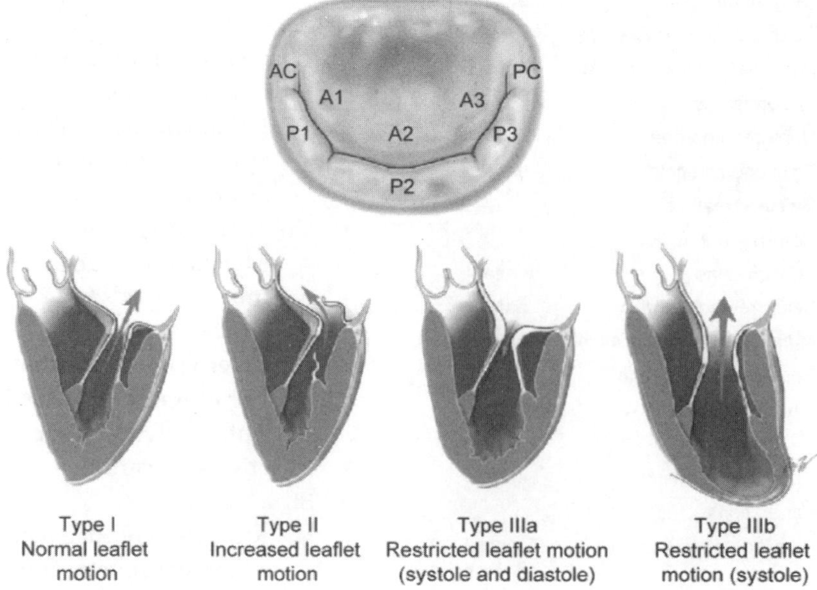

Fig. 39: Carpentiers types of mitral regurgitation.

- Massively dilated LA, protects pulmonary capillaries from pressure elevation
- Thus, pulmonary edema is an uncommon initial presentation in chronic MR
- However, over time, LA compliance decreases
- This results in an increase in LAP and simultaneous reduction in LA-LV gradient
- Pressure of regurgitant jet is transmitted to pulmonary ciculation causing pulmonary edema

❖ Left ventricular ejection fraction in chronic MR:
- Most often normal or supranormal
- This is because the LA serves as a low-pressure pathway during systolic ejection
- Thus, during systole, LV ejects blood:
  - Antegrade into aorta
  - Retrograde into left atrium
- This overestimates the LV systolic ejection fraction
- Ventricular dysfunction may be unmasked after valve repair/replacement
- LVEF becomes low when:
  - LV has decompensated with chronic MR
  - Acute LV ischemia

❖ Acute onset mitral regurgitation:
- LA pressure increased as there is no time for LA compensatory changes to occur
- *v wave* may be present on LAP/PAP/PCWP recordings

❖ Determinants of volume of mitral regurgitation:
- Volume of MR is determined by:
  - Regurgitant orifice area:
    - Regurgitant orifice area is increased by stretching of mitral valve
    - This can occur due to:
      - Increased preload causing stretching of mitral annulus
      - Depressed LV function causing increased LV size
  - LA–LV pressure differential which in turn depends on:
    - LA compliance
    - Systemic vascular resistance
- Regurgitant volume is reduced with:
  - Decrease in systemic vascular resistance
  - Increase in LA pressure

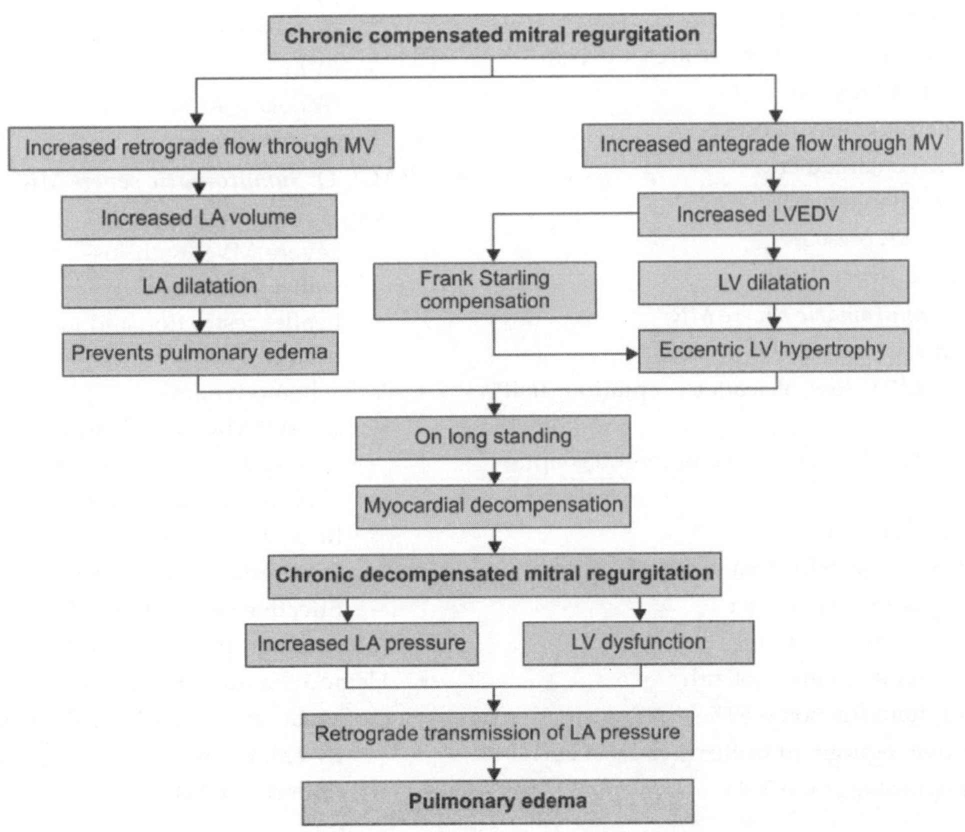

Stages of Mitral Regurgitation

- STAGE A: ***At risk for mitral regurgitation***:
  - Valve anatomy:
    - Mild MVP with normal coaptation
    - Mild valve thickening and leaflet restriction
  - Valve hemodynamics:
    - Absent MR jet
    - Central MR jet with area <20% of LA area
    - Vena contracta < 3 mm
  - Hemodynamic consequences: none
  - Symptoms: mild
- STAGE B: ***Progressive MR:***
  - Valve anatomy:
    - Severe MVP with normal coaptation
    - Leaflet restriction and loss of central coaptation
  - Valve hemodynamics:
    - Central MR jet with area 20–40% of LA area
    - Late systolic eccentric jet
    - Vena contracta 4–6 mm
    - Regurgitant volume < 60 mL
    - Regurgitant fraction < 50%
    - Effective regurgitant orifice area < 0.4 cm^2
    - Angiographic grade 1–2+
  - Hemodynamic consequences:
    - Mild LA enlargement
    - No LV enlargement
    - Normal PA pressure
  - Symptoms: absent
- STAGE C_1: ***Asymptomatic severe MR:***
  - Valve anatomy:
    - Severe MVP, loss of leaflet coaptation, flail leaflet
    - Leaflet restriction with loss of central coaptation
  - Valve hemodynamics:
    - Central MR jet with area > 40% of LA area
    - Holosystolic eccentric jet
    - Vena contracta > 7 mm
    - Regurgitant volume > 60 mL
    - Regurgitant fraction > 50%
    - Effective regurgitant orifice area > 0.4 cm^2
    - Angiographic grade 3–4+
  - Hemodynamic consequences:
    - Moderate-severe LA enlargement
    - LV enlargement
    - Pulmonary HTN at rest or with exercise
    - *LVEF > 60%*
    - *LVESD < 40 mm*
  - Symptoms: Absent
- STAGE C_2: ***Asymptomatic severe MR:***
  - Valve anatomy:
    - Severe MVP, loss of leaflet coaptation, flail leaflet
    - Leaflet restriction with loss of central coaptation
  - Valve hemodynamics:
    - Central MR jet with area > 40% of LA area
    - Holosystolic eccentric jet
    - Vena contracta > 7 mm
    - Regurgitant volume > 60 mL
    - Regurgitant fraction > 50%
    - Effective regurgitant orifice area > 0.4 cm^2
    - Angiographic grade 3–4+
  - Hemodynamic consequences:
    - Moderate-severe LA enlargement
    - LV enlargement
    - Pulmonary HTN at rest or with exercise
    - *LVEF < 60%*
    - *LVESD > 40 mm*
  - Symptoms: absent
- STAGE D: ***Symptomatic severe MR***:
  - Valve anatomy:
    - Severe MVP with loss of coaptation or flail leaflet
    - Leaflet restriction and loss of central coaptation
  - Valve hemodynamics:
    - Central MR jet with area > 40% of LA area
    - Holosystolic eccentric jet
    - Vena contracta > 7 mm
    - Regurgitant volume > 60 mL
    - Regurgitant fraction > 50%
    - Effective regurgitant orifice area > 0.4 cm^2
    - Angiographic grade 3–4+
  - Hemodynamic consequences:
    - Moderate-severe LA enlargement
    - LV enlargement
    - Pulmonary HTN

- Symptoms:
  - Decreased exercise tolerance
  - Exertional dyspnea

Clinical Features

- Chronic MR patients may remain asymptomatic for 20–40 years
- If acute MR:
  - Have normal or reduced LA compliance
  - Usually have sudden onset of:
    - Dyspnea on exertion
    - Pulmonary vascular congestion
    - Severe pulmonary edema
    - Congestive heart failure
- If chronic MR:
  - Usually show signs of low cardiac output and forward LV failure
  - Usually have gradual onset of:
    - Dyspnea on exertion
    - Paroxysmal nocturnal dyspnea
    - Fatigue
    - Atrial fibrillation
- Features of right heart failure on long standing:
  - Hepatic congestion and ascites
  - Pedal edema and anasarca
  - Raised JVP
- Examination:
  - Normal BP, arterial pulse with sharp upstroke
  - Raised JVP with:
    - Prominent *a waves* in patients with sinus rhythm
    - Prominent *v waves* if severe tricuspid regurgitation
  - Systolic thrill at apex
  - Hyperdynamic LV with brisk systolic impulse
  - Apex beat displaced laterally
  - S_1 absent
  - Wide splitting of S_2
  - Mitral regurgitation murmur:
    - Holosystolic murmur at apex, radiating to axilla
    - Increased intensity with squatting/hand grip
    - Reduced intensity with valsalva maneuver
    - If acute MR, ***seagull/cooing*** quality of murmur
- Complications:
  - Chest pain due to low diastolic pressure
  - Infective endocarditis
  - Arrhythmias
  - Embolic events

Characteristic	Chronic compensated	Chronic decompensated	Acute
Symptom onset	Absent	Gradual DOE	Abrupt DOE
Blood pressure	Normal	Normal	Hypotension
Pulmonary congestion	Absent	Variable	Severe
LA pressure	Normal	Increased	Increased
v wave	Absent	Variable	Increased
LV size	Increased	Increased	Normal
LA size	Increased	Increased	Normal

Investigations

- Complete blood count, BUN, SC, LFT
- Chest X-ray:
  - LA and LV are dominant chambers
  - LA might form right border of cardiac silhouette if massively enlarged
  - Calcification of mitral valve
  - ***Kerley A, Kerley B lines, Stag's antler signs*** if pulmonary edema
- ECG:
  - Normal in some
  - Inverted or biphasic T waves
  - ST segment changes in inferior leads
  - Arrhythmias:
    - *Supraventricular tachyarrhythmias most common*
    - Bradyarrhythmias
    - AV bypass tract especially with mitral valve prolapse ***(Barlows syndrome)***
  - Biatrial enlargement features
- Echocardiography:
  - Regurgitant fraction < 20% of total stroke volume: mild symptoms
  - Regurgitant fraction 20–50% of total stroke volume: moderate symptoms
  - Regurgitant fraction > 50% of total stroke volume: severe symptoms

Carpentier Classification of Mitral Regurgitation

Carpentier type	Leaflet motion	Jet direction
I	Normal, annular dilatation	Central
II	Excessive (prolapsed,flail)	Away from lesion
IIIa	Restricted, subvalvular fibrosis	Variable
IIIb	Restricted, tethering of leaflets	

- Flow volume curve
- Transesophageal echocardiography: Classification of MV leaflet motion

Treatment

Medical Therapy

- Digoxin
- Diuretics
- Vasodilators which cause reduction in SVR resulting in:
  - Increased forward stroke volume
  - Reduced regurgitant volume
- Afterload reduction maybe life-saving in acute MR

Surgical Therapy

- Considered for patients with moderate to severe symptoms
- Valve repair is preferred, to avoid problems associated with valve replacement like:
  - Thromboembolism
  - Hemorrhage
  - Prosthetic failure
- Mitral valve repair:
  - Recommended for all mitral regurgitations where possible
  - Mitral repair was initially restricted to posterior leaflet pathology
  - However, it is now being performed for pathologies in both leaflets
  - Isolated flail segment repair of PML is most favorable for successful repair
  - Repair is most often successful in:
    - Children and adolescents with pliable valves
    - Adults with MR secondary to MVP
    - Annular dilatation MR
    - MR due to chordal rupture
    - Perforated MV leaflet due to endocarditis
  - Repair is usually unsuccessful necessitating MV replacement in:
    - Old patients with rigid, calcified deformed valves
    - Radiation fibrosis
    - Severe sub-valvular chordal thickening
    - Major loss of leaflet substance
  - Repair techniques include:
    - Annuloplasty ring:
      - Used to provide support to the annulus and reduce annular size
      - Ring is usually incomplete along its circumference
      - Useful in pathologies involving annular dilatation
    - Quadrangular resection:
      - Quadrangular resection is used for isolated flail pathology of PML
      - Quadrangular segment of leaflet is resected
      - The resultant valvular defect is directly sutured
    - Sliding valvuloplasty:
      - Used for extensive myxomatous lesions of PML with flail
      - Resection of the redundant leaflet is carried out
      - Strip of leaflet along posterior mitral annulus is also resected
      - This reduces the length of posterior leaflet
    - Chordal replacement, shortening or transfer:
      - Used to repair AML prolapse or flail
      - Simple resection leaves AML with insufficient support
      - Thus, chordal transfer usually accompanies resection
      - Posterior chordae may be transferred to AML
      - The appropriate chordal length has to be ascertained to prevent:
        - Mitral restriction
        - Persistent mitral prolapse
    - Commissural plication:
      - Direct plication may be used for excessive leaflet tissue
      - This can be done in the commissural region
      - Middle scallops of AML and PML may be sewn together ***(Alfieri stitch)***

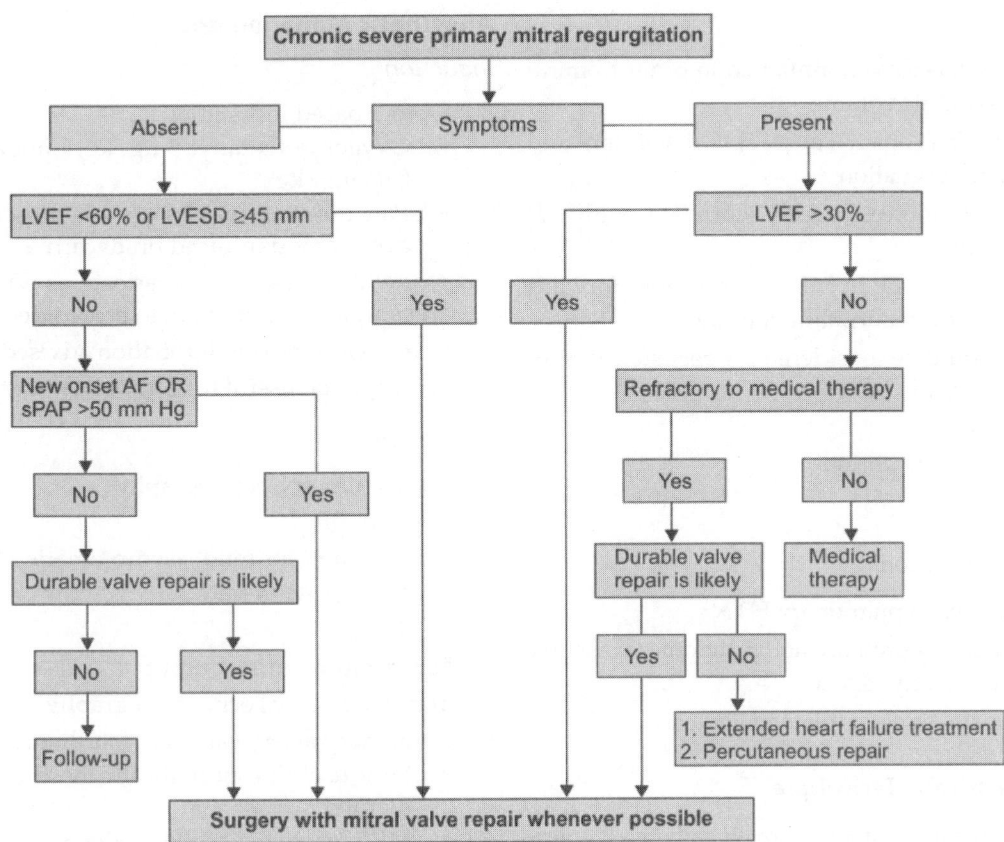

Anesthetic Goals

- *Faster, fuller and vasodilated* to maintain forward flow
- Rate: maintain slightly higher range (80–100 bpm)
- Rhythm:
  - Maintain sinus rhythm
  - If atrial fibrillation present, control ventricular rate
- Preload:
  - Maintain preload
  - Increase in preload worsens MR
- Afterload: reduced with anesthetics and vasodilators
- Contractility:
  - Maintain contractility
  - Avoid myocardial depression
  - Titrate myocardial depressants carefully
- M_VO_2: compromised if MR coexists with IHD

Rationale for Anesthetic Goals

Heart Rate and Rhythm

- Maintain sinus rhythm in high normal range (80–100 bpm)
- Bradycardia has dual detrimental effects:
  - Increased duration of systole prolongs regurgitation
  - Increased diastolic filling interval leads to more severe LV distension
- This in turn causes stretching of mitral annulus and further increases regurgitation

Preload

- Maintain preload
- Mitral regurgitation is a dynamic condition
- Increasing preload may cause LV distension
- Ventricular distension causes expansion of an already dilated MV annulus
- This may worsen MR

Afterload

- Lower SVR so that forward cardiac output is maximum
- Afterload reduction strategies:
  - Maintain adequate anesthetic depth
  - Systemic vasodilators and inodilators
  - Mechanical reduction of afterload with IABP
- Temporary use of ephedrine after which inotropic support needed to augment pressures
- Arteriolar dilators are effective as they reduce LA-LV gradient

Contractility

- Contractility has to be maintained in order to minimized end-systolic volume
- Increase in ESV again causes LV distention and aggravates regurgitation
- However, EF indices poorly correlate with LV systolic function
- This is because as EF in MR includes both forward systolic flow and regurgitant volume
- Inotropes should be considered for persistent hemodynamic instability:
  - Dobutamine
  - Low dose epinephrine
  - Milrinone

Pulmonary Hypertension

- Avoid increases in pulmonary HTN
- Pulmonary artery pressure and pulmonary vascular resistance is already raised
- Avoid hypoxia, hypercarbia and acidosis

Choice of Anesthetic Technique

- Spinal/epidural anesthesia are usually well tolerated
- This is because it reduces the SVR causing reduction in regurgitant fraction
- Bradycardia associated with spinal anesthesia is avoided as it increases regurgitant volume

Preoperative Preparation and Premedication

- Informed consent
- NPO orders
- Premedicate:
  - Premedicate with caution
  - Light premedication advised to prevent airway obstruction
  - Hypoventilation and asphyxia may exacerbate pulmonary HTN
  - Done in high dependency room under supervision
  - 0.5 mg midazolam IV titrated and given in increments
  - Supplemental oxygen can be given at this time
- Arrange for surgery-appropriate volume of blood
- Continue anti-arrhythmics until day of surgery
- Change warfarin to heparin preoperatively

Anesthetic Management

Induction

- Opioid based induction:
  - Oxygen + fentanyl 5 μg/kg + midazolam 0.03–0.05 mg/kg
  - Pancuronium may be used as muscle relaxant to avoid opiod induced bradycardia
- Acute increases in LV afterload, as after intubation and surgical stimulation, to be avoided
- Deep planes during intubation advised
- NTG may be useful to control increases in afterload

Monitoring

- Pulse oximetry, capnography
- Invasive BP:
  Not required for mild, asymptomatic MR
  Useful for severe MR
- ECG
- Temperature, urine output
- Transesophageal echocardiography
- Pulmonary artery catheter recording:
  - Very useful, especially for those on vasodilator therapy
  - MR recognized on PA wedge waveform as large *v wave with rapid y descent*
  - Especially prominent in acute MR or chronic MR with acute deterioration
  - Used for:
    - Assessment of intravascular filling
    - Measurement of cardiac output
    - Evaluation of effect of treatment
  - Suspect functional TR if raised PAP occurs
  - PCWP is poor indicator of LVEDP in chronic MR due to stiff, hypertrophied LV

Maintenance

- Balanced anesthesia with O_2 + air + volatile anesthetic is preferred
- Isoflurane, sevoflurane and desflurane may be used
- Volatile anesthetic agents have several beneficial effects:
  - Reduce SVR
  - Increase in heart rate
- Higher MAC values are preferred to lower SVR and maintain anesthetic depth
- Patients with severe LV dysfunction are very sensitive to volatile anesthetics
- Titrated doses of opioids are given to prevent bradycardia

- Pancuronium/vecuronium may be used to maintain NM blockade
- Avoid N_2O as it:
  - Increases pulmonary arterial pressure
  - Causes LV dysfunction

Ventilation

- Ventilation titrated to maintain near normal E_TCO_2 and pH
- Adequate time for expiration should be allowed to facilitate venous return
- Avoid factors causing increase in pulmonary arterial pressure:
  - Hypoxia
  - Hypercarbia
  - Acidosis
  - *High airway pressures*: Might constrict pulmonary capillaries and increase PAP
  - Excessive positive end expiratory eressure

Hemodynamics

Maintain Preload

- Judicious fluid administration
- Avoid fluid overload
- In case of hypotension: (especially acute MR)
  - Administer carefully titrated fluid boluses
  - Ephedrine boluses may be used for transient hypotension
  - Early inotropic support
  - Avoid vasoconstrictors such as phenylephrine
  - IABP useful in severe hypotension to reduce afterload and increase cardiac output

Maintain SVR

- NTG especially useful if any increase in SVR/PAP occurs
- Select agents which promote vasodilatation and tachycardia
- Dobutamine and milrinone are useful as inodilators

Reduce Pulmonary Vascular Resistance

- Avoid hypoxia and hypercarbia
- Check ABGs regularly
- Avoid acidosis
- Pulmonary vasodilatation if PAP > 2/3rd the systemic pressures with:
  - Nitric oxide 40 ppm is the agent of choice
  - Milrinone, amrinone, sildenafil, exoximone are alternatives
  - Inhaled PGE_1:
    - Dilates pulmonary smooth muscle
    - Almost complete first pass metabolism occurs in pulmonary endothelium
    - Therefore, it is pulmonary selective vasodilator

Extubation

- Extubation is carried out with caution to avoid hypoxia and hypercarbia
- Postoperative ventilation may be required for:
  - Prolonged surgery
  - Unexpected blood loss
- Extubate if:
  - Spontaneous ventilation with normal ABG
  - No bleeding and hemodynamically stable patient
  - Normothermia

Postoperative Period

Monitors

- ECG, pulse oximetry
- Invasive BP
- Urine output, CVP
- PA catheter
- ABG, temperature

Analgesia

- Multimodal analgesia
- Opioids: fentanyl or morphine
- Regional analgesia with epidural catheters
- Patient controlled analgesia

MITRAL STENOSIS

Introduction

- Valvular heart disease characterized by narrowing of the mitral valve orifice
- It is the most common lesion associated with Rheumatic Heart Disease (RHD)

Incidence

- Prevalence of rheumatic disease is higher in developing nations
- Incidence of rheumatic fever has been decreasing in industrialized countries
- Incidence of rheumatic disease in developed nations is 1 in 100,000

- Incidence of rheumatic disease in India is approximately 100–150 in 100,000
- Mitral stenosis is the most common manifestation of RHD:
  - 25% patients with RHD have isolated MS
  - 40% patients with RHD have mixed MS and MR
  - 38% patients with RHD have multivalvular disease
- Two thirds of patients with rheumatic MS are females
- The onset of symptoms usually occurs between the 3rd and 4th decade of life

Etiology

- *Rheumatic heart disease*: most common cause in developing countries
- Endomyocardial fibroelastosis
- Malignant carcinoid disease
- Systemic lupus erythematosus
- Rheumatoid arthritis
- Hunter-Hurler disease
- Fabrys disease
- Whipples disease
- Methysergide therapy
- ***Lutembacher syndrome***: ASD with rheumatic MS
- Congenital mitral stenosis

Pathology of Rheumatic Mitral Stenosis

- Stenosis begins decades after the first episode of acute rheumatic carditis
- Acute insult leads to the formation of multiple inflammatory foci called ***Aschoff bodies***
- Aschoff bodies are perivascular mononuclear infiltrates in the endocardium
- With time, thickening, contraction and commissural fusion of valve leaflets occurs
- Thickening typically begins at the tips and progresses towards commissures
- Fusion and contracture of chordae tendinae and papillary muscle heads is also seen
- This leads to restriction of diastolic motion with a ***diastolic doming*** of the leaflets
- The valve eventually becomes ***fish mouthed*** and may calcify on long standing
- This leads to reduction in the valve area and rheumatic mitral stenosis

Pathophysiology

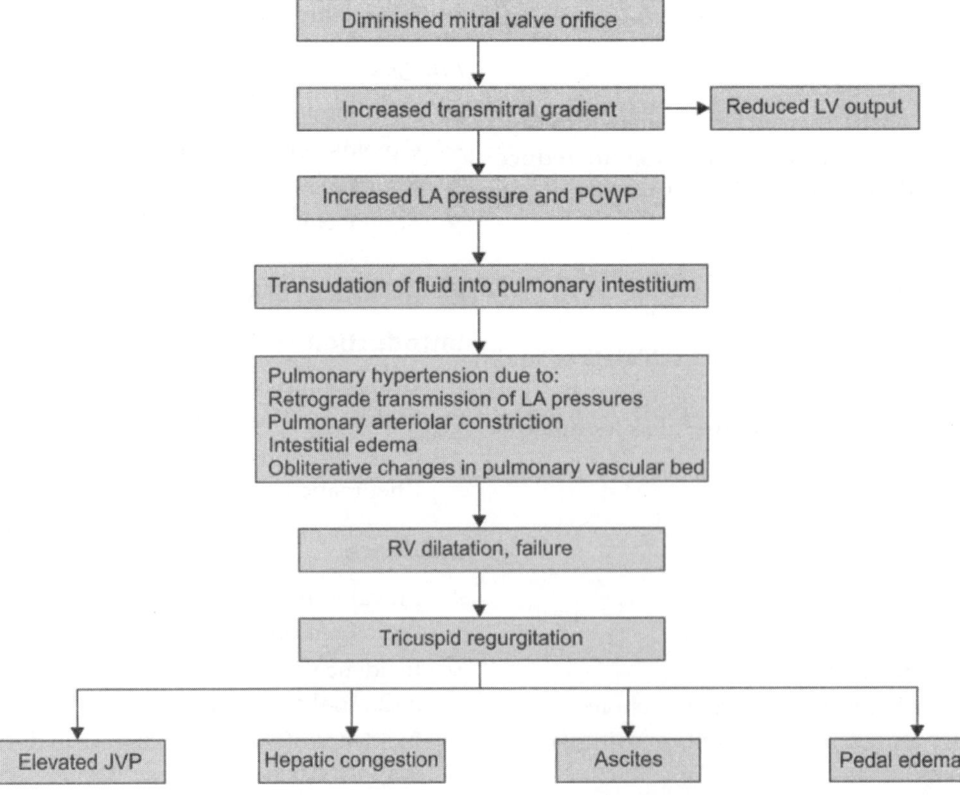

Clinical Features

- Symptoms of MS usually occur 10–20 years after acute rheumatic fever
- Most patients do not recall the history of acute rheumatic fever
- Patients are usually asymptomatic at rest during early stages of the disease

Symptoms

- Fatigue, dyspnea on exertion, PND, orthopnea
- Hemoptysis due to rupture of broncho-pulmonary varices
- Systemic/pulmonary arterial embolization
- Recurrent pulmonary infection: bronchitis, pneumonias
- Rapid decompensation occurs due to tachycardia caused by:
  - Infection, fever
  - Anemia
  - Thyrotoxicosis
  - Pregnancy
  - Atrial fibrillation

Signs

- Malar flush with pinched and blue facies: ***Mitral facies***
- Pulse:
  - Low volume pulse is typical in mitral stenosis
  - Extremities usually cold with associated peripheral cyanosis in severe MS
  - ***Delirium cordis***:
    - Irregularly irregular pulse
    - Typically seen with atrial fibrillation
- Increased respiratory rate and crackles due to pulmonary congestion
- ***Ascites precox***:
  - Name given to development of ascites, preceding limb edema in mitral stenosis
  - Liver is usually tender to palpate
  - Systolic pulsation of the liver may be seen if tricuspid regurgitation present
- ***Ortner syndrome***:
  - Also called cardiovocal syndrome
  - Hoarseness of voice occurring in mitral stenosis patients
  - This is due to compression of left RLN against LPA by the enlarged LA
  - Compression of bronchi by the enlarged LA can cause persistent cough
- Signs of right ventricular failure:
  - Ascites, anasarca, pleural effusion
  - Raised jugular venous pressure with:
    - Prominent 'a' wave indicating increased RA pressure
    - Prominent 'v' wave indicating tricuspid regurgitation
  - Parasternal heave
- Auscultation:
  - Normal sequence of sounds in mitral stenosis is S_1-S_2-OS-MDM
  - Loud S_1 due to:
    - This is due to wide closing excursion of mitral leaflets
    - This results in increased force during mitral valve closure
    - Loudness of S_1 depends on the pliability of mitral valve
    - Intensity of S_1 decreases as the valve becomes thick, fibrotic and calcified
  - Findings of pulmonary hypertension:
    - Accentuated P_2 component of second heart sound
    - Pulmonary ejection systolic click if pulmonary HTN is present
  - Opening snap (OS):
    - Heard after A_2 component of second heart sound
    - Heard along left sternal border/just medial to apex
    - This is due to sudden tensing of leaflets after they have completed opening
  - Mitral stenosis murmur:
    - Low pitched rumbling mid-diastolic murmur (MDM) at apex
    - Presystolic accentuation will be present if patient is in sinus rhythm
    - Best heart with bell of stethoscope
    - With patient in left lateral position
    - Breath to be held in expiration
    - Murmur usually radiates towards axilla
    - Accentuated by isometric exercise like squatting/handgrip

Clinical Assessment of Severity

- S_2 – OS gap:
  - Normal is 0.05 – 0.12 sec
  - If OS closer to S_2, MS is more severe
- Severity of MS increases as duration of MDM increases
- Can be assessed indirectly by assessing severity of pulmonary HTN
- Higher the RVSP, more severe is MS (Normal < 25 mm Hg)

Staging of Mitral Stenosis: ACC/AHA 2014 guidelines 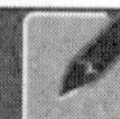

- Stage A: At risk of mitral stenosis
- Stage B: Asymptomatic with progressive mitral stenosis (mild-moderate)
- Stage C: Asymptomatic with echocardiographically severe MS
- Stage D: Symptomatic with echocardiographically severe MS.

Differential Diagnosis

- Infective endocarditis with large vegetation
- Mitral annular calcification
- Left atrial myxoma
- Ball valve thrombus
- Cor triatriatum

Prognosis

- Mitral stenosis is a progressive disease with slow, stable course in the early years
- This is followed by an accelerated course later on in the course of the disease
- Usually there is a latent period of 20–40 years from occurrence of rheumatic fever
- Symptoms begin to appear after this latent period in most cases
- Earlier presentation occurs due to:
  - More severe rheumatic insult
  - Repeated episodes of rheumatic carditis
- Once symptoms develop, within a decade, most patients become debilitated
- In patients with absent or minimal symptoms, 10-year survival is close to 80%
- Once limiting symptoms appear, 10-year survival drops to 15% in untreated patients

Complications

- Atrial fibrillation
- Systemic embolism:
  - LA thrombus formation occurs secondary to atrial fibrillation
  - The thrombus formed can embolize into systemic circulation
  - This can cause:
    - Myocardial infarction
    - Renal failure
    - Stroke
- Infective endocarditis
- Pulmonary hypertension
- Pulmonary edema

Investigation

- Chest X-ray:
  - Normal in early stages
  - ***Mitralization of left heart border***
  - LA enlargement: ***Double density sign***
  - RV enlargement later on and right ventricular apex
  - Pulmonary edema
  - Calcified valve, splaying of carina
- ECG:
  - May be normal
  - ***P-mitrale***:
    - Classic broad M-shaped P wave in lead II (LA enlargement)
    - P-wave may be more than 120 msec in duration
    - Biphasic P-waves may be seen in lead V_1
  - Right axis deviation, RBBB due to right ventricular hypertrophy
  - Atrial fibrillation
- Echocardiography:
  - Area of mitral valve, pressure gradient between left atrium and ventricle
  - Assessment of mitral valve anatomy—Wilkins score

- Size of LA, presence of LA thrombus
- Severity of associated lesions like mitral regurgitation
- Staging of the disease and to decide intervention of choice based on Wilkins score

❖ Holter monitoring

❖ Cardiac catherization:

- Not routinely done in mitral stenosis cases (Class I, LOE C)
- Indicated when:
  - Noninvasive tests are inconclusive
  - Discrepancy between noninvasive tests and clinical assessment of severity
- Uses of catheterization in mitral stenosis:
  - For calculation of MVA using ***Gorlins equation***
  - PCWP increases to 25–30 mm Hg when mitral valve area ≤ 2 cm^2
  - Valvular diastolic pressure gradients ≥ 25 mm Hg, if severe MS

❖ Exercise testing:

- Used to evaluate response of mean mitral gradient to exercise
- Useful in the presence of discrepancy between:
  - Noninvasive tests and
  - Clinical assessment of severity

❖ Pressure Volume Loop in MS

Echocardiographic Assessment of Severity of Mitral Stenosis

No.	Parameter	Mild	Moderate	Severe
1.	Mitral valve area	1.5–2 cm^2	1–1.5 cm^2	< 1 cm^2
2.	Pressure half time	< 150 msec	150–220 msec	> 220 msec
3.	Transmitral mean gradient	< 5 mm Hg	5–10 mm Hg	> 10 mm Hg
4.	Pulmonary artery systolic pressure	< 30 mm Hg	30–50 mm Hg	> 50 mm Hg
5.	Wilkins score	< 4	4–12	> 12
6.	LA size	< 45 mm	45–60 mm	> 60 mm
7.	Spontaneous echo contrast (SEC)	Absent	Usually present	Always present
8.	Proximal flow convergence	Absent	Usually present	Always present
9.	Deceleration time	< 517 msec	517–759 msec	> 759 msec

Assessment of Mitral Anatomy: *Wilkins Score*

Parameter	Grade 1	Grade 2	Grade 3	Grade 4
Mobility	Only tips restricted	Mid and base normal	Only base normal	No movement
Thickening	Normal	Thickened tip	Entire leaflet thick	Entire leaflet thick
	4–5 mm thickness	5-8 mm thickness	5-8 mm thickness	> 8–10 mm thickness
Calcification	Single area	Scattered areas	Midleaflet calcification	Calcification throughout
		Confined to margins		
Subvalvular Thickening	Minimal thickening	1/3 chordal length	2/3 chordal length	Entire chordal thickening
				Shortening of chordate
				Extends to papillary muscles

Management of Mitral Stenosis

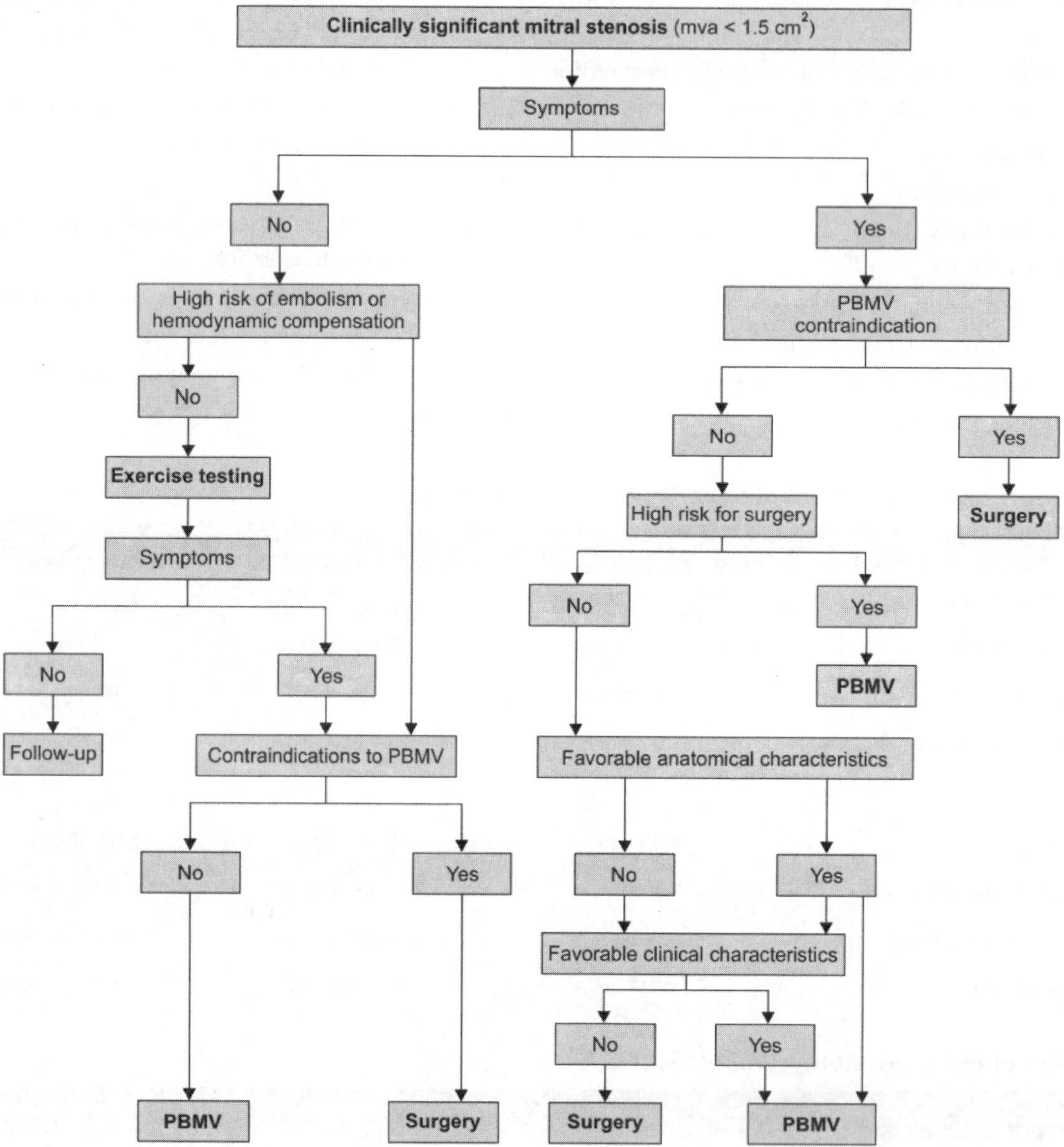

Medical Management

- Goals of medical management:
  - Improving symptoms
  - Preventing infective endocarditis
  - Decreasing recurrence of rheumatic fever-prophylaxis
  - Decreasing risk of thromboembolism
- Improving symptoms:
  - Diuretics are used to relieve pulmonary congestion
  - β blockers and calcium channel blockers used to prevent tachycardia
  - Atrial fibrillation with unstable hemodynamics:
    - Cardioversion is indicated to revert to sinus rhythm
    - Restoration of sinus rhythm improves functional capacity dramatically
    - In case of non-reversal to sinus rhythm, rate control is paramount
  - Atrial fibrillation with stable hemodynamics:
    - Requires aggressive treatment to control rate with:
      - Beta blockers
      - Calcium channel blockers
      - Digoxin

- Treat pulmonary edema with:
  - Bed rest, propped up nursing
  - Non-invasive or invasive ventilation
  - Administration of diuretics
  - Fluid restriction
- ❖ Infective endocarditis prophylaxis:
  - Given in high-risk patients prior to high-risk dental procedures
  - High risk patients include those with:
    - Prosthetic heart valve
    - Prosthetic material used for valve repair
    - Cardiac valvuloplasty
    - Previous history of infective endocarditis
  - High-risk dental procedures include:
    - Those that involve manipulation of gingival tissues
    - Those which involve perforation of oral mucosa
- ❖ Rheumatic fever prophylaxis:
  - Used in patients with streptococcal pharyngitis for primary prevention
  - Benzathine penicillin is used for primary prevention
- ❖ Anticoagulation:
  - Indicated in mitral stenosis with (Class I, LOE C):
    - Persistent or paroxysmal atrial fibrillation
    - Previous embolic events
    - Presence of left atrial thrombus
  - Warfarin is drug of choice at present for anticoagulation
  - Antiplatelet drugs are not approved to decrease thromboembolic risk
  - Warfarin monitored to target INR 2–3

PERCUTANEOUS BALLOON MITRAL VALVULOPLASTY

Introduction

- ❖ First described by K. Inoue in 1984
- ❖ Regarded as treatment of choice for isolated mitral stenosis with favorable anatomy

Indications

- ❖ Symptomatic moderate-severe mitral stenosis with: (Class I LOE B)
  - Stage D mitral valve disease
  - No contraindications
  - Favorable valve morphology
- ❖ *Asymptomatic moderate-severe mitral stenosis with:* (Class IIa LOE C)
  - PASP > 50 mm Hg at rest
  - PASP > 60 mm Hg with exercise
  - New onset atrial fibrillation
  - High-risk candidates for surgery
  - No contraindications
  - Favorable valve morphology
- ❖ Symptomatic mild mitral stenosis patients with: (Class IIb LOE C)
  - PASP > 60 mm Hg
  - PCWP > 25 mm Hg
  - Mean mitral valve gradient > 15 mm Hg

Contraindications

- ❖ Valve area over 1.5 cm^2 (Class III LOE C)
- ❖ Wilkins score > 10
- ❖ Presence of LA or LAA thrombus (Class III LOE C)
- ❖ Moderate-severe mitral regurgitation
- ❖ Unfavourable mitral valve anatomy:
  - Severe bicommisural calcification
  - Absence of commissural fusion
- ❖ Concomitant diseases:
  - Severe concomitant aortic valve disease
  - Severe combined tricuspid stenosis and regurgitation
  - Concomitant coronary artery disease requiring bypass surgery

Investigations

- ❖ Usually no specific laboratory studies are required in the absence of abnormal bleeding
- ❖ Complete blood counts, PT, INR however may be included as screening tests
- ❖ Transthoracic echocardiogram is done to assess mitral apparatus
- ❖ Exercise echocardiography can be useful in those with ambiguous symptoms
- ❖ Wilson score via TTE can be used to predict success of PBMV:
  - Score < 8:
    - Predicts excellent long-term results
    - Predicts a 5-year event free survival rate of 80%
  - Score 9–12 predicts intermediate results
  - Score more than 12 predicts poor outcomes
- ❖ Transesophageal echocardiogram is performed preoperatively to rule out LA clot
- ❖ Coronary angiogram recommended in:
  - Males > 35 years age
  - Women > 35 years age with either of:
    - Coronary risk factors
    - Postmenopausal

Techniques

- Inoue balloon technique
- Double balloon technique
- Multitrack technique
- Metallic commissurotomy

Choice of Anesthesia

- General anesthesia is preferred when TEE is being used to monitor dilatation
- Monitored anesthesia care may suffice when peri-procedural TTE is used
- Transseptal puncture may be painful in some patients and may require deeper planes

Monitors

- ASA monitors according to minimal monitoring standards
- Echocardiography:
  - Intraprocedural echocardiography is used to:
    - Guide the cardiologist during the procedure
    - Directing catheter and balloon across the mitral valve
    - Assess the results of valve dilatation
  - TEE preferred to TTE as it can provide more reliable peri-procedural imaging
  - TEE is more useful to reliably confirm transseptal needle position

Approaches

- Antegrade or transvenous approach:
  - This is the most commonly used approach
  - Approach is usually from the femoral vein
  - However jugular venous approach has also been described
  - Dilatation of the valve is done through trans-septal puncture
  - A balloon catheter is inserted from the femoral vein and advanced into the RA
  - The catheter is advanced across the atrial septum to access the mitral valve
- Retrograde or transarterial approach:
  - This is a rarely used approach
  - Mitral valve is approached retrograde from the aorta, across the aortic valve
  - Avoids the risk of persistent ASD seen with antegrade approach
  - This approach requires passing a large catheter across the aortic valve
  - Therefore it carries a risk of potential arterial damage
  - Due to its complexity it has been largely abandoned

Inoue Balloon

- This is the most commonly used device for balloon dilatation in PBMV
- Composed of a nylon and rubber micromesh which is pressure extensible
- Available in 4 sizes: 24, 26, 28 and 30 mm
- Balloon size is calculated using the patients height in cm
- Balloon size = (Patient height/10) + 10
- The device consists of a single balloon which inflates in three stages
- After crossing the mitral valve, distal portion of the balloon is first inflated
- The catheter is then pulled back to allow distal balloon to oppose the valve
- Proximal portion of the balloon is then inflated to engage the valve
- The middle portion of the balloon is inflated last to split the fused leaflets
- Repeated inflations are performed in larger balloon diameters
- This is titrated to achieve an optimal trans-mitral gradient reduction

Procedure

- Vascular access:
  - Obtained with a 7-French sheath in the femoral vein
  - Left femoral artery may be cannulated with a 5-French sheath
  - Femoral vein on the opposite side may be cannulated to measure PA pressures
- Transseptal puncture:
  - Goal of transseptal puncture is to cross over from the RA to LA via fossa ovalis
  - As viewed from the foot end, the atrial septum runs from 1 to 7 o'clock position
  - This is the most crucial step as many neighboring structures may be injured
  - The ***Brockenbrough needle*** is used for transseptal puncture
  - Successful entry into the LA is confirmed by recording LA pressure waveform
- Anticoagulation:
  - 5000 IU heparin is administered to ensure adequate anticoagulation
  - Blood samples are taken for ACT measurement after 3 minutes

- ❖ Hemodynamic assessment:
  - PA catheter is used to measure the hemodilution cardiac output and PA pressure
  - Pigtail catheter is used to measure left ventricular pressures
  - Trans-mitral gradient and valve area is then calculated
- ❖ Insertion of Inoue balloon:
  - The balloon is maneuvered across the mitral valve under fluoroscopic guidance
  - The balloon is inflated in 3 steps: distal, proximal and finally middle section
  - The balloon is then deflated and withdrawn into the left atrium
  - Echocardiographic assessment is done to ensure adequacy of valve dilatation

Complications

- ❖ Mitral regurgitation:
  - Moderate-severe MR occurs in up to 12% patients undergoing PBMV
  - Severe MR requiring surgery following PBMV occurs in 2.5% patients
  - Acute mitral regurgitation can occur due to:
    - Non-commissural tearing of anterior or posterior leaflet
    - Excessive commissurotomy
    - Leaflet perforation
    - Sub-chordal damage
- ❖ Residual iatrogenic ASD:
  - Iatrogenic ASD is present in all patients undergoing antegrade approach PBMV
  - However, this ASD almost always closes spontaneously within weeks

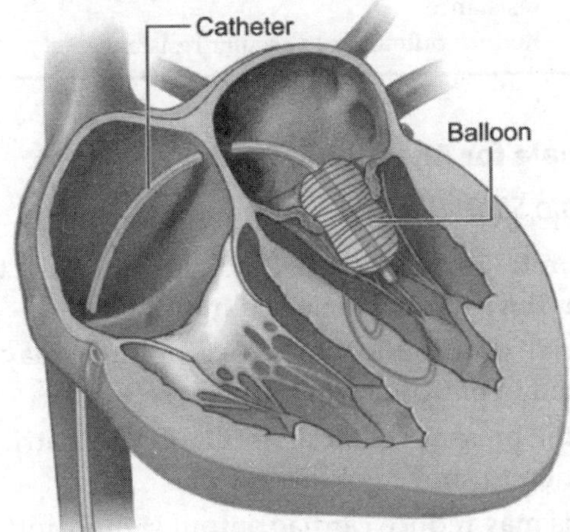

Fig. 40: Balloon mitral valvotomy.

  - Persistent ASDs are typically small and cause restrictive shunts
  - Less than 2% patients have a persistent shunt fraction greater than 1.5:1
  - This occurs when the LA pressures remain persistently elevated
- ❖ Transient ischemic attacks, stroke
- ❖ Cardiac perforation and hemopericardium
- ❖ Complete heart block
- ❖ Failure of PBMV

Prognosis

- ❖ Mitral valve area increases on an average from 1 cm^2 to 2 cm^2 after PBMV
- ❖ Mitral valve area reduction greater than 0.3 cm^2 occurs in 27% patients
- ❖ Enlarged mitral orifice results in:
  - Immediate decline in LA pressure
  - Decline in left atrial stiffness causing:
    - Improved LA contraction for patients in sinus rhythm
    - Increased LA reservoir for patients in atrial fibrillation
  - Trans-mitral pressure gradient
  - Immediate decline in pulmonary artery pressures (10–25%)
  - Increase in cardiac output
- ❖ Event free survival rates following PBMV:
  - 80% at 1 year
  - 71% at 2 years
  - 66% at 3 years
  - 60% at 4 years
- ❖ Mitral valve restenosis:
  - Defined as a loss of more than 50% of the initial gain following PBMV
  - Occurs in up to 2–20% of patients after PBMV
  - Time interval to restenosis can range from 3–10 years
  - Repeat PBMV or surgery can be considered based on the anatomy

Surgical Management

- ❖ Indications for surgery:
  - Stage D mitral stenosis: symptomatic with MVA < 1.5 cm^2
  - NYHA class III-IV symptoms
  - Poor mitral valve anatomy for PBMV
  - Failure of previous PBMV
  - MS associated with MR
  - Multivalvular disease
  - Associated CAD

- Options for surgical management include:
  - Closed mitral valvotomy
  - Mitral valve replacement
- Mitral valve replacement:
  - Prosthetic valves used can be mechanical or bioprosthetic valves
  - Mechanical valves preferred in:
    - Young age less than 65 years
  - Bioprosthetic valves preferred in:
    - Age above 65 years
    - Contraindications to anticoagulation

MITRAL STENOSIS PATIENT FOR NON-CARDIAC SURGERY

Preoperative Assessment

- Chest X-ray:
  - Normal in early stages
  - ***Mitralization of left heart border***
  - LA enlargement: ***Double density sign***
  - RV enlargement later on and right ventricular apex
  - Pulmonary edema
  - Calcified valve, splaying of carina
- ECG:
  - May be normal
  - ***P-mitrale***:
    - Classic broad M-shaped P wave in lead II (LA enlargement)
    - P-wave may be more than 120 msec in duration
    - Biphasic P-waves may be seen in lead V_1
  - Right axis deviation, RBBB due to right ventricular hypertrophy
  - Atrial fibrillation
- Echocardiography:
  - Area of mitral valve, pressure gradient between left atrium and ventricle
  - Assessment of mitral valve anatomy-Wilkins score
  - Size of LA, presence of LA thrombus
  - Severity of associated lesions like mitral regurgitation
  - Staging of the disease and to decide intervention of choice based on Wilkins score
- Holter monitoring
- Cardiac catherization:
  - Not routinely done in mitral stenosis cases (Class I, LOE C)
  - Indicated when:
    - Noninvasive tests are inconclusive
    - Discrepancy between noninvasive tests and clinical assessment of severity
  - Uses of catheterization in mitral stenosis:
    - For calculation of MVA using ***Gorlins equation***
    - PCWP increases to 25–30 mm Hg when mitral valve area ≤ 2 cm^2
    - Valvular diastolic pressure gradients ≤ 25 mm Hg, if severe MS
- Exercise testing:
  - Used to evaluate response of mean mitral gradient to exercise
  - Useful in the presence of discrepancy between:
    - Noninvasive tests and
    - Clinical assessment of severity
- Pressure volume loop in MS

Goals of Anesthesia

- Heart rate:
  - Maintain low heart rate
  - Prevent rapid ventricular rates
- Rhythm: maintain sinus rhythm
- Preload:
  - Judicious fluid loading, avoid fluid overload
  - Minimize increases in central blood volume
- Afterload:
  - Maintain afterload (SVR)
  - Avoid marked decreases in SVR
- Contractility: maintain contractility
- Systemic vascular resistance: maintain SVR
- Pulmonary vascular resistance:
  - Prevent sudden increases in pulmonary vascular resistance
  - Reduce pulmonary vascular resistance

Rationale for Anesthetic Goals

Maintain Sinus Rhythm

- In mitral stenosis, atrial kick is important to maintain flow across a stenosed mitral valve
- Atrial contribution to stroke volume may be elevated in patients with the stenosed valve
- In the presence of atrial fibrillation, this atrial contribution to stroke volume is lost
- This may reduce cardiac output significantly
- Thus, maintaining sinus rhythm is important in mitral stenosis

Prevent Rapid Ventricular Rates

- Stenosed MV causes stroke volume to be constant regardless of metabolic demand
- In this setting, heart may not be able to cope with situations demanding an increase in CO
- Any increase in heart rate will also reduce the diastolic filling time
- Thus stroke volume will reduce further and cause a decrease in cardiac output
- Sinus tachycardia and AF with FVR are the most common type of tachycardia
- Rate-control measures should aim to maintain ventricular rate < 110 bpm

Maintain Preload

- MS is associated with a higher than normal gradient between the LA and LV
- Thus, higher LA pressure is required to generate enough gradient across the MV
- Therefore, adequate preload is required to maintain high-normal LA pressure in MS
- However, sudden increase in central blood volume can precipitate pulmonary edema
- Thus, in mitral stenosis patients, avoid:
  - Over transfusion
  - Trendelenburg position
- CVP and PAP can be used to assess increase in central blood volume

Avoid Decreases in SVR

- Any decrease in SVR is compensated by an increase in heart rate
- This is because the stroke volume is fixed across the stenosed mitral valve
- Marked increase in heart rate causes rapid decompensation due to reduced diastolic time
- Thus, reduction in SVR causes a profound reduction in cardiac output
- SVR may be maintained with phenylephrine infusion

Prevent Increases in Pulmonary Arterial Pressure

- Avoid factors causing increase in PVR:
  - Hypercarbia
  - Hypoxia
  - Metabolic acidosis
  - Hypothermia
  - Lung hyperinflation
- If pulmonary HTN and RVF occurs:
  - IV dopamine (3–8 μg/kg/min) inotropic support
  - Pulmonary vasodilation with SNP (0.1–0.5 μg/kg/min)
  - Inhaled nitric oxide

Choice of Anesthetic Technique

- Neuraxial and regional anesthesia may be preferred where applicable
- Regional techniques such as peripheral nerve blocks are safer
- This is a particularly safe technique in the setting of anticoagulation
- Use of spinal anesthesia requires:
  - Avoidance of hypotension
  - Avoidance of tachycardia
  - Avoidance of sudden drop in SVR
  - Maintenance of adequate preload
- Epidural neuraxial techniques:
  - Associated with a more gradual onset of sympathetic blockade
  - This allows better control of the level of sympathectomy

Premedication

- Informed consent
- NPO orders:
  - 6 hours solids
  - 2 hours clear fluids
- Judicious fluid administration in the preoperative period to prevent pulmonary edema
- Avoid Trendelenburg position to avoid increasing central blood volume
- Drugs used for rate-control in mitral stenosis have to be continued until the surgery
- Discontinuation of anticoagulants prior to procedure at the appropriate time
- Diuretic induced hypokalemia has to be treated preoperatively

Monitors

- Pulse oximetry
- ECG
- NIBP
- Capnography
- Temperature
- Neuromuscular monitoring
- Urine output
- Invasive hemodynamic monitoring required in major surgery with fluid shifts:
  - Invasive arterial pressure
  - Central venous pressure
  - Pulmonary artery pressure

- Pulmonary capillary wedge pressure (represents the transmitral gradient in MS)
- LA pressure

❖ Caution with PA catheter PA rupture possible in those with chronic pulmonary HTN

❖ TEE useful in symptomatic MS patients undergoing major surgery

Induction

❖ Adequate preoxygenation is required to avoid hypoxia and increase in PVR

❖ Any induction agent can be used except for ketamine

❖ Ketamine causes tachycardia and should be avoided

❖ Neuromuscular blocking agents which cause histamine release (pancuronium) avoided

❖ β-blockers may be used to treat the tachycardia associated with intubation response

❖ Esmolol useful to obtain rate control owing to rapid onset and short duration of action

Maintenance

❖ Balanced anesthesia technique with low concentration of inhale anesthetic is used

❖ Nitrous oxide avoided as it causes pulmonary vasoconstriction and increased PVR

❖ O_2 + air + isoflurane 1 MAC is a useful balanced anesthesia technique

❖ Drugs used for maintenance should have minimal effects on:
- Heart rate
- Myocardial contractility
- Systemic vascular resistance
- Pulmonary vascular resistance

❖ Light anesthetic planes avoided as it causes detrimental tachycardia

Hemodynamics

❖ Fluid therapy carefully titrated to prevent volume overload

❖ Phenylephrine preferred to ephedrine as it lacks β-adrenergic agonist activity

❖ Vasopressin can be used in cases of intractable hypotension due to low SVR

❖ Intraoperative tachycardia:
- Treated with opioids to deepen the anesthetic plane
- β-blockers may be used to treat tachycardia unrelated to anesthetic plane
- Rate control agents used for new onset hemodynamically stable atrial fibrillation
- Cardioversion required for new onset hemodynamically unstable atrial fibrillation

❖ Inotropic support:
- May be required in those with secondary RV dysfunction
- Adrenaline and milrinone are useful choices

Extubation

❖ Postoperative ventilation may be advisable in patients with poor lung compliance

❖ This is common following major thoracic and abdominal surgery

❖ Reversal agents should be given slowly

❖ This is because tachycardia is associated with glycopyrrolate

❖ Thus, slow administration of reversal allows amelioration of drug-induced tachycardia

❖ Deep planes for extubation preferred to avoid tachycardia associated with extubation

Postoperative Management

Monitoring

❖ Pulse oximetry

❖ ECG

❖ NIBP

❖ Urine output

❖ Invasive BP and CVP in hemodynamically unstable patients

Management

❖ Anticoagulation is restarted as soon as the risk of postoperative bleeding has diminished

Analgesia

❖ Multimodal analgesia is preferred

❖ Adequate analgesia is paramount as it can lead to hypoventilation

❖ This in turn has a multitude of detrimental effects:
- Hypercarbia
- Tachycardia
- Increased pulmonary vascular resistance

MITRAL STENOSIS IN PREGNANCY

Introduction

Mitral stenosis is generally poorly tolerated during pregnancy due to physiological changes occurring during pregnancy.

Incidence

- Rheumatic MS forms 88% of heart disease associated with pregnancy in India
- 25% women with MS become symptomatic during pregnancy
- 67% of pregnant women with severe MS have complications in the peripartum period

Pregnancy Induced Changes on MS

- Moderate stenosis may become severe during pregnancy
- Pregnancy associated increase in central blood volume causes:
  - An increase in transmitral gradient which increases through pregnancy
  - This can cause a progression of symptoms from one NYHA class to another
  - The maternal outcome correlates well with the NYHA functional class
  - Mortality rates for class I and II amount to less than 1%
  - However for class III-IV, mortality rate ranges between 5% and 15%
- Increased heart rate of pregnancy reduces diastolic filling time:
  - This can increase left atrial pressures and PCWP
  - Also, tachycardia causes increased blood flow across the mitral valve
  - Therefore, there is increased likelihood of pulmonary edema
  - Women with asymptomatic MS before pregnancy tolerate pregnancy well
- Peripartum changes:
  - Rapid RV decompensation occurs during peripartum period in severe MS
  - This is due to limited ability to handle increases in central blood volume
  - This predisposes the parturient to pulmonary edema at the time of delivery
  - Factors causing increased risk of complications surrounding labor:
    - Pain
    - Tachycardia
    - Anxiety
    - Anemia
  - Morbidity and mortality is greatest during labor and immediate postpartum period
  - Most deaths occur between the 2nd and 9th days postpartum
- Autotransfusion:
  - Sudden increase in preload occurs following umbilical cord clamping
  - This is mainly due to autotransfusion from the uterus
  - Up to 500 mL of autotransfusion occurs with each uterine contraction
  - Also, there is a loss of fetal compression of the IVC after delivery
  - These factors increase the preload dramatically, causing severe pulmonary edema
  - Autotransfusion can continue for up to 24–72 hours after delivery
  - Thus, risk of pulmonary edema extends for several days after delivery
- Increased incidence of complications:
  - Pulmonary edema (35%)
  - Atrial fibrillation (7%)
  - Paroxysmal atrial tachycardia (3%)
- Factors predicting risk of maternal pulmonary edema in mitral stenosis:
  - Late antenatal presentation
  - Moderate-severe symptoms
  - Severity of mitral stenosis
  - Previously undiagnosed cardiac disease

Investigations

- Chest X-ray:
  - Normal in early stages
  - ***Mitralization of left heart border***
  - *LA enlargement*: ***Double density sign***
  - RV enlargement later on and right ventricular apex
  - Pulmonary edema
  - Calcified valve, splaying of carina
- ECG:
  - May be normal
  - ***P-mitrale***:
    - Classic broad M-shaped P wave in lead II (LA enlargement)
    - P-wave may be more than 120 msec in duration
    - Biphasic P-waves may be seen in lead V_1
  - Right axis deviation, RBBB due to right ventricular hypertrophy
  - Atrial fibrillation
- Echocardiography:
  - Area of mitral valve, pressure gradient between left atrium and ventricle

- Assessment of mitral valve anatomy—Wilkins score
- Size of LA, presence of LA thrombus
- Severity of associated lesions like mitral regurgitation
- Staging of the disease and to decide intervention of choice based on Wilkins score

❖ Holter monitoring

❖ Cardiac catherization:
- Not routinely done in mitral stenosis cases (Class I, LOE C)
- Indicated when:
  - Noninvasive tests are inconclusive
  - Discrepancy between noninvasive tests and clinical assessment of severity
- Uses of catheterization in mitral stenosis:
  - For calculation of MVA using ***Gorlins equation***
  - PCWP increases to 25–30 mm Hg when mitral valve area ≤ 2 cm^2
  - Valvular diastolic pressure gradients ≥ 25 mm Hg, if severe MS

❖ Exercise testing:
- Used to evaluate response of mean mitral gradient to exercise
- Useful in the presence of discrepancy between:
  - Noninvasive tests and
  - Clinical assessment of severity

❖ Pressure volume loop in MS

Echocardiographic Assessment of Severity of Mitral Stenosis

No.	Parameter	Mild	Moderate	Severe
1.	Mitral valve area	1.5–2 cm^2	1–1.5 cm^2	< 1 cm^2
2.	Pressure half time	< 150 msec	150–220 msec	> 220 msec
3.	Transmitral mean gradient	< 5 mm Hg	5–10 mm Hg	> 10 mm Hg
4.	Pulmonary artery systolic pressure	< 30 mm Hg	30–50 mm Hg	> 50 mm Hg
5.	Wilkins score	< 4	4–12	> 12
6.	LA size	< 45 mm	45–60 mm	> 60 mm
7.	Spontaneous echo contrast (SEC)	Absent	Usually present	Always present
8.	Proximal flow convergence	Absent	Usually present	Always present
9.	Deceleration time	< 517 msec	517–759 msec	> 759 msec

Assessment of Mitral Anatomy: *Wilkins Score*

Parameter	Grade 1	Grade 2	Grade 3	Grade 4
Mobility	Only tips restricted	Mid and base normal	Only base normal	No movement
Thickening	Normal	Thickened tip	Entire leaflet thick	Entire leaflet thick
	4–5 mm thickness	5–8 mm thickness	5–8 mm thickness	> 8–10 mm thickness
Calcification	Single area	Scattered areas	Midleaflet calcification	Calcification throughout
		Confined to margins		
Subvalvular Thickening	Minimal thickening	1/3 chordal length	2/3 chordal length	Entire chordal thickening
				Shortening of chordate
				Extends to papillary muscles

Medical Management

❖ Goals of medical management:
- Improving symptoms
- Preventing infective endocarditis
- Decreasing recurrence of rheumatic fever-prophylaxis
- Decreasing risk of thromboembolism

❖ Improving symptoms:
- Diuretics are used to relieve pulmonary congestion
- β blockers and calcium channel blockers used to prevent tachycardia
- Choice of beta blockers:
  - *Propranolol* is best as it has no teratogenic effects
  - Aenolol:
    - Associated with fetal growth retardation
    - Thus, it is avoided in the first trimester
  - Esmolol avoided as it is teratogenic

- Atrial fibrillation with unstable hemodynamics:
  - Cardioversion is indicated to revert to sinus rhythm
  - Restoration of sinus rhythm improves functional capacity dramatically
  - In case of non-reversal to sinus rhythm, rate control is paramount
- Atrial fibrillation with stable hemodynamics:
  - Requires aggressive treatment to control rate with:
    - Beta blockers
    - Calcium channel blockers
    - Digoxin
- Treat pulmonary edema with:
  - Bed rest, propped up nursing
  - Non-invasive or invasive ventilation
  - Administration of diuretics
  - Fluid restriction

❖ Rheumatic fever prophylaxis:
- Used in patients with streptococcal pharyngitis for primary prevention
- Benzathine penicillin is used for primary prevention

❖ Anticoagulation:
- Indicated in mitral stenosis with (Class I, LOE C):
  - Persistent or paroxysmal atrial fibrillation
  - Previous embolic events
  - Presence of left atrial thrombus
- Warfarin:
  - Warfarin is more efficacious than UFH for thromboembolic prophylaxis
  - However, warfarin is avoided during pregnancy
  - Maternal effects of warfarin anticoagulation during pregnancy:
    - Uteroplacental junction bleed and fetal wastage (30%)
    - Prematurity (45%)
    - Low birth weight (50%)
  - Fetal effects:
    - Warfarin can cross the placenta and cause fetal bleeding
    - Another risk during first trimester of pregnancy is teratogenicity
    - Warfarin is associated with ***Contradi or fetal warfarin syndrome***
- Anticoagulation protocol during pregnancy:
  - First 2 trimesters: LMW
  - SC or IV UFH heparin after 36 weeks till delivery

Surgical Management

❖ Surgery advised if:
- Moderate to severe MS is recognized before pregnancy
- If medical treatment is unsatisfactory during pregnancy
- Closed mitral valvotomy preferred to mitral valve replacement

❖ Percutaneous balloon mitral valvulotomy (PBMV):
- Done using Inoue balloon technique
- Method of choice for treating isolated severe symptomatic mitral stenosis
- Reserved for patients who do not respond to maximal medical therapy
- Success rate is nearly 100% in pregnant women
- Done under monitored anesthesia care with radiation shielding of the fetus

❖ Closed mitral valvotomy (CMV):
- Can be done at any stage of gestation if symptoms are severe
- Best done during 2nd trimester
- Maternal outcomes for PBMV and CMV are similar
- However, fetal loss is higher in CMV compared with PBMV

❖ Mitral valve replacement:
- Bioprosthetic heterogeneous porcine valve preferred
- Bioprosthetic valve avoids risk of warfarin related complications
- Best done in 2nd trimester
- Maternal mortality of 1.5–5% and fetal loss of 16–33%
- Indicated if:
  - MS is associated with significant MR
  - Calcified valve
  - Mural thrombus
  - Done only if critical MS with MVA < 1 cm^2 and NYHA class > III

CARPREG Risk Stratification *in MS with Pregnancy*

Risk factor	Score
Prior cardiac event or arrhythmia	1
NYHA III, IV or cyanosis	1
Left heart obstruction comprising of the following 3 classes:	1
• Mitral valve area < 2 cm^2	
• Aortic valve area 1.5 cm^2	
• LVOT gradient > 30 mm Hg	
Ejection fraction < 40%	1

CARPREG Score	Risk of cardiac complications
0 points	5%
1 point	27%
> 2 points	75%

Goals of Anesthesia

- ❖ Avoidance of aortocaval compression
- ❖ Prevention of acid aspiration
- ❖ Heart rate:
  - Maintain low heart rate
  - Prevent rapid ventricular rates
- ❖ *Rhythm*: maintain sinus rhythm
- ❖ Preload:
  - Judicious fluid loading, avoid fluid overload
  - Minimize increases in central blood volume
- ❖ Afterload:
  - Maintain afterload (SVR)
  - Avoid marked decreases in SVR
- ❖ *Contractility*: maintain contractility
- ❖ *Systemic vascular resistance*: maintain SVR
- ❖ Pulmonary vascular resistance:
  - Prevent sudden increases in pulmonary vascular resistance
  - Reduce pulmonary vascular resistance

Rationale for Anesthetic Goals

Maintain Sinus Rhythm

- ❖ In mitral stenosis, atrial kick is important to maintain flow across a stenosed mitral valve
- ❖ Atrial contribution to stroke volume maybe elevated in patients with the stenosed valve
- ❖ In the presence of atrial fibrillation, this atrial contribution to stroke volume is lost
- ❖ This may reduce cardiac output significantly
- ❖ Thus maintaining sinus rhythm is important in mitral stenosis

Prevent Rapid Ventricular Rates

- ❖ Stenosed MV causes stroke volume to be constant regardless of the metabolic demand
- ❖ In this setting, heart may not be able to cope with situations demanding an increase in CO
- ❖ Any increase in heart rate will also reduce the diastolic filling time
- ❖ Thus stroke volume will reduce further and cause a decrease in cardiac output
- ❖ Sinus tachycardia and AF with FVR are the most common type of tachycardia
- ❖ Rate-control measures should aim to maintain ventricular rate < 110 bpm

Maintain Preload

- ❖ MS is associated with a higher than normal gradient between the LA and LV
- ❖ Thus, higher LA pressure is required to generate enough gradient across the MV
- ❖ Therefore adequate preload is required to maintain high-normal LA pressure in MS
- ❖ However, sudden increase in central blood volume can precipitate pulmonary edema
- ❖ Thus, in mitral stenosis patients, avoid:
  - Over transfusion
  - Trendelenburg position
- ❖ CVP and PAP can be used to assess increase in central blood volume

Avoid Decreases in SVR

- ❖ Any decrease in SVR is compensated by an increase in heart rate
- ❖ This is because the stroke volume is fixed across the stenosed mitral valve
- ❖ Marked increase in heart rate causes rapid decompensation due to reduced diastolic time
- ❖ Thus, reduction in SVR causes a profound reduction in cardiac output
- ❖ SVR may be maintained with phenylephrine infusion

Prevent Increases in Pulmonary Arterial Pressure

- ❖ Avoid factors causing increase in PVR:
  - Hypercarbia
  - Hypoxia
  - Metabolic acidosis
  - Hypothermia
  - Lung hyperinflation
- ❖ If pulmonary HTN and RVF occurs:
  - IV dopamine (3–8 µg/kg/min) inotropic support
  - Pulmonary vasodilation with SNP (0.1–0.5 µg/kg/min)
  - Inhaled nitric oxide

Anesthetic Management

- ❖ Labor analgesia:
  - Segmental lumbar epidural anesthesia preferred as:
    - Eliminates pain and tachycardia accompanying uterine contraction
    - Does not alter patient hemodynamics significantly
    - Epidural analgesia can be administered in incremental doses
    - Total dose can be titrated to the desired sensory level (T_8-T_{10})
    - Prevents fatigue and deleterious effect of Valsalva maneuver

- Neuraxial opioids alone can be used in critical patients who cannot tolerate any degree of sympathectomy
- During the second stage, only the uterine contractile force should be allowed
- Maternal expulsive effort by Valsalva maneuver should be avoided
- Fetal descent during the second stage occurs by uterine contraction
- Second stage is usually expedited and delivery facilitated by:
  - Outlet forceps
  - Vacuum extraction
- Supplementary analgesia may be required during this stage
- This is usually provided with epidural fentanyl or low dose bupivacaine
- Invasive cardiac monitoring is required in NYHA III and IV patients
- Radial artery cannulation and PA catheter are useful in assessing cardiac output
- Supplemental oxygen useful to minimize increases in PVR
- Left uterine displacement and IV fluids are used to maintain venous return to heart
- Phenylephrine boluses (50 µg) is preferred for sudden drop in SVR

❖ Anesthesia for LSCS:
- Regional Anesthesia:
  - Has been proved to be a safer technique for cesarean section
  - *Spinal anesthesia is contraindicated*
  - But CSE may be better option in a situation like accidental dural puncture
  - Neuraxial block in anticoagulated parturient has risk of epidural hematoma
  - Useful for NYHA I and II patients
  - Preferred over GA as:
    - Induced sympathectomy decreases both preload and afterload
    - This relieves pulmonary congestion
    - Total dose can be titrated to achieve the desired sensory level
  - Anesthetic levels (T_4) established by slowly titrating LA through catheter
  - Epinephrine omitted from LA solution as it causes:
    - Tachycardia
    - Peripheral vasoconstriction
  - Treatment of hypotension during regional anesthesia:
    - *With decreased PCWP*: fluids to restore normal filling pressure
    - *With normal PCWP*: phenylephrine infusion
  - Contraindications to regional anesthesia:
    - Active heavy bleeding
    - Uncorrected coagulopathy:
      - HELLP syndrome
      - Thrombocytopenia
    - Local infection
- General Anesthesia:
  - Useful in:
    - Emergency situations
    - Failure of regional anesthesia
    - Sick patients who require elective intubation
    - NYHA III and IV patients
  - Advantages:
    - Provides airway control
    - Allows for TEE monitoring of mitral stenosis
  - Disadvantages:
    - Can cause tachycardia and hypotension during intubation
    - Positive pressure ventilation may reduce preload
    - Eventually low cardiac output results

Conduct of General Anesthesia

Premedication

❖ Avoid oversedation to avoid precipitants of pulmonary hypertension:
- Hypoxia
- Hypercarbia
- Acidosis

❖ Diazepam 0.1 mg/kg PO

❖ Anti-aspiration prophylaxis:
- 15–30 mL of 0.3M sodium citrate PO
- 1 mg/kg ranitidine IV
- 10 mg metaclopramide IV

❖ Drugs producing tachycardia to be avoided:
- Atropine
- Pancuronium
- Pethidine
- Ketamine

❖ Continue due dose of digoxin

❖ Large bore 16–18 G IV access mandatory

❖ Judicious IV crystalloid preloading prior to induction

Position

- Supine with left lateral tilt to avoid hypotension
- Avoid steep Trendelenburg:
  - Causes sudden increase in venous return
  - This can precipitate pulmonary edema

Induction and Intubation

- Preoxygenate with 100% O_2 for 3–5 minutes or for 4 maximal capacity breaths
- After abdominal preparation and draping, rapid sequence induction is carried out
- Etomidate, remifentanyl and succinylcholine is the ideal choice for induction
- IV fentanyl 1 µg/kg can be used as an alternative opioid analgesic
- High dose rocuronium can substitute succinylcholine
- Adequate opioid dose is important to provide analgesia and avoid tachycardia
- Fentanyl may cause fetal depression but benefits outweigh risks
- Opioid induction useful if frank pulmonary edema
- Xylocard used to decrease intubation response
- Deep planes preferred for intubation to avoid detrimental tachycardia
- Cricoid pressure is released only after ETT cuff is inflated and tube position checked
- Tachycardia due to intubation/incision treated by:
  - Deepening anesthetic plane
  - IV propranolol boluses

Hemodynamics

- IV fluids can be administered through large 16/18G cannula to maintain preload
- Avoid ephedrine as it causes tachycardia
- Phenylephrine is preferred vasopressor agent to treat sudden reductions in SVR
- RV dysfunction, if present, is managed by:
  - Optimizing acid base balance
  - Maintaining hypocapnea and hyperoxia
  - Using vasodilators (NTG 0.1–0.5 µg/kg/min) to decrease PVR
  - Inotropes like milrinone and dobutamine
- IV infusion of oxytocin may be administered after delivery of fetus:
  - 10–20 U of oxytocin taken in 1000 mL of saline
  - This is administered at a rate of 40–80 MU/min
- IV boluses of oxytoxin, ergometrine and PGF_{2a} ***contraindicated*** as it produces:
  - Severe hypotension
  - Tachycardia
  - Reduced SVR
  - Increased PVR
  - All these lead to low cardiac output eventually.

Maintenance

- Before delivery of fetus:
  - 100% O_2 + isoflurane 1 MAC
  - Vecuronium or cisatracurium boluses to maintain muscle paralysis
  - Nitrous oxide avoided as it increases PVR
- After delivery of fetus:
  - 100% O_2 + isoflurane 1 MAC
  - 1 µg/kg fentanyl + 0.05 mg/kg midazolam + 0.1 mg/kg vecuronium

Extubation

- At extubation, avoid inducing tachycardia
- Fully awake in left lateral Trendelenburg position to decrease chances of aspiration
- Slow administration of reversal to counter the tachycardia caused by glycopyrrolate

Intraoperative Problems

- Hypotension: dobutamine, milrinone
- New onset atrial fibrillation: cardioversion, digoxin and beta blockers
- Pulmonary edema: diuretics, PEEP
- Cardiac arrest

Postoperative

Complications

- Pulmonary edema
- Atrial fibrillation
- Aspiration
- Prolonged mechanical ventilation
- Respiratory depression

Monitoring

- Pulse oximetry
- BP
- ECG
- Urine output
- Temperature
- ABG
- Chest X-ray
- Fetal activity, APGAR score

Analgesia

- Opioids – fentanyl 1 µg/kg/hour infusion
- NSAIDs – Diclofenac 50 mg IV
- Resumption of anticoagulation as per ACCP guidelines
- Epidural analgesia if valve area >1.5 cm^2

AORTIC REGURGITATION

Introduction

- Aortic regurgitation is caused by inadequate closure of aortic valve leaflets
- This allows regurgitation of blood into LV during ventricular diastole

Incidence

- Prevalence or more than trace AR is approximately 13% in males and 8.5% in females
- Prevalence of AR varies with age
- Age more than 50 years is associated with increasing severity of AR

Types

- Primary aortic regurgitation:
  - Occurs due to disease of aortic valve apparatus per se
  - Can be due to:
    - Excessive movement of valve leaflets
    - Restrictive movement of valve leaflets
    - Perforation of valve leaflets
- Secondary aortic regurgitation:
  - Occurs due to marked dilatation of ascending aorta
  - When the aortic annulus dilates, aortic leaflets separate
  - This leads to loss of coaptation and aortic regurgitation
  - Secondary AR is the *most common cause* of aortic regurgitation

Etiology

- Primary aortic regurgitation:
  - Rheumatic heart disease
  - Myxomatous degeneration
  - Calcific aortic valve disease
  - Congenital heart disease:
    - Peri-membranous VSDs
    - Subaortic membrane
    - Sinus of Valsalva aneurysm
    - Bicuspid aortic valve due to incomplete closure of AV
    - Fenestrated aortic valve leaflet
  - Infective endocarditis:
    - Valve perforation
    - Valve destruction
    - Valve vegetation preventing leaflet movement
  - Genetic syndromes:
    - Marfans syndrome
    - Ehler-Danlos syndrome
    - Osteogenesis imperfecta
  - Systemic rheumatic disorders:
    - Systemic lupus erythematosus
    - Anti-phospholipid antibody syndrome
    - Rheumatoid arthritis
    - Ankylosing spondylitis
  - Drug induced valve disease
  - Iatrogenic:
    - Following percutaneous aortic valvuloplasty
    - Following device closure of peri-membranous VSDs
- Secondary aortic regurgitation:
  - Aortic root dilatation:
    - Degenerative aortic dilatation (age-related)
    - Cystic medial necrosis of aorta
    - Bicuspid aortic valve related root dilatation
    - Osteogenesis imperfecta
    - Arthritides:
      - Ankylosing spondylitis
      - Psoriatic arthritis
      - Reactive arthritis
    - Infective aortitis (syphilis)
    - Systemic HTN
    - Rare causes:
      - Behcet syndrome
      - Ulcerative colitis associated aortic dilatation
      - Relapsing polychondritis
  - Aortic dissection.
- Acute aortic regurgitation:
  - Acute rheumatic fever
  - Infective endocarditis
  - Aortic dissection
  - Ruptured sinus of Valsalva
  - Failure of prosthetic valve
- Chronic aortic regurgitation:
  - Rheumatic heart disease
  - Bicuspid aortic valve
  - Syphilis
  - Arthritides:
    - Reactive arthritis
    - Ankylosing spondylitis
    - Rheumatoid arthritis
  - HTN
  - Marfans syndrome
  - Osteogenesis imperfecta

Pathophysiology

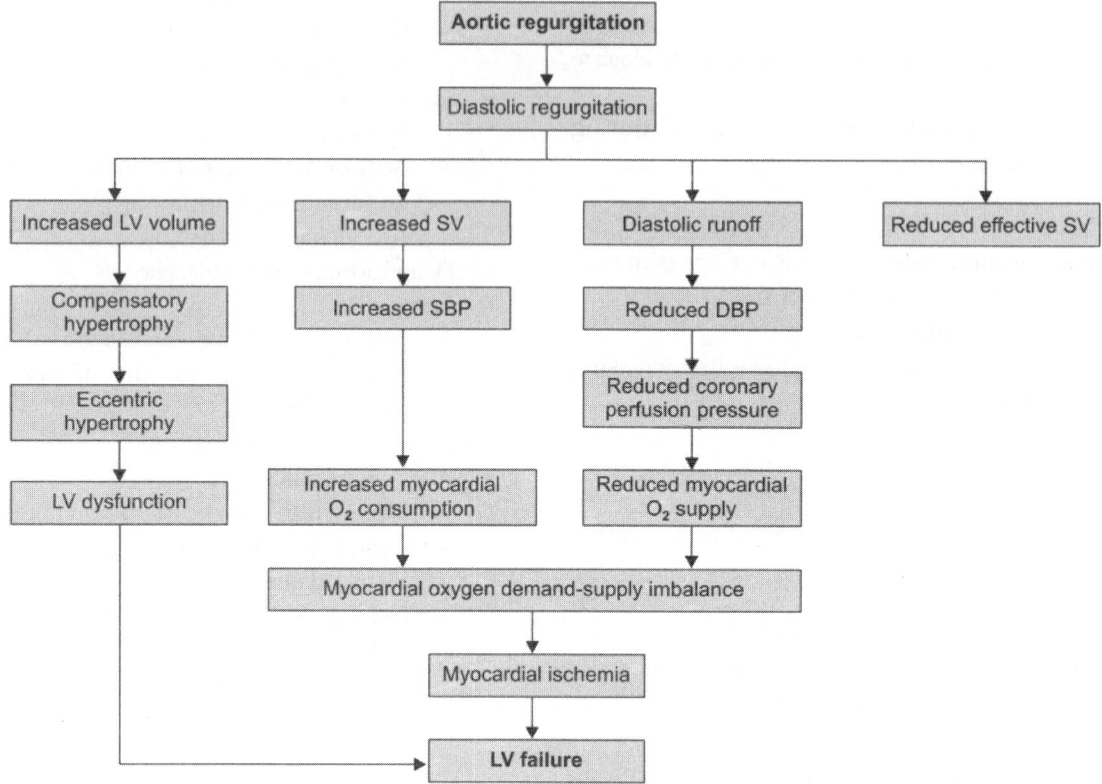

Clinical Features

- Symptoms:
  - Symptoms of chronic AR usually occur during 4th–5th decade of life
  - Common manifestations include:
    - Exertional dyspnea
    - Orthopnea
    - Paroxysmal nocturnal dyspnea
    - Palpitation (exacerbated in lying down position)
    - Nocturnal angina:
      - Occurs due to sleep induced reduction in heart rate and DBP
      - This exacerbates AR and reduces coronary perfusion pressure
      - Reduced coronary perfusion pressure causes angina
- Signs:
  - Arterial pulse:
    - Corrigans pulse:
      - Water hammer pulse
      - Characterized by rapid rise and rapid fall
      - Occurs due to rapid fall of arterial pressure during diastole
    - Demussets sign characterized by head nod with each heart beat
    - *Beckers sign*: Visible pulsations of retinal artery and pupils
    - *Muellers sign*: Systolic pulsations of uvula
    - *Maynes sign*: > 15 mm Hg fall in DBP with arm elevation
    - *Quinckes sign*: Capillary pulsations on fingertip
    - *Rosenbacks sign*: Systolic pulsations of liver
    - *Gerhadts sign*: Systolic pulsations of spleen
    - *Traubes sign*: Pistol shot sound over femoral artery
    - Duroziez sign:
      - Systolic and diastolic to-and-fro bruit on auscultation of femoral A
      - Heard on partial compression with stethoscope
    - Hills sign:
      - Popliteal BP exceeds brachial BP by more than 20 mm Hg
      - Is an exaggeration of normal physiological sign
    - Korotkoff sounds:
      - Measurement of DBP is difficult in AR

- On cuff deflation:
  - Systolic sounds are audible even on complete deflation
  - Thus, muffling of sounds (phase IV) is considered as DBP
- Precordial palpation:
  - Diffuse precordial pulse
  - Hyperdynamic in nature
  - Displaced inferiorly and laterally
- Auscultation:
  - Heart sounds:
    - S_1: Soft
    - S_2 Produced by AV closure is soft or absent
  - Murmur:
    - Murmur of AR:
      - Early diastolic murmur
      - Low intensity, high pitched
      - Has decrescendo pattern
      - Heard best in:
        - Left 3rd or 4th ICS along left sternal border
        - With patient sitting/leaning forward
        - Breath held in full expiration
    - Austin flint murmur:
      - Soft, low pitched, rumbling mid-late diastolic murmur
      - Heard at apex
      - Due to competing ante and retrograde flow across AV

Assessment of Severity

- Pulse pressure difference indicates severity of AR
- Duration of early diastolic murmur:
  - Duration of murmur increases with increasing severity
  - May be holosystolic murmur in severe AR

Investigations

- ECG:
  - Features of left ventricular hypertrophy may be present
  - ST depression (> 0.3 mV) and T-wave inversion indicates LV strain pattern
- Chest X-ray:
  - Cardiomegaly is frequently seen
  - Ascending aortic dilatation may be visible in chest X-ray
  - In later stages of the disease:
    - LA enlargement
    - Pulmonary artery enlargement
    - Pulmonary congestion and plethoric fields
- Echocardiography:
  - Transthoracic echocardiography is usually sufficient
  - TEE may be required for evaluation of aortic root
  - Surgery is usually indicated when LVESD > 50 mm
  - Useful to:
    - Identify cause of AR
    - Associated defects:
      - Other valvular lesions
      - Aortic pathology
      - Congenital defects (ruptured sinus of Valsalva, VSD)
    - Quantification of LV systolic function and LV dimensions
- Cardiac catheterization:
  - Contrast ventriculography is usually not done
  - Coronary angiography is done when:
    - Patient's age is more than 35 years to rule out coronary artery disease
    - Symptoms of CAD or LV dysfunction associated in younger patients
    - More than 2 risk factors for premature onset CAD

Echocardiographic Assessment of Severity of AR

Characteristic	Mild AR	Mild-moderate AR	Moderate-severe AR	Severe AR
LV size	Normal	Variable	Variable	Dilated
Jet height/LVOT height	≤ 24%	25–45%	46–64%	≥ 65%
Jet area/LVOT area	≤ 4%	5–20%	21–59%	≥ 60%
Vena contracta width	≤ 2 mm	3–5 mm	3–5 mm	≥ 6 mm
Regurgitant volume	≤ 29 mL	30–44 mL	45–59 mL	≥ 60 mL
Regurgitant fraction	≤ 29%	30–39%	40–49%	≥ 50%
EROA	≤ 0.09 cm^2	0.1–0.19 cm^2	0.2–0.29 cm^2	≥ 0.3 cm^2
Jet density	Faint	Dense	Dense	Dense
Regurgitant slope	Slow	> 2 m/s^2	> 2 m/s^2	> 3 m/s^2
Pressure half time	> 500 msec	200–500 msec	200–500 msec	< 200 msec
Diastolic flow reversal	Early diastolic	Intermediate	Intermediate	Holodiastolic

Stages of Aortic Regurgitation

- Stage A: ***At risk for AR:***
  - Anatomical lesions predisposing to AR:
    - Bicuspid aortic valve
    - Aortic valve sclerosis
    - Diseases of ascending aorta/aortic sinus
    - History of rheumatic fever
  - Absent or mild AR
  - No hemodynamic consequences
  - Absence of symptoms
- Stage B: ***Progressive AR***:
  - Mild- moderate AR on echocardiography:
    - Jet width/LVOT width < 64%
    - Vena contracta ≤ 5 mm
    - Regurgitant volume ≤ 59 mL/beat
    - Regurgitant fraction ≤ 49%
    - Effective Regurgitant Orifice Area (EROA) ≤ 0.29 cm²
    - Angiography grade ≤ 2+
  - Hemodynamic consequences:
    - Normal LV systolic function
    - Normal LV volume or mild LV dilatation
  - Absence of symptoms
- Stage C: ***Asymptomatic severe AR***:
  - Stage C_1:
    - Severe AR on echocardiography:
      - Jet width/LVOT width ≥ 65%
      - Vena contracta ≥ 6 mm
      - Regurgitant volume ≥ 60 mL/beat
      - Regurgitant fraction ≥ 50%
      - EROA ≥ 0.3 cm²
      - Angiography grade ≥ 3+
      - Holodiastolic flow reversal in proximal abdominal aorta
    - Hemodynamic consequences:
      - Normal LVEF (≥ 50%)
      - Mild-moderate LV dilatation (LVESD < 50 mm)
    - Absence of symptoms at rest
    - Symptoms on exertion
  - Stage C_2:
    - Severe AR on echocardiography:
      - Jet width/LVOT width ≥ 65%
      - Vena contracta ≥ 6 mm
      - Regurgitant volume ≥ 60 mL/beat
      - Regurgitant fraction ≥ 50%
      - EROA ≥ 0.3 cm²
      - Angiography grade ≥ 3+
      - Holodiastolic flow reversal in proximal abdominal aorta
    - Hemodynamic consequences:
      - Depressed LV systolic function (LVEF < 50%)
      - Severe LV dilatation:
        - LVESD ≥ 50 mm
        - Indexed LVESD ≥ 25 mm/m²
    - Absence of symptoms at rest
    - Symptoms on exertion
- Stage D: ***Symptomatic severe AR***:
  - Severe AR on echocardiography:
    - Jet width/LVOT width ≥ 65%
    - Vena contracta ≥ 6 mm
    - Regurgitant volume ≥ 60 mL/beat
    - Regurgitant fraction ≥ 50%
    - EROA ≥ 0.3 cm²
    - Angiography grade ≥ 3+
    - Holodiastolic flow reversal in proximal abdominal aorta
  - Hemodynamic consequences:
    - Associated with LV dysfunction:
      - Mild- moderate LVD: LVEF 41–50%
      - Severe LVD: LVEF ≤ 40%
    - Severe LV dilatation:
      - LVESD ≥ 50 mm
      - Body surface area indexed LVESD ≥ 25 mm/m²
  - Severe heart failure symptoms at rest.

Classification of Aortic Regurgitation

- Type I aortic regurgitation:
  - Characterized by normal cusp motion
  - Caused by functional aortic annular dilatation or cusp perforation
  - Techniques of repair:
    - Functional annular dilatation:
      - STJ remodelling techniques
      - Ascending aortic graft
      - Aortic annuloplasty
    - Cusp perforation:
      - Repaired commonly with:
      - Bovine pericardium
      - Autologous pericardial patch
- Type II aortic regurgitation:
  - Caused due to excessive movement of valve leaflets
  - Causes partial or total aortic cusp prolapse
  - Repaired commonly with:
    - Cusp plication
    - Triangular resection
    - Free margin resuspension
- Type III aortic regurgitation:
  - Caused due to restricted movement of aortic valve due to:
    - Cusp retraction
    - Cusp calcification

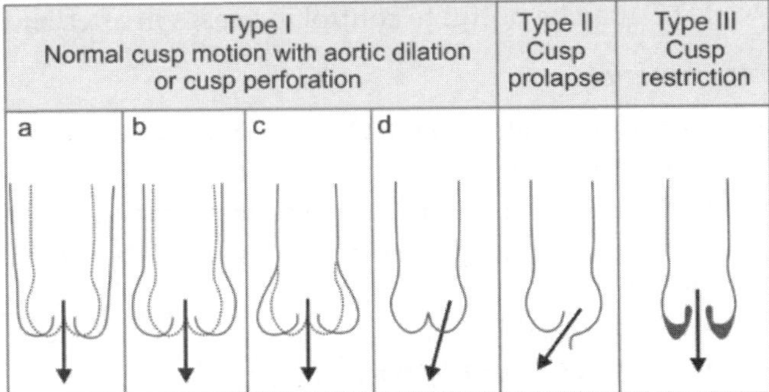

Fig. 41: Types of aortic regurgitation.

- Repaired commonly with:
  - Leaflet shaving
  - Leaflet decalcification
  - Patch repair.

Management

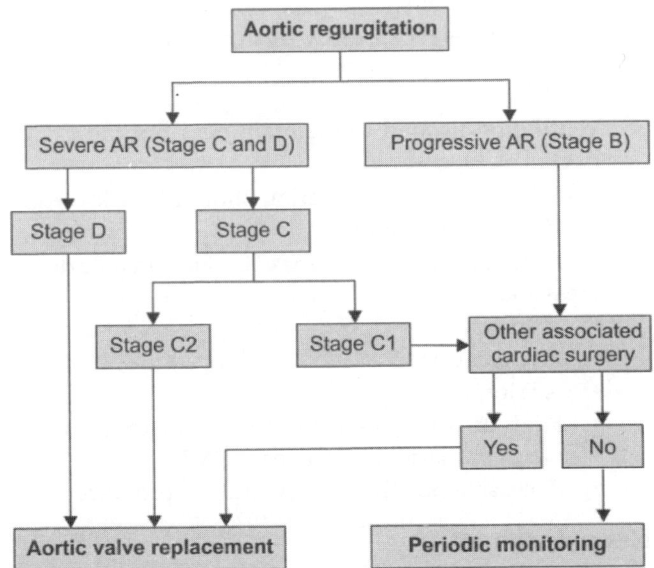

Anesthetic Goals

- ❖ Faster, fuller and vasodilated to augment forward flow
- ❖ Rate:
  - Avoid bradycardia
  - Maintain slightly higher range (80–100 bpm)
- ❖ Rhythm: Maintain sinus rhythm
- ❖ Preload: Maintain increased preload
- ❖ Afterload: Reduced with anesthetics and vasodilators
- ❖ Contractility:
  - Maintain contractility
  - Avoid myocardial depression
  - Inotropic supports may be required

Rationale for Anesthetic Goals

Heart Rate and Rhythm

- ❖ Maintain sinus rhythm in high normal range (80–90 bpm)
- ❖ Bradycardia increases duration of diastole
- ❖ Increased diastolic filling interval leads to more severe LV distension
- ❖ Thus, bradycardia produces acute LV volume overload

Preload

- ❖ Maintain preload
- ❖ Increasing preload abruptly may cause LV distension
- ❖ This may be detrimental to an already volume-overload LV

Afterload

- ❖ Abrupt increase in SVR reduces forward flow
- ❖ Thus, lower SVR is preferred so that forward cardiac output is maximum
- ❖ Afterload reduction strategies:
  - Maintain adequate anesthetic depth
  - Systemic vasodilators and inodilators
- ❖ Arteriolar dilators are effective in LV failure as they reduce afterload

Contractility

- ❖ Contractility has to be maintained in order to maximize forward flow
- ❖ Decreased contractility results in an increase in LV end systolic volume (LVESV)
- ❖ This may precipitate LV failure
- ❖ Thus inotropes may be used to minimize LDESV and LVEDV
- ❖ Inotropes should be considered for persistent hemodynamic instability:
  - Dobutamine
  - Low dose epinephrine
  - Milrinone

Choice of Anesthetic Technique

- ❖ Spinal/epidural anesthesia are usually well tolerated
- ❖ This is because it reduces the SVR causing reduction in regurgitant fraction
- ❖ Bradycardia associated with spinal anesthesia is avoided as it increases regurgitant volume

Preoperative Preparation and Premedication

- Informed consent
- NPO orders
- Premedicate:
  - Premedicate with caution, especially in patients with LVD
  - Light premedication advised to prevent bradycardia
  - Done in high dependency room under supervision
  - 0.5 mg midazolam IV titrated and given in increments
  - Supplemental oxygen can be given at this time
- Arrange for surgery-appropriate volume of blood

Monitoring

- Pulse oximetry, capnography
- Invasive BP monitoring:
  - Not required in asymptomatic AR
  - Useful in stage C and D aortic regurgitation for:
    - Beat-to-beat monitoring of BP
    - Sampling for ABG analysis
    - Titration of fluid therapy using SVV
- ECG
- Temperature, urine output
- For severe aortic regurgitation:
  - Transesophageal echocardiography
  - Pulmonary artery catheter:
    - PCWP may be used to guide preload augmentation
    - Especially useful when afterload reducing agents are used
    - This helps titrate fluid therapy in case of hypotension
    - PAC with pacing capability can be used to treat bradycardia

Anesthetic Management

Induction

- Adequate preoxygenation
- Opioid based induction:
  - Oxygen + fentanyl 2–5 μg/kg + midazolam 0.03–0.05 mg/kg
  - Ketamine may be used as an alternative induction agent
  - Pancuronium may be used as muscle relaxant to avoid opioid induced bradycardia
- Acute increases in LV afterload, as after intubation and surgical stimulation, to be avoided
- Deep planes during intubation advised
- NTG may be useful to control increases in afterload

Maintenance

- Balanced anesthesia with O_2 + air + volatile anesthetic is preferred
- Isoflurane, sevoflurane and desflurane may be used
- Volatile anesthetic agents have several beneficial effects:
  - Reduce SVR
  - Increase in heart rate
- Higher MAC values are preferred to lower SVR and maintain anesthetic depth
- Patients with severe LV dysfunction are very sensitive to volatile anesthetics
- In these patients, high-dose opioid anesthesia is preferred
- However, doses of opioids are titrated to prevent bradycardia
- Pancuronium/vecuronium may be used to maintain NM blockade
- Avoid N_2O as it causes LV dysfunction

Ventilation

- Ventilation titrated to maintain near normal E_TCO_2 PaO_2, $PaCO_2$ and pH
- Adequate time for expiration should be allowed to facilitate venous return
- Avoid factors causing increase in pulmonary arterial pressure:
  - Hypoxia
  - Hypercarbia
  - Acidosis
  - High airway pressures: might constrict pulmonary capillaries and increase PAP
  - Excessive positive end expiratory pressure

Hemodynamics

Maintain Preload

- Judicious fluid administration
- Avoid fluid overload in patients with LV dysfunction
- In case of hypotension:
  - Administer carefully titrated fluid boluses
  - Ephedrine boluses may be used for transient hypotension
  - Early inotropic support
  - Avoid vasoconstrictors such as phenylephrine

Reduce SVR

- NTG especially useful if any increase in SVR/PAP occurs

- Select agents which promote vasodilatation and tachycardia
- Dobutamine and milrinone are useful as inodilators

Maintain Contractility

- Early initiation of inotropes
- Inodilators may be preferred
- Drugs commonly used include:
  - Low dose adrenaline 0.05–0.1 μg/kg/min to reduce LVEDV and LVESV
  - Dobutamine 5–10 μg/kg/min

Considerations for CPB

- Initiation and termination of CPB may be problematic in these patients
- Prior to cross clamp placement, LV distention is possible if LV is not ejecting
- This can occur with:
  - Bradycardia
  - Ventricular fibrillation
  - Supra-ventricular tachycardia
- Thus, preventive measures on CPB include:
  - Allowance of LV ejection until aortic cross clamp is in place
  - Avoiding initiation of cooling until cross clamp has been applied
  - Intracardiac defibrillation to correct rhythm disturbances
- In case of LV distention with refractory causes, rapid application of LV vent is required
- Administration of cardioplegia:
  - In the presence of AR, CP administered into aortic root will be ineffective
  - This is because of AR-induced leak of CP into the LV
  - Thus, CP is administered:
    - Directly into coronary ostia after aortotomy
    - Retrograde in to coronary sinus
  - Aortotomy prior to CP may require induction of ventricular fibrillation
  - This may be done using fibrillators

Extubation

- Extubation is carried out with caution to avoid hypoxia and hypercarbia
- Postoperative ventilation may be required for:
  - Prolonged surgery
  - Unexpected blood loss
- Extubate if:
  - Spontaneous ventilation with normal ABG
  - No bleeding and hemodynamically stable patient
  - Normothermia

Postoperative Period

Monitors

- ECG, pulse oximetry
- Invasive BP
- Urine output, CVP
- PA catheter
- ABG, temperature

Analgesia

- Multimodal analgesia
- Opioids: fentanyl or morphine
- Regional analgesia with epidural catheters
- Patient controlled analgesia

AORTIC STENOSIS

Introduction

- Severe aortic stenosis is a clinical predictor of adverse cardiac outcomes
- In patients with severe AS undergoing intermediate-high risk surgeries:
  - Risk of MACE is close to 18.8%
  - Mortality rate is close to 6–10%
- Thus, surgery in a patient with AS puts the patient at high risk for major complications

Incidence

- AS occurs in 1–2% of individuals aged between 65 and 75 years
- Prevalence increases to close to 8% in patients more than 75 years old
- 50% of the patients with valvular AS more than 50 years old have associated CAD

Types of AS

- Supravalvar aortic stenosis: seen in association with ***Williams syndrome***
  - Type I supravalvar AS:
    - Thick fibrous ring present above the aortic valve
    - Fibrous ring is not mobile
    - Typical *hourglass appearance* of the ascending aorta
  - Type II supravalvar AS:
    - Thin, discrete fibrous membrane
    - Membrane is usually mobile
    - Valve leaflet may show doming during diastole
  - *Type III supravalvar AS*: diffuse narrowing

- Subvalvar aortic stenosis:
  - Dynamic subvalvar AS
  - Fixed subvalvar AS:
    - Type I: Discrete membrane
    - Type II: Fibromuscular ridge
    - Type III: Tunnel like narrowing
    - Type IV: Accessory/anomalous mitral valve tissue
- Valvar aortic stenosis

Etiology of Valvar Aortic Stenosis

- Congenital valvar aortic stenosis:
  - Unicuspid aortic valve
  - Bicuspid aortic valve
  - Tricuspid aortic valve due to unequal cusp size
  - Quadricuspid aortic valve
- Acquired valvar aortic stenosis:
  - Rheumatic heart disease
  - Calcific tricuspid aortic valve
  - Degenerative aortic stenosis
  - Systemic lupus erythematosus
  - Rheumatoid arthritis
  - Fabry's disease
  - Paget's disease
  - Ochronosis
  - Irradiation
  - Homozygous type II hypercholesterolemia
  - Obstructive vegetation

Pathophysiology of Aortic Stenosis

- Normal aortic valve area is 2.6–3.5 cm^2
- Normal aortic valve index is 2 cm^2/m^2

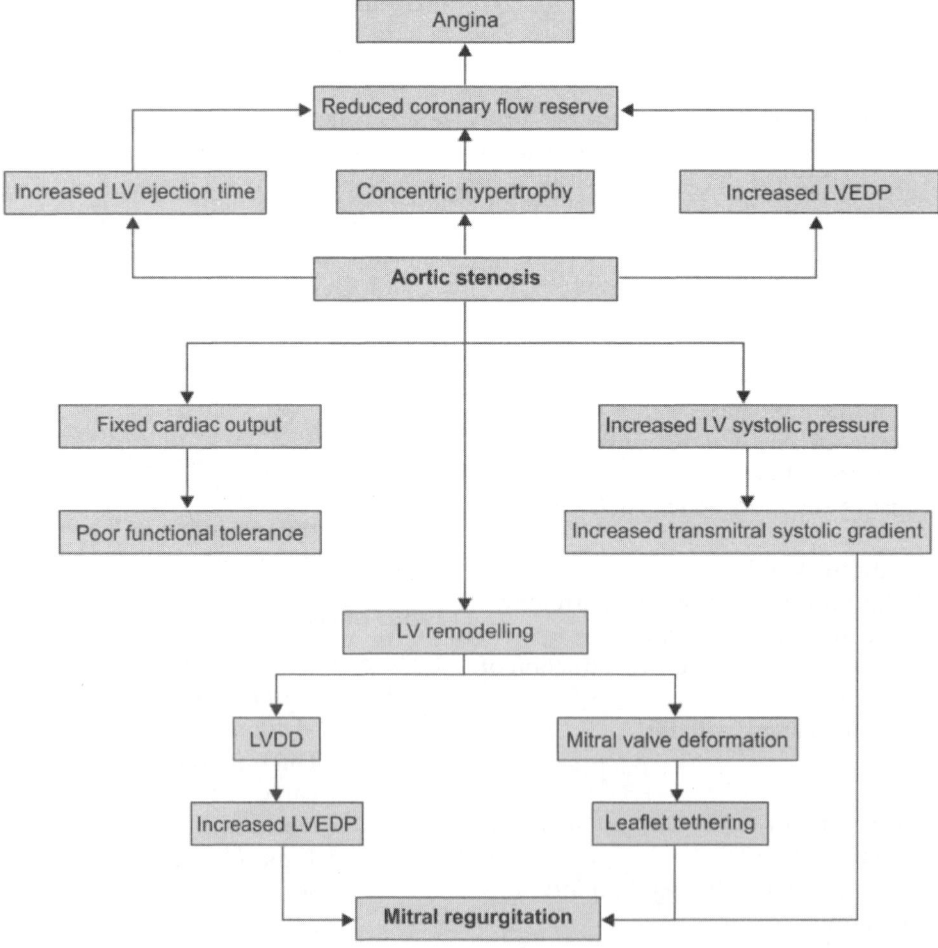

Clinical Features

Bicuspid Aortic Valve

- Commonly presents at 50–65 years of age
- Bicuspid aortic valve must undergo calcification to become stenotic
- *Most common* congenital valvular malformation of aortic valve

- *Most common* cause of AS in patients younger than 70 years of age
- Associated with:
  - Coarctation of aorta
  - Aortic root dilatation
  - Increased risk of aortic dissection
- Types of bicuspid aortic valve:
  - Fused right and left cusps (70–80%)
  - Fused right and non-coronary cusps (30–30%)
  - Fused left and non-coronary cusps (1–2%)

Degenerative Aortic Stenosis

- Commonly presents during 7th–8th decade
- *Most common* cause of aortic stenosis in the developed world
- Characterized by:
  - Calcification progressing from the base to edge of leaflets
  - Absence of commissural fusion
  - Usually does not involve the edge of the cusps
- Degree of calcification of the valve predicts clinical outcome
- Causes stellate shape of aortic valve orifice in systole

Rheumatic Aortic Stenosis

- *Most common* cause of aortic stenosis worldwide
- Associated with AR/MR
- Characteristics of rheumatic AS:
  - Calcification proceeds from edge to base
  - Associated with commissural fusion
- Causes triangular systolic orifice

Differences between Rheumatic and Calcific Aortic Stenosis

Characteristic	Rheumatic AS	Calcific AS
Commissures	Fused	Free
Leaflet involvement	Tips to base	Base to tips
Orifice in systole	Triangular	Stellate
Mitral valve involvement	30% cases have MS	Mitral annular calcification
Age of the patient	No particular age	Usually elderly
Others	Tips thickened	Tips are free
	Calcification of tips possible	Calcification of tips not seen

Symptoms

- Classical triad of symptoms:
  - Angina
  - Syncope
  - Dyspnea on exertion
- Valve area reduces 0.1–0.3 cm^2/year in aortic stenosis
- Systolic gradient increases 10–15 mm Hg per year
- In most patients symptoms appear only after:
  - Valve area drops to below 1 cm^2
  - Aortic velocity more than 4 m/sec
  - Mean gradient more than 40 mm Hg
- Latent period for symptom presentation in AS is around 10–20 years
- 75% of symptomatic patients with critical AS die within 3 years in the absence of surgery
- Paroxysmal nocturnal dyspnea and orthopnea indicate LV failure
- Angina:
  - Once angina appears, average life expectancy of the patient is 5 years
  - Causes of angina in aortic stenosis:
    - Increased myocardial oxygen demand with normal oxygen delivery
    - Reduced coronary flow reserve
    - Increased LVEDP, causing reduced coronary perfusion pressure
    - Reduced diastolic perfusion time during tachycardia
    - Associated coronary artery disease in 50% patients with AS
- Syncope:
  - Once syncope appears, average life expectancy is 3–4 years
  - Causes of syncope in aortic stenosis:
    - Exercise induced vasodilatation in the presence of fixed cardiac output
    - Transient bradycardia due to exertion
    - Abnormal baroreceptor response, causing failure to increase BP
    - Arrhythmias:
      - Atrial fibrillation common
      - Ventricular arrhythmias rare
- Exertional dyspnea:
  - *Most common* initial complaint in aortic stenosis patients
  - Appearance of exertional dyspnea represents impending LV failure
  - Once dyspnea appears, average life expectancy drops to 1–2 years
  - Causes of exertional dyspnea:
    - Inability of LV to increase CO across a fixed stenosis during exercise
    - LV diastolic dysfunction causing increased LV filling pressures with exercise

- Sudden cardiac death:
  - High risk of sudden death in aortic stenosis patients
  - In these patients, there is poor response to CPR
  - CPR is met with LVOTO, which renders systemic and coronary blood flow inadequate
- Other symptoms:
  - Gastrointestinal bleeding:
    - Also called ***Heydes syndrome***
    - Refers to the presence of intestinal angiodysplasia in the presence of AS
  - Calcific emboli to other organs like kidney and brain

Signs

- Palpation of pulse:
  - ***Pulsus parvus et tardus:***
    - Slow rising, low volume pulse
    - Low pulse pressure
    - Delayed peaking of pulse detected by simultaneously palpating apex beat
  - ***Pulsus alternans:***
    - Alternating amplitude of pulse with every heart beat
    - Occurs in the presence of left ventricular dysfunction
  - May be associated with carotid thrill/shudder
  - Pulse character is best appreciated in the carotids
- Precordial palpation:
  - Initially normal apex beat, which may then shift to left
  - Palpable S_4 due to vigorous LA contraction against a non-compliant LV
  - Systolic thrill may be palpable in second right ICS
  - Well sustained heave may be palpable in some cases
- Auscultation:
  - First heart sound:
    - First heart sound is essentially normal
    - Short ejection click may be heard after S_1 if the valve is bicuspid
  - Second heart sound:
    - S_2 is soft and single due to diminished and delayed A_2 component of S_2
    - S_2 may become split if AS is associated with severe LV dysfunction
  - S_4 may be heard due to forceful LA contraction against non-compliant LV
  - Ejection systolic murmur:
    - Characteristics:
      - Crescendo-decrescendo murmur
      - Murmur begins shortly after S_1
      - Increases in intensity towards midsystole
      - Then intensity reduces to end before S_2
      - Harsh quality
      - Heard at base of the heart (second RICS)
      - Heard best with patient leaning forward
      - Breath to be held in expiration
      - Radiates equally to carotid artery on both sides
    - Intensity of ESM:
      - Intensity is proportional to velocity of blood flow across the valve
      - Represents turbulence produced by the stenotic valve
      - Does not indicate the degree of stenosis of the valve
      - This is because as stenosis increases, blood flow across valve decreases
      - Maneuvers increasing intensity of ESM:
        - ESM intensity increases with maneuvers increasing LV contractility or volume like:
          - Leg raising
          - Squatting
          - Release of Valsalva
        - Peaking of ejection systolic murmur:
          - Correlates with severity of AS
          - Early peaking indicates mild-moderate AS
          - Late peaking indicates severe AS
        - Maneuvers decreasing intensity of ESM:
          - Valsalva maneuver (decreases LV volume)
          - Isometric handgrip (increases afterload)
- ***Bernheim effect:***
  - Term used when symptoms of RV failure precede those of LV failure in AS
  - Occurs due to bulging of interventricular septum into the RV during systole
  - This causes impedance in RV filling and elevated JVP
  - Eventually, features of RV failure develop

- *Gallavardin phenomenon:*
  - Refers to the murmur of AS being heard more prominently at the apex
  - Occurs due to radiation of high pitched frequencies of ESM towards apex of heart
  - This phenomenon may suggest associated mitral regurgitation

Clinical Assessment of Severity of Stenosis: Severe AS characterized by

- Longer duration of ESM
- Later peaking of ESM
- Slow rising pulse
- Narrow pulse pressure
- Left ventricular heave

Investigations

- B-type natriuretic peptide (BNP) levels:
  - Useful to:
    - Predict onset of symptoms in asymptomatic patients with severe AS
    - Diagnose cardiac causes of dyspnea on exertion
    - Assess functional status of the patient and left ventricular function
  - Allows prognostication of postoperative outcome post valve replacement
- ECG:
  - Left ventricular hypertrophy found in most patients with severe AS
  - ST depression (> 0.3 mV) and T-wave inversion indicates LV strain pattern
  - Atrial fibrillation can be seen during late stages of AS
  - Conduction block can occur due to calcification of conduction system
- Exercise stress test:
  - Contraindicated in symptomatic patients with severe AS
  - When being performed in AS patients, it requires strict surveillance
  - Dobutamine stress test may be more useful in low flow low gradient AS
- Chest X-ray:
  - Cardiac size is often normal
  - Prominent ascending aorta due to post-stenotic aortic dilatation
  - Valvular calcification common and better seen on lateral X-rays
  - In later stages of the disease:
    - LA enlargement
    - Pulmonary artery enlargement
    - Calcification of aortic valve
    - Pulmonary congestion
- Echocardiography:
  - For assessment of:
    - Severity of aortic stenosis
    - Degree of valve calcification
    - Ventricular function (systolic and diastolic)
    - Involvement of other valves, aortic pathology
- Cardiac catheterization:
  - Contrast ventriculography is usually not done
  - Coronary angiography is done when:
    - Patients age is more than 35 years to rule out coronary artery disease
    - Symptoms of CAD or LV dysfunction associated in younger patients
    - More than 2 risk factors for premature onset CAD
    - Severity of AS cannot be determined by echocardiography
- MRI:
  - Indications::
    - When echocardiography is suboptimal
    - To differentiate between bicuspid and tricuspid aortic valve
    - To evaluate aortic root and ascending aortic dimensions
    - To study the degree of calcification

Markers of Increased Rate of Progression in Asymptomatic AS

- Abnormal stress test
- Elevated B-natriuretic peptide (BNP)
- Moderate-severe valve calcification
- Very high aortic velocity (5–5.5 m/sec)
- Rapid increase in aortic velocity
- Increased hypertrophic left ventricular remodeling
- Reduced left ventricular longitudinal systolic strain
- Myocardial fibrosis
- Pulmonary hypertension

Markers of Increased Risk in AS Patients Undergoing Intervention:

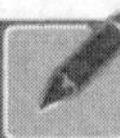

- Very high B-type natriuretic peptide
- Very low mean aortic valve gradient (< 20 mm Hg)
- Low ejection fraction
- Lack of contractile reserve in patients with low flow
- Severe ventricular fibrosis
- Very high STS score
- Oxygen dependent lung disease
- Advanced renal disease
- Frailty

Echocardiographic Assessment of Severity of Aortic Stenosis

Parameter	Mild	Moderate	Severe
Valve area (cm²)	≥ 1.5	1-1.5	≤ 1
AVA index (cm²/m²)	≥ 0.85	0.6-0.85	≤ 0.6
Aortic peak jet velocity (m/s)	2.6-2.9	3-4	> 4
Mean gradient (mm Hg)	< 20	20-40	> 40
Velocity ratio	> 0.5	0.25-0.5	< 0.25
Maximal cusp separation (mm)	> 20	10-20	< 10

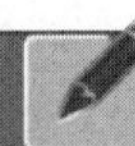

Stages of Valvular Aortic Stenosis

- Stage A: At risk for aortic stenosis (aortic sclerosis or bicuspid aortic valve)
- Stage B: Progressive aortic stenosis (mild-moderate)
- Stage C1: Asymptomatic severe aortic stenosis
- Stage C2: Asymptomatic severe AS with low LVEF
- Stage D1: Symptomatic severe AS
- Stage D2: Symptomatic severe low flow low gradient aortic stenosis with low LVEF
- Stage D3: Symptomatic severe low flow low gradient aortic stenosis

Stage	Name	Symptoms	LVEF	Hemodynamics
A	At risk	–	Normal	Vmax < 2 m/s
B	Progressive AS (mild)	–	Normal	Vmax 2–2.9 m/s
				Mean gradient < 20 mm Hg
	Progressive AS (moderate)	–	Normal	Vmax 3–3.9 m/s
				Mean gradient 20–39 mm Hg
C1	Asymptomatic severe AS	–	Normal	Vmax ≥ 4 m/s
				Mean gradient ≥ 40 mm Hg
				AVA ≤ 1 cm²
C2	Asymptomatic severe AS with low LVEF	–	Reduced	Vmax ≥ 4 m/s
				Mean gradient ≥ 40 mm Hg
				AVA < 1 cm²
D1	Symptomatic severe AS	Present	Normal or low	Vmax ≥ 4 m/s
				Mean gradient ≥ 40 mm Hg
				AVA < 1 cm²
D2	Symptomatic severe low flow low gradient AS with low LVEF	Present	Reduced	Vmax < 4 m/s
				Mean gradient < 40 mm Hg
				AVA < 1 cm²
D3	Symptomatic severe low flow low gradient AS	Present	Normal	Vmax < 4 m/s
				Mean gradient < 40 mm Hg
				AVA < 1 cm²

Management Options

Medical Management

- Limitation of physical activity to mild activity
- Management of concomitant diseases like hyperlipidemia and HTN
- Maintain intravascular volume status
- In patients with atrial fibrillation:
  - Rate control with digoxin and beta blockers
  - Anticoagulation with vitamin K antagonists

Balloon Aortic Valvotomy

- Aortic stenosis is relieved by inflating a balloon across the valve
- This occurs by:
  - Stretching of the valve annulus
  - Fracturing calcific deposits within the valve leaflets
  - Separation of calcified commissures
- Role is limited in older adults with AS as high risk of complications (10–20%) like:
  - Acute aortic regurgitation
  - Stroke
  - Myocardial infarction
  - Restenosis with clinical deterioration

Valve Replacement: SAVI/TAVI

- Indications:
  - Severe symptomatic stage D1 AS
  - Asymptomatic severe stage C2 AS with LVEF < 50%
  - Patients with stage C or D AS undergoing other cardiac surgery
- Valve replaced can be mechanical or bioprosthetic valve

Management

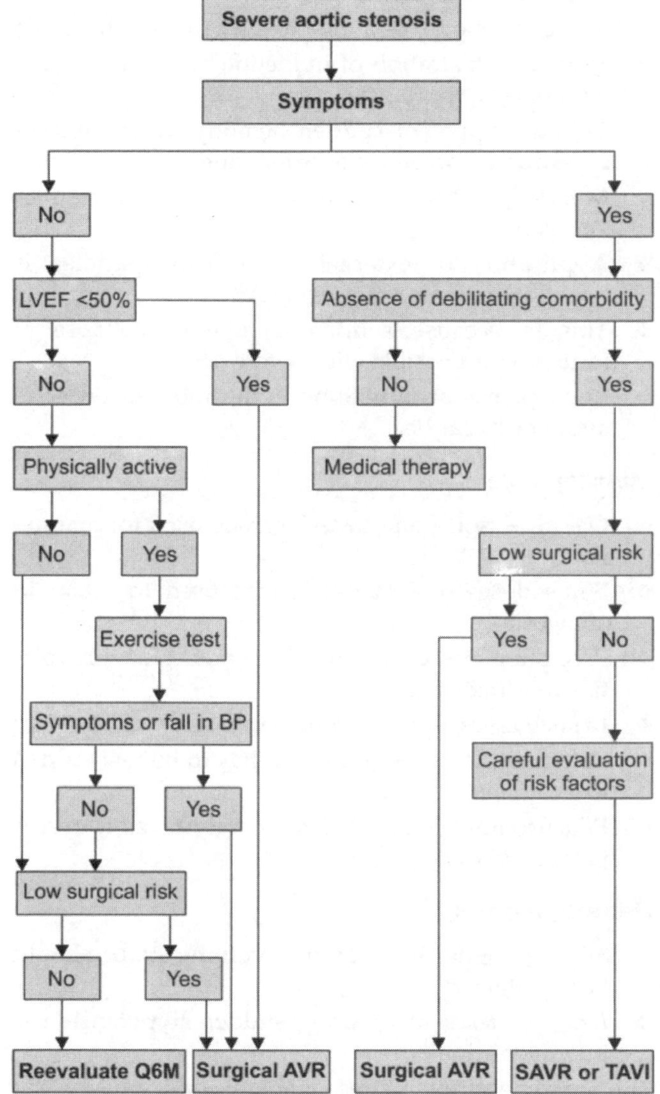

Choice of Anesthetic Technique

- Benefits of general anesthesia:
  - Can avoid vasodilatation seen with neuraxial blockade
  - Control of airway
  - Intraoperative TEE can be facilitated
- Benefits of regional anesthesia:
  - Avoids hemodynamic perturbations seen at the time of initiation of ventilation
  - Reduced bleeding
  - Better postoperative pain control
  - Reduced DVT incidence
- GA preferred over neuraxial techniques as AS patients tolerate reduction in SVR poorly
- Where regional anesthesia techniques are used, epidural anesthesia is preferred
- It is essential to avoid sudden reductions in SVR, irrespective of the anesthetic technique

Anesthetic Goals 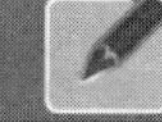

- Rhythm:
  - Maintain normal sinus rhythm
  - Sinus rhythm is important as LV is hypertrophied and less compliant
  - Thus, atrial kick is important to maintain preload on a poorly compliant LV
  - With a non-compliant LV, atrial contribution to cardiac output is almost 40%
  - Loss of sinus rhythm may produce dramatic reduction in stroke volume
- Rate:
  - Avoid tachycardia or bradycardia
  - Tachycardia:
    - To be avoided as it increases myocardial oxygen demand
    - Also, coronary perfusion is endangered as diastolic filling time is reduced
    - Thus, tachycardia increases the risk of myocardial ischemia manifold
  - Bradycardia:
    - To be avoided as cardiac output is fixed across the stenosed valve
    - Thus, with low heart rates, cardiac output may become unacceptably low
    - This may result in ventricular distension
- Preload:
  - Optimal preload involves maintaining a high normal fluid status
  - This is because in aortic stenosis, LV is hypertrophied
  - These patients are preload dependent to generate adequate cardiac output
  - Therefore, higher volume is required to keep the myofibrils stretched
  - Higher stretch is required to generate more contractile force from a non-compliant LV
- Afterload:
  - Avoid sudden reduction in afterload
  - Anesthetic technique is tailored to prevent fall in SVR
- *Contractility*: maintain contractility
- *Pulmonary vascular resistance*: maintain PVR

Preoperative Assessment and Preparation

- Goals of preoperative assessment:
  - Evaluation of signs of cardiac disease
  - Preoperative echocardiographic assessment of AS severity and LV function
  - Careful evaluation for coexisting coronary artery disease
  - Estimation of the risk of non-cardiac surgery
- Informed consent
- NPO orders:
  - 6 hours for solids
  - 4 hours for clear fluids

Premedication

- Light premedication is essential to avoid detrimental tachycardia
- Benzodiazepines can be used to provide anxiolysis
- β-blocker therapy can be continued on the morning of surgery

Monitors

- Pulse oximetry
- NIBP
- Capnography
- Neuromuscular monitoring
- Urine output
- ECG:
  - Leads II and V_5 to be monitored
  - Rhythm changes monitored with lead II
  - Ischemic changes are common and detected with lead V_5
- Invasive monitors:
  - Used based on the complexity of surgery and severity of disease
  - Useful monitors are:
    - Arterial line:
      - Useful in major surgeries with fluid shifts
      - Useful for repeated ABG sampling
    - Central venous access and PA catheter:
      - Care during insertion of catheter/guidewire
      - Triggering ectopics in these patients is avoided
      - This is because this can lead to cardiac arrest
    - TEE:
      - Routine use in non-cardiac surgery to be considered for severe AS
      - More useful compared with PA catheter as it allows a more comprehensive evaluation
- Invasive hemodynamic monitoring:
  - Monitoring should ideally:
    - Commence 12–24 hours preoperatively
    - Continue for 24–48 hours postoperatively
  - This is to cover the entire time period when major fluid shifts occur

Induction

- Presence of surgeon and perfusionist in the induction room prior to induction for cardiac surgery for severe aortic stenosis is mandatory
- Adequate preoxygenation for 3 minutes
- Etomidate is induction agent of choice in patients with moderate-severe AS
- Opioid induction preferred in those with significant LV dysfunction
- Propofol is avoided as it causes vasodilatation and acute drop in preload
- Ketamine should be avoided as it causes tachycardia
- Slow administration of induction agents in graded aliquots is important
- This is to prevent sudden hemodynamic compromise due to systemic vasodilatation
- Muscle paralysis is attained with rocuronium or vecuronium
- Application of external defibrillator paddles is useful in patients with severe AS
- This is because sudden circulatory collapse at induction is possible with severe AS
- Deep planes at intubation is desirable in order to avoid tachycardia

Maintenance

- O_2+ air + isoflurane 1 MAC can be used for maintenance
- Bolus doses of fentanyl can be used to maintain analgesia
- Precipitous reduction in SVR is possible with volatile anesthetic agents
- In such cases, opioid maintenance alone can be tried
- Sufficient depth of anesthesia has to be maintained to avoid tachycardia
- Pancuronium is avoided for paralysis, as it causes tachycardia

Hemodynamics

- Slightly higher intravascular volume status should be maintained
- *Drug of choice* for treating sudden hypotension is phenylephrine
- Norepinephrine is a reasonable second choice agent
- Hemodynamic goals:
  - Heart rate in isolated aortic stenosis patients between 50 and 60 beats/min
  - Peak systolic ventricular pressure < 200 mm Hg
  - Diastolic blood pressure above 60 mm Hg
  - Peak systolic ventricular pressure = (SBP + peak pressure gradient)
- Arrhythmias:
  - Persistent tachycardia is treated with β- blockers like esmolol
  - Supraventricular tachycardias are immediately cardioverted
  - Lidocaine, amiodarone and defibrillator should be readily available
  - This is because these patients develop ventricular arrhythmias commonly

- Bradycardia, junctional rhythm is aggressively treated with ephedrine and atropine

❖ Ischemic changes on the ECG:
- Caution when using NTG to treat ischemia in AS
- This is because NTG will reduce SVR further and also reduce preload
- This may worsen myocardial ischemia

❖ Cardiac arrest:
- Cardiopulmonary resuscitation in patients with aortic stenosis has poor outcomes
- This is because of the inability of external compressions to generate adequate flow across the stenotic valve

❖ Procedures that are at highest risk for perioperative MACE:
- Those involving increase in abdominal procedures (laparoscopic surgeries)
- Those involving quick increase in systemic blood pressure (vascular surgery)

Ventilation

❖ Initiation of positive pressure ventilation reduces the preload to the LV

❖ This acute fall in preload in patients with critical AS may result in hemodynamic collapse

❖ Therefore, initiation of positive pressure ventilation has to be gradual in severe AS

❖ Positive pressure ventilation, once initiated, is useful to assist ventricular function

Extubation

❖ Patient is extubated when warm, fully reversed and hemodynamically stable

❖ Deep planes at extubation desirable to prevent tachycardia

❖ Slow administration of the reversal agent preferred to avoid tachycardia associated with glycopyrrolate

Postoperative

Ventilation

❖ Short period of postoperative ventilation may be warranted in sick patients

❖ Gradual discontinuation of ventilation is warranted to prevent sudden increase in LV preload

Management

❖ Management in postoperative period involves the same hemodynamic goals

❖ Excessive fluid loss and hypovolemia is prevented to maintain preload

Monitors

❖ Pulse oximetry

❖ ECG

❖ NIBP

❖ Invasive monitors, if used during surgery

Analgesia

❖ Multimodal analgesia

❖ Opioid based analgesia most commonly used

❖ Epidural analgesia, where applicable, may be useful for postoperative pain

❖ NSAIDs are useful in reducing opioid comsumption

HYPERTROPHIC CARDIOMYOPATHY

Introduction

❖ Hypertrophic cardiomyopathy is an autosomal dominant inherited cardiomyopathy

❖ Characterized by histologically abnormal myocytes and myocardial hypertrophy

❖ This causes localized areas of LVH > 15 mm without any identifiable cause

❖ Hypertrophy develops in the absence of pressure/volume overload

❖ When hypertrophy results in LVOT obstruction, it is called hypertrophic obstructive CM

❖ Also called:
- ***Idiopathic hypertrophic subaortic stenosis***
- ***Asymmetrical septal hypertrophy***
- ***Hypertrophic obstructive cardiomyopathy***
- ***Muscular subaortic stenosis***

Incidence

❖ Most common genetic cardiovascular disease

❖ Most common primary cardiomyopathy

❖ Prevalence varies from 1 in 500 to as high as 1 in 200 in the general population

❖ Accounts for 50% of all sudden cardiac deaths in patients below 30 years age

❖ Incidence of sudden cardiac death of 1% per year in HCM patients

Etiology

❖ Autosomal dominant inheritance with variable penetrance

❖ Mutation of cardiac-β-myosin chain gene on chromosome 14 was 1st discovered mutation

❖ Gene codes for cardiac sarcomere proteins causing substitution of arginine by glutamine

- ❖ Currently mutations in at least 11 different genes have been attributed to cause HCM
- ❖ Most common mutations occur in:
  - β-myosin heavy chain (40%)
  - Myosin-binding protein C (40%)

Pathology

- ❖ Bizzare and disorganized arrangement of cardiac muscle cells
- ❖ Disorganized myofibrillar architecture
- ❖ Myocardial fibrosis and thickening of small intramural coronary arteries
- ❖ Systolic compression of intramyocardial segment of coronary artery

Regions of Hypertrophy

- ❖ Asymmetrical septal hypertrophy *most common* (60% of cases)
- ❖ Apical hypertrophy
- ❖ Hypertrophy of free wall of left ventricle
- ❖ Concentric LVH: < 10% patients
- ❖ Striking regional variations in hypertrophy occur
- ❖ This contrasts with secondary hypertrophy as in HTN where hypertrophy is more uniform

Pathophysiology

- ❖ HCM characteristically displays the following features:
  - Myocardial hypertrophy
  - Myocardial ischemia in the absence of CAD
  - Dynamic left ventricular tract obstruction
  - Systolic anterior motion of mitral valve
  - *Diastolic dysfunction*
  - Arrhythmias
- ❖ Dynamic LVOT obstruction in HCM:
  - Occurs in 20–30% patients of HCM
  - Etiology:
    - Hypertrophy of basal septum
    - Systolic septal bulging into LVOT
    - Hyperdynamic LV contraction causing ***Venturi effect***
    - Systolic anterior motion of mitral valve leaflet
    - Malposition of anterior papillary muscle
  - Characteristics of LVOT obstruction (LVOTO) in HCM:
    - The obstruction is dynamic and peaks in mid-late systole
    - Beat to beat variability of the degree of obstruction occurs
    - This is in contrast to aortic stenosis, where LVOT obstruction is fixed
    - LVOTO is accentuated by any intervention which reduces ventricular size
    - This is because it facilitates septal-leaflet contact
  - The interventions which increase obstruction are:
    - Increased contractility
    - Increased heart rate
    - Reduced preload/ventricular volume
    - Reduced afterload

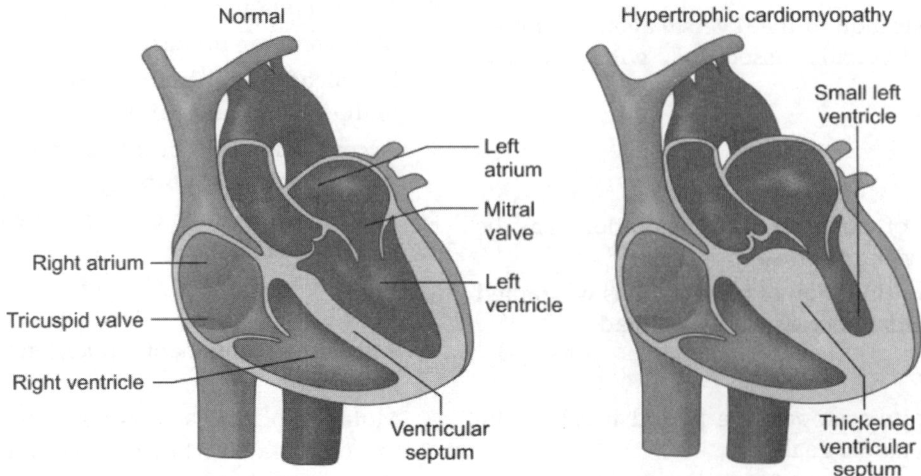

Fig. 42: Hypertrophic obstructive cardiomyopathy.

- Causes of myocardial ischemia in HCM:
  - Abnormal coronary arteries
  - Mismatch between ventricular mass and coronary size
  - Raised LVEDP which compromises subendocardial coronary perfusion
  - Decreased diastolic filling time
  - Increased oxygen consumption due to hypertrophy
- Causes of diastolic dysfunction in HCM:
  - Decreased ventricular wall compliance
  - Prolonged relaxation time
- Causes of arrhythmias in HCM:
  - Disorganized cellular architecture
  - Myocardial scarring from previous ischemia
  - Expanded interstitial matrix

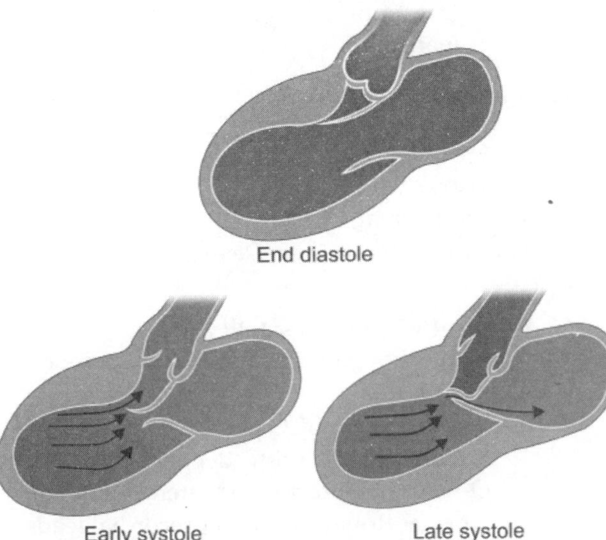

Fig. 43: Mechanism of LVOTO in HOCM.

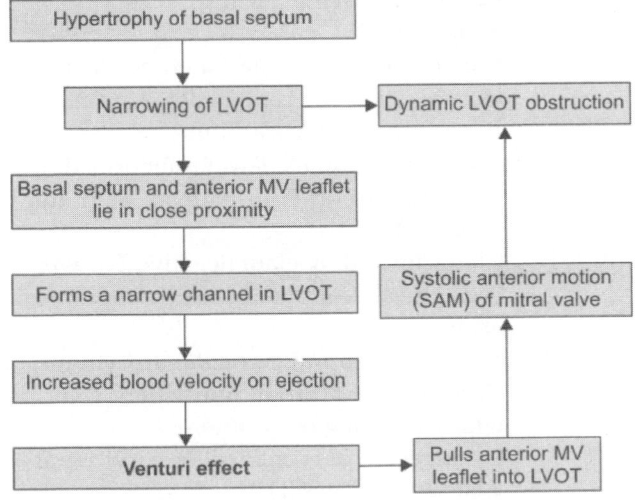

Factors Increasing LVOT Obstruction

- Decreased preload:
  - Hypovolemia
  - Vasodilators
  - Tachycardia
  - Positive pressure ventilation
- Decreased afterload:
  - Hypotension
  - Vasodilators
- Increased myocardial contractility:
  - Catecholamines
  - Digitalis

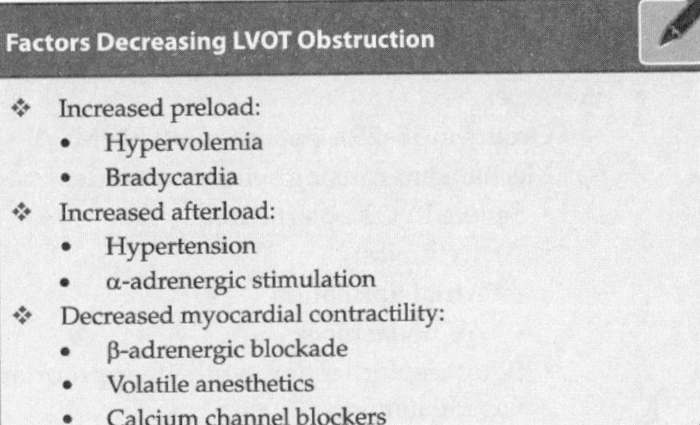

Factors Decreasing LVOT Obstruction

- Increased preload:
  - Hypervolemia
  - Bradycardia
- Increased afterload:
  - Hypertension
  - α-adrenergic stimulation
- Decreased myocardial contractility:
  - β-adrenergic blockade
  - Volatile anesthetics
  - Calcium channel blockers

Classification of Hypertrophic Cardiomyopathy

- Non-obstructive cardiomyopathy: Peak LVOT pressure gradient < 30 mm Hg
- Obstructive cardiomyopathy: Peak LVOT pressure gradient > 30 mm Hg
- Latent cardiomyopathy: Exercise-induced peak LVOT pressure gradient > 30 mm Hg

Clinical Features

- Symptoms:
  - Mostly asymptomatic and HCM is found as incidental finding on echocardiogram
  - Other symptoms commonly seen include:
    - Dyspnea on exertion
    - Fatigue
    - Atypical or anginal chest pain
    - Presyncope or syncope
    - Palpitations
  - Dyspnea on exertion:
    - Most common presenting manifestation
    - Occurs in > 90% of symptomatic patients
    - Causes of dyspnea in HCM include:
      - Diastolic dysfunction due to myocardial hypertrophy

- LVOTO causing:
  - Impaired LV emptying
  - Increased LVEDP
- Mitral regurgitation
- Systolic dysfunction in advanced stages

- Angina:
  - Occurs even in the absence of CAD in 25–30% patients
  - Commonly precipitated by heavy meals
  - Reduction in angina in recumbent posture is classical in HCM
  - This is because preload increases on lying down, augmenting the LV size
  - This reduces LVOTO and myocardial oxygen demand
- Syncope:
  - Occurs in 15–25% patients with HCM
  - Mechanisms causing syncope include:
    - Severe LVOT obstruction
    - Arrhythmias:
      - Atrial fibrillation
      - AV nodal block
    - Baroreceptor reflex with inappropriate vasodilatation
    - Exertional myocardial ischemia
- Sudden cardiac death (SCD):
  - HCM is the *most common* cause of SCD in young people (< 30 years)
  - This usually occurs during physical exertion
  - SCD may even be the 1st clinical manifestation
  - Most common autopsy finding in healthy athletes who die suddenly
- Arrhythmias:
  - Supraventricular and ventricular arrhythmias may be seen
  - These can present as dyspnea, presyncope or syncope

❖ Examination:
- Pulses bisferiens:
  - Mid-systolic LVOT obstruction occurs in HCM
  - This causes sudden deceleration of blood flow and a bifid pulse
- Double/triple forceful apical precordial in pulse
- Rapidly rising carotid pulse
- SVT/ventricular arrhythmias are common
- Normal first heart sound
- 3rd and 4th heart sound usually audible
- Systolic murmur:
  - Due to LVOTO:
    - Harsh crescendo-decrescendo systolic murmur
    - Begins slightly after 1st heart sound
    - Best heard at left lower sternal border and apex
    - May radiate to axilla and base
    - Does not radiate to the neck (as in AS)
    - Reduced by squatting and hand grip
    - Increased by Valsalva maneuver and standing
  - Due to mitral regurgitation:
    - Mid-late systolic murmur in posteriorly directed jet
    - May be holosystolic if centrally directed MR jet
    - Does not change intensity on Valsalva maneuver

Investigations

❖ Routine blood, BUN, SC, LFT

❖ Chest X-ray:
- May be normal
- Mild to moderate increase in cardiac silhouette

❖ ECG:
- Wide variation in ECG patterns
- None of the patterns are pathognomonic or highly specific
- Pseudo-infarction ECG pattern common:
  - Simulates MI with deeper than normal Q-waves in inferior and lateral leads
  - Normal R-wave in right precordial leads
  - Left ventricular hypertrophy pattern
- Abnormal broad Q waves:
  - Commonly seen in HCM
  - Simulates MI
  - Seen in lateral and inferior chest leads
  - Occurs due to septal depolarization of hypertrophied myocardium
- Primary and secondary T-wave abnormalities:
  - Occurs more often in patients with apical-type HCM
  - Characterized by giant negative T-waves
  - Seen most commonly in mid-precordial leads (V_2 to V_4)
- Ventricular and supraventricular arrhythmias:
  - Occurrence of atrial fibrillation coincides with worsening of symptoms
  - Occurrence of ventricular arrythmias is associated with SCD

- Holter monitoring:
  - Should be performed for 24–48 hours in all patients with HCM
  - Helps in risk stratification for SCD
- Echocardiogram:
  - Confirmatory test
  - LVH with wall thickness anywhere in ventricular wall > 15 mm is confirmatory
  - Used to evaluate:
    - Cardiac morphology
    - Systolic and diastolic dysfunction
    - Presence and severity of LVOTO
    - Degree of mitral regurgitation
  - Systolic function:
    - Visual assessment of ventricular function is often normal/hyperdynamic
    - LVEF is usually > 80%
    - Global longitudinal strain (GLS):
      - Impaired myocardial function may be present despite normal EF
      - GLS may therefore be useful to evaluate myocardial strain
  - Doppler echocardiogram:
    - Used to assess degree of LVOTO
    - Peak pressure gradient is determined from the peak velocity in LVOT
    - Can also be used to quantify the severity of mitral regurgitation
- Cardiac MRI:
  - Additional diagnostic modality in HCM
  - Provides high-resolution tomographic images of entire LV myocardium
  - Used to assess:
    - LV morphology
    - Maximal LV wall thickness
    - Risk stratification with late gadolinium enhancement (LGE)
  - Valuable in patients with:
    - Suboptimal echocardiographic studies
    - Hypertrophy of unusual locations (anterolateral free wall or LV apex)
- Catheterization studies:
  - Not done routinely in HCM
  - Reserved for HCM patients with associated:
    - Coronary artery disease
    - Restrictive cardiomyopathy
    - Fabry's disease/amyloidosis for endomyocardial biopsy
  - Information obtained from cardiac catheterization includes:
    - LVOT pressure gradient
    - Left ventricular end diastolic pressure
    - Left atrial pressure/PCWP
    - Coronary angiogram.

Treatment

Medical Therapy

- β blockers:
  - First line therapy for medical management of HCM
  - Uses of beta-blocker therapy:
    - Reduce inotropy and tachycardia
    - Allow longer diastolic filling time and increase stroke volume
    - Prevent increases in subaortic pressure gradient
- Calcium channel blockers (CCBs):
  - Used as second line agents
  - Commonly used agents include verapamil and diltiazem
  - Used when:
    - Beta-blocker intolerance
    - Suboptimal response with maximal beta-blockade
  - Uses of CCBs:
    - Reduce inotropy
    - Improve diastolic compliance by relaxing the heart
- Amiodarone: Used for SVT and ventricular arrhythmias
- Drugs avoided include:
  - ACE inhibitors (accentuate dynamic LVOTO)
  - Nitrates (reduce preload and afterload)
  - Diuretics (reduce preload)
- HOCM with pulmonary edema:
  - Diuretics and digoxin are avoided
  - Volume status is optimized
  - β blockers are preferred

Surgical Therapy

- Alcohol ablation of IV Septum, if septal thickness at site of injection ≤ 15 mm
- Pacing:
  - DDD (dual mode, dual chamber, dual sensing)
  - DDD pacing with short AV delay can be useful
  - Cannot be used in patients with atrial fibrillation
- Septal myectomy ***(Morrows procedure)***:
  - Performed through aortotomy on CPB
  - Involves resection of muscle from proximal basal ventricular septum
  - Tissue is removed up to 3 cm apically from the aortic valve

- Currently, Schaffs modification of Morrow procedure is used
- Here, extended resection up to 7 cm from the aortic valve is used
- This results in enlargement of LVOT
- May be combined with mitral valve replacement of repair
- Indications:
  - Severe drug refractory symptoms (NYHA III or IV)
  - Resting gradient ≥ 50 mm Hg
  - Exercise gradient ≥ 50 mm Hg

Nonsurgical Alternatives

- Dual chamber pacing:
  - Reduces the LVOTO and LVOT gradient in many patients
  - Occurs due to RV preexcitation altering the synergy of ventricular contraction
  - Largely abandoned as an alternative to surgery
- Percutaneous alcohol septal ablation:
  - Used for refractory HCM in poor surgical candidates
  - Done in the cardiac catheterization laboratory
  - Septal perforating branch of LAD supplying the culprit portion is identified
  - 1–3 mL alcohol is introduced into the target septal perforator branch of LAD
  - This produces a transmural MI within proximal ventricular septum
  - Localized infarction leads to subsequent necrosis and regression of basal septum
  - This mimics myectomy by reducing septal thickness and excursion
  - Associated with high risk of complications:
    - Complete heart block
    - Malignant ventricular arrhythmias
    - Repeat procedures due to therapeutic failure
  - Suboptimal in patients with:
    - Thick ventricles > 30 mm
    - Obstruction associated with generalized LV hypertrophy
    - Severe concomitant MR

Risk Prediction for SCD in HCM

- Major SCD risk factors
  - Family history of sudden cardiac death
  - Unexplained syncope
  - Severe LVH > 30 mm
  - Non-sustained ventricular tachycardia
  - Abnormal blood pressure response to exercise
- Potential SCD risk modifiers:
  - LVOT obstruction
  - Late gadolinium enhancement on cardiovascular MR imaging
  - Genetic mutations
  - LV apical aneurysm
  - End-stage phase of HCM (EF < 50%)
- Additional SCD risk factors:
  - Increased left atrial diameter
  - Young age at evaluation
- Putative SCD risk factors:
  - Paced ventricular electrogram fractionation
  - QRS fragmentation on ECG
  - Exercise induced NSVT/VF
  - Severe obstructive CAD
  - Microvascular ischemia
  - Midventricular obstruction
  - Atrial fibrillation
- Risk of SCD is below 0.5% per year if:
  - None of the 5 major risk factors exist
  - Absence or only mild symptoms of heart failure
  - Left atrium < 45 mm
  - LV wall thickness < 20 mm
  - LV outflow gradient < 50 mm Hg

Anesthetic Goals 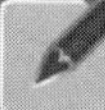

- Rate:
  - Maintain in normal range (60–80 bpm)
  - Avoid tachycardia
  - β blockers used to:
    - Reduce heart rate
    - Reduce LVOT gradient
    - Increase LVEDP
- Rhythm:
  - Maintaining sinus rhythm is important
  - These patients are poorly tolerant of loss in atrial kick
  - This is because of the presence of a poorly compliant LV muscle
  - Thus, relative contribution of atrial contraction to LV preload increases
  - Atrial pacing via pulmonary artery catheter may be useful
- Preload:
  - Maintain high preload
  - Saturated intravascular space is preferred perioperatively
  - This is because LV is thick and hypertrophied with a reduced compliance
  - Thus, outflow tract obstruction increases in hypovolemic conditions
  - Fluid challenge is one of the first steps to treat hypotension in HCM

Contd...

Contd...

- Afterload:
  - Maintain high systemic vascular resistance
  - Afterload reduction in HOCM increases LVOT obstruction and mitral regurgitation
  - Conversely, increasing the afterload reduces:
    - Outflow tract obstruction
    - Outflow gradient
    - Systolic anterior motion of MV
    - Mitral regurgitation
  - Thus, vasoconstrictors like phenylephrine and vasopressin are used
  - Severe hypotension is best treated with vasoconstrictors
- Contractility:
  - Prefer myocardial depression
  - This is because increased contractility results in an increase in dynamic LVOTO
  - Sympathetic stimulation and inotropic agents are avoided

Anesthetic Technique

- Neuraxial anesthesia is relatively contraindicated as it reduces SVR and preload
- When used, continuous spinal/epidural anesthesia may be preferable to bolus doses
- This is because continuous infusions allow better control of the level of sympathectomy
- Low dose combined spinal-epidural may be used for cesarean section
- Ropivacaine is *agent of choice* for cesarean sections
- Ephedrine and epinephrine are *contraindicated* for hypotension
- Maintaining euvolemia is important to avoid hypotension
- Phenylephrine is the agent of choice for treating severe persistent hypotension

Preoperative Evaluation and Preparation

- Patient is evaluated for:
  - Dynamic obstruction
  - Malignant arrhythmias
  - Myocardial infarction
- Functional status of the patient is noted (NYHA class)
- Immediate preoperative ECG is important as it acts as a baseline for further comparisons
- Echocardiography is reviewed for baseline LVOT gradient and severity of MR
- High risk patients for non-cardiac surgery include:
  - Significant LVOT pressure gradient:
    - > 30 mm Hg at rest
    - > 50 mm Hg on exercise
  - Moderate-severe mitral regurgitation
  - LV dysfunction with LVEF < 50%
  - Restrictive diastolic dysfunction
- Management of ICD:
  - ICDs should be reprogrammed to asynchronous mode preoperatively
  - Intraoperative electromagnetic interference causes inappropriate shock delivery
  - Thus, reprogramming is essential for any surgery where electrocautery is used:
    - Above umbilicus
    - Close to pulse generator
    - Close to leads of ICD

Premedication

- NPO orders
- Maintain euvolemia preoperatively by avoiding prolonged fasting
- Informed consent
- Large bore IV access is secured for intraoperative volume resuscitation
- Benzodiazepine premedication is used to avoid anxiety induced tachycardia
- Atropine is avoided during premedication (glycopyrrolate/scopolamine preferred)
- Chronically administered medications:
  - β blockade and calcium channel blockers are continued on the day of surgery
  - Anticoagulant therapy is discontinued after discussion with the cardiologist
  - Bridging therapy may be required for chronic anticoagulation.

Monitoring

- Pulse oximetry, capnography
- ECG:
  - Leads V5 and lead II used for monitoring
  - Lead II is useful for diagnosing SVT/junctional tachycardia
  - Lead V5 shows abnormal Q waves:
    - Occurs due to accentuation of normal septal depolarization
    - Should not be confused for old MI
  - Some patients may have short PR interval
- Invasive BP monitoring:
  - Indications for invasive BP monitoring includes:
    - History of arrhythmias
    - Likely need for intraoperative vasopressor support
    - Systolic dysfunction

- Large intraoperative volume shifts
- Planned volume expansion which may cause pulmonary edema
- Massive fluctuations in afterload (procedures with vascular clamping)
- Emergency surgeries
- Arterial line is used for:
  - Continuous IBP monitoring
  - Assessment of respirophasic variations to guide goal-directed fluid therapy
  - ABG sampling
- Arterial waveform in HCM shows pulsus bisferiens:
  - Initial rapid peak represents early unobstructed ventricular ejection
  - Subsequent downslope and second peak are a result of dynamic obstruction

❖ CVP line:
- Provides supplemental data regarding intravascular volume status
- However, it is an inaccurate guide to changes in LV volume
- Useful to administer vasoactive drugs intraoperatively

❖ PA catheter:
- PA catheter with pacing potential is preferred
- Useful for gauging intravascular volume
- PCWP is maintained in high normal to elevated range
- PCWP may overestimate patients true volume status

❖ Urine output

❖ Temperature

❖ Tranesophageal echocardiography for high risk surgeries.

Position

❖ Varies depending on the type of surgery

❖ Abrupt positioning changes are avoided

❖ This is because it can cause hemodynamic compromise due to changes in preload

Induction

❖ Adequate preoxygenation

❖ External defibrillator paddles may be used in patients with ICDs and frequent arrhythmias

❖ Agents avoided at induction include:
- Histamine releasing agents as they cause sudden fall in SVR
- Ketamine due to sympathomimetic properties

❖ Induction agents are selected to reduce likelihood of sympathectomy and hypotension

❖ Thiopentone or propofol may be given in graded, incremental doses

❖ Midazolam and fentanyl may be co-administered to reduce total dose of induction agent

❖ Propofol > 1.5 mg/kg is avoided to avoid reduction in SVR

❖ Deep planes of intubation preferred to:
- Minimize sympathetic stimulation
- Avoid tachycardia and increased contractility

Maintenance

❖ Balanced anesthesia with O_2 + N_2O+ sevoflurane

❖ High doses of inhalational agents are avoided as it may cause reduction in SVR

❖ Choice of volatile agent:
- Isoflurane can cause tachycardia and decreased SVR and is avoided
- Sevoflurane may be useful as it causes:
  - Mild myocardial depression
  - Minimal perturbations of heart rate and SVR
- Halothane and enflurane may be used as they cause myocardial depression
- High dose desflurane is avoided owing to its sympathomimetic action

❖ Opioids and NDMR given as intermittent boluses

❖ Vecuronium is the preferred NDMR:
- Pancuronium causes tachycardia
- Atracurium causes histamine release and reduces SVR

❖ Deep level of GA maintained to avoid tachycardia, especially to surgical incision

Hemodynamics

❖ Maintenance of euvolemia is important to prevent hypotension

❖ Prompt replacement of blood loss and careful titration of IV fluids is important

❖ Intraoperative hypotension is treated with volume and vasoconstrictors

❖ Volume overload is avoided as pulmonary edema is precipitated frequently

❖ This is due to the poor LV compliance causing rapid increase in LVEDP

❖ Infusions of phenylephrine/vasopressin may be used for persistent hypotension

❖ Agents causing increased contractility are avoided:
- Inotropes
- Calcium
- β agonists

- Short acting β blockers (IV esmolol 20–30 mg) may be used for persistent HTN
- Vasodilators (to treat HTN) are avoided
- Hypothermia is avoided as it causes tachycardia and increases myocardial oxygen demand
- Euthermia is maintained using:
  - Forced air warmers
  - IV fluid warmers
- Arrhythmias are treated with DC cardioversion rather than pharmacological methods
- Laparoscopic surgeries may cause further reductions in ventricular preload

Ventilation

- Positive pressure ventilation itself causes a reduction in ventricular preload
- This effect is accentuated by high tidal volumes and PEEP
- Thus, high tidal volume and PEEP are avoided
- Higher respiratory rate is preferred to prevent hypercapnia due to low tidal volumes

Emergence

- Postoperative ventilation may be required depending on intraoperative events
- Patient is extubated if:
  - Spontaneous ventilation with normal ABG
  - No bleeding and hemodynamically stable patient
  - Normothermia
- Sympathetic stimulation is avoided at extubation by ensuring:
  - Adequate analgesia using:
    - Systemic opioids
    - Intrathecal opioids/local anesthetic
  - IV boluses of short acting beta blockers (esmolol)

Postoperative Management

Monitors

- BP, ECG
- Pulse oximetry
- Temperature
- Urine output
- Arterial blood gas
- Echocardiography

Management

- ICD is reprogrammed to the original settings prior to discharge from PACU
- Defibrillator paddles are left in-situ until ICD reprogramming is completed
- Electrolytes are checked in patients with large intraoperative fluid shifts
- Beta-blockers and CCBs are resumed as soon as tolerated to prevent tachycardia
- Anticoagulation is resumed prior to discharge from PACU after cardiology consultation

Analgesia

- Multimodal analgesia used
- NSAIDs may be useful for their opioid sparing properties
- Intrathecal opioids are useful to prevent sympathectomy
- PCA may be used for severe pain

VENOUS AIR EMBOLISM

Introduction

- Venous air embolism can occur:
  - During any surgical procedure in which operative site is > 5 cm above RA
  - When pressure within an open vein is subatmospheric

Pathophysiology

- Two preconditions must exist:
  - Direct communication between a source of air and vasculature
  - Pressure gradient to favour passage of air into circulation
- Small amounts of air:
  - Broken up in capillary bed and absorbed
  - Does not produce symptoms
- Large amounts of air:
  - 20 mL of air intravenously can produce complications
  - 5 mL/kg of air in intravenous space required for significant injury: Shock/cardiac arrest
  - 2–3 mL of air in cerebral circulation can be fatal
  - 0.5 mL of air is left anterior descending artery can produce VF
- Transpulmonary passage of air:
  - Air can traverse pulmonary vascular bed to reach systemic circulation when a large volume of air is presented to pulmonary vascular filter
  - Pulmonary vasodilators including volatile anesthetics, reduce the threshold for transpulmonary passage

Pathogenesis

Can be caused by any open vein/sinus above the level of heart due to:

- Inability of vein to collapse:
  - Intracranial venous sinuses:
    - Transverse sinus
    - Sigmoid sinus
    - Posterior half of sagittal sinus
  - Diploic spaces
  - Emissary veins
  - Cervical epidural veins
  - Self retaining surgical retractors
  - Tracks formed around indwelling catheters (like central venous catheter)
- Level of venous pressure at the site:
  - *Posture*: sitting > supine > prone > lateral
  - Reverse Trendelenburg position:
    - At + 25° intracranial venous sinus pressure 0 cmH_2O
    - At + 90° produces a negative pressure of -12 ± 3 cmH_2O
  - Spontaneous ventilation:
    - Causes negative intrathoracic pressure
    - This potentiates negative pressure at operative site
  - In prone position, suction effect of pendulous abdomen can potentiate negative venous pressure within epidural veins

Etiology

I. Surgical Procedures

- Neurosurgery and otolaryngological surgery:
  - Most common cause
  - Especially common in ***Fowlers sitting position***
  - Also common in posterior fossa surgeries
- Craniofacial surgery
- Dental implant surgeries
- Liver transplantation
- Genitourinary surgery:
  - Those done in Trendelenburg position
  - Cesarean section
  - Compromised delivery
  - Surgeries involving tumors with high degree of vascularity
- Orthopedic surgeries:
  - Hip replacement
  - Spine surgery
  - Arthroscopy
- Vascular surgery:
  - End arterectomies
  - Lateral decubitus thoracotomy
- *Laparoscopic procedures*: incidence of VAE > 50%

II. Mechanical Insufflation

- Arthroscopic procedures
- Carbon dioxide hysteroscopy
- Laparoscopic surgeries
- Urethral procedures
- Orogenital sexual activity during pregnancy by entering myometrial veins
- Inadvertant infusion of air during IV contrast agent injection for:
  - CT angiography
  - Cardiac catheterization
  - Cardiac ablation procedures
- Positive pressure ventilation due to barotrauma (VILI) common in:
  - ARDS
  - Hyaline membrane disease
- Ingestion of hydrogen peroxide (rarely)

III. Iatrogenic Creation of Pressure Gradient

- Procedures causing pressure gradient:
  - During lumbar puncture
  - Inserion of CVP catheters
  - Thoracocentesis
  - Insertion of hemodialysis catheters/Hickmanns catheters
- Mechanisms of pressure differential:
  - Fracture/detachment of catheter connection
  - Failure to occlude needle hub
  - Presence of persistant catheter tract following removal of CVP catheter
  - Deep inspiration during insertion/removal which causes negative pressure
  - Hypovolemia which reduces CVP
  - Upright position which reduces CVP

IV. Diving

- Due to pulmonary barotrauma from voluntary breatholding
- Decompression sickness: air bubbles precipitate out into bloodstream if gas dissolved in blood at pressure, is not allowed sufficient time to outgas as ascent
- Rapid rewarming of following CPB

Clinical Features

Symptoms: In Awake Patient

- Dyspnea, nausea, dizziness
- Continous cough, substernal chest pain

- *Gasp reflex*:
  - Classic gasp at times
  - Reported when a bolus of air enters pulmonary circulation
- Agitation, disorientation
- Circulatory arrest if large amount of air blocks RVOT/TV/PV or PA (***Saddle embolus***)

Signs

Central Nervous System:

- Altered mental status
- Loss of consciousness
- Seizures, collapse, coma
- Transient focal neurodeficits
- Air bubbles in retinal blood vessels

Cardiovascular System:

- Raised JVP
- Nonspecific ST and T changes
- Hypotension
- Dysrhythmias, MI, cardiovascular collapse
- Pulmonary arterial HTN
- Mill wheel murmur:
  - Loud, machinery like churning murmur
  - Occurs due to blood mixing with air in right ventricle
  - Best heard over precordium

Respiratory System:

- Tachypnea, rales, wheeze
- Cyanosis, hemoptysis
- Reduced E_TCO_2, Low SpO_2
- Raised airway pressure
- Pulmonary edema
- Raised pulmonary vascular resistance.

Skin:

- Crepitus over superficial blood vessels
- ***Livedo reticularis***

Diagnosis

Arterial Blood Gas

- Hypoxia, hypercapnea
- Metabolic acidosis.

Chest X-ray

- May be normal
- Gas in pulmonary arterial system
- Pulmonary arterial dilatation
- Focal oligemia: ***Westermark sign***
- Pulmonary edema

ECG

- Low sensitivity
- Tachycardia, RV strain pattern
- ST depression, transient MI

CT Scan

- For emboli in central venous system:
  - Axillary and subclavian vein
  - Right ventricle
  - Pulmonary artery
- CT head for:
  - Intracerebral air
  - Cerebral edema/infarction

MRI

- Increased water concentration in affected tissues
- Not so reliable.

Transesophageal Echo

- *Highest sensitivity*, but invasive modality
- More sensitive than precordial Doppler
- Can detect air bubbles as small as 0.25 mL
- Can detect as less as 0.02 mL/kg of air
- Also evaluates cardiac function, right-left shunting of air

Precordial Dopper

- *Most sensitive non-invasive modality*
- Placed in right parasternal location between 2nd and 3rd or 3rd and 6th ribs
- Interruption of regular swishing of Doppler signal by sporadic roaring sounds indicates VAE
- Precordial Doppler along with E_TCO_2 is the current standard of care
- Transcranial Doppler useful for cerebral microemboli

End Tidal CO_2

- Sudden reduction in E_TCO_2 occurs
- This is due to sudden increase in pulmonary dead space causing V-Q mismatch
- Reduction of E_TCO_2 by 2 mm Hg is indicative of VAE

End Tidal Nitrogen

- Most sensitive gas sensing VAE
- Increased ETN_2 occurs if VAE is present
- Response time is much faster than E_TCO_2: changes occur 30–90 seconds earlier

Pulse Oximetry: Changes in SPO_2 Occur Very Late

Pulmonary Artery Catheter:
- Increase in PA pressure can occur
- Relatively insensitive indicator

Mean Airway Pressure: Increase in MAP is in direct proportion to amount of air entrained

Mass Spectrometry

Prevention of Venous Air Embolism

- Measures to reduce risk during surgery:
  - Nitrous oxide:
    - N_2O can be used provided it is eliminated when VAE occurs
    - If used, better to use 50% N_2O rather than 70%
  - Positive end expiratory pressure:
    - PEEP no longer used as even 10 cmH_2O PEEP is unlikely to increase CVP
    - PEEP increases chances of pulmonary artery embolism due to barotrauma
    - It also reduces preload, adding to hypotension
  - Head end elevation:
    - Elevate head end only as much as necessary
    - + 25° Trendelenburg causes 0 cmH_2O pressure in cerebral circulation
    - + 90° Trendelenburg causes +12 cmH_2O pressure in cerebral circulation
  - Reduce pressure gradient between site of potential entry and RA
  - Surgeons to be meticulous about:
    - Cauterizing
    - Tying blood vessels
    - Applying bone wax
  - Screening contrast ECHO to detect ASD before sitting position surgeries
- Measures to reduce risk during CVP placement:
  - Avoid and treat hypovolemia before catheter placement
  - During catheter insertion/removal:
    - Patient should be in supine position with head lowered
    - Insertion site should be 5 cm below RA
    - If patient is awake, he can hold breath to increase CVP
    - Doing Valsalva maneuver also increases CVP
  - Maintain all connections to central line, line closed/docked when not in use
- Measures to reduce risk during IPPV:
  - Prevent barotrauma by minimizing airway pressure during IPPV
  - Avoid PEEP

Treatment

- Prevent further air entry:
  - Surgeon should flood or pack surgical field with saline
  - Bone wax is applied to skull edges until entry site is identified
  - Intravascular volume infusion to increase CVP to 10–12 cmH_2O
  - Jugular vein compression:
    - Increases cranial venous pressure
    - Also slows air entrainment and cause back bleeding
    - This may help surgeon identify the source of embolus
  - Lower the head end to prevent cerebral embolization
  - Close wound quickly if none of measures help
  - Inflatable neck tourniquet available in case of VAE
- Treatment of intravascular air:
  - Aspirate right heart catheter: RA catheter mandatory in sitting craniotomies
  - Discontinue N_2O immediately
  - FiO_2 100% with inhalational anesthetic
  - Pressors and inotropes
  - ***Durants position***:
    - Lateral position with right side up
    - Allows air to remain in RA, where it wont contribute to airlock in RV
    - Air can then be aspirated from RA
  - Chest compressions:
    - Maintains cardiac output
    - Helps to break large air bubbles into smaller ones
    - Forces air out of RV into pulmonary blood vessels:improves cardiac output
  - Hyperbaric oxygen therapy:
    - In case of neurological manifestations/ cardiovascular instability
    - Helps by compression of existing bubbles
    - Establishes high diffusion gradient to speed up resolution of existing bubbles
    - Improves oxygenation of ischemic tissue and also reduces intracranial pressure
    - Good prognosis if initiated within 6 hours

Paradoxical Air Embolism

- Passage of air across patent foramen ovale which is present in 25% adults
- Necessary gradient to open foramen ovale may be 5 mm Hg

- ❖ Significant increase in right heart pressure must occur for PAE to occur
- ❖ Even when mean LAP > mean RAP, PAE can occur due to transient reversal of interatrial pressure gradient which occurs during each cardiac cycle
- ❖ PEEP and hypovolemia increase risk of PAE
- ❖ Avoid even small air bubbles in IV infusion
- ❖ Major cerebral and coronary morbidity: Causes MI/ stroke postoperatively

INFECTIVE ENDOCARDITIS

Introduction

- ❖ Refers to microbial infection of endocardial surface of the heart
- ❖ Infective endarteritis refers to proliferation of micro-organisms on:
  - Arterio-venous shunts
  - Arterio-arterial shunts (PDA)
  - Coarctation of aorta

Incidence

- ❖ Ranges from 3 to 10 episodes per 1,00,000 person-years
- ❖ Left sided IE most commonly occurs in patients with underlying heart disease
- ❖ Right sided IE occurs most commonly in intravenous drug abusers
- ❖ IV drug abuse accounts for almost 10% of all IE episodes
- ❖ Prosthetic valve endocarditis (PVE) occurs in 1–6% of patients with a prosthetic valve
- ❖ Almost 37% of PVEs occur due to extensive health-care exposure and are therefore nosocomial

Pathology

- ❖ Vegetations occur at the site of infection
- ❖ Vegetation consists of:
  - Platelets
  - Fibrin
  - Microcolonies of microorganisms
  - Scant inflammatory cells
- ❖ Sites of infection:
  - Heart valves (native/prosthetic)
  - On low pressure side of septum in VSD
  - Mural endocardium at sites of damage by aberrant jets of blood or foreign bodies
  - Intracardiac devices

Classification

- ❖ IE according to localization of infection:
  - Left sided native valve IE
  - Left sided prosthetic valve IE (PVE):
    - Early PVE: < 1 year after valve surgery
    - Late PVE: > 1 year after valve surgery
  - Right sided IE
  - Device related IE (permanent pacemaker or ICD)
- ❖ IE according to mode of acquisition:
  - Health care associated IE:
    - Nosocomial IE: In patient hospitalized > 48 hrs prior to onset of symptoms
    - Non-nosocomial IE:
      - ▪ Symptoms of IE starting < 48 hrs after admission
      - ▪ Associated with health care contact defined by:
        - Hospitalization in ICU < 90 days before onset of IE
        - Health care contact within 30 days of onset of IE for:
          - ○ Hemodialysis
          - ○ IV chemotherapy
          - ○ Intravenous therapy
          - ○ Home-based nursing
        - Residence in long-term care facility
  - Community acquired IE:
    - Symptoms of IE starting < 48 hours after admission
    - Without criteria for healthcare associated infection
  - Drug-abuse associated IE: In active IV drug user with no other source of infection
- ❖ Active IE:
  - IE with persistent fever and blood cultures
  - Active inflammatory morphology found at surgery
  - Patient still under antibiotic therapy for IE
  - Histopathological evidence of active IE
- ❖ Recurrent IE:
  - Relapse: Repeat episodes caused by same organism < 6 months after initial episode
  - Reinfection:
    - Infection with different microorganism
    - Repeat episode caused by same organism > 6 months after initial episode

Etiology

- ❖ Causative organisms:
  - Most commonly isolated organisms:
    - *Staphylococcus* species (31%):
      - ▪ Most common cause of healthcare associated IE

    - *S. aureus* (most common cause of IE)
    - Coagulase negative staphylococci (CoNS) such as *S. lugdunensis*
  - *Streptococcus* species (29%):
    - *S. viridans*
    - *S. gallolyticus* (associated with colon carci-noma and IBD)
    - *S. mitis*
    - *S. sanguis*
    - *S. mutans*
    - *S. milleri*
  - *Enterococcus* species (10%):
    - *E. faecalis*
    - *E. faecium*
- Infrequent pathogens:
  - Gram negative bacteria:
    - Adhere less readily to endocardium
    - Thus, they rarely cause IE
    - Gram negative organisms causing IE include:
      - *Enterobacteriaceae* (2%)
      - *Escherichia coli*
      - *Klebsiella pneumoniae*
  - HACEK group (2%):
    - *Haemophilus aphrophilus*
    - *Actinobacillus actinomycetemcomitans*
    - *Cardiobacterium hominis*
    - *Eikenella corrodens*
    - *Kingella kingae*
  - Other organisms:
    - *Streptococcus pneumoniae*
    - Fungi (2%):
      - *Candida albicans*
      - *Aspergillus* species
- Culture negative IE (8%):
  - *Abiotrophia* species (nutritionally variant streptococci)
  - *Bartonella* species
  - *Tropheryma whippelii*
  - *Coxiella burnetti*
  - *Brucella* species (in brucella-endemic regions)
  - *Legionella* species
  - Candida and aspergillus species

❖ Predisposing factors:
- Patient characteristics:
  - Age above 60 years
  - Male sex (3:2 ratio)
  - Drug addicts:
    - Most commonly results in right sided IE
    - May be due to valvular endothelial damage from illicit drugs
  - Poor dental hygiene
  - Prior history of IE
  - HIV infection
- Congenital heart disease:
  - Ventricular septal defect (most common)
  - Tetralogy of Fallot (second most common)
  - Congenital aortic stenosis (risk increases with increasing peak gradient)
  - Bicuspid aortic valve
  - Patent ductus arteriosus
  - Pulmonary stenosis (rare)
  - Coarctation of aorta
  - Tricuspid atresia
- Valvular heart disease:
  - Rheumatic heart disease:
    - Mitral stenosis/regurgitation
    - Aortic stenosis/regurgitation
  - Mitral valve prolapse (5–8 times higher than normal MV)
  - Mitral annular calcification
  - Risk of IE is low for:
    - Pulmonary regurgitation
    - Tricuspid valve regurgitation
- Surgical shunts:
  - Blalock-Taussig shunt
  - Peritoneovenous shunts
  - Ventriculo-atrial shunts
- Intracardiac devices:
  - Prosthetic heart valves:
    - Risk is highest during first 3 months after surgery
    - Risk of IE reduces after 12 months post-operatively
    - Incidence is equal during first year in:
      - Aortic and mitral positions
      - Mechanical and bioprosthetic valves
    - Risk of IE increases for bioprosthetic valves beyond 18 months
  - Transcatheter aortic valve replacement associated with higher risk in:
    - Younger age
    - Male gender
    - Diabetes mellitus
    - Moderate-severe aortic regurgitation
  - Cardiac implantable electronic devices (CIED):
    - Risk of IE is inversely proportional to duration since implantation
    - Risk is higher during the first year after implantation

- Risk factors for CIED infections causing IE include:
  - Recent manipulation of device
  - Device revision
  - Pulse generator change
  - Inadequate peri-procedural antibiotic prophylaxis
  - Post-procedure hematoma
- Chronic hemodialysis due to
  - Intravascular access
  - Immune impairment
- Transvenous pacemaker

❖ Precipitating factors:
- Dental procedures
- Use of oral irrigation devices
- Intravenous vascular access
- Ulcerative or inflammatory bowel disease
- Endotracheal intubation
- Hemodialysis
- IV chemotherapy
- Wound care

Clinical Features

❖ Features indicating infection:
- Fever:
  - Most common symptom of IE (seen in up to 90% patients)
  - Acute onset high fever 103–104°F
  - May be low grade in subacute infective endocarditis
  - Temporal pattern of fever or severity has no diagnostic utility
- Fever is often associated with:
  - Chills, rigors, night sweats
  - Arthralgia and diffuse myalgia
  - Weakness, malaise, loss of appetite, weight loss
- Amenorrhea in females

❖ Cardiac manifestations:
- New regurgitant murmur suggests infective endocarditis
  - Change in quality of preexisting murmur
  - Cardiac murmur is usually absent in right sided IE
- Manifestations due to cardiovascular complications:
  - Perivalvular abscesses and fistula
  - Myocardial infarction
  - Congestive cardiac failure
  - Suppurative and non-suppurative pericarditis
  - Complete heart block

❖ Immunological manifestations:
- Arthralgia, myalgia
- Petechiae:
  - Seen in 20–40% of patients
  - Seen over:
    - Skin of extremities
    - Mucous membranes:
      - Palate
      - Conjunctiva
- *Roth spots*:
  - Also called Litten spots
  - Rarely seen (2% of patients with IE)
  - Highly suggestive of IE
  - Represent petechiae in retina
  - Appear as exudative, edematous hemorrhagic lesions with pale centers
- *Oslers nodes*:
  - Rarely seen
  - Highly suggestive of IE
  - *Tender*, erythematous nodules on pulp of fingertips and toes
  - May also occur on thenar and hypothenar eminences
  - Occurs more commonly in the setting of prolonged sepsis
  - Occurs as a sequel of vascular occlusion by microthrombi
  - This leads to localized immune-mediated vasculitis presenting as nodules
- *Janeway lesions*:
  - Rarely seen
  - Highly suggestive of IE
  - More common in acute than subacute IE
  - *Non-tender* erythematous macules on palms and soles
  - Represent micro-abscesses with neutrophil infiltration of capillaries
- *Splinter hemorrhages*:
  - Non-blanching hemorrhagic spots under nails
  - Appear as linear reddish-brown lesions
  - Not diagnostic as they may be found in normal patients also
- Clubbing, splenomegaly, hematuria

Complications

❖ Cardiac complications:
- Heart failure:
  - More commonly associated with:
    - Aortic valve involvement
    - *Staphylococcus aureus* infections

- Usually occurs due to:
  - Aortic regurgitation due to valve dehiscence
  - Embolization of vegetations into coronary arteries
  - Obstruction of coronary ostia by abscess or vegetation
- Perivalvular abscess:
  - Occurs more commonly in large vegetations
  - Can lead to:
    - Conduction defects
    - Systemic embolization
- Other cardiac complications:
  - Pericarditis
  - Intracardiac fistula (aorto-atrial and aorto-ventricular)

❖ Metastatic infections causing:
- Septic embolization:
  - Risk factors are:
    - Left sided vegetations
    - Large vegetation size
    - Atrial fibrillation
  - Results in:
    - Stroke
    - Blindness
    - Ischemia of extremities
    - Splenic and renal infarction
    - Pulmonary embolism
- Metastatic abscess:
  - Occurs as a consequence of septic embolization
  - This can result in:
    - Splenic abscess
    - Renal abscess
    - Brain abscess
    - Psoas abscess
- Mycotic aneurysms:
  - Usually occurs at sites of vessel bifurcation
  - Infective metastasis into vasa vasorum causes arterial wall infection
  - This leads to arterial dilatation and aneurysms

❖ Neurological complications:
- Embolic stroke
- Brain abscess
- Aseptic/purulent meningitis
- Meningoencephalitis
- Cerebral hemorrhage due to ruptured mycotic aneurysm
- Seizures

❖ Renal complications:
- Renal infarction
- Renal abscess
- Immune complex mediated glomerulonephritis

❖ Musculoskeletal complications:
- Vertebral osteomyelitis
- Septic arthritis

❖ Pulmonary complications:
- Pneumonia
- Lung abscess
- Empyema thoracis

Investigations

❖ Tests for identification of the organism:
- Blood culture:
  - For diagnosis and detecting antibiotic susceptibility
  - *Sampling*: in the absence of prior antibiotic therapy:
    - Total of at least three blood culture sets
    - Optimal volume of blood for each blood culture is 20 mL
    - Ideally with first sample separated from the last by at least 1 hour
    - Obtained from different venipuncture sites over 24 hours
    - Patients with IE have continuous bacteremia
    - Thus, sampling need not be timed with occurrence of fever
    - Obtained prior to initiation of antibiotic therapy
  - If culture remains negative after 48–72 hours:
    - Two additional cultures may be obtained
    - Incubation period may be extended to 5 days
    - This is done to detect fastidious organisms such as HACEK
  - Blood cultures are repeated every 48–72 hours till clearance of bacteremia
  - Mainstay of diagnosis
- Serological tests:
  - *Brucella*
  - *Bartonella*
  - *Legionella*
  - *Coxiella burnetti*
- Special stains like Periodic Acid Schiff for *Tryponema whipleii*
- PCR to recover microbial DNA/RNA

❖ Echocardiography:
- Performed as soon as diagnosis of IE is suspected
- Transthoracic echocardiography has:
  - Low sensitivity of 75%
  - High specificity of 100%

- TEE is more sensitive (> 90%) compared to transthoracic echocardiography
- Uses:
  - Confirms IE in the presence of:
    - Vegetations
    - Abscesses
    - New dehiscence of prosthetic valve
  - Also useful to assess:
    - Valvular dysfunction
    - Size of vegetation
    - Underlying cardiac function
  - Detection of intracardiac complications
  - For follow up evaluation in the presence of clinical deterioration

❖ Other studies:
- Complete blood counts:
  - Normocytic normochromic anemia
  - Leukocytosis
  - Thrombocytopenia
- Chest X-ray is useful to diagnose:
  - Septic pulmonary emboli
  - Pulmonary infiltrates
  - Congestive cardiac failure
- ECG:
  - Abnormalities reflect paravalvular or myocardial extension of infection
  - Abnormalities include:
    - First degree AV node block
    - Bundle branch block
    - Complete heart block
- Elevated inflammatory marker (ESR, CRP) levels
- Other abnormalities:
  - Positive rheumatoid factors
  - Circulating immune complexes
  - Low complement levels
  - Cryoglobulinemia
  - Hypergammaglobulinemia
- Urinalysis:
  - Microscopic hematuria
  - Albuminuria
  - Pyuria
  - Red blood cell casts in glomerulonephritis
- Cardiac catheterization to check patency of coronary arteries
- Other imaging tools:
  - Cardiac MRI
  - Cardiac CT angiography
  - Fluorodeoxyglucose-PET with CT (FDG-PET/CT)

Modified Dukes Criteria for Diagnosis

Major Criteria

❖ Positive blood culture:
- Typical micro-organisms consistent with IE from 2 separate blood cultures:
  - Common organisms:
    - *Streptococcus viridans*
    - *Streptococcus gallolyticus*
    - HACEK group
    - *Staphylococcus aureus or*
  - Community acquired enterococci in the absence of primary focus or
  - All of 3 or a majority of 4 or more separate cultures with 1st and last drawn at least 1 hour apart
- Typical organisms consistent with IE from persistently positive blood cultures:
  - > 2 positive blood cultures of samples drawn > 12 hours apart
  - All of 3 or majority of 4 separate blood cultures
- Single positive culture for *Coxiella burnetii* or phase I IgG titer > 1: 800

❖ Imaging evidence of endocardial involvement:
- Positive echocardiogram for IE:
  - Vegetation
  - Intracardiac abscess, pseudoaneurysm
  - Valvular perforation or aneurysm
  - New partial dehiscence of prosthetic valve
- Abnormal activity around site of prosthetic valve detected by:
  - 18F-FDG PET/CT
  - Radiolabeled leukocytes SPECT/CT
- Definite paravalvular lesions on cardiac CT

Minor Criteria

❖ Predisposing heart conditions or injection drug abuse

❖ Fever ≥ 38°C (≥ 100.4°F)

❖ Vascular phenomena:
- Major arterial emboli
- Stroke
- Septic pulmonary infarcts
- Mycotic aneurysms
- Intracranial hemorrhage
- Conjunctival hemorrhages
- Janeway lesions

❖ Immunological phenomenon:
- Glomerulonephritis
- Oslers nodes
- Roths spots
- Rheumatoid factor

❖ Microbiology:
  - Positive blood culture not meeting major criteria/serology tests
  - Serological evidence of active infection with organism consistent with IE

Interpretation

❖ Definite infective endocarditis:
  • Pathological criteria:
    - Microorganisms demonstrated by cultures or histological examination of:
      ▪ Vegetation
      ▪ Intracardiac abscess specimen
    - Active IE shown by histological examination of pathological specimens:
      ▪ Vegetations
      ▪ Intracardiac abscess specimen
  • Clinical criteria:
    - 2 major criteria or
    - 5 minor criteria or
    - 1 major with 3 minor criteria
❖ Possible infective endocarditis:
  • One major criterion and one minor criterion or
  • Three minor criteria
❖ Rejected infective endocarditis:
  • Firm alternate diagnosis or
  • Resolution of symptoms with antibiotic therapy < 4 days or
  • No pathological evidence of IE at surgery with antibiotic therapy < 4 days or
  • Does not meet criteria for possible IE

Differential Diagnosis

❖ Intravascular catheter-related infections
❖ Cardiac device infections
❖ Prosthetic joint infections
❖ Hematogenous osteomyelitis
❖ Infected arterial aneurysm

Treatment

Empiric Antibiotic Therapy

❖ Empiric therapy is initiated for patients presenting with acute hemodynamic instability
❖ In the absence of acute symptoms, antimicrobial therapy is initiated after blood culture
❖ Empiric therapy is avoided in these circumstances as:
  • Non organism-specific therapy may not be curative
  • Drugs used for empiric therapy (aminoglycosides) may result in toxicity
❖ Empiric therapy is initiated after at least 2 blood culture samples have been obtained
❖ Vancomycin is an appropriate antibiotic:
  • IV 15–20 mg/kg Q8-12H
  • Maximum dose not to exceed 2 grams per dose

Specific Antibiotic Therapy

❖ Antibiotic therapy for IE is distinct:
  • Requires high doses of parenteral antibiotics
  • Bactericidal antibiotics are preferred
  • Needs prolonged therapy

Native Valve Bacterial Endocarditis			
Organism	*Drug*	*Dose*	*Duration*
		Streptococcus	
Penicillin sensitive		**Monotherapy**	
	Penicillin G	12–18 million U/day in 4–6 divided doses	4 weeks
	Ceftriaxone	2 g/day IV/IM in 1 dose	4 weeks
	Vancomycin	30 mg/kg/day IV in 2 divided doses	4 weeks
		Combination Therapy	
	Penicillin G Gentamicin	12–18 million U/day in 6 divided doses 3 mg/kg/day IV/IM in 1 dose	2 weeks
	Ceftriaxone Gentamicin	2 g/day IV/IM in 1 dose 3 mg/kg/day IV/IM in 1 dose	2 weeks
Moderately penicillin resistant		**Combination Therapy**	
	Penicillin G Gentamicin	24 million U/day IV in 4–6 divided doses 3 mg/kg/day IV or IM in 1 dose	4 weeks 2 weeks
		Monotherapy	
	Vancomycin	30 mg/kg/day IV in 2 divided doses	4 weeks

Contd...

Contd...

	Enterococci		
Penicillin and gentamicin sensitive	**Combination Therapy**		
	Penicillin G Gentamicin	18–30 million U/day IV in 6 divided doses 3 mg/kg/day IV in 3 divided doses	4–6 weeks 4–6 weeks
	Ampicillin Gentamicin	12 g/day IV in 6 divided doses 3 mg/kg/day IV in 3 divided doses	4–6 weeks 4–6 weeks
Penicillin sensitive and gentamicin resistant	**Combination Therapy**		
	Penicillin G Streptomycin	18–30 million U/day IV in 6 divided doses 15 mg/kg/day IV or IM in 2 divided doses	4–6 weeks 4–6 weeks
	Ampicillin Streptomycin	12 g/day IV in 6 divided doses 15 mg/kg/day IV or IM in 2 divided doses	4–6 weeks 4–6 weeks
Penicillin resistant and gentamicin sensitive	**Combination Therapy**		
	Vancomycin Gentamicin	30 mg/kg/day IV in 2 divided doses 3 mg/kg/day IV or IM in 3 divided doses	6 weeks 6 weeks
	Staphylococcus		
Oxacillin sensitive strains	**Monotherapy**		
	Nafcillin	12 g/day IV in 4–6 divided doses	6 weeks
	Oxacillin	12 g/day IV in 4–6 divided doses	6 weeks
	Cefazolin	6 g/day IV in 3 divided doses	6 weeks
Oxacillin resistant strains	**Monotherapy**		
	Vancomycin	30 mg/kg/day IV in 2 divided doses	6 weeks
	Daptomycin	> 8 mg/kg/dose	6 weeks
	HACEK Organisms		
	Monotherapy		
	Ceftriaxone	2 g/day IV or IM in 1 dose	4 weeks
	Ampicillin	12 g/day in 6 divided doses	4 weeks
	Ciprofloxacin	800 mg/day IV in 2 divided doses	4 weeks

Prosthetic Valve Bacterial Endocarditis			
Organism	*Drug*	*Dose*	*Duration*
	Streptococcus		
Penicillin sensitive	**Monotherapy**		
	Penicillin G	24 million U/day IV in 4–6 divided doses	6 weeks
	Ceftriaxone	2 g/day IV or IM in 1 dose	6 weeks
	Vancomycin	30 mg/kg/day IV in 2 divided doses	6 weeks
	Combination Therapy		
	Penicillin G	24 million U/day IV in 4–6 divided doses	6 weeks
	Gentamicin	3 mg/kg/day IV or IM in 1 dose	2 weeks
	Ceftriaxone	2 g/day IV or IM in 1 dose	6 weeks
	Gentamicin	3 mg/kg/day IV or IM in 1 dose	2 weeks
Penicillin resistant	**Combination Therapy**		
	Penicillin G	24 million U/day IV in 4–6 divided doses	6 weeks
	Gentamicin	3 mg/kg/day IV or IM in 1 dose	6 weeks
	Ceftriaxone	2 g/day IV or IM in 1 dose	6 weeks
	Gentamicin	3 mg/kg/day IV or IM in 1 dose	6 weeks
	Monotherapy		
	Vancomycin	30 mg/kg/day IV in 2 divided doses	6 weeks

Contd...

Contd...

		Enterococcus	
Penicillin and gentamicin sensitive		**Combination Therapy**	
	Penicillin G Gentamicin	18–30 million U/day IV in 6 divided doses 3 mg/kg/day IV in 3 divided doses	6 weeks 6 weeks
	Ampicillin Gentamicin	12 g/day IV in 6 divided doses 3 mg/kg/day IV in 3 divided doses	6 weeks 6 weeks
Penicillin sensitive and gentamicin resistant		**Combination Therapy**	
	Penicillin G Streptomycin	18–30 million U/day IV in 6 divided doses 15 mg/kg/day IV or IM in 2 divided doses	6 weeks 6 weeks
	Ampicillin Streptomycin	12 g/day IV in 6 divided doses 15 mg/kg/day IV or IM in 2 divided doses	6 weeks 6 weeks
Penicillin resistant and gentamicin sensitive		**Combination Therapy**	
	Vancomycin Gentamicin	30 mg/kg/day IV in 2 divided doses 3 mg/kg/day IV or IM in 3 divided doses	6 weeks 6 weeks
		Staphylococcus	
Oxacillin sensitive		**Combination Therapy**	
	Nafcillin Rifampicin Gentamicin	12 g/day IV in 6 divided doses 900 mg/day IV or PO in 3 divided doses 3 mg/kg/day IV or IM in 3 divided doses	≥ 6 weeks ≥ 6 weeks 2 weeks
	Cefazolin Rifampicin Gentamicin	6 g/day IV in 3 divided doses 900 mg/day IV or PO in 3 divided doses 3 mg/kg/day IV or IM in 3 divided doses	≥ 6 weeks ≥ 6 weeks 2 weeks
	Vancomycin Rifampicin Gentamicin	30 mg/kg/day IV in 2 divided doses 900 mg/day IV or PO in 3 divided doses 3 mg/kg/day IV or IM in 3 divided doses	≥ 6 weeks ≥ 6 weeks 2 weeks
Oxacillin resistant		**Combination Therapy**	
	Vancomycin Rifampicin Gentamicin	30 mg/kg/day in 2 divided doses 900 mg/day IV or PO in 3 divided doses 3 mg/kg/day IV or IM in 3 divided doses	≥ 6 weeks ≥ 6 weeks 2 weeks
		HACEK Organisms	
		Monotherapy	
	Ceftriaxone	2 g/day IV or IM in 1 dose	6 weeks
	Ampicillin	12 g/day in 6 divided doses	6 weeks
	Ciprofloxacin	800 mg/day IV in 2 divided doses	6 weeks

Fungal Endocarditis

- Induction therapy:
  - Amphotericin B (lipid formulation) 3–5 mg/kg IV daily and
  - Flucytosine 25 mg/kg PO Q6H
- Both antifungals are continued for 2–3 weeks
- After this, patient is taken up for surgical resection of vegetation when surgically feasible
- In patients unable to tolerate amphotericin B:
  - Caspofungin 150 mg IV daily
  - Micafungin 150 mg IV daily
  - Anidulafungin 200 mg IV daily
- Following surgery, long term suppressive therapy (6 weeks) is used with:
  - Fluconazole 400–800 mg (6–12 mg/kg) PO daily
  - Voriconazole
- Lifelong suppression with fluconazole is recommended in non-surgical candidate

Surgical Treatment

- Class I indications:
  - Early surgery (prior to completion of full antibiotic course) indicated for:
    - IE causing valve dysfunction resulting in heart failure
    - Left sided IE caused by:
      - *Staphylococcus aureus*
      - Fungi
      - Drug resistant organisms

  - IE complicated by:
    - Heart block
    - Annular of aortic abscess
    - Destructing penetrative lesions
  - Persistent infection indicated by:
    - Persistent bacteremia
    - Fever > 5–7 days after initiating antimicrobial therapy
- Prosthetic valve endocarditis with relapsing infection following antibiotic course
- Complete removal of CIED system for documented infections of device or leads

❖ Class IIa indications:
- Early surgery (prior to completion of full antibiotic course) indicated for:
- IE with recurrent emboli
- IE with persistent vegetations despite appropriate antibiotic therapy
- Complete removal of CIED systems for:
- *S. aureus*/fungal infections even in absence of CIED infection
- Patients undergoing valve surgery

❖ Class IIb indications:
- Early surgery indicated for native valve IE with mobile vegetations > 10 mm

Antithrombotic Therapy

❖ Anticoagulant and antiplatelet therapy are ineffective in reducing risk of embolism in IE
❖ Thus, they are not indicated to reduce risk of embolic complications
❖ They may be used for patients at risk for thrombotic complication of other coexisting diseases

Dental Care

❖ Patients with IE should undergo dental evaluation and treatment for:
- Periodontal infections and abscesses
- Pulpal infections

❖ Corrective dental care should be done under antibiotic cover.

Surgical Removal of Devices

❖ Intravascular catheters: Removal is recommended for prior indwelling catheters
❖ CIEDs: removal of both pulse generator and leads is recommended when:
- TEE demonstrates valve or lead vegetation
- Positive blood culture for *S. aureus* or candida
- High grade bacteremia with CoNS or Cutibacterium
- CIED pocket infection

❖ AV fistula:
- Excision of fistula is not required in most patients
- Alternate vascular access may be required for hemodialysis in these patients
- Thus, treatment for infected AV fistulas should be individualized
- Septic emboli from the AV fistula may however warrant surgical removal

Infective Endocarditis Prophylaxis

IE Prophylaxis Recommended for Following Procedures

❖ Dental procedures involving:
- Manipulation of gingival tissues
- Manipulation of periapical region of teeth
- Involving perforation or suturing of oral mucosa
- Tooth extractions
- Dental infections, drainage of dental abscess
- Apicoectomy

❖ Procedures involving incision or biopsy of respiratory mucosa:
- Incision or biopsy of respiratory tract mucosa
- Tonsillectomy
- Adenoidectomy
- Bronchoscopy with biopsy

❖ For elective surgeries, coexisting UTIs should be treated before surgery
❖ For emergent procedures involving infected tissues:
- IE prophylaxis is given for patients at high risk for IE
- Prophylactic antibiotic should cover enterococcal species

IE Prophylaxis no Longer Recommended for Following Procedures

❖ Gastrointestinal or genitourinary procedures
❖ For bronchoscopic procedures not involving incision of respiratory mucosa
❖ For low-risk dental procedures:
- Routine anesthetic injections through non-infected tissues
- Taking dental radiographs
- Placement of removable prosthodontic or orthodontic appliances
- Adjustment of orthodontic appliances
- Placement of orthodontic brackets
- Shedding of deciduous teeth and bleeding from trauma to lips or oral mucosa

❖ For non-dental procedures like:
- Transesophageal echocardiography
- Esophago-gastroduodenoscopy
- Colonoscopy

- In patients with screws/pins/plates
- In patients with previous bypass surgeries/stents

IE Prophylaxis Recommended for Following Cardiac Conditions

- High risk patients for infective endocarditis:
  - Prior history of infective endocarditis
  - Patients with prosthetic cardiac valves including:
    - Mechanical valves
    - Bioprosthetic valves
    - Homograft valves
  - Prosthetic material during 1st 6 months after placement including:
    - Annuloplasty rings
    - Chords
  - Unrepaired and palliated (including shunts and conduits) cyanotic CHD patients
  - Completely repaired CHD (during first 6 months) with:
    - Device implantation
    - Prosthetic material
  - Repaired CHD with residual lesions:
    - At the site of repair of CHD
    - Adjacent to site of prosthetic patch/device (preventing endothelialization)
  - Cardiac transplantation patients who develop valvulopathy

IE Prophylaxis not Recommended for Following Cardiac Conditions

- Patients with isolated secundum ASD
- 6 months or more after ASD/VSD/PDA repair with no deficits
- Patients with physiological, functional/innocent heart murmurs, including aortic sclerosis
- Physiological MR without murmur and structurally normal valves
- Physiological TR/PR without murmur and structurally normal valves

Drugs for Prophylaxis

No.	Situation	Drug	Adults	Children	Timing
1.	Oral	Amoxicillin	2 g PO	50 mg/kg	30–60 mins prior
2.	Unable to take orally	Ampicillin	2 g IV	50 mg/kg	30–60 mins prior
		Cefazoline	1 g IV	50 mg/kg	30–60 mins prior
		Ceftriaxone	1 g IV	50 mg/kg	30–60 mins prior
3.	Allergic to penicillin, oral	Cephalexin	2 g PO	50 mg/kg	30–60 mins prior
		Clindamycin	600 mg PO	15–20 mg/kg	30–60 mins prior
		Azithromycin	500 mg PO	15 mg/kg	30–60 mins prior
		Clarithromycin	500 mg PO	15 mg/kg	30–60 mins prior
4.	Allergic to penicillin	Cefazoline	1 g IV	50 mg/kg	30–60 mins prior
	Unable to take oral	Ceftriaxone	1 g IV	50 mg/kg	30–60 mins prior
		Clindamycin	600 mg	15–20 mg/kg	30–60 mins prior
5.	Allergic to penicillin, MRSA	Vancomycin	1 g IV	15 mg/kg	30–60 mins prior

PERIOPERATIVE MANAGEMENT OF PATIENTS WITH PACEMAKER

Introduction

- Electromagnetic interference (EMI) refers to the disruption of function of an electronic device when in the vicinity of an electromagnetic field generated by an external source
- Cardiac implantable electronic device (CIED) may be affected by EMI from the electrosurgery unit (ESU)

Types of CIED

- Permanent pacemaker (PPM): for conduction system disturbances
- Artificial implantable cardioverter-defibrillator (AICD): for life threatening arrhythmias
- Cardiac resynchronization therapy (CRT): for treatment of heart failure (HF)
- Cardiac resynchronization therapy with defibrillator (CRTD): for treatment of HF

Indications for CIED

- Indications for pacemaker:
  - Symptomatic bradycardia from:
    - Sinus node disease
    - AV-node disease
  - Long QT syndrome
  - Hypertrophic obstructive cardiomyopathy
  - Dilated cardiomyopathy

Contd...

Contd...

- ❖ Indications for AICD:
  - Prophylactic use in patients with ischemic cardiomyopathy with:
    - EF ≤ 30% and NYHA class I symptoms
    - EF ≤ 35% and NYHA class II-III symptoms
  - Non-ischemic cardiomyopathy with EF < 35% and NYHA class II-III symptoms
  - Ventricular fibrillation/VT from non-reversible cause
  - Brugada syndrome (RBBB with ST-elevation in V_1-V_3
  - Arrhythmogenic right ventricular dysplasia
  - Long QT syndrome
  - Hypertrophic cardiomyopathy
  - Infiltrative cardiomyopathy

Types of CIED Leads

- ❖ Unipolar leads:
  - Single electrode is present at the lead tip which serves as the cathode
  - The pulse generator serves as the anode
  - More susceptible to EMI than bipolar leads
- ❖ Bipolar leads:
  - Two electrodes are present at the distal end serving as cathode and anode
  - Have a lower risk of EMI due to close spacing between electrodes.

NASPE/BPEG Code for Pacemakers

Position I Pacing chamber	*Position II* Sensing chamber	*Position III* Response to sensing	*Position IV* Programmability	*Position V* Multisite pacing
O = None	O = None	O = None	O = None	O = none
A = Atrium	A = Atrium	I = Inhibited	R = Rate modulation	A = Atrium
V = Ventricle	V = Ventricle	T = Triggered		V = Ventricle
D = Dual (A+V)	D = Dual (A + V)	D = Dual (T + I)		D = Dual (A + V)

NASPE/BPEG Generic Defibrillator Code

Position I Shock chamber	*Position II* Anti-tachycardia pacing chamber	*Position III* Tachycardia detection	*Position IV* Anti-bradycardia pacing chamber
O = None	O = None	E = Electrogram	O = None
A = Atrium	A = Atrium	H = Hemodynamic	A = Atrium
V = Ventricle	V = Ventricle		V = Ventricle
D = Dual (A+V)	D = Dual (A+V)		D = Dual (A+V)

Sources of Interference with CIED

- ❖ Electromagnetic interference (EMI) with electrosurgery units (ESUs):
  - Most common source of EMI
  - Monopolar ESU causes EMI more often than bipolar electrocautery
  - Coagulation mode (high-voltage) causes more EMI than cutting (low-voltage) mode
  - Risk increases when ESU is used close to:
    - Pulse generator
    - Leads of ICD or pacemaker
- ❖ EMI due to other operative equipment:
  - Nerve stimulators for nerve blocks
  - Nerve stimulators for neuromuscular monitoring
  - Evoked potential monitors (SSEP, MEP)
  - Transcutaneous electrical nerve stimulation
  - Radiofrequency scanners used to find retained surgical instruments
  - Magnetic resonance imaging
  - Radiofrequency ablation devices
  - Extracorporeal shock wave lithotripsy
  - Electroconvulsive therapy
- ❖ Mechanical interference:
  - CVC guidewires may cause movement of CIED electrodes
  - Large tidal volumes
  - Shivering/fasciculations
  - Vibrating bone saws during craniotomy may cause mechanical interference

Risks of EMI

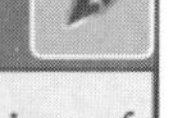

- ❖ Inhibition of pacing due to ventricular over-sensing of EMI
- ❖ Misinterpretation of EMI as tachyarrhythmia resulting in:
  - Delivery of inappropriate shocks
  - Anti-tachycardia pacing by AICD
- ❖ Direct damage to CIED altering ability to treat ventricular arrhythmias
- ❖ Myocardial burns
- ❖ Activation of noise reversion mode/electrical reset of device
- ❖ Total device failure with no output

Preoperative Evaluation

- Focused history:
  - History of:
    - HTN, DM, MI
    - Previous cardiac surgery
    - Cardiomyopathy
    - Peripheral vascular disease
    - Valvular heart disease
    - Congenital heart disease
  - History suggestive of pacemaker dysfunction: battery failure—
    - Vertigo
    - Syncopal attacks
- Focused examination:
  - Assess previous cardiac disease
  - Assess pacemaker function:
    - Type of pacemaker:
      - Demand: synchronous
      - Fixed: asynchronous
      - AICD
    - Determine pulse generator (PG) status:
      - Indication for placement
      - History of generator events
      - Last PG test date and battery status
      - Number and type of leads
    - Time of insertion:
      - Electrode displacement possible within 3 months of insertion
      - Battery failure if long term
    - Irregular heart rate: Competition of pacemaker with intrinsic heart rate
    - Check if pacing pulses are present and create paced beats
  - Device interrogation:
    - Patients should be examined for:
      - Underlying rhythm
      - Appropriate functioning of CIED
    - Device interrogation of CIED should be done:
      - Within 6 months prior to surgery for ICD
      - Within 12 months prior to surgery for conventional pacemaker
      - Within 3–6 months for cardiac resynchronization therapy device
  - Indications for CIED interrogation:
    - To disable anti-tachycardia shocks in ICDs when EMI is expected
    - Disable anti-tachycardia shocks when movement may be hazardous:
      - Intraocular surgery
      - Intracranial surgery
    - Produce asynchronous pacing in pacing-dependent patient
    - Increase paced heart rate in patients with bradycardia to augment CO
    - Disable mechanical sensor when surgery causes mechanical stimulation:
      - Breast surgery
      - Cardiac surgery
  - CIED reprogramming using magnet:
    - Magnets may be used for reprogramming if:
      - Response to magnet is known and effect is desirable
      - Patient is in supine position during surgery
      - Access to magnet is adequate:
        - Magnet may be observed
        - Magnet may be easily removed in case of arrhythmias
    - Responses to magnet application most commonly include:
      - Asynchronous pacing at fixed rate with fixed AV-delay for PM
      - Suspension of anti-tachycardia detection and therapy for ICDs
    - Advantages:
      - Changes in CIED function are reversible by removal of magnet
      - May not require placement of pacing/defibrillator pads
    - Disadvantages:
      - Does not result in asynchronous pacing with ICDs
      - Might fail to elicit response in obese patients
      - May be difficult to use in:
        - Lateral position
        - Prone position
      - Encroaches on surgical field if incision is close to pulse generator
  - Reprogramming using programming machine:
    - Useful to suspend anti-tachycardia therapy in ICDs
    - Advantages:
      - Allows change in pacing mode of ICD to asynchronous mode
      - Prevents intrusion of surgical field by magnet
    - Disadvantages:
      - Requires trained personnel
      - Requires transcutaneous pacing/defibrillator pads post-reprogramming
      - Changes in CIED function are not quickly reversible

- ❖ Cardiologists opinion of pacemaker function
- ❖ Investigations:
  - ECG:
    - For ischemia/previous MI
    - Confirm pacing capture: Pacing rate > intrinsic rate
    - No intrinsic rhythm: patient is pacemaker dependent
    - Only intrinsic rhythm: Test pacemaker function by converting to fixed mode with magnet
  - Chest X-ray:
    - Heart size, lung fields
    - Continuity of pacing leads, distal tip to be within cardiac cavity
    - Location of generator
    - Dual/single chamber
  - Serum potassium: Hyperkalemia increases pacing threshold
  - Acid base balance: May affect pacing threshold

Factors Affecting Pacing Function Perioperatively

- ❖ Electrolyte: Hypo/hyperkalemia
- ❖ Acid base balance: Acidosis/alkalosis
- ❖ Myocardial: Ischemia/acute infarction
- ❖ Drugs: Digoxin toxicity, catecholamines, antiarrhythmics
- ❖ Metabolic: Hypothermia, thyroid disturbances, hypoxia, hypoglycemia
- ❖ Factors which increase the pacing threshold:
  - Hyperkalemia
  - Acidosis, alkalosis
  - Hypoxia, hypoglycemia
  - Hypothermia
  - Anti-arrhythmic drugs
  - Thyroid disturbances

Preoperative Preparation

- ❖ Informed consent
- ❖ NPO orders
- ❖ Premedication with benzodiazepines/opioids
- ❖ Correct associated imbalances: potassium and acid base imbalances
- ❖ If electromechanical interference (EMI) unlikely, no special precaution is needed
- ❖ If EMI likely and CIED is a pacemaker:
  - Reprogram to asynchronous mode especially when pacing-dependent:
    - History of symptomatic bradycardia
    - Inadequate escape rhythm
    - History of AV-nodal ablation
  - Suspend rate adaptive functions
  - Reprogramming may be rarely done with a magnet placed over pulse generator
- ❖ If EMI likely and CIED is an AICD:
  - Suspend anti-tachyarrhythmia therapy function
  - Pacing mode may be changed to asynchronous mode in pacing-dependent patients
  - External pacing/defibrillator pads are placed prior to surgery

OT Preparation

- ❖ Suction apparatus
- ❖ Oxygen delivery apparatus
- ❖ Anesthetic drugs
- ❖ Monitors
- ❖ Chronotropic drugs kept ready
  - Atropine
  - Isoprenaline: 10–100 μg bolus or 0.05–0.2 μg/kg/min
  - Ephedrine
  - Adrenaline
- ❖ Temporary transcutaneous pacing should be made immediately available
- ❖ External cardioverter-defibrillator kept ready

Monitoring

- ❖ Pulse oximetry:
  - Continuous waveform display is important to detect mechanical systole
  - May be used as source of heart rate as ECG may display double-sensed values
- ❖ NIBP, urine output
- ❖ Continuous ECG:
  - Artifact filter is turned off to reduce high-frequency filtering
  - Selection of diagnostic mode preferred over monitor or filter modes
  - This allows display of high-frequency signals, including pacing spikes
  - Pacing artifacts may be misinterpreted as QRS complexes by the ECG monitor
  - This may result in display of erroneous heart rate
  - This occurs more commonly with unipolar leads
- ❖ Peripheral pulse to check cardiac output and pacemaker function
- ❖ Invasive monitoring if indicated for surgery
- ❖ Central venous catheterization:
  - Guidewire movement may cause:
    - Inhibition of pacemaker function
    - Delivery of inappropriate shock

- Thus, CIED should be reprogrammed prior to CVC placement:
  - Anti-tachycardia function suspended in ICDs
  - Asynchronous mode activated for pacemakers
- Continuous monitoring of ECG and pulse oximetry is required during insertion
- Displacement of CIED lead is common during first 3 months post-insertion
- Coronary sinus lead is the most prone to displacement during CVC insertion

❖ ABG for electrolytes

❖ Nerve stimulator: may interfere with pacing

❖ Beat to beat continuous CO monitor in HOCM

Choice of Anesthetic Technique

❖ Neuraxial blocks/regional anesthesia:
- Vasodilation may be poorly tolerated with fixed heart rate
- Avoid underhydration
- Caution during nerve blocks as nerve stimulator interferes with pacing

❖ General anesthesia:
- *Better preferred*
- TIVA is preferable when GA is used
- This is because:
  - Volatile agents in general increase AV delay and pacing threshold
  - Sevoflurane/isoflurane cause prolongation of QT interval

Considerations for GA in Patients with Pacemaker

❖ Placement of transcutaneous pacing/defibrillator pads:
- Placed before anti-tachycardia function of ICD has been disabled
- Allows treatment of malignant arrhythmias
- External defibrillator with pacing capability should be available
- Standard anterior-posterior location of pads preferred for left-sided CIEDs
- Anterolateral position may be used when AP position is not feasible

❖ Anesthetic agents:
- Anesthetic agents have minimal effect on CIED function
- Ketamine and etomidate cause myo-fasciculations which may interfere with pacing
- TIVA preferable as volatile anesthetics increase AV delay and pacing threshold
- N_2O accumulates in pacemaker generator pockets
- High doses of anesthetics which exacerbate bradycardia are avoided such as:
  - Dexmedetomidine
  - Opioids such as fentanyl
- In patients with prolonged QT-interval:
  - Agents prolonging QT-interval are avoided:
    - Haloperidol
    - High dose sevoflurane and isoflurane
    - Ondansetron
  - This reduces the risk of polymorphic VT due to QT prolongation
- Desflurane and enflurane do not have any effect on QT interval
- Caution with succinylcholine as:
  - Acute increase in potassium causes increase in pacing threshold
  - Myopotentials during fasciculations may be abnormally sensed

❖ Avoid underhydration as compensatory tachycardia to maintain CO is absent

❖ Considerations for diathermy/electrocautery interference:
- Risk of EMI with surgeries above the umbilicus are high
- Thus, anti-tachycardia therapy has to be suspended in above-umbilicus surgery
- Risk of EMI is negligible with surgeries below the umbilicus
- Unipolar cautery is the most common source of EMI
- Thus, it causes EMI especially in patients with unipolar CIED leads
- Therefore, use of bipolar cautery is recommended
- Ultrasonic/harmonic scalpel:
  - Avoids EMI
  - Also facilitates coagulation of tissue with minimal EMI
- Position of return plate/electrode pad of ESU:
  - Current path from ESU to pad should not cross CIED leads/generator
  - Plane described by return plate and active electrode of electrocautery is perpendicular to plane described by pacemaker and pacemaker electrode
- Similar considerations apply to pads of nerve stimulators and TENS
- Cutting mode (lower voltage) is used as it causes least EMI
- Smallest current intensity required for cutting is used

- ESU is used in short bursts: one second for every 10 seconds
- Avoid using electrocautery within 15 cm of the device/leads

Considerations for GA in Patients with AICD

- All ICDs have pacemakers incorporated into circuitry
- Preoperative assessment of cardiac condition
- Cardiology opinion for:
  - ICD interrogation
  - Programming device to no-response mode
- Preoperative preparation:
  - Signals from electrocautery may be misinterpreted as dysrhythmias
  - Convert AICD to no-response either by programming or using magnet
  - Once converted, device will not deliver therapy secondary to misinterpretation
  - Convert pacemaker to asynchronous mode so that it is not inhibited by cautery
  - Do not use electrocautery when AICD is programmed to sense and deliver therapy
  - AICDs must be programmed to respond to a magnet
  - Magnet will not change bradycardia related pacing parameters in the ICD
  - Apply patches for external defibrillation when ICD is programmed to no response
  - Ensure these pads are as far away as possible from device
  - Pads not to be in same plane as device and electrodes
- If PA catheter monitoring is required:
  - Discuss with the cardiologist
  - Document the need for PA catheter and discussion with cardiologist
  - Discuss possibility of dislodgement of ICD electrodes with patient
  - Maintain sterile technique, consider antibiotics before inserting lines
- Continue antiarrhythmic drugs until time of surgery
- No clear preferences of anesthetic technique between regional/general anesthesia
- If intraoperative arrhythmias occur:
  - Treat intraoperative causes to prevent recurrence
  - If dysrhythmia continues and *magnet has been used* to create no response mode:
    - Remove magnet from ICD
    - Allow ICD to charge and deliver a response
  - If dysrhythmia continues and ICD has been *programmed* to no response mode:
    - Reprogram ICD to deliver a response
    - Alternatively, use external defibrillation directly
    - Place external defibrillation paddles in antero-posterior location
    - Deliver sufficient shock
    - External pacing may be required if ICD is damaged with the shock
- While transporting the patient from OR:
  - Monitor patients ECG
  - Be prepared to deliver external defibrillation
  - Interrogate and reprogram ICD when patient has entered PACU

Postoperative Care

- Immediate postoperative period:
  - Check pacemaker functions, if procedure involved cardioversion and diathermy
  - Monitor cardiac rate and rhythm continuously
  - Back up pacing and cardioversion/defibrillation capability
- Postoperative restoration of CIED function:
  - Use cardiologist help
  - Interrogate to assess function
  - Reprogram appropriate setting
  - If CIED is AICD, restore all anti-tachycardia therapy

Treatment of Pacemaker Failure

Rate	Response
Adequate to maintain BP	Oxygen, airway control
	Place magnet over pacemaker
	Atropine, if sinus bradycardia
Severe bradycardia and hypotension	Oxygen, airway control
	Place magnet over pacemaker
	Transcutaneous/transvenous pacing if magnet fails
	Atropine if sinus bradycardia
	Isoproterenol to increase ventricular rate
No escape rhythm	Cardiopulmonary resuscitation
	Place magnet over pacemaker
	Transcutaneous/transvenous pacing if magnet fails
	Isoproterenol to increase ventricular rate

Emergency Cardioversion/Defibrillation

- Terminate all EMI sources
- Remove magnet to enable defibrillation pads

- ❖ Minimize current flow through pulse generator/ leads
- ❖ Defibrillation pads placed as far away from pulse generator as possible
- ❖ Defibrillation pads placed perpendicular to major axis pulse generator/leads
- ❖ To extent possible, pads placed in anterior-posterior location
- ❖ Use clinically appropriate energies

Complications

- ❖ Failure to fire
- ❖ Failure to capture
- ❖ ***Pacemaker syndrome*** seen with VVI mode
- ❖ Pacemaker tachycardia

Special Considerations

- ❖ TURP:
  - Use harmonic scalpel
  - Cutting mode may cause electromagnetic interference
  - Use cautery in short bursts
  - Coagulation mode does not interfere
  - May have to convert to fixed mode if diathermy plate placed around chest
  - Possibility of random reprogramming due to EMI
- ❖ Direct current electrical cardioversion:
  - Use lowest possible energy
  - Paddles placed as far away from generator as possible (> 10 cm)
  - Paddles placed perpendicular to line between generator and lead tip
  - Follow up with formal pacemaker interrogation
  - Modern CIEDs are fitted with Zener diodes to prevent damage from DC shocks
- ❖ MRI:
  - During MRI a large radiofrequency signal 30–3000 Hz is generated
  - This may induce lead heating of CIED up to 89°C leading to:
    - Myocardial thermal injury
    - Changes in pacing properties:
      - Inhibition of pacing
      - Rapid pacing induced by radiofrequency signal
  - For majority of older CIEDs, MRI is unsafe
  - Many modern CIEDs have been designed to be MRI conditional
  - MRI is contraindicated in pacing dependent patients
  - When MRI performed:
    - Imaging must be performed in 1.5 Tesla magnet
    - CIED is interrogated before and after the MRI
- ❖ Radiotherapy:
  - Ionizing radiation used in radiation therapy may result in pacemaker damage:
    - Temporary change resulting in oversensing
    - Reset to factory settings
    - Complete device failure
  - ≥ 1000 rads causes pacemaker damage
  - Non-neutron producing treatment is preferred to reduce risk of device reset
  - Pulse generator and leads should be outside radiotherapy field
  - Surgical relocation of pulse generator should be considered if EMI is inevitable
  - Verify pulse generator function before and after therapy
  - CIED is evaluated at weekly intervals in case of recurrent therapy
- ❖ Extracorporeal shock wave lithotripsy:
  - Used to treat upper urinary tract calculi
  - Piezoelectric crystals for rate-adaptive pacing may be damaged by ESWL waves
  - < 16 KV shock energy to be used
  - Do not focus lithotripsy beam near pulse generator
  - Pacing mode is changed to VOO or DOO to prevent EMI from ESWL waves

PERIOPERATIVE BETA-BLOCKADE

Introduction

Beta blockers are among the most commonly prescribed drugs and are frequently taken by patients about to undergo surgery.

Classification

- ❖ Nonselective beta blockers: act at β_1 and β_2 receptors
  - Propranolol, sotalol, timolol
  - Nadolol, oxprenolol
  - Pindolol, penbutalol
- ❖ Cardioselective β_1 blockers:
  - Atenolol, esmolol
  - Betaxolol, metaprolol
  - Bevantolol
- ❖ Selective β_2 blockers:
  - Butoxamine
  - ICI-118551

Intrinsic Sympathomimetic Activity

- Exert partial agonist effect at the receptor while blocking access to more potent agonist
- Thus, may behave like conventional beta blockers when sympathetic activity is high
- This property may protect against harmful effects of β blockers withdrawal
- β blockers with Intrinsic Sympathomimetic Acitivity (ISA):
    - Acebutalol, dilevalol, pindolol
    - Carteolol, oxprenolol
    - Celiprolol, penbutalol

Uses of Beta Blockers

- Treatment of essential HTN
- Treatment of angina pectoris and acute coronary syndromes
- Suppression of cardiac arrhythmias
- Treatment of congestive cardiac failure
- Prevention of excessive sympathetic nervous system activity: intubation, incision
- Preoperative preparation of hyperthyroid and pheochromocytoma patients
- Treatment of migraine, closed angle glaucoma
- Control of *tet spells*

Cardioprotective Effects of Perioperative Beta Blockade

- Reduction in heart rate and contractility
- Reduced myocardial oxygen demand and consumption
- Increased coronary flow due to increased diastolic time
- Redistribution of coronary blood flow to ischemic areas
- Enhanced plaque stability due to reduction in shear forces
- Anti-arrhythmic effects
- Possible anti-inflammatory effects:
    - Limit leukocyte recruitment
    - Reduce monocyte activation
    - Limit production of free radicals and metalloproteinase activity
    - Prevent release of growth factors
    - Antiapoptotic actions

Indications for Initiation of Perioperative Beta Blockade

- Patients with known CAD
- Patients with peripheral vascular disease
- Patients with more than 2 risk factors for CAD:
    - Age more than 65 years
    - Cigarette smoking
    - Diabetes
    - Hypertension
    - Cholestrol > 240 mg/dL
- Moderate to high risk surgery
- RCRI score of ≥ 3
- Vascular surgery with a positive stress test

Contraindications to Initiation of Perioperative Beta Blockade

- Low risk surgery
- RCRI score < 2
- Emergency surgery
- Beta blocker allergy
- Bradycardia (resting heart rate < 60 bpm)
- Second degree AV block
- Severe COPD

Current Guidelines: ACC-AHA 2014 guidelines

- Class I indications:
    - Beta blocker therapy should be continued in patients who have been on beta blockers chronically (LOE B)
- Class IIa indications:
    - Reasonable for beta blocker therapy management after surgery to be guided by clinical circumstances, independent of when the agent was started (LOE B)
- Class IIb indications:
    - Reasonable to begin preoperative beta blockers in:
        - Patients determined to be at intermediate or high risk for MI in preoperative risk stratification tests (LOE C)
        - Patients with 3 or more RCRI risk factors (LOE B)
    - In those in whom beta blocker therapy is initiated preoperatively, it is reasonable to begin therapy more than 1 day prior to surgery in order to give ample time to assess safety and tolerability (LOE B)
- Class III indications: Harm: LOE B
    - Beta blocker therapy should not be started on the day of surgery

Choice of Beta Blocker Therapy

- Cardioselective beta blockers are associated with better outcomes
- Atenolol and bisoprolol are preferred compared to metoprolol
- Long acting and fixed dose beta blockers not preferred due to difficulty in titration
- In anemic patients, selective β_2 blockade causes worse outcomes
- Patients using metoprolol may be more susceptible to bradycardia

Beta Blocker Dosages

No.	Drug	Oral Dose	IV Dose
1.	Atenolol	50–100 mg QID	
2.	Metoprolol	50–100 mg QID	5 mg Q5 min (up to 3 times)
3.	Propranolol	60 mg QID	0.1 mg/kg (maximum)
4.	Labetolol	100–600 mg QID	1–2 mg/kg
5.	Esmolol		50–300 µg/kg/min
6.	Carvedilol	25–50 mg BD	15 mg

Guidelines for Perioperative Beta Blockade

- Uses:
  - Beta blockers should be continued in those already taking them for:
    - Hypertension
    - Angina
    - Arrhythmias
  - β blockers like labetolol and esmolol can be used during intubation and preventing surgical stress response
  - Attempts to discontinue preoperative β blocker therapy causes:
    - Increased risk of rebound tachycardia, with or without AF
    - Myocardial infarction in patients with CAD
- Dosage:
  - Dosages for all individuals is not the same
  - Dosage is individualized according to patient and type of surgery
  - β blocker dose titrated to heart rate and blood pressure
  - Heart rate should be titrated to ***non-ischemia inducing heart rate***, 60–80 bpm
- Administration:
  - Initiation of beta blockers preoperatively should be done:
    - Ideally 1 month prior to surgery
    - At least 1 week prior to surgery
  - Continuation of beta blockers is recommended up to time of surgery
  - Therapy should be continued in IV form when GI absorption is in question
  - If β blocker has been omitted in preoperative regimen, esmolol and labetolol used
  - Beta blocker therapy should be continued for at least 30 days post surgery

Controversy of Perioperative Beta-Blockade

- Initial evidence for prophylactic beta blockade from studies in the 1990s were favourable
- Later studies showed no improvement or worse outcomes with β blocker therapy
- ***MSPIRG trial***: Positive result:
  - Enrolled 200 patients with, or at risk for CAD, undergoing non-cardiac surgery
  - Patients were randomized to receive atenolol or placebo
  - Atenolol was started PO or IV on the day of surgery and continued till discharge
  - 55% lower mortality was seen in patients treated with atenolol
  - Findings of the study:
    - Atenolol group had lesser incidence of perioperative ischemia
    - There was no difference in the short-term rates of MI or death
    - There was no improvement in in-hospital perioperative outcomes
    - However, mortality rate was lower at 6 months and 2 years post discharge
  - Concluded that:
    - Patients at risk for CAD had reduced mortality and MACE after treatment with atenolol
    - These beneficial effects lasted for up to 2 years after surgery
- ***DECREASE trial***: positive result:
  - 112 patients undergoing vascular surgery with abnormal stress echo were chosen
  - These patients were randomized into a study group and placebo group
  - Bisoprolol was started 1 month prior to surgery in the study group
  - Drug was continued for 1 month post surgery in the study group
  - Study was terminated prematurely
  - This was because the study group had 90% lower rate of MI and 30-day mortality
  - However, the study was criticized for:
    - Limited number of patients enrolled
    - Serious shortcomings in procedure used to obtain consent from patients
    - Scientifically inaccurate data collection
    - Publication based on unreliable data
- ***POBBLE study***: negative result:
  - Enrolled 103 patients who had no history of MI, undergoing vascular surgery
  - Metaprolol 50 mg given PO Q12H from time of admission till 7 days post surgery
  - Myocardial ischemia was seen in almost one-third of the patients after surgery
  - Study found no reduction in 30-day cardiovascular mortality rate
  - However, shorter duration of hospital stay was noted in the study

- *DIPOM study*: Negative result:
  - Diabetic Postoperative Mortality and Morbidity trial
  - Randomized 921 diabetic patients undergoing major non-cardiac surgery
  - 50 mg metoprolol PO started on the evening prior to surgery
  - Second dose given 2 hours prior to surgery
  - Metoprolol was continued Q24H till 8 days post surgery
  - Study found that there was no statistically significant effect on:
    - All cause mortality
    - Non-fatal cardiac morbidity
    - Acute myocardial infarction
    - Unstable angina
    - Congestive cardiac failure
  - Concluded that β-blocker therapy had no benefits in diabetics
- *POISE trial*: Mixed results:
  - Conducted in 8351 patients with atherosclerotic disease for non-cardiac surgery
  - Fixed dose SR-metaprolol 100 mg was started 2–4 hours prior to surgery
  - SR-metaprolol was continued once daily for 30 days post surgery
  - Outcomes were compared with a placebo treatment group
  - Significant reduction in outcome of cardiovascular events was seen
  - 30% reduction in rate of perioperative MI was reported
  - However, there was an increased risk of 30-day all cause mortality and stroke
  - The publication of negative results of this study caused a decline in β blocker use
  - Study was criticized for starting high doses shortly prior to surgery

Adverse Effects of Beta Blockade

- Stroke:
  - First statistically significant risk of stroke reported in POISE trial
  - Mechanisms:
    - As a side effect of hypotension and bradycardia seen with beta blockers
    - Cerebral vasodilatation may be blocked by beta blocker therapy precipitating ischemia
- Life threatening bradycardia/asystole
- Congestive cardiac failure
- Glucose intolerance/insulin resistance in diabetes
- Raynauds phenomenon precipitated if preexisting peripheral vascular disease
- MI on sudden withdrawal
- Uncontrolled HTN if used without prior α-blockade in pheochromocytoma
- Bronchospasm

ELECTIVE CARDIOVERSION AND DEFIBRILLATION

Introduction

- Cardioversion uses shock delivery synchronized with the QRS complexes on the ECG
- Defibrillation utilizes non-synchronized shock delivery randomly during cardiac cycle
- First used in 1952 by Gurvich using alternating current for transthoracic defibrillation
- Direct current defibrillators introduced into clinical practice by Lown in 1962

Mechanism

- Cardioversion delivers synchronized shock which depolarizes entire myocardium
- Tissue involved in re-entrant circuits is also depolarized
- This makes the reentrant circuit refractory to further depolarization
- Thus, the re-entrant circuit is no longer able to propagate or sustain re-entry
- This terminates arrhythmias resulting from a single re-entrant circuit such as:
  - Atrial flutter
  - Atrioventricular nodal re-entrant tachycardia (AVNRT)
  - Atrioventricular re-entrant tachycardia
  - Monomorphic ventricular tachycardia
- Controversy exists regarding mechanism for arrhythmias with multiple reentrant cicuits
- Critical mass hypothesis:
  - Certain mass of myocardium must be non-refractory to sustain arrhythmias
  - Defibrillation results in uniform depolarization of entire myocardium
  - This results in termination of the arrhythmia
  - Critical mass hypothesis proposes that critical mass of myocardium has to be depolarized simultaneously to achieve defibrillation
- Upper limit of vulnerability (ULV) hypothesis:
  - Low energy shocks may abolish small areas of localized re-entry

- However, they may stimulate other areas of myocardium during vulnerable period
- This results in new areas of localized re-entry which cause fibrillation
- Thus, for effective defibrillation, current above upper limit of vulnerability should be used

❖ Synchronization:
- Differentiates cardioversion from defibrillation
- Following contraction, myocytes become unresponsive to electrical stimulation
- This is known as the refractory period and is of 2 types:
  - Absolute refractory period: stimuli cannot initiate re-entry circuits
  - Relative refractory period:
    - Electrical stimuli can initiate re-entry circuits
    - Termed as the vulnerable period
    - Corresponds to upstroke and peak of T-wave on ECG
- Cardioversion shock is synchronized with R-wave of QRS complex
- Therefore, electrically vulnerable period is avoided

Indications

❖ Emergency re-establishment of an organized electrical rhythm:
- Hemodynamically unstable polymorphic VT
- Ventricular fibrillation
- Pulseless VT
- Narrow or wide QRS complex tachycardia associated with:
  - Hemodynamic instability
  - Chest pain
  - Pulmonary edema

❖ Elective re-establishment of sinus rhythm:
- Atrial fibrillation
- Atrial flutter
- Hemodynamically stable refractory VT

Contraindications

❖ Digitalis induced tachyarrhythmias due to risk of inducing ventricular fibrillation

❖ Sinus tachycardia

❖ Rhythms unresponsive to electric shock (multifocal atrial tachycardia)

❖ Stable atrial flutter with atrial clot

❖ Stable atrial fibrillation with atrial clot

❖ Specific advance directive such as do-not-resuscitate orders

Complications

❖ Post shock arrhythmias:
- Bradycardia, asystole
- Atrial/ventricular ectopics
- AV block
- Ventricular tachyarrhythmias

❖ Transient ST elevation with normal cardiac enzymes usually

❖ Unsuccessful cardioversion due to:
- Metabolic imbalance
- Hypovolemia
- Hypothermia
- Tension pneumothorax
- Hemothorax
- Tamponade

❖ Cutaneous burns at the paddle application site

❖ Myocardial damage

❖ Skeletal muscle injury, rhabdomyolysis, renal failure

❖ Systemic/pulmonary embolism in AF

Factors Affecting Defibrillation and Cardioversion

❖ Device related factors:
- Electrode position:
  - Two commonly used electrode positions are:
    - Anterolateral orientation
    - Anteroposterior orientation:
      - Requires lesser energy
      - Higher success rate
  - Electrode position should be individualized
  - Faulty electrode position may be a cause of defibrillation failure
- Pad size:
  - Important determinant of transthoracic current flow
  - Larger paddle is associated with:
    - Decrease in transthoracic resistance
    - Decreased myocardial necrosis
- Type of waveform:
  - Biphasic devices reverse polarity 5–10 seconds after discharge begins
  - Biphasic waveforms:
    - More efficient
    - Require lesser energy
- Defibrillation energy:
  - Biphasic defibrillators require lower energy for defibrillation
  - Thus, arrhythmia-appropriate energy has to be chosen for defibrillation
  - Ramping of energy levels is required in refractory arrhythmias

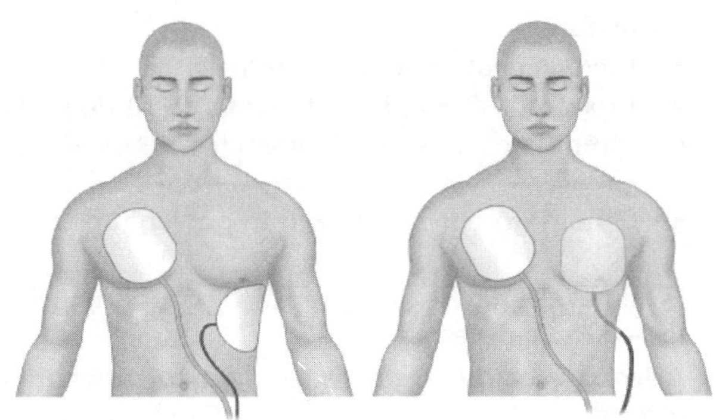

Fig. 44: Defibrillator pad position.

- Patient related factors:
    - Transthoracic impedance:
        - Impedance causes dissipation of energy to:
            - Thoracic cage
            - Lungs
            - Other organs of the chest
        - Impedance is determined by:
            - Electrode-skin interface
            - Inter-electrode distance
            - Electrode pressure
            - Phase of ventilation
            - Myocardial tissue properties
    - Type of arrhythmia:
        - Atrial flutter and ventricular tachycardia require lesser energy
        - Atrial fibrillation and ventricular fibrillation require higher energy
    - Duration of arrhythmia: Efficacy is reduced with prolonged duration
    - Use of antiarrhythmic drugs:
        - Drugs causing increased energy requirements: lidocaine
        - Drugs causing reduced energy requirements:
            - Adrenaline
            - Sotalol
            - Ibutilide

Preoperative Assessment

- Patient's associated conditions should be stabilized
- Patient may be hemodynamically unstable
- Serum electrolytes for hypokalemia
- Thyroid function tests as hyperthyroidism may cause AF
- ECG taken for detecting new arrhythmias
- Echocardiography to exclude LA clots especially if atrial fibrillation
- Digoxin therapy is commonly stopped prior to the procedure
- Ensure prior anticoagulation for 4 weeks duration for AF/flutter ≥ 2–3 days duration
- Anticoagulation continued for 4 weeks after cardioversion
- Preoperative antiarrhythmic drugs are continued on the day of procedure
- Antiarrhythmic drugs used are:
    - Procainamide
    - Amiodarone
    - Quinidine

Preoperative Preparation

- NPO guidelines:
    - Solids 6 hours
    - Clear fluids 2 hours
- IV access is secured for administration of drugs
- Sedative premedication is usually not required due to short duration of procedure
- Anti-aspiration prophylaxis:
    - Metaclopramide 0.1–0.2 mg/kg IV
    - Ranitidine 1–2 mg/kg IV
- Antiarrhythmic drugs started: procainamide, amiodarone
- Continue warfarin therapy

Dosage: Use only lowest possible energies

- Synchronized cardioversion:
    - Atrial fibrillation:
        - 120 to 200 J biphasic synchronized cardioversion
        - 200 J monophasic synchronized cardioversion
    - *Atrial flutter and PSVT*: 50–100 J biphasic synchronized cardioversion
    - VT: 100 J synchronized cardioversion increased in stepwise fashion
- VF: Unsynchronized defibrillation dose 200 J
- In pediatrics:
    - *Synchronized cardioversion*: 1 J/kg increased to 4 J/kg
    - *Unsynchronized defibrillation*: 4 J/kg

Equipment Preparation

- Defibrillator: Manual/semiautomated/fully automated
- Paddles, self-adhesive defibrillation pads
- Conductive gel or gel pads for defibrillation paddles
- Pacing wires: Transvenous and transcutaneous
- Resuscitation equipment:
    - Bag and mask device
    - Airway devices

- Suction
- IV cannulation
- Emergency drugs

Monitoring

- Pulse oximetry
- BP
- ECG:
  - Lead which produces large R/S wave and small T wave chosen
  - Obtain 12-lead ECG before and after delivery of shocks

Ideal Anesthetic Agent for Cardioversion

- Rapidly achieve the desired depth of anesthesia
- Allow early emergence
- Should not cause respiratory side effects
- Should not have arrhythmogenic potential

Anesthetic Agents Used

- No consistent difference exists between the anesthetic agents used for cardioversion
- Traditional anesthetic agents:
  - Propofol
  - Etomidate
  - Thiopentone
- Sedative agents:
  - Midazolam
  - Diazepam
- Inhalational agents:
  - Sevoflurane
  - Isoflurane

Position

- Supine position
- Propped-up position may be preferred in obese patients
- Chest is exposed and prepared to ensure adequate electrode contact
- Chest should be wiped dry to ensure absence of water following preparation
- Water/sweat reduces electrode adhesion on the chest

Procedure

- Synchronization mode of cardioverter is activated
- Markers on the R-waves indicating adequate R-wave recognition are identified
- Thus, proper R-wave synchronization is ensured prior to shock delivery
- Induction:
  - Preoxygenation for 3–5 minutes
  - Propofol 1–2 mg/kg with fentanyl 10–20 µg IV
  - Etomidate 0.3 mg/kg better choice as induction agent
  - Opioid dose is minimized to prevent apnea and PONV
- When eyelash reflex lost, apply the coupling gel followed by paddles
- Adequate coupling gel is applied to prevent fire hazard
- Approximately 12-kg pressure is applied to each paddle
- Position of paddles:
  - Antero-posterior position:
    - *Anterior*: apical area
    - *Posterior*: interscapular area
  - Antero-lateral position:
    - *Lateral*: 5th intercostal space along mid-clavicular line
    - *Anterior*: second intercostal space right of sternum
- Oxygen mask is adjusted to ensure delivery of oxygen away from patients chest
- The energy level of shock to be delivered is selected
- The charge button is pressed on the unit or the paddles
- Confirm that no one is touching the patient or cart before proceeding
- Synchronized shock of the selected strength is delivered by pressing discharge button
- Monitor is checked for return to sinus rhythm
- For persistent arrhythmias, energy level of shock is increased and procedure repeated
- 12-lead ECG is taken at the end of the procedure on successful return to sinus rhythm
- Ventilate patient with 100% O_2 until fully awake/able to maintain patient airway
- Nasopharyngeal airway may be used to maintain airway patency

Postoperative Management

Monitors

- Pulse oximetry
- ECG: obtain 12-lead ECG
- Noninvasive blood pressure.

Complications

- Post-shock arrhythmias
- VF and cardiac arrest
- Thromboembolism to cerebral emboli

- Pulmonary edema
- Aspiration pneumonia

NEGATIVE PRESSURE PULMONARY EDEMA

Introduction

- Phenomenon of alveolar capillary membrane injury after exposure of alveoli to subatmospheric pressures leading to abnormal accumulation of fluid in extravascular compartment of lung
- Also called:
  - ***Post-obstructive pulmonary edema***
  - ***Laryngospasm induced pulmonary edema***

Incidence

- 0.05–0.1% incidence
- Mortality as high as 40%
- Occurrence is under-recognized and often misdiagnosed

Risk Factors

- Patient related:
  - Male sex, young age
  - Athletes who can generate negative intrathoracic pressures up to -140 cmH_2O
  - Pediatric patients due to complaint chest wall
  - Obstructure sleep apnea, upper airway obstruction, obesity
  - Pharyngeal tumor mass, mediastinal tumor
  - Enlarged tonsils, epiglottitis, croup, Ludwigs angina
  - Vocal cord paralysis
  - Foreign body aspiration
- Surgery related:
  - Nasal, oral or pharyngeal surgeries
  - Chest tube suction
  - Temporo-mandibular joint arthroscopy
- Anesthesia related:
  - Anatomically difficult intubation
  - Laryngospasm
  - ET tube obstruction
  - ET tube and LMA biting
  - Tongue fall

Precipating Factors

- Upper airway obstruction
- Laryngospasm
- *Mullers maneuver*: Inspiration against closed glottis
- Sudden release of obstruction

Pathophysiology

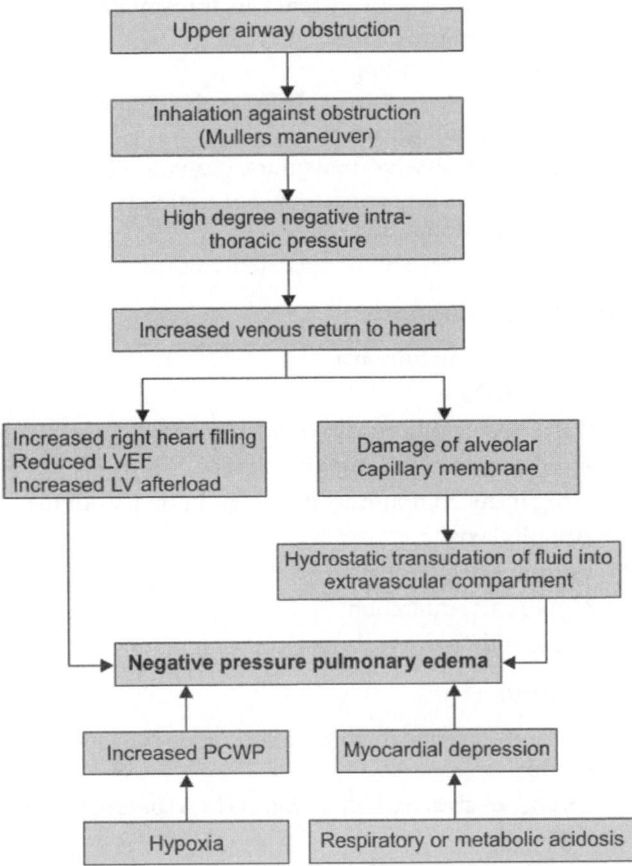

Clinical Features

- Usually presents immediately but may occur several hours later
- Rapid onset respiratory distress following occurrence of airway obstruction on emergence from general anesthesia
- Dyspnea and hemoptysis with pink frothy sputum is *hallmark*
- Tachycardia, hypertension and diaphoresis due to sympathetic activation
- Rales and wheeze (due to fluid compressed airway)
- Clinical and X-ray features usually resolve in 24 hours

Investigations

- Hypoxemia on pulse oximetry
- Hypoxia, metabolic, respiratory or combined acidosis on ABG
- Chest X-ray shows two phases of edema:
  - Intestitial edema
    - ***Kerley lines***
    - Peribronchial cuffing

- Subpleural effusion
- Occurs with increase in transmural arterial pressure of 15–25 mm Hg

• Alveolar flooding:
  - ***White-out areas***: Diffuse alveolar and interstitial infiltration
  - Occurs when transmural pressure > 25 mm Hg
  - Nodular opacities which coalesce into frank consolidation
  - Cardiac silhouette usually normal

Differential Diagnosis

- Aspiration pneumonia
- ALI/ARDS
- Cardiogenic pulmonary edema
- Fluid overload pulmonary edema
- Drug induced non-cardiogenic pulmonary edema
- Anaphylaxis
- Pulmonary embolism
- Myocardial infarction
- Pneumothorax

Prevention

- Prevent laryngeal stimulation and postoperative stridor
- *Laryngotracheal topical anesthesia* (LTA) before intubation with:
  - 4% lidocaine solution
  - 10% lidocaine spray
- IV lidocaine 1–1.5 mg/kg 90 seconds before intubation

Treatment

- Early diagnosis
- Oxygen supplementation:
  - 100% oxygen via face mask
  - CPAP/nasal bilevel positive airway pressure (BIPAP)
  - Apply early PEEP to promote alveolar expansion
  - Endotracheal intubation with positive pressure ventilation
- Diuretics:
  - Role is uncertain yet
  - Furosemide 1 mg/kg IV can be tried
- Break laryngospasm early:
  - ***Larsons maneuver***
  - Racemic epinephrine nebulization: 1 mg of 1: 1000 solution in 5 mL normal saline
  - Succinylcholine 0.5 mg/kg IV or 0.1–0.2 mg/kg if patient is biting ET tube
  - Dexamethasone/hydrocortisone

Prognosis: Self limited, with X-ray clearing and normalization of ABG occurring within 24–72 hours.

ANESTHESIA FOR OPCAB

Introduction

- Acronym for off pump coronary artery bypass (OPCAB) grafting
- Coronary artery stenosis is bypassed with an arterial or venous graft without using CPB
- Accounts for almost 22% of all coronary revascularization procedures

Key Surgical Features

- Operation on beating heart
- Absence of cardiopulmonary bypass
- Use of epicardial stabilizer (octopus/vortex stabilizer)
- Multiple vessel grafting
- Temporary interruption of coronary blood flow during anastomosis of distal vessels
- Use of intracoronary shunts
- Fast-track extubation either in OT/shortly thereafter

Surgical Steps

- Midline sternotomy
- Graft conduits are harvested and may include:
  - Internal mammary arteries (of both sides)
  - Saphenous veins
  - Radial artery of non-dominant hand
- Heparin 2 mg/kg before IMA clipping and isolation
- ACT is done after 3–5 minutes
- Pericardium is reflected to form the pericardial cradle
- Epicardial stabilizers are applied:
  - Used to stabilize the target vessel and surrounding myocardium
  - Currently used suction based stabilization devices include:
    - Octopus stabilizer (Medtronic Octopus system)
    - Starfish (Starfish Heart Positioner)
    - Octopus 3 Stabilizer (Medtronic inc., Minneapolis)
- Surgical visualization is optimized by using a blower or mister:
  - Sterile irrigation fluid is aerosolized and blown onto the site of anastomosis
  - This is done using carbon dioxide gas

- ❖ Arteriotomy is performed on the target coronary artery
- ❖ Intra-coronary shunts are used to maintain coronary flow as anastomosis is performed
- ❖ The distal anastomosis is completed on all the target coronary vessels
- ❖ Sequence of distal anastomosis depends upon the severity of disease
- ❖ Usually, the more severely stenosed coronary artery is anastomosed first
- ❖ This is because of the presence of collaterals from less severely diseased vessels which:
  - Maintain supply to area of more severe stenosis during anastomosis
  - Supply area of less severe stenosis after anastomosis due to pressure differential
- ❖ Distal anastomosis of coronaries on posterior aspect of heart requires lifting of the heart
- ❖ This results in verticalization of the heart and hemodynamic compromise
- ❖ This is followed by proximal anastomosis of the free end of conduits such as:
  - Saphenous vein graft
  - Radial artery graft
- ❖ The free ends are anastomosed to the ascending aorta using side-biting clamps
- ❖ Proximal anastomosis is not required for internal mammary artery grafts
- ❖ This is because the proximal end is not free and remains connected to the subclavian artery
- ❖ Heparin is reversal with protamine following proximal anasotmosis
- ❖ This is followed by hemostasis and chest closure in layers
- ❖ Surgical considerations during anastomosis include:
  - Adequate exposure of anastomosis site
  - Limit cardiac motion during anastomosis
  - Preserve myocardial viability during coronary flow interruption

Advantages of OPCAB

Feature	OPCAB	CABG
Intraoperative		
Ischemia	Transient, coronary	Global myocardial ischemia
Heparin dose	Less	More
Postoperative		
Arrhythmias (atrial fibrillation)	Rare	Common
Use of antiarrhythmics	Less used	More used
Post-procedure cardiac pacing	Less used	More used
Inotropic support	Fewer required	More required
Perioperative bleeding	Less	More
Perioperative transfusion	Less	More
Re-exploration for bleeding	Less	More
Metabolic disturbances	Less	More
Wound infection	Less	More
Length of ICU stay	Less	More
Length of hospital stay	Less	More
Cost	Less	More
Side Effects of CPB		
Drug pharmacokinetics	More predictable	Less predictable (on CPB)
Intraoperative awareness	Less	More
Hemodilution	Less	More
Complement activation, SIRS	Avoided	Present
Neuropsychiatric impairment	Reduced (< 1%)	More (2–3%)
Lung injury	Less	More
Troponin I	Less released	More released
Renal function	Better preserved	Impaired
Platelet dysfunction	Less	More

Patient Selection

- ❖ OPCAB can be performed in most patients who would be suitable for CABG
- ❖ However, it is preferred over CABG in patients at risk for injury with CPB like:
  - Advanced age
  - History of CVA/TIA/neuropsychiatric patient
  - Respiratory disease (COPD)
  - Impaired liver function
  - Impaired renal function/dialyzed patients
  - Immunosuppression
  - Severe myocardial dysfunction
  - Aortic diseases to avoid aortic cannulation and clamping:
    - Calcified aorta, aortic disease with increased risk of dissection, rupture
    - Atherosclerotic aorta

High Risk Patients for OPCAB

- ❖ High grade LMCA (left main coronary artery) lesions
- ❖ Proximal LAD (left anterior descending artery) lesions
- ❖ Triple vessel disease

Conversion from OPCAB to CABG

- Occurs in 3% surgeries
- Are associated with higher risk of adverse outcomes:
  - 30-day mortality
  - Stroke
  - Renal dysfunction
  - Wound infection
  - Respiratory failure
- Indications:
  - *Hemodynamic instability*: persistence for *more than 15 minutes* of:
    - Mean arterial pressure less than 50 mm Hg
    - Cardiac index less than 1.5 L/min/m_2
    - ST segment elevation more than 2 μV
    - Severe LV dysfunction or large new RWMA on TEE
    - $MvO_2 \leq 60\%$
  - Sustained malignant arrhythmias
  - Inability to access areas which require revascularization
  - Intra-myocardial coronary vessels
  - Need for coronary endarterectomy

Preoperative Assessment

- History:
  - Angina/recent MI
  - Cerebrovascular accident
  - *LV dysfunction*: prthopnea, paroxysmal nocturnal dyspnea
  - Diabetes mellitus, hypertension, smoking, hyperlipidemia
- Physical examination:
  - Raised JVP, basal crepitations
  - Pitting edema, S_3 gallop
  - Airway examination: Difficult airway anticipated due to DM/obesity
- Investigations:
  - Routine blood investigations, urine analysis, electrolytes
  - Renal function tests, liver function tests
  - Coagulation profile
  - ECG, chest X-ray
  - Echocardiography:
    - Localization of RWMA to identify new onset RWMA post-operatively
    - Associated valvular lesions and severity
    - Severity of LV dysfunction:
      - 40–50% EF: Mild LV dysfunction
      - 25–40% EF: Moderate LV dysfunction
      - Less than 25% EF: Severe LV dysfunction
  - Angiogram done within last 12 months
  - Depending on patient requirements:
    - Dobutamine stress test
    - Technetium 99m perfusion scan
- Assessment of comorbidities:
  - Carotid artery stenosis to determine need for a combined procedure
  - Peripheral vascular disease to determine risk of use of IABP
  - Pulmonary function tests in smokers for postoperative pulmonary complications

Preoperative Preparation and Premedication

- Optimize patient's preoperative DM, BP and lipid profile and heart rate
- Good patient communication necessary to avoid anxiety induced tachycardia
- PO lorazepam 1–2 mg may be given the night before surgery
- NPO orders
- Informed consent
- Two large (18 G) bore IV cannula inserted
- Arterial line as well as CVP access may be secured prior to induction under LA
- Premedication:
  - Midazolam 0.03 mg/kg IV
  - Morphine 0.05–0.1 mg/kg IV
  - Ranitidine 1 mg/kg IV or pantoprazole 20 mg IV
- Continue morning dose of β-blockers, CCB, and nitrates on day of surgery
- Stop ACE inhibitors and ARBs to prevent precipitous hypotension intraoperatively
- Oral hypoglycemic to be withheld on the morning of surgery

OT Preparation

- Anesthetic drugs
- Machine check
- Emergency medications: atropine, adrenaline, phenylephrine, calcium
- Airway equipment: ET tube, laryngoscope, airway, LMA, gum elastic bougie
- CPB machine and perfusionist on stand by
- IABP for:
  - Severe LV dysfunction
  - CAD with VSR
  - Acute mitral regurgitation
- Suction equipment
- External defibrillation pads before preparation and draping, defibrillator

Position: Supine

Monitoring

- ECG:
  - Lead II for rhythm disturbances
  - Lead V_5 with ST segment analysis for ischemia
  - V_4R and V_5R used if right ventricular ischemia
  - May show flatline during circumflex artery anastomosis due retraction of heart
- Pulse oximetry may be used for preoperative Allens test
- Capnography
- Invasive blood pressure monitoring:
  - Used for:
    - Continuous beat-beat monitoring of BP
    - Estimation of cardiac output by area under the curve
    - Stroke volume variation to monitor fluid responsiveness
  - Right radial artery cannulation is preferred
  - Left radial cannulation is avoided as it may be used as a conduit for grafting
  - Femoral artery cannulation:
    - Indications:
      - Severe LVD
      - Tight left main stenosis
    - Uses of femoral arterial cannulation:
      - Allows quick placement of IABP in case of emergencies
      - Allows percutaneous placement of cannulas for emergent CPB
      - Allows monitoring central-peripheral pressure gradient
- Bispectral index or entropy monitoring
  - For monitoring intraoperative awareness
  - Anesthetic dose may be reduced often due to hemodynamic perturbations
  - Thus, monitoring for awareness during surgery is important
- Neuromuscular monitoring
- CVP:
  - Inserted prior to induction, especially in severe LVD and tight left main stenosis
  - Acts as an auxillary guide to monitor fluid therapy
  - Useful for administration of vasoactive agents
  - Used to monitor central venous oxygen saturation
- PA catheter:
  - Routine use of PA catheter is not recommended
  - Indications for PAC in OPCAB include:
    - Severe LV dysfunction
    - Combined valve procedures
    - LV aneurysmectomy
    - Recent MI (< 30 days)
    - Renal dysfunction
    - Pulmonary HTN
    - Diastolic dysfunction
    - Ventricular septal rupture
- Temperature, urine output
- Periodic ABGs
- Continuous cardiac output monitoring, transcranial Doppler: Optional
- Transesophageal echocardiography:
  - Useful in:
    - Patients with raised LVEDP, to assess LV preload
    - Assessment of LV function
    - Detecting new RWMA
  - Views may be suboptimal during the distal graft anastomosis

Anesthetic Goals

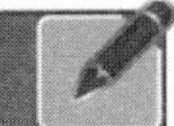

- *Cardiac protective anesthetic technique* used
- Heart rate:
  - Slow, 70–80 bpm for good LV function (*non-ischemia producing heart rate*)
  - 80–90 bpm for severe LV dysfunction
- Rhythm: Sinus rhythm
- Contractility: Myocardial depression preferred (if LV function is normal)
- Preload:
  - Judicious preload
  - Reduced preload preferred prior to anastomosis
  - Increased preload may be required during verticalization of heart
- Afterload: Maintain afterload (hypertension preferred to hypotension)
- Temperature: Keep patient warm
- MvO_2:
  - Maintain myocardial oxygen demand-supply ratio
  - Treat myocardial oxygen supply related disturbances
- Severe LMCA disease: Maintain diastolic pressure and heart rate at preoperative values

Induction

- Adequate preoxygenation for 3–5 minutes
- Induction in calm and relaxed manner
- Two methods of induction:
  - Patients with good LV function:
    - Normal doses of anesthetic agents as sympathetic response usually intact

- Thiopentone 3–5 mg/kg + vecuronium 0.1 mg/kg + fentanyl 5 µg/kg IV
- Propofol 2 mg/kg may be used as alternative
- Induction agents in titrated doses to prevent hypotension at induction
- β blockers and vasodilators kept ready to negate intubation response

- Patients with poor LV function:
  - Reduced doses of anesthetic as response to stimulation is suboptimal
  - Pancuronium 0.1 mg/kg + fentanyl 5 µg/kg + midazolam 0.05 mg/kg IV
  - Pancuronium is used to counter opioid induced bradycardia
  - Etomidate maybe used for induction to maintain hemodynamic stability
  - Vasopressors and inotropes kept ready

❖ Deep planes of anesthesia maintained at the time of intubation

❖ Prevention of intubation response:
- IV lignocaine 1.5 mg/kg 60–90 seconds prior to intubation
- Use of NTG/esmolol to blunt intubation response

❖ Ryles tube inserted to deflate stomach and left open

❖ Antibiotic prophylaxis as per hospital protocol

❖ NTG infusion started and continued throughout procedure

Maintenance

❖ Opioid based balanced anesthetic technique used

❖ O_2 + N_2O + isoflurane 1 MAC used for balanced anesthesia

❖ TIVA with propofol infusion is less preferred as it causes:
- Increased inotropic requirements
- Increase in postoperative troponin I levels

❖ Pure opioid based anesthesia technique preferred for severe LV dysfunction

❖ Vecuronium and fentanyl given as intermittent boluses during surgery

❖ Fentanyl bolus given before sternotomy to avoid hypertensive response

❖ Anticoagulation:
- Heparin 2 mg/kg (200 IU/kg) IV given before division of internal mammary A
- ACT maintained between 250 and 300 seconds
- ACT is checked at hourly intervals
- Heparin may be repeated in prolonged surgeries to maintain target ACT

❖ Protamine:
- May be given to reverse anticoagulation following proximal anastomosis
- Dose is titrated to maintain ACT around 150 seconds in postoperative period
- This may help in improving graft patency

Hemodynamics

❖ Rigid control of heart rate and blood pressure required

❖ Heart rate:
- Maintain heart rate of around 70 bpm (non-ischemia producing heart rate)
- Esmolol infusion/metaprolol boluses useful

❖ Dysrhythmias:
- Occurs due to:
  - Manipulation of heart
  - Myocardial ischemia
  - Reperfusion injury
  - Dyselectrolytemia
- Prevention of dysrhythmias:
  - Maintain normal electrolytes levels
  - Prior to manipulation of heart:
    - Infusion of magnesium sulphate
    - IV xylocard 1.5 mg/kg
    - Pacemaker to be readily available to treat bradyarrhythmias

❖ Hypotension:
- During distal anastomoses, especially distal RCA and obtuse marginal anastomosis
- Treatment:
  - IV fluids boluses
  - 20° Trendelenburg position
  - Phenylephrine 50–100 µg IV bolus or dobutamine infusion
  - Adjust stabilizer and reposition the heart

❖ Hypertension:
- Nitroglycerin 0.5–3 µg/kg/min IV
- β blockers: Labetalol/esmolol
- Calcium channel blockers

❖ Cardiac output:
- Maintaining cardiac output more important than BP
- May be reduced due to reduced contractility from ischemia/displacement of heart
- Dobutamine/dopamine used to maintain cardiac output
- Pre-anastomotic insertion of IABP may be necessary, especially in LMCA lesions

- Temperature: Prevent hypothermia:
  - Use warm IV fluids
  - Humidification of air
  - Maintain warm OT temperature
  - Position patient on heating mattress to prevent hypothermia
  - Forced air warmers

Hemodynamic Alterations during OPCAB

- Anastomosis of left anterior descending artery (LAD) and branches:
  - LAD lies on anterior aspect of heart in the interventricular grove
  - Positioning of heart for LAD anastomosis requires only slight traction on the heart
  - This positioning does not cause significant hemodynamic derangements
  - However, epicardial stabilizer is placed on actively contracting anterior wall
  - This may decrease the stroke volume and cardiac output
- Anastomosis of left circumflex (LCX) artery and branches:
  - Left circumflex artery runs in left AV groove and continues posteriorly
  - Exposure of LCX and its branches requires verticalization of the heart
  - This causes hemodynamic derangement by 2 mechanisms:
    - Atrial displacement:
      - Atria are displaced to lie below the ventricles
      - Thus, it requires higher filling pressures to maintain CO
    - Distortion of valvular anatomy:
      - Verticalization results in distortion of MV and TV anatomy
      - This may result in increased severity of MR and TR
  - Verticalization is also associated with changes in monitoring parameters:
    - Reduced amplitude of ECG waveforms
    - Unreliable CVP waveform and values
    - Loss of TEE imaging windows
  - Management of hemodynamic compromise:
    - Trendelenburg position
    - Fluid bolus to increase filling pressure
    - Vasopressors and inotropes to maintain perfusion pressure
- Anastomosis of right coronary artery (RCA) and branches:
  - RCA runs in the right AV groove and continues posteriorly
  - Exposure of distal RCA and PDA may require verticalization of heart
  - Exposure of proximal RCA requires only slight elevation with left displacement
  - Placement of epicardial stabilizer on the RV decreases the chamber volume
  - This may result in decreased RV filling and reduced cardiac output
  - Also, anastomosis of RCA may be accompanied by bradyarrhythmias and CHB
  - Management of hemodynamic compromise:
    - Trendelenburg position
    - Fluid bolus to increase filling pressure
    - Vasopressors and inotropes to maintain perfusion pressure
    - Epicardial pacing for bradyarrhythmias
- Proximal anastomosis:
  - Partial cross clamping of aorta done prior to proximal anastomosis
  - This requires rapid reduction of blood pressure:
    - Reverse Trendelenburg position beneficial
    - Volatile anesthetics/nitroglycerin useful
  - However, MAP should be maintained above 60 mm Hg
  - Watch for reperfusion injury on release of snuggers following anastomosis

Ventilation

- Lungs to be deflated at the time of sternotomy
- Hand ventilation may be required during:
  - Dissection of left internal mammary artery (LIMA)
  - Distal anastomosis to aid surgical exposure, especially for branches of LCX artery
- Recruitment maneuvres may be used to prevent atelectasis prior to chest closure

Extubation

- Usually ventilated postoperatively to assess for bleeding and persistent ischemia
- On-table extubation may be considered for single-graft OPCABs

Postoperative Management

Ventilation

- Extubation is termed as early extubation if performed *less than 6 hours postoperatively*

- Delayed extubation is preferred for:
  - Poor LV function
  - Emergency procedures
  - Obese patients
  - Combined procedures
  - Severe pulmonary disease
- Extubation done when:
  - Awake, normothermic
  - Hemodynamically stable
  - Minimal bleeding
  - Absence of acidosis
- Early institution of chest physiotherapy and early ambulation is preferred

Postoperative Analgesia

- IV opioids, patient-controlled analgesia
- Thoracic epidural
- Ketorolac + small dose opioids
- Multimodal approach

Monitors

- Pulse oximetry, temperature
- Blood pressure:
  - Maintained at less than 130 mm Hg to protect graft top-ends and reduce bleeding
  - Maintain nitroglycerine infusion to prevent graft spasm
- *Drains*: should be less than 100 mL/hour
- ACT, repeated ABG and blood sugar
- Echocardiography for:
  - LV ejection fraction
  - Regional wall motion abnormalities
  - Pericardial effusion and tamponade

Complications

- Pain
- Hypertension, tachycardia
- Bleeding, arrhythmias (atrial fibrillation)
- Myocardial ischemia due to graft occlusion
- Cognitive dysfunction, stroke
- Acute kidney injury
- LV dysfunction
- Low cardiac output syndrome (LCOS)

Regional Anesthesia

- Avoided when:
  - Severe LV dysfunction
  - Associated defects such as VSR, acute mitral regurgitation
  - Anticoagulation is continued up to surgery in patients with unstable angina
- Thoracic epidural anesthesia advantages:
  - Reduced stress response
  - Better analgesia
  - Allows early extubation
  - Better respiratory function postoperatively
  - Antianginal: reduces dynamic occlusion
  - Better distribution of coronary blood flow
  - Reduced oxygen demand
- Epidural anesthesia disadvantages:
  - More hypotension
  - Epidural hematoma, infection
  - Dural puncture with post-dural puncture headache
  - Spinal cord injury

Validation

- GOPCABE trial:
  - German off-pump CABG in elderly trial
  - Included patients > 75 years age
  - Study found increased need for repeat revascularizations
  - No significant difference was found between OPCAB and CABG for:
    - Death
    - Postoperative stroke
    - Postoperative renal replacement therapy
- ROOBY trial:
  - Randomized on/off bypass trial
  - OPCAB patients were associated with:
    - Worse 5-year survival rates
    - Worse 5-year event free outcomes including:
      - Death from any cause
      - Repeat revascularization
      - Non-fatal myocardial infarction
- In conclusion, OPCAB may be associated with:
  - Less bleeding
  - Less renal dysfunction
  - Less short-term neuro-cognitive dysfunction
  - Shorter hospital stay
  - Lower rates of long-term graft patency

ANESTHESIA FOR ON-PUMP CABG

Introduction

Most commonly performed cardiac surgical procedure where a coronary artery stenosis is bypassed with an arterial/venous graft using cardio-pulmonary bypass.

Preoperative Assessment

- History:
  - Angina/recent MI
  - Cerebrovascular accident
  - LV dysfunction: Orthopnea, paroxysmal nocturnal dyspnea
  - Diabetes mellitus, hypertension, smoking, hyperlipidemia
- Physical examination:
  - Raised JVP, basal crepitations
  - Pitting edema, S_3 gallop
  - *Airway examination*: difficult airway anticipated due to DM/obesity
- Investigations:
  - Routine blood investigations, urine analysis, electrolytes
  - Renal function tests, liver function tests
  - Coagulation profile
  - ECG, chest X-ray
  - Echocardiography:
    - Localization of RWMA to identify new onset RWMA post-operatively
    - Associated valvular lesions and severity
    - Severity of LV dysfunction:
      - 40–50% EF: Mild LV dysfunction
      - 25–40% EF: Moderate LV dysfunction
      - Less than 25% EF: Severe LV dysfunction
  - Angiogram done within last 12 months
  - Depending on patient requirements:
    - Dobutamine stress test
    - Technetium 99m perfusion scan
- Assessment of comorbidities:
  - Carotid artery stenosis to determine need for a combined procedure
  - Peripheral vascular disease to determine risk of use of IABP
  - Pulmonary function tests in smokers for post-operative pulmonary complications

STS Risk Assessment

- Can be used to assess risk of various adverse outcomes following CABG such as:
  - Risk of mortality
  - Renal failure
  - Permanent stroke
  - Prolonged ventilation
  - Reoperation
  - Long length of hospital stay

Contd...

Contd...

- Some of the variables used to calculate this outcome include:
  - Female gender, small size
  - Advanced age
  - Preoperative renal dysfunction
  - Extra-cardiac arteriopathy
  - Cerebral vascular disease
  - Peripheral vascular disease
  - Previous cardiac surgery/intervention
  - Chronic lung disease
  - Recent myocardial infarction
  - Emergency surgery
  - Poor LV function

Preoperative Preparation and Premedication

- Optimize patient's preoperative DM, BP and lipid profile and heart rate
- Good patient communication necessary to avoid anxiety induced tachycardia
- PO lorazepam 1–2 mg may be given the night before surgery
- NPO orders
- Informed consent
- Two large (18 G) bore IV cannula inserted
- Arterial line as well as CVP access may be secured prior to induction under LA
- Premedication:
  - Midazolam 0.03 mg/kg IV
  - Morphine 0.05–0.1 mg/kg IV
  - Ranitidine 1 mg/kg IV or pantoprazole 20 mg IV
- Continue morning dose of β-blockers, CCB, and nitrates on day of surgery
- Stop ACE inhibitors and ARBs to prevent precipitous hypotension intraoperatively
- Oral hypoglycemic to be withheld on the morning of surgery

OT Preparation

- Anesthetic drugs
- Machine check
- Emergency medications: Atropine, adrenaline, phenylephrine, calcium
- Airway equipment: ET tube, laryngoscope, airway, LMA, gum elastic bougie
- CPB machine and perfusionist on stand by
- IABP for:
  - Severe LV dysfunction
  - CAD with VSR
  - Acute mitral regurgitation

- ❖ Suction equipment
- ❖ External defibrillation pads before preparation and draping, defibrillator

Monitoring

- ❖ ECG:
  - Lead II for rhythm disturbances
  - Lead V_5 with ST segment analysis for ischemia
  - V_4R and V_5R used if right ventricular ischemia
- ❖ Pulse oximetry may be used for preoperative Allens test
- ❖ Capnography
- ❖ Invasive blood pressure monitoring:
  - Used for:
    - Continuous beat-beat monitoring of BP
    - Estimation of cardiac output by area under the curve
    - Stroke volume variation to monitor fluid responsiveness
  - Right radial artery cannulation is preferred
  - Left radial cannulation is avoided as it may be used as a conduit for grafting
  - Femoral artery cannulation:
    - Indications:
      - Severe LVD
      - Tight left main stenosis
    - Uses of femoral arterial cannulation:
      - Allows quick placement of IABP in case of emergencies
      - Allows percutaneous placement of cannulas for emergent CPB
      - Allows monitoring central-peripheral pressure gradient
- ❖ Bispectral index or entropy monitoring
- ❖ Neuromuscular monitoring
- ❖ CVP:
  - Inserted prior to induction, especially in severe LVD and tight left main stenosis
  - Acts as an auxillary guide to monitor fluid therapy
  - Useful for administration of vasoactive agents
  - Used to monitor central venous oxygen saturation
- ❖ PA catheter:
  - Routine use of PA catheter is not recommended
  - Indications for PAC in CABG include:
    - Severe LV dysfunction
    - Combined valve procedures
    - LV aneurysmectomy
    - Recent MI (< 30 days)
    - Renal dysfunction
    - Pulmonary HTN
    - Diastolic dysfunction
    - Ventricular septal rupture
- ❖ Temperature, urine output
- ❖ Periodic ABGs
- ❖ Continuous cardiac output monitoring, transcranial Doppler: optional
- ❖ Transesophageal echocardiography useful in:
  - Patients with raised LVEDP, to assess LV preload
  - Assessment of LV function
  - Detecting new RWMA

Anesthetic Goals 

- ❖ *Cardiac protective anesthetic technique* used
- ❖ Heart rate:
  - Slow, 70–80 bpm for good LV function (*non-ischemia producing heart rate*)
  - 80–90 bpm for severe LV dysfunction
- ❖ Rhythm: Sinus rhythm
- ❖ Contractility: Maintain contractility
- ❖ Preload: Maintain preload
- ❖ Afterload: Maintain afterload (hypertension preferred to hypotension)
- ❖ Temperature: Keep patient warm
- ❖ MvO_2:
  - Maintain myocardial oxygen demand-supply ratio
  - Treat myocardial oxygen supply related disturbances

Induction

- ❖ Adequate preoxygenation for 3–5 minutes
- ❖ Induction in calm and relaxed manner
- ❖ Two methods of induction:
  - Patients with good LV function:
    - Normal doses of anesthetic agents as sympathetic response usually intact
    - Thiopentone 3–5 mg/kg + vecuronium 0.1 mg/kg + fentanyl 5 µg/kg IV
    - Propofol 2 mg/kg maybe used as alternative
    - Induction agents in titrated doses to prevent hypotension at induction
    - β blockers and vasodilators kept ready to negate intubation response
  - Patients with poor LV function:
    - Reduced doses of anesthetic as response to stimulation is suboptimal
    - Pancuronium 0.1 mg/kg + fentanyl 5 µg/kg + midazolam 0.05 mg/kg IV
    - Pancuronium is used to counter opioid induced bradycardia
    - Etomidate may be used for induction to maintain hemodynamic stability
    - Vasopressors and inotropes kept ready

- Deep planes of anesthesia maintained at the time of intubation
- Prevention of intubation response:
  - IV lignocaine 1.5 mg/kg 60–90 seconds prior to intubation
  - Use of NTG/esmolol to blunt intubation response
- Ryles tube inserted to deflate stomach and left open
- Antibiotic prophylaxis as per hospital protocol
- NTG infusion started and continued throughout procedure

Position: Supine

Maintenance

PRE-Bypass

- Opioid based balanced anesthetic technique used
- O_2 + N_2O + isoflurane 1 MAC used for balanced anesthesia
- TIVA with propofol infusion is less preferred as it causes:
  - Increased inotropic requirements
  - Increase in postoperative troponin I levels
- Pure opioid based anesthesia technique preferred for severe LV dysfunction
- Fentanyl bolus given before sternotomy to avoid hypertensive response
- Fentanyl 1 µg/kg + vecuronium 0.05 mg/kg intermittent boluses to maintain analgesia
- Pump may be primed with anesthetic drug:
  - Vecuronium 0.1 mg/kg
  - Morphine 0.1–0.2 mg/kg
  - Fentanyl 250–500 µg
  - Midazolam 0.05 mg/kg
- Management of anticoagulation:
  - Heparin 3 mg/kg (300 IU/kg) is given prior to IMA clamping
  - Ensure that ACT is more than 480 seconds in sample taken 3 minutes thereafter
  - Once ACT values are confirmed, pump suction may be used to clear surgical field
- Make note of urine output once CPB ensues

During Bypass

- ABG and ACT are checked every half hour on CPB
- Heparin may be repeated at 1 mg/kg (100 IU/kg) every hour after the initial dose
- Volatile agent is added to the sweep gas being delivered to CPB oxygenator
- Hourly anesthetic supplementation to the venous reservoir with:
  - Vecuronium 0.05 mg/kg
  - Morphine 0.1 mg/kg
  - Midazolam 0.03 mg/kg
- Just prior to termination of CPB, following variables are noted:
  - Temperature
  - Mean arterial pressure
  - Hematocrit
  - Serum potassium
  - Urine output

Post-Bypass

- De-airing maneuvers once heart is being closed
- Defibrillate/cardiovert if VF/SVT
- Inotropes started once aortic cross clamp is removed
- Ventilation is started after:
  - PA perfusion is adequate
  - Last proximal graft is being sutured
  - Prominent pulsations are present on arterial line tracing
- Discontinue N_2O at this stage to prevent expansion of air bubbles
- Trouble shooting at weaning off CPB:
  - Hypotension associated with tachycardia, low CVP/PCWP: Fluid boluses
  - Hypotension with bradycardia, high CVP/PCWP: Inotropic support
  - Hypotension with high MvO2: inodilators
  - Hypotension with low MvO2: vasopressors
- Protamine (1:1 with heparin) given after venous decannulation
- Last internal suction done after half the protamine dose has been given
- ABG taken 5–10 minutes after protamine completed (for ACT and ABG)

Hemodynamics

- Goals:
  - Rigid control of heart rate and blood pressure required
  - Maintain heart rate around 70 bpm (esmolol/metaprolol useful)
  - Maintain systolic BP around 100–120 mm Hg during the procedure
  - Hypotensive anesthesia (SBP 80–100 mm Hg) is preferred during:

- Aortic cannulation to prevent aortic dissection
- Aortic decannulation following CPB termination
- Hemostasis

❖ Choice of fluids:
- Pre-CPB:
  - Isotonic crystalloids are preferred (lactated ringers or plasmalyte A)
  - Two units of cross matched and grouped PRBCs kept ready in OT
  - Blood is kept ready in redo cases as RV perforation may occur during sternotomy
- Post-CPB:
  - Isotonic fluids are preferred for maintenance
  - Volume of fluids may be guided by:
    - PCWP
    - TEE assessment of LVEDV
    - CVP
    - Stroke volume variations of arterial waveform
  - Blood products may be administered if required to ensure adequate hemostasis

❖ Dysrhythmias:
- Occurs due to:
  - Manipulation of heart
  - Myocardial ischemia
  - Reperfusion injury
  - Dyselectrolytemias
- Prevention of dysrhythmias:
  - Maintain normal electrolytes levels
  - Prior to manipulation of heart:
    - Infusion of magnesium sulphate
    - IV xylocard 1.5 mg/kg
    - Pacemaker to be available during weaning CPB

❖ Hypotension:
- IV fluids boluses
- 20° Trendelenburg position
- Phenylephrine 50–100 μg IV bolus or dobutamine infusion
- Adjust stabilizer and reposition the heart

❖ Hypertension:
- Nitroglycerin 0.5–3 μg/kg/min IV
- β blockers: labetalol/esmolol
- Calcium channel blockers

❖ Cardiac output:
- Maintaining cardiac output more important than BP
- May be reduced due to reduced contractility from ischemia/displacement of heart
- Dobutamine/dopamine used to maintain cardiac output

❖ Temperature: Prevent hypothermia:
- Use warm IV fluids
- Humidification of air
- Maintain warm OT temperature
- Position patient on heating mattress to prevent hypothermia
- Forced air warmers

Ventilation

❖ Lungs to be deflated at the time of sternotomy

❖ Hand ventilation may be required during:
- Dissection of left internal mammary artery (LIMA)
- Right atrial cannulation

❖ Once full flow on CPB is established, the lungs may be dropped

❖ Further gas exchange is maintained by the sweep gas delivered to oxygenator

❖ Ventilation is started after:
- PA perfusion is adequate
- Last proximal graft is being sutured
- Prominent pulsations are present on arterial line tracing

❖ If the pleura have been opened, both the lungs will be collapsed at termination of CPB

❖ Thus, manual reinflation at initiation of ventilation may be required to prevent atelectasis

❖ Re-expansion is done carefully to prevent IMA graft avulsion due to overzealous inflation

❖ Regular ventilation may be resumed following re-expansion of lungs

❖ Recruitment maneuvres may be used again to prevent atelectasis prior to chest closure

Checklist Prior to CPB Initiation

Item	Anesthetic Checklist
Anesthetic level	Narcotics, BZD, additional dose muscle relaxant
	Volatile anesthetic availability on pump
	Narcotics, benzodiazepines, relaxants added to pump prime
Monitors	To be visible to anesthetist and perfusionist
	Retrograde pressure monitored
	Swan-Ganz catheter pulled back 5–10 cm before CPB initiation
Anticoagulation	Heparin 300 IU/kg given
	ACT maintained above 480 seconds
Arterial line	Check for air
Venous line	Minimize air to prevent air-lock
Urine output	Maintained more than 0.5 mL/kg/hour
Retrograde cardioplegia line	Pressure displayed (usually RV trace)
	Position confirmed by TEE if available

Checklist Post CPB Initiation

Item	Objective	Problems	Solution
Arterial blood flow	Adequate pump flow	Low flow	Check line for kinks
	Normal pump pressure	High pump pressure	Check for aortic dissection
	MAP > 50 mm Hg	Low MAP	Check for innominate A cannulation
Arterial blood color	Bright	Dark color	Check O_2 supply to oxygenator
Venous return	Good return	Poor return	Check line for kinks
	Low venous pressure	High venous pressure	Check line for air
			Check table height is adequate
Heart filling	Heart to be empty	Distended ventricle	Check venous return
			Vent the heart
			If AR present, reduce flow
IV Fluids	Should be off	Still running	Stop IV fluids
Ventilation	Stopped	Ventilation on	Turn off unless partial CPB
	Deflated lungs	Lungs inflated	Check PEEP valve
Anesthesia	Adequate depth	Anesthesia too light	Add vapor to pump gas
			Repeat IV drugs every hour
Anticoagulation	ACT > 480 sec	Inadequate	Heparin 100 IU/kg every hour
Urine output	More than 2 mL/kg/hr	Inadequate	Diuretics

Checklist for Weaning from CPB

Item	Objective	Problem	Solution
Acid base status	Normal	Base deficit > 5 mmol/L ECF	Correct with bicarbonate
Electrolytes	Normal potassium	Hypo/hyperkalemia	Correct appropriately
	Normal magnesium	Hypo/hypermagnesemia	Use insulin if K+ very high
	Normal calcium	Hypo/hypercalcemia	
Hematocrit	≥ 7 g/dL	< 6.5 g/dL	Transfusion
			Hemoconcentration
Glucose	< 15 mmol/L	Hyperglycemia	Insulin
Anticoagulation	≤ 120 seconds	≥ 121 seconds	Additional protamine
			FFP/platelet concentrates
Transducer	Zeroed correct	Zero drift	Zero again at rewarming
Temperature	36–37°C	< 36°C	Inadequate rewarming
Blood pressure	Between 95 and 125 mm Hg	Less than 95 mm Hg	Inotropes
Heart rate	≥ 70 bpm	Bradycardia	Treat with anticholinergics
		Tachycardia	Treat hypovolemia/pain
Rhythm	Sinus rhythm	Heart block	Pacing (DDD is best)
		Atrial fibrillation	Cardioversion
		Ventricular fibrillation	Defibrillation, amiodarone
		Multiple VPCs	Check electrolytes
Cardiac output	Normal	Low	Inotropes ready
SVR	Normal	Inappropriate vasodilation	Vasopressors
		Inappropriate vasoconstriction	Vasodilators
Anesthesia	Adequate depth	Too light	Check infusion
			On vapourizer
IV fluids	Ready to run	Not ready	Prepare IV fluids
Ventilation	Ventilation on	Ventilation off	Switch on ventilation
	FiO_2 > 50%	FiO_2 < 50%	Increase FiO_2 > 50%
	No IMA stretching		
	Check pneumothorax		

Causes of Failure to Wean from CPB

- LV/RV dysfunction
  - Systolic ventricular dysfunction
  - Myocardial stunning:
    - Inadequate cardioplegia
    - Prolonged duration of cross clamping
- Myocardial ischemia:
  - Kinking/spasm of coronary artery bypass graft
  - *Coronary embolism*: air, atheromatous plaque, thrombus
  - *Hypoxia*: pulmonary edema, failure to restart ventilation
- Diastolic ventricular dysfunction:
  - Preexisting severe LVH
  - Volume overload due to excess volume intake from CPB circuit
- Hypovolemia:
  - Inadequate transfusion from CPB circuit
  - Occult blood loss
- Excess vasodilatation/vasoplegia:
  - Overdose of vasodilators
  - Sepsis
  - Systemic inflammatory response to CPB
- *Arrhythmias*: AF, CHB
- Exacerbation of valvular dysfunction:
  - Mitral regurgitation
  - Aortic regurgitation

Causes of Persistent Ischemia Following CABG

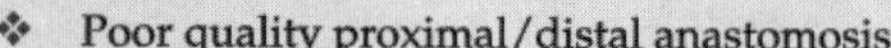

- Poor quality proximal/distal anastomosis
- Inadvertent incision of posterior coronary wall causing coronary dissection
- Deep suturing of coronary artery causing complete occlusion
- Inadequate graft length causing stretching of vein grafts post-CPB during filling of heart
- Excessive graft length leading to kinking of grafts
- Vein graft thrombosis
- Incomplete revascularization due to:
  - Diffuse distal disease
  - Ungraftable vessels
- Coronary embolization of air/atheromatous debris
- Coronary vasospasm
- Occlusion of IMA graft due to over-inflation of lung

Extubation

Usually ventilated postoperatively to assess for bleeding and persistent ischemia.

Postoperative Management

Ventilation

- Extubation is termed as early extubation if performed *less than 6 hours postoperatively*
- Delayed extubation is preferred for:
  - Poor LV function
  - Emergency procedures
  - Obese patients
  - Combined procedures
  - Severe pulmonary disease
- Extubation done when:
  - Awake, normothermic
  - Hemodynamically stable
  - Minimal bleeding
  - Absence of acidosis
- Early institution of chest physiotherapy and early ambulation is preferred

Postoperative Analgesia

- IV opioids, patient-controlled analgesia
- Thoracic epidural
- Ketorolac + small dose opioids
- Multimodal approach

Monitors

- Pulse oximetry, temperature
- Blood pressure:
  - Maintained at less than 130 mm Hg to protect graft top-ends and reduce bleeding
  - Maintain nitroglycerin infusion to prevent graft spasm
  - Calcium channel blockers may be started to prevent arterial graft spasm
- Drains: Should be less than 100 mL/hour
- ACT, repeated ABG and blood sugar
- Echocardiography for:
  - LV ejection fraction
  - Regional wall motion abnormalities
  - Pericardial effusion and tamponade

Complications

- Pain
- Hypertension, tachycardia
- Bleeding, arrhythmias (atrial fibrillation)
- Myocardial ischemia due to graft occlusion
- Cognitive dysfunction, stroke
- Acute kidney injury
- LV dysfunction
- Low cardiac output syndrome (LCOS)

FAST TRACK MANAGEMENT OF CABG

Introduction

- Fast tracking was introduced in late 1970s to reduce cost associated with cardiac surgery

- Term fast tracking in cardiac anesthesia was introduced in 1994 by Engelman
- Fast track management consists of:
    - Rapid postoperative extubation being the key component (within 6 hours)
    - Postoperative rehabilitation and discharge from hospital (within postoperative day 5)
- Ultrafast tracking consists of:
    - Extubation within 2 hours of surgery
    - Discharge from hospital within POD 4

Components of Fast Track CABG

- Altered anesthetic and surgical management
- Special recovery areas
- Early extubation
- Early mobilization
- Prophylactic/aggressive treatment of complications
- Discharge from ICU on postoperative day number 1
- Discharge from hospital on postoperative day number 5
- Out of hospital follow-up

Patient Selection for Fast Tracking

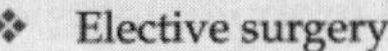

- Elective surgery
- Pre and postoperative cardiopulmonary stability
- Surgical procedures undertaken under mild-moderate hypothermia
- Absence of risk factors for postoperative bleeding
- Endocarditis
- Complex coagulation disorders
- Redo surgeries
- Absence of other associated surgical risk factors:
    - Acute ventricular septal rupture
    - Mitral regurgitation
    - LV aneurysm
    - Combined procedures involving valve surgery or aortic surgery

Exclusion Criteria for Fast Tracking

- Emergency surgery
- Large intraoperative blood loss
- High risk for postoperative bleeding
- Mechanical assist devices pre or post-operatively
- Complex surgery
- Endocarditis
- Psychiatric or neurological disorders
- Redo surgeries
- Intraoperative hypothermia < 32°C
- Severe LV dysfunction
- Preoperative renal impairment

Advantages of Early Extubation

- Earlier discharge
- Respiratory benefits:
    - Lesser endotracheal tube related complications
    - Improves mucus transport
- Cardiovascular benefits:
    - Improved cardiac output
    - Ventricular function returns to baseline within 24 hours after CABG in 90% patients

Perioperative Goals of Fast Track Management

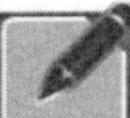

- Preoperative education and counseling
- Same day-admission when feasible
- Anesthetic technique tailored to facilitate early extubation
- Effective postoperative analgesia
- Protocol driven care
- Early ambulation
- Early discharge from ICU and hospital
- Regular follow-up following discharge (telephone/hospital visits)

Criteria for Fast Track Extubation

- Body temperature > 35.5°C
- Normal acid-base status
- Stable hemodynamics on minimal inotropic support
- Stable cardiac rhythm
- Adequate hemostasis with stable mediastinal drainage
- Adequate tidal volume and spontaneous respiratory rate
- Chest X-ray without major abnormalities
- Adequate urine output
- Adequate reversal of neuromuscular blockade
- Awake, alert, cooperative and moving all extremities

Anesthetic Considerations for Fast Track Cardiac Surgery

- Lower dose of opioids:
    - Fentanyl less than 5–15 μg/kg cumulative dose
    - Sufentanil less than 5–10 μg/kg cumulative dose
    - Remifentanil 0.2–0.75 μg/kg/min continuous infusion
- Supplementation with:
    - Inhalational agents: Sevoflurane or desflurane 0.6–1 MAC
    - Propofol infusion 25–100 μg/kg/min or less than 3 mg/kg/hour during surgery

- Avoidance of midazolam to prevent POCD
- Muscle relaxants:
  - Rocuronium:
    - 0.6–1 mg/kg for intubation
    - Repeat doses of 0.075–0.15 mg/kg boluses
  - Cis-atracurium:
    - 0.1–0.4 mg/kg intubation dose
    - Repeat doses of 0.03 mg/kg boluses

❖ Use of tranexamic acid during on-pump procedures
❖ Postoperative management:
- Goal directed fluid therapy
- Strict glycemic control (160–180 mg/dL) with insulin infusion
- Maintain chest tube patency through chest tube manipulation
- Pharmacological thromboprophylaxis begun on POD 1

❖ Postoperative ICU sedation:
- Propofol infusion continued
- Dexmedetomidine may be used for conscious sedation

❖ Postoperative analgesia:
- Multimodal analgesia preferred
- Morphine, NSAIDs
- Patient controlled analgesia
- Neuraxial techniques

CPB Considerations for Fast Track Cardiac Surgery

❖ Avoid excessive hemodilution (HCT< 24%)
❖ Minimal CPB prime volumes
❖ Vacuum assisted venous return
❖ Ultrafiltration
❖ Biocompatible CPB circuit and oxygenator
❖ Minimal systemic anticoagulation
❖ Prefer mild-moderate hypothermia
❖ Avoid hyperthermia at the time of rewarming (core temperature > 37.9°C)
❖ Adequate myocardial protection

Surgical Considerations for Fast Track Cardiac Surgery

❖ Appropriate patient selection
❖ Cardiac prehabilitation to augment preoperative functional capacity:
- Nutritional optimization
- Exercise training
- Anxiety reduction
- Chest physiotherapy

❖ Rehearsed, efficient surgical team
❖ Well planned, expeditious and technically superior surgery
❖ Meticulous myocardial protection
❖ Avoid intraoperative complications and residual structural defects
❖ Appropriate early use of inotropic support
❖ Surgical optimization of bleeding prior to chest closure
❖ Rigid sternal fixation
❖ Prevention of surgical site infections:
- Topical intranasal therapy to eradicate staphylococcal colonization
- Antibiotic to be administered within 60 minutes of skin incision
- Repeat antibiotic doses Q4H thereafter
- Dressing changes every 48 hours in the absence of soiling

Management in ICU

❖ Return to ICU:
- Reverse muscle relaxant as soon as stable to assess level of sedation
- Start fentanyl infusion at 0.01–0.03 µg/kg/min
- Continue propofol infusion at 10–30 µg/kg/min

❖ Awakening:
- If temperature <35°C, maintain propofol infusion
- If temperature 35–35.5°C, reduce propofol infusion
- If core temperature > 35.5°C:
  - Stop propofol infusion
  - Reduce fentanyl infusion by half
  - Give IV ketorolac 10–20 mg (0.5 mg/kg)

❖ Weaning:
- Wait for 10 minutes after discontinuing propofol infusion to start weaning
- 10–30 minutes taken to wean ventilatory support
- Place patient on CPAP when adequate spontaneous efforts
- Use E_TCO_2 and SpO_2 to assess adequacy of ventilation
- Maintain:
  - E_TCO_2 < 50 mm Hg
  - SpO_2 > 94%

❖ Extubation:
- Extubate once extubation criteria are met:
  - Body temperature > 35.5°C
  - Normal acid-base status
  - Stable hemodynamics on minimal inotropic support
  - Stable cardiac rhythm

- Adequate hemostasis with stable mediastinal drainage
- Adequate tidal volume and spontaneous respiratory rate
- Chest X-ray without major abnormalities
- Adequate urine output
- Adequate reversal of neuromuscular blockade
- Awake, alert, cooperative and moving all extremities
- Continue fentanyl infusion on as needed post-extubation
- Continue monitoring O_2 saturation, ABG, BP, ECG and urine output

PERIOPERATIVE MYOCARDIAL INFARCTION

Introduction

- Myocardial infarction is diagnosed when there is evidence of:
  - Acute myocardial injury along with
  - Clinical evidence of acute myocardial ischemia
- This is diagnosed by:
  - Atleast one troponin value (cTn) above 99th percentile upper range limit with
  - At least one of the following clinical changes:
    - Symptoms of myocardial ischemia
    - New ischemic changes on ECG
    - Development of pathological Q-waves
    - Imaging evidence of loss of viable myocardium or new RWMA
    - Identification of coronary thrombus by angiography or autopsy
- Myocardial injury is defined by at least one cTn value above upper limit of 99th percentile
- Myocardial injury during non-cardiac surgery (MINS):
  - Myocardial injury during 1st 30 days after non-cardiac surgery due to ischemia
  - Includes:
    - Myocardial ischemia (both symptomatic and silent)
    - Myocardial injury with:
      - Clinical evidence of ischemia not meeting diagnostic criteria
      - No evidence of non-ischemic etiology for cTn elevation

Definitions of Individual Diagnostic Criteria

- Roche fourth-generation Elecsys troponin-T level > 0.03 ng/mL is usually significant
- ECG criteria:
  - New Q-wave changes (≥ 30 msec) in any two contiguous leads
  - ST-segment elevation:
    - ≥ 2 mm in leads V_1, V_2 or V_3
    - ≥ 1 mm in other leads
  - ST-segment depression > 1 mm in at least 2 contiguous leads
  - Symmetric inversion of T-waves (≥ 1 mm) in at least 2 contiguous leads

Incidence

- Almost 35% of patients have cTn levels above 99th percentile URL
- 17% have an elevation in cTn values suggestive of evolving myocardial injury
- Incidence of perioperative MI in POISE trial was 5% at 30 days postoperatively
- Majority of these occurred within 48 hours post-surgery

Types of Perioperative MI

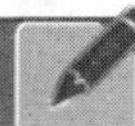

- Type I PMI: MI due to plaque disruption in athero-thrombotic CAD
- Type II PMI: MI due to myocardial oxygen demand-supply imbalance
- Type III PMI: Fatal MI with:
  - Symptoms suggestive of MI
  - Death prior to procurement of samples for cardiac biomarkers
- Type IV PMI: MI associated with percutaneous coronary intervention
- Type V PMI: MI associated with coronary artery bypass grafting

Causes

- Tachycardia:
  - More than 110 bpm associated with high risk
  - Most important determinant of myocardial oxygen consumption
  - Heart rate > 80–90 bpm in patients with preoperative resting heart rate 50–60 bpm increases risk
- Hypotension
- Hypertension
- Anemia with hematocrit < 28%
- Hypoxemia, hypercarbia
- Hypothermia
- Systolic and diastolic myocardial dysfunction

Pathophysiology

- Type I perioperative MI:
  - Occurs in the presence of an unstable coronary plaque
  - Plaque erosion or rupture occurs due to:
    - Sympathetic overactivity
    - Hemodynamic instability with hypotension and tachycardia
    - Coronary vasoconstriction
  - This leads to acute coronary thrombosis in the setting of:
    - Increased coagulability with decreased fibrinolysis
    - Recent PCI with stent
    - Premature cessation of Dual Antiplatelet Therapy (DAP)
  - This leads to acute coronary syndrome type of perioperative MI
- Type II perioperative MI:
  - Occurs in the presence of severe stable coronary artery disease
  - Occurs due to imbalance between myocardial oxygen demand and supply:
    - Increased myocardial oxygen demand may occur due to:
      - Increased heart rate due to:
        - Increased sympathetic activity
        - Withdrawal of β-blocker therapy
        - Arrhythmias
      - Increased myocardial wall stress due to:
        - Hypertension
        - Increased LVEDP
        - Pulmonary congestion
        - Atelectasis
    - Reduced subendocardial oxygen supply may occur due to:
      - Hypovolemia with hypotension
      - Systemic vasodilatation
      - Cardiac decompensation
      - Perioperative anemia
      - Hypoxemia
  - This leads to prolonged ST-depression (> 30 minutes) and type II perioperative MI
  - Demand myocardial ischemia is the predominant etiology of PMI

Diagnosis

- Rising patterns of cTn is key to making the diagnosis of PMI
- Thus, comparison of preoperative and postoperative values is important
- In the absence of cTn values, new pathological Q-waves can define PMI
- Persistent ischemic symptoms in the absence of biomarker and ECG changes require:
  - Echocardiographic evaluation for RWMA
  - Radionuclide myocardial perfusion imaging

Method	Information obtained	Problems	Sensitivity
TEE	New RWMA	Only one view at a time	Highest
	Severe hypokinesia		
	Akinesia/ dyskinesia		
	Transmural MI		
Coronary sinus lactate level	Myocardial lactate production		
PCWP	Raised PCWP	Poor sensitivity and specificity	
	a and c waves		
ST segment monitoring	ST depression	Requires V_4R for RCA	
	ST elevation, T wave changes	V_7,V_9 leads for post. wall ischemia	
Systemic pressures	Fall in arterial pressure	Low sensitivity and specificity	Lowest
	Increase in CVP		

Cardiac Biomarkers

- Troponin I
- CK-MB
- Lactate dehydrogenase
- Myoglobin
- Glycoprotein-BB
- AST, C-reactive protein, brain natriuretic peptide (BNP), myocardial lactate

Biomarker	Onset	Peak	Duration
Myoglobin	Immediate	2 hours	24 hours
GP-BB	1–3 hours	7 hours	36 hours
Troponin	2–4 hours	12 hours	7–10 days
CK-MB	4–8 hours	10–24 hours	48–72 hours
LDH	24–48 hours	72 hours	10–14 days

Differential Diagnosis

- Ischemic symptoms:
  - Anxiety
  - Esophageal reflux
- ECG changes:
  - Hyperventilation
  - Hypo/hyperkalemia
  - Pericarditis

- ❖ Elevated troponin levels:
  - Pulmonary embolus
  - Sepsis
  - Rapid atrial fibrillation
  - Chronic kidney disease

Perioperative MI Predictors

- ❖ Hemodynamically derived predictors:
  - None are reliable predictors
  - ***Rate pressure product (RPP) and triple index (TI):***
    - Rate pressure product = heart rate x systolic blood pressure
    - Triple index = Heart rate x systolic BP x PCWP
    - If *RPP ≥ 20,000*, patient is at increased risk of PMI
    - Both predictors are not reliable
  - ***Myocardial oxygen supply: demand ratio (DPTI: SPTI)***
    - DPTI:
      - Diastolic pressure time index
      - DPTI = (MDP – LVEDP) × (duration of diastole)
    - SPTI:
      - Systolic pressure time index
      - SPTI = MAP × duration of systole
    - MDP = mean diastolic pressure
    - MAP = mean arterial pressure
    - If *ratio < 0.5*, patient is at increased risk for subendocardial ischemia
    - Index is unreliable as increase in MvO_2 due to contraclility is not reflected
  - ***Mean arterial BP-heart rate quotient (pressure-rate quotient)***:
    - Pressure rate quotient = (Mean arterial pressure)/(Heart rate)
    - *PRQ less than 1* predicts increased risk of ischemia
    - Heart rate ≥ 110 bpm is *most important* determinant of PMI
- ❖ Revised cardiac risk index:
  - Predictors of MACE:
    - High risk surgical procedures:
      - Intra-peritoneal surgeries
      - Intra-thoracic surgeries
      - Supra-inguinal surgeries
      - Vascular surgery
    - Ischemic heart disease by any diagnostic criteria:
      - History of angina considered secondary to MI
      - History of myocardial infarction
      - Use of sublingual nitroglycerine
      - History of positive exercise test
      - Significant pathological Q waves on ECG
      - Patient who have undergone PTCA/CABG only if angina secondary to ischemia
    - History of congestive heart failure:
      - Pulmonary edema
      - Paroxysmal nocturnal dyspnea
      - Bilateral rales or S_3 gallop rhythm
      - Chest X-ray showing pulmonary vascular redistribution
    - History of cerebrovascular disease: TIA or stroke
    - Insulin dependent diabetes mellitus with preoperative insulin therapy
    - Preoperative serum creatinine ≥ 2 mg/dL
  - Rate of non-fatal myocardial infarction and cardiac arrest:
    - No risk factors: 0.4%
    - One risk factor: 1.0%
    - Two risk factors: 2.4%
    - Three or more risk factors: 5.4%
  - Rate of myocardial infarction and other MACE:
    - No risk factors: 0.5%
    - One risk factor: 1.3%
    - Two risk factors: 3.6%
    - Three or more risk factors: 9.1%

Screening for Perioperative MI

- ❖ Done using cardiac troponin levels
- ❖ Daily cTn measurements are recommended for 48–72 hours for:
  - Patients with high baseline risk (> 5%) at 30-postoperative days of:
    - Non-fatal MI
    - Cardiovascular death
  - Revised cardiac risk index score > 1
  - Age 45–64 years with significant cardiovascular disease
  - Age > 65 years

Prophylaxis

- ❖ Beta blockers:
  - Uses:
    - Beta blockers should be continued in those already taking them for:
      - Hypertension
      - Angina
      - Arrhythmias

- β blockers like labetalol and esmolol can be used to prevent stress response
- Attempts to discontinue preoperative β blocker therapy causes:
  - Increased risk of rebound tachycardia, with or without AF
  - Myocardial infarction in patients with CAD
- Dosage:
  - Dosage for all individuals is not the same
  - Dosage is individualized according to patient and type of surgery
  - β blocker dose titrated to heart rate and blood pressure
  - Heart rate is titrated to ***non-ischemia inducing heart rate***, 60–80 bpm
- Administration:
  - Initiation of beta blockers preoperatively should be done:
    - Ideally 1 month prior to surgery
    - Atleast 1 week prior to surgery
  - Continuation of beta blockers is recommended up to time of surgery
  - Therapy should be continued in IV form when GI absorption is in question
  - If β blocker has been omitted preoperatively, esmolol and labetalol are used
  - Beta blocker therapy should be continued for at least 30 days post-surgery

❖ Aspirin:
- Continuing aspirin perioperatively increases risk of bleeding
- This is associated with no additional benefits regarding:
  - Improved mortality
  - Incidence of non-fatal MI
- Thus, decision to continue aspirin has to be individualized
- It is usually stopped 5 days prior to elective surgeries
- The only exception is for CABG where it is continued on the day of surgery

❖ ACE inhibitors and ARBs: (Class IIa, LOE C)
- Continued in stable patients with ACEI therapy for:
  - Heart failure
  - LV systolic dysfunction
- Discontinued in stable patients with ACEI therapy for hypertension
- ACEI is initiated at least 1 week preoperatively in stable patients with:
  - Heart failure
  - LV systolic dysfunction

❖ Statins:
- Statins may reduce the incidence of perioperative MI
- Should be initiated in patients undergoing vascular surgery at least 2 weeks preoperatively (Class IIa, LOE B)
- Should be continued in patients already on statins (Class I LOE C)

❖ Calcium channel blockers:
- Not indicated in patients with heart failure and systolic dysfunction
- May be considered in patients with beta-blocker intolerance
- Should be continued perioperatively in patients with vasospastic angina

❖ Perioperative nitrates:
- No effect has been demonstrated on the incidence of perioperative MI
- May pose significant hemodynamic risk by reducing preload causing:
  - Hypotension
  - Tachycardia

❖ Clonidine:
- No evidence of benefit from prophylactic use of clonidine
- Thus, it is not given prophylactically for non-cardiac surgery (NCS)

❖ Dual antiplatelet therapy:
- Uninterrupted continuation of DAP should be considered for: (Class I, LOE C)
  - 4 weeks after BMS implantation
  - 3–12 months after DES implantation
- Discontinuation of $P2Y_{12}$ inhibitors is considered in patients with:
  - High risk of bleeding
  - Low risk of ischemic events
- Timing of discontinuation of $P2Y_{12}$ inhibitors: (Class IIa, LOE C)
  - 5 days for clopidogrel and ticagrelor
  - 7 days for prasugrel

❖ Preoperative prophylactic revascularization in stable IHD patients:
- Routine revascularization is not recommended for: (Class III, LOE B)
  - Low risk surgeries
  - Intermediate risk surgeries
- Revascularization is considered for: (Class IIb, LOE B)
  - High risk surgeries
  - Extensive of stress-induced perfusion defect

- Postoperative revascularization is considered in high risk patients
- Revascularization strategy:
  - CABG is preferred for:
    - Complex lesions with intermediate-high SYNTAX scores
    - Left main coronary artery disease
    - Urgent requirement of NCS (to avoid DAP-induced delays)
    - High risk of stent-restenosis:
      - Small diameter coronaries
      - Long lesions
      - Multiple stents
  - When PCI is used, BMS or newer generation DES are preferred

❖ Preoperative revascularization in patients with NSTEMI:
- Priority is given to the management of NSTEMI
- Elective surgery is postponed to facilitate treatment of NSTEMI (Class I, LOE A)
- Emergent surgeries are considered on individual basis (Class IIa, LOE C)
- Revascularization strategy (Class I, LOE B):
  - CABG is preferred for:
    - Complex lesions with intermediate-high SYNTAX scores
    - Left main coronary artery disease
    - Urgent requirement of NCS (to avoid DAP-induced delays)
    - High risk of stent-restenosis:
      - Small diameter coronaries
      - Long lesions
      - Multiple stents
  - When PCI is considered:
    - BMS/new-generation DES preferred
    - This is to limit delay in non-cardiac surgery to 1–3 months
    - Balloon angioplasty in low-risk patients

❖ Other intraoperative measures:
- Use of regional anesthesia where possible
- Use of volatile anesthetic agents to facilitate preconditioning
- Maintenance of hematocrit > 28%
- Maintenance of normothermia
- Use of postoperative sufentanyl 1 μg/kg/hour.

Goals of Perioperative Management

❖ Careful perioperative monitoring

❖ Low threshold for treating and preventing tachycardia

❖ Avoid hypotension, low cardiac output and cardiac decompensation

Perioperative Management

❖ Tight perioperative monitoring:
- ECG
- Echocardiography
- Transesophageal echocardiography
- Invasive blood pressure
- PA pressure monitoring

❖ Additional tests:
- Arterial blood gas, troponin I levels
- Treat any acid base disturbances
- Correct electrolyte imbalance

❖ Tachycardia treated aggressively:
- Tachycardia with hypotension:
  - Hypovolemia: IV fluid challenge
  - Anemia: Transfuse blood if:
    - Hematocrit less than 25% normally
    - Hematocrit less than 28% in patients with coronary artery disease
  - Low systemic vascular resistance:
    - Vasopressors added
    - Cut off volatile anesthetics
  - Cardiac failure: Inotropes, IABP
- Tachycardia with hypertension or normotension:
  - Beta blocker therapy:
    - Propranolol 0.5 mg boluses up to maximum of 0.1 mg/kg
    - Metaprolol 2.5 mg/kg increments up to maximum of 0.5 mg/kg
    - Esmolol 0.5 mg/kg bolus followed by 50 μg/kg/min
  - Calcium channel blockers or nitroglycerin
  - Check appropriate pain control, supplement opioids
  - If tachyarrhythmias, treat rate and rhythm

❖ Emergency coronary intervention/anticoagulation with GP-II_bIII_a antagonists only if:
- Persistent ST depression/elevation (lasting more than 30 minutes)
- Intractable cardiogenic shock

ANESTHESIA FOR PATIENTS WITH INTRACORONARY STENTS

Introduction

❖ Maintaining patency of intracoronary stents requires long-term dual anti-platelet therapy

❖ Therefore, perioperative management of these patients poses special issues

Types of Stents

❖ Bare metal stents (BMS):
- Eliminated acute vessel closure (occurs within 24 hours), seen with PTCA

- However, acute (< 24 hour) and subacute (24 hours–30 days) stent thrombosis can occur
- Incidence of stent rethrombosis is reduced with dual antiplatelet therapy
- Restenosis rate of the BMS is however high
- This is due to *neointimal hyperplasia* (medial hyperproliferation)
- This occurs due to endothelial damage from free ends of the stent

❖ Drug eluting stent (DES):
- Bare metal stent is coated with polymer containing sirolimus/paclitaxel
- Sirolimus and paclitaxel inhibit neointimal hyperplasia
- This lowers restenosis rate seen with bare metal stents
- However, DES when compared with BMS, have a higher incidence of:
  - Late stent thrombosis (> 30 days)
  - Very late stent thrombosis (> 1 year)
- This high incidence of late complications is due to delayed endothelialization
- Thus, DAPT is required during this time to allow complete endothelialization
- Therefore, patients treated with DES require longer duration of DAP therapy
- Risk factors for thrombosis after drug eluting stent:
  - Acute coronary syndrome
  - Diabetes mellitus, old age
  - Renal impairment
  - LVEF ≤ 30%
  - Premature discontinuation of dual antiplatelet therapy (DAP)

Dual Antiplatelet Therapy: *ACC-AHA 2014 Recommendations*

❖ Bare metal stents:
- Loading dose of 300–600 mg clopidogrel before implantation
- Aspirin 75–100 mg with clopidogrel 75 mg given for 4–6 weeks post-procedure to allow stent endothelialization
- Low dose aspirin continued thereafter, for life, as secondary prophylaxis
- Elective surgery postponed beyond 6 weeks of stent placement

❖ Drug eluting stent:
- Loading dose of 300–600 mg clopidogrel given before implantation
- Aspirin 75–100 mg with clopidogrel 75 mg given for 12 months post stent placement
- Thereafter, continue low dose aspirin life long, for secondary prophylaxis
- Postpone elective surgery for more than 12 months after stent placement

❖ Consider using BMS/PTCA rather than DES in patients due for urgent non-cardiac surgery within 12 months

Perioperative Anesthetic Problems

❖ Increased risk of bleeding: dangerous in closed compartment surgeries (neurosurgery)
❖ Acute perioperative stent thrombosis
❖ Complications arising due to simultaneous neuraxial blockade

Pathophysiology of Acute Perioperative Stent Thrombosis

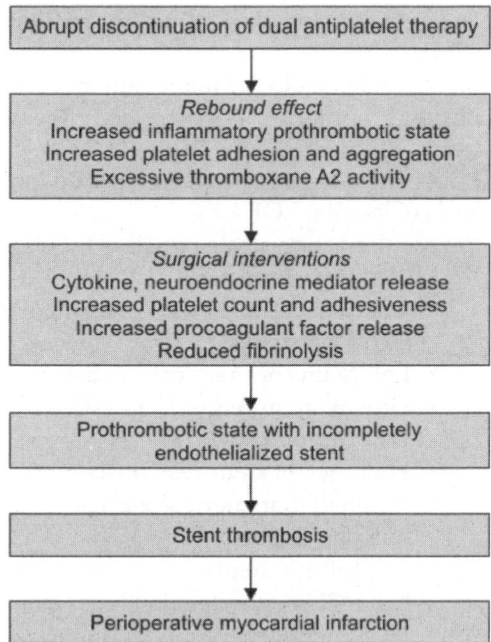

Risk Factors for Perioperative Thrombosis with DES

❖ Factors related to the stent:
- Left main coronary artery stent
- Stent in bifurcation/crossing arterial branch points
- Ostial stenting
- Small stent diameter (< 3 mm)
- Greater total stent length (> 18 mm)
- Multiple stents

❖ Factors relating to patient:
- Advanced age (> 80 years age)
- Previous stent thrombosis
- Heightened platelet activity:
  - Surgery
  - Cancer
  - Diabetes mellitus

- LV dysfunction
- Localized hypersensivity vasculitis (due to anti-proliferation drugs)
- Renal impairment
- Factors relating to dual anti-platelet therapy:
  - Resistance to anti-platelet therapy
  - Interruption of DAP therapy within 14 days of stent insertion is the *most important factor*
  - Inappropriate discontinuation of anti-platelet therapy

Preanesthetic Evaluation

- Evaluation to determine the risk of MACE can be done according to ACC- AHA 2014 guidelines for preoperative evaluation of cardiac patient for non-cardiac surgery
- History:
  - Duration since PCI
  - Type of stent: BMS/DES
  - Number, location of stents
  - Previous history of major adverse cardiac events or stent thrombosis
  - Drug regimen and any irregularities in the regimen
  - Urgency of surgery
  - Comorbidities: DM, CRF, low LVEF
  - History of conditions prone for thrombosis
  - Cardiology consultation
- Investigations:
  - Routine blood investigations
  - Platelet count and function
  - Bleeding and clotting time
  - Renal function tests
  - Arrange whole blood and platelet concentrates

Evaluating Risk of Bleeding

- Most of risk scores developed to predict bleeding risk do not apply to PCI patients
- ***HAS-BLED score:***
  - Developed using data collected 3978 patients in the Euro Heart Survey
  - Primarily used to predict 1 year major bleeding risk in those with AF on oral anticoagulants
  - But, the score can be used to predict risk of bleeding in most clinical situations
  - HAS-BLED mnemonic stands for:
    - Hypertension
    - Abnormal renal and liver function
    - Stroke
    - Bleeding
    - Labile INR
    - Elderly
    - Drugs or alcohol
  - Major bleeding is defined as:
    - Intracranial bleed
    - Hemoglobin decrease by > 2 g/dL
    - Bleeding requiring hospitalization
    - Bleeding requiring transfusion
  - Interpretation:
    - Calculated HAS-BLED scores usually range between 0–9
    - Total score > 3 implies a high risk of bleeding, which requires regular review
  - Disadvantages:
    - Type of anticoagulant:
      - Score was developed in patients treated with warfarin.
      - Thus, effectiveness with newer anticoagulants is not known
    - Score has limited use in predicting risk of hemorrhagic stroke

Mnemonic	Expansion	Criteria	Score
H	Hypertension	SBP > 160 mm Hg	1
A	Abnormal renal function	Dialysis	1
		Renal transplant patients	
		Serum creatinine > 2.26 mg/dL	
	Abnormal liver function	Cirrhosis	1
		Bilirubin > 2 times normal	
		AST/ALT/AP > 3 times normal	
S	Stroke	Prior history of stroke	1
B	Bleeding	Prior major bleeding (defined above)	1
L	Labile INR	Unstable or high INR	1
E	Elderly	Age > 65 yrs	1
D	Drugs	Prior alcohol/drug use (> 8 drinks/week)	1
		Other drugs (antiplatelets, NSAIDs)	

- ***The PRECISE-DAPT score***:
  - Simple 5-item risk score which predicts 1-year bleeding in those receiving DAPT following PCI
  - Score developed from a study of 14,963 patients with CAD who underwent PCI
  - Five item prediction algorithm includes:
    - Age
    - Prior history of spontaneous bleeding
    - Hemoglobin
    - White blood cell count
    - Creatinine clearance
  - PRECISE DAPT score higher than 25 was associated with high risk of bleeding
  - However, the score does not determine ischemic risk.

Evaluating Risk of Stent Thrombosis

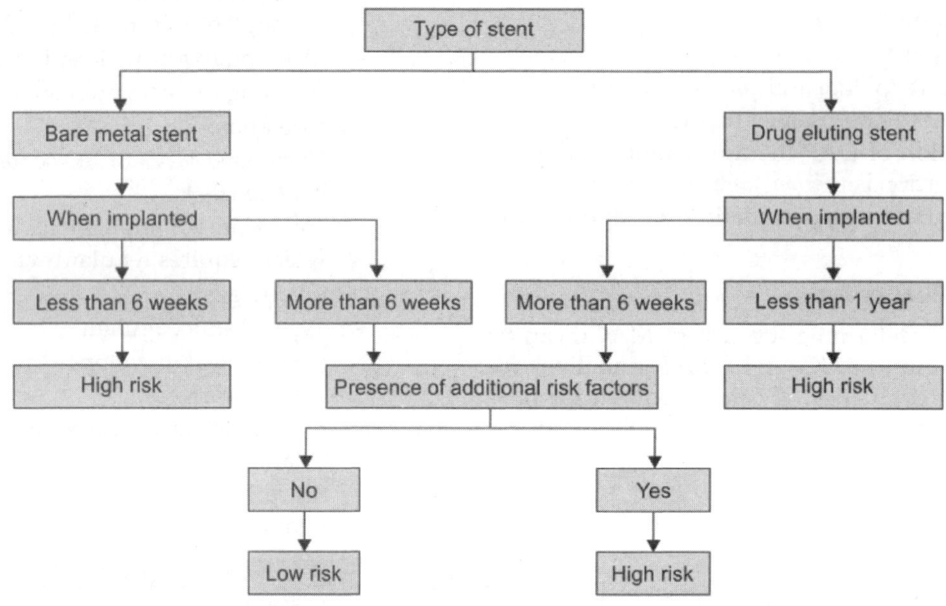

Perioperative Management: *2014 ACC- AHA Guidelines*

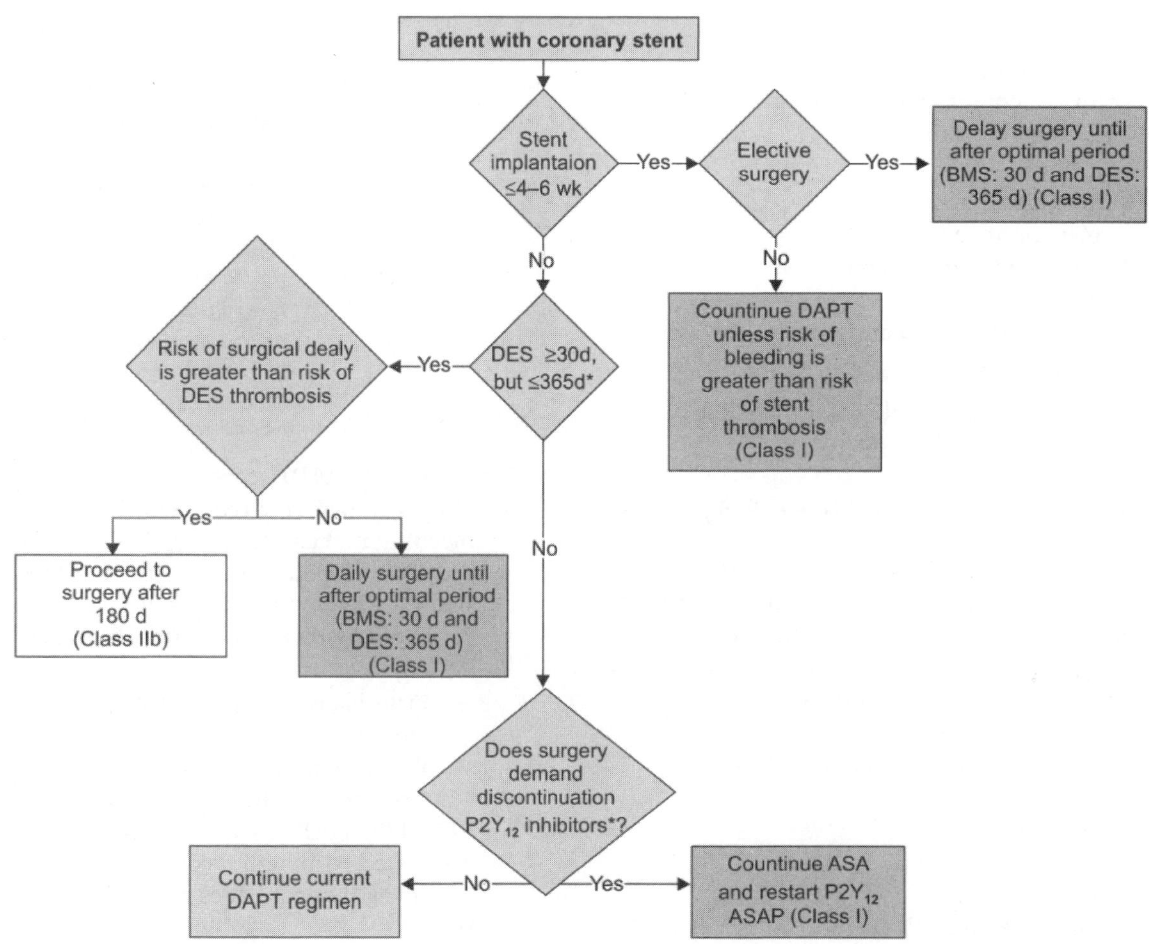

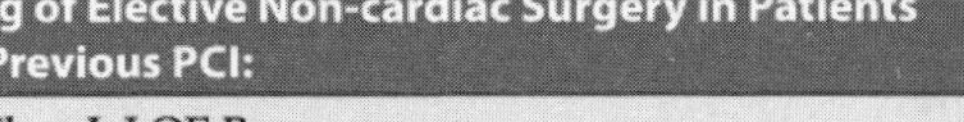

Timing of Elective Non-cardiac Surgery in Patients with Previous PCI:

- Class I: LOE B:
  - Elective non-cardiac surgery should be delayed for:
    - 14 days after balloon angioplasty
    - 30 days after BMS implantation
- Class IIa: LOE C:
  - When non-cardiac surgery is essential, discussion among treating physicians is required about:
    - Relative risks of surgery
    - Discontinuation or continuation of antiplatelet therapy
- Class IIb: LOE B:
  - Elective non-cardiac surgery after DES considered after 180 days if risk of further delay is greater than expected risks of ischemia and stent thrombosis
- Class III: Harm:
  - Elective non-cardiac surgery should not be performed:
    - Within 14 days of balloon angioplasty in those in whom aspirin will need to be discontinued preoperatively (LOE C)
    - Within 30 days of BMS implantation (LOE B)
    - Within 12 months after DES implantation in those in whom DAP will need to be discontinued preoperatively (LOE B)

Rationale of Continuing Aspirin

- Stent thrombosis is mainly a platelet-mediated phenomenon
- Therefore, antiplatelet agents play an important role in preventing stent thrombosis
- No difference was found in blood loss between aspirin users and non-users in OPCAB patients
- Protective effects of aspirin provided in vascular surgeries:
  - Improved long-term peripheral bypass graft potency
  - Reduced incidence of MI, TIA, stroke, death
- Aspirin however increases incidence of bleeding by a factor of 1.5
- In those with life-threatening perioperative bleeding platelet transfusion is recommended
- Aspirin does not increase severity or perioperative morbidity except in:
  - Intracranial surgeries
  - Spine surgeries
  - Intraocular surgeries
  - TURP (possibly)

Bridging Therapy

- Short acting GP-II_b/III_a antagonists (tirofiban/eptifibatide) is substituted for clopidogrel during perioperative period, if there is high risk of bleeding
- *Heparin has no antiplatelet action and is not protective against stent thrombosis*
- GP-II_b/III_a antagonists are used in:
  - Patients who have not completed dual antiplatelet therapy
  - Patients whose stent complexities increases risk of developing stent thrombosis

Dual Antiplatelet Therapy and Neuraxial Blockade

- Neuraxial block not recommended until:
  - Platelet function is within normal limits, or
  - Platelet transfusion is given before surgery
- If neuraxial blockade is planned:
  - Clopidogrel stopped 7 days before surgery
  - Ticlopidine stopped 14 days before surgery
  - Aspirin alone is not a contraindication for neuraxial blockade
  - Those receiving bridging therapy:
    - Discontinue abxicimab for 48 hrs before NAB
    - Discontinue eptifibatide and tirofiban for 48 hrs before NAB

PREOPERATIVE ASSESSMENT OF CARDIAC PATIENT FOR NON-CARDIAC SURGERY

Introduction

Preoperative risk assessment of the cardiac patient for non-cardiac surgery is done to help the health-care providers weigh the benefits and risks of the surgery and optimize the timing of surgery.

Goals

- To evaluate the presence and severity of already existing cardiac disease through:
  - Symptoms
  - Physical findings
  - Diagnostics tests
- To determine the need for preoperative intervention for existing cardiac disease
- To identify risk for perioperative heart disease based on risk factors
- To modify risk factors for perioperative adverse events
- Optimize timing of surgery

Historical Risk Indices

- Before 1990:
  - NYHA, ASA indices
  - Goldman, Cooperman
  - Detsky, Larsen
  - Penderson, Vanzetto
- After 1990:
  - ACC/AHA, ACP
  - Lee, ACC updated

Goldmans Cardiac Risk Index

Introduction

- First risk index, developed to predict risk of perioperative cardiac complications
- Developed by Goldman in 1977
- Also called the ***Original Cardiac Risk Index***

Characteristic	Criteria	Score
History	Age > 70 years	5
	Recent MI (within 6 months)	10
Cardiac exam	Signs of CHF	11
	Significant aortic stenosis	3
Electrocardiogram	Non-sinus arrhythmias or PVCs	7
	> 5 PVCs per minute	7
Laboratory findings	PO_2 < 60 mm Hg	3
	PCO_2 > 50 mm Hg	
	Serum potassium < 3 mEq/L	
	Bicarbonate < 20 mEq/L	
	BUN > 50 mg/dL	
	Creatinine > 3 mg/dL	
	Elevated SGOT	
	Chronic liver disease	
Surgical findings	Emergency surgery	4
	Intraperitoneal/intrathoracic/aortic surgery	3

Class	Goldmans score	Cardiac complication rate
Class I	0–5 points	1%
Class II	6–12 points	7%
Class III	13–25 points	14%
Class IV	26–53 points	78%

Lee's Revised Cardiac Risk Index (RCRI)

Introduction

- This is a tool used to estimate patients risk of perioperative cardiac complications, developed as a simplified modification of the Goldmans cardiac risk index
- It has been validated in several studies in the past, as one of the best scoring systems to predict perioperative cardiac risk in patients undergoing non-cardiac surgery

Importance

- Traditional risk factors for CAD are:
  - Smoking
  - Male gender
  - Hypercholesterolemia
  - Family history of CAD
- These are not the same factors which are associated with an increased incidence of perioperative cardiac events
- Therefore, separate scoring systems had to be developed for evaluating this risk
- Inclusions in the development of Lee's RCRI were:
  - Stable patients, more than 50 years of age
  - Undergoing major elective non-cardiac procedures
  - Expected length of stay more than 2 days
  - Done in a tertiary care hospital (*Brigham and Womens Hospital*)
- A total of 4315 patients were studied, out of which 2893 patients were used for deriving the index, which was prospectively validated in a further 1422 patients
- This was derived by looking for an association between preoperative variables and risk of cardiac complications in a selected cohort of surgical patients (the derivation cohort)

Components

- Six independent equally weighted risk factors were identified, which predicted risk of complications
- Each risk factor is assigned 1 point
- The risk factors are:
  1. High risk surgical procedures:
     - Intra-peritoneal surgeries
     - Intra-thoracic surgeries
     - Supra-inguinal surgeries
     - Vascular surgery
  2. Ischemic heart disease by any diagnostic criteria:
     - History of angina considered secondary to MI
     - History of myocardial infarction
     - Use of sublingual nitroglycerine
     - History of positive exercise test
     - Significant pathological Q waves on ECG
     - Patient who have undergone PTCA/CABG only if angina secondary to ischemia
  3. Congestive heart failure:
     - History of congestive heart failure
     - Pulmonary edema
     - Paroxysmal nocturnal dyspnea
     - Bilateral rales or S_3 gallop rhythm
     - Chest X-ray showing pulmonary vascular redistribution
  4. History of cerebrovascular disease: TIA or stroke
  5. Insulin dependent diabetes mellitus with preoperative insulin therapy
  6. Preoperative serum creatinine ≥ 2 mg/dL

Risk of Major Adverse Cardiac (MACE) Events

Class	Points	Mace risk
Class I	0 points	0.4%
Class II	1 point	0.9%
Class III	2 points	6.6%
Class IV	More than 3 points	11%

Major Adverse Cardiac Events Included in the Index

- Myocardial infarction
- Pulmonary edema
- Ventricular fibrillation
- Primary cardiac arrest
- Complete heart block

Disadvantages of Lee's RCRI

- Does not take into account all- cause mortality
- Only includes in-patient complications and not 30-day events

Validation

- Compared to the Goldmans index, Lee's RCRI was easier to use and more accurate
- Incorporated in the 2007 ACC-AHA preoperative risk evaluation guidelines
- *VISION STUDY*:
  - The Vascular events in non-cardIac Surgery patIents cOhort evaluatioN (VISION) study
  - Evaluated risk estimation performance of the RCRI in 34000 patients
  - Conducted in 29 hospitals in 15 countries, over 6 years
  - Validated the RCRI for perioperative risk assessment

Detsky Modified Multifactorial Index

Characteristic	Criteria	Score
Age	More than 70 years	5 points
Type of surgery	Emergency surgery	10 points
Myocardial infarction	No history	0 points
	Within 6 months	10 points
	Beyond 6 months	5 points
Angina	CCS class I-II	0 points
	CCS class III	10 points
	CCS class IV	20 points
	Unstable angina within 3 months	10 points
Pulmonary edema	No episodes	0 points
	Within 1 week	10 points
	Always present	5 points
Valvular disease	Possible critical aortic stenosis	20 points
Arrhythmias	Abnormal nonsinus rhythm	5 points
	More than 5 PVCs per minute	5 points
Lab findings	PO_2 < 60 mm Hg	5 points
	PCO_2 > 50 mm Hg	
	Serum potassium < 3 mEq/L	
	Serum bicarbonate < 20 mEq/L	
	BUN > 50 mg/dL	
	Creatinine > 3 mg/dL	
	Elevated SGOT	
	Chronic liver disease	

Class	Score	Risk of complications
Class I	0–5 points	6% complications
Class II	6–12 points	7% complications
Class III	13–25 points	20% complications
Class IV	26–100 points	100% complications

Eagles Criteria for Risk Assessment

Characteristic	Score
Age more than 70 years	1
Diabetes mellitus	1
Angina	1
Pathological Q waves	1
Ventricular arrhythmias	1

Score	Significance
Less than 1	No tests indicated
1–2	Non invasive testing warranted
More than 3	Angiography warranted

Preoperative Evaluation

- History:
  - Presence, severity and reversibility of CAD:
    - Risk factors:
      - Age
      - HTN, DM
      - Cholesterol
      - Smoking
    - Angina pattern:
      - Stable/unstable
      - Medications
      - Aggravating/relieving factors
    - Previous history of MI
  - Myocardial function:
    - Exercise capacity
    - Pulmonary edema
    - Orthopnea, PND, edema
    - NYHA classification:
      - Class 1:
        - No limitations of physical activity
        - On ordinary activity, no fatigue/syncope/palpitations
      - Class II:
        - Slight limitation of physical activity

        - Fatigue/palpitations/syncope on ordinary activity
    - Class III:
        - Marked limitation of activity
        - Fatigue on less than ordinary activity
    - Class IV: Symptoms occurring at rest
- Valvular heart disease:
    - Dyspnea, orthopnea, PND
    - History of medications
    - Hemoptysis
    - Embolic events
- Associated cerebral, cardiovascular, carotid, aortic vascular disease
- Prior cardiac evaluation: Non-invasive testing, angiography

❖ Physical examination:
- Vital signs: Pulse, blood pressure, respiratory rate
- Cardiac examination:
    - JVP, peripheral edema
    - Displaced apical impulse: cardiomegaly
    - S_3 gallop/S_4 gallop
    - Apical systolic murmur
    - Pulmonary edema

❖ Diagnostic tests:
- Routine blood tests, blood urea, serum creatinine
- Serum electrolytes: Especially in patients on diuretics
- If Hb ≤ 10 g%, transfuse blood in those with low cardiovascular reserve
- Brain natriuretic peptide ≥ 100 pg/mL indicates high risk of CCF
- Chest X-ray:
    - Cardiomegaly
    - Ventricular dysfunction: Increased vascular markings edema
    - Pleural/pericardial effusion
- ECG:
    - Should not be ordered simply because of advanced age
    - Only certain abnormalities are significant in preoperative assessment:
        - Q waves, especially if recent
        - Conduction abnormalities and arrhythmias
    - Establishing baseline for comparison is *most important* reason to obtain ECG preoperatively
    - If previous ECG is available and no change in risk factors/no new physical finding, it is unlikely that repeat ECG will be helpful
    - ***ACC-AHA 2014 recommendations***:
        - Class IIa recommendations: (LOE B)
            - May be excluded in those undergoing low-risk surgery
            - Reasonable to perform resting ECG in patients with:
                - Known CAD
                - Significant arrhythmias
                - Peripheral artery disease
                - Cerebrovascular disease
                - Other significant structural heart disease
        - Class IIb recommendations: (LOE B)
            - May be considered for asymptomatic patients without known CAD, except those undergoing low-risk surgeries
        - Class III recommendations: (LOE B)
            - No benefit
            - Routine preoperative resting 12-lead ECG not useful for asymptomatic patients undergoing low-risk surgeries
- Stress testing:
    - For patients with normal ECG who can exercise
    - Patients should be likely to achieve adequate heart rate response
    - Test is adequate when patient can achieve ≥ 85% of target heart rate
    - Target heart rate = 220 – age in years
    - Sensitivity and specificity of 70% and 70%
- Dobutamine stress test:
    - Useful for patients with normal ECG but unable to exercise
    - Avoided in:
        - Poorly controlled hypertension
        - Bradycardia
        - Aortic/cerebral aneurysm
        - Patients with pacemaker
    - ***2014 ACC-AHA recommendations:***
        - Class IIa recommendations: (LOE B)
            - Reasonable to perform dobutamine stress test or stress MPI in patients who are at elevated risk for non-cardiac surgery with poor functional reserve (< 4 METs)
        - Class III recommendations: (LOE B)
            - No benefits
            - Routine screening with noninvasive stress testing is not useful for patients undergoing low-risk non-cardiac surgery
- Nuclear perfusion imaging:
    - For patients unable to exercise and in whom dobutamine test is contraindicated
    - Myocardium said to have limited blood flow if it is normal at rest but shows reduced isotope uptake with exercise
- Echocardiography:
    - For evaluating RWMAs and LV function
    - Abnormal movement at rest indicates scar tissue

- Areas which are normal at rest but with abnormality which increases with increasing inotropy and chronotropy indicates stenotic lesions and limited blood flow
- Classification of LV dysfunction:
  - EF ≥ 50%: Normal
  - EF 41–49%: Mildly LV dysfunction
  - EF 26–40%: Moderate LV dysfunction
  - EF ≤ 25%: Severe LV dysfunction
- *2014 ACC-AHA recommendations:*
  - Class IIa recommendations: (LOE C)
    - Reasonable to perform preoperative evaluation of LV function in:
      - Patients with dyspnea of unknown origin
      - Patients with CHF and worsening dyspnea or other changes in clinical status
  - Class IIb recommendations: (LOE C)
    - Consider reassessment of LV function in clinically stable patients with previously documented LV dysfunction if no assessment has been done within the last one year
  - Class III recommendations: (LOE B)
    - Routine preoperative evaluation of LV function is not recommended

- Preoperative coronary angiography: Routine preoperative coronary angiography is not recommended (Class III: LOE B).

2014 ACC-AHA Guidelines for Perioperative Cardiac Assessment

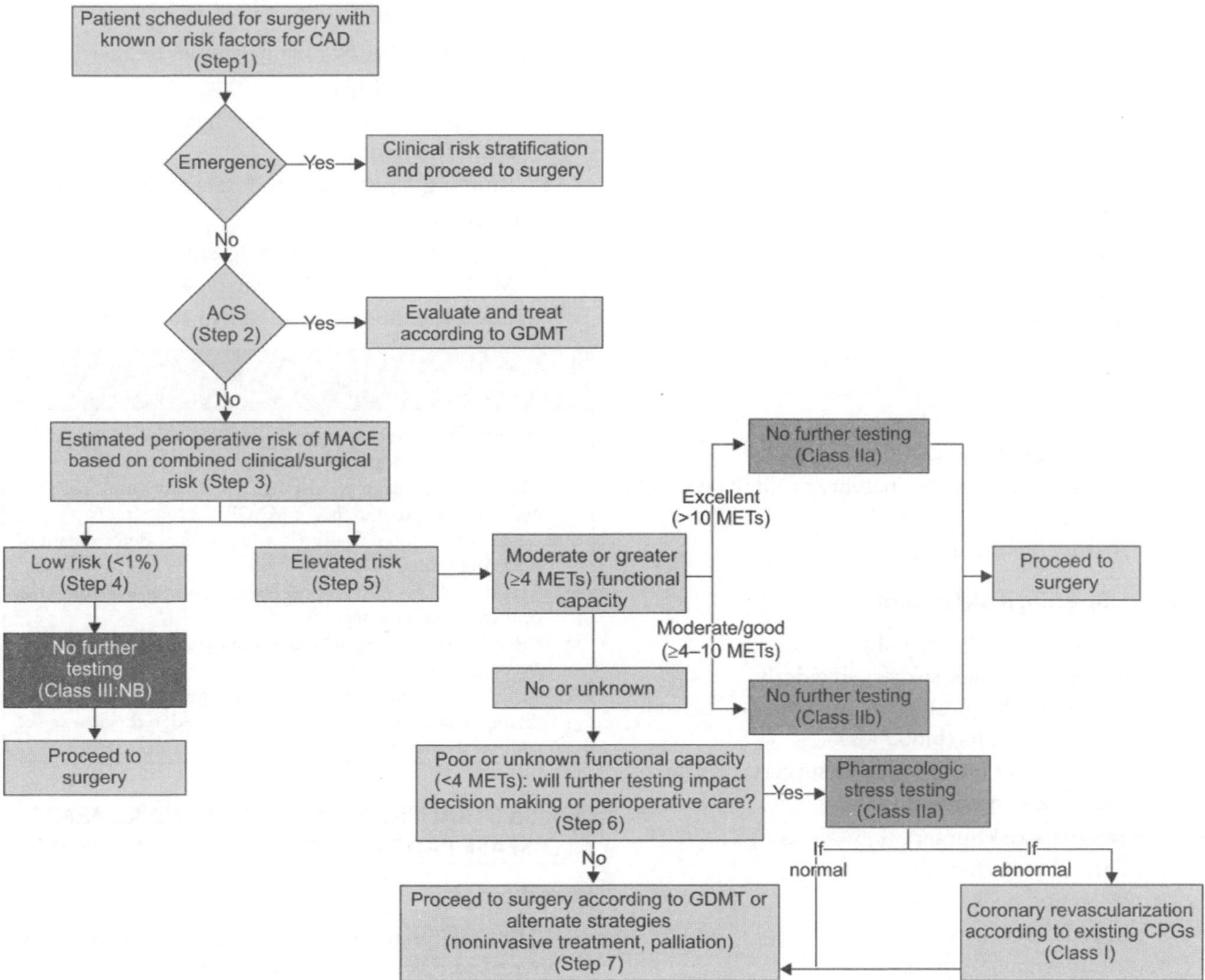

(ACS: acute coronary syndrome; GDMT: guideline directed medical therapy; MACE: major adverse cardiac event; CPG: clinical practice guideline)

Clinical Predictors of Perioperative Cardiovascular Risk

- Major predictors:
  - Unstable coronary syndromes:
    - Recent MI
    - Unstable angina
    - Severe angina CHA class III-IV
  - Decompensated CCF
  - Significant arrhythmias:
    - High grade AV block
    - Symptomatic ventricular arrhythmias in the presence of heart disease
    - Supraventricular arrhythmias with fast ventricular rate
  - Severe valvular heart disease
- Intermediate predictors:
  - Mild angina CHA class I-II
  - Prior MI based on:
    - History findings
    - Presence of pathological Q waves
  - Compensated or prior CHF
  - Diabetes mellitus
- Minor predictors:
  - Advanced age
  - Uncontrolled systemic HTN
  - Abnormal ECG findings:
    - Left ventricular hypertrophy
    - Left bundle branch block
    - ST-T abnormalities
  - Non-sinus rhythm
  - *Low functional reserve*: inability to climb one flight of stairs
  - History of stroke

Surgery Specific Risk Factors

- High risk surgery (> 5% risk):
  - Emergency major surgery in elderly
  - Prolonged surgical procedures associated with large fluid shifts/blood loss
  - Aortic/other major vascular surgery
  - Peripheral vascular disease
- Intermediate risk surgery (< 5% risk)
  - Carotid endarterectomy
  - Head and neck surgery
  - Intrathoracic surgery
  - Intraperitoneal surgery
  - Orthopedic surgery
  - Prostrate surgery
- Low risk (< 1% risk):
  - Superficial surgeries
  - Endoscopic surgeries
  - Breast, cataract surgery

Dukes Activity Status Index

1 MET is the oxygen consumption by a resting adult (3.5 mL/kg/min or 250 mL/min)

- Dukes status 1 MET:
  - Able to take care of self
  - Eat, dress, use toilet
  - Walk indoors or on level ground at 3.2–4.8 km/hr
- Dukes status 4 METs:
  - Light housework: Dusting, washing dishes
  - Climbs flight of stairs
  - Walks on level ground at 6.4 km/hr or 4 mph
  - Walks 1–2 blocks
- Dukes status 7 METs: Playing singles tennis, dancing
- Dukes status 10 METs:
  - Strenous sports: Swimming, singles tennis, basket ball, football
  - Running rapidly for moderate to long distances
- Significance:
  - Poor functional capacity: less than 4 METs
  - Moderate functional capacity: 4 to 7 METs
  - Good functional capacity: 7 to 10 METs

Recommendations 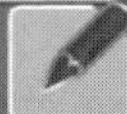

- All patients undergoing non-cardiac surgery should be assessed for perioperative MACE
- Clinical and surgery specific risk factors are used to estimate the patients risk of MACE
- Patients functional reserve is an important determinant of planning timing of surgery
- The 2014 ACC- AHA algorithm is used to determine the optimal timing for surgery
- Preoperative ECG is obtained to have a baseline available for comparison
- In those with known or suspected heart disease further testing is performed only if it is indicated in the absence of proposed surgery

RISK STRATIFICATION OF CONGENITAL HEART DISEASE PATIENT FOR NON-CARDIAC SURGERY

Introduction

- CHD children undergoing non-cardiac surgery have increased risk of morbidity and mortality
- However, the range of heart disease and surgical procedures make risk stratification difficult

Clinical Predictors of Perioperative Risk

- Factors associated with increased perioperative risk include:
  - Young age
  - Complexity of heart disease
  - Physiological status: 4 major risk factors:
    - Cardiac failure
    - Pulmonary hypertension
    - Arrhythmias
    - Cyanosis
  - Type of surgery
- The most important determinants of perioperative risk among these factors are:
  - Physiological status
  - Complexity of heart disease.

Influence of Age on Perioperative Risk

- Young age has a significant impact on the perioperative risk associated with CHD
- Some studies implicate age under 6 months with a substantial risk
- Other studies suggest higher perioperative risk up to 2 years age.

Influence of Complexity of Heart Disease on Perioperative Risk

- Highest risk of perioperative complications is seen in patients with:
  - Single ventricle physiology
  - Balanced circulation physiology
  - Patients with supra-systemic PA pressure
  - LVOT obstruction
  - Cardiomyopathy.

Influence of Physiological Status on Perioperative Risk

- Cardiac failure:
  - Cardiac failure may result due to volume overload, pressure overload, or both
  - Severe heart failure (stage C and D):
    - Children with severe cardiac failure are at a very high risk
    - This subset has a high incidence of perioperative morbidity:
      - Perioperative inotropic support 96%
      - Cardiac arrest 10%
    - These children are referred to specialist centres even for minor procedures
  - Mild heart failure (stages A and B):
    - This subset of children poses a lesser degree of perioperative risk
    - These children may be anesthetized with appropriate strategy at lower centres
    - Pertinent points during management include:
      - IV access may be difficult
      - Ketamine is the intravenous *induction agent of choice*
      - Propofol is avoided as it causes profound decrease in cardiac output
      - Induction times (both gaseous and IV) will be prolonged due to failure
      - Avoid prolonged use of 8% sevoflurane in the event of delayed induction
- Pulmonary hypertension (PHTN):
  - Pulmonary hypertension is defined as:
    - PA pressure > 25 mm Hg at rest
    - PA pressure > 30 mm Hg during exercise
  - Pulmonary HTN is a clear predictor of perioperative morbidity
  - The odds ratio for developing major perioperative complications is 8
  - These children also have other compounding factors like:
    - Reduced pulmonary compliance
    - Increased airway resistance
    - Increased work of breathing
    - Poor tolerance of respiratory tract infections
  - Thus, preoperative therapy for PHTN is an indication for referral to a higher center
- Arrhythmias:
  - RBBB is common in children with CHD
  - Ventricular ectopics however, is an ominous sign
  - Risk of perioperative death in children with ventricular ectopics is 30%
  - Incidence of fatal perioperative arrhythmias in single ventricle physiology is 30%
  - Thus, referral to a higher centre is warranted in CHD patients associated with:
    - Single ventricle circulation
    - Ventricular ectopics
    - Previous ventriculotomy
    - RV-PA conduits
- Cyanosis:
  - Cyanotic children are associated with:
    - Concurrent heart failure
    - Pulmonary hypertension
    - Arrhythmias
    - Thrombocytopenia, platelet dysfunction
    - Coagulopathy in 20% children
    - Cerebral venous thrombosis
  - Thus, children with cyanosis should be referred to higher centers.

Influence of Type of Surgery on Perioperative Risk

- Mortality of children with CHD undergoing major surgery is 16%
- Mortality of children with CHD undergoing minor surgery is however around 3%
- Thus, major surgery increases risk of death from 3% to 16%
- Major surgeries include:
  - Intraperitoneal surgeries
  - Intrathoracic surgeries
  - Vascular reconstructive surgeries
- Most common causes of cardiac arrest in CHD patients undergoing non-cardiac surgery are:
  - Hypovolemia
  - Massive transfusion
- Thus, children undergoing major surgery should be referred to a higher center.

Risk Categories

- High risk category:
  - Young age: Age under 2 years age
  - Complexity of heart disease: Complex lesions like:
    - Single ventricle physiology
    - Balanced circulation physiology:
      - Complete AV canal
      - Large VSDs
      - AP window
      - Truncus arteriosus
    - Cardiomyopathy
    - Aortic stenosis
  - Physiological status: Physiologically poorly compensated patients:
    - Cardiac failure
    - Pulmonary hypertension
    - Arrhythmias
    - Cyanosis
  - Type of surgery: Major surgery like:
    - Intraperitoneal surgery
    - Intrathoracic surgery
    - Emergency surgery
    - Anticipated major blood loss
  - Other factors:
    - Preoperative hospital stay more than 10 days
    - ASA physical status IV or V
- Intermediate risk category:
  - Young age: Age under 2 years old
  - Complexity of heart disease: Simple lesions with normal or series circulation like:
    - ASD
    - Small VSDs
    - PDA
    - TOF
  - Physiological status:
    - Physiologically normal
    - Physiologically well compensated lesions
  - Type of surgery: Major surgery like:
    - Intraperitoneal surgery
    - Intrathoracic surgery
    - Emergency surgery
    - Anticipated major blood loss
  - Others:
    - Preoperative hospital stay more than 10 days
    - ASA physical status IV or V
- Low risk category:
  - Age: Above 2 years old
  - Complexity of heart disease: simple lesions with normal or series circulation like:
    - ASD
    - Small VSDs
    - PDA
    - TOF
  - Physiological status:
    - Physiologically normal
    - Physiologically well compensated lesions
  - Type of surgery: Minor surgery like:
    - Body surface surgery Cataract, minor urological surgeries
    - Elective surgery
  - Others:
    - Preoperative hospital stay less than 10 days
    - ASA physical status I-III.

Risk Score

Feature	0	1	2
Congenital heart disease	Simple (ASD)	Moderate (ASD+PS)	Complex (TOF)
Congenital heart disease	Repaired, no residual	Repaired, residual	Palliated
Obstruction	None	Yes, Gdt < 40 mm Hg	Yes, Gdt > 50 mm Hg
Ventricle	2	1	1
	LV systemic	LV systemic	RV systemic
Ventricular dysfunction	Mild	Moderate	Severe
PVR	Normal, < 2 WU	2–4 WU	> 4 WU
SaO_2	> 90%	75–90%	< 75%
Hematocrit	30–45%	25–30% or 45–60%	< 25% or > 65%
Arrhythmia	Rare	Atrial	Ventricular
Drugs	1	2, 3	> 3

Score 0–5 = mild risk for perioperative complications
Score 6–13 = moderate risk for perioperative complications
Score 14–20 = high risk for perioperative complications

Preoperative Cardiac Assessment

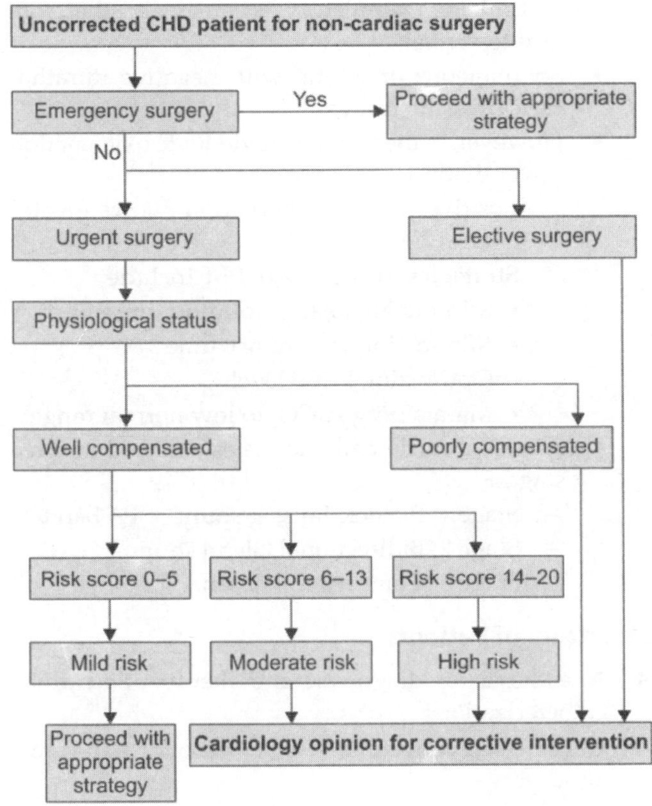

Preoperative Screening

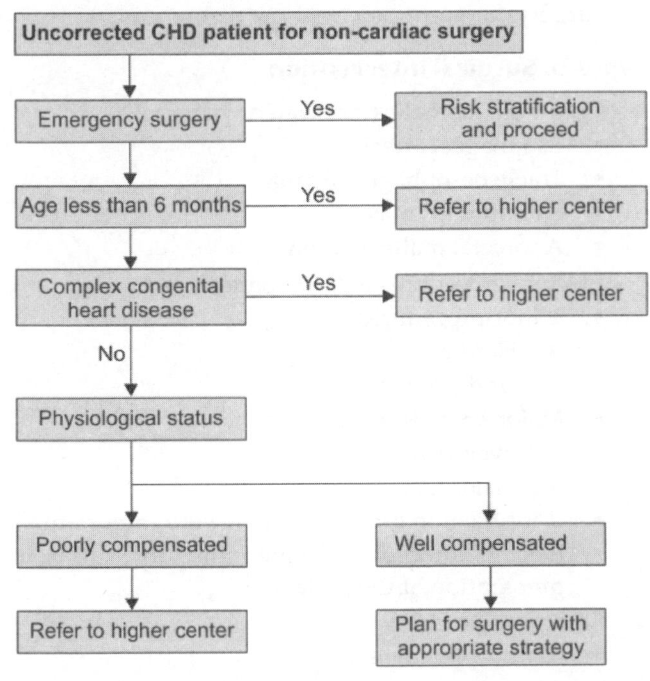

CONGENITAL HEART DISEASE PATIENT FOR NON-CARDIAC SURGERY

Introduction

- Incidence of congenital heart disease worldwide is 8–10/1000 live births
- Prevalence in India is 2.5–5.2/1000 live births
- Prevalence may be as high as 19.4/1000 live births
- Common congenital heart diseases between 0 and 5 years of age were:
  - VSD (33%)
  - ASD (19%)
  - Tetralogy of Fallot (16%)
- Intervention for associated extracardiac anomalies may be required in 10–15% of patients
- Children with CHD undergoing non-cardiac surgery have a higher risk of:
  - Morbidity
  - Anesthesia related cardiac arrest
  - 30-day mortality
- It is virtually impossible to have a single anesthetic technique owing to:
  - Complexity of defects
  - Variety of surgical procedures
  - Variety of surgical access

Limitations

- Evidence for risk stratifying patients is very limited
- Evidence base for perioperative management is limited

Classification of Congenital Heart Diseases

- Acyanotic/septal congenital heart disease:
  - ASD
  - VSD
  - PDA
  - AV canal defect
- Cyanotic congenital heart disease
  - Tetralogy of Fallot
  - Transposition of great arteries
  - Total anomalous pulmonary venous connection
  - Truncus arteriosus
  - Ebsteins anomaly
- Obstructive lesions:
  - Aortic stenosis
  - Coarctation of aorta
  - Interrupted aortic arch
  - Pulmonary stenosis

Types of Circulation in Congenital Heart Diseases

- Series or normal circulation:
  - Comprises of separate systemic and pulmonary circulations working together in series
  - Examples:
    - Most completely repaired CHD
    - Unrepaired CHD like:
      - ASD
      - VSD
      - PDA
      - TOF
  - Circulation and shunting in these lesions is determined by:
    - Size of defect
    - Pressure gradient
  - Large defects can exhibit circulation similar to balanced circulation
- Parallel or balanced circulation:
  - Pulmonary and systemic circulations communicate with each other
  - They do not function separately and do so physiologically, as being in parallel
  - Blood flow is determined by the relative resistance in each circuit
  - Thus, circulation is "balanced" by SVR and PVR
  - PVR and SVR determine magnitude and direction of shunt in this type of circulation
  - Excessive pulmonary blood flow causes:
    - Pulmonary edema
    - Poor systemic perfusion
  - Insufficient pulmonary blood flow produces profound cyanosis
  - Examples of balanced circulation:
    - Large VSD
    - AV canal defect
    - Truncus arteriosus
    - AP window
    - Hypoplastic left heart syndrome
    - Children with modified Blalock-Taussig shunt or with PA band
- Single ventricle circulation:
  - Used as a palliative strategy in CHDs not amenable to full anatomical correction
  - The functional single ventricle pumps blood into the systemic circulation
  - Pulmonary circulation occurs passively down a pressure gradient from PA to LA
  - PA-LA pressure gradient is the sole determinant of pulmonary blood flow
  - Therefore, increase in PVR and intrathoracic pressure will compromise PBF
  - Optimizing ventilatory strategy is therefore quintessential
  - Spontaneous breathing with negative intrathoracic pressure is ideal
  - However, in the event of inadequate oxygenation or ventilation:
    - Positive pressure ventilation allows greater control
    - Strategies to encourage PBF include:
      - Minimizing peak inspiratory pressure
      - Minimizing inspiratory time
      - Optimizing PEEP level
      - Maintaining $PaCO_2$ to low normal range
  - Single ventricle palliation is established in three stages:
    - Stage 1: Blalock Taussig shunt or PA band
    - Stage 2: Bidirectional Glenn shunt
    - Stage 3: Completion Fontan.

Spectrum of Patients

- Anesthesia for diagnostic and therapeutic cardiac catheterization
- Uncorrected congenital heart disease for non-cardiac surgery
- GUCHD (Grown Up CHD) patients for non-cardiac surgery
- Corrected CHD patients for non-cardiac surgery
- Partially palliated CHD patients for non-cardiac surgery.

Types of Surgical Intervention

- Common anomalies associated with CHD:
  - Esophageal atresia
  - Tracheoesophageal fistula
  - Exomphalos major
  - Anorectal malformations
- Elective procedures in CHD patients:
  - Minor procedures:
    - Hernia
    - Undescended testes
  - Major procedures:
    - Pyeloplasty
    - Major laparotomy
  - Prioritization of procedures is very important
  - Elective procedures allow time for sufficient preparation of the patient
- Emergency surgery:
  - Acute appendicitis

- Acute abdomen
- Trauma
- Insufficient time for preparation.

Preoperative Assessment

- Assessment of symptoms: 3 types of presentations:
  - Features of cyanosis in a cyanotic child:
    - Occurs when concentration of reduced Hb is more than 3–5 g/dL
    - Indicates a right to left shunt
    - Associated with cyanotic spells and squatting episodes
    - Effects of long standing cyanosis:
      - Coagulopathy
      - Paradoxical air embolism
      - Renal dysfunction
      - Hypertrophic osteoarthropathy
      - Cerebral abscess
      - Heart failure
      - Iron deficiency
  - Features of congestive failure in acyanotic child:
    - Occurs due to increased pulmonary blood flow
    - Recurrent respiratory tract infections
    - Sweating, reduced exercise tolerance
    - Tachypnea, chest retractions
    - Nasal flaring, use of accessory muscles of respiration
    - Difficulty feeding, poor growth
    - Pedal edema, raised jugular venous pulsations
    - Hepatomegaly, rales
    - Assessment of severity of failure:
      - Feeding habits
      - Extent of physical activity
      - Exercise tolerance
      - Degree of failure to thrive
  - Features of low cardiac output syndrome:
    - Usually occurs in:
      - Shones complex
      - LVOT obstruction
      - Hypoplastic left heart syndrome
    - Maybe associated with cardiac syncope
    - Cardiac syncope in children is usually caused by:
      - Arrhythmias
      - LVOT obstruction
    - Angina can be associated with:
      - LVOT obstruction
      - Anomalous origin of left coronary artery from PA (ALCAPA)
- Assessment of signs:
  - Height and weight of the patient has to be measured for failure to thrive
  - Peripheral pulses and blood pressure to be measured in all extremities for coarctation
  - Saturation to be measured in all limbs for differential cyanosis
  - Signs of breathlessness:
    - Tachypnea
    - Intercostal, subcostal retractions
    - Nasal flaring
    - Grunting
  - Signs of overt heart failure:
    - Jugular venous pulsations used in children above 5 years age
    - Below 5 years hepatomegaly is a reliable sign of heart failure
    - Up to 1 cm hepatomegaly is normal in neonates
    - Dependant peripheral edema is a late sign of cardiac failure
- Assessment of cardiac murmurs:
  - Ejection systolic murmur:
    - Aortic stenosis
    - Pulmonary stenosis
    - ASD
    - TOF
  - Pansystolic murmur:
    - VSD
    - Mitral regurgitation
  - Diastolic murmur: Aortic regurgitation
  - Continuous murmur:
    - PDA
    - Arteriovenous malformations
- Assessment of associated defects:
  - Specific features in syndromic associations:
    - Goldenhars syndrome (difficult intubation)
    - CHARGE syndrome (choanal atresia)
    - VACTERL syndrome (tracheoesophageal fistula)
    - Marfans syndrome (spontaneous pneumothorax)
    - Downs syndrome (atlanto-axial joint subluxation)
  - Subglottic stenosis to be suspected in patients with history of prolonged intubation
  - Avail history of implanted pacemakers, defibrillators.

Preoperative Investigations

Surgery	Blood	Examination	Investigation	Medication
Catheterization Minor surgery	Hemoglobin	BP all extremities	Chest X-ray	Continue all medicines
	Coagulation profile	Baseline saturation	Echo < 1 month	
	RFT	Effect due to exercise	Review CT/MRI	
	LFT	Edema		
	Blood group	Crackles		
	Save one adult unit of packed cells for any interventional procedure			
Major surgery Moderate-high risk	All blood investigations	BP all extremities	Chest X-ray	Continue all medicines
	Blood group	Baseline saturation	Recent echo	Stop ACE inhibitors
		Effect due to exercise		
		Edema		
		Crackles		
	Save *one cross matched* adult unit of packed cells			
GUCHD	All blood investigations	BP all extremities	Chest X-ray	Continue PHT medicines
	Blood group	Baseline saturation	Most recent echo	Stop ACE inhibitors
	Antibody screen	Effect due to exercise	Most recent MRI	
		Edema		
		Crackles		
	Save *at least one cross matched* adult unit of packed cells			

- Other investigations:
  - Electrolytes: Especially if the patient is on diuretics
  - Cardiology review:
    - Not required in fit and healthy CHD patients post complete repair
    - Required for:
      - Complex congenital heart lesions
      - Major surgery
- Anesthesia clearance is most important as cardiologist will not have full knowledge of anesthetic effects

Risk Prediction

- CHD children undergoing non-cardiac surgery are at an increased risk of morbidity
- However, the range of heart disease and surgical procedures makes risk stratification difficult
- Factors associated with an increased risk are:
  - Young age
  - Disease complexity
- Physiological status: 4 major risk factors:
  - Cardiac failure
  - Pulmonary hypertension
  - Arrhythmias
  - Cyanosis
- Type of surgery
- Highest risk patients are those with:
  - Functionally single ventricle
  - Patients with supra-systemic PA pressure
  - LVOT obstruction
  - Cardiomyopathy

Feature	0	1	2
Congenital heart disease	Simple (ASD)	Moderate (ASD+PS)	Complex (TOF)
Congenital heart disease	Repaired, no residual	Repaired, residual	Palliated
Obstruction	None	Yes, Gdt < 40 mm Hg	Yes, Gdt > 50 mm Hg
Ventricle	2	1	1
	LV systemic	LV systemic	RV systemic
Ventricular dysfunction	Mild	Moderate	Severe
PVR	Normal, < 2 WU	2–4 WU	> 4 WU
SaO_2	> 90%	75–90%	< 75%
Hematocrit	30–45%	25–30% or 45–60%	< 25% or > 65%
Arrhythmia	Rare	Atrial	Ventricular
Drugs	1	2, 3	> 3

Score 0–6 = Mild risk for perioperative complications
Score 6–14 = Moderate risk for perioperative complications
Score 14–20 = High risk for perioperative complications

Preoperative Cardiac Assessment

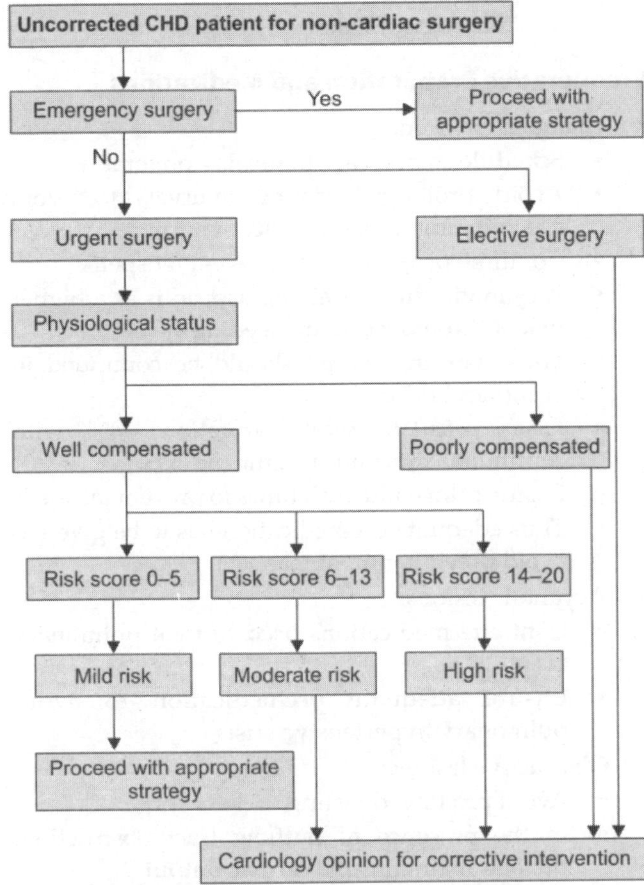

General Principles of Anesthesia in Children with CHD

- Expect an anxious patient due to multiple prior hospital visits
- Expect difficult IV access due to multiple admissions
- Plan for a lesion directed anesthetic management
- Preparation for lesion specific acute decompensation intraoperatively:
  - Hypercyanotic TET spell in TOF patients
  - Low cardiac output syndrome in:
    - Obstructive lesions:
      - Aortic stenosis
      - Coarctation of aorta
    - Cardiomyopathy
  - Pulmonary hypertensive crisis in:
    - AV canal defects
    - AP window
    - Large VSDs
- Plan the most appropriate surgical approach (laparoscopy/open)
- Ensure adequate antibiotic prophylaxis
- Infective endocarditis prophylaxis in indicated patients
- Evaluate associated chromosomal anomalies and syndromes
- Avoid air bubbles, particularly in right-left shunt lesion to prevent paradoxical air embolism

Chromosomal Anomalies Associated with CHD

- *Down's* syndrome:
  - Due to trisomy 21
  - Features include:
    - Mongoloid facies
    - Single simian palmar crease
    - Lax joints, atlanto-axial joint instability
    - Short stature, learning difficulties
    - Obstructive sleep apnea
    - Hypothyroidism, duodenal atresia
  - Associated with:
    - Cardiac defects in 40% of Down's syndrome patients
    - Complete AV canal defect
    - VSD
- *DiGeorge* syndrome:
  - Part of the spectrum of Catch 22 syndrome
  - Due to chromosome 22q11 deletion
  - Features include:
    - Learning difficulties
    - Hypocalcemia seen in 50% patients
    - Cleft palate seen in 11% patients
    - Absent thymus rarely seen
    - Frequent respiratory tract infections
  - Associated with:
    - Cardiac anomalies in almost 80% patients
    - Aortic arch abnormalities
    - VSD
- *Marfan's* syndrome:
  - Due to mutations in FBN1 gene
  - This reduces the amount of functional fibrillin-1 available to form connective tissue
  - Features include:
    - Abnormally tall stature
    - Long fingers
    - Scoliosis
    - High arched palate
    - Retinal detachment
    - Inguinal hernia
    - Spontaneous pneumothorax
  - Associated with:
    - Aortic root dilatation
    - Aortic dissection

- *CHARGE* association:
  - Due to CHD7 mutation
  - Features include:
    - **C**oloboma iris
    - **H**eart defects
    - **A**tresia choanae
    - **R**etarded growth
    - **G**enital abnormalities:
      - Hypogonadism
      - Undescended testes
      - Hypospadiasis
    - **E**ar deformity:
      - Abnormal bowl shaped and concave ears
      - Also known as *"lop ears"*
  - Associated with:
    - AV canal defect
    - VSD
- *VACTERL* association:
  - Due to interaction between multiple genetic and environmental factors
  - Features include:
    - **V**ertebral anomalies:
      - Fused vertebrae
      - Extra vertebrae
      - Hemivertebrae
    - **A**nal atresia
    - **C**ardiac defects
    - **T**racheoesophageal fistula
    - **R**enal abnormalities:
      - Absence of one or both kidneys
      - Ureteric obstruction
      - Early onset renal failure
    - **L**imb abnormalities:
      - Hypoplastic thumb
      - Polydactyly
      - Syndactyly
      - Radial aplasia
  - Associated with:
    - VSD
    - Tetralogy of Fallot
- *Goldenhar* syndrome:
  - Due to multiple factors
  - This causes disruption of development of 1st and 2nd pharyngeal arches
  - Features include:
    - Hemifacial microsomia
    - Poorly developed maxilla/mandible
    - Difficult intubation
    - Ear abnormalities:
      - Microtia
      - Anotia
    - Cleft palate
  - Associated with:
    - VSD
    - Tetralogy of Fallot

Preoperative Preparation and Medications

- Cyanotic children:
  - Schedule as first case in the day preferably
  - Avoid prolonged fasting intervals to avoid precipitating hyperviscosity syndrome
  - Continue propranolol to prevent tet spells
  - A cyanotic child receiving aspirin is at a higher risk of thrombosis than bleeding
  - Thus, aspirin therapy should be continued in cyanotic children
  - *Ensure patent BT shunt*: saturation > 85% with continuous murmur in right 2nd ICS
  - Ensure calm child at all times to prevent tet spells
  - Thus adequate premedication has to be given to avoid precipitation of tet spells
- Acyanotic lesions:
  - Continue medications used to treat pulmonary HTN
  - Ensure adequate premedication to avoid pulmonary hypertensive crisis
- Obstructive lesions:
  - Avoid prolonged fasting
  - In the presence of outflow tract obstruction, preload maintains the cardiac output
  - Thus, in the event of prolonged fasting, IV fluids have to be initiated
  - Ensure adequate premedication to avoid detrimental tachycardia

Role of Neuraxial Blockade

- Neuraxial blockade can be used in highly specific lesions for specific procedures
- CSE techniques can be used to titrate levels of anesthesia
- Contraindicated in:
  - Patients with right- left shunt lesions
  - Left sided obstructive lesions to avoid decrease in SVR
  - Failing Fontan circulation
- Low dose spinal can be used for:
  - Left-right shunts with normal ventricular function
  - Regurgitant lesions
- Advantages of neuraxial blockade:
  - Provides dense analgesia- reduces catecholamine response to surgery

- May be used for postoperative analgesia
- Maybe beneficial in patients with regurgitant lesions
- Facilitates spontaneous ventilation

Infective Endocarditis Prophylaxis

- Indicated in high risk patients undergoing high risk procedures
- High risk patients for infective endocarditis:
  - Prior history of infective endocarditis
  - Patients with prosthetic cardiac valves including:
    - Mechanical valves
    - Bioprosthetic valves
    - Homograft valves
  - Unrepaired and palliated (including shunts and conduits) cyanotic CHD patients
  - Prosthetic material during 1st 6 months after placement including:
    - Annuloplasty rings
    - Chords
  - Device implantation or stents during 1st 6 months after placement
  - Residual lesions at the site of repair of CHD
  - Residual lesions adjacent to prosthetic patch or device, preventing endothelialisation
- High risk procedures include:
  - High risk dental surgery:
    - Involving manipulation of gingival tissue or periapical region of teeth
    - Involving perforation or suturing of oral mucosa
    - Tooth extractions
    - Dental infections, drainage of dental abscess
  - Respiratory tract procedures:
    - Incision or biopsy of respiratory tract mucosa
    - Tonsillectomy
    - Adenoidectomy
    - Bronchoscopy with biopsy

Lesion Specific Anesthetic Goals

- Cyanotic lesions:
  - Ensure calm child at all times to prevent precipitation of tet spells
  - Good analgesia
  - Rate: Avoid bradycardia
  - Rhythm: Maintain sinus rhythm
  - Preload:
    - Maintain adequate preload
    - Avoid dehydration
  - Afterload/SVR:
    - Maintain or increase afterload to reduce R-L shunting
    - Avoid sudden reduction in afterload at induction
    - Neuraxial blockade avoided to prevent sudden fall in SVR
  - PVR: Avoid increases in PVR as it increases R-L shunting
  - Contractility: Avoid increase in contractility to prevent RVOT spasm
- Acyanotic lesions:
  - Ensure calm child if preoperative PHTN to avoid pulmonary hypertensive crisis
  - Ventilation:
    - Controlled ventilation preferred to reduce work of breathing
    - Avoid high FiO_2 to prevent increased pulmonary blood flow and cardiac failure
    - Saturation of 90–94% is adequate
  - Rate: Maintain age appropriate heart rate
  - Rhythm: Maintain sinus rhythm
  - Preload: Judicious preload
  - Afterload: Maintain or decrease SVR as increased SVR increases L-R shunt
  - PVR: Avoid decreases in PVR as it causes increased L-R shunt
  - Contractility: Maintain contractility
  - Avoid precipitating pulmonary hypertensive crisis by avoiding:
    - Hypoxia
    - Hypercarbia
    - Acidosis
    - Hypothermia
- Obstructive lesions:
  - Rate: Avoid tachycardia to prevent increases in myocardial oxygen demand
  - Rhythm: Maintain sinus rhythm as atrial kick contributes more to CO in the presence of LVOTO
  - Preload: Ensure adequate preload to attribute for reduced ventricular compliance
  - Afterload/SVR:
    - Maintain high/normal SVR in the presence of fixed LVOTO
    - Neuraxial blockade avoided to prevent sudden decrease in SVR
  - PVR: Maintain normal PVR
  - Contractility: Avoid decrease in contractility

Monitors

- Cyanotic lesions:
  - Pulse oximetry
  - ECG

- NIBP
- E_TCO_2
- Nasopharyngeal temperature
- BP and saturation on the side of prior BT shunt is usually inaccurate
- Invasive arterial and venous access:
  - Used in intermediate-high risk patients and major procedures
  - High risk of thrombus formation and embolic complications
  - Thus, regular flushing or autoflush systems of invasive lines are essential
  - Remove catheters as soon as possible in the postoperative period

❖ Acyanotic lesions:
- Pulse oximetry
- ECG
- NIBP
- E_TCO_2
- Nasopharyngeal temperature
- Invasive arterial and venous access in intermediate-high risk patients and procedure

❖ Obstructive lesions:
- Pulse oximetry
- ECG
- NIBP
- E_TCO_2
- Nasopharyngeal temperature
- Invasive arterial and venous access in intermediate-high risk patients and procedure

Induction

❖ Cyanotic lesions:
- Baseline SPO_2 has to be recorded to enable titration of FiO_2
- Gaseous induction with sevoflurane used in the absence of IV line
- Ketamine 2 mg/kg IV is *induction agent of choice* due to minimal effect on SVR
- Fentanyl and atracurium of vecuronium can be used to ensure muscle paralysis
- Ensure air bubble free IV lines to prevent paradoxical air embolism
- IV antibiotics to be administered 30–60 minutes prior to the procedure

❖ Acyanotic lesions:
- Inhalational induction with sevoflurane used in the absence of IV line
- Low dose propofol 0.5–1 mg/kg IV may be used for induction
- Ketamine may be used in the presence of ventricular dysfunction
- Fentanyl and atracurium of vecuronium can be used to ensure muscle paralysis
- Ensure air bubble free IV lines to prevent paradoxical air embolism
- Avoid light planes at intubation to avoid precipitation of pulmonary crisis
- Avoid high FiO_2 at induction to:
  - Minimize left-right shunt
  - Prevent increases in pulmonary blood flow
  - Maximize systemic perfusion
- IV antibiotics to be administered 30–60 minutes prior to the procedure

❖ Obstructive lesions:
- Inhalational induction with sevoflurane used in the absence of IV line
- Avoid prolonged use of high concentrations of sevoflurane
- Etomidate 0.2–0.3 mg/kg IV is *induction agent of choice*
- Fentanyl and atracurium of vecuronium can be used to ensure muscle paralysis
- Avoid light planes at intubation to prevent detrimental increases in heart rate
- IV antibiotics to be administered 30–60 minutes prior to the procedure
- *External defibrillation paddles* applied in those at high risk for arrhythmias

Maintenance

❖ Cyanotic lesions:
- Balanced anesthesia with volatile agents is the preferred technique
- O_2 + air + 1 MAC sevoflurane/isoflurane can be used for maintenance
- Fentanyl and atracurium/vecuronium boluses used to maintain analgesia and paralysis
- TIVA avoided due to risk of reduced SVR

❖ Acyanotic lesions:
- Balanced anesthesia with volatile agents is the preferred technique
- O_2 + air + 1 MAC sevoflurane/isoflurane can be used for maintenance
- Fentanyl and atracurium/vecuronium boluses used to maintain analgesia and paralysis

❖ Obstructive lesions:
- Balanced anesthesia with volatile agents is the preferred technique
- O_2 + air + 1 MAC sevoflurane/isoflurane can be used for maintenance

- Fentanyl and atracurium/vecuronium boluses used to maintain analgesia and paralysis
- TIVA avoided due to risk of reduced SVR

Ventilation

- Cyanotic lesions:
  - Titrate FiO_2 to maintain SpO_2 close to baseline values
  - Avoid hypoxia and hypercarbia
  - Significant $ETCO_2$-$PaCO_2$ gradient due to reduced pulmonary flow
  - Thus, periodic checking for adequacy of ventilation mandatory:
    - Tidal volume
    - Minute volume
    - Visualization of chest rise
    - Blood samples for $PaCO_2$ if arterial line is present
- Acyanotic lesions:
  - Avoid hyperoxia (LV failure) and hypoxia (pulmonary hypertensive crisis)
  - Avoid hypocarbia (LV failure) and hypercarbia (pulmonary hypertensive crisis)
  - In patients with severe PAH, $PaCO_2$ is maintained at 30–35 mm Hg to lower PVR
  - Avoid high FiO_2 to:
    - Minimize left-right shunt
    - Prevent increases in pulmonary blood flow
    - Maximize systemic perfusion
  - May require higher ventilator pressures due to pulmonary edema
- Obstructive lesions:
  - Mechanical ventilation itself acts as inotropic agent by increasing preload into LV
  - Thus, positive pressure ventilation is useful to reduce work of breathing
  - May require higher ventilatory pressures due to pulmonary edema

Hemodynamics

- Cyanotic lesions:
  - Maintain adequate preload with generous IV fluid volumes
  - Prefer a higher transfusion trigger of 30% hematocrit
  - Avoid fall in SVR- phenylephrine or vasopressin maybe used to treat hypotension
  - Vasopressin is the *agent of choice* as it increases SVR without increasing PVR
  - Avoid using inotropic agents to prevent increases in RVOT obstruction
- Acyanotic lesions:
  - Maintain judicious preload
  - In case of raised fluid requirements, colloids can be used to prevent fluid overload
  - Avoid high SVR as it increases left-right shunt
  - Avoid fall in PVR as it increases left-right shunt
  - Phenylephrine is *agent of choice* to treat hypotension as it increases SVR and PVR
- Obstructive lesions:
  - Avoid tachycardia to reduce myocardial oxygen demand
  - Maintain sinus rhythm as atrial kick contributes more to CO due to LVOTO
  - Cardioversion used to revert hemodynamically unstable SVT
  - Maintain intravascular volume taking into account pre-existing pulmonary edema
  - Maintain high- normal SVR:
    - Phenylephrine used to treat hypotension
    - Norepinephrine infusion is used to treat precipitous, sustained hypotension
  - Maintain contractility

Extubation

- Mild-moderate risk patients undergoing mild-intermediate risk procedures are extubated
- Postoperative ventilation preferred for high risk patients and major surgeries
- Cyanotic lesions:
  - Extubation in deep planes may be used as an effective strategy
  - This allows calm emergence and thus prevents precipitation of tet spells
- Acyanotic lesions:
  - Extubation in fully awake planes preferred to avoid post-extubation hypercarbia
  - Goals at extubation:
    - Minimize airway reactivity
    - Avoid coughing
    - Prevent sympathetic response to endotracheal tube
  - Dexmedetomidine infusion 0.2–0.7 µg/kg/min maintains sedation post extubation
- Obstructive lesions:
  - Extubation in deep planes may be used as an effective strategy
  - This allows the patient to emerge from anesthesia in a calm manner
  - This strategy avoids sympathetic response to extubation
  - Thus, myocardial oxygen demand is preserved

Postoperative Care

Monitoring

- Pulse oximetry
- ECG
- NIBP/IBP
- Careful monitoring for partial airway obstruction post extubation

Management

- Goals of management include:
  - Minimization of sympathetic stimulation: treat pain and anxiety
  - Encourage adequate ventilation and oxygenation
- Dexmedetomidine is a useful drug to maintain sedation and analgesia post extubation

Analgesia

- Multimodal analgesia used to treat pain
- NSAIDs
- Regional blocks
- IV- PCA can be employed in moderate- severe pain

Sequelae Post Congenital Cardiac Surgery

- ASD device closure:
  - Residual shunt
  - Device fracture
  - Device malposition
  - Septal aneurysm
- Surgical correction of coarctation of aorta:
  - Systolic hypertension
  - Residual gradient across coarctation
  - Aneurysm
  - Low left arm blood pressure due to subclavian flap
- Arterial switch operation for TGA:
  - Supravalvular AS, PS
  - Aortic regurgitation
  - Coronary artery stenosis
  - Ventricular dysfunction
- Rastelli procedure:
  - Residual VSD
  - Ventricular dysfunction
  - Outflow tract obstruction
  - Aortic, pulmonary regurgitation
- Tetralogy of Fallot:
  - Arrhythmias:
    - Right bundle branch block
    - AV block
  - Pulmonary valve regurgitation
  - RV dysfunction
  - Sudden death
- Single ventricle circulation:
  - Preload dependence
  - Ventricular dysfunction
  - Protein losing enteropathy

INTRA-AORTIC BALLOON PUMP

Introduction

- Most commonly used circulatory assist device (CAD) augmenting myocardial perfusion
- Consists of a double lumen balloon catheter placed in the descending thoracic aorta
- The balloon is inflated during diastole providing aortic counterpulsations
- Simplest and most readily available CAD
- Introduced in 1968.

Composition of IABP

- 25 mm sausage shaped balloon
- Mode of non-thrombogenic polyurethane
- Mounted on 90 cm long vascular catheter with:
  - One lumen for distal aspiration and flushing as well as pressure monitoring
  - Other lumen for periodic delivery and removal of helium gas
- Helium gas used for balloon distension
- Volume of balloon is 30–50 mL

Indications

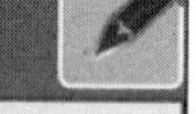

- Cardiogenic shock:
  - Post-ST-elevation myocardial infarction (Class IIa, LOE: B)
  - Myocarditis
  - Cardiomyopathy
  - Pharmacological
- Failure to wean from CPB:
  - Right/left ventricular failure
  - Increased inotropic requirements
  - Hemodynamic deterioration
- Stabilization for emergent cardiac surgery, delayed due to immediate inoperability:
  - MI with VSD
  - MI with mitral regurgitation
  - Unstable, refractory acute coronary syndrome
- Adjunctive therapy for high-risk angioplasty:
  - Prophylactically in hemodynamically unstable patients with:
    - Severe LV dysfunction (EF < 30%)
    - Complex, multivessel coronary artery disease

Contd...

Contd...

- Therapeutically for:
  - Prolonged hypotension
  - Pulmonary edema
  - Refractory ventricular arrhythmias
- Prophylactic use for coronary bypass in patients with left main coronary artery disease
- Refractory heart failure as a bridge to transplantation
- Intractable ventricular arrhythmias as a bridge to further therapy

Contraindications 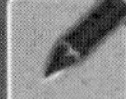

- Absolute contraindications:
  - Ascending aortic dissection/aneurysm
  - Severe calcific aorta
  - Peripheral vascular disease
- Relative contraindications:
  - Descending aortic dissection/aneurysm
  - Severe AR
  - Irreversible cardiac disease (not a transplant candidate)
  - Irregular rhythm
  - Sepsis
  - Uncontrolled bleeding diatheses
  - Irreversible brain damage
  - Severe non-cardiac systemic disease
  - Massive trauma, Do Not Resuscitate (DNR) patients
  - Local infection, inability to insert

Advantages of IABP

- Balloon deflation during ventricular systole:
  - Reduces LV afterload
  - Reduces peak LV stress and LV stroke work
  - Reduces myocardial oxygen demand
  - Reduces mitral valve regurgitation
  - Increases LV ejection
- Balloon inflation during ventricular diastole:
  - Increases coronary perfusion pressure
  - Augments coronary blood flow
  - Improves myocardial oxygen delivery
- Other effects:
  - Augments cardiac output
  - Reduces pulmonary capillary wedge pressure
  - Relieves pulmonary congestion

Insertion of IABP

- Inserted into femoral artery either percutaneously/ via surgical exposure
- Fluoroscopic guidance is preferred during insertion
- Length to be inserted calculated by measuring distance between:
  - Angle of Louis
  - Femoral artery
- Final position of the balloon should be such that:
  - Distal tip lies below left subclavian artery (to prevent emboli to brain)
  - Proximal tip lies above renal artery
- Pumping is initiated and controlled by the console using input from ECG and aortic pressure
- Alternate approaches:
  - Subclavian artery
  - Axillary artery
  - *Ascending aorta*: if PVD present
  - *Iliac artery*: in children where size of femoral artery is small
- Axillary approach is favoured for anticipated prolonged IABP use (>10–14 days).

Timing and Goal of Inflation and Deflation

- Inflation:
  - Timed to coincide with aortic valve closure
  - Inflated just prior to dicrotic notch
  - Inflation is continued throughout diastole
  - Produces rapid rise in diastolic BP
  - Balloon inflation creates a constant, increased pressure head between:
    - IABP balloon
    - Aortic valve
  - This constant pressure head improves coronary blood flow.

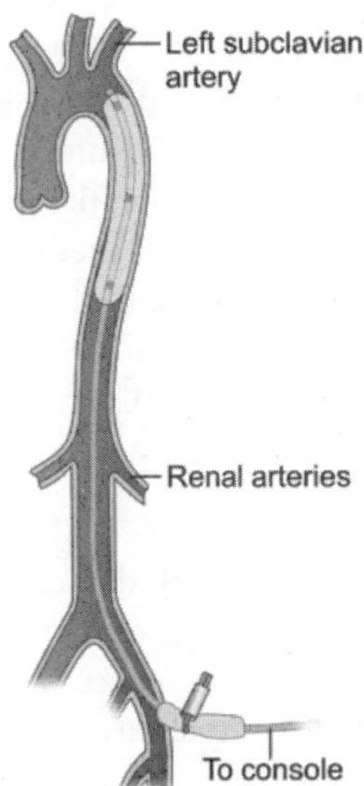

Fig. 45: Insertion of IABP.

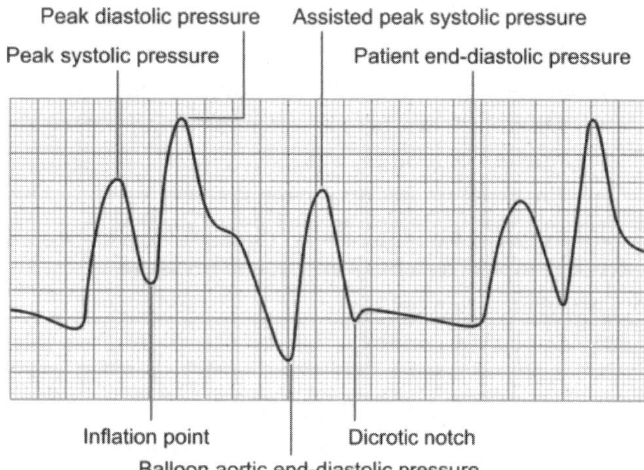

Fig. 46: Normal IABP waveform.

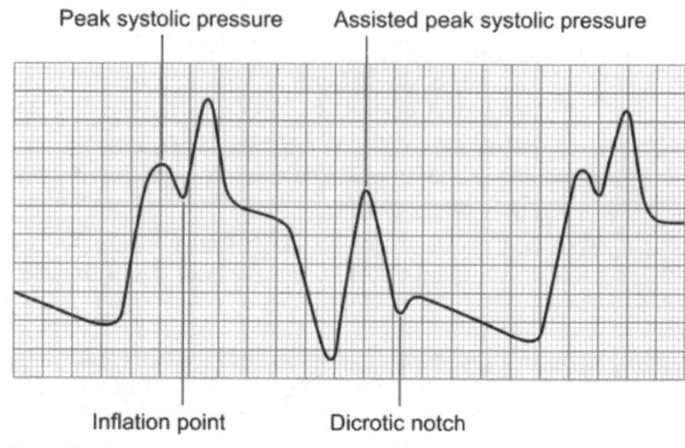

Fig. 48: Early inflation of IABP balloon.

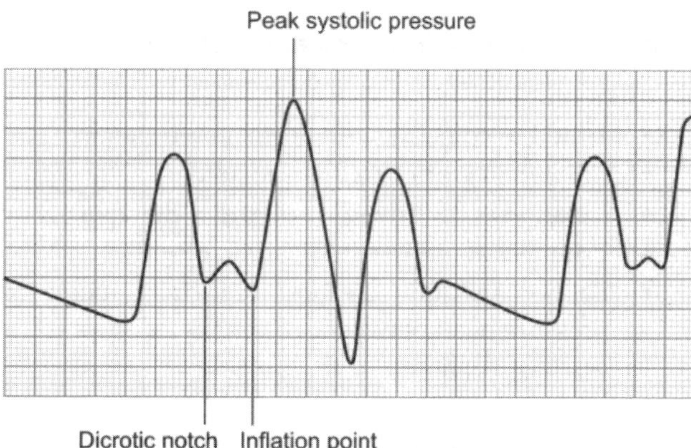

Fig. 47: Late inflation of IABP.

- Late inflation:
  - Results in delayed IABP balloon inflation after aortic valve closure
  - Thus, time for which the increased pressure head is maintained is reduced
  - This results in suboptimal performance of IABP
  - Therefore, IABP fails to augment coronary perfusion optimally.
- Early inflation:
  - Called early if inflation occurs more than 40 msec before dicrotic notch
  - Inflation therefore occurs before LV systolic ejection is completed
  - This results in:
    - Immediate closure of aortic valve
    - Premature termination of systolic ejection
  - Premature closure of aortic valve causes:
    - Decreased stroke volume for that cardiac cycle
    - Availability of increased preload for next cardiac cycle
  - Thus, detrimental effects of early inflation include:
    - Reduced cardiac output
    - Acute increase in end-diastolic volume stress
    - Increased LV wall tension and increased myocardial oxygen demand
    - Impaired perfusion with decreased myocardial oxygen supply
    - Acute aortic regurgitation.

❖ Deflation:

- Deflation should always occur:
  - Just at end-diastole
  - Immediately prior to next systolic ejection
- Deflation reduces afterload by reducing aortic end-diastolic pressure
- This reduces myocardial oxygen demand and increases cardiac output
- Early deflation:
  - IABP balloon is deflated before aortic valve opens for systolic ejection
  - This reduces the time for which the pressure head is maintained
  - Thus, it causes suboptimal performance of the IABP
  - It also allows aortic root pressure to return to baseline before LV ejection

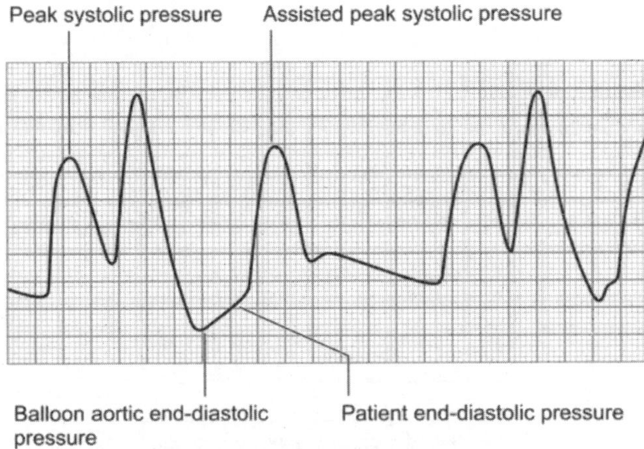

Fig. 49: Early deflation of IABP balloon.

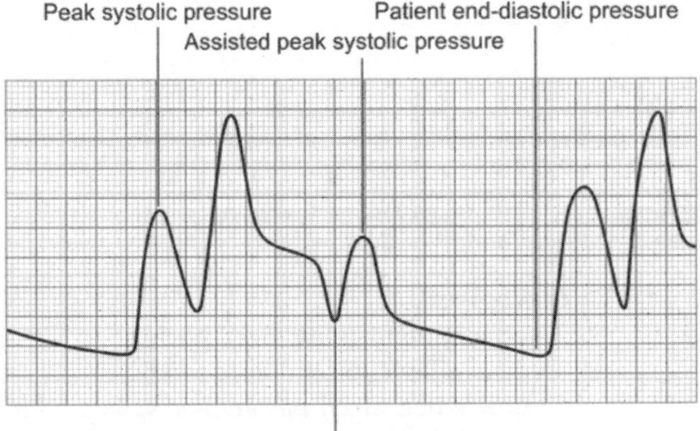

Fig. 50: Late deflation of IABP balloon.

  - This fails to decrease the impedance to aortic valve opening
  - Thus, it fails to decrease the myocardial oxygen demand
- Late deflation:
  - IABP balloon is deflated after aortic valve opening for LV ejection
  - Thus, balloon remains inflated during LV systole
  - This impeded LV ejection similar to application of an aortic clamp
  - Thus, the ventricle is forced to generate high pressure to open aortic valve
  - As a result, LV wall tension is increased causing increased LV work
  - This in turn leads to:
    - Increased myocardial oxygen demand
    - Impaired systemic perfusion
    - Metabolic acidosis
    - Aortic regurgitation.

Characteristics of IABP Waveform

- Balloon inflation point coinciding with location of patients dicrotic notch
- Steep slope of increasing pressure indicating rapid balloon inflation
- Assisted diastolic peak pressure perfusing coronary arteries while IABP is inflated
- Steep slope of pressure decline indicating rapid balloon deflation.

Care during IABP Therapy

- Nursed in 30–45° head end elevated position
- Chest radiograph should be obtained immediately after placement of IABP
- Hourly documentation of:
  - Bilateral distal pulses
  - Limb color and temperature
  - Capillary refill
  - Doppler evaluation
- Frequent evaluation of pressure waveform should be made
- Avoid standby mode for > 20 minutes due to risk of thrombus formation
- Daily evaluation for:
  - Insertion site infection
  - Insertion site bleeding/hematoma
  - Limb movement and sensation
- Daily measurement of:
  - Hematocrit
  - Platelet count (shear injury may cause thrombocytopenia)
  - Creatinine (backward balloon migration may occlude renal vessels).

Factors Influencing IABP Therapy

- *Location*: should be located immediately distal to left subclavian artery
- Inflation volume of 30–40 mL in adults
- Timing of inflation and deflation
- Patient related factors:
  - Heart rate
  - Rhythm
  - Mean arterial pressure
  - Aortic valve competence
  - Aortic wall compliance

Principles

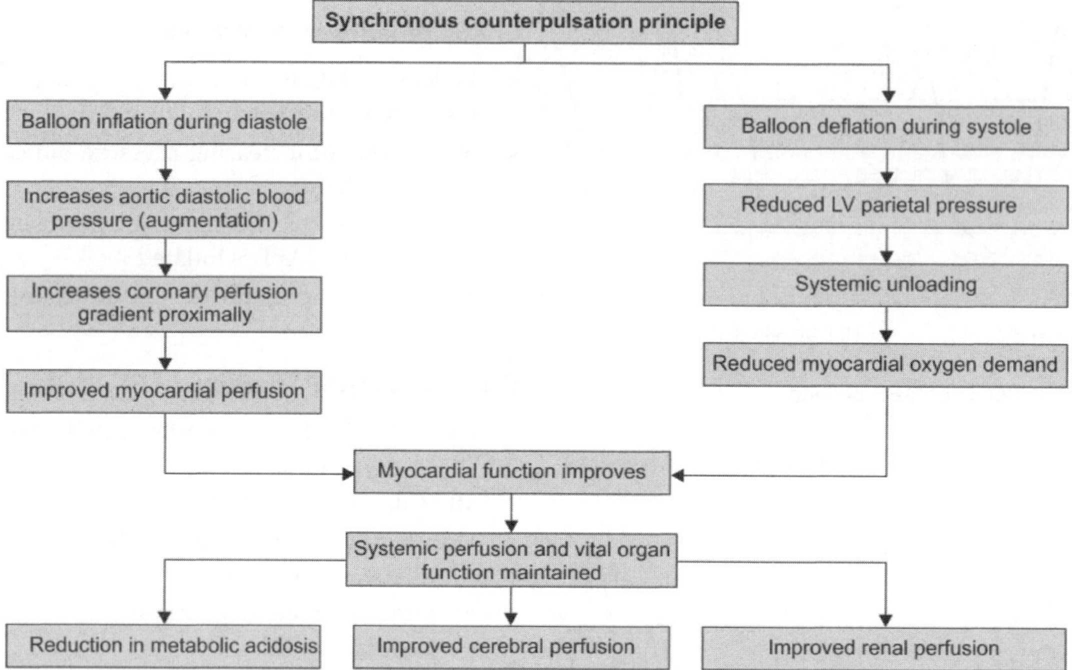

- Properly timed, optimally functioning balloon pump can:
  - Increase cardiac output by 20–30%
  - Decrease afterload by as much as 15%
- Other benefits include:
  - Decrease in myocardial oxygen demand
  - Reduction in systemic acidosis
  - Improvement in cerebral perfusion
  - Improvement in renal microcirculation

IABP Triggers

- Trigger refers to the source the IABP uses to identify the beginning of the cardiac cycle
- The IABP uses 5 triggering mechanisms:
  - ECG trigger:
    - R-wave is used to identify the beginning of cardiac cycle
    - This is the most commonly used trigger
    - More than 120 μV deflation/R wane
  - Pacemaker V spike:
    - Ventricular spike of pacing is the trigger event
    - This trigger is only available in semi-auto mode
    - Patient must be pacing-dependent for this trigger to be optimal
  - Pacer A spike:
    - Used in patients with atrial pacing
    - Only available in semi-auto mode
    - Useful when atrial pacemaker spikes interfere with R-wave detection
    - R-wave of the ECG trace is used to trigger IABP
  - Arterial pressure tracing:
    - With more than 15 mm Hg deflation
    - Inflation should always coincide with dicrotic notch of arterial tracing
  - Internal trigger:
    - Used when there is no mechanical cardiac cycle as in:
      - Asystole
      - Cardiopulmonary bypass
    - Allows asynchronous assistance via an internal signal at 80 bpm
    - Only available in semi-auto mode

Associated Therapies

- Heparin:
  - Used to prevent thrombus formation
  - Infusion may be started 4–6 hours post-operatively to prevent bleeding
- Increased inotropic support while weaning off IABP
- Antibiotic cover
- IV fluids to maintain preload

Weaning Criteria 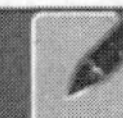

- Clinical criteria:
  - Absence of shock syndrome (hypotension, cool extremities)
  - Minimal need for vasopressors (< 5 µg/kg/min dopamine)
  - Cardiac catheterization/major surgery is planned
- Hemodynamic criteria:
  - Cardiac index more than 2.2 L/min/m^2
  - Wedge pressure < 18 mm Hg
  - Mean BP > 70 mm Hg
  - Less than 10% change in cardiac index, wedge pressure and heart rate during weaning

Methods of Weaning

- Weaning is typically carried out over 6–12 hours
- Two methods of IABP weaning exist:
  - Reducing the ratio of IABP inflation to heart rate
  - Reducing the volume inflation (augmentation strength) of the balloon
- However, reduction of augmentation is never preferred due to risk of thrombus formation
- Balloon augmentation is reduced in steps from 1:1 counter-pulsation to 1:2 and 1:3
- Appropriate intervals are required between reductions to assess:
  - Hemodynamic and neurological stability
  - Cardiac output and MvO_2
- After appropriate observation at 1:3 counter-pulsations, IABP can be removed

Complications

- Vascular complications:
  - Lower extremity ischemia:
    - *Most common complication*
    - Occurs in 9–25% of the patients
  - Arterial injury (perforation/dissection)
  - Aortic dissection
  - Femoral artery thrombosis and pseudo-aneurysm
  - Peripheral embolization
  - Compartment syndrome
  - Visceral ischemia (mesenteric infarction)
  - Femoral venous catheterization
- Miscellaneous:
  - Hemolysis
  - Thrombocytopenia:
    - Occurs in up to 50% of patients
    - This may be due to:
      - Mechanical trauma to platelets
      - Concomitant heparin induced thrombocytopenia
  - Infection, sepsis
  - Claudication pain (after removal)
  - Hemorrhage
  - Paraplegia, spinal cord ischemia
  - Entrapment of balloon
  - Left internal mammary artery occlusion
  - Coagulopathies
- Complications related to balloon:
  - Perforation of balloon(pre-insertion)
  - Balloon tear during insertion
  - Incorrect positioning
  - Balloon rupture post insertion:
    - Occurs rarely, in 1–2% of patients
    - Recognized by presence of blood in gas drive line
    - Dangerous as it results in direct gas embolism in systemic circulation
    - Results in gas embolism and cerebrovascular accidents
    - Warrants IABP balloon removal
  - Inadvertent removal

ANESTHESIA FOR ENDOVASCULAR AORTIC REPAIR

Introduction

- EVAR has become a standard treatment modality for thoracic and abdominal aortic aneurysms
- In EVAR, endovascular grafts are used to exclude the native aortic wall from blood flow
- Procedure is associated with low morbidity and mortality as it does not involve:
  - Surgical aortic exposure
  - Aortic cross clamping
  - Blood loss and fluid shifts
- First EVAR performed by ***Nicholas Volodos*** in 1987
- EVAR is associated with a 67% lower risk of 30-day mortality
- Latest techniques include:
  - FEVARs:
    - Fenestrated endovascular aortic repairs
    - Utilize fenestrations in graft to maintain perfusion via aortic branches
  - BEVARs:
    - Branched endovascular aortic repairs
    - Utilize branched grafts to maintain perfusion through aortic branches

Indications

- Thoracic EVAR (TEVAR):
  - Asymptomatic descending TAA with maximum diameter ≥ 5.5 cm
  - Rapid expansion ≥ 5 mm in 6 months
  - Maximum diameter < 5.5 cm in the presence of:
    - Saccular aneurysms
    - Thoracic aortic pseudoaneurysms
  - Blunt thoracic aortic injury with:
    - Complete transection of aortic wall
    - Pseudo-coarctation syndrome
  - Complicated type B aortic dissections with:
    - Persistent or recurrent pain
    - Uncontrolled HTN
    - Early aortic expansion
    - Signs of rupture:
      - Hemothorax
      - Peri-aortic and mediastinal hematoma
- Abdominal EVAR:
  - Abdominal aortic aneurysms:
    - Symptomatic AAA
    - Asymptomatic AAA with maximal diameter > 5.5 cm
    - Asymptomatic AAA in women with maximal diameter 5–5.4 cm
    - AAA associated with peripheral artery aneurysm:
      - Iliac aneurysm
      - Popliteal aneurysm
  - Abdominal aortic dissection

Patient Selection for EVAR

- For all aortic diseases, endovascular technique is used as the most feasible option
- However, benefits of EVAR are greatest in the short term
- Thus, EVAR is preferred over surgical repair for patients with:
  - Limited life expectancy
  - High perioperative risk
  - Anatomy suitable for endovascular repair (defined by the to-be-deployed device)
  - Following prior aortic repair with suture site aneurysms
- Surgical repair is preferred over TEVAR for:
  - Asymptomatic TAAs with maximum diameter of aneurysm > 5.5 cm in:
    - Ascending aorta
    - Arch of aorta
  - Asymptomatic descending TAA with maximal diameter > 6 cm

Contraindications

- Very short diseased segment
- Absence of adequate landing zone
- Aortic wall disease of proximal segment

Advantages of EVAR

- Reduced mortality and morbidity
- Reduced blood loss
- Reduced postoperative pain
- Reduced ICU stay
- Reduced postoperative pulmonary complications
- Can be done in very old/very sick patients in whom open surgery is contraindicated

Disadvantages of EVAR

- Risk of converting to open surgery exists
- Risk of bleeding, stroke, paraplegia, endovascular leaks and contrast nephropathy.

Surgical Technique

- Arterial access:
  - Most commonly bilateral femoral artery access:
    - One side is used for delivery of wide-bore sheath
    - Contralateral side is used for arteriography
  - No percutaneous devices are available for TEVAR
  - Thus, all TEVARs require vascular access through surgical cut-down
  - However, percutaneous approach devices are available for abdominal EVARs
  - Diameter and calcification of vessels may limit the use of percutaneous devices
  - Other vascular access procedures may be planned in complex repairs such as:
    - Creation of iliac artery conduit
    - Direct exposure of common iliac artery
    - Graft anastomosis to ascending aorta
- Graft deployment:
  - Deployment is done under fluoroscopic guidance or TEE
  - Anatomical suitability of the graft is confirmed prior to deployment with:
    - Adequate proximal graft landing-zone > 2 cm from LSCA
    - Adequate stent-graft diameter > 15% of landing zone diameter
  - Prior to graft deployment, BP is reduced to prevent:
    - Premature graft deployment
    - Distal migration of the graft due to pressure (wind-sock effect)

- Following deployment, the graft is ballooned at proximal and distal landing-zones
- Repeat aortography is performed at the conclusion to:
  - Ensure effective sac exclusion
  - Preservation of essential blood vessels
  - Detect presence of any endo-leaks
- Following confirmation of graft position, device sheath is removed
- The arteriotomy is repaired or closed with a closure device

Preoperative Evaluation

❖ History and examination of patient

❖ Chest X-ray, CT scan and MRI to delineate aortic anatomy

❖ Cardiovascular assessment:
- EVAR is associated with intermediate risk for perioperative cardiovascular events
- Patients with RV dysfunction have a higher risk of peri-procedural:
  - Cardiovascular mortality
  - Non-fatal cardiac arrest
  - Myocardial infarction
  - Development of CCF
  - Stroke
- Cardiovascular evaluation for EVAR should include:
  - Baseline ECG:
    - For comparison with postoperative ECGs
    - Presence of pre-operative Q-waves for myocardial infarction
    - Left ventricular hypertrophy, bundle branch block
    - QTc prolongation
    - Arrhythmias
  - Echocardiography
  - CT angiography for:
    - Aortic anatomy
    - Calcification of aorta
    - Delineation of landing zones
  - Additional evaluation in patients at high cardiovascular risks:
    - Recent MI
    - Decompensated heart failure
    - High-grade arrhythmias
    - Significant valvular heart disease

❖ Renal assessment:
- Patients undergoing EVAR have higher risk of severe renal dysfunction (0.7–2%)
- This is due to:
  - Intravenous contrast agents
  - Dislodgement of embolic debris by catheters into renal artery
  - Impingement of the graft on renal ostia
- Thus, creatinine is obtained following preoperative imaging (CT angiography)
- EVAR is deferred by at least 2 weeks if creatinine clearance is reduced

Anesthetic Considerations

❖ Remote site procedure

❖ Massive radiation necessitating proper radiation safety

❖ Prevention of contrast induced AKI:
- Maintenance of euvolemia
- Reduction of contrast load

❖ Preparation for sudden and major catastrophies such as aortic rupture

❖ Manipulation of surgical-step dependent hemodynamics

❖ Vital organ protection:
- Kidneys
- Spinal cord

❖ Management of peri-procedural anticoagulation with heparin

❖ Preparation for massive transfusion in the presence of inadvertent aortic trauma

❖ Preparation for immediate extubation due to absence of time taken for surgical closure

❖ Availability of cardiac surgical and perfusion team on standby for aortic emergencies

Anesthetic Goals

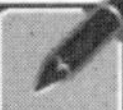

❖ Immobile patient to facilitate graft positioning

❖ Ensure adequate hydration to reduce risk of contrast nephropathy

❖ Control of peri-procedural hemodynamics according to surgical procedure

❖ Temperature control to prevent hypothermia

❖ Preservation of perfusion to:
- Splanchnic vessels
- Kidney
- Spinal cord
- Heart

Choice of Anesthetic Technique

❖ No sufficient data to indicate the best anesthetic technique

❖ However, LA with MAC may be preferred due to lesser postoperative complications

❖ Local anesthesia with MAC:
- Arterial access is secured under local anesthetic skin infiltration supplemented by:
  - Ilioinguinal nerve block
  - Iliohypogastric nerve block

- Anxiolysis and sedation may be accomplished using:
  - Midazolam
  - Fentanyl
  - Dexmedetomidine infusion
- May be preferred for emergency abdominal EVAR
- Advantages:
  - Reduced ICU and hospital stay
  - Avoidance of myocardial depression by general anesthetic agents
  - Reduced alteration of pulmonary mechanics
  - Avoids sympathetic stimulation during intubation and extubation
  - Early detection of aneurysm rupture due to retroperitoneal abdominal pain
  - Reduced 30-day mortality

❖ Neuraxial anesthesia:
- Single dose spinal, continuous spinal-epidural and epidural anesthesia may be used
- Catheter placement has to be timed with intraoperative heparin administration
- Level of anesthesia to be provided is T6-L3 lasting 3–4 hours
- Anxiolysis and sedation may be accomplished using:
  - Midazolam
  - Fentanyl
  - Dexmedetomidine infusion

❖ General anesthesia:
- Preferred for:
  - Anxious patients
  - Patients with anticipated poor MAC-compliance such as:
  - Heart failure (inability to lie supine)
  - Back pain
- Advantages:
  - Provides a motionless patient
  - Reduced patient anxiety
  - Less risk of movement during crucial endovascular steps
  - Complete suspension of respiration during graft deployment

Preoperative Preparation

❖ NPO guidelines

❖ Patient reassurance and informed consent

❖ Blood grouping and cross matching

❖ 10–15 units blood kept ready to cope with any emergencies

❖ Large bore IV cannula for rapid fluid administration

❖ Stabilize coexisting diseases and continue preoperative medications

❖ Immediate preprocedural addition of beta-blockers is not recommended

❖ Lumbar CSF drains may be placed preoperatively when indicated

Monitors

❖ Pulse oximetry, E_TCO_2

❖ ECG:
- Multi-lead ECG monitoring is important to detect myocardial ischemic insult
- Computerized ST-segment analysis should be used to identify change in trends

❖ Urine output

❖ Temperature, NIBP, TEE

❖ Radial arterial IBP:
- Advantages:
  - Hypotensive anesthesia may be required
  - Monitoring of intraoperative volume status
  - Repeated ABG analysis
- Right radial artery is preferred as the graft may cover LSCA
- The transducer is used to monitor distal limb perfusion after graft deployment

❖ CVP:
- Useful to guide fluid therapy
- Also used to administer vasopressor support

❖ PA catheter usually not required

❖ Transesophageal echocardiography:
- Useful for:
  - Thoracic aortic TEVAR
  - Emergency procedures
  - Complex EVARs
- Used to evaluate:
  - Aortic anatomy
  - Correct graft position
  - Endo-leaks
  - Intraoperative hemodynamic instability

❖ Monitoring for spinal cord ischemia:
- Risk of spinal cord ischemia increases with increasing length of the graft
- Increased risk is associated with graft length > 20 cm
- Ischemia can also arise from vascular exclusion due to graft position
  - *Monitoring can be done with*: somatosensory evoked potentials:
    - Stimuli applied to distal nerves of lower extremity such as:
      - Posterior tibial N
      - Peroneal N

- Resultant cortical potentials are monitored via scalp electrodes
- Monitors intactness of lateral and posterior columns

– Motor evoked potentials:
  - Electrical stimulation of scalp overlying motor cortex
  - Muscle action potentials in anterior tibialis are studies
  - Monitors intactness of corticospinal tract

Induction

- Adequate preoxygenation
- Induction with etomidate 0.3 mg/kg or propofol 1–2 mg/kg
- IV fentanyl 2 μg/kg and vecuronium 0.1 mg/kg may be used to intubate the patient
- IV lidocaine 1.5 mg/kg may be given 90 seconds prior to intubation to suppress response

Maintenance

- Balanced anesthesia with O_2 + air + volatile agent may be used
- Isoflurane or sevoflurane may be used
- The procedure is performed through groin incision and is thus less painful
- Thus, large and repeated doses of opioids are usually not required
- Vecuronium boluses may be used to maintain neuromuscular paralysis
- Dexmedetomidine may be used to:
  - Reduce anesthetic requirement
  - Facilitate early extubation
- Alternatively, TIVA with propofol and remifentanil may be used
- Anticoagulation:
  - Systemic anticoagulation with heparin is initiated prior to device insertion
  - IV heparin 5000–8000 IU is administered to achieve an ACT > 200 seconds
- Spinal cord protection:
  - Lumbar CSF drainage is rarely considered for abdominal EVAR
  - It may be used when:
    - History of prior repair of larger descending TAA or abdominal AA
    - Length of graft > 20 cms
  - When used, CSF drains are titrated to maintain CSF pressure 8–10 mm Hg
  - Drainage of CSF is limited to < 20 mL/hour during the first hour
  - Subsequent drainage should be limited to < 40 mL every 4 hours
  - Other mechanisms of spinal cord protection include:
    - Preoperative subclavian artery debranching using LCA-LSCA bypass
    - Minimizing occlusion of internal iliac arteries by using smaller sheaths

Hemodynamics

- Fluid therapy and renal protection:
  - Optimal volume status has to be maintained to prevent contrast induced AKI
  - Fluid depletion is corrected preoperatively using 1–1.5 mL/kg/hour isotonic saline for 6–12 hours
  - This is followed by intraoperative fluid administration
  - Fluid administration at this rate is continued postoperatively for 4–6 hours
  - There is no benefit for additional renal protective measures such as:
    - Acetylcysteine
    - Sodium bicarbonate
- Hemodynamics management:
  - Fastidious hemodynamic management is important as:
  - Hypertension may rupture the aneurysm
  - Persistent hypotension:
    - Defined as SBP < 90 mm Hg or 40% below baseline for > 10 minutes
    - Results in:
      - Myocardial ischemia
      - Postoperative renal dysfunction
      - SBP and DBP are maintained within 20% of the patients baseline
  - NTG infusion may be used to titrate hemodynamics in hypertensive patients
  - Additional infusions such as epinephrine and vasopressin should be immediately available
  - Hypotensive anesthesia:
    - Preferred during device deployment
    - Accomplished with administration of short acting agents:
      - IV propofol 10–30 mg boluses
      - IV esmolol 10–30 mg boluses
- Prevention of hypothermia:
  - Mild hypothermia up to 35°C may offer some degree of spinal cord protection
  - However, more severe hypothermia is prevented by:
    - Fluid warmers
    - Forced air warmers

Ventilation

- Conventional IPPV is used during the procedure with:
  - Tidal volume: 8 mL/kg body weight
  - Respiratory rate: 12–14 breaths per minute
  - FiO_2 minimal to maintain SpO_2 > 92%
  - I: E ratio: 1:2
  - PEEP: 5 cmH_2O
- Respiration is temporarily suspended during deployment of the stent

Extubation

- Early extubation is preferred to facilitate spinal cord evaluation
- Patient is usually extubated at the end of surgery when:
  - Fully awake
  - Hemodynamically stable
  - Fully reversed
- Hemodynamic alterations and bucking during extubation have to be minimized with:
  - Lidocaine
  - Esmolol
  - Nitroprusside/NTG

Postoperative Management

Management

- Postoperative ventilation may be indicated when:
  - Hemodynamic instability
  - Prolonged procedures
  - Hypothermia
- Fluid therapy is continued for 4–6 hours postoperatively
- CSF drainage may be continued for 48–72 hours postoperatively

Monitors

- Pulse oximetry
- ECG
- Urine output for renal function
- Spinal cord monitoring using SSEP and MEP

Analgesia

- Minimal pain due to limited surgical incision
- Multimodal analgesia preferred
- Local anesthetic infiltration
- Judicious opioid administration
- NSAIDs avoided due to risk of aggravating contrast induced AKI
- Epidural analgesia when present

Complications

- Endovascular leaks:
  - Type I: Leak occurs between graft and proximal/distal segment
  - Type II: Leak occurring through collateral (lumbar/inferior mesenteric A)
  - Type III: Due to structural faults with in-stent graft
- Migration of stent, kinking/leak around stent
- Paraplegia:
  - Common in thoraco-abdominal aneurysms
  - Consider CSF drainage to maintain cerebral perfusion pressure.
- Contrast nephropathy:
  - Risk factors:
    - Diabetes, hypertension, old age
    - Renal insufficiency
    - Repeated exposure at short intervals
    - Use of high osmolality non-ionic contrast
    - ACE inhibitor therapy
  - Treatment:
    - Hydration, N-acetyl cysteine
    - Antioxidants, vasodilators
    - Dopamine and phenoldopam tried
    - Dialysis
    - Diuretics not used during first 24 hours
- Stroke, abdominal pain, mesenteric ischemia

PHYSIOLOGICAL CHANGES DURING AORTIC CROSS CLAMPING

Introduction

- Aortic cross clamping is necessary for open infrarenal AAA surgery
- Location of the cross clamp may be:
  - Infra-renal (most common)
  - Juxtarenal
  - Rarely suprarenal
- Physiological response to aortic cross clamping is complex and depends upon:
  - Myocardial function
  - Presence of collateral circulation
  - Intravascular volume status of the patient
  - Function of sympathetic nervous system

Complications of Cross Clamping

- *30 day mortality*: 8–35%
- Complete/partial paraplegia (16–38%)
- Myocardial infarction (11%)
- Respiratory failure (36%)
- Renal failure (18–27%)
- *GI complications*: mainly hemorrhage: (7%)

Physiological Changes during Clamping

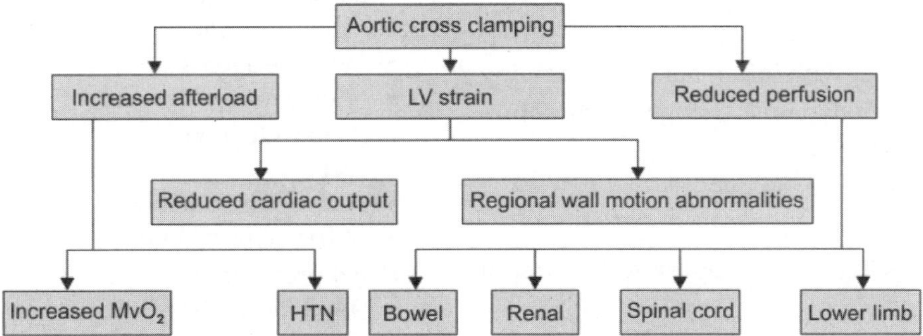

- Hemodynamic changes:
  - Hypertension above the cross-clamp
  - Hypotension below the cross-clamp
  - Increased afterload
  - Increased LV wall tension
  - Increased regional wall motion abnormalities
  - Reduced ejection fraction
  - Reduced cardiac output
  - Increased pulmonary capillary wedge pressure
  - Increased central venous pressure
  - Increased coronary blood flow
- Metabolic changes:
  - Reduced total body oxygen consumption
  - Reduced total body oxygen extraction
  - Increased mixed venous oxygen saturation
  - Reduced total body carbon dioxide production
  - Increased epinephrine and norepinephrine levels
  - Respiratory alkalosis
  - Metabolic acidosis
- Pulmonary changes:
  - Increased pulmonary vascular resistance
  - Increased pulmonary arterial pressure
  - Increased total lung water
- Renal changes:
  - 80% reduction in renal blood flow with suprarenal clamping
  - Redistribution of renal blood flow:
    - Increased blood flow to cortical and juxtamedullary layers
    - Reduced blood flow to ischemia-prone renal medulla
  - Renal changes persists for 60 min after systemic hemodynamics return to baseline
  - Increased chances of dialysis dependent ARF:
    - 2–3% incidence regardless of clamp position
    - 13% incidence if post-suprarenal clamping
    - 5% incidence if post-renal clamping
  - Causes of acute renal failure:
    - Reduced glomerular filtration rate
    - Reduced renal blood flow
    - Ischemia reperfusion injury
- Visceral and mesenteric changes:
  - Reduced blood flow occurs through superior and inferior mesenteric artery
  - Ischemia of left colon is more common due to reduced blood supply through inferior mesenteric artery
  - Gut ischemia also causes increased gut permeability and bacterial translocation
  - High dose methylprednisolone given at induction reduces this response
  - Visceral ischemia aggravated by:
    - Preexisting medical conditions
    - Renal dysfunction
    - Stage of aortic disease
    - Level of cross clamping
    - Duration of cross clamping
    - Perioperative hypotension
- CNS and spinal cord changes:
  - Reduced blood velocity in middle cerebral artery
  - Unclamping causes transient dilatation followed by sustained vasoconstriction of pial blood vessels due to:
    - Hemodynamic changes
    - Carbon dioxide accumulation and wash-out
    - Acidosis
    - TXA_2 release
  - Supraceliac cross clamping causes:
    - Reduced anterior spinal artery pressure
    - Increased CSF pressure
    - High CVP
- Coagulation changes:
  - Increased clotting factor activity occurs during cross clamping
  - Reduced speed of clot formation after unclamping

Factors Influencing Magnitude of Changes with Cross Clamping

- Level of aortic cross clamp:
  - Minimal changes with infrarenal cross clamping
  - Significant hemodynamic changes with supra-celiac clamping
- Anesthetic agents and technique
- Use of vasodilator therapy
- Use of diverting circulatory support in the form of bypass grafts
- Degree of pre-clamp collateralization
- Preclamping left ventricular function
- Patency of coronary circulation
- Intravascular volume status
- *Duration of aortic cross clamping*: increased SVR with longer cross clamping
- Body temperature

Therapeutic Interventions during Clamping

- Afterload reduction:
  - SNP, milrinone
  - Volatile agents
  - Aortofemoral bypass
- Preload reduction:
  - NTG
  - Controlled phlebotomy
  - Atrio-femoral bypass
- Renal protection:
  - Fluid administration
  - Distal aortic perfusion techniques
  - Selective renal artery perfusion
  - Mannitol
  - Drugs augmenting renal perfusion
- Other changes:
  - Induced hypothermia
  - Reduced minute ventilation
  - Sodium bicarbonate

Physiological Changes during Unclamping

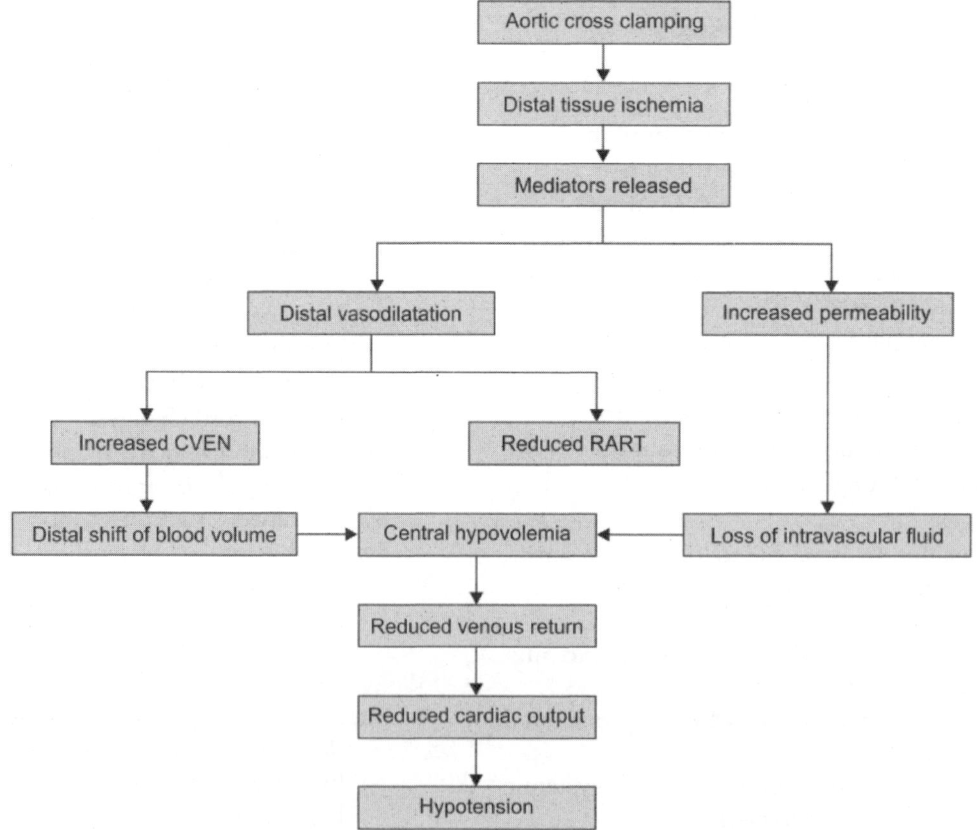

- Hemodynamic changes:
  - Reduced afterload
  - Distal pooling of blood
  - Reduced venous return
  - Reduced cardiac output
  - Reduced myocardial contractility

- Reduced arterial blood pressure
- Increased pulmonary artery pressure
- Reduced central venous pressure

❖ Metabolic changes:
- Increased total body oxygen consumption
- Increased total body oxygen extraction
- Reduced mixed venous oxygen saturation
- Increased serum lactate levels
- Reduced activated complement levels
- Increased prostaglandin levels
- Increased myocardial depressant factor levels
- Metabolic acidosis
- Hypothermia

Therapeutic Interventions at Unclamping

❖ Reduce volatile agents
❖ Increased IV fluid administration
❖ Increased vasoconstrictors
❖ Reduced vasodilators
❖ Reapply cross clamp if severe hypotension
❖ Consider mannitol
❖ Consider sodium bicarbonate administration

Humoral Factors which Cause Organ Dysfunction

❖ Acidosis
❖ Activation of RAS
❖ Activation of sympathetic nervous system
❖ Oxygen derived free radicals
❖ Prostaglandins
❖ Platelet and neutrophil sequestration
❖ Complement activation
❖ Cytokine release
❖ Myocardial depressant factor

Pulmonary Complications

❖ Pulmonary edema
❖ Pulmonary microembolization
❖ Complications due to one lung ventilation
❖ Atelectasis due to lung retraction
❖ Increased ARDS postoperatively due to remote reperfusion injury and capillary leak

Spinal Cord Protection

❖ Increase anterior spinal artery pressure:
- Aortofemoral shunting
- Maintain proximal hypertension
- ***Gott shunt***: between proximal thoracic ascending to descending thoracic aorta

❖ Reduce CSF pressure:
- Avoid cerebral vasodilators
- *CSF drainage*: role is controversial
- Corticosteroids, barbiturates

❖ Reduce central venous pressure:
- Controlled phlebotomy
- NTG, $MgSO_4$, calcium channel blockers
- Atriofemoral bypass

❖ Esoteric measures:
- Cooling (temperature drift)
- Selective spinal cord cooling using epidural cooling techniques
- Oxygen free radical scavengers:
  - N-acetyl cysteine
  - Mannitol
  - Superoxide dismutase
  - Allopurinol
- Limit cross clamp time to less than 30 minutes
- Application of sequential aortic cross clamp
- Enhanced spiral cord monitoring
  - Somatosensory Evoked Potentials
  - Motor Evoked Potentials
- Use EVAR where possible

❖ Avoid postoperative hypotension

Renal Protection

❖ Optimize oxygen demand/supply:
- Reduce tubular reabsorption (loop diuretics)
- Cooling (temperature drift)
- Maintain tissue oxygenation (heart, lung, hemostasis)
- Limit aortic cross clamp time to less than 30 minutes
- Sequential cross clamping

❖ Increase renal tubular flow:
- Fluid loading (most effective)
- Loop diuretics
- Mannitol 0.5–1 g /kg before reperfusion
- Dopamine 1–3 μg/kg/min
- Fenoldopam 0.1–0.3 μg/kg/min
- Maintain cardiac output

❖ Use endovascular techniques where possible (EVAR)
❖ Avoid nephrotoxins:
- NSAIDs
- ACE inhibitors
- Angiotensin receptor blockers
- Aminoglycosides

❖ Other techniques:
- Thoracic epidural for sympatholysis
- Prostaglandins

- Isovolemic hemodilution
- Maintain euglycemia
- Renal vasodilators:
  - Prostaglandin E1
  - Atrial natriuretic peptide
  - Theophylline

DEEP VEIN THROMBOSIS

Introduction

- The presence of a thrombus within a deep vein and accompanying inflammatory response in the vessel wall is called venous thrombosis/thrombophlebitis
- Superficial venous system in lower extremity includes greater and lesser saphenous veins and tributaries
- The deep veins are those which accompany major arteries

Etiology

Conditions associated with increased risk of DVT:

- Surgery:
  - Orthopedic, thoracic surgeries
  - Abdominal, genitourinary surgeries
- Neoplasms:
  - Pancreas (very common)
  - Genitourinary: ovary, testes
  - Lung carcinoma
  - Breast cancer
  - Stomach tumors
- Trauma:
  - Fracture spine, hip
  - Fracture of femur, tibia
  - Pelvic fractures
  - Traumatic brain injury:
    - Up to 25% patients with isolated brain injury develop DVT
    - Prophylaxis started 45 hrs after injury to prevent increased risk of bleeding
- Venulitis:
  - ***Burgers disease***
  - ***Behcets disease***
  - Homocysteinuria
- Immobilization: MI, CCF, stroke, postop convalescence
- Hypercoagulable states:
  - Pregnancy, OCP use
  - Myeloproliferative disorders, APLA syndrome, SLE
  - Multiple myeloma
  - DIC, factor V Leiden deficiency
  - Protein C and S deficiency, dysfibrinogenemia
  - Previous history of DVT

Pathogenesis

- ***Virchows triad*** describes factors which predispose to VTE:
  - Stasis of blood
  - Vascular endothelial damage
  - Hypercoagulability
- Initially, the thrombus contains principally platelets and fibrin
- RBCs then become interspersed within fibrin
- The thrombus then propogates along the direction of blood flow
- Inflammatory response in blood vessel is due to:
  - Granulocyte infilteration
  - Loss of endothelium and edema

Sites of Occurrence

- Lower extremity: Femoral vein, popliteal vein, iliac vein
- Pelvic vein
- Superior/inferior vena cava
- Upper extremites:
  - Due to increased use of subclavian or IJV catheters
  - More common in ICU population
  - Can result in pulmonary embolism in up to 2/3rd of cases
  - Also increases risk of post-thrombotic syndrome

Clinical Features

- 50% of cases develop within 1 week (usually within 4 days)
- Calf pain is *most common* complaint
- Edema is the *most specific* symptom
- Unilateral leg swelling, warmth, erythema
- Increased tissue turgor, prominent venous collaterals, distended superficial veins
- Tenderness along course of vein, cord may be palpable
- ***Phlegmasia alba dolens:***
  - Translates literally to painful, white inflammation
  - Refers to the pain, edema and blanched appearance of the affected limb
  - This is because intestitial pressure exceeds capillary perfusion pressure
  - This results in an extremely pale limb resembling acute arterial occlusion

❖ ***Phlegmasia cerulea dolens:***
  - Translates literally as painful, blue inflammation
  - The affected limb is markedly edematous, painful and cyanotic
  - Deoxygenated Hb in stagnant vein imparts cyanotic hue to the limb

❖ Bedside diagnosis may be difficult as only 1 of multiple veins may be involved allowing adequate venous return through remaining patent vessels

❖ ***Homans sign***:
  - Increased resistance or pain during foot dorsiflexion
  - It is present in less than one-third of patients with confirmed DVT
  - Sign can be found in more than 50% patients without DVT
  - Therefore, the sign is neither sensitive nor specific

❖ ***Moses sign***: Pain on squeezing calf muscles

Complications

❖ Short-term complications:
  - Prolonged hospitalization
  - Bleeding due to anticoagulation
  - Pulmonary embolism
  - Local extension of DVT
  - Embolization
  - Pulmonary embolism

❖ Long-term complications:
  - Post thrombotic syndrome
  - Pulmonary hypertension
  - Recurrent DVT
  - Embolic stroke through patent foramen ovale

Investigations

❖ Investigations to diagnose DVT:
  - D-dimer assay:
    - D-dimers are degradation products of cross-linked fibrin by plasmin
    - D-dimer levels are elevated in many conditions with clot formation like:
      - Recent surgery
      - Hemorrhage
      - Cancer
      - Sepsis
    - Therefore, the test is very sensitive (97%) but not specific (as low as 35%)
    - D-dimer levels remain increased in DVT patients for up to 7 days
  - Coagulation profile:
    - Done to evaluate for hypercoagulable state
    - Prolonged PT or aPTT can occur even in hypercoagulable states
  - Duplex venous ultrasonography:
    - Non invasive test
    - Most often used, current first line imaging examination
    - Low sensitivity in absence of symptoms
    - Thrombus detected by:
      - Direct visualization
      - By inference when vein does not collapse on compression
      - By flow abnormality
  - MRI:
    - Increasingly investigated for evaluation of suspected DVT
    - Diagnostic test of choice when:
      - DVT of SVC/IVC/pelvic veins
      - CT venography is contraindicated
  - Venography:
    - Contrast medium injected into superficial veins of foot
    - This is directed to deep venous system by application of tourniquet
    - Serial radiographs are taken subsequently
    - DVT is diagnosed by presence of filling defect
    - Confirmatory, *gold standard* test

❖ Investigation to rule out pulmonary embolism:
  - Spiral CT/HRCT
  - Pulmonary angiography: *Gold standard*
  - TEE:
    - Demonstrates RV performance, TR
    - May help to see thrombus in PA/right heart
  - V-Q scan: Defect in perfusion with normal ventilation

Wells Scoring System for DVT Probability

Findings	Criteria	Score
History	Paralysis, paresis, recent lower limb orthopedic cast	1 point
	Recently bedridden for > 3 days	1 point
	Major surgery within past 4 weeks	
	Active cancer or cancer treated within 6 months	1 point
Examination	Localized tenderness in deep vein system	1 point
	Swelling of entire leg	1 point
	Pitting edema greater in symptomatic leg	1 point
	Calf swelling > 3 mm compared with opposite leg	1 point
	Collateral non-varicose superficial veins	1 point

Contd...

Contd...

Findings	Criteria	Score
Alternate diagnosis more likely	Bakers cyst	-2 points
	Cellulitis	
	Muscle damage	
	Superficial vein thrombosis	
	Post phlebitis syndrome	
	Inguinal lymphadenopathy	
	External venous compression	

Wells Score	Interpretation
3–8 points	High probability of DVT
1–2 points	Moderate probability of DVT
-2–0 points	Low probability of DVT

Differential Diagnosis

- Achilles tendonitis
- Arthritis
- Muscle strain/tear/rupture
- Stress fracture
- Ruptured popliteal cyst
- Arterial occlusive disease
- Varicose veins
- Superficial thrombophlebitis
- Lymphedema
- Trauma/muscle hemorrhage

Treatment

- Criteria for hospital admission:
  - Pregnancy
  - Morbid obesity
  - Suspected or proven concomitant pulmonary embolism
  - Iliofemoral DVT
  - Significant cardiovascular or pulmonary comorbidity
  - Familial disorders of coagulation:
    - Antithrombin III deficiency
    - Protein C and S deficiency
    - Factor V Leiden deficiency
  - Renal failure (creatinine > 2 mg/dL)
- Anticoagulation:
  - Prevents thrombus propogation and allows lytic system to act
  - Unfractionated heparin:
    - Heparin prevents extension of the deep vein thrombus
    - It reduces, but does not eliminate the incidence of pulmonary embolism
    - UFH 80 IU/kg IV bolus dose given initially
    - This is followed by an infusion of 18 IU/kg/hr
    - aPTT level checked 6 hours after the initial bolus dose
    - Rate titrated to keep aPTT value 1.5 times that of control value
    - aPTT checked Q6H thereafter until 2 successive values are therapeutic
    - aPTT and platelet counts are then measured every 24 hours
  - Low molecular weight heparin:
    - LMWH is a non-inferior alternative to UFH for treatment of DVT
    - 1 mg/kg enoxaparin SC Q12H can be used effectively for anticoagulation
    - However, despite adequate therapy with LMWH, recurrence and pulmonary embolism rates are as high as 4.5%
  - Direct thrombin inhibitors:
    - Lepirudin 0.4 mg/kg followed by 0.15 mg/kg/hr
    - Argatroban 2 µg/kg/min
    - Bivalirudin 0.75 mg/kg followed by 1.75 mg/kg/hr
    - Used in patients with Heparin Induced Thrombocytopenia
  - Warfarin:
    - Warfarin is overlapped during the first 4–5 days of therapy with heparin
    - This is because of the initial hypercoagulable state induced by warfarin
    - Started as early as 1st day of heparin therapy if APTT is therapeutic
    - Therapy is kept overlapped with heparin until INR > 2 for at least 24 hours
    - Dosage of warfarin adjusted to maintain PT at INR of 2–3
  - Duration of therapy:
    - Continued for 3–6 months in acute first episode-DVT
    - Prolonged therapy is necessary to reduce chance of recurrence
    - Cessation of therapy after 3 months in those with:
      - Surgery associated acute proximal DVT
      - Acute proximal DVT provoked by non-surgical transient risk factor
      - High risk of bleeding
    - Long-term therapy is advocated for:
      - Recurrent DVT
      - Hypercoagulable states
      - Malignancy

- IVC filter/IVC plication:
  - Transvenous filter placement done through femoral venous access
  - Filters were developed to trap emboli and minimize venous stasis
  - SVC and IVC filters are available, to protect from pulmonary embolism
  - These act as a mechanical barrier to the flow of emboli larger than 4 mm
  - These are not recommended in patients with acute VTE on anticoagulant therapy
  - Filters are used when anticoagulants are contra-indicated
  - Filters do nothing to already formed thrombus
  - Some filters can be left permanently
  - Removable filters are removed once anti-coagulants are started
- Thrombolytics:
  - Used in:
    - Massive pulmonary embolism
    - Cor pulmonale
    - Hemodynamically compromised patients
  - Streptokinase/urokinase/t-PA used
  - Early administration of thrombolytics:
    - Accelerates clot lysis
    - Preserves venous valves
    - Reduces chances of developing post thrombotic syndrome
- Endovascular intervention:
  - Goals of endovascular intervention:
    - Reducing severity and duration of lower extremity symptoms
    - Preventing pulmonary embolism
    - Diminishing risk of recurrent venous thrombosis
    - Preventing postthrombotic syndrome
  - Transcatheter treatment consists of:
    - Catheter directed thrombolysis
    - Mechanical thrombectomy
    - Angioplasty
    - Stenting of venous obstruction
- Surgical thrombolysis:
  - Traditionally reserved for patients with phlegmasia cerulea dolens
  - Surgery is indicated when thrombus is extensive
  - In these cases, fibrinolysis alone is not enough to debulk the thrombus
  - Precisely defining location and extent of the thrombus is important
  - Traditional venous thrombectomy is perfomed using Fogarty catheter
  - Care must be taken to avoid dislodgement or fracturing the thrombus
- Ambulation:
  - Early ambulation is recommended as tolerated by the patient
  - Ambulation from day 2 of initiation of anticoagulant therapy
  - Use of elastic stockings is strongly recommended
- Management of pulmonary embolism:
  - Anticoagulation
  - Thrombolytic agents in patients with:
    - Severe hemodynamic compromise
    - Cardiac arrest unresponsive to resuscitative measures despite increased risk of hemorrhage
  - Symptomatic patients:
    - Intubate and positive pressure ventilation
    - Fluids and inotropes (amrinone)
    - Continuous IBP, CVP monitor
    - Pulmonary embolectomy with partial CPB

DVT PROPHYLAXIS

Introduction

- Venous TE is a major cause of death after surgery or trauma to lower limbs
- PE is the most common preventable cause of hospital death

Incidence

- DVT develops in 40–80% of orthopedic patients without prophylaxis
- Fatal pulmonary embolism occurs in 0.1–0.8% surgical patients
- Late initiation of prophylaxis (≥ 4 days after trauma) triples the risk of VTE
- Initiation of VTE prophylaxis within 8 hours of surgery had greatest preventive effect

Risk Factors for Development of DVT

Strong Risk Factors

- Fracture of hip/leg/spine injury
- Hip/knee replacement
- Surgeries of hip/pelvis
- Major trauma.

Moderate Risk Factors

- CNS disorders, paralytic stroke
- CVP lines, malignancy

- ❖ Thrombophilia, polycythemia
- ❖ Malignancy
- ❖ CCF, non-valvular atrial fibrillation with previous cerebral embolus
- ❖ Patients with prosthetic valves (Mitral > Aortic)
- ❖ Respiratory failure
- ❖ Irritable bowel disease/DM
- ❖ Pregnancy/postpartum
- ❖ Knee arthroscopy
- ❖ Chemotherapy, hormone replacement therapy, OCP, radiotherapy for pelvic neoplasm

Weak Risk Factors

- ❖ Bed rest more than 4 days
- ❖ Immobility due to sitting (car/plane travel)
- ❖ Increased age, obesity
- ❖ Laparoscopic surgery with duration of surgery more than 30 min
- ❖ Pregnancy/antepartum
- ❖ Varicose veins
- ❖ Trauma, severe infections

Other Risk Factors: Hypercoagulable States

- ❖ Factor V Leiden deficiency (most common disorder associated with VTE)
- ❖ Antithrombin III, protein C and S deficiency
- ❖ APLA, lupus anticoagulant, malignancy, OCP therapy.

Types of VTE Prophylaxis

- ❖ Primary prophylaxis:
  - Preferred method of prophylaxis
  - Comprises methods used to prevent DVT prior to its occurrence
  - Methods used include:
    - Low dose unfractionated heparin
    - Low molecular weight heparin
    - Fondaparinux
    - Intermittent pneumatic compression devices
    - Graduated compression stockings
    - Oral factors Xa inhibitors
- ❖ Secondary prophylaxis:
  - Secondary prophylaxis refers to early diagnosis and treatment of subclinical VTE
  - This is done by screening patients for the presence of DVT using:
    - Contrast venography
    - Venous ultrasound
    - MRI venography
  - It is not commonly used as the sensitivity of these tests are sub-optimal
  - May be useful for:
    - Patients in whom primary prophylaxis is contraindicated
    - Pregnant patients at high risk for DVT.

Risk Assessment for Thrombosis: Improve Thrombosis Score

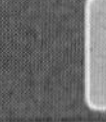

- ❖ Components:
  - Prior venous thromboembolism: 3 points
  - Diagnosed thrombophilia: 2 points
  - Current lower limb paralysis: 2 points
  - Current cancer: 2 points
  - Immobilized for at least 7 days: 1 point
  - Stay in ICU or coronary care unit: 1 point
  - More than 60 years old: 1 point
- ❖ Interpretation:
  - Absence of any risk factors: rate of VTE within 92 days of admission 0.4–0.5%
  - Score 1: Risk of VTE 0.6%
  - Score 2: Rate of VTE 1%
  - Score 3: Rate of VTE 3.1%
- ❖ Thromboprophylactic significance:
  - Total score 0–1:
    - Indicates low risk of DVT
    - Does not warrant thromoboprophylaxis
  - Total score ≥ 2 appropriate for thromboprophylaxis

Risk of Bleeding with Prophylaxis: Improve Bleeding Score

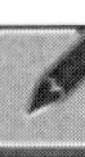

- ❖ Components:
  - Moderate renal failure: 1 point
  - Male sex: 1 point
  - Age 40–84 years: 1.5 points
  - Central venous catheter: 2 points
  - Rheumatic diseases: 2 points
  - Current cancer 2 points
  - Hepatic failure with INR > 1.5: 2.5 points
  - ICU/CCU stay: 2.5 points
  - Severe renal failure (CrCl < 30 mL/min): 2.5 points
  - Age > 85 years: 3.5 points
  - Gastroduodenal ulcer: 4 points
  - Bleeding in last 3 months: 4 points
  - Admission platelets < 50,000 cells/mm^3: 4 points
- ❖ Interpretation:
  - Score 1: 0.5% risk of bleeding
  - Score 4: 1.6% risk of bleeding
  - Score 7: 4.1% risk of bleeding
  - Score 15: 14% risk of bleeding
  - Thus, risk of bleeding is high when total score ≥ 7

Techniques of Thromboprophylaxis

Pharmacological Thromboprophylaxis

- ❖ Pharmacological prophylaxis is superior to mechanical prophylaxis

- Agents used include:
  - Low molecular weight heparin:
    - Most commonly used drug for thromboprophylaxis
    - More effective compared to UFH for VTE thromboprophylaxis
    - Doseage:
      - Enoxaparine 40 mg SC once daily
      - Dalteparin 5000 IU subcutaneous once daily
      - Tinzaparine 4500 anti-Xa units SC once daily
      - Nadroparin 3800–5700 anti-Xa units SC once daily
  - Low-dose unfractionated heparin:
    - Inferior to LMWH
    - Dose: UFH 5000 IU SC Q8-12H
  - Fondaparinux:
    - Very little data available to support routine use
    - May be as effective as LMWH
    - Dose: 2.5 mg SC once daily
  - Warfarin:
    - Not routinely used for immediate and short-term prophylaxis
    - This is because onset of action is delayed (36–72 hours)
  - Direct acting oral anticoagulants (DOACs):
    - Betrixoban and rivaroxaban are approved for use
    - Apixaban or dabigatran may be used as alternatives
    - Insufficient evidence limits routine use
    - Aspirin and clopidogrel do not reduce overall risk of VTE

Mechanical Thromboprophylaxis

- Mechanical thromboprophylaxis is less effective than pharmacological prophylaxis
- No mechanical method has shown a reduction in the incidence of pulmonary embolism
- Use of mechanical modalities alone is therefore, ineffective in moderate-high risk cases
- Therefore use of mechanical thromboprophylaxis is recommended primarily:
  - As adjunct to anticoagulant based prophylaxis
  - As alternative in patients at risk of bleeding
- Mechanical modalities available for prophylaxis include:
  - Passive devices: knee or thigh high graduated compression stockings (GCS)
  - Active intermittent pneumatic compression devices
  - Venous foot pumps
- Active intermittent pneumatic compression devices (AIPCD):
  - Designed to accomplish:
    - Decreased venous stasis
    - Improve blood flow velocity
    - Increase circulating fibrinolysins
  - Advantages of AIPCD:
    - Require no monitoring of anticoagulation levels
    - No increase in risk of bleeding
    - Well tolerated
- Graduated compression stockings (GCS):
  - Ineffective for VTE thromboprophylaxis when used alone
  - There is insufficient evidence to recommend routine use for VTE prophylaxis

Preoperative Considerations for Patients on VTE Prophylaxis

- Risk stratification for development of DVT is done for patients
- Patients with previous history of DVT:
  - Risk of recurrence:
    - Is 50% within 3 months of previous DVT without anticoagulant therapy
    - If 1 month of warfarin therapy is added, risk reduces to 10%
    - If 3 months therapy is added, risk is reduced to 5%
  - Elective surgery:
    - To be postponed in 1st month after episode of VTE
    - Ideally 3 months of anticoagulation is recommended before surgery
    - If urgent surgery is required, preoperative UFH given if INR < 2
    - Heparin not to be restarted for 12 hours after major surgery
    - aPTT is checked 12 hours after restarting therapy
- Patients on anticoagulant therapy:
  - Stop warfarin:
    - INR to be checked during preoperative visit
    - Withhold warfarin for at least 5 days prior to surgery
    - This allows PT/INR to normalize prior to surgery
    - Surgery is postponed till INR normalizes

- *Bridging therapy*:
  - During the time without warfarin, patients are at increased risk for VTE
  - UFH can be used to bridge anticoagulation therapy in perioperative period
  - LMWH can be used as it can be administered without need for monitoring
  - Chronic warfarin therapy > 1 month post-VTE episode:
    - Preoperative bridging not recommended
    - However postoperative heparin should be administered until:
      - Warfarin therapy is resumed
      - Documented INR is > 2

Anesthetic Considerations for Thromboprophylaxis

- Low risk procedures lasting < 30 minutes:
  - Comfortable position
  - Knees flexed at 5°
  - Avoid constriction and external pressure
  - Early mobilization
  - Prefer regional anesthesia
  - Good postoperative analgesia
  - Good physiotherapy
- Moderate risk procedures lasting > 30 minutes:
  - Proper positioning
  - AIPCD of calf and ankle (applied prior to sedation) and continued till patient is awake and moving
  - Compression stockings
  - Frequent alteration of OT table
  - Early mobilization
- High risk procedures:
  - Treated as per patients with moderate risk
  - Preoperative hematology consultation
  - Consider perioperative antithrombotic therapy

Thromboprophylaxis for Orthopedic Surgery

- High risk surgeries include:
  - Total hip arthroplasty
  - Total knee arthroplasty
  - Hip fracture surgery
- Drugs used include:
  - *LMWH (preferred agent)*: enoxaparin 40 mg SC OD
  - UFH 5000 IU SC Q12H
  - *Fondaparinux*: 2.5 mg 6–8 hours before surgery
  - Apixaban or dabigatran may be used as oral alternatives
  - Warfarin is avoided preoperatively
  - Sole use of aspirin for prophylaxis not recommended
- Prophylactic regimens:
  - High risk surgeries:
    - LMWH with AIPCD during hospital stay
    - Early mobilization
    - Neuraxial techniques
    - Extended LMWH prophylaxis postoperatively
    - Patients with high risk for bleeding:
      - AIPCD is used during hospital stay
      - Preoperative placement of IVC filter is not recommended
      - Early mobilization
      - LMWH is initiated once risk of bleeding reduces
  - Low risk surgeries: AIPCD alone
- Duration of VTE prophylaxis:
  - VTE prophylaxis should be
    - Initiated at least 12 hours prior to surgery
    - Resumed at least 12 hours postoperatively
  - VTE prophylaxis should be continued for at least 10–14 days
  - 28–35 days extended prophylaxis in high risk patients
- Elective spine surgery:
  - Routine use of VTE prophylaxis in low risk patients is not recommended
  - LMWH and AIPCD may be used for patients at high risk for VTE
- Role of neuraxial anesthesia:
  - Neuraxial anesthetic techniques are preferred as they reduce risk of VTE
  - Incidence of VTE is reduced through the following mechanisms:
    - Blood flow changes:
      - Causes rheological changes
      - Results in hyperkinetic lower limb blood flow due to vasodilation
      - This reduces venous stasis
    - Systemic effects of local anesthetics:
      - Anti-inflammatory property of LA
      - Circulatory effects of adrenaline used as adjuvant
    - Altered coagulation responses:
      - Prevents increases in Factor VIII and vWF levels
      - Attenuated postop reduction in antithrombin III levels
      - Reduced platelet reactivity
    - Avoids positive pressure ventilation and its effects on circulation.

Thromboprophylaxis for Non-orthopedic Surgery

Risk of VTE	Risk of bleeding	Thromboprophylaxis
Low risk (< 1.5%)	Moderate risk	None
Low risk (< 1.5%)	High risk	Mechanical prophylaxis
Moderate risk (3%)	Moderate risk	LWMH or AIPCD
Moderate risk (3%)	High risk	AIPCD
High risk (6%)	Moderate risk	LMWH and AIPCD or GCS
High risk (6%)	High risk	AIPCD till bleeding risk reduces and LMWH can be added
High risk cancer surgery	Moderate risk	Extended LMWH and AIPCD
High risk cancer surgery	High risk	AIPCD till bleeding risk reduces and LMWH can be added

Thromboprophylaxis in ICU

- High index of suspicion if:
  - Unexplained tachycardia, tachypnea, fever
  - Asymmetric limb edema
  - Increased dead space ventilation
- Anticoagulation:
  - LMWH used in high risk patients
  - UFH (low dose) used in moderate-low risk patients
  - Only TID regimens are effective for UFH
  - Fondaparinux use has not been studied in ICU
- IVC filters:
  - No evidence supporting preventive placement of filters
  - Can be placed in patients for whom LMWH is contraindicated
  - Removable filters available
- Other measures:
  - Flush catheter tips with heparin:
    - Heparin concentration should be 1 IU/ml
    - 3–4 mL of heparin added to 500 mL saline
  - Serial compression devices:
    - No evidence of benefit
    - Useful in patients in whom LMWH therapy is contraindicated

Latest Advances

- Newer factor Xa inhibitors:
  - Idraparinux:
    - Is is a metapentasaccharide
    - Usual dosage is once weekly administered subcutaneously
    - Phase II trials completed
  - *Razaxaban*: undergoing phase II trials
- Direct thrombin inhibitors: Ximelagatran:
  - Rapidly absorbed through the GI tract and converted to its active form melagatran
  - Has a rapid onset of action with predictable dose-response relationship
  - It does not affect aPTT or PT
  - Therefore, monitoring of anticoagulation is not required
  - Shown to be more effective than warfarin in preventing DVT
- Transcutaneous electrical nerve stimulation:
  - Intraoperative TENS prevents both venous stasis and blood hypercoagulability
  - Intraoperative TENS thus had significant, novel effect in preventing DVT

SUGGESTED READING

1. ACC/AHA 2008 guidelines: Warnes, C. A. et al., (2008). ACC/AHA 2008 guidelines for the management of adults with congenital heart disease: Executive summary. *Circulation*, 118(23), 2395–451.
2. ACCF/AHA task force practice guidelines: Fleisher, L. A. et al., (2009). ACCF/AHA focused update on perioperative beta blockade incorporated into the ACC/AHA 2007 guidelines on perioperative cardiovascular evaluation and care for noncardiac surgery. *Circulation*, 120(21), e169–276.
3. ACCP evidence-based Clinical Practice Guidelines: Hirsh,J., Guyatt, G., Albers, G. W., Harrington, R. and Schuneman, H. G. (2008). Antithrombotic and thrombolytic therapy. *Chest*, 133(6 Suppl), 110S–2S.
4. ACCP evidence-based Clinical Practice Guidelines: Kearon, C. et al., (2012). Antithrombotic therapy for VTE disease: Antithrombotic therapy and prevention of thrombosis. *Chest*, 141(2 Suppl), e419S–96S.
5. AHA 2007 guidelines: Wilson, W. et al., (2007). Prevention of infective endocarditis: Guidelines from the AHA. *Circulation*, 116(15), 1736–54.
6. AHA guidelines: Baddour, L. M. et al., (2015). IE in adults: Diagnosis, antimicrobial therapy and management of complications: a scientific statement for healthcare professionals from the AHA. *Circulation*, 132(15), 1435–86.
7. Ahlsson, A., Sobrosa, C., Kaijser, L., Jansson, E. and Bonfim, V. (2012). Adenosine in cold blood cardioplegia—a placebo-controlled study. *Interactive Cardiovascular and Thoracic Surgery*, 14(1), 48–55.
8. Al Kasab, S. M. et al., (1990). β-adrenergic blockade in the management of pregnant women with mitral stenosis. *American Journal of Obstetrics and Gynecology*, 163(1), 37–40.
9. AMISTAD 2 TRIAL: Ross, A. M., Gibbons, R. J., Stone, G. W., Kloner, R. A., Wayne Alexander, R. and AMISTAD-II Investigators. (2005). A randomized, double blinded, placebo-controlled multicenter trial of adenosine as an adjunct to reperfusion in the treatment of acute myocardial infarction (AMISTAD-II). *Journal of the American College of Cardiology*, 45(11), 1775–80.

10. Ammash, N. M. and Warnes, C. A. (2001). Ventricular septal defects in adults. *Annals of Internal Medicine*, 135(9), 812–24.
11. Anderson Jr, F. A. and Spencer, F. A. (2003). Risk factors for venous thromboembolism. *Circulation*, 107(23 Suppl 1), I9–16.
12. Anderson, R. H., Baker, E. J., Macartney, F. J., Rigby, M. L., Shinebourne, E. A. and Tynan, M. (2002). *Pediatric Cardiology*. 2nd ed. London: Churchill Livingstone.
13. Andropoulos, D. B., Stayer, S. A., Russell, I. A. and Mossad, E. B. (2010).*Anesthesia for Congenital Heart Disease*. 2nd ed. Oxford: Wiley Blackwell.
14. Anuar Abdul Aziz, K. and Meduoye, A. (2010). Is pH-stat or alpha-stat the best technique to follow in patients undergoingdeep hypothermic circulatory arrest? *Interactive Cardiovascularand Thoracic Surgery*, 10(2), 271–82.
15. Armstrong, R. A., Squire, Y. G., Rogers, C. A., Hinchliffe, R. J. and Mouton, R. (2019). Types of anesthesia for endovascular abdominal aortic aneurysm repair. *Journal of Cardiothoracic and Vascular Anesthesia*, 33(2), 462–71.
16. ARTS study: Costa, M. A. et al., (2001). Incidence, predictors, and significance of abnormal cardiac enzyme rise in patients treated with bypass surgery in the Arterial Revascularization Therapies Study (ARTS). *Circulation*, 104(22), 2689–93.
17. Asgeri, M., Ahmadpour, F., Negargar, S., Khadra, W. Z., Porhomayon, J. and Nader, N. D. (2011).The comparative myocardial protection by propofol and isoflurane in an in vivo model of ischemia reperfusion. *Seminars in Cardiothoracic and Vascular Anesthesia*, 15(1–2), 56–65.
18. Badgett, R. G., Lawrence, V. A. and Cohn, S. L. (2010). Variations in the pharmacology of beta-blockers may contribute to heterogenous results in trials of perioperative beta-blockade. *Anesthesiology*, 113(3), 585–92.
19. Bando, K et al., (1998). Effect of modified ultrafiltration in high-risk patients undergoing operations for congenital heart disease. *Annals of Thoracic Surgery*, 66(3), 821–7.
20. Barash, P. G. et al., (2017). *Clinical Anesthesia*. 8th ed.Philadelphia: Wolters Kluwer.
21. Barrett, K. E., Barman, S. M., Boitano, S. and Brooks, H. (2012). *Ganong's Review of Medical Physiology*. 24th ed. New York: McGraw Hill Lange.
22. Barron, D. J. (ed.) (2018). *Core Topics in Congenital Cardiac Surgery* 1st ed. Cambridge: Cambridge University Press.
23. Bates, S. M., Greer, I. A., Middeldorp, S., Veenstra, D. L., Prabulos, A.-M.and Vandvik, P. O. (2012). VTE, thrombophilia, antithrombotic therapy, andpregnancy: Antithrombotic therapy and prevention of thrombosis, 9th ed: American College of Chest Physicians evidence based clinical practice guidelines. *Chest*, 141(2 Suppl), e691S–736S.
24. Baum, V. C., Barton, D. M. and Gutgesell, H. P. (2000). Influence of congenital heart disease on mortality after noncardiac surgery in hospitalized children. *Pediatrics*, 105(2), 332–5.
25. Baumgartner, H. et al., (2009). Echocardiographic assessment of valve stenosis: EAE/ASE recommendations for clinical practice. *Journal of the American Society of Echocardiography*, 22(1), 1–23.
26. Baumgartner, H. et al., (2017). 2017 ESC/EACTS guidelines for the management of valvular heart disease. *European Heart Journal*, 38(36), 2739–91.
27. Beck, A. W.et al., (2016). Variations in abdominal aortic aneurysm care: A report from the International Consortium of Vascular Registries. *Circulation*, 134(24), 1948–58.
28. Belardinelli, L., Shrycock, J. C. and Fraser, H. (2006). Inhibition of late sodium current as a potential cardioprotective principle: effect of the late sodium current inhibitor ranolazine. *Heart*, 92(Suppl 4), iv6–14.
29. Berne, R. M. (1959). Cardiodynamics and the coronary circulation in hypothermia. *Annals of New York Academy of Sciences*, 80(2), 365–83.
30. Berqvist, D.and Hull, R. D. (2006). Effective thromboprophylaxis administered close to the time of major orthopedic surgery: A review. *American Journal of Orthopedics*, 35(5), 226–30.
31. Bhatla, N. et al., (2003). Cardiac disease in pregnancy. *International Journal of Gynaecology and Obstetrics*, 82(2), 153–9.
32. Birnie, D. H., Wang, J., Alings, M. and Philippon, F. (2019). Risk factors for infections involving Cardiac Implanted Electronic Devices. *Journal of the American College of Cardiology*, 74, 2845–54.
33. Bonow, R. O., Mann, D. L. and Tomaselli, G. F. (2019). *Braunwald's Heart Disease*. 11th ed. Philadelphia: Elsevier.
34. Boodhwani, M. et al., (2009). Repair-oriented classification of aortic insufficiency: impact on surgical techniques and clinical outcomes. *Journal of Thoracic and Cardiovascular Surgery*, 137(2), 286–94.
35. Born, D. et al., (1992). Pregnancy in patients with prosthetic heart valves: the effects of anticoagulation on mother, fetus, and neonate. *American Heart Journal*, 124(2), 413–7.
36. Bouabdallaoui, N. et al., (2018). Society of Thoracic Surgeons Risk Scoreand EuroSCORE-2 Appropriately Assess 30-day Post-operative Mortality in the STICH Trial and a Contemporary Cohort of Patients with Left Ventricular Dysfunction Undergoing Surgical Revascularization. *Circulation Heart Failure*,11(11), e005531.
37. Bramwell, C. and Jones, A. M. (1941). Coarctation of the aorta: The collateral circulation. *British Heart Journal*, 3(4), 205–27.
38. Brochard, L. Mancebo, J. and Pinsky, M. R. (2006). *Applied Physiology in Intensive Care Medicine*. Berlin: Springer.
39. Brown, T. A. (2012). *Rapid Review Physiology*. 2nd ed. Philadelphia: Elsevier.
40. Buckberg, G. D. (1991). Myocardial temperature management during aortic clamping for cardiac surgery. *Journal of Thoracic and Cardiovascular Surgery*, 102(6), 895–903.
41. Buckberg, G. D., Brazier, J. R., Nelson, R. L., Goldstein, S. M., McConnell, D. H. and Cooper, N. (1977). Studies of the effects of hypothermia on regional myocardial blood flow and metabolism during cardiopulmonary bypass. I. the adequately perfused beating, fibrillating, and arrested heart. *Journal of Thoracic and Cardiovascular Surgery*, 73(1), 87–94.

42. Butterworth, J. F., Mackey, D. C. and Wasnick, J. D. (2018). *Morgan and Mikhail's Clinical Anesthesiology*. 6th ed. New York: McGraw Hill Education.
43. Cahill, T. J. and Prendergast B. D. (2016). Infective endocarditis. *Lancet*, 387(10021), P882–93.
44. Cannon 3rd, R. O. (2005).Mechanisms, management and future directions for reperfusion injury after acute myocardial infarction. *Nature Clinical Practice Cardiovascular Medicine*, 2(2), 88–94.
45. Cardiac Society of Australia and New Zealand (2010). Guidelines for the management of antiplatelet therapy in patients with coronary stent undergoing non-cardiac surgery. *Heart Lung and Circulation*, 19(1), 2–10.
46. Carmosino, M. J., Friesen, R. H., Doran, A. and Ivy, D. D. (2007). Perioperative complications in children with pulmonary hypertension undergoing non-cardiac surgery or cardiac catheterization. *Anesthesia and Analgesia*, 104(3), 521–7.
47. Carrier, M. et al., (2002). Cardioplegic arrest with L-arginine improves myocardial protection: Results of a prospective randomized clinical trial. *Annals of Thoracic Surgery*, 73(3), 837–42.
48. Carvalho, E. M. F., Gabriel, E. A. and Salerno, T. A. (2008). Pulmonary protection during cardiac surgery: A systematic literature review. *Asian Cardiovascular Thoracic Annals*, 16(6), 503–7.
49. Cavalcante, J. L., Rodriguez, L. L., Kapadia, S. Murat Tuzcu, E. and Stewart W. J. (2012). Role of echocardiography in percutaneous mitral valve interventions. *Journal of the American College of Cardiology*, 5(7), 733–46.
50. CaVenT Study Group: Enden, T. et al., (2012). Long term outcome after additional catheter directed thrombolysis versus standard treatment for acute iliofemoral deep vein thrombosis (the CaVenT study): A randomized controlled trial. *Lancet*, 379(9810), 31–8.
51. Chaikoff, E. L. et al., (2018). The Society for Vascular Surgery Practice Guidelines on the Care of Patients With an Abdominal Aortic Aneurysm. *Journal of Vascular Surgery*, 67(1), e2–77.
52. Chakravarthy, M., Prabhakumar, P. andGeorge, A. (2017). Anesthetic considerations in patients with cardiac implantable electronic devices scheduled for surgery. *Indian Journal of Anaesthesia*, 61(9), 736–43.
53. Chandler, W. L.(2005). Effects of hemodilution, blood loss,and consumption on hemostatic factor levels during cardiopulmonary bypass. *Journal of Cardiothoracic and Vascular Anesthesia*, 19(4), 459–67.
54. Chassot, P.-G., van der Linden, P., Zaugg, M., Mueller, X. M. and Spahn, D. R. (2004).Off-pump coronary artery surgery: Physiology and anesthetic management. *British Journal of Anaesthesia*, 92(3), 400–13.
55. Chen, P. S., Wolf, P. D. and Ideker R. E. (1991). Mechanism of cardiac defibrillation: A different point of view. *Circulation*, 84(2), 913–9.
56. Chestnut, D. H. et al., (2019). *Chestnut's Obstetric Anesthesia: Principles and Practice*. 6th ed. Philadelphia: Mosby Elsevier.
57. CHILL-MI trial: Erlinge, D. et al., (2014). Rapid endovascular catheter core cooling combined with cold saline as an adjunct to percutaneous coronary intervention for the treatment of acute myocardial infarction: The CHILL-MI trial. *Journal of theAmerican College of Cardiology*, 63(18), 1857–65.
58. Cornelissen, A. J. M., Dankelman, J., Van Bavel, E. and Spaan, J. A. E. (2002). Balance between myogenic, flow-dependant, and metabolic flow control in coronary arterial tree: A model study. *American Journal of Physiology-Heart and Circulatory Physiology*, 282(6), 2224–37.
59. Corvera, J. S. et al., (2005). Polarized arrest with warm or cold adenosine/lidocaine blood cardioplegia is equivalent to hypothermic blood potassium cardioplegia. *Journal of Thoracic and Cardiovascular Surgery*, 129(3), 599–606.
60. Costa, F. et al., (2017). Derivation and validation of the predicting bleeding complications in patients undergoing stent implantation and subsequent dual antiplatelet therapy (PRECISE-DAPT) score: a pooled analysis of individual-patient datasets from clinical trials. *Lancet*, 389(10073), 1025–34.
61. Crossley, G. H. et al., (2011). The Heart Rhythm Society (HRS)/American Society of Anesthesiologists (ASA) Expert Consensus Statement on the Perioperative Management of Patients With Implantable Defibrillators, Pacemakers and Arrhythmia Monitors: Facilities and Patient Management. *Heart Rhythm*, 8(7), 1114–54.
62. Currigan, D. A., Hughes, R. J. A., Wright, C. E., Angus, J. A. and Soeding, P. F. (2014). Vasoconstrictor responses to vasopressor agents in human pulmonary and radial arteries: an in-vitro study. *Anesthesiology*, 121(5), 930–6.
63. Da Cruz, E., Dunbar, I. and James, J. (eds.) (2014). *Pediatric and Congenital Cardiology, Cardiac Surgery and Intensive Care*. 1st ed. London: Springer Reference.
64. Dai, N. et al., (2014). Different beta blockers and initiation time in patients undergoing non-cardiac surgery: A meta analysis. *American Journal of Medical Sciences*, 347(3), 235–44.
65. David Mazer, C. (1993). Calcium and stunned myocardium. *Journal of Cardiac Surgery*, 8(S2), 329–31.
66. Davies, M. R. and Cousins, J. (2009). Cardiomyopathy and anaesthesia. *Continuing Education in Anaesthesia Critical Care and Pain*, 9(6), 189–93.
67. Davis, M. D., Walsh, B. K., Sittig, S. E. and Restrepo, R. D. (2013). AARC clinical practice guidelines: blood gas analysis and hemoximetry: 2013. *Respiratory Care*, 58(10), 1694–703.
68. De Souza, J. A. et al., (2001). Percutaneous balloon mitral valvuloplasty in comparison with open mitral valve commissurotomy for mitral stenosis during pregnancy. *Journal of the American College of Cardiology*, 37(3), 900–3.
69. Deceppe, E. et al., (2017). Canadian Cardio-vascular Society guidelines on perioperative cardiac risk assessment and management for patients who undergo non-cardiac surgery. *Canadian Journal of Cardiology*, 33(12), 1735.
70. DECREASE Study Group: Poldermans, D. et al., (1999). The effect of bisoprolol on perioperative mortality and myocardial infarction in high-risk patients undergoing vascular surgery. *The New England Journal of Medicine*, 341, 1789–94.
71. Deitelzweig, S. and Jaff, M. R. (2004). Medical management of venous thromboembolic disease. *Techniques in Vascular and Interventional Radiology*, 7(2), 63–7.

72. Delaney, M. et al., (2013). Risk of extracorporeal life support circuit-related hyperkalemia is reduced by pre-bypass ultrafiltration. *Pediatric Critical Care Medicine*, 14(6), e263-7.
73. DELTA-MI trial: Bates, E. et al., (2008). Intracoronary KAI-9803 as an adjunct to primary percutaneous coronary intervention for acute ST segment elevation myocardial infarction. *Circulation*, 117(7):886–96.
74. Deswal, A. (2005). Diastolic dysfunction and diastolic heart failure: mechanisms and epidemiology. *Current Cardiology Reports*, 7, 178–83.
75. Detsky, A. S., Abrams, H. B., Fornath, N., Scott, G. and Hilliard, J. R. (1986). Cardiac assessment for patients undergoing noncardiac surgery a multifactorial cardiac risk index. *Archives of Internal Medicine*, 146(11), 2131–4.
76. Devereaux, P. et al., (2014). Aspirin in patients undergoing non-cardiac surgery. *The New England Journal of Medicine*, 370, 1494–503.
77. Devereaux, P. J. and Szczeklik, W. (2019). Myocardial injury after non-cardiac surgery: diagnosis and management. *European Heart Journal*. [Viewed 20 May 2020] Available from: https://doi.org/10.1093/eurheartj/ehz301.
78. Devereaux,P. J., Goldman, L., Yusuf, S., Gilbert, K., Leslie, K. and Guyatt, G. H. (2005). Surveillance and prevention of major perioperative ischemic cardiac events in patients undergoing non-cardiac surgery: A review. *Canadian Medical Association Journal*, 173(7), 779–88.
79. Diaz, L. K. and Andropoulos, D. B. (2005). New developments in pediatric cardiac anesthesia. *Anesthesiology Clinics of North America*, 23(4), 655–76.
80. DIPOM Trial group: Juul, A. B., et al. (2006). Effect of perioperative beta-blockade in patients with diabetes undergoing major non-cardiac surgery: Randomized placebo controlled, blinded multicenter trial. *British Medical Journal*, 332(7556), 1482.
81. Diprose, P. and Tom Pierce, J. M. (2001). Anaesthesia for patients with pacemakers and similar devices. *British Journal of Anaesthesia*, 1(6), 166–70.
82. Disque, K. (2016). *Advanced Cardiac Life Support Provider Handbook.* Las Vegas: Satori Continuum Publishing.
83. Dixit, R. et al., (2015). Epidemiology of congenital heart disease in India. *Congenital Heart Disease*, 10(5), 437–46.
84. Domenech, R. J. (1978). Regional diastolic coronary blood flow during diastolic ventricular hypertension. *Cardiovascular Research*, 12(11), 639–45.
85. Du, L.-J.et al., (2015). Association between ventricular end-diastolic pressure and coronary artery disease as well as its extent and severity. *International Journal of Clinical and Experimental Medicine*, 8(10), 18673–80.
86. Duebener, L. F. et al., (2002). Effects of pH management during deep hypothermic bypass on cerebral microcirculation: alpha-stat versus pH-stat. *Circulation*, 106(12 Suppl 1), I103–8.
87. El-Feky, M. and Gaillard, F. (2009). *Figure 3 sign*. Retrieved September 17, 2017, from Radiopaedia.org. [Viewed 20 May 2020] Available from: https://radiopaedia.org/articles/figure-3-sign.
88. Ellenbogen, K. A. and Wood, M. A. (2008). *Cardiac Pacing and ICDs*. 5th ed. New Jersey: Blackwell Publishing.
89. Ellis, R. J., Mavroudis, C., Gardner, C., Turley, K., Ullyot, D. and Ebert, P. A. (1980). Relationship between atrioventricular arrhythmias and the concentration of K+ion in cardioplegic solution. *Journal of Thoracic and Cardiovascular Surgery*, 80(4), 517–26.
90. Enhanced Recovery After Surgery Society Guidelines: Engelman, D. T. et al., (2019). Guidelines for perioperative care in cardiac surgery. *Journal of the American Medical Association*, 154(8), 755–66.
91. Estep, J. D. et al., (2013). Percutaneous placement of an intra-aortic balloon pump in the left axillary/subclavian position provides safe, ambulatory long-term support as bridge to heart transplantation. *Journal of the American College of Cardiology Heart Failure*, 1(5), 382–8.
92. Fedorow, C. A., Moon, M. C., Mutch, W. A. C. and Grocott, H. P. (2010). Lumbar cerebrospinal fluid drainage for thoracoabdominal aortic surgery: Rationale and practical considerations for management. *Anesthesia and Analgesia*, 111(1), 46–58.
93. Feldman, T. (2003). Core curriculum for interventional cardiology: Percutaneous valvuloplasty. *Catheterization and Cardiovascular Interventions*, 60(1), 48–56.
94. Ferro, G., Duilio, C., Spinelli, L., Spadafora, M., Guarnaccia, F. and Condorelli, M. (1991). Effects of beta blockade on the relation between heart rate and ventricular diastolic perfusion time during exercise in systemic hypertension. *American Journal of Cardiology*, 68(10), 1101–3.
95. Fleishar, L. A. et al. (2014). 2014 ACC-AHA guidelines on the perioperative cardiovascular evaluation and management of patients undergoing noncardiac surgery: Executive summary: A report of the American College of Cardiology/American Heart Association Task force on Practice Guidelines. *Circulation*, 130(24), 2215–45.
96. Fleisher, L. A. et al., (2014, December). *Onlinejacc*. Retrieved December 30, 2018, from www.onlinejacc.org. [Viewed 20 May 2020] Available from: http://www.onlinejacc.org/content/64/22/2373/F2.
97. Flick, R. P. et al., (2007). Perioperative cardiac arrests in children between 1988 and 2005 at a tertiary referral centre: A study of 92,881 patients. *Anesthesiology*, 106(2), 226–37.
98. Francis, C. W. et al., (2003). Comparison of ximelagatran with warfarin for the prevention of venous thromboembolism after total knee replacement.*The New England Journal of Medicine*, 1703–12.
99. Friesen, R. H. and Williams, G. D. (2008).Anesthetic management of children with pulmonary arterial hypertension. *Pediatric Anesthesia*, 18(3), 208–16.
100. Fuhrman, B. P. andZimmerman, J. J. (2017). *Fuhrman and Zimmerman's Pediatric Critical Care*. 5th ed. Philadelphia: Elsevier.
101. Gajewski, M. and Hillel, Z. (2012). Anesthesia management of patients with hypertrophic obstructive cardiomyopathy. *Progress in Cardiovascular Disease*, 54(6), 503–11.
102. Garson Jr., A et al., (1985). Prevention of sudden death after repair of tetralogy of Fallot: Treatment of ventricular arrhythmias. *Journal of the American College of Cardiology*, 6(1), 221–7.

103. Gay Jr, W. A. and Ebert, P. A. (1973). Functional, metabolic,and morphological effects of potassium-induced cardioplegia. *Surgery*, 74(2), 284–90.
104. Geerts, W. H. et al., (2008). Prevention of venous thromboembolism: American College of Chest Physicians Evidence-Based Clinical Practice Guidelines (8th Edition). *Chest*, 133(6 Suppl), 381S–453S.
105. Geissler, H. J., Mehlhorn, U., Laine, G. A. and Allen, S. J. (2003). Myocardial protection with esmolol during coronary artery bypass grafting surgery. *Anesthesiology*, 98, 164–7.
106. Gelman, S. (1995). The pathophysiology of aortic cross-clamping and unclamping. *Anesthesiology*, 82, 1026–57.
107. Gerotziafas, G. T. and Samama, M. M. (2005). Heterogeneity of synthetic factor Xa inhibitors.*Current Pharmaceutical Design*, 11(30), 3855–76.
108. Goldman L. et al., (1977). Multifactorial index of cardiac risk in noncardiac surgical procedures. *The New England Journal of Medicine*, 297(16), 845–50.
109. Gomar, C. and Errando, C. L. (2005). Neuroaxial anesthesia in obstetrical patients with cardiac disease. *Current Opinion in Anesthesiology*, 18(5), 507–12.
110. Goodwill, A. G., Dick, G. M., Kiel, A. M. and Tune, J. D. (2017). Regulation of coronary blood flow. *Comprehensive Physiology*, 7(2), 321–82.
111. GOPCABE study group: Diegeler, A. et al., (2013). Off-pump versus on-pump coronary-artery bypass grafting in elderly patients: *The New England Journal of Medicine*, 368, 1189–98.
112. Grabenwoger, M. et al., (2012).Thoracic Endovascular Aortic Repair (TEVAR) for the treatment of aortic diseases: a position statement from the European Association for Cardio-Thoracic Surgery (EACTS) and the European Society of Cardiology (ESC), in collaboration with the European Association of Percutaneous Cardiovascular Interventions (EAPCI). *European Heart Journal*, 33(13), 1558–63.
113. Gravlee, G. P., Davis, R. F., Hammon, J. and Kussman, B. (2015). *Cardiopulmonary Bypass and Mechanical Support: Principles and Practice*. 4th ed.Philadelphia: Wolters Kluwer.
114. Gropper, M., Eriksson, L., Fleisher, L., Wiener-Kronish, J., Cohen, N. and Leslie, K. (2020). *Miller's Anesthesia*. 9th ed. Philadelphia: Elsevier Health.
115. Habib, G. et al., (2009).Guidelines on the prevention, diagnosis, and treatment of infective endocarditis (new version 2009): The Task Force on the Prevention, Diagnosis, and Treatment of Infective Endocarditis of the European Society of Cardiology (ESC). *European Heart Journal*, 30(19), 2369–413.
116. Habib, G. et al., (2015).2015 ESC Guidelines for the management of infective endocarditis: The Task Force for the Management of Infective Endocarditis of the European Society of Cardiology (ESC). *European Heart Journal*, 36(44), 3075–128.
117. Hale, A. J. et al., (1996). Apoptosis: Molecular regulation of cell death. *European Journal of Biochemistry*, 236(1), 1–26.
118. Hall, J. E. (2016). *Guyton and Hall Textbook of Medical Physiology*. 13th ed. Philadelphia: Elsevier.
119. Hameed, A. et al., (2001). The effect of valvular heart disease on maternal and fetal outcome of pregnancy. *Journal of the American College of Cardiology*, 893–9.
120. Hammermeister, K., Sethi, G. K., Henderson, W. G., Grover. F. L., Oprian, C. and Rahimtoola, S. (2000). Outcomes 15 years after valve replacement with a mechanical vs bioprosthetic valve: Final report of Veterans Affairs randomized trial. *Journal of the American College of Cardiology*, 36(4), 1152–8.
121. Hayashi, Y. et al., (2004). Minimally-diluted blood cardioplegia supplemented with potassium and magnesium for combination of 'initial, continuous and intermittent bolus' administration. *Circulation Journal*, 68(5), 467–72.
122. Health, N. I. (2019, April 16). *Genetics home reference: your guide to understanding genetic conditions*. Retrieved April 28, 2019, from US National Library of Medicine. [Viewed 20 May 2020] Available from: https://ghr.nlm.nih.gov/condition/charge-syndrome#genes.
123. Healy, T. and Knight, P. (eds.) (2003). *Wiley and Churchill-Davidson's A Practice of Anesthesia. 7th ed. London: Hodder Arnold.*
124. Hennein, H. A., Mendeloff, E. N., Cilley, R. E., Bove, E. L. and Coran, A. G. (1994). Predictors of postoperative outcome after general surgical procedures in patients with congenital heart disease. *Journal of Pediatric Surgery*, 29(7), 866–70.
125. Hensley, F. A., Gravlee, G. P. and Martin, D. E. (2012). *A Practical Approach to Cardiac Anesthesia*. 5th ed. Philadelphia: Wolters Kluwer.
126. Hensley, N., Dietrich, J., Nyhan, D., Mitter, N., Yee, M.-S. and Brady, M. (2015). Hypertrophic cardiomyopathy: A review. *Anesthesia and Analgesia*, 120(3), 554–69.
127. Herring, N. and Paterson, D. J. (2018).*Levick's Introduction to Cardiovascular Physiology*. 6th ed.Boca Raton, FL: CRC Press.
128. Hill, E. E., Herijgers, P., Claus, P., Vanderschueren, S., Herregods, M.-C. and Peetermans, W. E.(2007). Infective endocarditis: Changing epidemiology and predictors of 6-month mortality: A prospective cohort study. *European Heart Journal*, 28(2), 196–203.
129. Hines, R. and Marschall, K. E. (ed.) (2018). *Stoelting's Anesthesia and Coexisting Disease*, 7th ed. Philadelphia: Elsevier.
130. Hoffman, J. I. and Christianson, R. (1978). Congenital heart disease in a cohort of 19, 502 births with long term follow up. *American Journal of Cardiology*, 42(4), 641–7.
131. Hoffman, J. I. E. (1990). Autoregulation and heart rate. *Circulation*, 82(5), 1880–1.
132. Hoffman, J. I. E. and Kalpan, S. (2002). The incidence of congenital heart disease. *Journal of the American College of Cardiology*, 39(12), 1890–900.
133. Hogue Jr., C. W., Palin, C. A. and Arrowsmith, J. E. (2006). Cardiopulmonary bypass management and neurological outcomes: an evidence-based appraisal of current practices. *Anesthesia and Analgesia*, 103(1), 21–37.
134. Hollenberg, S. M., (2017). Valvular heart disease in adults: etiologies, classification, and diagnosis. *FP Essentials*, 457, 11–6.

135. Holmes 4th, J. H. et al., (2002). Magnitude of inflammatory response to cardiopulmonary bypassand its relation to adverse clinical outcomes. *Inflammation Research*, 579–86.
136. Horlocker, T. T., Vandermeulen, E., Kopp, S. L., Gogarten, W., Leffert, L. R. and Benzon H. T. (2018). Regional anesthesia in the patient receiving antithrombotic or thrombolytic therapy: American Society of Regional Anesthesia and Pain Medicine Evidence-Based Guidelines (Fourth Edition). *Regional Anesthesia and Pain Medicine*, 43(3), 263–309.
137. Hornick, P. and Taylor, K. (1997). Pulsatile and non-pulsatile perfusion: The continuing controversy. *Journal of Cardiothoracic and Vascular Anesthesia*, 11(3), 310–5.
138. Horstkotte, D., Niehues, R. and Strauer, B. E. (1991). Pathomorphological aspects, aetiology and natural history of acquired mitral valve stenosis. *European Heart Journal*, 12(Suppl B), 55–60.
139. Hull, R. D. et al., (2001). Timing of initial administration of low-molecular-weight heparin prophylaxis against deep vein thrombosis in patients following elective hip arthroplasty: A systematic review. *Archives of Internal Medicine*, 161(16), 1952–60.
140. Iliceto, S. et al., (1996). Analysis of microvascular integrity, contractile reserve, and myocardial viability after acute myocardial infarction by dobutamine echocardiography and myocardial contrast echocardiography. *The American Journal of Cardiology*, 77(7), 441–5.
141. Inoue, K., Owaki, T., Nakamura, T., Kitamura, F. and Miyamoto, N. (1984). Clinical application of transvenous mitral commissurotomy by a new balloon catheter. *Journal of Thoracic and Cardiovascular Surgery*, 87(3), 394–402.
142. Izumi, M. et al., (2015). Less deep vein thrombosis due to transcutaneous fibular nerve stimulation in total knee arthroplasty: A randomized controlled trial. *Knee Surgery, Sports Traumatology, Arthroscopy*, 23(11), 3317–23.
143. Jensen, A. S. et al., (2015). Prevalence of cerebral and pulmonary thrombosis in patients with cyanotic congenital heart disease. *Heart*, 101(19), 1540–6.
144. Joseph, G. et al., (2005). Evaluation of a simplified transseptal mitral valvuloplasty technique using over-the-wire single balloons and complementary femoral and jugular venous approachesin 1,407 Consecutive Patients. *Journal of Invasive Cardiology*, 17(3), 132–8.
145. Joubert, I.A. and Dyer, R. A. (n.d.). Anesthesia for the pregnant patient with acquired valvular heart disease. *Update in Anaesthesia*. [Viewed 20 May 2020] Available from: https://www.wfsahq.org/components/com_virtual_library/media/9acd216d46c9c598fa147f9366841d51-a43ab3035f5ef3ca5c6f7d175d8ea850-Anaesthesia-for-the-Pregnant-Patient-with-Acquired-Valvular-.pdf.
146. Kakkar, V. V. and Adams, P. C. (1986). Preventive and therapeutic approach to venous thromboembolic disease and pulmonary embolism—can death from pulmonary embolism be prevented? *Journal of the American College of Cardiology*, 6(Suppl 2), 146B–58B.
147. Kambam, J. (ed.) (1994). *Cardiac Anaesthesia for Infants and Children*. St. Louis: Mosby.
148. Kaplan, J. A., Augoustides, J. G. T., Reich, D. L. and Manecke, G. R. (2017). *Kaplan's Cardiac Anesthesia*. 7th ed. Philadelphia: Elsevier.
149. Kavsak, P. A.et al., (2011). High sensitivity troponin T concentrations in patients undergoing non-cardiac surgery: a prospective cohort study. *Clinical Biochemistry*, 1021–4.
150. Kay, P. and Munsch, C. M. (2004). *Techniques in Extracorporeal Circulation*. 4th ed. Boca Raton, FL: CRC Press.
151. Kaya, C. T. and Erol, C. (2018). How to achieveinfective endocarditis prophylaxis. *E-journal of Cardiology Practice*, 16(3). [Viewed 20 May 2020] Available from: https://www.escardio.org/Journals/E-Journal-of-Cardiology-Practice/Volume-16/vol16no33.
152. Kearon, C. et al., (2006). Comparison of fixed-dose weight-adjustedunfractionatedheparin and low-molecular-weight heparin for acute treatment ofvenous thromboembolism. *Journal of the American Medical Association*, 296(8), 935–42.
153. Kearon, C. et al., (2016). Antithrombotic therapy for VTE disease: CHEST guideline and expert panel report. *Chest*, 149(2), 315–52.
154. Kim, M.-J.(2006). Long-term outcomes of significant mitral regurgitation after percutaneous mitral valvuloplasty. *Circulation*, 114(25), 2815–22.
155. Kishan, C. V., Wongpraparut, N., Adeleke, K., Frechie, P. O. and Kotler, M. N. (2000). Ortnery's syndrome in association with mitral valve prolapse. *Clinical Cardiology*, 23(4), 295–7.
156. Klavdios Steriotis, A. and Sharma, S. (2015). Risk stratification in hypertrophic cardiomyopathy. *European Cardiology Review*, 10(1), 31–6.
157. Knepp, M. D., Rocchini, A. P., Lloyd, T. R. and Aiyagiri, R. M. (2010). Long-term follow up of secundum atrial septal defect closure with amplatzer septal occluder. *Congenital Heart Disease*, 5(1), 32–7.
158. Knowles, P. R. and Press, C. (2017). Anaesthesia for cardioversion. *British Journal of Anaesthesia Education*, 17(5), 166–71.
159. Korbmacher, B., Simic, O., Schulte, S. D., Sons, H. and Schipke, J. D. (2004). Intermittent aortic cross-clamping for coronary artery bypass grafting: a review of a safe, fast, simple,and successful technique. *Journal of Cardiovascular Surgery*, 45(6), 535–43.
160. Krishna, M. and Zacharowski, K. (2009). Principles of intra-aortic balloon pumpcounterpulsation. *Continuing Education in Anaesthesia Critical Care and Pain*, 9(1), 24–8.
161. Kristen, S. D. et al., (2014). ESC/ESA guidelines on non-cardiac surgery: cardiovascular assessment and management. *European Heart Journal*, 35, 2383–431.
162. Kuczkowski, K. M. (2004). Labor analgesia for the parturient with cardiac disease: what an obstetrician needs to know? *Acta Obstetricia et Gynecologica Scandinavica*, 83(3), 223–33.
163. Kuczkowski, K. M. and Van Zundert, A. (2007). Anesthesia for pregnant women with valvular heart disease: the state of the art. *Journal of Anesthesia*, 21(2), 252–7.
164. Kumar, P. and Clark, M. (2017). *Kumar and Clark's Clinical Medicine*. 9th ed. Philadelphia: Elsevier.
165. Lake, C. L. and Booker, P. D. (2004).*Pediatric Cardiac Anesthesia*. 4th ed. Philadelphia: Lippincott Williams and Wilkins.

166. Lamy, A.et al., (2016). Five year outcomes after off-pump or on-pump coronary-artery bypass grafting. *New England Journal of Medicine*, 375(24), 2359–68.
167. Landesberg, G. (2003). The pathophysiology of perioperative myocardial infarction: Facts and perspectives. *Journal of Cardiothoracicand Vascular Anesthesia*, 17(1), 90–100.
168. Landesberg, G., Scott Beattie, W., Mosseri, M., Jaffe, A. S. and Alpert, J. S. (2009). Perioperative myocardial infarction. *Circulation*, 119(22), 2936–44.
169. Landoni, G., Bignami, E., Oliviero, F. and Zangrillo, A. (2009). Halogenated anaesthetics and cardiac protection in cardiac and non-cardiac anaesthesia. *Annals of Cardiac Anaesthesia*, 12(1), 4–9.
170. Lango, R. and Mrozinski, P. (2010). Clinical importance of anaesthetic preconditioning. *Anaesthesiology Intensive Therapy (Anestezjologia Intensywna Terapia)*, 42(4), 1206–12.
171. Larry Jameson, J., Fauci, A. S., Dasper, D. L., Hauser, S. L., Lomgo, D. L. and Loscalzo, J. (2018). *Harrison's Principles of Internal Medicine*. 20th ed. New York: McGraw Hill.
172. Le Manach,Y. et al., (2012). Impact of perioperative bleeding on the protective effect of b-blockers during infrarenal aortic reconstruction. *Anesthesiology*, 1203–11.
173. Lee, T. H. et al., (1999). Derivation and prospective validation of a simple index for the prediction of cardiac risk of major noncardiac surgery. *Circulation*, 100(10), 1043–9.
174. Lewis, S. R., Nicholson, A., Reed, S. S., Kenth, J. J., Alderson, P. and Smith, A. F. (2015). Anaesthetic and sedative agents used for electrical cardioversion. *Cochrane Database of Systematic Reviews*. [Viewed 20 May 2020] Available from: https://doi.org/10.1002/14651858.CD010824.pub2.
175. Liakopoulos, O. J. et al., (2008). Impact of preoperative statin therapy on adverse postoperative outcomes in patients undergoing cardiac surgery: A meta analysis of over 30,000 patients. *European Heart Journal*, 29(12), 1548–59.
176. Libby, P. P., Bonow, R. O., Mann, D. L. and Zipes, D. P. (2008). *Braunwald's Heart Disease: A Textbook of Cardiovascular Medicine*. 8th ed.Philadelphia: Saunders Elsevier.
177. Libby, R. P., Bonow, R. O., Mann, D. L. and Zipes, D. P.(eds.) (2007). *Braunwald's Heart Disease: A Textbook of Cardiovascular Medicine*. 8th ed. Philadelphia: Saunders.
178. Lill, M. C., Perloff, J. K. and Child, J. S. (2006). Pathogenesis of thrombocytopenia in cyanotic congenital heart disease. *American Journal of Cardiology*, 98(2), 254–8.
179. Link, M. S. et al., (2010). Part 6: Electrical therapies: automated external defibrillators, defibrillation, cardioversionand pacing. *Circulation*, 122(18 Suppl 3), S706–19.
180. Lip, G. Y. H., Frison, L., Halperin, J. and Lane, D. A. (2011). Comparative validation of a novel risk score for predicting bleeding risk in anticoagulated patients with atrial fibrillation: The HAS-BLED (Hypertension, Abnormal Renal/Liver Function, Stroke, Bleeding History or Predisposition, Labile INR, Elderly, Drugs/Alcohol Concomitantly) Score. *Journal of the American College of Cardiology*, 57(2), 173–80.
181. Luo, W., Li, B., Huang, R. and Lin, G. (2008). Effect of ischemic postconditioning in adult valve replacement. *European Journal of Cardiothoracic Surgery*, 33(2), 203–8.
182. Luthra, M. (2012). *Manual of Pediatric Cardiac Intensive Care*. 1st ed. Philadelphia: Elsevier.
183. Madazli, R., Sal, V., Cift, T., Guralp, O. and Goymen, A. (2009). Pregnancy outcomes in women with heart disease. *Archives of Gynecology and Obstetrics*, 281(1), 29–34.
184. Mainzer, G. et al., (2010). Morphologic, mechanical, conductive, and hemodynamic changes following trancatheter closure of atrial septal defect. *Congenital Heart Disease*, 5(1), 25–31.
185. Mangano, D. T., Layug, E. L., Wallace, A. and Tateo, I. (1996). Effect of atenolol on mortality and cardiovascular morbidity after noncardiac surgery. Multicenter Study of Perioperative Ischemia Research Group. *The New England Journal of Medicine*, 335(23), 1713–20.
186. Marber, M. S., Latchman, D. S., Walker, J. M. and Yellon, D. M. (1993). Cardiac stress protein elevation 24 hours after brief ischemia or heat stress is associated with resistance to myocardial infarction. *Circulation*, 88(3), 1264–72.
187. Marcus, R. H., Sareli, P., Pocock, W. A. and Barlow, J. B. (1994).The spectrum of severe rheumatic mitral valve disease in a developing country. Correlations among clinical presentation, surgical pathologic findings, and hemodynamic sequelae. *Annals of Internal Medicine*, 120(3), 177–83.
188. Maron, B. J., Rowin, E. J. and Maron, M. S. (2018). Global burden of hypertrophic cardiomyopathy.*Journal of the American College of Cardiology: Heart Failure*, 6(5), 6(5), 376–8.
189. Maron, M. et al., (2006). Hypertrophic cardiomyopathy is predominantly a disease of left ventricular outflow tract obstruction. *Circulation*, 114(21), 2232–9.
190. Martin. R., Fanaroff, A. and Walsh, M. (2011). *Fanaroff and Martin's Neonatal-Perinatal Medicine: Diseases of the Fetus and Infant*. 9th ed. Philadelphia: Elsevier Mosby.
191. Marulasiddappa, V. and Raghavavendra, B. S. (2015). Anesthesia for rare case of uncorrected pentology of Fallot undergoing craniotomy and drainage of brain abscess. *Journal of Clinical and Diagnostic Research*, 9(7): UD01–2.
192. Matte, G. S. (2015). Perfusion for Congenital heart surgery: Notes on cardiopulmonary bypass for a complex patient population. 1st ed. New Jersey: Wiley Blackwell.
193. Mick, S., Hilbertah, J. N., Davidson, M. J. and Fitzgerald, D. (2012). Zero balance ultrafiltration for the correction of acute acidosis after a period of prolonged deep hypothermic circulatory arrest. *Perfusion*, 27(1), 9–11.
194. Mohrman, D. E. and Heller, L. J. (2018). *Cardiovascular Physiology*. 9th ed.New York: Lange McGraw Hill.
195. Montalescot, G. et al., (2001). Platelet glycoprotein IIb/IIIa inhibition with coronary stenting for acute myocardial infarction. *The New England Journal of Medicine*, 344(25), 1895–903.
196. Moodie, D. S. (2014). *Clinical Management of Congenital Heart Disease from Infancy to Adulthood*. 1st ed. Minneapolis, MN: Cardiotext Publishing.

197. Moores, C. and Nimmo, A. F. (2012). *Core Topics in Vascular Anaesthesia*. Cambridge: Cambridge University Press.
198. Moorthy, R. K. and Rajshekhar, V. (2008). Management of brain abscess: An overview. *Neurosurgical Focus*, 24(6). [Viewed 20 May 2020] Available from: https://doi.org/10.3171/FOC/2008/24/6/E3.
199. Morris, C., Perris, A., Klein, J. and Mahoney, P. (2009). Anesthesia in haemodynamically compromised emergency patients: Does ketamine represent the best choice of induction agent? *Anaesthesia*, 64(5), 532–9.
200. Mosher, P., Ross Jr., J., McFate, P. A. and Shaw, R. F. (1964). Control of coronary blood flow by an autoregulatory mechanism. *Circulation Research*, 14(3), 250–9.
201. Mossad, E. B. (2013). Risk assessment of the congenital heart disease patient for noncardiac surgery. *Revista Mexicana de Anestesiologia*, 36(Suppl 1), S39–42.
202. Munoz, R., Morell, V., da Cruz, E. and Vetterly, C. G. (eds.) (2010). *Critical Care of Children with Heart Disease*. 1st ed. New York: Springer.
203. Murdoch, D. R. et al., (2009). Clinical presentation, etiology,and outcome of infective endocarditis in the 21st century: The International Collaboration on Endocarditis-Prospective Cohort Study. *Archives of Internal Medicine*, 169(5), 463–73.
204. Murry, C. E., Jennings, R. B. and Reimer, K. A. (1986). Preconditioning with ischemia: a delay of lethal cell injury in ischemic myocardium. *Circulation*, 74(5), 1124–36.
205. Murthy, T. W. G., Smith, J. H., Ranger, M. R. B. and Haynes S. R. (2011). General anesthesia for children with severe heart failure. *Pediatric Cardiology*, 32(2), 139–44.
206. Nayler, W. G. (1983). Calcium and cell death. *European Heart Journal*, 4(Suppl C), 33–41.
207. Neubauer, H. et al., (2018). Comparison of perioperative strategies in ICD patients: The perioperative ICD management study (PIM study). *Pacing and Clinical Electrophysiology*, 41(11), 1536–42.
208. Ng, C. S. H., Wan, S., Yim, A. P. C. and Arifi, A. A. (2002). Pulmonary dysfunction after cardiac surgery.*Chest*, 121(4), 1269–77.
209. Ngan Kee, W. D., Shen, J., Chiu, A. T., Lok, I. and Khaw, K. S. (1999). Combined spinal-epidural analgesia in the management of labouring parturients with mitral stenosis. *Anaesthesia and Intensive Care*, 27(5), 523–6.
210. Nishimura, R. A. et al., (2014). 2014 AHA/ACC Guideline for the Management of Patients With Valvular Heart Disease: A Report of the American College of Cardiology/American Heart Association Task Force on Practice Guidelines. *Journal of American College of Cardiology*, 63(22), e57–185.
211. O'Gara, P. T. et al., (2013). 2013 ACCF/AHA Guideline for the Management of ST-Elevation Myocardial Infarction: Executive Summary: A Report of the American College of Cardiology Foundation/American Heart Association Task Force on Practice Guidelines. *Catheterizations and Cardiovascular Interventions*, 82(1), e1–27.
212. O'Neil, M. P., Fleming, J. C., Badhwar, A., Ray Guo, L. (2012). Pulsatile versus nonpulsatile flow during cardiopulmonary bypass: Microcirculatory and systemic effects. *TheAnnals of Thoracic Surgery*, 94(6), 2046–53.
213. Okamoto, F., Allen, B. S., Buckberg, G. D., Bugyi, H. and Leaf, J. (1986).
214. Palacios, I. F., Sanchez, P. L., Harrell, L. C., Weyman, A. E. and Block, P. C. (2002). Which patients benefit from percutaneous mitral balloon valvuloplasty? Prevalvuloplasty and postvalvuloplasty variables that predict long-term outcome. *Circulation*, 105(12), 1465–71.
215. Park, M. K. (2008). *Pediatric Cardiology for Practitioners*. 5th ed. Philadelphia: St. Louis: Mosby Elsevier.
216. Park, M. K. (2014). *Park's Pediatric Cardiology for Practitioners*. 6th ed. St. Louis: Mosby Elsevier.
217. Perino Jr, A. C. and Reeves, S. T. (2020). *A Practical Approach to Transesophageal Echocardiography*. 4th ed. Philadelphia: Wolters Kluwer.
218. Perrault, L. P. and Menasche, P. (1999). Preconditioning: can nature's shield be raised against surgical ischemia-reperfusion injury? *Annals of Thoracic Surgery*, 68(5), 1988–94.
219. Peter Alston, R., Myles, P. S. and Ranucci, M. (eds.) (2015). *Oxford Textbook of Cardiothoracic Anaesthesia*. 1st ed. Oxford: Oxford University Press.
220. Peter Gorman, W., Davis, K. R. and Donnelly, R. (2000). Swollen lower limb—1: general assessment and deep vein thrombosis. *British Medical Journal*, 320(7247), 1453–6.
221. Piper, H. M., Garcna-Dorado, D. and Ovize, M. (1998). A fresh look at reperfusion injury. *Cardiovascular Research*, 38(2), 291–300.
222. POBBLE trial investigators: Brady, A. R., Gibbs, J. S. R., Greenhalgh, R. M., Powell, J. T. and Sydes, M. R. (2005). Perioperative beta-blockade (POBBLE) for patients undergoing infrarenal vascular surgery: Results of a randomized double-blind controlled trial. *Journal of Vascular Surgery*, 41(4), 602–9.
223. Podnar, T., Martanovic, P., Gavora, P. and Masura, J. (2001). Morphological variations of secundum-type atrial septal defects: Feasibility for percutaneous closure using Amplatzer septal occluders. *Catheterization and Cardiovascular Interventions*, 53(3), 386–91.
224. POISE study group: Devereaux, P. J. et al., (2008). Effects of extended-release metoprolol succinate in patients undergoing non-cardiac surgery (POISE trial): a randomised controlled trial. *Lancet*, 371(9627), 1839–47.
225. Poliac, L. C., Barron, M. E. and Maron, B. J. (2006).Hypertrophic cardiomyopathy. *Anesthesiology*, 104, 183–92.
226. PRESERVE Trial Group: Weisbord, S. D. et al., (2018). Outcomes after angiography with sodium bicarbonate and acetylcysteine. *The New England Journal of Medicine*, 378, 603–14.
227. Pridjian, A. K., Levitsky, S., Krukenkamp, I., Silverman, N. A. and Feinberg, H. (1987). Intracellular sodium and calcium in the postischemic myocardium. *Annals of Thoracic Surgery*, 43(4), 416–9.
228. Quinn, D. W. et al., (2006). Improved myocardial protection during coronary artery surgery with glucose-insulin-potassium: a randomized controlled trial. *Journal of Thoracic Cardiovascular Surgery*, 34–42.
229. Raha, A., Ganjoo, P. Singh, A. Tandon, M. S. and Singh, D. (2012). Surgery for brain abscess in children with cyanotic heart disease: an anesthetic challenge. *Journal of Pediatric Neurosciences*, 7(1), 23-6.

230. Ramamoorthy, C. et al., (2010). Anesthesia-related cardiac arrest in children with heart disease: Data from the Pediatric Perioperative Cardiac Arrest (POCA) registry. *Anesthesia and Analgesia*, 110(5), 1376–82.
231. Ramanathan, T. and Skinner, H. (2005). Coronary blood flow. *Continuing Education in Anaesthesia Critical Care and Pain*, 5(2), 61–4.
232. Ranucci, M. (2017). Anaesthesia and cardiopulmonary bypass aspects of fast track. *European Heart Journal Supplements*, 19(Suppl A), a15–7.
233. Registry, N. (1992). Complications and mortality of percutaneous balloon mitral commissurotomy. A report from the National Heart, Lung, and Blood Institute Valvuloplasty Registry. *Circulation*, 85(6), 2014–24.
234. Remadevi, K. S., Francis, E. and Krishna Kumar, R. (2009). Catheter closure of atrial septal defects with deficient inferior vena cava rim under transesophageal echo guidance. *Catheterization and Cardiovascular Interventions*, 73(1), 90–6.
235. Rezkalla, S. H. and Kloner, R. A. (2002). No-reflow phenomenon. *Circulation*, 105(5), 656–62.
236. Riambau, V. et al., (2017). Management of descending thoracic aortic diseases: clinical practice guidelines of European Society for Vascular Surgery. *European Journal of Vascular and Endovascular Surgery*, 53(1), 4–52.
237. Roshanov, P. S. et al., (2017). External validation of theRevised Cardiac Risk Index and update of its renal variable to predict the 30-day risk of major cardiac complications after non-cardiac surgery: rationale and plan for the analyses of the VISION study. *British Medical Journal Open*, 7(1), e013510.
238. Rozner, M. A., Kahl, E. A. and Schulman, P. M. (2017). Inappropriate implantable cardioverter-defibrillator therapy during surgery: an important and preventable complication. *Journal of Cardiothoracic and Vascular Anesthesia*, 31(3), P1037–41.
239. Salukhe, T. V., Dob, D. and Sutton, R. (2004). Pacemakers and defibrillators: Anaesthetic implications. *British Journal of Anaesthesia*, 93(1), 95–104.
240. Samanek, M. (1992). Children with congenital heart disease: probability of natural survival. *Pediatric Cardiology*, 13(3), 152–8.
241. Saxena, A. (2005). Congenital heart disease in India: A status report. *Indian Journal of Pediatrics*, 72(7), 595–8.
242. Saxena, A. et al, (2019). Indian guidelines for indications and timing of intervention for common congenital heart diseases: Revised and updated consensus statement of the working group on management of congenital heart diseases. *Annals of Pediatric Cardiology*, 12(3), 254–86.
243. Schermerhorn, M. L., James O'Malley, A., Jhaveri, A., Cortterill, P., Pomposelli, F. and Landon, B. E.(2008). Endovascular vs. open repair of abdominal aortic aneurysms in the medicare population. *The New England Journal of Medicine*, 358(5), 464–74.
244. Schulman, P. M. et al., (2019). Electromagnetic interference with protocolized electrosurgery dispersive electrode positioning in patients with implantable cardioverter defibrillators. *Anesthesiology*, 130, 530–40.
245. Schulman, P. M., Rozner, M. A., Sera, V. and Steckerm E. C. (2013). Patients with pacemaker or implantable cardioverter-defibrillator. *Medicine Clinics of North America*, 97(6), 1051–75.
246. Scott, D. A. and Denton, M. J. (2016). Spinal cord protection in aortic endovascular surgery. *British Journal of Anaesthesia*, 117(Suppl 2), i26–31.
247. Scott, T. and Swanevelder, J. (2009). Perioperative myocardial protection. *Continuing Education in Anaesthesia Critical Care and Pain*, 9(3), 97–102.
248. Sear, J. W. (2005). Kidney dysfunction in the postoperative period. *British Journal of Anaesthesia*, 95(1), 20–32.
249. Sechner, N. J., Arnsbo, P. and Wallin, L. (1978). Haemodynamic effects of oxytocin and methylergometrine (Syntocinon) on the systemic and pulmonary circulations of pregnant anaesthetized women. *Acta Obstetricia et Gynecologica Scandinavica*, 57(2), 97–103.
250. Sethi, S. and Kapil, S. (2014). Scalp block for brain abscess drainage in a patient with uncorrected tetralogy of Fallot. *World Journal of Clinical Cases*, 2(12), 934–7.
251. Sharma, S. K., Gambling, D. R., Gajraj, N. M., Truong, C. and Sidawi, J. (1994). Anesthetic management of a parturient with mixed mitral valve disease and uncontrolled atrial fibrillation.*International Journal of Obstetric Anesthesia*, 3(3), 157–62.
252. Silversides, C. K., Colma, J. M., Sermer, M. and Siu, S. C. (2003). Cardiac risk in pregnant women with rheumatic mitral stenosis. *American Journal of Cardiology*, 91(11), 1382–5.
253. Silvestry, F. E. et al., (2015). Guidelines for the echocardiographic assessment of atrial septal defectand patent foramen ovale: from the American Society of Echocardiography and Society for Cardiac Angiography and Interventions. *Journal of the American Society of Echocardiography*, 28(8), 910–58.
254. Singh, J. P. et al., (1999). Prevalence and clinical determinants of mitral, tricuspidand aortic regurgitation (The Framingham Heart Study). *American Journal of Cardiology*, 83(6), 897–902.
255. Siu, S. C. et al., (1997). Risk and predictors for pregnancy-related complications in women with heart disease. *Circulation*, 96(9), 2789–94.
256. Soliman, R., Fouad, E., Belghith, M. and Abdelmageed, T. (2016). Conventional hemofiltration duringcardiopulmonary bypass increases the serum lactate level in adult cardiac surgery. *Annals of Cardiac Anaesthesia*, 19(1), 45–51.
257. SOLSTICE trial: Kristin Newby, L. et al., (2014). Losmapimod, a novel p38 mitogen-activated protein kinase inhibitor, in non-ST-segment elevation myocardial infarction: A randomised phase II trial. *Lancet*, 384(9949), 1187–95.
258. Soto, B., Becker, A. E., Moulaert, A. J., Lie, J. T. and Anderson, R. H. (1980). Classification of ventricular septal defects. *British Heart Journal*, 43, 332–43.
259. Spyropoulos, A. C. and Mahan, C. (2009). Venous thromboembolism prophylaxis in the medical patient: controversies and perspectives. *American Journal of Medicine*, 122(12), 1077–84.
260. Sreedhar, R. (2017). Acyanotic congenital heart disease and transesophageal echocardiography. *Annals of Cardiac Anaesthesia*, 20(Suppl 1), S36–42.

261. Stone, M. E., Salter, B. and Fischer, A. (2011). Perioperative management of patients with cardiac implantable electronic devices. *British Journal of Anaesthesia*, 107(Suppl 1), i16–26.
262. Studies of controlled reperfusion after ischemia: XIV. Reperfusion conditions: Importance of ensuring gentle versus sudden reperfusion during relief of coronary occlusion. *Journal of Thoracic and Cardiovascular Surgery*, 613–20.
263. Surawicz, B. and Knilans, T.(2008). *Chou's Electrocardiography in Clinical Practice* 6th ed. Philadelphia: Saunders.
264. Sutton, S. W., Duncan, M. A., Chase, V. A., Marce, R. J., Meyers, T. P. and Wood, R. E. (2005). Cardiopulmonary bypass and mitral valve replacement during pregnancy. *Perfusion*, 20(6), 359–68.
265. Swerdlow, N. J., Wu, W. W. and Schermerhorn, M. L. (2019). Open and endovascular management of aortic aneurysms. *Circulation Research*, 124, 647–61.
266. Tabacova, S., Kimmel, C. A., Wall, K. and Hansen, D. (2003). Atenolol developmental toxicity: Animal to human comparisons. *Birth Defects Research Part A: Clinical and Molecular Teratology*, 67(3), 181–92.
267. Tashiro, T. et al., (2014). Perioperative risk of major non-cardiac surgery in patients with severe aortic stenosis: A reappraisal in contemporary practice. *European Heart Journal*, 35(35), 2372–81.
268. Therrien, J. and Webb, G. (2003). Clinical update on adults with congenital heart disease. *Lancet*, 362(9392), 1305–13.
269. Thygesen, K. et al., (2010). Recommendations for the use of cardiac troponin measurement in acute cardiac care. *European Heart Journal*, 31(18), 2197–204.
270. Thygesen, K. et al., (2018). Fourth universal definition of myocardial infarction (2018). *Circulation*, 138, e618–51.
271. Tintinalli, J. E., Stephan Stapczynski, J., John Ma, O., Yealy, D. M., Meckler, G. D. and Cline, D. M. (2016). *Tintinalli's Emergency Medicine*: A Comprehensive Study Guide. 8th ed. New York: McGraw Hill.
272. Tobis, J. and Shenoda, M. (2012). Percutaneous treatment of patent foramen ovaleand atrial septal defects. *Journal of the American College of Cardiology*, 60(18), 1722–32.
273. Topol, E. J. and Teirstein, M. D. (2008).*Textbook of Interventional Cardiology*. 5th ed. Philadelphia: Saunders Elsevier.
274. Tousoulis, D. (2018). *Coronary Artery Disease: From Biology to Clinical Practice*. Philadelphia: Elsevier.
275. Townsley, M. M., Windsor, J., Briston, D., Alegria, J. and Ramakrishna, H. (2018). Tetralogy of Fallot: Perioperative management and analysis of outcomes. *Journal of Cardiothoracic and Vascular Anaesthesia*, 33(2), 556–65.
276. Trial, BCIS-1 Investigators: Perera, D. et al., (2010). Elective intra-aortic balloon pump counterpulsation during high-risk percutaneous coronary intervention: a randomized controlled trial. *Journal of the American Medical Association*, 304(8), 867–74.
277. Trial, IMPROVE Investigators: Spyropoulos, A. C. et al., (2011). Predictive and associative models to identify hospitalized medical patients at risk for venous thromboembolism. *Chest*, 140(3), 706–14.
278. Trial, Veteran Affairs ROOBY-FS Group: Laurie Shroyer et al., (2017). Five-year outcomes after on-pump and off-pump coronary artery bypass. *The New England Journal of Medicine*, 377, 623–32.
279. Twite,M. D. and Ing, R. J. (2012). Tetralogy of Fallot: perioperative anesthetic management of children and adults. *Seminars in Cardiothoracic and Vascular Anesthesia*, 16(2), 97–105.
280. Urbankova, J., Quiroz, R., Kucher, N. and Goldhaber, S. Z. (2005). Intermittent pneumatic compression and deep vein thrombosis prevention: a meta-analysis in postoperative patients. *Journal of Thrombosis and Haemostasis*, 94(6), 1181–5.
281. Vahanian, A. et al., (2012). 2012 Guidelines on the management of valvular heart disease: the joint task force on the management of valvular heart disease of the European Society of Cardiology (ESC)and European Association for Cardio-Thoracic Surgery (EACTS). *European Heart Journal*, 33(19), 2451–96.
282. Valchanov, K., Jones, N. and Hogue, C. W. (eds.) (2018). *Core Topics in Cardiothoracic Critical Care*. 2nd ed. Cambridge: Cambridge University Press.
283. van Vonderen, J. J., Te Pas, A. B., Kolster-Bijdevaate, C. and van Lith, J. M. M. (2014). Non-invasive measurements of ductus arteriosus flow directly after birth. *Archives of Disease in Childhood: Fetal and Neonatal Edition*. [Viewed 20 May 2020] [Available from: 10.1136/archdischild-2014-306033]
284. van't Hof, A. W., Liem, A., Suryapranta, H., Hoorntje, J. C., de Boer, M. J. and Zijlstra, F. (1998). Angiographic assessment of myocardial reperfusion in patients treated with primary angioplasty for acute myocardial infarction: myocardial blush grade. Zwolle Myocardial Infarction Study Group. *Circulation*, 97(23), 2302–6.
285. Vegas, A. (2008). *Perioperative Transesophageal Echocardiography*. Toronto: University Health Network.
286. Verma, S. et al., (2002). Fundamentals of reperfusion injury for the clinical cardiologist. *Circulation*, 105(20), 2332–6.
287. Vijayalakshmi, I. B. (2013). *A Comprehensive Approach to Congenital Heart Diseases*. 1sted. New Delhi: Jaypee Brothers.
288. Vincent, J.-L.and Moore, F. (2017). *Textbook of Critical Care*. 7th ed. Philadelphia: Elsevier.
289. Vinten-Johansen, J. and Thourani, V. H. (2000). Myocardial protection: An overview. *The Journal of Extracorporeal Technology*, 32(1),38–49.
290. Wajekar, A. S., Shetty, A. N., Oak, S. P. and Jain, R. A. (2015). Anesthetic management for drainage of frontoparietal abscess in a patient of uncorrected Tetralogy of Fallot. *Indian Journal of Anaesthesia*, 59(4), 244–6.
291. Waldman, S., Krauss, A. N. and Auld, P. A. M. (1979). Baroreceptors in preterm infants: their relationship to maturity and disease. *Developmental Medicine & Child Neurology*, 21(6), 714–22.
292. Walji, S., Peterson, R. J., Neis, P., DuBroff, R., Gray, W. A. and Benge, W. (1999). Ultra-fast track hospital discharge using conventional cardiac surgical techniques. *Annals of Thoracic Surgery*, 67(2), 363–9.

293. Walker, I. (2008). Anaesthesia for non-cardiac surgery in children with congenital heart disease. *Update in Anaesthesia*, 46–56.
294. Wallace, A. W., Au, S. and Cason, B. A. (2011). Perioperative b-blockade: Atenolol is associated with reduced mortality when compared to metoprolol. *Anesthesiology*, 114(4), 824–36.
295. Walsh, S. R., Tang, T. Y., Kullar, P., Jenkins, D. P., Dutka, D. P. and Gaunt, M. E. (2008). Ischaemic preconditioning during cardiac surgery: a systematic review and meta-analysis of perioperative outcomes in randomised clinical trials. *European Journal of Cardiothoracic Surgery*, 34(5), 985–94.
296. Waman Junghare, S. and Desurkar, V. (2017). Congenital heart diseases and anaesthesia. *Indian Journal of Anaesthesia*, 61(9), 744–52.
297. Warner, M. A., Lunn, R. J., O'Leary, P. W., Schroeder, D. R., For the Mayo Perioperative Outcomes Group. (1998). Outcomes of noncardiac surgical procedures in children and adults with congenital heart disease. *Mayo Clinic Proceedings*, 73(8), 728–34.
298. Warren, O. J. et al., (2009). The inflammatory response tocardiopulmonary bypass: Part 1-mechanisms of pathogenesis. *Journal of Cardiothoracic and Vascular Anesthesia*, 23(2), 223–31.
299. Webb, C. A.-J., Weyker, P. D. and Flynn, B. C. (2015). Management of intra-aortic balloon pumps. *Seminars in Cardiothoracicand Vascular Anesthesia*, 19(2), 106–21.
300. Weerasinghe, A. and Taylor, K. M. (1998). The platelet in cardiopulmonary bypass. *Annals of Thoracic Surgery*, 66(6), 2145–52.
301. Well, P.S. et al., (1997). Value of assessment of pretest probability of deep-vein thrombosis in clinical management. *Lancet*, 350(9094), 1795–8.
302. White, M. C. (2010). Approach to managing children with heart disease for non-cardiac surgery. *Pediatric Anesthesia*, 21(5), 522–9.
303. White, M. C. and Peyton, J. M. (2011). Anesthetic management of children with congenital heart disease for non-cardiac surgery. *Continuing Education in Anaesthesia Critical Care & Pain*, 12(1), 17–22.
304. Wilkins, G. T., Weyman, A. E., Abascal, V. M., Block, P. C. and Palacios, I. F. (1988). Percutaneous balloon dilatation of the mitral valve: an analysis of echocardiographic variables related to outcome and the mechanism of dilatation. *British Heart Journal*, 60(4), 299–308.
305. Wilson, J., Russo, P., Russo, J. andTobias, J. D. (2005). Noninvasive monitoring of carbon dioxide in infants and children with congenital heart disease: end-tidal versus transcutaneous techniques. *Journal of Intensive Care Medicine*, 20(5), 291–5.
306. Wolman, R. L. et al., (1999). Cerebral injury after cardiac surgery: identification of a group at extraordinary risk. Multicenter Study of Perioperative Ischemia Research Group (McSPI) and the Ischemia Research Education Foundation (IREF) Investigators. *Stroke*, 30(3), 514–22.
307. Wright, G. (2001). Haemolysis during cardiopulmonary bypass: Update. *Perfusion*, 16(5), 345–51.
308. Wu, J. and Zipes, D. P. (2002). Mechanisms underlying atrioventricular nodal conduction and the reentrant circuit of atrioventricular nodal reentrant tachycardia using optical mapping. *Journal of Cardiovascular Electrophysiology*, 13(8), 831–4.
309. Xu,Y. et al., (2006). Activated platelets contribute importantly to myocardial reperfusion injury. *American Journal of Physiology-Heart and Circulatory Physiology*, 290(2), H692–9.
310. Yau, T. M. et al., (1993). Ventricular function after normothermic versus hypothermic cardioplegia. *Journal of Thoracic and Cardiovascular Surgery*, 105(5), 833–43.
311. Yellon, D. M., Alkhulaifi, A. M. and Pugsley, W. B. (1993). Preconditioning the human myocardium. *Lancet*, 342(8866), 276–7.
312. Yen, P. (2015). ASD and VSD flow dynamics and anesthetic management. *Anesthesia Progress*, 62(3), 125–30.
313. Yong, S. C. et al., (2011). Effect of remote ischemic preconditioning on renal dysfunction after complex valvular heart surgery: a randomized controlled trial. *Journal of Thoracic and Cardiovascular Surgery*, 142(1), 148–54.
314. Yoo, S.-J., MacDonald, C. and Babyn, P. (2010). *Chest Radiographic Interpretation in Pediatric Cardiac Patients*. 1st ed. New York: Thieme Medical Publishers.
315. Yurdakok, M. (2012). Fetal and neonatal effects of anticoagulants used in pregnancy: A review. *Turkish Journal of Pediatrics*, 54(3), 207–15.
316. Zaugg, M., Schaub, M. C., Pasch, T. and Spahn, D. R. (2002). Modulation of b-adrenergic receptor subtype activities in perioperative medicine: mechanisms and sites of action. *British Journal of Anaesthesia*, 88(1), 101–23.
317. Ziegler, J. W., Dunbar Ivy, D., KInsella, J. P. and Abman, S. H. (1995). The role of nitric oxide, endothelin, and prostaglandins in the transition of the pulmonary circulation. *Clinics in Perinatology*, 22(2), 387–403.
318. Zipes, D. P. and Jalife, J. (eds.) (1999). *Cardiac Electrophysiology: From Cell to Bedside*. 3rd ed. Philadelphia: WB Saunders.

4 CHAPTER

Anesthesia for Respiratory Disease

ANATOMY OF LARYNX

Introduction

- Larynx is the organ for voice production and phonation
- It is a sphincter at the inlet of lower respiratory passage

Situation and Extent

- Extends from root of tongue to trachea
- In adult males, it lies in front of C_5-C_6
- Lies higher in children and infants:
  - In infants: Level of C_3 vertebra
  - In children at 6 years age: Level of C_4-C_5 vertebrae

Size

- In males:
  - Length is 44 mm
  - Transverse diameter 36 mm
  - Sagittal diameter: 43 mm
- In females:
  - Length is 41 mm
  - Transverse diameter 36 mm
  - Sagittal diameter: 26 mm
- At puberty, male larynx grows rapidly, while female grows little

Bones of the Larynx

- Hyoid bone suspends the larynx during respiration
- Hyoid bone does not articulate with any other bone
- It is U-shaped and consists of 3 parts:
  - Body
  - Lesser cornu
  - Greater cornu
- Attachments of hyoid bone:
  - Ligamentous attachments:
    - Stylohyoid ligament to styloid process
    - Thyrohyoid membrane to thyroid cartilage
  - Muscular attachments:
    - Intrinsic muscles of tongue
    - Pharyngeal constrictors

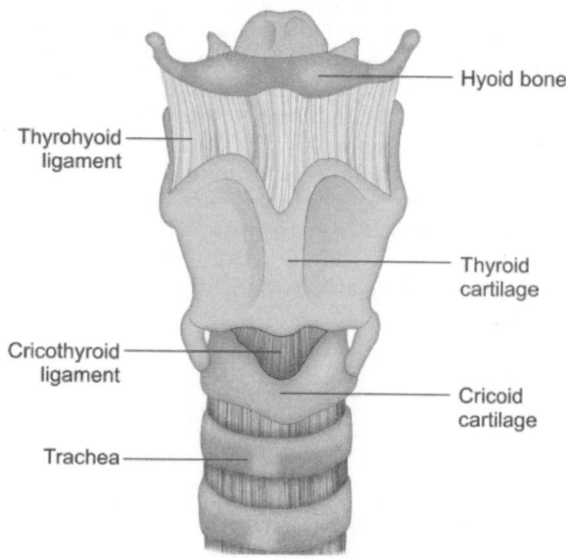

Fig. 1: Anterior view of larynx.

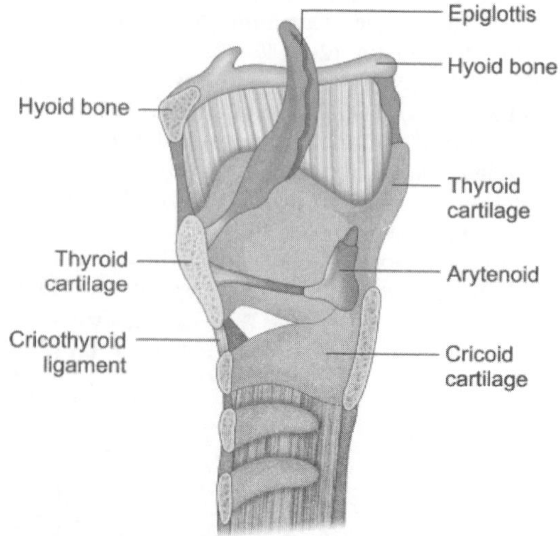

Fig. 2: Sagittal view of larynx.

Laryngeal Cartilages

- Laryngeal framework consists of 9 cartilages
- Types of cartilages:
  - Unpaired cartilages:
    - Thyroid
    - Cricoid
    - Epiglottis
  - Paired cartilages:
    - Arytenoid
    - Corniculate
    - Cuneiform
- Thyroid cartilage:
  - Longest laryngeal cartilage and largest structure in larynx
  - Consists of hyaline cartilage
  - Formed by 2 distinct quadrilateral laminae (alae)
  - Alae meet anteriorly forming:
    - 90° angle in males
    - 120° in females
  - Smaller angle in males results in:
    - Greater laryngeal prominence (Adams apple)
    - Longer vocal cords
    - Lower pitched voice
  - Vocal cords attached to middle of thyroid cartilage
  - Thyroid notch lies in the midline at the top of the alar fusion site
- Cricoid cartilage:
  - Represents anatomical lower limit of larynx
  - Consists of hyaline cartilage
  - Has signet ring shape
  - Thicker and stronger than thyroid cartilage
  - Only cartilage which forms a complete ring
  - Posterior part: Expanded and more bulky laminae
  - Anterior part: Narrow arch
  - Forms the narrowest part of pediatric airway
- Epiglottis:
  - Considered to be vestigial
  - Leaf like fibro-elastic cartilage
  - Found between larynx and base of tongue
  - Forms anterior wall of laryngeal inlet
  - Valleculae: Represents the space between:
    - Anterior surface of epiglottis
    - Posterior surface of oropharynx
- Arytenoid cartilage:
  - Pyramidal shaped
  - Consists of hyaline cartilage
  - Lie is posterior aspect of larynx
  - Has following parts:
    - Base: articulates with cricoid
    - Muscular process: Attached to intrinsic laryngeal muscle
    - Vocal process: Vocal cord
    - Apex: Supports corniculate cartilage
- Corniculate cartilage of ***Santorini***:
  - Consists of elastic cartilage
  - Articulates with apex of arytenoids
- Cuneiform cartilage of ***Wrisberg***:
  - Situated in front of corniculate cartilage
  - Consists of elastic cartilage
  - Provides passive support to aryepiglottic folds
  - Help in the movement of arytenoids.

Laryngeal Joints

- Cricoarytenoid joint:
  - Synovial joint
  - Two types of movements:
    - Rotatory: Abduction and adduction of vocal cords
    - Gliding: Closing and opening of posterior part of glottis
- Cricothyroid joint: Synovial joint

Laryngeal Membranes

- Extrinsic membranes:
  - Thyrohyoid membrane: Pierced by:

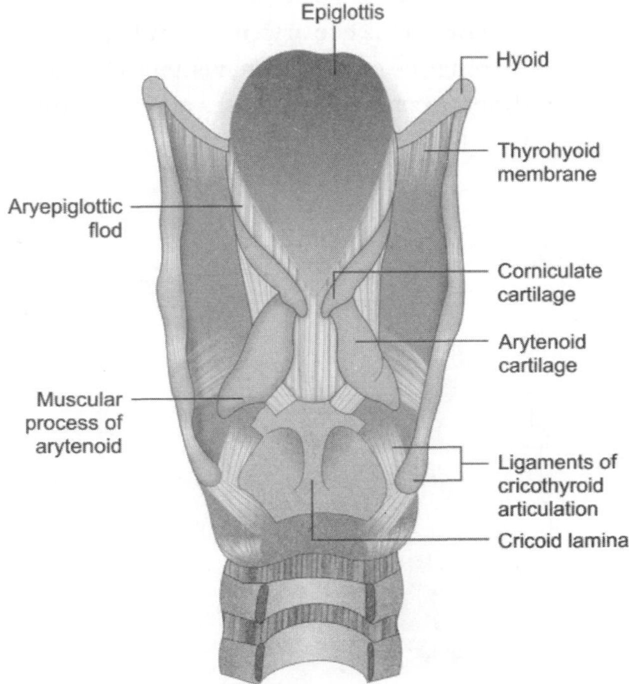

Fig. 3: Cartilages of the larynx.

- Superior laryngeal blood vessels
- Internal laryngeal nerve
- Cricothyroid membrane
- Cricotracheal membrane
- Intrinsic membranes:
  - Cricovocal membrane:
    - True vocal cord
    - Extends from midthyroid level to vocal process of arytenoids
    - Forms vocal ligament
  - Quadrangular membrane:
    - False vocal cord
    - Present between epiglottis and arytenoid
    - Lower border forms the vestibular ligament

Laryngeal Cavity

- Extends from laryngeal inlet to lower border of cricoid cartilage
- Vestibule or supraglottic larynx lies between:
  - Laryngeal inlet
  - Vestibular folds
- Space between the true cords is called rima glottidis or the glottis
- This is composed of 2 parts:
  - Anterior intermembranous part:
    - Situated between true vocal cords
    - Forms the anterior commissure
  - Posterior intercartilaginous part:
    - Between the two arytenoid cartilages
    - Forms the posterior commissure of the larynx
- At rest, space between the cords is normally around 8 mm
- Subglottic larynx lies between:
  - Free border of vocal cords
  - Cricoid cartilage
- Region between vestibular folds and glottis is called ventricle or sinus
- Ventricle may extend anterolaterally to a pouch-like area called laryngeal saccule.

Spaces of Larynx

- *Pre-epiglottic space of Boyer*:
  - Filled with fat, areolar tissue, lymphatics
  - Common site for *laryngeal carcinoma*
- Paraglottic space: continuous with pre-epiglottic space
- *Reinkes space:*
  - Potential space
  - Scanty connective tissue
  - Present under epithelium of vocal cords

Muscles of Larynx

- Intrinsic muscles:
  - Attach laryngeal cartilages to one another
  - Functions of intrinsic muscles:
    - Opening of glottis during inspiration
    - Closure of glottis during expiration
    - Altering tension of vocal cords during phonation
  - Those acting on vocal cords:
    - Abductors: Posterior cricoarytenoid
    - Adductors:
      - Lateral cricoarytenoid
      - Inter-arytenoid (also called transverse arytenoid)
      - Thyroarytenoid (external part)

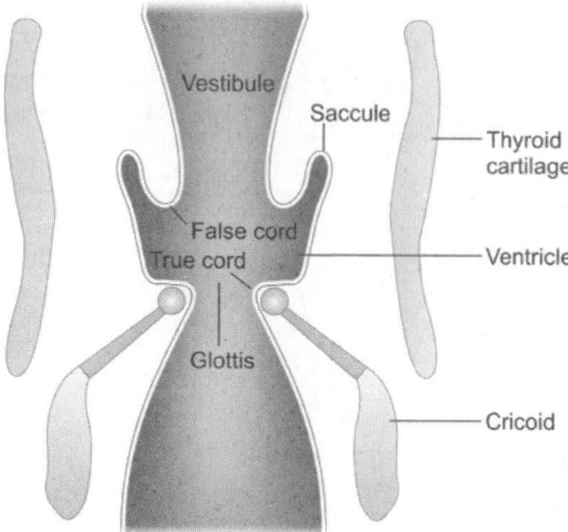

Fig. 4: Laryngeal cavity.

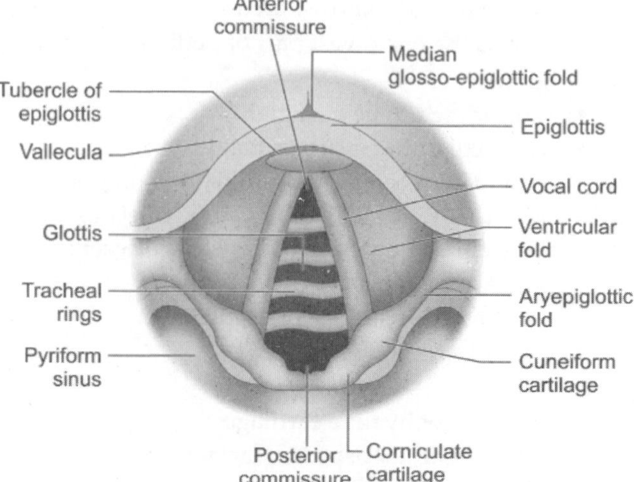

Fig. 5: Structures forming the laryngeal inlet.

- Tensors: Cricothyroid
- Vocalis: Internal part of thyroarytenoid
- Relaxors: Thyroarytenoid
- Those acting on laryngeal inlet:
  - Openers: Thyroepiglottis (part of thyroarytenoid)
  - Closers:
    - Interarytenoid (oblique part)
    - Aryepiglottic (posterior oblique part of interarytenoid)

❖ Extrinsic muscles:
- Attach larynx to surrounding structures such as hyoid bone
- Move larynx as a whole and help in laryngeal elevation and depression
- Elevators:
  - Primary elevators:
    - Stylopharyngeus
    - Salpingopharyngeus
    - Palatopharyngeus
    - Thyrohyoid
  - Secondary elevators:
    - Mylohyoid
    - Digastric
    - Stylohyoid
    - Geniohyoid
- Depressors: ***Strap muscles***:
  - Sternohyoid
  - Sternothyroid
  - Omohyoid
  - Thyrohyoid

Blood Supply

❖ Upto vocal cords:
- Superior laryngeal artery: Branch of superior thyroid artery (from external carotid artery)
- Superior laryngeal vein: Drains to superior thyroid vein

❖ Below vocal cords:
- Inferior laryngeal artery: Branch of inferior thyroid artery
- Inferior laryngeal vein: Drains into inferior thyroid vein

Lymphatic Drainage

❖ Above vocal cords: antero-superior group of deep cervical nodes

❖ Below vocal cords:
- Postero-inferior group of deep cervical lymph nodes
- Few into pre-laryngeal lymph nodes

Nerve Supply

❖ Motor nerve supply:
- All intrinsic muscles supplied by recurrent laryngeal nerve
- Except cricothyroid which is supplied by external laryngeal nerve (branch of superior laryngeal nerve)

❖ Sensory nerve supply:
- Above vocal cords: Internal laryngeal branch of superior laryngeal nerve
- Below vocal cords: Recurrent laryngeal nerve

Mucus Membrane of Larynx

❖ Lines larynx

❖ Loosely attached at most places

❖ Mucous glands distributed all over membrane except vocal folds

❖ Epithelium:
- Ciliated columnar epithelium
- Exception: Over vocal cords and upper vestibule where stratified squamous epithelium

VOCAL CORD PARALYSIS

Etiology

❖ In topographical manner:
- Supranuclear palsy: Rare
- Nuclear palsy:
  - Involves ***nucleus ambiguus*** in medulla
  - Vascular causes
  - Motor neuron disease
  - Neoplastic causes
  - Polio myelitis
  - Syringobulbia
- High vagal lesions:
  - Intracranial lesions:
    - Meningitis
    - Posterior fossa tumors
  - At jugular foramen:
    - Fractures
    - Nasopharyngeal carcinoma
    - Glomus tumors
  - At parapharyngeal space in neck:
    - Parapharyngeal tumors
    - Lymphomas
    - Penetrating injuries
- Low vagal/recurrent laryngeal nerve lesions:
  - Right sided palsy:
    - Neck trauma, thyroid diseases or surgery

- Esophageal carcinoma, cervical lymphadenopathy
- Subclavian artery aneurysms
- Carcinoma of right lung apex (Pancoasts tumor)
- Tuberculosis of cervical pleura
- Idiopathic causes

– Left sided palsy:
- Neck trauma, thyroid disease or surgery
- Bronchogenic carcinoma
- Esophageal carcinoma
- Aortic aneurysm
- Mediastinal lymphoma
- Intrathoracic surgery
- Idiopathic causes
- ***Ortners syndrome***

– Bilateral palsy:
- Thyroid surgery
- Thyroid carcinoma
- Carcinoma of cervical esophagus
- Cervical lymphadenopathy

- Systemic causes:
  - Diabetes, leprosy
  - Syphilis, lead poisoning
  - Diphtheria, mumps, typhoid
- Idiopathic in 30% cases

❖ Congenital causes:
- Birth trauma
- Congenital anomaly of great vessels/heart (great vein malformation of Galen)

Classification

❖ Recurrent laryngeal nerve palsy:
- Unilateral RLN palsy:
  - Partial RLN palsy
  - Complete RLN palsy
- Bilateral RLN palsy:
  - Partial RLN palsy
  - Complete RLN palsy

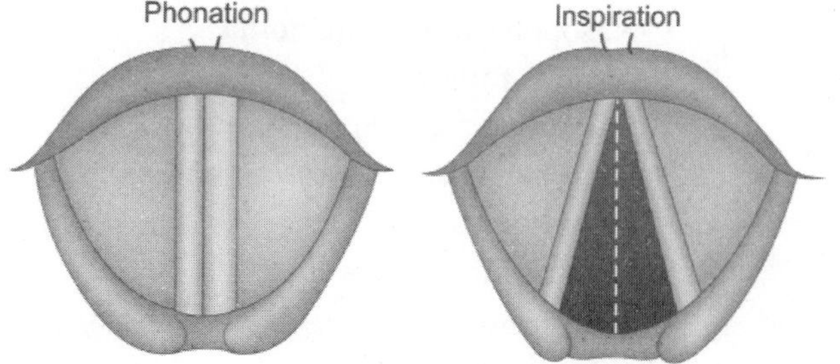

Fig. 6: Normal position of vocal cords.

❖ Superior laryngeal nerve palsy:
- Unilateral palsy
- Bilateral palsy

❖ Combined palsies:
- Unilateral palsy
- Bilateral palsy

❖ Vagal nerve palsy

Recurrent Laryngeal Nerve Palsy

Unilateral RLN Palsy

❖ Ipsilateral paralysis of all intrinsic muscles occurs, except cricothyroid

❖ ***Semons law***: In progressive lesions of RLN, only abductors of vocal cords(posterior cricoarytenoids) are first to be paralyzed and last to recover, compared to adductors

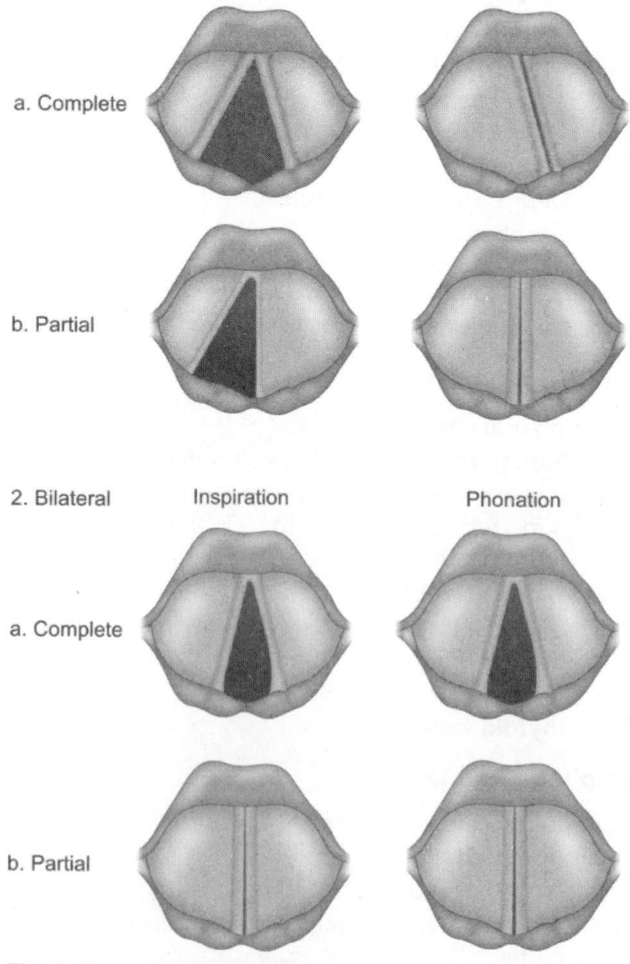

Fig. 7: Types of vocal cord palsy.

- ***Wagner-Grossman hypothesis***: Cricothyroid muscle, which receives innervation from SLN keeps cord in paramedian position due to its adductor function
- Clinical features:
  - One third of patients are asymptomatic
  - Vocal cord:
    - Takes median/paramedian position
    - Does not move laterally on deep inspiration
  - Changes in voice:
    - Gradually improves over time
    - This is due to compensation by healthy vocal cord, which crosses midline
  - No treatment is required
- Partial unilateral RLN palsy:
  - Only abductor fibres are impaired
  - Adductor fibres are intact
  - Vocal cord in *midline on affected side*
  - During inspiration, unaffected side fully abducts to compensate
  - During phonation, unaffected side is adducted
- Complete unilateral RLN palsy:
  - Both adductor and abductor affected
  - Vocal cord in *paramedian position on affected side*
  - During inspiration, unaffected vocal cord fully abducted and respiration not effected
  - During phonation, unaffected vocal cord crosses midline and comes in opposition with affected side

Bilateral RLN Palsy

- Acute condition
- Position of vocal cord is median/paramedian due to unopposed cricothyroid action
- Clinical features:
  - Dyspnea and stridor which worsen on exertion
  - Voice is good
- Treatment:
  - Emergency tracheostomy
  - Lateralization of vocal cords:
    - Arytenoidectomy
    - Endoscopic lateralization
    - Type II thyroplasty
    - Cordectomy
    - Nerve muscle implant
- Partial bilateral RLN palsy:
  - Only abductor fibres on both vocal cords are affected
  - Vocal cords remain in *midline position* as adductors take upper hand
  - Narrowing of glottis with severe impairment of respiration
  - Voice is good
  - Requires immediate tracheostomy
  - Lateralize vocal cords with surgery
  - More dangerous than complete bilateral RLN palsy
- Complete bilateral RLN palsy:
  - Bilateral abductor and adductor fibres affected
  - Both sides vocal cords remain in *paramedian position*
  - Respiration not affected as much as bilateral partial RLNP

Superior Laryngeal Nerve Palsy

Unilateral SLN Palsy

- SLN supplies cricothyroid which is tensor of vocal cord
- Palsy occurs in:
  - Thyroid surgery
  - Neuritis
  - Tumors, diphtheria
- Clinical features:
  - Weak voice
  - Increased risk of aspiration
  - Pitch cannot be raised
  - Vocal cords:
    - Askew position of glottis
    - Shortening of cord with loss of tension
    - Flapping of paralysed cord
    - *Cadaveric position*

Bilateral SLN Palsy

- Occurs in:
  - Trauma, cervical lymphadenopathy
  - Neuritis, neoplasia
- Clinical features:
  - Aspiration of food: Coughing and choking fits
  - Voice is weak and husky
- Treatment:
  - Neuritis cases recover spontaneously
  - Epiglottopexy maybe required to close inlet and protect lungs

Combined Paralysis

Unilateral Combined Paralysis

- Paralysis of all muscles in ipsilateral side except interarytenoid (as it receives bilateral innervation)

❖ Causes:
  - Thyroid surgeries
  - Lesions of ***nucleus ambiguus***/vagus nerve
❖ Clinical features:
  - Vocal cord in *cadaveric position*, 3.5 mm from midline
  - Healthy vocal cord unable to approximate paralyzed cord
  - Hoarseness of voice, aspiration
  - Ineffective cough
❖ Treatment:
  - Speech therapy
  - Medialization of vocal cords:
    - Teflon paste injection
    - Type I thyroplasty
    - Muscle/cartilage implant
    - Cricoarytenoid joint arthrodesis

Bilateral Combined Paralysis

❖ Occurs rarely
❖ Total anesthesia of larynx with both vocal cords in *cadaveric position*
❖ Clinical features:
  - Aphonia
  - Inability to cough
  - Aspiration
❖ Treatment:
  - Tracheostomy
  - Vocal cord plication
  - Epiglottopexy
  - Total laryngectomy

Congenital Vocal Cord Palsy

❖ Unilateral palsy:
  - Occurs more commonly
  - Causes:
    - Birth trauma
    - Congenital anomalies of heart/blood vessels
❖ Bilateral palsy:
  - Less common
  - Causes:
    - Hydrocephalus
    - ***Arnold-Chiari malformation***
    - Intracranial hemorrhage
    - Meningocele
    - Cerebral/nucleus ambiguus agenesis
❖ Treatment: Tracheostomy

AIRWAY ASSESSMENT

Definition

❖ Difficult intubation defined by need for more than 3 intubation attempts or attempts which last more than 10 minutes
❖ Difficult airway defined as the situation in which a conventionally trained anesthetist experiences difficulty with mask ventilation (unassisted anesthetist unable to maintain SpO_2 more than 90% using 100% oxygen) or inability to place endotracheal tube with conventional laryngoscopy after three attempts or attempts lasting more than 10 minutes

Objectives

❖ To provide safe anesthesia
❖ To facilitate successful management of difficult airway
❖ To reduce risk and likelihood of complications:
  - Airway trauma
  - CNS damage
  - Cardiopulmonary arrest

Airway Assessment

History

❖ Medical history:
  - Congenital/acquired facial (oropharyngeal) anomalies
  - Acromegaly, obstructive sleep apnea syndrome
  - Supraglottic tumors, laryngeal edema, radiotherapy, croup, epiglottitis, ***Ludwigs angina***
❖ Surgical history:
  - Unstable cervical spine
  - Faciomaxillary surgery
  - Vertebrobasillar insufficiency
  - Rheumatoid arthritis, ankylosing spondylitis
❖ Anesthetic history:
  - Previous difficult intubation
  - Pneumothorax, aspiration of gastric contents

General Examination

❖ Morbid obesity:
  - BMI more than 30 kg/m^2 suggests difficult intubation: use HELLP position
  - Neck circumference > 40 cm or 27 inches suggests difficult intubation
  - Causes of difficult intubation in obesity:
    - Short and thick neck
    - Limited atlanto-axial joint movement
    - Low cervical fat pads: reduced thyromental distance

- Thick suprasternal, presternal fat pads
- Excess soft tissue in pharynx and mouth

- Pregnancy, women with large breasts
- Abnormal posture
- Congenital anomalies:
  - Meningomyelocele
  - Faciomaxillary anomalies
  - Cystic hygroma
- Acromegaly:
  - Large jaw, tongue, lips, head
  - Generalized soft tissue swelling
  - Vocal cord thickening
  - Chondrocalcinosis of larynx
  - Subglottic narrowing
  - Enlarged thyroid gland

Local Examination

- Face:
  - ***Pierre-Robins syndrome***
  - ***Treacher-Collins syndrome***
  - ***Klippel-Feil syndrome***
  - ***Goldenhaar syndrome***
  - ***Downs syndrome***
  - Burns contractures
- Nose:
  - Deformities
  - Potency of nostril
- Teeth:
  - Dentures/edentulous
  - Long, loose/bucked teeth
- Oral cavity:
  - Macroglossia/glossoptosis
  - High arched palate/cleft palate
  - Limited mouth opening (less than 4 cm)
  - Micrognathia/retrognathia
  - Protruding/receding mandible
- Neck and cervical spine:
  - Neck: Increased thickness, abnormally long/short neck
  - Reduced range of movement, neck circumference more than 40 cm
- Distances:
  - Mouth opening:
    - Important as it determines space available for manipulating laryngoscope
    - Measured with mouth maximally opened
    - Inter-incisor distance for patients with teeth
    - Inter-alveolar distance for edentulous patients
    - Mouth opening more than 4 cm is sufficient
    - Mouth opening < 3 cms indicates reduced space for manipulation
  - Hyomental distance < 4 cms indicates difficult intubation
  - Thyromental distance:
    - Determined with the neck extended at atlan-to-occipital joint
    - Measured from tip of jaw (mentum) to superior thyroid notch
    - Indicative of adequacy of submental space
    - Submental space accommodates tongue during laryngoscopy
    - Distance more than 3 finger breadths or 6.5 cms is desirable
  - Sterno-mental distance:
    - Measured with neck in full extension
    - Distance between sternal notch and mandible
    - Surrogate measure of adequacy of neck extension
    - Distance more than 12.5 cms is optimal
    - Distance < 12 cms indicates inadequate neck extension
  - Horizontal length of mandible (9 cms)
- Temporomandibular joint:
  - Temporomandibular joint ankylosis
  - Masseteric spasm

Specific Tests

Mallampatti Score

- Mallampatti scoring is a measure of oral opening
- First described in 1985
- Evaluates degree of laryngeal exposure which would be possible on laryngoscopy
- Performed in sitting position without phonation
- Examines the ratio of size of tongue in relation to oropharynx
- Greater obstruction of pharyngeal structures by the tongue implies difficult intubation
- Sensitivity is low (49%) specificity is high (89%)
- Originally had 3 classes
- Four classes are present in modified Mallampatti score:
  - Class I:
    - Entire palatal arch seen
    - Bilateral faucial pillar and uvula seen
    - Faucial pillars seen up to their base
  - Class II: structures seen are:
    - Upper part of faucial pillars
    - Base of uvula
  - Class III: Only soft and hard palate seen
  - Class IV: Only hard palate seen

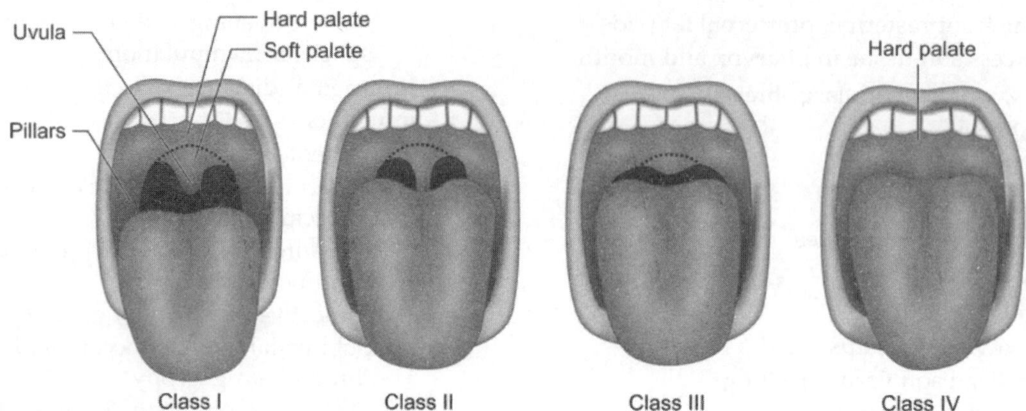

Fig. 8: Mallampatti classification.

Atlanto-occipital Joint Extension

- Evaluates ability to make sniffing/Magills position
- Normal is 35° with head held erect and facing directly to the front
- Measures angle traversed by occlusal surface of upper teeth on maximal extension

Mandibular Space

- Upper lip bite test (ULBT)
    - Patient is asked to move mandibular incisors as high on upper lip as possible
    - This is similar to biting the upper lip
    - Contact of teeth above the vermillion border is normal
    - This predicts ability to subluxate mandible during laryngoscopy
    - Grades:
        - Grade 1: Lower incisors fully covers upper lip
        - Grade 2: Lower incisors partially covers upper lip
        - Grade 3: Lower incisors do not reach upper lip
- ***Patils test***:
    - Measures thyromental distance
    - Interpretation:
        - Less than 6 cm suggests difficult airway
        - Between 6-6.5 cm suggests less difficult airway
        - More than 6.5 cm is normal
- ***Savvad test***: measures sternomental distance: more than 12.5 cm is normal
- ***Delilkan test***:
    - Index finger of left hand placed under jaw tip

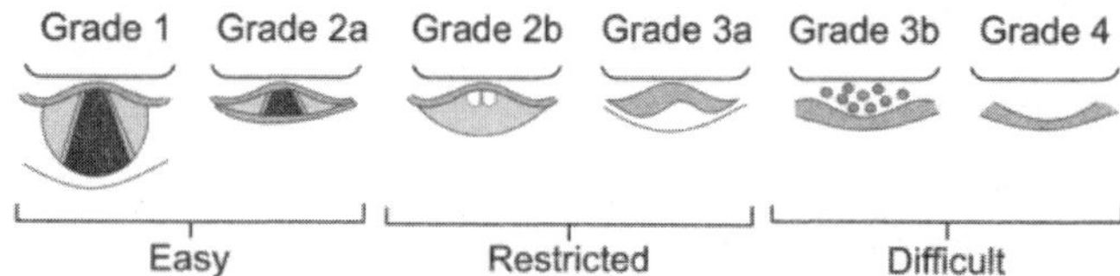

Fig. 9: Modified Cormack-Lehanes scoring system.

    - Index finger of right hand placed on occipital tuberosity
    - Patient asked to look at the ceiling
    - Interpretation:
        - If left finger higher than right: Normal neck extension
        - If left finger is at same height or lower than right finger: Abnormal extension

Modified Cormack and Lehanes Classification

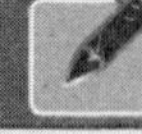

- Grade I: Full exposure of glottis
- Grade II:
    - Grade IIa: Partial exposure of glottis
    - Grade IIb: Only posterior portion of glottis or arytenoid cartilages
- Grade III:
    - Grade IIIa: Epiglottis can be lifted from posterior pharyngeal wall
    - Grade IIIb: Epiglottis cannot be lifted from posterior pharyngeal wall
- Grade IV: Neither glottis nor epiglottis is seen
- Difficulty of intubation:
    - Grades I and II: Adequate exposure
    - Grade III and IV: Inadequate exposure

Investigations

- Plain X-ray: Neck and chest
- Radiological assessment:

- Posterior mandibular depth (PMD): Distance between alveolus immediately behind third molar to lower border of mandible
- Effective mandibular length (EML):
  - Distance between tip of lower incisor to TMJ
  - Direct laryngoscopy is difficult if EML is less than 3-6 times PMD
- Reduced gap between occiput and C_1 vertebra

❖ Fluoroscopy for vocal cord mobility and emphysema
❖ Esophagogram for extrinsic mass/vascular ring
❖ Ultrasound for cellulitis, lymphadenopathy
❖ CT/MRI for congenital anomalies, mass, stenosis
❖ Pulmonary function tests: spirometry, pressure volume loops
❖ Indirect laryngoscopy
❖ Fibreoptic laryngoscopy

Difficult Mask Ventilation

❖ Criteria for difficult mask ventilation:
- Inability of one anesthetist to maintain SpO_2 more than 90%
- Need for > 4 L/min fresh gas flow
- Absence of chest movement
- Significant gas leak around face mask
- Requirement of two-handed mask ventilation
- Requirement of change of operator

❖ Predictors:
- Presence of a beard
- Obesity with BMI > 26 kg/m^2
- History of snoring
- Edentulous patients
- Old age > 55 years
- Other less important predictors:
  - Facial dressings/burns
  - Poor atlantooccipital joint extension
  - Pharyngeal pathology:
  - Lingual tonsil hypertrophy
  - Lingual tonsil abscess
  - Thyroglossal cyst

❖ OBESE score for predicting difficult mask ventilation:
- O: Obese (BMI > 26 kg/m^2)
- B: Bearded
- E: Elderly (> 55 years)
- S: Snorers
- E: Edentulous

❖ Hans mask ventilation grading scale:
- Grade 1: Ventilated by mask
- Grade 2:
  - Ventilated by mask with oral airway adjuvant
  - Muscle relaxants may be required
- Grade 3:
  - Difficult to mask ventilate with grade 2 maneuvers
  - Requires 2-person mask ventilation
- Grade 4: Unable to mask ventilate with or without muscle relaxants

Risk Factors for Difficult SGAD Ventilation

❖ Risk factors include:
- Male gender
- Obesity (BMI > 30 kg/m^2)
- Poor dentition
- Large incisors
- Neck radiation
- Reduced mouth opening
- Reduced cervical spine motion
- Tonsillar hypertrophy
- Hypopharyngeal and subglottic pathology

❖ RODS score for difficult SGAD placement:
- Reduced mouth opening limiting placement of SGAD
- Obstruction of airway at or below glottis not relieved by SGAD
- Distorted airway preventing SGAD seating
- Stiff lungs preventing ventilation following SGAD placement

Risk Factors for Difficult Videolaryngoscopy

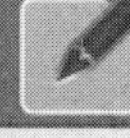

❖ ENT and cardiac surgery
❖ Difficult sniffing position
❖ Abnormal neck anatomy:
- Neck mass
- Radiation therapy

❖ Decreased cervical spine motion
❖ Decreased oral entry:
- Obesity
- Decreased mouth opening

❖ Decreased jaw mobility
❖ Restricted oropharyngeal space:
- Retrognathia
- Oropharyngeal bleeding and edema

Short Score for Difficult Cricothyroidotomy

❖ Surgery on neck
❖ Hematoma or infections in neck
❖ Obesity
❖ Radiation therapy
❖ Tumors of the neck

Scoring Systems for Difficult Intubation

Wilsons Score

Risk factor	Score
Weight	
Less than 90 kgs	0
90-110 kgs	1
More than 110 kgs	2
Head and neck movement	
More than 90°	0
Around 90°	1
Less than 90°	2
Protruding anterior maxillary/bucked teeth	
Absent (normal)	0
Moderate	1
Severe	2
Jaw movement (interincisor GAP and subluxation)	
IG > 5 cm or subluxation > 0	0
IG < 5 cm or subluxation = 0	1
IG < 5 cm or subluxation < 0	2
Receding mandible (retrognathia)	
Absent (normal)	0
Moderate	1
Severe	2

- Wilsons score less than 2 predicts normal intubation
- Wilsons score 3 predicts 75% difficult intubation cases
- Wilsons score 4 predicts 90% difficult intubation cases

Lemon Score

Physical signs	Less difficult airway	More difficult airway
Look externally	Normal face and neck	Abnormal face shape
	No face or neck pathology	Sunken cheeks
		Edentulous/bucked teeth
		Receding mandible
		Narrow mouth
		Bull neck, obesity
Evaluate 3-3-2-1	Mouth opening > 3 fingers or 6 cm	Less than 3 fingers or 5 cm
	Hyoid-chin distance > 3 fingers	Less than 3 fingers
	Thyromental distance > 3 fingers	Less than 3 fingers or 6 cm
	Lower jaw anterior subluxation > 1 finger	Less than 1 finger
Mallampatti score	Mallampatti I and II	Mallampatti II and III
Obstruction	None	Peritonsillar abscess
		Epiglottitis
		Retropharyngeal abscess
Neck mobility	Normal flexion and extension	Limited range of movement

LM-MAP Score

- L: Look for external face deformities
- M: Mallampatti score
- M: Measurements 3-3-2-1
- A: Atlanto-occipital extension
- P: Pathological obstruction – edema, tumors

Heaven Criteria for Difficult Emergency Intubation

- Hypoxemia: $SpO_2 < 93\%$ during initial laryngoscopy
- Extremes of size:
  - Pediatric patient < 8 years
  - Obesity > 26 kg/m^2
- Anatomical challenges limiting laryngoscopic view:
  - Trauma
  - Mass
  - Foreign body
- Vomit/blood/fluid in hypopharynx during laryngoscopy
- Exsanguination: Anemia causing desaturation during RSI associated apnea
- Neck: Limited range of motion

Four DS

- D_1: dentition: Prominent upper teeth, receding chin
- D_2: distortion: Edema/blood/vomitus/tumor/infection
- D_3: disproportion: Short chin/bull neck/large tongue
- D_4: dysmobility: Temporomandibular joints and cervical spine

Magboul 4Ms with Stop Sign

- 4Ms: Mallampatti, measurement, movement, malformation
- S: Skull (hydrocephalus/microcephalus)
- T: Teeth (bucked, protruded, loose, macro/micrognathia)
- O: Obstruction (obesity, short, bull neck, swelling in head/neck)
- P: pathology: Craniofacial anomalies, Treacher-Collins, Goldenhaar, Pierre-Robins syndromes

EXTUBATION OF DIFFICULT AIRWAY

Preparation of Extubation

- Fully awake extubation
- Sniffing/lateral/sitting position can be used
- Bite block should be in place to prevent biting the tube
- Remove throat pack if any
- Preoxygenate, fully reverse the patient
- Suction pharynx (trachea also if indicated)

- Extubate over guiding stylet:
  - *Cooks airway exchange catheter*
  - *Cardiomed endotracheal ventilation catheter*

Extubation Risk Assessment Tests

- *Leak test*
- Visualization of airway swelling
- Flexible fibreoptic scope visualization
- Neurological status assessment

Equipment Preparation

- Airways
- Ambubag, T-piece
- Laryngoscope blade
- ETT tube, LMAs
- Cricothyrotomy set

Routine Extubation Criteria

- Awake, alert, able to follow commands:
  - Sustained eye opening for pediatrics
  - Patient is able to understand commands for adults
- Protective reflexes returned:
  - Gag reflex
  - Swallow reflex
  - Cough reflex
- Adequate reversal of neuromuscular blockade:
  - Train of four 4/4
  - Sustained tetany at 50 Hz
  - Strong hand grip
  - Sustained head lift (more than 5 seconds)
- ABG reasonable with FiO_2 40%:
  - pH > 7.30
  - $PaO_2 \geq 60$ mm Hg
  - $PaCO_2 < 50$ mm Hg
- Respiratory mechanics adequate:
  - Respiratory rate 25-35 /min
  - Tidal volume > 5 cc/kg
  - Vital capacity ≥ 10–15 mL/kg
  - Negative inspiratory force ≥ –20 cmH_2O
  - Maximum Voluntary Ventilation > twice the minute volume
- For patients at risk of laryngeal edema:
  - Cuff leak test
  - Direct laryngoscopy and airway inspection
  - Fibreoptic bronchoscopic evaluation

Extubation of Patient with Difficult Airway

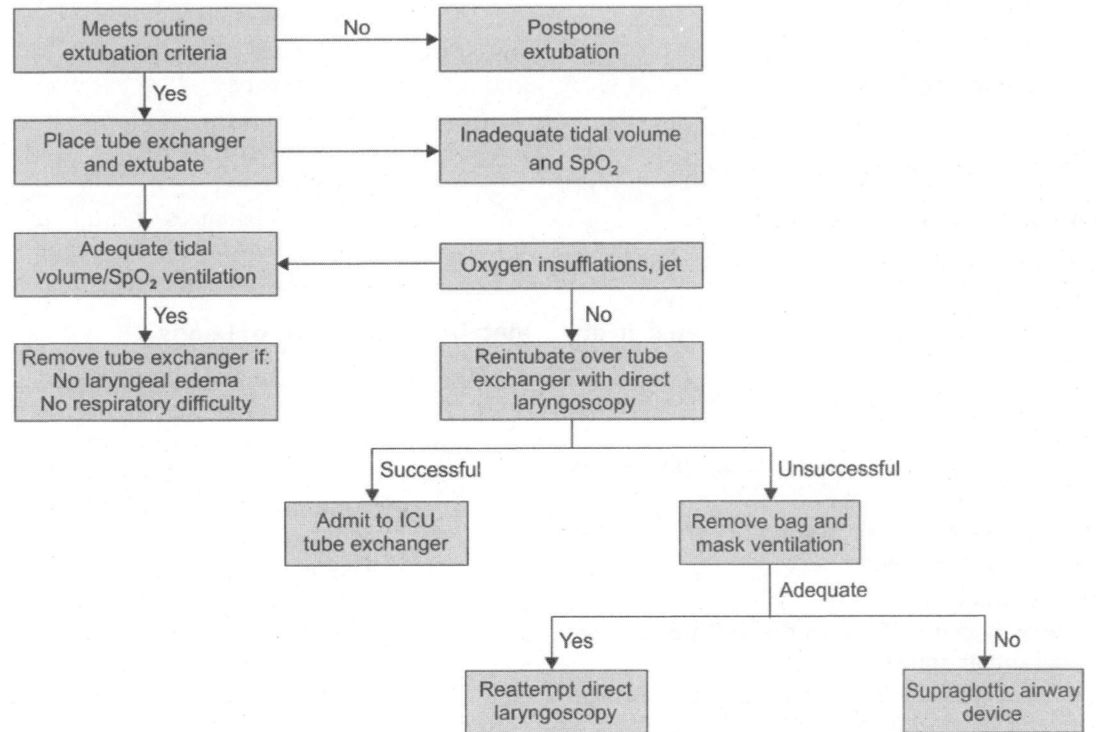

NON-RESPIRATORY FUNCTIONS OF LUNGS

Homeostatic Functions of Lungs

- Maintenance of acid-base balance:
  - Lungs are important determinants of blood pH by causing alterations in $PaCO_2$
  - This may result in respiratory acidosis/alkalosis
- Humidification:
  - Humidification occurs mainly in the nose and upper airway
  - Inhaled air is completely saturated with water vapour before it reaches trachea
  - Even at very high minute volumes most of the inhaled air is humidified
  - During exhalation however, some of the water vapour is reclaimed
  - However, in intubated patients, nasopharyngeal passage is bypassed causing:
    - Decreased humidification of delivered gases
    - Lack of reabsorption during exhalation
- Heat exchange:
  - Respiratory tract conserve heat by reclaiming it from expired air
  - Heat exchange occurs more prominently in the upper respiratory tract
  - Role of lungs in heat exchange becomes significant during:
    - Extreme cold
    - Dry conditions
    - Hyperventilation

Role as a Gas Reservoir

- Helps in voice production and phonation
- Helps in coughing, sneezing and hiccough

Defence Against Inhaled Substances

- The fate of inhaled particles depends largely on their size:
  - Particles 5–10 µm diameter are filtered in the upper airway
  - Particles 2–5 µm have a high likelihood of entering lower respiratory tract
  - Particles 0.5–2 µm are almost exclusively deposited in the alveoli
- Various mechanisms along respiratory tract protect against inhaled substances
  - Mucous blanket:
    - Airway is lined by pseudo-stratified ciliated columnar epithelium
    - The epithelium is covered by a viscous mucopolysaccharide gel
    - This is secreted by the goblet cells and forms the mucous blanket
    - The mucous blanket itself is 10 µm and consists of 2 layers:
      - Outer mucous gel layer
      - Inner periciliary sol layer
    - This forms the first line of defence against inhaled physical substances
  - Muco-ciliary escalator:
    - Epithelial cilia beat in the mucous blanket at a frequency of 10-15Hz
    - This action moves the overlying mucous towards the pharynx
    - This response is known as the muco-ciliary escalator
    - This propels the mucus blanket along with trapped particles outwards
  - Immune function: Immune function of the lung is mediated by:
    - Pulmonary alveolar macrophages (PAM):
      - PAM engulf particles which reach the alveoli
      - Further elimination occurs by:
        - Deposition into the muco-ciliary escalator
        - Removal via blood or lymph
      - PAMs are particularly effective against bacteria
    - Immune mediators:
      - Epithelial cells secrete multiple chemical mediators such as:
        - Mucins
        - Defensins
        - Lysozyme
        - Lactoferrin
        - Cytokines
      - These substances recruit inflammatory cells at the site of inflammation
      - This helps in maintaining mucosal integrity

Metabolic Functions of Lungs

- Handling of endogenous substances:
  - Various changes occur to hormones passing through pulmonary vasculature
  - Role in renin-angiotensin system (RAS):
    - Lung plays an important role in renin angiotensin system
    - This is due to high concentration of ACE in pulmonary endothelium
    - This enzyme catalyzes the conversion of AT-I to AT-II
    - AT-II is a powerful vasoconstrictor which acts to restore BP

- Changes to other hormones include:
  - Activation:
    - Angiotensin I
    - Arachidonic acid
  - Inactivation:
    - Amines:
      - Serotonin
      - Norepinephrine
    - Peptides:
      - Bradykinin
      - Atrial natriuretic peptide
      - Endothelin
    - Arachidonic acid derivatives:
      - PGD_2, PGE_2
      - PGF_2
      - Leukotrienes
    - Purine derivatives:
      - Adenosine
      - ATP
      - ADP
      - AMP
  - No change:
    - Amines:
      - Dopamine
      - Epinephrine
      - Histamine
    - Peptides:
      - Angiotensin II
      - Oxytocin
      - Vasopressin
    - Arachidonic acid derivatives:
      - PGI_2
      - PGA_2

❖ Pulmonary neuroendocrine system:
- Pulmonary neuroendocrine system comprises of:
  - Pulmonary neuroendocrine cells
  - Neuroepithelial bodies
- Functions of the pulmonary neuroendocrine system include:
  - Role in lung development:
    - These cells play an important role in lung development
    - This is done by potentiating:
      - Cell growth
      - Cell differentiation
      - Branching morphogenesis
  - Role as chemo-receptors:
    - These cells degranulate on exposure to hypoxic environment
    - They are connected to CNS by vagal afferent sensory fibres
    - Thus, they act as hypoxia sensitive chemoreceptors
  - Secretion of amines and peptides such as:
    - Serotonin
    - Bombesin

❖ Drug metabolism:
- Enzyme systems of the lungs includes:
  - Cytochrome P450 oxygenase
  - Sulfotransferase
  - Nitroreductase
  - N-methyltransferase
  - Glutathione-S-epoxide transferase
  - Glutathione-S-ARYL transferase
  - Epoxide hydrolase
  - Amine oxidase
- Lungs have substantial quantities of cytochrome P450 iso-enzymes
- Thus, lung has the capacity for drug metabolism via these enzymes
- Activity of these enzymes may increase up to 33% of that of the liver
- These enzymes are present in:
  - Type II pneumocytes
  - Clara cells
  - Endothelial cells
- Drugs with significant pulmonary metabolism include:
  - Theophylline
  - Salmeterol
  - Budesonide
  - Isoprenaline
- Most anesthetic drugs are taken up by the lungs to some extent
- However, they do not necessarily undergo significant metabolism in the lung
- Once systemic levels of the drug decrease, the drug is released from the lung
- Prilocaine is the only anesthetic drug metabolized within the lung
- However, in the clinical scenario pulmonary uptake is important because:
  - It may cause prolonged action of the drug
  - It may cause delayed onset of toxic manifestations (as in LAST)
- Anesthetic drugs with significant uptake in the lungs include:
  - Opioids:
    - Fentanyl 75%
    - Meperidine 65%
    - Alfentanil 10%
    - Morphine 4–7%
  - Induction agents:

        - Diazepam 30%
        - Propofol 28%
        - Thiopentone 14%
    - Local anesthetics:
        - Lidocaine 40–50%
        - Prilocaine 40%
        - Mepivacaine 20%
        - Bupivacaine 12%
    - Catecholamines:
        - Norepinephrine 16%
        - Dopamine 20%
    - Muscle relaxants: no significant uptake

Endocrine Functions of Lungs

- Mast cells and pulmonary neuroendocrine cells synthesize and secrete local hormones
- These hormones include:
    - Histamine:
        - Histamine is secreted by the mast cells
        - However, it has minimal uptake in the pulmonary circulation
        - Thus, metabolism of histamine within the lung is negligible
    - Serotonin:
        - Lungs contribute minimally to serotonin production
        - However, 5-HT secreted by the GIT is taken up by the lungs
        - This occurs primarily in the endothelial cells via active absorption
        - Pulmonary uptake is as high as 90%
        - Thus, very low quantities of 5-HT reach systemic circulation normally
        - Pulmonary uptake of 5-HT is important in carcinoid syndrome
        - Right heart receives a high concentration on 5-HT
        - Most of this is absorbed as it passes the pulmonary vasculature
        - Thus, valvular pathology is restricted to right heart in this syndrome
    - Prostaglandins:
        - Pulmonary endothelial cells secrete most prostaglandins
        - This function is modulated by changes in vascular flow
        - Prostaglandins produced include:
            - PGI_2 (continuously)
            - PGD_2
            - PGE_2, PGF_2

Role in Coagulation Cascade

- Lung is an important source of:
    - Endogenous procoagulants
    - Endogenous anticoagulants
    - Fibrinolytic agents
- Substances secreted in the lung include:
    - Thromboplastin
    - Heparin (mainly in mast cells)
    - Plasminogen activator

Role in Platelet Maturation

- Megakaryocytes undergo fragmentation within the lungs to produce platelets
- This is suggested by:
    - High concentration of megakaryocytes in the pulmonary circulation
    - Higher platelet count in the pulmonary vein compared with pulmonary artery
- Megakaryocytes bypassing the pulmonary vascular bed lodge in nail-bed capillaries
- This results in the release of various substance such as:
    - Platelet derived growth factor
    - Vascular endothelial growth factor
- This causes clubbing and hypertrophic osteoarthropathy via:
    - Vascular hyperplasia
    - Proliferation of periosteal layers

Non-respiratory Functions of Pulmonary Circulation

- Reservoir of blood:
    - Pulmonary vascular bed is a high capacitance vascular bed
    - It accommodates large blood volumes with minimal change in pressure
    - Approximately 10% of total blood volume is present in the lungs at any time
    - Thus, it acts as a vascular reservoir and is able to load and offload volume
    - The mechanisms involved in offloading volume include:
        - Recruitment of pulmonary vasculature:
            - At resting CO, pulmonary vascular bed is not fully perfused
            - Increase in CO, causes recruitment of under-perfused areas
            - These recruited areas accommodate the increased blood volume
        - Distention of pulmonary vasculature:
            - Walls of pulmonary vessels are thin with less smooth muscle

  - This enables it to distend with an increase in cardiac output
- These mechanisms help in altering pulmonary blood volume by 500-1000 mL
- Thus, preload requirements of the left heart are met

❖ Filter for blood borne substances:
- Lung acts as an important vascular filter due to its anatomical location
- It receives the entire right ventricular output
- Thus, it plays an important role in the uptake of:
  - Endogenous substances
  - Xenobiotics
- Mechanisms of filtration function include:
  - Physical filtration:
    - Pulmonary capillaries have a diameter of 7 μm
    - It has the ability to physically filter 99% of particles > 50 μm
  - Chemical filtration:
    - Pulmonary circulation acts as a chemical filter for thrombi
    - This is mainly through 2 mechanisms:
      - Pulmonary fibrinolytic system which breaks down clots
      - Production of heparin which inhibits coagulation
- Particles normally filtered by the lungs include:
  - Small thrombi
  - Fat cells
  - Amniotic fluid
  - Agglutinated white blood cells
  - Cancer cells
  - Bone marrow
  - Particles in IV fluids
- Conditions causing a disruption of this filter include:
- Patent foramen ovale due to intracardiac shunting
- Hepatopulmonary syndrome due to intrapulmonary vascular dilatation

❖ Drug absorption:
- Many medications are administered via inhalational formulations
- Drugs administered via inhalational route have high bioavailability due to:
  - Rapid absorption
  - Low pulmonary metabolism
- Main benefits of administration of inhaled drugs include:
  - Rapid onset of action due to:
    - Large surface area for absorption
    - High epithelial permeability
    - Increased vascularity
  - High local concentration by direct delivery
- Action of aerosolized drugs is completed in different steps:
  - Deposition:
    - Deposition in small airways is important to ensure drug action
    - Delivery into large airways results in muco-ciliary clearance
    - This results in poor drug delivery in COPD and asthma
  - Dissolution:
    - Dissolution of the drug is determined by drug hydrophobicity
    - Water soluble drugs dissolve in the fluid and are absorbed easily
  - Absorption:
    - Absorption of the drug occurs via different mechanisms:
      - Passive diffusion: Occurs along concentration gradient:
        - » Hydrophilic drugs through intercellular diffusion
        - » Hydrophobic drugs via transcellular diffusion
      - Active transport occurs for drugs with low passive permeability
  - Clearance: occurs mainly via:
    - Muco-ciliary clearance
    - Pulmonary alveolar macrophages
- Inhalational route aids systemic delivery of drugs with low oral bioavailability

FACTORS AFFECTING TISSUE OXYGENATION

Introduction

❖ Aerobic cellular respiration depends on efficient supply of oxygen and substrate to the mitochondria

❖ Normally oxygen content in mitochondria is 10 mm Hg

❖ Critical value of PO_2 in mitochondria is 1-2 mm Hg (***Pasteur point***) below which anaerobic respiration sets in

Physiology

❖ *Oxygen flux*:
- This is the amount of oxygen which leaves the left ventricle per minute (DO_2)
- The normal delivery of oxygen to tissues is 1000 mL/min
- DO_2 = cardiac output (Q) x arterial O_2 content

- $DO_2 = Q \times Hb\% \times SaO_2 \times 1.39$ ***(Huffners constant)***
- Since there are three variables which are multiplied to derive the DO_2, a small change in one variable may cause a large change in DO_2
- Huffners constant is the amount of O_2 (in mL), in 1 gm of Hb at sea level

❖ ***Supply independent oxygen consumption***:
- The normal delivery of oxygen to tissues is 1000 mL/min
- The normal consumption of O_2 at the tissue level is 250 mL/min (VO_2)
- Thus, oxygen is delivered in excess to the tissues
- This enables body to cope with a reduction in DO_2 without initially compromising aerobic respiration and oxygen consumption

❖ ***Supply dependant oxygen consumption***:
- When VO_2 falls with a reduction in DO_2, it is called supply dependent O_2 consumption
- Tissues are in dysoxia below this point

❖ Thus factors which decrease tissue oxygenation are:
- Reduced delivery (DO_2)
- Increased consumption (VO_2)
- Histotoxic hypoxia

Factors Causing Reduced Delivery (DO_2)

Macrovascular Level

❖ Factors affecting cardiac output:
- Hypovolemia
- Hemorrhage
- Congestive cardiac failure

❖ Factors affecting hemoglobin concentration (Hb%):
- Anemia:
  - Causes reduction in diffusive oxygen conductance
  - Causes reduction in number of binding sites for oxygen
  - Reduces surface area of RBC for effective oxygen diffusion
- Oxyhemoglobin dissociation curve:
  - Factors causing shift to right:
    - Acidosis (Bohr effect)
    - Hyperthermia
    - Hypercapnea
    - Increased 2,3-DPG
    - High altitude
    - Propranolol
    - Isoflurane
  - Factors causing shift to left:
    - Alkalosis
    - Hypothermia
    - Hypocapnea
    - Reduced 2,3-DPG
    - Fetal hemoglobin (HbF)
    - Carboxyhemoglobin
    - Methemoglobin
    - Carbon monoxide inhalation

❖ Factors affecting arterial oxygen saturation (SaO_2):
- Ventilation perfusion mismatch: lung collapse, chronic lung diseases
- Diffusion limitation: intestitial fibrosis
- Right to left shunting: Acute lung diseases (through inadequately oxygenated alveoli)

Microvascular Level

❖ Factors affecting microvascular tone:
- Central factors: Sympathetic vasoconstrictor tone reduces blood flow
- Local factors: Vasodilator tone:
  - Subject to autoregulation
  - Hypoxia causes vasodilation and increased blood flow by:
    - Increasing production of:
      - Nitric oxide (NO)
      - PGI_2
      - Endothelial derived humoral factor (EDHF)
    - Stimulation of ATP sensitive potassium channels

❖ Factors affecting oxygen diffusion from microvasculature to mitochondria:
- Capillary surface area
- Oxygen content
- Myoglobin facilitated diffusion of oxygen

Factors Affecting Oxygen Consumption

❖ Severe exercise
❖ Fever
❖ Thyrotoxicosis
❖ ***Halothane shakes***
❖ Pain
❖ Shivering

Histotoxic Hypoxia

❖ Oxygen delivery to mitochondria may be normal
❖ But mitochondria may be unable to utilize the oxygen due to some defect in the electron transport chain
❖ This can be due to:
- Carbon monoxide/cyanide poisoning
- Narcotics, alcohol poisoning
- Hydrogen sulphide poisoning (sewage byproduct used in leather tanning)

Oxygen Cascade

- Oxygen content of air (at sea level) is 160 mm Hg and falls to 10-15 mm Hg at the mitochondrial level. The transport of oxygen down this gradient is described as oxygen cascade
- Normally oxygen content in mitochondria is 10 mm Hg
- Critical value of PO_2 in mitochondria is 1-2 mm Hg (***Pasteur point***) below which anaerobic respiration sets in

OXYGEN CASCADE

Introduction

- Steps by which partial pressure of O_2 decreases from a higher level in inspired gas to a lower level in mitochondria is called O_2 cascade
- PO_2 reaches the lowest level (4-20 mm Hg) in the mitochondria

Steps of Oxygen Cascade

- Uptake in lungs
- Transport in blood
- Global delivery to tissues
- Regional distribution of O_2 delivery
- Diffusion from capillary to cell
- Cellular utilization of O_2

Oxygen Uptake in the Lungs

- In the pulmonary capillary, venous blood is exposed to higher PO_2 (100 mm Hg)
- Oxygen therefore diffuses down the partial pressure gradient into the capillaries
- This process is aided by low PCO_2 and H^+ ion concentration in pulmonary capillaries
- This causes ***Bohr shift*** of ODC in pulmonary capillaries and favours O_2 uptake
- Most of this oxygen is then transported in combination with hemoglobin
- Arterial oxygen tension is determined by:
  - Inspired oxygen concentration
  - Barometric pressure
  - Alveolar ventilation:
    - Alveolar ventilation maintains the alveolar O_2 pressure (P_AO_2)
    - This is determined by the tidal volume and respiratory rate
  - Diffusion of oxygen from alveoli to pulmonary capillaries:
    - P_AO_2 is the driving force for O_2 diffusion into pulmonary capillaries
    - Alveolar arterial O_2 gradient describes efficiency of O_2 uptake in lungs
  - Distribution and matching of ventilation and perfusion:
    - Ventilation and perfusion matching is required for efficient O_2 exchange
    - Ventilation-perfusion mismatch results in intrapulmonary shunting
    - This in turn may reduce arterial oxygen content

Oxygen Transport in Blood: Transported in Two Forms

- Hemoglobin bound oxygen:
  - 98% of the total O_2 in blood is carried within the RBCs as oxyhemoglobin

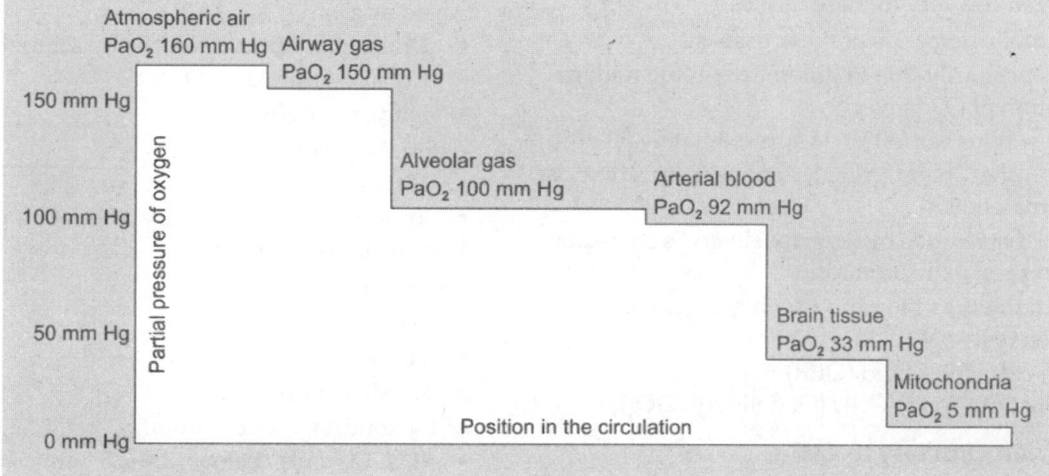

Fig. 10: Oxygen cascade.

- Each gram of hemoglobin can theoretically carry up to 1.39 mL of oxygen
- Dissolved oxygen:
  - Less than 2% of the total O_2 is circulated as dissolved oxygen in the plasma
  - For each mm Hg of PO_2, 0.003 mL of O_2 is dissolved per 100 mL of blood
  - This is called as the *solubility coefficient for oxygen* (0.003 mL/dL/mm Hg)
  - For a PaO_2 of 100 mm Hg dissolved oxygen is 0.3 mL in 100 mL of blood
  - This compares to approximately 20 mL of O_2 in the bound form to Hb
  - Thus, the amount of O_2 dissolved in plasma is negligible

Global Delivery to Tissues

- Global delivery refers to the amount of oxygen delivered to the tissues per minute
- This is also called *oxygen flux or oxygen dispatch*
- It is the product of the cardiac output and arterial oxygen content

  DO_2 = [Cardiac output (Qt)] × [Arterial oxygen content (CaO_2)]
- Normal O_2 flux amounts to 1000 mL oxygen/minute assuming:
  - Cardiac output of 5 litres
  - Hemoglobin of 15.6 g/dL
  - SpO_2 of 98%

Regional Distribution of Oxygen Delivery

- Oxygen saturation in blood draining out from different organs varies widely
- This reflects differences in both:
  - Oxygen delivery to these tissues
  - Metabolic demands of these tissues
- It occurs primarily due to differences in the regional distribution of O_2 delivery
- Hepatic venous saturation is approximately 30-40%
- On the other hand, renal venous saturation is approximately 80%
- Regional distribution of oxygen delivery is measured by the oxygen extraction ratio
- This is defined as the ratio of oxygen consumption to oxygen delivery

  Oxygen extraction ratio (OER) = {O_2 consumption (VO_2)}/{O_2 delivery (DO_2)}

Diffusion from Capillary to Cell

- As tissue PO_2 is low, O_2 diffuses down the partial pressure gradient and out of blood
- The blood PO_2 falls and oxygen is released from hemoglobin into physical solution
- This process continues till adequate oxygen has been released for aerobic metabolism
- It is aided by the high levels of PCO_2 and H^+ ions in the tissue level
- This causes a ***Bohr shift*** of ODC and aids unloading of O_2 into the tissues
- Each 100 mL of blood loses 5 mL of oxygen at the tissue level into interstitial fluid
- Thus, PO_2 falls from 100 mm Hg to 40 mm Hg

Cellular Utilization of Oxygen

- Oxygen constantly diffuses into the cells as it is constantly utilized by them
- Cellular metabolic rate determines the overall oxygen consumption
- This occurs via diffusion as intracellular PO_2 is lesser than interstitial fluid PO_2
- ***Pasteur point***:
  - Refers to mitochondrial PO_2 below which aerobic metabolism cannot occur
  - Usually around 1.4-2.3 mm Hg

Factors Affecting Cascade

- Dry atmospheric air:
  - Barometric pressure
  - FiO_2
  - Partial pressure of O_2 (PiO_2) = barometric pressure x FiO_2 = 760 × 0.21 = 160 mm Hg
- Humidification at 37°C:
  - Depends on saturated vapour pressure of water at body temperature
  - PO_2 = (atmospheric pressure – SVP) × FiO_2
  - PO_2 = (760 – 47) × 0.21 = 150 mm Hg
- Alveolar gas:
  - Dilution of atmosphere air by arterial air
  - Constant uptake of O_2
  - Diffusion defects
- Arterial O_2 tension:
  - V-P mismatch
  - True shunt of pulmonary arterial blood
  - Cardiac output
- Cellular PO_2:
  - Blood flow
  - Hb%
  - Cardiac output
- Mitochondria: ***Pasteur point:***
  - If DO_2 falls below 1.4-2.3 mm Hg, aerobic metabolism stops
  - This point is called Pasteur point

Causes of Failure of Cascade

- Stagnant hypoxia:
  - Low cardiac output
  - Peripheral vascular disease
  - Mechanical vascular occlusion
- Anemic hypoxia:
  - Anemia
  - Acute blood loss
  - Hemoglobinopathy
- Hypoxic hypoxia:
  - Inadequate ventilation
  - V-Q mismatch
  - Low FiO_2
- Shunt hypoxia:
  - Arteriovenous shunt
  - Congenital cardiac diseases

Clinical Implications

- When FiO_2 increased to 100%:
  - Small amount of O_2 dissolves in plasma at rate 0.3 mL O_2/100 mL plasma
  - But no significant increase in amount of oxygen carried by hemoglobin
  - This is because it is already 98% saturated with oxygen
- Any interference at any point of O_2 cascade causes significant changes downstream
- Changes at high altitude:
  - On ascent to higher attitude, barometric pressure reduces
  - Thus, even if FiO_2 is 21%, PiO_2 is only 70 mm Hg

OXYGEN FLUX

Introduction

- Refers to amount of oxygen leaving left ventricle per minute in arterial blood
- Also is the amount of oxygen delivered to peripheral tissues per minute

Measurement

Oxygen flux DO_2 = {Cardiac output (Q_t)} × {Arterial oxygen content (CaO_2)}

Arterial oxygen content = (O_2 bound to hemoglobin) + (dissolved O_2)

Where,

O_2 bound to Hb = Hb concentration × SpO_2 × K

Dissolved O_2 = cardiac output × pO_2 × 0.03

Components

- Hemoglobin bound oxygen:

Hemoglobin bound oxygen = (SpO_2) × (Hb) × (K) × (0.01)

Where:

SpO_2 is the percentage saturation of hemoglobin with oxygen

Hb is the hemoglobin concentration in g/dL

K = Huffners constant {amount of O_2 carried by 1 gm of Hb (around 1.39 mL)}

  - 98% of the total O_2 in blood is carried within the RBCs as oxyhemoglobin
  - Each gram of hemoglobin can theoretically carry up to 1.39 mL of oxygen
- Dissolved oxygen:

Dissolved oxygen = PO_2 × 0.03

  - Where PO_2 is the partial pressure of oxygen
  - Less than 2% of the total O_2 is circulated as dissolved oxygen in the plasma
  - The amount of dissolved oxygen in blood is derived from ***Henrys law***
  - This states that the concentration of any gas in solution is proportional to its partial pressure
  - Thus, the concentration of dissolved O_2 is proportional to its partial pressure
  - For each mm Hg of PO_2, 0.003 mL of O_2 is dissolved per 100 mL of blood
  - This is called as the *solubility coefficient for oxygen* (0.003 mL/dL/mm Hg)
  - For a PaO_2 of 100 mm Hg dissolved oxygen is 0.3 mL in 100 mL of blood
  - This compares to approximately 20 mL of O_2 in the bound form to Hb
  - Thus, the amount of O_2 dissolved in plasma is negligible and is ignored
  - The oxygen flux therefore simplifies to the equation:

Oxygen flux = CO × Hb × SpO_2 × 1.39

- However, dissolved oxygen may contribute to increasing oxygen transport when:
  - FiO_2 is increased to 100% (dissolved O_2 approaches 1.5 mL/100 mL blood)
  - Hyperbaric environments

Normal Values

- O_2 flux normally amounts to 1000 mL oxygen/minute assuming:
  - Cardiac output of 5 litres
  - Hemoglobin of 15.6 g/dL
  - SpO_2 of 98%
- Normally 250 mL/min of O_2 is taken up in the tissues

- This can increase with an increase in the metabolic rate
- The remaining 750 mL/min (or 75%) is returned to lung in mixed venous blood

Oxygen	Mixed venous	Arterial
Dissolved in plasma	0.13 mL/100 mL plasma	0.3 mL/100 mL plasma
Tension (PaO_2)	40 mm Hg	100 mm Hg
Amount combined with Hb (oxyhemoglobin)	14 mL/100 mL blood	19 mL/100 mL plasma
Saturation	75%	100%

Factors Affecting Oxygen Flux

- Factors affecting oxygen carrying capacity:
  - Anemia
  - Congestive cardiac failure
  - Metabolic/respiratory acidosis
  - Reduced alveolar ventilation
- Factors increasing oxygen demand:
  - Exercise
  - Pain
  - Shivering
  - Halothane shakes
  - Thyrotoxicosis
  - Metabolic acidosis

Clinical Relevance

- Maximal PaO_2 which can be achieved is 400-500 mm Hg
- For every 1% increase in SaO_2, PaO_2 increases by 40-50 mm Hg
- PaO_2 of 100 mm Hg indicates SaO_2 of 98%

PaO_2	SpO_2
100 mm Hg	98%
60 mm Hg	90%
50 mm Hg	80%
40 mm Hg	70%
27 mm Hg	50%

OXYGEN DISSOCIATION CURVE

Introduction

- Curve which mathematically equates:
  - Percentage saturation of hemoglobin and
  - Partial pressure of oxygen in blood
- It has a sigmoid shape and describes non-linear tendency of O_2 to bind to hemoglobin
- The sigmoid shape arises due to:
  - Increasing affinity of hemoglobin for O_2 with increasing PaO_2

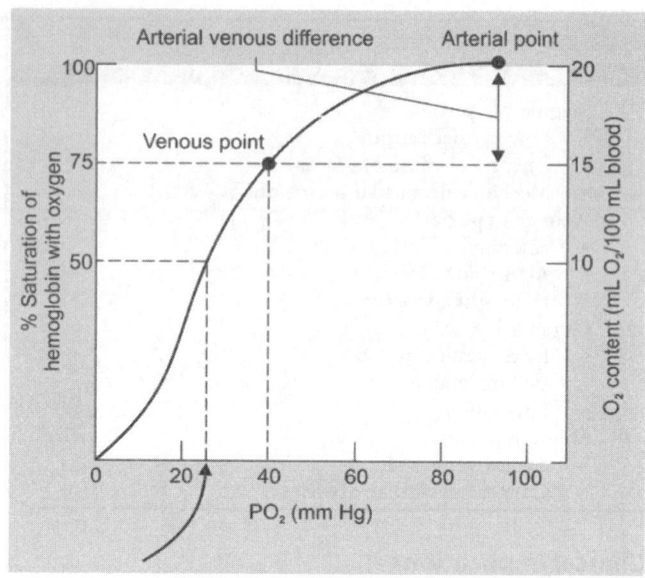

Fig. 11: Hemoglobin oxygen dissociation curve.

  - Decreasing affinity of hemoglobin for O_2 with decreasing PaO_2.

Rationale of ODC

- Oxygenation of hemoglobin:
  - Hemoglobin is a protein made of 4 subunits
  - Each subunit contains a heme moiety attached to a polypeptide chain
  - Normally, each hemoglobin molecule has two and two β chains
  - Heme is a porphyrin ring complex and includes one atom of ferrous (Fe^{2+}) iron
  - Each of the four Fe^{2+} iron atoms in Hb can bind to one O_2 molecule
  - Even after binding to oxygen iron remains in the ferrous form
  - Thus, its reaction with oxygen is called oxygenation and not oxidation
  - This reaction is represented as:

$$Hb + O_2 \rightarrow HbO_2$$

  - This is followed by the reaction of other ferrous atoms with oxygen
  - Thus, deoxyhemoglobin is converted to oxyhemoglobin represented by Hb_4O_8
- *Cooperativity*:
  - Binding of O_2 to one site on Hb molecule facilitates O_2 binding at other sites
  - This is referred to as cooperativity

- This is because of the quarternary structure of hemoglobin
- The first O_2 molecule which binds to Hb causes significant changes
- It releases the bonds holding globin molecules together
- Thus, the hemoglobin molecule transforms to a relaxed (R) configuration
- This results in the exposure of more O_2 binding sites on the Hb molecule
- This results in a 500-fold increase in the affinity of Hb to O_2
- This causes sigmoid shape of curve
- Conversely, as one molecule of O_2 becomes unbound, affinity for others also falls

Clinical Importance of ODC

- Role of Hb saturation:
  - Saturation of Hb with O_2 markedly increases on the steep part of the curve
  - This is especially pronounced between 10-60 mm Hg
  - At a PaO_2 of 60 mm Hg, hemoglobin saturation is 90%
  - Any further increase in PO_2 produces only a small increment in SpO_2
  - P_{50} refers to the PO_2 at which blood is 50% saturated with O_2
  - P_{50} can be used to describe the shift in position of ODC to left or right
  - Normal P_{50} is approximately 26 mm Hg
  - Reduction in P_{50} below 26 mm Hg results in leftward shift of ODC
  - Increases in P_{50} beyond 26 mm Hg results in rightward shift of ODC
- Rightward shift of ODC:
  - The affinity of Hb for oxygen reduces
  - Thus, higher PaO_2 is required for Hb to bind a given amount of O_2
  - The PaO_2 at which Hb is 50% saturated with oxygen increases
  - Conversely, oxygen is more easily released from hemoglobin
- Leftward shift of ODC:
  - The affinity of Hb for oxygen increases
  - Thus, lower PaO_2 is required for Hb to bind a given amount of O_2
  - The PaO_2 at which Hb is 50% saturated with oxygen reduces
- *Bohr effect*:
  - Refers to the decrease in O_2 affinity of Hb when the pH of blood falls
  - At tissue level (as in working muscle):
    - Affinity of hemoglobin to oxygen reduces at the tissue level due to:
      - Increase in $PaCO_2$
      - Increase in H^+ ion concentration
      - Higher temperature at tissue level
    - At tissue level, CO_2 produced enters blood and increases blood $PaCO_2$
    - This in turn raises levels of blood H_2CO_3 and H^+ ion concentration
    - This causes shift of ODC to the right
    - Thus, at the tissue level, unloading of O_2 occurs easily
  - In pulmonary capillaries:
    - Affinity of Hb to O_2 increases in pulmonary capillaries due to:
      - Reduced $PaCO_2$
      - Lower H^+ concentration
      - This causes shift of ODC to the left
    - Thus, in pulmonary capillaries, O_2 uptake into the blood occurs easily
- *Haldane effect*:
  - Refers to ability of deoxygenated hemoglobin to carry more CO_2
  - Oxygenation of Hb reduces its ability to transport CO_2
  - This is due to increased formation of carbamino compounds
  - Thus, in the lungs, oxygenation of blood causes unloading of CO_2
- Role of hemoglobin: Reduction of Hb % from 15 g% to 10 g% reduces PaO_2 from 100 to 40 mm Hg

Implications of Shape of Curve

- Allows Hb to load and unload O_2 efficiently as physiological condition dictates
- Beyond hemoglobin saturation ≥ 90% curve is flat
- Reflects 4 stage loading of O_2: Each Hb molecule binds four O_2 molecules
- O_2 unloading in tissues occurs over steep portion of curve

SpO_2	PaO_2
98%	100 mm Hg
90%	60 mm Hg
75%	47 mm Hg
50%	26.6 mm Hg
25%	15 mm Hg

Causes of Shift in ODC Curve

Shift to left	Shift to right
Causes:	Causes:
Alkalosis	Acidosis
Hypothermia	Hyperthermia
Hypocarbia	Hypercarbia
Reduced 2,3 – DPG	Increased 2,3-DPG
Fetal hemoglobin	High altitude
Carboxyhemoglobin	Isoflurane
Methhemoglobin	Propranolol
CO inhalation	
Results in reduced O_2 delivery to tissues	Results in increased O_2 delivery to tissues

Myoglobin Dissociation Curve (MDC)

- Myoglobin is important oxygen source for muscle
- Myoglobin resembles Hb but binds 1 rather than 4 molecules of O_2
- Thus, each myoglobin molecule has one site for O_2 binding
- The lack of cooperative binding results in the rectangular hyperbolic shape of MDC
- This is reflective of the one stage loading of myoglobin with O_2
- Also, compared to ODC, there is a leftward shift of MDC
- Thus, the P_{50} is 5 mm Hg implying a higher oxygen affinity at low PO_2
- This promotes a preferential transfer of O_2 from Hb rather than myoglobin.

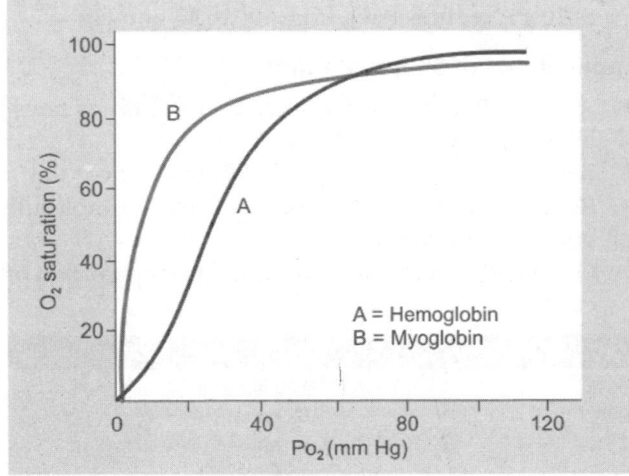

Fig. 12: Myoglobin dissociation curve

PULMONARY FUNCTION TESTS

Uses of PFTS

- Screen for type of lung disease:
  - Spirometry for obstructive lung disease
  - Flow-volume loops for restrictive disease
  - DLCO measurement for:
    - Pulmonary vascular disease
    - Interstitial lung disease
- Quantify severity of disease:
  - Severity of obstructive disease measured by FEV_1% predicted
  - Severity of restrictive disease measured by TLC% predicted
- Serial PFT measurements may be useful in asthma to:
  - Follow progression of disease
  - Observe response to therapy
  - Screen for transition from reversible to fixed obstruction:
    - Detected as a lack of response to bronchodilators
    - May require escalation of therapy
- Serial PFT measurements may also be useful to screen for:
  - Pulmonary effects of drug toxicity (amiodarone, bleomycin)
  - Progression of neuromuscular disease
  - Progression of diffuse parenchymal lung disease using TLC, FVC and DLCO
- Preoperative pulmonary function tests may be useful to:
  - Predict risk of postoperative complications for thoracic surgery
  - Obtain baseline information to guide perioperative management
  - Identify patients who may benefit from pulmonary rehabilitation therapy

Indications for PFTS

- In patients with signs suggestive of pulmonary disease:
  - Cough, wheeze
  - Breathlessness
  - Crackles, abnormal chest X-ray
- To monitor patients with known pulmonary disease for disease progression:
  - Interstitial fibrosis

- COPD
- Asthma
- Pulmonary vascular disease

❖ In diseases with respiratory complications:
- Connective tissue disorders
- Neuromuscular diseases

❖ Preoperative evaluation prior to:
- Lung resection
- Major abdominal surgeries
- Cardiothoracic surgeries

❖ Evaluation of patients at risk for lung disease: Exposure to pulmonary toxins:
- Radiation
- Medications:
  - Amiodarone
  - Bleomycin

❖ Surveillance following lung transplantation to assess for:
- Acute rejection
- Infections

❖ Obliterative bronchiolitis

Contraindications

❖ Myocardial infarction within 1 month
❖ Unstable angina within 1 month
❖ Recent thoraco-abdominal surgery
❖ Recent ophthalmic surgery
❖ Thoracic, abdominal or cerebral aneurysm
❖ Current pneumothorax

Classification of Pulmonary Function Tests

❖ Tests of mechanical ventilatory function:
- Bedside pulmonary function tests
- Spirometry:
  - Static lung volumes and capacities
  - Dynamic lung volumes

❖ Tests for gas exchange:
- Alveolar arterial gradient
- Diffusion capacity
- Gas distribution tests:
  - Single breath nitrogen test
  - Multiple breath nitrogen test
  - Helium dilution method
  - Radioactive xenon scintigram

❖ Tests of cardiopulmonary interaction:
- 6-minute walk test
- Stair climbing test
- Shuttle walk test
- Cardiopulmonary exercise testing

SPIROMETRY

Introduction

Spirometry is the measurement of airflow and lung volumes during various respiratory maneuvers.

Procedure

❖ The patient inhales as much air as possible and then exhales rapidly
❖ Exhalation should be done rapidly and forcefully for as long as flow can be maintained
❖ The patient should exhale for at least 6 seconds
❖ At the end of forced exhalation the patient inhales again fully and as rapidly as possible
❖ Characteristics of an acceptable spirometry effort includes:
- Begins from full inflation
- Shows minimal hesitation at the start of forced exhalation
- Shows explosive start of forced exhalation (time to peak flow < 0.12 seconds)
- Absence of coughing during the first second of forced exhalation
- Meets one of three criteria at the end of the test:
  - Smooth curvilinear rise of volume-time tracing to a plateau of at least 1 second duration
  - Forced expiratory time (FET) > 15 seconds in the absence of an expiratory plateau
  - Termination of the forced exhalation due to medical complications.

Static Lung Tests

❖ Tidal volume:
- Volume of air moving in and out of lungs during quiet respiration
- It is the volume inspired from resting lung volume reached at end-expiration
- Reduces with:
  - Decrease in lung compliance
  - Reduced respiratory muscle strength
- Normal values:
  - 500 mL in adults
  - 6-8 mL/kg in children

❖ Inspiratory reserve volume:
- Maximum volume of air inhaled from end-inspiratory tidal position
- 3.2 – 3.6 L

❖ Expiratory reserve volume:
- Maximum volume of air exhaled out from resting tidal end-expiratory position

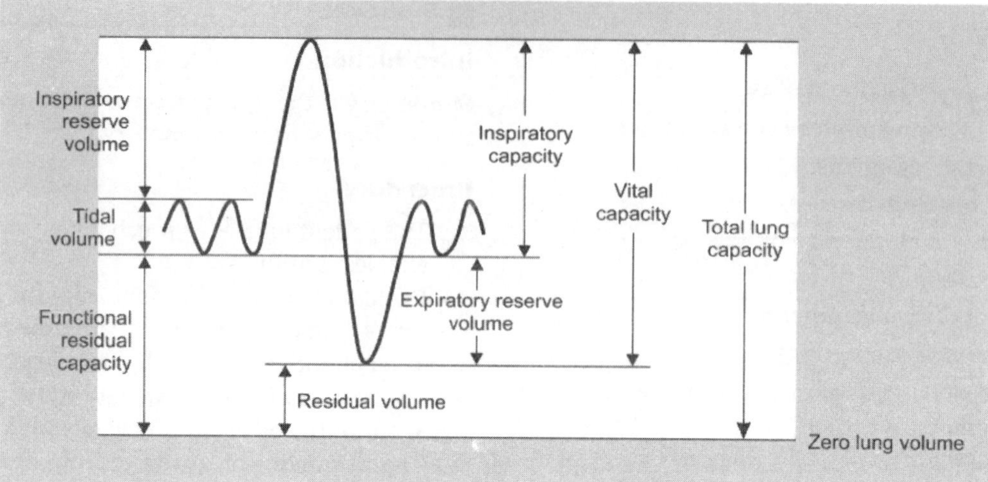

Fig. 13: Normal spirometry curve.

- Not of great diagnostic help
- Normally around 1.2 L

❖ Residual volume (RV):
- Normally following *maximal* expiratory effort, some air remains in the lung
- This volume of air remaining in lungs after maximal exhalation constitutes RV
- RV cannot be measured directly by spirometry
- It is indirectly measured as the difference between FRC and ERV
- Normal values:
  - 1.2- 2 L in adults
  - 20% of total lung capacity

Residual volume = (Functional residual capacity) – (Expiratory reserve volume)

❖ Vital capacity (VC):
- Refers to the maximum volume of air that can be inhaled and then exhaled
- This is calculated as the difference between TLC and RV
- Vital capacity is reduced in both obstructive and restrictive lung diseases
- In restrictive lung diseases:
  - Fibrosis limits the expansion of lung
  - Thus, TLC is reduced causing a reduction in VC
- In obstructive lung diseases:
  - Obstructive lung diseases cause impaired expiration and air trapping
  - This results in an increase in RV causing a reduction in VC
- Vital capacity correlates well with the ability for:
  - Deep breathing
  - Effective coughing
- Reduced vital capacity is seen in:
  - Pulmonary edema
  - Atelectasis
  - Mechanical extrapulmonary restriction:
    - Pleural effusion
    - Pneumothorax
    - Pregnancy
    - Large ascites
- Normal values:
  - 60 mL/kg in children
  - 4-6 L in adults

Vital capacity = (Total lung capacity) – (Residual volume)

❖ Inspiratory capacity:
- It is largest volume of gas that can be inspired from resting expiratory level
- Decreased in the presence of significant extra-thoracic airway obstruction
- Most PFTs measure only exhaled flows and volumes
- Extra-thoracic obstructions cause a delayed reduction in these volumes
- Thus, IC can be used to detect extra-thoracic airway obstruction early
- Changes in absolute values of IC parallel changes in VC
- Thus, IC correlates well with effective coughing
- Normal value: 3.6 L

Inspiratory capacity = (Tidal volume) + (Inspiratory reserve volume)

❖ Functional residual capacity:
- Volume of gas remaining in lung at the end of normal, passive expiration
- Influences ventilation perfusion relationships in lung
- Cannot be measured by a simple spirometer
- Normal value: 2.4 L

Dynamic Lung Tests

- Forced vital capacity:
  - Volume expired as forcefully and rapidly as possible after maximal inspiration
  - Measurement of FVC depends on patient effort and cooperation
  - In normal patients, FVC equals the VC
  - In obstructive lung diseases:
    - Forced expiration increases the intra-pleural pressure
    - However, the airway pressure is minimally affected
    - This triggers bronchiolar collapse and gas trapping
    - Thus, FVC may be reduced even though VC remains unchanged
  - In restrictive lung diseases:
    - Vital capacity is reduced due to a reduction in TLC
    - Thus, FVC also is reduced along with the reduction in VC
  - FVC < 15 mL/kg increases risk of postoperative pulmonary complications
- Forced expiratory volume (FEV_T):
  - Volume of gas expired over a given time interval during the FVC maneuver
  - T is the time elapsed in seconds from the onset of expiration
  - As FEV_T measures volume of gas exhaled over time, it is a measure of flow
  - Thus, severity of airway obstruction can be ascertained using FEV_T
  - However, FEV_T can be reduced in both obstructive and restrictive diseases
  - Measurement of FEV_T depends on patient effort and cooperation
  - Normal values of FEV_T:
    - $FEV_{0.5}$ = 50-60% of VC (within 0.5 seconds)
    - FEV_1 = 75-85% (within 1 second)
    - FEV_2 = 94% (within 2 seconds)
    - FEV_3 = 97% (within 3 seconds)
  - FEV_1/FVC:
    - Represents the ratio of FEV/VC during 1st second of FVC maneuver
    - Normally, at least 75% of VC is exhaled out during the 1st second
    - $FEV_1/FVC > 0.83$
    - $FEV_2/FVC > 0.94$
- Forced expiratory flow:
  - Measure of how much volume can be expired from lungs as a flow rate
  - Measured from FVC curve
  - Each quartile of FVC curve expressed as FEF value
  - $FEF_{25\%}$: Amount of air forcefully expelled out in first 25% of FVC test
  - $FEF_{50\%}$: Amount of air expelled out from lungs during first half of FVC test
  - Useful when detecting obstructive disease
  - $FEF_{50\%}$ lesser in obstructive airway disease
- Maximum mid-expiratory flow rate ($FEF_{25-75\%}$):
  - Amount of air expelled out during middle half of FVC maneuver
  - It is an early indicator of obstructive disease of medium sized airways
  - The $FEF_{25-75\%}$ is usually normal in restrictive lung diseases
  - Normal value:
    - Absolute values:
      - 4.7 L/second
      - 280 L/min
    - Percentage of predicted value: 100 + 25% of predicted value
  - Much more reliable and reproducible than FEV_1/FVC
- Peak expiratory flow rate:
  - Maximum flow rate achieved during FVC maneuver beginning with full inspiration and ending with maximal expiration
  - Useful measure of response to bronchodilator therapy
  - Normal value: 600 L/min
- Maximum voluntary ventilation:
  - Refers to maximum volume of gas that can be breathed in 1 minute voluntarily
  - Patient breathes in and out as maximally and rapidly for 10, 12 or 15 seconds
  - During the test, each breath is taken systematically:
    - At patients own ventilatory rate
    - Volume of air should be more than tidal volume
    - However, volume of air should be less than vital capacity
  - Total volume breathed is measured and results are extrapolated to 1 minute
  - Factors affecting MVV:
    - Strength of respiratory muscles
    - Lung-thoracic compliance
    - Airway resistance
  - This is the best test of respiratory muscle strength
  - Normal values: 170 L/minute in adults
  - Causes of reduced MVV:
    - Advanced age
    - Female sex
    - Neuromuscular disorders
    - Obstructive lung diseases

- MVV is usually normal in RLD
- Measurement of MVV depends on patient effort and cooperation
- It is a poor predictor of true pulmonary compliance and strength

Post-bronchodilator Spirometry

- Post-bronchodilator spirometry is used to determine reversibility of airflow limitation
- Indications:
  - Evidence of airway obstruction on baseline spirometry
  - Asthma
  - COPD
- Procedure:
  - Albuterol is administered via MDI (4 inhalations of 90–100 μg)
  - Equivalent short-acting β-agonist may be used via an MDI
  - Proper MDI technique is vital to prevent false negative results
  - Spirometry is then repeated after 10-15 minutes of bronchodilator therapy
- Increase in FEV_1 of > 12% or 200 mL suggests acute bronchodilator responsiveness

Limitations

- Not disease specific
- Cannot be used as sole screening tool
- Variable values depending upon age, sex, gender
- Effort dependant results
- Specific measurements do not predict post-op pulmonary complications

Interpretation of Spirometry

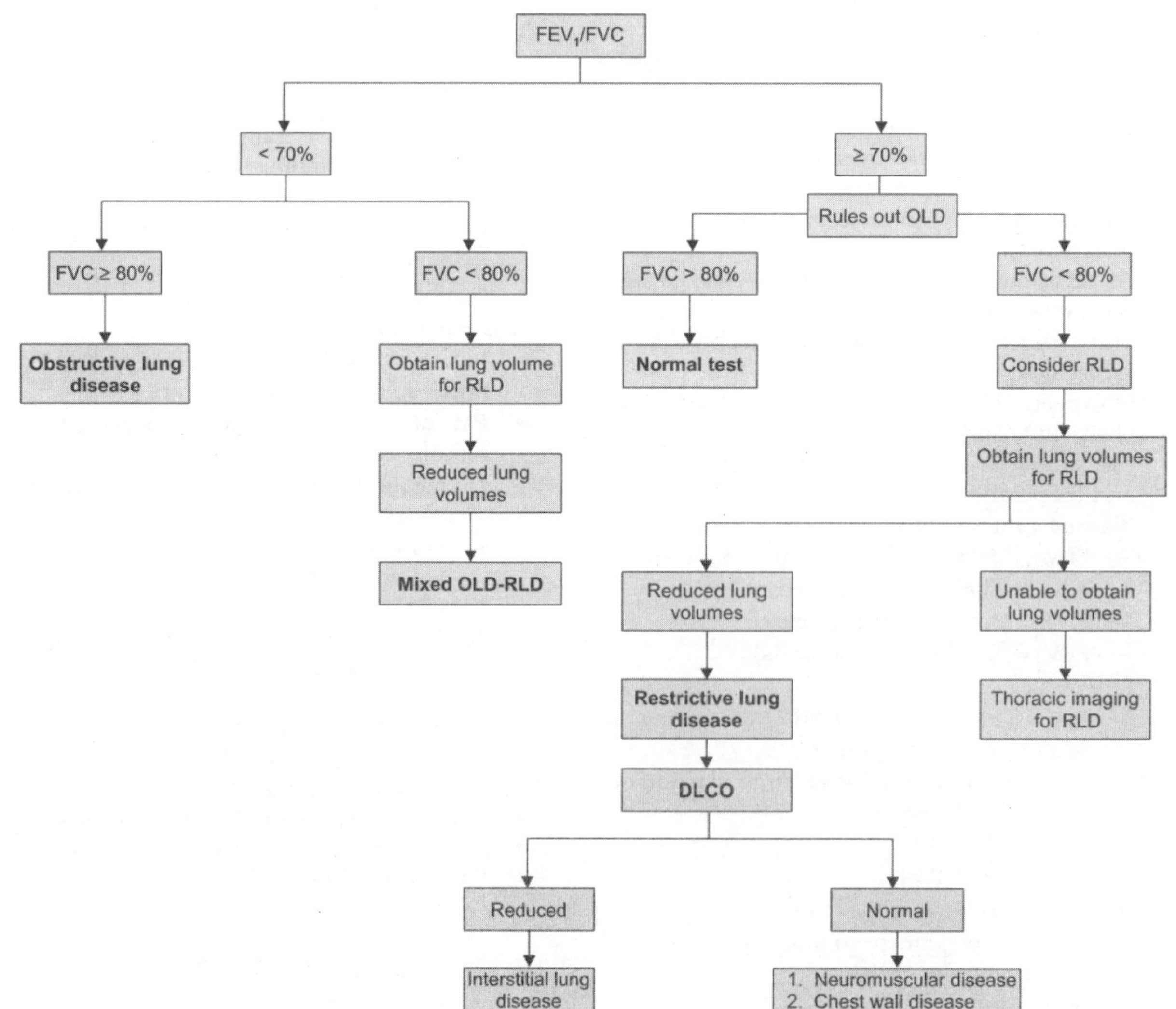

FUNCTIONAL RESIDUAL CAPACITY

Introduction

- It is the volume of air remaining in the lungs at passive end-expiration
- FRC = Residual Volume + Expiratory Reserve Volume (RV + ERV)

Normal Values

- Adults: Approximately 2400 mL for a 70-kg adult
- Children: 30-35 mL/kg
- Amounts to around 40% of total lung capacity

Measurement

- Body plethysmography:
  - ***Gold standard*** for measuring FRC
  - This technique measures FRC using Boyles law
  - Patient is placed in a ***body box or pneumotachometer***
  - This box is used to measure volume changes and FRC
  - Changes in volume are determined by changes in pressure within body box
  - Technique measures the total volume of gas at end expiration
  - This volume includes air which is trapped behind closed airways
  - Thus, it is useful when air spaces do not communicate with the bronchial tree
  - Other values derived by body plethysmography:
    - Specific airway resistance (sRaw)
    - Airway resistance (Raw)
    - Shift volume
  - However, this method requires sophisticated and expensive equipment
- Helium dilution method:
  - Measures dilution of air present in lungs at end-expiration by inhaled helium
  - Procedure:
    - Spirometer is filled with 10% helium in oxygen
    - Thus, the amount of helium is known at beginning of test (C_1)
    - Initial volume of helium-oxygen mixture in spirometer is taken as V_1
    - Patient is asked to breathe normally, starting from end-tidal expiration
    - The helium enters lungs and spreads to a new concentration C_2
    - V_2 is taken as the unknown volume in the lungs
    - Helium dilution is calculated by using conservation of mass principle

$$V_2 = \frac{V_1 (C_1 - C_2)}{C_2}$$

  - Technique does not measure air which is trapped behind closed airways
  - The technique is therefore older and simpler, but less accurate
- Nitrogen washout method:
  - Also called ***Fowlers method***
  - This is based on washing out nitrogen by breathing in 100% oxygen
  - Subject inhales 100% O_2 and exhales through a one-way valve
  - Total quantity of N_2 washed out of lungs by breathing in oxygen is measured
  - FRC is then determined by plotting N_2 concentration vs expired volume
  - More commonly used for anatomical dead space calculation
- Other methods:
  - CT scan
  - Multiple breath SF_6 procedure

Physiology

- FRC serves three primary physiological functions:
  - Reserve of oxygen:
    - FRC volume oxygenates blood passing through the lungs during apnea
    - Thus, it serves as a reserve of oxygen in the event of apnea
  - Prevention of airway collapse:
    - FRC volume keeps the alveoli partially inflated at end-expiration
    - This prevents airway collapse and atelectasis
  - Minimizes pulmonary vascular resistance:
    - FRC prevents airway collapse at end expiration
    - This helps in keeping small intra-alveolar vessels patent
    - Thus, FRC helps in minimizing pulmonary vascular resistance
- Effect on ventilation-perfusion relationship:
  - FRC also influences ventilation-perfusion relationship within the lung
  - Reduction in FRC causes atelectasis and lung collapse
  - This results in venous admixture and arterial hypoxemia

- Impact on intra-pleural pressure:
  - At FRC, inward recoil and outward expansion forces on lungs are equal
  - Thus, forces which retract and expand the lungs are exactly equal and opposite
  - This represents a balance between:
    - Inward forces of lung parenchyma
    - Outward forces of the chest wall
  - This creates a negative intrapleural pressure
  - In erect position, lung tissue gravitates towards the base
  - This creates a vertical gradient of intrapleural pressure
  - Intrapleural pressure at the apex = –10 cm H_2O (erect)
  - Intrapleural pressure at the base = –2.5 cm H_2O (erect)
  - Thus, alveoli are more distended at apex than at base

Factors Affecting Functional Residual Capacity

- Increased functional residual capacity:
  - Factors influencing lung size:
    - Increased height
    - Male gender
    - Peri-bronchial fibrosis
    - Bronchiolar obstruction
    - Obstructive lung disease
  - Factors influencing lung compliance:
    - Pathologically increased lung compliance as in asthma
    - Increased end expiratory pressure (auto-PEEP)
  - Factors influencing chest wall compliance:
    - Open chest
    - Uptight position
    - Prone position
- Decreased functional residual capacity:
  - Factors influencing lung size:
    - Short stature
    - Female gender
    - Restrictive lung diseases
  - Factors influencing lung compliance:
    - ARDS
    - Pulmonary edema
    - Tuberculosis
    - Sarcoidosis
  - Factors influencing chest wall compliance:
    - Increased intra-abdominal pressure:
      - Pregnancy
      - Ascites, hepatosplenomegaly
      - Major abdominal surgery
    - Decreased respiratory muscle tone:
      - Anesthesia/sedation
      - Neuromuscular diseases:
        - Myasthenia gravis
        - Lambert-Eaton syndrome
      - Bilateral diaphragmatic palsy
    - Others:
      - Supine position (decreases FRC by 20–25%)
      - Trendelenburg position
      - Obesity
      - Circumferential burns
      - Chest binder devices

Significance of Functional Residual Capacity

- Gas exchange:
  - Allows continuous exchange of gases
  - Some air is always present in lungs due to FRC
  - Therefore, O_2 and CO_2 concentrations are constant
- Dilutes inhaled toxic gases
- Load on right ventricle is reduced as collapsed lung increases PVR
- Preoxygenation:
  - Fills FRC (prior to induction) with oxygen
  - This increases oxygen reserve from 500 mL to 2400 mL
  - Thus, apneic periods are tolerated better
- Closing capacity (CC):
  - If CC = FRC, some airways remain closed, even with normal tidal volume breathing
  - If CC > FRC, airway closure causing V/Q mismatch
- Position: FRC reduces with:
  - Supine position
  - Trendelenburg position

Consequences of Decreased FRC

- Effects on lung mechanics:
  - Decreased lung compliance
  - Increased airway resistance due to loss of alveolar radial traction
  - Decreased tidal volume and increased respiratory rate
  - Increased work of breathing
  - Decreased tolerance of postural changes
- Effects on gas-exchange:
  - Decreased oxygen reserve causing reduced tolerance of apnea

- Increased resorption atelectasis
- Increased intra-pulmonary shunting

❖ Effects on pulmonary circulation:
- Increased pulmonary vascular resistance
- Increased right ventricular afterload

Effects of Anesthesia

❖ Reduced FRC:
- FRC reduced by around 20% (500-700 mL) post-induction
- This change is independent of NM paralysis and controlled ventilation
- Thus, reduction in FRC is seen in spontaneous and controlled ventilation
- FRC can be reduced by up to 50% in obese patients

❖ Mechanism: Reduced FRC occurs due to:
- Loss of inspiratory muscle tone:
  - This causes loss of outward recoil of chest wall
  - Thus, chest is drawn inwards, reducing the FRC
- Loss of tone of accessory muscles:
  - Scalene
  - Sternocleidomastoid
  - Intercostal muscles
- Loss of tone of diaphragm:
  - This causes a cephalad displacement of the diaphragm
  - Cephalad displacement is due to increase in abdominal blood volume
  - This causes a reduction in FRC
- Increased lung and chest wall recoil
- Absorption atelectasis due to high inspired FiO_2
- Supine/Trendelenburg position

❖ Consequences:
- Areas of low V/Q ratio
- Atelectasis
- Altered pulmonary mechanics
- Airway closure
- Postoperative hypoxemia

❖ Causes of postoperative reduction in FRC:
- Incisional pain
- Reflex diaphragmatic dysfunction: *main cause*
- Absence of spontaneous sighs
- Mechanical disruption of thorax and abdomen
- Stimulation of splanchnic and visceral afferents due to:
  - Bowel distention
  - Local irritation
  - Pneumo-peritoneum

❖ Prevention:
- 30° head up tilt
- Positive End Expiratory Pressure
- CPAP

❖ Restoration of FRC by:
- Early and active lung expansion manuvers:
  - Deep breathing and coughing
  - Incentive spirometry
  - CPAP
  - Recruitment manuvers
  - Sighs: Can generate upto 40 cm H_2O pressure
- Adequate postoperative analgesia:
  - Epidural: Very effective
  - Systemic opioids
  - Restoration of FRC by analgesia alone is limited and never complete

LUNG COMPLIANCE

Introduction

❖ Lung compliance is the change in lung volume (lung expansion) per unit pressure change

❖ Normal compliance of intact lung: 100 mL/cmH_2O

Calculation of Compliance

❖ Total lung compliance is calculated using the transthoracic pressure gradient

$$\text{Compliance CT (L/cm } H_2O) = \frac{\Delta V \text{ (litres)}}{\Delta P \text{ (cm } H_2O)}$$

Where,
C_T is total compliance
V is change in lung volume
P is change in pressure

❖ Total compliance is related to:
- Compliance of chest wall (C_{CW})
- Compliance of lungs (C_L)

❖ The lung and chest wall compliance are in series, analogous to electrical capacitance

❖ Thus, the reciprocal of total compliance is equal to sum of reciprocals of:
- Compliance of chest wall
- Compliance of lung

$$1/C_T = 1/C_L + 1/C_{CW} \text{ OR } C_T = \frac{(C_L)(C_{CW})}{(C_L + C_{CW})}$$

Where,
Total compliance = C_T
Lung compliance = C_L
Chest wall compliance = C_{CW}

❖ Compliance of the lung:
- Calculated using the transpulmonary pressure gradient
- Factors affecting lung compliance:

- Changes in lung volume
- Changes in pulmonary blood volume
- Extravascular lung water
- Pulmonary inflammatory processes and fibrosis

$$C_L\ (L/cm\ H_2O) = \frac{\Delta V\ (litres)}{P_A - P_{pl}\ (cm\ H_2O)}$$

Where,
C_L = compliance of the lung
P_A is the alveolar pressure
P_{pl} is the intrapleural pressure

- Compliance of the chest wall:
  - Calculated using the transmural pressure gradient
  - Factors affecting chest wall compliance:
    - Chest wall edema
    - Obesity
    - Pleural effusion
    - Pneumothorax
    - Diseases of costovertebral joints

$$CCW\ (L/cm\ H_2O) = \frac{\Delta V\ (litres)}{P_{pl} - P_{ambient}\ (cm\ H_2O)}$$

- Normal values are:
  - C_L = 200 mL/cmH_2O
  - C_{CW} = 200 mL/cmH_2O
  - C_T = 100 mL/cmH_2O
- In clinical practise only total lung compliance is measured

Measurement of Compliance

- Patient exhales out from a position of total lung capacity in steps of 500 mL
- Esophageal pressure is measured simultaneously
- The glottis is open and lung is allowed to stabilise for few seconds after each step
- A pressure volume curve is obtained from the spirometer
- Compliance of the lung is reflected by the slope of the curve

Types

- Static compliance
- Dynamic compliance
- Specific compliance

Static Compliance

- Refers to the lung compliance measured when there is no airflow
- Static compliance is a reflection of the elastic resistance of lung and chest wall
- Thus, components of static compliance are:
  - Chest wall compliance
  - Lung tissue compliance
- Measures between 40-60 mL/cm H_2O in critically ill patients

$$\text{Static compliance } (C_{ST}) = \frac{\text{Corrected tidal volume}}{(\text{Plateau pressure} - \text{PEEP})}$$

- Thus, static compliance is inversely related to plateau inspiratory pressure:
  - Obtained by applying inspiratory hold/occluding port at end inspiration
  - It is the pressure needed to maintain lung inflation in the absence of air flow
- Static compliance is usually higher than dynamic compliance
- This is because plateau pressure is usually lesser than peak inspiratory pressure
- Static compliance can be used to identify the ideal PEEP value

Dynamic Compliance

- Refers to the lung compliance measured when during normal tidal breathing
- Airway resistance is critical factor is measuring dynamic compliance
- Reflects condition of airway resistance and elastic properties of lung and chest wall
- Thus, components of dynamic compliance are:
  - Chest wall compliance
  - Lung tissue compliance
  - Airway resistance
- Measures between 30-40 mL/cm H_2O in critically ill patients
- Peak inspiratory pressure is pressure used to deliver tidal volume by overcoming non-elastic (airways) and elastic (lung parenchyma) resistance

Dynamic compliance (C_{DYN}) =

$$\frac{\text{Corrected tidal volume}}{(\text{Peak inspiratory pressure} - \text{PEEP})}$$

Specific Compliance

- It refers to the compliance that is normalized by a lung volume, usually the FRC
- Specific compliance is a measure of intrinsic elastic property of lung tissue
- It is used to compare the static lung compliance at different lung volumes
- Normally measures 50 mL/cm H_2O

- Similar value in both sexes and all ages including neonates

$$\text{Specific compliance} = \frac{\text{Compliance}}{\text{FRC (in mL)}}$$

Frequency Dependant Compliance

- An important determinant of dynamic compliance is airway resistance
- Airway resistance increases with airflow and a faster respiratory rate
- Therefore, there is a paucity of time for air to redistribute to slower lung units
- This causes an increased pressure measured per unit volume, ie, lower compliance
- Thus, any increase in airflow will decrease the dynamic compliance
- This is referred to as frequency-dependant dynamic compliance
- Static compliance is measured in the absence of any airflow
- Therefore, static compliance is frequency-independant

Factors Affecting Compliance

- Lung elastic recoil:
  - Surface tension in alveoli
  - Stretched elastic fibres in lung parenchyma
- Lung volume
- Diseased states

Variations in Compliance

- High compliance:
  - Increased lung compliance:
    - Surfactant therapy
    - Supine, upright posture
    - Ageing related loss of lung connective tissue
    - Emphysema
  - Increased chest wall compliance:
    - ***Ehler-Danlos syndrome***
    - Rib resection
    - Cachexia
    - Flail segment rib fractures
    - Open chest
- Low compliance:
  - Low static lung compliance:
    - Loss of surfactant: ARDS
    - Decreased lung elasticity:
      - Pulmonary fibrosis
      - Pulmonary edema
    - Decreased functional lung volume:
      - Pneumonectomy
      - Lobectomy
      - Pneumonia
      - Atelectasis
      - Small stature
    - Alveolar de-recruitment
    - Alveolar over-distension
  - Low dynamic lung compliance:
    - Increased airway resistance:
      - Bronchospasm
      - Asthma
      - COPD
      - Kinking of ETT
      - Airway obstruction due to retained secretions
    - Tachypnea causing reduced frequency-dependant dynamic compliance
  - Decreased chest wall compliance:
    - Structural abnormalities:
      - Kyphoscoliosis
      - Pectus excavatum
      - Circumferential burns
      - Surgical rib fixation
      - Chest binders
    - Functional abnormalities: Muscle spasm due to:
      - Seizures
      - Tetanus
    - Extra-thoracic causes:
      - Obesity
      - Abdominal compartment syndrome
      - Prone position

High Compliance

- Change in lung volume is large per unit change in pressure
- Exhalation is often inadequate due to lack of elastic recoil of lungs
- Related to conditions which increase patients FRC
- Characteristics:
  - Obstructive lung defect
  - Chronic air trapping
  - Destruction of lung tissue
  - Enlargement of terminal and respiratory bronchioles
  - Reduced minute ventilation

Low Compliance

- Change in volume is small per unit pressure change
- Work of breathing is high as lungs are stiff
- Low compliance causes refractory hypoxemia

- ❖ Condition compensated for by an increase in respiratory rate
- ❖ Characteristics:
  - Restrictive lung defect
  - Reduced lung volume
  - Reduced minute ventilation

Hysteresis Curve

- ❖ Different readings of the lung volume are taken at specific pressure points
- ❖ These are plotted on a curve to yield the pressure-volume curve
- ❖ This represents both the elastic and airway resistance properties of the lung
- ❖ Lung volume at any given pressure during inspiration is lesser than during expiration
- ❖ This is referred to as hysteresis and occurs due to:
  - Recruitment and de-recruitment of alveoli:
    - Collapsed alveoli require additional energy to re-expand
    - In contrast, well inflated alveoli are relatively elastic
    - These alveoli require lesser energy to inflate further
    - Thus, pressure-volume relationship of inflated alveoli are different
  - Alveolar surface tension:
    - Surface tension in collapsed alveoli is lower than inflated alveoli
    - This is because surfactant molecules are more closely packed in deflated alveoli
    - This increases the concentration at the air-fluid interface
    - This in turn decreases the surface tension in collapsed alveoli
- ❖ Interpretation of hysteresis curve:
  - The two meeting points in the curve represent:
    - End-inspiratory point
    - End-expiratory point
  - Line connecting the 2 meeting points measures the dynamic compliance.

Clinical Implications

- ❖ Work of breathing:
  - Lung compliance determines 65% of the work of breathing
  - Thus, decrease in compliance causes increased work of breathing (WOB)
  - The body adapts compensatory responses to negate this increased WOB
  - In the presence of a constant P_{PEAK} and P_{PLAT}:

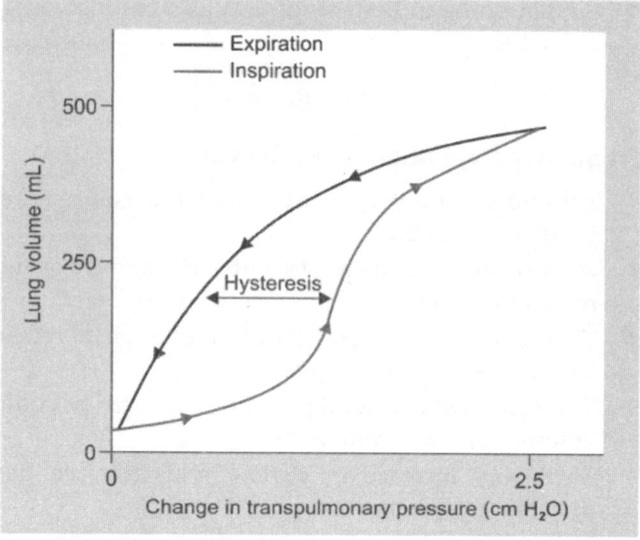

Fig. 14: Hysteresis curve.

    - Decrease in compliance causes a reduction in the tidal volume
    - This represents a compensatory response to low compliance
    - Since increase in WOB is avoided, TV reduces
    - Thus, compensatory response to low compliance comprises of:
      - Reduced tidal volume
      - Faster respiratory rate
- ❖ Effects on ventilation and oxygenation:
  - Reduced compliance results in:
    - Muscle fatigue
    - Ventilatory and oxygenation failure
  - Oxygenation failure causes reduction in delivery of O_2 needed for metabolism
  - Ventilatory failure occurs when tachypnea fails to eliminate carbon dioxide

Indicators of Compliance

- ❖ Hysteresis curve:
  - Line joining the 2 points of hysteresis curve measures dynamic compliance
  - Shift in slope towards volume axis indicates increase in compliance
  - Shift in slope towards pressure axis indicates low compliance
- ❖ Changes in peak inspiratory pressure:
  - When airway resistance increases:
    - Peak inspiratory pressure (PIP) increases
    - Plateau inspiratory pressure (P_{PLAT}) remains unchanged

- Thus, as PIP increases, dynamic compliance reduces
- As P_{PLAT} remains unchanged, static compliance remains the same
- When bronchospasm resolves, PIP and C_{DYN} return to normal

❖ Changes in plateau pressure:
- Changes in plateau pressure parallel changes in peak inspiratory pressure
- For e.g., atelectasis causes increased P_{PLAT} and PIP
- As P_{PLAT} and PIP are increased, static and dynamic compliance reduces
- When atelectasis resolves, P_{PLAT} and PIP return to normal

FLOW VOLUME LOOPS

Introduction

❖ Graphic analysis of inspiratory and expiratory flow rates against lung volume

❖ This is recorded during a maximally forced inspiratory and expiratory maneuver

❖ Lung volume is plotted on the X-axis and flow rate on Y-axis

❖ Expiratory flow rate is displayed above the horizontal baseline

❖ Inspiratory flow rate is displayed below the horizontal baseline

❖ Changes in contour of loop can aid in diagnosis and localization of airway obstruction

Procedure

❖ Patient is instructed to:
- Take a full inspiration to total lung capacity
- Exhale forcefully and maximally to residual volume (RV)
- Inspire forcefully and completely back to total lung capacity

❖ Thus, the maneuver typically involves 4 phases of breathing into spirometer:
- Tidal breathing for several breaths
- Maximum inspiratory effort to TLC
- Maximum expiration to residual volume as forcefully and as quickly as possible
- Maximum inspiration to TLC

Normal Curve

❖ Expiratory curve:
- Characterized by a rapid rise in the curve to peak flow rate
- This is followed by a linear fall in flow as the patient exhales towards RV
- The expiratory flow curve can be divided into quarters
- Flow rate at which 25% of VC has been exhaled is called FEF_{25}
- Flow rate at midpoint of VC (between TLC and RV) is known as FEF_{50}
- Flow rate at which 75% of the VC has been exhaled is called FEF_{75}
- During exhalation, maximal flow occurs during the first 25% of the maneuver
- Flow rates decrease progressively towards the RV
- Even with increasing effort, maximal flow rate decreases as RV is approached
- This is called expiratory flow limitation

❖ Inspiratory curve:
- Symmetrical saddle shaped curve
- Flow rate at midpoint of inspiration is called forced inspiratory flow-50 (FIF_{50})
- Normally FEF_{50} is less than FIF_{50} (FEF_{50}: $FIF_{50} < 1$)

❖ The flow volume loop yields information about:
- Forced vital capacity
- Tidal volume
- Peak inspiratory flow rate
- Peak expiratory flow rate
- Type of lung and airway pathology

❖ Parts of the normal expiratory curve:
- Effort dependent part (start of curve to V_{75}):
  - Refers to the first part of expiration
  - Upto approximately one third of vital capacity
  - Increasing the expiratory effort generates increased flow rate
  - Primarily due to subjects muscle effort rather than lung characteristics
- Effort independent part: (V_{75}-V_{25})
  - Linear part of curve after the first one-third of expiration
  - Increasing effort beyond this point will not cause increase in flow
  - Thus, it is effort-independent and flow-limited
  - Occurs due to dynamic compression of large airways.

Fixed Upper Airway Obstruction

❖ Can result in intra-thoracic or extrathoracic obstruction

❖ Examples:
- Tracheal stenosis

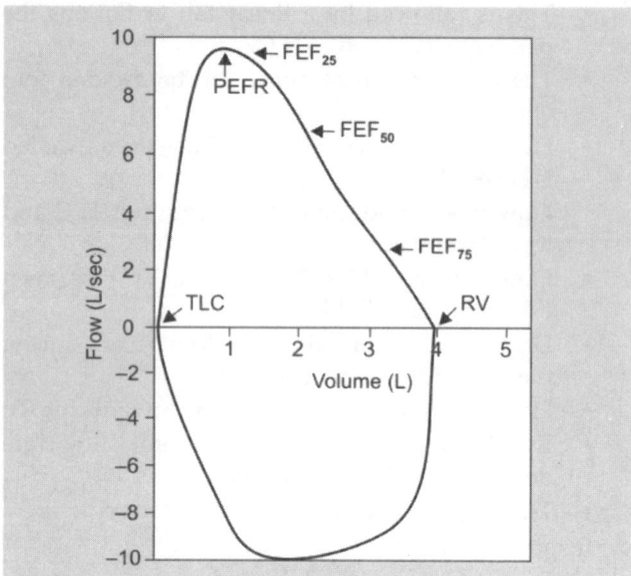

Fig. 15: Normal flow volume loop.

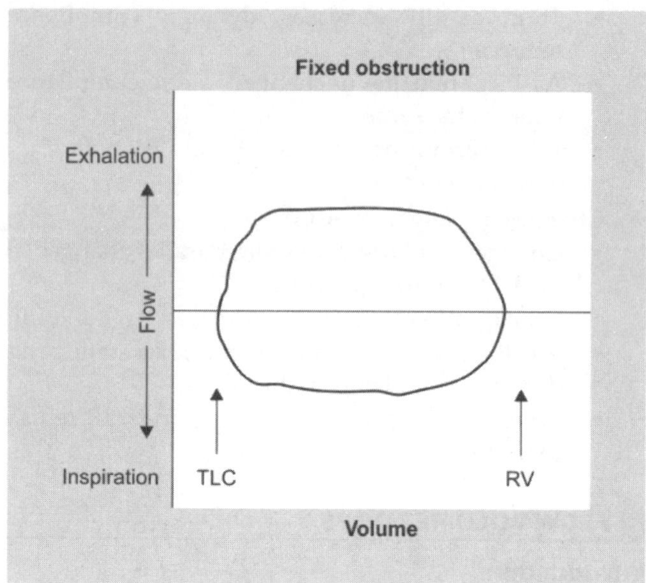

Fig. 16: Flow volume loop in fixed airway obstruction.

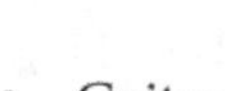

- Goitre
- Tumors

❖ Fixed obstruction limits modulating effect of transmural pressure on luminal diameter

❖ No significant change is seen in obstruction during inspiration and expiration

❖ Thus, airflow is limited equally during both inspiration and expiration

❖ This causes flattening of both inspiratory and expiratory limbs of flow volume loop.

❖ E/I = 1

❖ FEF_{50}: FIF_{50} = 1

Variable Extrathoracic Obstruction

❖ *E*xpiratory flow *N*ormal in *E*xtrathoracic obstruction

❖ Characterized by truncation or flattening of maximal inspiratory flow loop

❖ Thus, expiratory flow is normal while inspiratory flow reduces

❖ Examples:
- Vocal cord palsies
- Laryngomalacia
- Extra-thoracic tracheomalacia
- Obstructive sleep apnea syndrome
- Pharyngeal muscle weakness
- Neuromuscular disorders

❖ During inspiration:
- Upper airway is narrowed due to subatmospheric intra-luminal pressure

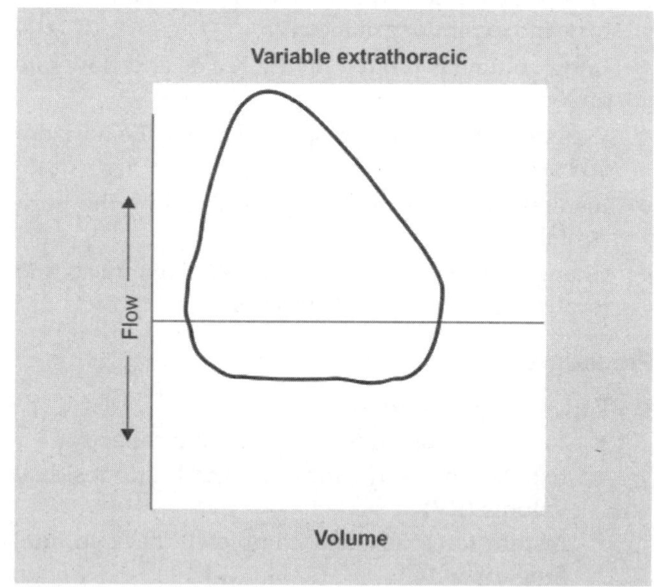

Fig. 17: Flow volume loop in variable extrathoracic obstruction.

- This results in inspiratory flow-limitation
- The effect is accentuated by sucking in of any obstructive lesions
- This may result in a Venturi effect, further reducing inspiratory flow

❖ Expiration is normal as the obstruction is pushed outwards by force of expiration

❖ E/I >1

❖ FEF_{50}/ FIF_{50} is elevated (> 1).

Variable Intrathoracic Obstruction

- Inspiratory limb is Normal in Intrathoracic obstruction
- Flattening or truncation of envelope of maximal expiratory curve occurs
- This is due to expiratory flow limitation
- Examples:
  - Retrosternal goitre
  - Intrathoracic tracheal tumors
  - Intrathoracic tracheomalacia
  - Bronchial tumors
  - Bronchogenic cysts
- Pleural pressure is negative compared with intratracheal pressure during inspiration
- Tumor is therefore sucked outwards during inspiration and does not cause obstruction
- Thus, no change is produced during inspiration and normal morphology is retained
- During expiration, pleural pressure becomes positive relative to tracheal pressure
- Thus, the tumor is pushed into the trachea causing partial obstruction
- This may lead to turbulent flow and Venturi effect adding to airway narrowing
- This produces an accentuated expiratory flow limitation
- Thus, expiratory part of flow volume loop is flattened or truncated
- E/I <1
- FEF_{50}: FIF_{50} is reduced.

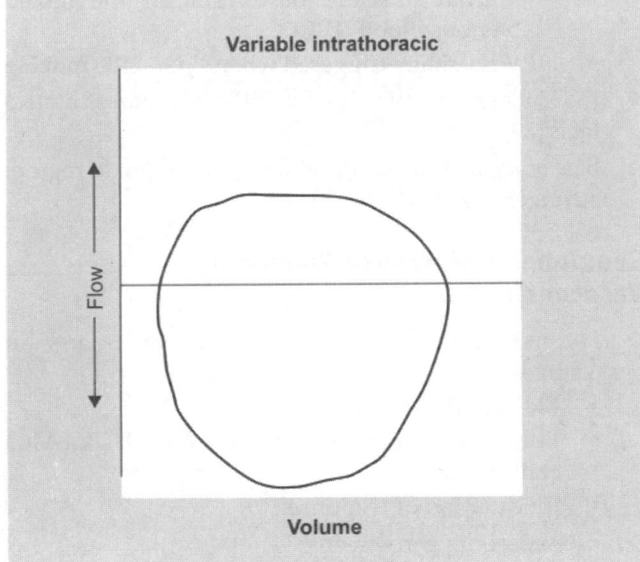

Fig. 18: Flow volume loop in variable intrathoracic obstruction.

Obstructive Lung Disease

- Examples:
  - Asthma
  - COPD
  - Bronchiectasis
  - Bronchiolitis
- Characterized by:
  - Increased TLC
  - Reduced peak inspiratory flow rate
  - Reduced peak expiratory flow rate
  - Failure of expiratory curve to reach zero
  - Scalloping of expiratory limb
- *Scalloping of expiratory limb of loop*:
  - Also called *coving or scooped out appearance*
  - Causes curvilinear expiratory limb with upward concavity
  - This is caused by reduction in flow rate in effort-independent part of curve
  - The reduction in flow rate occurs due to:
    - Compression of major central airways:
      - Seen only in severe emphysema
      - Airway support from surrounding parenchyma is lost
      - This results in large airway compression
    - Decreased elastic recoil of lung due to loss of lung parenchyma
    - Increased small airway resistance due to:
      - Narrowing of small airways
      - Bronchospasm
      - Airway secretions
  - Thus, normal reduction in expiratory flow rate is accentuated
  - *Airway collapse pattern*:
    - Seen in severe emphysema
    - Inward concavity becomes more accentuated
    - Results in the development of an inflection point
    - This is called airway collapse pattern of flow volume loop
- Initial part of expiratory curve represents the large airways
- Larger airways usually empty quickly without much obstruction
- Features seen in chronic bronchitis are:
  - Severe decrease in peak expiratory flow
  - Relatively mild scalloping.

Restrictive Lung Disease

- Examples:
  - Interstitial lung disease
  - Kyphoscoliosis

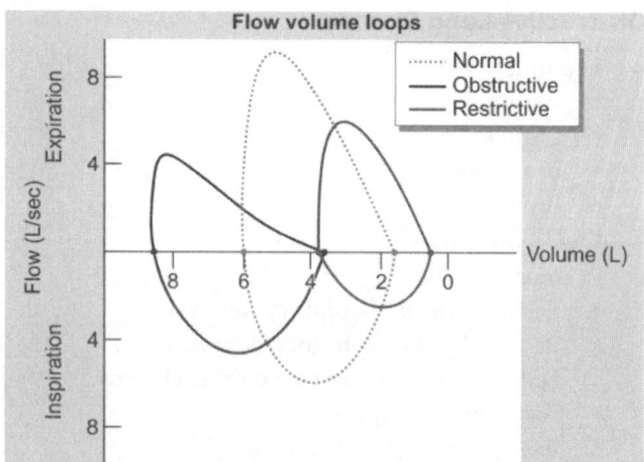

Fig. 19: Flow volume loop in pulmonary diseases.

- Characterized by:
  - Reduced TLC
  - Reduced vital capacity
  - Rapid decrease in inspiratory flow rate
  - Increased expiratory flow rate
  - Normal $FEF_{25-75\%}$ as no obstruction to airflow is present
- Thus, both the overall lung volume and peak flow rate are reduced
- However, when corrected for lung volume, the peak flow rate is supra-normal
- This is due to increased elastic recoil of the respiratory system
- This results in a tall and narrow flow volume loop
- The flow volume loop has a *witch-hat appearance* with a steep descending limb

  Mixed lung disease: Features of both OLD and RLD

HYPOXIC PULMONARY VASOCONSTRICTION

Introduction

- Refers to the reflex contraction of vascular smooth muscle in pulmonary circulation in response to low regional partial pressure of oxygen
- Is an auto-regulatory mechanism which reduces blood flow in hypoxic lung regions
- It is a distinguishing feature of pulmonary circulation from systemic circulation
- This is because in systemic circulation vasodilatation occurs in response to hypoxia

Role of Hypoxic Pulmonary Vasoconstriction

- In normal lung:
  - Ventilation and perfusion are not perfectly matched in the normal lung
  - Both ventilation and perfusion tend to increase towards the basal regions of lung
  - Perfusion tends to increase more, compared with ventilation at the lung bases
  - Thus, the V/Q ratio is lower at the basal regions
  - At the apical regions, ventilation is more than perfusion
  - Thus, V/Q ratio is more at the apical regions
  - However, role of HPV in normal lung is minimal
- In diseased lungs:
  - HPV is important to maintain respiratory homeostasis in:
    - COPD
    - Interstitial lung disease
    - Asthma
    - Pneumonia
    - Pulmonary edema
    - Pulmonary embolism
  - In these conditions, normal gas exchange depends on optimal V/Q matching
  - HPV plays a crucial role in redistributing blood flow to ventilated alveoli
  - Thus, it prevents intrapulmonary shunting and preserves gas exchange

Stimulus for HPV

- Partial pressure of oxygen in alveoli:
  - Partial pressure in O_2 in alveoli is the strongest stimulus
  - This in turn is determined by:
    - Partial pressure of oxygen in alveolus (P_AO_2)
    - Partial pressure of oxygen in the mixed venous blood (P_VO_2)
  - HPV is usually triggered when $P_AO_2 < 100$ mm Hg
- PvO_2: Primary stimulus for HPV in areas of atelectasis
- *Size of hypoxic segment*: Smaller the hypoxic region, stronger the HPV

Components of Hypoxic Pulmonary Vasoconstriction

- Hypoxic pulmonary vasoconstriction occurs in 3 stages:
  - Biological oxygen sensing
  - Pulmonary arterial smooth muscle cell (PASMC) contraction
  - Modulation of responses
- Biological oxygen sensing:
  - Primary stimulus is tissue partial pressure of oxygen in pulmonary arteriole

- This in turn is determined by:
  - Partial pressure of oxygen in alveolus (P_AO_2)
  - Partial pressure of oxygen in the mixed venous blood (P_VO_2)
- P_VO_2 is the primary stimulus in non-ventilated areas of the lung
- The stimulus in turn initiates PASMC contraction by:
  - Direct modulation of potassium channels
  - Mitochondrial reactive oxygen species (ROS) production
  - Alteration in membrane bound protein function
  - Alteration of cyclooxygenase and lipoxygenase pathways

❖ Pulmonary arterial smooth muscle cell (PASMC) contraction:
- Following initiation of HPV, PASMC membrane depolarization occurs
- This leads to an increase in cytosolic calcium ion concentration
- Calcium ions bind to calmodulin thereby activating myosin light-chain kinase
- This leads to contraction of pulmonary arterial smooth muscle cells

❖ Modulation of responses:
- Modulation refers to the inhibition or enhancement of HPV responses
- This occurs primarily through:
  - Direct physiological means via local mediators:
    - This is the principal modulating mechanism
    - Occur due to changes in intracellular pH or temperature
    - Local mechanisms involved in response modulation include:
      - Reduction in nitric oxide
      - Reduction in prostacyclin levels
      - Increased endothelin-1 production
  - Humoral mechanisms occurring primarily via angiotensin II
  - Neuronal modulation through sympathetic activation: Less important

Mechanisms of HPV

❖ Sensor mechanism:
- Occurs within mitochondria of pulmonary arterioles in a hypoxic environment
- During electron transfer, uncoupled electrons produce ROS
- This forms the basis of sensor mechanism of HPV stimulation
- Other theories of sensing mechanism:
  - Smooth muscle microsomal NADPH oxidoreductase
  - Sarcolemmal NADPH oxidase

❖ Effector mechanism:
- Core effector mechanism for HPV resides in the PASMC
- This mechanism triggers the closure of voltage-gated L-type calcium channels
- This leads to an increase in cytosolic calcium ion concentration
- This in turn leads to PASMC contraction and HPV

Phases of Hypoxic Pulmonary Vasoconstriction

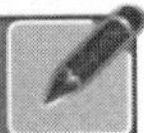

❖ Phase 1:
- Begins within the first few seconds of hypoxic insult
- Maximal at 15 minutes
- Mediated by potassium channels

❖ Phase 2:
- Occurs when hypoxia is sustained (more than 30-60 minutes)
- Maximal at 2 hours
- Mediated by increased release of endothelin

Characteristics

❖ Occurs when $P_AO_2 < 100$ mm Hg
❖ Maximal at $P_AO_2 < 30$ mm Hg
❖ Reduces blood flow to non-ventilated lung by around 50%
❖ Rapid onset over first 30 minutes
❖ Slowly increases to maximum response at around 2 hours
❖ Response to second hypoxic challenge will be greater than the first challenge

Factors Affecting HPV

❖ Physiological factors:
- Age: HPV is more intense in fetal and neonatal circulation
- Acidosis:
  - HPV can be caused by both metabolic and respiratory acidosis
  - Vasoconstriction is mainly due to alteration in extracellular H^+ ions
  - Thus, this effect is independent of hypoxic stimuli

- Respiratory diseases:
  - Respiratory diseases cause heterogenous changes in the lung
  - Thus, HPV plays an important role in optimizing V/Q matching
  - Thus, inhibition of HPV in this scenario may worsen hypoxemia
- Drugs:
  - Causing inhibition of HPV:
    - Catecholamines at low doses:
      - Adrenaline
      - Dopamine
      - Dobutamine
      - Isoprenaline
    - Acetazolamide
    - Inhaled nitric oxide
    - Corticosteroids
    - Phosphodiesterase inhibitors:
      - Sildenafil (PDE_5)
      - Milrinone (PDE_3)
    - Prostacyclin:
      - Epopostenol
      - Iloprost
    - Endothelin receptor antagonists:
      - Bosentan
      - Ambrisentan
      - Sitaxsentan
      - Macitentan
    - ACE inhibitors
    - Calcium channel blockers
    - Volatile anesthetic agents
  - Causing potentiation of HPV:
    - Catecholamines at high doses:
      - Adrenaline
      - Dopamine
      - Dopexamine
      - Noradrenaline
      - Phenylephrine
    - Inhaled β_2-agonists
    - Almitrine

Effects of Anesthesia on HPV

- During general anesthesia:
  - Ventilation-perfusion matching is altered during general anesthesia due to:
    - Absorption atelectasis due to use of high FiO_2
    - Changes in diaphragmatic shape and position with supine position
    - Changes in regional lung compliance
    - Effect of general anesthetic agents:
      - HPV is inhibited by all volatile agents when MAC > 1
      - Older agents such as halothane have a more profound effect
      - Nitrous oxide increases PVR although effect on HPV is unclear
      - Propofol has no effect on HPV
    - Positive pressure ventilation
    - Changes in cardiac output
  - During TLV, maintenance of oxygenation does not rely on HPV
  - This is because high FiO_2 prevents alveolar hypoxia in areas with low V/Q ratio
- During epidural analgesia:
  - HPV is not modulated significantly by central neurogenic control
  - Thus, neuraxial blockade may not have any impact on HPV
  - Reduction in PaO_2 during epidural anesthesia may be due to:
    - Associated one lung ventilation
    - Decrease in cardiac output
    - Decrease in mixed venous oxygen saturation due to vasodilatation
    - Anemia due to blood loss causing reduced oxygen carrying capacity

Effect of OLV on HPV

- At the onset of OLV, decrease in mean airway pressure of non-ventilated lung occurs
- This redistributes the pulmonary blood flow to non-ventilated lung
- On persistent lung collapse, blood is diverted away from non-ventilated lung by:
  - Hypoxic pulmonary vasoconstriction
  - Collapse of intra-alveolar blood vessels
- Relative contributions of each of these factors is unknown
- Effect of volatile agents on HPV during OLV:
  - During TLV, VAs are delivered to the pulmonary vasculature by alveoli
  - In contrast, during OLV, VAs are delivered through mixed venous blood
  - Effect of VA on HPV is more potent when delivered through the alveolus
  - Thus, VAs have minimal effect on HPV during OLV
- Effect of sustained hypoxia during OLV on HPV:
  - During sustained hypoxia, HPV is maximal at 2 hours following stimulus

- Once phase 2 of HPV sets in, offset of HPV is also delayed
- Thus, during subsequent lung collapse and expansion, HPV reflex is augmented
- Thus, during subsequent periods of OLV, desaturation is less pronounced
- This may be important during bilateral thoracic surgical procedures

❖ Other determinants of HPV during OLV:
- Metabolic and respiratory acidosis
- Alterations in cardiac output
- Changes in mixed venous oxygen saturation

Effects of Hypoxic Pulmonary Vasoconstriction

❖ Redistributes pulmonary blood flow from hypoxic to ventilated lung

❖ Maintains PaO_2 by reducing shunt flow through hypoxic lung

❖ Reduces shunt flow by almost 10-20%

DEAD SPACE/WASTED VENTILATION

Introduction

❖ Dead space is the amount of air inhaled, which does not take part in gaseous exchange

❖ It refers to volume which does not take part in gas exchange due to lack of perfusion

❖ Dead space ventilation:
- Is the condition when ventilation is in excess of perfusion
- It is that part of the tidal volume which does not contribute to gas exchange

❖ Minute alveolar ventilation:
- Refers to the volume reaching the respiratory zone where gas exchange occurs
- Minute alveolar ventilation depends on TV, RR and dead space volume
- Minute alveolar ventilation is an important determinant of alveolar CO_2 levels
- Normally minute volume is around 4 L/minute

Alveolar minute ventilation = {(Tidal volume) × (Respiratory rate)} – {Dead space volume}

Types

❖ Anatomic dead space

❖ Alveolar dead space

❖ Physiological dead space

❖ Apparatus dead space

Anatomical Dead Space

❖ Volume of air in conducting airways, which does not take part in gaseous exchange

❖ Refers to the air present in:
- Trachea
- Bronchi up to respiratory bronchiole

❖ Volume of anatomical dead space is measured by Fowlers method

❖ Normal values:
- In general, anatomical DS equals the patients weight in pounds
- Around 2 mL/kg of ideal body weight
- Amounts to one-third of tidal volume
- For a tidal volume of 500 mL, around 150 mL is the anatomical dead space

❖ Increased anatomical dead space:
- Anatomical dead space increases with large inspiration
- This is because of radial traction on bronchi by surrounding lung parenchyma
- It is also increased with neck extension and jaw protrusion

❖ Anatomical dead space-tidal volume ratio:
- Reduction in V_T causes a higher anatomic dead space to V_T ratio
- If V_T is reduced from 500 to 300 mL, DS to TV percent would increase from 30% (150/500) to 50% (150/300)

Alveolar Dead Space

❖ Refers to alveoli which are ventilated but not perfused in the lung parenchyma

❖ Constitutes lung volume which is unable to take part in gaseous exchange due to lack of pulmonary perfusion

❖ Alveolar dead space is obtained by subtracting anatomical DS from physiological DS

❖ Etiology:
- Occurs due to overdistension of alveoli or lack of pulmonary perfusion
- Occurs due to:
  - Overdistension of alveoli: COPD
  - Reduced perfusion: low cardiac output:
    - Congestive cardiac failure
    - Blood loss
  - Obstruction of pulmonary blood vessels:
    - Vasoconstriction
    - Pulmonary embolism

Physiological Dead Space

- This is sum of anatomical and alveolar dead space
- Physiological dead space is measured using Bohrs method
- Physiological dead space-tidal volume ratio:
  - Normal value of physiological DS-tidal volume ratio is 0.2-0.3
  - In healthy individuals, alveolar dead space volume is negligible
  - Thus, anatomical DS equals physiological DS
  - However, in diseases with altered V/Q ratios, alveolar DS increases
  - In these conditions, physiological DS exceed anatomical DS
  - $\frac{V_D}{V_T}$ less than 60% predicts weaning success from mechanical ventilation

Apparatus Dead Space

- Refers to the dead space volume contributed by the use of airway equipment
- Constitutes the fraction of the tidal volume that is rebreathed
- Thus, apparatus dead space does not contribute to carbon dioxide elimination
- Devices which increase apparatus dead space include:
  - Junction of Y-piece connectors
  - Catheter mounts
- This dead space is usually 50- 100 mL and may increase up to 300 mL
- Contribution of apparatus dead space to rebreathing may be significant in neonates
- Thus, minimal connections are warranted in this population to reduce rebreathing

Factors Increasing Physiological Dead Space

Type of change	Clinical condition
Low tidal volume	Causes relative increase in V_D/V_T: Drug over dose Neuromuscular disease
Increased alveolar dead space	Low cardiac output: Congestive cardiac failure Blood loss
	Obstructive of pulmonary blood vessels: Pulmonary vasoconstriction Pulmonary embolism

Implications of Increased Dead Space

- Carbon dioxide elimination:
  - Elimination of carbon dioxide is inversely proportional to dead space volume
  - Thus, when dead space increases, carbon dioxide elimination reduces
- Effect on minute ventilation:
  - Pulmonary diseases result in an increase in alveolar dead space
  - This triggers an increase in minute ventilation to maintain $PaCO_2$ levels
  - This is accomplished mainly by an increase in respiratory rate
- Apparatus dead space:
  - Apparatus dead space contributes significantly to rebreathing in neonates
  - MV has to be increased proportionately to ensure adequate gas exchange
  - Persistent hypercarbia necessitates minimization of apparatus DS

Causes of Wasted Ventilation

- Insufficient ventilation
- Muscle fatigue
- Ventilatory failure
- Oxygenation failure

Measurement

- Fowlers method:
  - Technique described by Fowler in 1948 to measure anatomical dead space
  - Based on washout of N_2 from lung and is also called nitrogen washout method
  - Patient is asked to inhale tidal volume of 100% O_2 starting from FRC
  - On inhalation, anatomical dead space first fills up with 100% oxygen
  - Patient then exhales through a one-way valve
  - Nitrogen content of exhaled air is measured by a nitrogen analyser
  - The nitrogen content is plotted as a function of time to obtain a graph
  - On expiration, N_2 concentration starts at 0 and increases slowly
  - Nitrogen concentration then reaches a plateau
  - The gas volume exhaled prior to reaching the plateau is the anatomical DS
  - Total volume of N_2 washed out on exhalation is also measured

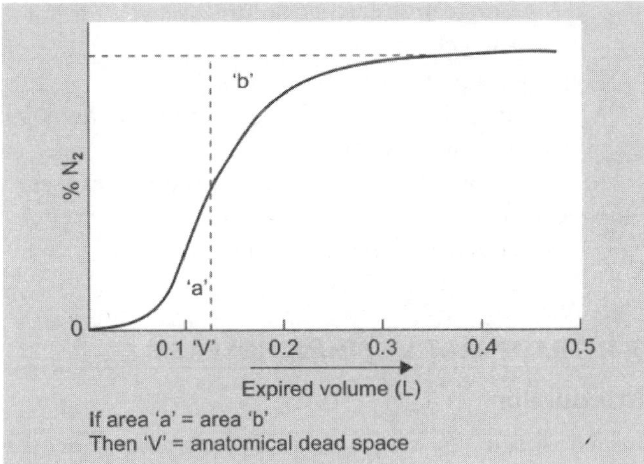

Fig. 20: Fowlers method.

- This volume can be measured with single breath/multiple breaths
- Bohrs method:
  - This is based on the assumption that carbon dioxide is absent in:
    - Anatomical dead space gas
    - Alveolar dead space gas
  - This is because there is no gas exchange in these areas
  - Thus, only the ideal alveolar gas contains carbon dioxide
  - Carbon dioxide content of mixed expired gas is equal to product of:
    - Alveolar ventilation
    - Concentration of carbon dioxide in ideal alveolar gas
  - Physiological dead space is calculated using the formula:

$$\text{Physiological dead space } V_D = \frac{(PaCO_2 - PECO_2) \times V_T}{PaCO_2}$$

Where,

$PaCO_2$ = arterial CO_2 levels

$PECO_2$ = CO_2 in mixed alveolar gas

V_T = tidal volume

- Volume capnogram:
  - Carbon dioxide is used as a marker instead of nitrogen
  - Exhaled carbon dioxide is plotted against the volume of air exhaled
  - Arterial CO_2 concentration ($PaCO_2$) is plotted on the Y-axis
  - A line is drawn at this point, parallel to the X-axis
  - A vertical line is drawn at the end tidal carbon dioxide point
  - This represents the end of expiration
  - The area under the curve represents effective alveolar ventilation
  - Area between line from $PaCO_2$ level to capnogram is the physiological DS

ALVEOLAR-ARTERIAL OXYGEN GRADIENT

Introduction

- This measures difference between oxygen concentration in alveoli and arterial system
- It is calculated as the difference between:
  - Calculated pressure of O_2 in alveolar sacs
  - Measured pressure of O_2 in blood

Calculation

$P(A\text{-}a)\ O_2$ =

(calculated P_AO_2) – (measured PaO_2) = $P_AO_2 - PaO_2$

Where:

$P(A\text{-}a)\ O_2$ = alveolar-arterial O_2 gradient in mm Hg

P_AO_2 = alveolar O_2 tension in mm Hg

P_aO_2 = arterial oxygen tension in mm Hg

Calculation of Alveolar Oxygen Pressure

- Arterial oxygen pressure is directly assessed using arterial blood gas analysis
- However, P_AO_2 is not easily measurable
- It is calculated using the alveolar gas equation:

$$P_AO_2 = [P_B - PH_2O)\ FiO_2] - \frac{[PaCO_2]}{RQ}$$

Where:

P_B = atmospheric pressure (≅ 760 mm Hg)

PH_2O = water vapour pressure (≅ 47 mm Hg)

P_aCO_2 = arterial CO_2 tension

RQ = respiratory quotient = 0.8

Physiological Alveolar Arterial Oxygen Gradient

- In an ideal system, no alveolar-arterial gradient would exist
- Thus, oxygen would diffuse and equalise across the alveolar basement membrane
- Thus, in an ideal system, $P(A\text{-}a)\ O_2$ would be zero
- However, physiological ventilation- perfusion mismatch causes a minimal $P(A\text{-}a)\ O_2$
- Thus, alveoli with low V/Q ratio and shunt cause a low PaO_2 without altering P_AO_2

- This causes an increase in the $P(A-a) O_2$
- In the presence of lung disease, A-a gradient increases with the number of unventilated alveoli

Values

- Normal $P(A-a) O_2$ ranges from 6- 10 mm Hg on room air
- On an average, $P(A-a) O_2$ increases by 4 mm Hg every decade
- Normal $P(A-a) O_2$ should be less than $\frac{[\text{patients age}]}{4} + 4$
- On 100% FiO_2, every 50 mm Hg difference in $P(A-a) O_2$ approximates a 2% shunt

Importance

- Used to estimate degree of hypoxemia:
  - $P(A-a) O_2 < 10$ mm Hg = normal
  - $P(A-a) O_2$ 10–30 mm Hg = mild impairment of gas exchange
  - $P(A-a) O_2$ 20–30 mm Hg = moderate impairment of gas exchange
  - $P(A-a) O_2 > 30$ mm Hg = severe impairment of gas exchange
- Used to locate source of hypoxemia
- To estimate degree of physiological and right-left shunt
- To predict success of weaning

Alterations in Alveolar-Arterial Gradient

- Physiological increase in $P(A-a) O_2$:
  - Old age
  - Obesity
  - Fasting
  - Supine patient
  - Heavy exercise
- Hypoxemia with increase in $P(A-a) O_2$:
  - Arises from impaired gas exchange across alveolar membrane
  - Diffusion defects:
    - Pulmonary fibrosis
    - Emphysema
    - Asbestosis
  - V/Q mismatch:
    - Pulmonary embolism
    - Airway obstruction
    - Interstitial lung disease
  - Shunting:
    - Intracardiac shunts (VSD, PDA)
    - Intrapulmonary shunts:
      - Pulmonary arterio-venous malformation
      - Pneumonia
    - Congestive cardiac failure
    - Atelectasis
- Hypoxemia with normal $P(A-a) O_2$:
  - Occurs when gas exchange across the alveolar membrane is normal
  - This is usually due to extra-pulmonary causes
  - Causes:
    - Alveolar hypoventilation
    - Low $FiO_2 < 21$ %

INTRAOPERATIVE BRONCHOSPASM

Introduction

Bronchospasm is an abnormal contraction of the smooth muscle of bronchi, resulting in acute narrowing and obstruction of the respiratory airway.

Etiology: According to cause:

Respiratory Causes

- Upper airway:
  - Tumours of pharynx and larynx
  - Tracheomalacia
  - Laryngeal edema/infection
  - Foreign body
- Lower airway:
  - COPD
  - Bronchial Asthma
  - Bronchitis
  - Bronchiectasis
  - Cystic fibrosis
- Pulmonary:
  - Infection
  - Pulmonary edema
  - Pneumonia

Mechanical Irritation

- Airway manipulation
- Endotracheal intubation
- Endobronchial intubation
- Secretions in large airway
- Aspiration of gastric contents

Drugs

- Anesthetics:
  - Desflurane in smokers
  - Isoflurane inhalation induction
- Others:
  - Morphine
  - Mivacurium, atracurium, rapacuronium, doxacurium
  - Beta blockers

- Aspirin, NSAIDs
- Cholinesterase inhibitors: neostigmine
- Atropine > 1 mg
- Glycopyrrolate > 0.5 mg

Allergy

❖ Allergens, latex allergy, anaphylaxis
❖ Drugs:
  - Antibiotics
  - IV contrast
  - Transfusion reactions

Others

❖ Light anesthetic plane
❖ Distended urinary bladder
❖ Peritoneal retractions
❖ Smoke inhalation
❖ Carcinoid tumour

Etiology: As per anesthetic stages:

❖ Causes during induction:
  - Airway irritation
  - Aspiration
  - Anaphylaxis
  - Pulmonary edema
  - Displaced ETT
  - Unknown
❖ Causes during maintenance: *Most common*:
  - Anaphylaxis
  - Aspiration
  - Airway irritation
  - Pneumothorax
  - Endobronchial intubation
  - Pulmonary edema
  - Drug induced:
    - Vancomycin
    - Protamine
❖ Causes at extubation:
  - Airway irritation
  - Extubation spasm
  - Pulmonary edema
  - Aspiration
  - Anaphylaxis/allergy
  - Accidental extubation

Pathophysiology

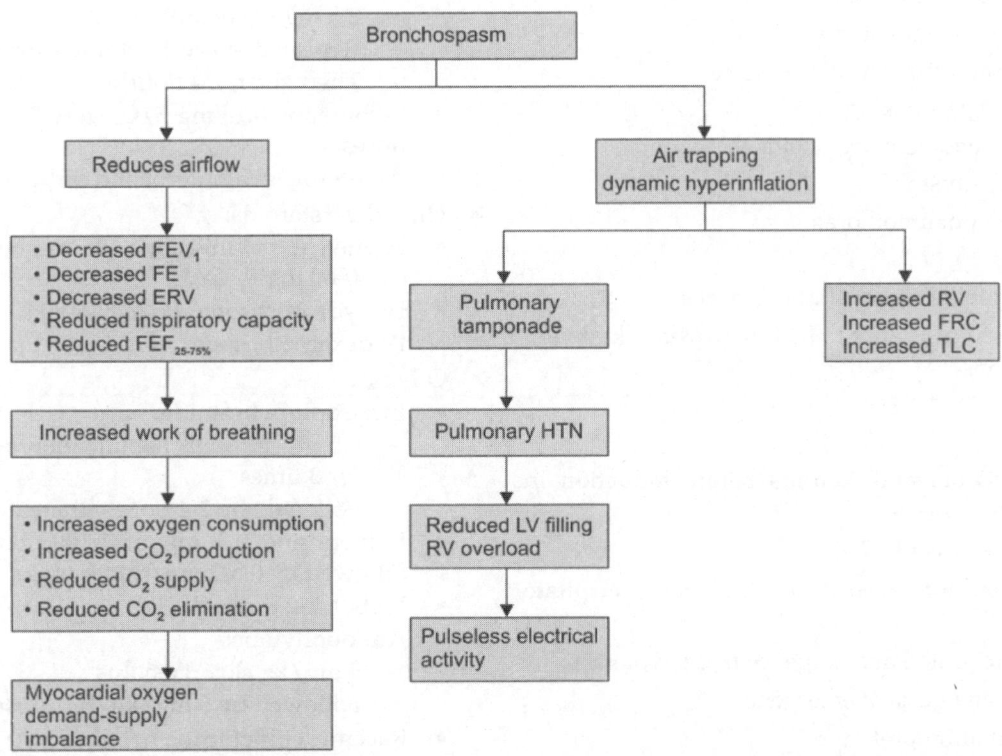

Clinical Features

- Signs and symptoms:
  - Reduced chest excursion
  - Coughing
  - Reduced breath sounds
  - Prolonged expiratory phase
  - Wheezing/rhonchi
  - *Silent chest*: Critically reduced air entry
- Monitors:
  - Hypoxia, hypercarbia
  - Reduced phase II slope on capnograph
  - Reduced compliance of reservoir bag
  - Reduced tidal volume
  - Increased peak inspiratory pressure

Differential Diagnosis

- Causes of unilateral rhonchi:
  - Endobronchial intubation
  - Foreign body: Dislodged tooth
  - Tension pneumothorax
  - Kinked endotracheal tube
  - Obstructed endotracheal tube (ETT)
  - Intestitial pulmonary edema
- Causes of raised peak airway pressure:
  - Increased inspiratory flow rate
  - Excessive tidal volume
  - Increased intrapleural pressure
  - Coughing/ bucking
  - Steep Trendelenburg position
  - Pleural effusion
  - Tension pneumothorax
  - Ascites
  - Abdominal gas insufflation/packs
  - Increased resistance in ETT: narrowing/kinking/secretions

Prevention

- Bronchodilators and steroids before induction in susceptible patients
- Prefer LMAs over ETT
- Neostigmine for reversal of NMB may precipitate spasm
- Careful suctioning at emergence in deep planes
- Adequate analgesia at emergence
- Deep extubation preferred
- Postoperative period:
  - Adequate analgesia
  - Bronchodilator therapy
  - Incentive spirometry
  - Deep breathing exercises
  - Early mobilization

Treatment

- Monitors:
  - Pulse oximetry
  - E_TCO_2, ECG
  - NIBP, ABG
  - Peak inspiratory pressure
  - Frequent auscultation
  - Auscultate chest and respiratory limb of anesthesia circuit to confirm wheeze
- Ventilation:
  - Turn to manual bag ventilation
  - Switch to 100% FiO_2
  - Heliox mixture with 21-30% O_2 (low viscosity of 0.52 kg/m^3)
- Deepen anesthetic plane:
  - Increase concentration of isoflurane/sevoflurane
  - Ketamine *agent of choice* for asthmatics
  - Propofol also can be used
- β_2 agonists:
  - Through nebulization/MDI via airway adaptor
  - Salbutamol:
    - 2.5 mg via nebulisation
    - Repeated every 20 minutes for 3 times
    - Then given 2-4 hourly
  - Terbutaline 0.25 mg S/C every 20 minutes for 3 doses
  - Albuterol, levalbuterol and pirbuterol are others
- High dose steroids:
  - IV methyl-prednisolone 125 mg bolus followed by 40-60 mg IV Q6H
  - IV hydrocortisone 200 mg Q4-6H
  - IV dexamethasone
- Others:
  - Ipratropium bromide:
    - 0.5 mg through nebulization every 30 mins for 3 times
    - Followed by 2-4 hourly thereafter
  - Epinephrine 0.3 mL of 1:1000 solution bolus followed by 0.5-2 mg/min infusion
  - $MgSO_4$ 1-2 gms gIV
  - Aminophylline:
    - 5 mg/kg slow IV bolus
    - Followed by 5 mg/kg/hr infusion
  - Racemic epinephrine nebulization

INTRAOPERATIVE HYPERCARBIA

Introduction

Hypercarbia exists when $PaCO_2 > 45$ mm Hg.

Etiology

Increased CO_2 Production

- Fever
- Sepsis
- Thyrotoxicosis
- Pheochromocytoma
- Malignant hyperthermia
- IV infusion of dextrose containing solutions
- Total parenteral nutrition

Impaired CO_2 Transport

- Reduced cardiac output
- Hypotension
- Hypovolemia
- Pulmonary embolism
- Occlusion of blood vessels: V/Q mismatch

Impaired Ventilation

- *Anesthesia related*: Respiratory muscle weakness due to:
  - Muscle relaxants
  - High spinal
  - Epidural
  - Phrenic nerve palsy due to peripheral nerve block
  - Depressants: Volatile agents/sedatives
- Ventilator related:
  - Disconnection/kinked ETT
  - Faulty inspiratory/expiratory valves
  - Exhausted soda-lime
  - Low tidal volume/respiratory rate
  - Spontaneous ventilation with low flow of gases
  - Leaks in breathing circuit
- Pulmonary causes:
  - Atelectasis
  - Pulmonary embolism
  - Bronchospasm
  - Pneumothorax
- Surgery related:
  - Laparoscopic surgery with CO_2 insufflation
  - Upper abdominal surgeries: Pain and reduced FRC
  - One lung ventilation associated surgeries
- Respiratory tract infections:
  - Pneumonia
  - COPD
  - Pleural effusion

Effects of Hypercarbia

Central Nervous System

- For each 1 mm Hg rise in $PaCO_2$, CBF increases by 1.8 mL/100g/min
- Increased CO_2 crosses BBB causing:
  - Reduced pH of CSF
  - Vasodilation of cerebral blood vessels
  - Raised ICP
- $PaCO_2 > 90$ mm Hg reduces seizure threshold (***CO_2 narcosis***)

Respiratory System

- Hypercarbia increases pulmonary vascular resistance
- Potentiates hypoxic pulmonary vasoconstriction
- Maximal stimulation occurs at $PaCO_2$ around 100 mm Hg

Cardiovascular

- Increases plasma epinephrine and norepinephrine
- Increases heart rate and BP
- Very high level causes hypotension and bradycardia

GIT and Renals

- Increases hepatic and portal venous blood flow
- Causes retention of HCO_3^- in renal tubules
- Metabolic alkalosis: Compensatory

Metabolic effects: Increases potassium leakage from cells into plasma

Treatment

- Supportive:
  - Antibiotics for any pathological states/infections preoperatively
  - Avoid dextrose solutions if increased chances of hypercarbia
  - Treat hypotension and hypovolemia promptly
- Anesthesia related:
  - Titrate volatile anesthetics, NMBA and sedatives
  - Avoid high spinal/epidural
  - Caution during nerve block: ultrasound guided blocks better
  - Use NM monitoring to avoid excess muscle relaxation
  - Give adequate dose of reversal
  - Adequate intraoperative analgesia to reduce BMR
  - Insufflation pressure kept at <20 mm Hg in laparoscopic surgeries

❖ Ventilator related:
  - Thorough machine check preoperatively
  - Correct kink/disconnection in ETT
  - Leaks in breathing circuit corrected
  - Increase FGF during spontaneous ventilation according to minimum volume needed
  - Adjust tidal volume and respiratory rate according to $PaCO_2/E_TCO_2$
  - If soda lime exhausted, increase FGF and change to open circuit

❖ Treat cause:
  - Pheochromocytoma: SNP/NTG/$MgSO_4$
  - Thyroid storm: maintain HR < 90 bpm, esmolol, antithyroid medications
  - Malignant hyperthermia: Dantrolene
  - Pulmonary edema:
    - Diuretics
    - Positive pressure ventilation with PEEP
  - Pneumothorax:
    - 14 gauge needle inserted in 2nd ICS, midclavicular line
    - ICD in 4th ICS, midaxillary line
  - Air embolism:
    - 100% oxygen
    - Inotropes
    - Trendelenburg or Durants position
    - Hyperbaric oxygen therapy
  - Bronchospasm:
    - 100% oxygen
    - Deepen anesthetic plane
    - Salbutamol inhaled
    - IV aminophylline and hydrocortisone

SURFACTANT THERAPY

Introduction

❖ These are complex lipoprotein molecules secreted by the lungs

❖ They contain a polar and non polar portion, and maintain stability of pulmonary tissue

❖ Surfactants reduce surface tension of fluids lining lung, thereby preventing atelectasis

❖ Exogenous surfactant therapy is effective in reducing morbidity in preterm infants

Structure: Has ***amphipathic*** structure with:

❖ Tail/hydrophobic group:
  - Can be linear/branched
  - Has little affinity for bulk solvent

❖ Head/hydrophilic group:
  - Strong affinity for bulk solvent
  - Can be neutral/charged

Components of Natural Surfactant

❖ Phospholipid:
  - Makes up 70- 80% of surfactant
  - Dipalmitoyl phosphatidylcholine (DPPC) is the principal phospholipid (85%)
  - Remaining 15% contains:
    - Phosphatidyl-inositol
    - Phosphatidyl-glycerol

❖ Neutral lipids:
  - Make up 10% of surfactant
  - Predominantly cholesterol

❖ Proteins:
  - Make up 8- 10% of surfactant
  - Responsible for spreading of DPPC as a monolayer to reduce surface tension
  - Four types of proteins are present in surfactant:
    - SP-A
    - SP-B
    - SP-C
    - SP-D

Metabolism

❖ Surfactant is synthesized by:
  - Type II alveolar epithelial cells
  - Airway epithelial cells
  - ***Clara cells***

❖ They are synthesized in the endoplasmic reticulum of these cells

❖ Surfactant is stored in lamellar bodies as closely packed bilayers

❖ Surfactant is transported through the Golgi apparatus through multivesicular bodies

❖ It is then secreted into the liquid lining of alveoli by exocytosis

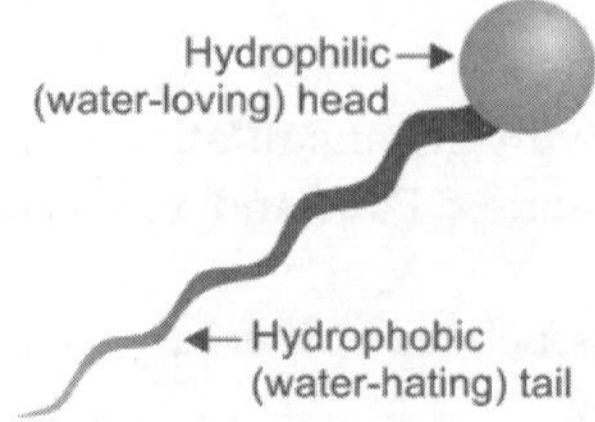

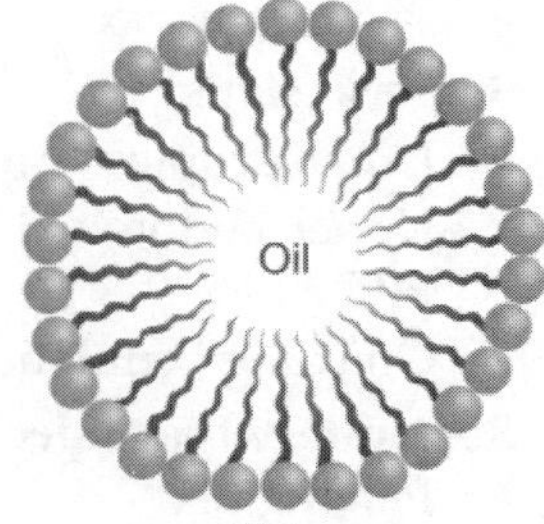

Fig. 21: Surfactant molecule.

- Following secretion, DPPC is organized into a lattice called tubular myelin
- This results in a mono-layer at air-liquid interface to reduce surface tension
- DPPC is then taken back into type-II cells in the form of small vesicles
- These are transported for storage in the form of lamellar bodies for recycling

Functions

- Prevents end expiratory collapse of alveoli
- Regulates size of alveoli
- Increases pulmonary compliance
- Keeps alveoli dry
- Plays role in pulmonary host defence mechanisms

Indications

- Neonatal respiratory distress syndrome (RDS):
  - Prophylactic use: in infants at high risk for RDS like:
    - Preterm infants < 29 weeks
    - Birth weight < 1250 grams
    - Congenital surfactant deficiency
    - Pulmonary alveolar proteinosis
    - $PaO_2/P_AO_2 < 0.22$
  - Early rescue therapeutic use: in infants with established RDS like:
    - Symptomatic infants within first hour of life
    - Persistent severe RDS with $FiO_2 > 0.4$ to maintain $SpO_2 > 90\%$
    - $PaO_2/P_AO_2 < 0.22$
- Other indications where surfactant *may be* considered:
  - Meconium aspiration syndrome
  - Group B streptococcus pneumonia
  - Massive pulmonary hemorrhage
- Role of prophylactic surfactant therapy:
  - Reduces neonatal mortality and incidence of pneumothorax
  - However, there is no change in the incidence of bronchopulmonary dysplasia
  - This approach is usually avoided in favour of antenatal steroid therapy

Contraindications

- Congenital anomalies incompatible with life beyond the neonatal period
- Respiratory distress in infants with laboratory evidence of lung maturity
- CDH: surfactant may cause a clinical deterioration if pulmonary hypoplasia is severe
- Hemodynamically unstable patient
- Active pulmonary hemorrhage

Classification

Class	Origin	Example
Natural	Amniotic fluid extract	Human amniotic fluid
		Surfactant
Modified natural	Bovine lung	BLESS
		Infasurf
		Survanta
		Alveofact
	Porcine lung	Curosurf
Synthetic	Synthetic	KL_4 surfactant
		ALEC
		Venticute
		Exosurf
		Lucinactant (FDA approved)

Dosage

Name	Feature	Dosage
Synthetic surfactants		
KL_4 surfactant	With proteins	Not yet available
ALEC (Pumactant)	With proteins	Not yet available
Venticute	With proteins	Not yet available
Exosurf (Colfosceril palmitate)	No proteins	*Prophylactic dose:*
		5 mL/kg Q12H for upto 3 total doses
		First dose within 15 mins of birth
		Rescue dose:
		5 mL/kg Q12H upto 2 total doses
Modified natural surfactants		
Infasurf/ Calfactant	Bovine (calf lung)	3 mL/kg Q12H up to 3 doses
Survanta/ Beractant	Minced bovine lung	4 mL/kg Q6H up to 4 doses in first 48 hours
		Usually requires Q12H doses during first 48 hours
Curosurf/ Poractant alfa	Porcine lung lavage	Initial dose 2.5 mL/kg (200 mg/kg)
		Upto two additional doses can be given
		Repeat dose: 1.25 mL/kg (100 mg/kg) Q12H
		Maximum total dose: 5 mL

Complications

- Procedural complications resulting from the administration of surfactant:
  - Plugging of ETT by surfactant:
    - Hemoglobin desaturation and increased need for supplemental O_2
    - Bradycardia due to hypoxia
  - Tachycardia due to agitation, with reflux of surfactant into the ETT
  - Pharyngeal deposition of surfactant
  - Inadvertent unilateral administration of surfactant:
    - Surfactant is administered to only one lung
    - Common with right mainstem intubation
  - Administration of suboptimal dose
- Physiologic complications of surfactant replacement therapy:
  - Apnea
  - Pulmonary hemorrhage
  - Marginal increase in retinopathy of prematurity
  - Volutrauma due to increase in lung compliance after surfactant replacement
  - Nosocomial infections

Monitoring During Therapy

- Position of patient
- Oxygen saturation by pulse oximetry
- Blood pressure, heart rate, ECG
- FiO_2 and ventilator settings
- Breath sounds, chest-wall movement
- Proper placement and position of delivery device and ETT
- Pulmonary mechanics and tidal volumes
- Following administration, monitor:
  - Reflux of surfactant into ETT
  - Invasive and/or noninvasive measurements of arterial blood gases
  - Chest radiograph

Modes of Administration

- INSURE (Intubation, Surfactant, Extubation)
  - Neonates are intubated with ETT according to gestational age and weight
  - Surfactant is administered in 2 divided bolus aliquots
  - The patient is allowed to stabilize in between administration of the 2 aliquots
  - Patient is promptly extubated to nasal CPAP following administration
  - Reserved for:
    - Neonates with good respiratory effort
    - With minimal resuscitation
    - Absence of other associated congenital issues
  - Associated with:
    - Less need for mechanical ventilation
    - Lower incidence of bronchopulmonary dysplasia
    - Lesser air leak syndromes
    - Lesser mechanical ventilation
    - Extubation from lower ventilator settings
- Selective surfactant replacement therapy:
  - Surfactant is administered through the ETT
  - Trachmac device may be used for administration
  - Prescribed surfactant volume is withdrawn and 1 mL of air is added
  - The ETT connecter is removed prior to administration
  - Appropriate adaptor for the Trachmac device is attached to the ETT
  - Trachmac catheter is inserted to the appropriate distance in the ETT
  - Syringe with preloaded surfactant is attached to the Trachmac device
  - Initial half-dose is instilled over 5-10 seconds
  - The Trachmac device is slowly withdrawn with manual inflation of lung
  - Routine ventilation is resumed with observation for chest rise/fall
  - Ventilation may be complicated by transient airway occlusion
  - This may be associated with sudden onset desaturation
  - Vital signs are thus allowed to stabilize prior to next dose
  - The second half dose is then administered followed by the drawn-up air
  - Air serves to clear the residual surfactant from the Trachmac device
  - Patient is reconnected to ventilator and ventilated following replacement
  - Child is subsequently extubated from lower ventilator settings
  - This technique is initiated upon clinical evidence of RDS, such as:
    - Radiological findings
    - Increased FiO_2 requirement
    - Increased work of breathing

- Pharyngeal instillation before first breath:
  - Done as soon as the infants head appears on:
    - Perineum for vaginal delivery
    - Operative incision site for cesarean delivery
  - The mother stops pushing
  - The pharynx and stomach are suctioned with a catheter
  - Surfactant solution is instilled into the posterior pharynx through a catheter
  - This is done without direct laryngoscopy
  - Infant is then stimulated to breathe as soon as the shoulders are delivered
  - Less preferred method
- Laryngeal mask airway (LMA) administration:
  - LMA requires less skill to place than traditional intubation with an ETT
  - Surfactant delivery can be accomplished sooner with LMA
  - Efficacy in reducing severity of RDS is similar to ETT administration
  - Also, LMA reduces proportion of neonates requiring mechanical ventilation
- Bronchoalveolar lavage:
  - Bronchoalveolar lavage with surfactant is another alternative
  - Surfactant lavage is a safe and effective alternative treatment for MAS
  - Synthetic surfactant lucinactant is used
  - This is because it resists inactivation by oxidants present in inflamed lungs
- Aerosolized surfactant:
  - Called non-invasive surfactant therapy (NIST)
  - Aerosolized surfactant and nasal CPAP therapy reduces need for intubation
  - Ideal preparation, dose and route of delivery are still being researched
  - 200 mg/kg poractant alfa is aerosolized
  - This is done using a customized vibrating nebulizer (eFlow Neonatal)
  - 100 mg/kg dose is repeated after 12 hours in the presence of persistent RDS

Outcome

- Surfactant replacement therapy helps to:
  - Reduce severity of RDS
  - Reduce pulmonary intestitial emphysema (PIE)
  - Improves lung function
  - Has beneficial long term effects on airway resistance
  - Reduce pulmonary vascular resistance
  - Reduce severity of epithelial necrosis
  - Reduce incidence of intraventricular hemorrhage
  - Reduce mortality rate in RDS patients
- No benefit is seen however, in adult ARDS

Current Recommendations European Consensus Guidelines 2019

- Early administration of animal-derived surfactant preparations in infants with RDS
- Most effective when given within the first 30–60 minutes of life
- Poractant alfa (curosurf) is preferable to beractant (survanta)
- Dosage:
  - Initial dose 200 mg/kg preferred over lower doses
  - Repeat doses may be administered for:
    - Persistent evidence of RDS (FiO_2 requirement > 0.30)
    - Preterm infants < 30 weeks gestation with RDS

OXYGEN THERAPY

Introduction

- Refers to the administration of oxygen as a therapeutic modality
- O_2 therapy in patients with normal SpO_2 has been associated with increased mortality
- Thus, O_2 should be administered conservatively to maintain SpO_2 no more than 96%

Physical Properties

- Colourless, odourless and tasteless gas
- Molecular weight 32
- Specific gravity 1.105
- Boiling point at 760 mm Hg = –183°C
- Melting point -218°C
- Solubility in plasma at 37°C = 0.003 mL/100 mL blood/mm Hg PaO_2
- Solubility in water at 37°C = 2.4 mL/100 mL water
- Cannot be ignited but supports combustion
- Below –183°C it is transparent blue liquid and slightly heavier than water
- Critical temperature = –118°C

Preparation and Storage

- By fractional distillation of liquid air
- CO_2 removed air is first derived
- O_2 and N_2 are separated using their boiling points
- Stored in the liquid form in 1500 kg capacity tanks

- Tanks are insulated by vacuum shell
- Temperature is maintained between –175 to 150°C

Cylinders

- Black with white shoulders in India
- Green colour cylinders in USA
- Pin index = 2, 5
- Capacity:
  - E cylinder = 660 L /1900 PSI
  - M cylinder = 3450 L/ 2200 PSI
  - H cylinder = 6900 L/ 2200 PSI
- Pressure at pipeline/ circuit = 4 bar/ 60 PSI
- Pressure at pressure regulator = 400 KPa/ 60 PSI

Indications

- Alveolar hypoventilation:
  - Reduced central drive:
    - Anesthetic overdose
    - Inadequate NMBA reversal
    - Chest injuries
    - Central hypoventilation syndrome
  - Peripheral causes:
    - Reduced diaphragmatic movement
    - Postoperative pain
    - Upper airway obstruction
- Intrapulmonary shunt:
  - Pulmonary arteriovenous communication
  - Congenital heart disease
  - Endobronchial intubation
  - COPD
  - Atelectasis
  - Airway obstruction
  - Pneumothorax/hemothorax
- Wasted ventilation:
  - Pulmonary embolism
  - Pulmonary obstruction
  - Pulmonary HTN
  - Cardiac failure
- Diffusion defects:
  - Pulmonary edema
  - Retained secretions
- Increased demand:
  - Convulsions
  - Postoperative shivering
  - Hyperthermia

Goals

- Increase oxygen content of blood
- Increase oxygen delivery to tissues
- Achieve PaO_2 > 60 mm Hg with FiO_2 < 0.5
- Achieve SpO_2 > 90% with FiO_2 < 0.5
- Decrease myocardial and respiratory workload

Recommendations for Oxygen Therapy

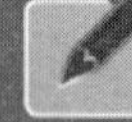

- For patients with MI/stroke:
  - Routine use of oxygen therapy is not recommended
  - O_2 therapy may be initiated when:
    - SpO_2 < 90%
    - PaO_2 < 60 mm Hg
    - Respiratory distress
    - Cardiac failure
  - Oxygen therapy should not be initiated when SpO_2 > 92%
  - Oxygen therapy is titrated to maintain SpO_2 < 96%
- For acutely ill medical patients:
  - O_2 therapy is initiated when SpO_2 < 90%
  - O_2 therapy is titrated to maintain SpO_2 < 96%
  - Exceptions to these recommendations include those requiring high SpO_2:
    - Carbon monoxide poisoning
    - Cluster headaches
    - Sickle cell crisis
    - Pneumothorax
- For patients at risk for hypercapneic respiratory failure:
  - O_2 therapy is initiated when SpO_2 < 88% in hypercapneic patients
  - O_2 therapy is titrated to maintain SpO_2 < 92%
  - Examples:
    - COPD
    - Obesity hypoventilation
    - Obstructive sleep apnea
    - Neuromuscular respiratory distress
    - Decreased central respiratory drive:
      - Sedative overdose
      - Encephalitis

Oxygen Delivery Devices

- Low flow delivery devices/variable performance equipment:
  - Nasal cannula
  - Nasal catheter
  - Facemask:
    - Simple Hudsons facemask
    - Partial rebreathing mask
    - Non rebreathing mask
- High flow/fixed performance equipment:
  - Venturi mask
  - Nebulizers
  - Oxygen hood
  - Hyperbaric oxygen
- Intravenous oxygen therapy
- Humidified high flow oxygen cannula (HFNC)

No.	Low flow system	High flow system
1.	FiO_2 for given flow rate varies with RR and TV	Not influenced by tidal volume/respiratory rate
2.	Variable performance	Fixed performance
3.	FiO_2 not predictable	FiO_2 fixed and accurate
4.	FiO_2 depends on capacity of anatomical reservoir	Does not depend on capacity of reservoir
5.	FGF inadequate to meet total inspiratory flow	FGF is adequate
6.	Rebreathing occurs	No rebreathing
7.	Temperature of gas not controlled	Can be controlled
8.	Humidity of gas not controlled	Can be controlled
9.	Used in patients with stable breathing patterns:	In dyspneic patients:
	• Postoperative ward	• Pulmonary edema
	• Anemic patients	• Asthma COPD
10.	Examples:	Examples:
	• Nasal cannula	• Venturi mask
	• Nasal catheter	• Anesthetic bag and mask
	• Face mask	• Hyperbaric oxygen

NASAL CANNULA

Introduction

- Most widely used device
- Ideal for long-term oxygen therapy

Design

- Contains 2 prongs protruding 1 cm into the nose
- These are held in place with an adjustable head strap

Usage

- Prongs are inserted 1 cm inside nares
- Continuous O_2 flow fills the anatomical reservoir (50 mL)

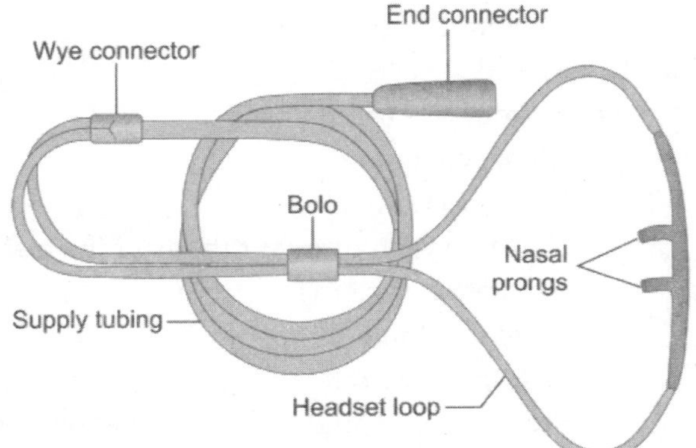

Fig. 22: Nasal cannula.

- Ambient air is also entrained through the nostrils
- With mouth breathing, Venturi effect occurs in the posterior pharynx
- This entrains oxygen into the lung from the anatomical reservoir
- Reservoir therefore empties into the lungs with each inspiration
- Recommended flow rate = 1-6 L/min

Delivered FiO_2

- Calculated using ***Sharpies and Harrisons*** formula:

  Reservoir O_2 + Nasal O_2 + Room air O_2 = Final O_2
- Precise FiO_2 cannot be calculated as air mixes with 100 % O_2
- Delivered FiO_2 depends upon:
  - Oxygen flow rate
  - Volume of oxygen reservoir (nasopharynx)
  - Respiratory pattern:
    - Tidal volume
    - Respiratory rate

No.	Flow rate	FiO_2
1.	1 Liter	24 %
2.	2 Liters	28 %
3.	3 Liters	32 %
4.	4 Liters	36 %
5.	5 Liters	40 %
6.	6 Liters	44 %

Indications

- Patients with low O_2 requirement
- Stable breathing pattern
- Home oxygen therapy

Advantages

- Simple and cheap
- Comfortable for patients
- Well tolerated with increased patient compliance
- Can be worn during eating , drinking , etc

Disadvantages

- Cannot be used in patients with blocked nasal passage
- Irritates nasal mucosa at FGF flows above 2 L/min
- Drying of nasal cavity
- Higher flow rates are uncomfortable
- Unpredictable FiO_2

NASAL CATHETERS

Design

- Comprises a single lumen catheter lodged in the anterior nares
- Appears like suction catheter with multiple openings at distal end
- Foam collar helps to lodge the catheter in the anterior nare
- Sizes 8-14 Fr

Use

- Tip of the catheter to be inserted up to fold of soft palate
- Catheter is slowly pulled back so that the tip lies beyond posterior nares above uvula
- Has to be changed from 1 nostril to the other every 8 hours
- Flow rates up to 3 L/min in conscious patients
- Flow rates up to 6L/min in unconscious patients
- Up to 40% FiO_2 may be delivered

Advantages

Gas flow does not impinge on 1 area of nostril due to multiple openings.

Disadvantages

- Avoided in patients with nasal mucosal tears due to risk of surgical emphysema
- FiO_2 delivered is unpredictable
- Causes nasal irritation

SIMPLE FACE MASK

Introduction

Variable performance device as the performance varies from breath-to-breath.

Design

- Plastic body of mask with side holes
- Port to connect to a source of oxygen supply
- Elastic band to connect mask to the patient

Principle

- Oxygen flows into mask through tubing
- Body of the mask acts as the reservoir for oxygen:
  - 70–100 mL in pediatric masks
  - 175–200 mL in adult masks

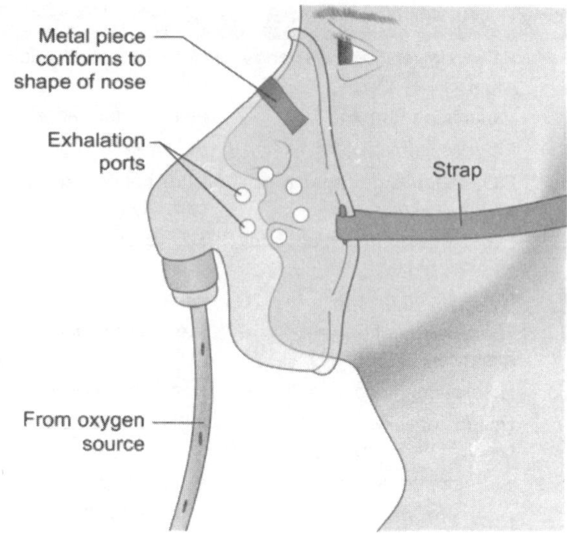

Fig. 23: Simple face mask.

- Ambient air is entrained through the holes on the side of the mask
- During expiratory pause:
  - Fresh gas flow vents the expired gases through the side holes
  - FGF also fills the reservoir with fresh oxygen supply during the pause
  - Thus, fresh oxygen is available at the start of the next inspiration
- Thus the holes in the side of the mask serve to:
  - Entrain ambient air to control the FiO_2
  - Vent exhaled gases
- In the absence of expiratory pause:
  - Fresh gas flow does not vent expired gases
  - Thus, rebreathing may occur
  - Reservoir does not get time to fill with fresh oxygen
  - Thus, delivered FiO_2 may reduce
- Minimum flow rate of 4 L/min to avoid rebreathing
- Usually flow rate of 6-10 L/min
- FiO_2 delivered:
  - Varies from 35 – 65 %
  - FiO_2 depends upon:
    - Fresh gas flow rate
    - Size of oxygen reservoir (body of the mask)
    - Ventilation pattern:
      - Tidal volume
      - Respiratory rate
    - Presence of expiratory pause to allow refilling of mask reservoir
    - Mask size and fit

Disadvantages

- Has to be removed during eating, drinking, etc
- CO_2 can collect in mask and add to dead space if flow rate < 5 L/min
- Flow rate > 10 L/min vented out through openings and does not increase FiO_2

Advantages

- Lower cost
- Greater patient comfort
- Ability to change FiO_2 by altering fresh gas flow rate

PARTIAL REBREATHING MASK

Design

- Combines the facemask with a collapsible O_2 reservoir bag
- The reservoir bag usually has a capacity > 1 litre
- Inspired gas therefore contains:
    - Oxygen from continuous fresh oxygen supply
    - Oxygen from reservoir bag
    - Air entrained through side-ports
    - Air from space between mask and skin of face
- If O_2 flow rate is adjusted to prevent collapse of the bag, minimal rebreathing occurs
- FiO_2 of 60 – 80 % can be attained with flow rates 5-7 L/min

Disadvantages

- Some amount of rebreathing still possible

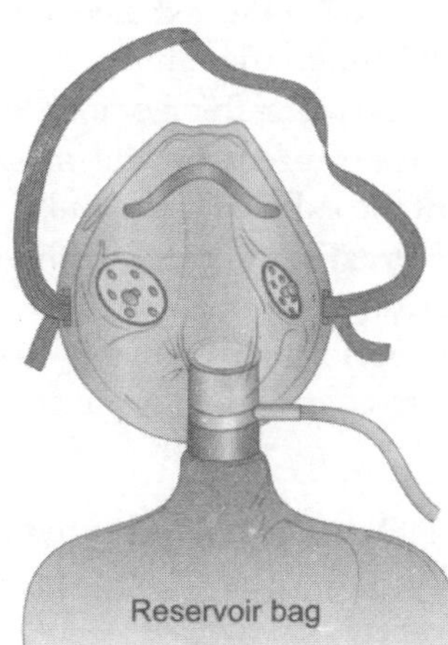

Fig. 24: Partial rebreathing masks.

NON-REBREATHING MASK

Design

- Combines facemask with reservoir bag and unidirectional valves
- One unidirectional valve is fitted between the mask and reservoir bag
- This valve ensures that patient inhales air preferentially from the reservoir bag
- Thus this valve functions to:
    - Prevent rebreathing
    - Ensure delivery of 100% O_2 to the reservoir bag
- A second valve is present which seals side holes of mask during inhalation
- Thus, ambient air is not entrained into the inspired gas
- This augments the inspired FiO_2
- Flow rates of upto 6 – 10 L/min
- Reservoir bag volume = 750 – 1250 mL
- FiO_2 : 60 – 80 % but up to 95 – 100 % achievable with adequate seal

Indications

- When FiO_2 > 60% needed at low flows
- When patient needs NPPV but does not tolerate it
- Failed NPPV
- Patients with hypoxemia and spontaneous ventilation
    - Trauma
    - Poisoning
    - Myocardial infarction

Advantages

- Higher delivered FiO_2
- Low fresh gas flow rates
- No rebreathing

Disadvantages

- Needs airtight fitting
- To be removed during feeding
- Needs close observation

VENTURI MASK

Introduction

- High-airflow fixed-performance oxygen enrichment device
- Also called high air flow oxygen enrichment device (HAFOE)

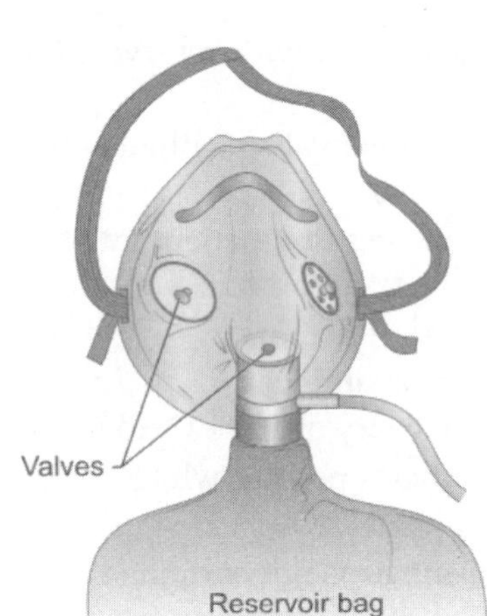

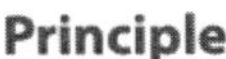

Fig. 25: Non-rebreathing mask.

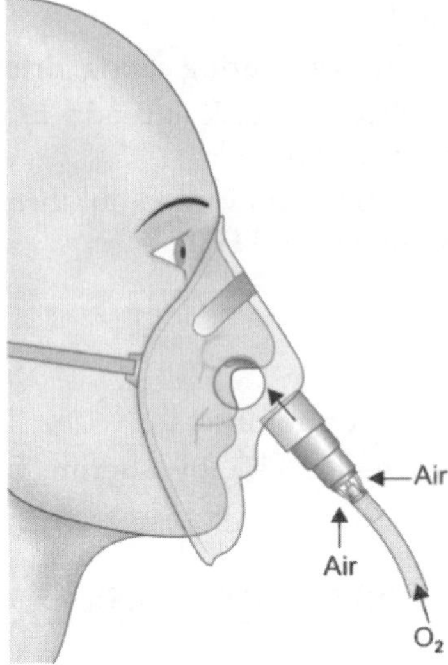

Fig. 26: Functioning of Venturi mask.

Principle

- Bernoullis principle:
  - Described in 1778
  - In order to maintain a flow, a fluid must increase its velocity as it flows through a constriction
- Venturi effect:
  - Based on the Bernoullis principle
  - Pressure of gas/liquid is inversely proportional to its velocity in laminar flow
  - Thus, narrowing of tube diameter causes:
    - Increase in velocity of gas flowing through the tube
    - Reduction of pressure at that point in the tube
  - If the constriction is suitably sized:
    - Negative pressure develops surrounding the narrowed orifice
    - Ambient air from side holes will be entrained into mainstream flow
  - Delivered FiO_2:
    - FiO_2 generated is dependent on the degree of air entrainment
    - This in turn depends upon the size of the narrowed aperture
    - Narrower apertures create more negative pressure
    - This results in entrainment of more ambient air and lesser FiO_2
    - Conversely, less entrainment ensures delivery of a higher FiO_2
    - Delivered FiO_2 can therefore be fixed and predetermined

Design

- Proximal end or base of the mask consists of the colour-coded Venturi device
- Specified flow of pure oxygen enters the device through a narrow orifice
- Oxygen velocity increases at the narrowing and hence pressure drops
- Just past this orifice are the openings on Venturi device
- Room air enters these openings on the device and mixes with oxygen
- Critical feature is size of opening through which oxygen enters the device
- FiO_2 can be calibrated by varying the aperture controlled by colour-coded nozzles
- Holes are present on both sides of the plastic body of the mask
- Due to high FGF rate, exhaled gases are rapidly flushed out through these holes
- Thus, there is no rebreathing or increase in dead space
- The side holes present on the mask are therefore used to vent the exhaled gases only
- This is in contrast to the function these holes serve in variable performance masks
- In variable performance masks the holes entrain ambient air to control the FiO_2

Indications

- To control FiO_2 in patients with hypoxic respiratory drive (COPD)
- Unstable respiratory pattern
- Inadequate ventilator efforts
- Pulmonary edema

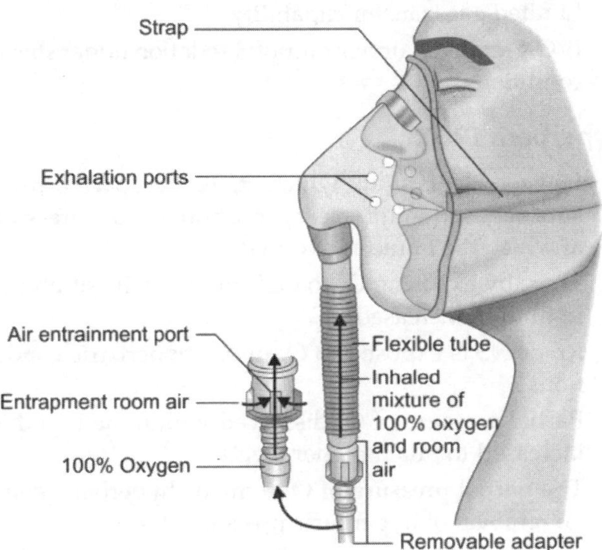

Fig. 27: Venturi mask design.

- Pulmonary consolidation
- ARDS

Advantages

- No need of airtight fit
- FiO_2 predictable and accurate
- Fixed enrichment ratio independent of patients ventilator pattern
- No apparatus dead space
- No rebreathing
- Easy to use
- Economical due to low oxygen flows
- Can be used as an attachment to tracheal tube or SGOD as a part of T-piece system

Disadvantages

- Facial discomfort
- Cannot be worn during feeding, drinking, coughing, etc
- FiO_2 can be increased if enrichment ports are obstructed by patients hands or bedsheets

FiO_2 Delivered

No.	O_2 flow rate	Air entrained	Total flow to patient	Colour	Fio_2
1.	2 L/min	51 L/min	53 L/min	Blue	0.24
2.	4 L/min	41 L/min	45 L/min	White	0.28
3.	8 L/min	37 L/min	45 L/min	Yellow	0.35
4.	10 L/min	32 L/min	42 L/min	Red	0.40
5.	15 L/min	15 L/min	30 L/min	Green	0.60

INTRAVENOUS OXYGEN THERAPY

Introduction

- Involves direct administration of dissolved oxygen into the vascular system
- Method of improving oxygenation independent of alveolar gas exchange
- IVOX introduced by ***Regelsberger***

Physiology

- Oxygen delivery at the tissue level depends upon the oxygen content of blood
- Arterial oxygen content in turn is determined by:
  - Concentration of oxygen bound to hemoglobin
  - Dissolved oxygen content
- Under normal circumstances, most of the oxygen is bound to hemoglobin
- Only a small fraction is transported as dissolved oxygen
- IVOX aims at increasing the quantity of dissolved O_2 to meet cellular requirements
- Similar principle is involved with hyperbaric O_2 therapy, using advanced equipment

Indications

- ARDS/ALI
- Acute respiratory failure
- Acute exacerbation of lung disease
- Patients awaiting lung transplants
- Lung surgery

Contraindications

- Narrow vein size
- Left sided SVC
- Absent/duplicate/hypoplastic IVC
- Peripheral vein thrombosis/infection
- Refractory cardiac failure
- Coagulopathies
- MODS

Design

- Available in sizes 7-10 mm outer diameter
- Basic functional component is hollow fibers furled into a bundle
- Houses around 1000 fibres with numerous pores of 0.3 mm diameter
- 6 FDA-6 FAP membrane selectively permeable to gases covers the pores
- Lies freely inside the lumen of SVC/IVC without impairing the blood flow

- Pulsating balloon within the bundle directs the blood flow within
- Size selected by calculating venous size using Doppler USG

Method of Insertion

- Obdurator with J tipped wire is introduced into right femoral vein/IJV
- Position is checked with C-arm
- Device is advanced to occupy entire length of IVC and lower portion of SVC
- Device is then unfurled to lie within the lumen
- Blood shunts between the hollow fibres
- Bacterial filter is connected to the oxygen inlet
- Venotomy is subsequently repaired
- 100% oxygen is introduced through the central conduit of coaxial tube
- Gases are drawn along the length of fiber under subatmospheric pressure
- This negative pressure prevents gas embolization in the event that fiber ruptures
- Can be used for upto 28 days without complications

Complications

- Thrombocytopenia
- Blood loss
- Ipsilateral pedal edema
- Femoral vein thrombosis
- Limb ischemia

Factors Affecting Performance

- Device surface area for gas exchange
- PaO_2
- PvO_2
- $PvCO_2$
- Cardiac output
- Duration of implantation

Advantages

- Reduces pulmonary workload
- Permits reduction in ventilatory support
- Reduces airway pressure
- Prevents ventilator induced barotrauma
- Prevents ventilator induced cardiac derangements

Disadvantages

- Supplies only 30-40 % of total metabolic requirement of oxygen
- Limited gas transfer capability
- IVOX removed under propofol sedation under sterile conditions

Hyperbaric IVOX

- Utilizes Henrys law which states that partial pressure of gas in solution is proportional to the pressure at which the liquid is exposed
- Thus, by exposing O_2 to high pressure, its solubility in fluid in increased
- RL or NS is exposed to O_2 under hyperbaric conditions
- Partial pressure of O_2 dissolved within the liquid is increased to much higher levels
- The partial pressure of O_2 remains hyperbaric even on removal of hyperbaric pressure
- This hyperbaric pressure is maintained in solution for at least 4 hours
- When this solution is transfused, dissolved O_2 content of arterial blood increases
- Deoxygenated Hb will bind to the dissolved O_2 and become oxygenated
- This results in an increase in the SpO_2 relative to amount of O_2 delivered

Polymeric Microparticle Based Oxygen Delivery

- Polymer hollow microparticles (PHM) are used
- These are thin-walled, hollow polymer microcapsules with nanoporous shells
- These are easily charged with oxygen prior to intravenous infusion
- PHMs release this oxygen when exposed to deoxygenated blood
- Still in experimental stages

COMPLICATIONS OF OXYGEN THERAPY

Pulmonary Complications

- Progressive hypercapnia:
  - Occurs if respiratory drive is dependent on hypoxic stimulus
  - Inhaling high FiO_2 causes hypoventilation and hypercarbia
  - Common in COPD patient (respiratory center insensitive to hypercarbic drive)
  - Prevented by controlling FiO_2 to 24-30% in COPD patients
- Absorption atelectasis:
  - Occurs when 100% oxygen administered in COPD

- O_2 displaces all the N_2 in airway
- O_2 has high solubility and thus gets absorbed
- O_2 remaining in airway gets fully absorbed causing alveolar collapse
- Changes occur within 6 minutes of 100% O_2

- Drying and crusting of secretions: Dry O_2 administration
- Nitrogen narcosis: Hyperbaric O_2 therapy

Cardiovascular Complications

- Rare complication of cardiovascular depression
- Hyperbaric oxygen has direct myocardial depressant actions
- Especially in patients with increased sympathetic activity
- Sudden relief of hypoxia abolishes sympathetic overactivity
- Causes hypotension and circulatory collapse

Other Complications

- Fire hazard
- Depression of hematopoiesis
- Oxygen toxicity–free radical mediated injury

OXYGEN TOXICITY

Introduction

Results from overproduction of free radicals from oxygen molecule.

Molecules Formed

- Superoxide ions
- Hydrogen peroxide
- Singlet oxygen

Structures Damaged

- DNA
- Lipids
- -SH containing proteins

Protective Enzymes

- Superoxide dismutase
- Catalase
- Antioxidants
- Free radical scavengers:
  - Glutathione peroxidase
  - Vitamins C and E
  - Acetyl cysteine
  - Mannitol

Factors Affecting Toxicity

- Inspired oxygen consentration
- Time of exposure
- Humidity
- Circulating catecholamine levels
- Circulating corticosteroid levels
- Circulating endotoxins
- Leucocyte accumulation in lungs
- Drugs:
  - Bleomycin
  - Mitomycin C

Measurement of Toxicity

Unit Pulmonary Toxic Dose (UPTD) = $t \cdot \sqrt[m]{\frac{0.5}{(P-0.5)}}$

t = exposure time in minutes

P = inspired PO_2

M = slope constant (empirical value = 1.2)

No.	UPTD	Change
1.	< 1425	10% fall in vital capacity
2.	>2190	20% fall in vital capacity

Manifestations

- Pulmonary toxicity: ***Lorren – Smith*** effect
- CNS toxicity: ***Paul – Bert*** effect
- Retrolental fibroplasia in neonates (RFN)
- Retinopathy of prematurity (ROP)

Paul Bert Effect

Mechanism

- Inactivation of –SH containing enzymes controlling GABA levels
- Occurs on exposure to oxygen at 2 ATM pressure
- Increased incidence with
  - Acute hyperbaric oxygen administration
  - High dose penicillin
  - Hypoglycemia and sepsis

Clinical Features

- Twitching of periocular and perioral muscles
- Pupillary dilatation
- Visual dazzle
- Vertigo/nausea
- Numbness, seizures

Treatment

- Gradual withdrawal of high pressure oxygen
- Inhalation of room air
- Anticonvulsants – phenytoin phenobarbitone barbiturates

Lorren Smith Effect

Mechanism

- P_AO_2 more important than P_aO_2
- Occurs when oxygen administration at pressures between 0.7-3 ATM
- Occurs after 30 hrs exposure to PiO_2 of 100 kPa
- Patient can tolerate 100% oxygen upto 10-12 hrs

Pathophysiology

- Due to peroxidation of lipids-resulting lipid peroxides inhibit cell function
- Oxidation of –SH groups in essential enzymes
- Reversal and inhibition of electron transport chain
- Loss of pulmonary surfactant
- Absorption, collapse and alveolar edema

Pathology

- Exudative phase:
  - Interstitial edema
  - Destruction of type I pneumocytes
- Proliferative phase:
  - Proliferation of type II pneumocytes
  - Thickened blood air barrier
  - Hyaline membrane formation

Clinical Features

- Substernal discomfort
- Chest pain, cough – *earliest* signs
- Reduced vital capacity *most sensitive* indicator
- Respiratory rate, minute volume and compliance falls
- Frank ARDS

Retrolental Fibroplasia

Etiology

- Due to oxygen induced retinal vasoconstriction
- Occurs in premature infants with:
  - < 30 wks gestation
  - <1200 g birthweight
  - Exposure to high oxygen concentration, e.g., 150mm Hg > 2 hrs
- PaO_2 < 140 mm Hg is safe

Staging

No.	Stage	Changes
1.	I	Thin white line separates anterior avascular and posterior avascular parts of retina
2.	II	White line increases in volume and called *Ridge*
		5-10 % progress to stage III
		80 % regress to normal
3.	III	Tissue proliferates posteriorly from ridge
		Can be mild/moderate/ severe
		Can regress by 6 mths
4.	IVa	Partial retinal detachment with macula attached
		Macula gets detached
5.	V	Total retinal detachment

Prevention of Oxygen Toxicity

- Use lowest FiO_2 for shortest time
- Reduction of oxygen consumption
- *Air Breaks* – intermittent air breathing periods
- Early use of PEEP to reduce shunt
- -SH compounds , glutathione and cysteine
- Antioxidants – Vitamins C and E
- Maintain acid base balance

LARYNGOSPASM

Introduction

It is an exaggerated glottic closure reflex which persists long after the removal of the stimulus.

Etiology

- More common after upper airway procedures especially ENT surgeries
- More common in pediatric age group
- Intraoperative causes:
  - Respiratory tract infections, chronic smokers
  - Drugs: Morphine, barbiturates: increase parasympathetic activity
  - Volatile anesthetics: Ether > isoflurane > halothane > enflurane
  - Procedures:
    - Endoscopy
    - Esophagoscopy, upper abdominal manipulation
  - Lighter planes with stimulation of visceral nerve endings in pelvis, abdomen, thorax, larynx
  - Presence of nasogastric tube
  - Local airway irritation, nasal irritation
- Postoperative causes:
  - Immediate postoperative causes: Extubation especially after halothane anesthesia
  - Delayed postoperative causes:
    - Local airway irritation by:
      - Collected secretions, regurgitated gastric contents after bout of coughing

    - Silent regurgitation by the sides of nasogastric tube
    - Presence of oropharyngeal or naropharyngeal airway
  - Hypoxia producing vomiting and regurgitation
  - Epiglottitis

Pathophysiology

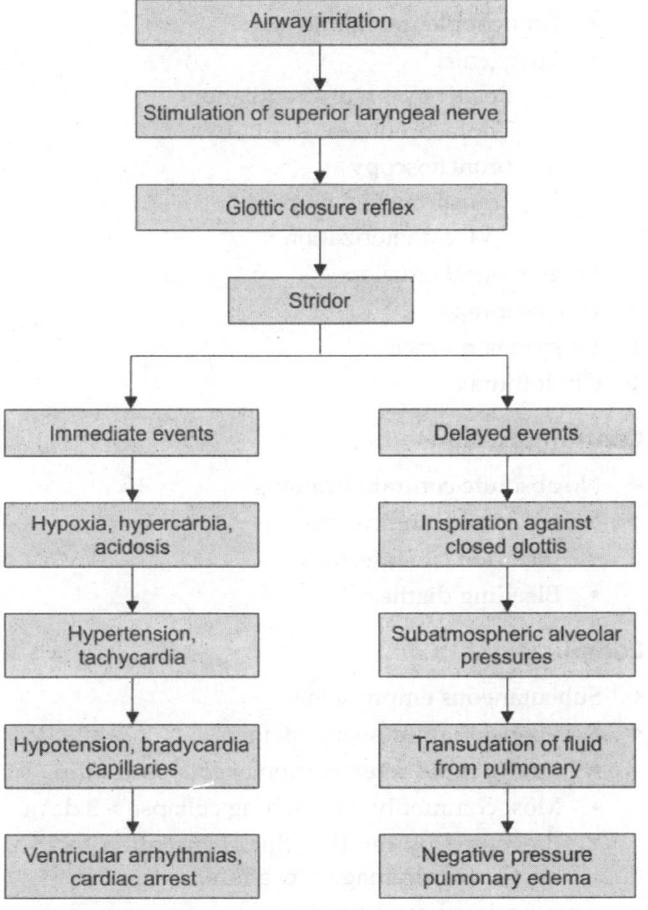

Clinical Features

- More common in children especially after ENT surgeries
- Acutely dyspneic and tachypneic
- Intercostal and suprasternal notch indrawing
- Abdominal wall rises but chest sinks during inspiration and vice versa
- Stridor, tracheal tug and paradoxical respiratory movements as obstruction worsens
- On auscultation, inspiratory and expiratory sounds best heard with precordial stethoscope in children which ceases on complete obstruction (***silent chest***)

Management

Intraoperative Management

- Remove noxious and irritant stimulant:
  - Stop surgical stimulation of visceral nerve endings
  - Suctioning of larynx
  - Removal of artificial airway
- Deepen anesthetic plane:
  - Intravenous propofol or other IV drugs preferred
  - 1-2 mg/kg propofol IV maybe given
  - Caution while using volatile anesthetics as they may increase laryngospasm
  - *Sevoflurane* may be used: *Least irritant*
- Facilitate ventilation:
  - Gentle positive end expiratory pressure
  - Continuous positive airway pressure (CPAP) of 40 cm H_2O with 100% O_2 via tightly sealed face mask
  - Acts as pneumatic splint to break the spasm
  - Forcible jaw thrust with bilateral digital pressure on body of mandible just anterior to mastoid process: ***Laryngospasm point: Larsons maneuver***
  - If complete obstruction avoid CPAP as stomach distension occurs
- Heliox mixture:
  - Mixture of 70% helium and 30% oxygen
  - Turbulent airflow depends on gas density
  - Since helium makes gas mixture less dense, air flow is improved
  - Concentration of helium titrated according to hypoxia
  - Improved tidal volume and reduced airway resistance occurs
- Racemic epinephrine:
  - 1 mg of 1:1000 solution in 5 mL of normal salilne nebulized every 30 minutes
  - Droplet deposition on inflamed swollen mucosa causes intense vasoconstriction
  - This reduces cord edema
- Steroids:
  - Dexamethasone 0.1 mg/kg IV Q6H
  - Takes 4-6 hrs to act
- Succinylcholine:
  - If all maneuvers fail succinylcholine in a dose of 0.1-0.5 mg/kg IV used
  - IM dose: 4-5mg/kg
  - Intralingual/intraosseus routes also can be used
- Deepen plane of anesthesia before resuming noxious stimulus

- If all these methods fail to relieve spasm, percutaneous airway should be considered
- Management of complications: Negative pressure pulmonary edema
  - 100% oxygen
  - Head end elevation
  - Positive airway pressure
  - Diuretics

Postoperative Management

- Remove noxious stimuli:
  - Thorough oropharyngeal and nasopharyngeal suctioning before shifting to ward
  - Nasogastric tube aspiration at 1 hour intervals
  - Removal of airway
- Facilitate ventilation:
  - Ensure proper oxygenation after extubation
  - Good topical anesthesia for larynx
  - Anesthetic plane cannot be deepened as it will delay extubation
  - Facilitate ventilation with CPAP and Larsons maneuver
- Drugs:
  - Racemic epinephrine, steroids, heliox mixture
  - Succinylcholine if all other measures fail
- Securing airway:
  - Reintubate patient if desaturation continues with standby expert
  - Forceful intubation against closed glottis not advised
  - Percutaneous airway preferred in such cases

Prevention of Post-Extubation Laryngospasm

- IV lidocaine 1 mg/kg
- Topical lidocaine
- IV magnesium sulphate
- Deep extubation, lateral position
- Adequate suctioning before extubation

Differential diagnosis: If laryngospasm fails to resolve with all these maneuvers, think of other causes of post extubation stridor like:

- Laryngomalacia
- Tracheomalacia
- Vocal cord palsy
- Airway edema
- Hematoma
- Soft tissue obstruction
- Presence of foreign materials like packs

INTERCOSTAL DRAIN

Introduction

Thoracostomy tube connects intercostal space with drainage system for removal of air and fluid.

Indicatons

- Large pneumothorax > 25%
  - Ruptured bleb
  - Chest trauma
  - Bronchopleural fistula
  - Iatrogenic:
    - Positive pressure ventilation
    - Thoracocentesis
    - Bronchoscopy
    - Transbronchial biopsy
    - CVP catheterization
- Large pleural effusion
- Hemothorax
- Empyema thoracis
- Chylothorax

Contraindications

- No absolute contraindications
- Relative contraindications:
  - Insertion site infection
  - Bleeding diathesis

Complications

- Subcutaneous emphysema
- Reexpansion pulmonary edema:
  - Due to rapid re-expansion of collapsed lung
  - Most commonly seen in lung collapse > 3 days
  - Prevented by limiting fluid evacuation to 1500 mL during drainage procedure
- Access related complications:
  - Hemorrhage at insertion site
  - Hematoma
  - Infections with long-standing ICDs causing empyema
  - Laceration of lung parenchyma
  - Laceration of surrounding organs:
    - Heart
    - Diaphragm
    - Esophagus
    - Stomach
    - Liver
    - Spleen

- Avulsion of neurovascular structures:
  - Phrenic nerve
  - Intercostal artery and nerve
  - Sympathetic chain
- Technical complications:
  - Blood clot within ICD preventing further drainage
  - Kinking of ICD preventing lung re-expansion
  - Rare complications:
    - Pleuro-cutaneous fistulas
    - Partially retained catheter

Types of Chest Tubes

- Chest tubes are usually made of polyvinylchloride and silicon
- They may be straight or curved, trocar or non-trocar
- Small bore ICDs:
  - Are < 20 Fr external diameter
  - Include:
    - Flexible silicon drains (Blake drain)
    - Pigtail catheters
    - Indwelling pleural catheters
  - Not indicated for:
    - Loculated or complex pleural effusion
    - Hemothorax
    - Chest trauma
- Large bore ICDs:
  - Are > 20 Fr external diameter
  - Conventionally preferred for pleural effusion
  - Large size prevents occlusion of the ICD and inadequate drainage

Chest Tube Size

- Neonates: 12-14 Fr
- Children: 18 Fr
- Small adults: 28-32 Fr
- Large adults: 36-40 Fr
- Large size tubes are preferred for:
  - Hemothorax (18-40 Fr)
  - Chylothorax (16-28 Fr)
  - Empyema (16- 28 Fr)
  - Bronchopleural fistulas (20- 28 Fr)
- Smaller size tubes (16- 20 Fr) are adequate for adult pneumothorax

Site of Insertion

- Pneumothorax: 2nd or 3rd intercostal space anteriorly along MCL or MAL
- Pleural effusion: 4th to 6th ICS along MAL (usually a line lateral to nipple)
- Point of entry is directly over body of rib to avoid injury to neurovascular bundle
- Skin is punctured just above the rib as the neurovascular bundle lies below each rib

Method of Placement

- Operative tube thoracostomy:
  - Done under strict asepsis
  - Adequate LA infiltration at the incision site
  - Incision is made just above and parallel to rib
  - Pleura is entered via blunt dissection
  - Pleural space is inspected with the index finger
  - Chest tube guided into space with finger and hemostat
  - Safer than trocar method
  - Finger inspection avoids ICD placement between parietal pleura and chest wall
  - Incision required is larger to allow digital manipulation
- Trocar tube thoracostomy:
  - Done under strict asepsis
  - Adequate LA infiltration at the incision site
  - Incision is made just above and parallel to rib
  - Chest tube with trocar inside is inserted into the incision
  - Trocar insertion is limited to 1-2 cm to avoid puncture of lung
  - Once inside the pleural space, the tube is advanced over trocar
  - ICD is clamped before complete withdrawal of trocar
  - Requires smaller incision
  - Causes less pain and patient discomfort

Drainage Systems

One Chamber System

- This is a one-chamber water-seal system
- Drains fluid from pleural cavity using gravity
- The system is without an active intrinsic suction source
- However, an active suction source may be connected to aid evacuation
- Design:
  - Following placement of the ICD, it is connected to the flexible ***Creech*** tubing
  - This is done using a clear, rigid plastic connector flange

- The Creech tube drains into the chamber system
- The chamber initially contains 100 mL sterile water
- The chamber has a short air vent tube which prevents build-up of pressure
- Creech tubing is submerged 2 cm inside the sterile water
- This submersion minimizes the risk of air entering pleural cavity
- This acts as a water seal system which allows air to escape but prevents return

❖ Depth of submersion in water:
- This determines hydrostatic pressure to be overcome to evacuate air
- Thus, fluid accumulation increases resistance to drainage of fluid from pleura
- This in turn increases the work of breathing (WOB)
- This system is therefore no longer preferred

❖ Bubbling from the Creech tubing:
- This is normal and indicates the presence of air in the pleural space
- Absence of bubbling from the tubing suggests:
  - ICD obstruction
  - Clearance of air from pleural space

❖ Disadvantages:
- Dead space:
  - Dead space of the collection system is represented by:
    - Volume of tubing
    - Volume of collection chamber
  - Increased dead space results in increased WOB
  - Thus, the tubing volume has to be minimized to reduce WOB
- Fluid accumulation:
  - Causes more of Creech tubing to be submerged
  - This can result in laboured breathing
  - WOB is proportional to depth of submersion of tube
- Kinking/obstruction of tube:
  - Can cause absence of bubbling
  - This may be confused with clearance of pneumothorax

Two Chamber System

❖ Drains fluid from pleural cavity using gravity

❖ The system is usually without an active intrinsic suction source

❖ However, an active suction source may be connected to aid evacuation

❖ Chamber 1:
- Both tubes are above the fluid level and not submerged
- Collects pleural fluid via gravity
- Amount of pleural drainage is measured from the 1st chamber
- The pleural air evacuated escapes into the second chamber with the water seal

❖ Chamber 2:
- Longer tube:
  - Submerged in 2 cm of sterile water
  - Acts as the water seal system
- Shorter tube:
  - Not submerged in water
  - Allows air to escape and prevents pressure build up
  - Can be connected to suction system to aid active evacuation

❖ Advantages:
- Submersion depth of long tube in chamber 2 remains unchanged
- Thus, WOB is unaffected by volume of fluid collected in chamber 1.

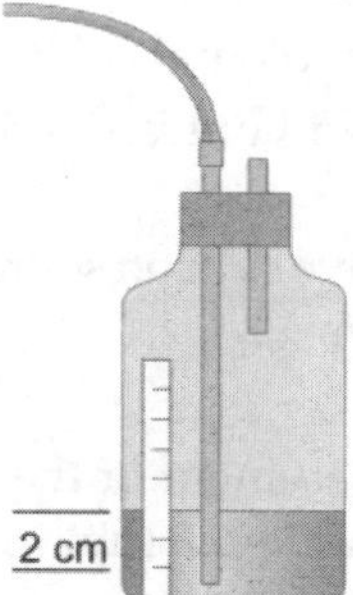

Fig. 28: One chamber system for ICD.

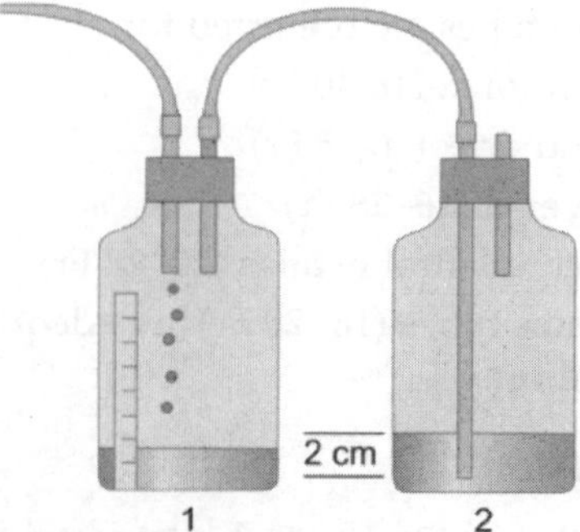

Fig. 29: Two chamber system for ICD.

Three Chamber System

- Most commonly used system and is most versatile
- Drains fluid from pleural cavity using low-level suction
- Use of suction reduces the resistance to pleural fluid outflow and WOB
- Chamber 1:
  - Collection chamber
  - Both tubes are above the fluid level and not submerged
  - Collects pleural fluid/evacuates pleural air
  - Amount of pleural drainage is measured from the 1st chamber
- Chamber 2:
  - Water seal chamber
  - Longer tube:
    - Submerged in 2 cm of sterile water
    - Acts as the water seal system
  - Shorter tube:
    - Not submerged in water
    - Allows air to escape and prevents pressure build up
- Chamber 3:
  - Suction chamber
  - Water level in chamber regulates amount of suction in the system
  - Water level of 15 cm height attains suction of –15 cm H_2O
  - Low level suction (–10 to –20 cm H_2O) is recommended for ICD
  - Overfilling of water increases suction
  - Underfilling reduces suction
- Working principle:
  - Vacuum draws air into fluid through venting tube in chamber 3
  - This causes a constant bubbling effect
  - Too much bubbling indicates high vacuum level
  - Water level in chamber 3 should therefore be kept at an appropriate level
  - Evaporation lowers submersion depth

Care of ICD

- Water level in chamber 2 and creech tube to vary with respiration
- If drainage holes on ICD become visible reposition or reinsert immediately

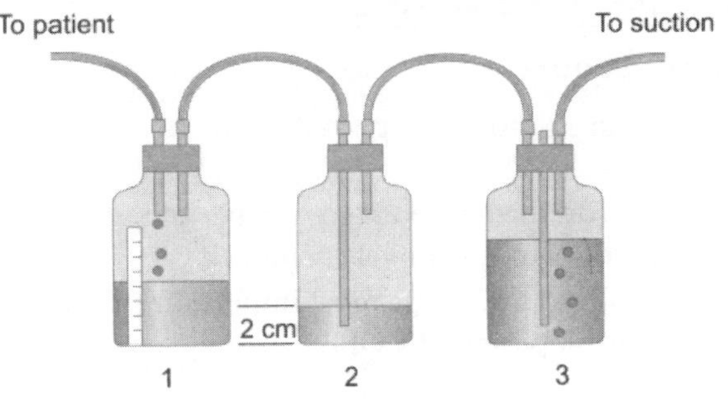

Fig. 30: Three chamber system for ICD.

- If ICD disconnected from patient:
  - Apply occlusive vaseline gauze over incision
  - Monitor for respiratory distress
- If ICD disconnected from drain:
  - Clamp ICD for not more than 1 min
  - Reconnect to new drainage system
- If excessive bubbling through chamber 2:
  - Maybe air leak in drainage system
  - Large pneumothorax

Transport with ICD

- Oxygen source, emergency drugs and airway equipment to be ready
- Chest tube must be functional
- Ensure stable vital signs prior to transport
- Drainage system not to be dropped/tipped
- Drainage system to be lower than patient's chest at all times (else fluid may flow back into pleural cavity and cause infection)
- ICD not to be clamped at any time (may cause tension pneumothorax)
- ICD to be connected to water seal system during transport

Removal of ICD

- ICD is removed when:
  - Drainage has completely stopped
  - < 100 mL drain in 24 hours
  - Pneumothorax has resolved with no air leak (bubbling in chamber)
  - No air leak on Valsalva/forceful cough
- Procedure:
  - Suture removed
  - Valsalva maneuver before pulling out ICD
  - Petroleum gauze and pressure dressing to opening immediately
  - Follow up chest X-ray after 4 hrs

CIGARETTE SMOKING

Introduction

- Smoking history is reported by the number of pack-years
- This is defined as average number of packs per day times the number of years smoked
- Smoking is the single most important risk factor for the development of COPD

Preoperative Effects of Smoking

- Acute effects:
  - Carbon monoxide effects:
    - Carboxyhemoglobin (COHb) levels:
      - Normal patients: 1%
      - Smokers: 8-10%
    - Effects of carboxyhemoglobin:
      - Causes absolute reduction in blood oxygen content
      - Shift of oxy-hemoglobin dissociation curve to left
      - Reduced delivery of oxygen to tissues
  - Nicotinic effects:
    - Blood levels of nicotine ranges between 15-50 mg/mL
    - Induces hepatic enzymes
    - Stimulates sympatho-adrenal system causing:
      - Raised epinephrine, norepinephrine levels
      - Raised cortisol levels
- Chronic effects:
  - Respiratory system:
    - Increased sputum volume due to:
      - Increased sputum production
      - Reduced ciliary motility
    - COPD characterized by:
      - Increased synthesis of elastolytic enzymes from macrophages
      - Increased lung compliance
      - Limited elastic recoil
      - Increased airway reactivity
      - Flattened diaphragmatic configuration
    - Increased reactive oxygen metabolites: OH^-, peroxide radicals
    - Immunoregulatory changes: altered antigen presentation
    - Increased epithelial permeability, changed pulmonary surfactant
    - V/Q mismatch, gas trapping, increased dead space ventilation
    - Inefficient carbon dioxide elimination, arterial hypoxemia
  - Changes in pulmonary function:
    - Increased minute ventilation: 1.5–2 times normal
    - FEV_1 and VC may be normal
    - FEV_1/VC and RV/TLC may be reduced
    - Impaired diffusion capacity (due to CO)
  - Cardiovascular system:
    - Increased SBP and DBP
    - Increased heart rate
    - Increased myocardial oxygen demand
    - Coronary vasospasm, variant angina and MI
  - Gastrointestinal system:
    - Increased gastric volume
    - Lax LES tone
    - Increased chances of preoperative acid peptic disease
    - Increased risk of aspiration

Postoperative Effects of Smoking

- Postoperative pulmonary function:
  - Primarily restrictive changes:
    - Proportional reduction in all lung volumes
    - No change in airway resistance
    - Severity is gauged by reduction in FRC
    - Rapid and shallow respiration occurs
  - Operative site is *single most important determinant*:
    - Upper abdominal surgeries: 40-50% reduction in FRC
    - Lower abdominal and thoracic surgeries: 30% reduction in FRC
    - Intracranial, vascular ENT surgeries: 15-20% reduction in FRC
- Postoperative pulmonary complications (PPC):
  - Mainly pneumonia and segmental atelectasis occurs
  - Sometimes ventilatory failure can occur
  - Most important postoperative pulmonary care is to ambulate the patient
  - Predictors of postoperative pulmonary complications in smokers:
    - Smoking history: Risk increases with > 60 pack years
    - Operative duration: PPC increases if surgical duration > 3 hours
    - Analgesic technique: PPC reduced by postoperative epidural analgesia
    - Associated comorbidities
  - Operative site is important predictor of PPC:
    - Open upper abdominal surgeries increase risk of PPC at least 2-fold
    - Lesser risk for lower abdominal, thoracic and ENT surgeries

- Associated comorbidities:
  - Smokers with COPD are at increased risk for PPC
  - Asthma does not increase risk of postoperative pneumonia and atelectasis but can be exacerbated
- Postoperative Nausea and Vomiting (PONV):
  - Smokers have reduced risk of PONV
  - This is due to low postoperative CNS dopamine levels in smokers
  - This causes desensitization of CTZ to nausea
- Total postoperative complications:
  - Increased risk of postoperative complications in smokers
  - Smoking cessation > 6 months prior to surgery reduces all-cause mortality
  - Benefits of preoperative smoking cessation include:
    - Reduced volume of sputum
    - Reduced incidence coughing
    - Reduced incidence of pneumonia and respiratory failure
    - Reduced incidence of wound infections and general infections
    - Reduced duration of hospital stay

Consequences of Smoking Cessation

- Nicotine withdrawal syndrome:
  - Refers to the craving for cigarettes in the absence of nicotine
  - Symptoms peak in the first 3 days following cessation
  - Symptoms subside over next 3-4 weeks
  - Craving for cigarettes however, may persists for many years
  - Symptoms include:
    - Increased appetite
    - Dysphoria, depressed mood
    - Insomnia
    - Irritability, frustration, anger
    - Difficulty concentrating
    - Restlessness
- Weight gain:
  - Occurs following smoking cessation due to:
    - Decreased metabolic rate
    - Increased activity of lipoprotein lipase
    - Increased appetite
  - Weight gain of 1–2 kgs occurs within first 2 weeks of cessation
  - Average total weight gain is approximately 4–5 kgs
- Depression:
  - Occurs as a component of nicotine withdrawal syndrome
  - May be more pronounced in those with psychiatric disorders
  - However, benefits of smoking cessation outweigh the risks in these patients
- Cough and mouth ulcers:
  - Increased cough and mouth ulcers occur following cessation
  - This is temporary and peaks in first few weeks after cessation

Smoking Reduction

- Few data are available to support smoking reduction over complete cessation
- PPCs are increased even with consistent low-level smoking
- Reduction of smoking by even 50% does not reduce risk of all-cause mortality
- This may be due to modification in the style of smoking including:
  - Increased number of puffs from one cigarette
  - Increase puff-volume causing increased smoke intake
- Thus, complete smoking cessation is preferable preoperatively to smoking reduction

Preoperative Cessation Strategies GOLD Recommendations 2018

- Timing of smoking cessation:
  - Currently no recommendations exist for optimal timing for smoking cessation
  - Cessation ≥ 6 months prior to surgery equalizes risk for PPC to non-smokers
  - Cessation ≥ 8 weeks before surgery reduces risk of PPC four-fold because:
    - Mucociliary function normalizes within 2-3 weeks of quitting smoking
    - Carboxyhemoglobin levels normalizes within 8-24 hours
  - Effects of preoperative smoking cessation:
    - Reduced CO levels:
      - Increased oxygen delivery
      - Reduced myocardial work
    - Reduced level of coronary vasoconstrictors
    - Improved exercise capacity
    - Improved mucociliary activity
    - Reduced airway reactivity
    - Improved pulmonary immune function
    - Better wound healing
    - Reduced incidence of general infections
    - Reduced neurological complications
    - Reduced hospital stay

- Cessation strategies:
  - Behavioral management in addition to nicotine substitutes is recommended
  - Behavioral management: '5a' approach:
    - Ask: Identify all tobacco users
    - Advice: Urge smoking cessation in tobacco users
    - Assess: Determine willingness to quit tobacco use
    - Assist: Aid in quitting:
      - Practical counselling
      - Provide social support
      - Recommend use of pharmacotherapy
      - Provide supplementary materials
    - Arrange: regular follow up
  - Nicotine substitutes:
    - Nicotine transdermal patch:
      - Has long-acting, slow onset pattern of action
      - Produces relief from nicotine withdrawal upto 24 hours
      - Patch is applied to non-hairy skin site
      - Patch is applied at night usually
      - This is because 1-3 hours is required to attain adequate levels
      - Daily change in application site is recommended
      - Dose cannot be titrated to prevent symptoms
      - Dose:
        - > 10 cigarettes/day:
          - 10 weeks course
          - 21 mg/day for 6 weeks
          - 14 mg/day for 2 weeks
          - 7 mg/day for 2 weeks
      - 10 cigarettes/day:
        - 8 weeks course
        - 14 mg/day for 6 weeks
        - 7 mg/day for 2 weeks
    - Nicotine chewing gum:
      - Short acting nicotine replacement therapy
      - Can be used to treat cravings during patch therapy
      - May be used Q1-2H in the absence of patch therapy
      - Dose:
        - 22-24 mg/day for person who smokes 1 pack/day
        - Therapy is continued for 6 weeks
        - Following this, gradual reduction in dose is attempted
        - Therapy may be continued for 3 months total duration
    - Other substitutes:
      - Nicotine lozenges
      - Nicotine inhalers
      - Nicotine nasal spray
      - Nicotine mouth spray
      - Nicotine sublingual tablets
  - Pharmacological adjuncts:
    - Adjuncts increase success of cessation of smoking
    - Adjuncts may increase risk of graft rejection
    - Various adjuncts available:
      - Varenicline:
        - Blocks nicotine from binding to its receptor
        - Acts at the mesolimbic dopamine system
        - This system is associated with nicotine addiction
        - Stimulates nicotine activity but to lesser extent
        - Smoking cessation is advised 1 week after initiating therapy
        - This is to attain stable blood levels of varenicline
        - Dose:
          - Treatment course of 12 weeks
          - 0.5 mg daily for first 3 days
          - 0.5 mg Q12H for next 4 days
          - 1 mg Q12H for 11 weeks
      - Buproprion hydrochloride:
        - Acts by enhancing NE and dopamine release in CNS
        - Less effective compared to varenicline
        - Smoking cessation is advised 1 week after initiating therapy
        - This is to attain stable blood levels of bupropion
        - Dose:
          - Treatment course is 12 weeks
          - 150 mg daily for 3 days
          - 150 mg Q12H for remaining duration of course
      - Less commonly used adjuncts:
        - Nortriptyline
        - Cytisine
        - Selective serotonin reuptake inhibitors
        - Clonidine
        - Other strategies:
          - Bronchodilation, chest physiotherapy, forced oral fluids
          - Deep breathing exercises, incentive spirometry
          - Stir-up regimes are as effective as incentive spirometry
          - Intermittent CPAP mask

No.	Time of cessation	Benefits
1.	12-24 hrs before surgery	Reduced CO, nicotine levels
		Increase in P_{50}
2.	48-72 hrs before surgery	COHb levels normalized
		Improved ciliary function
3.	1-2 weeks before surgery	Decreased sputum production
4.	3-4 weeks before surgery	Wound healing normalizes
5.	4-6 weeks before surgery	Improved PFTs
6.	6-8 weeks before surgery	Immune function, metabolism normalizes
7.	8-12 weeks before surgery	Reduced postoperative morbidity and mortality
		4 times reduced risk of PPC
8.	> 6 months before surgery	Equal risk of PPC as non-smokers

CHRONIC OBSTRUCTIVE PULMONARY DISEASE

Introduction

- COPD is a disease characterized by:
  - Airflow limitation which is not fully reversible
  - Less than 12% reversibility post-bronchodilator therapy
- COPD is a challenge to the anesthesiologist due to high risk of:
  - Intraoperative pulmonary complications
  - Postoperative pulmonary complications:
    - Pneumonia
    - Reintubation after initial extubation
    - Prolonged intubation > 48 hours
- COPD includes 3 components:
  - Chronic Bronchitis: Defined as productive cough on most days for ≥ 3 months duration for ≥ 2 consecutive years or recurrent excessive sputum which severely impairs expiratory flow
  - Emphysema: Anatomically defined as condition characterized by destruction and enlargement of airways distal to respiratory bronchioles (including respiratory bronchioles, alveolar ducts and alveoli)
  - Small airway disease: Chronic airflow obstruction within small bronchioles

Etiology

- Risk factors:
  - Smoking > 60 pack years associated with COPD, passive smoking
  - Occupational exposure:
    - Coal mining
    - Gold mining
    - Cotton and textiles industry
  - Low birth weight
  - Ambient air pollution:
    - M allele: Normal α_1 antitrypsin (AT) levels
    - S allele: Slightly reduced α_1 antitrypsin levels
    - Z allele: Severely reduced α_1 antitrypsin levels
  - Recurrent childhood respiratory tract infection
  - Previous history of tuberculosis
  - Poor socioeconomic status
  - Malnutrition
- Pathological changes:
  - Collapse during expiration due to:
    - Deterioration in elasticity or recoil within lung parenchyma
    - Decreased rigidity of bronchiolar wall
  - Enlargement of air sacs due to:
    - Increased gas flow velocity in narrowed bronchiole
    - Active bronchospasm
    - Obstruction due to pulmonary secretions

Pathophysiology

- Flow limitation:
  - Flow limitation occurs usually during forced expiratory maneuver
  - It occurs even at rest for tidal volume expiration in severe COPD
  - In normal patients:
    - Elastic recoil pressure of alveoli is transmitted to intrathoracic airways
    - Thus, pressure in airway lumen always exceeds intrapleural pressure
  - However, in COPD, elastic recoil pressure of alveoli is low
  - This results in development of equal pressure point (EPP) in the airway lumen
  - This causes airway luminal flow limitation during expiration
- Right ventricular dysfunction:
  - RV dysfunction may occur in upto 50% patients with COPD
  - RV dysfunction occurs because of increased PA pressures in COPD
  - Chronic recurrent hypoxemia causes RV dysfunction and cor-pulmonale
  - Thus, supplemental oxygen is administered to maintain PaO_2 60-65 mm Hg
- Effect of oxygen therapy on respiratory drive and hypercarbia:
  - Patients with COPD have elevated $PaCO_2$ levels at rest
  - This is due to mechanically inefficient pulmonary function

- Thus, lungs are unable to maintain WOB proportionate to metabolic rate
- Elevated $PaCO_2$ level causes raised bicarbonate levels in CSF
- Medullary chemoreceptors become reset to higher blood levels of CO_2
- Chemoreceptor sensitivity to CO_2 is reduced in such patients
- Thus, respiratory control mechanisms become insensitive to $PaCO_2$
- In these patients respiratory drive is maintained by hypoxic stimulus
- On administration of higher FiO_2, CO_2 retention occurs
- This is because of 2 mechanisms:
  - Respiratory drive mechanism:
    - High FiO_2 removes hypoxemic stimulation of respiratory drive
    - This may result in:
      - Hypoventilation
      - Precipitation of hypercapneic coma
    - However, this mechanism plays only a minor role
  - Reversal of hypoxic pulmonary vasoconstriction (HPV):
    - Administration of high FiO_2 results in removal of HPV
    - This causes:
      - Increase in intrapulmonary shunting
      - Increase in $PaCO_2$
    - This is the major mechanism by which hypercapneic coma develops

Clinical Features

- Symptoms:
  - Episodic dyspnea/dyspnea on exertion (emphysema)
  - Chronic, productive cough (chronic bronchitis)
  - Orthopnea, wheezing
  - Personal history of smoking and atopy
  - Family history of allergies
  - Past history of respiratory illness
  - Sleep induced hypoxemia due to hypoventilation during REM sleep
- Signs:
  - Nasal polyps
  - Rhonchi on auscultation
  - Prolonged expiration lasting more than 6 seconds
  - Early inspiratory/end inspiratory/expiratory crackles
  - Reduced or absent breath sounds
  - ***Barrel shaped chest***
  - ***Tripod sign***:
    - Patient sits in tripod position
    - Done to facilitate use of:
      - Sternocleidomastoid
      - Scalenei muscles
      - Intercostal muscles
  - ***Hoovers sign***: Paradoxical inward movement of ribcage with inspiration
  - Signs of right heart failure:
    - Raised CVP
    - Hepatic congestion
    - Peripheral edema

Characteristic	Cardiac dyspnea	Respiratory dyspnea
Onset	Dyspnea followed by cough	Cough followed by dyspnea
Predominant symptom	Dyspnea	Cough
Cardiac symptoms	Chest pain, palpitations, syncope	Rare
PND, orthopnea	*Pathognomonic*	Orthopnea may be present
		PND absent
Relieving factors	Diuretics and inotropes	Rest and bronchodilators

Feature	Chronic bronchitis	Emphysema
Also called	Blue bloaters	Pink puffers
Characteristic	Combination of cyanosis and edema	Lack of cyanosis with ***pursed lip breathing***
Pathophysiology	Mucus and inflammation	Loss of elastic recoil
	Thickening of bronchial wall	Destruction of lung parenchyma
Elastic recoil	Normal	Reduced
Airway resistance	Increased	Normal or slightly increased
Built	Often obese	Thin built, cachexic
Consciousness	Drowsy	Alert
Respiratory drive	Poor	Good
Dyspnea	Moderate	Severe
Cough	Frequent	With exertion
Sputum	Copious	Scanty
Respiratory failure	Early onset, Type II failure	Late onset, usually Type I failure
Hematocrit	Increased, polycythemia	Normal, normocythemia
PaO_2	Reduced	Reduced
$PaCO_2$	More than 40 mm Hg	Usually normal, < 40 mm Hg
Spirometry	Moderate airway obstruction	Severe airway obstruction
Total lung capacity	Normal	Reduced
DLCO	Normal	Reduced

Contd...

Contd...

Feature	Chronic bronchitis	Emphysema
FEV_1	Reduced	Reduced
Cor pulmonale	Marked and early	Mild and late
Chest X-ray	Increased vascular markings	Hyperinflation
		Reduced pulmonary markings
CT scan	Normal	Emphysematous changes
Prognosis	Poor	Good
Anesthetic management	More complications	Less complications

Collateral Ventilation in COPD

- Refers to ventilation of alveolar structures through passages or channels which bypass normal airways
- Pathways for collateral ventilation are:
  - Interalveolar pores: ***Pores of Kahn***
  - Accessory bronchioles:
    - ***Channels of Lambert***
    - Alveolar passage
  - Accessory respiratory bronchioles connecting bronchiole to bronchiole
  - Across fissures
- In normal lungs, resistance to collateral flow is 50 times greater than resistance to flow in normal airways
- This resistance is markedly reduced in emphysema with low resistance collateral channels with pressure gradients across them
- This is proven by the fact that selective lobar intubation and ventilation does not lead to collapse of other lobes

Investigations

- Bedside pulmonary function tests:
  - ***Sabrasez breath holding*** more than 30 seconds
  - ***Match blowing test***
  - Limitation indicates limited cardio-respiratory reserve
- Complete blood count:
  - Leucocytosis due to infection
  - Polycythemia
  - Raised serum α_1-AT levels
  - COHb levels $\geq$ 8-10 %
- ECG:
  - RV strain pattern
  - R: S ratio > 1 in lead V1
  - Low voltage QRS
  - Poor R wave progression
  - P pulmonale in lead II: Indicates right atrial hypertrophy
- Chest X-ray:
  - Normal lung fields in early COPD
  - Characteristic features include:
    - Hyperlucency due to:
      - Arterial vascular insufficiency in peripheral zones
      - Hyperinflation of alveoli
    - Flattening of diaphragm with loss of domed appearance
    - Vertical tubular cardiac silhouette
    - Emphysematous bullae: rare but confirms diagnosis
  - Hyperinflation, increased vascular markings: Chronic bronchitis
  - Hyperinflation, reduced vascular markings (more at lung base): emphysema
  - Retrosternal air space more than 2 cm diameter in lateral chest X-ray
  - Consolidation if LRTI
- CT scan:
  - More sensitive than chest X-ray for diagnosis of COPD
  - Not routinely used for diagnosis
  - Indications:
    - Screening for lung cancer
    - Evaluation of lungs prior to lung surgery
  - Findings on CT-scan:
    - Bronchial wall thickening
    - Alveolar septal destruction
    - Airspace enlargement
- ABG:
  - Usually normal until COPD becomes severe
  - PaO_2 and $PaCO_2$ may not increase until $FEV_1 < 50\%$
  - Hypoxemia with (A-a) O_2 gradient $\geq$ 10 mm Hg
  - Awake hypercapnea more than 45 mm Hg indicates increased risk of POPC
- Pulmonary function tests:
  - If abnormal, indicates a 20-40% risk of POPC
  - No threshold value beyond which risk of surgery is prohibitive
    - FVC: Normal or slightly elevated
    - FEV_1: Normal or slightly reduced
    - FEV_1/FVC: Confirmatory of COPD and characterized by:
      - Reduced below 70% of predicted
      - Not reversible with bronchodilator therapy
    - $FEF_{25-75\%}$:
      - Reduced to less than 70% of predicted value
      - May be first and only abnormality

- FRC: Normal or increased if gas trapping
- TLC: Normal or increased if gas trapping
- MV: 1.5-2.5 times normal

- Exercise testing $VO_{2(max)}$ < 1 Litre indicates 75% mortality risk
- Bronchodilator therapy:
  - 15% improvement in PFT following bronchodilator therapy indicates positive response
  - Improvement indicates that this therapy should be started before surgery

- Flow volume loops
- Echocardiography if pulmonary HTN or cor-pulmonale
- Overnight oximetry/formal sleep studies if central apnea present

Gold Classification of Severity

Category	Name	FEV1
GOLD 1	Mild	FEV_1 > 80% predicted
GOLD 2	Moderate	FEV_1 50-80% predicted
GOLD 3	Severe	FEV_1 30-50% predicted
GOLD 4	Very severe	FEV_1 < 30% predicted

Bode Index for COPD Survival Prediction

Variable	Points on bode index			
	0	1	2	3
Body mass index	> 21	< 21		
FEV1 % predicted	≥ 65	50-64	36-49	≤ 35
Medical research council dyspnea scale	0-1	2	3	4
6-minute walk test	≥350 mts	250-349 mts	150-249 mts	≤149 mts

- BODE index has been found to be better predictor of survival than FEV_1 alone
- 4-year survival rates:
  - 0-2 points: 80%
  - 3-4 points: 67%
  - 5-6 points: 57%
  - 7-10 points: 18%

American Thoracic Society Classification of Severity

- Stage I:
  - FEV_1 more than 50% predicted (includes mild and moderate COPD)
  - No significant dyspnea, hypoxia or hypercarbia
- Stage II: FEV_1 between 35-50% of predicted value
- Stage III: FEV_1 ≤ 35% of predicted value
- Life expectancy ≤ 3 years in patients 60 years age with stage III COPD

Risk Factors for Postoperative Pulmonary Complications

- Patient related:
  - Advanced age more than 60 years
  - Smoked > 40 pack years
  - Morbid obesity
  - Current respiratory symptoms
- Procedure and anesthesia related:
  - Surgery related:
    - Emergency surgery
    - Thoracic/upper abdominal surgery
    - Head and neck surgery
    - Neurosurgery
    - Vascular/ aortic aneurysm surgery
  - Anesthesia related:
    - Anesthetic duration > 2.5 hours
    - General anesthesia > spinal anesthesia > epidural anesthesia
- Test predictors:
  - Inability to walk 500 feet in 6 minutes
  - Inability to ascend 2 flights of stairs (12 steps per flight of stairs)
  - PaO_2 < 50 mm Hg on room air
  - $PaCO_2$ > 45 mm Hg
  - Postoperative FEV_1 < 40% of predicted normal
  - FEV_1 < 800 mL or $PaCO_2$ > 45 mm Hg indicates very high risk of POPC
  - Less than 15 mL/kg/min oxygen consumption on exercise testing (VO_{2max})
  - Combined predicted FEV_1 and DLCO postoperatively < 35% of normal
  - Serum albumin < 3.5 g/dL
  - BUN > 0.3 mg/dL

Ariscat Risk Index for POPC Prediction

No.	Feature	Score
1.	Age	
	< 50 years	0
	51-80 years	3
	> 80 years	16
2.	Preoperative SpO_2	
	> 96%	0
	91-95%	8
	< 90%	24
3.	Respiratory infection in last 1 month	17
4.	Preoperative hemoglobin < 10 g/dL	11
5.	Type of surgery	
	Upper abdominal	15
	Intrathoracic	24

Contd...

Contd...

No.	Feature	Score
6.	Duration of surgery	
	< 2 hours	0
	2-3 hours	16
	> 3 hours	23
7.	Emergency surgery	8

- Low risk category:
  - < 26 points
  - Risk of postoperative pulmonary complications: 1.6%
- Intermediate risk category:
  - 26-44 points
  - Risk of postoperative pulmonary complications: 13.3%
- High risk category:
  - > 45 points
  - Risk of postoperative pulmonary complications: 42%

POPC Risk Reduction Strategy

- Preoperative strategies:
  - Smoking cessation at least 6 weeks prior to surgery
  - Treat evidence of expiratory airflow obstruction
  - Treat RTI with antibiotics
  - Lung volume expansion maneuvers:
    - Deep breathing exercises
    - Incentive spirometry
    - Chest physiotherapy
    - Intermittent CPAP
- Intraoperative strategies:
  - Minimal invasive techniques for surgery: Laparoscopy preferred
  - Use regional anesthesia where possible
  - Avoid long acting neuromuscular blockers
  - Avoid prolonged surgery lasting more than 3 hours
- Postoperative strategies:
  - Lung expansion maneuvers:
    - Deep breathing exercises
    - Incentive spirometry
    - Continuous positive airway pressure
    - Chest physiotherapy
  - Optimal analgesia:
    - Patient controlled analgesia
    - Neuraxial opioids
    - Regional techniques for analgesia
    - Nerve blocks

Choice of Anesthetic Technique

- Regional anesthesia:
  - Preferred over general anesthesia for:
    - Lower abdominal surgeries
    - Procedures on extremities
  - Regional anesthesia preferred over GA as:
    - Avoids airway instrumentation
    - Reduces risk of:
      - Laryngospasm
      - Bronchospasm
      - Barotrauma
    - Better pain control which improves pulmonary function
    - Eliminates need for opioids
    - Reduces risk of DVT
    - Allows early mobilization: reduces risk of POPC
  - Level of neuraxial blockade is restricted to T_6 sensory level only
  - This is because extension of block above this level causes:
    - Respiratory muscle dysfunction
    - Impairment of ventilatory function resulting in:
      - Reduced ERV
      - Reduced PEFR
      - Reduced maximum minute ventilation
  - Interscalene blocks are avoided to prevent ipsilateral phrenic nerve palsy
- General anesthesia:
  - Indications:
    - Severe dyspnea
    - Inability to lie supine
    - Persistent coughing
    - Upper abdomen and intrathoracic procedures
    - Prolonged surgeries
  - Avoid use of histamine releasing agents:
    - Ester group of local anesthetics
    - Drugs with preservatives of amide group
  - Use of LMA is associated with lower risk of bronchospasm

Preoperative Patient Preparation and Premedication

- Smoking cessation:
  - Smoking cessation for at least 6 weeks is recommended
  - Cessation for more than 8 weeks reduces risk of POPC
  - Cessation for more than 4-8 weeks improves mucociliary clearance
- Optimize dosage and continue use of bronchodilators:
  - Increase frequency of inhalers/nebulization to Q4H
  - β_2 agonists are *drugs of choice*
  - Ipratropium bromide reported to produce more bronchodilation than β_2 agonists

- Addition of bronchodilator therapy:
  - Added if 15 % improvement in PFT after bronchodilator trial
  - Nebulization:
    - Salbutamol:
      - 0.5% respirator solution used
      - 0.5 mL salbutamol + 1.5 mL saline nebulized Q6H
      - Dose can be increased to 1 mL of salbutamol
      - Salbutamol respule 2.5 mg Q4-6H
    - Ipratropium bromide:
      - Respirator solution used
      - 0.5 mL ipratropium + 1.5 mL saline Q4-6H
      - Ipravent respule 500 µg Q4-6H
  - Inhalers:
    - Budesonide respule 0.5 mg or 1 mg Q12H
    - Salbutamol inhaler 2 puffs QID
    - Tiotropium bromide inhaler 2 puffs OD
    - Ipratropium bromide 2 puffs QID
- Steroids:
  - Cause only 15-20 % reduction in inflammation in COPD patients
  - Steroids given only if adequate response to bronchodilator therapy is not seen
  - Inhalational agents: Fluticasone/beclomethasone dipropionate/budesonide/mometasone
  - Short course of oral prednisolone 30-40 mg/day to be reduced in 7-10 days
- Aminophylline:
  - 5-7 mg/kg IV over 20 minutes loading dose
  - Followed by 0.5-0.7 mg/kg/hr to maintain serum aminophylline levels of 5-20 µg/mL
- Antibiotics:
  - Given preoperatively if active infection: amoxicillin with clavuronic acid 625 mg TID
  - Sepsis prophylaxis with appropriate antibiotics
- Other drugs:
  - Acetylcysteine (mucolytic) and oral expectorants to patients with viscous secretions
  - Cromolyn sodium/nedocromil/roflumilast as oral anti-inflammatory agents
  - Caution with sedative drugs in patients with severe obstruction/hypercapnea
  - DVT prophylaxis (as polycythemia usually present)
- Lung expansion strategies:
  - Cough and deep breathing exercises
  - Incentive spirometry, stir up regimens
  - Intermittent CPAP
  - Postural drainage and chest percussion if secretory chest
- Pulmonary rehabilitation:
  - Comprises of education in breathing exercises and nutrition
  - Done for 2-4 wks prior to surgery
  - Helps to reduce risk of POPC
  - Used for non-malignant resection in patients with severe COPD
- Adequate hydration:
  - Forced oral fluids more than 3 L/day
  - Prevents dehydration and drying up of secretions
- Correct conditions which contribute to respiratory muscle weakness:
  - Malnutrition
  - Electrolyte imbalance
  - Metabolic and endocrine disorders
- If COPD with cor-pulmonale:
  - Inhaled NO with O_2 1 L/min can be used for 3 months
  - Portable inspiratory pulsing device used
  - This causes greater increase in pulmonary hemodynamics than oxygen alone
  - NO relieves pulmonary vasoconstriction and also increases blood supply to poorly ventilated areas
  - This causes reduction in PaO_2
  - Thus, NO should always be combined with low O_2 flows
- Premedication:
  - Benzodiazepines
  - Antisialogogues:
    - Glycopyrrolate and ipratropium bromide used
    - Use is controversial as it may dry up secretions

Monitors

- Pulse oximetry:
  - Detects significant desaturation
  - PaO_2 is important to detect subtle changes in intrapulmonary shunting
- E_TCO_2, NIBP
- ECG: For arrhythmias/MI (due to hypercapnea)
- Baseline ABG:
  - Recommended for ATS stage II and III COPD
  - Important as postoperative ventilation aims to keep $PaCO_2$ at baseline levels
  - Increased $PaCO_2$-E_TCO_2 gradient may be present
- CVP may be used if RVF present but will not indicate intravascular volume in such cases

- Urine output, neuromuscular monitoring
- Temperature monitoring

Induction

- Adequate preoxygenation as FRC may be increased
- Inhalational induction is usually avoided due to:
  - Pungent odour of volatile agents
  - Slower induction due to V/Q mismatch
- Intravenous induction is therefore preferred
- Propofol (2 mg/kg), ketamine (1.5 mg/kg), etomidate or midazolam maybe used
- Avoid long acting muscle relaxants: vecuronium/rocuronium
- Avoid long acting opioids and NMB to prevent prolonged respiratory depression
- Opioids like fentanyl/pethidine/alfentanyl/remifentanyl preferred
- Avoid histamine releasers:
  - Morphine, pancuronium
  - Atracurium and cisatracurium, mivacurium
- Prevent bronchospam at intubation:
  - Deep planes at intubation
  - IV lidocaine 1.5-2 mg/kg 90 seconds prior to intubation
  - Local anesthetic spray on vocal cords may help

Maintenance

- Balanced anesthesia with O_2 + air + 1 MAC volatile anesthetic preferred
- Volatile agent based anesthesia is preferred as:
  - They can be rapidly eliminated
  - This facilitates early and more complete recovery
  - This prevents residual postoperative ventilatory depression
- However, in very severe airflow obstruction, delayed recovery may result
- This is because of air-trapping causing retention of volatile agents
- Isoflurane and sevoflurane are the preferred agents
- Desflurane is avoided as it causes bronchial irritation and bronchospasm
- Nitrous oxide should be avoided as it may cause:
  - Expansion and rupture of bullae
  - Tension pneumothorax
  - Limitation of inspired FiO_2
  - Aggravation of pulmonary hypertension
- Halothane sensitizes patients to catecholamines and is avoided in:
  - Patients with hypercarbia
  - Preoperative β_2 agonist and aminophylline therapy
- Avoid long acting opioids and NMB (alfentanil/remifentanyl/vecuronium preferred)
- Propofol and remifentanyl based TIVA may be used as an alternative

Hemodynamics

- Adequate hydration important to prevent drying up of secretion.
- Judicious fluid therapy in patients with corpulmonale
- Titrated to maintain urine output more than 0.5 mL/kg/hour

Ventilation

- Avoid spontaneous ventilation as hypercapnea results
- Avoid hyperventilation:
  - Can cause prolonged apnea
  - CO_2 production reduces under GA due to low BMR
  - $PaCO_2$ levels as it is will be low under GA
  - Thus, CO_2 levels have to build up considerably before baseline $PaCO_2$ levels are reached to trigger ventilation
- Ventilatory settings:
  - FiO_2 titrated to maintain $SpO_2 > 90\%$
  - Tidal volume 6-8 mL/kg
  - Respiratory rate 8-10 /min: Allows enough time for expiration and also for venous return
  - Increased expiratory time
  - Peak airway pressure < 30 cm H_2O
  - Plateau airway pressure < 20 cm H_2O
  - Avoid PEEP/sighs:
    - Adverse cardiovascular effects
    - Also, increased risk of bulla rupture
  - Slow inspiratory flow rate preferred
- Humidification of gases:
  - Presence of ETT bypasses natural humidification system
  - Thus, inspired gases should be humidified to prevent drying up of secretions
  - Especially useful if duration of surgery more than 2 hours
  - Done with HME filter
- Goals of mechanical ventilation:
  - PaO_2: 60–100 mm Hg

- $PaCO_2$ maintained at preoperative levels
- pH 7.35-7.45

Intraoperative Complications

- Bronchospasm
  - Deepen anesthetic plane:
    - Increase MAC of volatile anesthetic
    - IV ketamine supplementation
  - Increase FiO_2
  - ETT suction, check for kinking/obstruction
  - Stop surgical stimulation
  - IV corticosteroids
  - Nebulized β_2 agonists or racemic epinephrine
  - IV epinephrine in refractory cases
  - Use ICU ventilators to control airway pressure
- Rupture of bulla
- Pneumothorax: Needle in IInd ICS in mid-clavicular line
- Myocardial infarction: due to comorbidities
- Arrhythmias: due to hypercarbia
- Laryngospasm

Extubation

- Deep and early extubation after thorough suctioning as ET tube:
  - Increases airway resistance
  - Causes reflex bronchoconstriction
  - Reduced ability to clear secretions
  - Increases risk of iatrogenic infections
- Reversal of NMB controversial as neostigmine may cause bronchoconstriction
- Recovery in sitting position improves FRC

Postoperative Care

Postoperative Management

- Propped up recovery position: improves FRC
- Oxygen therapy:
  - Hypoxemia in COPD is defined as:
    - $PaO_2 < 55$ mm Hg or $SpO_2 < 88\%$
    - When COPD is associated with cor-pulmonale or polycythemia:
      - PaO_2 55-60 mm Hg
      - $SpO_2 < 88\%$
  - Thus, oxygen therapy should be titrated to maintain SpO_2 90-92%
- Early mobilization:
  - Single most important aspect of postoperative pulmonary care
  - Increases FRC and improves oxygenation
  - Improves ventilation-perfusion matching
- Antibiotic prophylaxis
  - Salbutamol 2.5 mg nebulization QID
  - Ipratropium 500 μg nebulization QID
  - Convert to inhalers at least 24 hours prior to discharge.
- Avoid smoking as it causes delayed wound healing and reduces resistance to infection
- Chest physiotherapy:
  - Lung expansion maneuvers
  - Incentive spirometry
  - Use of intermittent CPAP:
    - Indicated in patients unable to perform:
      - Deep breathing exercises
      - Incentive spirometry
    - Returns FRC to normal within 72 hours
  - FRC returns to normal after 3-7 days if CPAP is not used
- Administration of steroids after 3rd postoperative day does not delay wound healing

Postoperative Ventilation

- Routine postoperative mechanical ventilation is seldom beneficial
- However, postoperative ventilation may be indicated in patients with:
  - Preoperative $FEV_1 < 50\%$
  - Preoperative FEV_1/ FVC < 0.5
  - Baseline $PaCO_2 > 50$ mm Hg
- Ventilatory goals:
  - Maintain normal pH 7.35-7.45
  - Maintain SpO_2 90-92%
  - Maintain preoperative baseline $PaCO_2$ levels
  - Minimize risk of air-trapping:
    - Reduce I:E ratio
    - Low respiratory rate
- Weaning from postoperative ventilation:
  - Gradual weaning of ventilatory support
  - T-piece trial beneficial prior to extubation
  - Use of bronchodilators pre-extubation to minimize airway resistance
  - Reduce work of breathing post-extubation using:
    - Continuous positive airway pressure (CPAP)
    - Bilevel positive airway pressure (BIPAP)
  - Indications for NIV: At least one of the following:
    - Respiratory acidosis with:
      - pH 7.35
      - $PaCO_2 > 45$ mm Hg

- Persistent hypoxemia despite supplemental oxygen therapy
- Severe dyspnea with:
  - Clinical signs of respiratory fatigue
  - Increased work of breathing
  - Use of accessory muscles of respiration
  - Paradoxical movement of abdomen
  - Intercostal retraction

Monitors

- Pulse oximetry, NIBP
- Periodic ABGs especially in stage II and III patients
- Urine output, ECG

Postoperative Analgesia

- Epidural/regional nerve blocks
- Morphine avoided
- Fentanyl, pethidine and tramadol can be used
- Avoid aspirin in asthmatic bronchitis

Complications

- Pneumonia
- Atelectasis
- Bronchospasm
- Prolonged mechanical ventilation
- Pneumothorax
- Prolonged bronchopleural fistula

ONE LUNG VENTILATION

Introduction

- Refers to the mechanical separation of the 2 lungs to allow ventilation of only 1 lung
- It is a technique used to facilitate surgery for thoracic and pulmonary surgeries
- First double lumen tube was designed by ***Head*** in 1889 with 2 tracheal cannulas:
  - Short tracheal cannula
  - Longer endobronchial cannula
- This was mainly used in experimental studies on dogs and rabbits
- The first use of endobronchial anesthesia in humans was by ***Gale and Waters*** in 1932
- They used an endobronchial tube with carinal cuff which would block both bronchi
- The first right and left sided endobronchial tubes were designed by ***MacGill*** in 1936

Goals of OLV

- Provide quiet field for performance of surgery
- Maintain adequate gas exchange:
  - Oxygen saturation of hemoglobin > 90%
  - PaO_2 > 60 mm Hg
- Maximize pulmonary vascular resistance in non-ventilated lung
- Minimize pulmonary vascular resistance in ventilated lung
- Protect ventilated lung from over-distension injury:
  - *Protective lung ventilation*
  - Plateau airway pressure < 25 cm H_2O
  - $PaCO_2$ around 35 + 3 mm Hg
  - Tidal volume 6-8 mL/Kg

Indications Based on Requirement of OLV

- Absolute indications:
  - Isolation of lungs to prevent spillage/contamination:
    - Infection, abscess
    - Massive hemorrhage
    - Unilateral infected cyst/bulla
  - Surgical opening of major conductive airway
  - Control of distribution of ventilation to one lung:
    - Broncho-Pleural Fistula (BPF)
    - Broncho-pleural-cutaneous fistula
    - Unilateral cyst/bulla
    - Major disruption/trauma to bronchus
  - Unilateral bronchoalveolar lavage
  - Video assisted thoracoscopic surgery (VATS)
- Relative indications:
  - Surgical exposure: High priority:
    - Upper lobectomy
    - Pneumonectomy
    - Lung volume reduction surgery
    - Minimally invasive cardiac surgery
    - Thoracic aortic aneurysm
  - Surgical exposure: Low priority:
    - Middle/lower lobe lobectomy
    - Thoracoscopy
    - Esophageal resection
    - Mediastinal mass resection
    - Thymectomy
    - Bilateral sympathectomy
    - Thoracic spine surgery
  - ***Differential lung ventilation*** in reperfusion injury:
    - After lung transplant
    - After unilateral pulmonary thromboembolectomy
    - Unilateral lung trauma

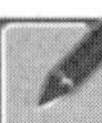

Indications Based on Techniques of Isolation

- Specific indications for DLT:
  - Protection of lung from contralateral contamination:
    - Lung abscess
    - Lung cyst
    - Pulmonary hemorrhage
    - Bronchoalveolar lavage
  - Control and continuity of gas exchange:
    - Bronchopleural fistula
    - Bronchial disruption
    - Pneumonectomy
- Indications with the use of DLT or bronchial blocker: surgical exposure for:
  - Video assisted thoracoscopic surgery
  - Lobectomy
  - Bilobectomy
  - Mediastinal mass resection
  - Esophageal surgery
  - Orthopedic procedures
  - Minimally invasive cardiac surgeries
- Specific indications for bronchial blockers:
  - Difficult airway:
    - Limited mouth opening
    - Nasotracheal intubation
    - Awake orotracheal intubation
  - Already intubated patients requiring lung isolation
  - Tracheostomy patients requiring lung isolation
  - Selective lobar blockade
  - Potential for mechanical ventilation in postoperative period

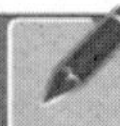

Indications Based on Purpose of Lung Isolationy

- Lung separation for surgical procedures:
  - Pulmonary resection:
    - Lobectomy
    - Pneumonectomy
    - Wedge resection
  - Mediastinal surgery
  - Esophageal surgery
  - Thoracic vascular surgery
  - Thoracic spine surgery
  - Video assisted thoracoscopic surgery
  - Minimally invasive cardiac surgery
- Lung isolation for prevention of cross contamination:
  - Pulmonary hemorrhage
  - Purulent pulmonary secretions
  - During whole lung lavage for pulmonary alveolar proteinosis
- To decrease airway pressure on the side of pathology:
  - Bronchopleural fistula
  - Unilateral cyst/bullae

Contraindications

- Dependence on two-lung mechanical ventilation
- Questionable ability to tolerate OLV:
  - Severe pulmonary disease
  - Prior pulmonary resection
- Procedural difficulty:
  - Intraluminal airway mass may restrict the access to tracheobronchial tree
  - The mass may be dislodged during airway manipulation
  - This may eventually result in complete airway occlusion

Techniques

Technique	Advantages	Disadvantages
Double lumen tubes:		
Direct laryngoscopy	Quickest technique	Size selection difficult
Via tube exchanger	Placement possible without bronchoscopy	Difficult to use if difficult airway
Fibreoptically	Repositioning rarely required	Potential laryngeal trauma
	Bronchoscopy to isolated lung possible	Potential bronchial trauma
	Suction to isolated lung possible	Not optimal for postoperative ventilation
	CPAP can be easily added	
	Can alternate OLV to either lung easily	
	Best device for lung absolute isolation	
Bronchial blocker (BB):		
Arndts system	Size selection not an issue	More time required for positioning
Cohen blocker	Easily added to regular ETT	Repositioning required more often
Fuji uniblocker	Allows ventilation during placement	Bronchoscopy required for positioning
	Easier in difficult airway and children	Right lung isolation suboptimal
	Postoperative ventilation by removing BB	Bronchoscopy to isolated lung impossible
	Selective lobar isolation possible	Minimal suction to isolated lung
	CPAP to isolated lung possible	Difficult to alternate OLV to either lung
Univent	Same as bronchial blocker	Same as for BB
	Less repositioning compared to BB	ETT portion has higher airflow resistance
	Rarely used	
Endobronchial tube	Like regular ETT	Bronchoscopy necessary for placement
	Easier use in difficult airway	Does not allow suction to isolated lung
	Longer than regular ETT	Difficult right lung OLV
	Short cuff for lung isolation	
	Indicated in difficult airway	
ETT in bronchus	Easier in difficult airway	Does not allow suction to isolated lung

Contd...

Contd...

Technique	Advantages	Disadvantages
		Does not allow CPAP to isolated lung Cuff not designed for lung isolation Difficult right lung OLV

Techniques of Lung Separation

- Double lumen tubes:
  - ***Carlens*** left sided DLT
  - ***Whites*** right sided DLT
  - ***Robertshaws*** left/right sided DLT
  - ***Brice Smith*** left/right sided endobronchial tube
  - Bronchocath-portex type DLT
- Single lumen tube with endobronchial blockers:
  - Modified SLT with enclosed BB:
    - Integrated Torque Control Blocker (***Univent***)
    - ***Fogarty*** arterial embolectomy catheter
  - Conventional SLT with enclosed BB:
    - Hybrid wire-guided BB (***Arndt Endobronchial System***)
    - ***Cohens*** tip deflecting endobronchial blocker
    - ***Fuji Uniblocker***
- Single lumen endobronchial tubes:
  - ***Gordon-Greene*** (right side) with carinal hook
  - ***Macintosh-Lethersdale*** (left side)
  - ***Pallistor-Brompton*** triple cuff tube: Two bronchial and one tracheal cuff
- Single lumen ETT advanced into the bronchus

Anesthetic Management

Monitors

- Pulse oximetry: After initiation of OLV, PaO_2 falls for up to 45 minutes
- E_TCO_2, shape of capnogram, differential capnography
- Peak airway pressure
- Pressure volume loop
- Actual tidal volume (V_T) delivered: measured with spirometer
- Frequent ABGs
- Ausculation of dependant lung frequently
- DLT position checked once lateral position assumed

Position

- Mostly lateral position
- In lateral position:
  - PaO_2 levels are better than supine position
  - Dead space and arterial E_TCO_2 gradient increases
  - This requires a 20% increase in minute volume to maintain same $PaCO_2$

Maintenance

- Both TIVA and volatile agent based balanced anesthetic techniques may be used
- TIVA technique *is theoretically more advantageous* as:
  - It preserves hypoxic pulmonary vasoconstriction
  - Thus, it helps in reducing the shunt fraction
  - Also, propofol is less dependent on pulmonary elimination
  - Since VAs are eliminated via the lung, emergence may be delayed
  - Balanced anesthesia or TIVA may be used to maintain anesthesia
- Multiple studies between the 2 techniques have shown insignificant differences in:
  - Oxygenation
  - Shunt fraction
  - Markers of inflammation
  - Clinical outcomes
- Thus, currently there is insufficient evidence to support either technique
- Balanced anesthesia with 0.5-1 MAC isoflurane/sevoflurane is most commonly used

Hemodynamics

- Restrictive fluid therapy strategy is preferred as excessive IV fluids can cause:
  - Increased intrapulmonary shunting
  - Pulmonary edema of dependant lung
  - Occurs especially if prolonged surgery
- Ringers lactate or plasmalyte is the *maintenance fluid of choice*
- Fluids are administered only for replacing intraoperative losses
- Replacement of third space fluid loss is avoided
- Judicious fluid administration is important as it reduces risk of postoperative ALI
- Vasopressors are used instead of fluids to maintain hemodynamic instability
- During left thoracotomy surgical manipulation can cause:
  - Pericardial manipulation
  - Arrhythmias
  - Cardiac compression
  - Hypotension

Ventilation

- Protective lung ventilation strategy is preferred with:
  - Smaller tidal volume
  - PEEP
  - Lower airway pressure

- $FiO_2 < 100\%$
- Permissive hypercapnia

❖ Mode of ventilation:
- Pressure-controlled ventilation is recommended over volume control modes
- This is especially important for:
  - Patients at high risk of Acute Lung Injury (ALI)
  - Bullae, pneumonectomy
  - Post lung transplantation

❖ Fraction of inspired oxygen:
- Minimum FiO_2 to maintain $SpO_2 \geq 90\%$
- This helps to prevent absorption atelectasis

❖ Tidal volume:
- 4-6 mL/kg for OLV
- 6-8 mL/kg for TLV
- Adjust tidal volume to maintain:
  - Peak airway pressure ≤ 35 cm H_2O
  - Plateau airway pressure ≤ 25 cm H_2O

❖ Respiratory rate:
- Rate is adjusted to maintain E_TCO_2 close to patients baseline E_TCO_2
- Rate of 12-20 breaths/minute is usually required

❖ Positive end expiratory pressure:
- PEEP of 5-10 cm H_2O is required if low tidal volume ventilation (5-7 mL/kg)
- PEEP is limited to 0-5 cm H_2O in patients with COPD

❖ Continue two lung ventilation for as long as possible

❖ Permissive hypercapnia:
- Permissive hypercapnia is advantageous for OLV
- This is because:
  - It potentiates HPV
  - Causes rightward shift of ODC
  - Enhances oxygen delivery to the tissues
  - Improves wound healing
- $PaCO_2$-E_TCO_2 is usually high during OLV
- Thus, regular arterial blood gas sampling is necessary

❖ Continuous Positive Airway Pressure (CPAP):
- Applied to non-ventilated, non-dependent upper lung
- 1-2 cm H_2O CPAP to fully inflated lung is usually sufficient
- However, even 5-10 cm H_2O CPAP may increase volume of lung
- This results in encroachment into the surgical field and hampers surgery
- Considered as *most effective therapy* to treat severe hypoxia
- Mechanism of action:
  - Reduces shunt flow through collapsed lung
  - Diverts blood to ventilated lung due to increase in vascular resistance in non-ventilated lung
  - Improves V/Q ratio
- Applied after delivering an inspiratory V_T to non-dependent lung to keep it slightly expanded
- Disadvantages:
  - Reduces surgeons view
  - Increases chance of air leak if stapler placed on partially deflated lungs
  - Hemodynamic changes and over-distension if CPAP ≥ 15 cm H_2O
- Apply frequent recruitment manuvers

❖ Positive end expiratory pressure:
- Applied to dependant lung
- Useful in patients with low dependant lung volume
- Mechanism of action:
  - Restores alveoli
  - Recruits alveoli
  - Improves gas exchange
- If PEEP applied along with large V_T:
  - Over-distension of alveoli occurs
  - Compression of intra-alvelolar blood vessels
  - May worsen V/Q mismatch
- Reduce intrinsic/auto PEEP by:
  - Reducing V_T, RR and I:E time ratio
  - Treat bronchospasm
  - Clear secretions
  - Applying extrinsic PEEP

Improving Deflation of Non-ventilated Lung

❖ Denirogenate both lungs prior to OLV:
- Denitrogenation with 100% oxygen replaces the nitrogen present in air
- Since nitrogen is poorly soluble it is absorbed very slowly into circulation
- Oxygen is more soluble compared with nitrogen
- Thus, replacement with oxygen hastens lung collapse

❖ Disconnection of anesthetic circuit:
- Anesthetic circuit is disconnected and expiration is allowed for 20-30 seconds
- This results in prolonged expiration and fall of E_TCO_2
- OLV is then begun through the ventilated side of DLT

- Use of pressure-controlled ventilation:
  - Use of pressure-controlled ventilation avoids peaking of airway pressures
  - This reduces likelihood of gas being forced past the inflated cuff of the DLT
  - This decreases the chance of inadvertent reinflation of the non-ventilated lung
- Application of low-pressure suction:
  - Low-pressure suction (20 cm H_20) to the non-ventilated lung aids collapse
  - Suction also prevents passive entrainment of sir in the non-ventilated lung

Re-expansion of the Non-Ventilated Lung

- This is done at the end of the surgical procedure to reinflate all atelectatic areas
- It is accomplished with a sustained inflation at low levels of positive airway pressure:
  - 20-30 cm H_2O
  - 10-15 seconds
- Higher pressures are avoided due to risk of creation of new air leaks after resection
- This maneuver may be repeated to maintain optimal recruitment of lung tissue

Postoperative

Ventilation

- Indications:
  - Facial edema
  - Secretions
  - Laryngeal trauma
  - Hypothermia
  - Inadequate NMJ reversal
  - Unexpected blood loss/fluid shift
- Management of individual tubes:
  - Univent tube: Blocker is withdrawn and the tube is used as SLT
  - Bronchial blocker:
    - Blocker is withdrawn
    - Single lumen tube is left in place
  - Double lumen tube:
    - Leave DLT in place if difficult airway/facial edema
    - In such cases, withdraw DLT to place the 19-20 cm mark at teeth
    - Change to single lumen tube in other cases
    - Change to SLT with tube exchanger/video laryngoscope
    - Extubate after diuresis and steroid therapy to reduce facial and airway edema

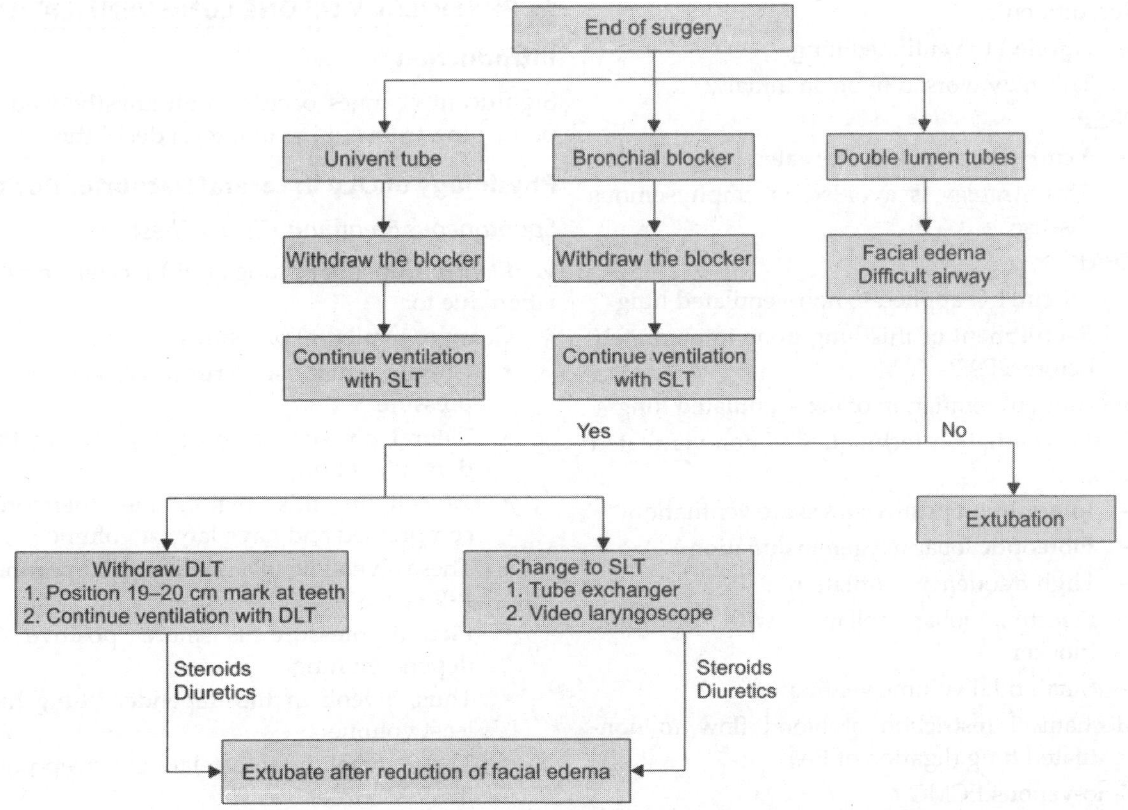

Hypoxia During OLV

Prediction of Hypoxia During OLV

- Side of surgery: Common during right thoracotomy as:
  - Right lung is larger and 10% better perfused than left
  - Increased shunt and reduced $PaCO_2$ during right side thoracotomy
- Two lung oxygenation:
  - If PaO_2 levels are good during TLV in lateral position, they will be better during OLV
  - Thus, chances of hypoxia is less if PaO_2 is good with two lung ventilation
- Preoperative ventilation-perfusion scan: to study shunting and PaO_2

Treatment of Hypoxia during OLV

- Severe/precipitous desaturation: resume two lung ventilation
- Gradual desaturation:
  - Ensure delivered FiO_2 is 1
  - Ensure cardiac output is optimal
  - Reduce volatile anesthetics to < 1 MAC
  - Check position of DLT/BB with fibreoptic bronchoscopy
  - Hand ventilate to check for lung compliance
  - Recruitment:
    - Applied to ventilated lung
    - This may worsen hypoxia initially
  - PEEP:
    - 5 cmH_2O applied to ventilated lung
    - This strategy is avoided in emphysemous disease
  - CPAP:
    - 1-2 cmH_2O applied to non-ventilated lung
    - Recruitment of this lung done immediately before CPAP
  - Intermittent reinflation of non-ventilated lung
  - Partial ventilation techniques to non-ventilated lung
    - Intermittent positive pressure ventilation
    - Fibreoptic lobar oxygen insufflation
    - High frequency ventilation
    - Selective lobar collapse with bronchial blocker
    - Small tidal volume ventilation
  - Mechanical restriction of blood flow to non-ventilated lung (ligation of PA)
  - Veno-venous ECMO
- Other manuvers:
  - Pressure controlled ventilation instead of volume control in patients with significant restrictive lung disease (preoperative FVC < 77% of predicted value)
  - Deepen anesthetic plane if light
  - Bronchodilator therapy if bronchospasm
  - Suction secretions with bronchoscope and check position of tube
  - Do not hyperventilate dependant lung as hypocapnea causes:
    - Increased shunt fraction and decreased $PaCO_2$
    - Increased vascular resistance in dependant lung
- Newer interventions:
  - Eliminate vasodilators: NTG, halothane
  - Selective administration of PGE_1 to ventilated lung
  - Nitric oxide synthetase inhibitor (***L-Name***) to hypoxic lobe
  - Almitrine with nitric oxide 20 ppm to non-ventilated lung
- If all the manuvers fail, institute two lung ventilation

PHYSIOLOGY OF ONE LUNG VENTILATION

Introduction

Significant changes occurs in an anesthetized patient on turning from supine to lateral decubitus.

Physiology of OLV in Lateral Decubitus Position

Spontaneous Breathing, Closed Chest

Ventilation: Dependant lungs (DL) receives more ventilation due to:

- Changes in pleural pressure:
  - Gravity causes a vertical gradient in pleural pressure
  - Pleural pressure is more negative in the non-dependent lung
  - Alveoli in this region are therefore least compressed and have largest volume
  - These alveoli lie in a relatively flat portion of the P-V curve
  - Pleural pressure is more positive in the dependent lung
  - Thus, alveoli in the dependent lung have the least volume
  - These alveoli lie in a relatively steep portion of the P-V curve

- ❖ Changes in diaphragmatic contour:
  - Lower diaphragm is pushed higher inside chest than upper diaphragm
  - This occurs due to abdominal contents pushing the lower hemidiaphragm
  - Owing to the more sharply curved lower diaphragm, it is able to contract better
  - This results in better ventilation

Perfusion: Increased perfusion to dependant lung due to gravity.

V/Q Ratio

- ❖ Non-dependant lung (NDL) alveoli have the maximum volume
- ❖ Alveoli in the dependant lung have least volume
- ❖ V/Q ratio decreases from non-dependant to dependant lung
- ❖ However, due to gravity, dependant lung receives more perfusion
- ❖ Thus, the V/Q ratio is not greatly altered

Spontaneous Breathing, Open Chest

Ventilation

- ❖ In the open hemithorax, pleural interface of non-dependent lung is disrupted
- ❖ Thus, no negative pressure is generated in the pleural cavity in response to:
  - Spontaneous breathing
  - Chest wall expansion
- ❖ In dependent lung, however, closed hemithorax results in negative pleural pressure
- ❖ This results in 2 important phenomena:
  - *Mediastinal shift*
  - *Pendelluft*
- ❖ Mediastinal shift:
  - The negative pleural pressure of DL is equally applied to mediastinum

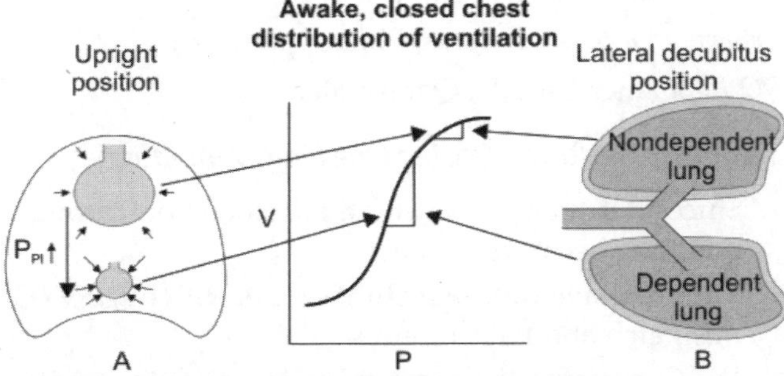

Fig. 31: Spontaneous breathing closed chest.

  - Thus, the mediastinum is pulled away from NDL during inspiration
  - During expiration, positive intrathoracic pressure pushes mediastinum into NDL
  - Thus, mediastinum is:
    - Pulled towards DL during inspiration
    - Pushed into NDL during expiration
  - This mediastinal shift results in:
    - Reduction of tidal volume in dependent lung
    - Increase in tidal volume to the NDL
- ❖ Pendelluft:
  - There is a loss of negativity of the pleural pressure of non-dependant lung
  - Thus, this lung is free to collapse due to surgical pneumothorax
  - Pleural pressure of dependent lung however remains negative
  - Thus, with each inspiration, the dependent lung receives air from:
    - Atmosphere via the trachea
    - Non-dependent lung via the bronchi
  - This results in pulmonary steal of air from the NDL to DL
  - Inspiration therefore results in:
    - Dependant lung expansion
    - Non-dependent lung collapse
  - During expiration, gas from dependent lung escapes via:
    - Mainstem bronchus into trachea
    - Bronchi into non-dependent lung
  - This results in a pendular motion of the lung with respiration called pendelluft
- ❖ This results in the following changes:
  - DL is poorly ventilated as FRC is decreased by mediastinal weight
  - NDL is better ventilated as it has no restriction to movement by chest wall
- ❖ Thus, in a spontaneously breathing patient with open chest:
  - Ventilation is increased in NDL
  - Ventilation is decreased in DL

Perfusion: Dependant lung is better perfused

V/Q Ratio:

- ❖ Dependant lung is poorly ventilated and over-perfused
- ❖ Non-dependant lung is over inflated and under-perfused
- ❖ Therefore, V/Q mismatch occurs

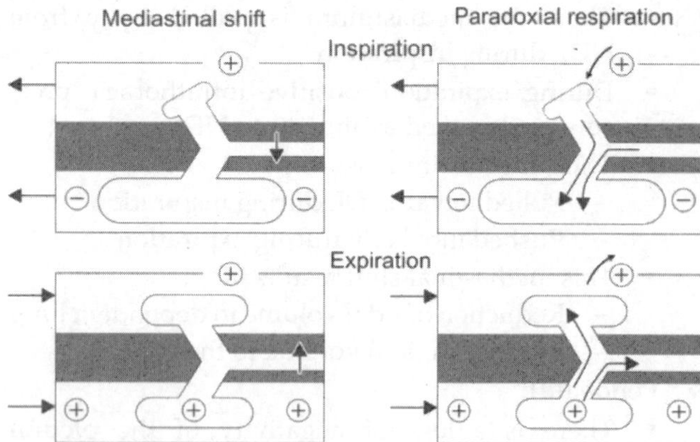

Fig. 32: Spontaneous breathing open chest.

Anesthetized, Closed Chest

Ventilation

- Most of the tidal volume delivered (55%) goes to non-dependant lung
- This is because of reduced expansion of DL due to:
  - Mediastinal shift:
    - Mediastinal shift impeding expansion of DL
    - FRC of NDL becomes 15 times that of dependant lung
  - Shift in abdominal contents:
    - Abdominal contents are pushed cephalad in DL hemithorax
    - However, diaphragm is paralysed and flaccid
    - Thus, it does not contribute to increased ventilation as in awake state
  - Other factors in DL:
    - Poor mucociliary clearance
    - Absorption atelectasis in DL
    - Suboptimal positioning
- Thus, majority of ventilation is shifted to NDL
- This is in contrast with what happens during spontaneous ventilation
- Thus, in an anesthetized patient with closed chest:
    - Ventilation to NDL is increased
    - Ventilation to DL is decreased

Perfusion: Dependant lung gets more perfusion

V/Q Ratio

- Non-dependant lung moves from initial flat portion to steep portion of P-V curve
- Dependant lung moves from steep portion to lower flat portion of P-V curve

Anesthetized, Open Chest

Ventilaton

- Open hemithorax reinforces and increases the changes seen in NDL with anesthesia

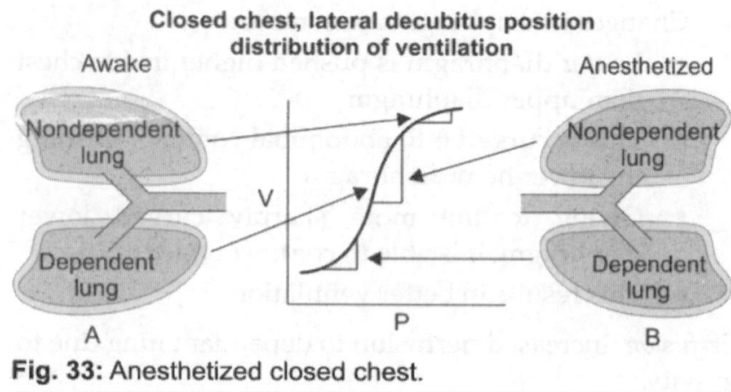

Fig. 33: Anesthetized closed chest.

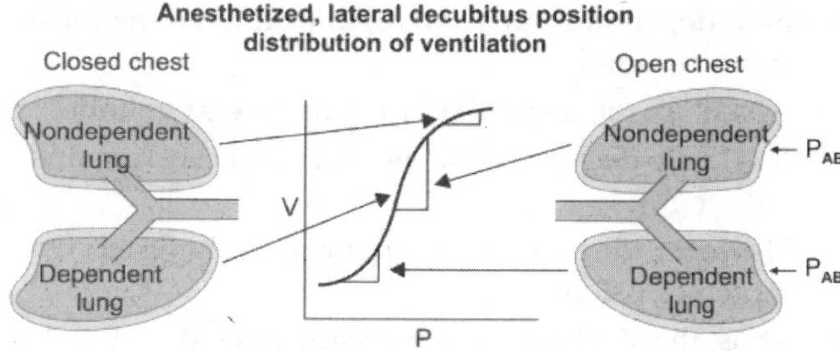

Fig. 34: Anesthetized open chest.

- More ventilation occurs in non-dependant lung as:
  - Pressure of abdominal contents pressing on upper diaphragm is minimal
  - Thus, resistance to diaphragmatic movement by abdominal contents is minimal
  - Also, the open chest wall minimizes resistance to NDL movement
- Ventilation of dependant lung continues to be poor owing to:
  - Mediastinal shift impeding expansion of diaphragm
  - Pressure of abdominal contents (P_{AB}) resisting diaphragmatic expansion
- Thus, in an anesthetized patient with open chest:
  - Ventilation is maximum in NDL
  - Ventilation is minimum in DL

Perfusion: Dependant lung is better perfused

V/Q Ratio: Increased V/Q mismatch

Changes in Perfusion During One Lung Ventilation

- Since NDL lung is not ventilated, blood flow through that lung becomes a shunt
- Thus massive right-left stunt occurs with huge V/Q mismatch and PaO_2 reduces
- $PaCO_2$ remains the same provided minute ventilation is maintained

- Perfusion to non-dependant lungs reduces due to:
  - Passive mechanisms:
    - Gravity
    - Surgical retraction
    - Pre-existing disease
  - Active mechanism: Hypoxic pulmonary vasoconstriction
- Perfusion to dependant lung increases due to:
  - Gravity
  - Hypoxic pulmonary vasoconstriction

Factors Which Counter Effects of Lateral Decubitus Position

- Kinking of pulmonary artery in operated lung
- Gravity dependant reduction in dependant lung perfusion
- Progressive atelectasis due to mechanical compression
- Reduces perfusion of non-dependant lung
- Obligatory right-left transpulmonary shunt due to increased $A\text{-}aDO_2$
- Hypoxic pulmonary vasoconstriction
- Surgical retraction and mechanical compression of non-dependent lung

DOUBLE LUMEN TUBES

Introduction

- DLT is currently the most widely used means for achieving lung separation and OLV
- Widely used technique for:
  - Lung isolation
  - Selective ventilation
  - Intermittent suctioning of either lung
- First DLT was designed by ***Carlens*** in 1950
- However, owing to the narrow lumina of these tubes, flow resistance was higher
- Thus, ***Robertshaw*** in the 1960s introduced design modifications in the Carlens DLT

Indications

- Specific indications for DLT:
  - Protection of lung from contralateral contamination:
    - Lung abscess
    - Lung cyst
    - Pulmonary hemorrhage
    - Bronchoalveolar lavage
  - Control and continuity of gas exchange:
    - Bronchopleural fistula
    - Bronchial disruption
    - Pneumonectomy
- Indications with the use of DLT or bronchial blocker: surgical exposure for:
  - Lobectomy
  - Bilobectomy
  - Video assisted thoracoscopic surgery
  - Minimally invasive cardiac surgeries
  - Mediastinal mass resection
  - Esophageal surgery
  - Orthopedic procedures

Indications for Right Sided DLT

- Distorted anatomy of the entrance of left main bronchus by:
  - Intra/extra bronchial tumor compression
  - Descending thoracic aortic aneurysm
- Surgery involving left mainstem bronchus:
  - Left sided tracheobronchial tree disruption
  - Left sided pneumonectomy
  - Left sided single lung transplantation
  - Left sided sleeve resection

Contraindications

- Absolute contraindication: carinal/proximal mainstem endobronchial lesions
- Relative contraindications:
  - Difficult upper airway anatomy causing anticipated difficult intubation
  - Full stomach requiring rapid intubation to avoid aspiration
  - Critically ill patients dependent on two-lung ventilation

Types

- Carlens left sided DLT
- Whites right sided DLT
- Robertshaw right/left sided DLT
- Bronchocath-Portex type DLT
- Silibroncho DLT
- Brice-Smith left/right sided endobronchial tube

Design

- All the DLT are essentially based on the design suggested by ***Carlens and Bjork***
- The central shaft of the DLT is ellipsoid and contains a septum
- The septum divides the tube into 2 symmetric D-shaped lumens to:
  - Minimize diameter
  - Minimize turbulent airflow

- Thus, DLTs essentially consist of two endotracheal tubes bonded together:
  - One lumen is long enough to reach the mainstem bronchus
  - The other is short and ends with an opening in the distal trachea
- At the proximal end of each lumen is a standard 15-mm ETT adapter
- To this is attached a short length of tubing which creates a Y-shape
- This permits independent attachment for:
  - Ventilatory apparatus
  - Clamping
  - Opening to atmospheric air
  - Suctioning
- At the distal end of the DLT, the shaft is surrounded by two inflatable cuffs
- Lung separation is achieved by the inflation of these 2 cuffs:
  - Proximal tracheal cuff located in the distal trachea
  - Distal bronchial cuff located in the mainstem bronchus
- Right sided DLTs:
  - The right upper lobe bronchus arises close to the tracheal bifurcation
  - The orifice of right upper lobe (RUL) bronchus is 1-2.5 cm from the carina
  - Thus, right sided DLTs must have a separate portal to ventilate RUL bronchus
  - A right sided DLT employs a proximal ventilation port on endobronchial side
  - This is in order to facilitate ventilation of the right upper lobe bronchus

Advantages

- Quickest technique
- Placement possible without bronchoscopy
- Preformed curve which allows preferential entry into a bronchus
- Requires lesser degree of skill
- Repositioning rarely required
- Suction to isolated lung possible
- Bronchoscopy to isolated lung possible
- CPAP can be easily added
- Can alternate OLV to either lung easily
- Allows conversion to two lung ventilation

Disadvantages

- Expensive
- Size selection difficult
- Difficult to use in difficult airway/abnormal trachea
- Not optimal for postoperative ventilation
- Potential laryngeal trauma
- Potential bronchial trauma
- Trauma to vocal cord, larynx and arytenoids
- Difficult to place as larger cross-sectional area

Selection of DLT Size

- Properly sized DLT is one in which:
  - Main body of the DLT passes through the glottis without resistance
  - The tube advances easily within the trachea
  - Bronchial component passes into the intended bronchus without difficulty
  - Has a bronchial tip 1-2 mm smaller than diameter of patients left bronchus
  - Tube leak is present with a deflated bronchial cuff
  - Tube leak disappears after bronchial cuff inflation with < 3 mL air
- Complications of DLT- patient size mismatch:
  - Undersized tubes:
    - Associated with:
      - Inadequate lung isolation
      - Increased airway resistance
      - Overinflation of bronchial cuff as a trouble-shooting maneuver
      - Accidental distal migration of DLT
    - Pneumothorax and pneumomediastinum can occur due to:
      - Distal migration of endobronchial tip:
        - Endobronchial tip may migrate into left lower bronchus
        - This causes delivery of entire TV to left lower bronchus
      - Higher resistance to gas flow of smaller tubes
      - Presence of intrinsic auto-PEEP
    - Bronchial rupture can occur by distal migration of tracheal lumen
  - Oversized tubes: Bronchial rupture in smaller patients
- Selection of DLT using chest X-ray:
  - Useful to select appropriate size of DLT
  - Preoperative postero-anterior chest X-ray may be used
  - Tracheal diameter is measured at the level of clavicle
  - This can be used to predict the size of DLT
  - However, the method has limited predictive value in:
    - Patients of smaller stature
    - Women
    - Patients of Asian descent

- Thus, this method is not frequently used to predict the required DLT size

Tracheal width	Predicted left bronchial width	Recommended DLT size
≥ 18 mm	≥ 12.2	41
≥ 16 mm	≥ 10.9	39
≥ 15 mm	≥ 10.2	37
≥ 14 mm	≥ 9.5	35

❖ Selection of DLT using CT scan:
- 3-dimensional reconstruction of tracheobronchial anatomy is done
- This is then superimposed on the transparent DLT to match the correct size

❖ Selection of DLT size based on patients sex and height:

Patient height	Tube size		Depth of insertion
	Male	Female	
136-164 cm	37 Fr	35/ 32 Fr	27 cm
165-179 cm	39 Fr	37 Fr	29 cm
180- 194 cm	41 Fr	39 Fr	31 cm

❖ Depth of insertion of DLTs:

Formula for depth of insertion =

$$12 + \frac{[\text{patient height in cm}]\ \text{cm}}{10}$$

❖ In patients with height < 155 cm, height is not good predictor of adequate depth

Complications

❖ Malposition of DLT:
- One of the most common complications
- Causes of malpositioning include:
  - Dislodgement of endobronchial cuff due to overinflation
  - Surgical manipulation of the bronchus
  - Extension of the head during positioning

❖ Airway trauma and tracheobronchial tree rupture:
- Risk factors:
  - Direct trauma:
    - Insertion with too much force
    - Oversized DLT (too large for bronchus)
    - Advancement of DLT with stylet in place
    - Movement of tube with inflated cuffs
  - Cuff over-inflation:
    - Too rapid inflation of cuffs
    - Inflation of too large volume of cuff
    - Undersized DLT requiring large cuff volume for adequate seal
    - Cuff distension due to use of nitrous oxide
  - Pre-existing airway pathology:
    - Congenital airway problems
    - Airway wall weakness from tumor infiltration/infection
    - Airway distortion due to intrabronchial tumors
    - Patients receiving long term steroid therapy
    - Hypotension with hypoperfusion to the airway
- Presents as:
  - Unexpected air leak
  - Subcutaneous emphysema
  - Airway bleeding
  - Protrusion of cuff into surgical field
- Prevention of airway rupture:
  - Routine review of chest X-rays for airway abnormalities
  - Removal of DLT stylet after passing the vocal cords
  - Use FOB guidance when resistance is encountered during intubation
  - Upsizing DLTs when bronchial cuff volume required is > 3 mL
  - Avoidance of nitrous oxide

❖ Hypoxemia due to:
- Tube malposition
- Tube occlusion
- Excessive shunting during OLV

❖ Tension pneumothorax of dependant lung

❖ Inadvertent suturing of DLT to bronchus during surgery

❖ Traumatic laryngitis

❖ Hoarseness of voice

Preparation of the DLT

❖ Tracheal and bronchial cuffs are inflated and checked for:
- Cuff leaks
- Symmetrical cuff inflation

❖ Verify whether each inflation tube is associated with the proper cuff

❖ Cuff should be lubricated with a water-soluble lubricant

❖ Stylet is lubricated with a water-soluble lubricant and place inside the bronchial lumen

❖ The stylet should not extend beyond the tip of the DLT

❖ The connectors are assembled so that it can be affixed to the DLT after intubation

Blind Technique of DLT Insertion

❖ Endobronchial tip of DLT is inserted through vocal cords with direct laryngoscopy

❖ DLT tip should pass the glottis without any resistance

❖ The stylet is then removed and DLT is rotated 90° to the left for left sided DLT

❖ DLT is slowly advanced to the correct depth

- Too deep insertion may cause left mainstem bronchial rupture
- Left sided DLTs are easier to place than right DLTs
- During insertion of left sided DLTs:
  - Maneuvers which help in avoiding right mainstem bronchus are:
    - Turning the patients head to the right
    - Tilting the head towards right shoulder while advancing the DLT
  - This results in correct positioning of left DLTs in 92% cases

Cuff Inflation

- Tracheal cuff inflation:
  - Inflated in a manner similar to that of a tracheal tube
  - Usually inflated with 20 mL of air
- Bronchial cuff inflation:
  - More difficult to inflate bronchial cuff correctly
  - Bronchial cuff should be inflated with less than 3 mL of air
  - Over-inflation may result in:
    - High cuff pressure transmitted onto bronchial wall
    - Cuff herniation into carina
  - Bronchial cuff is therefore inflated with small incremental volumes
  - Inflation is continued until airtight seal is attained
  - The total bronchial cuff volume should be restricted to less than 3 mL
  - Techniques of identifying cuff inflation volume:
    - Water immersion test:
      - The proximal end of the tracheal lumen is immersed in water
      - Patient is ventilated through the bronchial lumen
      - With a deflated bronchial cuff, ventilation causes bubbling on PPV
      - Bronchial cuff is then inflated in small increments
      - This is continued until no air bubbles are seen on PPV
    - Other similar tests include:
      - Connecting balloon to tracheal lumen
      - Connecting capnograph to tracheal lumen

Techniques of Confirmation of DLT Position

- Auscultation
- Fibreoptic bronchoscope:
  - Through tracheal lumen
  - Through endobronchial lumen
- Chest X-ray
- Fluoroscopy
- Radiopaque marker
- Water seal test
- Selective capnography

Confirmation by Auscultation

- 3 step method is followed to confirm position of the DLT
- This method however, is not reliable
- Step 1:
  - During bilateral ventilation, tracheal cuff is inflated to seal air leak at glottis
  - Bilateral ventilation is confirmed by auscultation
- Step 2:
  - Tracheal lumen of DLT is clamped proximally
  - Port distal to clamp is opened
  - DLT is ventilated via the bronchial lumen
  - Bronchial cuff is inflated to minimum volume
  - This seals air leak from open tracheal lumen port
  - Correct left-unilateral ventilation is confirmed by auscultation
- Step 3:
  - Tracheal lumen clamp is released and port closed
  - Resumption of bilateral breath sounds is confirmed by auscultation
- Step 4:
  - Each side is clamped selectively
  - Absent sounds are confirmed on the unilateral clamped side
  - Contralateral side should have clear breath sounds

Confirmation by Fibreoptic Bronchoscope

- *Gold standard* for confirmation of DLT position
- Through tracheal lumen:
  - Inflated blue bronchial cuff should lie just beyond carina on the left
  - Ensure endobronchial cuff is around 5 mm below carina in left bronchus
  - This prevents bronchial cuff herniation over the carina after inflation
  - Identify take-off of right upper lobe (RUL) bronchus
  - Also identify take- off of RML and RLL bronchi from bronchus intermedius

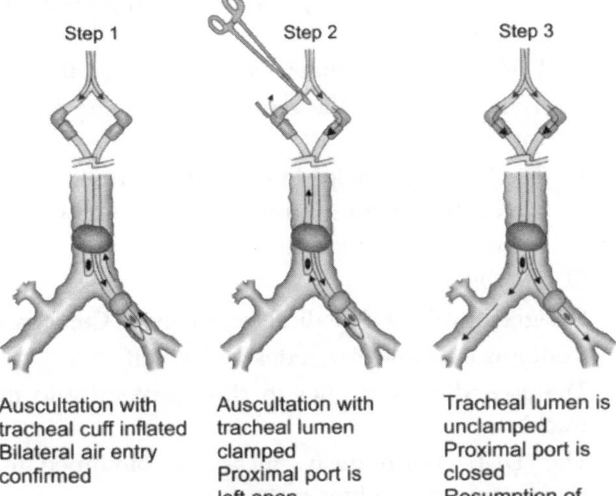

Fig. 35: Auscultatory confirmation of DLT position.

- Through endobronchial lumen:
  - Check for endobronchial luminal patency
  - Identify both LUL and LLL orifices

Confirmation with Radio-Opaque Marker

- Radio-opaque line surrounds ***Mallinckrodt's Bronchocath tube***
- Line is proximal to bronchial cuff
- Marker is 4 cm from distal tip of endobronchial lumen
- Marker reflects white during fibreoptic visualization

Modifications of DLT

- Silibroncho DLT:
  - Introduced by Fuji Systems, Tokyo
  - Made of silicone and has a wire-reinforced endobronchial tip
  - The D-shaped wire reinforces the lumen to maintain the tip at 45°
  - Reinforcement prevents kinking of lumen and maintains flexibility at same time
  - Advantages include:
    - Presence of a bevelled bronchial tip
    - Reduced bronchial cuff length which increases the margin of safety
  - Especially useful if left mainstem bronchus is perpendicular to trachea:
    - Occurs if patient has already undergone left upper lobectomy
    - Expansion of LLL, in this case displaces left main bronchus upwards

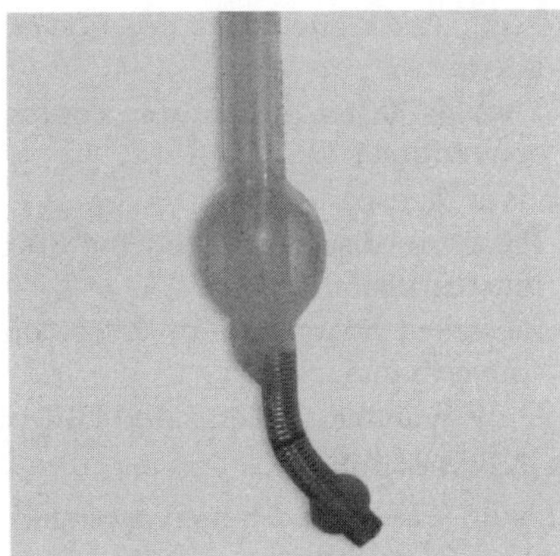

Fig. 36: Silibroncho tube.

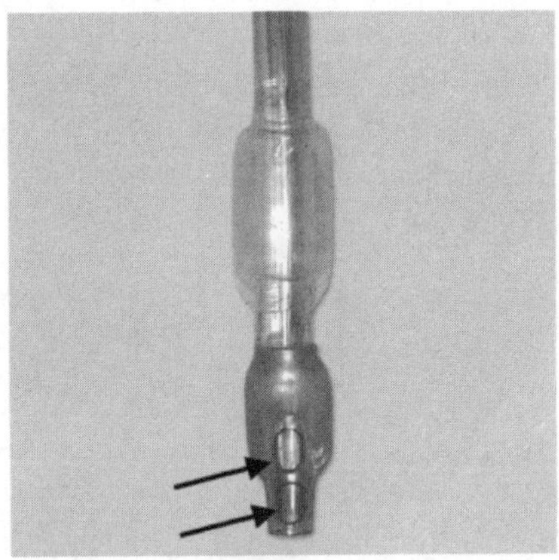

Fig. 37: Cliny DLT.

- Cliny right sided DLT
  - Designed by Create Medic Company Ltd, Yokohama, Japan
  - Specially designed as a right sided DLT
  - Has a long oblique bronchial cuff with 2 ventilation ports for the RUL
  - Proximal bronchial cuff is located immediately opposite tracheal orifice
  - Useful in patients with a very short right mainstem bronchus
- VivaSight DLT:
  - It is designed by ET View Medicals, Misgav, Israel
  - The DLT has an integrated high-resolution camera
  - The camera is embedded at the end of the DLT
  - This allows continuous monitoring of the tracheal carina and DLT position
  - The DLT also has an integrated flush system for in-situ camera lens cleaning
  - Advantages:
    - Allows continuous airway monitoring

- Facilitates immediate correction of DLT malpositions
- Enables faster intubation compared with conventional DLTs

- Disadvantages:
  - Presence of secretions on the tip of camera impairs vision
  - Increased hoarseness of voice compared to conventional DLTs
  - Only available for left sided DLT placement

❖ Papworth BiVent Tube:

- DLT with 2 D-shaped lumen arranged in a side-by-side configuration
- Characteristics of the tube are:
  - Preformed single posterior concavity

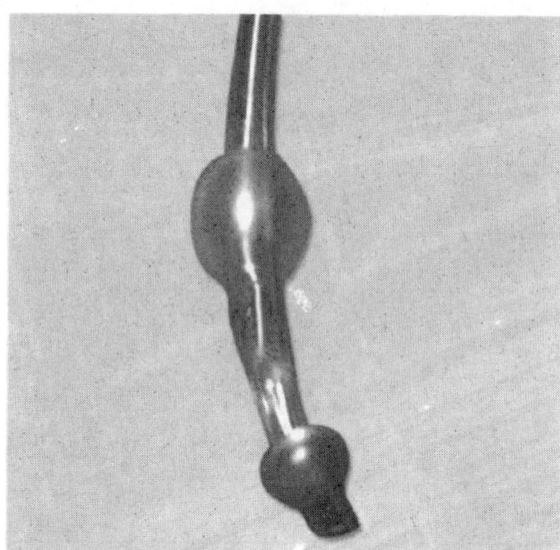

Fig. 38: VivaSight DLT.

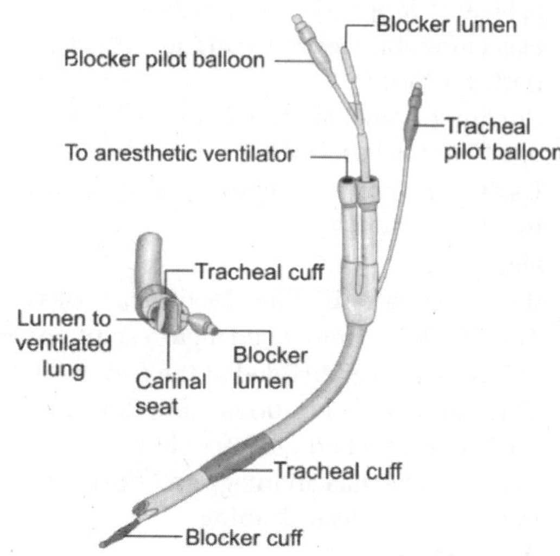

Fig. 39: Papworth BiVent tube.

  - Single inflatable, low volume, high pressure tracheal cuff
- Distal end has 2 pliable crescent shaped flanges
- They arise from the central portion and form a forked tip
- The forked tip helps to seat at the carina
- This tube can be used without the requirement of endoscopic guidance

❖ ECOM DLT:

❖ Designed by ECOM Medical Inc, San Juan, Capistrano

❖ Contains multiple electrodes on the cuff

❖ The ascending aorta lies in close proximity to the trachea

❖ The DLT continuously measures bioimpedance signals from ascending aorta

❖ Device is connected to ECOM monitor in conjunction with an arterial catheter

❖ This provides continuous cardiac output measurements

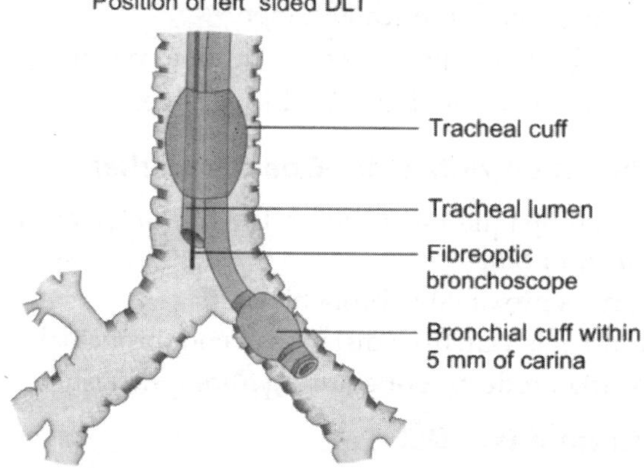

Fig. 40: Correct positioning of left sided DLT.

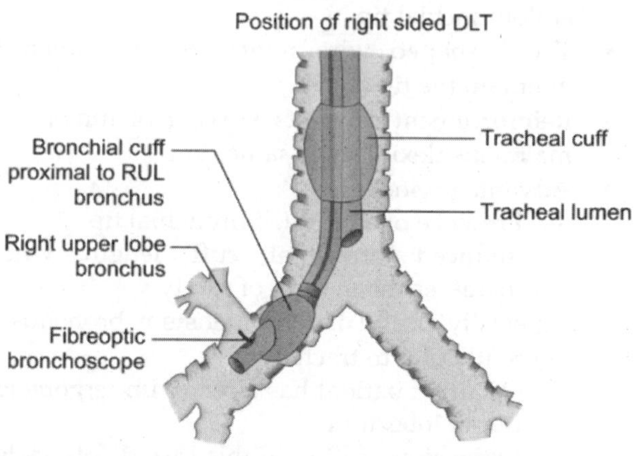

Fig. 41: Correct positioning of right sided DLT.

Trouble Shooting DLT Malposition

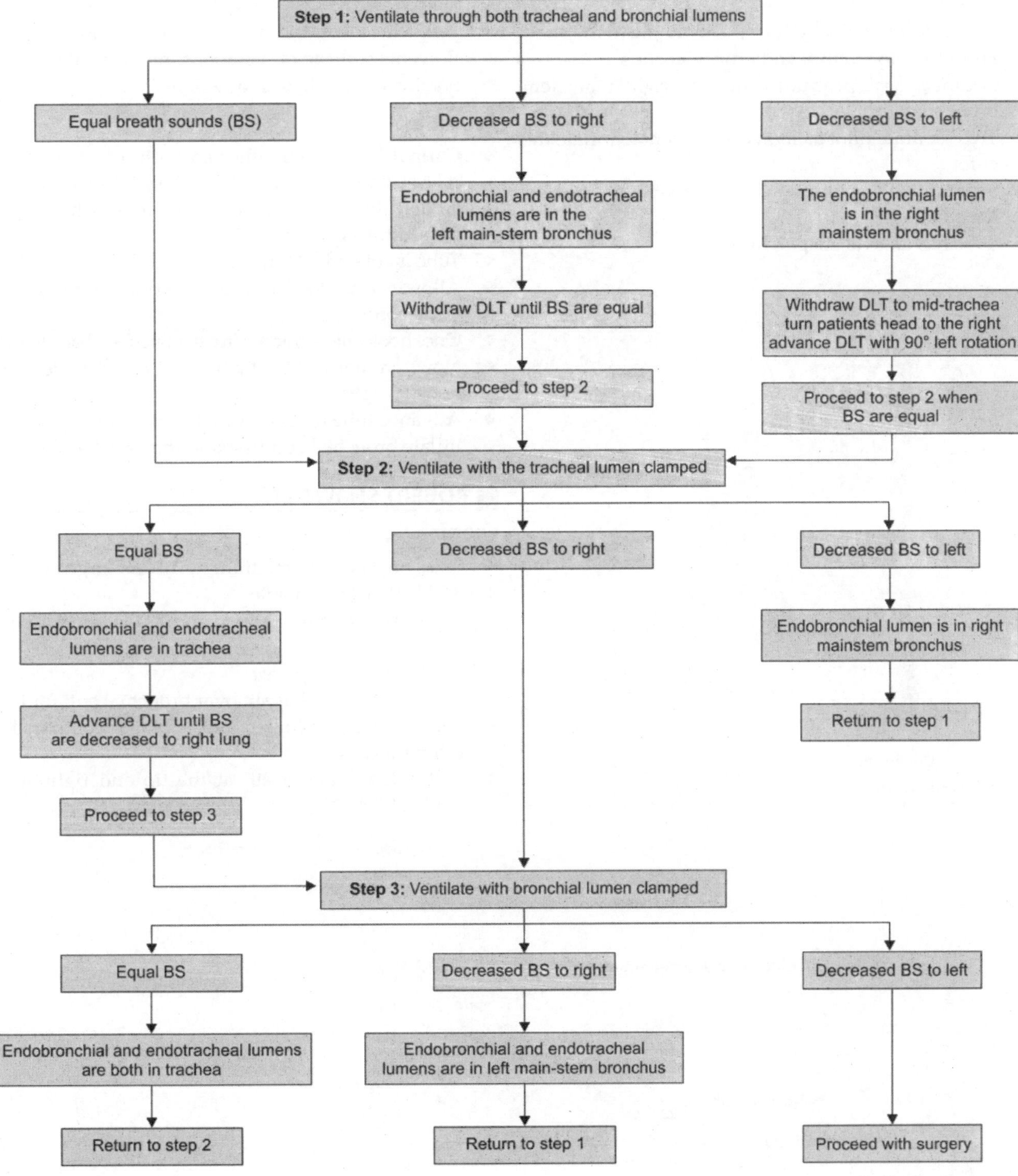

CARLENS TUBE

Introduction

- First clinically used DLT designed by Carlens in 1950
- Originally used by pulmonologists for split function spirometry
- Useful for massive hemoptysis when verification of DLT position is difficult

Features

- Sizes 35,37,39,41 French
- The endobronchial tip forms a 45° angle to the shaft
- Has separate tracheal and bronchial cuffs
- A *carinal hook* protrudes into the right mainstem bronchus
- Two separate pilot balloons are present to inflate the cuffs
- Separate ETT connections are available for each of the channels
- Tube has an oval shaped lumen

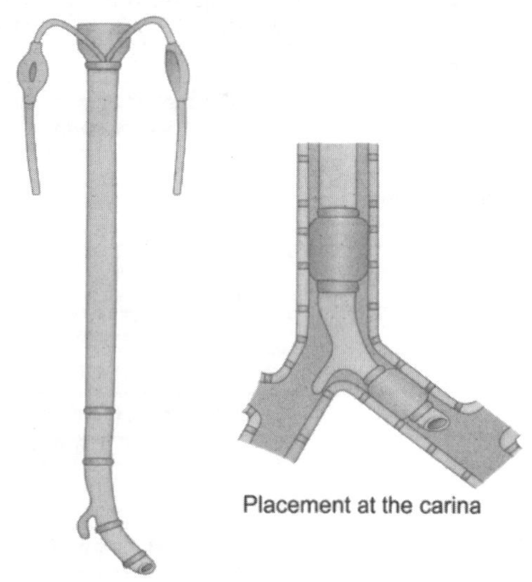

Fig. 42: Carlens DLT.

Advantages

- Helps in OLV
- Helps to isolate and collapse operative lung
- Prevents spillage of secretions into normal lung
- Suction can be done at any time

Procedure

- Carinal hook is initially tied with a knot which is released after positioning, for easy intubation
- Under direct laryngoscopy, endobronchial tip is passed through cords
- Tube is rotated 180° to left
- Allow carinal look to pass anterior commissure of vocal cords
- Once hook enters trachea, tube rotated 90° back to right
- Now, endobronchial tip is positioned to left and hook to right
- Advance tube till resistance felt at carina
- Inflate bronchial cuff first and then tracheal cuff

ROBERT SHAW DLT

Features

- Sizes no.8 (small), medium no.10 and large no. 12
- 35,37,39,41 Fr available
- 32 Fr used for small adults and 28 Fr used for pediatrics
- *No carinal hook is present*
- Right sided tube has slit over bronchial cuff for RUL
- Has a D-shaped lumen and is bigger compared to other tubes
- Left sided angle of 40° at the tip and right sided angle of 20° at tip

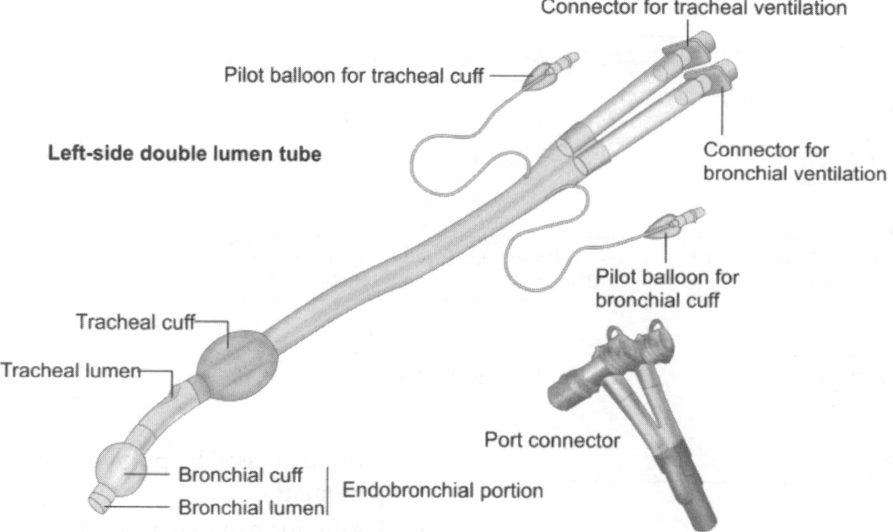

Fig. 43: Robertshaws DLT.

Procedure

- Tube inserted between vocal cords with concavity facing upwards
- Rotate the tube through 90°
- Once tube passes vocal cords, remove laryngoscope
- Support the jaw and advance tube
- Endobronchial portion directed towards the bronchus which has to be intubated

Advantages

- Absence of carinal hook
- Left and right sided tubes are available
- Larger diameter and D-shaped lumen:
  - Allows easy passage of suction catheter
  - Low resistance to gas flow
- Has fixed curvature which facilitates easy positioning
- Decreased chances of kinking

Whites DLT

- Sizes 37, 39,41 Fr available
- This is the right sided version of Carlens tube with a carinal hook
- The tube has both tracheal and bronchial cuffs
- Separate pilot balloons are present to inflate each of the cuffs
- Slit is present in the endobronchial cuff to ventilate RUL bronchus
- For right lung anesthesia, clamp left side to allow left lung surgery

BRONCHIAL BLOCKERS

Introduction

- Bronchial blockers are inflatable devices that are passes through a SLT to selectively occlude a bronchial orifice
- First used by ***Sir Ivan Magill***

Characteristics of Ideal Blockers

- Balloon shaped to stabilize it in bronchus
- Low pressure and high-volume characteristics of balloon preferred
- Flexible and easy to manipulate into mainstem/lobar branches
- Balloon to have channel for deflation and suction distal to it
- Be adaptable to use internal and external to standard ETT
- Wide variety of sizes

Indications

- Patients with difficult airway:
  - Avoids the need for tube exchange
  - Following laryngeal surgery
  - Patients with tracheostomy
  - Patients with distorted bronchial anatomy due to compression by:
    - Tumors
    - Aneurysm
  - Patients requiring nasotracheal intubation
- For OLV management:
  - Facilitates segmental blockade in patients who cannot tolerate OLV
  - Morbid obesity
  - Pediatric patients
  - Already intubated patients
- For surgical procedures not involving the lung:
  - Esophageal surgery
  - Spine surgery requiring transthoracic approach
  - Minimally invasive cardiac surgery

Technique

- Trachea intubated with SLT
- BB may pass within/outside the ETT
- When BB is inflated, that lung will not be ventilated
- Suction catheter element which passes to the tip allows the isolated lung to be deflated and suctioned
- Blocker therefore allows continued inflation of one lobe of operated lung
- For e.g., if placed in right bronchus intermedius, it will allow RUL ventilation when surgery is on RLL

Types of Bronchial Blockers

- ***Thomsons***
- ***Magills***
- ***Macintosh-Lethersdale***

Use of Brochial Blockers

- Modified SLT with enclosed BB:
  - ***Integrated Torque Control Blocker: Univent***
  - ***Fogarty Arterial Embolectomy catheter***
- Conventional SLT with enclosed BB:
  - ***Hybrid Wire Guided BB***
  - ***Cohens Tip deflecting endobronchial blocker***
  - ***Fuji Uniblocker***

Advantages

- Size selection is not an issue
- Easily added to regular ETT

- Allows ventilation during placement
- Easier to place in difficult airway
- Postoperative two lung ventilation (TLV) is possible by removing BB
- Selective lobar lung isolation possible
- CPAP to isolated lung possible

Disadvantages

- More time for positioning and repositioning is often required
- Bronchoscope is essential for positioning
- Right lung isolation is suboptimal due to RUL anatomy
- Bronchoscopy to isolated lung is impossible
- Minimal suction is possible to isolated lung
- Difficult to alternate OLV to either lung

Size Selection

- Most commonly used intra-luminally (coaxially) with SLT
- Maybe used separately through glottis/tracheostomy, external to SLT
- For 9 Fr BB, ETT > 7 mm ID used with FOB < 4 mm diameter
- Larger bronchoscopes require ETT > 7.5 mm ID

Complications

- Failure to achieve lung separation
- Inclusion of distal wire loop to stapling line during right upper lobectomy
- Displacement of BB with lodgement above carina
- Shearing of balloon

Comparison

Feature	DLT	Univent	ARNDT
Time to position	2 minutes	2 minutes	3 minutes
Time for lung collapse	17 minutes	19 minutes	26 minutes
Suction	±	±	Majority require
Surgical exposure	Excellent	Excellent	Excellent

UNIVENT BRONCHIAL BLOCKER

Introduction

- It is a single lumen ETT with a moveable endobronchial blocker
- ***Torque Control Blocker Univent*** (TCBU) is latest version of Univent
- Manufactured by Fuji Systems Corporation, Tokyo, Japan

Design

- This is a cuffed silicone tube with small additional internal lumen along concave side
- The internal channel present within the Univent, encloses a moveable BB
- The uninvent has a shape similar to standard ETT
- This BB can be used to block left/right/any secondary bronchi
- Thus, in essence the tube has two compartments:
  - A large lumen for passage of oxygen/air
  - A smaller lumen in the middle for the enclosed BB
- Characteristics of the bronchial blocker:
  - Made of flexible, non-latex material
  - Has a blue high-pressure and low-volume cuff
  - Has a flexible shaft which is easy to guide into a bronchus
  - A slight bend is present in the BB just above the cuff
  - Tip of the BB is radio-opaque
  - Has external depth markings to determine blocker position in relation to tube
  - A grip is present which allows rotation of the blocker
  - A locking clamp fixes the depth of BB below the tip of the tube
- First generation Univent tube was difficult to direct into selected bronchus
- This was mainly because the BB would spin on its long axis
- Second generation Univent tubes (TCBU) have a high friction coefficient
- This facilitates direction of the BB into the target main stem bronchus

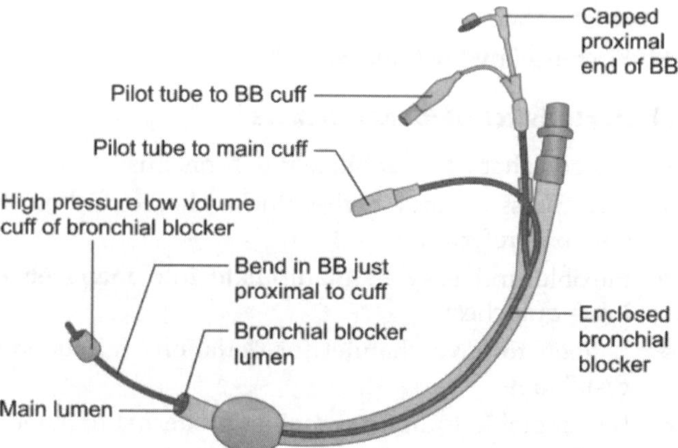

Fig. 44: Univent tube.

Preparation of the Tube

- Before use, the BB and tube cuffs should be inflated and checked for leaks
- Both the tube and blocker should be well lubricated
- Following cuff deflation, BB is pushed back and forth in the tube
- This is done to ensure free movement of the BB within the tube
- The BB is then fully retracted into the tube lumen and fixed in place using the clamp

Technique

- Enclosed BB is fully retracted into the lumen of the tube
- Technique used for conventional ETT intubation is used
- In case of difficult airway, the tube may be inserted over airway exchange catheters
- The bronchial blocker itself can be used as an introducer for the tube
- Once the tube is inserted, the tracheal cuff is inflated and patient is ventilated
- Confirmation of tube and BB position:
  - FOB is passed into the main lumen through the adaptor with a port for FOB
  - Under direct vision, BB is advanced into targeted bronchus
  - In case of malposition, the BB position may be changed under FOB guidance
  - The direction of the tip of the BB can be changed by twisting the shaft
  - The tracheal tube cuff has to be deflated prior to any change in direction
  - A guidewire may be inserted into the BB lumen to aid in positioning
  - This may be used to direct the BB into place, especially for smaller airways

Bronchoscopic Insertion of Univent Tube

- FOB is passed through the tracheal tube into the bronchus to be blocked
- The tracheal tube is then advanced into the bronchus to be blocked
- The BB is advanced into the bronchus and tube is withdrawn into the trachea
- This leaves the blocker in the bronchus to be blocked
- However, this technique may result in trauma to the airway

Size Selection of Univent Tubes

Internal diameter	Outer diameter	Age
3.5 mm (uncuffed)	7.5/8	6-10 years
4.5 mm	8.5/9	10-14 years
6 mm	9.7/11	14-16 years
6.5 mm	10.2/12	16-18 years
7 mm	11.6/12.5	Adult
7.5 mm	11.2/13	Adult
8 mm	11.7/13.5	Adult
8 mm	12.2/14	Adult
9 mm	12.7/14.5	Adult

Procedure for Lung Isolation

- Prior to cuff inflation, lung is deflated with the BB open to the atmosphere
- The BB cuff is inflated using the least amount of air that will provide a seal
- The typical cuff inflation volume is 5-6 mL
- Methods to confirm optimal cuff volume and adequate seal are:
  - Bubble test:
    - Proximal end of bronchial lumen is placed in water within a beaker
    - When the bronchus is sealed, no bubbling is observed in the water
    - This gives us the optimal volume required to maintain cuff seal
  - Carbon dioxide analyser method:
    - Sample line from the carbon dioxide analyser is used
    - This is attached to the proximal end of the BB
    - Waveform is traced for the point of disappearance
    - This gives us the optimal volume required to maintain cuff seal

Advantages

- Easier to insert and position compared with a DLT
- Provides lung isolation equivalent to DLV
- Useful in patients with:
  - Difficult airway
  - Tracheostomy
  - Nasal intubation
  - Planned postoperative ventilation
  - Following mediastinoscopy/thoracotomy when tube exchange is difficult
  - Following bilateral lung transplant
- Other advantages include:
  - Use of suction
  - Application of CPAP
  - Allows insufflation of oxygen through the blocker lumen

- BB with the cuff deflated may be used for jet ventilation during carinal resection
- Can be converted to SLT by deflating and withdrawing the BB

Disadvantages

- Large external diameter: Difficult to negotiate the vocal cords
- Not recommended for use in children below 6 years of age
- Shape of the tube is fixed which may make intubation difficult while using FOB
- May distort neck anatomy and make IJV cannulation difficult
- Greater incidence of malpositioning during patient positioning compared with DLT
- Presence of BB reduces the size of lumen which may be blocked easily by secretions
- Low-volume, high-pressure cuff may cause bronchial mucosal injury
- Deflation of lung is usually slower
- More expensive compared with DLT

Complications

- Dislodgement of cap from the tip of the blocker
- Fragmentation of the inner wall of the tube and connector
- Failure to achieve lung separation
- Inclusion of BB into stapling line
- Bronchial perforation
- Inflation of BB cuff near tracheal lumen causing respiratory arrest
- Risk of negative pressure pulmonary edema

ARNDT ENDOBRONCHIAL BLOCKER

Introduction

- It is a bronchial blocker assembly used in patients with a SLT already in place
- It is a wire guided endobronchial blocker with a loop snare
- Manufactured by Cook Critical Care

Structure

- It consists of 2 parts:
  - Blocking catheter
  - Special airway adapter
- Blocking catheter:
  - An independent BB is attached to a 5, 7 or 9 Fr catheter
  - Available in 65 and 78 cm length
  - Inner lumen measures 1.4 mm in diameter
  - Side holes are present at distal end of catheter to enable lung deflation
  - Has high-volume and low-pressure cuff
  - The cuff can be elliptical or spherical in shape
  - The spherical balloon becomes elliptical when inflated in the small bronchus
  - Inner lumen has flexible nylon wire passing from the proximal to distal end
  - The wire ends as a small loop which can be coupled with the FOB
  - The size of the loop may be increased or decreased
  - This is done by advancing or retracting the loop assembly
  - The loop serves as a guide wire to introduce the blocker
- Airway adapter:
  - Multiport adapter which has 4 ports:
    - 15-mm female connector which attaches to the tracheal tube
    - Side port with 15-mm male connector for connecting the breathing system
    - Port angles 30° for the bronchial blocker
    - A port for the flexible endoscope
  - The bronchoscopy port has a plastic sealing cap

Size Selection of ARNDT Blockers

Size	Smallest SLT internal diameter	Length	Cuff shape	Cuff volume
9 Fr	7.5 mm	78, 65 cm	Elliptical	6-12 mL
9 Fr	7.5 mm	78, 65 cm	Spherical	4-8 mL
7 Fr	6 mm	65 cm	Spherical	2-6 mL
5 Fr	4.5 mm	65, 50 cm	Spherical	0.5-2 mL

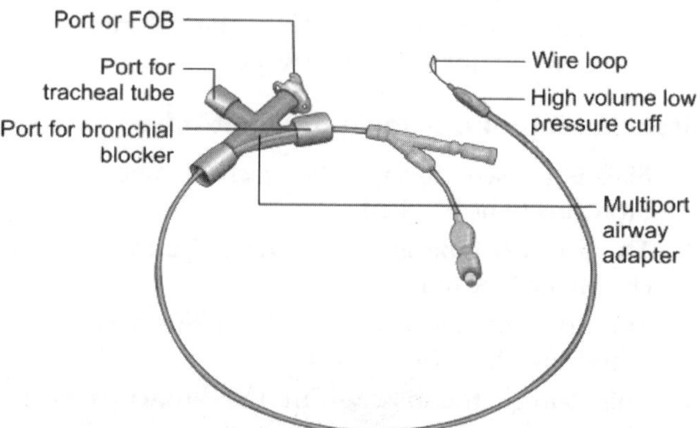

Fig. 45: Arndts endobronchial blocker.

Preparation of the Tube

- The outer sides of the blocker and the bronchoscope are lubricated with silicon
- Wire loop is adjusted to closely approximate the outer diameter of the FOB
- Blocker balloon is inflated to test for leaks and then fully deflated

Methods of Placement

- Following intubation, the multiport adapter is attached to the breathing system
- The tracheal tube is connected to the appropriate port on the adapter
- FOB is advanced through the guidewire loop
- This allows the BB to follow the bronchscope
- FOB is advanced distally into the airway to be blocked
- The guidewire is then slid out over the end of the bronchoscope
- The blocker is slid distally over the FOB into the selected bronchus
- The bronchoscope is withdrawn slightly to visualize the blocker
- The blockers position is then adjusted under bronchoscopic guidance
- The balloon is then inflated under direct vision to fill the entire bronchial lumen
- Cuff inflation usually requires 4-8 mL of air to obtain total bronchial blockade
- Optimal position of the cuff is confirmed:
  - Balloons outer surface is present 5 mm below the tracheal carina
  - Proper seal with no air leak from the targeted bronchus
- The balloon may then be deflated until OLV is required
- The wire loop is removed following satisfactory positioning of the BB
- This is because retention of the loop may damage the airway
- Also, the loop may be included while stapling during bronchial closure
- The open channel created by wire removal can be used for application of CPAP

Advantages

- Has been used in children up to 2 years of age
- Useful in patients:
  - Who are already intubated
  - With tracheostomy
  - Requiring nasotracheal intubation
  - Requiring awake intubation
- Useful in patients requiring selective lobar blockade for severe pulmonary bleeding
- The open channel created by wire removal can be used for:
  - Administration of oxygen therapy
  - Application of CPAP
  - Suctioning

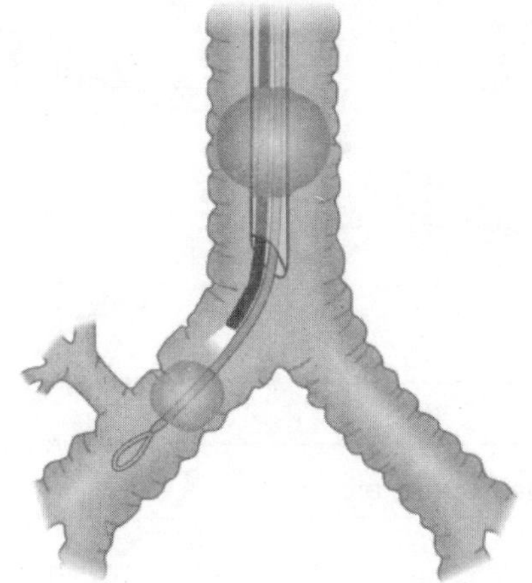

Fig. 46: Placement of Arndt blocker.

Disadvantages

- Once the wire is removed, it cannot be reinserted to allow repositioning of the blocker
- Placement of the blocker compulsorily requires availability of FOB
- Takes more time to position compared with DLT or Univent tubes
- Tip of the blocker may get caught in the side holes of the tracheal tube

Complications

- Shearing of balloon while removal through the blocker port
- More prone to dislodgement during positioning
- Inclusion of loop in suture line

FOGARTY EMBOLECTOMY CATHETER

Introduction

- Designed as a vascular tool for embolectomy but can be used for lung isolation
- Can be used as rescue device when DLT placement is difficult

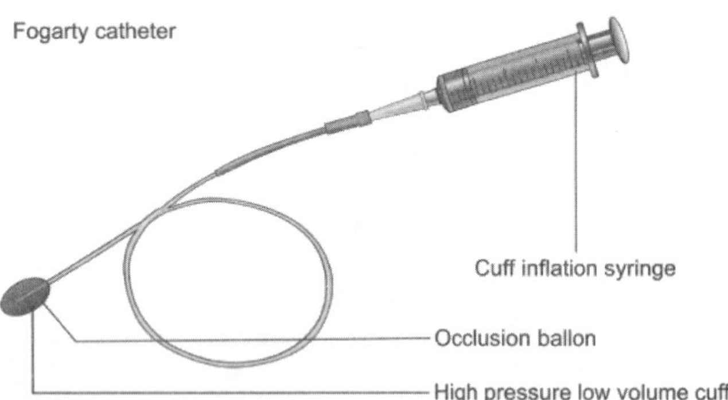

Fig. 47: Fogarty catheter.

Design

- Embolectomy catheter with a stylet in place
- Stylet facilitates formation of a curvature in the distal tip
- This aids guidance of the catheter into the target bronchus
- The occlusion balloon has a high-pressure, low-volume cuff
- Adult bronchi can be blocked with 7 Fr catheters
- 2-5 Fr catheters can be used for pediatric blockade

Preparation of the Catheter

- Balloon is tested for any leaks by inflation with air followed by deflation
- The blocker is then lubricated with silicone jelly to facilitate easy passage

Method of Placement

- The catheter may be positioned in different ways:
  - Placed through the tracheal tube
  - Placed alongside the tracheal tube
  - Placed through a hole made in the side of the tracheal tube
- The Arndt multiport adapter may be used to facilitate easy passage
- FOB is advanced into the SLT through the adapter for FOB
- The catheter along with stylet is guided into appropriate bronchus under FOB vision
- Once the tip is advanced into proper position, the stylet is removed
- The catheter balloon is inflated with air under vision and FOB is withdrawn

Disadvantages

- Made of natural rubber latex: *Contraindicated in latex allergy*
- Does not have a hollow/open channel for suctioning/oxygen insufflation
- Lack of guide wire device to aid positioning
- Lung collapse takes longer and may not be complete as with:
  - DLT
  - BB with hollow lumen
- Balloon is high-pressure and low-volume causing increased risk of mucosal injury
- Obstructed lung segment cannot be re-expanded until catheter is removed

Complications

- Airway rupture by forceful introduction
- Bronchial rupture due to over-inflated balloon
- Can be included in stapling line

COHENS FLEXITIP ENDOBRONCHIAL BLOCKER

Introduction

- It is an independent endobronchial blocker
- Has a wheel in its most proximal part which deflects tip of BB into desired bronchus
- Manufactured by Cook Critical Care

Design

- Available only in size 9 Fr and 65 cm length with inner lumen of 1.4 mm diameter
- The device has a spherically shaped balloon
- Side holes are incorporated at the distal end of the catheter between the tip and balloon
- This can be used to:
  - Evacuate gas from the lung and facilitate lung deflation
  - Insufflation of oxygen
- The bronchial blocker has a high-volume, low-pressure cuff
- A wheel-turning device is present at the most proximal part of the unit
- This enables deflection of the tip of the blocker by > 90
- This can be used to guide the entry of BB into the desired bronchus
- The distal tip of the device is pre-angled to facilitate entry into the targeted bronchus
- The cuff is blue in colour to enable easy visualization through the FOB
- A torque grip is present at the 55-cm mark to allow rotation of the blocker

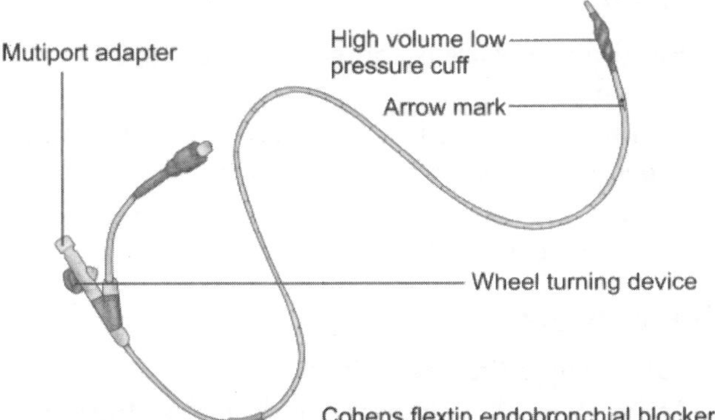

Fig. 48: Cohens flexitip endobronchial blocker.

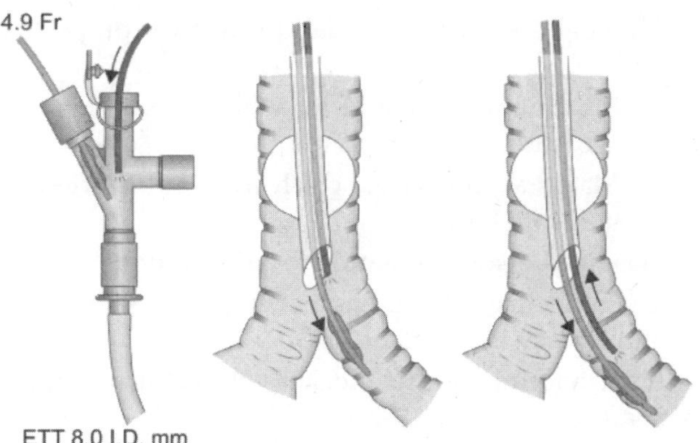

Fig. 49: Placement of Cohens blocker.

- An arrow is marked on the distal tip above the balloon
- This indicates the direction in which the tip will deflect when seen with FOB
- A multiport adapter is present which ensures air-tight seal when in place

Preparation of the Tube

- Blocker balloon is inflated to test for leaks and then fully deflated
- The outer side of the blocker balloon and FOB is lubricated with silicon
- This facilitates easy passage through the tracheal tube

Methods of Placement

- The Cohen blocker is advanced through an 8-mm ID SLT
- FOB guidance is used to visualize passage of the BB into the mainstem bronchus
- Right bronchial blockade:
  - The arrow on the BB is aligned with the right main bronchus
  - Proximal wheel is turned to deflect the tip towards the right main bronchus
  - FOB is positioned at least 5 mm below the tracheal carina in right bronchus
  - The tip of the BB is then advanced under FOB guidance
  - Optimal position provides a view of the outer surface of fully inflated balloon
  - This usually requires 4-8 mL of air
- Left bronchial blockade:
  - Tip of the SLT is positioned near entrance of the left main bronchus (LMB)
  - Cohens blocker is twisted towards the left bronchus and advanced
  - Once the blocker is in the LMB, the tracheal tube is withdrawn
  - Optimal position is when balloon is seen at least 5 mm below carina in LMB

Advantages

- Useful in patients:
  - Who are already intubated
  - With tracheostomy
  - Requiring nasotracheal intubation
  - Requiring awake intubation
- The central main lumen can be used for:
  - Administration of oxygen therapy
  - Application of CPAP
  - Limited suctioning

Disadvantages

- Requires 2 personnel to manipulate into position:
- One person to deflect the tip
- Second person to rotate and advance the catheter

FUJI UNIBLOCKER

Introduction

This is an independent bronchial blocker made of silicon.

Design

- Available in 4.5 and 9 Fr sizes, and is 65 cm in length
- It has a high-volume balloon with a gas barrier property
- This prevents diffusion of gas into or out of the cuff

- The balloon has mucosal protective properties as:
  - Maximum volume of air which can be injected is 6 mL
  - Maximal pressure which can be exerted is < 30 mm Hg
- Has fixed distal angulation to aid insertion
- The bronchial blocker has a swivel connector which allows easy insertion of FOB
- It has a torque control blocker with an incorporated shaft
- This enables easy guidance into the desired bronchus

Preparation of the Blocker

- The blocker is inflated and tested for any leaks prior to deflation
- The outer surface of the balloon is then lubricated with silicon jelly

Method of Placement

- Endobronchial blocker is advanced through the tracheal tube under FOB guidance
- Torque control shaft with the BB enables guidance into the desired target bronchus
- Right main bronchial (RMB) blockade:
  - FOB is positioned at least 5 mm below the tracheal carina in right bronchus
  - The tip of the BB is then advanced under FOB guidance
  - Optimal position provides a view of the outer surface of fully inflated balloon
  - This usually requires 4-8 mL of air
- Left main bronchial (LMB) blockade:
  - Blocker is twisted towards the left bronchus and advanced
  - Optimal position is when balloon is seen 5-10 mm below carina in LMB

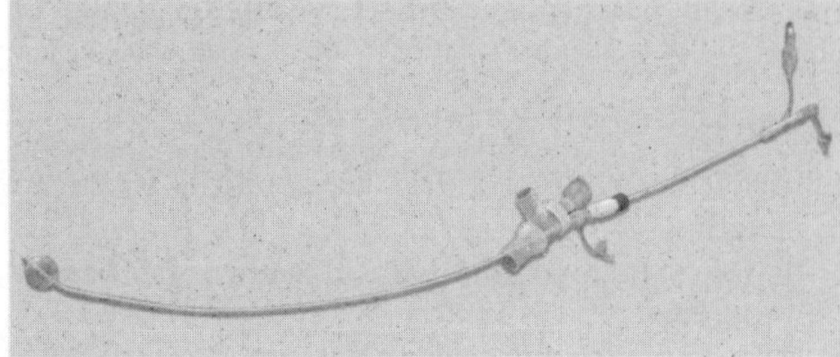

Fig. 50: Fuji uniblocker.

Advantages

- Surgical exposure is equivalent to that provided by left sided DLTs
- Can easily negotiate the glottis and tracheostomy tubes compared with Univent tubes
- More easily used in small stature patients compared with Univent tubes

Disadvantages

- Takes longer time to position
- More chances of intraoperative malposition compared to DLTs
- Better for left sided surgeries when compared to right sided surgeries

E-Z BLOCKER

Introduction

- It is an independent BB with a Y-shaped bifurcation made of polyurethane
- Designed by Teleflex, Morrisville

Design

- Available in 7 Fr size and is 75-cm long
- It is manufactured with a Y-shaped distal end
- Both limbs of the distal end are fitted with:
  - An inflatable balloon
  - Central channel to allow suction
- Each limb is colour coded (yellow/blue)
- This allows easy identification with the matching pilot balloon
- The blocker also has a multiport adapter with 3 different ports:
  - For connection to the SLT
  - To allow advancement of the blocker
  - To allow advancement of the FOB

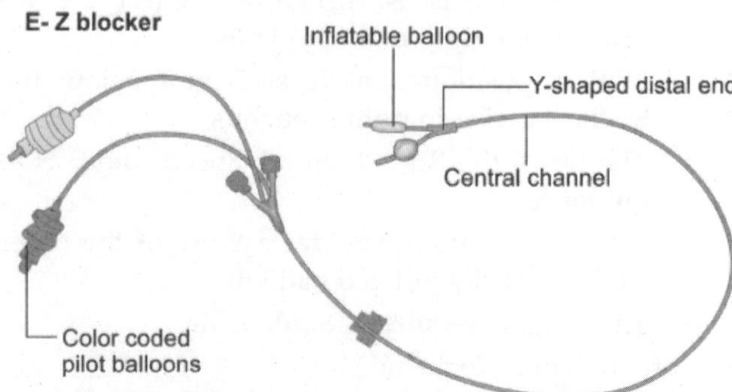

Fig. 51: E-Z Bronchial blocker.

Preparation of the Blocker

- The blocker is inflated and tested for any leaks prior to deflation
- The outer surface of the balloon is then lubricated with silicon jelly

Method of Placement

- The BB is advanced through the lumen of the SLT
- The Y-shaped end is seated at the tracheal carina
- Each independent tip should be located in the entrance of the RMB and LMB
- The balloon on the targeted bronchus side is inflated under FOB guidance
- This may require up to 10-14 mL of air to obtain adequate seal
- Optimal position is when outer surface of balloon is 5-10 mm within the bronchus
- FOB is withdrawn following verification of BB position

Advantages

- Useful in bilateral procedures as it does not require repositioning of the BB

Disadvantages

- Both limbs may enter into the same bronchus (usually right)
- Malpositioning is common during surgery
- Risk of airway trauma

PREOPERATIVE EVALUATION FOR THORACATOMY

Goals

- To recognize patients ability to tolerate procedure
- To identify high risk patients
- To risk stratify perioperative management
- To focus resources on high risk patients to improve outcome
- To assess the risk of postoperative pulmonary complications (POPC)

Initial Assessment

- All patients:
  - Cardiopulmonary tests
  - Concomitant illnesses
- Cancer patients:
  - Mass effect
  - Metastasis effect
  - Metabolic effect
  - Medication effect
- COPD patients:
  - Baseline ABG
  - History of bronchodilator, steroid and physiotherapy
- Renal dysfunction:
  - Blood urea nitrogen
  - Serum creatinine

Components of Preoperative Evaluation

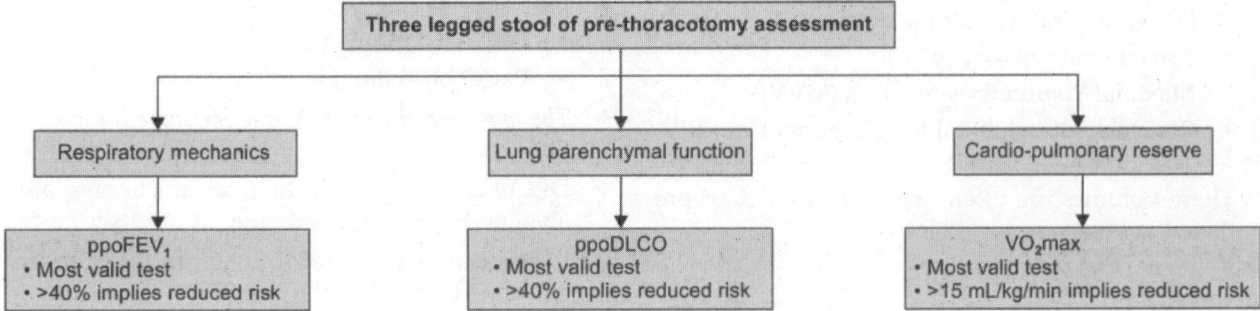

History

- Dyspnea: Onset, severity, positional variation
- Orthopnea which relieves on upright position
- Cough, hemoptysis, wheeze
- Exercise tolerance
- Cigarette smoking: > 20 pack-years increases the risk of POPC
- History of bronchodilator and steroid therapy for perioperative supplementation

Examination

- Cyanosis, clubbing, osteoarthropathy
- Respiratory rate and pattern
- ***Hoovers sign, Tripod sign***
- Tracheal deviation, wheeze, crackles, decreased or absent sounds
- Signs of right ventricular failure:
  - Split S_2 with increased P_2
  - Edema
  - Raised JVP
  - Congestive hepatomegaly

Routine Investigations

- Complete blood count, BUN, serum, creatinine, electrolytes
- ABG on room air, coagulation profile
- Chest X-ray, CT/MRI to localize lesion
- ECG: Signs RV overload

Assessment of Respiratory Function

- This is done to assess the 3 basic functions of the respiratory system:
  - Transport of oxygen into the alveoli- respiratory mechanics
  - Transport of oxygen into the blood- lung parenchymal function
  - Transport of oxygen into the tissues- cardiopulmonary interaction

A. *Respiratory Mechanics*

- Many tests of pulmonary volumes show correlation with post-thoracotomy outcomes:
  - Forced expiratory volume in 1 second (FEV_1)
  - Forced vital capacity (FVC)
  - Maximal Voluntary Ventilation (MVV)
  - Residual volume/total lung capacity ratio (RV/TLC ratio)
- These volumes are often expressed as a % of predicted volumes, corrected for:
  - Age
  - Sex
  - Height
- *Predicted postoperative FEV1 (ppoFEV1):*

$$ppoFEV_1\ (\%) = \text{preoperative } FEV_1 \times \frac{[1 - (\text{percentage of functional tissue removed})]}{100}$$

- *ppo FEV1 is the most valuable test for respiratory mechanics*
- Calculation of percentage of functional tissue removed:
  - This is based on number of functioning subsegments of lung removed
  - The lung is taken to have 19 segments in total:
    - 3 segments in both the upper lobes
    - 2 segments in both the middle lobes and lingula
    - 5 segments in the right lower lobe
    - 4 segments in the left lower lobe
  - Number of remaining segments following resection is calculated
  - This is multiplied by the preoperative FEV_1 measurements
  - Thus, the equation for calculation changes to:

$$ppoFEV_1\ (\%) = \text{preoperative } FEV_1 \times \frac{[1 - (\text{resected segments})]}{19}$$

- Interpretation:
  - ppo FEV_1 > 40% indicates low risk of POPC
  - ppo FEV_1 30-40% indicates moderate risk of POPC
  - ppo FEV_1 <30% indicates high risk of POPC

B. *Parenchymal Function*

- Traditional values which contraindicate lung resection include:
  - $PaO_2 < 60$ mm Hg
  - $PaCO_2 > 45$ mm Hg
- *The most useful test of the gas exchange capacity of the lung is the DLCO*
- DLCO correlates with the total functioning area of alveolar basement membrane
- Postresection predicted DLCO (ppoDLCO) can be calculated similar to the $ppoFEV_1$
- ppoDLCO: The minimal values compatible with successful outcome are:
  - ppoDLCO < 40% predicts increased risk of POPC and cardiac complications
  - ppoDLCO < 20% predicts an unacceptably high perioperative mortality rate

C. *Cardio-pulmonary Interactions*

- *Gold standard for assessment of cardio-pulmonary function*
- Metabolic equivalents (METS)
  - Exercise capacity is described in metabolic equivalents of task
  - 1 MET is the metabolic equivalent required for sitting quietly
  - 4 METS is the metabolic equivalent required to climb 1 flight of stairs
  - Ability to climb 2 flights of stairs without stopping is required for resection
  - 10 feet is the commonly used standard for the height of the flight of stairs
  - Patients with a limited ability to climb stairs require further testing
- VO_{2MAX}:
  - *Most useful predictor of post-thoracotomy outcome*
  - VO_2max > 20 mL/kg/min implies low risk of POPC
  - VO_2max < 15 mL/kg/min implies high risk of POPC
  - VO_2max < 10 mL/kg/min implies very high risk of morbidity and mortality
- ***Brunellis*** stair climbing test:
  - 20 steps to be present per flight
  - Done at patients own pace but without stopping
  - Ability to climb 5 flights of stairs implies VO_{2MAX} is more than 20 mL/kg/min
  - Ability to climb 2 flights implies VO_{2MAX} of around 12 mL/kg/min
  - Inability to climb 2 flights predicts high risk of POPC
- Anaerobic threshold (AT) during exercise testing:
  - Anaerobic threshold during exercise predicts postoperative complications
  - This is the exercise level at which lactate begins to accumulate in the blood
  - It is measured by repeated lactate measurements taken during exercise
  - Normal anaerobic threshold values:
    - Approximately 55% of VO_2max in untrained patients
    - More than 80% of VO_2max in trained patients
  - AT values of < 11 mL/kg/min is associated with increased risk of POPC
- 6-minute walk test (6MWT):
  - Is the most valid simple exercise test
  - It is the maximal distance a patient can walk in 6 minutes
  - 6MWT shows excellent correlation with maximal O_2 consumption (VO_2max)
  - VO_2max can be calculated from the distance covered during 6MWT in meters

$$VO_2max = \frac{\text{distance covered in meters during the 6MWT}}{30}$$

  - 6 MWT < 2000 feet or 610 mts implies VO_2MAX < 15 mL/kg/min
  - Exercise oximetry > 4% during 6 MWT or stair climbing predicts high risk of POPC

D. *Others*

- Ventilation-perfusion scintigraphy:
  - Useful to assess the contribution of the to-be-resected lobe to lung function
  - If the preoperative contribution of the lobe is minimal, postoperative function will be minimally altered
  - Test should be performed for any patient with:
    - Preoperative FEV_1 < 80% of predicted
    - Preoperative DLCO < 80% of predicted
- Split lung function tests:
  - Test simulates postoperative respiratory situation
  - Done using BB/endobronchial tube

Assessment for Malignancies

A. Mass effect:

- Tracheal distortion
- RLN/phrenic nerve palsy
- Pancoasts tumor
- Obstructive pneumonia
- Lung abscess

B. Metastasis:

- Brain
- Bone
- Liver
- Adrenals

C. Medications:

- Pulmonary toxicity:

- Bleomycin
- Mitomycin

❖ Cardiotoxicity: Doxorubicin

❖ Nephrotoxicity: Cisplatin

D. Metabolic:

❖ Hypercalcemia due to hyperparathyroidism

❖ Cushing syndrome: ACTH

❖ SIADH, GH

❖ Lambert Eaton syndrome

❖ Hypertrophic pulmonary osteoarthropathy

Factors Associated with Increased Perioperative Morbidity

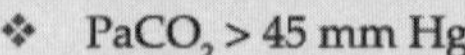

❖ $PaCO_2 > 45$ mm Hg

❖ $PaO_2 < 50$ mm Hg on room air

❖ Inability to walk 2000 feet in 6 minutes

❖ Inability to ascend 2 flights of stairs

❖ Inability to attain 7.5 mL/kg/min oxygen consumption

❖ $ppoFEV_1 < 30\%$ of expected normal value for the patient

❖ Measures of right heart catheterization after balloon occlusion of PA:
- Mean PA pressure > 35 mm Hg
- $PaO_2 < 45$ mm Hg
- $PaCO_2 > 60$ mm Hg

Assessment of Cardiac Function

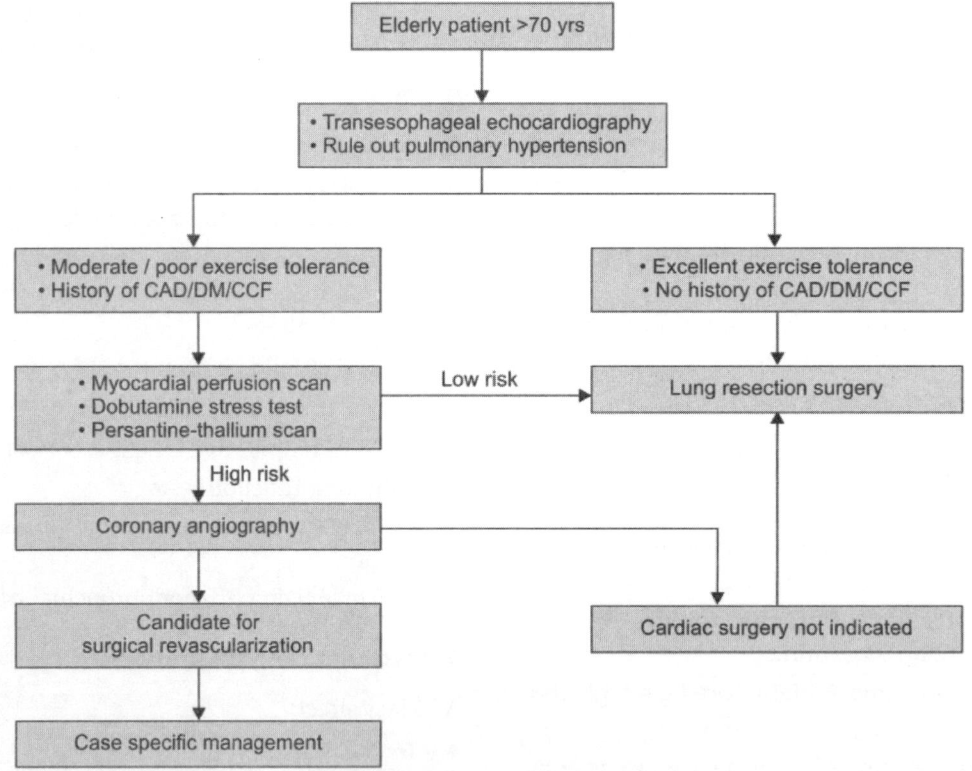

TRCRI score	Risk
0 points	< 5%
1–1.5 points	5–10%
≥ 2 points	11–20%

Component	Points
Pneumonectomy	1.5
Coronary artery disease	1.5
Cerebrovascular disease	1.5
Serum creatinine > 2 mg/mL	1

Preoperative Thoracic Revised Cardiac Risk Index (TRCRI)

❖ Cardiac complications are the second most common cause of perioperative morbidity in thoracic surgical population

❖ Commonest cardiac complications are:
- Myocardial ischemia
- Arrhythmias
- Heart failure

❖ Thoracic RCRI was developed specifically for thoracic surgery patients

❖ However, predictive risk of this score in prospective studies has been suboptimal

Implications of Preoperative Assessment

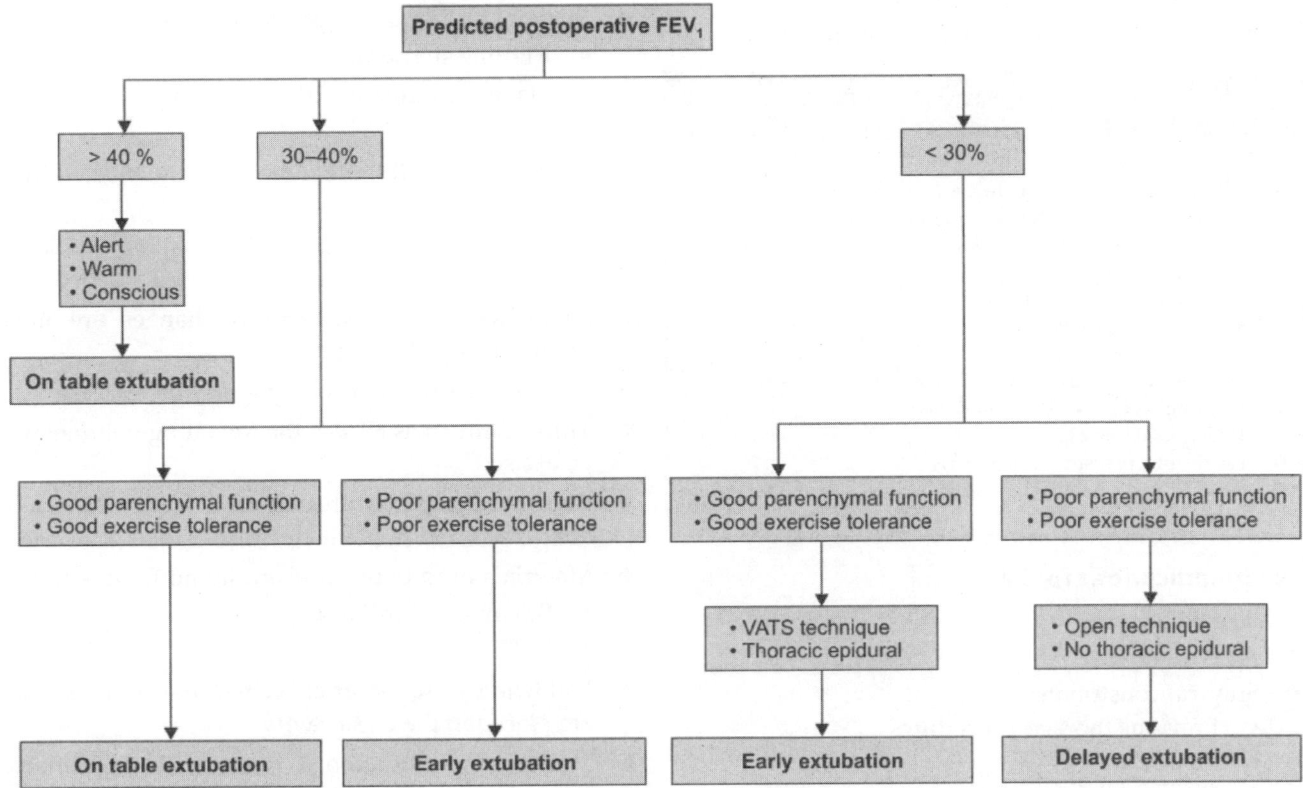

LUNG VOLUME REDUCTION SURGERY

Introduction

- LVRS is used to improve exercise tolerance and relieve dyspnea in severe emphysema
- Aims at reducing lung volume by multiple wedge resections of emphysematous tissue
- This reduces lung volume and improve symptoms in severely symptomatic patients
- Initially performed in 1957 by ***Brantigan and Mueller***
- However, due to high operative rate of 18%, the procedure was not widely adopted
- ***Cooper*** modified the technique resecting 20-30% of lung tissue in 1995
- This resulted in lower mortality rates with wider acceptance
- Also called reduction pneumoplasty or bilateral pneumonectomy

Rationale

- Increases elastic recoil of bronchioles:
  - LVRS reduces the size mismatch between hyperinflated lung and chest cavity
  - This restores the outward circumferential pull on the bronchioles
  - Thus, elastic recoil is increased, improving expiratory airflow
- Improvement in diaphragmatic function:
  - LVRS reduces the FRC of the lung
  - This returns the diaphragm to the more normal curved configuration
  - This helps in improving diaphragmatic function
  - Thus, efficiency of diaphragmatic breathing is increased
- Improved cardiac function:
  - LVRS reduces the intrathoracic pressure and improves venous return
  - Thus, LV filling, end-diastolic volume and cardiac output increase
- Other mechanisms include:
  - Improved vascular endothelial function
  - Reduced dynamic hyperinflation due to reduced lung volume during exercise

Indications

- Severe heterogeneous emphysema
- Rare indications:
  - Resection for stage 1 lung cancer
  - To wean ventilator dependant COPD patients

- To reduce hyperinflation of native lung after unilateral lung transplantation
- To serve as a bridge to lung transplantation

Inclusion Criteria for LVRS

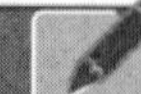

- Age < 75 years
- Smoking cessation for more than 1 month (6 months ideally)
- No previous thoracotomy or pleurodesis
- Absence of respiratory infections for 3 weeks prior to surgery
- Absence of comorbidities:
  - Coronary artery disease
  - Chronic asthma
  - Bronchitis
- Prednisolone requirement < 20 mg/day
- FEV1 between 15-35% of predicted
- $PaCO_2$ < 50 mm Hg
- PA systolic pressure < 50 mm Hg
- Able to complete preoperative pulmonary rehabilitation program for 6 weeks

Contraindications for LVRS

- Age > 75 years
- Active smoking
- Surgical constraints:
  - Previous thoracic procedures
  - Pleurodesis
  - Chest wall deformity
- Significant comorbidity:
  - Clinically significant bronchiectasis
  - Clinically significant coronary artery disease
  - Heart failure with EF < 45%
  - Uncontrolled HTN
  - Obesity
- High dose systemic steroids
- Pulmonary hypertension with:
  - PASP > 50 mm Hg
  - Mean PA pressure > 35 mm Hg
- Physiological parameters:
  - PaO_2 < 45 mm Hg on room air
  - $PaCO_2$ > 60 mm Hg
  - Low DLCO < 30% of predicted
  - Low FEV_1 < 20% of predicted
  - Poor exercise tolerance (shuttle walk < 150 meters)

Predictors for High Risk LVRS

- Age > 70 years
- Diffuse homogenous emphysema
- Non-upper lobe predominant emphysema
- 6-minute walk test distance 200 metres
- $PaCO_2$ > 45 mm Hg
- FEV_1 < 20% along with DLCO < 30%

Technique

- Bilateral LVRS may be performed via:
  - Midline sternotomy
  - Staged anterolateral thoracotomy
  - VATS
- For bilateral LVRS, the more severely affected lung is reduced first
- Volume reduction is achieved by making a series of wedge excisions
- Areas where emphysematous changes are most severe are serially resected
- Typically, 20-30% of each lung may be resected
- Thus, as much as 60% of the total lung volume may be excised
- Buttressed staple sutures are used to close the resultant defects and prevent air leaks
- Materials used to buttress anastomotic sites are:
  - Bovine pericardial strips
  - PTFE strips
- Following completion of wedge resections, 2 ICDs are placed in the chest cavity
- Mechanical ventilation is resumed to the deflated lung
- This is followed by chest closure

Anesthetic Goals

- Ensuring preoperative optimization of the patient
- Providing optimal surgical field with lung separation and OLV
- Maintenance of normothermia for prolonged surgeries
- Rapid emergence and early extubation to avoid postoperative ventilation
- Optimal postoperative analgesia to encourage spontaneous ventilation

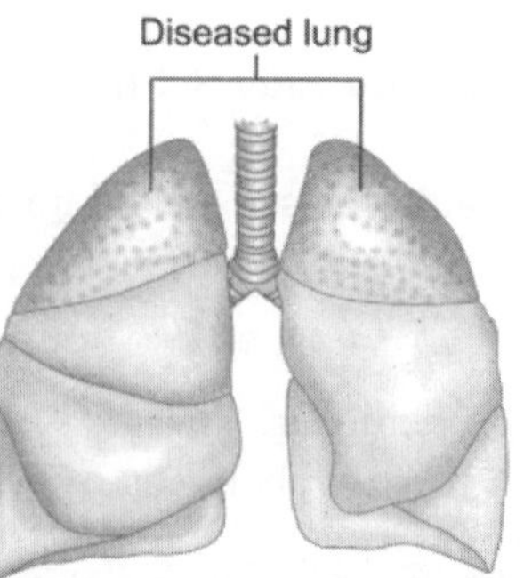

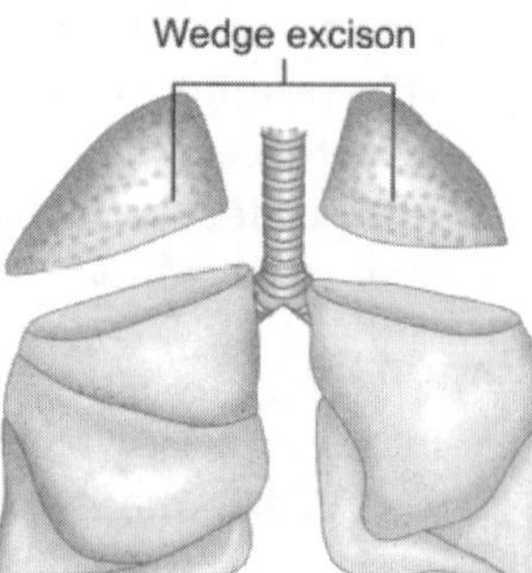

Fig. 52: Lung volume reduction surgery.

Anesthetic Considerations 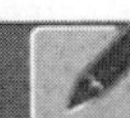

- Deliberate hypoventilation and permissive hypercapnia intraoperatively
- Intraoperative gas trapping:
  - PPV in emphysema patients leads to intraoperative gas trapping
  - This can cause dynamic hyperinflation, auto-PEEP and pneumothorax
- Restrictive fluid strategy
- Occult coronary artery disease:
  - Most LVRS surgeries are done in smokers with advanced age
  - These patients have severely restricted physical activity
  - Thus, there is increased risk of occult coronary artery disease
- Early postoperative extubation:
  - Postoperative air leak due to disruption of suture lines is a significant risk
  - Thus, rapid emergence and early extubation are the primary goals

Preoperative Preparation and Optimization

- Cessation of smoking for at least 6 months prior to LVRS
- Pulmonary rehabilitation is recommended prior to LVRS and comprises:
  - Optimization of medical therapy with bronchodilators
  - Aggressive management of infections with antibiotics
  - Exercise training
- Most patients lead a sedentary lifestyle due to poor functional capacity
- Thus, exercise training is recommended for at least 6 weeks prior to surgery
- Exercise training has several advantages:
  - Tests endurance and exercise tolerance
  - Increases maximal oxygen consumption
  - Tests for dormant coronary artery disease
- Training includes:
  - Bicycle ergometer training
  - Distance walking on flat surfaces
  - Weight lifting
- Long term oxygen therapy may be established prior to LVRS
- Patient should preferably be free of respiratory infections for 3 weeks prior to surgery
- Prophylactic immunization against pneumococcus and influenza is recommended

Premedication

- NPO orders
- Informed consent
- A large bore IV cannula is secured on the ipsilateral side in unilateral LVRS
- 2 units of blood should be kept cross matched and ready
- Sedation:
  - Avoided if the patient is calm and cooperative
  - This is because these patients already have compromised respiratory function
  - IV midazolam 0.03 mg/kg may be given in anxious patients
  - Doses are minimized to prevent delayed extubation postoperatively
- IV glycopyrrolate 0.01 mg/kg as an anti-sialogogue especially if FOB is planned
- Perioperative steroid supplementation is given as patient is often on steroids
- Airway blocks can be given if awake intubation is planned
- Cardiac and respiratory medicines are continued in perioperative period
- Theophylline therapy should be withheld if:
  - Serum levels > 20 ng/mL
  - Side effects such as:
    - Nervousness, tremors
    - Tachycardia
- Thoracic epidural can be inserted preoperatively for postoperative pain management
- Antibiotic therapy to be given as per hospital protocol
- Chest physiotherapy is essential for mobilization of secretions
- DVT prophylaxis necessary as increased risk of DVT due to polycythemia

Monitors

- Pulse oximetry, E_TCO_2
- ECG, NIBP
- Arterial line:
  - Essential for beat-to-beat monitoring of blood pressure
  - Also useful for repetitive ABG sampling
- Urine output, temperature
- CVP:
  - Essential as large fluid shifts may occur
  - Also useful for administration of vasopressors

- However, it may not be an accurate indicator of fluid status as:
  - Chest cavity is open following sternotomy
  - Inaccurate in the lateral position for thoracotomy
  - Significant pulmonary HTN may be present
- Placed following induction due to poor tolerance of Trendelenburg position

❖ BIS and neuromuscular monitoring:
- Doses of anesthetic agents are minimized during the procedure
- Thus, BIS monitoring is useful to prevent intraoperative awareness

❖ Continuous spirometry

❖ Monitor airway pressure and tidal volume

❖ PA catheter:
- Not routinely indicated
- May be helpful in patients with mild PAH as OLV increases PA pressure

Induction

❖ GA with DLT and OLV is preferred to ensure lung *separation*

❖ Prolonged preoxygenation is usually required:
- Necessary in these patients as they have:
  - Poor alveolar ventilation
  - Increased airflow resistance
  - Increased FRC
- Preoxygenation is done for 10-12 minutes

❖ Preoxygenation may have to be done in sitting position in severe dyspnea

❖ IV induction is preferred with thiopentone or propofol

❖ High preoperative sympathetic tone causes:
- Slow intravenous induction
- Profound hypotension at the time of induction

❖ Inhalational induction is avoided as:
- Severe bullous disease delays uptake of inhalational agents
- Also, bullae may make uptake of volatile agents unpredictable

❖ Intermediate acting NMBAS with absence of histamine liberation are preferred

❖ Thus, vecuronium or cisatracurium are used for neuromuscular blockade

❖ DLT inserted following NMB with fibreoptic bronchoscopic (FOB) guidance

Position

❖ *Bilateral LVRS through sternotomy*: Supine with arms to the sides

❖ *Thoracotomy approach*: Lateral decubitus position as for lung pneumonectomy

Maintenance

❖ TIVA and balanced anesthesia with volatile agents may be used for maintenance

❖ TIVA is *preferred technique* as:
- It preserves hypoxic pulmonary vasoconstriction
- Thus, it helps in reducing the shunt fraction
- Also, propofol is less dependant on pulmonary elimination
- Since VAs are eliminated via the lung, emergence may be delayed

❖ Propofol with remifentanil infusion may be used to maintain anesthesia

❖ If balanced anesthesia used, isoflurane 0.5-1 MAC can be used

❖ N_2O contraindicated if balanced anesthesia is used

❖ Volatile anesthetics have increased alveolar-arterial gradient

❖ Prophylactic ICD insertion is not recommended as it may rupture bulla

Ventilation

❖ LVRS patients are at high risk for barotrauma and gas trapping

❖ Thus, pressure controlled/ pressure limited ventilation is preferred

❖ Volume control modes of ventilation are avoided

❖ Ventilatory strategy:
- Deliberate hypoventilation and permissive hypercapnea
- One lung ventilation during resection
- Restricted tidal volumes:
  - < 5 mL/kg for OLV
  - < 9 mL/kg for TLV
- Low respiratory rate:
  - < 16 breaths/ min for OLV
  - < 12 breaths/ min for TLV
- Prolonged expiratory time: I: E ratio 1:3 for OLV and TLV
- Peak airway pressure < 35 cm H_2O

❖ Permissive hypercarbia is usually well tolerated if the pH is maintained above 7.20

❖ In case of hypercarbia with pH < 7.20 strategies used are:
- Gradual increase in respiratory rate
- Suctioning of airway secretions
- Optimization of muscle relaxation
- Inhaled bronchodilator therapy

- In the presence of bullae, IPPV is avoided until the bulla is surgically isolated
- If IPPV is used prior to bulla isolation:
  - Increased anatomical deadspace occurs due to increased size of bulla
  - Air leak, bulla rupture and tension pneumothorax possible
- Reduce auto-PEEP:
  - Intermittently disconnect from ventilator to allow lungs to empty
  - Manual compression of chest to empty auto-PEEP

Hemodynamics

- Precipitous hypotension most commonly occurs on induction due to:
  - Dynamic hyperinflation leading to auto-PEEP
  - Sudden loss of high preoperative sympathetic tone
  - Activation of thoracic epidural anesthesia
- Restrictive fluid strategy is preferred to enable early extubation
- Large intraoperative fluid shifts are treated with:
  - Judicious use of IV fluids to prevent postoperative ALI
  - Use colloids to reduce the risk of pulmonary edema
  - Inotropic support may be used to reduce fluid administration
- Maintain normothermia:
  - IV fluids warmers
  - Forced air warmers
  - Heat-moisture exchangers

Extubation

- Early extubation is preferred to avoid postoperative IPPV
- IPPV may increase airway pressure and disrupt anastomotic sites
- This may lead to air leak syndromes postoperatively
- Extubation criteria following LVRS:
  - Awake and cooperative patient
  - Stable hemodynamic parameters
  - Rapid shallow breathing index < 70
  - Adequate oxygenation with spontaneous breathing (SpO_2 > 92%, FiO_2 35%)
  - Adequate analgesia
  - Core temperature > 35.5 °C
  - Absence of shivering
- Patient may be ventilated for 1-2 hours postoperatively if the criteria are not met
- DLT is changed to SLT if postoperative ventilation is planned

Postoperative Care

Management

- In case of postoperative ventilation:
  - Airway pressures are minimized
  - FiO_2 is adjusted to maintain SpO_2 between 90-92%
  - Permissive hypercarbia with $PaCO_2$ up to 60 mm Hg
- Care of ICD:
  - ICDs are connected to a water seal system to detect air leaks
  - Suction on ICD is usually avoided
  - This is because suction increases the trans-pulmonary pressure
  - Lung tissue in these patients is fragile
  - Thus, suction on the chest tubes may result in overdistension of the lungs
  - This may result in magnification and prolongation of air leaks
- Pulmonary rehabilitation post-extubation:
  - Chest physiotherapy resumed as early as 1-hour post-surgery
  - Incentive spirometry
  - Early mobilization

Analgesia

- Multimodal analgesia
- Opioids:
  - Dose is minimized to prevent respiratory depression
  - Administered via systemic/neuraxial/PCA routes
- Thoracic epidural analgesia especially for bilateral LVRS sone through sternotomy
- Intercostal, intrapleural, paravertebral blocks
- NSAIDs

Complications

- Air leak and pneumothorax:
  - *Most common* complication
  - Can be avoided by the use of appropriately sized and positioned ICD
- Respiratory failure:
  - Can be due to:
    - Bronchospasm
    - Pneumothorax
    - Accumulation of airway secretions
    - Inadequate analgesia
    - Infections causing pneumonia
  - Treated with non-invasive positive pressure ventilation

- Other postoperative complications include:
  - Persistent air leaks and bronchopleural fistula
  - Pulmonary embolism
  - Arrhythmias
  - Myocardial infarction

Prognosis

- LVRS is a major thoracic surgery performed in patients with:
  - Limited pulmonary reserve
  - Significant comorbidities
- LVRS is associated with significant mortality and morbidity
- Reported mortality rate is 5.5% and major pulmonary morbidity rate is 29.5%
- Intermediate postoperative improvement occurs in symptoms and PFTs
- Occurs due to:
  - Decompression of airways
  - Reduction in airway resistance
  - Reduction in work of breathing
  - Reduction in auto-PEEP
  - Increase in dynamic compliance
- Used as an alternative to lung transplant

PNEUMONECTOMY

Introduction

- Pneumonectomy refers to complete surgical removal of the ipsilateral lung
- Right pneumonectomy refers to removal of entire right lung including:
  - Upper lobe
  - Middle lobe
  - Lower lobe
- Left pneumonectomy refers to removal of entire left lung including:
  - Upper lobe
  - Lower lobe

Incidence

- First single-stage pneumonectomy done as early as 1933 by Dr. Evarts Graham
- Right pneumonectomy is associated with higher incidence of:
  - Bronchopleural fistula
  - Higher mortality
- Mortality rates for other lung resections like lobectomy is 1–2%
- For pneumonectomy, mortality rates increase to 8–10%
- Pneumonectomy is also associated with higher risk of complications such as:
  - Cardiac complications
  - Acute lung injury
  - ARDS

Indications

- Primary indication is bronchial carcinoma *not amenable to alternative resection*
- Indications for malignant lesions:
  - Tumours originating from main stem bronchus
  - Tumours proximal to bronchus intermedius
  - Tumours with hilar involvement
- Indications for non-malignant lesions:
  - Traumatic injury to lung with uncontrolled hemorrhage
  - Chronic infective diseases of the lung
  - Fungal infections causing destroyed lung
- Quality of life in general is poorer when compared with lobectomy or bilobectomy
- Thus, pneumonectomy is considered as the last option
- It is usually performed only when all other options are deemed inappropriate

Procedure

- Pneumonectomy:
  - Surgery is done through a standard posterolateral incision
  - Mediastinal pleura is incised
  - Main blood vessels are stapled first and include:
    - Pulmonary artery
    - Superior and inferior pulmonary veins
  - This is followed by stapling of the mainstem bronchus
  - The entire lung is then taken out of the chest
  - Tests are then done for any air-leaks
  - Reconstruction of bronchial stump is completed
  - Bronchial stump is minimized to prevent accumulation of secretions.

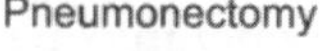

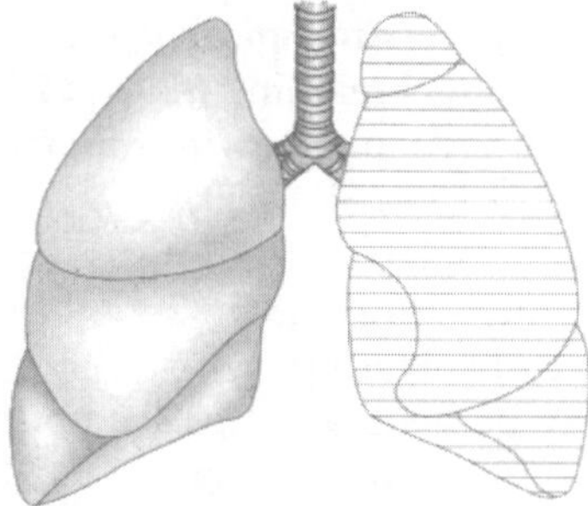

Fig. 53: Pneumonectomy.

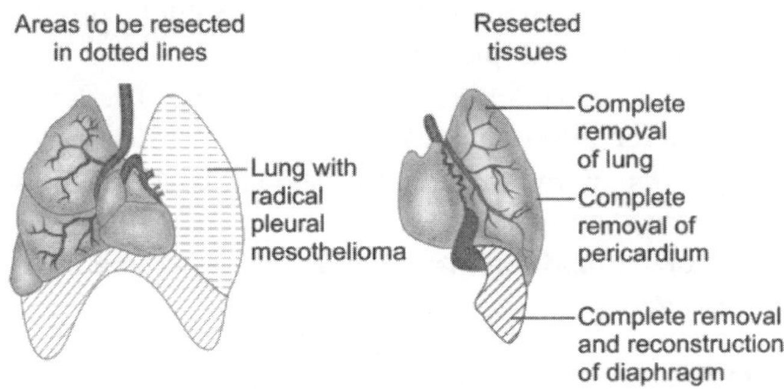

Fig. 54: Extrapleural pneumonectomy.

- ❖ Extrapleural pneumonectomy:
  - Radical type of resection for patients with malignant pleural mesotheliomas
  - This comprises of excision of:
    - The affected lung
    - Ipsilateral pleura
    - Ipsilateral hemidiaphragm
    - Ipsilateral hemipericardium
  - Rarely done as mortality is worse compared with medical management
  - Increased blood loss occurs due to involvement of chest wall blood vessels.
- ❖ *Completion pneumonectomy*: Excision of residual lung tissue after previous resection
- ❖ Carinal pneumonectomy:
  - Rarely performed
  - Done for tumours of distal trachea or carina
  - Refers to excision of lung and carina
- ❖ Sleeve pneumonectomy:
  - Mostly done for right sided tumours via right thoracotomy
  - Done for tumours of most proximal parts of mainstream bronchus and carina
  - Surgery is done in two stages:
    - First stage: Left thoracotomy and pneumonectomy
    - Second stage:
      - Right thoracotomy
      - Mobilization of tracheobronchial bifurcation
      - Carinal excision along with involved main bronchus
      - Circumferential anastomosis
  - Resected specimen consists of:
    - Involved lung
    - Carina
    - Distal trachea
    - Proximal involved bronchus

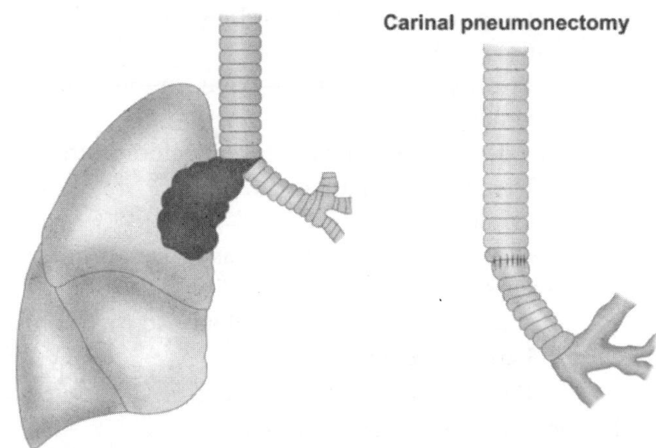

Fig. 55: Carinal pneumonectomy.

  - Operative mortality is up to 4 times that of standard pneumonectomy

Anesthetic Considerations

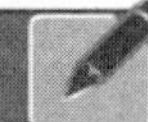

- ❖ Determine suitability for resection using 3-legged stool approach:
  - Respiratory mechanics
  - Parenchymal function
  - Cardio-respiratory interaction
- ❖ Preoperative optimization:
  - Smoking cessation
  - Pulmonary rehabilitation
  - Treatment of lung infection
  - Treatment of bronchospasm
- ❖ Intraoperative management:
  - Lung isolation
  - Thoracic epidural analgesia
  - Restrictive fluid strategy
  - Lung protective ventilation
  - Avoidance of hypothermia

Preoperative Evaluation and Risk Assessment

- ❖ Preoperative risk assessment for all lung resections should be along 3 domains:
  - Operative mortality
  - Perioperative myocardial events
  - Postoperative dyspnea
- ❖ Operative mortality:
  - Postoperative mortality for thoracic surgery is calculated using ***Thoracoscore***
  - Thoracoscore incorporates 9 factors:
    - Age (< 55, 55-65, > 65 years)
    - Sex
    - ASA score (< 2, > 3)
    - Performance status according to Zubrod scale (< 2, > 3)

- Dyspnea severity according to MRC scale (< 2, > 3)
- Priority of surgery (elective, urgent, emergency)
- Extent of resection (pneumonectomy, others)
- Diagnosis (malignant, benign)
- Comorbidity score
- However, Thoracoscore has been found inaccurate in predicting mortality
- Thus, preoperative assessment should focus on:
  - Patients exercise capacity
  - Physiological reserve

❖ Perioperative myocardial events:
- Cardiologist opinion is sought in all patients with an active cardiac condition:
  - Unstable angina
  - Heart failure
  - Significant arrhythmias
  - Severe valvular heart disease
- Revised Cardiac Risk Index may be used to assess risk for cardiac morbidity
- Thoracic RCRI may be used as an alternative
- However, predictive risk of both these scores has been found to be suboptimal
- All patients undergoing pneumonectomy should undergo echocardiography

❖ Postoperative dyspnea:
- Evaluation for postoperative dyspnea entails evaluation of:
  - Respiratory mechanics
  - Parenchymal function
- Thus, most important determinants of postoperative dyspnea include:
  - ppoFEV_1
  - ppoDLCO

High Risk Patients

❖ Age > 70 years
❖ FVC < 50% predicted
❖ FEV_1 < 50% predicted or < 2 litres
❖ MVV < 50% predicted
❖ DLCO < 50% predicted
❖ $PaCO_2$ > 45 mm Hg on room air
❖ Abnormal ECG

Premedication

❖ Continue all cardiovascular and respiratory drugs
❖ IV midazolam 0.03-0.15 mg for anxiolysis
❖ IV glycopyrrolate 10 μg/kg
❖ DVT prophylaxis with LMWH
❖ Appropriate preoperative surgical antibiotic prophylaxis as per hospital protocol
❖ Large bore IV access is secured in case of requirement for blood transfusion
❖ 2 units of red blood cells should be kept cross matched and ready
❖ Thoracic epidural may be inserted for perioperative analgesia

Monitor

❖ Pulse oximetry, E_TCO_2
❖ NIBP, ECG
❖ Urine output, nasopharyngeal temperature
❖ Tidal volume, airway pressure
❖ Continuous display of airway pressure volume loops
❖ Invasive arterial cannulation recommended for:
- Frequent ABG sampling
- Continuous monitoring of IBP

❖ CVP placement is recommended for:
- Guiding perioperative fluid management
- Administration of vasoactive drugs

❖ However, CVP may be unreliable as a monitor of intravascular fluid status due to:
- Lateral position of patient
- Open chest

❖ Invasive cardiac output monitoring has not been validated due to presence of an open thorax

Induction

❖ GA with OLV and DLT is technique of choice
❖ Prolonged preoxygenation is required as rapid desaturation may occur
❖ IV induction is done with *thiopentone or propofol*
❖ Slow induction occurs due to high preoperative sympathetic tone
❖ Profound hypotension can occur at the time of induction
❖ DLT/BB/SLT can be used to ensure lung isolation
❖ DLT which does not interfere with ipsilateral airway is chosen for pneumonectomy
❖ Thus, for a right sided pneumonectomy, left DLT is preferred
❖ If a left DLT is used for left pneumonectomy, it has to be withdrawn before stapling
❖ This is to prevent accidental inclusion of the DLT/BB into the suture line
❖ DLT inserted following NMB with fibreoptic bronchoscopic (FOB)

Position

- ❖ Patient is placed in the left or right lateral decubitus position with a table break
- ❖ Fastidious checking is required of:
  - Eye protection
  - Pressure points
  - Neck position
- ❖ DVT prophylaxis may be provided using graduated compression stockings
- ❖ Normothermia is maintained with:
  - Forced air warmer
  - Fluid warmer

Maintenance

- ❖ TIVA or balanced anesthesia can be used
- ❖ 0.5-1 MAC isoflurane is preferred if balanced anesthesia is used
- ❖ N_2O and halothane are avoided
- ❖ NMBAs are carefully titrated in the presence of Eaton Lambert syndrome

Ventilation

- ❖ Operative lung may be collapsed as soon as skin disinfection and draping is completed
- ❖ Problems with oxygenation may occur early during the procedure itself
- ❖ This may improve when the pulmonary artery is clamped and shunting is interrupted
- ❖ Lung protective OLV/HFPPV with DLT is useful:
  - Tidal volume 5-6 mL/kg is ideal
  - Limit peak airway pressure to < 35 cm H_2O
  - Limit plateau airway pressure to < 25 cm H_2O
  - PEEP 5 cm H_2O
  - Target normal $PaCO_2$
  - Avoid hyperoxia: target SpO_2 between 94-98%
- ❖ DLT/BB is withdrawn just before bronchus is stapled
- ❖ This avoid accidental inclusion of the DLT/ BB into the suture line
- ❖ *Leak-test* of bronchial stump suture line is then performed:
  - Performed once bronchial stump is closed and hemostasis achieved
  - Clamp on the DLT to the operated side is released
  - The bronchial stump is submerged under warm saline
  - Airway pressure is slowly increased to 25-40 cm H_2O
  - This, tests the integrity of the stump by detecting any air-leaks
- ❖ Airway is suctioned to collapse the lung before reinflation
- ❖ Once the chest drains have been inserted, the remaining lobe is reinflated
- ❖ Observing the pleural surface confirms if superficial lung tissue is reinflated
- ❖ At the time of chest closure, suction is applied to the ICD through an underwater seal
- ❖ Air leak during this time is suggested by:
  - Collapse of the ventilator reservoir
  - Reduction in the expired minute volume
- ❖ Suction is then disconnected and reapplied once spontaneous breathing is established
- ❖ ICDs are then left unclamped until the remaining lung has re-expanded fully
- ❖ DLT is replaced with SLT at the end of surgery

Hemodynamics

- ❖ Usually blood loss varies between 200-800 mL
- ❖ Rarely massive blood loss requiring blood transfusion occurs
- ❖ Risk factors associated with post-pneumonectomy pulmonary edema are:
  - Increased perioperative fluid administration
  - Right sided pneumonectomy
  - Increased postoperative urine output
- ❖ Thus, judicious fluid administration is important:
  - Reduces risk of postoperative Acute Lung Injury (ALI)
  - Administration of < 3 L in first 24 hrs is associated with reduced risk of ALI
  - Vasopressors are used instead of fluids to maintain hemodynamic instability
- ❖ Supplementation for third space loss has to be avoided
- ❖ Surgical manipulation can cause cardiac compression and hypotension
- ❖ Significant blood loss is possible in extra-pleural pneumonectomy

Clamping of the Pulmonary Artery

- ❖ Final test for pneumonectomy is the clamping of the pulmonary artery (PA)
- ❖ Once clamped, entire pulmonary blood supply is shunted to the non-operative lung
- ❖ Thus, excess fluid administration is associated with a high risk of pulmonary edema
- ❖ Post-pneumonectomy pulmonary edema has a high mortality rate, up to 50%

- Indicators of a postoperative cardiac complications following clamping include:
  - Excessive rise in CVP
  - Significant cardiovascular collapse
- Goals of fluid administration during the first 24 hours are:
  - Fluid administration less than 3 L in first 24 hours
  - Maximal urine output of 0.5 mL/kg/hour
  - Positive fluid balance < 20 mL/kg

Extubation

- May require postoperative ventilation if:
  - Long duration surgery
  - Large fluid shifts
- Patients are extubated when they are:
  - Awake
  - Warm
  - Comfortable

Postoperative Care

Management

- Nurse in sitting up position to allow expansion of remaining lung
- Humidified oxygen is supplemented via face mask
- Judicious fluid administration is continued during postoperative period
- Use of respiratory adjuncts such as incentive spirometry are useful
- Repeated chest X-rays are taken for pneumothorax

Analgesia

- Adequate analgesia is important to allow:
  - Effective cough
  - Clearance of secretions
  - Early mobilization
- Multimodal analgesia is preferred
- Opioids: Systemic/neuraxial/PCA opioids can be used
- Thoracic epidural
- Paravertebral/intercostal/intrapleural blocks

Complications

- Hemorrhage
- Retention of secretions
- Infection
- Atelectasis
- Respiratory failure
- *Acute Lung Injury (ALI)*: Increased risk if:
  - Preoperative alcohol abuse
  - Right sided pneumonectomy
  - Increased intraoperative ventilatory pressure index
  - Increased perioperative IV fluid administration
  - Increased urine output in postoperative period
- Arrhythmias: Usually atrial arrhythmias
- Pulmonary HTN and RV dysfunction due to increased afterload from increase in PVR occurring postoperatively
- Cardiac herniation if right sided pericardial resection is done
- Post-pneumonectomy pulmonary edema especially in sleeve pneumonectomy

Management of ICD

- Different practises exist with regards to postoperative ICD management
- There is no consensus as yet for best management of post-pneumonectomy space
- Single basal ICD is usually used
- ICD is left clamped but connected to an underwater seal
- It is unclamped for 1-2 minutes every hour to:
  - Assess for hemorrhage
  - Release air
  - Centralize the mediastinum
- Prolonged unclamping is avoided to prevent mediastinal shift into empty hemithorax
- Suction is also contraindicated for the same reason
- If ICD is not placed intraoperatively:
  - Air is aspirated from post-pneumonectomy space at the end of surgery
  - Cannula is placed through chest wall in supine position
  - Air is aspirated till there is negative pressure in the space
  - This will centralize mediastinum
- ICD is removed after 12-24 hours in the absence of any drains

BRONCHOPLEURAL FISTULA

Introduction

- BPF are airleaks occurring via connections between the airways and pleural space
- Can involve:
  - Mainstem bronchus
  - Lobar bronchus
  - Segmental bronchus

- If there is additional communication to the surface of chest, it is called cutaneous BPF

Incidence

- Most commonly seen following lung resection surgery
- Incidence ranges from:
  - 4.5- 20% following pneumonectomy
  - 0.5-1% following lobectomy
- Morbidity ranges from 25-71 %

Etiology

- Bronchopleural fistulas:
  - Penetrating trauma:
    - Iatrogenic trauma:
      - Most commonly due to rupture of bronchial stump post-pneumonectomy
      - Instrumentation from inside the airway
    - Non-iatrogenic penetrating trauma:
      - Gunshots
      - Penetrating chest wounds
      - Impalement
  - Blunt trauma:
    - Crush injuries
    - Acceleration-deceleration injuries
  - Medical disorders:
    - Erosion of bronchus by carcinoma or chronic inflammation
    - Spontaneous rupture of lung abscess/ empyema cavity into bronchus
- Alveolar-parenchymal fistulae: Traumatic rupture of bulla/cyst during ventilation (by barotrauma/ PEEP).

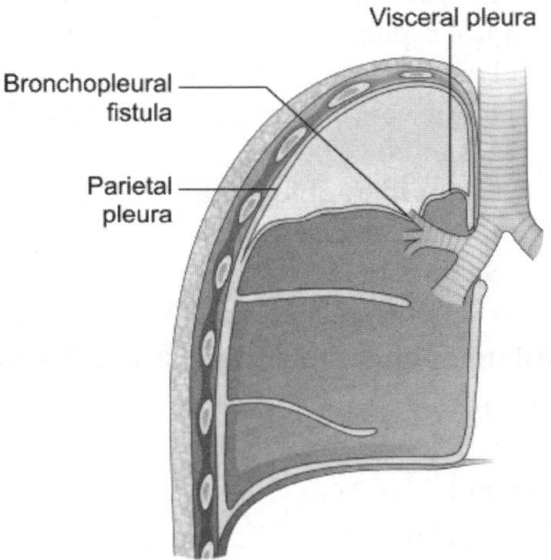

Fig. 56: Bronchopleural fistula.

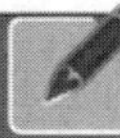

Risk Factors for APF in Lung Resection Surgery

- Advanced age
- Female gender
- History of:
  - Smoking
  - Diabetes mellitus
  - Chronic steroid use
  - COPD or other underlying lung disease
- Large bullae
- Low FEV_1/DLCO
- Marked pleural adhesions during surgery
- Upper lobe/diffuse emphysema

Types

- Alveolar parenchymal-pleural fistulas (APF):
  - Originates from lung parenchyma
  - Pathological communication between:
    - Pulmonary parenchyma distal to segmental bronchus (alveoli)
    - Pleural space
  - Usually presents as pneumothorax
  - Called Prolonged Air Leak (PAL) if it persists beyond 5 days
- Bronchopleural fistulas (BPF): Originating from tracheobronchial tree

Classification of Postoperative BPF

- Early onset/acute BPF:
  - Occurs 1-7 days following surgery
  - Usually due to surgical dehiscence
  - May be life threatening due to:
    - Tension pneumothorax
    - Asphyxiation from pulmonary flooding
  - Requires prompt surgical intervention
- Intermediate onset/subacute BPF:
  - Occurs 8-30 days following surgery
  - Insidious in onset and presentation
  - Primarily related to secondary infection
- Late onset/chronic BPF:
  - Occurs more than 30 days following surgery
  - Usually associated with:
    - Infections
    - Debilitated status
    - Fibrosis of pleural space

Diagnosis

- Clinical features:
  - Sudden onset dyspnea which is severe in nature
  - Cough with hemoptysis or purulent sputum
  - Fever
  - Subcutaneous emphysema
  - Contralateral deviation of trachea

- Sepsis, ARDS
- Persistent airleak, empyema
- In lobectomy patients:
  - Persistent air leak
  - Purulent drainage from chest tube are diagnostic

❖ Investigations:
- Preoperative BT, CT, creatinine, urea, LFTs, ECG
- Neutrophilia, raised total counts
- ABG: hypoxia, hypercarbia, metabolic acidosis
- Chest X-ray:
  - Air filled pleural space, new air-fluid level
  - Shifting of trachea, collapse of lung
  - Reducing fluid level on serial chest X-ray following pneumonectomy
- Bronchography and sinogram: Used as *confirmatory tests*
- Bronchoscopic exploration for evaluation of stump
- Inhalation of radionuclide:
  - Mixture of radiolabelled xenon and O_2-N_2O is inhaled
  - Radionuclide accumulates in pleural space in the presence of BPF
- Methylene blue injection into pleural space and recovering it in sputum

Surgical Management of BPF

❖ Usually done via VATS approach

❖ Steps of surgical repair include:
- Revision of the stump with debridement of necrotic tissue
- Suture reclosure of bronchial stump with vascularized flap tissue such as:
  - Omentum
  - Muscle tissue

Conservative Management of BPF

❖ Small bronchopleural fistulas can be conservatively managed by:
- Adequate ventilation
- Appropriate antibiotic therapy

❖ Ventilatory strategies:
- One lung ventilation:
  - Bronchus of normal lung intubated and ventilated
  - This allows BPF to rest and heal with help of antibiotics
  - However, this may lead to an intolerable intrapulmonary shunt
  - PEEP may be needed to maintain PO_2
- Differential lung ventilation:
  - Each lung is managed with different types of ventilation
  - Done through DLT and two synchronized ventilators
  - Healthy lung is ventilated with normal ventilator
  - Affected lung is exposed to smaller tidal volume or HFJV
  - CPAP with oxygen at pressures below the *critical opening pressure* of the BPF can be used
  - Critical opening pressure is determined by assessing lowest level of CPAP which must be applied to the bronchus on affected side to produce continuous bubbling through the underwater seal
- High frequency jet ventilation:
  - Used for larger BPF or multiple BPFs
  - This causes minimal gas loss through fistula as V_T is low
  - Thus, BPF may heal more quickly
  - Also, hemodynamic effects are usually minimal
- Unidirectional chest tube valve:
  - Usually, inspiratory cycle of ventilator triggers closure of chest tube valve
  - Valve again opens during expiration
  - This reduces gas flows across BPF during positive pressure ventilation
  - Flow across fistula is reduced by increasing pleural pressure during positive pressure breaths
  - This reduces the pressure gradient across the BPF
- Other strategies for BPFs not amenable to surgical repair:
  - Large fistulas (> 8 mm):
    - Airway stents (silicone/covered metallic stents)
    - Angiographic coils
    - Amplatzer devices
  - Small fistulas (< 8 mm):
    - Occlusive materials:
- Albumin-glutaraldehyde tissue adhesive
- Fibrin glue
    - Sclerosants:
- Ethanol
- Tetracycline
    - Ablative therapy with Nd:YAG laser
    - Endobronchial valves

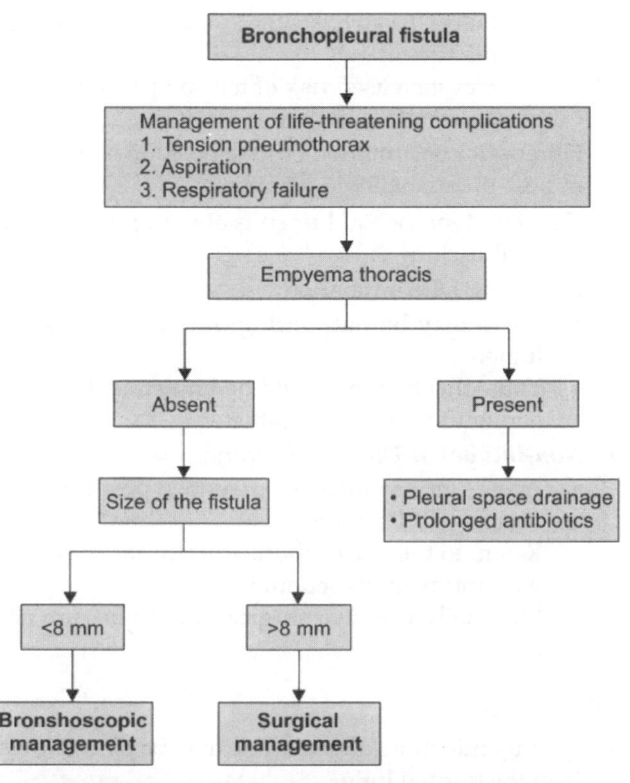

Anesthetic Considerations

- Air leak:
  - Effective ventilation is difficult in these patients
  - This is due to large air leak through the BPF
  - Tidal volume is preferentially delivered into the pleural space
  - This leak occurs through the low resistance BPF
- Risk of positive pressure ventilation (PPV):
  - PPV may increase air leak across the BPF
  - This can cause tension pneumothorax and delayed healing of fistula
- Difficulty in ventilation:
  - This occurs due to difference in compliance between the 2 lungs
  - This can cause reduced alveolar ventilation and intrapulmonary shunting
  - This in turn causes carbon dioxide retention and increased acidosis
- Lung isolation:
  - Essential to ensure lung isolation prior to initiation of PPV
  - This prevents contamination of healthy lung in the presence of empyema

Preoperative Preparation

Drainage of Empyema

- Empyema if present, should be drained before surgery to close the BPF
- This is to avoid risk of tension pneumothorax during positive pressure ventilation
- Drainage is done with person sitting up and leaning towards affected side
- A drain to underwater seal system is left behind in the pleural cavity prior to induction
- Chest X-ray should be taken to determine the efficacy of the procedure

Estimation of Size of BPF

- Important as it determines the amount of air leak through the BPF
- This can be done in two ways:
  - Amount of ICD drain after pneumonectomy:
    - Continuous drainage/ bubbling implies that BPF is large
    - Intermittent drainage/bubbling implies small size of BPF
  - Loss of tidal volume (TV):
    - Difference between inspired and expired TV estimates size of BPF
    - Small difference between inspired and expired TV implies small sized BPF
    - This is measured by connecting spirometer to:
      - A tightly fitting face mask in non-intubated patients
      - ETT in intubated patients

Premedication

- NPO orders
- Informed consent
- Premedication is not required in case of emergency surgery
- IV midazolam 1-2 mg can be used
- Glycopyrrolate 10 µg/kg IV as antisialogogue
- Anti-aspiration prophylaxis if awake intubation is planned
- Ensure a patent, functioning ICD prior to induction
- Thoracic epidural may be placed prior to induction of anesthesia

Monitors

- Pulse oximetry, capnography, ECG
- Blood pressure: IBP preferred
- CVP, urine output
- Temperature

Induction and Intubation

- 100% oxygen with face mask of appropriate size
- Sitting up position preferred pre-induction to prevent spill over of infected secretions
- Priority is to isolate the affected side in terms of contamination and ventilation

- ❖ Endobronchial tube is placed and position confirmed before initiation of PPV
- ❖ Care of ICD:
  - Chest tube patency is reconfirmed
  - Chest tube has to be left unclamped during induction to:
    - Avoid any bouts of coughing
    - Prevent build-up of a tension pneumothorax in case a preexisting valve mechanism exists
  - During induction, suction of ICD is avoided to prevent loss of tidal volume
- ❖ Choice of ETT:
  - Single lumen ET tube:
    - Can be used for small sized BPF
    - Positioned proximal to expected location of the BPF
    - Bronchial blocker can be used to ensure lung isolation thereafter
  - Double lumen tube:
    - Used for larger sized BPF
    - Best choice for delivering PPV
    - Advantages of DLT:
      - Allows adequate ventilation of normal lung
      - Prevents air leak through BPF
      - Avoids contamination of normal lung during lateral positioning
    - Largest possible tube selected so that it provides a close fit in trachea
- ❖ Intubation techniques:
  - Awake intubation of an anesthetized airway:
    - Done with the help of fibreoptic bronchoscopy and double lumen tube
    - Is the *safest and most ideal* technique
    - Neuroleptanalgesia with topical airway anesthesia may be required
    - Not always feasible as it requires:
      - A very cooperative patient
      - Excellent topical anesthesia
  - Intubation under deep anesthetic plane:
    - Intubation carried out with the patient breathing spontaneously
    - Done using IV propofol 2 mg/kg or thiopentone 5 mg/kg
    - Spontaneous ventilation is maintained until lung isolation is secured
    - Avoids the risk of air leak during positive pressure ventilation
    - Usually not well tolerated in older patients with comorbidities
  - Rapid sequence induction:
    - Done with IV ketamine/thiopentone and succinylcholine
    - Direct bronchoscopy is used to guide DLT placement
    - Has increased risk of tension pneumothorax and contamination
- ❖ Fibreoptic confirmation of tube position is preferred in post-pneumonectomy patients
- ❖ Tip of endobronchial lumen is always positioned in the healthy lung
- ❖ Following DLT intubation:
  - There may be outpouring of pus from tracheal lumen
  - Thus, this lumen should be immediately suctioned with a large bore catheter
- ❖ ***Non-intubated Thoracic Surgery***:
  - Avoids airway instrumentation in post-pneumonectomy BPF patients
  - Refers to the use of thoracic epidural anesthesia with intravenous sedation
  - Minimally invasive surgical techniques are preferred

Positioning

- ❖ During induction, affected side may be placed lower than the normal lung
- ❖ This is achieved by tilting the table towards the affected side
- ❖ This allows gravitational drainage of pus/infected material in the pleural cavity
- ❖ This minimizes the risk of contamination of healthy lung during lateral positioning
- ❖ Lateral decubitus position is used during surgery
- ❖ Water-tight seal of the DLT or BB is confirmed prior to lateral positioning
- ❖ Deflation of bronchial cuff prior to lateral positioning is avoided
- ❖ Lung with BPF is placed in non-dependent position (on the upper side)

Maintenance

- ❖ Nitrous oxide is avoided
- ❖ *TIVA is the preferred technique*
- ❖ This is because delivery of volatile agents may be unreliable in the presence of BPF
- ❖ Oxygen + air + isoflurane/sevoflurane may be used to ensure balanced anesthesia
- ❖ Fentanyl + vecuronium are given in intermittent boluses

Ventilation

- ❖ Lung protective OLV with DLT is useful
- ❖ Pressure control or volume control modes may be used

- Tidal volume 5-6 mL/kg is ideal
- Increased I-time
- Limit peak airway pressure to < 35 cm H_2O
- Limit plateau airway pressure to < 25 cm H_2O
- Minimal PEEP 5 cm H_2O
- Target normal $PaCO_2$
- Avoid hyperoxia: Target SpO_2 between 94-98%

Approaches to Positive Pressure Ventilation

Technique	Advantages	Disadvantages
SLT, conventional ventilation	Simple to perform	Effective only with small BPF
		Difficult to maintain low airway pressure
SLT intubation of healthy lung	Simple to perform	Difficult in severe pulmonary disease
	Protects against contamination	
Differential lung ventilation	Protects against contamination	Difficult to perform
	Allows optimal mode for each lung	
	Can be combined with HFO/ BB	
Bronchial blockers	Allows highly selective isolation	Requires skilful placement
	Maximizes volume of ventilated lung	May be dislodged during surgery
	Can be combined with HFO	
HFO ventilation	May be combined with other techniques	Requires special equipment
	Airway pressures are minimized	
	Minimizes expiratory gas trapping	
	Can be used for prolonged ventilation	
HF jet ventilation	May be combined with other techniques	Requires special equipment
		Control of TV difficult
		Warming and humidification difficult
		Associated with gas trapping

Management of Massive Air Leak

- Prior to airway isolation:
  - Railroading of DLT:
    - Patient in intubated with a smaller diameter ETT
    - Fibreoptic bronchoscope is guided into the intact mainstem bronchus
    - DLT is then railroaded into the bronchus to isolate the healthy lung
  - Rigid bronchoscopy:
    - Rigid bronchoscope is passed into the intact mainstem bronchus
    - COOKs airway exchange catheter is passed into the healthy bronchus
    - Rigid bronchoscope is then removed
    - Single lumen tube is railroaded into the healthy mainstem bronchus
  - Arndt endobronchial blocker:
    - This may be passed into the BPF via rigid bronchoscopy
    - This may control the air leak temporarily
    - Alternatively, a large Fogarty embolectomy catheter can be used
- After chest is opened:
  - Ventilation can be improved by lung packing
  - Manual control of air leak restores delivered tidal volumes

Extubation

- Early extubation is preferred
- This is to avoid barotrauma to the surgical stump from positive pressure ventilation
- Extubated fully awake, warm and fully reversed

Postoperative Management

- Double lumen tube is changed to SLT if postoperative ventilation is planned
- Shifted to ICU in sitting position once spontaneous ventilation is adequate
- Respiratory failure is common postoperatively in these patients

PLEURECTOMY AND DECORTICATION

Introduction

- Pleurectomy refers to the procedure where parietal pleura is stripped over all but diaphragmatic and mediastinal surface of lung
- Decortication refers to removal of restrictive layer of fibrous tissue overlying the lung, chest wall and diaphragm, thereby allowing the lung to expand

Indications

- Decortication:
  - Symptomatic fibrothorax with:
    - Severe lung symptoms
    - Presence of thick, fibrous pleural peel for > 4-6 weeks
    - Radiological evidence of trapped lung with restricted lung expansion

- Failure of other interventions in clearance of hemothorax or empyema
- Refractory tuberculous empyema

❖ Pleurectomy:
- Malignant pleural mesothelioma (most commonly)
- Less common indications include:
  - Primary pneumothorax
  - Pneumothorax secondary to COPD
  - Traumatic pneumothorax
  - Malignant pleural effusions

Contraindications

❖ There are no absolute contraindications to decortication/ pleurectomy

❖ Relative contraindications:
- Conditions with questionable surgical benefit:
  - Severe lung disease where decortication will not ensure lung expansion
  - Presence of active pleural space infections
  - Large airway stenosis/obstruction
- Uncontrolled pulmonary infections
- Contralateral lung disease
- Chronically debilitated patients
- Coagulopathy
- Chest wall infections
- Terminal disease

Procedure

❖ Open approach:
- Patient is placed in the lateral decubitus position
- Chest cavity is breached at the 5th or 6th intercostal space
- Axillary thoracotomy may be used for apical disease
- In most chronic cases, the parietal and visceral pleura are fused
- In these patients pleurectomy is preferred to decortication
- In other patients, plane of dissection is created carefully between the 2 pleura
- Fibrin peel is removed in a piecemeal fashion from parietal and visceral pleura
- Care should be taken not to injure the lung parenchyma and cause air leaks
- Following complete removal of the peel, lungs are checked for:
  - Complete re-expansion
  - Air leaks
- Two chest tubes are inserted along:
  - Base of the diaphragm
  - Apex of the lung
- The chest is then irrigated and all blood suctioned out before closure

❖ Thoracoscopic approach:
- Associated with lesser pain, better outcomes and quicker recovery
- Currently regarded as the gold standard for treatment of early empyema
- Early in the disease process the fibrin peel is thin and easily removable
- Once the disease process becomes chronic, the fibrous peel becomes thick
- Thus, thoracoscopic removal of the peel becomes difficult
- Procedure differs from the open technique only in the instruments used
- 3-4 ports are used during the procedure to ensure adequate surgical access
- Fibrin peel is removed in a piecemeal fashion from parietal and visceral pleura
- Following removal of the peel and suctioning of pus, the cavity is irrigated
- Two chest tubes are inserted at the port sites
- The skin is closed following removal of the scope

Anesthetic Considerations

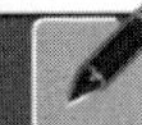

❖ Preoperative considerations:
- High incidence of preoperatively compromised respiratory function due to:
  - Associated infective lung diseases such as lung abscess/ bronchiectasis
  - Prior lung resections
- Thus, preoperative optimization of the patient is important:
  - Smoking cessation
  - Pulmonary rehabilitation
  - Treatment of associated lung infections

❖ Intraoperative considerations:
- Lateral decubitus position
- Perfect lung *isolation* to prevent soiling of healthy lung during OLV
- Thoracic epidural analgesia
- Restrictive fluid strategy
- Lung protective ventilation
- Avoidance of hypothermia
- Possibility of intraoperative modification of surgical technique such as:
  - Pleurodesis
  - Lobectomy (if severe lung parenchymal damage)

❖ Postoperative considerations:
- Failure of lung expansion at the end of surgery causing difficult ventilation
- Life threatening complications post operatively:
  - Sepsis
  - Bronchopleural fistula

Anesthetic Technique

- GA with DLT and OLV is the preferred technique to provide:
  - Lung isolation in case of associated infective lung diseases
  - Lung separation for VATS procedures
  - To ensure OLV in case of emergency conversion to lobectomy
- Single lumen tubes may be considered in:
  - Pediatric patients
  - Pleural drainage procedures with limited resection

Preoperative Assessment

- Similar to pre-thoracotomy evaluation
- Preoperative risk assessment for decortication should focus on:
  - Patients exercise capacity and physiological reserve
  - Risk of postoperative complications and dyspnea
  - Risk of perioperative myocardial events
- Risk of postoperative dyspnea:
  - Evaluation for postoperative dyspnea entails evaluation of:
    - Respiratory mechanics
    - Parenchymal function
  - Thus, most important determinants of postoperative dyspnea include:
    - $ppoFEV_1$
    - ppoDLCO
  - Other causes of postoperative dyspnea are:
    - Failure of lung expansion following decortication
    - Presence of large persistent air leaks due to parenchymal injury
    - Recurrent empyema
  - Thus, evaluation should include assessment of risk for these conditions:
    - Extent of fibrothorax and amount of fibrin peel to be removed
    - Associated pulmonary diseases
    - Discussion with surgeon regarding risk of parenchymal injury
- Perioperative myocardial events:
  - Cardiologist opinion is sought in all patients with an active cardiac condition:
    - Unstable angina
    - Heart failure
    - Significant arrhythmias
    - Severe valvular heart disease
  - Revised Cardiac Risk Index may be used to assess risk for cardiac morbidity
  - Thoracic RCRI may be used as an alternative
  - However, predictive risk of both these scores has been found to be suboptimal
- Also, in the presence of a pneumothorax:
  - Estimate the size of existing pneumothorax
  - Confirm the presence of a functioning ICD

Premedications

- NPO orders
- Informed consent
- Large bore IV access is secured in case of requirement for blood transfusion
- 2 units of red blood cells should be kept cross matched and ready
- IV midazolam 0.03 -0.15 mg can be given for anxiolysis
- Appropriate preoperative surgical antibiotic prophylaxis as per hospital protocol
- Most patients are debilitated, septic and already on antibiotic therapy
- Preoperative antibiotic therapy has to be continued in the perioperative period
- ICD placement:
  - ICD should be placed 12 hours prior to surgery in the presence of:
    - Large pleural effusion > 2/3rd of hemithorax
    - More than 200 mL pleural collection
  - Slow drainage of the pleural fluid is recommended
  - This is to avoid rapid reinflation of the collapsed lung
  - This in turn can precipitate ipsilateral ***reexpansion pulmonary edema***
- All cardiovascular and respiratory drugs are to be continued
- Thoracic epidural may be inserted for perioperative analgesia

Monitor

- SpO_2, E_TCO_2
- NIBP, ECG
- Temperature, urine output for procedures expected to last more than 2 hours
- Tidal volume, airway pressure
- IBP/CVP is usually recommended except for minor procedures with limited resection

Induction

- GA with OLV and DLT is technique of choice
- Prolonged preoxygenation is required as rapid desaturation may occur

- IV induction is done with *thiopentone or propofol*
- Induction agents are given slowly as profound hypotension can occur at this time
- DLT can be used to ensure lung isolation
- DLT is inserted following NMB with fibreoptic bronchoscopic (FOB) guidance

Position

- Patient is placed in the left or right lateral decubitus position with a table break
- Axillary roll is essential and a sandbag may be used for support
- Fastidious checking is required of:
  - Eye protection
  - Pressure points
  - Neck position
- DVT prophylaxis may be provided using graduated compression stockings

Maintenance

- Balanced anesthesia and TIVA are alternatives for maintenance of anesthesia
- TIVA is preferred for patients receiving OLV
- This is because volatile anesthetics inhibit HPV
- Balanced anesthesia can be used for small procedures with SLT
- This is achieved with:
  - 0.5- 1 MAC isoflurane
  - Opioid boluses
  - Judicious boluses of intermediate acting NMBAs
- Halothane and N_2O are avoided

Ventilation

- OLV is rarely required for decortication
- This is because lung on affected side is already compressed from fibrothorax
- Collapse of ipsilateral lung may be necessary in severe cases to aid surgical exposure
- Lung protective OLV with DLT is useful:
  - Tidal volume 5-6 mL/kg is ideal
  - Limit peak airway pressure to < 35 cm H_2O
  - Limit plateau airway pressure to < 25 cm H_2O
  - PEEP 5 cm H_2O
  - Target normal $PaCO_2$
  - Avoid hyperoxia: Target SpO_2 between 94-98%
- *Leak-test* can be performed at the end of the procedure:
  - Clamp on the DLT to the operated side is released
  - Airway pressure is slowly increased to 25-40 cm H_2O
  - Integrity of the lung parenchyma is tested by:
    - Visible air-leaks
    - Loss of tidal volume
- At the end of surgery:
  - Observing the pleural surface confirms if superficial lung tissue is reinflated
  - Lung can be fully expanded at using CPAP therapy
  - This helps to oppose parietal and visceral pleura
  - DLT may be replaced with SLT prior to extubation

Hemodynamics

- Precipitous hypotension can occur on induction
- Restrictive fluid administration is important:
  - Reduces risk of postoperative Acute Lung Injury (ALI)
  - Administration of < 3 L in first 24 hrs is associated with reduced risk of ALI
  - Vasopressors are used instead of fluids to maintain hemodynamic instability
  - Supplementation for third space loss has to be avoided
- Surgical manipulation can cause cardiac compression and hypotension
- Blood loss:
  - Usually blood loss varies between 500–2000 mL
  - Significant blood loss possible if pleura is extensively diseased
  - Thus, blood transfusion may be required intra-operatively
- Circulatory collapse is possible when the patient is turned *effusion side up*
- This occurs due to mediastinal shift which in turn reduces the venous return
- Patient is turned supine to drain the pleural effusion if this occurs
- Normothermia is maintained with:
  - Forced air warmer
  - Fluid warmer

Extubation

- Patient can be extubated at the end of procedure when fully awake and reversed
- Postoperative ventilation may be required if:
  - Bilateral pleurectomy
  - Generalized lung disease
  - Large intraoperative fluid shifts

Postoperative Care

Management

- Usually require 12-24 hours of ICU care
- Patient is nursed in the sitting up position

- Humidified oxygen via face mask
- Fluid therapy is minimized in the postoperative period
- Early resumption of oral feeds accelerates recovery
- Pleural space is continuously drained with ICD
- Suction on ICD aids lung expansion
- Postoperative chest X-ray is taken to confirm full lung expansion
- Postoperative *lung volume replacement therapy* is essential:
  - Deep breathing
  - Incentive spirometry
  - Intermittent CPAP

Analgesia

- Decortication/pleurectomy is a very painful surgery, especially if done bilaterally
- Multimodal analgesia:
  - Thoracic epidural
  - Paravertebral/intercostal/intrapleural blocks
  - Opioids: Systemic/neuraxial/PCA
  - NSAIDs

Complications

- Pneumothorax
- Atelectasis
- Empyema
- Trauma to vital structures

POSTOPERATIVE ANALGESIA FOR THORACIC SURGERY

Introduction

- No single technique is preferred and sufficient
- Multimodal analgesia is used

Aims

- To reduce distress of patient
- To make early mobilization possible
- To improve lung function
- Reduce postoperative complications
- Reduce mortality and morbidity
- Reduce length of hospital stay

Causes of Pain

Acute Pain

- Incision pain: Caused by intercostal nerve (T_4-T_6)
- Chest drain: Pain caused by intercostal nerves (T_7- T_8)
- Diaphragm pleural pain caused by phrenic nerve (C_3- C_5)
- Mediastinal pleural pain caused by vagus nerve (CN X)
- Shoulder joint pain caused by brachial plexus (C_5- C_7)

Chronic Pain

- Chronic incisional pain
- Chronic post-thoracotomy neuralgia

Ipsilateral Shoulder Pain

- Position during surgery
- Exacerbation of chronic arthralgia due to position
- ICD in lung apex causing irritation of parietal pleura
- Referred pain from diaphragmatic irritation
- Transection of major bronchus
- Posterior end of posterolateral thoracotomy incision is not blocked by thoracic epidural. This can be described as shoulder pain.

Analgesic Alternatives

Regional Blocks

- Intercostal nerve block
- Extrapleural nerve block
- Intrapleural nerve block
- Paravertebral block
- Thoracic epidural

Opioids

- Parentral
- Intrathecal
- Epidural
- Patient controlled analgesia

Others

- Cryoanalgesia
- Ketamine
- Dexmedetomidine
- NSAIDs
- TENS

Regional Blocks

Intercostal Nerve Block

- Useful for incisional pain
- Block given at lower border of rib at lateral edge of sacrospinalis muscle
- Total bupivacaine dose per session to be less than 1 mg/kg
- Simple to perform
- Short duration of action of bupivacaine necessitates indwelling catheter

- Indwelling catheters are difficult to position percutaneously
- Does not act on diaphragmatic/mediastinal pleura

Extrapleural Block

- Indwelling catheter is placed in pocket of retracted pleura
- Tip of catheter lies at the costo-vertebral joint
- Good analgesia
- LA may spread to paravertebral space

Intrapleural Block

- Catheter placed between parietal and visceral pleura
- Causes widespread intercostal nerve block
- Does not spread to paravertebral space
- Unpredictable action as local anesthetic may be drained through ICD
- Causes rapid systemic absorption of local anesthetic

Paravertebral Block

- Good analgesia of anterior and posterior primary ramii
- Allows local anesthetic spread to multiple levels from the insertion site
- Indwelling catheter is difficult to place and frequent dislodgement of catheter possible
- Causes fewer side effects than thoracic epidural

Thoracic Epidural

- Given at T_3–T_8 level with bupivacaine + fentanyl/hydromorphone infusion
- *Gold standard* of analgesia for thoracic surgeries
- Provides for excellent analgesia with raised FRC
- Causes extensive sympathetic block and motor weakness
- Respiratory depression and hypotension may occur if bolus injections used
- Foleys catheter mandatory to differentiate urinary retention from oliguria

Opioids

- Generally poor analgesia even with PCA, as MEAC produces sedation and hypoventilation
- Can be used as adjuvant to reduce local anesthetic dose

Others

Cryoanalgesia

- Implies the application of extreme cold –60°C to intercostal nerve
- Produces disruption of nerve impulse transmission for upto 6 months
- Associated with:
  - ***Chronic post-thoracotomy pain syndrome***
  - Higher failure rates

NSAIDs

- Inadequate when used alone
- Synergistic action with regional anesthesia and opioids
- Reduces opioid consumption by 30%
- Good for shoulder pain
- Paracetamol upto 4g/day PO or PR
- COX-II inhibitors are better

Ketamine

- Low dose ketamine effective at doses of 1mg/kg IM
- Continuous low dose infusion can be given for refractory pain

Dexmedetomidine

- Reduces opioid consumption
- 0.3-0.4 *μg/kg/hr* IV infusion

Transcutaneous Electrical Nerve Stimulation (TENS)

- Useful for mild to moderate pain
- Insufficient pain relief if used alone

VIDEO ASSISTED THORACOSCOPIC SURGERY

Introduction

- VATS is a minimally invasive (key-hole) surgical procedure
- Involves creation of an intentional pneumothorax
- This is followed by introduction of the thoracoscope through chest wall
- This allows direct vision into thoracic cavity without a big incision
- Thoracoscope was first used as early as 1910 for the treatment of tuberculosis
- Procedure regained popularity in the 1990s with advances in technology

Indications

- General intrathoracic cavity:
  - Chest wall surgery: Nuss procedure for pectus excavatum
  - Laser application for treatment of tumours
  - Retrieval of foreign body

- Parenchymal disease:
  - Diagnostic:
    - Fibrosis
    - Pneumonitis
    - Solitary nodule
  - Therapeutic:
    - Wedge resection, segmentectomy, lobectomy
    - Resection of bleb/ bullae
    - Identification and closure of bronchopleural fistula (BPF)
    - Removal of bronchogenic cysts
    - Lung Volume Reduction Surgery (LVRS)
- Pleural disease:
  - Diagnostic:
    - Biopsy
    - Thoracocentesis
  - Therapeutic:
    - Adhesiolysis
    - Pleurodesis
    - Decortication
- Mediastinum:
  - Diagnostic:
    - Thymoma
    - Lymphoma
    - Germ cell tumors
    - Sarcoma
  - Therapeutic:
    - Removal of mediastinal cysts
    - Thymectomy
    - Resection of tumours
- Esophagus and diaphragm:
  - Repair of esophageal perforation
  - Esophagectomy
  - Vagotomy
  - Anti-reflux surgery
  - ***Hellers*** cardiomyotomy
  - CDH repair
- Cardiovascular:
  - Diagnostic:
    - Pericarditis
    - Tumors
    - Diagnosis of cardiac herniation post-pneumonectomy
  - Therapeutic:
    - Pericardiectomy
    - Pericardial window
    - MIDCAB
    - Minimally invasive valve procedures
    - PDA ligation
- Spine surgery:
  - Dorsal thoracic sympathectomy
  - Splanchnicolysis
  - Drainage of spinal abscess
  - Discectomy
  - Fusion and correction of spinal deformity
- Trauma:
  - Assessment of injury
  - Treatment of hemorrhage
  - Evacuation of clot
- Staging of lung, pleural and esophageal cancer

Contraindications

- Previous surgery or radiotherapy
- Extensive pleural disease
- Central/ endobronchial lesions
- Large tumors > 6 cm

Advantages of Vats

- Small and cosmetic incision
- Ribs are not spread resulting in:
  - Less postoperative pain
  - Reduced shoulder dysfunction
- Benefits to the respiratory system:
  - Reduced risk of respiratory dysfunction
  - Reduced risk of atelectasis produced by splinting
  - Reduction in respiratory secretions
  - Better PFTs compared with open thoracotomy
- Lower risk of complications:
  - Atrial fibrillation
  - Prolonged air leaks
  - Pneumonitis
- Lesser blood loss
- Better postoperative outcomes:
  - Earlier mobilization
  - Faster postoperative recovery
  - Lesser overall morbidity
  - Reduced duration of hospital stay
- Reduced OT time for some procedures
- Reduced hospital stay and costs

Procedure

- Surgery is done in the lateral decubitus position
- 3-5 entry ports are created in the chest wall on the side of the pathology
- Video camera is inserted through the entry port
- This is used to allow direct visualization of the entrance of trocar into thoracic cavity
- Ipsilateral lung is collapsed through lung isolation prior to trocar insertion

- Pneumothorax may be created occasionally to aid in:
  - Collapsing the lung
  - Breaking of adhesions
- The surgery is then completed by using the other ports for introducing instruments
- Uniportal VATS refers to the use of VATS through only 1 utility incision
- This may be accomplished through the transaxillary or subxiphoid regions.

Anesthetic Considerations

- CO_2 insufflation may be done during VATS causing:
  - Raised airway pressure
  - Increased E_TCO_2
  - Mediastinal shift with hypotension
  - Reduced SpO_2
- Lung *separation* using DLT and one lung ventilation
- Protective lung ventilation
- Restrictive fluid strategy intraoperatively
- Potential for massive, sudden hemorrhage
- Sudden mediastinal shift and hypotension possible
- Lateral position during surgery

Choice of Anesthetic Technique

- Local anesthesia:
  - Usually well tolerated for simple, brief diagnostic procedures
  - LA is infiltrated into lateral thoracic wall and parietal pleura
  - Topical local anesthetic is applied on visceral pleura
  - Mild sedation may be given to enhance patient cooperation
  - Stellate ganglion block can be given concomitantly

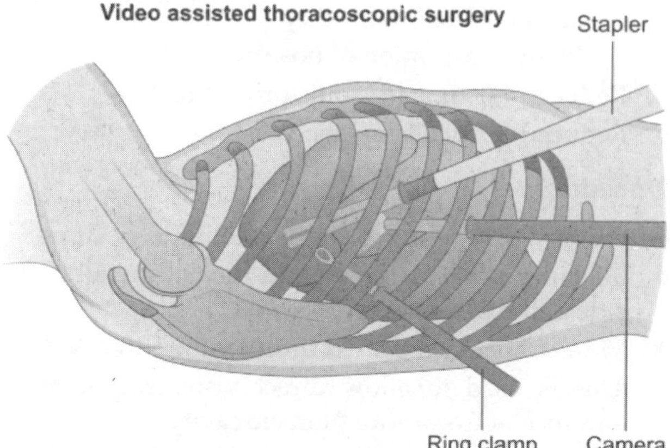

Fig. 57: Video-assisted thoracoscopic surgery.

  - This inhibits cough reflex from hilar manipulation
  - Partial collapse of the operated lung occurs when air enters pleural cavity
  - Insufflation of CO_2 to create pneumothorax should be avoided
  - High FiO_2 is given via facemask to overcome shunt due to loss of lung volume
  - Changes in PaO_2, $PaCO_2$ and cardiac rhythm are minimal under LA
- Regional anesthesia:
  - Usually well tolerated for simple, brief diagnostic procedures
  - Intercostal N block given at the level of incision and two spaces above and below
  - Other alternatives include:
    - Thoracic epidural
    - Paravertebral block
    - Intrapleural blocks
  - IV stellate ganglion block accompanies RA always to inhibit cough reflex
  - Supplemental oxygen and sedation is given as required
  - Better compared to local anesthesia as it provides postoperative analgesia
- GA with OLV:
  - *Technique of choice*
  - DLT/BB can be used to collapse lung
  - DLT is better as it allows selective ventilation of contralateral lung
  - DLT allows rapid collapse of lung
  - Thus, CO_2 insufflation may not be required to optimize surgical conditions
- GA with two lung ventilation:
  - Requires CO_2 insufflation
  - Useful in small children where lung isolation is not possible

Anesthetic Management

Preoperative Evaluation

- Same as for thoracotomy
- Also evaluate for congenital heart disease and airway compression
- 50% compression of trachea indicates increased perioperative risk

Preoperative Preparation

- Preparation for airway control:
  - Endotracheal tubes, double lumen tubes, bronchial blockers
  - Video laryngoscope

    - Flexible fibreoptic bronchoscope
    - Separate circuit for delivery of CPAP to non-ventilated lung
- Preparation of appropriate monitoring equipment
- Preparation of warming devices to prevent hypothermia
- Preparation for regional anesthetic technique as planned:
    - Thoracic epidural analgesia
    - Paravertebral analgesia

Preoperative Optimization and Premedication

- IV access:
    - At least one large bore IV access is required routinely
    - Two large bore cannulas are secured when there is high risk of blood loss:
        - Surgeries involving hilar dissection
        - Adhesions due to prior radiation therapy
        - Prior lung surgery
    - Antecubital veins are avoided as they may be distorted during positioning
- Intranasal (0.3 mg/kg) or IV midazolam (0.03-0.15 mg/kg) can be used for anxiolysis
- Adequate blood is kept ready as massive bleeding is possible intraoperatively
- Perioperative bronchodilator and steroid therapy are continued
- Antibiotic prophylaxis, chest physiotherapy given preoperatively

Monitors

- Pulse oximetry
- E_TCO_2:
    - Aids in detection of displacement of DLT intraoperatively
    - Large E_TCO_2-$PaCO_2$ gradients may occur during OLV
    - Thus, frequent ABG monitoring is required to detect hypercarbia
- NIBP, ECG
- Neuromuscular monitor
- Temperature, urine output in procedures expected to last more than 2 hours
- Airway pressure
- ***Differential capnography***
- Invasive blood pressure monitoring is indicated for:
    - Patients undergoing extensive pulmonary resection such as lobectomies
    - Patients with high risk of significant bleeding:
        - Hilar involvement
        - Extensive adhesions
- Radial artery of dependant arm may be used for:
    - Continuous monitoring of arterial BP
    - Intermittent sampling for ABGs
    - Respirophasic variations in waveform to guide goal directed fluid therapy
- Central venous catheter:
    - Usually not indicated in patients with normal cardiac function
    - Placed on the side of thoracoscopy when required
    - This is recommended to avoid inadvertent bilateral pneumothorax
    - Indications for CVC access:
        - Patients with difficult vascular access
        - Anticipated need for intraoperative vasopressor infusion
        - Vascular access in children

Induction

- IV or inhalational induction can be used
- Selection of agents and techniques is based on the coexisting disease
- Short acting agents are preferred to allow rapid emergence and recovery
- Intermediate acting NMBAs can be used depending on duration of surgery
- Fibreoptic bronchoscopy is performed after intubation to:
    - Verify DLT position
    - Remove secretions which may impair oxygenation during OLV
    - Identify endobronchial lesions which might change surgical plan
- Rigid bronchoscope may be used to stent distal airway obstructions

Position

- Supine/slight lateral (15-30°) position for anterior mediastinal surgeries
- 90° lateral position for hilar masses and lobectomy
- Nearly prone position for posterior mediastinal masses
- Lateral decubitus positioning:
    - Elbows are flexed to bring forearms parallel to face
    - Upper arm placed in gutter support
    - Adequate padding of extremities and pressure points to be ensured

Maintenance

- Balanced anesthesia or TIVA may be used to maintain anesthesia
- There is currently insufficient evidence to support either technique
- Balanced anesthesia with 0.5–1 MAC isoflurane/sevoflurane is most commonly used
- TIVA may be advantageous as volatile anesthetics inhibit HPV
- Halothane and N_2O are avoided
- Intermittent boluses of fentanyl may be used to provide analgesia
- Intermediate acting NMBAs are used to maintain neuromuscular paralysis

Ventilation

- OLV is initiated before introduction of the trocar
- Lung protective ventilation is preferred during both OLV and two lung ventilation
- Goals of OLV:
  - FiO_2 100%
  - Tidal volume 6–7 mL/kg
  - Respiratory rate 12–20 cycles/min
  - E_TCO_2 32–38 mm Hg
  - Peak airway pressure < 35 cm H_2O
- Following initiation of OLV PaO_2 continues to fall for 45 minutes
- Constant monitoring for increase in airway pressures is required
- This is due to dislodgement of DLT/bronchial blocker during surgical manipulation
- CPAP for upper lung is avoided as distended lung interferes with surgical exposure

Reasons for Inadequate Lung Collapse during OLV

- Displaced DLT/bronchial blocker
- Pleural adhesions/disease
- Fibrosis
- Chronic bronchitis causing gas trapping
- Emphysema
- Tumor causing narrowing of airways and gas trapping

Improving Lung Collapse during VATS

- Ensure complete denitrogenation prior to initiation of lung collapse:
  - Poorly soluble nitrogen in air delays collapse in non-ventilated alveoli
  - Thus, presence of air in non-ventilated lung at onset of OLV delays collapse
  - Ventilation with 100% FiO_2 for 3-5 minutes prior to initiation of OLV ensures denitrogenation
- Avoid entrainment of room air into non-ventilated lung during OLV:
  - This occurs when lumen of DLT to non-ventilated lung is open during OLV
  - Passive paradoxical ventilation of the non-ventilated lung will occur
  - This results in inspiration during the expiratory phase of the ventilated lung
  - The tidal volumes generated may reach up to 130 mL/breath
  - Thus, air is drawn into the non-ventilated lung and prevents collapse
- Application of suction to the nonventilated lung at the onset of OLV:
  - Low suction (–20 cm H_2O) improves rate of lung collapse at the start of OLV
  - This ensures better lung collapse during the procedure

Management of Desaturation during VATS

- Severe/acute desaturation: Resumption of two lung ventilation
- Gradual desaturation:
  - Ensure 100% FiO_2
  - Position of DLT/bronchial blocker is checked with fibreoptic bronchoscopy
  - Recruitment maneuver of the ventilated lung
  - Application of PEEP 5 cm H_2O to the ventilated lung
  - Optimization of cardiac output
  - Partial ventilation of the non-ventilated lung:
    - Segmental reinflation with fibreoptic bronchoscope
    - High frequency jet ventilation

Hemodynamics

- Ringers lactate or plasmalyte is *fluid of choice*
- Minimal blood loss occurs usually
- Restrictive fluid therapy strategy is preferred as excessive IV fluids can cause:
  - Increased intrapulmonary shunting
  - Pulmonary edema of dependant lung
  - Occurs especially if prolonged surgery
- Intraoperative crystalloid administration is restricted to < 6 mL/kg/hour
- Fluids are administered only for replacing intraoperative losses

- ❖ Replacement of third space fluid loss is avoided
- ❖ Hypothermia is prevented by using forced air warmers and fluid warmers

Extubation

- ❖ Functional ICD with under water seal is inserted prior to extubation
- ❖ Preextubation bronchoscopy is performed to:
  - Ensure patent bronchial passages
  - Remove residual blood and secretions
  - Examine newly created bronchial stump
- ❖ Bilateral air entry has to be checked at the time of extubation
- ❖ Patient is extubated in semi-Fowlers position when fully awake and reversed
- ❖ Avoid coughing/straining at extubation

Indications for Conversion to Open Thoracotomy

- ❖ Intraoperative complications (most commonly hemorrhage)
- ❖ Technical considerations:
  - Poor visualization
  - Inability to isolate the lung through OLV
  - Inability to tolerate OLV
- ❖ Oncological considerations:
  - Upstaging of tumors
  - Unexpected chest wall involvement
- ❖ Anatomical considerations:
  - Difficult anatomy
  - Poor interlobar fissure
  - Diffuse pleural adhesions
  - Central tumor location with the need for more complex reconstruction

Postoperative Care

Management

- ❖ Nursed in sitting up position
- ❖ Encourage early mobilization of patient
- ❖ Avoid high airway pressures, to prevent rupture, if postoperatively ventilated

Analgesia

- ❖ Pain is usually minimal after VATS
- ❖ LA infiltration at the incision site
- ❖ Intrapleural block, paravertebral, thoracic epidural
- ❖ NSAIDs
- ❖ Opioid sparing analgesic techniques are preferred to prevent respiratory depression

Complications

- ❖ Complications of thoracic surgery:
  - Subcutaneous emphysema, empyema, recurrent pneumothorax
  - Infection, pneumonia, empyema, abscess
  - Pulmonary edema
  - Persistent air-leaks
  - Arrhythmias: AF, SVT
  - ***Down lung syndrome***
  - ***Horners syndrome***
- ❖ Complications specific to thoracoscopy:
  - Hemorrhage:
    - Incidence ranges from 0.4-2%
    - May require emergent conversion to thoracotomy
  - Visceral damage:
    - Recurrent laryngeal nerve
    - Aorta or SVC
    - Trachea
    - Diaphragm
    - Liver
    - Spleen
  - Lung herniation through chest wall
  - Air embolism
  - Port site recurrence of pulmonary and esophageal tumors
  - Dissemination of metastasis to thoracostomy tube site
  - Chronic pain due to compression of intercostal nerves with thoracoscope

BRONCHOALVEOLAR LAVAGE

Introduction

- ❖ This is a minimally invasive procedure performed during flexible bronchoscopy
- ❖ It provides important information about immunological and inflammatory processes

Indications

- ❖ Symptomatic pulmonary alveolar proteinosis: BAL is *treatment of choice*
- ❖ Diagnostic indications:
  - Viral, bacterial and fungal pneumonias
  - Quantitative cultures for ventilator associated pneumonias
  - Infiltrates in an immunocompromised host
- ❖ Evaluation of:
  - Diffuse lung infiltrates
  - Interstitial lung disease

- Suspected pulmonary hemorrhage
- Suspected malignancies
- Can be used as an alternative therapy in: (questionable benefit)
  - Cystic fibrosis
  - Asthmatic bronchitis
  - Lipid pneumonitis
  - Radioactive dust inhalation
  - Silicosis
  - Alveolar microlithiasis

Contraindications

- There is no absolute contraindication for BAL
- Relative contraindications include:
  - Acute respiratory distress syndrome with hypoxemia: risk of desaturation
  - Bronchopleural fistulas: non-return of adequate fluid
  - Life threatening arrhythmias
  - Refractory hypoxemia

Techniques

- Bronchoalveolar lavage:
  - The fibreoptic bronchoscope is advanced into the lavage site bronchus
  - 100-240 mL fluid is instilled into the subsegmental bronchus
  - This is done in 20- 50 mL aliquots
  - The fluid is then recovered via gentle suction and specimen is sent for analysis
- Bronchial washings:
  - 10- 30 mL of saline is instilled into the selected pulmonary segment
  - Secretions are then aspirated directly from large airways and sent for analysis
- Protected specimen bronchial brushing:
  - Similar to BAL
  - Uses an endobronchial catheter wedged in the tracheobronchial tree
  - The brush is rubbed against areas of suspected infection
  - It is then removed from the procedure port of the bronchoscope
  - The brush is then aseptically cut into the sterile diluent and sent for analysis
- Whole lung lavage (WLL):
  - Used as a therapeutic modality for pulmonary alveolar proteinosis
  - 10-15 liters of fluid are instilled via the DLT under general anesthesia
  - This is then drained out in 500–100 mL aliquots

Procedure of Whole Lung Lavage

- Procedure is usually done in supine position
- First lung lavage is done on the lung with worse PaO_2 on OLV
- If both lungs are equally involved, left lung is lavaged first
- This is because gas exchange is better with a larger right lung
- Thus, patient may tolerate right lung lavage with a relatively less diseased left lung
- GA is induced and OLV is instituted to the non-lavage lung
- Irrigation system is connected to the non-ventilated tube of DLT
- First lung lavage:
  - 1 Litre NS (37°C) is introduced in non-lavage lung
  - Irrigating fluid is placed 30 cm above mid-axillary line
  - Collection container is placed 60 cm below patient
  - Small level suction can also be used (<20 cm H_2O)
  - Cycle is repeated till the collected effluents are clear
  - Usually 10-20 L of fluid is instilled and more than 90% is recovered
  - If cumulative dose of in-fluid exceeds out-fluid by more than 1000 mL:
    - Suspect hydrothorax
    - Immediate chest X-ray taken
  - Vibration and percussion are applied during the filling and drainage phase
  - Lavage lung is suctioned at the end of procedure
  - 10 mg furosemide IV is given to increase diuresis
- Recovery phase:
  - Protective bilateral lung ventilation is continued
  - Fluid balance is evaluated and diuretic therapy may be considered
  - IV furosemide 10 mg may be used to increase diuresis
  - Recovery phase usually lasts for 45 minutes to 1 hour
- Second lung lavage:
  - Patient is evaluated for feasibility for second lung lavage
  - Lavage is then continued similar to the first lung lavage
- Landing phase: Comprises of transition from OLV to DLV
- Emerging phase: From the time of onset of DLV to extubation

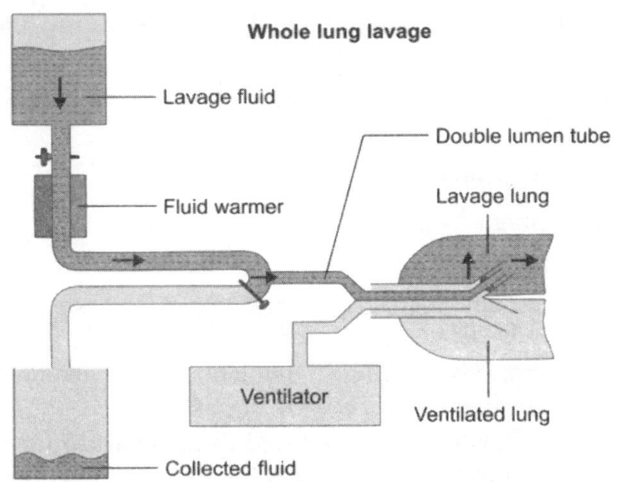

Fig. 58: Whole lung lavage.

- Observation phase: Patient is observed post extubation in the ICU.

Preoperative Investigations and Premedication

- Routine blood investigations
- Chest X-ray, CT scan, V-P scan to determine most impaired lung
- If recent lung biopsy has been done, ICD is placed as BPF maybe present
- Light premedication with benzodiazepines is usually sufficient

Monitors

- SpO_2, E_TCO_2
- NIBP, ECG
- Precordial stethoscope on ventilated lung to check fluid leak
- Tidal volume, pulmonary compliance
- Airway pressure-volume loop (spirometry):
  - Allows breath-to-breath monitoring of respiratory dynamics
  - Useful to detect any loss of lung isolation
  - Thus, it helps to prevent flooding of the ventilated lung
- IBP:
  - Recommended for invasive blood pressure monitoring
  - Also helps in repeated arterial blood gas analysis
- PAC *may be* used:
  - For continuous monitoring of mixed venous oxygen saturation
  - As a therapeutic aid to diverge blood away from the lavaged lung
- TEE *may be* used to assess RV function in the presence of pulmonary HTN
- Fluid which is moved in and out with each BAL cycle
- ABG: BAL is terminated if the (A-a)DO_2 increases

Induction

- Adequate preoxygenation required prior to induction
- IV induction with thiopentone/propofol/etomidate
- Atracurium used to ensure muscle relaxation
- Left sided DLT is placed with FOB confirmation of tube position
- Left DLT with carinal hook is used for WLL as it offers better DLT stability
- DLT is secured and maintain hand on DLT throughout procedure
- This is necessary to prevent tube dislodgement under pressure of saline during BAL
- Adequacy of cuff seal is checked at 50 cm H_2O for perfect lung separation

Position

- Procedure is usually conducted in the supine position
- Reverse Trendelenburg position is used during the filling phase
- After fluid instillation, chest percussion is done during the fluid dwell time
- Trendelenburg position is used during the drainage phase to aid recovery of fluid

Maintenance

- Volatile anesthetic agents are generally avoided
- TIVA is the preferred technique as:
  - Frequent need for airway access during the procedure for:
    - Suction
    - Bronchoscopy
  - This may lighten the anesthetic plane if VA is used
- If necessary 0.5–1 MAC isoflurane can be used
- Halothane and N_2O are contraindicated

Hemodynamics

- Minimal intravenous fluids are used
- This is because high volumes of fluid are absorbed from the alveolar space
- This results in a high trans-alveolar fluid flux
- IV furosemide may be used at the end of lavage to ensure optimal fluid balance
- Warming blankets are used to ensure normothermia as WLL usually lasts 5–6 hours

Prelavage Evaluation

- Conventional ventilation is continued for 5 minutes
- This is followed by ABG evaluation
- Right sided OLV is initiated for 5 minutes followed by an ABG analysis
- This is followed by left sided OLV for 5 minutes and ABG analysis
- This allows estimation of severity of individual lung involvement

Ventilation

- During lavage:
  - OLV with lung protective ventilation is used with:
    - Highest possible FiO_2
    - Usually, 100% FiO_2 is required during lavage
    - Tidal volume 6-8 mL/kg
    - PEEP 7-12 cm H_2O
  - Changes in oxygenation occurring during lavage:
    - Increases during filling phase
    - Decreases during drainage phase
  - This is because of transmission of hydrostatic pressure from lavage lung
  - This itself acts similar to HPV and improves oxygenation
  - If severely hypoxemic during OLV:
    - Nitric oxide administration to ventilated lung
    - Inflation of PAC balloon in PA of lavage lung
    - ECMO
- During resting phase:
  - Bilateral lung protective ventilation is used
  - Minimal tolerable FiO_2
  - Tidal volume 6-8 mL/kg
  - Minimal tolerable PEEP
  - Target $PaO_2 > 70$ mm Hg
- OLV with lung protective strategy is continued during subsequent lavages

Interlavage Evaluation

- The freshly lavaged lung is placed on OLV for 5 minutes followed by ABG
- If PaO_2 is above 70 mm Hg, second lung lavage is resumed
- If PaO_2 is below 70 mm Hg, techniques to improve oxygenation are considered:
  - Inhaled nitric oxide
  - Inflation of PA catheter

Landing Phase

- Fibreoptic bronchoscopic evaluation is performed at the end of lavage
- This is to rule out any undetected leaks during the procedure
- Post procedure, DLT is replaced by SLT for postoperative ventilation

Postoperative Care

Management

- Emerging phase:
  - Usually managed in the post-anesthesia care unit/ICU
  - Protective lung ventilation is required postoperatively, usually for 2-4 hours
  - FiO_2 is gradually reduced to minimal required, as tolerated by the patient
  - De-recruitment is possible during this phase requiring recruitment maneuvers
  - ABG and a check X-ray has to be taken during this phase
  - Patient is extubated at the end of this phase when fully awake and warm
- Observation phase:
  - Patient is observed in the ICU for 24 hours post procedure
  - ABG and chest X-ray is repeated prior to shifting out of ICU
  - Alveolar infiltrates if, present on chest X-ray, usually clear within 24 hours
  - Cough and lung volume expansion strategies should be followed post procedure
  - Non-invasive ventilatory support may be required

Monitors

- ECG, SpO_2, $ETCO_2$
- Repeated ABGs, chest X-ray

Complications

- Common complications:
  - Cough
  - Transient infiltrates which typically resolve in 24 hours
  - Transient decrease in PaO_2
  - Leakage
- Infrequent complications:
  - Transient fever
  - Chills
  - Myalgia
- Serious complications:
  - De-recruitment and hypoxemia
  - Pneumothorax

MEDIASTINAL ANATOMY

Anatomy

- Parts of mediastinum:
  - Superior mediastinum
  - Inferior mediastinum:
    - Anterior mediastinum
    - Posterior mediastinum
    - Middle mediastinum
- Boundaries:
  - Trans-thoracic plane:
    - Extends from sternal angle to lower border of T_4 at upper level of pericardium
    - Divides into superior and inferior mediastinum
  - Inferior mediastinum is divided into anterior, middle and posterior mediastinum by heart and pericardial sac

Contents

- Anterior mediastinum:
  - Extends between anterior pericardial reflection and sternum
  - Contains:
    - Thymus
    - Aortic arch
    - Superior vena cava
    - Areolar tissue
    - Lymph nodes
- Middle mediastinum contains:
  - Heart and pericardium
  - Tracheal bifurcation
  - Main bronchi
  - Hila of lung
  - Phrenic nerve
  - Lymphatics
  - Lymph nodes

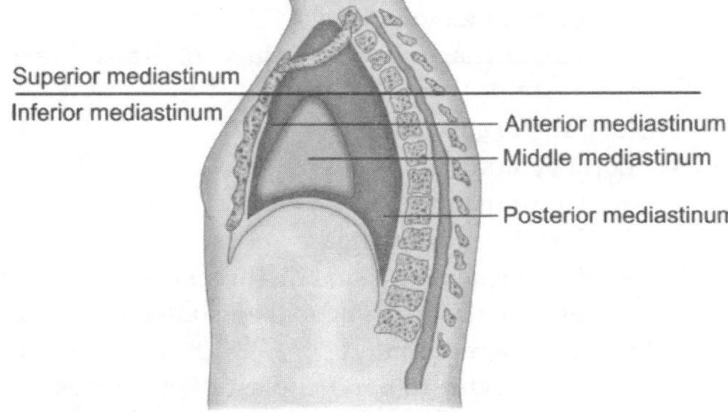

Fig. 59: Parts of the mediastinum.

- Posterior mediastinum:
  - Extends between posterior pericardial reflection and vertebral column
  - Contains:
    - Esophagus, thoracic duct
    - Descending aorta
    - Azygous and hemiazygous vein
    - Vagus nerve
    - Sympathetic chain
    - Paravertebral lymph nodes

Mediastinal Masses

- Superior mediastinum:
  - Retrosternal thyroid
  - Thymoma
- Anterior mediastinum:
  - Benign lesions:
    - Thymic tumors:
      - Thymoma
      - Thymic cyst
      - Thymic hyperplasia
    - Intrathoracic thyroid:
      - Substernal goitre
      - Ectopic thyroid tissue
    - Parathyroid adenoma
    - Teratomas/dermoid cyst
    - Others:
      - Hemangioma
      - Lipoma
      - Fibroma
  - Malignant lesions:
    - Thymic carcinoma
    - Thyroid carcinoma
    - Germ cell tumors:
      - Seminomas
      - Mixed germ cell tumors
    - Non-seminoma tumors:
      - Yolk sac tumor
      - Embryonal carcinoma
    - Others:
      - Choriocarcinoma
      - Liposarcoma
      - Fibrosarcoma
- Middle mediastinum:
  - Benign lesions:
    - Benign adenopathy
    - Cysts:
      - Bronchogenic cyst
      - Pericardial cyst
      - Enteric cyst
    - Hiatus hernia
    - Vascular masses and enlargement

- Malignant lesions:
  - Lymphoma
  - Esophageal cancer
  - Metastatic lung cancer
- ❖ Posterior mediastinum:
  - Benign lesions:
    - Neurogenic lesions:
      - Neurofibroma
      - Neurilemmoma
      - Chemodectoma
      - Meningoceles
      - Pheochromocytomas
    - Foramen of Bochdalek hernia
    - Thoracic spine disease: Potts spine
  - Malignant lesions:
    - Neurogenic tumors:
      - Neurosarcoma
      - Ganglioneuroblastoma
      - Neuroblastoma
    - Esophageal carcinoma

ANESTHESIA FOR MEDIASTINAL MASS

Introduction

- ❖ Mediastinal masses present the anesthesiologist with unique challenges
- ❖ Key to successful perioperative management of these patients is:
  - Knowledge of:
    - Mass anatomy
    - Its relationship with surrounding structures:
      - Tracheobronchial tree
      - Heart
      - Major blood vessels
    - Pathophysiology of the mass
  - Careful preoperative assessment
  - Discussion and perioperative planning with the surgeon
  - Preparation to manage cardiorespiratory complications

Pathophysiology

- ❖ Mediastinum is in close proximity to the airway and other cardiovascular structures
- ❖ Thus under GA, extrinsic compression of these structures by the mass may result
- ❖ Most complications arise due to masses in the anterior mediastinum
- ❖ However, middle and posterior mediastinal masses can also cause complications
- ❖ Reasons for increased complications under general anesthesia include:
  - Reduction in lung volume by 500-1000 mL under GA
  - Relaxation of bronchial smooth muscle leading to greater compressibility
  - Loss of spontaneous diaphragmatic movement with paralysis:
    - This reduces the normal transpleural pressure
    - Thus, forces which keep the airways dilated are obtunded
    - This in turn causes airway collapse
  - Extrinsic airway compression by the mediastinal mass
- ❖ Complications are more commonly seen during:
  - Changing patient posture from upright to supine
  - Transitioning from awake to anesthetized state
  - Moving from spontaneous ventilation to positive pressure ventilation
  - Changing muscle tone from unparalysed to paralyzed state

Preanesthetic Evaluation

- ❖ Goals of anesthetic assessment:
  - Assess risk of airway compromise/hemodynamic instability due to:
    - Mass effect on airway and lungs
    - Mass effect on major cardiovascular structures and circulation
  - Assess risk for complications due to loss of compensatory mechanisms:
    - Shifting mass effects with positional changes
    - Loss of airway patency due to relaxation of airway muscles
    - Increased intrathoracic pressure due to NM paralysis and IPPV
  - Assess risk for complications due to surgical manipulation and resection:
    - Compression of airway structures and great vessels
    - Loss of airway continuity or patency due to unplanned injuries
    - Hemorrhage due to injury of heart/great vessels
- ❖ History and examination:
  - Local symptoms:
    - Chest pain
    - Dyspnea, dysphagia
    - Headache and visual disturbances
    - Syncopal/near syncopal episodes
  - Systemic symptoms:
    - Mainly due to paraneoplastic syndromes
    - Eaton-Lambert syndrome has important anesthetic considerations

- Assess for:
  - Degree of severity of symptoms
  - Exacerbating factors: change in position
  - Actions which alleviate symptoms
- Examination:
  - Look for features of SVC syndrome such as:
    - Facial/upper extremity edema
    - Hoarseness of voice due to vocal cord edema
  - Hypotension suggests cardiac compression/tamponade

❖ Investigations:
- Imaging studies:
  - Include:
    - Chest X-ray
    - CT scan
    - MRI (rarely indicated)
  - Useful for providing anatomical details of the lesion
  - Performed on awake patient
  - Thus, they do not predict changes possible with anesthetic induction
- Pulmonary function tests:
  - Not routinely performed for mediastinal masses
  - Spirometry and flow volume loops may be used
  - However, these correlate poorly with airway obstruction
  - Thus, PFTs have minimal utility for patient management
- Transthoracic and transesophageal echocardiography:
  - Can be done in supine and lateral position
  - This helps in detecting cardiovascular compression preoperatively
- Other useful investigations include:
  - Preoperative awake fibreoptic bronchoscopic examination:
  - This can be done in the supine and lateral positions
  - Helps in assessing dynamic airway compression
  - PET scans for tumor staging

Grading of Symptoms

❖ Asymptomatic

❖ Mildly symptomatic: Can lie supine with some cough or pressure sensation

❖ Moderately symptomatic: Can lie supine for short periods but not indefinitely

❖ Severely symptomatic: Cannot tolerate supine position

Preoperative High-Risk Criteria

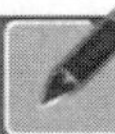

❖ Cardiopulmonary signs at presentation:
- Dyspnea in supine position
- Increased cough in supine position
- SVC syndrome
- Pericardial effusion
- Syncopal episodes

❖ Combined obstructive and restrictive picture on PFTs

❖ PEFR < 40%

❖ Tracheal compression to < 50% of predicted cross sectional area (in children)

Risk Stratification for General Anesthesia

Stage	Risk class	Description
A	Safe	Asymptomatic *adult or child*
		Tracheobronchial (TB) diameter on CT > 50% of normal
B	Unsafe	Severely symptomatic *adult or child*
		Child with TB diameter < 50% of normal regardless of symptoms
C	Uncertain	Mild to moderate symptoms in *child* with TB diameter > 50% of normal
		Mild to moderate symptoms in *adult* with TB diameter < 50% of normal
		Adult or child unable to give history

Preoperative Preparation

❖ Tumor size may be reduced preoperatively with:
- Anterior chemotherapy
- Steroids
- Radiation therapy

❖ However, preoperative chemo-radiotherapy may distort the histological diagnosis

❖ Tracheobronchial stenting may be performed via flexible/rigid bronchoscopy

❖ However, this may worsen hemodynamics by displacing the mass into vascular structures

❖ In the presence of SVC syndrome:
- Head end elevated nursing
- Steroids and diuretics

Anesthetic Considerations

❖ Tracheo-bronchial tree compression causing airway obstruction

❖ Compression of intrathoracic superior vena cava causing:
- Tongue and orofacial swelling leading to difficult mask ventilation
- Laryngeal edema leading to extubation failure
- Distension of veins:
  - Increased chances of bleeding during intubation
  - Altered consciousness causing delayed extubation
  - Raised ICP

❖ Cardiac compression by large tumors causing:

Contd...

Contd...

- Arrhythmias due to extended dissection
- Cardiac arrest post- induction

❖ Systemic coexisting diseases:
- Patients usually have an advanced ASA grade
- Associated paraneoplastic syndromes:
  - ACTH
  - ADH
  - Parathyroid hormone

❖ Coexisting Eaton Lambert syndrome causing increased sensitivity to NDMR

Contd...

Contd...

❖ Preoperative chemotherapy and radiotherapy-related complications:
- Bleomycin Lung
- Cisplatin: renal complications
- Anthracycline, doxorubicin: Cardiac complications

❖ Intraoperative vital organs damage: Left RLN or bilateral RLN injury:
- Postoperative stridor
- Phrenic nerve injury
- SVC, aorta

Choice of Anesthetic Technique

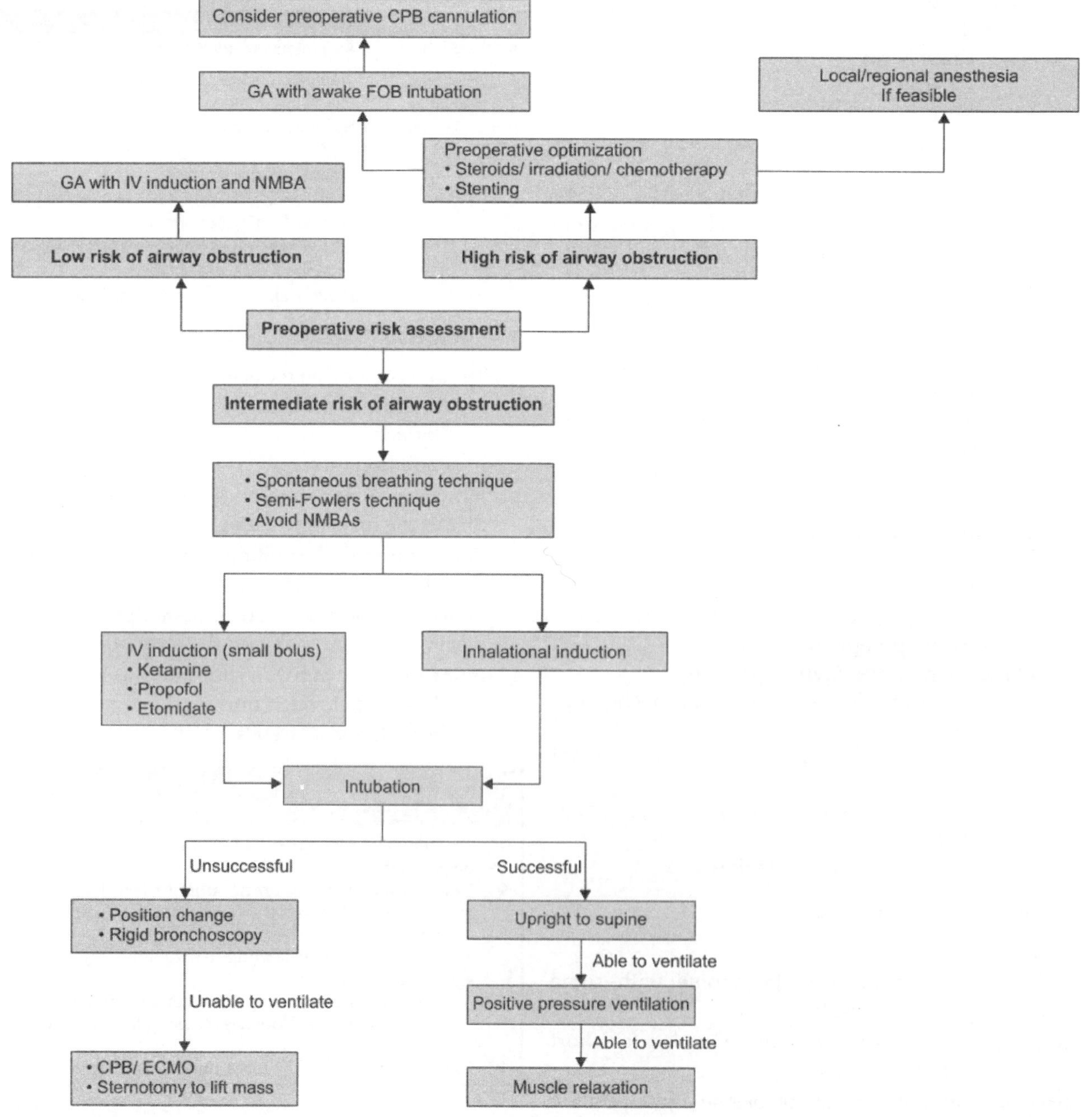

Premedication

- IV cannulation:
  - 2 large bore IV cannulae are secured prior to induction
  - In the presence of SVC syndrome:
    - Mass effect causes occlusion of venous drainage of upper body
    - Thus, venous cannulae are secured in veins which drain into the IVC
    - 2 large bore cannulae are usually secured in the lower limb
    - Alternatively, femoral vein is cannulated with a multi-lumen CVC
    - In patients with difficult venous access:
      - Dual CVCs may be secured
      - One catheter drains into the SVC and the other into IVC
      - The IVC catheter is used until mass resection is complete
      - SVC catheter can be used in the postoperative period
- Blood availability:
  - Preoperative discussion with the surgeon about anticipated blood loss
  - Risk of massive blood loss exists for large masses in critical locations
  - Thus, cross matched blood has to be kept readily available
- Premedication:
  - Anti-sialogogues may be used to:
    - Reduce airway secretions prior to awake bronchoscopy
    - Reducing vagal responses to airway manipulation
  - Adequate local anesthetic instillation if fibreoptic bronchoscopy is planned
  - Sedation:
    - Sedation is avoided in the presence of airway obstruction
    - IV midazolam 0.05 mg/kg can be given if airway obstruction is absent
- Patient is shifted in head elevated position in the presence of significant dyspnea
- Placement of thoracic epidural catheters can be accomplished prior to induction

Monitors

- Pulse oximetry
- E_TCO_2, ECG
- IBP monitoring
  - Placed depending on the size and location of the mediastinal mass
  - Patients with SVC syndrome may have ipsilateral subclavian A compression
  - In case of unilateral involvement, catheters are placed in both upper limbs
  - In case of bilateral involvement, femoral artery is catheterized
- CVP monitoring necessary to guide fluid and inotropic therapy
- Neuromuscular monitoring especially in the presence of Eaton-Lambert syndrome
- Airway pressure for tracheal/bronchial compression
- In the presence of cardiac/PA compression, consider:
  - PA catheter: Rarely used as:
    - Risk of vascular perforation during PAC placement
    - Technically challenging in the presence of vascular compression
    - Lack of convincing evidence for PAC monitoring
  - Cardiac output monitors
  - Transesophageal echocardiography:
    - Allows continuous visualization of the left and right ventricles
    - Thus, dynamic obstruction can be detected immediately
    - It also allows estimation of ventricular volume and cardiac function
    - This aids in titration of fluid and vasopressor therapy

Induction

- Adequate preoxygenation
- Ensure presence of surgical and perfusion team (for CPB) at the time of induction
- Patient is induced in sitting position in the presence of cardiac compression
- Induction agents generally used are:
  - Ketamine
  - Etomidate
- These agents are preferred for their safe hemodynamic profile
- Drug administration in upper limb is avoided in the presence of SVC syndrome
- This is because action of the drug may become unpredictable
- Spontaneous ventilation may be maintained with boluses of ketamine or propofol

- Neuromuscular blockade is preferably avoided until the airway is secured
- Intubation:
  - Flexible bronchoscopy may be done prior to intubation to:
    - Assess endobronchial invasion of the tumor
    - Presence of airway obstruction and severity
    - Dynamic airway collapse with change in position
  - LMAs are used during flexible bronchoscopy as:
    - They provide a conduit for FOB insertion
    - They allow better control of ventilation
  - Tubes used for intubation may include:
    - Reinforced ETT are usually preferred
    - Microlaryngoscopy tubes for distal lesions causing compression
    - DLT may be used in case intraoperative lung isolation is required
- ETT may be used to stent the airway obstruction if it is located proximally
- Rigid bronchoscope with JV may be used in cases of distal airway obstruction
- Video laryngoscope may be used for placement of the DLT
- Activation of thoracic epidural:
  - Usually avoided until resection of the tumor is complete
  - This is to avoid inducing sympathectomy during the surgical procedure
  - Epidural opioids may be used prior to incision to ensure adequate analgesia
  - When activated, doses are minimized and given in small aliquots
  - Thus, thoracic epidurals (T_2-T_5 level) are mainly used for postoperative pain

Rescue Operations for Airway Obstruction

- Microlaryngeal tube advanced distal to airway obstruction
- Double lumen tube
- Repositioning patient to position of comfort (lateral or prone)
- Resumption of previously tolerated state:
  - Upright position
  - Spontaneous ventilation
  - Awaken from anesthesia
- Rigid bronchoscopy beyond stenosis
- Initiation of cardiopulmonary bypass/ECMO

Maintenance

- Balanced anesthesia with volatile anesthetic agents is the preferred method
- Opioid analgesics may be administered as boluses or continuous infusion
- Maintain deep planes to avoid coughing as it can cause venous engorgement in chest
- Neuro-muscular blocking agents (NMBAs):
  - Use of NMBAs during the procedure is controversial
  - Spontaneous ventilation carries the risk of coughing and air embolism
  - Neuromuscular paralysis carries the risk of loss of airway control
  - Spontaneous ventilation is preferred when the airway obstruction is significant
  - In the presence of minimal airway obstruction NMBAs may be used
  - Short acting muscle relaxants are usually preferred
  - NMBAs are avoided/limited in the presence of Lambert Eaton syndrome

Ventilation

- Continuous monitoring of oxygenation, ventilation and airway pressures is necessary
- Intraoperative complications which can compromise ventilation include:
  - Shifting of mass effect due to surgical compression
  - Surgical trauma causing inadvertent breach of the airway
  - Airway collapse due to tracheomalacia
  - Malposition of the ETT
- In mechanically ventilated patients:
  - Pressure controlled ventilation used to detect early increase in airway pressure
  - High airway pressures may be required due to:
    - Compression of lungs by the mediastinal mass
    - Surgical packing and manipulation
  - Sanders injector/jet ventilator used if rigid bronchoscopy is required
  - Low FiO_2 is used if patient has had recent bleomycin therapy

Hemodynamics

- Hemodynamic compromise may occur during:
  - Induction of anesthesia
  - Change in patient position
  - Transition from spontaneous ventilation to IPPV

- Fluid restrictive strategy is preferred intraoperatively:
  - Perioperative fluid restriction to < 3 mL/kg/hour of crystalloids
  - Avoidance of fluid therapy to reverse intraoperative oliguria
  - Intraoperative crystalloid is limited to 1.5-2 L in the absence of hemorrhage
  - Fluid therapy is directed to maintain cardiac output when it is monitored
  - Transfusion trigger generally used is 25%
- Techniques to maintain intraoperative hemodynamic stability include:
  - Optimizing volume status with goal directed fluid therapy
  - Administering inotropes and vasopressors
  - Use of short acting, rapidly titratable anesthetic agents
  - Replacement of blood loss with colloids/blood

Extubation

- Fibreoptic bronchoscopy is performed prior to extubation to:
  - Assess airway patency
  - Assess airway continuity following tumor resection
  - Rule out tracheomalacia
  - Perform suction and lavage in patients with excessive secretions
- Coughing and bucking are avoided during extubation especially for:
  - Patients with significant tracheomalacia
  - Inadvertent intraoperative injury to the tracheobronchial tree
- Coughing increases airway pressure, compromising tracheal anastomosis
- This may lead to airway bleeding and air leak syndromes postoperatively
- Patient is extubated only after:
  - Full recovery of reflexes
  - Full recovery of neuromuscular function
  - Fully awake
- Consider postoperative ventilation if:
  - Long duration of surgery
  - Accidental resection of major nerves
  - Airway patency absent

Postoperative Care

Management

- Nursing in sitting up position
- Check X-ray for pneumothorax is mandatory
- Monitor for postoperative airway obstruction

Analgesia

- Multimodal analgesia
- LA infilteration of wound
- Thoracic epidural analgesia (T_2-T_5 levels)
- Intercostal blocks
- Paracetamol and NSAIDs
- IV patient-controlled analgesia

Complications

- Hemorrhage
- Airway obstruction post-induction due to:
  - Loss of lung volume due to compression by the mediastinal mass
  - Obstructed tip of ETT by wall of tracheobronchial tree
  - Loss of pleural pressure and transmural pressure gradient
- Airway obstruction post extubation due to:
  - Increased mass size due to surgical manipulation causing edema and hematoma
  - Creation of turbulent gas flow by PPV
  - Tracheomalacia
  - RLN injury
- Air leak syndromes:
  - Pneumothorax
  - Hemothorax
  - Chylothorax
  - Pneumomediastinum
- Nerve injury:
  - RLN injury, phrenic N, injury
  - Initiation of autonomic reflexes by:
    - Stimulation of tracheal/aortic arch receptors
    - Vagal reflexes
- Others:
  - Acute tracheal collapse
  - Esophageal tear, thoracic duct injury
  - Mediastinitis

ANESTHESIA FOR MEDIASTINOSCOPY

Introduction

- Diagnostic procedure first described by ***Eric Carlens*** in 1959
- Surgical procedure is performed with a mediastinoscope to examine the mediastinum
- Essential in staging of lung cancer despite availability of other imaging methods
- Morbidity related to medistinoscopy ranges from 2–8%

Indications

- Staging of bronchogenic carcinoma: has a high sensitivity > 80% and specificity 100%
- Mediastinal mass biopsy (when other investigations are inconclusive)
- Diagnosis of mediastinal lymphadenopathy:
  - Sarcoidosis
  - Lymphomas
  - Tuberculosis
  - Fungal infections
- Diagnosis and treatment of mesotheliomas
- Excision of small mediastinal tumors

Contraindications

- Absolute contraindications:
  - Previous mediastinoscopy:
    - This results in extensive scar formation and adhesions
    - The plane of dissection is eliminated, making dissection impossible
  - Previous recurrent laryngeal nerve injury
  - Ascending aortic aneurysms
- Relative contraindications:
  - Cerebrovascular disease
  - Severe cervical spine disease with limited neck extension
  - Tracheal deviation
  - Superior vena caval obstruction due to risk of bleeding from distended veins
  - Thoracic aortic aneurysm
  - Previous chest radiotherapy

Procedure

- Cervical mediastinoscopy:
  - Done via midline transverse incision
  - 3 cm incision is made above suprasternal notch
  - Pretracheal plane is identified by careful dissection
  - Mediastinoscope is then advanced along this plane
  - It is advanced along the anterior aspect of trachea
  - Blunt dissection is used to develop the plane distally
  - Biopsy forceps are used to sample nodal tissue or remove small intact nodes
  - Frozen section biopsy of the samples may be performed intraoperatively
  - The strap muscles are then closed in serial layers prior to cutaneous closure
  - Resection of lung cancers may be performed in the same setting
- Transthoracic mediastinoscopy or ***Chamberlain procedure:***
  - Also called anterior mediastinotomy
  - More invasive compared to cervical medastinoscopy
  - Transverse incision is made lateral to left sternal border at the angle of Louie
  - The incision is carried through the pectoralis fibres to the IInd costal cartilage
  - The IInd costal cartilage is incised from the sternum to costochondral junction
  - The costal cartilage is excised flush with:
    - Sternum medially
    - Costochondral junction laterally
  - After identifying the tumor, biospies are performed with scissors/scalpel
  - This is followed by serial closure of the dissected layers.

Preoperative Assessment

- Clinical assessment:
  - Mostly done in smokers with pulmonary disease

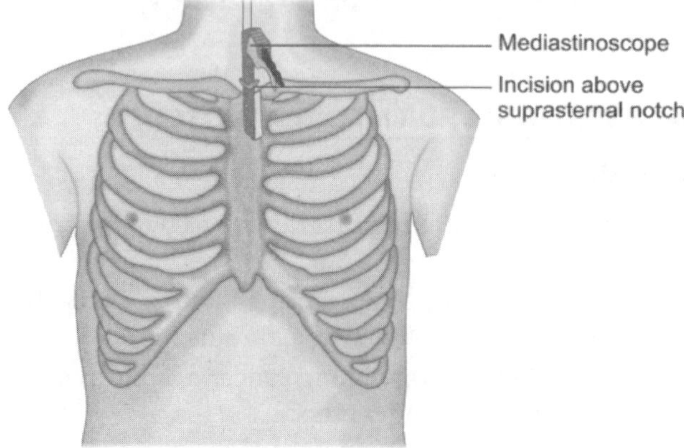

Fig. 60: Cervical mediastinoscopy.

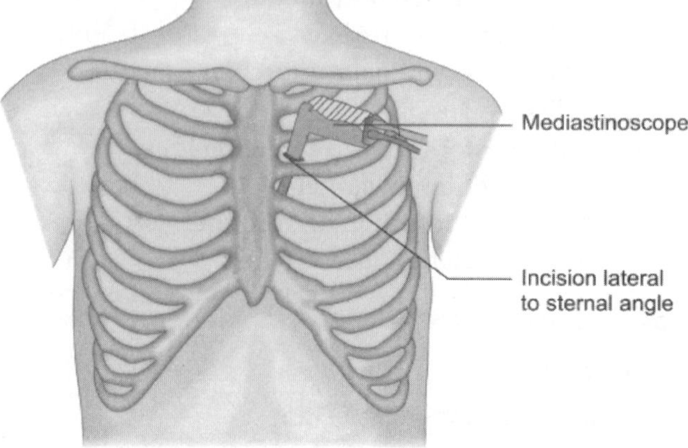

Fig. 61: Chamberlains procedure.

- History suggestive of airway obstruction:
  - Unilateral wheeze
  - Dyspnea, stridor
  - Cough, cyanosis
  - Recurrent RTI due to tracheobronchial compression
- History of comorbidities:
  - HTN, coronary disease
  - Peripheral vascular disease
  - Stroke or TIA
- Evidence of Eaton Lamberts syndrome with proximal myopathy
- Syncope on Valsalva maneuver is suggestive of cardiac compression
- Positional variation: Orthopnea reduces on sitting up

❖ Investigations:
- Complete blood count
- Blood urea, serum creatinine, electrolytes
- Baseline ABG on room air
- Chest X-ray may show mediastinal widening due to SVC syndrome
- Pulmonary function tests:
  - Done in upright and supine position
  - Disproportionate reduction in MEFR: Increased chances of tracheomalacia
  - Combined OLD and RLD pattern suggests increased incidence complications
  - If cyanosis occurs with good PFTs:
    - Indicates PA occlusion
    - Pulmonary angiography should be done
- Flow volume loops in supine and upright position
- CT scan/MRI of airway to study:
  - Extent of tumour
  - Effect on surrounding structures
- ECG may show signs of pulmonary HTN
- Echocardiography: Done in supine and upright position for cardiac compression

Anesthetic Considerations

❖ Tracheo-bronchial tree compression causing airway obstruction

❖ Limited access to airway intra-operatively

❖ Persistence of tracheo-bronchial obstruction postoperatively:
- If the procedure is diagnostic, airway compression is not relieved
- Compression may be aggravated due to injury and edema

❖ Compression of intrathoracic superior vena cava causing:
- Tongue and orofacial swelling leading to difficult mask ventilation
- Laryngeal edema leading to extubation failure
- Distension of veins:
  - Increased chances of bleeding during intubation and mediastinoscopy
  - Altered consciousness causing delayed extubation
  - Raised ICP

❖ Cardiac compression by large tumors causing:
- Arrhythmias due to extended dissection
- Cardiac arrest post-induction

❖ Systemic coexisting diseases:
- Patients usually have an advanced ASA grade
- Associated paraneoplastic syndromes:
  - ACTH
  - ADH
  - Parathyroid hormone

❖ Coexisting Eaton Lambert syndrome causing increased sensitivity to NDMR

❖ Preoperative chemotherapy and radiotherapy-related complications:
- Bleomycin Lung
- Cisplatin: renal complications
- Anthracycline, doxorubicin: cardiac complications

❖ Potentially life-threatening complications:
- Torrential hemorrhage
- Pneumothorax
- Airway disruption
- Air embolism

❖ Intraoperative vital organs damage: left RLN or bilateral RLN injury:
- Postoperative stridor
- Phrenic nerve injury
- SVC, aorta

Anesthetic Goals 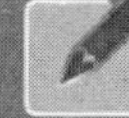

❖ Optimize surgical conditions:
- Deep anesthetic planes
- Adequate neuromuscular paralysis

❖ Prevent partial airway obstruction from being made complete by:
- Securing airway in an awake, spontaneously breathing patient
- Ensuring spontaneous ventilation after induction of GA
- Passing ETT/bronchoscope/stent past the site of airway obstruction
- Lateral/semi-Fowlers position if extreme airway compromise

Contd...

Contd...

- Prepare for distal airway obstruction using:
  - Standby rigid bronchoscope (RB)
  - Jet ventilation
- Prepare for sudden complete airway loss using standby CPB
- Prepare for massive transfusion:
  - Large bore IV access
  - Readily available cross matched blood
  - Lower extremity IV access in the presence of SVC syndrome

High Risk Patients for Mediastinoscopy

- Cardiopulmonary signs at presentation:
  - Dyspnea in supine position
  - Increased cough in supine position
  - SVC syndrome
  - Pericardial effusion
  - Syncopal episodes
- Combined obstructive and restrictive picture on PFTs
- PEFR < 40%
- Tracheal compression to < 50% of predicted cross sectional area (in children)

Preoperative Preparation and Premedication

- Preoperative stabilization:
  - Consider preoperative chemotherapy or radiotherapy to shrink the tumour size
  - Tracheobronchial stenting is performed in severely dyspneic patients
  - In the presence of SVC syndrome:
    - Head end elevated nursing
    - Steroids and diuretics
- IV cannulation:
  - 2 large bore IV cannulae are secured prior to induction
  - In the presence of SVC syndrome:
    - 2 large bore cannular are secured in the lower limb
    - Alternatively, femoral vein is cannulated with a multi-lumen CVC
- Cross matched blood to be kept readily available
- Premedication:
  - Anti-sialogogues may be used to:
    - Reduce airway secretions prior to awake bronchoscopy
    - Reducing vagal responses to airway manipulation
  - Adequate local anesthetic instillation if fibreoptic bronchoscopy is planned
  - Sedation:
    - Sedation is avoided in the presence of airway obstruction
    - IV midazolam 0.05 mg/kg can be given if airway obstruction is absent
- Patient is shifted in head elevated position in the presence of significant dyspnea

Choice of Anesthetic Technique

- Local anesthesia is preferred for minor procedures in cooperative patients with:
  - Small mediastinal masses
  - Compromised airway
- General anesthesia:
  - Preferred for prolonged procedures in anxious patients
  - Techniques include:
    - Awake intubation:
      - Preferred in the presence of significant airway obstruction
      - Conducted with FOB with adequately anesthetized airway
      - Allows visualization of the exact level of airway obstruction
      - Endotracheal tube is placed distal to the obstruction
      - RB should be available for distal airway obstructions
    - Inhalational induction with spontaneous ventilation:
      - Used in the absence of airway obstruction
      - Muscle relaxants are avoided
      - Deep anesthetic plane is ensured to prevent coughing
      - Less preferred as:
        - Coughing results in damage to surrounding structures
        - Spontaneous ventilation increases risk of air embolism
        - This is because of head-elevated position during surgery
    - Intravenous induction with muscle paralysis:
      - Used in the absence of airway obstruction
      - Muscle relaxants are administered once airway is secured
      - Preferred as it reduces the risk of coughing and air embolism

Risk Stratification for General Anesthesia

Stage	Risk class	Description
A	Safe	Asymptomatic *adult or child*
		Tracheobronchial (TB) diameter on CT > 50% of normal
B	Unsafe	Severely symptomatic *adult or child*
		Child with TB diameter < 50% of normal regardless of symptoms
C	Uncertain	Mild to moderate symptoms in *child* with TB diameter > 50% of normal
		Mild to moderate symptoms in *adult* with TB diameter < 50% of normal
		Adult or child unable to give history

Monitors

- Pulse oximetry:
  - SpO_2 probes can be placed on both the hands
  - This is because right innominate A compression may occur during procedure
  - This is identified as a decrease in amplitude of SPO_2 signal
  - Thus, right sided probe can be used to identify RI artery compression
- E_TCO_2, ECG
- NIBP/ IBP monitoring:
  - Usually NIBP monitoring is sufficient
  - BP monitoring is preferably done on the left hand/ radial artery
  - This is because RIA compression by mediastinoscope can give low readings
  - Additional IBP on right hand may be placed to check for compression of RIA
- Neuromuscular monitoring especially in the presence of Eaton-Lambert syndrome
- Airway pressure for tracheal/bronchial compression by the mediastinoscope
- PA catheter and cardiac output monitors in the presence of cardiac/PA compression

Induction

- Adequate preoxygenation
- Ensure presence of surgical and perfusion team (for CPB) at the time of induction
- Patient is induced in sitting position in the presence of cardiac compression
- Induction agents may be chosen depending on the hemodynamic status:
  - Propofol
  - Ketamine
  - Etomidate
- Drug administration in upper limb is avoided in the presence of SVC syndrome
- This is because action of the drug may become unpredictable
- Spontaneous ventilation may be maintained with boluses of ketamine or propofol
- Neuromuscular blockade is preferably avoided until the airway is secured
- Intubation:
  - *Single lumen tubes are sufficient* to secure the airway for mediastinoscopy
  - Reinforced tube is preferred to reduce risk of ETT kinking intraoperatively
  - Longer microlaryngoscopy tubes may be used if distal trachea is compressed
- ETT may be used to stent the airway obstruction if it is located proximally
- Rigid bronchoscope with JV may be used in cases of distal airway obstruction

Rescue Operations for Airway Obstruction

- Microlaryngeal tube advanced distal to airway obstruction
- Double lumen tube
- Repositioning patient to position of comfort (lateral or prone)
- Resumption of previously tolerated state:
  - Upright position
  - Spontaneous ventilation
  - Awaken from anesthesia
- Rigid bronchoscopy beyond stenosis
- Initiation of cardiopulmonary bypass/ECMO

Position

- Supine with slightly head up (20°) position to relieve venous congestion
- Neck extended with shoulder bolsters
- Arms positioned by the side of the patient

Maintenance

- Balanced anesthesia with volatile anesthetic agents is the preferred method
- Opioid analgesics may be administered as boluses or continuous infusion
- Maintain deep planes to avoid coughing/bucking as:
  - Increased risk of trauma by medistinoscope
  - Can cause venous engorgement in chest
- Neuro-muscular blocking agents (NMBAs):

- Use of NMBAs during the procedure is controversial
- Spontaneous ventilation carries the risk of coughing and air embolism
- Neuromuscular paralysis carries the risk of loss of airway control
- Spontaneous ventilation is preferred when the airway obstruction is significant
- In the presence of minimal airway obstruction NMBAs may be used
- Short acting muscle relaxants are usually preferred
- NMBAs are avoided/limited in the presence of Lambert Eaton syndrome

Ventilation

- Spontaneous ventilation is preferred in the presence of significant airway obstruction
- In mechanically ventilated patients:
  - Pressure controlled ventilation used to detect early increase in airway pressure
  - High airway pressures may be required due to:
    - Compression of lungs by the mediastinal mass
    - Surgical packing and manipulation
  - Sanders injector/jet ventilator used if rigid bronchoscopy is required
  - Low FiO_2 is used if patient has had recent bleomycin therapy

Hemodynamics

- Cardiac compression:
  - Commonly occurs during the procedure
  - Watch for arrhythmias, factitious cardiac arrest
  - Vasopressors/inotropes used if hypotension occurs due to compression
- Hemorrhage:
  - Hemorrhage is the *most common* complication
  - Blood loss may be substantial
  - If venous bleeding occurs, induced hypotension may be used
  - Fluids, if given in upper limb, may enter mediastinum
  - Therefore, if venous bleeding occurs, use lower limb large bore angiocatheter

Extubation

- Fibreoptic bronchoscopy is performed prior to extubation to rule out tracheomalacia
- Coughing and bucking are avoided during extubation
- Patient is extubated only after:
  - Full recovery of reflexes
  - Full recovery of neuromuscular function
  - Fully awake
- Consider postoperative ventilation if:
  - Long duration of surgery
  - Accidental resection of major nerves
  - Airway patency absent

Postoperative Care

Management

- Nursing in sitting up position
- Check X-ray for pneumothorax is mandatory
- Monitor for stridor due to RLN injury or paratracheal hematoma

Analgesia

- LA infilteration of wound
- Paracetamol and NSAIDs are usually sufficient for postoperative analgesia
- IV patient-controlled analgesia may be used for severe pain

Complications

- Hemorrhage:
  - *Most common* complication
  - Temporarily stopped by surgical packing
  - Direct hemostasis following median sternotomy may be required
- Airway obstruction post-induction due to:
  - Loss of lung volume due to compression by the mediastinal mass
  - Obstructed tip of ETT by wall of tracheobronchial tree
  - Loss of pleural pressure and transmural pressure gradient
- Airway obstruction post extubation due to:
  - Increased mass size due to surgical manipulation causing edema and hematoma
  - Creation of turbulent gas flow by PPV
  - Tracheomalacia
  - RLN injury
- Air leak syndromes:
  - Pneumothorax
  - Hemothorax
  - Chylothorax
  - Pneumomediastinum
- Nerve injury:
  - RLN injury, phrenic N, injury

- Initiation of autonomic reflexes by:
  - Stimulation of tracheal/aortic arch receptors
  - Vagal reflexes
- Factitious cardiac arrest:
  - Absent right radial pulse but present on left side
  - Occurs due to compression of innominate A by mediastinoscope
  - Transient left hemiparesis possible postoperatively
- Others:
  - Acute tracheal collapse
  - Esophageal tear, thoracic duct injury
  - Mediastinitis
  - Air embolism:
    - Common in spontaneously breathing patient due to inadvertent venous rent
    - Risk is increased in sitting position

RIGID BRONCHOSCOPY

Introduction

- Rigid bronchoscopy (RB) is an invasive surgical technique used to visualize:
  - Oropharynx
  - Larynx
  - Vocal cords
  - Trachea
  - Proximal pulmonary branches
- First reported use of bronchoscopy was in 1897 by ***Gustav Killian***
- It was first used to remove a pork bone from the right mainstem bronchus

Indications for Rigid Bronchoscopy

- Diagnostic:
  - Stridor
  - Chronic cough
  - Airway trauma
  - Severe hemoptysis
  - Tracheostomy surveillance
  - Interval evaluation after laryngo-tracheal reconstruction
  - Assessment of toxic inhalation or aspiration
  - Evaluation of laryngeal pathology
- Therapeutic:
  - Foreign body evaluation and management
  - Management of severe laryngotracheal infections
  - Management of mass lesions of airway, including recurrent respiratory papillomatosis
  - Placement of stents
  - Assisting in laser therapy

High Risk Patients

- Adults:
  - Presence of foreign body
  - Neoplastic disease
  - Carinal involvement
- Pediatrics:
  - History of foreign body aspiration
  - Tetralogy of Fallot
  - Need for biopsy or drainage of lesions during bronchoscopy

Instrumentation

- The bronchoscope is a hollow rigid metal tube which is bevelled at the distal end
- Side holes are present at the end to allow ventilation proximal to the tip
- Bevelled edge of the tip is used to facilitate introduction of the bronchoscope
- The ports which are usually present on the bronchoscope are:
  - Main port:
    - Working channel used for aspiration
    - Also used for insertion of instruments such as:
      - Telescopes
      - Biopsy forceps
      - Laser fibres
      - Balloon devices
      - Cryotherapy probes
      - Stents
  - Superior port: Connected to the prismatic light deflector and light source
  - Inferior port: Ventilation port connected to the anesthesia circuit
- The size of the bronchoscope should be tailored to the individual patient
- The size chosen should:
  - Maximize the surgeons view
  - Minimize the risk of airway trauma

Size	Length	ID (mm)	OD (mm)	Age
2.5	20	3.5	4.2	Premature
3	20, 26	4.3	5	Premature, newborn
3.5	20, 26, 30	5	5.7	Newborn- 6 months
3.7	26, 30	5.7	6.4	6 months- 1 year
4	26, 30	6	6.7	1-2 years
5	30	7.1	7.8	3- 4 years
6	30, 40	7.5	8.2	5- 7 years
6.5	43	8.5	9.2	Adult

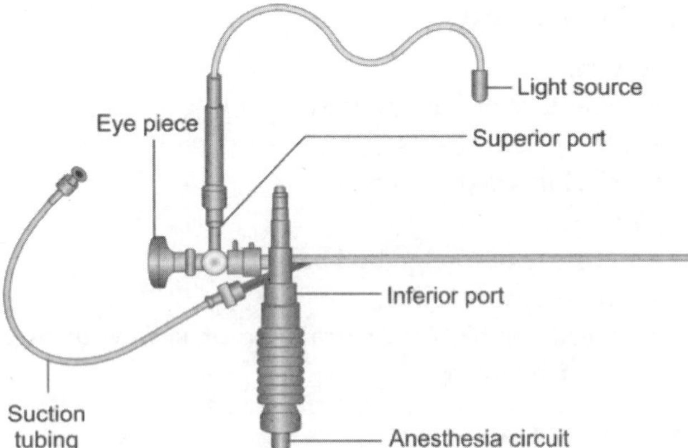

Fig. 62: Parts of a rigid bronchoscope.

Anesthetic Considerations

- Sympathetic stimulation: Highly stimulating requiring deep anesthetic planes
- Unprotected airway:
  - Risk of aspiration
  - Potentially challenging ventilation
  - Potential for loss of airway access
- Technical considerations:
  - Shared airway with the surgeon
  - Open circuit leading to OT contamination with volatile agents
  - Need for total intravenous anesthesia
- Considerations of jet ventilation: Risk of barotrauma and pneumothorax
- Postoperative considerations:
  - High risk of laryngeal edema
  - Requires immediate arousal from deep planes to maintain patent airway
- Potential for procedure specific complications:
  - Airway fire especially in laser surgeries
  - Airway hemorrhage
  - Gas embolism
  - Traumatic injuries

Preoperative Assessment

- Thorough history to assess:
  - Previous cardiac disease
  - Recent myocardial infarction
  - Documented dysrhythmias
  - Asthma/COPD
- Evaluate for clinical signs of airway obstruction
- Preoperative ECG for patients with history of:
  - Smoking
  - Diabetes mellitus
  - Hypertension
  - Hypercholesterolemia
- Preoperative chest X-ray may show signs of:
  - Congestive cardiac failure
  - Pulmonary consolidation
  - COPD
  - Foreign body
  - Pneumothorax
  - Atelectasis
- Preoperative coagulation profile in the presence of:
  - Prior history of coagulopathy
  - Renal dysfunction
  - History of antiplatelet use
- Pulmonary function tests:
  - Not routinely indicated
  - Predictors of postoperative pulmonary complications on PFTs include:
    - FVC < 20 mL/kg
    - FEV < 50%
- Arterial blood gas analysis for patients with coexisting pulmonary diseases
- Assessment for difficult intubation:
  - Obesity
  - High Mallampatti score
  - Bucked teeth
  - Restricted head and neck movement
  - Receding mandible
  - Reduced thyromental distance
  - Reduced sternomental distance
- Assessment for difficult mask ventilation:
  - Age > 55 years
  - Edentulous patients
  - Presence of a beard
  - History of snoring
  - BMI > 26 kg/m^2

Premedication

- Anti-aspiration prophylaxis:
  - Omeprazole 40 mg PO can be given on the night before surgery
  - Dose can be repeated on the day of surgery 2-6 hours prior
- Pulmonary therapy for patients with severe stridor:
  - Cool saline mist
  - Racemic epinephrine nebulization
  - Systemic steroids
- All cardiac and respiratory drugs are avoided
- No sedation if significant airway obstruction
- IV glycopyrrolate 10 μg/kg given to reduce the secretions during bronchoscopy
- IV midazolam 0.03-0.15 mg/kg

Monitors

- Pulse oximetry, NIBP, ECG
- E_TCO_2:
  - Cannot be monitored
  - This is because the airway is open to atmosphere
  - Transcutaneous pCO_2 monitoring can be used as an alternative
- BIS monitoring as high risk of awareness due to use of TIVA
- Neuromuscular monitoring
- CVP/IBP according to patient condition
- ABGs if prolonged procedure

Induction

- Adequate preoxygenation
- IV induction:
  - Preferred in elderly patients
  - Propofol/short acting IV agents are used
  - Short acting muscle relaxants are preferred for intubation:
    - Succinylcholine
    - Mivacurium
  - NDMRs such as atracurium may be used for prolonged procedures such as:
    - Stent placement
    - Tumor resection
- Inhalational induction:
  - Used when there is uncertainty about securing the airway with bronchoscope
  - Indications:
    - Children
    - Upper airway obstruction such as tracheal stenosis
    - Presence of foreign body
  - NMBAs are avoided post induction to maintain spontaneous ventilation
  - Opioid doses are minimized to prevent hypoventilation and apnea
- Insertion of the metal endoscope precludes placement of an ETT
- Mouth guard may be used prior to insertion of the bronchoscope to protect the teeth
- Lidocaine may be sprayed on the vocal cords during insertion of the bronchoscope

Position

- Supine with cervical extension
- Shoulder rolls can be used to ensure adequate neck extension

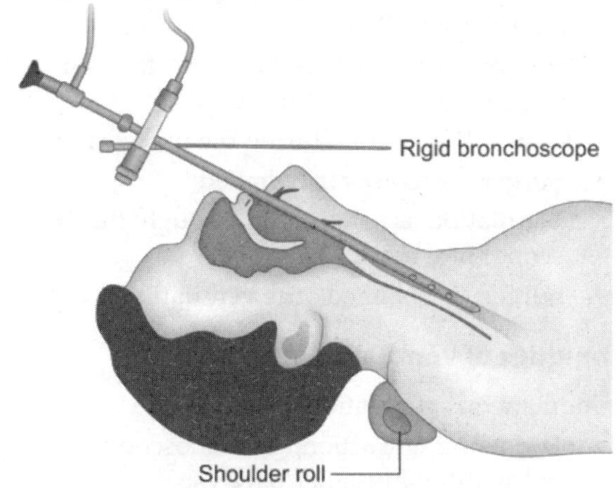

Fig. 63: Position for rigid bronchoscopy.

- Other adjuncts to enable passage of bronchoscope include:
  - Removal of pillow
  - Lowering the head of the operating table

Maintenance

- Deep anesthetic planes are required as the procedure is very painful
- TIVA with propofol and remifentanyl is the preferred technique
  - Propofol 75-150 µg/kg/min
  - Remifentanil:
    - Loading dose 1 µg/kg
    - Maintenance dose 0.1-0.2 µg/kg/min
- Balanced anesthesia:
  - May be used in children
  - If balanced anesthesia is used, loss of VA around the bronchoscope can occur
  - This can cause rapid lightening of the anesthetic plane
  - Isoflurane is one of the most soluble volatile agents
  - This minimizes changes in anesthetic depth when respiration is interrupted
  - Thus, 1.5-2 MAC isoflurane is the preferred volatile anesthetic agent
- Vecuronium/atracurium may be used if prolonged surgery is anticipated
- Lowest possible FiO_2 (< 40% if possible) is used if procedure involves Nd-YAG laser
- This is to reduce the risk of airway fire

- ❖ Throat packs may be placed if increased loss of tidal volume during PPV
- ❖ Continuous communication with the surgeon is required in case of desaturation
- ❖ If desaturation occurs during the procedure:
  - Surgery is temporarily halted
  - Ventilation is continued through the bronchoscope/face mask
  - Surgery is resumed once ventilation is optimized

Techniques of Ventilation

- ❖ Spontaneous ventilation:
  - Following induction, bronchoscopy is carried out without muscular paralysis
  - Topical anesthesia/nerve blocks can be used to prevent coughing
  - However, spontaneous ventilation techniques are not preferred as:
    - It increases risk of traumatic complications
    - It causes technical difficulties to the surgeon
    - Placement of the bronchoscope requires extreme extension
    - This may not be tolerated by a spontaneously breathing patient
- ❖ Apneic ventilation:
  - Adequate preoxygenation is ensured
  - Following induction and NMB, patient is hyperventilated with 100% FiO_2
  - Relative hypocapnia and complete de-nitrogenation is targeted
  - Adequate preoxygenation allows brief periods of apnea to be tolerated
  - $PaCO_2$ increases 6 mm Hg during first minute and at 3 mm Hg/min thereafter
  - O_2 may be insufflated via catheter placed above the carina at 10-15 L/min
  - This technique limits the duration of surgical exposure to 5-minute intervals
  - Thus, it cannot be used for procedures requiring extended airway manipulation
- ❖ Ventilating bronchoscope:
  - Ideal for infants and children
  - Mechanical ventilator is connected to the ventilating port of the bronchoscope
  - Child is ventilated intermittently using a reservoir bag
  - However, ventilation is possible only when the eye-piece is in place
  - Gases may leak through the space between the bronchoscope and vocal cords
  - Thus, higher fresh gas flows may be required to maintain a full reservoir bag
  - Advantages:
    - Requires lighter planes
    - Facilitates conventional ventilation
    - Allows better control over ventilation
    - Better immobilization of airway and better exposure
    - FiO_2, lung compliance and tidal volume monitored constantly
    - Avoids barotrauma seen with HFJV
  - Disadvantages:
    - Limits period of instrumentation as ventilation possible only when eyepiece is in place
    - Gas leakage:
      - The sides of the bronchoscope should approximate the airway
      - A smaller size bronchoscope results in gas leaks around it
      - This can result in hypoxia and hypercarbia
    - Leak of VA and light anesthetic plane possible if discrepancy between size of bronchoscope and airway
- ❖ High frequency jet ventilation:
  - Upto 150-300 breaths/min can be delivered
  - Oxygenation and ventilation is comparable to low frequency jet ventilation
  - Tracheobronchial wall is immobilized during ventilation
  - This results in better surgical exposure
- ❖ Jet ventilation using Sanders Venturi Injector:
  - Technique:
    - High pressure O_2 (50 PSIG) is injected intermittently
    - This is done through a needle at the proximal end of bronchoscope
    - Needle used is 16-18 G, 2.5-3.5 cm long
    - It is placed parallel to the long axis of bronchoscope
    - Injector needle size is matched with:
      - Type of bronchoscope
      - Oxygen pressure required
    - O_2 delivered using controllable pressure relief value and toggle switch
    - When toggle switch is depressed, room air is entrained along with O_2
    - Proximal end of bronchoscope remains open to allow gas exchange
  - Physiology:
    - Uses Venturi principle to ensure ventilation

- Delivery of oxygen at high pressures creates a negative pressure
- This entrains air from outside the injector to flow into airways
- This results in expansion of the lungs
- Exhalation is passive and relies on lung collapse following removal of pressure
- Sufficient time must be allowed for egress of entrained air to prevent:
  - Breath stacking
  - Progressive hyperinflation

- Advantages:
  - Allows continuous ventilation
  - Presence of the eye-piece is not necessary for ventilation
  - Duration of bronchoscopy is minimized
  - Permits extended bronchoscopy
- Disadvantages:
  - Entrainment of air causes variable FiO_2 at the distal end
  - Poor alveolar ventilation can result if:
    - Compliance of lungs is poor
    - Size mismatch between bronchoscope and tracheal wall
  - Difficult to assess adequacy of ventilation
  - Uncertain FiO_2 and volatile anesthetic dose
  - Barotrauma
  - Spillage of blood into tracheobronchial tree
  - May cause dislodgement and distal migration of foreign bodies

Emergence

- ❖ Airway is thoroughly suctioned at the end of the procedure
- ❖ All anesthetic agents are turned off and neuromuscular blockade completely reversed
- ❖ Patient is ventilated until spontaneous respirations resume
- ❖ This may be done with a face mask or LMA
- ❖ Topical lidocaine may be used to prevent coughing and laryngospasm
- ❖ Postoperative ventilation may be required if airway is edematous

Postoperative Care

- ❖ Intubated patients may be extubated when fully awake and after full reversal
- ❖ O_2 is administered following extubation by mask in sitting position
- ❖ Sitting up position is preferred for nursing
- ❖ In the presence of post-operative airway edema:
  - Racemic epinephrine nebulization
  - Steroids

Complications

- ❖ Immediate complications:
  - Hypoxia and hypercarbia
  - Traumatic injury to oropharyngeal structures:
    - Teeth
    - Lips
  - Arytenoid dislocation
  - Airway perforation
  - Complications due to hyperextension:
    - Spinal cord injury: Especially in patients with osteoporosis
    - Vasovagal reactions
    - Cerebral ischemia due to occlusion of vertebral arteries
  - Airway hemorrhage
  - Bronchospasm due to inadequate anesthetic plane
  - Arrhythmias due to:
    - Inadequate depth of anesthesia
    - Sympathetic stimulation
    - Hypoxia
    - Hypercarbia
    - Vasovagal reaction
    - Bronchodilators
  - Gas embolism
  - Aspiration:
    - Airway is never completely secured during rigid bronchoscopy
    - Thus, patient is at risk for aspiration of:
      - Oropharyngeal secretions
      - Blood clots
    - Defer bronchoscopy in patients at risk for aspiration
- ❖ Delayed complications:
  - Laryngeal and subglottic edema:
    - Occurs due to manipulation of laryngeal structures
    - More detrimental in children owing to small airway diameter
    - Can be prevented by administration of steroids
  - Barotrauma, especially if HFJV is used resulting in:
    - Pneumothorax
    - Pneumomediastinum
    - Perforation of esophagus
  - Atelectasis

FLUID MANAGEMENT IN THORACIC SURGERY

Introduction

- Maintaining optimal fluid balance is a crucial element of thoracic anesthesia
- Extreme limitation of fluid administration risks hypovolemia and organ dysfunction
- On the other hand, excess fluid results in pulmonary edema, ALI and anastomotic leaks

Causes of Intravascular Volume Derangements

- Preoperative factors:
  - Preoperative fasting
  - Preoperative dehydration
  - Mechanical bowel preparation
- Anesthesia related factors:
  - Anesthetic drug induced vasodilatation
  - Sympathetic blockade due to neuraxial anesthesia
  - Positive pressure ventilation
- Surgery related factors:
  - Hemorrhage
  - Coagulopathy
  - Prolonged surgery causing insensible losses
  - Delayed resumption of feeds post-surgery

Effects of Intravascular Volume Derangements

- Hypovolemia:
  - Hypotension during induction of anesthesia
  - Decreased tissue perfusion
  - Shock
  - Multiorgan failure
- Hypervolemia: Causes tissue edema resulting in:
  - Postoperative pulmonary edema
  - Postoperative respiratory failure
  - Gastrointestinal edema
  - Decreased gastrointestinal motility
  - Postoperative ileus
  - Dilutional coagulopathy
  - Impaired wound healing
  - Anastomotic leaks

Pathophysiology

- Multiple hit hypothesis:
  - A number of insults accumulate to cause ARDS post thoracic surgery
  - The first insult is usually activation of the systemic inflammatory response by:
    - Surgical trauma
    - Atelectasis
    - Manipulation of tissue
  - The first hit prepares the lung to subsequent hits or insults
  - The subsequent hits can be:
    - Liberal fluid administration
    - FFP transfusion
    - Mediastinal lymphatic damage
    - Non- protective ventilation strategy
- Role of the endothelial glycocalyx layer (EGL):
  - The EGL is present on the luminal surface of capillaries and acts as a sieve
  - Endothelial glycocalyx layer comprises of:
    - Endothelial glycocalyx
    - Retained plasma proteins
  - Thus, the EGL prevents entry of plasma proteins into the sub-glycocalyx layer
  - Thus, the EGL plays a crucial role in modulating trans-vascular fluid flux
  - Pulmonary edema is caused by increased permeability of capillary vasculature
  - This allows for the egress of protein rich fluid into the interstitial compartment
  - One of the primary reasons for egress of fluid is the breakdown of the EGL
  - This can occur due to multiple factors:
    - Ischemia reperfusion injury
    - Inflammation
    - Infection
    - Atrial natriuretic peptide (ANP)
  - Liberal fluid strategy during thoracic surgery results in the release of ANP
  - This in turn causes breakdown of the EGL and pulmonary edema

Factors Damaging Endothelial Glycocalyx Layer

- Inflammation (TNF- α)
- Ischemia- reperfusion
- Infection/sepsis
- Hypervolemia (ANP)
- Surgical trauma
- Hyperglycemia
- Low-density lipoproteins
- Cardiopulmonary bypass
- High tidal volumes
- Hypoxia
- Hypertension

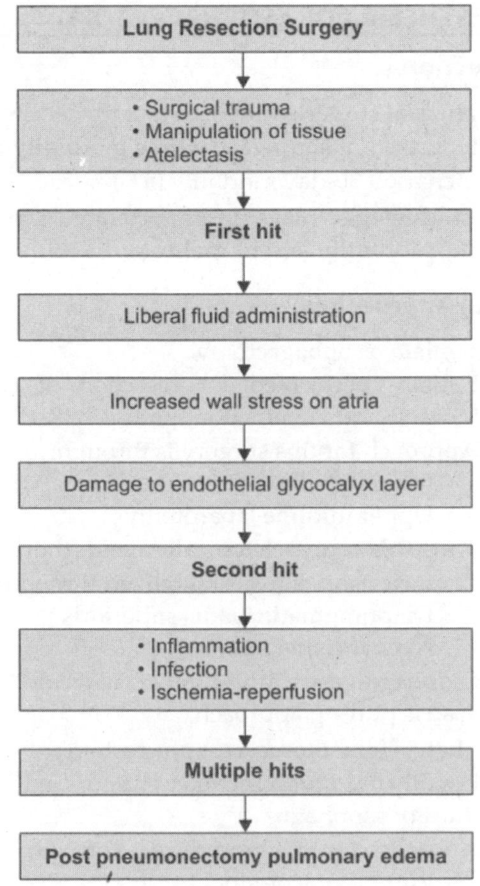

Fluid Management Strategies

- Liberal fluid management strategy:
  - Comprises the traditional fixed-volume approach to fluid therapy
  - This included administration of fluid to account for:
    - Presumed preoperative deficits
    - Intraoperative blood loss
    - Intraoperative urinary loss
    - Non-anatomical third space loss
  - It has since been established that third spaces do not exist
  - Also, crystalloids were replaced for blood loss in a 3:1 ratio
  - High volume fluid preloading is recommended prior to neuraxial techniques
  - Disadvantages:
    - Use of large volumes of crystalloid fluid
    - Increased perioperative tissue edema
    - Increased likelihood of post pneumonectomy pulmonary edema
- Restrictive fluid management strategy:
  - With this strategy, only fluid lost during surgery is replaced
  - Crystalloids are administered at a rate of 1-3 mL/kg/hour
  - Additional fluids may be administered for blood loss during surgery
  - Crystalloids are replaced for blood loss in a 1.5:1 ratio
  - Colloids are replaced in a 1:1 ratio
  - Patients do not receive preloading prior to neuraxial blockade
  - Replacement of non-anatomical third-space losses are avoided
  - Deep planes of anesthesia with BIS values < 40 are avoided
  - Advantages:
    - Decreased risk of pulmonary edema
    - Reduced hospital stay
    - Improved clinical outcomes
  - Disadvantages:
    - Increased risk of perioperative AKI
    - Increased incidence of hypovolemia and hypotension
- Goal directed fluid management strategy:
  - Fluid therapy is titrated to achieve pre-defined goals with this strategy
  - Intravascular volume status is optimized prior to initiating vasopressor therapy
  - Goals to which fluid replacement is titrated include:
    - Pulse pressure variation
    - Stroke volume variations
    - Stroke volume
    - Cardiac index
  - Advantages:
    - Lower risk of mortality
    - Reduced acute kidney injury
    - Improved clinical outcomes
    - Shorter length of hospital stay
  - Disadvantages:
    - Requires more invasive monitoring techniques
    - Variable clinical measures/endpoints

Choice of Fluids

- Ideal fluid for perioperative volume replacement is not definitively known
- Crystalloids:
  - Normal saline:
    - Causes hyperchloremic metabolic acidosis

- Volumes more than 1.5-2 L are associated with:
  - Renal injury/failure
  - Increased length of hospital stay
  - 30-day mortality
- Balanced salt solutions:
  - Includes lactated Ringers and plasmalyte
  - Associated with decreased incidence of AKI compared with NS
  - However, excessive balanced salt solutions may results in:
    - Hyperlactatemia
    - Metabolic alkalosis
    - Hypotonicity

❖ Colloids:
- Include:
  - Albumin (preferred)
  - Hydroxyethyl starch (avoided)
  - Gelatins
- Associated with:
  - Renal injury
  - Anaphylaxis, anaphylactoid reactions
  - Coagulopathy

❖ With respect to the risk of pulmonary edema (PE):
- No outcome benefits have been identified for colloids over crystalloids
- In the absence of fluid overload choice of fluid does not affect incidence of PE

❖ Thus, based on current evidence, use of crystalloids is recommended for maintenance

❖ Colloids should be reserved for active bleeding in the absence of:
- Sepsis
- Renal dysfunction
- Coagulopathy

Recommendations 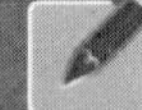

❖ *Encourage* clear fluid consumption up to 2 hours prior to the surgery
❖ Maintenance fluids at 1.5 mL/kg/hour of balanced salt solution
❖ Replacement of evaporative losses at 1 mL/kg/hour
❖ Replacement of blood loss to maintain haematocrit > 25%
❖ Restrict fluid administration in the first 24 hours to less than 2 mL/kg/hour
❖ Restrict perioperative positive fluid balance to less than 1.5 L
❖ Prefer vasopressors/ inotropes to treat:
- Anesthesia induced vasodilation
- Ongoing hypoperfusion

❖ Use goal-directed therapy for moderate- high risk patients
❖ Encourage early transition from intravenous to oral fluid therapy
❖ Lung protective mechanical ventilation strategies

ANESTHESIA FOR ESOPHAGECTOMY

Introduction

❖ Esophageal surgeries are high risk procedures with:
- Increased major perioperative morbidity (65%)
- Increased 30-day mortality (4%)

❖ Anesthesiologist plays an important role in reducing the morbidity and mortality

Surgical Approaches

❖ Trans-hiatal esophagectomy:
- Usually performed for resection of cervical, thoracic and EG junction tumors
- Approach for this surgery is through:
  - Incision in the left neck
  - Upper midline laparotomy
- Thus, this approach typically avoids thoracotomy
- Thoracic esophagus is mobilized through:
  - Diaphragmatic hiatus superiorly
  - Neck incision inferiorly
- Esophago-gastric anastomosis is created with a gastric pull-up approach

❖ Ivor-Lewis transthoracic esophagectomy:
- Usually used for resection of tumors in the lower third of esophagus
- Approach for this procedure is through:
  - Right thoracotomy
  - Upper midline laparotomy
- Esophago-gastric anastomosis is performed through thoracotomy under vision

❖ Modified Ivor-Lewis transthoracic esophagectomy:
- Usually performed for tumors of GE junction
- Performed via a single left thoracoabdominal incision
- Esophago-gastric anastomosis is completed via gastric pull-up in the left chest

❖ McKewan 3-stage procedure:
- Combines transhiatal and transthoracic approaches
- Procedure consists of 3 steps:
  - Total transthoracic esophagectomy
  - Thoracic lymphadenectomy
  - Cervical esophago-gastric anastomosis
- The procedure therefore requires 3 incisions:
  - Right posterolateral thoracotomy for en-bloc resection of esophagus
  - Upper midline laparotomy for:
    - Mobilization of stomach
    - Preparation of gastric conduit
  - Left neck exposure for esophago-gastric anastomosis

No.	Approach	Lesion	Incision
1.	***Ivor-Lewis*** Laparotomy and right thoracotomy		2 incisions: • Upper abdominal midline • Right 5th and 6th ICS thoracotomy
2.	Left thoracoabdominal (modified Ivor-Lewis)	Lower esophagus	• Right lateral thoracotomy • Extended to left upper lateral abdomen • One incision
3.	***Orringer*** Transhiatal	Lower esophagus Mid esophagus	2 incisions: • Upper abdomen midline • Left neck
4.	***McKewan 3 stage*** Combined chest neck and abdomen	Upper esophagus Mid esophagus	3 incisions: • Right thoracotomy • Laparotomy • Left cervical anastomoses
5.	Minimally invasive thoracoscopy and laparoscopy		1 or 2 incisions: • Avoids blunt dissection in chest • Neck incision in end

Anesthetic Goals

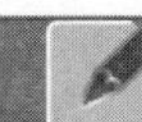

- Optimize nutritional status prior to surgery
- Minimize risk of aspiration: Rapid sequence induction preferred
- Consider one lung ventilation to improve surgical exposure for:
  - Thoracotomy
  - Minimal access thoracoscopic procedures
  - Robotic procedures
- Protective lung ventilation
- Judicious fluid administration especially when OLV is used
- Adequate postoperative pain management with:
  - Thoracic epidural analgesia
  - Paravertebral block
  - Erector spinae block

Anesthetic Considerations

- In all patients:
  - Remote airway
  - Poor preoperative nutritional status
  - Increased risk of aspiration:
    - Consider rapid sequence induction
    - Awake fiberoptic intubation used in high risk patients
  - Hypothermia due to extensive resection
  - Large intraoperative fluid shifts
  - Avoid intraoperative hypotension to prevent:
    - Gastric tube ischemia
    - Postoperative anastomotic leaks
  - Preoperative chemotherapy which reduces immunity
  - Postoperative TPN
- For transthoracic approach (Ivor-Lewis):
  - One lung ventilation
  - Thoracic epidural analgesia
  - Intra-operative ETT exchange:
    - OLV is required during thoracotomy
    - Since laparotomy may be done initially, SLT may be used initially
    - SLT may be replaced by DLT prior to thoracotomy
    - This approach is useful in patients with:
      - High risk of aspiration due to:
  - High-grade obstruction
  - Gastroparesis
      - Emergency surgeries
  - Intraoperative position change from supine/prone to right/left lateral
  - Consider early extubation and ERAS
- For trans-hiatal approach:
  - Double lung ventilation:
    - Risk of intra-operative tracheal injury is high
    - Thus, only long-length uncut ETT is used
  - Thoracic epidural analgesia
  - During surgical dissection:
    - Surgical dissection is usually blind and done via the abdominal hiatus
    - Thus, great vein and cardiac compression are common during dissection
    - This can precipitate:
      - Hypotension
      - Cardiac arrhythmias
    - Thus, volume status has to be optimized prior to dissection
    - Other complications include:
      - Pneumothorax
      - Mediastinal bleeding from injury to aorta or azygous vein
      - Injury to membranous trachea
  - Risk of massive hemorrhage necessitating emergency open thoracotomy
- For minimally invasive approach:
  - One lung ventilation with lung separation is essential

- Thoracic epidural analgesia optional as pain may be minimal
- Pneumoperitoneum causing:
  - Hypercarbia
  - Hemodynamic changes
- For robotic esophagectomy:
  - Limited access to the patient following robotic docking:
    - Secure all vascular access and confirm line patency
    - Arterial line and central venous access may require long extensions
  - Limited access to airway due to position of the robotic chassis:
    - Confirm ideal position of DLT or bronchial blocker
    - Use of newer DLTs with cameras such as VivaSight preferable
  - Risks associated with patient positioning:
    - Brachial plexus injuries
    - Robotic arm collision with patients body
  - Use of carbon dioxide to improve surgical exposure can cause:
    - Hypercarbia
    - Gas embolism
    - Bradycardia and hemodynamic compromise

Preoperative Evaluation and Optimization

- Thorough history and physical examination is important during anesthetic evaluation
- Signs and symptoms of GERD, esophageal obstruction and aspiration are to be evaluated
- Patients nutritional status should be assessed as malnutrition increases morbidity
- Comorbid conditions should be evaluated and optimized prior to surgery
- Preoperative 12-lead ECG should be taken for all patients:
  - Screens for myocardial ischemia and arrhythmias
  - Serves as a baseline for comparison in the event of complications
- Preoperative chest X-ray is important to detect:
  - Silent aspiration
  - Coexisting pulmonary/cardiac disease
- Echocardiography should be done when:
  - Suspicion of:
    - Wall motion abnormalities
    - Valvular heart diseases
  - Cardiac effects of chemoradiation
- PFTs should be done in patients undergoing thoracotomy with associated:
  - Obesity
  - COPD
- GERD prophylaxis:
  - Indicated in patients with:
    - Severe GERD
    - Risk of aspiration pneumonia
  - Drugs used include H_2-receptor antagonists and proton pump inhibitors
  - Definitive evidence of risk reduction with GERD prophylaxis is lacking
- Management of malnutrition:
  - Dietician should be consulted to optimize weight, fat and protein status
  - Restoration of protein status is important as:
    - It improves wound healing
    - Prevents infections
    - Prevents anastomotic breakdown
- Pulmonary rehabilitation is recommended as most patients are smokers:
  - Optimization with bronchodilators
  - Aggressive management of infections with antibiotics
  - Preoperative chest physiotherapy
- Bone marrow suppression:
  - Seen in patients undergoing neoadjuvant chemotherapy
  - Bone marrow suppression leads to anemia and thrombocytopenia
  - Need for preoperative optimization has to be individualized based on:
    - Risk of aspiration pneumonia
    - Urgency of surgery
  - In severe cases thrombocytopenia may preclude epidural analgesia
- *P-POSSUM score*:
  - Used for calculating the risk of perioperative mortality and morbidity
  - Parameters used in the scoring system include:
  - Physiological parameters:
    - Age
    - Cardiac signs
    - Respiratory history
    - Systolic blood pressure
    - Pulse rate
    - Glasgow coma scale
    - Hemoglobin
    - White cell count
    - Urea
    - Sodium
    - Potassium
    - ECG

- Operative parameters:
  - Operative severity
  - Multiple procedures
  - Total blood loss
  - Peritoneal soiling
  - Presence of malignancy
  - Mode of surgery

Premedication

- NPO for 6-8 hours:
  - Optimal NPO period is not known for severe gastroesophageal pathology
  - Longer fasting interval is recommended in patients with:
    - Severe gastroesophageal pathology
    - Dysmotility syndromes
    - Paraesophageal hernias
    - Esophageal diverticula
    - Achalasia cardia
- Informed consent
- 2 large-bore IV cannulae are placed as massive fluid shifts may be anticipated
- IV midazolam 1-2 mg can be administered in preoperative holding area for anxiolysis
- IV glycopyrrolate 0.01 mg/kg especially if awake intubation is planned
- Preoperative medications for GE reflux are continued on the morning of surgery
- *Anti-aspiration prophylaxis* especially for patients with symptomatic GERD:
  - IV ranitidine 1 mg/kg
  - IV metaclopramide 0.15 mg/kg
  - 30 mL of 0.3M sodium citrate 10 minutes prior to induction
- Anti-aspiration prophylaxis with sodium citrate is avoided in patients with:
  - Significant esophageal obstruction
  - Esophageal motility disorders
- Thoracic epidural may be placed in patients with no contraindications to TEA

Monitors

- Pulse oximetry
- ECG:
  - Both leads II and V_5 are continuously monitored for:
    - Myocardial ischemia
    - Arrhythmia
  - Arrhythmias are common during manipulation of mediastinal structures
- E_TCO_2, core temperature
- Urine output
- Invasive blood pressure monitoring:
  - Essential for monitoring when:
    - Transthoracic approach is planned
    - Large fluid shifts are possible intraoperatively
    - Coexisting comorbidities of CVS/ RS
  - Also, hypotension may occur during manipulation of mediastinal structures
- Central venous access:
  - Important to assess the fluid status of the patient
  - Also useful for delivery of vasoactive medications perioperatively
  - Left IJV is avoided as esophageal anastomoses may be done in left neck
- BIS, neuromuscular monitoring
- Point-of-care ABG analysis helps in maintenance of:
  - Perioperative oxygenation
  - Acid base balance
  - Blood glucose levels
  - Hemoglobin and electrolyte balance

Induction

- Adequate preoxygenation is necessary
- *Rapid sequence induction* with cricoid pressure is the preferred technique
- Induction agents are based on hemodynamic status and underlying comorbidities:
  - Thiopentone/propofol
  - Ketamine/etomidate
- Succinylcholine or rocuronium are used to facilitate RSI
- Fentanyl can be administered for analgesia at induction
- Head-end elevation to 30° is important to minimize risk of regurgitation
- Airway obstruction at induction:
  - Airway compromise may manifest in patients with:
    - Posterior and superior mediastinal masses
    - Achalasia cardia
  - Trachea is easily compressed posteriorly due to lack of cartilaginous support
  - Thus, esophageal dilatation causes near-complete tracheal occlusion
- Nasogastric tube:
  - Should be inserted at induction and is removed during resection

- Inserted prior to induction in patients at high risk of GER such as achalasia
- It is reinserted with surgical guidance following anastomoses

❖ Intubation:
- Awake intubation is planned in patients with difficult airway
- DLT with OLV is used in patients undergoing thoracotomy/thoracoscopy
- Alternatively, SLT may be inserted and BB may be used for lung separation
- FOB is used for confirmation of the DLT and BB
- In case of SLT, BB may be used for OLV when:
  - Unexpected change in surgical plan to include thoracotomy
  - Inadvertent injury to trachea during surgery

Maintenance

❖ GA may be maintained using balanced anesthesia techniques/TIVA

❖ Use of TIVA may offer additional immunological techniques due to:
- Anti-inflammatory and anti-oxidant properties of propofol
- Ability to preserve natural killer cell function

❖ NMBAS are used to aid surgical exposure and prevent diaphragmatic movement

❖ Thoracic epidural may be activated to augment intraoperative analgesia

Ventilation

❖ One lung ventilation during thoracotomy

❖ Left sided DLT is usually preferred to ensure lung separation

❖ Goals of OLV:
- Minimal FiO_2 to maintain $SpO_2 > 92\%$
- Tidal volume 6-7 mL/kg
- Respiratory rate 12-20 cycles/min
- E_TCO_2 32-38 mm Hg
- Peak airway pressure < 35 cm H_2O

❖ DLT may be changed to SLT to improve surgical access prior to cervical anastomoses

Hemodynamics

❖ Preoperative fluid deficits may be substantial in these patients due to:
- Poor preoperative intake
- Prolonged fasting intervals

❖ Restrictive fluid strategy is usually preferred especially when OLV is used

❖ Cardiac compression may occur during surgical mobilization causing hypotension

❖ Causes of intraoperative hypotension include:
- Compression of IVC and other intrathoracic vessels
- Blood loss
- Arrhythmias

❖ Persistent hypotension in the presence of euvolemia necessitates inotropic therapy

❖ Fluid challenge test may be used to aid clinical decision-making regarding inotropes

❖ Colloids and PRBCS may be used to replace blood loss depending upon hematocrit

❖ Sudden, torrential hemorrhage is possible and therefore blood should be kept ready

❖ Avoid hypothermia:
- Fluid warmer
- Forced air blankets

❖ Vasopressors may be avoided during surgery as:
- They are associated with vasoconstriction of blood vessels in gastric tube
- This may lead to poor tissue perfusion at the anastomotic site
- This may contribute to postoperative anastomotic leaks

Extubation

❖ Early extubation is preferred when extubation criteria are met:
- Patient is fully conscious
- Able to maintain ventilation and oxygenation
- Adequate muscle strength
- Stable hemodynamics
- Minimal risk of aspiration

❖ Head up tilt of 30° is recommended during extubation to minimize aspiration

❖ If postoperative ventilation is planned, DLT is replaced with SLT

❖ Postoperative ventilation if cold or hemodynamically unstable

Postoperative Management

Management

❖ Enteral feeding with jejunostomy/nasoduodenal tube is initiated after 24 hours

❖ Total parenteral nutrition

❖ Early ambulation and chest physiotherapy to avoid pulmonary complications

- Pleural drains may be removed once drainage is minimal
- Mediastinal drains are left until anastomotic integrity is confirmed
- Contrast study of esophagus is performed prior to initiation of oral feeds

Analgesia

- Multimodal analgesia
- Thoracic epidural analgesia:
  - Is the gold standard for postoperative analgesia
  - Drugs used for thoracic epidurals include a mixture of:
    - 0.1% bupivacaine
    - Fentanyl 5 µg/mL
    - Epinephrine 2 µg/mL
  - This mixture is administered at a rate of 5-8 mL/hour
  - Epidural catheters are left in-situ until removal of pleural drains
- Regional blocks:
  - Paravertebral blocks: Analgesic efficacy comparable with TEA
  - Intercostal nerve blocks used in combination with PCA
  - Erector spinae block
- *Patient Controlled Analgesia* with morphine
- NSAIDs

Complications

- Intraoperative complications:
  - Perioperative arrhythmias (especially atrial fibrillation)
  - Hypotension
  - Trauma to major blood vessels
  - Inadvertent injury to trachea during surgery
  - Tension pneumothorax due to inadvertent disruption of pleural layer
- Postoperative complications:
  - Pulmonary complications:
    - Atelectasis
    - Respiratory failure
    - Pneumonia, sepsis
  - Recurrent laryngeal nerve injury
- Leakage and rupture of esophageal anastomosis

SUGGESTED READING

1. Aboussouan, L. S. and Stoller, J. K. (1994). Diagnosis and management of upper airway obstruction. *Clinical Chest Medicine*, 15(1), 35–53.
2. Ahmed-Nusrath, A. and Swanevelder, J. (2007). Anesthesia for mediastinoscopy. *Continuing Education in Anaesthesia Critical Care & Pain*, 7(1), 6–9.
3. Aitkenhead A., Thompson, J., Rowbotham, D. and Moppett, I. (2013). *Smith and Aitkenhead's Textbook of Anaesthesia*. 6th ed. London: Churchill Livingstone Elsevier.
4. Al-Shaikh, B. and Stacey, S. (2019). *Essentials of Equipment in Anaesthesia, Critical Care and Perioperative Medicine*. 5th ed. London: Elsevier.
5. Amizuka, T., Shimizu, H., Niida, Y. and Ogawa, Y. (2003). Surfactant therapy in neonates with respiratory failure due to hemorrhagic pulmonary edema. *European Journal of Pediatrics*, 162(10), 697–702.
6. Arslantas, M. K. et al., (2015). Effect of the amount of intraoperative fluid administration on postoperative pulmonary complications following anatomic lung resections. *Journal of Thoracic and Cardiovascular Surgery*, 149(1), 314–20.
7. Atkinson, S. and Fox, S. B. (2004). Vascular endothelial growth factor (VEGF)-A and platelet derived growth factor play a central role in the pathogenesis of digital clubbing. *Journal of Pathology*, 203(2), 721–8.
8. Attar, A.S., Taghaddomi, R. J. and Bagheri, R. (2013). Anesthetic management of patients with anterior mediastinal masses undergoing Chamberlain procedure. *Iranian Red Crescent Medical Journal*, 15(4), 373–4.
9. Aveyard, P. and Lindson-Hawley, N. (2014). Should smokers be advised to cut down as well as quit? *British Medical Journal*, 348, f7535.
10. Aziz, M. F., Bayman, E. O., Van Tienderen, M. M., Todd, M. M., StAGE Investigator Group and Brambrink, A. M. (2016). Predictors of difficult videolaryngoscopy with GlideScope or C-MAC with D-blade: secondary analysis from a large comparative videolaryngoscopy trial. *British Journal of Anaesthesia*, 117(1), 118–23.
11. Barash, P. G. et al., (2017). *Clinical Anesthesia*. 8th ed. Philadelphia: Wolters Kluwer.
12. Barrett, K. E., Barman, S. M., Boitano, S. and Brooks, H. (2012). *Ganong's Review of Medical Physiology*. 24th ed. New York: McGraw Hill Lange.
13. Baughman, R. P. (2007). Technical aspects of a bronchoalveolar lavage: recommendations for a standard procedure. *Seminars in Respiratory and Critical Care Medicine*, 28(5), 475–85.
14. Bechard, P., Letourneau, L., Lacasse, Y., Cote, D. and Bussieres, J. S. (2004). Perioperative cardiorespiratory complications in adults with mediastinal mass. *Anesthesiology*, 100(4), 826–34.
15. Biere, S. S. A. Y. et al., (2012). Minimally invasive versus open esophagectomy for patients with esophageal cancer: a multicentre open labelled randomized controlled trial. *Lancet*, 379(9829), 1887–92.
16. Boer, F. (2003). Drug handling by the lung. *British Journal of Anaesthesia*. 91(1), 50–60.
17. Brandstrup, B. (2018). Finding the right balance. *New England Journal of Medicine*, 378, 2335–6.
18. Brister, N. W., Barnette, R. E., Kim, V. and Keresztury, M. (2008). Anesthetic considerations in candidates for lung volume reduction surgery. *Proceedings of the American Thoracic Society*, 5(4), 432–7.

19. Brodsky, J. B. and Lemmens, H. J. (2003). Left double lumen tubes: clinical experience with 1170 patients. *Journal of Cardiothoracic and Vascular Anesthesia*, 17(3), 289–98.
20. Brown, T. (2012). *Rapid Review Physiology*. 2nd ed. Philadelphia: Elsevier.
21. Bussieres, J. S. (2016). Bronchial blocker versus left double-lumen endotracheal tube in video-assisted thoracoscopic surgery: a randomized-controlled trial examining time and quality of lung deflation. *Canadian Journal of Anesthesia*, 63(7), 818–27.
22. Butterworth, J., Mackey, D. and Wasnick. J. (2018). *Morgan and Mikhail's Clinical Anesthesiology*. 6th ed. New York: Lange.
23. Canet, J. et al., (2010). Prediction of postoperative pulmonary complications in a population-based surgical cohort. *Anesthesiology*, 113(6), 1338–50.
24. Cattaneo, S. M. et al., (2008). Use of video-assisted thoracic surgery for lobectomy in elderly patients results in fewer complications. *Annals of Thoracic Surgery*, 85(1), 231–6.
25. Celli, B. R. et al., (2004). The body-mass index, airflow obstruction, dyspnea, and exercise capacity index in chronic obstructive pulmonary disease. *New England Journal of Medicine*, 3501(10), 1005–12.
26. Chandrashekhar Shelgaonkar, V., Sonowal, J., Badwaik, M. K., Manjrekar, S. P. and Pawar, M. (2015). A study of prediction of difficult intubation using Mallampatsi and Wilson score correlating with Cormack Lehane grading. *Journal of Evidence Based Medicine and Healthcare*, 23(2), 3458–66.
27. Chang, D. W. (2014). *Clinical Application of Mechanical Ventilation*. 4th ed. Boston: Delmar Cengage Learning.
28. Chu, D. K. et al., (2018). Mortality and morbidity in acutely ill adults treated with liberal versus conservative oxygen therapy (IOTA): a systematic review and meta-analysis. *Lancet*, 291(10131), 1693–705.
29. Committee on Fetus and Newborn and American Academy of Pediatrics. (2014). Respiratory support in preterm infants at birth. *Pediatrics*, 133(1), 171–4.
30. Crawley, S. M. and Dalton, A. J. (2015). Predicting the difficult airway. *British Journal of Anaesthesia Education*, 15(5), 253–7.
31. CureNeb Study Team, Minocchieri, S., Berry, C. A. and Pillow, J. J. (2019). Nebulised surfactant to reduce the severity of RDS: a blinded, parallel, randomised controlled trial. *Archives of Disease in Childhood, Fetal & Neonatal Edition*, 104(3), F313–9.
32. Cutz, E., Yeger, H., Pie, J. and Ito, T. (2008). Pulmonary neuroendocrine cell system in health and disease. *Current Respiratory Medicine Reviews*, 4(3), 174–86.
33. da Silva Sardenberg, R. A., Younes, R. N. and Deheizelin, D. (2010). Lung volume reduction surgery: an overview. Revista da Associacao Medica Brasiliera, 56(6). [Viewed 20 May 2020] Available from: https://doi.org/10.1590/S0104-42302010000600025
34. Davey, A. and Diba, A. (2012). *Ward's Anesthetic Equipment*. 6th ed. Philadelphia: Saunders Elsevier.
35. de Lima, A., Kheir, F., Majid, A. and Pawlokski, J. (2018). Anesthesia for interventional pulmonology procedures: a review of advanced diagnostic and therapeutic bronchoscopy. *Canadian Journal of Anesthesia*, 65(7), 822–36.
36. Dhingra, P. L. (2017). *Diseases of Ear, Nose and Throat*. 7th ed. Gurgaon: Elsevier.
37. Dorsch, J. A. and Dorsch, S. E. (2008). *Understanding Anesthesia Equipment*. 5th ed. Philadelphia: Wolters Kluwer.
38. Dunn, J.-O. C. and Grocott, M. P. (2016). Physiology of oxygen transport. *British Journal of Anaesthesia Education*, 16(10), 341–8.
39. Eberhart, L. H. J., Arndt, C., Cierpka, T., Schwanekamp, J., Wulf, H. and Putzke, C. (2005). The reliability and validity of upper lip bite test compared with the Mallampati classification to predict difficult laryngoscopy: an external prospective evaluation. *Anesthesia & Analgesia*, 101(1), 284–9.
40. Elayaperumal, A. K. and Jackson, R. E. (2018). Anesthesia for lung volume reduction surgery and endobronchial valves. *British Journal of Anaesthesia Education*, 18, 193–8.
41. Elston, W. J., et al., (2004). Safety of research bronchoscopy, biopsy and bronchoalveolar lavage in asthma. *European Respiratory Journal*, 24, 375–7.
42. Erdos, G. and Tzanova, I. (2009). Perioperative anesthetic management of mediastinal mass in adults. *European Journal of Anaesthesiology*, 26(8), 627–32.
43. Fessler, H. E., Schwarf, S. M., Ingenito, E. P., McKenna Jr, R. J. and Sharafkhaneh, A. (2008). Physiological basis for improved pulmonary function after lung volume reduction. *Proceedings of the American Thoracic Society*, 5(4), 416–20.
44. Flood, P., Rathmell, J. P. and Shafer, S. (2015). *Stoelting's Pharmacology & Physiology in Anesthetic Practice*. 5th ed. Philadelphia: Wolters Kluwer.
45. Gehlbach, J. A., Rehder, K. J., Gentile, M. A., Turner, D. A., Grady, D. J. and Cheifetz, I. M. (2017). Intravenous oxygen: a novel method of oxygen delivery in hypoxemic respiratory failure? *Expert Review of Respiratory Medicine*, 11(1), 73–80.
46. GOLD. (2018). Pocket guide to COPD diagnosis, management, and prevention: 2018 report. [Viewed 19 May 2020] Available from: https://goldcopd.org/wp-content/uploads/2018/02/WMS-GOLD-2018-Feb-Final-to-print-v2.pdf.
47. Gonzalez-Rivas, D., Fierira, E. Delgado, M., Mendez, L., Fernandez, R. and de la Torre, M. (2014). Evolving from conventional video-assisted thoracoscopic lobectomy to uniportal: the story behind the evolution. *Journal of Thoracic Disease*, 6(Suppl 6), S599–603.
48. Gopel, W. et al., (2011). Avoidance of mechanical ventilation by surfactant treatment of spontaneously breathing preterm infants (AMV): an open-label, randomized, controlled trial. *Lancet*, 378(9803), 1627–34.
49. Gropper, M., Eriksson, L., Fleisher, L., Wiener-Kronish, J., Cohen, N. and Leslie, K. (eds.) (2020). *Miller's Anesthesia*. 9th ed. Philadelphia: Elsevier Saunders.
50. Grønkjær, M. et al., (2014). Preoperative smoking status and postoperative complications: a systematic review and meta-analysis. *Annals of Surgery*, 259(1):52–71.
51. Gu, W.-J., Wang, F. and Liu, J.-C. (2015). Effect of lung-protective ventilation with lower tidal volumes on clinical outcomes among patients undergoing surgery: a meta-analysis of randomized controlled trials. *Canadian Medical Association Journal*, 187(3), e101–9.

52. Hackett, S., Jones, R. and Kapila, R. (2019). Anesthesia for pneumonectomy. *British Journal of Anaesthesia*, 19(9), 297–304.
53. Hagberg, C. (2013). *Benumof and Hagberg's Airway Management*. 3rd ed. Philadelphia: Elsevier Saunders.
54. Hall, J. E. (2016). *Guyton and Hall Textbook of Medical Physiology*. 13th ed. Philadelphia: Elsevier.
55. Hammound, Z. T. (1999). The current role of mediastinoscopy in the evaluation of thoracic disease. *Journal of Cardiovascular Surgery*, 118(5), 894–9.
56. Han, R., Tremper, K. K., Kheterpal, S. and O'Reilly, M. (2004). Grading scale for mask ventilation. *Anesthesiology*, 101(1), 267.
57. Hartigan, P. M., Ng, J.-M. and Gill, R. R. (2018). Anesthesia in a patient with a large mediastinal mass. *New England Journal of Medicine*, 379(6), 587–8.
58. Hausman Jr, M. S., Jewell, E. S. and Engoren, M. (2015). Regional versus general anesthesia in surgical patients with chronic obstructive pulmonary disease: does avoiding general anesthesia reduce the risk of postoperative complications? *Anesthesia & Analgesia*, 120(6), 1405–12.
59. Herting, E. et al., (2000). Surfactant treatment of neonates with respiratory failure and group B streptococcal infection. *Pediatrics*, 106(5), 957–64.
60. Hillier, J. and Gillbe, C. (2003). Anesthesia for lung volume reduction surgery. *Anaesthesia*, 58(12), 1210–9.
61. Hines, R. (ed.) (2017). *Stoelting's Anesthesia and Co-existing Disease*. 7th ed. Philadelphia: Elsevier.
62. Imperatori, A. et al., (2008). Perioperative complications of video-assisted thoracoscopic surgery. *International Journal of Surgery*, 6(Suppl 1), S78–81.
63. Isaacs, R.S. and Sykes, J. M. (2002). Anatomy and physiology of the upper airway. *Anesthesiology Clinics of North America*, 20(4), 733–45.
64. Jaffe, R. A., Schmlesing, C. A. and Gollanu, B. (2009). *Anesthesiologist's Manual of Surgical Procedures*. Baltimore: Lippincott Williams Wilkins.
65. Janssens, M. and Hartstein, G. (2001). Management of difficult intubation. *European Journal of Anaesthesiology*, 18(1), 3–12.
66. Joseph, D., Puttaswamy, R. K. and Krovvidi, H. (2013). Non-respiratory functions of the lung. *Continuing Education in Anaesthesia Critical Care & Pain*, 13(3), 98–102.
67. Kacmarek, R., Stoller, J. and Huer, A. (2017). *Egan's Fundamentals of Respiratory Care*. 11th ed. St Louis: Elsevier.
68. Kam, P. and Power, I. (2015). *Principles of Physiology for the Anaesthetist*. 2nd ed. Boca Raton, FL: CRC Press.
69. Kiefer, T. (2017). *Chest Drains in Daily Clinical Practice*. Konstanz: Springer.
70. Konstantinos Katsoulis, T., Kostikas, K. and Kontakiotis T. (2016). Techniques for assessing small airways function: possible applications in asthma and COPD. *Respiratory Medicine*, 119, e2-e9.
71. Kreit, J. W. (2018). *Mechanical Ventilation: Physiology and Practice*. 2nd ed. Oxford: Oxford University Press.
72. Lacaze-Masmonteil, T. (2003). Exogenous surfactant therapy: newer developments. *Seminars in Neonatology*, 8(6), 433–40.
73. Landsberg, J. (2018). *Manual for Pulmonary and Critical Care Medicine*. 1st ed. Philadelphia: Elsevier.
74. Langeron, O. et al., (2000). Prediction of difficult mask ventilation. *Anesthesiology*, 92(5), 1229–36.
75. Larry Jameson, L., Fauci, A. S., Kasper, D. L., Hauser, S. L., Longo, D. L. and Loscalzo J. (2018). *Harrison's Principles of Internal Medicine*. 20th ed. New York: McGraw Hill.
76. Lim, B. E. (2010). Guidelines on the radical management of patients with lung cancer. *Thorax*, 65(Suppl 3), iii1–27.
77. Longnecker, D. E., Mackey, S. C., Newman, M. F., Sandberg, W. S. and Zapol, W. M. (2017). *Anesthesiology*. 3rd ed. New York: McGraw Hill Education.
78. Lumb, A. B., (2017). *Nunn's Applied Respiratory Physiology*. 9th ed. London: Elsevier.
79. Lumb, A. B. and Slinger, P. (2015). Hypoxic pulmonary vasoconstriction: physiology and anesthetic implications. *Anesthesiology*, 122(4), 932–46.
80. Martinez, F. J. (2005). Surgical therapy for chronic obstructive pulmonary disease. *Seminars in Respiratory and Critical Care Medicine*, 26(2), 167–91.
81. Maturana, A. Torres-Pereyra, J., Salinas, R., Astudillo, P., Moya, F. R. and The Chile Surf Group. (2005). A randomized trial of natural surfactant for moderate-severe meconium aspiration syndrome. *Pediatric Academic Societies*, 57, 1545.
82. McCall, P., Steven, M. and Shelley, B. (2019). Anesthesia for video-assisted and robotic thoracic surgery. *British Journal of Anaesthesia Education*, 19(12), 405–11.
83. McFadden, E. R. (1992). Heat and moisture exchange in human airways. *American Review of Respiratory Disease*, 146(5 Pt 2), S8–10.
84. McGrath, B., Tennuci, C. and Lee, G. (2017). The history of one lung anesthesia and the double-lumen tube. *Journal of Anesthesia History*, 3(3), 76–88.
85. McQuillan, P. M., Allman, K. G. and Wilson, I. H. (2007). *Oxford American Handbook of Anesthesiology*. 2nd ed. Oxford: Oxford Medical Publications.
86. Meyer, K. C. et al., (2012). An official American Thoracic Society clinical practice guideline: the clinical utility of bronchoalveolar lavage cellular analysis in interstitial lung disease. *American Journal of Respiratory and Critical Care Medicine*, 185(9), 1004–14.
87. Miller, T. E. and Myles, P. S. (2019). Perioperative fluid therapy for major surgery. *Anesthesiology*, 130, 825–32.
88. Miller, T. E. and Myles, P. S. (2019). Perioperative fluid therapy for major surgery. *Anesthesiology*, 130, 825–32.
89. Modolo, N. S. P. et al., (2013). Intravenous versus inhalation anesthesia for one-lung ventilation. *Cochrane Database Systematic Reviews*, 2013(7), CD006313.
90. Murray, M. J., Harrison, B. A., Mueller, J. T., Rose, S. H., Wass, C. T. and Wedel, W. J. (2015). *Faust's Anesthesiology Review*. 4th ed. Philadelphia: Elsevier.
91. Nagahiro, I., Aoe, M., Date, H., Andou, A. and Shimizu, N. (2007). Bronchopleural fistula after lobectomy for lung cancer. *Asian Cardiovascular and Thoracic Annals*, 15(1), 45–8.
92. Naunheim, K. S. et al., (2006). Predictors of operative mortality and cardiopulmonary morbidity in the National Emphysema Treatment Trial. *Journal of Thoracic and Cardiovascular Surgery*, 131(1), 43–53.
93. Nausheen F. et al., (2019). The HEAVEN criteria predicts laryngoscopic view and intubation success for both direct

and video laryngoscopy: a cohort analysis. *Scandinavian Journal of Medicine*, 27(1), 50.

94. Okuda, M., Go, T. and Yokomise, H. (2017). Risk factor of bronchopleural fistula after general thoracic surgery: review article. *General Thoracic and Cardiovascular Surgery*, 65, 679–85.
95. Ozcan, P. E. et al., (2007). Effects of thoracic epidural anesthesia on pulmonary venous admixture and oxygenation during one-lung ventilation. *Acta Anaesthesiologica Scandinavica*, 51(8), 1117–22.
96. Patton, J. S., Fishburn, C. S. and Weers, J. G. (2004). The lungs as a portal of entry for systemic drug delivery. *Proceedings of the American Thoracic Society*, 1(4), 338–44.
97. Pavel C. R., Morris, M. J., Nicholson, K. L. and Haues, J. A. (2008). Inspiratory flow volume loops and the diagnosis of upper airway obstruction. *Clinical Pulmonary Medicine*, 15(5), 274–82.
98. Pellegrino, R. et al., (2005). Interpretative strategies for lung function tests. *European Respiratory Journal*, 26(5), 948–68.
99. Pfister, R. H. (2012). Initial respiratory support of preterm infants: the role of CPAP, the INSURE method, and noninvasive ventilation. *Clinical Perinatology*, 39(3), 459–81.
100. Pierre, S, et al., (2017). Guidelines on smoking management during the perioperative period. *Anaesthesia Critical Care & Pain Medicine*, 36(3), 195–200.
101. Pinheiro, J. M. B., Santana-Rivas, Q. and Pezzano, C. (2016). Randomized trial of laryngeal mask airway versus endotracheal tube for surfactant delivery. *Journal of Perinatology*, 36(3), 196–201.
102. Polin, R. A., Carlo, W. A. and Committee on Fetus and Newborn and American Academy of Pediatrics. (2014). Surfactant replacement therapy for preterm and term neonates with respiratory distress. *Pediatrics*, 133(1), 156–63.
103. Rajaram, S. (2015). *Critical Care Procedure Book*. New York: Nova Biomedical.
104. Ramachandran, S. K., Mathis, M. R., Tremper, K. K., Shanks, A. M. and Kheterpal, S. (2012). Predictors and clinical outcomes from failed Laryngeal Mask Airway UniqueTM: a study of 15,795 patients. *Anesthesiology*, 116(6), 1217–26.
105. Ranu, H., Wilde, M. and Madden, B. (2011). Pulmonary function tests. *Ulster Medicine Tests*, 80(2), 84–90.
106. Raphael, J., Regali, L. A. and Thiele, R. H. (2017). Hemodynamic monitoring in thoracic surgical patients. *Current Opinion in Anesthesiology*, 30(1), 7–16.
107. Rath, L., Gullahorn, G., Connolly, N., Pratt, T., Boswell, G. and Cornelissen, C. (2012). Anterior mediastinal mass biopsy and resection: anesthetic techniques and perioperative concerns. *Seminars in Cardiothoracic and Vascular Anesthesia*, 16(4), 235–42.
108. Rau, B., Hunerbein M., Below, C. and Schlag, P. M. (1998). Video-assisted thoracic surgery: staging and management of thoracic tumours. *Surgical Endoscopy*, 12(2), 133–6.
109. Reed, M. J., Dunn, M. J. G. and McKeown, D. W. (2005). Can an airway assessment score predict difficulty at intubation in the emergency department. *Emergency Medicine Journal*, 22(2), 99–102.
110. Rigotti, N. A. (2002). Clinical practice: treatment of tobacco use and dependence. *The New England Journal of Medicine*, 346(7), 506–12.
111. Roberts, J. T. (1990). Functional anatomy of the larynx. *International Anesthesiology Clinics*, 28(2), 101–5.
112. Scott Harris, R. (2005). Pressure-volume curves of the respiratory system. *Respiratory Care*, 50(1), 78–99.
113. Seekell, R. P. et al., (2016). Oxygen delivery using engineered microparticles. *Proceedings of the National Academy of Sciences of the USA*, 113(44), 12380–5.
114. Senturk, M., Orhan Sunger, M. and Sungur, Z. (2017). Fluid management in thoracic anesthesia. *Minerva Anestesiologica*, 83(6), 652–9.
115. Shin, C. H. et al., (2018). Effects of intraoperative fluid management on postoperative outcomes: a hospital registry study. *Annals of Surgery*, 267(6), 1084–92.
116. Siemieniuk, R. A. C. et al., (2018). Oxygen therapy for acutely ill medical patients: a clinical practice guidelines. *British Medical Journal*, 363, k4169.
117. Slinger, P. (2009). Update on the anesthetic management for pneumonectomy. *Current Opinion in Anesthesiology*, 22(1), 31–7.
118. Slinger, P. (ed.) (2019). *Principles and Practice of Anesthesia for Thoracic Surgery*. 2nd ed. Toronto: Springer.
119. Slinger, P. and Karsli, C. (2007). Management of the patient with a large anterior mediastinal mass: recurring myths. *Current Opinion in Anesthesiology*, 20(1), 1–3.
120. Smetana, G. W. (1999). Preoperative pulmonary evaluation. *New England Journal of Medicine*, 340(12), 937–44.
121. Smith, T., Pinnock, C., Lin, T. and Jones, R. (eds.) (2006). *Fundamentals of Anaesthesia*. 3rd ed. Cambridge: Cambridge University Press.
122. Solaini, L., Prusciano, F., Bagioni, P., di Francesco, F., Solaini, L. and Poddie, D. B. (2008). Video-assisted thoracic surgery of the lung: analysis of intraoperative and postoperative complications over 15 years and review of literature. *Surgical Endoscopy*, 22(2), 298–310.
123. Sterner, J. B., Morris, M. J., Sill, J. M. and Hayes, J. A. (2009). Inspiratory flow-volume curve evaluation for detecting upper airway disease. *Respiratory Care*, 54(4), 461–6.
124. Suresh, G. K. and Soll, R. F. (2005). Overview of surfactant replacement trials. *Journal of Perinatology*, 25, S40–4.
125. Sweet, D. G. et al., (2019). European Consensus Guidelines on the Management of Respiratory Distress Syndrome: 2019 update. *Neonatology*, 115(4), 432–50.
126. Talbot, N. P. Balanos, G. M., Dorrington, K. L. and Robbins, P. A. (2005). Two temporal components within the human pulmonary vascular response to 2 hours of isocapnic hypoxia. *Journal of Applied Physiology*, 98(3), 1125–39.
127. Tan, Z., Tan, K. T. J. and Poopalalingam, R. (2016). Anesthetic management for whole lung lavage in patients with pulmonary alveolar proteinosis. *A & A Case Reports*, 6(8), 234–7.
128. Tarry, D. and Powell, M. (2017). Hypoxic pulmonary vasoconstriction. *British Journal of Anaesthesia Education*, 17(6), 208–13.
129. Theadom, A. and Cropley, M. (2006). Effects of preoperative smoking cessation on incidence and risk of intraoperative and postoperative complications in adult smokers: a systematic review. *Tobacco Control*, 15(5), 352–8.

130. Treacher, D. F. and Leach, R. M. (1998). Oxygen transport—1. Basic principles. *British Medical Journal*, 317(7168), 1302–6.
131. Tucker, H. M. and Harvey, M. (1993). *The Larynx*. 2nd ed. New York: Thieme Medical.
132. Varoli, F., Roviaro, G., Grignani, G. Vergani, C. Maciocco, M. and Rebuffat, C. (1998). Endoscopic treatment of bronchopleural fistulas. *Annals of Thoracic Surgery*, 65(3), 807–9.
133. Veelo, D. P. and Geerts, B. F. (2017). Anesthesia during esophagectomy. *Journal of Thoracic Disease*, v.9(Suppl 8), S705–12.
134. Vincent, J.-L. and Moore, F. (eds.) (2017). *Textbook of Critical Care*. 7th ed. Philadelphia: Elsevier.
135. Vlahu, T. and Vigneswaran, W. T. (2017). Pleurectomy and decortication. *Annals of Translational Medicine*. 5(11), 246.
136. West, J. B. (2012). *Respiratory Physiology: The Essentials*. 9th ed. Baltimore: Wolters Kluwer.
137. Wigmore, T. J., Mohammed, K. and Jhanji, S. (2016). Long term survival for patients undergoing volatile versus IV anesthesia for cancer surgery: a retrospective analysis. *Anesthesiology*, 124(1), 69–79.
138. Wilde, M., Nair, S. and Madden, B. (2007). Pulmonary function tests-a review. *Care of The Critically Ill*, 23(6), 173–7.
139. Yang, M. et al., (2011). Does a protective ventilation strategy reduce the risk of pulmonary complications after lung cancer surgery? A randomized controlled trial. *Chest*, 139(3), 530–7.
140. Yao, S., Mao, T., Fang, W., Xu, M. and Chen, W. (2013). Incidence and risk factors for acute lung injury after open thoracotomy for thoracic diseases. *Journal of Thoracic Disease*, 5(4), 455–60.
141. Yentis, S. M. and Lee, D. J. (1998). Evaluation of an improved scoring system for the grading of direct laryngoscopy. *Anesthesia*, 53(11), 1041–4.
142. Yoneda, K. Y. and Shelton, L. S. (2001). Mediastinal tumors. *Current Opinion in Pulmonary Medicine*, 7(4), 226–33.

5 CHAPTER

Anesthesia for Endocrine Disorders

ACROMEGALY

Introduction

Clinical syndrome which occurs due to overproduction of growth hormone (GH) from anterior pituitary, causing overgrowth of bone, connective tissue and viscera.

Etiology

- Pituitary adenomas (90%)
- Extrapituitary tumors:
  - Hypothalamic hamartoma, choristoma, ganglioneuroma
  - Medullary carcinoma of thyroid
  - Bronchial carcinoid
  - Small cell lung cancer
  - Pancreatic islet cell tumor
  - Adrenal adenoma
  - Pheochromocytoma
- Iatrogenic: Use of recombinant GH to prevent ageing

Clinical Features

- Neuromuscular:
  - Visual field defects
  - Proximal myopathy
  - Nerve entrapment syndrome (Carpal Tunnel syndrome, ulnar artery compromise)
  - Kyphoscoliosis
- Cardiovascular: Major cause of mortality and morbidity
  - Hypertension
  - Cardiomegaly, LV hypertrophy, diastolic dysfunction
  - CAD, congestive cardiac failure
  - Arrhythmias: SVT/PVCs on stress/exercise
  - Valvular abnormalities
  - Cardiomyopathy
- Respiratory system:
  - Somnolence, central and obstructive sleep apnea (60% patients)
  - Deep and hollow voice
  - Hoarseness of voice due to:
    - Vocal cord thickening
    - Recurrent laryngeal nerve palsy due to stretching
  - Dyspnea/stridor due to subglottic narrowing
  - Increased lung volumes
  - Ventilation–perfection mismatch
- Endocrines:
  - Impaired glucose tolerance
  - Diabetes mellitus (25% patients)
  - Hypo/hyperthyroidism
  - Hypopituitarism (due to tumor compressing pituitary gland)
  - Hypercalcemia, hypercaliciuria
  - Diabetes insipidus
- Gastrointestinal:
  - Colonic polyps
  - Colon carcinoma
- Skin:
  - Acanthosis nigricans
  - Hyperhydrosis, oily skin
  - Skin tags
- Soft tissue:
  - Increased heel pad thickness
  - Coarse facial features
  - Large, fleshy, nose
  - Carpal Tunnel syndrome
  - Increased pharyngeal and laryngeal soft tissues, macroglossia, enlarged epiglottis
- Musculoskeletal:
  - Frontal bossing
  - Increased space between lower incisors
  - Macrognathia, prognathism
  - Increased size of feet and hands
  - Arthropathy
- Due to parasellar extension:
  - Headache
  - Visual field defects
  - Rhinorrhea

Pathogenesis

- Hyerptension occurs due to:
  - Prolonged OSAS
  - Antinatriuretic effect of GH: Stimulates renin angiotensin increases blood volume
  - Positive inotropic effect of IGF – I
- LVH occurs due to interstitial fibrosis

Investigations

- Complete blood count urea, serum creatinine, thyroid profile, blood sugar
- Electrolytes and serum calcium, baseline ABG
- Preoperative direct laryngoscopy for:
  - Subglottic stenosis
  - Enlarged tongue and mandible
  - Enlarged epiglottis and vocal cords: Reduced-laryngeal aperture
- Indirect laryngoscopy for vocal cord involvement
- Chest X-ray
- ECG: SVT/PVC, bundle branch block, ST-T wave changes, LVH
- Echocardiography:
  - Left ventricular hypertrophy
  - Ejection fraction
  - Regional wall motion abnormalities
  - Diastolic dysfunction
- Lateral X-ray/CT scan of neck
  - For pharyngeal tissue overgrowth
  - Glottic involvement
- CT/MRI for suprasellar enlargement and enlarged sellaturcica
- Diagnostic:
  - Increased IGF_1 levels
  - Random GH level > 5 ng/mL
  - Glucose tolerance test:
    - 75 gms anhydrous glucose given orally
    - Failure of GH level to fall below 1 μg/L within 1–2 hours of glucose challenge is *confirmatory*

Treatment

- Medical management:
  - Uses:
    - Preoperative shrinkage of large adenomas
    - Relief of symptoms
    - Reduction of GH levels
  - Indications:
    - Elderly patients with increased morbidity
    - Patients who decline surgery
    - Failure of surgery to achieve biochemical control
  - Drugs used are:
    - Bromocriptine:
      - Reduces GH levels by decreasing secretion
      - More than 20 mg/day given in 3–4 divided doses
      - Not favourable for long term use
    - Octreotide:
      - Somatostatin analogue
      - 50 mg subcutaneous TID increased up to 1500 μg/day
      - Depot preparation 30 mg IM once a month can be used
      - Provides good palliation in 50% patients
    - *Pegvisomant*:
      - Growth hormone analogue
      - Binds to GH receptor and prevents GH action
      - Withdraw GH if being used
  - Symptomatic therapy for Carpal Tunnel syndrome and other manifestations
- Radiotherapy:
  - Sterotactic ablation of adenoma by gamma knife radiotherapy useful
  - Can be given if complete removal of tumor by surgery is not possible
  - Disadvantages:
    - High rate of late hypopituitarism
    - Slow rate of biochemical response (5–15 years)
    - Ineffective in normalizing IGF levels
    - External pituitary radiation used commonly
- Surgery:
  - Transphenoidal and resection is *treatment of choice*
  - Transfrontal hypophysectomy used if suprasellar extension
  - Advantages:
    - Soft tissue swelling improves immediately
    - GH levels normalize within 1 hour
    - IGF-I levels normalize within 3–4 days
    - LV size usually returns to normal
    - Failure for LV to do so may indicate persistent interstitial fibrosis

PREOPERATIVE ASSESSMENT

- History:
  - Chest pain, dyspnea on exertion
  - Numbness, polydipsia, headache/visual disturbances: For spinal anesthesia

- Hoarseness of voice: Vocal cord palsy thickening/ RLN palsy
- Stridor: Subglottic narrowing

❖ Drug history:
  - Octreotide may cause nausea, vomiting and diarrhea
  - Bromocriptine causes severe postural hypotension on induction

❖ Examination:
  - Blood pressure, murmurs, edema
  - CNS findings, other systems

❖ Airway assessment:
  - Difficult airway common due to:
    - Large jaw, tongue, lips and head
    - Generalized soft tissue swelling of pharynx and larynx
    - Vocal cord thickening, chondrocalcinosis of larynx: Small glottis aperture
    - Subglottic narrowing
    - Enlarged thyroid gland may compress trachea
  - 30% incidence of difficult airway
  - Difficult airway maybe clinically unpredictable

Preoperative Preparation and Premedication

❖ Informed consent, discuss possibility of awake fiber-optic intubation

❖ Discuss need to breathe through mouth post-extubation, if trans-sphenoidal hypophysectomy

❖ NPO guidelines
  - 6 hours: Solids
  - 2 hours: Clear fluids and water

❖ Avoid respiratory depressants

❖ Glycopyrrolate 20 µg/kg IV especially if awake fiber-optic intubation is planned

❖ Somatostatin analogues sometimes used

❖ Glucose with insulin infusion started if glucose intolerance present

❖ Continue all medications on the morning of surgery, except insulin

Role of Regional Anesthesia

❖ Is the preferred technique where applicable

❖ May be technically difficult and unreliable due to skeletal changes

OT Preparation

❖ Skilled assistant

❖ Difficult airway cart:
  - Selection of long armoured ET tubes
  - Fibreoptic laryngoscope, tracheostomy tube
  - Large sized face mask, long bladed laryngoscope
  - Oral airways

❖ Anesthetic drugs thiopentone, fentanyl, vecuronium, succinylcholine

❖ Suction apparatus

❖ Monitors

❖ Emergency drugs:
  - Atropine, adrenaline
  - Phenylephrine, NTG, SNP
  - Dopamine, dobutamine

Monitors

❖ Pulse oximeter: Probe may be too small for patients fingers

❖ E_TCO_2, temperature

❖ ECG, urine output

❖ Invasive blood pressure monitoring:
  - For prolonged surgery or for repeated ABGs
  - Do Allens test before inserting radial line, as collateral circulation at wrist may be inadequate
  - Arterial line preferred at brachial/femoral sites

❖ CVP/PAC if cardiovascular disease is significant

❖ Blood glucose at frequent intervals

❖ Peripheral nerve stimulator:
  - Has altered sensitivity to neuromuscular blockers
  - This is due to hypercalcemia/neuromuscular abnormalities

Induction

❖ Adequate preoxygenation for 3–5 minutes

❖ IV thiopentone (3–4 mg/kg) + fentanyl 1–2 µg/kg + vecuronium 0.1 mg/kg

❖ Check adequacy of ventilation before administering paralyzing agent

❖ Anticipate difficult mask ventilation: Use large masks with gauze packing if difficult mask ventilation

❖ Avoid hypertensive response at intubation: Lidocaine 1.5 mg/kg IV 90 seconds before intubation

❖ Oral intubation preferred as nasal mucosa maybe thickened

❖ Awake fiber-optic intubation is *technique of choice*

❖ Use smaller diameter ET tube as vocal cords may be thickened with subglottic stenosis

❖ Lidocaine 1.5 mg/kg and alfentanyl 10 µg/kg to suppress intubation response

- Elective tracheostomy done if:
  - Awake fiber-optic not possible
  - Those patients with vocal cord involvement
  - History of sleep apnea

Maintenance

- Avoid nitrous oxide if air pneumo-encephalography planned
- O_2 + air + isoflurane 1 MAC used to maintain balanced anesthesia
- Fentanyl and vecuronium given as intermittent boluses
- Hypotensive anesthesia techniques preferred

Positioning

- Size of patient makes positioning difficult
- Long tables may be required owing to tall stature of patient
- Protect against nerve injuries:
  - Ulnar nerve at elbow
  - Common peroneal nerve below knee
  - Median nerve at wrist

Hemodynamics

- Judicious fluid therapy in those with poor LV function
- Treat hypertension with antihypertensives
- Hypotensive anesthesia preferred in those undergoing trans-sphenoidal hypophysectomy
- Monitor blood sugar for hyperglycemia

Extubation

- Fully awake extubation in propped up position when:
  - Conscious and obeys commands
  - Stable hemodynamics
  - Normal temperature
  - TOF ratio ≥ 0.7
- Neostigmine 0.05 mg/kg with glycopyrrolate 0.02 µg/kg to reverse the patient
- Elective postoperative ventilation considered in those with severe airway obstruction

Postoperative Care

Management

- Propped up position
- Supplemental oxygen therapy
- Encourage oral breathing in case of trans-sphenoidal hypophysectomy
- ACTH and TSH replacement post-hypophysectomy

Monitors

- Pulse oximetry
- E_TCO_2, NIBP
- ABG, blood glucose
- Urine output, ECG
- Temperature, adequacy of ventilation

Analgesia

- Caution with the use of opioid analgesics: Respiratory depression
- Patient controlled analgesia useful
- NSAIDs preferred
- Use regional analgesia where possible
- Multimodal analgesia preferred

Complications

- Airway obstruction
- Negative pressure pulmonary edema
- Hypoglycemia as insulin requirements reduce postoperatively
- Temporary/permanent diabetes insipidus: Treat with DDAVP (especially after hypophysectomy)

HYPERTHYROIDISM

Introduction

Clinical syndrome resulting from excessive production of thyroid hormones T_3 and T_4.

Incidence

- Most common cause is Graves disease (60–80% cases)
- Most common between 20–50 years and more frequent in women

Normal Values

Hormone	Conventional units	SI units
TSH	0.5–4.7 µU/mL	0.5–4.7 mU/L
Total T4	4.5–10.9 µg/dL	58–140 nmol/L
Free T4	0.8–2.7 ng/dL	10.3–35 pmol/L
Total T3	60–181 ng/dL	0.92–2.78 nmol/L
Free T3	1.4–4.4 pg/mL	0.22–6.78 pmol/L

Etiology

- Primary thyrotoxicosis:
  - Graves disease 90%
  - Toxic multinodular goiter
  - Toxic adenoma
  - ***De-Quervains thyroiditis***

- Postpartum thyroiditis: Can persist for 3–6 months post-partum
- Carcinoma thyroid
- ***Struma ovarii***
- ***McCune-Albright syndrome***

❖ Secondary thyrotoxicosis:
- Pituitary adenoma secreting TSH
- Trophoblastic tumors:
  - Choriocarcinoma
  - Hydatiform mole
- Functioning follicular carcinoma
- Extrathyroidal: Factitious hyperthyroidism (increased iodine intake)

❖ Iatrogenic causes:
- Thyroid replacement therapy
- Iodine therapy: ***Jod-Basedowsphenomenon***
- Amiodarone
- Radiation therapy

Clinical Features

❖ Central nervous system:
- Insomnia, impaired concentration, nervousness
- Fine, resting tremors
- Periodic paralysis and chorea: Rare
- Depression and withdrawal: *Apathetic thyrotoxicosis*
- Intolerance to heat, fatigue, apathy

❖ Ocular signs:
- ***Von Graeffes***: Upperlid lags as patient looks down
- ***Joffroys***: Nowrinkling of forehead
- ***Stellwags***: Staring look, infrequent blinking
- ***Moebius***: Inability to converge eyeballs
- ***Dalrymple:*** Upper sclera visible due to retraction of upper lid

❖ Goitre: Diffuse, nodular

❖ Cardiovascular system:
- Hypertension:
  - Increased SBP, reduced DBP
  - Widened pulse pressure
- Increased stroke volume and cardiac output
- Reduced SVR and PVR
- Increased blood volume
- Bounding pulse, palpitation
- High output cardiac failure
- ***Thyrotoxic cardiomyopathy***
- Mitral valve prolapse, aortic systolic murmur
- Arrhythmias:
  - Sinus tachycardia
  - Atrial fibrillation, SVT
  - Complete heart block
  - Ventricular arrhythmias

❖ Respiratory system:
- Hypercarbia and increased oxygen consumption due to increased BMR
- This causes high minute volume: High tidal volume and increased respiratory rate
- Vital capacity decreases due to respiratory muscle weakness
- Dyspnea on exertion
- Exacerbation of asthma

❖ Gastrointestinal:
- Weight loss despite increased appetite
- Decreased GI transit time
- Secretory diarrhea
- Anorexia, vomiting

❖ Genitourinary:
- Amenorrhea/oligomenorrhea
- Infertility, loss of libido
- Gynecomastia, spontaneous abortion

❖ Hematological:
- Anemia
- Neutropenia
- Thrombocytopenia

❖ Dermatological:
- *Pretibial myxedema*
- Increased sweating, warm and moist skin
- Palmar erythema
- Onycholysis, diffuse alopecia
- Pruritus and urticaria
- Clubbing, *thyroid acropachy*

❖ Neuromuscular:
- Muscle weakness
- Muscle stiffness and wasting
- *Proximal myopathy*
- Hyperactive reflexes, osteopenia

Investigations

❖ Complete blood count:
- Anemia
- Thrombocytopenia
- Neutropenia

❖ Renal function tests, blood glucose, electrolytes (hypercalcemia)

❖ Increased serum alkaline phosphatase

❖ Thyroid function tests:
- Low TSH levels
- High T_3, T_4 levels

- Increased uptake of radioactive iodine 24 hours after its administration
- Tests done within last 6 months are usually adequate if symptoms or therapy has not been changed significantly

❖ ECG: LVH, arrhythmias
❖ ECHO: LVH, RWMA, EF
❖ *Indirect laryngoscopy*: For preoperative vocal cord movement (medicolegal importance)
❖ X-ray (AP and lateral): Neck and thoracic inlet
❖ CT scan for degree of tracheal compression if retrosternal extension
❖ Pulmonary function tests
❖ Flow volume loops

Treatment

❖ Medical management: Takes 6–8 weeks to make patient pharmacologically euthyroid
- Antithyroid drugs for 6–8 weeks:
  - Propylthiouracil:
    - 200–300 mg PO Q8–12H
    - Inhibits peripheral T_4 to T_3 conversion
  - Methimazole:
    - 10–20 mg Q12H
    - Faster response, once daily dosing
  - Carbimazole 30–45 mg/day
  - Not effective until 6–8 weeks when thyroid stores are depleted and hence new thyroid hormones are not synthesized
- Saturated solution of potassium iodide (SSKI):
  - Antithyroid drugs should precede SSKI
  - This is because iodide given alone will act as substrate for new thyroid hormone synthesis and worsen thyrotoxicosis
  - 3 drops orally Q8H for 7–14 days
  - Reduces gland vascularity and hormone release (***Wolff-Chaikoff effect***)
  - Continuing SSKI beyond 14 days does not have any beneficial effects
  - Onset of action within 24 hours
  - Contraindication:
    - Children
    - Pregnancy and breastfeeding
  - Safe to become pregnant 4 months or more after iodide therapy
  - Lugols iodine is an effective alternative
- β blocker therapy:
  - Non-selective β blockers better than selective β blockers
  - Selective β-blockers are good only for treatment of tachycardia
  - Non-selective blockers also block peripheral conversion of T_4 to T_3 via β action over 1–2 weeks
  - This reduces tachycardia, anxiety, tremors and heat intolerance
  - β blockers relieve signs and symptoms but do not reduce thyrotoxicosis
  - Propranolol 40–80 mg Q6-8H

❖ Radioiodine therapy:
- Destroys thyroid cell function
- Used for initial treatment of relapses after trial of antithyroid drugs
- Antithyroid drugs to be stopped at least 3 days before radioactive I^{131} therapy to optimize iodine uptake
- May cause hypothyroidism
- Not recommended in pregnancy due to risk of fetal hypothyroidism

❖ Surgical management:
- Subtotal thyroidectomy
- Now less commonly used as alternative
- Indicated in:
  - Large toxic multinodular goiter
  - Solitary toxic adenoma
  - Failed medical therapy
  - Underlying carcinoma

Anesthetic Management for Thyroid Surgery

Preoperative Evaluation

❖ Elicit history of goitre, history of drugs and anesthetic exposure
❖ Systemic examination
❖ Airway assessment: Anticipate difficult intubation if:
- History of positional dyspnea/dysphagia
- Infilterating carcinoma is independent risk factor
- History of dyspnea/stridor for trachea compression
- More than 50% tracheal narrowing on chest X-ray

❖ Difficult intubation as:
- Increased chances of cord palsy in malignancy
- Distortion and rigidity of structures
- Intraluminal spread of malignancy
- Displaced larynx

❖ SVC syndrome: Venous engorgement of face and arms

- May cause laryngeal edema: Use smaller ET tube
- Preoperative endocrinologist consultation

Preoperative Preparation for Elective Surgery

- T~kes 6–8 weeks to make patient pharmacologically euthyroid
  - Antithyroid drugs for 6–8 weeks:
    - Propylthiouracil:
      - 200–300 mg PO Q8–12H
      - Inhibits peripheral T_4 to T_3 conversion
    - Methimazole:
      - 10–20 mg Q12H
      - Faster response, once daily dosing
    - Carbimazole 30–45 mg/day
    - Not effective until 6–8 weeks when thyroid stores are depleted and hence new thyroid hormones are not synthesized
  - Saturated solution of potassium iodide (SSKI) :
    - Antithyroid drugs should precede SSKI
    - This is because iodide given alone will act as substrate for new thyroid hormone synthesis and worsen thyrotoxicosis
    - 3 drops orally Q8H for 7–14 days
    - Reduces gland vascularity and hormone release (***Wolff-Chaikoff effect***)
    - Continuing SSKI beyond 14 days does not have any beneficial effects
    - Onset of action within 24 hours
    - Contraindication:
      - Children
      - Pregnancy and breastfeeding
    - Safe to become pregnant 4 months or more after iodide therapy
    - Lugols iodine is an effective alternative
  - β blocker therapy:
    - Non-selective β-blockers better than selective β-blockers
    - Selective β-blockers are good only for treatment of tachycardia
    - Non-selective blockers also block peripheral conversion of T_4 to T_3 via β-action over 1–2 weeks
    - This reduces tachycardia, anxiety, tremors and heat intolerance
    - β blockers relieve signs and symptoms but do not reduce thyrotoxicosis
    - Propranolol 40–80 mg Q6–8H
- Current trend is:
  - Preoperative preparation with propranolol and NaI alone
  - Advantages:
    - This is a much quicker approach (1–2 weeks vs 6–8 weeks)
    - It shrinks thyroid gland as well as traditional approach
    - It reduces peripheral conversion of T_4 to T_3
    - Also treats symptoms of LVF (but does not correct LVF)

Preoperative Preparation for Emergency Surgery

- Antithyroid drugs:
  - Propylthiouracil 200–400 mg Q6H PO or via NGT
  - Methimazole 20–40 mg Q6H PO/NGT/rectally
- Saturated solution of potassium iodide:
  - Given after 1 hour of administering antithyroid drugs
  - 5 drops given PO/via NGT Q6H
  - Lugols iodine 30 drops PO/via NGT Q6H
- β blockers:
  - Propranolol 0.5–1 mg/kg IV bolus
  - Esmolol 500 μg/kg IV bolus followed by infusion
  - β blockers titrated to restore heart rate < 90 bpm
- Sodium iopanoate:
  - 500 mg Q12H
  - Effects similar to iodide therapy
  - Releases iodine which inhibits synthesis and also blocks peripheral conversion of T_4 to T_3
- Steroids:
  - Dexamethasone 2 mg IV Q6H (8–12 mg/day)
  - Reduces hormone release and peripheral conversion of T_4 to T_3
  - Hydrocortisone 40 mg Q6H is an alternative

Adequacy of Patient Preparation

- Heart rate less than 90 bpm in normal sinus rhythm
- Normal pulse pressure
- Resolution of new cardiac murmur
- Relief of tremors, anxiety, palpitation, dyspnea and heart intolerance

Role of Regional Anesthesia

- Preferred technique
- Avoid epinephrine containing local anesthetics
- Bilateral superficial cervical plexus block maybe used for limited thyroidectomy

Premedication

- Elective surgery postponed until euthyroid state has been achieved

- Correct preoperative dehydration if diarrhea is severe
- NPO guidelines:
    - 6 hours solids
    - 2 hours clear fluids
- Informed consent
- Preoperative sedation:
    - Avoid excess sedation
    - Mild sedation with benzodiazepines (0.1 mg/kg diazepam PO)
    - Avoid opioids as muscle fatigue and hypotonicity increases risk of respiratory depression
- Avoid atropine and scopolamine as:
    - It causes tachycardia
    - Interferes with heat regulation
- Use glycopyrrolate 0.02 mg/kg IV, if necessary, as antisialogogue
- Continue antithyroid and β blockers on day of surgery
- PONV and antibiotic prophylaxis

Anesthetic Goals

- Achieve depth of anesthesia which inhibits sympathetic response to surgical stimuli
- Avoid administration of any drug which stimulates sympathetic nervous system:
    - Ketamine, pancuronium
    - Atropine, ephedrine
    - Epinephrine
- Adequate eye protection

Monitors

- Pulse oximetry, E_TCO_2
- NIBP, IBP if LV dysfunction
- CVP/PAC in unstable patients
- ECG, urine output
- Airway pressure if thyroid surgery
- Temperature especially in emergency surgeries
- Esophageal stethoscope
- Neuromuscular monitoring important as increased incidence of myasthenia gravis in thyrotoxic patients

Induction

- Adequate preoxygenation for 3–5 mins as oxygen requirement is high
- If there is no anticipated airway obstruction:
    - Thiopentone 3–4 mg/kg + vecuronium 0.1 mg/kg + fentanyl 1–2 µg/kg
    - Thiopentone is *agent of choice* as thiourylene nucleus inhibits peripheral T_4 to T_3 conversion
    - Unanticipated airway obstruction may occur after muscle relaxant is administered
- If airway obstruction is anticipated:
    - Awake fiber-optic intubation/inhalational induction preferred
    - Ask attendant to lift gland upwards and laterally
    - Tip of ETT to be advanced beyond any area of tracheal compression
    - Use armoured flexometallic tube to avoid kinking under drapes
    - Tube firmly taped in position and all connection secured as access during surgery is limited
    - Inhalational induction may be delayed if stridor/reduced minute volume preoperatively
- Ensure adequate anesthetic depth for intubation, rapid lightening of consciousness at intubation may occur
- Also prone for hypotensive response which is exaggerated during induction of anesthesia as they are chronically hypovolemic and vasodilated
- Reduced doses of initial neuromuscular blocking agent
- Topical local anesthesia of larynx is useful to reduce sympathetic response

Maintenance

- $N_2O + O_2$ + isoflurane 1 MAC
- Avoid halothane as:
    - Increased chances of hepatic necrosis
    - Adrenaline may be used with LA solution at the time of skin infilteration
- Fentanyl 1 µg/kg and reduced doses of vecuronium given as intermittent boluses
- Reduced fentanyl doses to ensure patient can maintain patent airway post extubation
- Carefully titrate muscle relaxation as thyrotoxicosis patients have increased incidence of myasthenia gravis
- Muscle relaxants cannot be used after intubation if repeat surgery is being performed as surgeon may use nerve stimulator to identify recurrent laryngeal nerve

Position

- Neck extended fully with head uptilt up to 15–20° to reduce venous bleeding
- Venous air embolism is a complication in this position

- Neck extension may change the ET tube position
- Thus, recheck tube position after final positioning of patient
- Patient prone for corneal abrasion owing to:
  - Exophthalmos
  - Eyelid retraction

Hemodynamics

- Profound hypotension may occur at time of induction
- Treat any hypotension with fluids and vasopressors
- Phenylephrine ornorepinephrine used commonly
- Avoid sympathomimetics like ephedrine as it may cause exaggerated response
- Carotid sinus manipulation may cause bradycardia and hypotension:
  - Administer atropine
  - Stop stimulating the carotid sinus
  - Administrative of lidocaine in that area may prevent recurrence

Ventilation

- ET intubation with CMV preferred
- Avoid hyperventilation as the resultant alkalosis and hypokalemia may aggravate muscle weakness
- Excess airway pressure may occur during manipulation of trachea
- Head down tilt and Valsalva maneuver before wound closure helps in identifying bleeding points
- LMA is nowadays being used without the use of neuromuscular blocking agents
- Since patient is spontaneously breathing, it allows real time recurrent laryngeal nerve function monitoring

Extubation

- Full reversal with neostigmine 0.05 mg/kg and glycopyrrolate 0.02 mg/kg IV
- Deep planes at extubation preferred as:
  - It avoids risk of coughing
  - Wound hematoma is avoided which may cause airway obstruction postoperatively
- Direct laryngoscopy and visualization of vocal cord movement post-extubation may be done to check RLN function
- In cases of suspected tracheomalacia:
  - Fiber-optic bronchoscope used to assess for airway collapse as ET tube and bronchoscope are pulled back
  - If tracheal collapse is noted, ET tube and FOB is immediately advanced
  - ET tube is left in place if questionable ability to protect airway
  - Mechanical ventilation is continued postoperatively

Postoperative Care

Management

- Continue postoperative antithyroid regimen until T_4 levels reduce
- Calcium supplementation if low Ca^{2+} levels due to accidental excision of parathyroid gland
- Check calcium levels at 6 and 24 hours post surgery
- Nasal fibreoptic laryngoscopy post extubation for documentation of RLN injury
- If hematoma formation occurs:
  - Intubate early before airway edema occurs (due to reduced venous return from cords)
  - 45° head up tilt to increase venous return
  - Remove alternate sutures and inform surgeon
  - Steroids and racemic epinephrine to reduce laryngeal edema

Complications

- Immediate complications:
  - Airway obstruction due to:
    - Hemorrhage
    - RLN injury
    - Tracheal collapse
    - Tracheomalacia especially if long standing goiter
  - Thyroid storm
- Delayed complications:
  - Thyroid storm
  - Recurrent laryngeal nerve injury
  - Hematoma from coughing
  - Bullous glottic edema
  - Tracheoesophageal fistula
  - Pneumothorax if dissection of sternum and mediastinum occurs
  - Phrenic nerve injury
  - Pneumomediastinum
  - Hypocalcemia and parathyroid gland damage: Presents within 12–72 hours
  - Superior laryngeal nerve injury: Causes increased risk of aspiration

Pain

- NSAIDs
- Opioids – low dose
- PCA
- Multimodal analgesia
- Superficial cervical plexus block/S/C/LA

THYROID STORM

Introduction

Life-threatening hypermetabolic state in a patient whose hyperthyroidism has been severly exacerbated by illness/surgery.

Incidence

- Rare but associated with 20–30% mortality
- May occur up to 18 hours after surgery

Precipitating Factors

- Thyroid related:
  - Vigorous thyroid manipulation
  - Palpation of thyroid gland, ingestion of thyroid hormone
  - Thyroid surgery
  - Radioactive iodine therapy, iodine therapy
  - Iodinated contrast dyes
  - Withdrawal of antithyroid drug therapy
- Non-thyroid illnesses:
  - Infections
  - Cerebrovascular accidents
  - Congestive cardiac failure, myocardial infarction
  - Bowel infarction, pulmonary embolism
  - Non-thyroid surgery
  - Diabetic ketoacidosis, trauma
- Most commonly precipitated by operating on an acutely hyperthyroid gland

Clinical Features

- Can occur intraoperatively, like malignant hyperthermia, or up to 6–24 hours postoperatively
- Presents with:
  - Nausea, vomiting, diarrhea, jaundice
  - Altered consciousness: agitation, delirium, coma, confusion, seizures
- Sinustachycardia (> 140 bpm), fever (≥ 40 °C), sweating
- Myocardial infarction, cardiac failure and dysrhythmias common
- No muscle rigidity/increase in CPK/metabolic or respiratory acidosis as in malignant hyperthermia

Differential Diagnosis

- Malignant hyperthermia
- Neuroleptic malignant syndrome
- Pheochromocytoma
- Hypoxic encephalopathy/hypothalamic stroke
- Light anesthesia, sepsis
- Drug overdose: Cosine, amphetamine
- Delirium tremens
- Heat stroke

Investigations

- Lab analysis usually not useful
- TFTs are not routinely available to emergency physician
- Leukocytosis, hyperglycemia, increased transaminases and bilirubin seen
- ECG, chest X-ray, urinalysis and blood culture used to identify cause

Treatment

- Treat precipitating cause:
  - Antibiotics for infection
  - Digoxin for CCF especially if AF with fast ventricular rate
  - Treat diabetic ketoacidosis
- Non-specific treatment:
  - Antithyroid drugs:
    - Initiated as first line of therapy
    - Propylthiouracil:
      - 1 gm loading dose
      - Followed by 250–500 mg Q6H PO/via NGT
      - Acts within 1 hour
    - Methimazole 40 mg PO followed by 25 mg Q6H PO
  - Iodine therapy:
    - Sodium iodide 1 gm IV over 12 hours
    - KI 5 drops TID PO/via NGT
    - Lugols iodine 5–10 drops TID PO/NGT
    - Start 1 hour after administration of PTU
    - Iapanoic acid 1 gm IV Q8H for 24 hours then 500 mg IV BD
    - $LiCO_3$ 800–1200 mg PO/day
  - β blocker therapy:
    - IV propranolol:
      - 0.5 mg/kg IV Q5 min till heart rate is below 90/min
      - Followed by 2 mg IV Q4H

- IV esmolol:
  - 0.5 mg/kg IV bolus
  - Followed by 50–100 μg/kg/min infusion
- Alternatives:
  - Combined α + β blocker
  - α_2 antagonists
  - Reserpine 2.5–5 mg IM Q6H
  - Guanethidine 30–40 mg Q6HPO

❖ Steroids:
- Hydrocortisone 100–200 mg IV Q8H
- Dexamethasone 2 mg IV Q6H

❖ Supportive therapy:
- Oxygen therapy, Foleys catheter
- Ventilation if required, NGT inserted as most medication are PO
- IV saline and glucose to correct electrolytes and blood sugar levels
- Inotropes, diuretics if CCF present
- Monitor temperature, IBP and CVP

❖ Surface cooling:
- Cold lavage of body cavity
- Ice packs, cooling blankets
- Reduced ambient temperature, tepid sponging
- Paracetamol preferred: 650 mg PO Q4H
- Avoid aspirin/NSAIDs as they displace thyroid hormones from serum proteins
- Pethidine 25–50 mg IV Q4–6H to reduce shivering
- Hemodialysis and plasmapheresis used if refractory

HYPOTHYROIDISM

Introduction

Clinical syndrome resulting from deficiency of thyroid hormones T_3 and T_4.

Incidence

❖ Relatively common
❖ Incidence 0.5–0.8% of adult population
❖ More common in females
❖ Incidence is 4:1000 in females and 1:1000 in males

Etiology

❖ Primary hypothyroidism (95% cases) with increased TSH levels:
- Iodine deficiency
- Hashimotos disease, auto-immune
- Radiation therapy
- I^{131} therapy
- Surgical removal
- Drugs:
  - Iodine
  - Propylthiouracil, methimazole
  - Lithium, amiodarone
- Hereditary defects in biosynthesis
- Congenital defects in gland development

❖ Secondary hypothyroidism with reduced TSH levels:
- Hypothalamic disease
- Pituitary disease

Clinical Features

❖ Clinical features of hypothyroidism present when TSH > 10 mU/L
❖ Slow onset, insidious and progressive course
❖ Central nervous system:
- Reduced BMR: Lethargy, cold intolerance
- Slow, dull speech, hoarse voice
- Slow mental function, slow movements
- Fatigue, lethargy, listlessness
- Stiffness, cramps, pain, pseudomyotonia
- Cerebellar ataxia
- Depression, apathy, psychosis
- ***Hashimoto encephalopathy***
- Slow relaxation of deep tendon reflexes: *Hung up reflexes*
- Arthralgias

❖ Cardiovascular system:
- Bradycardia
- Low stroke volume and cardiac output: hypotension
- Increased PVR: Hypertension
- Reduced blood volume: Pale skin
- Pericardial effusion which is rich in triglycerides and cholesterol
- Reduced myocardial contractility
- *Hypothyroid cardiomyopathy*
- Cardiac failure (rare in the absence of coexisting cardiac disease)
- Angina: Rare but may occur at the time of T_4 replacement
- Predisposed to MI
- ECG:
  - Low voltage complexes (due to pericardial effusion)
  - T wave flattening/inversion
  - Ventricular arrhythmias (due to amyloid in conduction system)
  - Predisposed to MI
- ***Amyloid cardiomyopathy***

- Respiratory system:
  - Reduced ventilatory response to hypoxia and hypercarbia
  - Pleural effusion
  - Large tongue, sleep apnea
  - Hoarseness of voice, acute respiratory obstruction
  - Maximum breathing capacity, minute volume and CO transfer factor reduced
- Gastrointestinal:
  - Weight gain with loss of appetite
  - Ileus, constipation
  - Increased gastric emptying time
  - Ascitis and peritoneal effusion
- Genitourinary system:
  - Glomerulonephritis
  - Nephrotic syndrome
  - Amyloid nephropathy
  - Menorrhagia
- Skin:
  - Myxedema
  - Cool, mottled skin due to peripheral vasoconstriction
  - Dry hair, alopecia, vitiligo
  - Dry, pale and thick skin with reduced sweating
  - ***Carpal Tunnel syndrome***
  - *Myxedema:* Non-pitting edema due to mucopolysaccharide (MPS) deposition
  - Periorbital edema
- Hematology:
  - Anemia: Normochromic, normo/macrocytic
  - Associated with pernicious anemia
  - Platelet dysfunction
  - Coagulation factor (VIII) dysfunction
  - Hypercholesterolemia
  - Hypertriglyceridemia

Investigation

- General investigations:
  - Complete blood count, renal function tests, blood sugar levels (hypoglycemia)
  - Electrolytes: Hyponatremia common
  - Hb, peripheral smear: Anemia
  - Coagulation profile: BT, CT, PT, INR for coagulopathy
  - Increased cholesterol, triglycerides, CPK and LDH
  - ECG:
    - Low voltage QRS complexes
    - Sinus bradycardia
    - Flattened/inverted T waves
  - Chest X-ray:
    - Cardiomegaly due to pericardial effusion
    - Pleural/pericardial effusion
    - Thoracic inlet X-ray to diagnose tracheal involvement
  - Indirect laryngoscopy for preoperative vocal cord dysfunction
  - Screen for other autoimmune disorders
- Thyroid specific investigations:
  - Thyroid function tests:
    - Reduced FT4 and FT3 with raised TSH if primary hypothyroidism
    - Reduced FT4, FT3 and TSH if secondary hypothyroidism
    - *Single best predictor* at cellular level is TSH levels
  - Thyroid scan with I^{131}/Tc^{99m}: cold, hypofunctioning nodule
  - Thyroid USG: Cystic/solid/mixed lesions
  - CT/MRI if tracheal compression
  - TPO antibodies screen

Classification of Severity

- Subclinical hypothyroidism:
  - Normal T_3 and T_4 levels
  - Raised TSH levels (5–10 mU/L)
  - No clinical features
- Mild hypothyroidism:
  - Reduced or normal T_3 and T_4
  - Mean TSH of 18 mU/L
  - Some clinical features
- Severe hypothyroidism:
  - Reduced T_3 and T_4
  - Mean TSH of 90 mU/L
  - Full clinical profile

Anesthetic Considerations

- Anemia and coagulation abnormalities: Increased blood loss
- Increased sensitivity to sedatives NMBA
- Increased gastric emptying time: Increased chances of aspiration
- Profound hypotension on anesthetic induction
- Prone for hypothermia as BMR is low
- Muscular weakness: Controlled ventilation preferred
- Hypoglycemia and hyponatremia
- Anticipate difficult intubation as
  - Large tongue
  - Edematous vocal cords
  - Edematous oral cavity
  - Goiter: Tracheal compression, tracheomalacia

Preoperative Optimization

- Choice of patients:
  - Mild-moderate hypothyroidism: No need to postpone elective surgery
  - Severe hypothyroidism: Postpone surgery when possible till these patient are at least partially treated
  - Also for pregnant patients and myxedema coma
- Hypothyroidism with coronary artery disease:
  - Need for thyroid replacement therapy to be weighed against risk of precipitating MI
  - In asymptomatic patients/unstable patients with cardiac ischemia:
    - Delay in T_4 replacement considered
    - Urgent myocardial revascularization planned
    - Plan to start thyroid replacement therapy in ICU
- Optimization in elective surgery:
  - Delay surgery if $T_4 < 1$ µg/dL or severe hypothyroidism until patient is euthyroid
  - Start T_4 with 50 µg/day (1.6 µg/kg)
  - Gradually increase to 100 µg/day over weeks through 12.5–25 µg increments
  - In elderly with CAD, start 25 µg/day and increase monthly by 25 µg/day
  - Alternate preparations:
    - Animal thyroid extract
    - L-triodothyronine
    - Liotrix: combination of T_4 and T_3 (4:1)
  - Patient may not experience full relief in symptoms until 3–6 months after normal TSH levels are reached
- Optimization in emergency surgery:
  - IV L-thyroxine 300–500 µg over 1–5 minutes or
  - IV L-tri-iodothyronine 25–50 µg IV followed by T_3 25 µg IV Q8H
  - Steroid coverage with dexamethasone/cortisol
  - Milrinone:
    - Used in the presence of CCF:
    - Phosphodiesterase III inhibitor
    - *Most effective* inotrope in hypothyroidism
    - Does not depend on β receptors which are low in number and sensitivity in hypothyroidism

Premedication

- NPO status:
  - 6 hours solids
  - 2 hours clear fluids
- Informed consent
- No preoperative sedation as drug induced respiratory depression is common
- Adequate IV fluid loading preoperatively as they tolerate hypovolemia poorly
- Antiaspiration prophylaxis:
  - IV ranitidine 1 mg/kg
  - IV metoclopramide 10 mg
- Continue thyroid hormones on the day of surgery
- Omission of thyroid dose may be tolerated as T_4 has long $T_{½}$ of 8 days
- Hydrocortisone 100 mg IV as associated adrenocortical insufficiency present
- Antibiotic prophylaxis as per hospital protocol

Regional Anesthesia

- Regional anesthesia (RA) preferred where possible if no contraindication
- Adequate intravascular volume to be established to prevent precipitous hypotension
- Difficult landmarks if associated obesity
- Caution exercised if coexistent coagulopathy

Induction

- Give all anesthetic drugs slowly
- Ketamine is induction *agent of choice* as other drugs associated with hypotension
- Reduced doses of NMBA used as muscle weakness already present
- Rapid sequence induction with ketamine and succinylcholine if full stomach picture
- If airway obstruction is anticipated:
  - Awake fiber-optic intubation
  - Ask attendant to lift gland upwards and laterally
  - Tip of ETT to be advanced beyond any area of tracheal compression
  - Use armoured flexometallic tube to avoid kinking under drapes
  - Tube firmly taped in position and all connection secured as access during surgery is limited

Maintenance

- $O_2 + N_2O$ + isoflurane for balanced anesthesia
- No significant reduction in MAC
- Avoid halothane as it has myocardial depressant action
- Fentanyl 1 µg/kg and small doses of vecuronium given intermittantly
- Ketamine also can be used for maintenance, as an infusion

Monitors

- Pulse oximetry, E_TCO_2
- BP: NIBP/IBP based on cardiovascular status
- ECG: MI/arrhythmias
- Urine output, temperature
- Precordial stethoscope if thyroid surgery
- Neuromuscular monitoring: Interference with excitability in hypothyroid patients
- ABG and blood sugar regularly: Hypoglycemia, hyponatremia
- Airway pressure if thyroid surgery

Ventilation

- ET tube with CMV preferred due to:
  - Preexisting muscular weakness
  - Reduced response to hypoxia and hypercarbia
- Hypocapnea may be present due to reduce BMR
- Excess airway pressure during manipulation of thyroid gland common

Hemodynamics

- IV fluids containing dextrose used to prevent hypoglycemia
- Intraoperative hypotension common due to:
  - Reduced cardiac output
  - Blunted baroreceptor reflexes
  - Reduced intravascular volume
- Hypotension is:
  - Less responsive to catecholamines
  - Ephedrine/dopamine/epinephrine used if severe hypotension
  - *Best inotrope* is milrinone
  - Supplemental steroids given if refractory hypotension
- Actively warm patient to avoid hypothermia (more common as low BMR present)

Extubation

- Fully awake extubation in semirecumbent position
- Neostigmine 0.05 mg/kg + glycopyrollate 0.02 mg/kg IV for reversal
- May require prolonged mechanical ventilation as ↑ incidence of myasthemia grows in hypothyroidism
- Deep planes at extubation preferred if thyroid surgery has been done, as:
  - It avoids risk of coughing
  - Wound hematoma is avoided which may cause airway obstruction postoperatively
- Direct laryngoscopy and visualization of vocal cord movement post-extubation may be done to check RLN function
- In cases of suspected tracheomalacia:
  - Fiber-optic bronchoscope used to assess for airway collapse as ET tube and bronchoscope are pulled back
  - If tracheal collapse is noted, ET tube and FOB is immediately advanced
  - ET tube is left in place if questionable ability to protect airway
  - Mechanical ventilation is continued postoperatively

Postoperative Care

Management

- Nurse in propped up position
- Continue thyroid medications postoperatively
- IV hydrocortisone 100 mg Q6H given
- Calcium supplementation if low Ca^{2+} levels due to accidental excision of parathyroid gland
- Check calcium levels at 6 and 24 hours post surgery
- Nasal fiber-optic laryngoscopy post extubation for documentation of RLN injury
- If hematoma formation occurs:
  - Intubate early before airway edema occurs
  - 45° head up tilt to increase venous return
  - Remove alternate sutures and inform surgeon
  - Steroids and racemic epinephrine to reduce laryngeal edema

Monitors

- Pulse oximetry, BP, ECG
- Temperature, urine output
- Electrolytes and sugar
- ABG

Analgesia

- Avoid opioids/use low dose to avoid respiratory depression
- Non-opioids: Ketolac as adjuvant
- Regional anesthesia
- Local anesthetic infilteration
- Multimodal analgesia preferred

Complications

- Myxedema coma
- Delayed recovery owing to:
  - Hypothermia
  - Muscle weakness

- Slow drug biotransformation
- Low BMR

- Respiratory depression/failure
- Sleep apnea
- Reduced free water clearance with dilutional hyponatremia
- Hypothermia
- Prolonged postoperative ileus, bleeding

MYXEDEMA COMA

Introduction

- Rare and severe form of hypothyroidism in which patients with preexisting long standing hypothyroidism present with life-threatening decompensation
- It is a medical emergency

Predisposing Factors

- Infection, trauma, surgery
- Cold exposure, drugs
- CNS depressants/sedatives
- Lithium, amiodarone
- Cerebrovascular accident
- Congestive cardiac failure
- Inadequate thyroid replacement therapy
- Previously undiagnosed hypothyroidism

Clinical Features

- Mortality rate of 25–30%
- Hypoventilation
- Hypothermia (80% patients) *is cardinal feature*
- Altered sensorium: Delirium, unconsciousness, coma
- Bradycardia with hypotension and cardiovascular collapse
- Severe dilutional hyponatremia due to SIADH
- Hypoglycemia, acidosis, hypercapnea
- Periorbital non-pitting edema, hung up DTR
- Drug toxicity from medications common due to reduced drug clearance

Investigations

- Anemia, hyponatremia, hypoglycemia
- Raised serum transaminases, CPK and LDH, hypercholesterolemia
- ABG: Hypoxemia, hypercapnea, acidosis
- ECG:
  - Sinus bradycardia
  - Increased corrected QT interval
  - Low voltage complexes
  - Flat/inverted T waves
- Chest X-ray: Pericardial effusion
- Blood culture and urine analysis for detecting cause

Treatment

- ICU admission
- Monitor:
  - ECG, SpO_2, E_TCO_2
  - BP, drug levels
  - Urine output, electrolytes and sugar
  - Temperature, ABG
- Treat precipitating cause:
  - Empirical antibiotic therapy
  - Only life saving surgery to be done
- Supportive therapy:
  - ET intubation with CMV may be required for first 48 hours
  - Avoid sedatives/use lower dose
  - Cardiovascular support:
    - Milrinone is *best inotrope*
    - Dopamine/norepinephrine can be tried
- Thyroid replacement therapy:
  - L-thyroxine:
    - 200–300 μg IV loading dose over 5–10 minutes
    - Followed by 50–200 μg/day IV
  - L-triodothyronine:
    - 25–50 μg IV loading dose
    - Followed by 25 μg Q8H IV
  - Combined replacement:
    - 200 μg T_4 + 25 μg T_3 as bolus
    - Followed by 50–100 μg/day T_4 and 10 μg Q8H T_3
- Steroid replacement therapy:
  - IV hydrocortisone 100 mg QID
  - Continued until normal adrenal function can be confirmed
- Hypothermia:
  - Prevent additional heat loss
  - Cautious passive external rewarming done
  - Sudden rewarming may cause peripheral vasodilation and cardiovascular collapse
  - External warming done only if temperature < 30 °C
- Electrolytes and sugar:
  - IV fluid restriction to correct hyponatremia
  - 3% saline used if severe hyponatremia

- IV glucose containing fluids used for maintenance
- Avoid hypotonic IV fluids as they cause water retention

CUSHING'S SYNDROME

Introduction

- It refers to the clinical state of increased free circulating glucocorticoids
- Cushing's disease refers to only those patients with ACTH secreting pituitary tumors
- Cushing's syndrome refers to patients with all causes of raised cortisol levels

Incidence

- Most common in third and fourth decades
- 3 times more common in females

Etiology

- ACTH dependent disease:
  - Pituitary adenomas
  - Ectopic ACTH producing tumors:
    - Bronchial adenoma
    - Bronchogenic carcinoma
    - Pancreatic carcinoma
    - Medullary carcinoma thyroid
    - Carcinoid tumor of thymus
    - Carcinoid tumor of ovary
  - Exogenous ACTH administration
- Non-ACTH dependant disease:
  - Adrenal adenoma
  - Adrenal carcinoma
  - Adrenal micronodular dysplasia:
    - Sporadic
    - Familial (***Carney's syndrome***)
  - Adrenal macronodular hyperplasia
  - Exogenous glucocorticoid administration: *Most common* cause
- Others: Pseudo-Cushing's syndrome
  - Alcoholism
  - Chronic depression
- Cushing's syndrome in patients more than 60 years old is most commonly due to adrenal carcinoma/ ectopic ACTH production

Pathogenesis: Main actions of glucocorticoids are

- Suppression of pituitary ACTH secretion
- Glycogen deposition
- Increased gluconeogenesis
- Fat deposition
- Protein catabolism and reduced protein synthesis
- Immunosuppression
- Mineralocorticoid actions:
  - Sodium retention
  - Potassium loss
  - Increased free water retention
- Uric acid production

Clinical Features

- Central nervous system:
  - Labile mood
  - Depression, confusion, psychosis, apathy
- Cardiovascular:
  - Hypertension
  - Hypervolemia
  - Fluid retention
  - Congestive cardiac failure
- Genitourinary:
  - Oligomenorrhea/amenorrhea
  - Decreased libido, virilizing signs
  - Hypertrophied clitoris
  - Kidney stones (due to high uric acid)
  - Polyuria
  - Increased reflux esophagitis
- Metabolic:
  - Glucose intolerance
  - Diabetes mellitus
  - Hypernatremia, increased bicarbonate levels, hypocalcemia
  - Hypokalemic metabolic alkalosis (especially if ectopic ACTH production)
- Skin:
  - Acne, hirsuitism, frontal balding
  - Easy bruising, violaceous striae
  - Hyperpigmentation
  - Thin and fragile skin with poor wound healing
  - Florid complexion (telangiectasis)
  - Plethoric facies
  - Increased chances of infection
- Subcutaneous tissue:
  - Lemon on matchstick appearance
  - Fat deposition in:
    - Upper face (***moon face***)
    - Interscapular area (***buffalo hump***)
    - Mesenteric bed (***truncal obesity***)
    - Supraclavicular area
    - Mediastinal widening

- Edema
- Growth arrest in children

❖ Musculoskeletal:
- Proximal muscle wasting
- Myopathy, asthenia
- Proximal weakness

❖ Bone:
- Osteoporosis, osteopenia
- Pathological rib fractures
- Vertebral collapse, kyphosis

Investigations

❖ General:
- Complete blood count (leucocytosis)
- Renal function tests, blood glucose, electrolytes
- ECG: Ischemia, hypokalemia, LVH
- Chest X-ray:
  - Kyphoscoliosis, osteoporosis
  - LVH, lower lobe collapse
  - Carcinoma bronchus
- Lung function tests
- CT scan/MRI abdomen: Tumor localization
- Pituitary MRI with gadolinium contrast

❖ Confirmatory tests:
- High plasma cortisol levels with loss of diurnal variation:
  - Absence of normal reduction at 12 AM
  - Absence of peaking at 6 AM
  - Normal value: 165–680 nmol/L
- Increased 24 hour urinary cortisol secretion:
  - More than 50 µg/day
  - Failure to fall to less than 10 µg/day
- Failure of plasma cortisol to fall less than 5 µg/dL after low dose dexamethasone suppression test (0.5 mg Q6H for 48 hours) is *diagnostic*
- ACTH levels in plasma:
  - Normal (less than 60 pg/mL) or high levels (30–150 pg/mL) indicates pituitary disease
  - Low levels (less than 10 pg/mL) indicates:
    - Adrenal disease
    - Exogenous cortisol production
  - Very high levels (more than 200 pg/mL) indicates ectopic ACTH production

Treatment

❖ Surgical therapy:
- Trans-sphenoidal microadenomectomy for pituitary tumors
- Excision of adrenal tumor by laparoscopy/open excision
- Adrenelectomy for bilateral hyperplasia has cure rates up to 100%
- Most patients with carcinoma, however, die within 3 years despite surgery
- Metastasis to liver and lung most common

❖ Medical therapy:
- Medical adrenelectomy:
  - Done when:
    - Surgery not feasible
    - Severe syndrome prior to surgery
  - Aim is to produce complete adrenal gland suppression
  - Done with steroid synthesis inhibitors:
    - Ketoconazole 600–1200 mg/day
    - Mitotane 2–3 g/day
    - Aminoglutethemide 1 g/day
    - Metyrapone 2–3 g/day
- Mifepristone is a competitive glucocorticoid antagonist and an alternative form of therapy
- Platinum is an alternative form of therapy

❖ Radiation therapy:
- For osseous mets as these are refractory to drug therapy
- Pituitary gamma radiation reserved for tumor recurrence
- Side effects:
  - Ocular motor palsy
  - Hypopituitarism
- Remission rate < 50% with long time lag between therapy and remission

❖ Treatment modalities for adrenal hyperplasia:
- Therapy to reduce ACTH production:
  - Transphenoidal resection of microadenoma
  - Radiation therapy
- Therapy to reduce adrenocortical cortisol secretion:
  - Bilateral adrenelectomy
  - Chemical adrenelectomy

Anesthetic Considerations

❖ OSAS and obesity
❖ GERD: Aspiration
❖ Osteoporosis: Careful positioning
❖ Easy skin bruising on IV access: Difficult access
❖ Electrolyte imbalances preoperatively
❖ Hypertension
❖ Impaired glucose tolerance
❖ Increased intravascular volume state
❖ Muscle weakness: Judicious administration of neuromuscular blockers

- Intraoperative steroid replacement therapy
- Postoperative infections common

Preoperative Assessment

- Routine history, history of drug intake and exercise tolerance
- All investigations, especially electrolytes
- Assess airway for difficult intubation (obese, DM)
- Assess ease of local anesthetic technique
- Check for preoperative weakness: Increased sensitivity to NMB
- Assess ease of IV line placement: Obesity and fragile skin
- Preoperative orthostatic hypotension warns against interoperative hypovolemia

Preoperative Preparation and Premedication

- Optimal control of:
  - DM, hypertension, CCF
  - Electrolyte abnormalities: Postpone surgery if K^+ lesser than 2.8 mEq/L
  - Restrictive lung disease
- Normalize intravascular volume status and electrolytes preoperatively
- Spironolactone 25–100 mg Q8H (up to 400 mg/day) started preoperatively
- NPO orders:
  - 6 hours for solids
  - 2 hours for clear fluids
- Informed consent
- Difficult IV access due to obesity and fragile skin: Good care of IV lines
- Premedication:
  - Midazolam 0.05–0.15 mg/kg IV
  - Diazepam 0.1 mg/kg PO
- Continue all medications including inhibitors of cortisol synthesis, steroids and antihypertensives
- Discontinue morning dose of insulin and diuretics
- Start glucose insulin drip if necessary
- Antibiotic and DVT prophylaxis before surgery
- Antiaspiration prophylaxis:
  - Ranitidine 1 mg/kg IV
  - Metaclopramide 10 mg IV

Monitors

- Pulse oximetry, E_TCO_2
- NIBP/IBP, ECG
- CVP: Patients tend to have higher CVP
- Peripheral nerve stimulator
- Urine output, temperature
- ABG, blood glucose, hematocrit

Position

- Careful positioning due to osteoporosis
- Increased risk of corneal abrasion due to exophthalmos: Proper eye cover
- Protect against nerve injury especially if lateral position used during adrenelectomy

Induction

- Adequate preoxygenation for 3–5 minutes
- *Rapid sequence induction* preferred for obese patients
- Etomidate 0.3 mg/kg *induction agent of choice* as it transiently reduces synthesis and release of cortisol
- Reduced dosage of NMB initially if weakness present preoperatively
- Administer anesthetic agents slowly and carefully as patients are sensitive to cardio depressant effects
- Neuromuscular monitoring before intubation as reduced doses of muscle relaxants administered
- Prepare for difficult intubation
- Avoid laryngoscopic response at induction

Maintenance

- O_2 + N_2O + isoflurane 1 MAC to maintain balanced anesthesia
- Fentanyl 1 μg/kg and vecuronium (low doses) given as intermittent boluses
- Cortisol replacement therapy:
  - Started at the time of starting tumor resection
  - Hydrocortisone 100 mg/day IV for unilateral and bilateral adrenelectomy
- Frequent blood glucose monitoring: Abnormal glucose tolerance intraoperatively

Ventilation

- ET tube with IPPV preferred as muscle weakness present
- High FiO_2 may be required
- Avoid hyperventilation as it causes alkalosis and hypokalemia

Hemodynamics

- Avoid IV fluids containing sodium
- Hemodynamic changes not as profound as for pheochromocytoma

- Hypertensive surges at the time of tumor manipulation treated with IV phentolamine 1 mg given every 5 minutes
- Major blood loss may occur during resection of highly vascular tumors: Keep blood ready

Extubation

- Extubate when:
  - Fully awake
  - Hemodynamically stable
  - Adequately reversed, TOF ratio > 0.7
  - Good ABG
- Neostigmine 0.05 mg/kg and glycopyrrolate 0.02 mg/kg IV prior to extubation
- Fully awake extubation in propped up position after TOF ratio ≥ 0.7
- Delayed extubation possible owing to residual neuromuscular weakness

Postoperative Care

Management

- Avoid excessive administration of Na^+ containing IV fluids as mineralocorticoid action of fludrocortisone will increase Na^+ resorption
- Continuous humidified oxygen therapy
- Physiotherapy, spirometry and early mobilization
- Steroid synthesis inhibitors started if surgery does not reduce effect of carcinoma
- Steroid replacement:
  - Hydrocortisone dose reduced by 50% every day till 20–30 mg/day on third postoperative day
  - Fludrocortisone 0.05–0.1 mg/day PO started on third postoperative day
  - Fludrocortisone continued lifelong in bilateral adrenelectomy patients
  - If unilateral adrenelectomy, fludrocortisone therapy individualized based on status of contralateral adrenal gland
  - Dosage reduced if HTN/CCF/hypokalemia
- DVT prophylaxis continued
- Vitamin D (therapy before surgery may cause hypercalcemia and renal stones)
- Insulin infusion and electrolyte correction
- Topical administration of Vitamin A to wound site to increase tensile strength of healing wounds which reduces in the presence of glucocorticoids

Monitors

- Pulse oximetry, capnography
- NIBP/IBP, CVP
- Temperature, urine output
- Neuromuscular monitoring

Complications

- Delayed awakening
- Hypoxemia, OSAS
- Adrenal insufficiency
- Transient DI/meningitis if pituitary resection
- Blood loss, pneumothorax
- Persistent hypertension due to permanent changes in vasculature
- ***Nelson's syndrome***: If pituitary tumor not diagnosed preoperatively and only adrenelectomy is done
- Respiratory complications due to:
  - Muscle weakness
  - Obesity
  - Kyphosis and rib fractures
- Delayed wound healing
- Postoperative stroke, MI, pulmonary thromboembolism
- Electrolyte abnormalities, pancreatitis
- High mortality: 5–10% if bilateral adrenelectomy

Analgesia

- Opioid infusion: Lower dose to prevent respiratory depression
- Patient controlled anesthesia
- Epidural analgesia where applicable
- Local anesthesia
- Multimodal analgesia

Role of Regional Analgesia

- Advantages:
  - Good analgesia
  - Rapid mobilization
  - Reduced DVT incidence
  - Reduced stress response
  - Reduced opioid requirement
- Disadvantages:
  - Technically difficult due to obesity
  - Consider osteoporosis with vertebral body collapse

CONN'S SYNDROME

Introduction

Syndrome arising due to primary hyperaldosteronism.

Incidence

- Rare occurrence
- Accounts for 1% of patients with hypertension
- More common between 30–50 years
- Occurs twice as commonly in females

Etiology

- Adrenal adenomas (called aldosteronomas) – 60%
- Bilateral adrenal hyperplasia (30%)
- Adrenal carcinoma
- Secondary hyperaldosteronism:
  - Increased aldosterone secretion due to increased renin activity
  - Causes are:
    - Congestive cardiac failure
    - Nephrotic syndrome
    - Cirrhosis
    - Some forms of hypertension (e.g., renal artery stenosis)

Pathophysiology

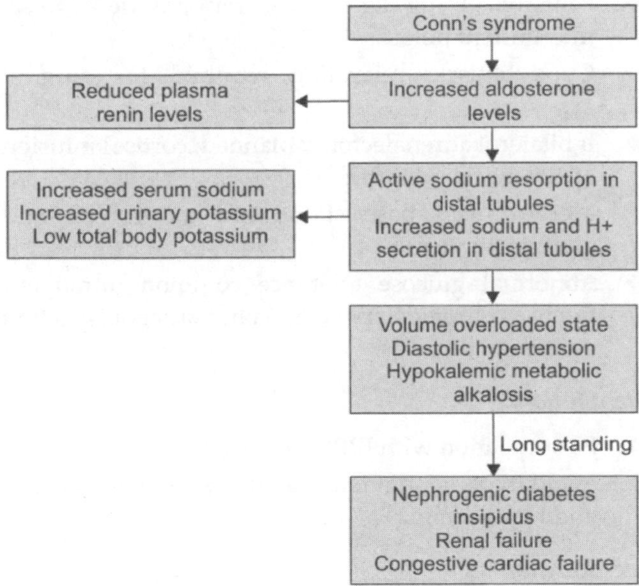

Clinical Features

- Cardiovascular:
  - Refractory hypertension: Mainly diastolic HTN (≥ 100–125 mmHg)
  - Renal and retinal damage from hypertension
  - Cardiomyopathy: From chronic potassium depletion
  - Congestive cardiac failure: Due to increased catecholamine levels
  - Arrhythmias, hypervolemia
- Metabolic:
  - Hypokalemic metabolic alkalosis (usually K^+ ≤ 3 mEq/L)
  - Abnormal glucose tolerance (50% patients)
  - Hypocalcemia and tetany due to alkalosis
  - Hypomagnesemia
  - Hypernatremia rarely
- Renal:
  - Nephropathy, proteinuria
  - Nephrogenic diabetes insipidus due to tubular damage
  - Renal failure due to hypertension
  - Polyuria, nocturia due to impaired renal concentrating ability
  - *Characteristic absence of edema*
- Neuromuscular:
  - Increased incidence of stroke
  - Skeletal muscle weakness from hypokalemia
  - Skeletal muscle cramps

Diagnostic Criteria

- Severe diastolic hypertension without edema
- Hyposecretion of renin which fails to increase during volume depletion
- Hypersecretion of aldosterone which does not reduce in response to volume expansion

Investigations

- General:
  - Complete blood count, renal function tests, blood glucose
  - ABG:
    - Hypernatremia
    - Hypokalemic alkalosis
    - Electrolytes (Ca^{2+} and mg^{2+})
  - ECG:
    - Arrhythmias LVH
    - T-wave flattening, U waves suggestive of hypokalemia
  - ECHO for LVH, RWMA, EF
  - Chest X-ray: Cardiomegaly
  - Fundoscopy for retinal hypertensive changes
  - USG, CT, MRI for tumor localization
  - Blood grouping and cross matching
  - Selective adrenal venous sampling
  - Urinary K^+ levels: Raised
- Diagnostic:
  - Raised plasma aldosterone levels:
    - More than 15 ng/dL when salt intake not restricted
    - More than 9.5 ng/dL after saline infusion is confirmatory

- Plasma renin activity:
  - If suppressed: Primary aldosteronism
  - If elevated: Secondary aldosteronism
- Adrenal venous sampling for aldosterone:
  - High on ipsilateral tumor side
  - Low on contralateral side
- Aldosterone-renin ratio:
  - More than 400 in primary aldosteronism
  - Normal in secondary aldosteronism

Treatment

- Primary aldosteronism due to adenoma:
  - Surgical excision for unilateral adenoma
  - Medical therapy:
    - Used for bilateral adenomas
    - Consists of:
      - Dietary salt restriction
      - Spironolactone 25–100 mg Q8H (up to 400 mg/day)
      - Oral K^+ replacement
      - Antihypertensives: CCB and ACE inhibitors are effective
- Idiopathic bilateral hyperplasia: Surgery done only when:
  - Significant and symptomatic hypokalemia
  - Not controlled by medical therapy (spironolactone/triamterene/amiloride)

Anesthetic Management

Preoperative Optimization and Premedication

- Spironolactone 25–100 mg TID (up to 400 mg/day) started preoperatively
- K^+ infusion (e.g. 6–20 mmol/hr) for at least 24 hours preoperatively
- Glucose insulin infusion if necessary
- Evaluate volume status: Preoperative orthostatic hypotension may warn against intraoperative hypovolemia
- NPO guidelines:
  - 6 hours: Solids
  - 2 hours: Clear fluids and water
- Informed consent
- Continue antihypertensives on day of surgery
- Diazepam 0.1 mg/kg PO for sedation
- Antibiotic prophylaxis as per hospital protocol

Monitors

- Pulse oximetry, E_TCO_2
- ECG, NIBP
- IBP useful for ABG, blood glucose and hematocrit
- CVP for guiding fluid therapy
- PAC for intravascular volume status and response to IV fluids
- Temperature and urine output

Induction

- Adequate preoxygenation for 3–5 minutes
- Thiopentone 3–4 mg/kg + fentanyl 1–2 µg/kg + vecuronium (low dose) for induction
- Slow injection of anesthetic agents to avoid hypotension
- Deep planes of intubation to avoid hypertensive surges

Maintenance

- $O_2 + N_2O$ + isoflurane 1 MAC
- MAC value of inhalational agents increase in the presence of hypernatremia
- Avoid sevoflurane if hypokalemic nephropathy and polyuria present
- Fentanyl 1 µg/kg + vecuronium (low dose) intermittent boluses
- Good muscle relaxation required for surgical exposure
- If bilateral adrenalectomy planned, cortisol infusion at 100 mg/day started
- Monitor acid base status and electrolytes and glucose frequently
- Abnormal glucose tolerance common intraoperatively as chronic hypokalemia has antagonist action on insulin secretion

Ventilation

- ET intubation with IPPV preferred
- Avoid hyperventilation to avoid increasing alkalosis and hypokalemia

Hemodynamics

- Avoid Na^+ containing fluids
- Massive blood loss may occur from injury to nearby blood vessels
- Treat hypertensive surges with:
  - Phentolamine 2.5–5 mg IV every 5 min
  - Labetolol 10–20 mg IV
- Avoid hypo and hypertensive episodes
- Extubation Neostigmine 0.05 mg/kg + glycopyrrolate 0.02 mg/kg IV
- Watch for residual NMB action potentiated by

hypokalemia

- Extubate when:
  - Fully awake
  - Hemodynamically stable
  - Adequately reversed, TOF ratio > 0.7
  - Good ABG

Postoperative Care

Management

- Respiratory support maybe required as:
  - Increased sensitivity to respiratory depressants and NMBS
  - Compensatory respiratory acidosis for metabolic alkalosis
- Postoperative fludrocortisone as in Cushing's syndrome for bilateral adrenalectomy
- Avoid excessive Na^+ containing fluids
- Insulin infusion for blood sugar control
- Correction of electrolyte abnormalities
- Na^+ and K^+ levels return to normal within a week

Monitor

- Pulse oximetry, ECG
- NIBP/IBP, CVP
- Urine output, temperature
- ABG, blood glucose, electrolytes
- Chest X-ray

Complications

- Mineralocorticoid/glucocorticoid deficiency
- Persistant hypertension due to permanent changes in vascular resistance
- Pneumothorax
- Electrolyte abnormalities

Pain

- Opioids as patient controlled analgesia
- NSAIDs as adjuvants
- Thoracic epidural: Best pain relief
- Multimodal analgesia

CARCINOID SYNDROME

Introduction

- Carcinoid tumor is a slow growing, benign, small intestinal tumor arising from enterochromaffin cells capable of metastasis but with good prognosis
- Carcinoid syndrome occurs when a metastatic carcinoid tumor releases vasoactive peptides into systemic circulation which leads to signs and symptoms collectively called carcinoid syndrome

Apudomas: Tumors of amine precursor uptake and decarboxylation:

- Pheochromocytoma
- Carcinoid tumor
- Gastrinoma
- VIPoma
- Isulinoma

Sites of Occurrence

- Gastrointestinal tract (75%):
  - Appendix *most common* but rarely metastasizes to cause syndrome
  - *Ileocecal* region causes *highest incidence of metastasis*
  - Colon, rectum
- Head and neck
- Lung and bronchus
- Gonads: Testes and ovary
- Thymus, breast
- Pancreas, genitourinary tract

Substances secreted: Up to 20 peptides and amines including:

- Serotonin, bradykinin
- Histamine, prostaglandins
- Vasoactive intestinal peptide
- Catecholamines: Dopamine
- Substance P, neurotensin
- Tachykinin, neuropeptide K
- Motilin

Pathophysiology

- 20% of patients with carcinoid tumor exhibit carcinoid syndrome
- As most tumors are located in GIT, their products are released into portal circulation and destroyed by the liver before they can cause systemic effects
- Carcinoid syndrome therefore manifests only in:
  - Patients with hepatic metastasis, who cannot metabolize the products
  - Those in whom products are directly released into systemic circulation like:
    - Carcinoid of thymus
    - Carcinoid of gonads

- Cardiac disease:
  - Substances which escape hepatic metabolism undergo pulmonary metabolism
  - Thus, right sided heart disease is more common than left sided disease
- Serotonin:
  - Little direct effect on heart
  - Positive inotropic and chronotropic effect
  - Vasoconstriction and vasodilation
  - Increased GI motility
  - Increased net intestinal water, Na^+, Cl^- and K^+ secretion
  - Bronchoconstriction
- Bradykinin:
  - Vasodilation of small resistance blood vessels
  - Stimulates histamine release from mast cells
  - Increases vascular permeability and causes edema
  - Does not affect myocardium directly
- Histamine:
  - Vasodilation of small blood vessels
  - Reduces total peripheral resistance
  - Bronchoconstriction

Clinical Features

- Most commonly asymptomatic
- Most commonly found as incidentaloma during appendicular surgery
- Skin:
  - Flushing:
    - Affects neck and torso
    - Is the *most common* symptom (90%)
  - Venous telangiectasia
- Gastrointestinal:
  - Diarrhea:
    - Very common
    - Watery diarrhea (up to 30 times/day)
    - Causes malabsorption state and steatorrhea
  - Chronic abdominal pain, intestinal obstruction
  - Hepatomegaly, hyperglycemia
- Cardiovascular:
  - Hemodynamic instability:
    - Tachycardia
    - Hypotension more common
    - Uncontrolled hypertension
  - ***Carcinoid heart disease***:
    - Components:
      - Right heart lesions: Tricuspid regurgitation, pulmonary stenosis
      - Premature atrial complexes, supraventricular tachycardia
    - Results in right heart failure with hepatomegaly and edema
    - Occurs due to:
      - Myocardial plaque formation
      - These are deposits of fibrous tissue on endocardium of right sided valve cusps
      - This is due to action of serotonin and tachykinin on platelets and endocardium
- Others:
  - Bronchoconstriction (20%), pruritus, lacrimation, facial edema
  - Hypoalbuminemia, hyponatremia, hypokalemia, hypochloremia
  - ***Pellagra***: diarrhea, dementia, dermatitis
  - Hemoptysis due to bronchial carcinoid
- ***Carcinoid triad:***
  - Cardiac involvement (usually tricuspid regurgitation/pulmonary stenosis)
  - Flushing
  - Diarrhea
- Carcinoid crisis:
  - Clinical features:
    - Intense flushing
    - Diarrhea, abdominal pain
    - Cardiovascular instability
  - Precipitating factors:
    - Stress and anxiety
    - Biopsy
    - Drugs: Catecholamines, pentagastrin, SSRI
    - Tumor debulking surgery
    - Chemotherapy with octreotide
    - Biotherapy
    - Hepatic artery embolization
    - Exercise, alcohol and cheese

Location	Presentation
Small intestine	Abdominal pain
	Intestinal obstruction
	Gastrointestinal bleeding
	Tumor
Rectal	Bleeding
	Constipation/diarrhea
Bronchial	Asymptomatic (31%)
Thymic	Anterior mediastinal mass
Ovarian and testicular	Mass on physical examination
Metastatic	Hepatomegaly

Drugs Associated with Crises

- Succniylcholine, mivacurium
- Atracurium, d-tubocurarine
- Epinephrine, norepinephrine
- Isoprenalin, dopamine
- Thiopentone, morphine

Diagnosis

- 5-hydroxyl indole acetic acid (5HIAA) :
  - Metabolite of serotonin
  - Normally 3–15 mg/24 hour urine sample
  - ≥ 30 mg in 24 hour urine sample is diagnostic
  - False positive test: Coffee/chocolate, banana, avocado, walnut, pineapple
  - False negative test: Phenergan, methyldopa, epinephrine and norepinephrine
- Chromograffin levels in plasma

Preoperative Evaluation

- History and examination:
  - Dyspnea, orthopnea, wheezing
  - Edema, arrhythmia, murmur
- If diarrhea present:
  - Orthostatic blood pressure
  - Serum electrolytes, BUN, serum creatinine, albumin
- If cardiac involvement:
  - ECG, echocardiography
  - Electrolytes
- Others:
  - LFTs and clotting profile if metastatic lesions
  - Chest X-ray and pulmonary function tests
- Increased perioperative risk with:
  - Increased levels of 5-HIAA
  - Carcinoid heart disease
- Preoperative endocrinologist consultation

Treatment

- Medical management:
  - Avoid conditions which precipitate flushing
  - Dietary nicotinamide supplementation
  - Treatment of right heart failure and wheezing
  - $H_1 + H_2$ blockers for flushing: Diphenhydramine + ranitidine
  - Antidiarrheals: Loperamide/diphenoxylate
  - 5-HT_3 blockers for vomiting: Ondansetron
  - Octreotide and lanreotide to reduce tumor size
- Surgey: Only potentially curative therapy for non-metastatic tumors
- Hepatic artery embolization: Used alone or with chemotherapy (*chemoembolization*)
- Biotherapy: Done with interferons

Preoperative Optimization

- Octreotide:
  - Synthetic somatostatin analogue
  - Somatostation is a GI regulatory peptide which reduces production and release of gastropancreatic hormones
  - It reduces the amount of serotonin secreted from carcinoid tumor
  - *Drug of choice* for preop, intraop and postop management of carcinoid symptoms
  - 50–500 μg (usually 100 μg) S/CQ8H
  - Dose titrated to relief of symptoms and prevention of hypotension
  - Given for 2 weeks preoperatively
  - Half life of 25 hrs, duration of action is 12 hrs
  - IM formulation also available
  - Side effects:
    - Bradycardia and complete heart block following IV bolus
    - Somnolence
    - Hyperglycemia
- $H_1 + H_2$ antagonists: H_2 antagonists more important than H_1 antagonists
- Serotonin antagonists:
  - Cyproheptidine and methysergide for GI features
  - Ketanserin for vasoconstriction/bronchospasm, platelet aggregation and hypertension
- Bradykinin antagonists:
  - Aprotinin and steroids
  - Used for treatment of flushing and hypotension refractory to octreotide
  - Aprotinin inhibits kallikrein cascade
  - Steroids:
    - Reduce synthesis of prostaglandin which mediate actions of bradykinin
    - Effective in bronchial carcinoids
- Bronchodilators and treatment of right heart failure

Anesthetic Considerations

- Asymptomatic carcinoid tumor does not present anesthetic difficulties
- Hypovolemia and electrolyte abnormalities
- Use somatostatin analogues to prevent mediator release

- ❖ Avoid factors which precipitate crises:
  - Anxiety
  - Hypercarbia, hypoxia
  - Hypothermia, hypotension
- ❖ Prepare for resistant bronchospasm and sudden variation in BP at induction and when tumor is handled
- ❖ Avoid histamine releasing agents

Preoperative Medication

- ❖ Correct fluid and electrolyte abnormalities
- ❖ Nutritional support required if severe malabsorption
- ❖ NPO orders:
  - 6 hours for solids
  - 2 hours for clear fluids
- ❖ Informed consent
- ❖ Continue antagonists of serotonin, bradykinin and histamine preoperatively:
  - Octreotide 10–100 µg IV slowly 1 hour prior to surgery
  - Promethazine, ranitidine
  - Ondansetron is *antiemetic of choice*
- ❖ Anxiolysis with benzodiazepines: Midazolam 0.05–0.15 mg/kg IV

OT Preparation

- ❖ Anesthetic drugs
- ❖ Suction apparatus
- ❖ Monitors
- ❖ Emergency drugs:
  - Atropine, phenylephrine, NTG, SNP
  - Dopamine, dobutamine
- ❖ All antimediator drugs kept ready in OT:
  - Ketanserin
  - Cyproheptidine
  - Somatostatin
  - Aprotinin
  - Antihistaminics

Monitors

- ❖ Pulse oximetry, E_TCO_2
- ❖ NIBP used if short duration surgery
- ❖ IBP/CVP inserted preinduction as induction can cause large BP swings
- ❖ ABG and blood sugars
- ❖ Temperature, urine output
- ❖ Airway pressures
- ❖ PA catheter: Caution while floating if right heart valves are damaged
- ❖ TEE if right heart is involved

Induction

- ❖ Adequate preoxygenation for 3–5 minutes
- ❖ Smooth anesthetic technique with avoidance of major hemodynamic changes
- ❖ Etomidate and vecuronium are *drugs of choice*
- ❖ Propofol/etomidate used as induction agents
- ❖ Vecuronium/rocuronium can be used as muscle relaxants
- ❖ Sufentanyl/fentanyl/alfentanyl/remifentanyl can also be used
- ❖ Topical laryngeal LA spray and xylocard to avoid pressor response at intubation
- ❖ Avoid:
  - Ketamine for induction
  - Succinylcholine as scholine induced fasciculations can precipitate crisis
  - Histamine releasers like morphine, pethidine and thiopentone

Maintenance

- ❖ O_2 + air + isoflurane 1 MAC for balanced anesthesia
- ❖ Desflurane *is drug of choice* in cases of hepatic metastasis as it is less metabolized
- ❖ Vecuronium and fentanyl given as intermittent boluses
- ❖ Octreotide infusion at 50–100 µg/hr during surgery with 100–150 µg IV bolus prior to manipulation of tumor
- ❖ Fluid resuscitation and electrolyte correction important as carcinoid tumors have high gastric output and gastric fluid losses during surgery

Intraoperative Complications

- ❖ Severe hypo/hypertension
- ❖ Fluid and electrolyte shifts
- ❖ Bronchospasm
- ❖ Hypo/hyperglycemia
- ❖ Hyperglycemia more common as octreotide inhibits insulin secretion

Hemodynamics

- ❖ Hypotension:
  - IV fluid boluses
  - Octreotide 10–20 µg IV bolus dose
  - Aprotinin/vasopressin/angiotensin boluses if refractory hypotension
  - Phenylephrine, calcium chloride, and milrinone relatively safe
  - Avoid vasopressors as they stimulate amine release

- Hypertension treated with:
  - Ketanserin, octreotide
  - Increased volatile agents
  - Labetolol/clonidine
- Tachycardia: Esmolol/propranolol
- If tricuspid regurgitation present, avoid factors causing pulmonary hypertension:
  - Angiotensin, vasopressin
  - Hypoxia, hypercarbia
  - Acidosis, hypothermia

Extubation

- Glycopyrrolate 0.02 mg/kg + neostigmine 0.05 mg/kg for reversal
- Extubated once patient is:
  - Hemodynamically stable
  - Fully awake
  - TOF ≥ 0.7
  - Adequately warmed

Choice of Regional Anesthesia

- Relatively contraindicated as hypotension can precipitate bradykinergic crisis
- Graded epidural can be used in a patient adequately treated with octreotide
- Avoid hypotension by:
  - Using diluted LA solution
  - Epidural opioids to reduce LA use
  - Graded epidural
  - Adequate preloading with IV fluids

Postoperative Care

Monitoring

- Pulse oximetry
- Intense hemodynamic monitoring: IBP/CVP/PAC
- ECG, repeated ABG and blood sugar
- Pain scale, urine output and temperature

Management

- Delayed recovery may occur due to serotonin release
- Octreotide slowly weaned over 7–10 days following resection
- IV octreotide 10–20 µg boluses for hypotension

Analgesia

- Adequate analgesia to reduce amine release
- Reduce opioid dose as increased somnolence and respiratory depression common
- NSAIDs as adjuvants
- Regional anesthesia, epidural safe
- Local anesthetic infilteration can be used to supplement analgesia
- Multimodal analgesia

DIABETES MELLITUS

Introduction

- Diabetes mellitus diagnosed if:
  - FBS ≥ 126 mg/dL
  - RBS ≥ 200 mg/dL with symptoms of diabetes
  - 2 hour PPBS ≥ 200 mg/dL
- Called impaired fasting glucose if FBS between 100–125 mg/dL
- Called impaired glucose tolerance if 2 hour PPBS is between 140–199 mg/dL
- Called critical illness induced hyperglycemia if:
  - Blood glucose ≥ 200 mg/dL
  - In the absence of known DM
  - Occurs frequently in elderly

Classification

- Primary:
  - Type 1 diabetes mellitus/insulin dependent diabetes mellitus (IDDM)
    - Type IA: Immune mediated
    - Type IB: Idiopathic
  - Type II diabetes mellitus/non-insulin dependent diabetes mellitus (NIDDM)
    - Non-obese NIDDM
    - Obese NIDDM
    - Maturity onset diabetes of young (MODY)
  - Gestational diabetes mellitus
- Secondary:
  - Pancreatic disease:
    - Pancreatitis, pancreatic carcinoma
    - Pancreatectomy, cystic fibrosis
  - Endocrinological:
    - Acromegaly, Cushing's syndrome
    - Pheochromocytoma, glucagonoma
    - Hyperthyroidism
  - Genetic syndromes:
    - ***Downs, Klinefelters syndrome***
    - ***Turners, Prader-Willi syndrome***
  - Insulin receptor abnormalities:
    - ***Leprechaunism***, Type A insulin resistance
    - ***Robson-Mendelhall syndrome***

- Infection: Congenital rubella, CMV
- Drug induced:
  - Glucocorticoids, thyroid hormones
  - β blockers, pentamidine
  - Phenytoin, thiazides

Incidence

- Most common endocrine disorder
- 8 to 17 per 100, 000 per year incidence
- Prevalence 20.1% in patients > 65 years

Types

Type I diabetes mellitus	Type II diabetes mellitus
IDDM	NIDDM
Absence of insulin in the body	Peripheral insulin resistance
Plasma glucagon is high and suppressible	Plasma glucagon is high and resistant
Age at onset less than 40 years	Age at onset more than 40 years
Chromosome 5	Chromosome 2
Body habitus normal/wasted	Obese
Susceptible to DKA	Resistant to DKA
Resistant to HONC	Susceptible to HONC
Unresponsive to sulfonylurea therapy	Respond to sulfonylurea therapy
Associated with autoimmune diseases	Not associated with autoimmune diseases

Risk Factors for Type II Diabetes Mellitus

- Family history of DM
- Overweight, physical inactivity
- Excess abdominal fat (even if BMI is normal)
- Native Americans, Asians, Hispanics
- Female: Male: 2:1
- Polycystic ovarian disease, history of vascular disease
- Previous IGT/IFG
- Long standing HTN ≥ 140/90 mmHg
- Patients on steroids

Actions of Insulin

Increased anabolism	Decreased catabolism
Carbohydrate metabolism	
Glucose transport	Reduced gluconeogenesis
Glucose phosphorylation	Reduced glycogenolysis
Increased pyruvate dehydrogenase	
Increased pentose phosphate shunt	
Glycogenesis	
Glycolysis	
Fat Metabolism	
Triglyceride synthesis	Reduced lipolysis
Fatty acid synthesis	Reduced fatty acid oxidation
Increased lipoprotein lipase	Reduced ketogenesis
Protein metabolism	
Increased amino acid transport	Reduced protein breakdown
Increased protein synthesis	

Pathogenesis

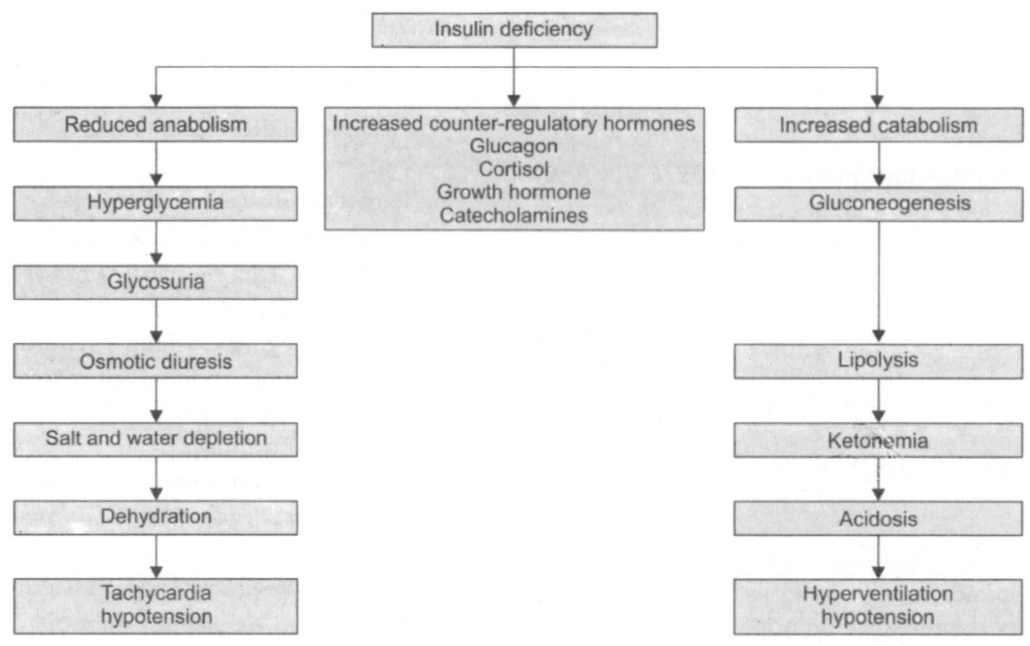

Complications

- Acute complications:
  - Diabetic ketoacidosis (DKA)
  - Hyperosmolar non-ketotic coma (HONC)
  - Hypoglycemia (*Bloodglucose ≤ 50 mg/dl*)
- Chronic complications:
  - Microvascular:
    - Eye disease:
      - Retinopathy
      - Macular edema
    - Neuropathy:
      - Sensory and motor neuropathy
      - Autonomic neuropathy
    - Nephropathy
  - Macrovascular:
    - Coronary artery disease
    - Cerebrovascular accidents
    - Peripheral vascular disease
  - Others:
    - Cataract, glaucoma
    - Gastrointestinal:
      - Gastroparesis, constipation
      - Diarrhea
    - Genitourinary:
      - Uropathy
      - Erectile dysfunction
    - Dermatological
    - Infection
- Complications of therapy:
  - ***Dawn phenomenon***:
    - Occurs in Type 1 DM
    - Due to increased requirement of insulin post midnight
    - This is because of glucagon surgeca using hyperglycemia
  - ***Somagyi phenomenon***: Compensatory hyperglycemia following hypoglycemia

Preoperative Evaluation

- History:
  - Central nervous system:
    - Peripheral neuropathy (glove and stocking neuropathy)
    - Headache, syncope
    - TIA/stroke
  - Cardiovascular:
    - MI: Increased chances if erectile dysfunction present
    - Silent MI: Increased chances if autonomic neuropathy
    - Hypertension
    - Congestive cardiac failure: Especially if poor glycemic control
    - Dyspnea on exertion/reduced exercise tolerance
  - Respiratory:
    - Frequent infections
    - Reduced VC, FVC, FEV, DLCO
  - Gastrointestinal:
    - Gastroparesis due to ganglion cell damage
    - Postprandial vomiting, early satiety
    - Delayed gastric emptying
  - Genitourinary:
    - Erectile dysfunction
    - Renal failure especially if age ≥ 55 years and diabetes and hypertension coexist
  - Medication history, history of anesthetic exposure
  - Episodes of hypoglycemia/hyperglycemia
- Examination:
  - Document vitals, orthostatic vital signs and skin breakdown points
  - Sensory examination
  - Airway examination:
    - ***Stiff joint syndrome***:
      - Seen in poorly controlled DM
      - Reduced mobility of cervical, atlanto-occiptal and TM joint occurs
    - ***Prayer sign***: Inability to approximate palmar surface of interphalangeal joints
    - ***Palm print sign***:
      - Alteration in palm print when it is taken on paper
      - Indicates interphalangeal joint stiffness
- Fundoscopy for retinopathy
- Tests for autonomic dysfunction
- Back for edema and infection: Difficult to perform subarachnoid block

Investigations

- Routine blood: Hb, TC, DC, ESR
- Renal function tests
- Preoperative FBS ≤110 mg% in non-critically ill patients: ***ACE recommendations***
- ECG, treadmill test for silent MI
- Chest X-ray: Cardiomegaly
- Pulmonary function tests
- Glycated hemoglobin:
  - Called HbA1c
  - Best evidence of glucose control over last 1–2 months
  - Level < 2% recommended by ADA

- Microalbuminuria ≥ 29 mg/day with HbA1c ≥ 8.1% predicts 80% risk of CRF
- HbA1c 8.5–9% predicts increased chances of retinopathy

Glucotoxicity

- Delayed wound healing:
  - Due to abnormal glycosylation of proteins
  - This causes reduced elastance and tensile wound healing strength
- Intracellular swelling due to macromolecules like sorbitol
- Impaired oxygen transport
- Endothelial dysfunction
- Adverse effect on CNS recovery after ischemia:
  - Common if blood glucose ≥ 150–250 mg/dL
  - Blood glucose should be <200 mg/dL in a diabetic patient about to undergo surgeries in which hypotension or reduced cerebral blood flow may occur
- Disruption of autoregulation:
  - Causes vasodilation
  - This prevents target organs from protecting against increase in systemic BP
- Osmotic dieresis: Dehydration and electrolyte imbalance

Anesthetic Consideration

- Difficult intubation due to stiff joint syndrome
- Increased risk of aspiration due to gastroparesis: Treat all diabetics as full stomach
- Increased risk of hypothermia due to autonomic dysfunction causing vasodilation
- Poor response to atropine/catecholamines if autonomic neuropathy
- Increased risk of nerve injury
- Increased perioperative complications:
  - Perioperative MI in those with erectile dysfunction
  - CCF due to both systolic and diastolic dysfunction
  - Perioperative renal failure
  - Increased risk of wound infections
- Reduced oxygen saturation and transport in pregnancy due to glycosylation of Hb

Glycemic Goals: ***ACE recommendations*:**

- ICU care: 110–180 mg/dL
- Intraoperative control: Less than 150 mg/dL
- Perioperative control: 90–130 mg/dL

GLYCEMIC REGIMENS

Sliding Sale

- Advantages: Easy to calculate
- Disadvantages:
  - Not used in major surgery
  - Blood glucose not optimally controlled

Blood glucose	Insulin
Less than 150 mg/dL	Nil
150–200 mg/dL	2 IU
200–250 mg/dL	4 IU
250–300 mg/dL	6 IU
300–350 mg/dL	8 IU
More than 350 mg/dL	10 IU + blood sugar monitoring

Modified Sliding Scale

Blood glucose	Insulin
< 60 mg/dL	Selected dose withheld for 1 hour
	IV 50% dextrose at 0.01–0.02 mL/kg/min
	Hourly blood sugar monitoring
≥ 125 mg/dL without supplemental dextrose	Next dose should be 20–40% lesser
≤ 100 mg/dL or < 125 mg/dL and decreasing	Scheduled dose maintained till BS ≥ 125 mg/dL
100–200 mg/dL and stable	Current dose continued
200–350 mg/dL	Increase scheduled dose by 10–20%
≥ 350 mg/dL	Increase dose by 20–40%

Classic Non-Tight Control Regimen

- NPO from 12 midnight with glass of orange juice kept by the side for emergency
- At 6 AM on day of surgery, IV 5% dextrose at 125 mL/hr/70 kg body weight
- After starting IV infusion, half the usual morning dose of usual type of insulin given S/C
- Continue 5% dextrose intraoperatively at at least 125 mL/hr/70 kgs
- Monitor blood glucose postoperatively and treat as per sliding scale

Tight Control Regimen

Aim: To maintain blood sugar between 79–120 mg/dL

Indications for Tight Glycemic Control

- Type 1 DM (as they need insulin to avoid DKA)
- Pregnant diabetics
- Major surgery or bowel anastomosis

- Those requiring post-procedure ICU stay
- Diabetics undergoing CPB
- Those with global CNS ischemia (e.g., following cardiac arrest)
- Surgery in those with DKA
- Type II DM do not benefit from tight perioperative control unless ICU stay is required according to current data

Regimen I

- Determine preprandial blood glucose on evening before surgery
- IV infusion of 5 and dextrose at 50 mL/hr/70 kg body weight
- *Piggy back* regular insulin:
  - 50 IU added to 250 mL NS
  - Flush infusion line with first 60 mL of infusate
- Rate of infusion:
  - (Blood glucose)/150 normally
  - (Blood glucose)/100 if:
    - Patient on steroids (except inhaled)
    - Obese with BMI ≥ 35
- Repeat blood glucose Q4H and adjust insulin to obtain blood glucose 100–200 mg/dL
- On morning of surgery:
  - Administer non-dextrose containing fluids
  - Insulin startedwith insulin infusion rate (BG/150 or BG/100)
- Determine blood glucose at the start of surgery and Q2H for rest of 24 hour period
- Treat hypoglycemia (< 50 mg/dL) with 15 mL 50% dextrose with termination of infusion

Regimen II

- Obtain feedback mechanism pancreas and set controls for desired blood glucose levels
- Start 2 IV lines

Advantages

- Improves CNS outcome after global/focal ischemic event
- Decreased incidence of polyneuropathy
- Improves weaning from CPB
- Decreased renal dysfunction and need for dialysis
- Reduced need for blood transfusion
- Reduces deaths in ICU and duration of ICU stay
- Improved oxygen transport
- Prevents wound infection
- Improves wound healing

Disadvantages

- Increased incidence of hypoglycemia
- Lack of potassium supplementation

GIK Regimen

Blood sugar	IV Insulin	KCL	IV Fluids 100 mL	Subcutaneous
< 100	1 IU	2 mEq	10% D	Nil
101–200	2 IU	2 mEq	10% D	4 IU
201–300	3 IU	2 mEq	10% D	6 IU
301–400	4 IU	2 mEq	5% DNS	8 IU
≥ 400	4 IU	2 mEq	NS	10 IU

- Combination of 10% dextrose and insulin is added to 500 mL fluid bag
- This provides 250 gms glucose and 50 U insulin in 24 hours
- Advantage: Prevents hypo/hyperglycemia
- Disadvantage: New bag of fluid is required every time glucose falls outside range

Vellore Regimen

Advantages: Simple, safe and inexpensive
Disadvantages: Potassium levels are not corrected

Blood glucose	Insulin	IV fluid
Less than 70 mg/dL	Nil	D5 100 mL IV rapidly
		Measure blood sugar after 15 min
70–100 mg/dL	Nil	D5 at 100 mL/hr
110–150 mg/dL	1 IU	100 mL D5
150–200 mg/dL	2 IU	100 mL D5
200–250 mg/dL	3 IU	100 mL D5
250–300 mg/dL	4 IU	100 mL D5
More than 300 mg/dL	6 IU	NS

Alberti Regimen

- Initial insulin solution: 500 mL 10% dextrose with 10 mmol KCL and 15 IU insulin
- Infuse at 100 mL/hr (i.e., 3 IU/hr)
- Check blood glucose second hourly
- Adjust infusion rate according to result:

Blood glucose	Infusion
Less than 117 mg/dL	2 IU/hr
117–200 mg/dL	3 IU/hr
More than 200 mg/dL	4 IU/hr

Watt-Hirsch Regimen

- Also called ***variable rate insulin regimen***
- Infuse glucose at 5 gm/hr, K^+ at 2–4 mEq/hr and insulin at 0.5–1 IU/hr

- Measure blood glucose hourly
- Insulin is either piggy backed with glucose or given as separate infusion

Blood glucose	Action
Less than 80 mg/dL	Stop infusion for 30 minutes
	25 gms glucose given IV
	Restart insulin 0.3–0.6 IU/hr when blood glucose more than 120 mg/dL
80–120 mg/dL	Reduce insulin by 0.3 IU/hr
120–180 mg/dL	No change
180–240 mg/dL	Increase insulin infusion by 0.3 IU/hr
More than 240 mg/dL	Increase insulin infusion by 0.5 IU/hr

Computer Controlled Insulin Infusion

- Computer adjusts rate of infusion according to blood sugar levels
- Baseline blood glucose and initial parameters entered into computer
- Insulin per hour = multiplier x (blood glucose - 60)
- Blood glucose monitored every 20 minutes

Preoperative Preparation

- Postpone elective surgery if:
  - HbA1c 7–9% for ≤ 5 years old
  - HbA1c 6–8% for ≥ 5 years old
  - Abnormal electrolytes
  - Ketonuria
- Posted usually as first case of day to avoid hypoglycemia
- NPO orders:
  - Kept NPO for 12 hours
  - Increased risk of gastroparesis causes delayed emptying
  - Glucose tablet/clear juice kept at bedside in the event of hypoglycemia
- Correct any fluid deficit/electrolyte disturbances
- VBG/blood sugar and ketones on morning of surgery
- Monitor glucose:
  - Immediately perioperatively
  - Every 3 hours till oral intake has resumed for minor surgery
  - Every 1–2 hour till oral intake has resumed for major surgery
- Control of blood sugar:
  - Type I DM:
    - Discontinue long acting insulin 1–2 days before surgery
    - Change to subcutaneous short acting insulin Q4-6H according to blood sugar
    - Not necessary to change intermediate acting insulin to short acting insulin preoperatively
    - If insulin pump is present:
      - Continue pump for short surgeries
      - Switch to IV insulin infusions for major surgery
  - Type II DM:
    - Stop long acting OHAs (chlorpropamide) at least 48 hours before surgery
    - Metformin:
      - Stopped 24 hours before surgery
      - Stopped for 48 hours after any procedure using IV contrast dye
    - Discontinue morning dose of all other OHAS except thiazolidines which can be taken as they do not predispose to hypoglycemia
  - On the morning of surgery:
    - For type I DM, continue usual insulin as half the usual morning dose
    - 5% dextrose given at 2 mg/kg/min
    - This is followed by insulin at (BG/150 or BG/100) IU/hr
    - Monitor blood glucose hourly intraoperatively
    - Maintain blood sugar with the help of selected protocol
- Sedation:
  - IV midazolam 0.05–0.15 mg/kg for sedation
  - IV glycopyrrolate 0.02 mg/kg
- Antiaspiration prophylaxis:
  - IV metoclopramide 10 mg
  - IV ranitidine 1 mg/kg
- Appropriate IV antibiotics as per hospital protocol
- Consider β blocker therapy on morning of surgery if CAD is present with DM

Choice of Anesthetic Technique

Regional anesthesia: Technique of choice where applicable:

- Advantages:
  - Avoids aspiration
  - Better if difficult airway
  - Patient is awake: Easy to recognize hypoglycemia
  - Reduced incidence of DVT
  - Reduced stress response to surgery
  - Good postoperative analgesia
  - Reduced chances of pulmonary infection

- Disadvantages:
  - Exaggerated hypotension especially if autonomic neuropathy present
  - Increased risk of epidural abscess
  - Caution if preexisting neuropathy
  - Increased risk of nerve injury
- Guidelines:
  - Local anesthetic requirement is lower
  - Combination of LA with adrenaline may increase risk of ischemic or edematous nerve injury
  - Bradycardia may be unresponsive to atropine
  - Isoprenaline/1:10, 000 adrenaline used in such cases
  - Chart preexisting nerve damage as increased chance of nerve injury
  - Technique: May be difficult if edema is present
- Contraindications:
  - Autonomic neuropathy
  - Infections

General Anesthesia

- Advantages:
  - Better cardiovascular stability
  - Airway is protected from silent aspiration
- Disadvantages:
  - Difficult intubation
  - Difficult to recognize hypoglycemia
  - Altered elimination of drugs due to renal involvement
  - Increased stress response

Anesthetic Management

Induction

- Adequate preoxygenation for 3–5 minutes
- Anticipated difficult intubation: Awake intubation preferred
- If not, *rapid sequence induction* used to avoid aspiration
- Etomidate is *drug of choice* as it inhibits adrenal steroidogenesis
- Etomidate, fentanyl and vecuronium used for induction
- Reduce dose of induction agent and give drugs slowly to avoid hypotension
- Atracurium/cisatracurium if renal fuction tests are altered
- β blockers and lidocaine used to reduce intubation response as BP is labile

Monitors

- Pulse oximetry, blood sugar second hourly
- E_TCO_2, electrolytes and ABG Q4-6H
- BP, ECG
- Urine output, temperature
- IBP/CVP if cardiovascular instability

Maintenance

- TIVA is good alternative but care to avoid lipid overload
- Avoid volatile anesthetics as it impairs glucose tolerance
- Narcotic based anesthetic techniques best to reduce cardiovascular depression
- Prophylactic NTG used if increased risk of CAD
- Nasogastric tube inserted to empty stomach
- Midazolam in high doses reduces cortisol secretion
- Clonidine and dexmedetomidine give good glycemic control

Hemodynamics

- Non-dextrose containing IV fluids used
- Avoid Ringer's lactate as it causes hyperglycemia
- In event of sudden bradycardia and hypotension which is unresponsive to atropine (give up to 40 µg/kg) try adrenaline 1:10, 000 or isoprenaline
- If intraoperative hypoglycemia occurs, 20 mL 50% dextrose given and sugars checked after 1 hour
- Bank blood may contain ACD which may aggravate hyperglycemia
- One unit insulin reduces glucose by 25 mg/dL
- 1 mL 25% dextrose increases glucose by 1 mg/dL

Extubation

- Prolonged duration of action of muscle relaxants and delayed recovery may occur if RFTs are elevated
- Extubate only if:
  - Full neuromuscular recovery
  - Good hemodynamic stability

Postoperative

- Check blood sugar Q2-6H, serum creatinine and electrolytes Q4-6H
- Continue infusion till oral feeding is established
- If feeding is delayed add glucose to IV fluid as required
- Once patient resumes oral intake and insulin requirement < 20 IU/day treatment is changed to patients chronic regimen
- Metformin is reinstituted only after RFTs found to be normal

Treatment of Diabetes Mellitus

Exogenous Insulin

Type	Preparation	Onset	Peak	DOA
Fast acting	Insulin-lispro	15 mins	30–90 min	3–4 hrs
	Regular	30–60 mins	2–4 hrs	6–8 hrs
	Semilente	1–3 hrs	5–10 hrs	16 hrs
Intermediate acting	Isophane (NPH)	2–4 hrs	6–12 hrs	18–26 hrs
	Lente	2–4 hrs	6–12 hrs	18–26 hrs
Long acting	Protamine–zinc	4–8 hrs	14–24 hrs	28–36 hrs
	Ultralente	4–8 hrs	14–24 hrs	28–36 hrs

Insulin Analogue

Analogue	Onset	Peak	DOA
Lispro insulin	5–15 mins	1–2 hrs	2–3 hrs
Glargine insulin	1–3 hrs	No peak	24 hrs
Aspart	5–15 mins	1–2 hrs	2–3 hrs

Oral Hypoglycemic Agents

- Sulfonylureas:
  - Tolbutamide, chlorpropamide
  - Glibenclamide, glipizide, glimepiride, glyburide, glyclazide
  - Insulin secretogogues with increased insulin secretion
  - Duration of action: 12–18 hrs (48 hours for chlorpropamide)
- Biguanides:
  - Metformin mechanism of action:
    - Increases peripheral responsiveness to insulin
    - Reduces hepatic gluconeogenesis
    - Potentiates insulin release
  - Duration of action of 6–8 hours
  - Can cause lactic acidosis
  - Contraindicated if serum creatinine >1.5, liver failure, alcoholics, etc
- Thiazolidine diones:
  - Mechanism of action: Releases insulin and increases peripheral responsiveness to insulin
  - Roglitazone, pioglitazone
  - Duration of action: 3–5 hours
- α-glucosidase inhibitors:
  - Acarbose and miglitol
  - Reduces absorption of glucose from GIT
  - Can cause GI flatulence
- Non-insulin secretogogues: Repaglinide, nateglinide, sitagliptin
- Ingap peptides:
  - Islet neogenesis associated protein (INGAP)
  - Causes regrowth of normally functioning islet cells
- Inhaled insulin:
  - 1 mg = 3U of subcutaneous insulin
  - Has a rapid onset of action
  - Causes sore throat and dry mouth

Diabetic Patient for CABG

- Perioperative mortality of 5% vs 1.5% for non-diabetics
- Tight glucose control regimen advocated conventionally
- Recent studies show no difference in mortality and morbidity than those who received conventional glucose management (treatment of blood glucose ≥ 200 mg%)
- In fact, statistically insignificant increase in incidence of stroke and death noted with tight control regimen
- Marked hyperglycemia may occur during CPB which may be unresponsive to insulin until rewarming
- Increased inotropic support and IABP may be required post-bypass
- Administration of washed cells advocated as ACD or adenine supplemented blood may cause hyperglycemia
- Ill effects during surgery:
  - Reduced vasodilation in response to ischemia
  - Reduced coronary collateral circulation
  - Increased levels of reactive oxygen species, low NO levels
  - Diminished response to ischemic and anesthetic preconditioning

DIABETIC KETOACIDOSIS

Introduction

- Acute life-threatening complication of diabetes mellitus
- Insulin is the *only anabolic hormone produced by pancreas*

Incidence

- 15 episodes per 1000 diabetics
- More common in Type I diabetes mellitus
- Can also occur in Type II diabetes mellitus

Diagnostic Criteria

- Blood glucose ≥ 250 mg/dL
- Osmolality ≥ 300–320 mosm/L
- Arterial pH ≤ 7.3
- Serum bicarbonate ≤ 15 mEq/L
- Moderate ketonemia

Etiology

- About 25% patients have no clear precipitating cause
- Omission of daily insulin injection
- Infections:
  - Pneumonia
  - Gastroenteritis
  - Urinary tract infection
  - Pancreatitis
  - Sepsis
- Infarction:
  - Myocardial infarction
  - Cerebrovascular accident
  - Mesenteric infarcts
  - Peripheral infarct
- Trauma, surgery
- Hyperthyroidism
- Pregnancy
- Pulmonary embolism
- Drugs:
  - Steroid use
  - Cocaine abuse

Ketones Produced

- Acetone
- Acetoacetic acid
- β-hydroxy butyric acid

Pathophysiology

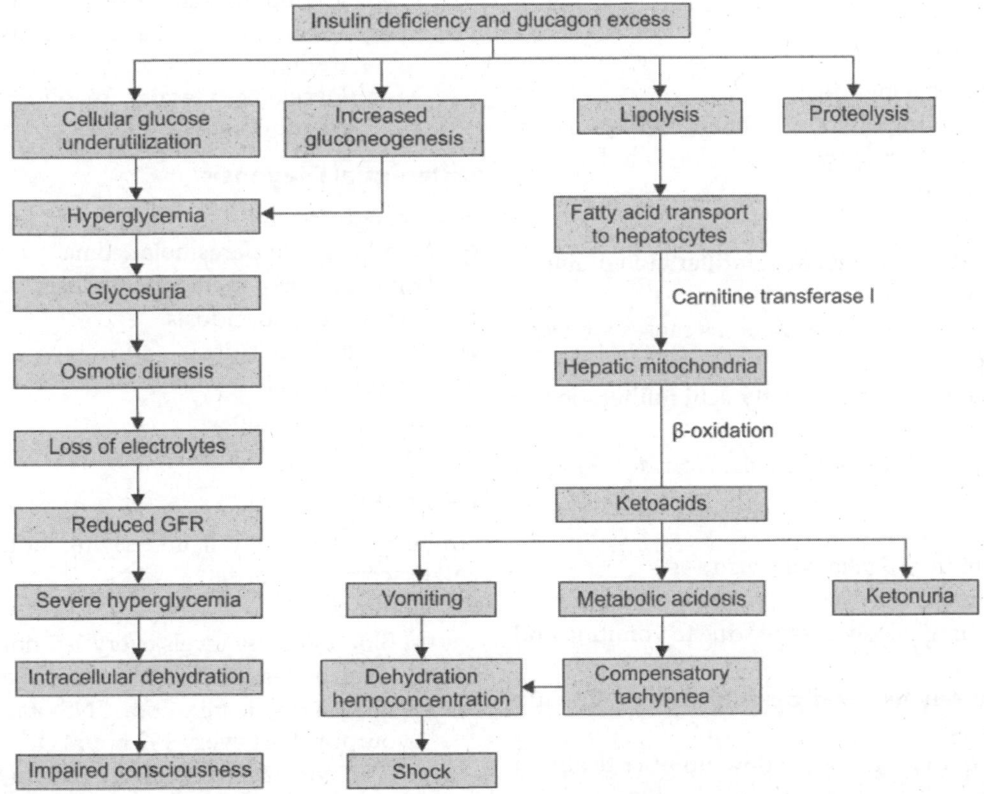

Clinical Features

- Hyperglycemia:
  - Causes increased serum osmolality
  - Osmotic diuresis
  - Hyponatremia, hypokalemia, hypocalcemia, hypomagnesemia
  - Hypochloremia, hypophosphatemia
- Acidosis:
  - Hyperventilation, shortness of breath
  - ***Kussmauls breathing if severe*** (fruity odor): *Classic presentation*
  - Nausea, vomiting (also caused by raised PGE^2 and PGI^2)

- Abdominal pain due to ileus, gastric distension/ pancreatitis
- Weakness, lethargy, obtundation, cerebral vasodilatation and edema, coma
- Hypothermia due to peripheral vasodilatation (even if infection present)
- Impaired myocardial contractility: reduced cardiac output

❖ Volume contraction:
- Compensatory polyuria and polydipsia: *earliest symptom*
- Orthostatic hypotension
- Hypotension and tachycardia
- Poor skin turgor, dry mucous membrane
- Dehydration
- Frank hypovolemic shock

Investigations

❖ Leukocytosis due to hemoconcentration

❖ ECG: Sinus tachycardia/hypokalemia features

❖ Blood glucose:
- Usually $\geq$ 300 mg/dL
- Lower if impaired gluconeogenesis, as in alcoholics/liver failure

❖ Urinary glucose

❖ Renal function tests:
- Increased due to fatty acid infilteration of liver
- Prerenal azotemia
- Interference from ketone bodies causes spurious elevation

❖ Liver function tests due to fatty acid infilteration of liver

❖ Raised serum CPK, amylase, triglycerides, lipoproteins

❖ ABG/VBG:
- Wide anion gap metabolic acidosis
- Compensatory hypocapnea may occur
- Metabolic alkalosis possible due to vomiting and diuresis
- Usually venous blood gas suffices for follow up of therapy
- ABG required only for follow up of critically ill patients
- (ABG pH – VBG pH) = 0.3
- Anion gap is *most accurate* determinant of recovery

❖ *Nitroprusside stick test*:
- For blood and urine ketone bodies
- Only detects acetoacetic acid
- May increase after treating DKA as β-hydroxy butyric acid gets converted to acetoacetic acid
- Thus only initial ketone detection in urine is necessary as subsequent measurement may yield spurious results

❖ Serum electrolytes:
- Potassium:
  - Initial potassium at presentation maybe normal or high due to:
    - Metabolic acidosis causing extracellular shift of K^+ ions
    - Increased intravascular osmolarity
    - Prerenal azotemia
  - Initial hypokalemia at presentation indicates severe total body potassium depletion due to osmotic renal losses
- Others:
  - Hyponatremia
  - Hypomagnesemia
  - Hypocalcemia
  - Hypochloremia
  - Hypophosphatemia
  - These may be masked due to hemoconcentration
  - Dyselectrolytemias manifest on initiating therapy, usually after 24 hours

Differential Diagnosis

❖ Hypoglycemia

❖ Non-ketotic hyperosmolar coma

❖ High anion gap metabolic acidosis

❖ Starvation ketoacidosis

❖ Alcoholic ketoacidosis

❖ Lactic acidosis

❖ Uremic ketoacidosis

❖ Ingestion of salicylates, ethanol, ethylene glycol

Treatment

Surgery is done only if underlying surgical condition will exacerbate acidosis

❖ Monitors:
- Blood glucose levels every 1–2 hours
- Electrolytes, ABG and anion gap every 4 hours
- Vital signs, respiration, CNS status and intake-output chart every 1–2 hours
- CVP considered if elderly patient/heart disease present
- Continuous ECG monitoring

❖ General:
- 1 or 2 large bore IV cannula 16–18G inserted
- Nasogastric tube inserted if vomiting/altered mental status
- ET intubation and CMV if significant respiratory distress present

- Active warming if hypothermia
- Foleys catheterization

❖ Goals of therapy: DKA has resolved if:
- pH> 7.3
- HCO^{3-} > 18 mEq/L
- Blood glucose < 200 mg/dL

❖ Fluids:
- Average fluid deficit in DKA is 50–100 mL/kg (5–10 L)
- This is the *first priority in treatment* of DKA
- Choice of fluid:
  - NS recommended for initial resuscitation
  - Hypotonic D½ NS:
    - Reduces tendency to develop hyperchloremic MA following treatment with NS
    - Added if blood glucose < 300 mg/dL after initial resuscitation
  - D5 added when blood glucose is 250 mg/dL to be given at 100 mL/hr
- Rate of administration:
  - 250–500 mL/hr depending on degree of hypovolemia
  - One third of fluid deficit corrected over first 6–8 hours
  - Remaining two thirds given over next 24 hours
  - Alternative regimen:
    - 2 liters over first 2 hours
    - 2 liters over next 2–6 hours
    - 2 liters over next 6–12 hours
    - Remaining deficit corrected over next 12 hours
    - If volume depletion is not severe, 500 mL/hr given for 4 hours

❖ Insulin:
- Second priority unless K+ < 3.3 mEq/L
- Goal of therapy: Blood glucose 150–200 mg/dL
- Rate of infusion:
  - Initial bolus of 0.15 IU/kg or 0.4 IU/kg IM
  - Rate of infusion after bolus dose:
    - (Blood glucose)/150 IU/hr
    - (Blood glucose)/100 IU/hr, if:
      - Infection
      - Concurrent steroids
      - BMI ≥ 35
- Duration of infusion: Continued until:
  - pH ≥ 7.3
  - Anion gap normalized (at least 12 hours usually)
  - Ketonemia resolved (at least 12–48 hours)
- Method of infusion:
  - Continuous IV infusion of regular insulin
  - Prepared as 100 U insulin in 100 mL of NS
  - Insulin binds to plastic tubing
  - So, first 25 mL of this solution should be discarded
  - Drip is placed at a port closest to skin
  - IM/SC insulin avoided as absorption is erratic due to vasoconstriction in response to hypovolemia
- Insulin resistance:
  - Occurs due to infection usually
  - Suspected if blood glucose reduces by ≤ 50–70 mg/in first hour
  - Increasing infusion rate, IV bolus of 0.2–0.4 U/kg tried
  - Volume expansion with IVF also makes cells more responsive to insulin
- Stopping infusion:
  - Overlap period:
    - When S/C intermediate/long acting insulin given along with infusion of regular insulin
    - Usually started when patient resumes oral feeds
  - If adequate insulin levels are not reached by S/C route before stopping infusion, DKA relapses
- Maximum rate of decline of blood glucose is 75–100 mg/dL/hr
- Delay insulin therapy by 30 min after K^+ correction if serum K^+ < 3.3 mEq/L

❖ Potassium:
- Third priority for treatment unless K^+ <3.3 mEq/L
- Usually K^+ deficit of 3–5 mEq/kg is present
- For each 0.1 change in pH, serum K^+ changes 0.5 mEq/L inversely
- Goal is to maintain K^+ between 4–5 mEq/L during acute phase of treatment
- Intracellular deficit is replaced over many days

Serum potassium	Rate of administration
More than 5 mEq/L	Nil until less than 5 mEq/L with good urine output
3.3–5 mEq/L, urine > 0.5 mL/kg/hr	10 mEq/hr for at least 4 hours
Less than 3.3 mEq/L	15–20 mEq/hr IV
	Insulin therapy initiated 30 minutes later

- Potassium phosphate/potassium acetate used to prevent hyperchloremia
- Oral K^+ supplements started as soon as patient takes oral feeds

- Phosphate:
  - Monitored on presentation and 24 hours into therapy
  - Corrected only if serum serum phosphate ≤1 mg/dL
  - Usually oral phosphate supplementation is enough
  - No established role of IV phosphate supplementation in emergency department
  - IV dose: 0.2–0.68 mmol/kg IV over 12 hours
  - PO dose: 30 mmol/day (1 g/day)
- Magnesium:
  - Monitored on presentation and 24 hours into treatment
  - Treated only if serum mg^{2+} < 1.2 mEq/L or patient is symptomatic
  - Oral mgO 60–90 mEq/day
  - IV $mgSO_4$ (1–2 g over 15 min followed by 250–500 mg/hr)
- Bicarbonate:
  - Routine use in DKA not recommended
  - Indications: ***ADA recommendations***:
    - If pH< 7 after initial resuscitation 50 mEq/L in 200 mL ½ NS over 1 hour
    - If pH< 6.9, 100 mEq/L in 400 mL ½ NS over 2 hours
  - Advantages of bicarbonate:
    - Improved myocardial contractility
    - Elevated VF/VT threshold
    - Improved catecholamine tissue response
    - Reduced work of breathing
  - Disadvantages of bicarbonate:
    - Worsens hypokalemia
    - *Paradoxical CNS acidosis* due to conversion to CO_2 in CSF
    - Worsening intracellular acidosis
    - Na+ overload and hypertonicity
    - Shift to left of oxy-hemoglobin dissociation curve
    - Impaired tissue oxygenation
    - Delayed recovery from ketosis
    - Increased serum lactate levels
    - Precipitates cerebral edema
- Others:
  - Treat precipitating cause
  - DVT prophylaxis in high risk patients

Prognosis

- Less than 5% mortality
- Increased mortality if:
  - Precipitating cause is MI/infection
  - Increased BUN
  - Increased blood glucose
  - Blood HCO_3^- < 10 mEq/L

Complications

- Aspiration in comatose patients
- Vascular stasis, DVT and pulmonary embolism
- ARDS due to fluid therapy
- Cerebral edema (very common) and intracranial hemorrhage
- Sepsis, upper GI bleed
- Complications of therapy:
  - Hypoglycemia
  - Hypokalemia
  - Hypophosphatemia
  - Resistant metabolic acidosis
  - Hyperchloremic non-anion gap metabolic acidosis (common)

Risk of General Anesthesia in Uncorrected DKA

- Increased risk of cardiac arrest due to:
  - Hyperkalemia
  - Severe myocardial depression due to metabolic acidosis
  - Depressant action of anesthetics
- Increased risk of hypotension and arrest if SAB given due to severe hypovolemia
- Myocardial depression is unresponsive to catecholamine therapy

HYPEROSMOLAR NON-KETOTIC SYNDROME

Introduction

- Syndrome of severe hyperglycemia, hyperosmolality and lack of ketonemia in patients with poorly controlled or undiagnosed type II DM
- Also called:
  - Hyperosmolar hyperglycemic state (HHS)
  - Hyperosmolar hyperglycemic non-ketotic syndrome (HHN)

Definition

- Serum glucose ≥ 600 mg/dL
- Plasma osmolality ≥ 315 mosm/kg
- Serum bicarbonate ≥ 15 mEq/L
- Arterial pH ≥ 7.3
- Serum ketones negative/mildly positive in a 1:2 dilution

Precipitating Factors

- Central nervous system:
  - Cerebrovascular events
  - Infections

- Cardiovascular:
  - Myocardial infarction
  - Congestive cardiac failure
- Respiratory system:
  - Pulmonary emboli
  - Pneumonia
- Gastrointestinal:
  - GI hemorrhage
  - Parenteral/enteral feeds
  - Pancreatitis
  - Mesenteric ischemia
- Genitourinary:
  - Renal insufficiency
  - Peritoneal/hemodialysis
  - Urinary tract infections
- Drugs:
  - Diuretics, lithium
  - β-blockers, mannitol
  - Cimetidine, glucocorticoids
- Others:
  - Infections, burns
  - Rhabdomyolysis, heat related illness

Pathophysiology: Three main causes of HONC

- Reduced insulin utilization
- Increased hepatic gluconeogenesis and glycogenolysis
- Impaired renal glucose excretion

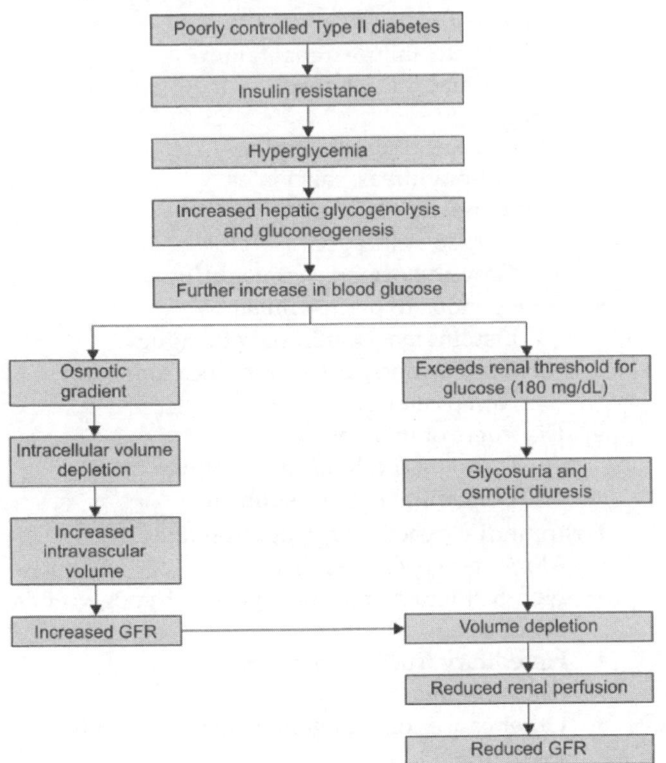

Characteristic	DKA	HONC
Plasma glucose	More than 250	More than 600
Arterial pH	Less than 7.3	More than 7.3
Serum bicarbonate	Less than 15	More than 15
Urine ketones	Moderate	Small
Serum ketones	Moderate	Small
Serum osmolarity	300–320	More than 320
Anion gap	More than 10	Less than 12
Alteration in sensorium	Alert to stuporous	Stuporous/comatose

Clinical Features

- Symptoms:
  - Insidious onset of polyuria, weight loss and reduced oral intake
  - Elderly patient with history of poorly controlled type II DM
  - Weakness, anorexia, fatigue, cognitive impairment
  - Dyspnea, cough, pneumonia, UTI
  - History of underdosing/non-compliance with insulin
- Signs:
  - Poor skin turgor, dry mucous membrane, sunken eyes
  - Hypotension, tachycardia, shock
  - Seizures (focal/generalized) coma, altered mental status
  - Tremors, clonus, hypo/hyperreflexia, positive plantar response
  - Hemiplegia/hemisensory defects
  - Normothermia/hypothermia due to vasodilation
- Notably absent symptoms:
  - Nausea and vomiting
  - Abdominal pain
  - Kussmauls respiration

Investigations

- Definitive investigations:
  - Blood glucose ≥ 600 mg/dL
  - Serum osmolarity ≥320 mOsm/L with absent ketone bodies
  - Increased BUN and serum creatinine due to prerenal and renal azotemia
  - Electrolytes:
    - Hypo/hyper/normal Na^+
    - Hypokalemia
    - Hypomagnesemia
    - Hypophosphatemia
  - ABG: Anion gap metabolic acidosis in 50% patients
  - Complete blood count

- Ancillary investigations:
  - Blood/sputum/urine culture
  - Liver function tests, pancreatic enzyme determination
  - Cardiac enzymes, ECG
  - Chest X-ray, CT head
  - Thyroid function, coagulation profile
  - Lumbar puncture

Treatment

- Goals:
  - Treat underlying cause
  - Correct hypovolemia
  - Restore tissue perfusion
  - Correct electrolyte abnormalities
  - Gradual correction of hyperglycemia and osmolarity
- Monitor:
  - Central venous pressure, urine output
  - BP, ECG, pulse oximetry
  - Serum K^+ every hour until steady state achieved
  - Blood glucose hourly
  - CT brain and mental status assessment for cognitive impairment
- Fluid resuscitation:
  - Fluid deficits on an average 20–25% of TBW or 8–12 liters
  - Normal saline most appropriate for replacement initially
  - Once hemodynamically stable, use ½ NS
  - One half of deficit replaced over 12 hours and balance over next 24 hours
  - Rate of correction according to associated renal and cardiac impairment
  - Rate of correction:
    - 500–1500 mL/hr during first 2 hours followed by 250–500 mL/hr if mild hypotension
    - 4–14 mL/kg/hr if moderate-sever hypotension
- Electrolytes:
  - K^+ replacement done once urine output is adequate
  - Replaced as potassium phosphate to prevent hypophosphatemia
  - Replace at 10–20 mEq/hr, until $K^+ \geq 3.3$ mEq/L
  - Phosphate and magnesium usually self correct and require no treatment
- Insulin:
  - Volume replacement to precede insulin therapy
  - On administration of insulin, intravascular volume may decrease further
  - Continuous infusion after bolus of 0.1 U/kg at 0.1 U/kg/hr
  - Blood glucose reduces at steady rate of 50–70 mg/dL/hr
  - Once BG < 250 mg%:
    - IV solution changed to D5½ NS
    - Insulin infusion reduced to half or 0.05 U/kg/hr
  - Continue insulin until patient mentally alert and osmolarity < 315 mOsm/L
  - Maintain blood glucose between 250–300 mg/dL
- Postoperative care:
  - If patient is NPO, continue IV insulin
  - Supplement with subcutaneous insulin as needed
  - When patient can eat give S/C insulin or shift to previous insulin regimen
  - Look for precipitating causes

HYPOGLYCEMIA

Introduction

Diagnosed by **Whipples triad** which consists of:

- Symptoms consistent with diagnosis
- Usually occurs at serum glucose < 50 mg/dL
- Resolves following glucose administration

Etiology

- Fasting hypoglycemia:
  - Critical illness:
    - Hepatic failure, renal failure
    - Cardiac failure, sepsis
  - Drugs:
    - Insulin, ethanol, quinine
    - Sulfonylureas, salicylates
  - Hormone deficiencies:
    - Cortisol, glucagon
    - Growth hormone, epinephrine
  - Endogenous hyperinsulinism:
    - Insulinoma, insulin secretogogue
    - β cell tumors, auto-antibodies to insulin
    - Non β cell tumors
  - Disorders of infancy:
    - Transient intolerance of fasting
    - Congenital hyperinsulinism
- Postprandial (reactive) hypoglycemia:
  - Alimentary/post-gastrectomy
  - Non-insulinoma pancreatogenous hypoglycemia syndrome
  - Hereditary fructose intolerance
  - Galactosemia
  - Other causes of endogenous hyperinsulinism
  - Idiopathic

Clinical Features

- *Hyperepinephrinemic/autonomic/sympathomimetic*:
  - Sympathetic symptoms:
    - Anxiety, irritability, palpitations, nervousness
    - Tremors, nausea and vomiting, tachycardia, HTN
  - Cholinergic symptoms:
    - Sweating, salivation
    - Bradycardia, paresthesias
    - Changes in pupillary size
- *Neuroglycopenic*:
  - Altered consciousness, lethargy, unresponsiveness
  - Behavioural changes, confusion, agitation
  - Seizures, focal neurodeficits

Differential Diagnosis

- Stroke/TIA
- Traumatic brain injury
- Seizure disorder
- Brain tumors
- Psychosis, hysteria
- Sympathomimetic drug ingestion

Prevention

- Stop/reduce dose of offending drugs
- Treat critical illness
- Replace GH/cortisol if deficient
- Surgery/chemotherapy/radiotherapy for tumors
- Frequent feeding and avoidance of fasting
- Intake of uncooked corn starch at bed time
- Overnight intragastric infusion of glucose in some patients

Treatment

- Glucose supplementation:
  - Intravenous supplementation:
    - Initially 1 gm/kg body weight dextrose as D50W
    - Followed by D10W infusion to maintain serum glucose > 100 mg/dL
    - Each 50 gm D50W solution increases blood glucose by 60 mg/dL
    - Repeat glucose every 30 minutes for first 2 hours to detect ***rebound hypoglycemia***
  - Oral supplementation:
    - Useful in conscious and oriented patients
    - 300 gms/1200 Kcal of carbohydrates given as snacks
- Glucagon:
  - 1 mg given IM/IV
  - Response is slower and short lived (mental status normalizes after 7–10 min)
  - Useful in diabetes/if IV access not available
  - Ineffective in alcoholics, elderly and others with low glycogen stores
- Steroids:
  - 100–200 mg hydrocortisone IV
  - Especially useful if resistant hypoglycemia/signs of adrenal insufficiency
- Octreotide:
  - Somatostatin analogue
  - Used for sulfonylurea induced hypoglycemia
  - 50–125 µg S/C initially followed by 125 µg/hr infusion
  - Only recommended after glucose therapy has been initiated
- Thiamine:
  - 100 mg IV thiamine given with glucose in severe nutritional deficiency as it could precipitate ***Wernickes encephalopathy***
  - Thiamine acts as coenzyme in conversion of pyruvate to -ketoglutarate which is important to generate ATP (main source of ATP to CNS)
  - Depletion of thiamine causes Wernickes syndrome

SUGGESTED READING

1. Barash, P.G. (2017). *Clinical Anesthesia*. 8th ed. China: Wolters Kluwer.
2. Butterworth, J., D. Mackey, D., Wasnik, J. (2018). *Morgan and Mikhails Clinical Anesthesiology*. 6th ed. New York: McGraw-Hill Education/Medical.
3. Flood, P. (2015). *Stoeltings Pharmacology and Physiology in Anesthetic Practice*. 5th ed. China: Wolters Kluwer.
4. Gropper, M., Eriksson, L., Fleisher, L., Wiener-Kronish, J., Cohen, N., Leslie, K. (2020). *Millers Anesthesia*. 9th ed. Philadelphia: Elsevier Saunders.
5. Marino, P.L. (2017). *The little ICU book of facts and formulas*. 2nd ed. China: Wolters Kluwer.
6. Marschall, K., Hines, R.L. (2017). *Stoeltings Anesthesia and Coexisting Disease*. 7th ed. New York: Elsevier.
7. Miller, R.D., Eriksson, L., Fleisher, L, Wiener-Kronish, J., Cohen, N., Young, W. (2014). *Millers Anesthesia*. 8th ed. New York: Elsevier Health.
8. Miller, T.E., Myles, P.S. (2019). Perioperative fluid therapy for major surgery. *Anesthesiology*, 130(5), 825-32.
9. Tintinalli, J., Stapczynski, J., John Ma, O., Yealy, D., Meckler, G., Cline, D. (2016). *Tintinallis Emergency Medicine*. 8th ed. New York: McGraw Hill.

6

CHAPTER

Anesthesia and the Kidney

ANATOMY OF THE NEPHRON

Introduction

- Nephron is the *structural and functional unit* of the kidney
- It is also called the ***uriniferous tubule***
- Histologically, each kidney is composed of approximately 1 million nephrons

Parts of a Nephron:
Each Nephron has 2 Major Portions

- Renal corpuscle:
  - Glomerulus
  - Glomerular capsule
- Renal tubule:
  - Proximal convoluted tubule
  - Loop of Henle
  - Distal convoluted tubule
  - Collecting duct
  - Juxtaglomerular apparatus

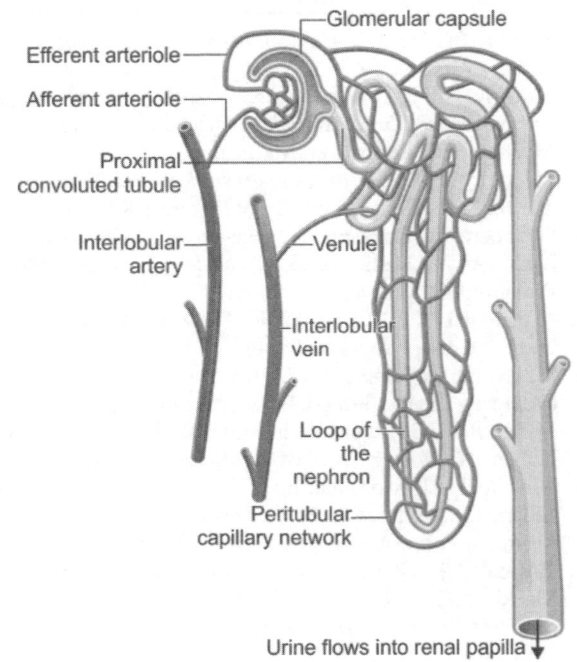

Fig. 1: Nephron.

Renal Corpuscle

- Also called ***Malphigian body***
- Consists of a glomerulus surrounded by a glomerular capsule (Bowmans capsule)
- Glomerulus:
  - Name given to the capillary network within the renal corpuscle
  - All glomeruli are present within the renal cortex
  - Glomerulus arises from the afferent arteriole, which is of larger diameter
  - It empties into the efferent arteriole, which is of smaller diameter
  - This difference in diameters helps maintain a high pressure within the glomerulus
  - Thus, the glomerulus, is in essence, a high pressure capillary bed
  - Wall of the glomerulus consists of a single layer of flattened endothelial cells
  - Large fenestrations are present between the endothelial cells
  - It is here, that blood is initially filtered to form the filtrate
  - Efferent arterioles:
    - Receives the blood exiting from the glomerulus
    - Efferent arteriole forms a second capillary network around the renal tubule
    - This network is called the ***peritubular capillaries***
    - In juxtamedullary nephrons, peritubular capillaries are long
    - The capillaries that follow the loop of Henle are called the ***vasa recta***
    - As the glomerular filtrate passes through the tubule, the capillary network reabsorbs most of the solutes and water
    - Thus, this represents a capillary bed draining into a second capillary bed
    - Thus, it is an example of portal system

- Glomerular capsule:
  - Also called ***Bowmans capsule***
  - Double walled cup like structure, which encloses the glomerulus
  - This represents the first part of the nephron
  - This is from where the fluid filtered from the glomerulus enters into the nephron
  - Wall of the capsule is made of a single layer of flattened epithelial cells
  - Glomerular capsule consists of 3 layers:
    - Outer parietal layer:
      - Consists of simple squamous epithelial cells
      - This layer has minute fenestrations of 12 nm diameter
    - Inner visceral layer:
      - Outer parietal layer cells continue and transform into the inner layer
      - This layer consists of large nucleated cells called podocytes
      - The finger like projections of the podocytes are called pedicels
      - These pedicels cover the glomerular capillaries
      - The pedicels interdigitate to form small ***filtration slits***
    - Middle basement membrane:
      - This membrane lies between the glomerular endothelium and the podocytes
      - This membrane is selectively permeable
      - It forms an important part of the ***filtration membrane***
      - Components of the filtration membrane are:
        - Endothelial fenestrations
        - Glomerular basement membrane
        - Filtration slits of the podocytes

Functioning of the Renal Corpuscle

- Ultrafiltration occurs in the renal corpuscle
- Negatively charged particles, however, are not filtered across into the renal tubule
- This is because most of the proteins in the filtration membrane are negatively charged
- Thus, negatively charged molecules are repelled back
- The glomerular filtrate therefore consists of predominantly positively charged molecules

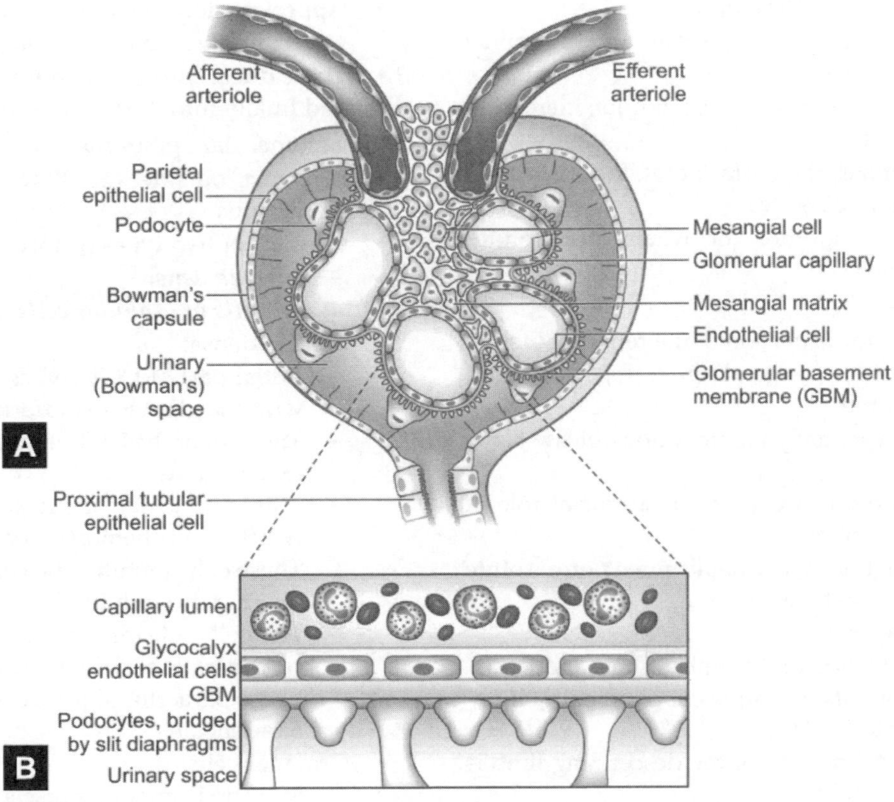

Figs. 2A and B: Glomerulus.

- Filtration membrane therefore prevents the passage of:
  - Blood cells
  - Large proteins
  - Most negatively charged molecules more than 8 nm

Renal Tubules

- Renal tubule is the continuation of the Bowmans capsule
- The parts of the renal tubule are:
  - Proximal convoluted tubule
  - Loop of Henle
  - Distal convoluted tubule
  - Collecting ducts
  - Juxtaglomerular apparatus
- Proximal convoluted tubule (PCT):
  - Fluid filtrate collected in the Bowmans capsule enters into the PCT
  - PCT is lined by simple cuboidal cells
  - Selective reabsorption occurs here
  - These cells have a high concentration of mitochondria
  - This is because most of the ions are transported actively across these cells
  - Thus, the requirement of energy as adenosine triphosphate (ATPP) is high
  - Prominent microvilli are present on the luminal surface of these cells
  - These microvilli form a brush border, increasing the surface area
  - This maximizes the surface area for absorption and secretion of solutes
  - Maximal reabsorption of water and solutes occurs in the PCT
- Loop of Henle:
  - U-shaped middle portion of the renal tubules
  - Consists of a descending limb, loop and ascending limb
  - These are essentially continuations of the same tubule
  - Counter current mechanism is a crucial role of the loop of Henle
  - Osmoregulation and establishment of a solute gradient occurs here
  - Descending limb:
    - Initial portion of the limb is short and thick
    - This consists of simple cuboidal epithelium, similar to the PCT
    - The distal portion of the descending limb is long and thin
    - This part is permeable to water
  - Ascending limb:
    - Consists of a long and thin initial portion
    - The distal portion is long and thick
    - The distal part is impermeable to water
    - This consists of simple cuboidal epithelium, similar to the distal convoluted tubule (DCT)
- Distal convoluted tubule:
  - Formed by simple cuboidal epithelium
  - Selective reabsorption occurs here
  - Solute exchange in this part of the tubule is also an active process
  - Therefore, these cells have high concentration of mitochondria
  - However, these cells have fewer microvilli, compared to those on the PCT
- Collecting ducts:
  - These ducts represent a continuation of the nephron
  - They are lined by simple cuboidal epithelium, to facilitate water transport
  - Thus, osmoregulation or water retention occurs here
  - Each duct collects filtrate from different nephrons for final modification
  - These ducts merge as they descend into the medulla, to form terminal ducts
  - Approximately 30 terminal ducts are formed, which empty into the papillary duct
  - These ducts empty into minor calyx, major calyx and finally into the renal pelvis
- Juxtaglomerular apparatus:
  - Lies just outside the Bowmans capsule and glomerulus
  - Consists of two types of specialized cells:
    - ***Macula densa***
    - ***JG cells or granular cells***
  - Macula densa:
    - Initial part of DCT comes into direct contact with the glomerular arterioles
    - The wall of the DCT at that point is called the macula densa
    - This is a cluster of cuboidal epithelial cells, which form chemoreceptors
    - These cells monitor the composition of fluid flowing through the DCT
    - The cells release signals in response to Na^+ concentration in the filtrate
    - These paracrine signals consist of either ATP or adenosine
  - Granular cells:
    - Modified smooth muscle cells, which line the afferent arteriole

- These cells contract or relax in response to paracrine signals from the macula
- Thus, the JG apparatus regulates blood flow into the glomerulus
- JG cells also produce renin

Types of Nephrons

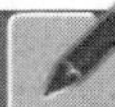

- ❖ Cortical nephrons:
  - Have short loops of Henle
  - These do not dip far beyond the renal cortex
  - These nephrons do not contain vasa recta
  - Approximately 85% of nephrons are cortical nephrons
- ❖ Juxtamedullary nephrons:
  - Have long loops of Henle
  - These extend deep into the renal medulla
  - These long loops of Henle are accompanied by the vasa recta
  - These nephrons are responsible for creating the ***corti-copapillary osmotic gradient***
  - Approximately 15% of nephrons are juxtamedullary nephrons

RENAL FUNCTION TESTS

Introduction

- ❖ Renal function tests include a spectrum of tests to analyze:
  - Severity of renal impairment
  - Cause of renal impairment
  - Rapidity of progression of kidney disease
- ❖ Assessment of the glomerular filtration rate (GFR) is most commonly used to assess severity of kidney injury

Assessment of Glomerular Function

- ❖ The GFR is the best measure of glomerular function
- ❖ Normal GFR is approximately 125 mL/min
- ❖ Manifestations of reduced GFR are not seen till the GFR falls to 50% of normal
- ❖ Commonly used methods to assess the GFR include:
  - Blood urea nitrogen (BUN):
    - Not a direct correlate of GFR
    - BUN is usually not elevated until the GFR falls below 75% of normal
    - Non-renal causes of elevated BUN:
      - Reduced circulating blood volume (pre-renal azotemia)
      - Catabolic states:
        - Exercise
        - Bleeding
        - Steroids use
      - High protein diets
      - Massive tissue breakdown
      - Tetracycline
    - Non-renal causes of reduced BUN:
      - SIADH
      - Malnutrition
      - Sickle cell anemia
      - Liver disease
  - Creatinine:
    - Serum creatinine provides valuable information as a marker for GFR
    - Measured using *Jaffe alkaline picric acid reaction*
    - This is because:
      - Creatinine is freely filtered at the glomerulus
      - It is neither absorbed nor secreted
    - Thus, creatinine levels more or less reflect glomerular filtration
    - Calculation of creatinine clearance using creatinine:

$$C = \frac{(U \times V)}{P}$$

C = creatinine clearance
U = urinary creatinine concentration
V = urinary flow rate
P = plasma creatinine concentration

    - However, the creatinine levels are also affected by:
      - Turnover of muscle tissue
      - Dietary intake of proteins
    - Non-renal conditions causing elevated serum creatinine levels:
      - Ketoacidosis
      - Drugs:
  - Cephalothin, cefoxitin
  - Flucytosin, aspirin
  - Cimetidine, trimethoprim
    - Non-renal causes of decreased serum creatinine:
      - Advanced age
      - Cachexia
      - Liver disease
  - Cystatin C:
    - It is a low-molecular weight protein produced by all nucleated cells
    - Cystatin C is filtered at the glomerulus and not reabsorbed
    - However, it may be metabolized in the tubules
    - This may result in lower than actual measurements
    - Since it is freely filtered, serum values correlate inversely with GFR

- Thus, low values indicate higher GFR and better renal function
- High values indicate lower GFR and poor renal function
- Advantages of cystatin C:
  - Correlates more closely with the GFR than creatinine
  - More accurate than serum creatinine
  - Values are not affected by:
    - Muscle mass
    - Diet
- It is more accurate in patients with low creatinine production:
  - Old age
  - Children
  - Kidney transplant recipients
  - Cirrhosis
- Higher levels of cystatin C may be associated with:
  - Male gender
  - Advanced age
  - Diabetes, fat mass

- Measurement of creatinine clearance
  - GFR estimation equations:
    - ***Cockroft- Gault equation***:
      - Estimates the creatinine clearance from serum creatinine
      - For women, the value obtained is multiplied by 0.85
      - This is to account for the lower muscle mass
      - More accurate in patients with GFR 10-100 mL/min
      - Less accurate in patients with near normal GFR
      - Disadvantages:
        - » Formula is not adjusted for body surface area
        - » Overestimates creatinine clearance by 10–40%

$$\text{GFR in mL/min} = \frac{(140 - \text{age}) \times \text{lean body weight}_{(kg)}}{\text{Creatinine}_{(mg/dL)} \times 72}$$

    - Modification of diet in renal disease (MDRD) equation:
      - Clearance of iothalamate was used to derive this equation
      - For women, the value obtained is multiplied by 0.742
      - Used only for CRF patients with stable creatinine levels
      - Cannot be used in acute renal failure
      - Less accurate in patients with near normal/ high GFR
      - May underestimate GFR in healthy subjects by up to 29%

$$\text{GFR in mL/min/1.73 m}^2 = 175 \times (\text{S. creatinine})^{-1.154} \times (\text{age})^{-0.203}$$

    - Chronic kidney disease epidemiology (CKD EPI) equation:
      - More accurate when GFR is normal/ slightly reduced
      - Estimates the GFR more accurately at higher levels of GFR
      - For women, the value obtained is multiplied by 1.018
      - Prediction of GFR with CKD EPI equation results in:
        - » Lower prevalence of CKD
        - » Better risk prediction

$$\text{GFR} = 141 \times \min(\text{Scr}/\kappa, 1)^{\alpha} \times \max(\text{Scr}/\kappa, 1)^{-1.209} \times 0.993^{\text{Age}}$$

κ = 0.7 if female
κ = 0.9 if male
α = –0.329 if female
α = –0.411 if male
min = the minimum of Scr/κ or 1
max = the maximum of Scr/κ or 1
Scr = serum creatinine

- Choice of equations:
  - CKD EPI equation is used owing to its improved performance
  - This equation is useful at both high and low levels of GFR
- Other equations used:
  - Lund malmo revised equation (LMR)
  - Full age spectrum equation (FAS)

Assessment of Tubular Function

- Urine concentration:
  - Urinary specific gravity is an index of renal tubular function
  - It increases with concentrated urine and decreases with diluted urine
  - Determination of the urine osmolality is a similar, more specific test
  - Excretion of concentrated urine is indicative of excellent tubular function
  - A urinary osmolality > 750 mOsm/kg H_2O implies normal concentrating ability

- Urinary proteins:
  - Protein excretion in normal patients may be as high as 150 mg/day
  - Massive proteinuria (> 750 mg/day) is always abnormal and indicates renal disease
- Urinary glucose:
  - Glucose is freely filtered in the glomerulus
  - It is subsequently reabsorbed in the proximal tubule
  - Glycosuria signifies that tubular reabsorption capability has been exceeded
  - The renal glycosuric threshold is 180 mg/dL
- Dipstick assays:
  - Uses dry chemistry methods to detect the presence of abnormal substances
  - Substances which can be detected include:
    - Protein
    - Glucose
    - Ketones:
      - Useful to detect ketones in:
        - DKA
        - Starvation ketoacidosis
        - Severe vomiting
      - Detects only acetoacetate and acetone
      - Does not detect beta-hydroxy butyrate
    - Bilirubin
    - Urobilinogen
    - Nitrite
    - Leukocyte esterase

Nonspecific Tests

- Urine volume
  - Intraoperative urine output is a controversial marker of renal function
  - Pre and postoperative oliguria (<0.5 mL/kg/hour) has been used to define AKI
  - But, in the intraoperative scenario, many non-renal factors influence urine volume
  - These include:
    - Hemodynamic instability
    - Decreased blood volume
    - Decreased cardiac output
    - Fluctuating hormone levels (aldosterone, renin, ADH)
  - Thus, it may not be a reliable sign of impending renal dysfunction
- Urinary sodium concentration:
  - Traditionally urinary Na^+ level < 20 mEq/L is consistent with prerenal azotemia
  - However, other non-renal factors may affect urinary sodium levels:
    - Secretion of aldosterone
    - Secretion of ADH
    - Diuretic therapy
    - Sympathetic nervous system tone
  - Thus, urine sodium alone cannot be used to distinguish pre-renal ARF from ATN
- Fractional excretion of sodium:
  - Fe_{Na} reflects the percentage of Na^+ filtered by the kidney which is excreted

$$FE_{Na} = \frac{\text{Excreted Na}}{(\text{Filtered Na}) \times 100} = \frac{U_{Na}P_{Cr}}{U_{Cr}P_{Na} \times 100}$$

P_{Cr} = plasma creatinine level
P_{Na} = plasma sodium level
U_{Cr} = urinary creatinine level
U_{Na} = urinary sodium level

  - Interpretation:
    - Fe_{Na} < 1% implies pre-renal azotemia
    - Fe_{Na} > 2% implies acute tubular necrosis

Measurement of Renal Blood Flow

- Renal blood flow can be measured by clearance of infused para-aminohippurate (PAH)
- PAH is almost entirely cleared from plasma by filtration and secretion
- Thus, PAH clearance approximates rate of renal plasm flow (RPF)
- Although available, this test is rarely used in clinical practice

Additional Diagnostic Tests

- Urinalysis:
- Gross and microscopic observation of urine is a readily available and inexpensive test
  - Gross appearance of urine may indicate bleeding or infection of the urinary tract
  - Microscopic examination may reveal:
    - RBCs-indicates renal injury
    - WBCs-indicates infection
    - RBC casts-indicates glomerulonephritis
    - WBC casts-indicates pyelonephritis
- Serum and urine electrolytes:
  - Serum sodium, potassium, chloride and bicarbonate may be altered in renal disease
  - Urinary sodium and chloride levels help differentiating causes of hyponatremia

Imaging Studies

- CT scan of the kidneys:
  - Modality of choice to evaluate kidney stones

- Can detect all kinds of stones including uric acid stones and non-obstructing stones
- Can also be used to evaluate masses in the kidney

- CT angiography:
  - Used for evaluation of renal artery stenosis
  - However, requirement of contrast material increases the risk of renal insult
- MRI and MR angiography:
  - Useful for the evaluation of:
    - Renovascular disease
    - Renal masses
  - It is advantageous as it does not require contrast material

Reference Values of Common Tests

Test	Range
Urea nitrogen	5–25 mg/dL
Creatinine	0.5–1.5 mg/dL
Uric acid	2.5–7.5 mg/dL
Urine analysis	
Color	Straw-amber
Appearance	Clear-hazy
Proteins	0 mg/dL
Blood	Negative
Glucose	0 mg/dL
Ketones	0 mg/dL
pH	4.5-8
Specific gravity	1.002-1.030
Bilirubin	Negative
Microscopic urinalysis	
RBCs	0-3 per high power field
WBCs	0-5 per high power field
Casts	0-2 per low-power field

Recent Biomarkers of AKI

- Markers for glomerular filtration:
  - Cystatin C
  - Beta-2 microglobulin
- Biomarkers for tubular function:
  - α1- microglobulin
  - β2- microglobulin
  - Albumin
  - Retinol-binding protein
  - Immunoglobulin C
  - Transferrin
  - Ceruloplasmin
  - Lambda and kappa light chains
  - Total protein
- Biomarkers reflecting tubular cell response to stress:
  - Neutrophil gelatinase associated lipocalin
  - Urinary interleukin 18
  - Kidney injury molecule 1 (KIM 1)
  - Liver fatty acid binding protein

TURP SYNDROME

Introduction

Term used to describe the signs and symptoms which occur with excessive absorption of irrigating solution during TURP, primarily due to circulatory overload, water intoxication and occasionally toxicity from the irrigating fluid.

Etiopathogenesis

- Resection of the gland opens up the prostatic venous sinuses
- This causes absorption of fluids across the venous sinuses
- This causes:
  - Fluid overload resulting in:
    - Hypertension, bradycardia
    - Pulmonary edema, CCF, MI
    - Hypoosmolality and hyponatremia
  - Hypoosmolality resulting in:
    - Cerebral edema, Cushings reflex
    - Hypertension, bradycardia
  - Dilutional hyponatremia resulting in:
    - Confusion, restlessness
    - Seizures, coma
- Syndrome occurs due to absorption of large amounts of hypotonic fluids
- About 20 mL/min of fluids is absorbed
- This can go upto 200 mL/min
- When 2 litres of fluid is absorbed, TURP syndrome results

$$\text{Volume absorbed} = \frac{\text{Preoperative Na}^+}{\text{Postoperative Na}^+} \times \text{ECF} - \text{ECF}$$

Predisposing Factors

- Hydrostatic pressure of irrigating fluid (> 60 cmH_2O)
- Duration of surgery ≥ 60 minutes
- Size of gland ≥ 45 g
- Hemorrhage: Causes opening of sinuses
- Irrigation fluid: Distilled water increases risk
- Poorly controlled preoperative CCF

Clinical Features

CNS and RS	CNS	Metabolic	Others
Hypertension (SBP and DBP)	Agitation	Hyponatremia	Hemolysis
Brady/tachyarrhythmias	Confusion	Hyperglycinemia	ARF
CCF	Restlessness	Hyperglycemia	
Pulmonary edema	Seizures	Hyperammonemia	
MI	Coma	Hypoosmolarity	
Shock	Transient visual disturbances		

Sodium level	CNS disturbance	ECG findings
120 mEq/L	Confusion Restlessness	Occasionally QRS widening
115 mEq/L	Somnolence Nausea	Widening of QRS complexes ST segment elevation
110 mEq/L	Seizures Coma	Ventricular tachycardia Ventricular fibrillation

Prevention

- Optimize preoperative Na^+ levels 130 mEq/L
- Treat CCF preoperatively adequately
- Conservative treatment of BPH in critically ill (medical therapy/balloon dilatation)
- Avoiding distilled water for irrigation
- Limit hydrostatic pressure by reducing height of pole to:
  - 60 cm during initial half of surgery
  - 30 cm in the last part of surgery
- Avoid over-distension of bladder
- Restrict duration of surgery to ≤ 1 hour
- Microdrip set for IV fluids in cardiac/renal patients
- Use of vasopressors to control regional anesthesia induced hypotension instead of fluids

Management

- Ensure adequate oxygenation with face mask or nasal cannula
- Terminate surgery as soon as possible
- Consider insertion of invasive monitor if cardiovascular instability present
- Attach 12 lead ECG
- Collect blood for estimation of:
  - Creatinine, glucose
  - Serum electrolytes, ABG
- Correction of hyponatremia:
  - If asymptomatic, (Na^+ > 120 mEq/L): fluid restriction with diuretics
  - If symptomatic hyponatremia:
    - Amount of Na^+ required = TBW (desired Na^+ - present Na^+)
    - Correction rates:
      - Mild symptoms: 0.5 mEq/L/hr
      - Moderate symptoms: 1 mEq/L/hr
      - Severe symptoms: 1.5 mEq/L/hr
      - Avoid rapid correction to prevent ***central pontine demyelination***
    - Choice of fluids:
      - Isotonic saline for mild-moderate symptoms
      - 3% saline (or 5%) if severe symptoms or serum Na^+ < 110 mEq/L
      - Stop hypertonic saline when symptoms cease or Na^+ > 120 mEq/L
      - Rate of 3% NaCL should be < 100 mL/hr
    - Treatment of complications:
      - Seizures:
        - Midazolam 2–4 mg IV
        - Diazepam: 3–5 mg IV
        - Thiopentone: 50–100 mg IV
        - Phenytoin: 15–20 mg/kg at ≤ 50 mg/min
      - Pulmonary edema:
        - Diuretics
        - CPAP ventilation
        - Intubation and positive pressure ventilation

CHRONIC RENAL FAILURE

Introduction

Chronic renal failure is a clinical syndrome characterized by progressive and irreversible decline in renal function for more than 3 months causing GFR to reduce below 60 *mL/min/1.73 m²*.

Etiology

- Diabetes mellitus (45%)
- Glomerulonephritis
- Pyelonephritis
- Polycystic kidney disease
- Hypertension
- Systemic lupus erythematosus

Calculation of GFR: *Cockroft-Gault Formula*

$$\text{GFR/creatinine clearance (mL/min)} = \frac{(140\text{-age}) \times (\text{weight in kgs}) \text{ in males}}{72 \times (\text{serum creatinine})}$$

$$\text{GFR/creatinine clearance (mL/min)} = \frac{(140\text{-age}) \times (\text{weight in kgs}) \times 0.85 \text{ in females}}{72 \times (\text{serum creatinine})}$$

Classification: *KDOQI Staging System* (NKF-KDOQI 2013 Guidelines)

Stage	Description	GFR (mL/min/1.73 M_2)
Stage 1	Kidney damage with normal or increased GFR	> 90 mL/min/1.73 m²
Stage 2	Mild reduction in GFR	60–89 mL/min/1.73 m²
Stage 3a	Moderate reduction in GFR	45–59 mL/min/1.73 m²
Stage 3b	Moderate reduction in GFR	30–44 mL/min/1.73 m²
Stage 4	Severe reduction in GFR	15–29 mL/min/1.73 m²
Stage 5	Kidney failure	< 15 mL/min/1.73 m²

In stage 1 and 2, with normal or borderline GFR, the following markers aid diagnosis:

- Albuminuria:
  - Albumin excretion > 30 mg/ 24 hours
  - Albumin: Creatinine ratio > 30 mg/g
- Urine sediment abnormalities
- Dyselectrolytemias due to tubular disorders
- Structural abnormalities detected by imaging

Clinical Features

- Clinical features generally become manifest with CKD stages 4–5
- Central nervous system:
  - Peripheral neuropathy, uremic encephalopathy
  - Autonomic neuropathy, asterixis, myoclonus
  - Muscle twitching, confusion, seizures, coma
  - ***Restless legs syndrome***
- Cardiovascular system:
  - Hypertension, LVH
  - Arrhythmias, conduction block
  - Fluid overload, CCF, cardiomyopathy
  - Uremic pericarditis, accelerated atherosclerosis
  - Calciphylaxis and vascular calicification resulting in:
    - Valvular heart disease
    - Calcified atherosclerotic lesions
  - Complications of AV fistula shunts:
    - Congestive failure
    - Limb ischemia
    - Steal syndrome
    - Pulmonary atheroembolism
- Respiratory system:
  - Intestitial/alveolar edema
  - Pleural effusion
- Gastrointestinal system:
  - Anorexia, nausea, vomiting
  - Hiccoughs
  - Mucosal ulcerations, acid peptic disease
  - GI hemorrhage
  - Delayed gastric emptying, adynamic ileus
- Endocrine system:
  - Glucose intolerance, diabetes mellitus
  - Secondary and tertiary hyperparathyroidism
  - Vitamin D deficiency
  - Hypertriglyceridemia
- Metabolic:
  - Hyponatremia (hypernatremia rare)
  - Hyperkalemia (hypokalemia rare)
  - Hypocalcemia, hypoalbuminemia
  - Hypermagnesemia, hyperphosphatemia, hyperuricemia
  - High anion gap metabolic acidosis/hyperchloremic normal anion gap metabolic acidosis
- Hematological:
  - Anemia: Due to reduced renal erythropoietin synthesis
  - Platelet dysfunction or ***uremic thrombocytopathy***
  - Leukocyte dysfunction
- Musculoskeletal system:
  - Renal osteodystrophy
  - Periarticular calcification
  - Rhabdomyolysis after major surgery
- Skin: Hyperpigmentation, pruritus, ecchymosis

Pharmacological Considerations

- Effects of CRF on drug disposition:
  - Dose adjustment usually required if GFR < 50 mL/min
  - Absorption of drugs: Delayed due to delayed gastric emptying
  - Distribution:
    - V_d increased or decreased depending on TBW
    - Time since last dialysis influences V_d of certain drugs like remifentanil
  - Protein binding:
    - Acidic drugs:
      - Acidic drugs bind to albumin
      - Protein binding is reduced for acidic drugs in CKD
      - This is due to hypoalbuminemia seen in CKD
      - Also, acids like uric acid compete for binding sites with albumin
      - This results in increased free drug levels of acidic drugs
    - Basic drugs:
      - Basic drugs mainly bind to 1 acid glycoprotein (AAG)
      - Protein binding is increased for basic drugs in CKD
      - This is due to increase in AAG levels associated with CKD
      - This results in reduced free drug levels of basic drugs
  - Elimination: Increased T½ for drugs eliminated by kidney
- Volatile anesthetics:
  - Sevoflurane:
    - Releases ***compound A (sevo-olefin)*** which is nephrotoxic
    - It also increases fluoride levels

- Isoflurane and desflurane are safe
- Enflurane avoided as it is nephrotoxic

❖ Neuromuscular blockers:
- Succinylcholine:
  - Causes transient increases in serum potassium levels of 0.5–1 mEq/L
  - Maybe used in CKD provided preoperative potassium levels are normal
  - Avoid repeated administration
  - *Avoid succinylcholine if serum $K^+ > 5.5$ mEq/L*
- Atracurium and cisatracurium are better choices
- Cisatracurium is *drug of choice* due to:
  - Reduced incidence of histamine release
  - Drug is more potent
  - Less production of laudanosine
  - Has shorter duration of action
- Vecuronium and rocuronium have long duration of action

❖ Induction agents:
- Thiopentone requires lesser dose and lower rate of administration as:
  - Volume of distribution is increased
  - Reduced plasma protein binding
- Propofol: Dose is unchanged but causes profound hypotension

❖ Anticholineesterases:
- Neostigmine clearance reduced: causes prolonged parasympathetic activity
- Use glycopyrollate instead of atropine

❖ Non-opioid analgesics:
- *Contraindicated* including COX 2 inhibitors
- Paracetamol is safe

❖ Opioids analgesics:
- Morphine:
  - Metabolized to:
    - Morphine-3-glucuronide which reduces seizure threshold
    - Morphine-6-glucuronide which causes:
- Delayed onset of sedation
- Respiratory depression
  - Reduce dose and frequency of morphine
- Fentanyl: Reduced clearance
- Tramadol:
  - Forms O-demethyl tramadol which is excreted by kidneys
  - This may be epileptogenic: reduce dose and increase dosing interval
- Pethidine: Forms nor-meperidine which causes seizures, altered mentation
- Alfentanil and remifentanyl are safe

❖ Local anesthetics:
- Shorter duration of action due to altered protein binding
- Reduce dose by 25% as altered protein binding reduces seizure threshold

Regional Anesthesia Considerations

❖ Advantages of regional anesthesia techniques:
- Effective anesthesia
- Good postoperative analgesia
- Minimal physiological disturbances
- Improves vascular flow via regional sympathectomy

❖ Reasons to avoid neuraxial blockade in CRF:
- Uremic encephalopathy:
  - Raised ICT
  - Uncooperative patient
- Hemodynamically unstable
- Platelet dysfunction common: Possibility of hematoma
- Heparin administered during hemodialysis: Possibility of hematoma

Anesthetic Management

Preoperative Evaluation

❖ History:
- Establish cause and duration of CRF
- Evaluate the level of renal function impairment
- Evaluate and explain possible need for dialysis postoperatively
- History of comorbidities: HTN, DM, IHD, SLE and details of therapy

❖ Examination:
- Blood pressure: Standing and sitting position
- Flow murmur due to anemia
- Pericardial rub

❖ Ankle edema due to CCF/hypoproteinemia

❖ Investigations:
- Complete blood count: anemia, thrombocytopenia
- Serum electrolytes for hyperkalemia/ hyponatremia/hypocalcemia
- BUN and serum creatinine for assessing severity
- Blood glucose for glucose intolerance
- BT and CT especially if regional anesthesia considered
- ABG for acid base status and hypoxemia
- ECG: For hyperkalemia (***sigma waves***) and hypocalcemia (prolonged QT_c)
- ECHO: for cardiac function and pericardial effusion

- Chest X-ray: For signs of fluid overload, pleural effusion, cardiomegaly
- Arteriogram/renal Doppler: if renal artery stenosis is suspected

❖ ***Residual renal function:***
- Defined as the 24-hour urine volume > 100 mL
- Presence of residual renal function is associated with:
  - Lower risk of mortality
  - Reduced intradialytic weight gain
  - Improved solute clearance in HD patients

Preoperative Risk Assessment

❖ Euvolemic patients:
- Usually responsive to diuretic therapy
- Have no significant electrolyte abnormalities or bleeding tendencies
- Usually have uncomplicated perioperative courses
- Do not require dialysis perioperatively

❖ Patients with volume overload:
- Require further cardiovascular evaluation
- Fluid overload attributed to CKD in the absence of cardiovascular disease
- Combination diuretic therapy administered to achieve euvolemia
- Diuretic resistance may develop in those with chronic, progressive edema
- Perioperative dialysis considered in these patients

❖ Patients already on dialysis:
- Determine the following prior to surgery:
  - Adequacy of dialysis
  - Preoperative dialysis needs
  - Postoperative dialysis timing
  - Dosage requirements for all medicines
- Effects of preoperative dialysis:
  - Fluid depletion:
    - Redistribution of extravascular fluid occurs during dialysis
    - This results in depletion of intravascular fluid volume
  - Electrolyte disturbances, especially hypokalemia
  - Residual anticoagulation from heparinization of the circuit
- Preoperative dialysis scheduled 12–24 hours prior to surgery to reduce risk of:
  - Volume overload
  - Hyperkalemia
  - Bleeding due to anticoagulation during dialysis

Preoperative Optimization

❖ NPO orders

❖ Informed consent

❖ Preoperative sedation:
- Given only if patient is stable
- Avoid sedation if unstable hemodynamics
- Reduced dose of benzodiazepines used for sedation
- Midazolam is relatively safe

❖ Promethazine 2.5–25 mg IM used for sedation and antiemesis

❖ Antiaspiration prophylaxis as gastroparesis associated with CKD:
- 30 mL of non-particulate sodium citrate
- 50 mg ranitidine IV
- 10 mg metoclopramide or 8 mg ondansetron IV

❖ Continue all drugs on the day of surgery, especially antihypertensives

❖ Stop morning dose of oral hypoglycemics and insulin on day of surgery

❖ Preoperative blood transfusion:
- Avoid unnecessary blood transfusions
- Transfuse if Hb < 6-7 g/dL
- Target Hb > 10 g/dL
- But difficult to maintain Hb levels above 10 g/dL

❖ Preoperative dialysis:
- Done within 24 hrs of surgery, to optimize fluid and electrolyte status
- Hemodialysis is more effective than peritoneal dialysis
- Optimize BP and serum potassium levels post-dialysis
- Optimize ACT as heparin is used during dialysis
- Serum potassium < 5.5 mEq/L preferred on the day of surgery

Care of Arteriovenous Fistula

❖ Made between:
- Radial artery and cephalic vein
- Brachial artery and basilic vein
- Usually made on non-dominant hand

❖ Purpose is to improve venous access for subsequent dialysis

❖ Complications of AV fistula:
- Infection
- Stenosis
- Thrombosis
- Aneurysm
- Limb ischemia

- ❖ Done under GA/local infilteration/brachial plexus block
- ❖ If patient is dialysis dependant:
  - Dialysis to finish 4–6 hrs preoperatively to allow fluid shift
  - Heparin to be eliminated
  - Full blood count, BU, SC, BT and CT should be measured post-dialysis
  - Protect limb with fistula carefully
  - BP cuff and IV line to be on other hand/leg
  - Avoid application of pressure on the fistula
  - Pad the fistula adequately at the time of positioning to avoid pressure
  - Give slow and titrated doses of induction agents

Monitoring

- ❖ Pulse oximetry and capnography
- ❖ ECG for hyperkalemia/hypocalcemia
- ❖ Blood pressure: NIBP cuff not to be tied in arm with AV fistula as occlusion may occur
- ❖ Neuromuscular monitoring, precordial stethoscope
- ❖ Urine output: Maintain > 0.5 mL/kg/hr
- ❖ IBP if major fluid shifts expected
- ❖ CVP, PA monitoring for fluid optimization in unstable patients
- ❖ Regular ABGs for acid base status

Induction

- ❖ Preoxygenate for 5–6 minutes as anemia with increased cardiac output increases oxygen demand
- ❖ Opioids:
  - Avoid morphine as high levels of M-6-G may cause respiratory depression
  - Fentanyl is relatively safe
- ❖ Induction agents:
  - Induction agents given slowly to avoid hypotension
  - Thiopentone, propofol and etomidate relatively safe
  - Reduced dose of thiopentone (2–3 mg/kg) as V_d is increased in CKD
  - Dose reduction is required for etomidate (0.2–0.4 mg/kg)
  - Induction with inhalational agents is safe as reversal is easy
- ❖ Muscle relaxants:
  - Succinylcholine safe if serum K^+ levels is below 5.5 mEq/L
  - K^+ release following succinylcholine administration is not exaggerated in CKD
  - Atracurium, cisatracurium and mivacarium safe
  - Vecuronium and rocuronium duration of action prolonged 1½ times
  - Atracurium/cisatracurium preferred: Cistracurium is better
- ❖ *Rapid sequence induction* with cricoid pressure if history of nausea, vomiting/GI bleed
- ❖ Beta blocker (esmolol, propranolol) or lidocaine used to blunt intubation response
- ❖ Hypotension common during induction of anesthesia
- ❖ Use of LMA is safe and advantages as:
  - It avoids intubation response
  - Avoids need for paralysis

Position

- ❖ Gradual positional changes in those with autonomic neuropathy
- ❖ Care taken while positioning to adequately pad pressure areas

Maintenance

- ❖ Avoid:
  - Morphine and alfentanyl as action is prolonged
  - Meperidine as it causes prolonged CNS excitation
- ❖ Fentanyl and remifentanyl:
  - Pharmacokinetics is unaffected
  - Can be used safely
- ❖ Volatile anesthetics:
  - Avoid sevoflurane and enflurane
  - Isoflurane, desflurane best preferred as least effect on renal blood flow and CO
- ❖ Nitrous oxide:
  - Used with caution in:
    - Patients with ventricular dysfunction
    - Severe anemia with Hb < 7 g/dL
  - Otherwise can be used safely
- ❖ Controlled ventilation preferred as inadequate spontaneous ventilation with progressive hypercarbia can cause respiratory acidosis circulatory depression and hyperkalemia
- ❖ Reversal of neuromuscular blockade requires no change in dose

Hemodynamics

- ❖ Maintenance of cardiac output essential as in the presence of anemia, reduction of cardiac output may be deleterious
- ❖ Superficial operation requires only correction of insensible fluid loses with 5% dextrose

- Choice of fluids:
  - Ringer lactate avoided as it contains:
    - 5 mEq/L of potassium
    - 29 mmol/L of lactate
  - Normal saline is the *best maintenance fluid*
  - Glucose free solutions to be used as glucose intolerance might be worsened
  - Avoid starches as it can accumulate and worsen CRF
  - Gelatin containing fluids are safe
  - Replacement of blood loss with packed cells is best
- Management of hypotension:
  - Judicious fluid therapy to treat hypotension
  - Avoid precipitating fluid overload and CCF
  - If inadequate response with fluid therapy:
    - β-receptor agonists or dopamine used
    - Phenylephrine useful as vasopressor
- Antihypertensives:
  - Furosemide and thiazide action is prolonged
  - Propranolol, esmolol and labetolol: no change
  - Nifedipine, diltiazem and verapamil: no change
  - Nitroglycerine is safe
  - Sodium nitroprusside less desirable as cyanide toxicity occurs on prolonged use
  - Hydralazine:
    - Duration of action is prolonged
    - Cautious use advised

Postoperative Care

Complications

- Bleeding and infections more common: Due to lymphocyte and platelet dysfunction
- Worsening renal function
- Worsening acidosis
- Electrolyte imbalance/anemia
- Recurarization

Monitors

- SpO_2, ECG, BP
- Frequent ABGs
- Check BUN, creatinine, Hb
- Urine output

Analgesia

- Avoid NSAIDs, morphine, pethidine
- Fentanyl, remifentanyl effective
- Epidural analgesia if normal coagulation profile
- Early mobilization

RENAL REPLACEMENT THERAPY

Introduction

- Renal replacement therapy (RRT) is the term used to describe all approaches to the mechanical support of non-endocrine functions of the kidney
- This was the first technique to replace the function of an organ
- The first human application of the artificial kidney was by ***Kohler*** during World war II
- In 1960, ***Scribner and Quinton*** developed the arteriovenous shunt
- This allowed the initiation of intermittent hemodialysis as the first line therapy for ESRD

Indications

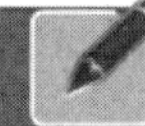

- RRT should be considered in the presence of 1 criterion
- RRT is strongly recommended in the presence of 2 criteria
- Criteria include:
  - Urine volume:
    - Oliguria (urine output < 200 mL/ 12 hours)
    - Anuria (urine output 0–50 mL/12 hours)
  - Renal function tests:
    - Blood urea > 35 mmol/L or 98 mg/dL
    - Serum creatinine > 400 µmol/L or 4.5 mg/dL
    - Serum potassium > 6.5 mEq/L or rapidly rising
    - Uncompensated metabolic acidosis (pH < 7.1)
    - Serum sodium < 110 mEq/L and > 160 mEq/L
  - Others:
    - Pulmonary edema unresponsive to diuretics
    - Temperature > 40°C
  - Uremic complications:
    - Encephalopathy
    - Myopathy
    - Neuropathy
    - Pericarditis
  - Overdose with dialyzable toxin such as lithium

Principles of Renal Replacement Therapy

- Diffusion principle:
  - Main principle used during conventional hemodialysis
  - A semipermeable membrane separates two aqueous solutions
  - Comprises of movement of small molecular weight solutes across the membrane
  - Movement occurs from higher to lower concentration compartment
  - Ineffective for larger molecular weight substances (> 5000 Da)
  - Substances moving from the blood to dialysate compartment:
    - Creatinine
    - Urea

- Potassium
- Phosphorous
- At the same time bicarbonate moves from the dialysate to blood
- This helps in simultaneous correction of AKI induced acidosis
- Water elimination is negligible when diffusion is uniquely applied

❖ Convection principle:
- Main principle used during hemofiltration
- A semipermeable membrane separates two aqueous solutions
- Comprises of the movement of water by mass transport across pressure gradient
- Forces driving the movement of water include:
  - Hydrostatic pressure
  - Transmembrane pressure
- This fluid transport across the membrane is called *ultrafiltration*
- During convection, a small amount of solute moves along with the fluid
- This solute removal depends on the sieving coefficient of the membrane

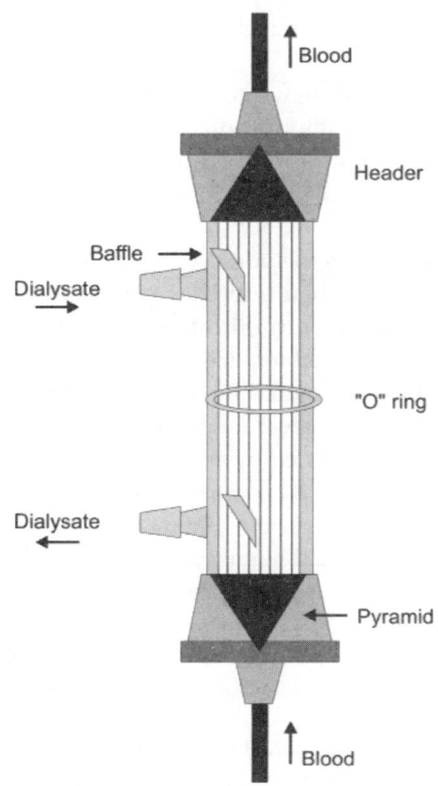

Fig. 3: Hollow fibre dialyzer.

Dialyzers

❖ Types of dialyzers:
- Hollow fiber dialyzers:
  - Most commonly used dialyzers currently
  - Contain numerous hollow fibers, similar in structure to a human capillary
  - These capillary-like fibers are bundled together within the dialyzer shell
  - This serves as the dialyzer membrane across which blood and dialysate flow
- Parallel plate dialyzers:
  - These are no longer in common use
  - Designed with flat sheets of membrane material arranged in parallel
  - Each membrane sheet is laid on top of the other
  - Blood and dialysate flow in parallel through separate spaces between the sheets
  - Exchange of solutes and water occurs across the pores within each sheet

❖ Types of membranes:
- Different types of membranes available are:
  - Unmodified cellulose:
  - Substituted cellulose
  - Synthetic cellulose membranes
  - Synthetic non-cellulose membranes
- Cellulose membranes are less permeable and bioincompatible
- Thus, the membranes most commonly used now are:
  - Synthetic cellulose membranes
  - Synthetic non-cellulose membranes

❖ Important characteristics of membranes are:
- Priming volume:
  - Prime volume is lesser with hollow-fiber dialyzers
  - Priming volume usually ranges from 160-270 mL
  - Low priming volumes are preferred to minimize risk of hemodynamic compromise

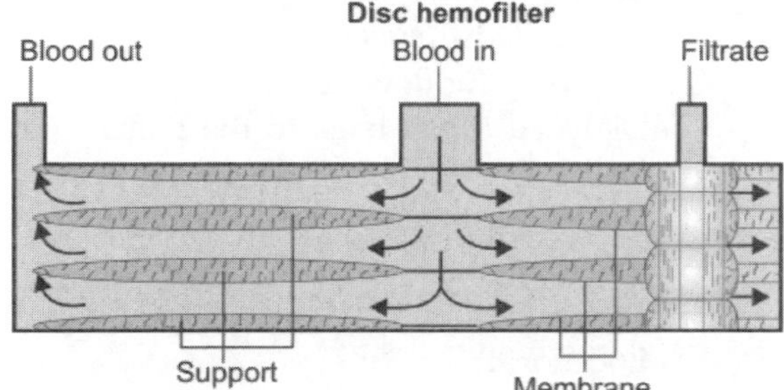

Fig. 4: Parallel plate dialyzer.

- Clearance:
  - Clearance of solutes determines the dialyzer efficiency
  - Dialyzer clearance is measured in terms of:
    - Urea clearance (small molecules)
    - Creatinine clearance (small molecules)
    - Vitamin B12 clearance (large molecules)
  - Dialyzer clearance is measured by the ***mass transfer coefficient*** KoA
  - KoA determines the dialyzer's efficiency of clearance
  - KoA is defined by:
    - Membrane porosity
    - Membrane thickness
    - Solute size
    - Flow rate of blood and dialysate
  - Preferred values of KoA for different clinical scenarios:
    - Between 300–600 for chronic hemodialysis
    - More than 600 for those requiring high efficiency dialysis
- Surface area: dialyzers with higher surface areas have higher urea clearances
- ***Ultrafiltration coefficient*** (KUf):
  - Ultrafiltration coefficient correlates directly with membrane permeability
  - It refers to volume of fluid transferred across per mm Hg pressure gradient
  - High KUf values denote higher permeability to water
  - Low KUf values denote lower permeability to water

Dialysis Machines and Tubings

- The dialysis machine includes:
  - Blood pump to move blood between patient and dialyzer
  - Delivery system to transport dialysis solution
- Tubing systems:
  - Inlet tubing:
    - For flowing undialyzed blood from the patient to the dialyzer
    - Also called *arterial line*
  - Outlet tubing for flowing:
    - Dialyzed blood back to the patient *(venous line)*
    - Dialysis effluent (spent dialysate)
- Monitoring devices:
  - Pressure monitors:
    - Locations:
      - Proximal to the blood pump
      - Distal to the dialyzer
    - Purpose:
      - To guard against excess suction of blood from the patient
      - To guard against excessive resistance to return of blood to patient
  - Venous air trap monitor
  - Temperature sensor for measuring temperature of the dialysate

Composition of Ideal Dialysate

- For intermittent hemodialysis:
  - Sodium 150 mmol/L
  - Bicarbonate 31 mmol/L
  - Potassium 3-4 mmol/L
  - Calcium 1.75 mmol/L
  - Glucose 5.5 mmol/L
  - Temperature: 35 C
- For CRRT:
  - Sodium 140 mmol/L
  - Bicarbonate 30 mmol/L
  - Potassium 3-4 mmol/L
  - Calcium 1.25 mmol/L
  - Phosphate 1
  - Magnesium 0.6 mmol/L
  - Chloride 115 mmol/L

Types of RRT

- Intermittent renal replacement techniques:
  - Most common technique used for chronic renal failure
  - Blood and dialysate circulated in countercurrent manner without contact
  - Ultrafiltration rate = scheduled weight loss
  - Typically performed 3-4 hours thrice weekly or daily
  - Techniques include:
    - Hemodiafiltration
    - Isolated ultrafiltration
- Continuous renal replacement therapy techniques:
  - Represents modalities which provide continuous support for severely ill patients
  - Usually defined by duration above 24 hours
  - Advantages over intermittent renal replacement techniques:
    - Enhanced hemodynamic stability
    - Lesser incidence of dialysis disequilibrium syndrome
    - More consistent salt and water removal
    - Enhanced clearance of inflammatory mediators
  - Techniques include:
    - Slow continuous ultrafiltration
    - Hemofiltration: CAVH, CVVH

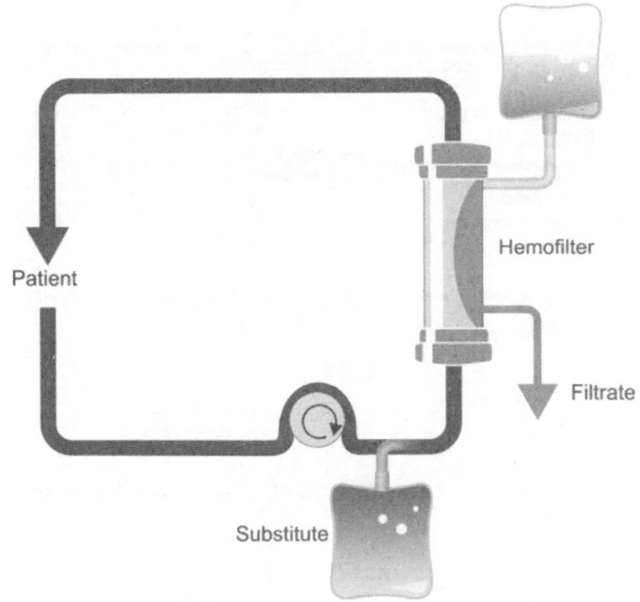

Fig. 5: CRRT setup.

- Hemodialysis: CAVHD, CVVHD
- Hemodiafiltration: CAVHDF, CVVHDF
- Extended daily dialysis

❖ Hybrid techniques:
- Slow low efficiency daily dialysis (SLEDD)
- Sustained low efficiency daily dialysis with filtration (SLEDD-F)

Techniques of Continuous RRT

❖ Slow continuous ultrafiltration (SCUF):
- Technique used for fluid control only
- Not useful in patients who are uremic/hyperkalemic as solute removal is minimal
- Blood is driven through a highly permeable filter using *convective* mechanism
- Uses extracorporeal circuit in arterio-venous or veno-venous mode
- Does not use dialysate/ replacement fluid
- Rate of arterial flow is 50–100 mL/min
- Ultrafiltration rate is 2–8 mL/min
- Ultrafiltration rate is controlled and low compared to CVVH
- Ultrafiltrate volume produced = weight loss
- Up to 8 L of fluid can be safely removed per day
- Used only for fluid control in volume overloaded patients

❖ Continuous veno venous hemofiltration (CVVH):
- Blood is driven through a highly permeable filter
- Usually uses extracorporeal circuit in veno-venous mode
- Can be used in arterio-venous mode also
- Purifies blood using *convective principle* through a high permeability membrane
- Uses hydrostatic pressure to filter plasma water across the membrane
- Thus, it does not use dialysate fluid as solutes are entirely removed by convection
- Rate of ultrafiltration is controlled and high (20-25 mL/hour)
- Due to this high rate, replacement fluid is given to prevent volume depletion
- Volume of ultrafiltrate is therefore replaced by the replacement solution
- The amount of replacement fluid is determined by the desired net volume balance
- Small and middle molecular weight molecules are removed in the same concentration as plasma water
- Thus, there is no change in the plasma concentration of these solutes by CVVH
- However, the replacement fluid administered may dilute solutes such as creatinine
- Types of CVVH based on volume replacement:
  - Predilution hemofiltration: Replacement fluid delivered before filter
  - Post-dilution hemofiltration: Replacement fluid delivered after filter

❖ Continuous veno venous hemodialysis (CVVHD):
- Purifies blood via *diffusion* principle using low permeability dialyzer
- Uses extracorporeal circuit in veno-venous mode
- Blood is driven through a low permeability dialyzer
- Dialysate solution is circulated in countercurrent flow in dialysate compartment
- Rate of flow of the dialysate fluid is 1–2 L/hour
- Dialysate flow rate amounts to approximately 20–25 mL/kg/hour
- In contrast to CVVH, rate of ultrafiltration is only 2–8 mL/min
- Therefore, replacement fluid is not used in this method
- Ultrafiltrate produced = weight loss

❖ Continuous veno venous hemo dia filtration (CVVHDF):
- Uses *diffusive and convective* principles for blood purification

- Requires infusions of both dialysis fluid and replacement fluid
- A high permeability membrane is used
- Thus, small and medium sized molecules are removed
- Dialysate solution is circulated in countercurrent direction
- Rate of filtration 8–12 mL/min
- Volume of ultrafiltration is variable, similar to CVVH
- Replacement fluid is usually required to maintain euvolemia
- The volume of replacement fluid is determined by the desired net volume balance

❖ Continuous high flux dialysis (CVVHFD):
- Blood purification via diffusive and convective principles
- Uses highly permeable membrane
- Back diffusion occurs in the membrane
- Dialysate solution is circulated in countercurrent direction
- Accessory pumps are used to control ultrafiltration
- Rate of filtration is 2–8 mL/min

❖ Continuous plasma filtration adsorption (CPFA):
- Uses a highly permeable plasmafilter to filter fluid plasma
- This is allowed to pass through a bed of adsorbent material such as carbon/ resins
- Can be coupled with CVVH or CVVHDF

❖ Hemoperfusion (HP):
- Patient's blood is circulated on a bed of coated charcoal powder
- Removes solutes by adsorption
- Indicated in cases of poisoning and intoxication with agents removed by charcoal
- Causes platelet and protein depletion

❖ Plasmapheresis (PP):
- Uses specific plasma filters to filter plasma as a whole
- Blood reconstituted by infusion of plasma products like albumin/frozen plasma
- Used to remove proteins and protein bound solutes

❖ High volume hemofiltration:
- Hemofiltration with a high-volume setting > 45 mL/kg/hour
- Uses highly permeable membrane

❖ High permeability filtration: Uses high cutoff permeable membranes

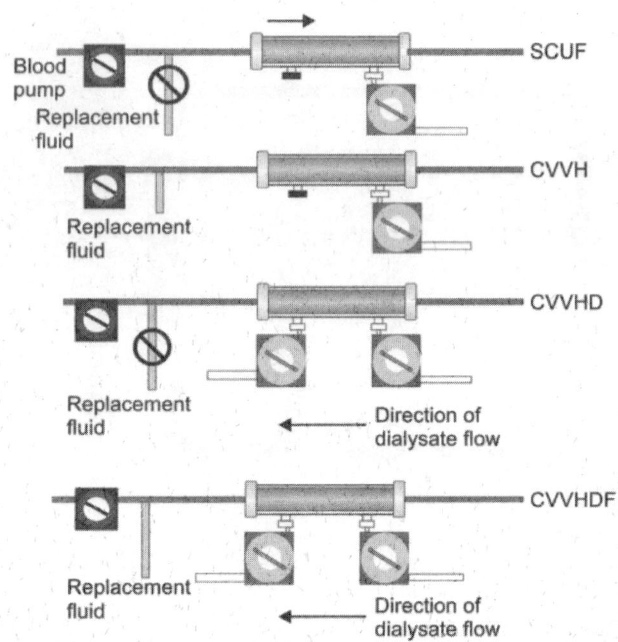

Fig. 6: Types of CRRT.

Clinical Characteristics of RRT Techniques

	Intermittent	Continuous		
	IHD	*CVVH*	*CVVHDF*	*CVVHD*
Solute clearance	Diffusion	Convection	Both	Diffusion
Duration (h)	4–6	> 24	> 24	> 24
Blood flow (mL/min)	200–350	100–250	100–250	100–250
Diffusion	++++	–	++	++++
Convection	+	++++	++	+
Urea clearance (mL/min)	150–200	20–45	20–45	20–45
Filtration fraction	< 5%	20–25%	15–20%	< 5%
Fluctuations of ICP	++++	–	–	–
Hemodynamic stability	–	++++	++++	++++
Fluid balance control	++	++++	++++	++
pH stability	+ =	++++	++++	++++
Need for anticoagulation	+	+++	++	++
Membrane	Synthetic	Synthetic	Synthetic	Synthetic

(IHD: intermittent hemodialysis; CVVH: continuous veno venous hemofiltration; CVVHDF: continuous veno venous hemo dia filtration; CVVHD: continuous veno venous hemodialysis; SLED: slow low efficiency daily dialysis)

Dose of RRT (KDIGO 2012 Guidelines)

❖ Intermittent hemodialysis:
- Dosing in IHD is based upon:
  - Dose delivered per session
  - Frequency of sessions
- The recommended Kt/V for patients undergoing IHD is 3.9 per week
- Thus, if IHD is targeted thrice a week, target Kt/V should be 1.2 per treatment

Contd...

Contd...

- ❖ Continuous renal replacement therapy:
  - Recommended effluent flow rate is 25 mL/kg/hour
  - This is in order to achieve a minimum effluent rate of 20 mL/kg/hour over 24 hours
  - Higher intensity dialysis does not result in improved survival/ clinical benefits
  - Therapy is usually discontinued once creatinine clearance exceeds 20 mL/min

Anticoagulation during RRT

- ❖ During dialysis, contact occurs between the blood and tubing of the circuit
- ❖ This results in the activation of coagulation cascade
- ❖ This becomes a major concern during continuous methods
- ❖ Techniques used:
  - Mechanical methods:
    - Adequate sized vascular access:
      - 13.5–15.5 French catheters
      - Length of catheter 15–20 cm
    - Optimal site of vascular access:
      - Right IJV preferred site
      - Femoral veins are a good alternative
      - Subclavian vein is avoided
    - Avoid kinking/torsion of circuit tubing
    - Blood flow rate > 100 mL/min
    - Continuous monitoring of venous bubble trap
    - Maintain plasma filtration fraction < 25%
  - Pharmacological:
    - Unfractionated heparin:
      - Given at 5–10 IU/kg/hour
      - This technique is effective, cheap and widely available
      - Disadvantages:
        - Development of HIT
        - Development of heparin resistance
      - Efficiency is monitored by:
        - ACT
        - Anti-Xa activity
    - LMWH: Cannot be used for continuous methods
    - Citrate:
      - Excellent and effective anticoagulation with minimal risk to patient
      - Recommended as the first choice in many centers
      - Sodium citrate is infused into the inflow limb of the circuit
      - This chelates the calcium and prevents clotting
      - Citrate returning back to the patient is metabolized to bicarbonate
      - A Ca^{2+} infusion may be required to replace Ca^{2+} lost in the effluent
      - However, this technique is still not FDA approved for CRRT
      - Contraindications:
        - Acute liver failure with transaminase levels > 1000 IU/L
        - Cardiogenic shock with blood lactates > 8 mmol/L
      - Disadvantages:
        - Special dialysate is required
        - Calcium infusion is required
        - More expensive

CONTINUOUS RENAL REPLACEMENT THERAPY

Introduction

Represents modalities which provide continuous renal support for severely ill patients, usually defined by a duration above 24 hours.

Indications

- ❖ The major indication for choosing continuous renal replacement therapy (CRRT) over IHD is hemodynamic instability
- ❖ Hypotension with CRRT is less common as the rate of fluid removal is slower
- ❖ CRRT is preferred over IHD for:
  - Patients requiring ongoing large volume fluid replacement
  - Acute brain injury
  - Raised ICP
- ❖ However, IHD is preferred over CRRT for patients hyperkalemic requiring RRT
- ❖ Indications can be classified according to the cause as:
  - Renal causes:
    - Severe hyperkalemia (serum K^+ > 6.5 mEq/L)
    - Signs of uremia:
      - Pericarditis
      - Encephalopathy
      - Declining mental status
    - Severe metabolic acidosis (pH < 7.1)
    - Alcohol and drug intoxications
  - Non-renal causes:
    - SIRS
    - Crush syndrome
    - Lactic acidosis

- Refractory fluid overload
- Congestive heart failure

Modalities of CRRT

- Slow continuous ultrafiltration (SCUF):
  - Technique used for fluid control only
  - Not useful in patients who are uremic/ hyperkalemic as solute removal is minimal
  - Blood is driven through a highly permeable filter using *convective* mechanism
  - Uses extracorporeal circuit in arterio-venous or veno-venous mode
  - Does not use dialysate/ replacement fluid
  - Rate of arterial flow is 50–100 mL/min
  - Ultrafiltration rate is 2–8 mL/min
  - Ultrafiltration rate is controlled and low compared to CVVH
  - Ultrafiltrate volume produced = weight loss
  - Up to 8 L of fluid can be safely removed per day
  - Used only for fluid control in volume overloaded patients
- Continuous veno venous hemofiltration (CVVH):
  - Blood is driven through a highly permeable filter
  - Usually uses extracorporeal circuit in veno-venous mode
  - Can be used in arterio-venous mode also
  - Purifies blood using *convective principle* through a high permeability membrane
  - Uses hydrostatic pressure to filter plasma water across the membrane
  - Thus, it does not use dialysate fluid as solutes are entirely removed by convection
  - Rate of ultrafiltration is controlled and high (20-25 mL/hour)
  - Due to this high rate, replacement fluid is given to prevent volume depletion
  - Volume of ultrafiltrate is therefore replaced by the replacement solution
  - The amount of replacement fluid is determined by the desired net volume balance
  - Small and middle molecular weight molecules are removed in the same concentration as plasma water
  - Thus, there is no change in the plasma concentration of these solutes by CVVH
  - However, the replacement fluid administered may dilute solutes such as creatinine
  - Types of CVVH based on volume replacement:
    - Predilution hemofiltration: replacement fluid delivered before filter
    - Post-dilution hemofiltration: replacement fluid delivered after filter
- Continuous veno venous hemodialysis (CVVHD):
  - Purifies blood via *diffusion* principle using low permeability dialyzer
  - Uses extracorporeal circuit in veno-venous mode
  - Blood is driven through a low permeability dialyzer
  - Dialysate solution is circulated in countercurrent flow in dialysate compartment
  - Rate of flow of the dialysate fluid is 1–2 L/hour
  - Dialysate flow rate amounts to approximately 20–25 mL/kg/hour
  - In contrast to CVVH, rate of ultrafiltration is only 2–8 mL/min
  - Therefore, replacement fluid is not used in this method
  - Ultrafiltrate produced = weight loss
- Continuous veno venous hemo dia Filtration (CVVHDF):
  - Uses *diffusive and convective* principles for blood purification
  - Requires infusions of both dialysis fluid and replacement fluid
  - A high permeability membrane is used
  - Thus, small and medium sized molecules are removed
  - Dialysate solution is circulated in countercurrent direction
  - Rate of filtration 8–12 mL/min
  - Volume of ultrafiltration is variable, similar to CVVH
  - Replacement fluid is usually required to maintain euvolemia
  - The volume of replacement fluid is determined by the desired net volume balance

Vascular Access

- Currently only veno-venous modalities are being used
- Arterio-venous modalities are no longer used due to risk of arterial cannulation:
  - Embolization
  - Bleeding
  - Hematoma
  - Limb ischemia
- Requires reliable vascular access capable of blood flows of at least 200–250 mL/min
- Standard catheters are double-lumen tunneled or non-tunneled dialysis catheters

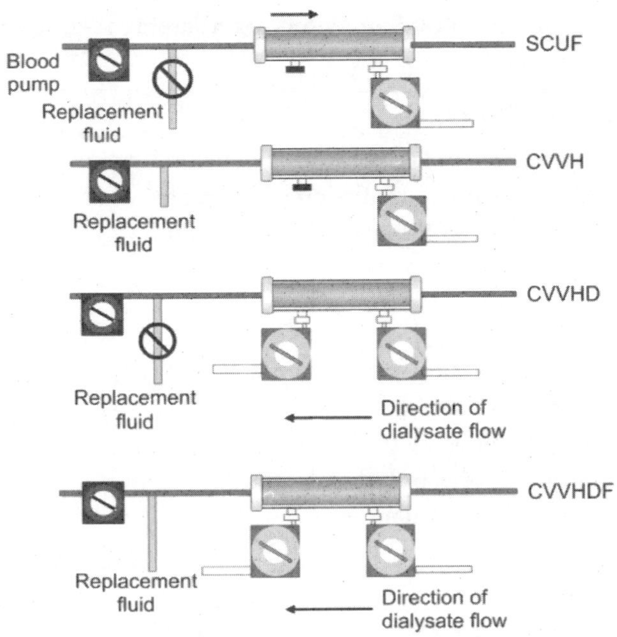

Fig. 7: Types of CRRT.

- In those patients with indwelling AV fistulas, the fistulas should not be used for CRRT
- This is to avoid the risk of causing injury to the AV fistula or graft
- Preferred sites in order of preference:
  - Right IJV
- Femoral vein Subclavian vein is usually avoided as:
  - They are associated with subclavian stenosis
  - This may prevent future placement of catheters/ AV fistulas and AV grafts

Equipment

- Multiple integrated systems are available for CRRT
- The basic components of all machines are similar and include:
  - Roller pumps controlling blood flow and dialysate inflow
  - Balancing systems to provide ultrafiltrate control
  - Microprocessor driven control of dialysate inflow and outflow

Components of Dialysate

- Sodium 140 mmol/L
- Bicarbonate 30 mmol/L
- Potassium 3–4 mmol/L
- Calcium 1.25 mmol/L
- Phosphate 1 mmol/L
- Magnesium 0.6 mmol/L
- Chloride 115 mmol/L

CRRT Parameters

- Modality:
  - The modality is selected based upon the CRRT device availability at the institute
  - There are no studies which show better clinical outcomes with a specific modality
  - CVVH and CVVHDF can remove larger molecular weight solutes
- Dose:
  - The dose is defined by the effluent flow rate
  - Recommended effluent flow rate is 25 mL/kg/hour
  - This is in order to maintain a minimum effluent rate of 20 mL/kg/hr over 24 hours
  - Higher rates are used for severe metabolic derangements requiring urgent correction
  - Effluent rates up to 40–70 mL/kg/hour are used until acidosis is partially corrected
  - Once acidosis is partially corrected, flow rate can be reduced to 25 mL/kg/hour
- Filtration fraction:
  - Defined as the proportion of plasm water entering the dialyzer which is filtered
  - Filtration fraction is usually maintained below 20%
  - Higher filtration fractions are associated with hemoconcentration and circuit clotting

$$\text{Filtration fraction} = \frac{\text{Ultrafiltration flow rate}}{\text{Plasma water flow rate}}$$

- Blood flow rate:
  - For patients on anticoagulation, blood flow rate in maintained at 200 mL/min
  - A higher flow rate of 200–300 mL/min is maintained if anticoagulation is not used
  - Low flow rates of 100–150 mL/min can cause blood stasis and clotting
  - Thus, clinically optimized flow rates are important

Anticoagulation During CRRT (KDIGO 2012 Guidelines)

- Anticoagulation is recommended for all CRRT modalities
- However, anticoagulation free CRRT may be considered when:
  - Filter life can be maintained for more than 24 hours
  - Platelet count < 50000/mm^3
- Options for anticoagulation include:
  - Unfractionated heparin:
    - Given at 5–10 IU/kg/hour

  - This technique is effective, cheap and widely available
  - Disadvantages:
    - Development of HIT
    - Development of heparin resistance
  - Efficiency is monitored by:
    - ACT
    - Anti-X_a activity
- Regional citrate anticoagulation:
  - Excellent and effective anticoagulation with minimal risk to patient
  - Recommended as the first choice in many centers
  - Sodium citrate is infused into the inflow limb of the circuit
  - This chelates the calcium and prevents clotting
  - Citrate returning back to the patient is metabolized to bicarbonate
  - A Ca^{2+} infusion may be required to replace Ca^{2+} lost in the effluent
  - However, this technique is still not FDA approved for CRRT
  - Contraindications:
    - Acute liver failure with transaminase levels > 1000 IU/L
    - Cardiogenic shock with blood lactates > 8 mmol/L
  - Disadvantages:
    - Special dialysate is required
    - Calcium infusion is required
    - More expensive
- Less common methods such as:
  - Low molecular weight heparin
  - Thrombin antagonists:
    - Bivalirudin
    - Argatroban
  - Heparinoids
  - Platelet inhibiting agents

❖ Continuous anticoagulation causes increased risk of bleeding and thrombocytopenia

Advantages

❖ Useful in hemodynamically unstable patients as lower rates of fluid removal
❖ Provides excellent control of azotemia, electrolyte and acid base balance
❖ Efficient removal of fluid in special circumstances like ARDS and pulmonary edema
❖ Helps in administration of parenteral nutrition, IV medication and inotropes
❖ Hemofiltration reduces intracranial tension
❖ Removes proinflammatory mediators: IL-1, IL-6, IL-8, TNF

Disadvantages

❖ Requires regular monitoring of hemodynamic status
❖ Requires regular infusion of dialysate
❖ Requires continuous anticoagulation
❖ Expensive

Complications

❖ Vascular access site malformation
❖ Air embolism
❖ Circuit blood clotting
❖ Fluid and electrolyte imbalance
❖ Acid-base imbalances
❖ Bleeding
❖ Thrombosis
❖ Infection/ sepsis
❖ Membrane bio-incompatibility
❖ Hypothermia
❖ Nutrient losses

RRT IN SEPSIS

Introduction

❖ Severe sepsis is associated with AKI in 5–50% of patients
❖ Almost 45–70% of all AKI occurring in the ICU is due to sepsis
❖ Thus, RRT is a frequently used adjuvant therapy in sepsis
❖ Dialysis requiring AKI in the septic scenario has a high mortality of 40–50%
❖ This increases to 60–80% in the presence of other associated organ dysfunction

Indications 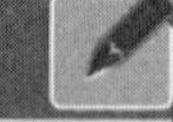

❖ Indications in sepsis are similar to other indications of CRRT in AKI
❖ These include:
- Progressive azotemia
- Volume overload
- Metabolic acidosis
- Severe dyselectrolytemias

❖ Compared to conventional indications, early initiation is recommended in sepsis
❖ This is in order to provide immunomodulation along with replacement of renal function
❖ CRRT is preferred over IHD in stable patients as well as those with septic shock

Factors to Consider Prior to Initiation of CRRT In Sepsis

- Severity of illness:
  - AKI severity and trend
  - Levels of BUN and creatinine
  - Electrolyte imbalance and acid base status
  - Fluid balance and evidence of fluid overload
  - Presence of associated organ dysfunction
- Necessity of procedure:
  - Likelihood of recovery of function without CRRT
  - Nature and timing of renal insult
  - Presence of oliguria
  - Concurrent use of vasopressors
  - Ventilatory requirement
- Risks associated with the procedure:
  - Complications of vascular access:
    - Hemorrhage
    - Thrombosis
    - Bacteremia
  - Complications of CRRT:
    - Hypersensitivity to extracorporeal circuit
    - Intradialytic hypotension
  - Prolongation of AKI

Role of CRRT in Sepsis

- For inflammation and metabolic adaptation:
  - High cytokine concentration in sepsis is associated with:
    - Slow renal recovery
    - Increased mortality
  - Thus, extracorporeal removal of cytokines affects the immune pathology
  - It reduces the excessive metabolic adaptation seen in septic AKI
  - Metabolic adaptation leads to:
    - Hyperglycemia
    - Immunosuppression
    - Secondary infection
  - During CRRT, clearance of cytokines improves the sensitivity to insulin
- Alteration of energy balance in septic AKI:
  - Sepsis causes an alteration in energy balance by:
    - Causing mitochondrial injury
    - Reducing intracellular ATP stores
  - CRRT affects the energy balance in sepsis by:
    - Regulating the metabolic adaptation
    - Providing a continuous source of energy during extracorporeal circulation

Mechanisms of CRRT in Sepsis

- *Peak concentration hypothesis*:
  - Removes cytokines from blood during proinflammatory phase of sepsis
  - This resets the septic process to a lower level of dysregulation
  - This eventually restores immune homeostasis
- *Threshold immunomodulation hypothesis*:
  - CRRT results in the removal of proinflammatory mediators
  - When the levels fall below a threshold, proinflammatory processes are halted
  - This is responsible for immunomodulatory effects of CRR
  - However, the threshold levels are unclear
- *Mediator delivery hypothesis*:
  - HVHF increases the lymphatic flow by 20-40 times
  - Mediators and cytokines are eventually 'dragged' with lymph
  - This pulls cytokines from tissues to blood from where it is removed by CRRT
  - This results in immunomodulation

Vascular Access

- Site of vascular access in order of preference:
  - Right internal jugular vein
  - Femoral vein
  - Left internal jugular vein
  - Right subclavian vein
- Ultrasound guided placement of catheters
- Chest X-ray confirmation of placement
- Avoid topical antibiotics over skin insertion site

Modalities of CRRT in Sepsis

- Standard dose CRRT:
  - The turnover rate of inflammatory mediators in sepsis is very high
  - The volume of mediators removed by conventional CRRT may not be clinically significant
  - Thus, use of standard dose CRRT for septic AKI cannot be recommended
- High adsorption hemofiltration:
  - Uses a PMMA membrane with a symmetric microporous structure
  - This membrane removes cytokine molecules by adsorption
  - It has greater dialysance for middle and high molecular weight substances
  - However, due to clogging, the membrane has to be replaced every 24 hours

- High volume hemofiltration (HVH):
  - This uses continuous ultrafiltration to produce high ultrafiltrate volumes
  - Definition of HVH is controversial (> 50 mL/kg/hour)
  - Removes medium sized molecules by convection
  - Currently there is no evidence for the use of this modality in sepsis
- High cut off hemofiltration (HCO):
  - This technique utilizes membranes with a cut-off of up to 60 kD in human blood
  - This results in increased clearance of mediators which increase mortality risk
  - However, it also results in the removal of high volumes of albumin
  - Although initially developed for use in sepsis, it has also been used for myeloma
  - No large RCT has been conducted and its efficacy is yet to be established
- Coupled plasma filtration adsorption (CPFA):
  - Involves plasma separation followed by an adsorptive step
  - The adsorptive step is done over activated charcoal sorbent
  - This allows the non-specific removal of mediators
  - After the return of purified plasma to the circuit, standard hemodialysis is applied
- Renal artificial device (RAD):
  - Utilizes non-autologous renal human renal tubular cells
  - These cells are grown along the inner surface of hollow fibers aligned in a cartridge
  - This is incorporated in an extracorporeal perfusion circuit
  - Ultrafiltrate is pumped through the RAD, allowing elimination of substances from the circuit

Dose of CRRT

- Optimal intensity of CRRT in sepsis patients remains controversial
- Earlier studies suggested better outcomes with high flow rates (40 mL/kg/hour)
- At present there is no evidence to suggest a dose above 20 mL/kg/hour

Anticoagulation for CRRT in Sepsis

- Inflammatory cytokines can activate the coagulation system
- This can lead to the formation of microvascular thrombosis
- This process leads to multiorgan dysfunction in sepsis
- Anticoagulant therapy is therefore associated with survival benefit in severe sepsis
- Heparin is associated with an increased risk of hemorrhage in sepsis
- Thus, regional citrate anticoagulation is recommended in these patients

PERITONEAL DIALYSIS

Introduction

- Procedure using peritoneum as a membrane for fluid exchange therapy in azotemic patients
- First performed in 1923 by ***Georg Ganter*** at university of Wurzburg

Physiology

- Peritoneal dialysis uses the peritoneal membrane as a filter
- Peritoneal membrane is a semi-permeable membrane
- This allows water and solute transport from the vascular system to peritoneal cavity
- The peritoneal cavity can hold up to 3 liters of fluid
- Only 1.5–2.5 liters of peritoneal fluid is used clinically for peritoneal dialysis
- Multiple processes take place simultaneously during peritoneal dialysis:
  - Diffusion:
    - Process which is responsible for removal of solutes
    - Concentration gradient between dialysate and blood is the driving force
    - Solutes move from high concentration areas to low concentration areas
    - Small solutes move quickly through the membrane
    - Larger solutes move slowly across the peritoneal membrane
    - Thus, reaching equilibrium point with larger solutes takes longer time
  - Osmosis and ultrafiltration:
    - Refers to the movement of solvent from low to high solute concentration
    - Glucose present in the dialysate acts as an osmotic agent
    - Thus, glucose creates an osmotic gradient
    - This aids removal of fluid from the peritoneal cavity
- Factors influencing solute diffusion:
  - Surface area
  - Peritoneal permeability
  - Solute characteristics

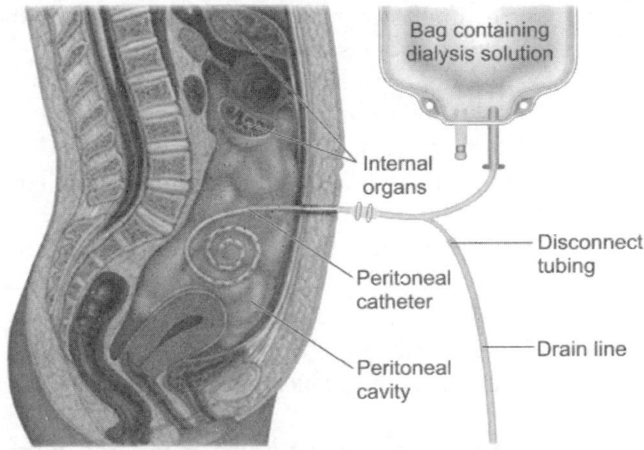

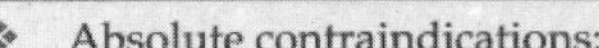

Fig. 8: Peritoneal dialysis.

- Concentration gradient
- Temperature of dialysis solution
- Blood flow
- Dwell time

❖ Factors influencing fluid osmosis:
- Surface area
- Peritoneal membrane permeability
- Pressure gradients:
  - Hydrostatic pressure
  - Oncotic pressure

Goals of Peritoneal Dialysis

❖ Remove uremic toxins and metabolic waste
❖ Maintain positive nitrogen balance
❖ Reverse symptoms of uremia
❖ Reestablish normal fluid and electrolyte balance

Indications

❖ Renal indications: CKD or AKI (requiring renal replacement therapy) with:
- Vascular access failure or difficult vascular access
- Intolerance to hemodialysis:
  - Severe peripheral vascular disease
  - Ischemic heart disease
  - Cardiomyopathy
- Children aged 0–5 years
- Bleeding diathesis as no need of anticoagulation
- Multiple myeloma
- Chronic infections
- Labile diabetes mellitus

❖ Non-renal indications:
- Refractory congestive cardiac failure
- Hepatic failure
- Hypothermia, hyperthermia
- Pancreatitis

Contraindications

❖ Absolute contraindications:
- Severe inflammatory bowel disease
- Ischemic bowel disease
- Acute active diverticulosis
- Peritoneal fibrosis and adhesions
- Abdominal abscess

❖ Relative contraindications:
- Severe malnutrition
- Obesity
- Hernias
- Colostomy

Peritoneal Dialysis Catheters

❖ Parts of the catheter:
- Intraperitoneal section:
  - This part of the catheter has numerous openings
  - Open tip allows free flow of dialysate
- Subcutaneous section:
  - Passes from the peritoneal membrane to the skin
  - Tunnels through the muscle and subcutaneous fat
  - This section is around 5–10 cm long
  - This tunneled section protects against infections
- External section:
  - Allows connection to the dialysate section

❖ Cuffs:
- Two cuffs are present, made of Dacron
- Locations of the two cuffs:
  - Subcutaneous tissue
  - Pre-peritoneal space
- Functions of the cuff:
  - Stabilize the catheter
  - Limit movement of the catheter
  - Prevents fluid leaks

❖ Types of catheters:
- ***Straight Tenckhoff catheter***
- Curled Tenckhoff catheter
- Swan neck catheter
- Toronto Western catheter

Composition of PD Solution

1. pH 5.2
2. Osmolarity 363 mOsmol/L
3. Sodium 130 mmol/L (hyponatremic compared to plasma which aids removal of sodium)
4. Calcium 1.5 mmol/L
5. Magnesium 0.75 mmol/L
6. Chloride 100 mmol/L
7. Bicarbonate 35 mmol/L (buffering agent)
8. Glucose 1.36–4.25 g/dL (osmotic agent)

Procedure

- Infusion: Refers to the time taken for infusion of the dialysate into the cavity
- Dwell time: Refers to the time during which dialysate is present in the peritoneal cavity
- Drainage time: Refers to the time taken for draining the dialysate after exchange

Conduct of Peritoneal Dialysis: *ISPD 2014 Guidelines*

- Catheter type and insertion:
  - Tenckhoff catheter remains the *gold standard* for peritoneal dialysis
  - Catheter size chosen in order to maximize:
    - Dialysate dwell time
    - Contact with peritoneal membrane
- Prevent peritonitis:
  - Strict asepsis recommended during insertion
  - Prophylactic antibiotics need to have adequate tissue levels prior to insertion
- Fluid exchange system:
  - Closed system fluid exchange preferred
  - Collapsible bags with integral transfer tubings form a closed system
  - These are recommended as the *gold standard* for fluid exchange during PD
- PD solutions:
  - PD solution using lactate as buffer is the *gold standard*
  - Standard PD solutions do not contain potassium
  - After 4–6 hour exchanges, serum and dialysate potassium concentrations are similar
  - Serum potassium levels, therefore, have to be checked atleast once daily
  - Potassium supplementation is recommended when serum $K^+ < 4$ mmol/L
  - 4 mmol/L is added to the dialysate solution to correct hypokalemia
- Fluid exchange therapy:
  - Duration of cycle time is dictated by clinical circumstances
  - Short cycle times (every 1–2 hrs) are preferred during the initial 24 hours
  - This is targeted to correct hyperkalemia, fluid overload and acidosis
  - Usual cycles during initial therapy:
    - Body weight < 50 kg: 1.5 liters 2 hours cycles
    - Body weight 50–80 kg: 2 liters 2 hours cycles
    - Body weight > 80 kg: 2 liters 1.5 hours cycles
  - Cycle time is increased to 4-6 hours once the following have resolved:
    - Pulmonary edema
    - Metabolic acidosis
    - Hyperkalemia
  - Fluid overload is avoided to maintain euvolemic states
  - Once euvolemic, dextrose concentration and cycle time is adjusted to maintain neutral fluid balance
- Drug clearance during PD:
  - Enhanced antibiotic clearance may occur during PD
  - Antibiotic levels have to be monitored where possible
  - Dose of antibiotics have to be adjusted to maintain therapeutic levels

Clinical Applications

- Removal of solutes can be maximized by:
  - Maximizing time on peritoneal dialysis
  - Maximizing concentration gradient:
    - Larger dwell volumes
    - Frequent exchanges
  - Maximizing effective peritoneal surface area
  - Maximizing fluid removal
- Removal of fluid by ultrafiltration can be maximized by:
  - Maximizing osmotic gradient:
    - Higher tonicity fluids
    - Shorter dwell times
  - Larger dwell volumes
  - Increasing urine output (diuretics)

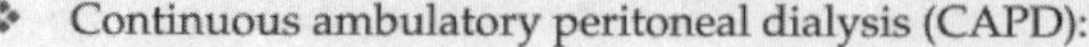

Types of Peritoneal Dialysis

- Continuous ambulatory peritoneal dialysis (CAPD):
  - Machine free and exchanges are done manually by the patient
  - Dialysis fluid is infused in to the peritoneal cavity
  - Dwell time is usually 3–5 hours
  - Up to 5 cycles can be done in a day, each lasting 30–40 minutes
- Automated peritoneal dialysis (APD):
  - Exchanges are done using a cycler machine
  - Usually done at night, when the patient is asleep
- Intermittent peritoneal dialysis (IPD):
  - Usually used in patients who are hemodynamically unstable
  - Used as a means to tide over crisis scenarios in children with AKI
  - Performed in short cycles (10 min infusion, 30 min dwell time, 20 min drain time)

Advantages of Peritoneal Dialysis

- Gentle, sustained fluid removal
- Better preservation of residual renal function
- Lower risk of bacteremia
- Better hemodynamic stability as no need for extra-corporeal circulation
- Useful in hemodynamically unstable patients
- Solute removal is gradual leading to:
  - Less potential for disequilibrium syndrome
  - Less potential for intracranial fluid shifts
- More physiological:
  - Less exposure to synthetic membranes
  - Less incidence of inflammatory responses
- Earlier recovery of renal function
- Minimal infrastructure
- Lower cost
- Cosmesis: Catheters concealed under clothing
- Patient satisfaction

Disadvantages

- Precise prediction of ultrafiltrate volume not possible
- Greater dependence on patient

Complications

- Complications of catheter placement:
  - Early complications:
    - Bowel perforation
    - Bleeding
    - Wound infection
    - Outflow failure
    - Peritonitis
  - Late complications:
    - Exit site infection
    - Cuff protrusion
    - Hernias
- Complications of the dialysis procedure:
  - Protein loss
  - Hyperglycemia
  - Hypertriglyceridemia
  - Weight gain
  - Shoulder pain
  - Raised intra-abdominal pressure

CONTRAST INDUCED NEPHROPATHY

Introduction: *KDIGO Clinical Practice Guidelines 2012*

- Contrast induced nephropathy (CIN) is defined as acute impairment in renal function occurring within 48–72 hours after IV contrast administration
- Impairment in renal function for CIN is defined as:
  - Increase in absolute serum creatinine level by 0.5 mg/dL
  - 25% increase in serum creatinine level from the basiline

Incidence

- CIN is the *third leading cause* of hospital acquired AKI
- Actual incidence of CIN is unclear due to use of different diagnostic criteria
- Incidence of 2% in patients without any risk factors
- Incidence of CIN increases to 9% in diabetics
- Diabetic nephropathy patients have a CIN risk of almost 90%

Physiology

- Contrast media (CM) exert adverse effects through multiple mechanisms on the kidney:
- Direct cytotoxic effect:
  - Direct cytotoxic effect is exerted on the renal proximal tubular cells
  - This effect is primarily through the action of reactive oxygen species
  - This can precipitate acute tubular necrosis (ATN)
- Renal vasoconstriction:
  - Renal vasoconstriction is precipitated by inhibiting nitric oxide synthesis
  - Principal molecule causing this is asymmetrical dimethylarginine (ADMA)
  - Direct action of ADMA on vascular smooth muscle leads to vasoconstriction
  - Vasoconstriction is predominantly seen in the deeper portions of outer medulla
  - This in turn reduces GFR and can cause AKI
- Change in rheological properties of blood:
  - CM can increase blood viscosity and decrease RBC deformability
  - This can result in intravascular sludging and local ischemia

Types of Contrast Agents

- High osmolar monomers (HOCM) (ionic):
  - Diatrizoate (Renografin)
  - Ioxitaalamate (Telebrix)
- Low osmolar monomers (LOCM) (nonionic):
  - Iohexol (Omnipaque)
  - Iopamidol (Isovue)
  - Iomeprol (Iomeron)
  - Ioversol (Optiray)

- Iopromide (Ultravist)
- Iopentol (Imagopaque)

❖ Low osmolar dimers (LOCM) (ionic): Ioxaglate (Hexabrix)

❖ Isoosmolar dimers (IOCM) (nonionic):
- Iodixanol (Visipaque)
- Iotrolan (Isovist)

Characteristics of Contrast Agents

❖ Osmolarity:
- Defines the osmolarity of the CM with respect to the osmolarity of blood
- HOCM are 5–7 times more osmolar than blood (> 1500 mOsm/kg)
- LOCM are 2–3 times more osmolar than blood (600-900 mOsm/kg)
- LOCM are less nephrotoxic compared with HOCM

❖ Molecular structure:
- Refers to the number of benzene rings in the molecule
- Dimeric CM are nonionic and have higher viscosity
- This influences renal tubular blood flow and may precipitate ATN

Risk Factors

❖ Patient related:
- Advanced age > 60 years
- Preexisting chronic kidney disease (most significant)
- Diabetes mellitus
- Hypertension
- Metabolic syndrome
- Anemia
- Hypoalbuminemia
- Multiple myeloma
- Chronic heart failure

❖ Procedure related:
- Concomitant IABP use has higher risk of CIN
- Intervention related CM use has higher incidence compared with diagnostic use

❖ Contrast related:
- Volume of contrast: High volume contrast (>100 mL) associated with higher risk
- Repeat contrast: Administration within 48-72 hours associated with high risk
- Intra-arterial contrast administration associated with higher risk
- Contrast characteristics:
  - Osmolarity: IOCM preferred over LOCM and HOCM: RECOVER trial
  - Ionicity: Non-ionic agents associated with lesser risk
  - Viscosity: Low viscosity agents associated with lesser risk

Mehran Risk Stratification Score

No.	Characteristic	Score
1.	Hypotension	5 points
2.	IABP use	5 points
3.	Congestive heart failure	5 points
4.	Serum creatinine > 1-5 mg/dL	4 points
5.	Age > 75 years	4 points
6.	Anemia	3 points
7.	Diabetes mellitus	3 points
8.	Contrast colume	1 point for every 100 mL used

No.	Risk Category	Total Score	CIN Risk
1.	Low risk	≤ 5	7.5%
2.	Moderate risk	6-10	14%
3.	High risk	11-15	26.1%
4.	Very high risk	≥ 16	57.3%

Differential Diagnosis

❖ Atheroembolic renal failure

❖ Prerenal and postrenal azotemia (AKI)

❖ Acute interstitial nephritis

❖ Acute tubular necrosis

Findings

❖ Oliguria is rare in CIN

❖ Serum creatinine levels:
- Begin to increase within 24 hours of contrast administration
- Peak levels between days 3 and 5
- Return to baseline within 14 days

❖ Serum cystatin C (surrogate marker) elevated in CIN

❖ Urine analysis:
- Osmolality < 350 mOsm/kg
- Fractional excretion of sodium (FENa) varies widely
- Other findings:
  - Renal tubular epithelial cells
  - Pigmented granular casts
  - Urate crystals

❖ Renal biopsy: ***Osmotic nephrosis*** of renal tubular epithelial cells:
- Cell vacuolization
- Interstitial inflammation
- Cellular necrosis

Prevention and Treatment

❖ Hydration

❖ Prevention of CIN centers around avoiding volume depletion

- Forced diuresis found to be inferior to hydration with saline
- Volume expansion with normal saline preferred to 0.45% saline
- Oral fluids not as effective as intravenous fluids
- 1–1.5 mL/kg/h NS started 6 hrs prior and continued for 6–24 hrs post pre-procedure
- Post procedure volume expansion more important than pre-procedure hydration
- *Renal guard system*:
  - System designed to optimize fluid therapy in order to minimize incidence of CIN
  - Comprises a console and RenalGuard single use set for infusion and urine collection
  - The urine collection set is connected to the patients Foleys catheter
  - The infusion set connects to the standard IV catheter
  - The console measures the volume of urine collected in the collection set
  - Equal volume of fluid is infused to match the patients urine output
  - Thus, euvolemia and adequate hydration status is maintained
  - ***REMEDIAL II trial***:
    - The system was evaluated by the REMEDIAL II trial
    - Concluded that the RenalGuard system along with N- acetylcysteine is effective renoprotective strategy for patients at high risk for CIN
- Diuretics:
  - Not recommended for use in the absence of hydration
  - However, diuretic therapy along with matched hydration reduces incidence in high risk cases
- Forced diuresis:
  - Forced diuresis with mannitol and furosemide have been attempted
  - These strategies have been found to worsen CIN by causing dehydration
  - Forced diuresis is no longer recommended
- Statin therapy:
  - Favourable in CIN due to anti-inflammatory and pleiotropic properties
  - Reduced incidence of CIN in those patients pretreated with high dose statins
  - Multiple studies have reported benefits of using statin therapy to prevent CIN
- Intravenous bicarbonate:
  - Alkalinizes renal tubular fluid and prevents free radical injury
  - 3 mL/kg/hr started 1 hr prior and continued at 1 mL/kg/hr for 6 hrs post procedure
  - Found to be un beneficial, compared with placebo therapy in the PRESERVE trial
- N-acetyl cysteine:
  - Useful due to antioxidant and free radical scavenger properties
  - 600 mg PO Q12H for 24 hours before and on the day of the procedure
  - Found to be un beneficial, compared with placebo therapy in the PRESERVE trial
- Optimize imaging procedure:
  - Use of alternate imaging modalities
  - Minimizing use of contrast to less than 100 mL
  - Maximal Allowable Contrast Dose

$$= \frac{5\ \text{mL/kg body weight}}{\text{Baseline creatinine}}$$

  - Use of iso-osmolar non-ionic contrast agents
  - Avoid repeat contrast exposure for 72 hours after initial procedure
- Withhold other nephrotoxic agents:
  - Withdrawal recommended 24 hours prior to contrast administration:
  - Agents maybe started 48–72 hours post exposure
  - Agents withheld include:
    - ACE inhibitors
    - NSAIDs
    - Metformin
- Preemptive hemodialysis:
  - Not shown to be of any benefit
  - Not recommended for prophylactic use
- Renal replacement therapy:
  - CM clearance is reduced in those with CIN
  - This can cause damage in a two pronged fashion:
    - Increased contrast load
    - Prolonged tubular exposure
  - This can potentiate toxicity to remaining functional tissue and non-renal tissues
  - Thus, dialysis may be required on emergent basis in those with severe CIN
  - Also immediate post-procedure dialysis recommended in:
    - Patients already on long term hemodialysis
    - Those at very high risk for CIN
  - CM can be effectively removed by hemodialysis
  - 70–80% of CM can be removed by a 4-hour hemodialysis

- Other therapies:
  - Ascorbic acid:
    - Useful due to its antioxidant properties
    - 3 gm given pre-procedure and 2 grams Q12H for 24 hours post procedure
  - Theophylline and aminophylline:
    - Vasodilators which counteract intra-renal vasoconstriction
    - Useful in preventing CIN in very high risk cases
  - Other vasodilators:
    - Calcium channel blockers
    - Atrial natriuretic peptide
    - L-arginine
  - Prostaglandin E_1

Prognosis

- Following contrast administration, creatinine levels usually peak between 2–5 days
- Values usually return to normal within 14 days
- Less than one third of CIN patients develop residual renal impairment
- Of these, less than 1% patients with CIN require dialysis
- CIN is however, associated with a higher risk of in-hospital and 1-year mortality
- Mortality in CIN patients requiring dialysis may reach up to 36%
- Most patients with CIN die from a non-renal or procedural complication

Validation *Preserve Trial*

- Randomized controlled prospective trial enrolling 5177 patients undergoing angiography
- Divided into 2 groups:
  - Oral placebo group
  - Those receiving IV sodium bicarbonate and 5 days of oral acetylcysteine
- Primary end points:
  - Need for dialysis
  - Persistent increase in serum creatinine of at least 50% from baseline
  - Death
- The study concluded that there was no benefit of IV sodium bicarbonate or oral acetylcysteine in preventing any of the primary end points

PERIOPERATIVE ACUTE KIDNEY INJURY

Introduction

- AKI is defined as any one of the following:
  - Urine output less than 0.5 mL/kg/hr for more than *6 hours*
  - Increase in serum creatinine by more than 0.3 mg/dL within *48 hours*
  - Increase in serum creatinine to more than 1.5 times baseline within last *7 days*
- Surgery-associated AKI (SA-AKI) increases perioperative morbidity significantly

Incidence of SA-AKI

- Overall incidence of SA-AKI is 57%
- Incidence of Aki within the first week of ICU admission was:
  - 52% in patients undergoing elective surgery
  - 56% in those undergoing emergency surgery
  - 62% in medical ICU patients

Etiology of Perioperative AKI

- Pre-renal causes of SA-AKI:
  - Hypovolemia:
    - Bleeding
    - Dehydration
    - Extravasation
  - Vasodilatory hypotension:
    - Sepsis
    - Low cardiac output states
  - Acute and chronic heart failure
  - Locally impaired renal circulation:
    - Medications
    - Renovascular disease
  - Chronic liver disease
  - Abdominal compartment syndrome
- Intrinsic renal causes of SA-AKI:
  - Acute tubular injury due to:
    - Prolonged ischemia
    - Malignant hypertension
    - Systemic inflammation:
      - Major surgery
      - Cardiopulmonary bypass
      - Sepsis
  - Nephrotoxins:
    - Aminoglycosides, amphotericin
    - ACE inhibitors
    - NSAIDs
    - Chemotherapeutic agents
    - Contrast agents (CI-AKI)
  - Rhabdomyolysis:
    - Post crush injury
    - Drug overdose
    - Status epilepticus
    - Malignant hyperthermia

- Hemolysis including cardiopulmonary bypass
- Hypercalcemia

❖ Post-renal causes of SA-AKI:
- Nephrolithiasis
- Prostatic hypertrophy
- Retroperitoneal fibrosis
- Pelvic masses
- Bladder tumors

Perioperative AKI Syndromes

❖ Hemodynamic mediated AKI:
- AKI can result from various hemodynamic perturbations during surgery
- Decreased perfusion pressure:
  - Reduced perfusion pressure hampers perfusion by reducing blood flow
  - Reduced perfusion pressure occurs due to various causes:
    - Due to anesthetic associated reduction in arterial tone
    - Also, reduction in preload can occur during surgery due to:
      - Hypovolemia
      - Anesthetic associated venodilation
      - Positive pressure ventilation reducing venous return
- High venous pressure causing organ congestion:
  - High venous pressure causes blood accumulation in the organs
  - This causes congestion within the kidney, an organ which cannot expand
  - This predisposes the patient to SA-AKI
  - Causes of high venous pressure are:
    - Hypervolemia or fluid overload
    - High pleural pressure
    - Abdominal compartment syndrome

❖ DAMP- induced AKI:
- Stands for Danger Associated Molecular Protein-induced AKI
- Various molecules are released during ischemia reperfusion
- Tissue injury associated with surgery itself releases various DAMPs
- These molecules include:
  - Myoglobin
  - Uric acid
  - High mobility group protein B1 (HMGB1)

❖ Inflammatory AKI:
- Surgery is associated with the release of a number of inflammatory mediators
- These inflammatory mediators may damage the nephrons and cause AKI
- Inflammatory mediators include:
  - Tumor necrosis factor
  - Cytokines and chemokines

❖ Nephrotoxic AKI:
- Nephrotoxic drugs administered perioperatively predisposes the kidney to AKI
- Hydroxyethyl starch in higher doses has been linked with AKI
- Saline increases incidence of major adverse kidney events
- Bacterial death with bactericidal antibiotics predisposes to endotoxemia and AKI

❖ Obstructive AKI:
- Urinary retention post surgery can arise during:
  - Colorectal surgeries
  - Urological/ gynecological surgery
- Retention can also occur due to:
  - Drug-associated urinary retention
  - Injury to urethra during catheterization
  - Malfunctioning or misplacement of Foleys catheter
  - Clogging of the catheter with urinary casts

Rifle Classification

❖ Older system used to define and classify AKI

❖ RIFLE is an acronym for risk, injury, failure, loss of function and ESRD

❖ The patient can be classified according to either GFR or urine output criteria

❖ The criterion which supports the more severe classification should be used

❖ The RIFLE criteria uses changes in renal function within *7 days* to classify patients

❖ Superimposition of acute on chronic failure is indicated by RIFLE-F

❖ The risk stage has more sensitivity and includes patients who actually do not have failure

❖ Progression through the more severe stages is marked by:
- Decreasing sensitivity
- Increasing specificity

1. RISK stage:
   - Serum creatinine increased by 1.5–2 times the baseline
   - GFR decreased by more than 25%
   - Urine output less than 0.5 mL/kg/hr for less than 6 hours
2. INJURY stage:
   - Serum creatinine increased 2–3 times the baseline

- GFR decreased by more than 50%
- Urine output less than 0.5 mL/kg/hr for more than 12 hours

3. FAILURE stage:
   - Serum creatinine increased more than 3 times the baseline value
   - Serum creatinine > 4 mg/dL
   - Acute rise in serum creatinine > 0.5 mg/dL
   - GFR decreased by more than 75%
   - Urine output less than 0.3 mL/kg/hr for more than 24 hours
   - Anuria for 12 hours
4. LOSS OF FUNCTION:
   - Persistent acute renal failure
   - Complete loss of kidney function more than 4 weeks requiring dialysis
5. END STAGE RENAL DISEASE:
   - Dialysis dependant patient
   - Complete loss of renal function more than 3 months requiring dialysis

Staging of Acute Kidney Injury: KDIGO Consensus Classification

- Stage I:
  - Serum creatinine 1.5–1.9 times the baseline
  - Increase in serum creatinine by more than 0.3 mg/dL
  - Urine output less than 0.5 mL/kg/hour for more than 6 hours
- Stage II:
  - Serum creatinine 2–2.9 times the baseline
  - Urine output less than 0.5 mL/kg/hour for more than 12 hours
- Stage III:
  - Serum creatinine more than 3 times the baseline
  - Increase in serum creatinine to more than 4 mg/dL
  - Urine output less than 0.3 mL/kg/hour for more than 24 hours
  - Persistent anuria for more than 12 hours
  - Initiation of renal replacement therapy

Risk Factors for Perioperative AKI

- Patient related factors:
  - Older age
  - Male sex
  - Diabetes mellitus
  - Limited cardio-respiratory reserve
  - Chronic cardiac failure
  - Chronic kidney disease
  - Chronic liver disease
  - Sepsis
- Surgery related factors:
  - Emergency surgery
  - Cardiac surgery
  - Liver transplant surgery
  - Vascular surgery
  - Intraperitoneal surgery
  - Prolonged duration of surgery
  - Major hemorrhage
  - Blood transfusion
  - Intraoperative hypovolemia and hypotension
- Pharmacological factors:
  - NSAIDs
  - ACE inhibitors
  - AT II receptor blockers
  - Aminoglycosides, glycopeptide antibiotics
  - Immunosuppressive drugs
  - Hydroxyethylstarch solutions
  - Contrast agents

Risk Stratification for Perioperative AKI

SL. Nos.	Risk Factors	Score
1.	Age > 56 years	1
2.	Male sex	1
3.	Active congestive cardiac failure	1
4.	Hypertension	1
5.	Ascites	1
6.	Emergency surgery	1
7.	Intraperitoneal surgery	1
8.	Preoperative serum creatinine > 1.2 mg/dL	1
9.	Diabetes mellitus on oral or insulin therapy	1

Risk Index Class	Risk Factors
Class I	0-2 risk factors
Class II	3 risk factors
Class III	4 risk factors
Class IV	5 risk factors
Class V	≥ 6 risk factors

Prevention of Perioperative AKI

- General measures:
  - Consider ICU admission
  - Consider renal replacement therapy
  - Avoid subclavian catheters if possible
  - Avoid hyperglycemia
  - Consider functional hemodynamic monitoring
- Ensure adequate perfusion pressure:
  - Adequate perfusion pressure is essential to maintain renal blood flow
  - Reduced renal blood flow leads to renal hypoxia, inflammation and fibrosis

- Prolonged episodes of hypotension reduces renal perfusion, causing AKI
- In patients undergoing non-cardiac surgery, higher incidence of AKI seen with:
  - Mean arterial pressure < 60 mm Hg for > 20 minutes
  - Mean arterial pressure < 55 mm Hg for > 10 minutes
- Individualized blood pressure control reduces occurrence of AKI

❖ Ensure adequate volume status:
- Judicious fluid loading is required to avoid hyper or hypovolemia
- Hypovolemia reduces the perfusion pressure to the kidneys and thus the GFR
- Hypervolemia increases venous pressure and causes renal congestion
- Therefore, optimal fluid state is paramount to maintain renal perfusion
- Fluid restrictive strategy more detrimental compared with fluid liberal strategy
- Goal directed fluid therapy protocols offers best method of minimizing AKI
- Goal directed therapy(GDT) end points can include titration towards optimal:
  - Cardiac output
  - Arterial lactate
- Avoid excess blood loss and unnecessary blood transfusions

❖ Role of balanced crystalloids:
- Large amounts of normal saline leads to hyperchloremic acidosis
- This produces renal vasoconstriction and increases risk of AKI
- Thus, saline based fluid strategy results in higher incidence of SA-AKI
- Use of saline in critically ill patients resulted in higher rate of all-cause mortality
- Thus, use of balanced crystalloids in the perioperative period is recommended

❖ Monitor serum creatinine and urine output:
- Intensive monitoring of urine output in hospitalized patients:
  - This is defined as no gaps in UO data for more than 3 hours
  - Intensive monitoring leads to:
    - Improved AKI detection
    - Decreased incidence of fluid overload
    - Improved survival in those who develop AKI
- Perioperative oliguria:
  - Oliguria is an ominous sign in the perioperative period
  - Causes of perioperative oliguria:
    - Intravascular volume depletion
    - Systemic hypoperfusion
    - Perioperative ADH release which can occur due to:
      - Pain
      - Nausea and vomiting
      - Neurosurgery

❖ ***Furosemide stress test (FST)***:
- Furosemide requires several parts of the nephron to be intact for its action
- Therefore it is an ideal drug to interrogate renal function
- FST is done in patients with stage I and II AKI
- FST involves the administration of 1–1.5 mg/kg furosemide IV
- Urine output is documented over the next 2 hours
- UO less than 100 mL/hr over the 2 hours following furosemide dose is positive
- These patients have a higher risk of progression to stage III AKI
- This test has a specificity of 84.1% and sensitivity of 87.1%

❖ Nephrotoxic AKI prevention:
- Consider alternatives to radiocontrast procedures to prevent CI-AKI
- Discontinue all nephrotoxic agents when possible
- Consider non-invasive and invasive diagnostic workup
- Check frequently for changes in drug dosing

❖ Remote ischemic preconditioning (RIPC):
- RIPC is triggered by brief periods of transient ischemia and reperfusion
- Protective effects are not limited to the tissue receiving the preconditioning stimulus
- Protective effects can be traceable even in remote organs
- RIPC may be effective in triggering endogenous protection against renal damage
- BP cuff around the arm is inflated 50 mm Hg above the SBP to induce ischemia
- After 5 minutes, the cuff is deflated and reperfusion of the tissue is allowed
- These cycles are repeated several times to provide RIPC

- Other therapies:
  - Renal vasodilators:
    - Agents used include dopamine and dopexamine
    - No evidence to show that they prevent onset or halt AKI progression
    - Such agents are not recommended outside clinical trial settings
  - Diuretics:
    - Diuretics limited to controlling fluid balance and prevent fluid overload
    - No evidence to show that preemptive diuresis reduces onset of AKI
    - Inappropriate diuretic use predisposes to prerenal AKI
    - Other therapies attempted with insufficient evidence include: Atrial natriuretic peptide
    - Theophylline

Perioperative AKI Prevention Bundle: KDIGO 2012 Guidelines 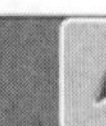

- Maintenance of volume status
- Maintenance of perfusion pressure
- Monitoring serum creatinine and urine output
- Discontinuation and avoidance of nephrotoxic agents
- Use of alternatives to radiocontrast agents
- Maintenance of normoglycemia
- Functional hemodynamic monitoring

Management

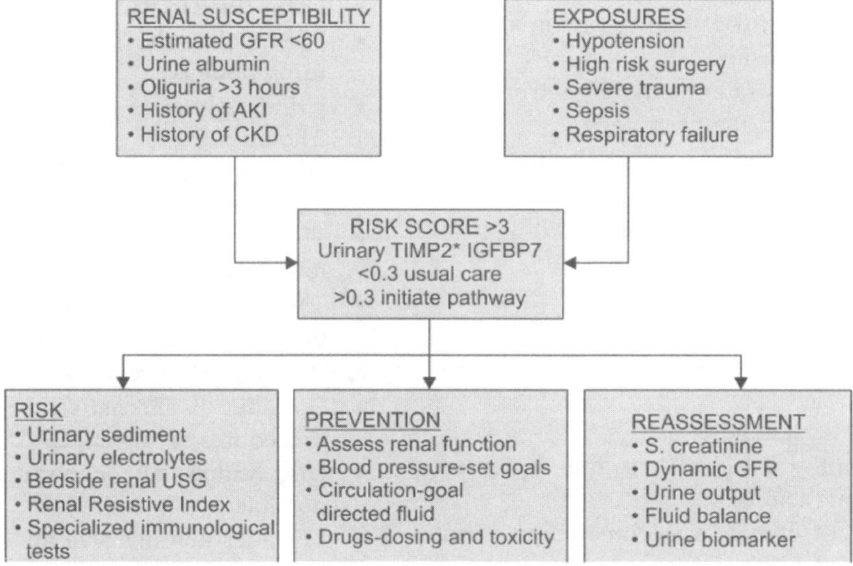

Prognosis

- SA-AKI is associated with worse patient outcomes, hospital morbidity and mortality
- Most cases of community acquired AKI (CA-AKI) are secondary to volume depletion
- Thus, up to 90% cases of CA-AKI have a potentially reversible cause
- Mortality rate of CA-AKI may be as low as 7%
- Hospital acquired AKI (HA-AKI) occurs more often as a part of multi-organ failure
- Therefore, hospital acquired AKI generally has a poorer prognosis
- Mortality rate of HA-AKI may be as high as 70%

SURGERY FOR VASCULAR ACCESS IN RENAL DIALYSIS

Introduction

Vascular access surgeries in ESRD patients are amongst the commonest surgeries done by vascular surgeons.

Types of Vascular Access

- Indwelling dialysis catheters:
  - Consists of indwelling dialysis catheters sited in a central vein
  - Advantages:
    - Can be used for dialysis immediately after insertion
    - Do not require maturation time as for AV fistulas and grafts

- Disadvantages:
  - Risk of infection
  - Risk of central venous thrombosis
- Thus, they are only used for short term indications such as during:
  - Wait period for arterio-venous access surgery
  - Wait period for graft maturation

❖ Arterio-venous fistulas:
- Consists of a direct surgical anastomosis between an artery and a vein
- These are the commonest forms of access for hemodialysis
- These are usually created in the non-dominant arm
- Three sites in the upper limb where it is commonly done are between:
  - Radio-cephalic fistula at the wrist:
    - Also called ***Brescia-Cimino fistula***
    - Often offered as the initial site of choice
    - Preserves the proximal locations for later use
    - Provides the lowest flow rate amongst all other sites
  - Brachio-cephalic fistula in the upper arm:
    - More proximally located fistula
    - Thus, higher flow rates are achievable
    - However, it increases the incidence of steal effect
  - Brachio- basilic fistula in the upper arm:
    - More difficult to create due to relative inaccessibility
    - Has a reduced frequency of prior venous access
    - Thus, the vein is often better preserved at the formation of fistula
    - This is therefore used after multiple failed distal fistulas
- Site of fistula creation is determined by the condition of the vessels
- The fistula is usually created as distally as possible
- This is in order to reduce the risk of limb ischemia postoperatively

❖ Arterio-venous grafts:
- Consists of an interposing length of graft placed between the artery and vein
- Usually used grafts are made of polytetrafluoroethylene or PTFE
- Dialysis needles are subsequently inserted directly into the graft
- Advantages:
  - Ease of cannulation
  - Shorter maturation times
  - Large surface area
- However, long term patency is inferior compared with AV grafts
- Sites of insertion of AV grafts are:
  - In the forearm between radial artery and vein in antecubital fossa
  - Between brachial artery and axillary vein in the upper arm
  - *Looped thigh graft* between femoral artery and vein
  - *Necklace graft* between axillary artery and contralateral axillary vein

Maturation Time

❖ This refers to the time taken for vessel wall thickening and enlargement to occur

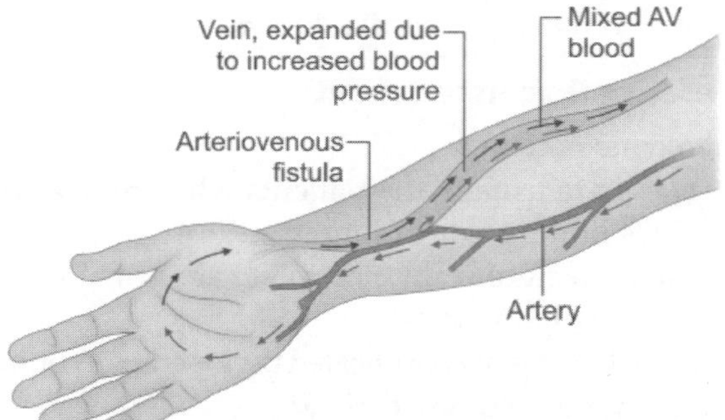

Fig. 9: Arteriovenous fistula.

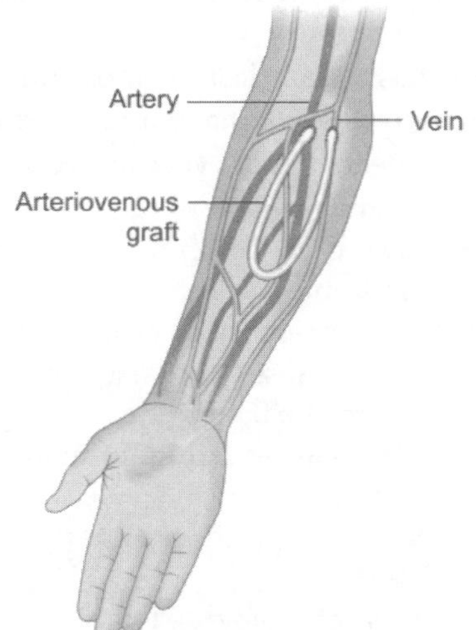

Fig. 10: Arteriovenous graft.

- Maturation time is required in order to allow repetitive cannulation for dialysis
- Changes occurring during maturation:
  - Typically, the artery increases in diameter by 50%
  - Retrograde blood flow in artery distal to the anastomosis
  - Increase in venous diameter by about 150%
  - Increase in blood flow through the vein up to 500 mL/min
- Fistula maturation time:
  - Between 4–6 weeks for upper arm fistulas
  - 8 weeks for radio-cephalic fistulas
- Graft maturation time:
  - Usually taken as 2–3 weeks
  - Synthetic polyurethane grafts may be used as early as 24 hours after creation

Characteristics of an Ideal Vascular Access

- Good blood inflow through the feeding artery
- Should provide blood flow rate of at least 300 mL/min without recirculation
- Should be able to be used up to 3 times a week
- Must be superficial (< 0.6 cm skin deep)
- Must have a thick wall
- Must have a long straight segment to allow 2 needle punctures 2.5 cm away
- Diameter should be >0.6 cm
- Good venous outflow without causing distal limb ischemia

Complications of AV Fistulas and Grafts

- Graft failure:
  - High failure rates are seen with both AV fistulas and grafts
  - AV fistulas usually last for approximately 5 years
  - AV grafts on the other hand usually last for 2–3 years
  - Failure rate in the first year can be as high as 30%
  - Causes of graft failure:
    - Primary graft failure due to failure of graft maturation:
      - Due to presence of venous tributaries:
        - This causes diversion of blood away from the fistula site
        - This causes failure of maturation of the graft
      - Due to the presence of peripheral vascular disease
    - Late graft failure due to:
      - Graft stenosis
      - Graft thrombosis
- Aneurysm formation:
  - Aneurysm formation can lead to skin necrosis in severe cases
  - The aneurysmal segment has to be shortened, bypassed or excised
- Infection:
  - Infections are more common (up to 10 times higher) in AV grafts than fistulas
  - Infections occur due to the repeated punctures during dialysis
- Thrombosis: Up to 6 times higher in AV grafts compared with fistulas
- Claudication:
  - Seen in both AV fistulas and grafts
  - This is due to the steal phenomenon causing ischemic symptoms in the distal limb
  - Symptoms are more commonly associated with upper arm fistulas

Anesthetic Considerations

- Due to ongoing dialysis:
  - Timing the patients routine hemodialysis is important
  - IHD is usually scheduled on the day prior to surgery, within 24 hours
  - Surgery done on the day of IHD predisposes to dialysis disequilibrium syndrome
  - IHD is not done earlier to avoid hypervolemia due to delay in surgery
- Due to complications associated with ESRD:
  - Risk of IHD is almost twice that of the general population
  - Uncontrolled HTN
  - Associated diabetes
  - Autonomic neuropathy
  - Anemia of chronic disease
- Due to the planned surgical procedure:
  - Minimize vascular access attempts
  - Avoid side of planned fistula/indwelling fistula for monitoring/vascular access

Preoperative Risk Assessment

- Euvolemic patients:
  - These are usually the patients who are dialyzed 12–24 hours prior to surgery
  - Have no significant electrolyte abnormalities or bleeding tendencies
  - Usually have uncomplicated perioperative courses
- Patients with volume overload:
  - These are usually the patients who present with surgical emergencies

- Thus, routine IHD cannot be optimally timed
- Require further cardiovascular evaluation
- Fluid overload attributed to CKD in the absence of cardiovascular disease
- Have a high rate of perioperative complications

❖ Patients already on dialysis:
- Determine the following prior to surgery:
  - Adequacy of dialysis
  - Preoperative dialysis needs
  - Postoperative dialysis timing
  - Dosage requirements for all medicines
- Effects of preoperative dialysis:
  - Fluid depletion:
    - Redistribution of extravascular fluid occurs during dialysis
    - This results in depletion of intravascular fluid volume
  - Electrolyte disturbances, especially hypokalemia
  - Residual anticoagulation from heparinization of the circuit
- Preoperative dialysis scheduled 12–24 hours prior to surgery to reduce risk of:
  - Volume overload
  - Hyperkalemia
  - Bleeding due to anticoagulation during dialysis

Preoperative optimization

❖ NPO orders

❖ Informed consent

❖ Preoperative sedation:
- Given only if patient is stable
- Avoid sedation if unstable hemodynamics
- Reduced dose of benzodiazepines used for sedation
- Midazolam is relatively safe

❖ Promethazine 2.5–25 mg IM used for sedation and antiemesis

❖ Anti-aspiration prophylaxis as gastroparesis associated with CKD:
- 30 mL of non-particulate sodium citrate
- 50 mg ranitidine IV
- 10 mg metoclopramide or 8 mg ondansetron IV

❖ Continue all drugs on the day of surgery, especially antihypertensives

❖ Stop morning dose of oral hypoglycemics and insulin on day of surgery

❖ Preoperative blood transfusion:
- Avoid unnecessary blood transfusions
- Transfuse if Hb < 6–7 g/dL
- Target Hb > 10 g/dL
- But it is usually difficult to maintain Hb levels above 10 g/dL

❖ Preoperative dialysis:
- Done within 24 hours of surgery, to optimize fluid and electrolyte status
- Hemodialysis is more effective than peritoneal dialysis
- Optimize BP and serum potassium levels post-dialysis
- Optimize ACT as heparin is used during dialysis
- Serum potassium < 5.5 mEq/L preferred on the day of surgery

Monitors

❖ Care should be taken to preserve current fistulas

❖ Blood pressure cuffs are tied on the opposite arm or leg

❖ All current fistulas should be padded in the absence of surgical intervention on them

❖ Arterial cannulation should be avoided to preserve the vessels for future surgeries

Vascular Access (UK Renal Association Guidelines 2015)

❖ Avoid accessing the fistula or the limb with the fistula

❖ Wide bore cannulas are usually not required

❖ This is because the source of bleeding can be easily controlled in fistula surgery

❖ Cannulation attempts should be minimized

❖ This is in order to preserve the veins for potential future fistula creation

❖ Use of indwelling dialysis lines are avoided except in emergencies

❖ This is because they contain high dose heparin which may be accidentally injected

Anesthetic Technique

❖ Local anesthesia:
- Least physiologically intrusive method
- Least well tolerated

❖ General anesthesia:
- Induction should be smooth with minimal influence on cardiovascular function
- IV etomidate may be a safe agent in hemodynamically unstable patients
- IV propofol may be used in hypertensive patients
- Remifentanil may be used for intraoperative analgesia

- Initiation of positive pressure ventilation reduces cardiac preload and cardiac output
- This may in turn lead to precipitous hypotension
- Thus, neuromuscular paralysis should be avoided in these patients
- Fluid loading in these patients also cannot be used due to the pre-existing ESRD
- Thus, careful titration of anesthetic agents is necessary to prevent hypotension
- Airway can be secured with a laryngeal mask airway (LMA)
- Maintenance of anesthesia should be with:
  - Short acting drugs
  - Minimal renal metabolism
- Remifentanil and propofol infusion can be used to maintain the anesthetic plane

❖ Regional anesthesia:
- Techniques used:
  - Supraclavicular nerve block
  - Infraclavicular block
- Advantages:
  - Prolonged duration of action- useful for postoperative analgesia
  - Blocks the musculocutaneous nerve, thus allowing tourniquet use
  - Sympathectomy like effect leading to:
    - Venous dilatation and shorter maturation times
    - Lower failure rates
    - Higher patency rates
    - Avoids side effects of GA such as airway manipulation
    - Better hemodynamic stability
    - Postoperative analgesia
    - Faster recovery
- Disadvantages:
  - Local anesthetic systemic toxicity
  - Peripheral nerve injury
  - Block failure
  - Hematoma
  - Infections

SUGGESTED READING

1. Bagshaw, S.M., et al. (2016). Precision continuous renal replacement therapy and solute control. *Blood Purification*, 42(3), 238–47.
2. Barrett, B.J., Carlisle,E.J. (1993). Meta-analysis of the relative nephrotoxicity of high and low osmolality iodinated contrast media. *Radiology*, 188(1), 171–8.
3. Bellomo, R., Chapman, M., Finfer, S., Hickling, K., Myburgh, J. (2000). Low dose dopamine in patients with early renal dysfunction: a placebo controlled randomized trial. *Lancet*, 356(9248), 2139-43.
4. Bellomo, R., et al. (2004). Acute renal failure- definition, outcome measures, animal models, fluid therapy and information technology needs: the second international consensus conference of the Acute Dialysis Quality Initiative (ADQI) group. *Critical Care*, 8(4), 204–12.
5. Bihorac, A., (2015). Critical connections guiding AKI prevention using biomarkers. *Critical Connections*, 14(2), 1–11.
6. Bradley, T., Teare, T., Milner, Q. (2017). Anesthetic management of patients requiring vascular access surgery for renal dialysis. *British Journal of Anesthesia*, 17(8), 269–74.
7. Briasoulis, A., Mallikethi-Reddy, S., Sharma, S., Briasouli, A.A., Afonso, L. (2015). 3-hydroxy-3-methylglutaryl CoA reductase enzyme inhibitors for the prevention of contrast induced nephropathy: a metaanalysis of prospective RCTs. *American Journal of Therapeutics*, 22(6), 158–66.
8. Briguori, C., Visconti, G., Ricciardelli, B., Condorelli, G. (2011). Renal insufficiency after contrast media administration trial II (REMEDIAL II): RenalGuard system in high risk patients for CI-AKI. *Circulation*, 6(9), 1260–9.
9. Brown, J.R., et al. (2010). Does safe dosing of iodinated contrast prevent contrast induced AKI. *Circulation: Cardiovascular Interventions*, 3(4), 346–50.
10. Butterworth, J., Mackey, D., and Wasnick, J. (2013). *Morgan and Mikhails Clinical Anesthesiology*. 6th ed. New York: McGraw Hill Education.
11. Chawla, L.S., et al. (2013). Development and standardization of a furosemide stress test to predict the severity of acute kidney injury. *Critical Care*, 17(5), R207.
12. Cullis, B., et al. (2014). ISPD Guidelines for peritoneal dialysis for AKI. *Journal of The International Society for Peritoneal Dialysis*, 34(5), 494–517.
13. Deinum, J., Derkx, F.H. (2000). Cystatin for estimation of glomerular filtration rate? *Lancet*, 356(9242), 1624–5.
14. Eknoyan G., et al. (2013). Clinical Practice Guideline for the evaluation and management of chronic kidney disease. *Kidney International Supplements*, 3(1), 1–138.
15. From AM, Bartholmai, B.J., Williams, A.W., Cha, S.S., McDonald, F.S.(2008). Mortality associated with nephropathy after radiographic contrast exposure. *Mayo Clinic Proceedings*, 83(10), 1095–100.
16. Gabriel D.P., Caramori, J.T., Martim, L.C., Barretti, P., BalbiA.L. (2008). High volume peritoneal dialysis vs daily hemodialysis: a randomized controlled trial in critically ill patients with acute kidney injur: a pilot study. *Kidney International*, 587–93.
17. Goergen S.K., Rumbold, G., Compton, G., Harris, C. (2010). Systematic review of current guidelines,and their evidence base, on the risk of lactic acidosis after administration of contrast medium for patients receiving metformin. *Radiology*, 254(1), 261–9.
18. Gomez H., et al. (2014). A unified theory of sepsis induced acute kidney injury: inflammation, microcirculatory dysfunction, bioenergetics, and the tubular cell adaptation to injury. *Shock*, 41(1), 3–11.
19. Gross, J.L., Prowle J.R. (2015). Perioperative acute kidney injury. *British Journal of Anesthesia*, 15(4), 213–8.
20. Hattori, N., Oda, S. (2016). Cytokine adsorbing hemofilter: old but new modality for septic acute kidney injury. *Renal Replacement Therapy*, 41, 2.

21. Hoste E.A., et al. (2015). Epidemiology of acute kidney injury in critically ill patients: the multinational AKI-EPI study. *Intensive Care Medicine*, 41(8), 1411–23.
22. Ichai, C., Quintard,H.,and Orban, J. (2012). Metabolic disorders and critically ill patients. Nice: Springer.
23. Jin, K., et al. (2017). Intensive monitoring of urine output is associated with increased detection of acute kidney injury and improved outcomes. *Chest*, 152(5), 972–9.
24. Joannes-Boyau O., et al. (2013). High volume vs standard volume hemofiltration for septic shock patients with AKI (IVOIRE study). *Intensive Care Medicine*, 39(9), 1535–46.
25. Kellum J.A.,et al. (2012). Kidney disease improving global outcomes (KDIGO)—clinical practise guidelines for acute kidney injury. *Kidney International*, 2(1), 1–115.
26. Kline J.A., Gordon B.E., Williams, C., Blumenthal, S., Watts, J,A., Diaz-Buxo, J. (1999). Large pore hemodialysis in acute endotoxic shock. *Critical Care Medicine*, 27(3), 588–96.
27. Kumwenda, M., et al. (2015). Clinical practice guidelines: Vascular access for hemodialysis. *Journal of Kidney Care*, 281–94.
28. Lameire, N.H., (2006). Contrast induced nephropathy: prevention and risk reduction. *Nephrology Dialysis Transplant*, 21(1), 11–23.
29. Levey A.S., Bosch, J.P., Lewis, J.B., Greene, T., Rogers, N., Roth, D. (1999). A more accurate method to estimate GFR from serum creatinine: a new prediction equation: MDRD group. *Annals of Internal Medicine*, 130(6), 461–70.
30. Levey A.S., et al. (2003). National Kidney Foundation practice guidelines for chronic kidney disease: evaluation, classification and stratification. *Annals of Internal Medicine*, 139(2), 137–47.
31. Levey A.S., et al. (2009). A new equation to estimate glomerular filtration rate. *Annals of Internal Medicine*, 150(9):604–12.
32. Liu X., et al. (2016). Non-GFR determinants of low molecular weight serum protein filtration markers in CKD. *American Journal of Kidney Diseases*, 68(6), 892–900.
33. Macedo, E, Mehta, R. (2016). Continuous dialysis therapies: Core curriculum. *American Journal of Kidney Disease*, 68(4), 645–57.
34. Marini, J.J., Dries, D.J. (2019). *Critical Care Medicine: The Essentials and More*. 5th ed. Philadelphia: Lippincott Williams and Wilkins.
35. Marschall, K.,Hines, R.E.(2018). *Stoeltings Anesthesia and Coexisting Disease*. 7th ed. Philadelphia: Elsevier.
36. Mehran R., et al. (2004). A simple risk score for prediction of CIN after percutaneous coronary intervention: development and initial validation. *Journal of American College of Cardiology*, 44(7), 1393–9.
37. Mehta R.L., et al. (2004). Spectrum of acute renal failure in the intensive care unit: the PICARD experience. *Kidney International*, 66(4), 1613–21.
38. Menting T.P., Wever K,E., Brunschot, D., Van der Vliet, D., Rovers, M.M., Warle, M.C. (2017). Ischemic preconditioning for the reduction of renal ischemia reperfusion injury. *Cochrane Database of Systematic Reviews*.
39. Miller, R.D., Eriksson, L., Fleisher, L, Wiener-Kronish, J., Cohen, N., Young, W. (2015). *Millers Anesthesia*. 8th ed. Philadelphia: Elsevier Saunders.
40. Mohammed, N.M., Mahfouz, A., Achkar, K., Rafie, I.M., Hajar, R. (1998). Radiocontrast induced nephropathy. *Seminars in Nephrology*, 14(3), 551–7.
41. Moores C., Nimmo, A.F. (2012). Core Topics in Vascular Anesthesia. *Cambridge: Cambridge University Press*.
42. Myles, P.S., et al. (2018). Restrictive Versus Liberal Fluid Therapy for Major Abdominal Surgery Trial. *New England Journal of Medicine*, 378(24), 2263-74.
43. Nissenson, A., Fine, R. (2017). *Handbook of Dialysis*. 5th ed. Philadelphia: Elsevier.
44. Nolin T.D., Frye, R.F., Matzke, G.R. (2003). Hepatic drug metabolism and transport in patients with kidney disease. *American Journal of Kidney Disease*, 42(5), 906–25.
45. Peng Z.Y., et al. (2012). Bactericidal antibiotics temporarily increase inflammation and worsen acute kidney injury in experimental sepsis. *Critical Care Medicine*, 40(2), 538–43.
46. Peppelenbosch, A., van Kuijk, W., Bouvy, N.D., van der Sande, F.M.,Tordoir, J.H. (2008). Peritoneal dialysis catheter placement technique and complications. *Nephrology Dialysis Transplantation Plus*, 1(Suppl 4), iv23–iv28.
47. Ronco, C. (2017). Evolution of technology for CRRT: forty years of improvements. *Contributions to Nephrology*, 189, 114–23.
48. Ronco, C., et al. (2002). A pilot study of coupled plasma filtration with adsorption in septic shock. *Critical Care Medicine*, 30(6), 1250–5.
49. Ronco, C., et al. (2003). Interpreting the mechanisms of CRRT in sepsis: the peak concentration hypothesis. *Artificial Organs*, 27(9), 792–801.
50. Ronco, C., Kellum, J.A., Bellomo, R., House, A.A. (2008). Potential interventions in sepsis related AKI. *Clinical Journal of American Society of Nephrology*, 3(2), 531–44.
51. Self, W.H., et al. (2018). Balanced crystalloids versus saline in non-critically ill adults. *New England Journal of Medicine*, 378(9), 819–28.
52. Semler, M.W., (2018). Balanced crystalloids versus saline in critically ill adults. *New England Journal of Medicine*, 378(20), 829–39.
53. Shemesh, D., et al. (2006). Sympathectomy like effects of brachial plexus block in arteriovenous access surgery. *Ultrasound in Medicine and Biology*, 32(6), 817–22.
54. Shemesh, D., Raikhinstein, Y., Orkin, D., Goldin, I., Olsha, O. (2014). Anesthesia for vascular access surgery. *The Journal of Vascular Access*, 15(Suppl 7), 38–44.
55. Shemin, D., Bostom, A.G., Laliberty, P., Dworkin L.D. (2001). Residual renal function and mortality risk in hemodialysis patients. *American Journal of Kidney Disease*, 38(1), 85–90.
56. Shetty, A., Oreopoulos, D.G. (2000). Peritoneal dialysis: its indications and contraindications. *Dialysis and Transplantation*, 29(2), 71–7.
57. Shoker, A., Hossain, M.A., Koru-Sengul, T., Raju, D.L., Cockcroft, D. (2006). Performance of creatinine clearance equations on the original Cockroft-Gault population. *Clinical Nephrology*, 66(2), 89–97.
58. Sieberth, H.G., Kierdorf, H. (1999). Is cytokine removal by continuous hemofiltration feasible? *Kidney International Supplements*, 56(72), S72–S79.

59. Spargias, K., et al. (2004). Ascorbic acid prevents contrast mediated nephropathy in patients with renal dysfunction undergoing coronary angiography or intervention. *Circulation*, 110(18), 2837–42.
60. Sun, L.Y., Wijeysundera, D.N., Tait, G.A., Beattie, W.S. (2015). Association of intraoperative hypotension with acute kidney injury after elective noncardiac surgery. *Anesthesiology*, 123(3), 515–23.
61. Thapa, S., Brull, S. (2000). Succinylcholine induced hyperkalemia in patients with renal failure: an old question revisited. *Anesthesia Analgesia*, 91(1), 237–41.
62. Toprak, O. (2007). Risk markers for contrast induced nephropathy. *American Journal of Medical Sciences*, 334(4), 283–90.
63. Trainor, D., Borthwick, E., Ferguson, A. (2011). Perioperative management of the hemodialysis patient. *Seminars in Dialysis*, 24(3), 314–26.
64. Tumlin, J., et al. (2008). Efficacy and safety of renal tubule cell therapy for acute renal failure. *Journal of American Society of Nephrology*, 19(5), 1034–40.
65. Vincent, J., Morre, F. (2017). *Textbook of Critical Care*. 7th ed. Amsterdam: Elsevier.
66. Weisbord, S.D., et al. (2018). Outcomes after angiography with sodium bicarbonate and acetylcysteine. *The New England Journal of Medicine*, 378(7), 603–14.
67. Yamakawa, K., et al. (2016). Benefit profile of anticoagulant therapy in sepsis: a nationwide multicentre registry in Japan. *Critical Care*, 20, 1–12.
68. Ympa, Y.P., Sakr, Y., Reinhart, K., Vincent, J. (2005). Has mortality from acute renal failure decreased? A systematic review of literature. *American Journal of Medicine*, 118(8), 827–32.
69. Zhang J., et al. (2018). How does CRRT affect septic acute kidney injury. *Blood Purification*, 46(4), 326–31.

7

CHAPTER

Anesthesia and Liver

FUNCTIONS OF THE LIVER

Introduction

Liver is a vital organ and performs myriad metabolic functions.

I. Reservoir for Blood Volume

- Vasculature of the liver:
  - Most vascular organ in the body
  - Receives almost one-third of the total cardiac output
  - 1 mL blood is supplied per gram of liver tissue
  - This large volume of blood forms the splanchnic reservoir
  - Low resistance of the hepatic sinusoids allows it to store large volumes of blood
  - Has a *unique dual blood supply*
  - Approximately 75% of the total hepatic flow is through the portal vein
  - Remaining 25% of the blood flow is supplied through hepatic artery
  - Hepatic artery originates in the celiac trunk of abdominal aorta
  - Portal vein is formed by union of superior mesenteric vein and splenic vein
  - Portal vein transmits entire venous drainage of pre-portal splanchnic beds to the liver
- Mechanisms of intrinsic regulation of hepatic blood flow:
  - ***Hepatic arterial buffer response (HABR):***
    - Most important intrinsic mechanism
    - Changes in portal vein flow cause reciprocal changes in hepatic artery flow
    - Mediated through adenosine from periportal system
    - Adenosine in a potent vasodilator
    - By manipulating levels of adenosine, hepatic arterial tone can be altered
    - At its maximum, HABR can double hepatic arterial flow
    - Endotoxemia and splanchnic hypoperfusion can abolish HABR
  - Metabolic control:
    - Mediated by changes in pH or pO_2 of portal venous blood
    - This causes increase or decrease in hepatic arterial flow
    - Metabolic and respiratory changes in acid base balance also can modulate hepatic blood flow
  - Pressure-flow autoregulation:
    - Myogenic responses of vascular smooth muscle also regulate hepatic flow
    - Hypertensive responses cause an increase in myogenic tone
    - This regulates detrimental increases in hepatic flow
    - Hypotensive responses likewise cause a decrease in myogenic tone
    - This regulates decreases in hepatic flow
    - Thus, hepatic flow is maintained during hypotensive episodes

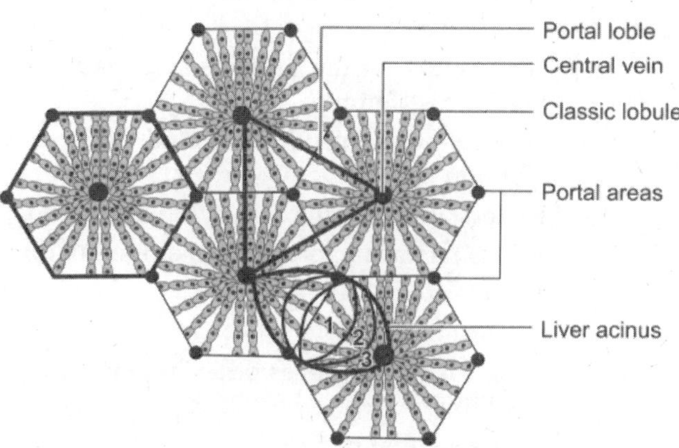

Fig. 1: Portal microstructure.

- Mechanisms of extrinsic regulation of hepatic blood flow:
  - Neural control:
    - Neural control is exerted via:
      - Vagus nerve
      - Phrenic nerve
      - Splanchnic nerve (post-ganglionic sympathetic fibres from T_5-T_{11})
    - Decreases in sympathetic tone increases splanchnic reservoir volume
    - Increases in sympathetic tone decreases splanchnic reservoir volume
    - Hepatic arterial system has α_1, α_2, β_2 and D_1 receptors
    - Portal venous system has only α_1 and D_1 receptors
  - Humoral control:
    - Exerted via glucagon, angiotensin II and vasopressin
    - Glucagon causes relaxation of hepatic arterial smooth muscle
    - Angiotensin II causes constriction of hepatic and portal beds
    - Vasopressin increases hepatic arterial and decreases portal venous resistance
    - Due to this profile, vasopressin maybe used in treating portal hypertension

II. Role in Metabolism

- Protein metabolism:
  - Protein breakdown:
    - Liver plays central role in production and breakdown of amino acids
    - Amino acids are broken down to ketoacids, glutamine and ammonia by transamination
    - ***Krebs- Henseleit cycle*** removes ammonia and other nitrogenous wastes from the body
  - Protein synthesis:
    - Almost 15% of the proteins synthesized by the liver is albumin
    - Healthy adults produce around 12–15 g of albumin per day
    - Factors affecting albumin synthesis include:
      - Plasma oncotic pressure (main regulator)
      - Dietary amino acids
      - Hormones
    - Liver also synthesizes other important proteins like:
      - Procoagulants
      - Hormones
      - Cytokines and chemokines
      - Acute phase reactants
      - Transport proteins
- Carbohydrate metabolism:
  - Glycogen:
    - Liver regulates carbohydrate metabolism mainly through glycogen
    - In the fed state, glucose is polymerized to glycogen and stored
    - This is mediated through glycogen synthase
    - In the starving state, glycogen is depolymerized to glucose
    - This is mediated via glycogen phosphorylase
  - Gluconeogenesis:
    - When glycogen stores are exhausted, hepatic gluconeogenesis is used
    - Substrates for gluconeogenesis:
      - Lactate
      - Glycerol from hydrolysis of triglycerides
      - Alanine, glutamine from protein catabolism
- Lipid metabolism:
  - Fatty acid synthesis:
    - Dietary fatty acids reach liver in the form of chylomicrons
    - These are processed into triglycerides through esterification
    - These maybe stored in the liver, in the form of triglycerides
    - Alternatively, they can be transported to other organs as lipoproteins
    - In the presence of sufficient glycogen, even glucose may be stored as triglycerides
  - Fatty acid metabolism:
    - Mainly via β-oxidation pathways
    - Glucagon activates this pathway and stimulates lipolysis
    - Insulin inhibits β-oxidation and fatty acid metabolism
    - Fatty acids are sequentially cleaved through β-oxidation to yield acetyl-CoA.

III. Enterohepatic Circulation

- Bile is formed by hepatocytes and is secreted eventually into the duodenum
- Bile plays an important part in absorption of molecules with minimal acqueous solubility

- Constituents of bile:
  - Water (97%)
  - Conjugated bile salts (< 1%)
  - Cholesterol, fatty acids, phospholipids
  - Lecithin
  - Conjugated bilirubins
  - Electrolytes, inorganic salts
  - Alkaline phosphatase
- Bile salts are formed from cholesterol by hepatocytes
- Primary bile salts are chenodeoxycholic acid and cholic acid
- These are secreted into the duodenum and travel through the intestine
- These are then absorbed from the terminal ileum and metabolized to secondary bile acids
- Both types of bile acids reach the liver again via portal venous blood
- This forms the enterohepatic circulation
- Through this system, about 95% of the bile acids are conserved

IV. Coagulation System

- Procoagulants:
  - Most of the procoagulants are synthesized in the liver
  - Factors synthesized in the liver are Factors I, II, V, VII, IX, X, XI, XII, XIII
  - *Exceptions* are factors III, IV (calcium) and VIII (von-Willebrand factor)
- Regulators of coagulation:
  - Liver also synthesizes regulators of coagulation
  - These are:
    - Protein C
    - Protein S
    - Protein Z
    - Plasminogen activator inhibitor (PAI)
    - Antithrombin III
- Posttranslational modification:
  - Vitamin K dependent factors undergo post translational modification in the liver
  - This involves γ-carboxylation of glutamate residues at the amino terminus
  - This process creates procoagulants capable of forming complexes with calcium
  - Thus, procoagulants are primed for participation in the coagulation cascade
  - Vitamin K dependent factors include:
    - Factor II
    - Factor VII
    - Factor IX
    - Factor X
    - Protein C and S

V. Bilirubin Metabolism

- Main source of bilirubin is heme metabolism
- Approximately 300 mg of bilirubin is produced by the body everyday
- 80% of bilirubin is derived from the phagocytosis of RBCs
- This is done by macrophages in the liver, spleen and bone marrow
- Reticuloendothelial cells extract protein from hemoglobin and convert heme to bilirubin
- Bilirubin is transported to the liver in conjugation with albumin
- Hepatocytes extract the bilirubin and conjugate it with glucuronic acid
- These conjugates are secreted in the bile for excretion via the gut

VI. Regulation of Hematogenous Endocrine Mediators

- Liver plays an important role in metabolism of hormones and hormone binding proteins
- *Synthesis*: Hormones synthesized by hepatocytes are:
  - Angiotensinogen
  - Thrombopoietin
  - Insulin like growth factor I (IGF-I)
  - Activation of thyroxine (T4) to triiodothyronine (T3)
- *Inactivation*: Hormones inactivated by the liver are:
  - Aldosterone
  - Anti-diuretic hormone
  - Estrogens, androgens
  - Insulin
  - Thyroxine (T4)

VII. Modulator of Immune and Inflammatory Processes

- Liver is the largest reticuloendothelial organ in the body

- Kupffer cells play an important role in immune modulation
- Kupffer cells form almost 10% of the total liver mass
- Functions of Kupffer cells are:
  - Degradation of toxins
  - Phagocytosis of bacteria
  - Processing antigens
  - Attenuation of inflammatory response by removing inciting agents from bloodstream
  - Inciting inflammatory response by releasing cytokines, chemokines and leukotrienes

VIII. Metabolism and Excretion of Xenobiotic Molecules

- Hepatocytes eliminate drugs through 3 phase reactions:
- Phase I:
  - Uses CYP and mixed function oxidases
  - This increases polarity of the drugs by insertion of polar groups
  - Groups inserted include:
    - Hydroxide group
    - Amine group
    - Sulfhydryl group
- Phase II:
  - Conjugates phase I metabolites with water soluble substrates
  - This increases polarity of the drugs
  - Substrates used are:
    - Glucuronic acid
    - Glutathione
    - Sulphates
    - Acetates
- Phase III:
  - Involves excretion of the metabolites into biliary canaliculi
  - Uses specific molecules called *ATP-Binding Cassette (ABC) transport proteins*

LIVER FUNCTION TESTS

Introduction

- Refers to standard test panels used to detect hepatobiliary status
- Misnomer as none of the tests measure any specific liver function

I. Detection of Hepatic Injury

- Aminotransferases:
  - Refers to two enzymes:
    - Alanine aminotransferase (ALT, SGPT)
    - Aspartate aminotransferase (AST, SGOT)
  - These enzymes are involved in gluconeogenesis
  - ALT is highly specific, compared with AST as it is a cytoplasmic liver enzyme
  - AST isoenzymes are found in extrahepatic tissues like:
    - Brain, heart
    - Skeletal muscle
    - Kidney, pancreas
  - Both these enzymes are localized to acinar zone 1
  - These enzymes are released into circulation as a result of hepatocellular injury
  - Normal levels of these enzymes are:
    - AST 10–40 U/L
    - ALT 7–56 U/L
  - Mild elevation:
    - Levels between 100–249 IU/L
    - Causes of mild elevation:
      - Steatosis, alcohol consumption
      - Medications
      - Hemochromatosis
      - Cholestasis
      - Chronic viral hepatitis
      - Neoplasms, cirrhosis
  - Moderate elevation:
    - Levels between 250–999 IU/L
    - Causes of moderate elevation:
      - Acute viral hepatitis
      - Drug induced liver injury
      - Acute exacerbations of chronic liver disease
  - Severe elevation:
    - Levels between 1000- 1999 IU/L
    - Often due to acute hepatitis superimposed on chronic active liver disease
  - Extreme elevations:
    - Levels above 2000 IU/L
    - Often due to massive hepatic necrosis
    - Causes of extreme elevation:
      - Fulminant viral hepatitis
      - Paracetamol poisoning
      - Shock liver, hypoxic hepatitis
      - Autoimmune hepatitis
      - Acute biliary obstruction

- Lactate dehydrogenase:
  - Normal levels 70–250 IU/L
  - Elevation in LDH levels can be due to hepatic and extrahepatic causes
  - Concomitant elevation of ASL and ALT when due to hepatocellular injury
  - Thus, rarely yields more information than that provided by AST and ALT levels
  - Hepatic causes of elevated LDH:
    - Fulminant hepatitis
    - Paracetamol poisoning
    - Hypoxic hepatitis
    - Malignancies
  - Extrahepatic causes of elevated LDH:
    - Hemolysis, rhabdomyolysis
    - Tumor necrosis, renal infarction
    - Acute cerebrovascular accident
    - Myocardial infarction
- Glutathione-S-transferase:
  - Specific for some patterns of drug induced liver injury
  - Released rapidly after hepatocellular injury
  - Has a brief plasma $T_{1/2}$ of 90 minutes
  - GST localizes in acinar zone 3 (centrilobular region)
  - This zone has cells with highest susceptibility to injury from hypoxia or drugs
  - More sensitive than AST and ALT for centrilobular necrosis

II. Assessment of Protein Synthesis

- Serum albumin:
  - Indicates effectiveness of protein synthetic function of the liver
  - Normal serum concentration is 3.5-5.5 g/dL
  - In chronic liver diseases, protein synthetic function is diminished
  - This causes low plasma albumin levels
  - Plasma albumin has a $T_{1/2}$ of nearly 3 weeks
  - Changes in albumin level is seen days after cessation of protein synthetic function
  - Other causes of hypoalbuminemia:
    - Increased albumin catabolism
    - Circulatory overload states
    - Maldistribution of albumin
    - Renal albuminuria (nephrotic syndrome)
    - Protein losing enteropathies
- Prothrombin time:
  - Prothrombin time is used to monitor patients with acute liver dysfunction
  - Only 20–30% of normal factor activity is required for normal coagulation
  - Thus prolonged PT usually reflects severe liver disease
  - Procoagulants derived from the liver have a shorter $T_{1/2}$ compared with albumin
  - Factor VII has the shortest $T_{1/2}$ among hepatic procoagulants (4–6 hours)
  - This is reflected as a high PT, occurring soon after onset of hepatic dysfunction
  - Thus, PT start to fall within 24 hours of onset of severe liver dysfunction
  - Prolongation of PT more than 3–4 sec from control is significant
  - This usually corresponds to an INR> 1.5

III. Detection of Cholestatic Disorders

- Alkaline phosphatase:
  - Lacks specificity for hepatobiliary diseases
  - Normal values range from 40–112 IU/L
  - Extrahepatic sources of ALP are:
    - Bone, leukocytes
    - Intestines, kidneys
    - Placenta, neoplasms
  - Usually is only mildly elevated or normal in liver parenchymal diseases
  - Marked elevation of ALP suggests conditions causing biliary obstruction
  - ALP has a $T_{1/2}$ of almost 1 week
  - Thus, serum ALP levels remain elevated for days after bile flow has normalized
- Gamma glutamyl transpeptidase (GGT):
  - It is a canalicular enzyme
  - Normal range between 10–48 IU/L
  - Compared with ALP, it remains normal in disorders of the bone
  - Thus, elevated GGT suggests that elevated ALP is of hepatic origin
  - Conditions causing elevated GGT levels:
    - Alcoholism
    - Medications: anticonvulsants, H2 receptor blockers
    - Prostrate disease
    - Obesity, diabetic nephropathy, HTN

❖ Bilirubin:
- Normal serum bilirubin is less than 1.5 mg/dL
- Jaundice is readily discernible at serum bilirubin levels above 4 mg/dL
- Scleral icterus can be demonstrated at bilirubin levels above 3 mg/dL
- Conjugated hyperbilirubinemia:
  - Occurs when conjugated bilirubin is not effectively eliminated
  - Conjugated bilirubin is water soluble
  - Thus, this is associated with presence of urinary urobilinogen
  - Causes:
    - Dubin- Johnson syndrome
    - Rotor syndrome
    - Acquired intrahepatic cholestasis
    - Extrahepatic biliary obstruction
- Unconjugated hyperbilirubinemia:
  - Seen when bilirubin production exceeds ability of liver to conjugate it
  - Unconjugated bilirubin is not water soluble
  - Thus, urinary urobilinogen is absent
  - Causes:
    - Gilbert syndrome
    - Crigler-Najjar syndrome
    - Hemolysis
    - Acquired defects in bilirubin conjugation

IV. Quantitative Liver Function Tests

❖ Hepatic clearance:
- Hepatic clearance of a substance reflects the total hepatocellular mass
- Substances used are indocyanine green and bromsulphalein

❖ Caffeine clearance:
- Patients take an oral dose of caffeine (150- 300 mg)
- Caffeine metabolites in saliva are measured for upto 24 hours

❖ Aminopyrine breath test:
- Not commonly used in clinical practice
- Patient is asked to inhale ^{14}C- labeled aminopyrine
- Amount of ^{14}C-labelled CO_2 in patients breath is measured for 2 hours
- Low levels of carbon dioxide indicates impaired liver function

❖ Monoethylglycinexylidide (MEGX) assay:
- IV lidocaine is given in a dose of 1mg/kg
- 15 minutes later, a blood sample is obtained and assayed for MEGX

❖ Other tests:
- Galactose elimination capacity
- Antipyrine clearance

V. Measurement of Hepatic Blood Flow

❖ Clearance techniques:
- Uses indirect Ficks principle to approximate hepatic blood flow
- Valid for substances with a high hepatic clearance
- Substances used to study clearance are:
  - Indocyanine green dye
  - Propranolol
  - Lidocaine
  - Colloidal particles- gold 198
- Indocyanine green extraction is one of the *most reliable* techniques
- After injection of the substance, time- radioactivity curve is plotted
- Area under the curve is used to estimate hepatic blood flow
- Severe liver disease renders these tests as unreliable

❖ Indicator dilution techniques:
- Unlike clearance techniques, these tests are reliable in a severe liver disease
- Radiolabeled indicator like iodinated albumin is injected into the spleen
- Indicator dilution is measured from samples obtained from the hepatic vein
- Indicator dilution curve is used to estimate hepatic blood flow

❖ Direct measurements:
- Uses electromagnetic flow probes placed on hepatic A or portal V
- Surgical access is used to place the probes
- Probe is left in-situ after implantation procedure
- Telemetry is then used to measure hepatic blood flow

VI. Radiological and Endoscopic Methods

- Procedures used commonly to evaluate hepatobiliary disorders are:
  - Percutaneous transhepatic cholangiography (PTHC)
  - Endoscopic retrograde cholangiopancreatography (ERCP)
- Percutaneous transhepatic cholangiography (PTHC):
  - Evaluates intrahepatic bile ducts of patients with unexplained hepatic cholestasis
  - Dilated intrahepatic ducts suggest mechanical occlusion of these ducts
  - When dilatation is absent, most likely cause is parenchymal disease
- Endoscopic retrograde cholangiopancreatography (ERCP)
  - ERCP provides intraductal access to biliary tree and pancreatic duct
  - Mainly used to diagnose and treat extrahepatic biliary disorders
  - Less invasive compared with surgery
- Esophagogastroscopy:
  - Used to evaluate submucosal varices in those with portal hypertension
  - Varices may be treated with banding if indicated
- Splenoportography:
  - Evaluates splenic and portal veins
  - Allows evaluation of extent of portosystemic shunts

VII. Tests for Specific Diseases

- Serological tests to identify microbial and autoimmune causes:
  - Viral etiology:
    - Hepatitis A, B, C, D, E and F
    - Hepatotropic viruses A, B, C, E
    - Cytomegalovirus
    - Epstein-Barr virus
  - Autoimmune etiology:
    - Anti-asialoglycoprotein antibodies useful for autoimmune hepatitis
    - Anti-mitochondrial antibodies characteristic in primary biliary cirrhosis
    - Primary sclerosing cholangitis:
      - Anti-smooth muscle antibodies
      - Anti-nuclear antibodies
- Genetic tests to identify hereditary metabolic disorders
- Tumor marker assays for malignancies:
  - Plasma α-fetoprotein (AFP):
    - Highly specific for hepatocellular carcinoma (HCC)
    - Sensitivity ranges from 50–90%
  - Plasma γ-carboxylated prothrombin levels:
    - HCC cells make procoagulants without γ-carboxylating them
    - High levels of des-γ-carboxylated, vitamin K dependent procoagulants occurs in HCC

POSTOPERATIVE JAUNDICE

Introduction

- Most cases of postoperative jaundice manifest within 3 weeks of surgery
- Most common causes of postoperative jaundice are:
  - Resorption of hematomas
  - Hemolysis following blood transfusion

Etiology

- Prehepatic causes:
  - Transfusion related:
    - Senescent RBC breakdown
    - Hemolytic reactions
    - Multiple blood transfusions
  - Hemolysis due to prosthetic valves:
    - Caged ball valves- Starr- Edwards valve
    - Multiple prosthetic valves
    - Prosthetic valve endocarditis
    - Periprosthetic leaks
  - Resorption of massive hematomas:
    - Retroperitoneal hematomas
    - Intraabdominal hematomas
  - Drug induced erythrocyte lysis:
    - Thiopentone
    - Acetaminophen, ibuprofen
    - Penicillin and derivatives
    - Cephalosporins
    - Ranitidine
    - Procainamide, hydralazine
    - Insulin
    - Intravenous contrast media
- Hepatic causes:
  - Preexisting liver disease

- Gilberts syndrome, Crigler-Najjar syndrome
- Dubin- Johnson syndrome, Rotor syndrome
- Drug induced hepatitis:
  - Allopurinol, bleomycin, cyclosporine, cisplatin
  - Amiodarone, phenytoin, propylthiouracil
  - Amoxicillin, erythromycin, ketoconazole
  - Diclofenac, naproxen, indomethacin, piroxicam
  - Statins
  - Halothane hepatitis
  - Total parenteral nutrition
- Ischemic or hypoxic injury
- Viral hepatitis
- Intrahepatic cholestasis:
  - Sepsis
  - Total parenteral nutrition
  - Acalculous cholecystitis

❖ Posthepatic causes:
- Postoperative cholecystitis
- Extrahepatic cholestasis:
  - Retained common bile duct stone
  - Bile duct injury
- Postoperative pancreatitis

Pathophysiology

❖ Three events lead to postoperative jaundice

❖ Overproduction of bilirubin:
- Prehepatic cause of postoperative jaundice
- Occurs as bilirubin production exceeds livers ability to conjugate it
- Thus, associated with unconjugated hyperbilirubinemia
- Hemolysis can lead to anemia, hemoglobinuria and renal failure
- Usually occurs as a result of:
  - Drug induced erythrocyte destruction
  - Mechanical RBC destruction
- Laboratory findings:
  - Anemia
  - Peripheral smear shows:
    - Fragmented RBCs
    - Reticulocytosis
  - Indirect hyperbilirubinemia
  - Positive direct antiglobulin test
  - Low serum haptoglobin
  - Urinary haptoglobin

❖ Direct hepatocellular injury:
- Hepatic cause of postoperative jaundice
- It is associated with conjugated hyperbilirubinemia
- Marked elevations in serum aminotransferases is also seen
- Usually occurs as a result of:
  - Drug induced hepatitis
  - Cardiogenic, non-cardiogenic shock
  - Sepsis, systemic inflammatory response syndrome
  - Viral hepatitis
- Laboratory findings:
  - Grossly elevated serum transaminases
  - Conjugated hyperbilirubinemia
  - Increased GGT, 5′ nucleotidase
  - Increased alkaline phosphatase

❖ Extrahepatic obstruction:
- Posthepatic cause of postoperative jaundice
- Occurs due to obstruction of the bile duct, preventing bilirubin excretion
- Ability of the liver to conjugate bilirubin, however, is preserved
- Thus, it is associated with conjugated hyperbilirubinemia
- Ultrasonography useful in diagnosing extrahepatic obstruction
- Acute renal failure:
  - High incidence of acute renal failure seen with obstructive jaundice
  - Seen in almost 8- 10% patients with postoperative obstructive jaundice
  - Incidence of ARF coincides with the degree of hyperbilirubinemia
  - Obstructive jaundice results in low levels of intestinal bile acids
  - This causes increased resorption of gut endotoxins
  - This stimulates release of inflammatory mediators like endothelin
  - Endothelin causes potent renal vasoconstriction
  - Thus, renal perfusion is reduced, causing ARF

- Laboratory findings:
  - Conjugated hyperbilirubinemia
  - Increased GGT, 5′ nucleotidase
  - Increased alkaline phosphatase
  - Minimal or no elevation in Transaminases
  - Presence of bilirubin in urine

Grading of Severity 

- ❖ Mild postoperative jaundice: Serum bilirubin < 4 mg/dL
- ❖ Severe postoperative jaundice: Serum bilirubin >4 mg/dL.

Classification of Postoperative Jaundice

- ❖ Early postoperative jaundice (< 3 weeks):
  - Hemolysis
  - Blood transfusions
  - Resorption of hematoma
  - Gilberts syndrome
  - Hypotension, hypovolemia
  - Infection, sepsis
  - Drug induced
  - Acute viral hepatitis
  - Bile duct injury
  - Hepatic artery ligation
  - Postoperative cholecystitis
  - Postoperative pancreatitis
- ❖ Delayed postoperative jaundice (> 3 weeks):
  - Drugs
  - Blood transfusion
  - Total parenteral nutrition.

Treatment

- ❖ Prehepatic causes: Treat underlying cause
- ❖ Hepatic causes:
  - Broad spectrum antibiotics
  - Adjustment of TPN
  - Restoration of hepatic perfusion
  - Removal of offending medications
  - Antiviral agents
  - Supportive care
- ❖ Posthepatic causes:
  - ERCP, sphincterotomy and stone removal for common bile duct stones
  - ERCP, balloon dilatation, stent placement for biliary strictures
  - Surgical correction for those strictures not amenable to endoscopic interventions

HALOTHANE HEPATITIS

Definition

Jaundice occurring in a patient who is previously exposed to halothane within 3 weeks with fever, rashes and lab evidence of raised liver enzymes like SGOT, SGPT and antibodies.

Incidence

- ❖ Male:female: 1:2
- ❖ Most commonly seen in middle age group
- ❖ Relatively rare in children
- ❖ Incidence in children: 1:1,00,000–2,00,000 patients
- ❖ Type I halothane hepatitis: 25–30%
- ❖ Type II halothane hepatitis: 1:6000–35000 patients

Classification 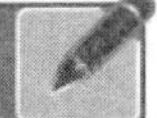

- ❖ Type I halothane hepatitis:
  - Mild form
  - Relatively common (25–30% of those who receive halothane)
  - Results from reductive (anaerobic) biotransformation of halothane
  - Benign features
  - Self limiting disease
  - Mild rise in serum transaminase and glutathione-S-transferase
  - Altered postoperative drug metabolism
  - Not characterized by jaundice or clinically evident hepatocellular disease
  - Does not occur after exposure to other inhalational agents
- ❖ Type II halothane hepatitis:
  - Severe form
  - Relatively uncommon
  - Appears to be immune mediated
  - Occurs due to antibody formation to oxidative metabolites of halothane
  - Fulminant features
  - Causes massive centrilobular necrosis
  - Clinically fever, jaundice, grossly elevated serum transaminases
  - Results in fulminant liver failure
  - Fatality rate of 50%
  - Can occur after exposure to other volatile anesthetics like enflurane.

Metabolism and Mechanism

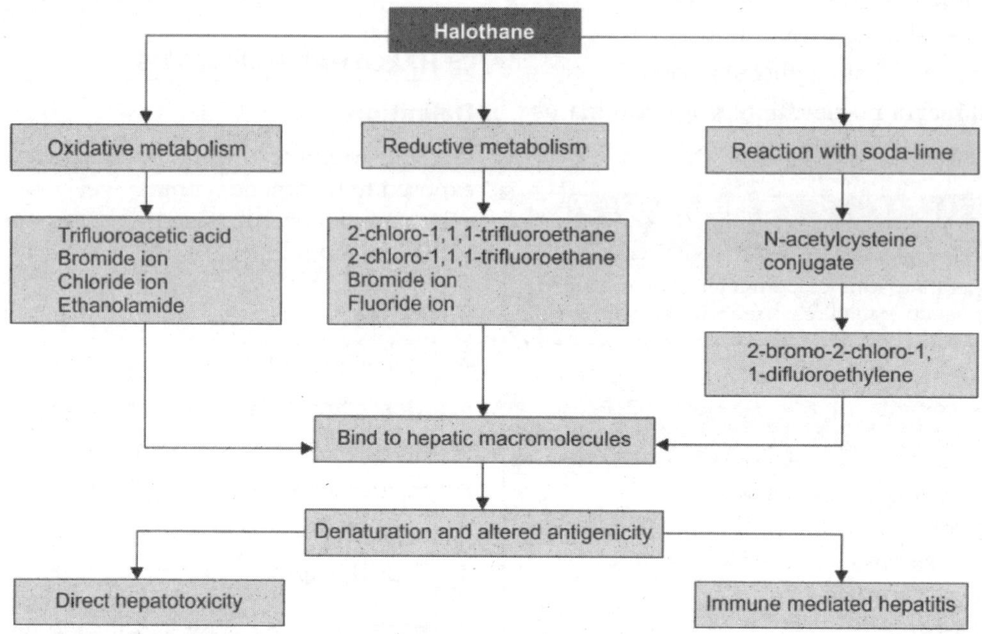

Risk Factors

- Multiple exposures at intervals < 6 weeks (most important)
- Prior history of post anesthetic fever/jaundice
- Duration: prolonged exposure, major surgeries
- Obesity, middle age, pregnancy
- Female sex
- Genetic predisposition
- Enzyme induction (alcohol/barbiturate abuse)
- Drug allergy, recent viral hepatitis.

Predisposing Factors

- Pregnancy
- Viral hepatitis
- Burns
- Hypoxia, hypercarbia.

Clinical Features

- Type I hepatotoxicity is usually clinically silent
- Type II hepatotoxicity:
  - Onset 5-7 days following exposure
  - Onset can occur upto 4 weeks post surgery
  - High grade fever lasting for 3–14 days
  - Jaundice:
    - Onset usually occurs 7–10 days after exposure
    - Onset can occur earlier within 1-2 days, if prior exposure to halothane
  - Nausea, vomiting, anorexia
  - Chills, myalgia, rash
  - Moderate liver enlargement with tenderness
  - Fulminant liver failure ensues.

Lab Findings

- Leucocytosis, eosinophilia
- Raised serum bilirubin
- Raised serum ALT, AST and alkaline phosphatase
- Increased prothrombin time
- Increased GST > 2 is specific index
- ELIZA may detect halothane related antibodies
- Liver biopsy: widespread centrilobular hepatocellular necrosis.

Guidelines for Safe Use

- Prefer TIVA
- Avoid halothane if:
  - Age more than 70 years
  - Obese females
  - Preexisting liver disease/biliary surgery
  - If family history of unexplained jaundice after halothane
  - Recent halothane exposure within 6 weeks.

Differential Diagnosis

- Blunt abdominal trauma
- Acute liver failure
- Alcoholic hepatitis
- Infective hepatitis
- Biliary obstruction
- Cirrhosis

Prognosis

- In the absence of fulminant liver failure, full recovery occurs
- If fulminant liver failure occurs, mortality rate of 50%
- Concomitant hepatic encephalopathy results in mortality rate of 80%

Treatment

- Medical therapy:
  - Supportive therapy:
    - Restrict protein intake
    - Oral neomycin/lactulose
    - Maintain fluid and electrolyte balance
    - Support ventilation if necessary
    - Correct coagulopathies, hypoglycemia
  - Molecular adsorbent recirculating system (MARS)
- Surgical therapy: Orthotopic liver transplantation

ANESTHETIC MANAGEMENT OF PATIENT WITH LIVER DISEASE

Preoperative Evaluation and Preparation

Preoperative Evaluation

History taking:

- History of platypnea (dyspnea in upright position)
- Risk factors:
  - Blood transfusion
  - Alcohol abuse
  - Illicit drug use
  - Tattoos
  - Personal/family history of jaundice

Physical Examination

- Encephalopathy
- Altered sleep wake cycles
- Jaundice
- Scleral icterus
- Halitosis
- Parotid enlargement
- Gynecomastia
- Spider angioma
- Clubbing
- Leuconychia
- Palmar erythema
- Asterixis
- Hepato-splenomegaly

Investigations

- Complete blood count: anemia
- Blood urea nitrogen, serum creatinine: prerenal azotemia or hepatorenal syndrome
- Blood sugar levels
- Liver function tests
- Serum albumin, globulin, albumin: globulin ratio
- Serum electrolytes: hypokalemia due to diuretic use
- Coagulation profile: altered PT INR very sensitive indicator
- ECG: dyselectrolytemias
- Chest X-ray: pleural effusion more commonly on right side
- Echocardiography

Classification Systems

Child Pugh classification of severity of liver disease:

No.	Parameter	1 point	2 points	3 points
1.	Bilirubin (mg/dL)	<2	2–3	>3
2.	Albumin (g/dL)	>3.5	2.8–3.5	<2.8
3.	Increase in prothrombin time (s)	1–3	4–6	>6
4.	Ascites	None	Slight	Moderate
5.	Encephalopathy	None	1–2	3–4

Child Pugh grades:
5–6 points : Grade A
7–9 points : Grade B
10–15 points : Grade C

Preoperative Preparation

Goals

- Optimize nutritional status
- Optimize cardiopulmonary function

- Medical control of ascites
- Correct dyselectrolytemias.

Preparation

- Fluid restriction, diuretics
- Paracentesis for large volume ascites
- Preoperative antibiotics to reduce infection
- Prophylactic H_2 blocker for 4-6 wks
- Fresh frozen plasma and Vitamin K to correct coagulopathy
- Cryoprecipitate and DDAVP if bleeding time prolonged
- Lactulose and Neomycin if encephalopathy
- Antiaspiration prophylaxis :
  - Ranitidine 1 mg/kg IV
  - Metaclopramide 10 mg IV

INTRAOPERATIVE MANAGEMENT

Anesthetic Considerations

Preoperative Considerations

- Antiaspiration prophylaxis
- Increased chances of infection – antibiotic coverage
- Poor preoperative nutritional status
- Electrolyte imbalances
- Avoid preoperative sedation
- Coagulopathy:
  - Avoid regional anesthesia
  - Avoid intramuscular injections
  - Adequate blood ready
  - Blood conservation strategies

Intraoperative Considerations

- Universal precautions if indicated
- Increased risk of aspiration:rapid sequence induction
- Avoid traumatic intubation
- Careful nasogastric tube placement as esophageal varices possible
- Altered drug metabolism:
  - Increased volume of distribution
  - Reduced plasma protein levels
  - Reduced drug metabolism
  - Reduced excretion
  - Increased duration of action of succinylcholine , cisatracurium ***relaxant of choice***
- Titrated dose NMBAS and sedatives
- Avoid halothane , nitrous oxide
- Drug interactions:
  - Neomycin increases duration of neuromuscular blockade
  - Cimetidine potentiates relaxant drug action
- Massive intraoperative fluid shifts—invasive BP monitor mandatory
- Profound hypotension on induction—graded doses of induction agents
- *Increased third spacing*: Hypotension on draining ascitic fluid
- Careful to avoid fluid overload
- Titrate fluids to maintain urine output >0.5 mL/kg/hr and CVP between 2–5 mm Hg
- Use sodium free fluids : albumin is fluid of choice
- Increased blood loss due to coagulopathy
- Careful blood transfusion to avoid encephalopathy
- Citrate toxicity possible due to reduced liver function
- *Large operative field exposure:* hypothermia common

Postoperative

- Expect delayed recovery
- Avoid NSAIDs for pain
- Increased chances of complications :
  - Hepatic encephalopathy
  - Hepatorenal syndrome
  - Hepatopulmonary syndrome.

Monitors

- Pulse oximetry
- Capnography
- NIBP
- Temperature probe
- ECG
- Neuromuscular monitoring
- Arterial line: for invasive BP/repeated blood sampling
- Central venous access: for prolonged procedures with potential for blood loss
- Pulmonary artery catheterization for:
  - Anticipated prolonged vascular exclusion
  - Preoperative sepsis
- Periodic arterial blood gas analysis

- Periodic blood sugar as prone for hypoglycemia
- Point of care testing:
  - Blood chemistry for anemia
  - Coagulation analysis

Induction

- *Rapid sequence induction* as high risk for aspiration
- Reduced induction dosage of thiopentone
- Propofol maybe preferred as it avoids phase II metabolism
- Two large bore intravenous cannulas to be available
- Restrict fluid administration during induction of anesthesia

Maintenance

- O_2 + air + isoflurane/sevoflurane/desflurane
- Avoid halothane
- Supplemental narcotic agent – fentanyl is ***opioid of choice***
- Atracurium ***muscle relaxant of choice***
- Pass anesthetic gases through large capacity heat moisture exchanger
- Fluids passed through warmer
- Forced warm air devices on upper and lower parts of body

Hemodynamics

Goals:
- Avoid undesired hypovolemia
- Avoid vasodilation to prevent low peripheral perfusion pressures
- Autologous blood donation and intraoperative blood recovery systems where necessary
- Judicious use of norepinephrine or vasopressin to restore perfusion pressures
- Maintain CVP around 2–5 mm Hg
- Maintain urine output > 0.5 mL/kg/hour

Colloids:
- Reduces extravascular translocation of fluids
- Improves mesenteric perfusion
- Rapid restoration of postoperative gut function
- Preferred fluids:
  - 5% albumin
  - 20% albumin
  - Hetastarch in a balanced salt solution

Crystalloids:
- Intraoperative use restricted to minimum
- Causes fluid extravasation

Blood products:
- Fresh frozen plasma: Used as maintenance fluid in coagulopathy
- Packed red cells: *Transfusion trigger* 25%

Extubation

- Fully awake and warm with stable vital signs
- Fully reversed and extubated

ANESTHETIC MANAGEMENT OF PATIENTS WITH OBSTRUCTIVE JAUNDICE

Introduction

Obstructive jaundice refers to the increase in serum bilirubin levels due to bile flow obstruction.

Etiology

- Extrahepatic causes:
  - Benign:
    - Cholelithiasis- most common
    - Chronic pancreatitis
    - Parasitic infections:
      - Ascariasis
      - Clonorchiasis
    - Biliary atresia
    - Choledochal cysts
  - Malignant:
    - Pancreas
    - Ampulla
    - Bile duct
    - Gall bladder
- Intrahepatic causes:
  - Hereditary:
    - Dubin Johnson syndrome
    - Rotor syndrome
    - Cholestatic jaundice of pregnancy
    - Recurrent intrahepatic cholestasis
  - Acquired:
    - Cholestatic drugs
    - Sclerosing cholangitis
    - Biliary cirrhosis.

Pathophysiology

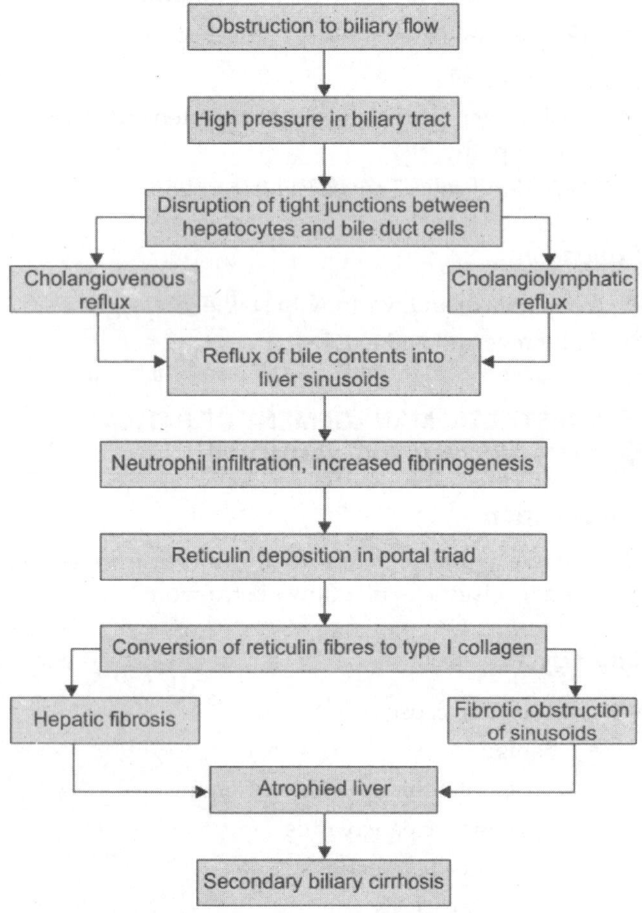

Pathophysiological Effects of Obstructive Jaundice

- Cardiovascular system:
  - Bradycardia due to direct effects of bile acids on SA node
  - Impaired cardiac contractility causing ventricular depression
  - Redistribution of blood volume into splanchnic circulation
  - Impaired response to beta adrenergic agents
  - Decreased peripheral vascular resistance
  - This results in a hypotensive patient prone for circulatory collapse
  - Also, bleeding causes an exaggerated hypotensive response
- Gastrointestinal system:
  - Malabsorption steatorrhea
  - Decreased absorption of fat soluble vitamins A, D, E, K
  - Intestinal mucosal barrier dysfunction
  - Bacterial translocation
  - Portal vein endotoxemia
  - Gastritis, stress ulcers
- Renal system:
  - Renal vasoconstriction and hypoperfusion
  - Shunting of blood away from cortex to medulla
  - Tubular and renal cortical necrosis
  - Hepatorenal syndrome
- Hemostatic system:
  - Decreased clotting factor synthesis- prolonged PT
  - Vitamin K deficiency due to biliary obstruction- impedes γ-carboxylation
  - Hypersplenism causing thrombocytopenia
  - Endotoxemia causing:
    - Increased fibrinolysis
    - Low grade DIC
  - All these factors contribute to coagulopathy in obstructive jaundice
  - Loss of calcium
- Immune system:
  - Depressed RE system function
  - Impaired T-cell proliferation
  - Decreased neutrophil chemotaxis
  - Defective phagocytosis
- Wound healing:
  - Delayed wound healing
  - High incidence of wound dehiscence
  - Pruritis due to high serum bile acid levels
  - Incorporation of prolene in collagen causing defective collagen synthesis

Anesthetic Considerations

- Surgical considerations:
  - Usually involves prolonged surgery (like Whipples or distal gastrectomy)
  - Increased blood loss and fluid shifts
  - Wide incision made during surgery warrants good postoperative analgesia
- Pharmacological considerations:
  - Low levels of serum proteins causing:
    - Increased free drug levels
    - Increased chances of toxicity
    - Prolonged action of drugs
- Nutritional considerations:
  - Increased incidence of hypoglycemia
  - Increased incidence of electrolyte imbalance

Contd...

Contd...

- Hematological considerations:
  - Anemia, thrombocytopenia, coagulopathy- increased transfusion requirements
  - Leucopenia- increased chances of infections
- Cardiovascular considerations:
  - Less tolerance to hypovolemia
  - Increased chances of circulatory collapse
- Renal considerations:
  - Increased incidence of perioperative acute renal failure 8–10%
  - Prerenal azotemia, renal insufficiency

Choice of Anesthetic Technique

- Thoracic epidural anesthesia:
  - Recommended site is T_6-T_8 level
  - Useful in patients undergoing upper abdominal surgeries:
    - Gastrectomy
    - Hepatectomy
    - Whipples procedure
  - Advantages:
    - Provides stable hemodynamics
    - Protective effect on intestinal barrier function
    - Reduces endotoxin induced intestinal barrier dysfunction
    - Improves intestinal microcirculation
    - Can be used for postoperative analgesia
  - Disadvantages:
    - Hypotension may occur if blood volume is low
    - Traction on gall bladder may cause bradycardia
    - Coagulopathy may contraindicate insertion
- General anesthesia:
  - Advantages:
    - Better anesthetic effect compared with thoracic epidural
    - Lower incidence of hypotension, compared with thoracic epidural
    - Good response to inotropes, compared with thoracic epidural
    - Safer compared with thoracic epidural
  - Disadvantages:
    - Delayed awakening
    - Poor postoperative analgesia compared with thoracic epidural

Administration of General Anesthesia

Preoperative Assessment and Preparation

- Ensure adequate NPO status
- Obtain informed consent
- Reassess PT and electrolyte status on the morning of surgery
- Consider short acting BDZ (midazolam) and H_2 receptor antagonist for premedication
- Coagulopathy:
  - Intravenous Vitamin K 1–10 mg used to correct coagulopathy
  - Vitamin K given twice daily is initiated 3 days prior to surgery
  - Fresh frozen plasma used when vitamin K is not useful
- Endotoxemia:
  - Preoperative antibiotic therapy to counter endotoxemia
  - Use of oral lactulose to reduce translocation
  - Early reestablishment of enteral nutrition to protect intestinal flora
- Protection of renal function:
  - Prevent hypovolemia- judicious fluid loading
  - Avoid nephrotoxic drugs:
    - Aminoglycosides
    - NSAIDs
  - Low dose dopamine
- Optimize nutritional status:
  - High protein, high carbohydrate, low fat diet
  - Nasojejunal feeding in those who cannot tolerate enteral feeds
  - In those with severe malnutrition, parenteral nutrition initiated
  - Overnight intravenous fluid therapy may be used to optimize intravascular volume

Induction

- Adequate preoxygenation for 3 minutes
- Propofol can be used for induction, given slowly, to avoid precipitous hypotension
- Etomidate can be used in lower doses, in hemodynamically unstable patients
- Succinylcholine is avoided as it stimulates vagus nerve causing bradycardia
- Atracurium or cisatracurium are the muscle relaxants of choice

- Fentanyl can be used for analgesia in reduced doses
- Avoid hypotension at induction using ephedrine boluses

Monitoring

- Pulse oximetry
- ECG
- Capnography
- NIBP
- Temperature
- Neuromuscular monitoring
- Urine output
- Blood loss
- BIS/entropy for depth of anesthesia monitoring
- CVP may be used to guide fluid therapy
- Invasive blood pressure monitoring in major surgeries, with large fluid shifts
- ABG and blood sugar at frequent intervals for hypoglycemia and dyselectrolytemia
- Thromboelastogram for point-of-care coagulation monitoring

Maintenance

- Balanced anesthesia techniques preferred
- Dosage of inhalational anesthetics should be reduced due to enhanced neurotoxicity
- Choice of inhalational agent:
  - Halothane avoided in view of hepatotoxicity
  - Isoflurane:
    - Sensitivity to isoflurane is enhanced in obstructive jaundice
    - This can cause hypotension and bradycardia with isoflurane use
  - Desflurane effects are similar to isoflurane
  - Sevoflurane is best suited for maintenance of anesthesia
- Spasm of sphincter of Oddi:
  - Incidence is very low
  - Morphine avoided due to its propensity to cause spasm of the sphincter
  - This effect can last up to 2 hours following the drug administration
  - Intraoperative manipulation of the sphincter can contribute to spasm
- O_2+ air + sevoflurane can be used for maintenance of balanced anesthesia
- Fentanyl and atracurium/cisatracurium boluses to maintain anesthetic plane

Ventilation

Prevent increases in hepatic venous pressure by:

- Avoiding large tidal volumes
- Avoiding high airway pressures
- Maintaining eucapnia

Hemodynamics

- Fluid administration should be judicious to maintain LV stroke volume
- Stroke volume variation (SVV) and pulse pressure variation (PPV) useful indices
- Static variables like MAP and CVP are inferior to SVV and PPV in predicting fluid responsiveness
- Fresh frozen plasma maybe used to tackle excessive bleeding
- Maintain renal protection with:
  - Mannitol
  - Furosemide
  - Low dose dopamine

Extubation

- Hemodynamically stable patients can be extubated on table
- Consider postoperative ventilation for:
  - Malignant dyselectrolytemias
  - Cardiovascular instability
  - Hypothermia
- Caution while administering neostigmine as its cholinergic action can cause arrhythmias

Postoperative Care

Management

- Oxygen supplementation
- Antibiotics and H_2 receptor antagonist therapy continued
- Early reinstitution of enteral feeds advocated
- Mannitol may be used to maintain urine output in adequately fluid loaded patients
- Maintain urine output > 1 mL/kg/hour

Monitor

- Pulse oximetry
- ECG

- ❖ NIBP/IBP
- ❖ CVP for fluid therapy
- ❖ CNS status for hepatic encephalopathy
- ❖ Urine output for hepatorenal syndrome

Analgesia

- ❖ Compared with normal people, pain threshold is increased in obstructive jaundice
- ❖ This reduces the analgesic requirement by up to 50%
- ❖ NSAID use is avoided
- ❖ Multimodal analgesia useful
- ❖ Concomitant regional anesthesia useful in reducing opioid requirements

HEPATORENAL SYNDROME

Introduction

- ❖ Refers to the development of functional renal failure, with histologically normal kidneys, in patients with advanced chronic liver disease
- ❖ Severe complication of cirrhosis which is almost always irreversible
- ❖ Survival in HRS patients is measured in weeks-months

Predicting Factors

- ❖ Hepatomegaly, history of ascites
- ❖ Esophageal varices
- ❖ Poor nutritional status
- ❖ Serum sodium and potassium
- ❖ Glomerular filtration rate
- ❖ Blood urea nitrogen
- ❖ Serum, urinary osmolality
- ❖ Urinary sodium excretion
- ❖ Free water clearance after water load

Precipitating Factors

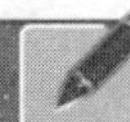

- ❖ Spontaneous bacterial peritonitis (most common)
- ❖ Rapid correction of ascites without plasma expansion
- ❖ Large volume paracentesis (4–6 L/day) without albumin replacement
- ❖ Gastrointestinal bleeding
- ❖ Injudicious diuretic therapy
- ❖ NSAID therapy in patients with borderline renal function

Contd...

Contd...

- ❖ Major surgery, major bleeding
- ❖ Other infections:
  - Urinary tract infections
  - Gastrointestinal infections
  - Biliary infections
  - Sepsis.

Pathophysiology

- ❖ ***Peripheral vasodilatation theory***:
  - Most widely accepted theory
  - Portal hypertension results in splanchnic vasodilatation
  - This is the inciting event for development of HRS
  - Splanchnic vasodilatation is mediated by:
    - Nitric oxide (principally)
    - Carbon monoxide
    - Glucagon
    - Vasodilator peptides
  - Vasodilatation sequesters blood in splanchnic vascular bed
  - This leads to reduced effective arterial blood volume (*arterial underfilling*)
  - Due to coexisting cirrhotic cardiomyopathy, cardiac output reduces
  - Compensatory neurohormonal vasoconstrictor systems get stimulated and include:
    - Renin angiotensin aldosterone system (RAAS)
    - Sympathetic nervous system (SNS)
    - Arginine vasopressin (AVP)
  - This causes:
    - Sodium and water retention
    - Ascites, hyponatremia
    - Renal vasoconstriction
  - Renal vasoconstriction produces a decline in renal blood flow and GFR
  - This ultimately results in renal failure and hepatorenal syndrome
- ❖ ***Hepatorenal reflex theory:***
  - Abnormal hepatic blood flow directly alters renal hemodynamics
  - Acute increases in portal venous pressure causes reflex renal vasoconstriction
  - Phenomenon is not seen when the liver is denervated

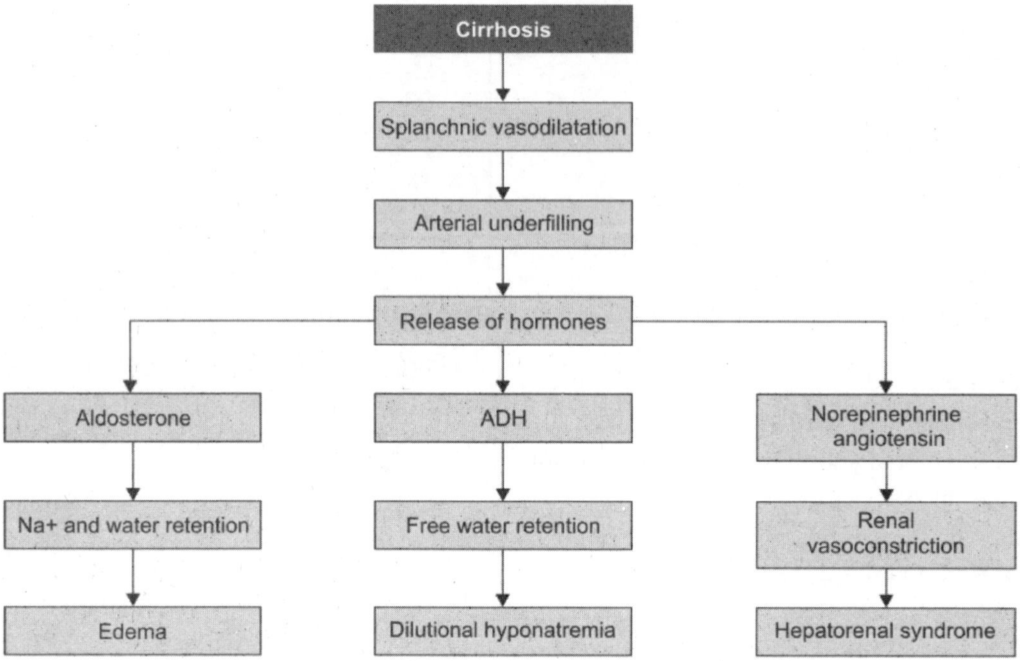

TYPES: ***International Ascites Club classification:***

No.	TYPE I HRS	TYPE II HRS
1.	Rapidly progressive	Insiduous symptoms
2.	Usually occurs within 2 weeks	Evolves over weeks to months
3.	Severe renal impairment	Moderate renal function impairment
4.	Serum creatinine > 2.5 mg/dL	Serum creatinine 1.5- 2.5 mg/dL
5.	Commonly precipitated by Spontaneous bacterial peritonitis	Occurs de novo
6.	Poor prognosis	Better prognosis
7.	Median survival approximately 2 weeks	Median survival approximately 6 months

Diagnostic Criteria: HRS is Essentially a Diagnosis of Exclusion

I. International Ascites Club (IAC) Criteria

Major criteria:

- Chronic or acute liver disease with portal HTN and advanced hepatic failure
- Low GFR as indicated by:
  - 24 hour creatinine clearance < 40 mL/min
  - Serum creatinine >1.5 mg/dL
- Absence of parenchymal disease as suggested by:
  - Normal renal ultrasound
  - Proteinuria < 500 mg/dL
- Absence of infections, nephrotoxins and shock
- Absence of sustained improvement (decrease in serum creatinine < 1.5 mg/dL or increase in creatinine clearance to > 40 mL/min following:
  - Diuretic therapy withdrawal
  - 1.5 L fluid load

Minor criteria: Not necessary for diagnosis and only provide additional information:

- Oliguria <500 mL/day
- Urinary Na^+ <10 mEq/L
- Serum Na^+ < 130 mEq/L
- Urine RBCs < 50 per high power field
- Urinary osmolality greater than plasma osmolality

II. Revised IAC Diagnostic Criteria for HRS

- Cirrhosis with ascites
- Serum creatinine > 1.5 mg/dL
- Absence of parenchymal kidney disease as indicated by:
  - Normal renal ultrasound
  - Proteinuria > 500 mg/day
  - Microscopic hematuria > 50 RBCs per high power field
- Absence of shock
- No current or recent treatment with nephrotoxic drugs

- ❖ Absence of improvement in serum creatinine (to less than 1.5 g/dL) following:
  - More than 2 days diuretic withdrawal
  - Volume expansion with albumin (1–100 g/kg body weight/day)

Laboratory Findings

- ❖ Hyponatremia, hyperkalemia
- ❖ Elevated blood urea nitrogen
- ❖ Decreased plasma osmolality
- ❖ Elevated urinary osmolality
- ❖ Decreased urinary sodium excretion
- ❖ Elevated plasma renin activity
- ❖ Elevated plasma noradrenaline activity

Treatment

Supportive Therapy

- ❖ Support Airway Breathing
- ❖ *Avoid nephrotoxins*: NSAIDs, IV contrast agents
- ❖ Protein restriction
- ❖ Plasma volume expansion:
  - Increasing total plasma volume increases the central blood volume
  - Intravenous albumin infusions used to increase central blood volume
  - This improves preload, mean arterial pressure and kidney perfusion

Vasopressors

- ❖ Is the primary medical treatment for type I HRS
- ❖ Forms first line of treatment along with volume expansion with albumin
- ❖ Help by causing splanchnic vasoconstriction and reducing renal vasoconstriction
- ❖ Unlikely that vasopressors improve survival beyond short term
- ❖ Drugs used:
  - Terlipressin:
    - Vasoconstrictor of choice ***(EASL guidelines)***
    - Acts on V_1 receptors on vascular smooth muscle cells
    - Used in combination with albumin
    - Improves renal function in 40–50% patients with type I HRS
  - Vasopressin, ornipressin
  - Norepinephrine, dopamine
  - Midodrine (α_1 agonist) 5–10 mg TID per orally
  - Octreotide 100 µg subcutaneously BD

III. Others

- ❖ Transjugular intrahepatic portosystemic shunt (TIPS):
  - TIPS is considered if vasopressor therapy fails
  - Avoided as first line therapy due to lack of data (ADQI recommendations)
  - Intrahepatic stent inserted, which connects portal vein and hepatic vein
  - This shunts blood away from portal vein into systemic vein
  - Thus, portal pressure is reduced and systemic volume is augmented
  - TIPS can however, aggravate liver failure and precipitate encephalopathy
  - Contraindications for TIPS:
    - Serum bilirubin > 5 mg/dL
    - Child- Pughs score > 11
    - INR > 2
    - Cardiopulmonary disease
- ❖ Extracorporeal support systems:
  - Renal replacement therapy:
    - Hemodialysis is generally ineffective in HRS
    - Continuous veno-venous hemofiltration is preferred in unstable patients
    - Indications:
      - Failure of vasoconstrictor therapy
      - Presence of contraindications for TIPS
      - As a bridge for liver transplantation
      - To treat specific complications of renal impairment:
  - Metabolic acidosis
  - Hyperkalemia
  - Volume overload
  - Uremic symptoms
    - Complications:
      - Hypotension
      - Coagulopathy
      - Infections
  - ***Molecular adsorbent recirculating system (MARS)***:
    - Modified dialysis technique
    - Combines functions of dialysis machine with closed-loop albumin circuit
    - Used to extract albumin-bound, water-soluble substances from blood

- Removes vasodilators involved in pathogenesis of HRS like:
  - Nitric oxide
  - Tumor necrosis factor
  - Cytokines
- Not widely used
- Not supported by any large studies

• *Prometheus:*
- Extracorporeal technique
- Uses fractional plasma separation and adsorption, with hemodialysis
- Removes water soluble, albumin bound substances
- Current use limited

IV. Liver Transplantation

❖ Only definitive therapy
❖ Reverses HRS if performed early
❖ 5 year survival of 60% for HRS patients who underwent liver transplantation
❖ Orthotopic liver conventionally used
❖ Living donor liver transplant (LDLT) also used in some centres

V. Treat Complications

❖ Hyponatremia
❖ Hyperkalemia
❖ Hypokalemia

Prevention

❖ Avoiding hypovolemic states:
  • Avoid high dose diuretics
  • Slow treatment of ascites
  • Coloading with albumin during paracentesis
  • Avoidance of nephrotoxic agents:
    - NSAIDs
    - Aminoglycosides

❖ Early management of infections , hemorrhage and dyselectrolytemia
❖ Albumin when used with cefotaxime, to treat SBP, reduces risk of developing HRS
❖ Oral norfloxacin administration may reduce incidence of HRS
❖ Pentoxyfylline may be useful due to its beneficial effects on renal function

Differential Diagnosis

No.	Investigation	Prerenal ARF	HRS	ARF
1.	Urine sodium	< 10 mEq/L	< 10 mEq/L	>30 mEq/L
2.	Urine:plasma creatinine	>30:1	>30:1	<20:1
3.	Urine-plasma osmolarity	100 mOsm	100 mOsm	0 mOsm
4.	Urinary sediment	Normal	Unremarkable	Casts, debris

HEPATOPULMONARY SYNDROME

Introduction

❖ Pulmonary vascular disorder occurring in patients with liver disease
❖ *Defined as a triad of:*
  • Liver disease
  • Abnormal arterial oxygenation, with abnormal alveolar-arterial gradient:
    - $PaO_2 < 80$ mm Hg
    - $AaDO_2 > 15$ mm Hg
  • Evidence of intrapulmonary vascular dilatation (IPVD)

Pathophysiology

❖ Occurs in patients with chronic liver disease
❖ Severe liver disease is not a prerequisite for development of HPS
❖ HPS can occur even in patients with mild liver dysfunction
❖ Different mechanisms explain development of HPS
❖ ***Intrapulmonary vascular dilatation:***
  • Hallmark in HPS is formation of microscopic intrapulmonary arteriovenous dilations
  • This may be due to decreased hepatic clearance of vasodilators
  • This results in accumulation of excess vasodilators
  • Vasodilators with a contributory role include:
    - Nitric oxide
    - Tumor necrosis factor α
    - Vasoactive intestinal peptide
    - Substance P
    - Atrial natriuretic peptide
  • Intrapulmonary vessels are usually 8-15 μm
  • In HPS, the vessels dilate to 15-500 μm
  • Two patterns of IPVD can occur:
    - Type I lesions:
      ▪ More common (85%)

- *Diffuse* vascular dilatations at precapillary level
- Located close to gas exchange units of the lung
- Respond well to oxygen therapy, to attain PaO_2 > 200 mm Hg

– Type II lesions:
- Less common (15%)
- *Discrete*, localized dilatations
- Located distant from the gas exchange units of the lung
- Respond poorly to oxygen therapy
- Unable to raise PaO_2 > 200 mm Hg with supplemental oxygen

❖ ***Alveolar- capillary oxygen disequilibrium theory***:
- Proposes that pulmonary capillaries are grossly dilated
- Oxygen molecules are thus unable to permeate to the center of the dilated vessels
- The center of these dilated capillaries carry the erythrocytes and hemoglobin
- Thus, inability to adequately oxygenate hemoglobin occurs, leading to hypoxemia

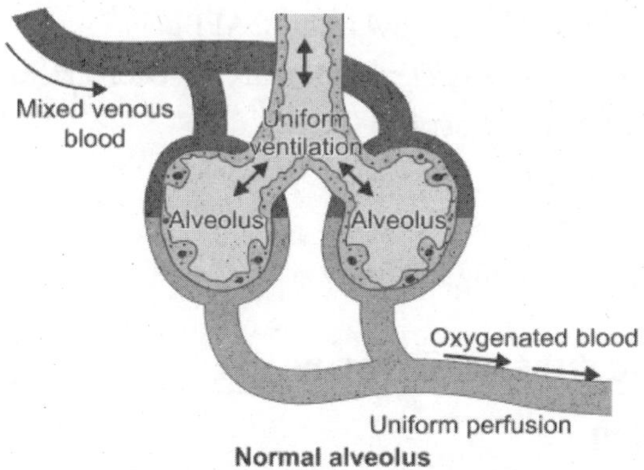

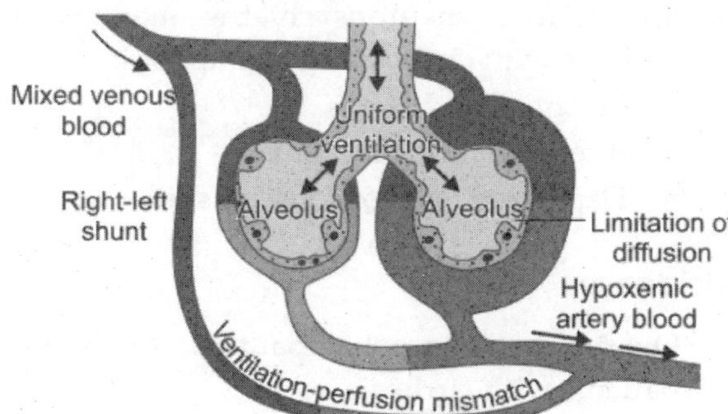

Fig. 2: Hepatopulmonary syndrome.

Risk Factors

Other conditions associated with HPS include:
- ❖ Post- Fontan procedure
- ❖ Non- cirrhotic portal hypertension
- ❖ Ischemic hepatitis
- ❖ Acute liver failure

Clinical Features

❖ Hypoxic symptoms:
- Dyspnea on exertion or at rest
- Platypnea:
  - Occurs in 25% of patients
  - Dyspnea occurs when patient stands upright
  - Dyspnea improves on assuming supine posture
- Weakness and easy fatigueability
- Peripheral cyanosis and digital clubbing can also occur
- Orthodeoxia:
  - Decreased oxygen tension when upright
  - Oxygen tension improves on assuming supine posture

❖ Hepatic symptoms:
- Jaundice, ascites
- Gastrointestinal bleeding
- Esophageal varices
- Spider angioma
- Palmar erythema
- Gynecomastia
- Splenomegaly

Classification:

- ❖ *Mild HPS:* PaO_2 > 80 mm Hg
- ❖ *Moderate HPS:* PaO_2 60–79 mm Hg
- ❖ *Severe HPS:* PaO_2 50-59 mm Hg
- ❖ *Very severe HPS:* PaO_2 < 50 mm Hg.

Investigations

❖ ***Orthodeoxia test:***
- Patient asked to lie down from standing position
- Positive test suggested by:
  - Decrease in PaO_2 by > 4 mm Hg
  - Decrease in oxygen saturation by > 5%

❖ Arterial blood gas analysis:
- Hypoxemia with PaO_2 < 70 mm Hg with an FiO_2 = 0.21

- Respiratory alkalosis along with hypoxemia is characteristic of HPS
- Abnormal alveolar-arterial gradient > 15 mm Hg

❖ ***Hyperoxia test***:
- ABG is measured on the patient, while breathing room air
- Then, patient is made to breathe 100% oxygen for 10 minutes
- If PaO_2 is < 150 mm Hg, it confirms the presence of intrapulmonary shunt

❖ Chest X-ray:
- Maybe normal in most patients
- Bibasal 1.5–3 mm medium sized nodular or reticulonodular opacities

❖ Transthoracic echocardiography:
- Contrast enhanced TTE is useful
- Considered gold standard for detecting IPVD
- Delayed filling of contrast on left side of the heart is pathognomonic of IPVD
- 10 mL agitated saline is injected into a peripheral vein
- Presence of microbubbles in left heart > 3 cardiac cycles after their appearance in right heart suggests delayed filling of contrast

❖ Computed tomography:
- May show peripheral arteriolar dilatation
- Maybe useful to differentiate the types of HPS

❖ Pulmonary perfusion scan:
- Scan done with albumin microaggregates labeled with technetium- 99 m
- Extrapulmonary uptake of the macroaggregates is studied
- This allows us to quantify the percentage of intrapulmonary dilatations
- It is considered pathological with values > 6%

Differential Diagnosis

❖ Hepatic hydrothorax

❖ Portopulmonary hypertension

Poor Prognostic Factors

❖ PaO_2 < 50 mm Hg on room air

❖ Shunt fraction > 20% on pulmonary perfusion scan

❖ Severe pulmonary HTN

❖ Positive hyperoxia test.

Management

❖ Supportive therapy:
- Long term oxygen therapy:
  - Indicated in those with severe HPS with PaO_2 < 60 mm Hg
- Oxygen therapy given to maintain oxygen saturation above 88%

❖ TIPS:
- Helps in reducing portal pressure and decongesting portal venous system
- Offers uncertain benefits

❖ Liver transplantation:
- Indicated in those with progressive hypoxemia (PaO_2 < 60 mm Hg), poorly responsive to medical management
- Only definitive treatment for those with HPS
- Offers complete resolution of gas exchange in most patients with HPS
- PaO_2 < 50 mm Hg is a contraindication to liver transplantation
- Resolution of IPVD has been observed from 3 months post transplant

❖ Other experimental therapies:
- Somatostatin analogues
- Caffeic acid phenethyl ester (CAPE)
- *Almitrine bismesylate:* Pulmonary vasoconstrictor
- Indomethacin, aspirin
- Norfloxacin
- Corticosteroids
- Plasma exchange therapy

HEPATIC ENCEPHALOPATHY

Introduction

❖ Spectrum of neuropsychiatric manifestations in patients with cirrhosis and comprises:
- Personality changes
- Intellectual impairment
- Depressed level of consciousness

Incidence

❖ Overt hepatic encephalopathy occurs in 30–45% of patients with cirrhosis

❖ Is the second most common cause for admission following cirrhosis (MC cause is ascites)

Classification

- Type A: Encephalopathy associated with *A*cute liver failure
- Type B:
  - Encephalopathy associated with porto-systemic *B*ypass
  - No intrinsic hepatocellular disease
- Type C:
  - Encephalopathy associated with *C*irrhosis
  - Can be minimal, episodic or persistent

Precipitating Factors

- Related to decreased ammonia clearance or increased ammonia load
- Dietary protein overload: increased ammonia load
- Renal failure: decreased ammonia clearance
- GI bleeds: increased ammonia load
- Infections:
  - Increased tissue catabolism causing increased ammonia load
  - Impaired renal function causing ammonia retention
- Constipation: increases production of ammonia
- Medications:
  - Opioids
  - Benzodiazepines
  - Antidepressants
  - Antipsychotic agents
- Diuretic therapy:
  - Diuretic therapy causes contraction alkalosis
  - This facilitates conversion of ammonium ion to ammonia
  - This increases ammonia load

Pathogenesis

- ***Ammonia hypothesis***:
  - Encephalopathy occurs due to hyperammonemia in cirrhosis
  - Hyperammonemia occurs due to 2 main factors:
    - Loss of hepatocytes:
      - Cirrhosis is associated with the loss of hepatocytes
      - Thus, decrease in mass of functioning liver occurs
      - This prevents detoxification of ammonia
    - Shunting of blood:
      - Cirrhosis causes the formation of porto-systemic shunts
      - Ammonia containing blood is therefore shunted into the systemic circulation
  - Neurotoxic effects of ammonia include:
    - Impairs amino acid metabolism
    - Impairs energy utilization in the brain
    - Inhibits generation of excitatory post-synaptic potentials
- ***GABA hypothesis***:
  - Traditionally encephalopathy was attributed to raised neural GABA activity
  - Later studies showed no change in sensitivity of GABA receptors

Clinical Features

- Asterixis
- Hyperventilation
- Decreased body temperature
- ***Fetor hepaticus***:
  - Sweet musty aroma
  - Due to exhalation of mercaptans
- ***Hepatic myelopathy***:
  - Rarely seen
  - Rapidly progressive
  - Neurological deficits are refractory to medical therapy
  - Symptoms include:
    - Lower extremity weakness, difficulty in walking
    - Spastic paraparesis, hyperreflexia
- Extrapyramidal symptoms:
  - Rarely seen in patients with porto-systemic shunting
  - Due to manganese deposition in basal ganglia
  - Symptoms include:
    - Tremors, bradykinesia
    - Cog-wheel rigidity, shuffling gait

Grades of Hepatic Encephalopathy

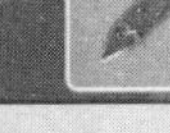

West Haven classification system:
- Grade 0: Covert hepatic encephalopathy
  - Minimal hepatic encephalopathy
  - Previously known as subclinical hepatic encephalopathy

Contd...

Contd...

- Lack of detectable changes in personality or behavior
- Minimal changes in memory and concentration
- Asterixis is absent

❖ Grade 1: Covert hepatic encephalopathy
- Trivial lack of awareness
- Shortened attention span
- Hypersomnia, insomnia, inversion of sleep pattern
- Euphoria, depression or irritability
- Slowing of ability to perform mental tasks
- Asterixis is absent

❖ Grade 2: Overt hepatic encephalopathy
- Lethargy or apathy
- Disorientation, inappropriate behavior
- Slurred speech, asterixis, drowsiness
- Gross deficits in ability to perform mental tasks
- Obvious personality changes, inappropriate behavior
- Intermittent disorientation- ***characteristic***
- Asterixis is present- ***characteristic***

❖ Grade 3: Overt hepatic encephalopathy
- Somnolent, but can be aroused
- Unable to perform mental tasks
- Disorientation with time and place
- Marked confusion, incomprehensible speech
- Amnesia, fits of rage

❖ Grade 4: Overt hepatic encephalopathy
- Coma, with or without response to painful stimuli.

Lab Findings

❖ Blood ammonia levels:
- Elevated blood ammonia levels diagnostic
- Arterial and free venous samples preferred
- Tourniquet use may yield falsely elevated results

❖ EEG:
- High amplitude, low frequency, triphasic waves are characteristic

❖ Visual evoked responses:
- Not commonly used

❖ CT:
- Important to rule out intracranial lesions

❖ MRI:
- Hyperintensity of globus pallidus seen in HE
- Maybe due to manganese deposition in globus pallidus

Differential Diagnosis

❖ Intracranial lesions:
- Subdural hematoma
- Intracranial bleeds

❖ Infections:
- Meningitis
- Encephalitis

❖ Metabolic encephalopathy
❖ Toxic encephalopathy
❖ Uremic encephalopathy

Management

❖ Correct precipitating factors:
- Hypovolemia
- Constipation
- Metabolic disturbances
- Infections
- Gastrointestinal bleeding
- Avoid CNS depressants

❖ Supportive therapy:
- Endotracheal intubation in patients with severe grade 3-4 encephalopathy
- Regularize sleep pattern
- H_1 blockers maybe used to improve sleep disturbances

❖ Decrease ammonia production:
- Dietary protein intake:
  - Consider vegetable source of proteins
  - Consider using branched chain amino acids
  - Can tolerate upto 1.2 g/kg/day or proteins
- Cathartics: lactulose:
  - Mechanism of action:
    - Acts by inhibiting intestinal ammonia production
    - Lactulose gets converted to lactic acid in intestine
    - This creates an acidic environment
    - Acidic environment favors conversion of ammonia to NH_4^+ ion
    - Ammonium ions are not absorbed form the intestines
    - Ammonia is thus excreted eventually
  - Dose:
    - Initial dose 30 mL PO once or twice daily
    - Dose maybe increased as tolerated
    - Dose titrated such that patient has 2-4 loose stools per day
    - High doses (30 mL q2-4H) in severe encephalopathy
- Antibiotics:
  - Commonly used antibiotics are:
    - Neomycin
    - Metronidazole
    - Oral vancomycin
    - Oral quinolones
    - Rifaximin

- Neomycin:
  - Commonly used as second line of management
  - Therapy considered after initiating treatment with lactulose
  - Mechanism is by reducing colonic load of ammoniagenic bacteria
  - Initial dose of 250 mg P.O q6-12H
  - Dose can be increased to maximum of 4 g per day

❖ Increase ammonia clearance:

- Hepa-Merz granules:
  - Can be used to improve ammonia clearance
  - It is a stable salt of 2 constituent amino acids:
    - L- ornithine
    - L- aspartate
  - L- ornithine stimulates urea cycle, thus clearing ammonia
  - L- aspartate acts as a substrate for glutamate, which clears ammonia
- Zinc:
  - Zinc administration increases urea cycle enzyme activity
  - This accelerates ammonia clearance
  - Zinc sulphate used in dose of 600 mg PO q24H
- Other agents used:
  - Sodium benzoate
  - Sodium phenylbutyrate
  - Sodium phenylacetate
  - L- carnitine

SUGGESTED READING

1. Ahboucha, S., Butterworth, R.F. (2004). Pathophysiology of hepatic encephalopathy: a new look at GABA from the molecular standpoint. *Metabolic Brain Disease*, 19(3–4), 331–43.
2. Arroyo, V., et al(1996). Definition and diagnostic criteria of refractory ascites and hepatorenal syndrome in cirrhosis. *Hepatology*, 23(1), 164–76.
3. Betrosian, A.P., Agarwal, B., Douzinas, E.E. (2007). Acute renal dysfunction in liver diseases. *World Journal of Gastroenterology, 13(42), 5552–9.*
4. Bjornsson, E., Olsson, R. (2005). Outcome and prognostic markers in severe drug-induced liver disease. *Hepatology*, 42(2), 481–9.
5. Blei A.T., Córdoba, J. (2001). Practise parameters committee of the American COllege of Gastroenterology- hepatic encephalopathy. *American Journal of Gastroenterology*, 96(7), 1968–76.
6. Butterworth, J., Mackey, D., and Wasnick, J. (2013). *Morgan and Mikhails Clinical Anesthesiology*, 6th ed.. New York: McGraw Hill Education.
7. C, E. (2010). *World Journal of Gastroenterology*.
8. Davis, H.H., Schwartz, D.J., Lefrak, S.S., Susman, N., Schainker, B.A. (1978). Alveolar capillary disequilibrium in hepatic cirrhosis. *Chest*, 73(4):507–11
9. Delcker, A.M., Yang, Z., Qi, X., Fan, D., Han, G. (2000). L-ornithine-l-aspartate vs placebo in the treatment of hepatic encephalopathy: a meta analysis of randomized placebo-controlled trials using individual data. *Hepatology*, 28(5), 783–92.
10. Feldman, M., Friedman, L.S., Sleisenger, M.H. (2002). *Sleisenger and Fordtran's gastrointestinal and liver disease pathophysiology, diagnosis and management*. St. Louis: Saunders.
11. Ferenci, P., Lockwood, A., Mullen, K., Tarter, R., Weissenborn, K., Blei, A.T. (2002). Hepatic encephalopathy- definition, nomenclature, diagnosis and quantification. *Hepatology*, 35(3), 716–21.
12. Garcia-Tsao, G., Parikh, C.R., Viola, A. (2008). Acute kidney injury in cirrhosis. *Hepatology*, 48(6), 2064–77.
13. Gines, A. et al. (1993). Incidence, predictive factors and prognosis of HRS in cirrhosis with ascites. *Gastroenterology*, 105(1), 229–36.
14. Gines, P., et al. (1988). Randomized comparative study of therapeutic paracentesis with and without intravenous albumin in cirrhosis. *Gastroenterology*, 94(6), 1493–502.
15. Gonwa, T.A., Klintmalm, G.B., Levy, M., Jennings, L.S., Goldstein, R.M., Husberg, B.S . (1995). Impact of pretransplant renal function on survival after liver transplantation. *Transplantation*, 59(3), 361–5.
16. Green, J., Better, O.S. (1995). Systemic hypotension and renal failure in obstructive jaundice- mechanistic and therapeutic aspects. *Journal of American Society of Nephrology*, 5(11), 1853–71.
17. Guy, S., et al. (1995). Does nasoenteral nutritional support reduce mortality after liver transplant. *Hepatology*, 22, 144A.
18. Irwin M.G., Trinh, T., Yao, C. (2009). Occupational exposure to anesthetic gases: a role for TIVA. *Expert Opinion on Drug Safety*, 8(4), 473–83.
19. Krowka, M. (2000). Hepatopulmonary syndromes. *Gut*, 1–4.
20. Krowka, M.J., Cortese, D.A. (1990). Hepatopulmonary syndrome: an evolving perspective in the era of liver transplantation. *Hepatology*, 11(1), 138–42.
21. Kwo, P.Y., Cohen, S.M., Lim, J.K. (2017). Evaluation of abnormal liver chemistries. *American Journal of Gastroenterology*, 112(1), 18–35.
22. Lee, W.S., Wong, S.Y., Ivy, D.D., Sokol, R.J (2018). Hepatopulmonary syndrome and portopulmonary hypertension in children: recent advances in diagnosis and management. *The Journal of Pediatrics*, 14–21.
23. Low, G., Alexander, G.J., Lomas, D.J.. (2015). Hepatorenal syndrome: aetiology, diagnosis and treatment. *Gastroenterology Research and Practice*, 207012.

24. Machicao, V. I., Balakrishnan, M., Fallon, M.B. (2014). Pulmonary complications in chronic liver disease. *Hepatology*, 59(4), 1627–37.
25. Marchesini, G., Fabbri, A., Bianchi, G., Brizi, M., Zoli, M. (1996). Zinc supplementation and amino acid-nitrogen metabolism in patients with advanced cirrhosis. *Hepatology*, 23(5), 1084–92.
26. Miller, R.D., Eriksson, L., Fleisher, L, Wiener-Kronish, J., Cohen, N., Young, W. (2015). *Millers Anesthesia*. 8th ed. Amsterdam: Elsevier Health.
27. Moller S., Becker U. (1992). Insulin-like growth factor 1 and growth hormone in chronic liver Disease. *Digestive Diseases*, 10, 239–48.
28. Mushlin P.S., Gelman, S. (2010). *Hepatic physiology and pathophysiology*. 7th ed. Philadelphia: Churchill Livingstone.
29. Nadim, M.K., et al. (2012). Hepatorenal syndrome: the 8th international consensus conference of the acute dialysis quality initiative (ADQI) group. *Critical Care*, 16(1), R23.
30. National Halothane Study: Possible association between halothane anesthesia and postoperative hepatic necrosis. (1966). *Journal of American Medical Association*, 197(10), 775–88.
31. Parks, R.W., Diamond, T., McCrory, D.C., Johnston, G.W., Rowlands, B.J. (1994). Prospective study of postoperative renal funstion in obstructive jaundice & the effect of perioperative dopamine. *British Journal of Surgery*, 81(3), 437–9.
32. Poordad, F.F. (2007). The burden of hepatic encephalopathy. *Alimentary Pharmacology and Therapeutics*, 25(Suppl 1), 3–9.
33. Rodríguez-Roisin, R., Krowka, m.J., Hervé, Ph., Fallon, M.B. (2004). ERS Task Force Pulmonary- Hepatic Vascular disorders. *European Respiratory Journal*, 861–80.
34. Salerno, F., Gerbes, A., Ginès, P., Wong, F., Arroyo V. (2007). Diagnosis, prevention and treatment of hepatorenal syndrome in cirrhosis. *Gut*, 56(8), 1310–8.
35. Scahper, J., et al. (2013). Regional sympathetic blockade attenuates activation of intestinal macrophages and reduces gut barrier failure. *Anesthesiology*, 118(1), 134–42.
36. Schafer, D.F., Jones, E.A. (1982). Hepatic encephalopathy and the GABA neurotransmitter system. *Lancet*, 319(8262), 18–20.
37. Seki E., Schnabl, B. (2012). Role of innate immunity and the microbiota in liver fibrosis: crosstalk between the liver and gut. *Journal of Physiology*, 590(3), 447–58.
38. Shawcross, D.L., et al. (2016). How to diagnose and manage hepatic encephalopathy: a consensus statement on roles and responsibilities beyond the liver specialist. *European Journal of Gastroenterology and Hepatology*, 28(2), 146–52.
39. Tyagi, P., Sharma, P., Sharma, B.C., Puri, A.S., Kumar, A., Sarin, S.K. (2011). Prevention of hepatorenal syndrome in patients with cirrhosis & ascites: a pilot RCT between pentoxifylline and placebo. *European Journal of Gastroenterology and Hepatology*, 23(3), 210–7.

Pain and Regional Anesthesia

ASSESSMENT OF PAIN

Introduction

- Pain is what the patient says it is: ***John Bonica***
- Biggest problem in the assessment of pain is that it is subjective
- While patients with postoperative pain may require significantly lesser evaluation, those with chronic pain may require more extensive evaluation
- WHO (1996) stated that upto 80% of patients may be inadequately treated for pain

History

- History of presenting illness:
  - Onset: Sudden (fracture pain)/insidious (migraine)
  - Duration: Acute or chronic
  - Type of pain:
    - Neuralgic (shooting/stabbing)
    - Deafferentiation pain (burning)
    - Malignancy (dull and boring)
  - Site: May be referred pain
  - Radiation of pain
  - Continuous/intermittent/occasional
  - Aggravating/relieving factors
  - Associated bowel and bladder disturbances, numbness and weakness
  - Previous history of interventions and the efficacy of such treatment
- Personal history:
  - Job satisfaction, work compensation
  - Habits: Tobacco chewing, smoking, alcohol
  - Marital life, family disputes, children, menstrual history

Physical Examination

- Pallor, icterus, cyanosis, clubbing
- Lymphadenopathy, edema, rashes
- Vital signs
- Central nervous system:
  - Higher mental functions: Sensory and motor system
  - Cranial nerve examination: Reflexes and gait
- Trigger point detection
- Straight leg raising test for back pain with radiculopathy
- Paraspinal tenderness for facetal problems
- Tinels test for nerve compression

Evaluation of Severity of Pain

Categorical Evaluation

- Pain graded as absent, mild, moderate, severe and excruciating
- Simple but not sensitive test

Numerical Scale

- 11 point scale where 0 is no pain and 10 represents worst pain
- Unidimensional scale

Visual Analogue Scale

- Most popular scale as it is easiest and simplest
- Pain assessment done as self report on single dimension
- Consists of a 10 cm scale with digits from 1 to 10
- There are no gradations on the side which the patient sees
- The 100 gradations are only visible to the person evaluating the pain
- Person asked to compare current pain to worst pain he has ever faced in life (like labor pain, surgical pain/fracture pain, etc.)
- Useful for pain relief follow up by asking the patient to compare pre-treatment and post-treatment pain

McGill Pain Questionnaire

- Assesses pain in a multimodal way
- Measures pain in three ways:
  - Sensory: Discriminative (nociceptive pathway)
  - Motivational: Affective (reticular and limbic pathway)
  - Cognitive: Evaluative (cerebral cortex)

- Contains a checklist of words describing symptoms
- Checklist contains 20 sets of descriptive words:
  - Aspects 1–10 represents sensory aspects of pain
  - Aspects 11–15 represent affective aspects
  - Aspect 16 represents evaluative aspect
  - Aspects 17–20 other miscellaneous aspects
- Patient selects the sets which apply to his/her pain and circles the words in each set which best describe his pain
- A numerical value is attached to each word
- The sum of all points gives a rank value which is called ***Pain Rating Index (PRI)***
- Each aspect of pain can also be evaluated individually
- Can also be used as a diagnostic tool

Breakthrough Questionnaire: To Assess Breakthrough Pain in Cancer Patients

Body Chart:

- Different sites of pain are marked at the time of evaluation
- Marking is done along with the nature of each, so that it is available at the time of review
- Duration, intensity, effect of movement, superficial/deep nature of pain and effect on sleep recorded on chart

Evaluation of Etiology of Pain

- Plain radiography: Inexpensive, quick and can be done without preparation
- Ultrasonography: Evaluation of abdominal organs
- Doppler: Evaluates arterial and venous systems
- CT scan:
  - Detects acute hemorrhage
  - Gives excellent bony detail
- MRI:
  - Good for soft tissue characterization
  - Useful for diagnosis of nerve entrapment syndromes
- Scintigraphy: For functional status of an organ
- Epiduroscopy:
  - Fibreoptic camera is inserted through sacral hiatus into lower epidural space
  - Camera guided upwards towards lower lumber discs and nerve roots
  - Allows color visualization of dura, blood vessels, fat, areolar tissue and pathological changes in epidural space
- Electromyography:
  - Employs needle electrodes to record potentials in individual muscles
  - Muscle potentials are recorded while at rest and then as the patient is asked to move the muscle
  - Triphasic motor unit action potential is usually seen when the patient moves his muscle
  - Abnormal findings, as in denervation, include:
    - Persistent insertion potentials
    - Presence of sharp positive waves
    - Fibrillatory activity
    - Fasciculation potentials
  - Abnormalities in muscles produces:
    - Changes in amplitude and duration of action potential
    - Polyphasic action potentials
  - Can be used to:
    - Distinguish between neurogenic and myogenic disorders
    - Confirm diagnosis of entrapment syndrome, neural trauma and polyneuropathies
    - Localize lesion to spinal cord/nerve root/limb plexus/peripheral nerve
- Nerve conduction studies:
  - Peripheral motor or sensory nerve is supramaximally stimulated
  - Needle electrodes record potentials in the appropriate muscles
  - Characteristics studied:
    - Latency:
      - Time between stimulation and onset of muscle potential
      - Measures fastest conducting motor fibers in the nerve
    - Amplitude: Indicates number of functional motor units
    - Duration: Reflects range of conduction velocities in the nerve
  - Can distinguish between mononeuropathy and polyneuropathy:
    - Mononeuropathies due to trauma/compression
    - Polyneuropathies can be:
      - Demyelination neuropathies:
        - Due to inherited and autoimmune neuropathies
        - Causes slow nerve conduction with prolonged latency
      - Axonal neuropathy:
        - Causes reduction in amplitude of action potential with preservation of conduction velocities
        - This neuropathy occurs due to toxic, inherited, traumatic and ischemic diseases
      - Diabetic neuropathy: is mixed type.

- Other investigations:
  - Arthrography
  - PET scan
  - Arteriography
  - Myelography

Psychological Evaluation

- Important as patients with chronic pain often have psychological problems like:
  - Somatization disorder
  - Conversion disorder
  - Hypochondriasis
  - Depression
- Determines contribution of affective and behavioral factors to perception of pain

Waddells Nonorganic Signs

- Consists of a group of physical signs which may indicate non-organic/psychological component of low backache
- These are:
  - Tenderness: Superficial sensitivity to light touch over lumbar spine/tenderness over large area
  - Simulation: Axial loading where light pressure is applied to skull in upright position, simulated rotation of lumbar spine with shoulders
  - Distraction: More than 40 difference in sitting vs supine straight leg raising test
  - Regional disturbances:
    - Motor: Generalized giving way
    - Sensory: N-dermatomal loss of sensation to pin prick in lower limbs
  - Overreaction: Disproportionate pain response to testing
- Any individual sign marks its category as positive
- When three or more categories are positive, the finding is considered clinically significant
- Detects non organic component to pain but does not exclude organic cause

Minnesota Multiphasic Personality Inventory

- Consists of a 566 item true-false questionnaire
- Defines patient's personality on 10 clinical scales
- Three validity scales identify patients who are deliberately trying to hide traits or alter results
- Test is lengthy and some questions may be insulting
- Cannot reliably distinguish organic and functional pain but gives an idea about the role of psychological factors

Beck's Depression Inventory: Used to Identify Patients with Major Depression

Symptom check List 90:

- 90 items problems checklist
- Allows examinee to rate symptoms of physical and emotional distress on a 5 point scale

Multidimensional Pain Inventory (MPI)

Medical Outcomes Survey 36 Item Short Form (SF 36)

Pain Disability Index (PDI)

Oswestry Disability Questionnaire (ODQ)

Evaluation of Outcome of Pain

- Success of treatment regime can be decided only if a positive response lasts for more than 3 weeks
- Evaluation graded in terms of quality of life too and not just with the pain score

PAIN EVALUATION IN CHILDREN

Introduction

- Evaluation of pain in children is tricky as:
  - Pediatric patient may not be able to express pain in suitable words
  - Children may not reveal pain for fear of injections
- Physiological fetal pain perception systems develop at around 26 weeks of gestation
- Babies have a mature nervous system, able to feel pain and which is unfortunately coupled with an immature ability to produce neurochemicals which can inhibit pain

Clinical Assessment

- Mostly indirect assessment in neonates by observing physiological changes or behavioral responses of neonate/infant to pain
- Physiological changes:
  - Tachycardia
  - Tachypnea
  - Hypertension
  - Palmar diaphoresis
  - Behavioral changes:
    - Changes in facial expressions:
      - Eyebrow bulge
      - Eye squeeze
      - Nasolabial furrow
      - Pursing of lips
      - Taut tongue
      - Chin quivering
    - Changes in body movement: Diffuse body movement to noxious stimuli
    - Changes in type of cry

Pain Measurement in Preschool Children

Happy-Sad Face Scale

- Also useful in illiterate people
- Shows child's face in different moods
- Child asked to select facial expression which best reflects pain expression
- Assesses affective and fear component of pain

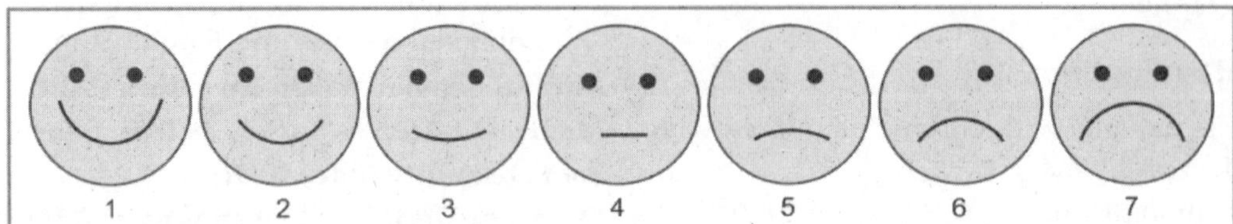

Oucher Scale

- Shows photos of a Caucasian child face with increasing levels of discomfort
- Child selects facial expression which best reflects their experience of hurt
- These photos are used for children who cannot count
- On the left is a numerical scale for older children who can count till 100

Nancy-Hesters Poker Chip Pain Rating Scale

- Four red poker chips are aligned horizontally in front of child
- Child is told that the chips are pieces of hurt and that the 1st chip is just a little hurt, 2nd a little more hurt, and 4th is most hurt
- Ask the child how many pieces of hurt do you have and assess according to the response

Color Scale

- Child asked to select a color using marker/crayons which is like their worst hurt, then a color like a little less hurt, even less hurt and finally no hurt
- A numerical value can be placed on each color
- Asking the child to select a color which is most like the pain they are currently experiencing can then assess pain intensity

Wong Bakers Faces Scale: Consists Six Faces Ranging from Very Happy to Tearful Face

Description	Alert Smiling	No humour Serious face	Furrowed brow Pursed lips Breath holding	Wrinkled nose Raised upper lip Rapid breathing	Slow blink Open mouth	Eyes closed Moaning Crying
Category	No pain	Pains little bit	Pains little more	Pains even more	Pains whole lot	Pains worst
Score	0	1	2	3	4	5
Alternate score	0	2	4	6	8	10

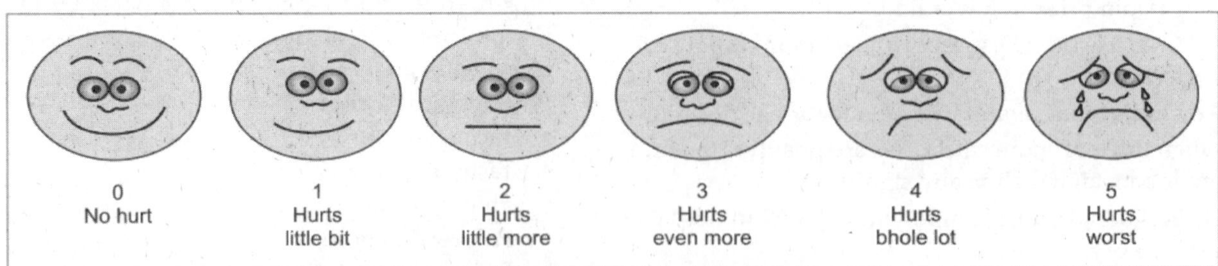

Activity Tolerance Scale

Pain	Score
No pain	0
Can be ignored	2
Interferes with tasks	4
Interferes with concentration	6
Interferes with basic needs	8
Bed rest required	10

Comfort Scale

- 8 indicators used:
  - Alertness
  - Calmness/agitation
  - Muscle tone
  - Blood pressure
  - Respiratory response
  - Physical movement
  - Facial tension
  - Heart rate

- Each indicator scored between 1–5 based on behavior exhibited
- Patient observed for 2 minutes and total score is calculated
- Ranges between 8–40
- Range between 17–26 indicates adequate sedation and pain control
- Useful in ICU environment

FLACC Behavioral Pain Assessment Tool

- Uses Faces, Legs, Activity, Cry and Consolability (FLACC)
- Each of these is scored between 0–2 to provide a score ranging 0–10

Cheops Scale (Children Hospital of Eastern Ontario Pain Scale)

- *Gold standard* for comparative purposes
- Has 6 categories of behavior which are scored individually (0.2 or 1.3)
- These are then totalled for a score between 4–13
- Complicated and impractical to use

Chipps Scale (Children Infants Postoperative Pain Scale)

- Includes 5 behavioral items found to be consistently indicative of pain in children
- These items are:
  - Crying
  - Facial expression
  - Posture of trunk
  - Posture of legs
  - Motor restlessness

Others

- Ladder scale
- Linear analogue scale
- Objective pain scale
- ***Abu-Saad*** pediatric pain assessment tool
- ***Varini-Thompson*** pediatric pain questionnaire
- Premature Infant Pain Profile (PIPP)

Pain Measurement in School Aged Children

- Able to read and write and comprehend what is explained to them
- Scales used are:
  - Six point (0–5) numerical verbal pain score: used in children > 9 years to assess headache
  - 0–100 numerical scale
  - Visual analogue scale
  - Macgills pain questionnaire
  - Wong bakers FACES pain rating scale
  - Comfort scale
  - Activity tolerance scale

PHANTOM LIMB PAIN

Introduction

- Phenomenon occurring in an amputated limb where sensation persists that the amputated limb is still there and moving like the other parts of body
- In case of the limb, most of these sensations are painful and is made worse by stress, anxiety and weather changes
- ***Phantosmia***: Perception of an odorant where none is there
- ***Phantogeusia/dysgeusia***:
  - Distortion in the perception of a taste
  - Perception of a taste where there has been no tastant ingested

Incidence: Occurs in Upto 80% of Amputations

Location of Pain

- Peripheral limb following amputation
- Tooth pain following tooth extraction
- Breast pain following mastectomy
- Appendix following appendicectomy

Pathogenesis

- Phantom limb pain occurs due to ***law of projection*** which states that no matter where a particular sensory pathway is stimulated along its course to the cortex, the conscious sensation produced is referred to the location of receptor
- The ends of the nerve cut at the time of amputation form nerve tangles called neuromas
- These may discharge spontaneously or when pressure is applied on them
- The impulses generated in them are in the nerve fibres which previously came from sense organs of the amputated limb
- Thus sensations are projected to where the receptors used to be

Mechanism

- Peripheral mechanisms:
  - Caused by central and peripheral mechanisms
  - Due to formation of neuromas
  - Increased C fibre activity in amputated limb
  - Increased Na^+ channel activation
- Central mechanism: ***Reorganization of Somatosensory Cortex theory***:
  - Abnormal firing of internuncial neurons occurs, due to development of new synaptic connections in cerebral cortex
  - Area of somatosensory cortex representing the hand lies in close proximity to that representing the arm and face

- Thus, when the hand is amputated, new synaptic connections are formed between the areas representing arm, hand and face
- Thus, sensations from arm and face are transmitted to the amputated stump where the hand used to be

Manifestations

- Pain may be immediate, occurring at the time of amputation
- Most commonly, pain occurs within first few days following amputation
- Pain is not felt all the time, only few days in a month
- Most sensations are of warmth, itching, squeezing, tingling
- Aggravated by stress, anxiety and weather changes
- 50% patients experience reduction in pain over time
- In remaining 50% patients, pain increases or remains unchanged

Prophylaxis

- Preemptive analgesia is important as brain seems to implant sensation from preoperative state
- This can be done by:
  - Perioperative epidural infusion of opioids/local anesthetics/clonidine
  - Continuous brachial plexus block with memantine (an NMDA antagonist)
  - Opioids/neuroleptanalgesia

Treatment

- Pharmacological methods:
  - Antidepressants
  - Neuroleptics
  - Sodium channel blockers
  - Opioids
  - Gabapentin (NMDA antagonist)
- Non-pharmacological methods:
  - Heat application
  - Relaxation techniques: Reduce stress
  - Massage of amputated area
  - Transcutaneous Electrical Nerve Stimulation (TENS)
  - Biofeedback
  - Spinal cord stimulation
    - Electrical stimulator is implanted under skin
    - Electrode is placed next to spinal cord
    - The nerve pathway in the spinal cord is stimulated
    - This interferes with pain impulses projected to the brain, which cause phantom limb pain

POST DURAL PUNCTURE HEADACHE

Introduction

Headache resulting from any breach of the dura mater, occurring with an incidence as high as 25%.

Etiology

- Diagnostic lumbar tap
- Myelogram
- Spinal anesthesia
- Epidural wet tap

Pathophysiology

- Dura is under longitudinal strain
- Thus, a slit which is oriented perpendicular to this longitudinal tension will be pulled open
- A slit oriented parallel to this tension will be pulled to close the slit

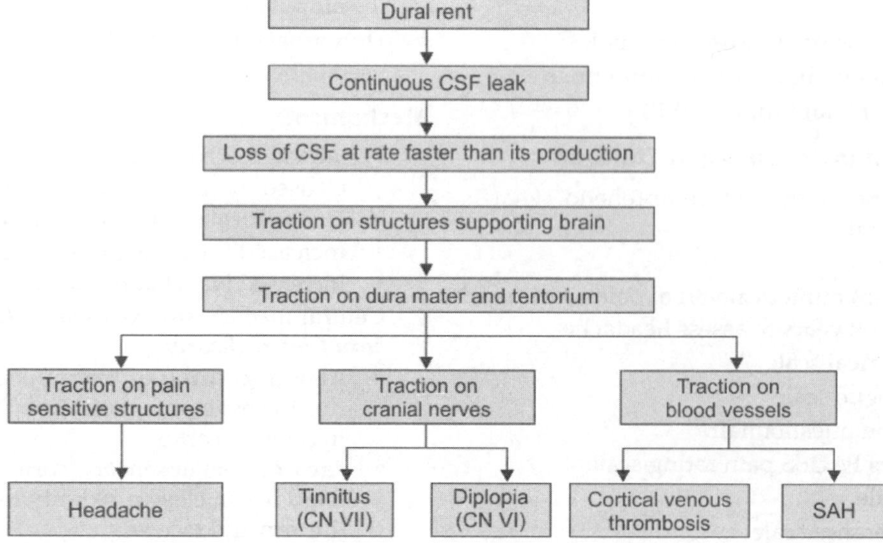

Factors Increasing Incidence 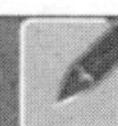

- Age: More common in young patients
- Gender: Female more affected than males
- Pregnancy: More common in pregnant patients
- Needle size: More common with larger needles (27 or 25 G preferred)
- Needle bevel: Less when needle bevel is parallel to long axis of dura
- Needle type: More common with cutting tip than pencil tip (*Whitacres needle preferred*)
- Dural punctures: More common with multiple punctures

Clinical Features

- Headache:
  - Occurs 12–72 hours following procedure
  - Usually occurs immediately after procedure
  - Bilateral, frontal/retro-orbital headache
  - May be occipital and extend into neck and shoulder
  - Associated with nausea and photophobia
  - *Hallmark* association with body position where headache increases with sitting/standing and reduced on lying down
  - Increased during coughing/staining
- Associated features:
  - Tinnitus (CN VIII traction)
  - Diplopia (CN VI traction)
  - Cortical venous thrombosis
  - Subarachnoid hemorrhage rarely
  - Subdural hemorrhage rarely

Management

- Conservative management:
  - Bed rest decreases the hydrostatic pressure which drives CSF leak
  - Adequate IV or oral fluid administration
  - Analgesics: NSAIDs, sumatriptan
  - Caffeine:
    Stimulates CSF production and also causes vasoconstriction of intracranial vessels
    300–500 mg P.O/IV Q12H
  - Stool softeners and soft diet to minimize Valsalva straining
- Invasive management:
  - Epidural blood patch:
    - Very effective in treating PDPH
    - 90% patients respond to single patch
    - 90% of initial non-responders obtain relief from second patch
    - Done after giving a trial of conservative therapy for 12–24 hours
    - Mechanism of action:
      - Forms a clot over the dural rent
      - This prevents further CSF leaks
    - Injected blood spreads over spinal segments more in the cranial direction
    - Technique requires two clinicians
    - Epidural puncture is done at same space or one space lower
    - Once in epidural space, 15–20 mL of blood is drawn from forearm under aseptic conditions
    - Blood is slowly injected through the back until pain is felt in the back
    - Patient placed supine for 1–2 hours following procedure to reduce CSF leak from dural rent
    - Prophylactic epidural patch not very effective in preventing PDPH
    - Side effects of blood patch:
      - Backache
      - Radicular pain
      - Epidural hematoma
      - Bradycardia
      - Cranial nerve palsies
  - Epidurally administered fibrin glue is an effective alternative
  - Epidural saline bolus/ACTH hormone requires further investigation
  - Surgical closure of dural rent: Last resort

PAIN THERAPY IN CANCER PATIENTS

Introduction

Management of cancer pain is multifaceted and includes:

- Antineoplastic treatment
- Pharmacological management
- Interventional management
- Behavioral and psychological management
- Hospice care

Mechanism of Cancer Pain

I. Somatic/Nociceptive Pain:

- Originates from skin, muscle and bone
- Through Aδ and C fibres
- Eg-Due to tumor infilteration of bone/joints

II. Visceral Pain:

- Originates from solid or hollow visceral organs
- Mediated by visceral sympathetic efferent fibres
- Eg-Due to obstruction of hollow viscus

III. Sympathetic Pain:

- Occurs after nerve or limb injury
- Associated with allodynia, hyperpathia, sudomotor dysfunction

- ❖ Poorly responsive to opioids
- ❖ Eg-Radiation nerve injury

IV. Neuropathic Pain:

- ❖ Sharp lancinating pain
- ❖ Poorly responsive to opioids
- ❖ Eg-Vinca alkaloid induced neuropathy

Causes

I. Cancer itself

II. Cancer therapy pain:

- ❖ Chemotherapy:
  - Mucositis
  - Constipation
  - Abdominal cramps
  - Peripheral neuropathy
  - Diarrhea
- ❖ Radiotherapy:
  - Mucositis
  - Peripheral neuropathy
- ❖ Surgical treatment:
  - Postoperative pain Phantom limb pain
  - Stump pain Post mastectomy pain

Assessment

- ❖ Simple Descriptive Pain Distress Scale
  - None
  - Annoying
  - Uncomfortable
  - Dreadful
  - Horrible
  - Agonizing
- ❖ Numerical Pain Distress Scale
  - 0 – no pain
  - 5 – distressing pain
  - 10 – agonizing pain
- ❖ Visual Analogue Scale
  - 0 – no pain
  - 10 – unbearable pain

Modalities of Management

I. Pharmacological:

- ❖ Analgesics:
  - NSAIDs
  - Opioids
- ❖ Adjuvants:
  - Antidepressants
  - Anticonvulsants
  - Neuroleptics
  - Corticosteroids
  - Systemic local anesthetics
  - $\alpha 2$ adrenergic agonists
  - Botulinum toxin

II. Nonpharmacological:

- ❖ Injection Techniques:
  - Somatic and sympathetic nerve blocks
  - Intrathecal and epidural neurolytics
  - Cryoanalgesia
- ❖ Neuroablative techniques:
  - Radiofrequency denervation
  - Pituitary injection of alcohol
- ❖ Neurostimulatory techniques:
  - Transcutaneous Electrical Nerve Stimulation - TENS
  - Spinal Cord Stimulation–SCS
  - Intracerebral Stimulation–ICS
- ❖ Complementary/Alternative approaches:
  - Massage
  - Hot/cold sponges
  - Paraffin baths
  - Fluidotherapy
- ❖ Psychological interventions:
  - Lifestyle changes
  - Yoga
  - Biofeedback relaxation
- ❖ Palliative:
  - Deep X-rays
  - Tumor excision
  - Radiotherapy
- ❖ Rehabilitation approaches

I. Pharmacotherapy:

I. PCT and NSAIDs:

No.	Drug	Dosage	Side effects
1.	Acetaminophen	650 mg Q4H PO	
		10 – 15 mg/kg Q4H PO	
		15 – 20 mg/kg Q4H PR	
2.	Ibuprofen	400 – 600 mg Q6H PO	Peptic ulceration
		10 mg/kg Q6H PO	Gastric erosions
			Nausea vomiting
3.	Ketorolac	60 mg initially	Bleeding diathesis
		30 mg Q6H IM	Thrombocytopenia
		Not to exceed 5 days	Hepatorenal dysfunction

II. Opioids:

No.	Drug	Oral	Parenteral	Side effects
1.	Morphine	30 mg Q3–4H	10 mg Q3–4H	Sedation
2.	Morphine SR	90 – 120 mg Q12H	NA	Nausea constipation
3.	Hydromor-phone	6 mg Q3–4H	1.5 mg Q3–4H	Respiratory depression
4.	Methadone	20 mg Q6–8H	10 mg Q6–8H	Myoclonus
5.	Codeine	60 mg Q3–4H	60 mg Q2H IM or SC	Tolerance
6.	Oxycodone	10 mg Q3–4H	NA	Physical dependance
7.	Fentanyl	Trandermal 25/50/100 μ (lasts for 72 hrs)		GI toxicity

III. Adjuvant Analgesics:

No.	Drug	Dose	Indications
1.	Dexamethasone	High dose regimen – 100 mg/day	Acute severe pain
		Low dose regimen–10–20 mg/day PO/IV	Bone pain
			Raised ICT, visceral pain
2.	Prednisone	40–100 mg PO	Bone pain
			Raised ICT, visceral pain
3.	Carbamazepine	200–1600 mg PO	Trigeminal neuralgia
			Neuropathic pain
4.	Phenytoin	300–500 mg PO	Neuropathic pain
5.	Amitriptyline	25–150 mg PO	Neuropathic pain with depression
6.	Lidocaine	5 mg/kg IV/SC	
7.	Mexiletine	450–600 mg PO	
8.	Dextroamphetamine	5–10 mg PO	
9.	Methylphenidate	10–15 mg PO	
10.	Ketamine	0.15 mg/kg/hr IV	Refractory pain resistant to opioids
11.	Gabapentin	100–300 mg/day upto 3600 mg/day	Trigeminal neuralgia
			Post herpetic neuralgia
			Diabetic peripheral neuropathy
12.	Pregabalin	75–150 mg Q12H PO	Trigeminal neuralgia
			Post herpetic neuralgia
			Diabetic peripheral neuropathy

II. Non-pharmacological Approaches

- Physical modalities:
  - Rehabilitation
  - Heat application
  - TENS
  - Therapeutic exercise and massage
- Behavioural interventions:
  - Meditation
  - Hypnosis
  - Music therapy
  - Systemic desensitization
- Complementary medicine:
  - Acupuncture

III. Radiation and Chemotherapy

IV. Palliative Surgeries

V. Special Procedures

Neurolytic Neural Blockade

No.	Type of pain	Type of block
Peripheral nerve blocks		
1.	Facial and neck pain	Trigeminal nerve, Glossopharyngeal nerve
2.	Chest and abdominal wall	Intercostal/paravertebral nerve block
3.	Intrathoracic malignancy	Intercostal nerve block
4.	Perineal	Sacral nerve
Sympathetic nerve blocks		
1.	Head, neck, arm pain	Stellate ganglion block
2.	Pancreas, upper abdominal pain	Celiac plexus block
3.	Pelvic pain	Hypogastric plexus block
4.	Leg pain	Lumbar sympathetic block

Transcutaneous Electrical Nerve Stimulation

- Stimulates larger afferent fibres
- May provide pain relief in neuropathic cancer pain
- Electrodes are placed in the same dermatome as the pain
- Stimulated periodically by direct current from a generator

Spinal Cord Stimulation

- Activates descending modulating systems
- Inhibits sympathetic outflow
- Most effective for neuropathic pain
- Electrodes placed in epidural space and connected to subcutaneous generator

Intracerebral Stimulation

- Electrodes implanted into periacqueductal and periventricular grey matter
- May cause infections and hemorrhage

Intrathecal Pumps

- Used in patients with unmanageable side effects of opioids
- Should have life expectancy >3 months
- 1/10th IV dose required for epidural pumps
- 1/100th IV dose required for intrathecal pumps
- Expensive procedure

Radiofrequency Ablation

- Radiofrequency current into affected nerve destroys it
- Used for intercostal N, trigeminal N, paravertebral N

PATIENT CONTROLLED ANALGESIA

Introduction

Technique of pain management which allows patient to administer their own analgesics on demand

Types

- Patient Controlled Intravenous Analgesia (PCA)
- Patient Controlled Epidural Analgesia (PCEA)
- Patient Controlled Intranasal Analgesia (PCINA)
- Patient Controlled Transdermal Analgesia (PCTA)
- Patient Controlled Regional Analgesia (PCRA)
- Subcutaneous Patient Controlled Analgesia

Variables

I. Bolus dose/demand dose

- Dose which is delivered when patient activates PCA due to severe pain
- Optimal dose to be chosen
- Optimal dose causes good analgesia with minimal side effects
- High dose can cause respiratory depression

II. Lockout interval

- Time from end of delivery of first dose until machine responds to another demand
- Effectively, a safety feature of PCA pumps
- Ranges from 5–20 minutes
- Affects efficacy of PCA
- Too long lockout: Inadequate analgesia
- Too short lockout: Increased side effects

III. Background infusion

- Improves analgesia and prevents arousal with severe pain
- Usually reserved for opioid tolerant patient with chronic pain
- Also used in pediatric population
- Opioids will be delivered regardless of level of sedation

IV. Dose limits

- Safety feature
- Limits maximum amount of drug that can be delivered over a certain period
- 1 hr and 4 hr limits present
- Commonly 10 mg in 1 hr and 30 mg in 4 hours for morphine
- Prevents overdose of analgesics

V. Loading dose

- Total opioid dose initially required to provide analgesia
- Administered by pre-setting PCA pump

Assessment During PCA

- Analgesia levels: VAS scores
- Sedation levels: ***Richmond Agitation Sedation Scale*** (RASS Score)
- Respiratory assessment:
- Pulse oximetry: Especially for obesity, OSAS, old patient
- Capnography: For respiratory depression

Indications

- Postoperative pain management
- Chronic pancreatitis
- Post-trauma
- Burns
- Sickle cell crisis

Contraindications

- Pulmonary disease
- Obstructive sleep apnea
- Renal/hepatic dysfunction
- Congestive cardiac failure
- Closed head injury
- Altered mental status
- Lactating mothers
- Very young children (< 5 yrs)
- If > 2 risk factors are present, PCA avoided in standard dosing regimens

Advantages

- Superior pain relief with less medications
- Reduces delay between request for pain medication and administration

- Improves postoperative pulmonary function
- Reduces postoperative pulmonary complications
- Less potential for overdose when smaller doses are prescribed
- Lesser daytime sedation
- Higher patient acceptance and satisfaction
- Improved sleep pattern
- Earlier postoperative mobilization

Disadvantages

- Narcotic dependence
- High cost – requires special equipment
- Patient factors:
  - Requires mental alertness
  - Physical ability to press the button
  - Ability to understand concept of PCA
  - Caution required in patients with liver/renal/pulmonary disease

Complications

- Nausea, vomiting
- Constipation
- Pruritis
- Excessive sedation
- Faulty equipment:
  - Failure of antireflux valve
  - Faulty programme
  - Patient tampering
  - Use of pump close to MRI machine

Drugs Used

- Most commonly morphine
- Hydromorphone
- Fentanyl
- Sufentanyl
- Tramadol

Regimens

IV. PCA:

No.	Opioid	Demand dose	Lockout	Basal infusion
1.	Morphine	1–2 mg	6–10 min	0–2 mg/hr
2.	Hydromorphone	0.2–0.4 mg	6–10 min	0–0.4 mg/hr
3.	Fentanyl	20–50 µg	5–10 min	0–50 µg/hr
4.	Sufentanyl	4–6 µg	5–10 min	0–8 µg/hr
5.	Tramadol	10–20 mg	6–10 min	0–20 mg/hr

PCEA

No.	Drug	Continuous	Demand dose	Lockout interval
1.	0.05% bupivacaine	4 mL/hr	2 mL/hr	10 min
	5 µg/ml fentanyl			
2.	0.0625% bupivacaine	4–6 mL/hr	3–4 mL/hr	10–15 min
	5 µg/mL fentanyl			
3.	0.1% bupivacaine	6 mL/hr	2 mL/hr	10–15 min
	5 µg/mL fentanyl			
4.	0.2% ropivacaine	5 mL/hr	2 mL/hr	20 min
	5 µg/mL fentanyl			

Adjuvants to PCA

- Ketamine maybe added to reduce side effects and improve analgesia
- Antiemetics like droperidol and cyclizine added to reduce nausea

PREEMPTIVE ANALGESIA

Introduction

Antinociceptive treatment that prevents establishment of altered central processing of afferent input from injuries.

Pathophysiology

- Tissue injury produces biphasic response
- *Peripheral sensitization* –
  - Due to local release of neurotransmitters
  - Substance-P, prostaglandins, bradykinins, serotonin, histamine
- *Central sensitization:*
  - Continued barrage of afferent input from site of injury
  - Activation of NMDA receptors in spinal cord occurs
- Noxious stimuli sensitize nervous system to subsequent stimuli
- Normal pain response curve shifts to left
- Causes hyperalgesia and allodynia
- Preemptive analgesia aims to prevent sensitization
- 2 essential requirements:
  - Establishment of effective level of analgesia
  - Inhibition of inflammatory mediators

Preemptive Analgesia Strategies

- Infilteration with local anesthetics
- Nerve blocks

- Epidural block with catheter
- Subarachnoid block
- Drugs:
  - NSAIDs, COX-2 inhibitors: Paracetamol, ketorolac, etoricoxib
  - NMDA antagonists: Ketamine, magnesium
  - Alpha 2 agonists: Clonidine, dexmedetomidine
  - Glucocorticoids: Dexamethasone
  - Cholinergic drugs: Nicotine
  - Gabapentin, pregabalin

Principles of Preemptive Analgesia

- Depth of analgesia must be adequate to block nociceptive input
- Technique of analgesia should be extensive enough to include entire surgical field
- Duration of analgesia should include both surgery and postsurgery

Use

- Preemptive epidural analgesia effective in reducing analgesic consumption
- Preincision infilteration with local anesthetics beneficial
- Multimodal approach addressing multiple sites along pain pathway needed to prevent central sensitization

No.	Drug	Route	Initial dose	Continuous dose
	Epidural analgesia			
1.	Morphine	Epidural	3 mg	1-2 mg/hr
2.	Buprenorphine	Epidural	0.1 mg	0.02–0.03 mg/hr
	Supraspinal analgesia			
3.	Ketamine	Intravenous	1 mg/kg	0.5 mg/kg/hr

Efficacy

- Controversy surrounding use in clinical setting despite being effective in animal models
- Not all clinical trials demonstrate efficacy
- May reduce risk of developing chronic postoperative pain
- Reduces incidence of phantom limb pain post limb amputation

POSTOPERATIVE PAIN RELIEF

Adverse Effects of Acute Pain

- Cardiovascular:
  - Tachycardia
  - Hypertension
  - Increased cardiac workload
- Respiratory:
  - Respiratory muscle spasm
  - Atelectasis
  - Hypoxia
  - Increased risk of LRTI
- Gastrointestinal: Increased postop ileus
- Renal:
  - Increased risk of oliguria
  - Urinary retention
- Coagulation: Increased risk of thromboemboli
- Immunological: Impaired immune function
- Muscular: Muscle weakness and fatigue
- Psychological: Anxiety, fear and frustration

Clinical Assessment

- Categorical Rating Scale
- Visual Analogue Scale
- Verbal Numerical Rating Scale

Management

- Preemptive analgesia: Started before onset of pain
- Balanced analgesia: By multimodal approach

PHARMACOLOGICAL SYSTEMIC OPIOIDS

Codeine

- Weak opioid
- Combined with paracetamol

Dextropropoxyphene

- Weak opioid
- Combined with paracetamol

Methadone

- Used in maintenance therapy in opioid addicts
- Used for chronic pain
- Limited use in acute pain

Fentanyl

- Strong opioid
- Fast onset
- No active metabolites
- 1–5 μg/kg IV bolus dose
- Infusion 0.5–2 μg/kg/hr

Morphine

- Morphine 6 glucuronide stronger than morphine
- 0.1–0.2 mg/kg IV bolus dose
- 20–30 µg/kg/hr infusion

Pethidine

- Accumulation of norpethidine occurs
- Nausea, vomiting common
- 0.1–1 mg/kg IV bolus dose
- 200–300 µg/kg/hr infusion

Tramadol

- Atypical centrally acting analgesic
- Opioid agonist
- Nausea and vomiting common
- 0.5–1 mg/kg IV bolus
- 0.1–0.2 mg/kg/hr infusion

Buprenorphine

Routes of Administration

- Intravenous
- Subcutaneous – unpredictable blood levels in hypovolemia
- Intramuscular
- Transdermal – fentanyl patch 25–100 µg/hr
- Patient Controlled Analgesia
- Intrathecal opioids:
  - Fentanyl 5–25 µg
  - Morphine 100–500 µg
  - Sufentanyl 2.5–10 µg
- Epidural opioids:
  - Morphine 1–6 mg bolus, 0.1–1 mg/hr infusion
  - Fentanyl 25–100 µg bolus, 25–100 µg/hr infusion

NONOPIOID ANALGESICS

Local Anesthetics

- Local infilteration
- Peripheral N/plexus block
- Continuous neuraxial block
- Safe, effective and reduces side effects of opioids

NSAIDs

- Paracetamol 10–15 mg/kg PO Q6H
- Paracetamol 15–20 mg/kg PR Q6H
- Ibuprofen 6–10 mg/kg PO Q6H
- Ketorolac 30 mg IM Q6H
- Diclofenac 12.5–100 mg IV
- Rofecoxib 20–50 mg PO
- Parecoxib 20–40 mg IM/IV

Analgesic Adjuvants

- Ketamine – 0.5 mg/kg /hr
- α2 agonists –
  - Clonidine 1–2 µg/kg intrathecal
  - Clonidine 2–3 µg/kg epidural
  - Clonidine 0.5 µg/kg intravenous
  - Dexmedetomidine 1 µg/kg IV over 1 minute
- Neostigmine – 25–100 µg intrathecal
- Corticosteroids – dexamethsone 2–4 mg IV
- Gabapentin 900 mg PO 1–2 hr prior to surgery

NONPHARMACOLOGICAL

Cryoanalgesia

- Intense cooling of peripheral nerves to <–5 to –20 °C
- Causes disintegration of axon and myelin sheath
- Does not disrupt perineurium and epineurium
- Cause interruption of nerve conduction for several weeks
- Intercostal N frozen in thoracotomy
- Ilioinguinal N frozen in hernia repair

Electroanalgesia

- Transcutaneous Electrical Nerve Stimulation
- Acupuncture Like TENS (ALTENS)
- Percutaneous Neuromodulation Therapy
- Transcutaneous Acupoint Electrical Stimulation

Others

- Ultrasound therapy
- Hypnotherapy
- Lazer stimulation

Latest Advances

Capsaicin

- Can be used as cream form or injectable
- Acts on C-fibre nerve endings
- Has opioid sparing effect
- Cautious use in those with liver disease and ACE inhibitors

Tapentadol

- New receptor antagonist
- 18 times affinity of morphine
- Inhibits norepinephrine uptake
- Contraindicated in asthma and paralytic ileus

Liposome Encapsulated Local Anesthetic

Extended Release Epidural Morphine

- Acts for upto 48 hours

PERIOPERATIVE PAIN MANAGEMENT IN OPIOID DEPENDANT PATIENT

Introduction

Physiological state of adaptation to opioids characterized by emergence of a withdrawal syndrome during abstinence which maybe relieved in total or part by readministration of the substance.

Problems

- Require higher doses of opioids perioperatively
- Experience higher incidence of sedation
- Tolerance to other side effects of opioids
- Higher incidence of intraoperative awareness
- Ketamine interaction with depth of anesthesia monitors
- Disruption of sleep/altered sleep cycle
- Require longer duration of postoperative analgesia

Goals

- Promote adequate perioperative analgesia
- Prevent drug withdrawal syndromes
- Maintain collaborative multidisciplinary approach
- Assist with psychiatric and behavioral issues

Principles of Management

Multimodal Analgesia

- Local anesthetics
- Anticonvulsants
- NSAIDs
- Acetaminophen
- Nitrates
- Opioids
- α2 agonists
- Tricyclic antidepressants
- Selective serotonin reuptake inhibitors

Preoperative Management

- Evaluation:
  - For early recognition and high index of suspicion
  - Evaluate what opioid and nonopioid analgesic is being used preoperatively
  - Assess patients chronic baseline requirement
  - Calculate total opioid requirement
  - Mode of administration
- *Fentanyl challenge test:*
  - Fentanyl given to levels which cause respiratory depression
  - Pharmacokinetic modeling done
  - Uses:
    - To predict intraoperative and postoperative opioid requirements
    - Calculation of PCA bolus dose and infusion rate
- Assess history of:
  - Previous surgery or trauma resulting in undermedication
  - Inadequate analgesia or relapsing episodes
  - Patients fears and expectations
  - Reassure patient regarding pain control and anxiety
  - Patient education about management plan
- Management:
  - Anxiolytics as indicated
  - Consultation with pain specialist
  - Patient instructed to take normal opioid dose
  - Maintain fentanyl patch already present only if:
    - No significant fluid shift
    - No hypovolemia/peripheral vasoconstriction
    - No sweating affecting adhesion of patch
    - No pyrexia
  - Consider nonopioid analgesics preoperatively:
    - Acetaminophen 1 g 1–2 hours preoperative
    - Celecoxib 1–2 hours preoperative
    - Gabapentin/pregabalin preoperative

Intraoperative Management

- Monitor intraoperative vital signs
  - Heart rate
  - Blood pressure
  - ECG
  - Pupil size
  - Respiratory rate
  - BIS/entropy
- Place warming devices away from transdermal patch to avoid excess absorption
- Opioid strategies:
  - Maintain baseline opioids
  - Increase intraoperative and postoperative opioid dose to compensate for tolerance
  - Opioid rotation – dose of new opioid < 50% of calculated equianalgesic dose
  - Ensure adequate intraoperative loading with long acting opioid if remifentanyl infusion used intraoperatively

- Titrate fentanyl and morphine to respiratory rate of 8–10 breaths/min
- Titrate opioids to moderately miotic pupils

❖ Peripheral neural or plexus blockade

❖ Neuraxial analgesia when clinically indicated

❖ Adjuvant medications:
- Use nonopioids as analgesic adjuvants
- Ketamine 0.5 mg/kg followed by 2 μg/kg/min infusion
- Ketorolac 0.5 mg/kg IV if not given preoperatively
- Acetaminophen 1 g per rectally if not given preoperatively

Assessment of Pain

❖ Dynamic measures of pain to be considered-ability to deep breathe and cough

❖ *Functional Activity Score* useful:
- A: No limitation of relevant activity due to pain
- B: Mild limitation of physical activity
- C: Severe limitation of physical activity

Postoperative Management

❖ Plan preoperatively for postoperative analgesia

❖ Use multimodal analgesia techniques

❖ Regional analgesia:
- Removes need for additional systemic analgesia
- Consider continuous catheter techniques
- Neuraxial opioids may not prevent opioid withdrawal
- Difficult to estimate appropriate safe dose as requirements maybe higher
- Increases risk of respiratory depression if used concurrently with systemic opioids

❖ Opioid strategies:
- Maintain baseline opioid level
- Incremental dosing regimens
- Transdermal buprenorphine- 480 μg/day for 20 μg/hour delivery system
- PCA with basal infusion used as primary therapy
- PCA can be used to supplement epidural analgesia techniques
- Use synergistic opioid mixtures (morphine and oxycodone):
  - Better pain control
  - Reduced side effects
  - Reduces individual drug dosage
- Continue neuraxial opioids (intrathecal/epidural infusion)
- Tramadol good choice due to lower abuse potential

❖ *Opioid rotation*:
- Switching from one opioid to another
- Use of opioid different from preadmission opioid
- Improves analgesia and reduces opioid related side effects
- Mechanisms:
  - Incomplete opioid cross tolerance
  - Differing receptor activity
  - Presence of active metabolites
- Opioid doses converted with opioid conversion ratios
- Drugs commenced with 30–50% calculated equi-analgesic dose

❖ Nonopioid co-analgesic for opioid sparing properties:
- Low dose ketamine:
  - 0.25–0.5 mg/kg bolus
  - 2–4 μg/kg/min infusion
- Acetaminophen 1 g every 6 hrs
- NSAIDs or COX-2 inhibitors
- Gabapentin/pregabalin
- α_2 agonists-clonidine also prevents withdrawal symptoms

❖ During transition phase:
- Period of transition from regional/parenteral techniques to oral opioids/adjuvants
- Allow on demand use of short acting opioids every 3 hours
- Taper opioid doses towards preoperative doses

❖ Prevention of withdrawal syndrome:
- Maintain usual opioid dose equivalent
- Continue other CNS depressants/stimulants
- High index of suspicion
- Methadone maintenance therapy (MMT):
  - Given once a day
  - Suppresses withdrawal symptoms for 24 hrs
  - Can be given PO/IV/IM/subcutaneously
- Buprenorphine maintenance therapy (BMT):
  - Usually given once a day
  - Given as transdermal patch
  - 2–24 mg per day generally required

Discharge Criteria

Reverse Pain Ladder

STEP I
Paracetamol
± NSAIDs
± Tramadol
± Additional opioids

STEP II
Paracetamol
± NSAIDs
± Tramadol

STEP III
Paracetamol
± NSAIDs

INTRAVENOUS REGIONAL ANESTHESIA (IVRA)

Introduction

- It is a method of producing analgesia of part of a limb with an IV injection of local anesthetic while the circulation to the limb is occluded
- Also called ***Biers block***
- First used by ***August Bier*** in 1908

Indications

- For short procedures lasting less than 90 minutes
- Surgeries of forearm and hand:
  - Closed reduction of fractures
  - Carpal tunnel syndrome
- Surgeries of foot
- ***Rydings*** method of digital IVRA: For paronychia

Contraindications

- Obese patients: As tourniquet would be ineffective
- Where prolonged tourniquet time is contraindicated:
  - Sickle cell disease
  - Cellulitis
- Hypersensitivity of local anesthetics
- Untreated heart block:
  - Relative contraindication
  - Sudden release of LA may convert partial block to complete block/precipitate asystole
- Patients with cardiac diseases like uncompensated CCF as lidocaine reduces contractility

Mechanism of Action

- This method uses vascular bed to bring LA to the nerve endings as well as nerve trunk
- The vascular channels in the core of the nerve lie close to nerve fibrils
- These channels carry the drug to the nerve from which it diffuses to the periphery causing nerve blockade

Technique

- Fasting as for general anesthesia:
  - 6 hours for solids
  - 4 hours for liquids
  - 2 hours for clear liquids
- IV sedation:
  - Useful as:
    - Improves patient comfort
    - Increases threshold for toxic effects
  - But prevents early identification of CNS toxic effects if patient is deeply sedated
- Check BP on operative side: Enables cuff inflation to correct pressure after exsanguination
- Resuscitation equipment kept ready
- Cannulation of vein:
  - Cannula removed if duration of surgery less than 1 hour
  - Kept in-situ and flushed with heparinized saline if duration more than 1 hour
  - Veins on dorsum of hand preferred
  - Cannulation of more proximal veins results in patchy block
  - Inflate cuff to above diastolic BP to make veins prominent and cannulate vein
  - Cannulate vein in other hand too, to administer fluids and drugs in case of toxicity
  - Long IV cannula not used as cannula tip may lie beyond tourniquet cuff
  - This may cause direct LA injection into systemic circulation
  - Exsanguinate limb using ***Esmarch bandage***/limb elevation for 3 minutes
- Tie tourniquet:
  - Double tourniquet is usually used
  - Cuff is inflated to above *occlusion pressure*:
    - It is the pressure at which radial pulse disappears
    - Usually *150 mm Hg more than systolic BP*
  - If double tourniquet used:
    - First inflate proximal tourniquet and wait for anesthetic effect to take place
    - Then inflate distal tourniquet so that the area of tourniquet inflation is anesthetized
- Local anesthetic injection:
  - 25 mL of 0.5% lidocaine for forearm
  - 50 mL of 0.5% lidocaine for arm
  - 100 mL of 0.5% lidocaine for thigh
  - Other local anesthetics: Lidocaine 1.5–3 mg/kg with prilocaine 3–4 mg/kg
  - LA solution to be preservative free as it can cause thrombophlebitis
  - LA solution should be without adrenaline
  - More concentrated LA results in use of lower volume causing patchy block
- Release of tourniquet:
  - Minimum duration:
    - Tourniquet kept inflated for minimum of 30 minutes
    - Release of tourniquet before this would be akin to directly injecting LA into systemic circulation

- If it was kept inflated for 30–40 minutes:
  - Deflate the cuff and then immediately reinflate within 30 seconds
  - This releases a test dose of LA slowly into circulation
  - Tourniquet can then be completely deflated after 1 minute
- If tourniquet was inflated for more than 40 minutes:
  - Tourniquet released directly
  - If tourniquet pain occurs, deflate proximal tourniquet while keeping distal tourniquet inflated

❖ Monitor:
- Blood pressure
- ECG, pulse oximetry
- CNS status

❖ Prolonging IVRA effect:
- Leave IV catheter in situ
- Reinjection of local anesthetic:
  - After 1 hour, tourniquet deflated and bleeding vessels are cauterized
  - Tourniquet is then reinflated and LA solution reinjected into vein
  - Half the initial dose of LA is usually sufficient
- Other techniques:
  - Dilute solution of levo-bupivacaine (0.125%) can be used
  - Adjuvants like tramadol, ketorolac and clonidine used after cuff deflation

Advantages

❖ High success rate (96% success rate)
❖ Ease of performance
❖ Quicker onset: Within 5 minutes
❖ Controllable duration (duration governed by time for which tourniquet remains inflated and not on duration of action of local anesthetic)
❖ Controllable extent with tourniquet
❖ Rapid recovery after cuff release: Ideal for day care anesthesia
❖ Minor risk only, of systemic toxicity, if safely performed

Disadvantages

❖ Tourniquet related complications: Pain and neuropathy
❖ Exsanguination of limb required
❖ Inability to provide bloodless field due to gradual venous engorgement due to intraosseous blood flow
❖ Rapid recovery: No postoperative analgesia possible
❖ Toxic reaction: LA toxicity

Complications

❖ LA toxicity: CNS and CNS toxicity, methemoglobinemia
❖ Peripheral nerve damage: tourniquet palsy
❖ Compartment syndrome
❖ Thrombophlebitis with chlorprocaine
❖ Absence of postoperative analgesia

Factors Influencing La Toxicity

❖ Leakage of LA before tourniquet release:
- Leakage through intraosseus veins
- Leakage through ordinary veins when venous pressure exceeds cuff pressure (as can happen during rapid LA injection)
- Malfunctioning tourniquet

❖ Incomplete exsanguination results in release of reservoir of LA on cuff deflation
❖ Arm movements after tourniquet release discouraged
❖ Repeated deflation and inflation of cuff reduces toxicity

Regional Sympathetic Block

❖ Described by ***Hannington-Kiff***
❖ Monitor BP, secure IV line
❖ Patient placed on table which can be tilted
❖ Guanethidine 20 mg in 25 mL normal saline with 0.5% prilocaine (to reduce pain on injection)
❖ Reserpine 1–1.5 mg or bretylium 5 mg/kg also used
❖ Postural hypotension possible for 48 hours after block
❖ Effect can last as long as 4–6 weeks
❖ Advantages:
- Can be used after *post-sympathectomy escape phenomenon*
- Useful for patients on anticoagulants
- Avoids complications of stellate ganglion block
- Prevents adhesions due to phenol in lumbar plexus block

STELLATE GANGLION BLOCK

Introduction

❖ Stellate ganglion belongs to the ortho-sympathetic system and is formed by the fusion of *first thoracic and inferior cervical ganglion*

- Sympathetic block produced; covers thorax, axillary region and upper limb
- Also called ***cervicothoracic sympathetic block***

Regional Anatomy

- Cervical sympathetic chain lies between:
  - Anteriorly: Carotid sheath
  - Posteriorly: Prevertebral muscles
- Stellate ganglion extends from:
  - Transverse process of C_7 (*Vertebra prominens*) to neck of first rib
  - Between longus colli posteriorly and carotid and vertebral artery anteriorly
- Ganglion lies in close contact with:
  - Subclavian artery
  - Recurrent laryngeal nerve
  - Inferior thyroid artery
  - Right side apical pleura
- Usually blocks upper thoracic and all cervical ganglia

Indications

- In children:
  - Severe circulatory disturbances of upper limb
  - Ventricular tachyarrhythmias due to familial prolonged QT interval syndromes
  - Treatment of pediatric herpes zoster ophthalmicus
- In adults:
  - Circulatory in sufficiency due to occlusive vascular diseases:
    - Chronic:
      - Raynauds disease
      - Scleroderma
      - Frostbite
    - Acute:
      - Traumatic/embolic vascular occlusion
      - Accidental intra-arterial thiopentone injection
  - Pain:
    - Post-traumatic syndrome *(causalgia)*
    - Causalgia following abdominal injury
    - Phantom limb, ***Pagets disease***, neoplasms
    - Herpes zoster, trophic skin changes
  - Others:
    - Hyperhidrosis, ***Sudecks dystrophy***
    - ***Shoulder–hand syndrome***
    - Stroke, ***Menieres disease***, amblyopia due to poisoning with quinidine

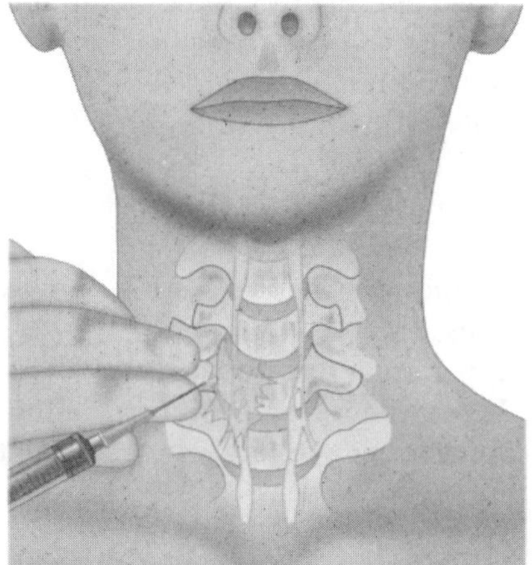

Fig. 1: Stellate ganglion block.

Procedure

Paratracheal Approach

- Called ***anterior approach of Leriche***
- Patient should not talk during procedure
- Patient lies supine with head slightly lifted forward and tilted dorsally
- Done to stretch esophagus away from transverse cervical process on left side
- Palpate trachea and carotid pulse between sternocleidomastoid and trachea
- Palpate Chassaignac's tubercle at the level of cricoid cartilage
- Raise a skin wheal over this tubercle
- Two fingers now pressed down to the C_6 tubercle, pushing away carotid artery laterally and trachea towards midline
- 22 G, short bevelled, 4.5 cm long needle with 20 mL syringe attached is advanced till it hits the C_6 tubercle
- Hand holding needle is kept braced against the patient and needle is withdrawn 2 mm to clear from longus colli muscle
- Aspirate and check for CSF/blood
- Inject 2 mL of local anesthetic if no aspirate
- If high resistance occurs on injection: prevertebral muscle present
- If radiating pain occurs on injection: needle has penetrated nerve root
- 15–20 mL of bupivacaine/ropivacaine is injected
- Patient may feel lump in the throat and may be temporarily hoarse
- Food and fluids to be withheld till laryngeal reflexes become intact

Continuous Technique

- Done with radio-opaque Teflon catheter
- This is introduced with X-ray control using paratracheal technique
- Stylet is withdrawn and catheter is fixed for continuous injection

Chemical Stellate Ganglion Block

- 1–2 mL of 6% acqueous phenol/10% phenol in Conray dye used
- Complete cervicothoracic sympathetic blockade is not assured
- The arm might partially escape in which case injection at T_2-T_3 can be used as supplement
- This is rarely used owing to its close proximity to pleura
- Dural sheath may be entered and LA may migrate to medulla oblongata

Signs of Successful Block

- Horners syndrome:
  - Ptosis
  - Miosis
  - Anhydrosis
  - Unilateral nasal stuffiness
  - Unilateral skin and conjunctival flushing
- *Cobalt blue sweat test* also useful
- Increase in temperature of ipsilateral arm also suggests successful block

Complications

- Nerve injuries:
  - Horners syndrome
  - Recurrent laryngeal nerve palsy
  - Neuralgia along chest wall and inner arm
  - Brachial plexus, phrenic nerve block
- Inadvertent injection:
  - Intravascular injection: vertebral artery, carotid artery, subclavian artery
  - Epidural, subarachnoid injection
  - Intradural injection: Slow onset of symptoms
- Soft tissue:
  - Pneumothorax
  - Osteitis of transverse process
  - Mediastinitis due to esophageal puncture

INTERSCALENE BLOCK

Introduction

Developed as an alternative to supraclavi-cular approach to brachial sheath.

Advantages

- Can be used when proximal block is required: Shoulder surgeries
- Can be performed with arm in any position
- Pneumothorax risk is reduced
- Landmarks are usually clear, even in stout patients

Disadvantages

- Essential to elicit paraesthesias
- Supplementary ulnar nerve block may be required
- Common but serious side effects
- Spares lowest branches of plexus (C_8 and T_1) which innervate ulnar forearm

Indications: Shoulder, humerus and forearm surgeries

Anatomy

- Cervical nerves of brachial plexus after leaving the respective intervertebral foramen pass laterally into a deep gutter/groove in superior surface of transverse process of cervical vertebrae
- This groove separates transverse process into anterior and posterior tubercles, which give rise to scalenus anterior and scalenus medius respectively
- After leaving transverse process, nerve roots of plexus pass into a plane between two scalenei called *paravertebral/interscalene groove or space* as trunks of brachial plexus
- This interscalene groove lies at level of cricoid cartilage
- The gutter on cervical transverse process is directed laterally downwards (45) and forwards

Position

- Supine with neck straight, but head turned slightly to opposite side
- Arm is placed by the side with shoulder depressed as for supraclavicular nerve block

Stimulation

- Deltoid: For shoulder surgery
- Elbow flexion: For humerus surgery

Volume of Local Anesthetic

- 10–20 mL: For upper root analgesia
- 20–40 mL: For lower root analgesia
- 1% lidocaine or 1% prilocaine used
- 0.25–0.5% bupivacaine/levobupivacaine also can be used
- Use of long acting analgesics may provide analgesia for 12–14 hours

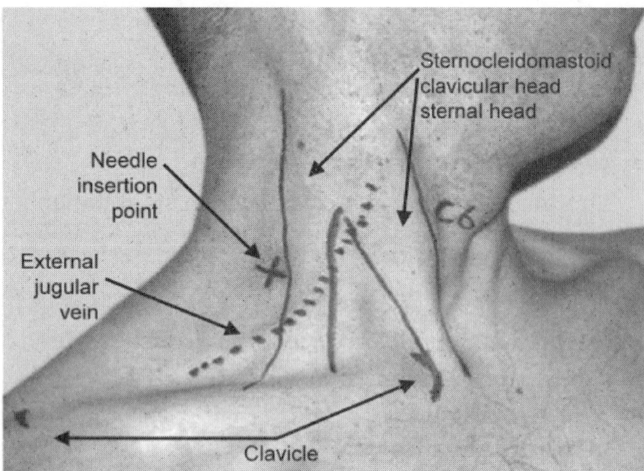

Fig. 2: Interscalene block.

Techniques

- *Winnies technique*:
  - Landmarks:
    - Cricoid cartilage
    - Posterior border of sternocleidomastoid
    - Interscalene groove
  - Depth of insertion: 1–2 cm (very near surface)
  - Procedure:
    - Identify posterior border of sternocleidomastoid: Patient lifts head
    - Identify interscalene groove over belly of scalenus
    - Line drawn from cricoid cartilage to intersect interscalene groove
    - This is point of entry at the level of C_6 transverse process
    - External jugular vein might overlie this point
    - Digital pressure and massage might help in distant spread of LA
  - Direction of needle:
    - Inward, 45 caudal and slightly backwards
    - Towards contralateral elbow/nipple
- *Mieirs approach*:
  - Indications:
    - Shoulder and humerus surgery
    - Difficult anatomy: Short neck resulting in poor identification of groove
    - Continuous catheter technique
  - Depth of insertion: 3.5–5 cm
  - Landmarks:
    - Posterior border of sternocleidomastoid
    - Thyroid cartilage prominence (C_4)
    - Subclavian artery above clavicle
  - Procedure:
    - Mark posterior border of sternocleidomastoid at level of thyroid prominence
    - Palpate subclavian artery over first rib behind clavicle
    - Line joining reduced these two, marks approximate groove
  - Direction of needle: Caudally, passing along long axis of interscalene groove towards subclavian artery
  - Advantages:
    - Reduced risk of epidural/intrathecal injection
    - Easier to place catheter due to angle of approach
    - Catheter placed using insulated Tuohy needle for shoulder arthroplasty
- ***Posterior interscalene block: Pippas approach***
  - Anatomical landmarks:
    - C_7 spinous process
    - C_6 spinous process
    - Cricoid cartilage
    - Sternocleidomastoid
  - Technique:
    - Seated position with cervical spine flexed backwards
    - Puncture site 3 cm away from midline between spinous processes of C_6 and C_7
    - Direction of needle 5–10° lateral and aimed at height of cricoid
  - Puncture depth: 6–8 cm
- Ultrasound guided interscalene block

Side Effects

- Nerve blocks:
  - Phrenic nerve block (100%)
  - Recurrent laryngeal nerve block (15%)
  - Stellate ganglion block (Horners syndrome)
- Epidural/spinal injection/spinal cord injury:
  - Easily detected if nerve stimulator is used
  - Avoid injecting when current responses are present at less than 0.4 mA
  - This suggests subarachnoid position of needle tip
- Vertebral artery injection: Even 1–3 mL of LA solution can precipitate seizures as direct entry into brain occurs
- Intravenous injection: Slower onset LA toxicity
- Bilateral spread of interscalene block
- Pneumothorax due to advancing needle too far especially in a lateral direction

- C_6 neuropathy:
  - Occurs as needle may pin nerve root against tubercle
  - Suspect C_6 neuropathy if first injection of LA produces crampy pain sensation
  - This suggests intraneural position of needle tip
  - Withdrawal needle if so, as intraneural injection produces neuropathy

Contraindications

- Not to be done in anesthetized patients
- Caution in patient with COPD or unilateral phrenic nerve palsy

SUPRACLAVICULAR BRACHIAL PLEXUS BLOCK

Introduction

The brachial plexus is blocked at a point where it is most compactly arranged, at the level of the 3 trunks.

Advantages

- Brachial plexus blocked at a patient where it is most compactly arranged
- Whole brachial plexus is blocked: Excellent anesthesia of entire arm including hand
- Technique can be performed with arm in virtually any position
- Low volume of local anesthesia solution required

Disadvantages

- Risk of pneumothorax
- Considerable experience required to master it

Indications: Elbow, wrist, Hand Surgeries

Contraindications

- Uncooperative patient
- Inexperienced practitioner
- Difficult stature patients in whom landmarks are not clear
- Respiratory cripples in whom pneumothorax or phrenic nerve palsy causes dyspnea
- Bilateral supraclavicular block not performed to avoid risk of bilateral phrenic nerve palsy

Anatomy

- At the lateral border of anterior scalenii muscle, plexus passes between the first rib and clavicle to enter axilla
- Trunks are tightly oriented vertically on top of first rib, just posterior to subclavian artery
- Faster onset block due to perivascular sheath narrowing at this level
- Motor block faster than sensory as Mantle fibres are motor at this level
- Ulnar border of hand missed in 5% cases

Techniques

- Paresthesia technique
- Nerve stimulator technique
- USG guided block

Position

- Patient is positioned supine without pillow
- Head is turned to 30 to contralateral side
- The ipsilateral shoulder should be depressed downwards (caudal) and posteriorly by gentle pressure on the shoulder

Approaches

- Classic approach:
  - Interscalene groove palpated at its most inferior point
  - This is just posterior to subclavian artery pulsation
  - The pulsation is felt in a plane just medial to midpoint of clavicle
  - Skin wheal raised with local anesthetic solution
  - 22G, 15 inch needle is directed caudally
  - Shaft of needle and syringe kept parallel to the plane of head and neck
  - Needle is directed, aiming at ipsilateral toe
  - Needle is advanced till paresthesia is felt or muscle contraction of forearm is seen
  - If muscle contraction still present with voltage of nerve stimulator decreased to 0.5 mA, 25–40 mL of LA is injected
- Another technique:
  - Identify and measure width of clavicular head of sternocleidomastoid
  - Double the width and measure that distance from medial end of clavicle
  - The terminal part of interscalence groove should lie at this point, one finger breadth posterior to clavicle
  - Volume injected: 0.5 mL/kg upto 40 mL local anesthetic
- *Patrick technique*:
  - Used if no paresthesias are elicited, but the rib is contacted
  - LA solution is injected between skin and rib, behind the artery

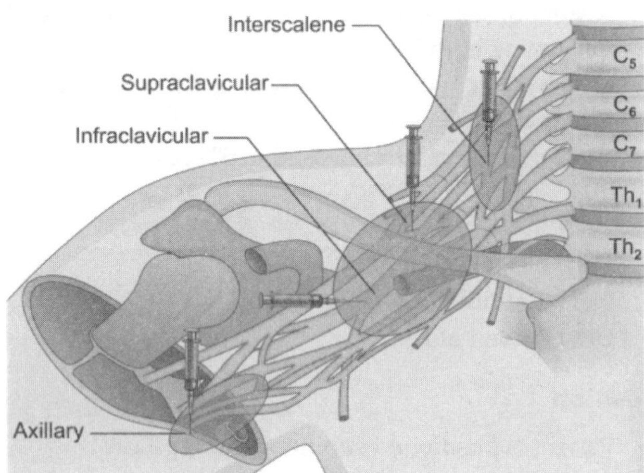

Fig. 3: Supraclavicular block versus other brachial plexus approaches.

- If subclavian artery pulsation and landmarks are not felt:
  - The point where straight portion of EJV crosses the clavicle used to identify the midclavicular point
  - Asking patient to blow out his cheeks will make EJV prominent
  - Needle is inserted 1–2 cm behind midpoint of clavicle

End Points

- Motor activity of forearm and hand: Inject LA solution
- Flexion and extension of wrist and fingers: inject LA solution
- Blood in needle: Redirect needle more posteriorly and laterally
- Bone: Redirect needle and walk the needle more posteriorly and laterally
- No motor activity and depth of needle is equal to width of clavicle: Withdraw needle and reassess land marks
- Caution: Absolutely no medial angulation of needle

Complications

- Pneumothorax/hemothorax:
  - Incidence 0.5–6%
  - Tall and thin patients with high apical pleura more at risk
  - Due to:
    - Needle puncturing pleura
    - More commonly needle pierces lung and lung surface gets torn by needle
    - Pneumothorax is then caused by air escaping from lung
  - Suspect when cough/dypnea/pleuritic chest pain
  - Confirmed by chest X-ray
  - Majority take *upto 24 hrs to develop*
  - If extensive (50% involvement), continuous drainage occurs for 24–48 hrs
  - If lesser degree, air is removed, only if symptoms present with simple syringe aspiration
  - Takes weeks for complete absorption
- Phrenic nerve palsy:
  - Occurs in 40–60 % cases
  - If bilateral palsy in patients with underlying chest disease, signs of hypoxia may occur
- ***Horners syndrome (Stellate ganglion block)***:
  - Occurs in 70–90% cases when large volume of LA used (50 mL)
  - No treatment is necessary
- Nerve damage/neuritis:
  - Uncommon complication
  - Occurs due to:
    - Faulty position of arm during surgery
    - Trauma by needle
    - Prolonged ischemia of nerve due to vasoconstrictor drug
    - Too concentrated LA solution
- Local anesthetic toxicity:
  - Due to inadvertent intravascular injection/use of excessive LA
  - Prevented by repeated aspiration while injecting LA

AXILLARY NERVE BLOCK

Introduction

Provides excellent operative condition for surgeries of forearm and hand with reduced risk of major complications

Indications

Surgeries of elbow, forearm, hand

Limitations

- Arm must be abducted to perform the block
- Extent of anesthesia insufficient for shoulder/upper arm surgery without using large volume of solution
- Circumflex and musculocutaneous nerve are missed in single shot injection as they leave the axillary sheath proximal to the point of injection
- Radial nerve missed in 25% cases

Anatomy

- Neurovascular bundle lies 1–2 cm below skin surface
- Subclavian artery becomes axillary artery just below clavicle where trunks of brachial plexus split into anterior and posterior divisions at lateral border of pectoralis minor

- In the axilla, musculocutaneous nerve has already left the sheath and lies within coracobrachialis muscle
- The fascial sheath in axilla might be multi-compartmental with one compartment covering each nerve and the fascial septa may be responsible for patchy anesthesia
- Medial aspect of sheath (superficial): Subcutaneous tissue covering lies behind biceps/coracobrachialis and in front of triceps
- Relations in the sheath:
  - Median nerve: Lies anterior to axillary artery (above)
  - Ulnar nerve: Posterior to axillary artery (below)
  - Radial nerve: Posterior and lateral (below and laterally)
  - Musculocutaneous nerve: Anterior and lateral (within coracobrachialis)
  - Axillary vein: Medial to artery

Landmark

- Axillary artery pulsations
- Pectoralis major insertion

Depth of Insertion: 10–15 mm

Volume of Local Anesthetic

- 0.5 mL/kg upto 50 mL can be used
- 40 mL of LA solution reaches upto coracoid process thus blocking musculocutaneous nerve
- Increasing volume of solution above 40 mL does not improve spread to musculocutaneous nerve

Techniques

- Perivascular technique:
  - Pulse of axillary artery identified as high in axilla as possible
  - Using immobile needle technique 22 G, 1.5 inch needle is directed parallel to neurovascular bundle, i.e. at apex of axilla
  - Oscillation of needle produced by arterial pulsations indicates that needle is at least near the artery and thus probably within the sheath
  - Local anesthetic solution (15–20 mL) injected at this point
  - Same procedure applied for injection below pulsation
- Transarterial technique:
  - Axillary artery pulsations identified
  - 22 G, 1.5 inch needle advanced till bright red blood aspirated
  - Needle advanced or withdrawn till aspiration ceases
  - LA injected (40 mL at once or 20 mL anterior and 20 mL posterior to artery)
- Paresthesia technique:
  - Useful if pulsations are not felt (fat patient)
  - Needle directed towards axillary artery to elicit single specific or multiple paresthesias
  - If concerned about septation, paraesthesias elicited in ulnar, median and radial nerve distribution and LA injected separately at these sites
  - Paresthesia only at surgical site also may be elicited
  - Regardless of whether single or multiple paresthesias are elicited, injected volume should be 40 mL
- Nerve stimulator technique:
  - 2 inch and 22 G insulated simulating needle inserted proximal to hand palpating pulses, and appropriate muscle twitches are sought
  - Once identified and after reducing stimulation to less than 0.5 MA, witnessing fade of motor activity after 1 mL of LA is injection and negative aspiration of blood, local anesthetic is delivered
  - Nerve stimulation causes the following:
    - Median nerve: Flexion of index/middle finger
    - Ulnar nerve: Thumb adduction, little finger flexion
    - Radial nerve: Thumb extension
    - Musculocutaneous nerve: Elbow flexion
- Loss of resistance technique: Click/pop is felt on entering fascial sheath
- Continous axillary block:
  - 17/18 G needle, 20/22 G catheter used
  - Continuous infusion of 0.25% bupivacaine at 20–30 mg/hr is effective
  - First bolus dose given and then infusion started 1 hour after bolus
  - Not many toxic reactions
  - Used for long surgeries like reimplantation
- Ultrasound guided axillary block: using high frequency (10–15 MHZ) linear probe
- Tourniquet block:
  - Few mL of LA solution is deposited in subcutaneous tissues from biceps to triceps on medial surface of upper arm on withdrawal to block intercostobrachial nerve and its communication with medial cutaneous nerve of arm
  - This communication may cause tourniquet pain inspite of a successful axillary block

Testing Block: Pull-push-pin-pin test

Pull (flexion of arm): Test musculocutaneous nerve

Push arm against resistance: Tests radial nerve

Pin: the thenar prominence: Tests median nerve

Pin: fifth digit: Tests ulnar nerve

Promoting Proximal Flow within Sheath

- Important to increase chances of musculocutaneous nerve block
- Techniques of promoting proximal flow:
  - Digital pressure applied immediately distal to needle with index and middle fingers both during and immediately after injection
  - Tourniquet application
  - Adduct arm as soon as injection is completed: this removes effect of pressure of humeral head which may be limiting proximal spread

Complications: Very low rate of complications:

- Intravascular injection
- Repeated elicitation of paresthesias cause neuropathy postoperatively: Ultrasound guidance and careful attention to injection pressures during block reduces incidence of neuropathy
- Hematoma if axillary artery is punctured (self-limiting)
- Infection

PARAVERTEBRAL BLOCK

Introduction

Potential space deep to endothoracic fascia that intercostal N traverses, on route to intercostal space.

Anatomy

- Wedge shaped space adjacent to vertebral body
- Spinal roots emerge and divide into dorsal and ventral rami
- Boundaries:
  - Anterolaterally: Pleura
  - Superiorly: Inferior aspect of upper rib
  - Inferiorly: Superior aspect of lower rib
  - Medially: Adjacent vertebra, intervertebral foramen
  - Posteriorly: Costotransverse ligament

Indications

- Lower thoracic surgery
- Lumbar surgery
- Pelvic surgery
- Groin surgery (herniorrhaphy)
- Upper leg surgery
- Treatment of chronic pain syndromes:
  - Post thoracotomy
  - Post mastectomy
  - Nerve entrapment syndrome following herniorrhaphy

Contraindications

- Local infections
- Mentally unstable patients
- LA sensitivity
- Surgery at site of block

OT Preparation

- Emergency medications
- Airway equipment
- Antiseizure drugs
- Connect pulse oximeter, ECG, NIBP, Nerve stimulator if required

Technique

I. Lumbar Paravertebral:

- Prone position
- Aseptic precautions
- Palpate and mark each lumbar spinous process

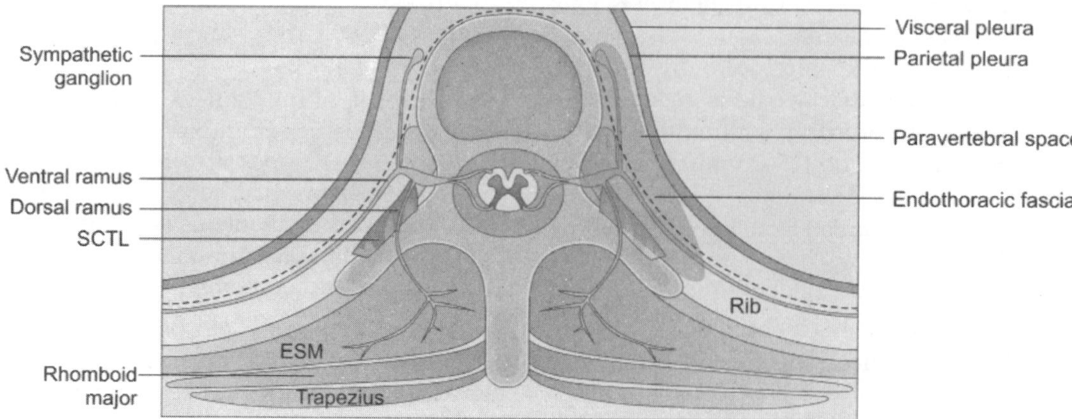

Fig. 4: Paravertebral block.

- Draw horizontal line @ cephalad edge of each process
- 2 vertical lines drawn parallel to and 3–5 cm from midline
- Raise skin wheal at points of intersection of the 2 lines
- 22 G, 8 cm needle perpendicular to skin until it touches transverse process @ depth of 3–5 cm
- Withdraw slightly and redirect to slide off caudal edge of transverse process
- Advance 1–2 cm deeper and inject 6–10 mL of local anesthetic

II. Thoracic Paravertebral:

- Prone position
- Aseptic precautions
- Palpate cephalad aspect of each spinous process
- 22 G 8 cm needle inserted perpendicular to skin and 2–3 cm lateral to spinous process
- Once transverse process is hit, withdraw needle little
- Advance it to pass cephalad to transverse until LOR is felt
- Inject 5 mL of LA per level

III. Open Vision Technique:

- Epidural catheter passed into open hemithorax via tuohy needle
- Small incision on parietal pleura and fascia covering paravertebral gutter
- Thread tip of catheter close to neurovascular bundle of cephalad intercostal space
- Suture to reduce spread of LA

Continuous Paravertebral Block

- 0.1 mL/kg/hr of 0.5% bupivacaine
- 1 mL/10 kg/hr of 1% lidocaine (maximum 7 mL/hr)
- Can be combined with NSAIDs/opioids

Complications

- LA toxicity
- Pneumothorax
- Subarachnoid/epidural space injection
- Intraperitoneal injection
- Puncture of retroperitoneal/intraabdominal organs
- Infection/hematoma
- Paravertebral muscle pain/quadratus lumborum weakness
- Nerve injury

Advantages Over Epidural

- Comparable analgesia
- Reduced neuraxial hematoma
- Reduced hypotension
- Fewer failed blocks
- Reduced nausea and urinary retention

LUMBAR PLEXUS BLOCK

Introduction

- Comprises of injection of local anesthetic into lumbar plexus in fascial plane within the posterior aspect of psoas major
- Also called *psoas compartment block*

Anatomy

- Derived from ventral ramii of lumbar nerve roots L_1-L_4
- Contribution from T_{12} in 50% cases
- Made up of 7 nerves
  - Iliohypogastric T_{12}-L_1
  - Ilioinguinal L_1
  - Genitofemoral L_1-L_2
  - Lateral femoral cutaneous L_2-L_4
  - Obturator L_2-L_4
  - Accessory obturator L_3L_4
  - Femoral L_2-L_4
- After leaving intervertebral foramina courses via psoas compartment bounded:
  - Aneriorly: Psoas muscle fascia
  - Posteriorly: Quadratus lumborum fascia
- Plexus blocked in psoas compartment

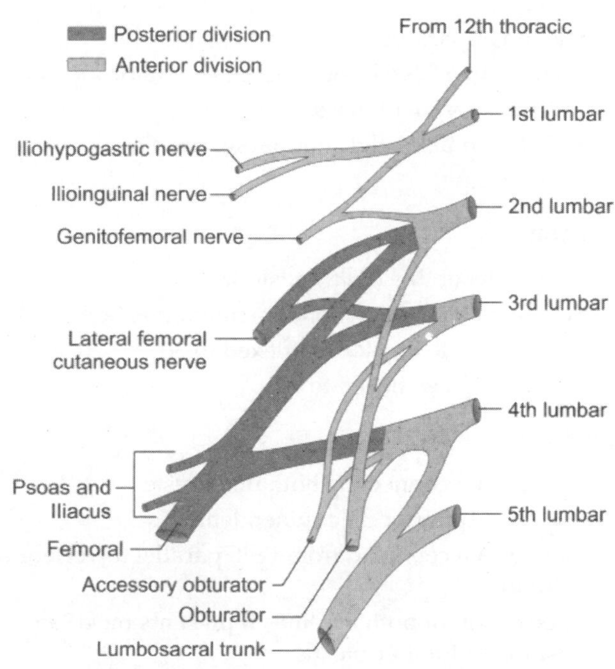

Fig. 5: Lumbar plexus.

Indications

- Analgesia:
  - Neuralgias of thigh
  - Fascia lata pain syndrome
  - Total knee replacement
  - Total hip replacement
  - Revision hip arthroplasty
  - Hemiarthroplasty
  - Surgeries on neck/shaft femur
- Anesthesia:
  - Anterior cruciate ligament repair
  - Knee arthroscopy
  - Patellar tendon repair
  - Surgeries of thigh- skin graft/biopsy
  - Saphenous vein stripping

Patient Preparation

- NPO status confirmed
- Consent taken
- Venous access secured
- IV midazolam 0.03–0.05 mg/kg can be administered
- Standard monitors applied – ECG, blood pressure, pulse oximetry

OT Preparation

- Emergency drugs kept ready (thiopentone, adrenaline, atropine)
- Airway equipment (facemask, endotracheal tube, airways)
- Suction apparatus
- 1% lidocaine 0.5% bupivacaine in equal proportions
- Around 25 – 30 mL used
- 21 G 4 inch insulated stimulating needle
- 20 cc syringe

Position

- Lateral decubitus (*Sims*) position
- Side to be blocked in nondependent position
- Hip on side to be blocked flexed to 30°
- Ipsilateral knee flexed to 90°

Technique

- Line drawn connecting both iliac crests
- Posterior superior iliac spine identified
- Line drawn cephalad from PSIS parallel to vertebral column
- Intersection of both the lines represents most lateral position of lumbar plexus
- Insertion point 4 cm from midline
- Needle advanced perpendicularly at insertion point
- Loss of resistance felt on entry into psoas compartment
- When needle enters psoas compartment (70–90 mm) quadriceps twitch noted
- Reduce stimulation to < 0.5 mA while witnessing activity
- Witness fade of motor activity after injection of 1 mL of local anesthetic
- After negative aspiration of blood 25–40 mL local anesthetic injected

Advantages

- Lower pain scores
- Less morphine consumption
- Less hypotension/nausea/vomiting
- Reduces postoperative blood loss
- Greater patient satisfaction
- Earlier hospital discharge

Disadvantages

- Deep anatomical location of plexus
- Needs large volumes of local anesthetic owing to size of plexus
- Serious complication rate
- Safer alternatives – femoral nerve block

Complications

- Epidural/subdural injection
- Total spinal anesthesia
- Peripheral nerve damage
- Intravascular injection
- Puncture of renal pelvis
- Retroperitoneal hematoma
- Infection
- Neuropraxia/neurolysis
- Sympathetic block secondary to extravasation of local anesthetic

THREE IN ONE BLOCK

Introduction

Technique to block 3 of the 4 nerves of leg with single injection of local anesthetic:

- Femoral nerve
- Obturator nerve
- Lateral cutaneous nerve

Also called *Inguinal Paravascular Technique* of lumbar plexus anesthesia

Anatomy

- Nerves emerging from lumbar plexus lie between:
  - Anteriorly: Psoas major
  - Posteriorly: Quadratus lumborum
- Compartment formed extends beneath inguinal ligament
- Single femoral sheath forms closed space
- Sheath encloses all nerves involved in lumbar plexus
- Drugs injected into this sheath travel upwards
- Sufficient volume (> 25 mL) to be injected

Supply

- Femoral nerve:
  - Anterior and medial portion of thigh and knee
  - Cutaneous innervation of medial and lateral portion of thigh
  - Periosteum of femur
- Lateral femoral cutaneous nerve
  - Sensory to lateral buttock
  - Sensory supply to lateral thigh and knee joint
- Obturator nerve:
  - Medial thigh
  - Hip joint
  - Adductor muscles

Indications

- Analgesia:
  - Post-total knee arthroplasty
  - Post-anterior cruciate ligament repair
  - Plaster applications femoral fractures
  - Fracture neck/shaft of femur
  - Above/below knee amputations

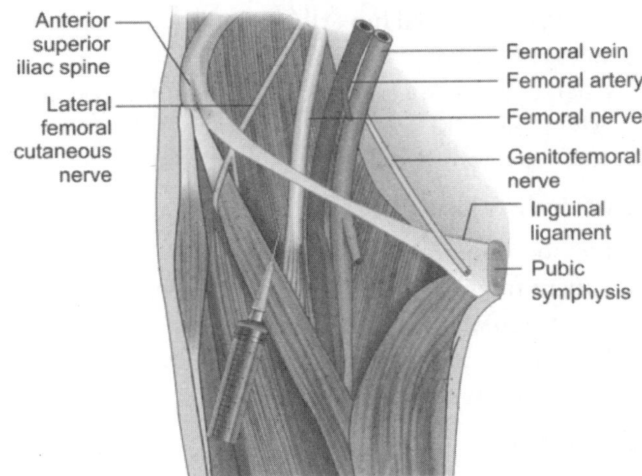

Fig. 6: Femoral nerve block.

- Anesthesia:
  - Skin graft/muscle biopsy anterior aspect of thigh
  - Knee surgery in combination with sciatic N block
  - Procedures on lower leg/foot in combination with lower leg

Contraindications

- Burn/infection at injection site
- Local anesthetic allergy
- Coagulopathy
- Presence of prosthetic vascular graft of femoral artery
- Preexisting neurological disease
- Patient refusal

Complications

- Intravascular injection
- LA toxicity
- Femoral Nerve trauma
- Prolonged motor blockade
- Hematoma formation
- Block failure

Patient Preparation

- NPO status confirmed
- Consent taken
- Venous access secured
- IV midazolam 0.03–0.05 mg/kg can be administered
- Standard monitors applied – ECG, blood pressure, pulse oximetry

OT Preparation

- Emergency drugs kept ready (thiopentone, adrenaline, atropine)
- Airway equipment (facemask, endotracheal tube, airways)
- Suction apparatus
- 1% lidocaine 0.5% bupivacaine in equal proportions
- Around 25 – 30 mL used
- 21–23 G 3–5 cm blunt needle
- 20 cc syringe

Technique

- Supine position
- Stand opposite to side of block
- Aseptic precautions
- Site of insertion is 2 cm below line joining ASIS and pubic tubercle

- Needle inserted perpendicularly 2 cm lateral to femoral artery pulsations
- Needle advanced till 2 pops are felt (fascia lata and fascia iliaca)
- Paresthesias maybe felt along femoral N innervation
- Quadriceps contractions identifies femoral N if nerve stimulator used
- Needle immobilized and pressure applied below needle
- 25–30 mL local anesthetic injected in graded aliquots after negative aspiration
- Distal pressure applied to ensure cephalad spread
- Needle removed and area massaged
- Lateral femoral cutaneous N often partially blocked with single injection
- Can be blocked simultaneously at anterior superior iliac spine

Advantages

- Single injection used
- Lesser local anesthetic needed
- High success rate
- Simple technique
- Can be used in geriatric population

Disadvantages

- Lateral cutaneous femoral N sparing
- Obturator N sparing
- Risk of permanent nerve injury

FASCIA ILIACA BLOCK

Introduction

Delivery of sufficient volume of local anesthetic behind fascia iliaca causes compartment block

Anatomy

- Fascia Iliaca Compartment
- Potential space bounded by:
  - Anterior: Fascia Iliaca (overlaid by Fascia Lata)
  - Posterior: Iliopsoas muscle
  - Medial: Vertebral column
  - Craniolaterally: Inner lip of iliac crest
  - Craniomedially: Continuous with space between quadratus lumborum and its fascia
  - Contents:
    - Femoral nerve
    - Lateral femoral cutaneous nerve
    - Obturator nerve
    - Genitofemoral nerve

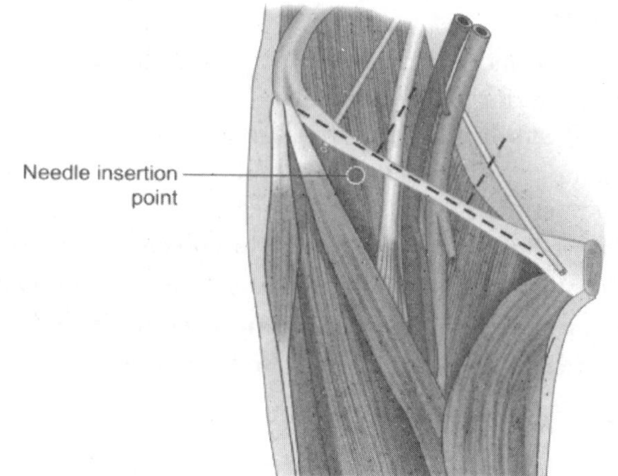

Fig. 7: Fascia iliaca block.

Supply

- Femoral nerve:
  - Anterior and medial portion of thigh and knee
  - Cutaneous innervation of medial and lateral portion of thigh
  - Periosteum of femur
- Lateral femoral cutaneous nerve
  - Sensory to lateral buttock
  - Sensory supply to lateral thigh and knee joint
- Obturator nerve:
  - Medial thigh
  - Hip joint
  - Adductor muscles

Indications

- Perioperative analgesia or fracture neck or shaft of femur
- Adjuvant analgesia for hip surgeries
- Analgesia for total hip arthroplasties
- Analgesia for above knee amputation
- Analgesia for knee surgeries (in combination with sciatic N block)
- Analgesia for lower leg tourniquet pain

Contraindications

- Previous femoral bypass surgery
- Patient refusal
- Anticoagulation
- Infection or inflammation over injection site
- Local anesthetic allergy

Complications

- Block failure
- Intravascular injection

- LA toxicity
- Infection
- Perioperative injury secondary to numbness

Patient Preparation

- NPO status confirmed
- Consent taken
- Venous access secured
- Standard monitors applied – ECG, blood pressure, pulse oximetry

OT Preparation

- Emergency drugs kept ready (thiopentone, adrenaline, atropine)
- Airway equipment (facemask, endotracheal tube, airways)
- Suction apparatus
- 1% lidocaine 0.5% bupivacaine in equal proportions
- Around 25–30 mL used
- 3.5 inch 22 G Whitacre spinal needle
- 20 cc syringe

Position

- Supine position
- Stand same side of block

Technique

- Aseptic precautions
- Landmarks similar to femoral N block
- Line drawn from anterior superior iliac spine to pubic tubercle
- Junction of outer and middle thirds is identified
- 2 cm distal to junction is needle entry site
- Block does not require nerve stimulator
- Needle inserted perpendicular to skin till two 'pops' are felt
- First pop occurs as needle passes through fascia lata
- Second pop felt as needle passes through fascia iliaca
- Following negative aspiration 25–30 mL of local anesthetic injected
- Injection at 30° angle to skin in superior direction
- Pressure applied over injection site for 10 seconds following procedure

Advantages

- Does not require nerve stimulator
- Can be performed very quickly
- Not very painful
- Patients often do not require sedation
- Avoids injury to nerve and artery
- Catheter can be placed for continuous postoperative analgesia

Disadvantages

- Inconsistent block success
- Femoral nerve blocked more consistently compared with lateral cutaneous femoral nerve and obturator nerve

LATERAL FEMORAL CUTANEOUS BLOCK

Introduction

Superficial nerve block providing sensory anesthesia and analgesia to lateral thigh.

Anatomy

- Originates from lumbar plexus, dorsal divisions of L2–L3
- Traverses laterally from psoas muscle
- Courses anterolaterally along iliacus muscle
- Emerges inferior and medial to ASIS
- Passes between inguinal ligament and sartorius muscle
- Divides into anterior and posterior branches

Supply

- Sensory to lateral buttock
- Sensory supply to lateral thigh and knee joint

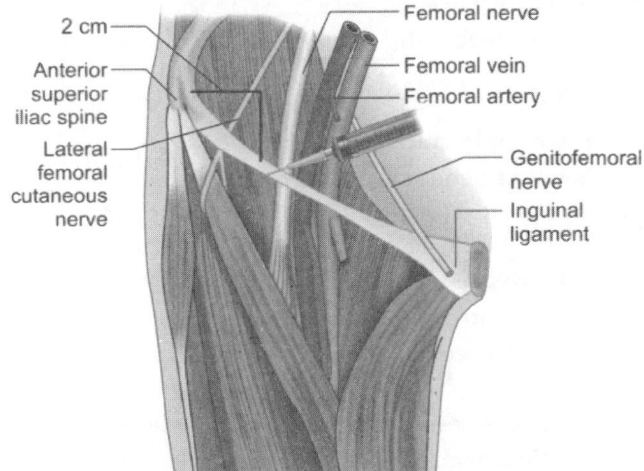

Fig. 8: Lateral cutaneous nerve block.

Indication

- Skin or muscle biopsy from lateral thigh
- Harvest site for skin graft
- In concurrence with femoral N block or fascia iliaca block
- Evaluation of lateral thigh pain
- Meralgia paresthetica

Contraindication

- Preexisting peripheral neuropathy
- Previous femoral bypass surgery
- Patient refusal
- Anticoagulation
- Infection or inflammation over injection site
- Local anesthetic allergy

Patient Preparation

- NPO status confirmed
- Consent taken
- Venous access secured
- IV midazolam 0.03–0.05 mg/kg can be administered
- Standard monitors applied – ECG, blood pressure, pulse oximetry

OT Preparation

- Emergency drugs kept ready (thiopentone, adrenaline, atropine)
- Airway equipment (facemask, endotracheal tube, airways)
- Suction apparatus
- 1% lidocaine, 40 mg methylprednisolone if indicated
- Around 10–12 mL used
- 22 G 2 inch needle
- 10 cc syringe

Position

- Supine or lateral
- Stand on same side of block

Technique

- Strict asepsis
- As a field injection technique
- Point of injection 2 cm distal and 2 cm medial to ASIS
- Pop felt as needle passes through fascia lata
- Needle advanced slightly beyond resistance
- Needle repeatedly reinserted above and below fascia in lateral to medial direction
- Local anesthetic injected in fanwise technique as needle is reinserted
- Pressure applied over injection site for 10 seconds post injection to prevent ecchymosis

Advantages

- Nerve stimulator not required
- Minimal complication rate
- Well tolerated
- Absence of motor block

Disadvantages

- No continuous technique as catheter insertion not indicated

Complications

- Low complication rate
- Post-block ecchymosis/hematoma
- Neuritis secondary to needle trauma or drug toxicity
- Inadvertant femoral N block
- Perforation of colon – intra-abdominal abscess

OBTURATOR NERVE BLOCK

Introduction

Provides anesthesia to medial thigh and relaxation to adductor muscles of hip.

Anatomy

- Mixed nerve derived from anterior primary rami of L_2, L_3 and L_4
- Runs within psoas major muscle during initial course
- Crosses close to bladder wall on its inferior/lateral portion
- Nerve exits pelvis and enters medial thigh through obturator foramen
- Divides into anterior and posterior divisions to supply adductors of thigh

Supply

- Sensory:
  - Medial thigh
  - Hip joint
- Motor:
  - Adductor muscles of thigh
  - Articular branch to hip and knee

Indications

- Adductor release procedure – adductor tenotomy
- Treatment of spasticity of thigh adductors due to hemiplegia/cerebral palsy

- To suppress "***Obturator Reflex***" during TURBT
- As a supplement to femoral/sciatic N block
- Chronic pain secondary to knee arthrosis/pelvic tumors
- Diagnosis of hip pain

Contraindications

- Burn/infection/inguinal lymphadenopathy at injection site
- Presence of prosthetic vascular graft of femoral artery
- Preexisting obturator neuropathy
- Paresis of adductor group of muscles
- Local anesthetic allergy
- Coagulopathy
- Patient refusal

OT Preparation

- Emergency drugs kept ready (thiopentone, adrenaline, atropine)
- Airway equipment (facemask, endotracheal tube, airways)
- Suction apparatus
- 1% lidocaine or 0.5% bupivacaine
- Around 15–20 mL used
- 21 G 4 inch needle
- 10 cc syringe

Patient Preparation

- NPO status confirmed
- Consent taken
- Venous access secured
- IV midazolam 0.03–0.05 mg/kg can be administered
- Standard monitors applied – ECG, blood pressure, pulse oximetry

Position

- Supine position
- Thigh slightly abducted and externally rotated
- Stand on the side of block

Technique

- *LABATS* classical technique
- Aseptic precautions
- Needle inserted perpendicular to skin, 1.5 cm lateral and 1.5 cm inferior to pubic tubercle
- Needle advanced posterior direction towards superior pubic ramus
- Local anesthetic injected as needle is advanced
- On contacting bone needle redirected in lateral and caudal direction and advanced
- Needle enters obturator foramen at 2–4 cm depth
- Adductor motor response of thigh elicited
- Reduce stimulation to < 0.5 mA
- Witness fade of motor activity after injection of 1 mL local anesthetic
- 15–20 mL local anesthetic injected in graded aliquots after negative aspiration of blood

Advantages

Prevents bladder perforation during TURBT

Disadvantages

- Technically difficult
- Lack of clear landmarks
- Block complexity
- Inconsistent results
- High complication rate

Complications

- Adductor muscle spasm
- Hematoma
- Perforation of bladder/rectum/spermatic cord
- Peripheral nerve damage–obturator neuropathy due to:
  - Needle trauma
  - Intraneural injection
  - Nerve ischemia
  - LA toxicity
- Intravascular injection
- LA Systemic Toxicity - LAST
- Infection
- Neuropraxia/neurolysis

SCIATIC NERVE BLOCK

Introduction

Sciatic nerve, the terminal branch of sacral plexus is the largest nerve in the body.

Anatomy

- Originates from lumbo-sacral trunk
- Terminal branch of sacral plexus
- Formed by anterior primary rami of spinal roots L_{4-5} S_{1-3}
- Exits pelvis through greater sciatic notch
- Travels between gluteus maximus and piriformis muscle

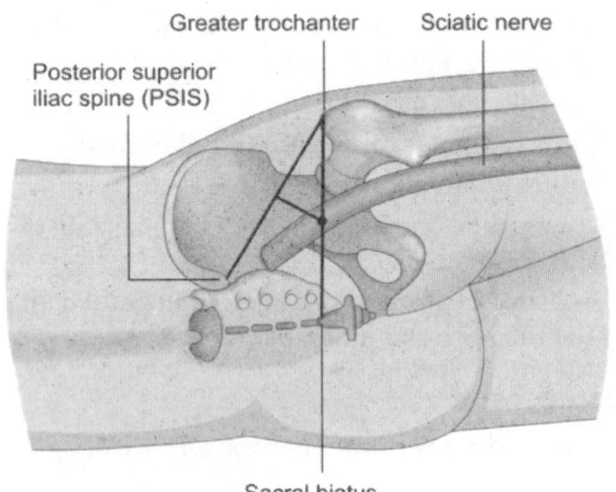

Fig. 9: Sciatic nerve block.

- Continues towards posterior thigh between greater trochanter and ischial tuberosity
- Divides into 2 branches in superior aspect of popliteal fossa:
  - Tibial nerve
  - Common peroneal nerve

Supply

- Sensory:
  - Posterior hip capsule
  - Knee joint
  - Lower extremity distal to knee except along antero-medial aspect
- Motor:
  - Hamstring muscles
  - All lower extremity muscles distal to knee

Indications

- Diagnosis and treatment of sciatic nerve entrapment
- Pyriformis syndrome
- In combination with femoral or lumbar plexus blocks
- Below knee amputations
- Foot and ankle surgeries

Contraindications

- Burn/infection at injection site
- Local anesthetic allergy
- Coagulopathy
- Preexisting neurological disease

OT Preparation

- Emergency drugs kept ready (thiopentone, adrenaline, atropine)
- Airway equipment (facemask, endotracheal tube, airways)
- Suction apparatus
- 1% lidocaine 0.5% bupivacaine in equal proportions
- Around 15–25 mL used
- 21 G 4 inch insulated needle
- 10 cc syringe

Patient Preparation

- NPO status confirmed
- Consent taken
- Venous access secured
- IV midazolam 0.03–0.05 mg/kg can be administered
- Standard monitors applied – ECG, blood pressure, pulse oximetry

Technique

I. **Classic Posterior Approach of *Labat:***

Position

- Lateral decubitus position (Sims position)
- Operative extremity non-dependant

Technique

- Strict asepsis
- Line drawn from greater trochanter to posterior superior iliac spine (GT-PSIS line)
- Second line drawn from greater trochanter to sacral hiatus (GT-SH line)
- Line drawn perpendicular to midpoint of GT-PSIS line in caudal direction
- Intersection of this perpendicular and GT-SH line is needle insertion point
- Needle advanced perpendicular to skin
- After eliciting gluteal stimulation, needle advanced further
- Motor response of distal ankle, foot or toes elicited
- Reduce stimulation to < 0.5 mA
- Witness fade of motor activity after injection of 1 mL local anesthetic
- 20–25 mL local anesthetic injected in graded aliquots after negative aspiration of blood
- Pressure applied for 10 seconds and patient made to lie supine immediately after injection

II. **Lithotomy Approach of *Raj*:**

Position

- Lithotomy position

Technique

- Strict asepsis
- Midpoint between greater trochanter and ischial tuberosity identified

- Needle inserted at this point and advanced perpendicular to skin
- Motor response elicited in distal ankle, foot or toes
- Reduce stimulation to < 0.5 mA
- Witness fade of motor activity after injection of 1 mL local anesthetic
- 15–20 mL local anesthetic injected in graded aliquots after negative aspiration of blood

III. Anterior Approach of *Meier*:

Position

- Supine position
- Legs in slight internal rotation

Technique

- Strict asepsis
- Line drawn between pubic tubercle and anterior superior iliac spine
- Second line drawn parallel to inguinal ligament starting from greater trochanter and going medially across anterior thigh
- First line is divided into 3 parts and perpendicular drawn from junction of middle and inner thirds
- Point of intersection of perpendicular and second line is point of insertion of needle
- Needle inserted perpendicular to skin
- Advanced till motor response of distal ankle or foot or toes noted
- Reduce stimulation to < 0.5 mA
- Witness fade of motor activity after injection of 1 mL local anesthetic
- 15–20 mL local anesthetic injected in graded aliquots after negative aspiration of blood

Advantages

- Multiple approaches

Disadvantages

- Block takes long onset time as it is resistant to LA penetration
- Difficult positioning especially in lower limb fractures
- Block crosses multiple muscle planes – painful
- Risk of injury to major vessels
- Incomplete sensory block below knee – requires supplemental saphenous N block
- Almost always requires a supplemental block
- Anterior approach is very distal – sparing of posterior cutaneous nerve of thigh

Complications

- Partial block – injection distal to branching of sciatic nerve
- Intra-neural injection - neuropraxia/neurolysis
- Hematoma – damage to inferior gluteal vessels
- Intravascular injection
- LA Systemic Toxicity - LAST
- Infection

POPLITEAL BLOCK

Introduction

Involves blocking sciatic nerve in the popliteal fossa

Anatomy

Boundaries of popliteal fossa:

- Lateral: Biceps femoris tendon
- Medial:
  - Semimembranosus
  - Semitendinosus
- Contents:
  - Popliteal artery (immediately lateral to semitendinosus)
  - Popliteal vein (lateral to artery)
  - Tibial nerve
  - Common peroneal nerve (lateral to vein, medial to biceps femoris)
- Tibial nerve continues deep to gastrocnemius muscle
- Common peroneal nerve passes between head and neck of fibula to supply lower leg

Indications

- Tourniquet analgesia for calf tourniquet
- Sural nerve biopsy

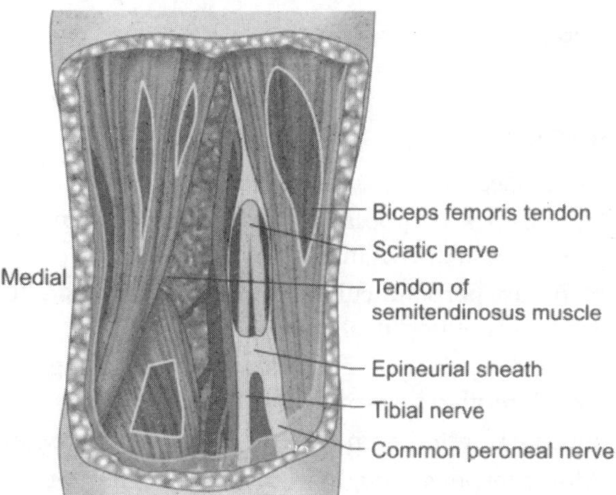

Fig. 10: Popliteal nerve block.

- Short saphenous nerve stripping
- Foot and ankle surgeries
- In conjunction with saphenous nerve block for complete anesthesia distal to knee

Contraindications

- Burn/infection at injection site
- Local anesthetic allergy
- Coagulopathy
- Preexisting neurological disease

OT Preparation

- Emergency drugs kept ready (thiopentone, adrenaline, atropine)
- Airway equipment (facemask, endotracheal tube, airways)
- Suction apparatus
- 1% lidocaine 0.5% bupivacaine in equal proportions
- Around 25–30 mL used
- 22 G 2 inch insulated stimulating needle
- 20 cc syringe

Patient Preparation

- NPO status confirmed
- Consent taken
- Venous access secured
- IV midazolam 0.03–0.05 mg/kg can be administered
- Standard monitors applied – ECG, blood pressure, pulse oximetry

Technique

I. Posterior Approach:

Position

Prone position

Technique

- Strict asepsis
- Boundaries of popliteal fossa identified and popliteal crease drawn inferiorly
- 8–10 cm perpendicular line drawn cephalad from midpoint of popliteal crease
- Insertion point is 1 cm below apex of triangle and 1 cm lateral to perpendicular line
- Needle inserted perpendicular to skin and advanced
- Motor response sought in distal ankle, foot or toes
- Reduce stimulation to <0.5 mA while witnessing activity
- Witness fade of motor activity after injection of 1 mL of local anesthetic
- After negative aspiration of blood 30–40 mL local anesthetic injected

II. Lateral Approach

Position

Supine position

Technique

- Palpate inter-tendinous groove between vastus lateralis and biceps femoris
- Groove present 10–12 cm proximal to superior notch of patella
- Needle advanced at 30° to skin, posteriorly angled
- Motor response elicited in distal ankle, toes or foot
- Reduce stimulation to < 0.5 mA while witnessing activity
- Witness fade of motor activity after injection of 1 mL of local anesthetic
- After negative aspiration of blood 25–40 mL local anesthetic injected

Advantages

- Preserves hamstring function
- Allows early mobilization of postoperative patient
- Prolonged postoperative analgesia

Disadvantages

- Variable success rate

Complications

- Block failure
- Heel necrosis
- Intraneural injection
- Intravascular injections – LA Systemic Toxicity (LAST)
- Hematoma
- Infection

SAPHENOUS NERVE BLOCK

Introduction

Allows rapid anesthetization of antero-medial lower extremity, including medial malleolus.

Anatomy

- Largest terminal sensory branch of femoral nerve
- Derived from L3L4 nerve roots
- Travels through femoral triangle, lateral to vessels

- Beyond femoral triangle, it lies between sartorius and gracilis
- Distal to knee, it proceeds caudally along medial aspect of leg, with saphenous vein
- Provides sensory innervation to medial aspect of lower leg between knee and medial malleolus

Indications

- Saphenous vein harvesting
- Knee arthroscopy
- Anterior cruciate ligament reconstruction
- Analgesia following medial meniscectomy
- Wound exploration/abscess drainage medial malleolus
- Usually in conjunction with popliteal block for medial foot/ankle surgery
- Usually not performed alone

Contraindications

- Preexisting peripheral neuropathy
- Patient refusal
- Anticoagulation
- Infection or inflammation over injection site
- Local anesthetic allergy

OT Preparation

- Emergency drugs kept ready (thiopentone, adrenaline, atropine)
- Airway equipment (facemask, endotracheal tube, airways)
- Suction apparatus
- 1% lidocaine
- Around 10–12 mL used
- 22 G 10 cm needle
- 10 cc syringe

Patient Preparation

- NPO status confirmed
- Consent taken
- Venous access secured
- IV midazolam 0.03–0.05 mg/kg can be administered
- Standard monitors applied – ECG, blood pressure, pulse oximetry

Position

- Supine position
- Thigh abducted and externally rotated

Technique

I. Below Knee Field Block Approach:

- Strict asepsis
- Subcutaneous infilteration of local anesthetic (7–10 mL)
- Infilteration starts from tibial tuberosity, directed medially
- Infiltration completed near posterior aspect of leg

II. Transsartorial Approach:

- Strict asepsis
- Identify sartorius muscle on medial aspect of leg, just above knee
- Needle inserted 2 cm above patella, slightly posterior and caudal to coronal plane
- Needle advanced through body of sartorius until it reaches subsartorial plane
- 7–10 mL local anesthetic injected

III. Paravenous Approach:

- Strict asepsis
- Tourniquet placed proximal to knee
- Leg placed over side of bed to make vein palpable
- Injection site along medial side of leg, just below patella
- 5 mL local anesthetic deposited on either side of vein in subcutaneous tissue

Complications

- Block failure
- Post-block ecchymosis/hematoma
- Neuritis secondary to needle trauma or drug toxicity
- Intravascular injection – Local anesthetic systemic toxicity (LAST)
- Infection

ANKLE BLOCK

Introduction

Ankle block accomplished by blocking 5 nerve trunks:

- Tibial nerve (L_{45},S_{123})
- Sural nerve
- Deep peroneal nerve (L_{45},S_{12})
- Superficial peroneal nerve (L_{45},S_{12})
- Saphenous nerve (L_{234})

Indications

- Heal spur excision
- Mortons neuroma excision
- Lacerations of foot
- Heal spur excision

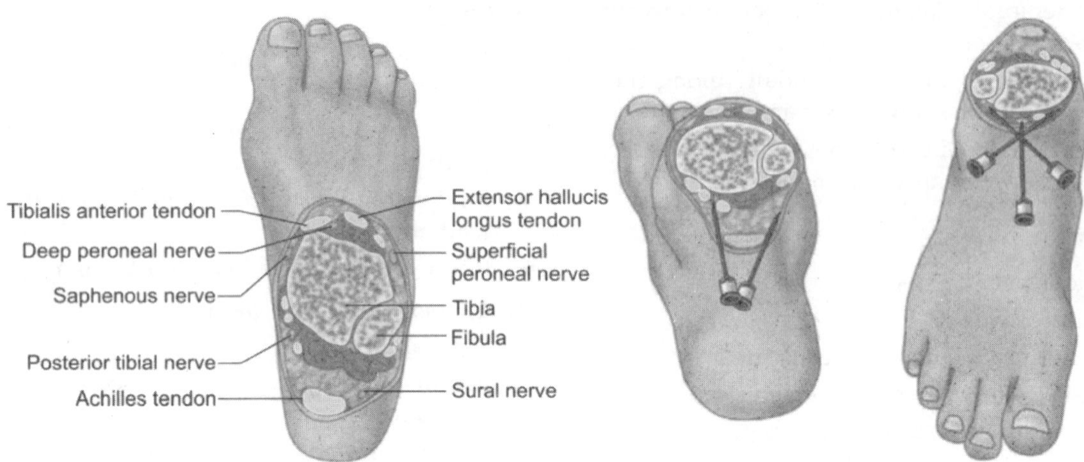

Fig. 11: Ankle block.

- Diabetic foot
- Toe amputation

Contraindications

- Localized infection of foot
- Young children
- Allergy to local anesthetics
- Patient noncompliance

Advantages

- Ease of administration
- Safe technique
- Rapid onset of anesthesia
- Avoids neuraxial or general anesthetic complications

Disadvantages

- Purely sensory
- Requires at least 3 separate injections
- Uncomfortable for patient

Complications

- Infection
- Residual paresthesias
- Hematoma
- Vascular puncture
- Nerve injury
- Block failure

Patient Preparation

- NPO status confirmed
- Consent taken
- Venous access secured
- IV midazolam 0.03–0.05 mg/kg can be administered
- Standard monitors applied–ECG, blood pressure, pulse oximetry

OT Preparation

- Emergency drugs kept ready (thiopentone, adrenaline, atropine)
- Airway equipment (facemask, endotracheal tube, airways)
- Suction apparatus
- 1% lidocaine 0.5% bupivacaine in equal proportions
- Around 30 mL used
- 25 G 3–5 cm needle
- 10 cc syringe

Position

- Supine
- Blanket/pillow under lower leg

Tibial Nerve

Anatomy

- Lies behind posterior tibial artery
- Anteromedial to Achilles tendon
- Deep to flexor retinaculum

Supply

- Sole and plantar portion of toes upto nails

Technique

- 3–5 cm 25G needle
- Directed at right angle to tibia
- Medial to Achilles tendon at level of upper border of medial malleolus

- Advanced until paresthesia elicited or bone contacted
- 5–7 mL local anesthetic injected near posterior aspect of tibia
- Equal volume injected during withdrawal

Sural Nerve

Anatomy

- Located posterior to lateral malleolus
- Resides in superficial plane
- Accompanies short saphenous vein
- Extends to third digit

Supply

- Cutaneous sensation of lower posterolateral ankle, lateral foot, fifth toe

Technique

- Subcutaneous infilteration from lateral malleolus to Achilles tendon
- Given at upper border of lateral malleolus
- 5–10 mL of local anesthetic injected

Deep Peroneal Nerve

Anatomy

- Courses midway between malleoli
- Assumes position between anterior tibial and extensor hallucis longus tendons
- Present beneath extensor retinaculum at dorsum of foot
- Lies lateral to deep peroneal artery

Supply

- Innervates short extensors of toe
- Skin sensations to interdigital cleft between great and second toes

Technique

- Patient dorsiflexes foot
- Tendon of extensor hallucis longus identified
- 25G 3–5 cm needle used
- Needle inserted perpendicular to skin along line joining malleoli
- Point of insertion lateral to dorsalis pedis artery
- LOR felt during passage through extensor retinaculum
- Advanced until tibia is felt
- Paresthesia maybe felt between great and second toe
- 3–5 mL local anesthetic injected

Superficial Peroneal Nerve

Anatomy

- Located on dorsal lateral aspect of foot
- Lie superficially above fascial plane

Supply

- Cutaneous sensation to dorsum of foot and toes
- All areas supplied except between great and second toes

Technique

- Inject local anesthetic subcutaneously
- Injected laterally from site of injection of deep peroneal nerve
- Directed towards superficial aspect of lateral malleolus
- 5–10 mL local anesthetic solution injected

Saphenous Nerve

Anatomy

- Runs anterior to medial malleolus near long saphenous nerve
- Lies deep and posterior to great saphenous vein

Supply

- Cutaneous innervation to anteromedial side of lower leg
- Medial foot midway to toes

Technique

- 3–5 mL local anesthetic injected subcutaneously
- Medially posterior to great saphenous vein
- Local anesthetic injected at anterior aspect of medial malleolus

COMPLEX REGIONAL PAIN SYNDROME

Introduction

CRPS formerly known as *reflex sympathetic dystrophy*, is a debilitating neuropathic pain disorder causing severe burning pain and vasomotor instability, due to autonomic nervous system dysfunction, usually in an extremity.

Types

CRPS Type I

- ***Reflex sympathetic dystrophy***
- Minor injuries/fractures of limb precede onset of symptoms

CRPS Type II

- ***Causalgia***
- Develops after injury to major peripheral nerve

Etiology

Highest incidence between 50–70 years age
More frequently in women

- Trauma affecting distal part of extremity
- Postsurgical condition
- Contusions
- Strain/sprain
- CNS lesions:
  - Spinal cord injuries
  - CVA
  - Cardiac ischemia

Pathophysiology

Various theories:

- Genetic predisposition
- Immobilization of limb
- Unregulated sympathetic nervous system
- Exaggerated neurogenic inflammation

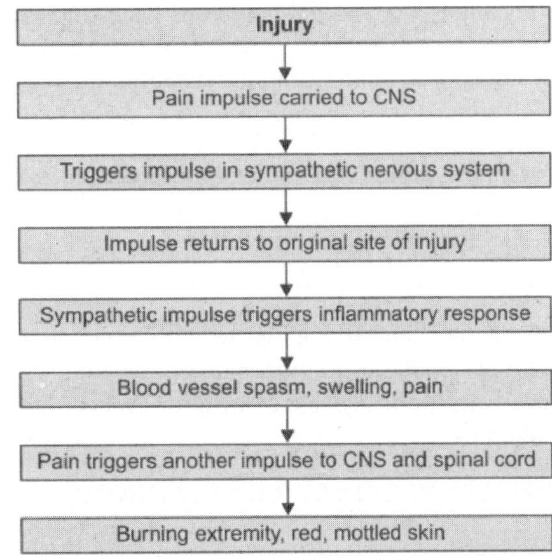

Clinical Features

Pain

- Poorly controlled
- Distal extremity
- Burning, spontaneous pain
- Disproportionate intensity to the inciting event
- Increases with limb in dependant position

Autonomic Disturbances

- Swelling, sweating in the distal extremity
- Affected limb warmer than normal limb
- Hyper or hypohydrosis of affected limb

Trophic Changes

- Abnormal nail growth
- Increased/decreased hair growth
- Thin, glossy skin
- Osteoporosis in chronic cases
- Restriction of passive limb movements
- Weakness of all muscles of extremity
- Movement disorders:
  - Loss of voluntary control
  - Bradykinesia
  - Dystonia
  - Myoclonus, tremors

CRPS type II has all these features in addition to focal deficits due to lesions of peripheral nerve

Stages

- *Warm stage*: With initial vasomotor symptoms
- *Intermediate stage*: With sudomotor symptoms
- *Cold stage*: With dystrophic and motor changes

Diagnosis

Modified IASP Diagnostic Criteria (Budapest Criteria)

I. Continuing pain disproportionate to inciting event

II. At least one symptom in each category of:

Sensory:

- Hyperesthesia
- And/or allodynia

Vasomotor:

- Temperature asymmetry
- And/or skin color changes
- And /or skin color asymmetry in affected region

Sudomotor/edema:

- Edema
- And/or sweating changes
- And/or sweating asymmetry in affected region

Motor/trophic:

- Decreased range of motion
- And/or motor dysfunction (weakness, tremor, dystonia)
- And/or trophic changes (hair, nails, skin) in affected region

III. At least one sign in 2 or more categories:

Sensory: Evidence of:

- Hyperalgesia to pin prick
- And/or allodynia to light touch and/or deep somatic pressure and/or joint movement

Vasomotor: Evidence of:

- Temperature asymmetry
- And/or skin color changes and/or asymmetry

Sudomotor/edema: Evidence of:
- ❖ Edema
- ❖ And/or sweating changes
- ❖ And/or sweating asymmetry

Motor/trophic: Evidence of:
- ❖ Decreased range of motion
- ❖ And/or motor dysfunction (weakness, tremor, dystonia)
- ❖ And/or trophic changes (hair, skin, nails)

IV. No other diagnosis better explains the signs and symptoms

Treatment

Options

- ❖ Anti-inflammatory agents:
  - Naproxen
  - Ketorolac
  - Prednisone
  - Intravenous immunoglobulins
  - Anti-TNF monoclonal antibodies
- ❖ Free Radical Scavengers:
  - Topical DMSO
  - Vitamin C
- ❖ Inhibition of pain sensitization:
  - Intrathecal baclofen
  - Topical capsaicin
  - Carbamazepine oral
  - Gabapentin oral
  - Nifedipine oral
  - Ketamine oral
  - Intrathecal glycine
  - Intravenous lidocaine
  - Intrathecal morphine
- ❖ Sympatholytic agents:
  - Topical clonidine
  - Intravenous lidocaine + guanethidine
  - Phenoxybenzamine
  - Reserpine

Goals

- ❖ Relative pain reduction of at least 50%
- ❖ Reduction of VAS score by 30 mm on 100 mm scale

Guidelines

- ❖ General;
  - Immobilize affected limb
  - Careful contralateral physiotherapy – ***acute treatment of choice***
  - Assume passive physical therapy of affected limb once resting pain subsides
  - Active isometric strengthening in combination with sensory desensitization programmes till restoration of complete motor function
- ❖ Analgesics:
  - NSAIDs: COX-2 inhibitors (etodolac, aceclofenac) ***first line analgesics***
  - Gabapentin, pregabalin: ***First line coanalgesics***
  - Opioids
  - Antidepressants
  - Calcium regulation agents: If refractory pain
- ❖ Anti-inflammatory
  - Corticosteroids
- ❖ Muscle relaxants:
  - Tizanidine
  - Baclofen
  - Clonazepam
- ❖ Sympatholytic procedures:
  - Sympathetic ganglion blocks:
    - Stellate ganglion blocks
    - Lumbar sympathetic blocks
  - Continuous intrathecal drug delivery systems:
    - ***Continuous Intrathecal Pump Implantation (CIPI)***
    - With intrathecal baclofen
    - Exorbitant cost
  - ***Radiofrequency neurolysis (RFN):***
    - Decreased incidence of neuritis
    - Avoids tinnitus
    - Avoids blindness
    - Avoids urethral stricture
  - ***Spinal cord stimulation:***
  - ***Endoscopic thoracic sympathectomy (ETS)***
  - ***Motor cortex stimulation***
- ❖ Psychological support:
  - Cognitive behavioral therapy
  - Transcedental meditation

SUGGESTED READING

1. Barash, P.G., et al. (2017). *Clinical Anesthesia*. 8th ed. China: Wolters Kluwer.
2. Butterworth, J., Mackey, D., Wasnik, J. (2018). *Morgan and Mikhails Clinical Anesthesiology*. 6th ed. New York: McGraw-Hill Education/Medical.
3. Dorsch, J.A., Dorsch, S.E. (2008). *Understanding Anesthesia Equipment*. 5th ed. Philadelphia: Wolters Kluwer/LWW.
4. Gropper, M., Eriksson, L., Fleisher, L., Wiener-Kronish, J., Cohen, N., Leslie, K. (2020). *Millers Anesthesia*. 9th ed. Philadelphia: Elsevier Saunders.
5. Horlocker, T.T., Vandermeuelen, E., Kopp, S.L., Gogarten, W., Leffert, L.R., Benzon, H.T. (2018). Regional anesthesia in the patient receiving antithrombotic or thrombolytic therapy. *Regional Anesthesia and Pain Medicine*, 43(3), 263-309.
6. Miller, R.D., Eriksson, L., Fleisher, L, Wiener-Kronish, J., Cohen, N., Young, W. (2014). *Millers Anesthesia*. 8th ed. New York: Elsevier Health.

9

CHAPTER

Machine and Monitors

MINIMUM MONITORING STANDARDS

Introduction

- Emphasizes importance of regular and frequent measures and integration of clinical judgment with experience and the potential for extenuating circumstances which can influence accuracy of monitoring systems
- Emphasizes melding of physical signs with instrumentation

Objectives

- Intended to encourage quality patient care
- Applied to all GA, RA and MAC
- Standards may be exceeded at any time based on judgment of anesthetist

Standard I

Objective

- Emphasizes importance of clinical observation
- To modify anesthesia care based on clinical observations

Requirement

- Qualified personnel to be in OT during GA/RA/MAC to monitor patient continuously
- If known direct hazard to anesthetist, e.g. radiation, some provision for remote observation to be made
- If emergency requires temporary absence of anesthetist, judgment exercised to compare emergency with anesthetized patients condition and in selection of substitute during temporary absence

Standard II

- Constitutes standards for evaluation of patients oxygenation ventilator, circulation and temperature
- Mandates the following:

1. Oxygenation

   Objective:
   - To ensure adequate O_2 concentration in inspired gas and blood during all anesthetics

   Methods:
   - Use of O_2 analyzer with low concentration alarm limit during GA
   - Assess blood oxygenation using pulse oximetry
   - Adequate illumination and exposure of patient to assess color
2. Ventilation

   Objective:
   - To ensure adequate ventilation of patient during all anesthetics

   Methods:
   - Clinical signs:
     - Chest excursion
     - Movement of reservoir breathing bag
     - Auscultation of breath sounds
   - Sufficient ventilation assessed by clinical signs and exhaled CO_2
   - Ensure correct placement of ETT/LMA with clinical assessment and identification of CO_2 is expired gas
   - Continuous E_TCO_2 monitored from time of ETT/LMA placement till extubation
   - Monitor tidal volume and E_TCO_2
   - When using mechanical ventilator, use a device which is able to detect disconnection of circuits
   - Device to give audible alarm on disconnection.
3. Circulation

   Objective:
   - To ensure adequacy of patients circulatory function during all anesthetics

   Methods:
   - Continuous display of ECG
   - Determine BP and HR at least at 5 min interval
   - In addition to these, at least one of:
     - Palpation of peripheral pulse
     - Evaluation of quality of pulse
     - Auscultation of heart sounds
     - Pulse plethysmography/oximetry
     - Monitoring IBP trace
     - Ultrasound peripheral pulse monitoring

4. Temperature
   Objective:
   - To aid in maintenance of appropriate body temperature during all anesthetics

   Methods:
   - Continuously monitor patients temperature and record on anesthesia record

PULSE OXIMETRY

Introduction

- Non-invasive method of measuring hemoglobin saturation with oxygen using a light signal transmitted through tissue
- ***Fifth vital sign***

Principle

- Estimates SpO_2 from differential absorption of red and infrared light in tissues
- ***Beer Lambert law***: Relates concentration of solute to intensity of light transmitted through the solution
- Oxyhemoglobin absorbs more infrared light (940 nm)
- Deoxyhemoglobin absorbs more red light (660 nm)
- Ratio of absorption of red and infrared wavelength analyzed by microprocessor

Physics

- Combines two technologies:
  - *Spectrophotometer*: Measures oxyhemoglobin saturation
  - *Optical plethysmography*: Measures pulsatile changes in arterial blood volume at sensor site
- Differentiation between arterial blood and other components by determining change in transmitted light caused by pulsatile flow of arterial blood

Types of Pulse Oximetry

1. Transmission pulse oximetry:
   - Most common type

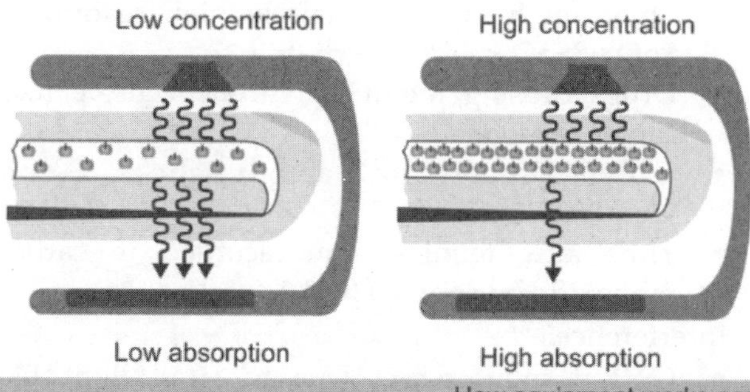

Fig. 1: Pulse oximeter.

   - Light beam transmitted through a vascular bed and detected on the opposite side of that bed
2. Reflectance pulse oximetry:
   - Relies on light reflected back from blood
   - Probe has both the LED and photodiode on same side
   - Disadvantages:
     - Can be errors due to light reflected from skin
     - Signal weaker than that in transmission pulse oximetry
     - Vasoconstriction may overestimate SpO_2
3. Co-oximetry:
   - ***Gold standard*** for measuring SaO_2
   - Traditional blood gas analyzer capable of measuring:
     - Concentration of oxyhemoglobin
     - Reduced hemoglobin
     - Carboxyhemoglobin
     - Methemoglobin
4. Transcutaneous oximetry:
   - Two wavelengths of light used to measure quantity of oxygenated and deoxygenated blood
   - Measures SaO_2 instead of PO_2

Results Displayed

- Percentage saturation of hemoglobin
- Arterial pulse waveform
- Heart rate

Other Variables

- Fractional O_2 saturation (% HbO_2) is ratio of oxyhemoglobin to sum of all hemoglobin species present
- Functional O_2 saturation (SaO_2) is ratio of oxyhemoglobin to all functional hemoglobin

Sites of Application

- Finger, toe
- Ear
- Cheek, forehead
- Tongue, pharynx, esophagus
- Thenar, hypothenar eminence, palm, wrist
- Lower calf, ankle, foot
- Penis

Uses of Pulse Oximetry

Anesthetic Procedures

- Mandatory for any anesthetic procedure including moderate sedation cases
- Particularly useful in:
  - Pre-existing lung diseases

- Special anesthetic techniques (one lung ventilation)
- OSAS and polysomnography

Controlling Oxygen Administration

- Allows lowest safe oxygen flow
- Prevents development of retinopathy in premature infants by setting high SpO_2 alarms at 95% (avoids hyperoxia)

Monitoring Vascular Volume and Peripheral Circulation

- Skipped beats/waxing and waning pattern indicates hypovolemia
- Reduction in plethysmographic amplitude indicates hypovolemia
- Dicrotic notch descends to baseline with increasing vasodilation and gets higher with vasoconstriction
- Can detect arm positions which compromise circulation (during shoulder surgery)
- Patients with limb fractures may have compromised circulation distal to fracture
- Evaluating effectiveness of palmar collateral circulation

Determining SBP: By placing pulse oximeter on same side as BP cuff

Locating Artery

When axillary artery not palpable, place pulse oximeter on a ipsilateral finger

Apply pressure on axilla till pulse wave disappears

Evaluate epidural: Increase in amplitude of pulse oximeter waveform by 10% indicates successful block

Adequacy of CPR: Amplitude of pulse oximetry waveform indicates adequacy of CPR

Complications

- Corneal abrasions: On recovery from GA, if patient rubs eye with finger having probe
- Pressure and ischemic injury:
  - On prolonged application
  - Ranging from persistent numbness to ischemic injury
- Burns:
  - Due to incompatibility between probe of one manufacturer and pulse oximeter of another
  - During MRI
- Electrical Shock:
  - Rare
  - Due to diathermy

Advantages

- Light weight and compact
- Accurate, non invasive fast response time
- Not affected by other gases/vapors
- Tone modulation with change in saturation
- Continuous measurement displayed
- Determines respiratory and circulatory variables:
  - If BP low and pulse signal good, patient is vasodilated with good CO
  - If BP and pulse signal low, patient has low CO

Recent Advances

- Error correction of inaccuracies due to motion sensitivity and hypoperfusion
- Multiwavelength pulse oximeters: 8 wavelength pulse oximeters capable of measuring several species of Hb
- Reflectance pulse oximetry: Useful if poor signal transmission during hypoperfusion

Contraindications

Limitations/Disadvantages

- Failure to detect:
  - External pressure: CPB
  - Hypotension, hypovolemia: Hypothermia
  - Raynauds phenomenon: Improper position
  - Low cardiac output
- Inaccurate:
  - Sickle cell anemia: Onychomycosis
  - High amounts of fetal Hb: Too large/too small a probe
  - Low saturation levels: Long finger nails
  - Dark skinned people: Dyes: methylene blue, indocyanin green
  - Nail polish: Poor peripheral pulsations
- Methemoglobinemia:
  - Methemoglobin absorbs light equally at both red and infrared wavelengths
  - As a result of this, the 1:1 absorption ratio corresponds to saturation reading of 85%
  - Thus, methHb causes falsely high reading of SpO_2 if $SaO_2 < 85\%$
  - Drugs causing methHb: Nitrobenzene, benzocaine, dapsone
  - CarboxyHb and HbO_2 absorb light at 660 nm identically
  - Thus false readings are recorded in carbon monoxide poisoning (100%)
- Interference:
  - Optical interference: Due to stray light like sunlight/fluorescent light/OR light/IR radiant warmers causing inaccurate readings

- Electrical interference: Due to electrocautery
- Motion artefacts: In shivering/Parkinsons
- Erractic performance in dysrhythmias
- May not function in IABP patients

❖ Delayed hypoxic event detection:
- Does not detect hypoventilation and hypercarbia with reduction in SpO_2
- Especially if patient is receiving supplemental O_2

CAPNOGRAPHY

Definitions

❖ Capnography is defined as continuous monitoring of CO_2 concentrations versus time in a gas mixture
❖ Capnogram is the tracings of waveforms obtained on the monitor
❖ Capnography is the machine that generates the wave form
❖ Capnometer is the device that performs the measurement and displays the readings in numerical form

Types of Capnographs

I. Side Stream Analyzer

Technique

❖ Sample is removed from circuit to be evaluated
❖ Withdraws gas 50-150 mL/min via sampling tube near ETT
❖ Sample transported to a distant device for evaluation
❖ Sampled gas is then released into atmosphere/returned to circuit through a second tube

Sites of Sampling

❖ Endotracheal tube
❖ Facemask (placed in patients nares/attached to upper lip)
❖ LMA (can be inserted through elbow connector)
❖ Mask outlet in non-intubated patients
❖ Jet ventilator (connected to sampling lumen)

Advantages

❖ Allows for unobstructive sampling near patient
❖ Calibration usually automatic
❖ Patient interface is light
❖ Sampling port can be used to administer bronchodilators

Disadvantages

❖ Prone to gas leak, sample tube obstruction and moisture problems
❖ Hypoventilation if sampling rate > fresh gas flow rate
❖ Error if sampling rate > expiratory flow rate: causes inspired gas to be sampled

Sources of Error

❖ Water vapor condensation in sample tubing
❖ Liquids and particulate matter entering cell
❖ Delayed response time
❖ Multiple sites for damage/gas leakage
❖ CO_2 can diffuse out of sample tube
❖ Longer tubing increases chances of error

II. Main Stream/Direct Flow Through

Technique

❖ Total volume of inspired and expired gas passes through sensing device
❖ Sensing device located at endotracheal tube (sensor)
❖ Measuring chamber warmed to 40°C to prevent condensation of water vapor on sensor window
❖ Eg: *Siemens Sirecrust 300* and *FEF ETCO$_2$* detector

Advantage

❖ Allows for analysis of multiple gases
❖ Very accurate and stable
❖ Avoids sampling system
❖ No delay in response time
❖ Reduces sample tubing dead space

Disadvantages

❖ Large and bulky
❖ Adds more dead space in pediatric patients
❖ Can cause kinking of ETT due to weight
❖ Requires frequent calibration
❖ Prone to soiling with mucus/saliva due to proximity to patient
❖ Leak/circuit disconnection can occur
❖ Can measure only O_2 and N_2O
❖ Difficult to use in intubated patients
❖ *Siemens 300 Sirecrust* uses a heated sensor which may cause thermal burns

Side Stream vs Mainstream Capnography

No.	Main stream/non-diverting	Side stream/diverting
1.	Sensor located between breathing circuit and ETT	Sensor located in main vent
2.	No sampling required	Sample tubing aspirates gas
3.	Have fast response time	Slow response time
4.	Standard gas not required for calibration	Supply of calibration gas is needed
5.	Frequent calibration required	Automatically calibrated
6.	Increased dead space due to use of adaptor	No such problem

Contd...

Contd...

No.	Main stream/non-diverting	Side stream/diverting
7.	Patient interface heavy due to weight of adaptor	Patient interface is light
8.	Adaptor causes kink in ETT/ disconnection of circuit	No such problem
9.	Difficult to use in unintubated patients	Relatively easy
10.	Cannot be used for this	Sampling port: to administer bronchodilator
11.	Water and secretions are seldom a problem	Secretions can occlude sample tubing
12.	Damaged by inhaled drugs like inhaled β blockers	Not so
13.	May cause thermal burns	Not so
14.	Not possible	*Hyperventilation*: If sampling rate > FGF

Principles: Three methods available:

- Infrared analysis: Quantitative
  - Blackbody radiation technology
  - Microstream technology
- Chemical colorimetric analysis: Semiquantitative
  - Hygroscopic
  - Hydrophobic
- Mass spectroscopy

INFRARED ANALYSIS

Introduction

- Most common technology
- Used most commonly with side stream sampling

Principle

- Gases with 2 or more dissimilar atoms in a molecule have specific IR light absorption spectra (E.g.: CO_2, N_2O)
- Amount of IR absorbed proportional to concentration of absorbing molecules
- Concentration determined by comparing IR light absorbance in sample with known standard

Technologies

I. Blackbody Radiation Technology

- Most commonly used
- Heated element called blackbody emitter is source of IR
- Filter present to block radiation which is outside the desired range
- Analyzer selects appropriate IR wave length to maximize absorption by selected gas
- Sensor detects transmitted IR light and converts it to electrical signals
- Electrical signal amplified and concentration is displayed

II. Microstream Technology

- Laser based technology to generate IR light
- Uses smaller sample cell and low flow rates (50 mL/min)
- IR light precisely matches absorption spectrum of CO_2
- Emitted electrons excite nitrogen molecules
- These molecules collide with CO_2 molecules and excite them
- IR light of signature wavelength of CO_2 emitted as excited CO_2 molecules drop back to ground state
- Amplitude of signal depends on amount of IR radiation absorbed which is proportional to CO_2 concentration

Advantages

- Rapid response time
- Require low sample flow
- Not affected by pressure of other gases
- Small sample cell required which is useful in:
  - Small patient
  - High respiratory rates
  - Low flow applications
  - Non- intubated patient

Disadvantages

- Continuous withdrawal of gas from RS (if used with side stream)
- Propensity to leak/occlude
- Sensitive to water accumulation

CHEMICAL COLORIMETRIC ANALYSIS

Principles

- Consists of a pH sensitive indicator enclosed in a housing
- When indicator is exposed to carbonic acid (formed by reaction CO_2 and H_2O), it becomes acidic

Technologies

I. Hygroscopic

- Can detect CO_2 concentration in range 0.25-0.6 %
- Minimum CO_2 concentration to produce color change is 0.54 %

- Life span of detector depends on humidity of expired gas
- Reduced humidity prolongs detectors life
- Color changes are:
  - Purple: Low CO_2 (< 0.5% or < 2.3 mm Hg)
  - Beige: Moderate CO_2 (0.5-2% or 3.7-7.6 mm Hg)
  - Yellow: High CO_2 (>2% or > 15.2 mm Hg)
  - Changes color back to purple after removal of CO_2

II. Hydrophobic

- Color changes from blue to green to yellow as CO_2 concentration increases
- Faster response time
- Less affected by humidity
- Performs better at higher respiratory rate

Advantages

- Cheaper, easy to use, disposable
- Small in size, portable
- Useful in remote site resuscitative evaluation
- Not affected by N_2O or anesthetic vapor
- Require no other equipment

Disadvantages

- May be several breaths before conclusion is drawn–
- Wait for six breaths with colorimetric methods
- False positive results in:
  - Ingested carbonated drinks/antacids
  - Mask ventilation
- False negative results in:
  - Low tidal volume
  - Low E_TCO_2 concentration
  - Compromised lung perfusion

Mass Spectrometry

- Gas withdrawn continuously through capillary lines
- Sample directed into mass spectrometer
- Sample is ionized and then exposed to magnetic field in a vacuum chamber
- Ionized molecules separated by mass–charge ratio
- Collectors in vacuum chamber determine concentration of each gas component

CAPNOGRAPH

Types of Capnographs

- Time volume capnograph
- Volume capnograph

Description

- Height depends on E_TCO_2 concentration
- Frequency depends on respiratory rate
- Rhythm shows regularity of breathing
- Normal shape is ***Top Hat/Sine Wave***
- Baseline is normally zero (EA)

Phases of Capnograph

Phase I: EA

- *Inspiratory Baseline*
- Usually is zero
- Reflects inspired gas devoid of CO_2

Phase II: BC

- *Expiratory upstroke*
- Rapid S-shaped upswing
- Represents transition gas from anatomical dead space
- Prolonged in:
  - Partial endotracheal tube obstruction
  - COPD, bronchospasm
  - Upper airway obstruction

Phase III: CD

- *Plateau phase*
- Represents gas coming from alveoli
- End of phase III at point D is *End tidal point*

Phase IV: DE

- *Inspiratory downstroke*
- Represents patient inhalation
- CO_2 levels abruptly falls to zero

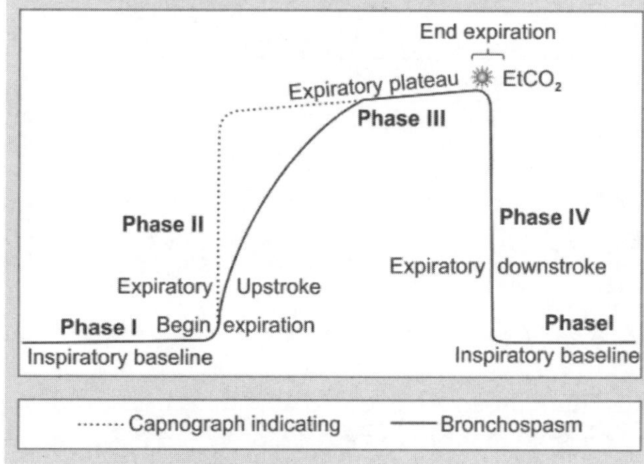

Fig. 2: Normal capnograph.

Angles of Capnograph

α *Angle*

- *Take off/elevation angle*
- Angle between phase II and phase III
- Normally between 100–110
- Decreased in obstructive lung diseases
- Increased in:
  - Airway obstruction
  - PEEP

β *Angle*

- Angle between phase III and descending limb of capnogram
- Normally around 90
- Decreased in airway obstruction and PEEP
- Increased in rebreathing

Variation in Shape of Waveform

- *Cardiogenic oscillations*
  - Due to heart beating against lungs
- Incompetent inspiratory uni-directional valve
  - Prolonged plateau with slanting inspiratory downstroke
- Irregular plateau/baseline
  - Displacement of ETT into upper larynx/lower pharynx with intermittent ventilation of stomach and lungs
  - Pressure on chest
- Leak in sample line during IPPV
- Biphasic expiratory plateau
  - Severe kypho-scoliosis
  - One lung ventilation
  - Single lung transplantation
  - Very high airway resistance
- Obstruction/sample contamination
- Contamination of sample with fresh gas or ambient air
  - Occurs due to sampling site being too close to fresh gas flow inlet
  - Leak in sample tube

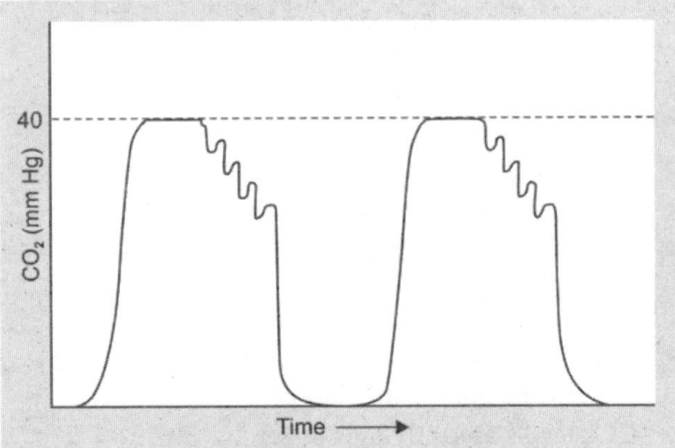

Fig. 3: Cardiogenic oscillations on capnogram.

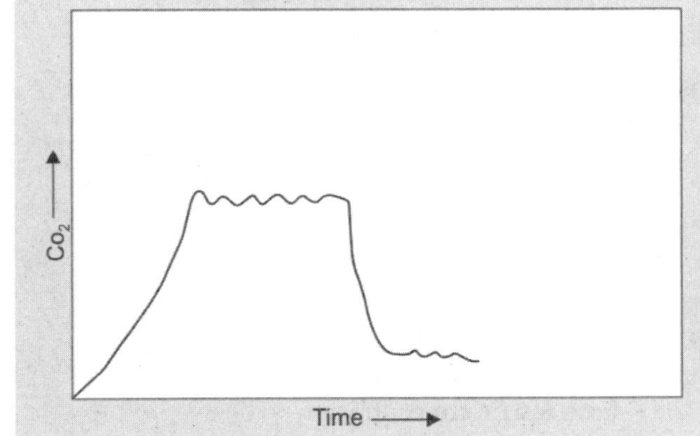

Fig. 5: Irregular baseline.

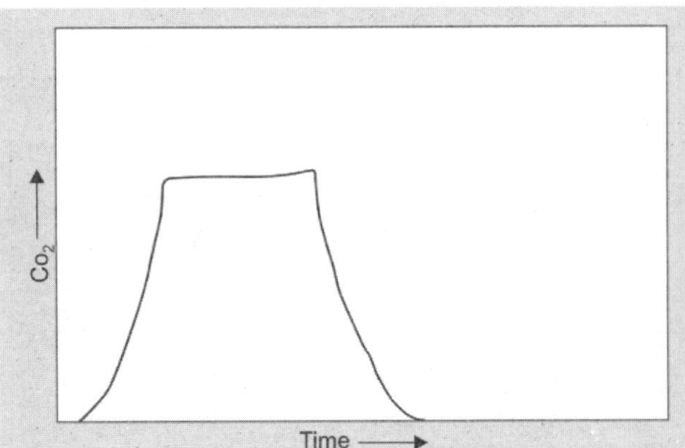

Fig. 4: Incompetent inspiratory unidirectional valve.

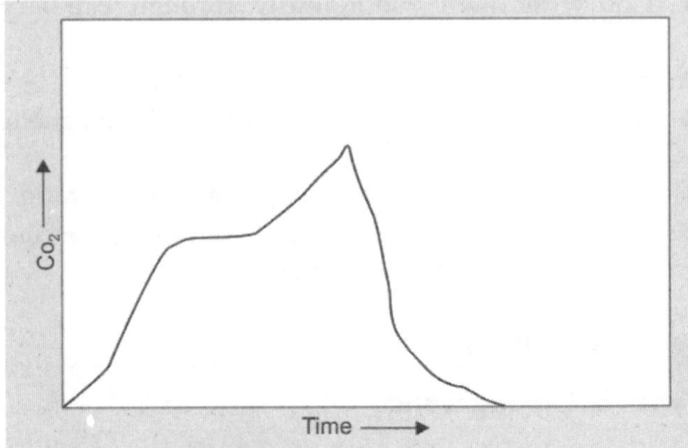

Fig. 6: Leak in sample line.

Too low sampling rate in side stream analyzer

❖ Curare cleft/notch
  - Depression is last third of plateau
  - Occurs if patient is spontaneously breathing
  - Due to lack of synchronous action between intercostal muscles and diaphragm
  - Also seen in:
    - Flail chest
    - Hiccough
    - Pneumothorax
    - Spontaneous breaths in a patient on ventilator

❖ Rebreathing with elevated base line

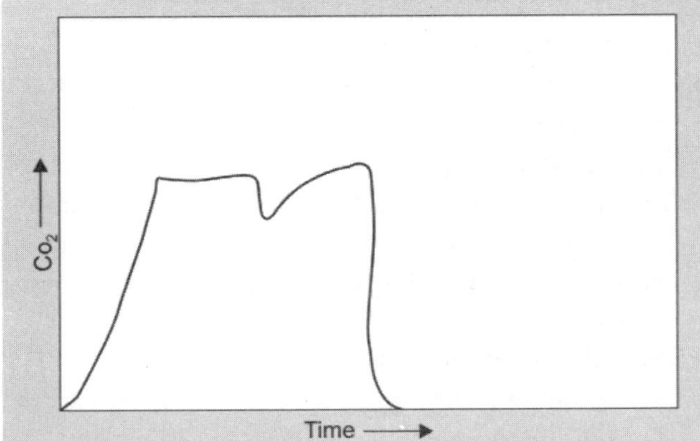

Fig. 7: Biphasic expiratory plateau.

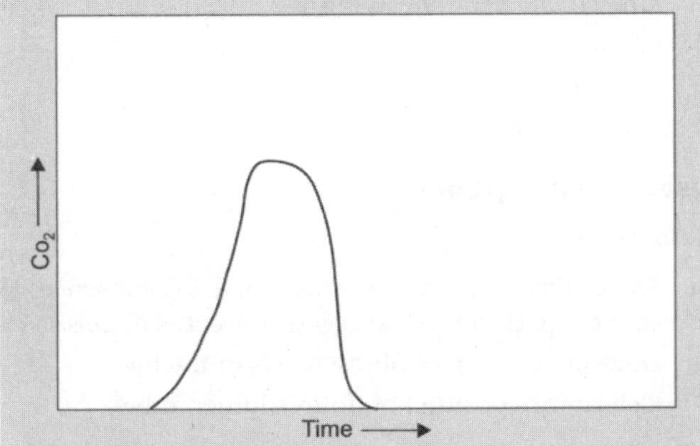

Fig. 8: Obstruction.

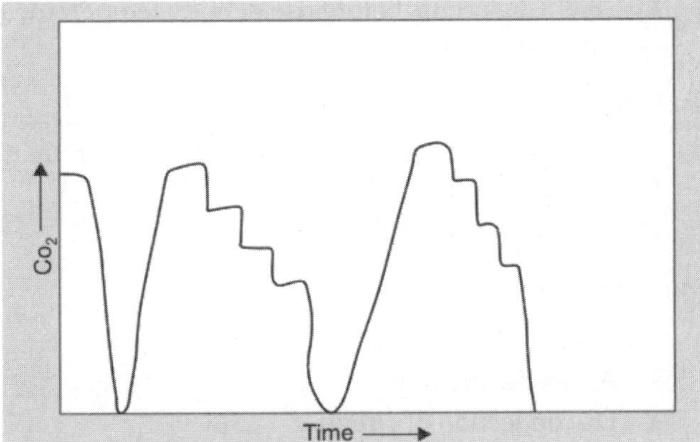

Fig. 9: Sampling contamination.

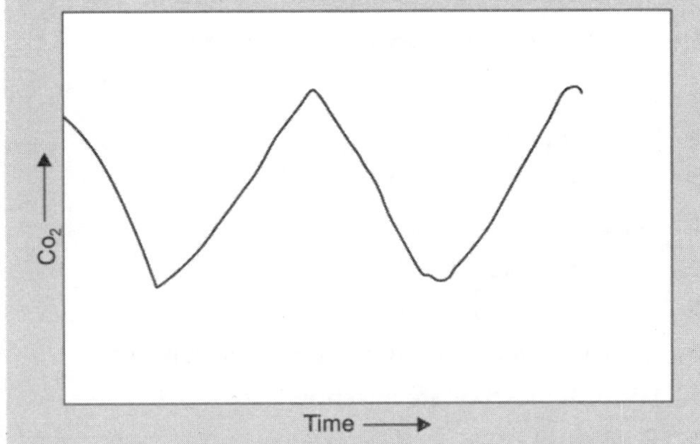

Fig. 10: Low sampling rate.

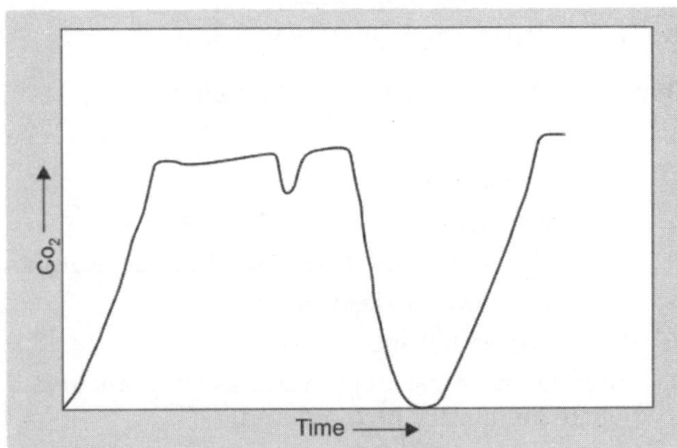

Fig. 11: Curare cleft.

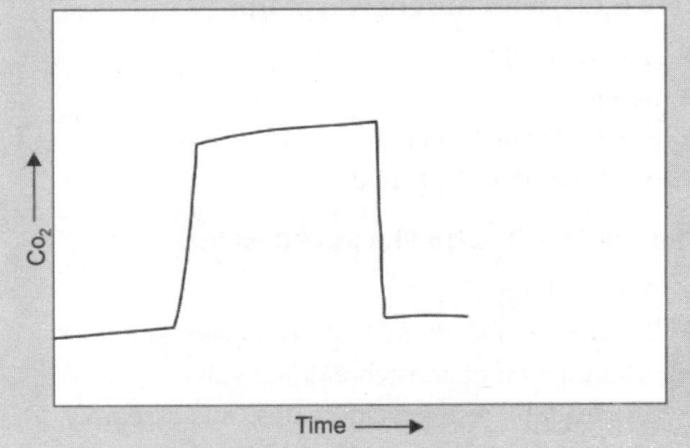

Fig. 12: Rebreathing with elevated baseline.

CAPNOMETRY

Normal Values

- E_TCO_2: 35-45 mm Hg
- $PaCO_2 - E_TCO_2$ gradient: 1–5 mm Hg ($PaCO_2 > E_TCO_2$)
- $PaCO_2 - E_TCO_2$ gradient during general anesthesia: 5–10 mm Hg

Elevated E_TCO_2 with Normal Waveform

- Hypoventilation
- Hyperthermia
- Malignant hyperthermia
- Sepsis
- Hyperthyroidism
- Pain, anxiety, shivering
- Increased skeletal muscle tone, convulsion
- Sodium bicarbonate injection
- Reperfusion:
  - Tourniquet release
  - Aortic cross clamp release
- During laparoscopic surgery with CO_2

Decreased E_TCO_2 with Normal Waveform

- Hyperventilation
- Hypothermia, shock
- Hypothyroidism
- Increased depth of anesthesia, use of muscle relaxants
- Increase anatomical dead space
- Pulmonary embolism
- Surgeries on heart lung and dissecting aneurysm (where pulmonary BF is reduced)
- Wedging of PA catheter
- Leakage in sample line

Zero E_TCO_2 with Absent Waveform

- Disconnection
- Apnea
- Ventilator malfunction
- Blockage of sample line

Elevated E_TCO_2 with Elevated Baseline

- Rebreathing
- Exhausted absorbent, bypassed absorbent
- Malfunction of non-rebreathing valve
- Inadequate fresh gas flow rates, mis-assembly
- Problem with inner tubing in Bain circuit
- Increased apparatus dead space

Elevated E_TCO_2 with Abnormal Waveform

- Prolonged expiratory upstroke seen
- Upper airway obstruction
- COPD
- Bronchospasm

Causes of Increased $PaCO_2$ -E_TCO_2 Gradient

- Right-left cardiac shunt
- Endobronchial/esophageal intubation
- Decreased cardiac output states
- Increased dead space ventilation:
  - Air/amniotic fluid/fat pulmonary embolism
  - Bronchospasm
- Hypoperfusion states with decreased pulmonary blood flow
- Sample contamination:
  - Disconnection
  - Cuff leaks
  - Sample tube leaks
- Shallow tidal breaths
- Uneven alveolar emptying
- COPD
- Smoking
- Advanced age

Uses of Capnography

Respiration

- To confirm correct placement of ETT: Presence of stable E_TCO_2 for > 3 successive breaths (*Barash*)
- Determines if tip of fibrescope is in trachea
- Determines position of double lumen tube

Metabolism

- Diagnosis of malignant hyperthermia
- Rise is E_TCO_2 occurs before rise of body temperature in malignant hyperthermia

Circulation

- Assessment of Effectiveness of CPR - better than ECG, pulse and BP (DORSH)
- Detects pulmonary embolism

Equipment Function

- Indicates:
  - Apnea/extubation
  - Disconnection of circuit
  - Ventilator malfunction
  - Leaking ETT cuff/circuit

- Incompetent inspiratory/expiratory valve
- Assessment of functioning of soda lime canister

Others

- Detection of tracheo-esophageal/broncho-esophageal fistula
- Guides blind intubation
- Detects tracheo-bronchial injury during thoracoscopy
- Confirm placement of needle in cricothyroidotomy
- Correct positioning of Ryles tube

TEMPERATURE MONITORING

Introduction

Objective of temperature monitoring and perioperative thermal management is to detect normal disturbances and maintain appropriate body temperature during anesthesia.

Uses

- Monitor intraoperative hypothermia
- To estimate mean body temperature and total body heat content
- Prevent overheating (as during rewarming)
- Facilitates detection of malignant hyperthermia
- Rough measure of peripheral perfusion and cardiac output (peripheral temperature)
- To evaluate vasomotion and adequary of neuromuscular monitoring through muscle/skin surface monitoring

Types

- Mercury thermometer
- Electrical thermometers:
  - Thermistor
  - Thermocouple
- Deep tissue thermometers
- Infrared monitors
- Liquid crystal thermometry

Indications

- When duration of surgery ≥ 1 hr
- For office based sedation, RA/GA in pediatric patients (ASA)
- During regional anesthesia when changes in body temperature are intended/anticipated/suspected
- Core temperature when duration of GA ≥ 30mins
- When ambient OT temp ≥ 21°C
- In PACU when intraoperative hypothermia occurs

Mechanism

- Mercury thermometers:
  - Slow, cumbersome
  - Largely obsolete, used only in calibration laboratries
- Thermocouple:
  - Two dissimilar metals contact each other at one or more points
  - Produces voltage when temperature of one metal differs from other parts of circuit
  - Two junctions are created in the circuit
  - First junction is maintained at a known temperature
  - Second junction is placed on temperature probe tip
  - The temperature difference produces a current
  - Voltage of the current depends on temperature difference across the junctions
  - The voltage of current is then recorded as temperature
- Thermistor:
  - Type of resistor whose resistance varies significantly with temperature
  - Change in resistance of thermistor is recorded as a temperature
- Infrared monitors:
  - Evaluate IR energy emitted from surfaces above absolute zero degrees
  - Too large to fit onto tympanic membrane
  - Extrapolate tympanic membrane temperature from outer ear temperature
  - Unreliable
- Deep tissue thermometers:
  - Creates a region of zero heat flow under the probe
  - Based on actively reducing cutaneous heat flux to zero
  - Newly developed system: *CTM-205*
  - Derives core temperature from temperature of forehead and sole of foot
- Liquid crystal thermometry:
  - Organic crystals existing in a state between solid and liquid-*Liquid Crystal*
  - Suspension of microencapsulated liquid crystals used
  - Suspensions are set into thin polymer sheets with black substrate, usually adhesive
  - This is placed on skin surface to monitor temperature

Sites

Core Temperature

- Tympanic membrane:
  - Difficult to position due to curvature of aural canal
  - Occlude canal with wool after positioning to avoid cooling by ambient wind
  - Good reflection of core temp
  - Theoretically measures brain temperature as TM is close to ICA
  - Risk of TM perforation
  - Minimal lag time
- Nasopharynx:
  - Accurate if placed adjacent to nasopharyngeal mucosa
  - Causes epistaxis
  - Altered by respiratory gases, but close to ICA
- Oral and axillary temperature:
  - Axillary 0.5-1°C lesser than oral temperature
  - Oral 0.5-1°C lesser than rectal temperature
- Esophageal:
  - Incorporated intoesophageal stethoscope
  - Placed at point of maximal heart sounds/even more distally
  - Positioned behind heart in lower third of esophagus
  - 24 cm below larynx
  - Position avoids measuring temperature of tracheal gases
  - Reliable even during rapid temperature changes
- Tracheal temperature:
  - Thermistor placed within anterior surface of specially designed tracheal tube
  - Inaccurate even at fresh gas flows < 1L/min
- PA blood temperature:
  - Accurate core temperature
  - ***Gold standard*** for core temperature monitoring
  - Approximates jugular bulb temperature
- Urinary bladder:
  - Difficult to probe
  - Temperature influenced by urinary flow
  - Considered as *intermediate temperature*
- Rectal temperature:
  - Affected by cystoscopy, lavage, stools
  - Considerably lags behind core temperature
  - Considered an *"intermediate temperature"*
  - Slow responses to change in core temperature

Peripheral Temperature

- Considerably lower than core temperature
- Forehead temperature 2°C lower than core temperature
- Does not increase rapidly during malignant hyperthermia
- Indicates cardiac output

NONINVASIVE BLOOD PRESSURE MONITORING

Indications

- Use of any anesthetic no matter how trivial, is absolute indication
- As an indicator of organ perfusion

Contraindications

- Extremities with vascular abnormalities
- On limbs with AV shunts created for dialysis
- On limbs with IV line

Techniques

I. Palpation: Riva-Rocci method/Return to Flow method

- Locate palpable peripheral pulse
- Inflate BP cuff proximal to pulse until flow is occluded
- Release cuff by 2-3 mm Hg per heart beat
- Measure cuff pressure at which pulsations are again palpable
- Disadvantages:
  - Underestimates SBP due to:
    - Insensitivity of touch
    - Delay between flow under cuff and distal pulsations
  - Does not provide DBP/MAP

II. Doppler Probe

- Indicated in:
  - Obese patients
  - Pediatric patients
  - Shock
- Doppler probe transmits ultrasound signals which is reflected by tissues
- As RBC move through artery, Doppler frequency shift is detected by the probe
- Difference between transmitted and recorded frequency creates swishing sound
- Probe to be positioned directly above an artery
- Interference from probe movement/electrocautery
- Shift in frequency of sound waves when their source moves relative to the observer: ***Doppler effect***

III. Piezo Electric Crystal

- Variation of Doppler technology
- Detects lateral arterial wall movement
- Detects both SBP and DBP

IV. Auscultation

- Inflate cuff to pressure between SBP and DBP
- Partially collapses artery and produces turbulent flow with ***Korotkoff sounds***
- Stethoscope placed under/distal to distal third of BP cuff
- Appearance of first sound taken as SBP
- Disappearance of sound/muffled sound: DBP
  - Phase I:
    - Snapping sound
    - Clear tapping sounds for at least 2 consecutive beats is the systolic BP
  - Phase II: Murmurs heard between systolic and diastolic BP
  - Phase III: Loud, crisp tapping sound
  - Phase IV: Thumping sounds heard within 10 mm Hg of diastolic BP
  - Phase V: Disappearance of sound considered as diastolic BP
- Disadvantages:
  - ***Auscultatory gap***:
    - When sounds not heard between SBP and DBP
    - Common in hypertensive patients
    - Underestimation of diastolic BP
  - Difficult to auscultate sounds during hypotension/vasoconstriction
  - Motion artefacts and electrocautery interferes with measurement
  - Quick deflation underestimates BP
  - Unreliable in low flow states as flow will be non-pulsatile

V. Oscillometry

- Types:
  - Automated intermittent
  - Automated continuous
- Variations in cuff pressure due to arterial pulsations during cuff deflation used
- Arterial pulsations cause oscillations in cuff pressure
- Oscillations are small if cuff is inflated above systolic BP
- Oscillation are maximal at mean arterial pressure, after which they decrease
- Pressure at which oscillation amplitude changes is taken as SBP
- Pressure at which peak amplitude of pulsations occurs corresponds to MAP
- SBP and DBP derived from formula which examine rate of change of pressure pulsations
- Disadvantages:
  - Unreliable during arrhythmias (AF)
  - Not used on patients on CPB
  - May underestimate systolic BP
  - Shivering, motion artefacts may overestimate BP

VI. Arterial Tonometry

- Measures beat to beat BP
- Senses pressure required to partially flatten superficial artery against a bony structure
- Contains several pressure transducers applied to skin over artery
- Contact stress between transducers and skin reflects intraluminal pressure
- Produces tracing similar to invasive BP waveform
- Sensitive to movement artefact and frequent calibration required

VII. Other Methods:

- Photo oscillometry
- Motion of arterial wall

Prerequisites

- Cuff bladder should extend at least half way around extremity
- Width of cuff should be 40% of circumference of extremity
- Bladder length should encircle at least 80% of extremity

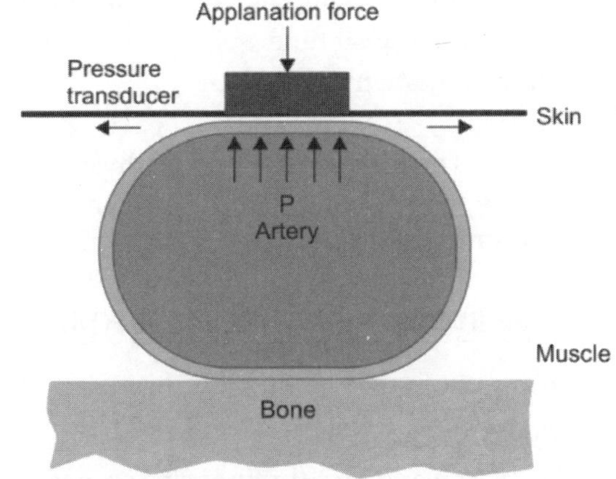

Fig. 13: Arterial tonometry.

Complications

- Pain
- Petechiae and ecchymoses
- Hematomas beneath and distal to cuff
- Venous stasis and thrombophlebitis
- Extravasation of intravenous fluids
- Nerve palsies on frequent use:
  - *Ulnar neuropathy*
  - Avoided by applying cuff proximal to ulnar groove
- Compartment syndrome due to prolonged inflation cycle

Sources of Error

- Equipment failure in obese patients
- False high readings in:
  - Small cuffs
  - Cuff applied too loose
  - Extremity below heart level
- False low readings in:
  - Large cuffs
  - Extremity above heart level
  - Quick deflation
- Hydrostatic error:
  - When cuff is placed on extremity above/below level of RA
  - Corrected by adding/subtracting 0.7 mm Hg for every centimeter that the cuff is off the horizontal plane of heart

Automated Continous Techniques

- Allow continuous assessment of BP without arterial cannulation
- Techniques:
  - Arterial volume clamp method for finger BP
  - Using pulse transit time
  - Arterial tonometry
  - ***Finapres:***
    - Based on oscillometry and plethysmography
    - Cuff tied around middle phalanx/base of thumb

INVASIVE BLOOD PRESSURE MONITORING

Indications

During Surgery

- Cardiac/vascular/chest/brain/spine surgeries
- Unstable patients undergoing surgery
- Induced hypotension/hypotensive anesthesia
- Anticipation of wide blood pressure swings
- Planned mechanical/pharmacological cardiovascular manipulation
- Failure of NIBP

Others

- Need for multiple arterial blood gas analysis
- Supplementary diagnostic information from waveform
- Determination of volume responsiveness from systolic BP and pulse pressure variations
- End organ disease necessitating precise BP regulation

Contraindications

- Arteries without documented collateral blood flow
- Extremities with PVD (***Raynauds phenomenon***)

Sites of Cannulation

Radial Artery

- Preferred site as superficial collateral flow
- Collateral flow verified by:
  - ***Allens test***
  - Doppler probe
  - Plethysmography
  - Pulse oximetry
- Disadvantage includes a large difference between aortic root and radial artery pressure after separation from CPB

Allens Test

- Unreliable
- Exsanguinate hand by making a fist while occluding radial and ulnar A with fingertips
- Patient relaxes blanched hand
- Flushing of thumb:
  - Within 5 sec: Good collateral flow
  - 5-10 sec: Equivocal
  - > 10 sec: Insufficient collateral

Ulnar Artery

- More difficult as deeper and more tortuous course
- Prime source of blood flow to hand

Brachial Artery

- Insertion site medial to biceps tendon
- Predisposed to kinking
- Large and easily identifiable

- Close to aorta: Less waveform distortion
- Damage to median nerve, can accommodate 18 G needle

Axillary Artery

- Can cause nerve damage from hematoma/traumatic cannulation
- Insertion site at junction of pectoralis and deltoids
- Air and thrombi can embolize to brain during flushing

Femoral Artery

- Prone to:
  - Pseudoaneurysm: Retroperitoneal hemorrhage
  - Atheroma
  - Increased incidence of infection and arterial thrombosis
- Aseptic necrosis of head of femur in children
- Easy access possible in low flow states
- Longer catheters preferred

Dorsalis Pedis and Post Tibial Artery

- Have most distorted waveforms as farthest from aorta
- higher systolic BP estimates
- modified Allens test for collateral flows

Complications

- Hematoma: Bleeding
- Vasospasm: Arterial thrombosis
- Air embolism: Skin necrosis
- Abnormal blood flow which normalizes in 3–70 days
- Nerve damage: Axillary N/ulnar N/median N
- Infection
- Unintentional intraarterial drug injection
- Potential for thromboembolism during catheter placement
  - Reduced by compressing proximal and distal arterial segment
  - Aspirate cannula during withdrawing
- Loss of digits
- Volume overload due to continuous flush system in pediatrics

Increased Risk of Complication in:

- Prolonged cannulation: Female gender
- Hyperlipidemia: Use of vasopressor
- Repeated insertion attempts: Extra corporeal circulation

Reduced Risk of Complications in

- Small sized catheter used
- Heparinized saline continuously infused at 2–3 mL/hr
- Flushing of catheter is limited
- Meticulous attention to asepsis

Technique of Radial Artery Cannulation

- Direct arterial puncture
- ***Seldinger*** technique–guidewire assisted cannulation
- Transfixation – withdrawal method

Direct Arterial Puncture

- Supinate hand, extend wrist
- Pressure-tubing-transducer system to be ready nearby
- System flushed with heparinized saline (0.5-2 IU/mL of saline)
- Palpate radial pulse
- Tip of index middle finger identifies area of maximal impulse
- Prepare skin with bactericidal agent
- 0.5 mL lidocaine infilterated directly above artery with 27 G needle
- 18 G needle used as skin punch
- 20/22 G IV catheter through skin at 45° angle directed toward point of palpation
- Upon blood flashback, lower needle to 30°
- Advance catheter 1-2 mm to make sure tip of catheter is in lumen of artery
- *Spin* catheter to advance it off the needle which is withdrawn
- Connect pressure tubing
- Water proof tape/suture to hold catheter in place

Prerequisites

- Tubing of catheter to be stiff: Remove air bubbles
- Limit number of stop cocks: Connecting tube not very long
- Mass of fluid is small

Position of Transducer

- Diaphragm at the level of mid-axillary line/right atrium in supine position
- In sitting position craniotomies, transducer placed at level of ear
- This approximates BP in *Circle of Willis* as arterial BP in brain is different from left ventricular pressure

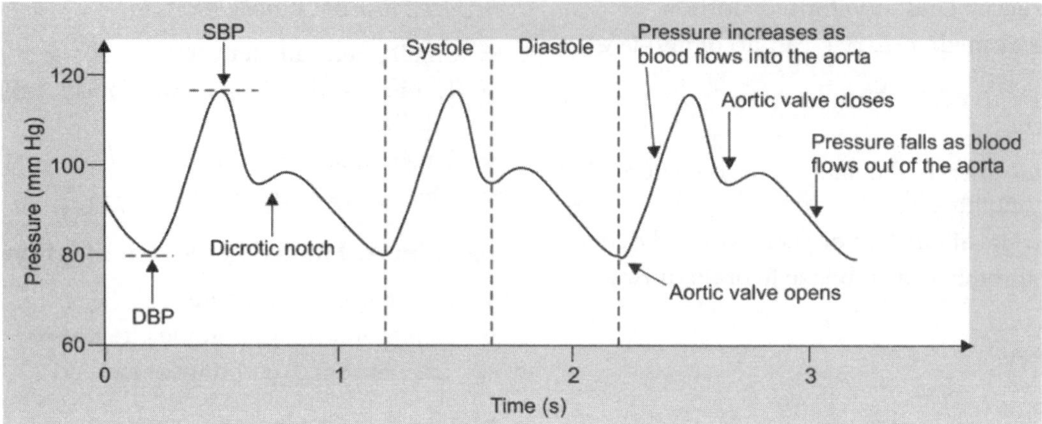

Fig. 14: Arterial pressure waveform.

Components of System

Mechanical Coupling

- Achieved by connecting fluid filled tubing to intravascular space
- Mechanical motion of fluid in tubing converted to electrical signals by mechanoelectrical transducer

Pressure Transducer

- Converts mechanical energy to electrical signals
- Contains diaphragm which forms base of fluid filled dome
- Pressure of fluid on tubing moves diaphragm
- Sensing elements in diaphragm converts movement into electrical signal
- Based on ***Strain Gauge principle*** where stretching a wire/silicon crystal changes its electrical resistance
- Sensing elements arranged as a ***Wheatstone bridge circuit*** so that voltage output is proportional to pressure on diaphragm
- When pressure applied on diaphragm, strain on number 2 and 3 resistor is increased while that on number 1 and 4 is reduced
- Change in resistance across the bridge was proportional to change in BP

Amplifier and Processing Unit

- Amplifies small electrical signals
- Processes waveforms and derives ABP using ***Fourier analysis***

Display: Can be via:

- Oscilloscope
- Digital read out
- Galvanometer

Waveform Analysis

1. Systolic upstroke
2. Systolic peak pressure
3. Systolic decline
4. Dicrotic notch
5. Diastolic runoff
6. End diastolic pressure
   - Rate of upstroke indicates contractility
   - Rate of down stroke indicates peripheral vascular resistance
   - Variations in size during respiratory cycle indicates hypovolemia
   - Area under pressure curve equals mean arterial pressure

Physics of IBP

Accuracy of transducing system affected by two properties:

- Damping (ζ): *Zeta*
  - Represents tendency of fluid in measuring system to extinguish motion
  - Damping coefficient of 0.6- 0.7 optimal
  - Under damping falsely overestimates systolic BP and vice versa
- Natural frequency: (*Fn*)
  - Represents tendency of measuring system to resonate
  - *Fn* of transducer (usually > 200 Hz) must exceed *Fn* of arterial pulse (16-30 Hz)
  - Addition of tubing, stopcocks and air bubbles reduces *Fn* of system
  - If *Fn* is very low, system will be over-damped and SBP will be underestimated
  - Optimize ζ and *Fn*

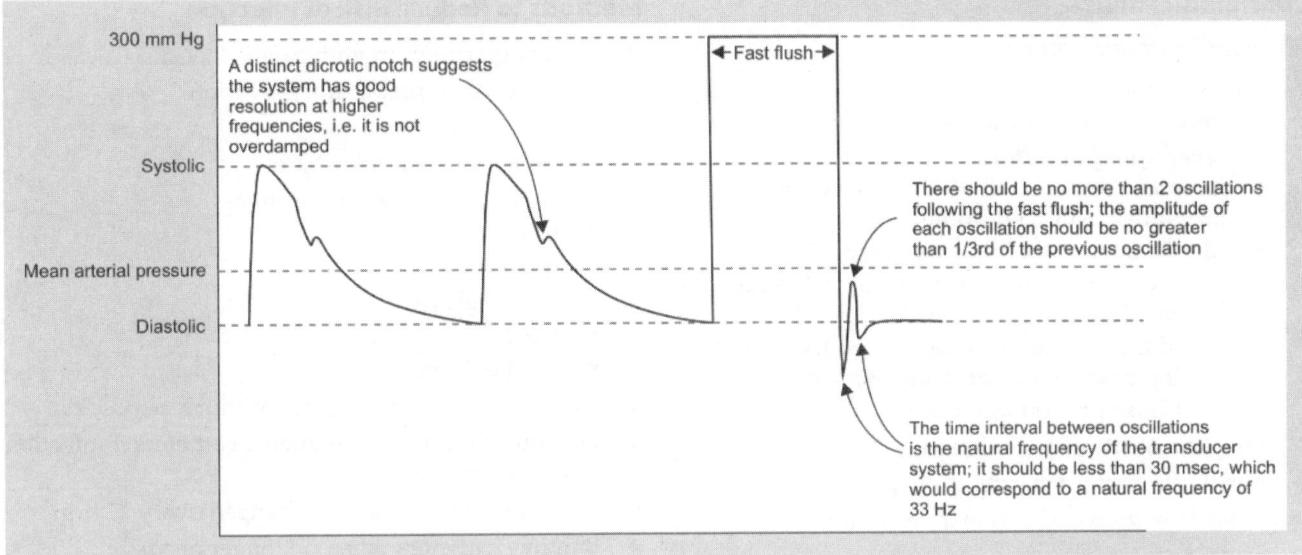

Fig. 15: Fast flush test.

- Fast flush test:
  - Bedside method to determine ζ and *Fn* of transducing system
  - Examine characteristics of resonant waves recorded after release of a flush
  - Damping estimated by amplitude ratio of first pair of resonant waves
  - *Fn* estimated by dividing paper speed by interval cycle

Sources of Error

- Hydrostatic error:
  - Sudden increase in BP as position of transducer not adjusted
  - Commonly occurs after change in OT table height
- Transducer system to be rezeroed multiple times
- ***Whip effect***:
  - Especially seen in intracardiac catheters
  - Due to oscillation of free tip of catheter in whip like fashion
  - Column of fluid in measuring system also oscillates
- Over damping/under damping
- Thrombi/air in tubing

CENTRAL VENOUS PRESSURE

Introduction

Important procedure for intravascular volume status monitoring and also administration of drugs in presence of poor peripheral line.

Uses

- Gives estimate of intravascular volume status
- Assesses venous tone
- Assess right ventricular function and right ventricular filling pressure
- Useful in diagnosing pathological cardiac conditions like constrictive pericarditis
- Approximates LV filling pressure in healthy heart

Indications

- Assessment of volume status:
  - For major surgeries involving:
    - Large fluid shifts
    - Blood loss in patients with good heart function
    - Major trauma
  - IV volume assessment when urine output is unreliable or unavailable:
    - Chronic renal failure
    - Radical cystectomy
- Frequent venous blood sampling
- Drug/fluid infusions:
  - Inadequate peripheral IV access
  - Chronic drug administration/administration of vasoactive and irritant drugs
  - Rapid infusion of IV fluids
  - Total parenteral nutrition
- Hemodialysis
- Placement of temporary transvenous pacing wire
- Surgeries with high risk of air embolism like sitting position posterior fossa craniotomies

Contraindications

Absolute Contraindications

- *SVC syndrome*:
  - Venous cannula not to be put in neck/subclavian area/upper extremity
  - Venous pressures of SVC does not reflect RA pressure in SVC syndrome
  - Medications administered through IJV will reach central circulation through collaterals in a delayed fashion
  - Rapid fluid administration trough IJV will:
    - Increase venous pressure even more
    - Cause pronounced edema
- Infection at site of cannulation
- Renal cell carcinoma extending into RA
- Fungating tricuspid valvular vegetation

Relative Contraindications

- Coagulopathies: Can cause:
  - Hemorrhage
  - Hematoma and infection
  - Hemothorax
  - Airway obstruction
- Newly inserted pace maker:
  - Pace maker wires may get dislodged during insertion of CVP catheter
  - A wait of 4-6 wks in patients with newly inserted pacemaker wires is required
- Ipsilateral carobid endarterectomy due to possibility of carotid artery puncture

Sites of Cannulation

- Depends of skill of operator
- Avoid sites involving:
  - Infection
  - Burns
  - Other dermatological processes
- Preferred sites:
  - Internal Jugular Vein
  - Subclavian Vein
  - External Jugular Vein
  - Antecubital Vein
  - Femoral Vein
- Risk of infection: Femoral v. > internal jugular v. > subclavian v
- IJV better in patients with:
  - Coagulopathies: bleeding at subclavian artery if punctured is difficult to control
  - Acute lung injury where risk of pneumothorax is high

Methods to Reduce Risk of Infection

- Education program with safety checklist
- Chlorhexidine preparatory solution
- Use subclavian vein site
- Avoid femoral puncture site
- Use maximal barrier precautions:
  - Cap
  - Mask
  - Sterile gloves
  - Gown
  - Sterile drape
- Avoid guidewire exchanges as much as possible
- Use antimicrobial impregnated catheters if infection rates remain high
- Fluid administration sets changed every 72 hrs
- Remove catheters when no longer needed

Use of Ultrasound Guidance

Advantages

- Allows better visualization of anatomy and exact vessel location
- Avoids preexisting thrombus
- Reduces failure rates and multiple attempts at catheterization
- Reduces infection rates

Indications of USG Guided Access

- Anatomically difficult:
  - Morbid obesity, short and thick neck
  - Local scarring
  - Radiation therapy
  - Transplant patients
  - Edema
- Associated comorbidities:
  - Coagulopathies
  - Bullons emphysema
  - Maximal ventilatory support

Techniques of Cannulation

Three techniques of cannulation:

- Catheter over needle
- Catheter through needle
- Catheter over guidewire (***Seldingers technique***)

IJV Cannulation

Central/Middle Approach

- Positioned at 15° Trendelenburg position, head turned to contralateral side

- Using maximal barrier precautions after LA infilteration, operator punctures skin with 22 G finder needle with a syringe attached at apex of triangle formed by:
  - Two bellies of sternocleidomastoid muscle
  - Clavicle
- Internal Carotid Artery pulsations are felt 1–2 cm medial to this point
- Finder needle directed at 45° angle towards ipsilateral nipple with constant aspiration
- After successful puncture, large bore needle is introduced in identical place
- After cannulation, guidewire is introduced
- Depth of guidewire insertion limited to 15–20 cm to avoid arrhythmias
- Scalpel used to enlarge skin invision
- A dilator is advanced over guidewire to dilate the tract and is removed
- The central venous catheter is then threaded over the guidewire
- Dressing catheter with chlorhexidine impregnated sponge reduces infection

Anterior Approach

Needle inserted 0.5 to 1 cm lateral to carotid artery pulsations at level of cricoid cartilage directed at ipsilateral toe.

Posterior Approach

- Needle inserted 1 cm dorsal to point where external jugular vein crosses posterior border of sternocleidomastoid and directed caudally and ventrally towards suprasternal notch
- Incidence of carotid artery puncture is high as needle is aimed in the direction of the carotid artery

Subclavian Vein Cannulation

Position

- Patient is 15–30° Trendelenburg with bedroll between scapulae
- Patients head turned to contralateral side, arms are by the side

Infraclavicular Approach

- Skin puncture with 18G needle, attached to syringe
- Puncture done 2–3 cm caudal to midpoint of clavicle
- Direction of insertion towards suprasternal notch until it abuts the clavicle
- The needle is walked down the clavicle until inferior edge is cleared
- As needle is advanced, it is kept as close to inferior edge of clavicle as possible, to avoid puncturing dome of pleura
- When blood return is established:
  - Needle bevel is turned 90 towards heart
  - Syringe is removed and guidewire inserted
  - Needle is removed and dilator is advanced over guidewire
- The central venous catheter is advanced over guidewire to appropriate depth

Supraclavicular Approach

- Skin puncture just superior to clavicle and lateral to insertion of clavicular head of SCM
- Needle advanced towards contralateral nipple just under
- It should enter subclavian vein at depth of 1–4 cm
- Approach has 90–95% success rate

Confirmation of Proper Position of Cannula

- Comparison of color/PaO_2 of blood sample and arterial sample drawn simultaneously
- Attach cannula to transducer via sterile tubing to observe pressure waveform
- Retrograde flow:
  - Attach cannula to sterile tubing and allow retrograde flow into upright tubing
  - If in vein, blood level in tubing will stop rising at level consistent with CVP
  - Also,the blood level will demonstrate respiratory variation
- Ultrasonography
- Chest X-ray is *confirmatory*

Complications

- Complications during central venous cannulation:
  - Arterial puncture with hematoma and infection/airway obstruction
  - Arteriovenous fistula
  - Air emboli if negative pressure within venous system
  - Nerve injury:
    - Phrenic nerve
    - Brachial plexus
    - Stellate ganglion
  - Hemothorax if subclavian artery lacerated
  - Chylothorax if injury to thoracic duct

- Pneumothorax which is most common with subclavian artery cannulation
- Catheter/wire shearing: may require:
  - Removal with surgery
  - Removal through percutaneous transvenous technique

❖ Complications of catheter presence:
- Thrombosis, thromboembolism
- Infection, sepsis, endocarditis
- Arrhythmias:
  - Extrasystoles
  - Ventricular fibrillation
  - Transient atrial/ventricular arrhythmias
  - Complete heart block
  - Prevented by limiting guidewire insertion to 22 cm
- Hydrothorax:
  - Due to erosion of catheter into pleural cavity
  - Fluid infused via catheter will then accumulate in pleural cavity
- RA/RV perforation and tamponade:
  - Increased incidence with long dilators/catheters and inflexible guidewire
  - Reduced incidence by reducing angle of puncture to 40
  - Use single orifice polyurethane/silicon catheters/pigtail tip catheters

Normal CVP Waveform

Waveform component	Phase of cardiac cycle	Mechanical event
Upstrokes		
a wave	Atrial systole	Atrial contraction
c wave	Isovolumetric contraction	Tricuspid valve "doming" into RA
	Carotid impact wave	Due to early systolic pressure transmission from adjacent carotid artery
v wave	Last part of isovolumetric relaxation	Systolic filling of RA
Downstrokes		
x descent		Atrial relaxation, descent of base, systolic collapse
x' descent		
y descent		Early ventricular filling diastolic collapse
		TV opens and blood from RA enters RV

Waveform Abnormalities

❖ Loss of A wave: Atrial flutter/fibrillation

❖ Canon A waves: Occurs when:
- RA contracts against closed tricuspid valve as in:
  - Junctional rhythm
  - Complete heart block
  - Ventricular arrhythmias
- Increased resistance to RA emptying:
  - Tricuspid stenosis
  - Right ventricular hypertrophy
  - Pulmonary stenosis
  - Pulmonary arterial HTN

❖ *Canon V waves*/C-V waves:
- Tricuspid regurgitation
- Right Ventricular failure
- RV papillary muscle ischemia
- Constrictive pericarditis/tamponade

❖ Constrictive pericarditis: M configuration with:
- Prominent A and V waves
- Steep X and Y descents

❖ Atrial fibrillation:
- Loss of a wave
- Prominent c wave

❖ Tricuspid regurgitation:
- Tall systolic c-v wave
- Loss of x descent

❖ Tricuspid stenosis:
- Tall a wave
- Attenuation of y descent

❖ Right ventricular ischemia:
- Tall a and v waves
- Steep x and y descents
- M/W configuration

❖ Constrictive tamponade:
- Dominant x descent
- Attenuated y descent

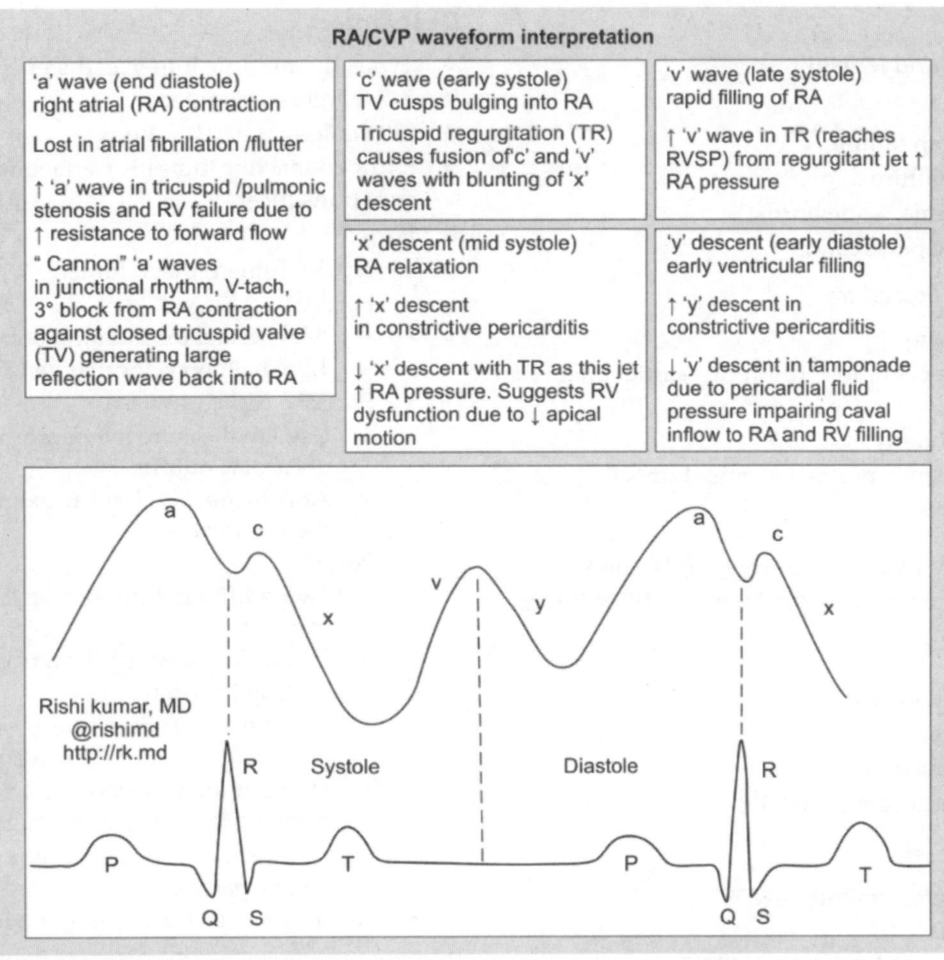

Fig. 16: Normal CVP waveform.

PULMONARY ARTERY PRESSURE MONITORING

Introduction

- PAC catheters is a very useful monitor of:
  - LV and RV function
  - Hemodynamic status
  - Guides therapy with pharmacological and non-pharmacological agents

Uses

- Guides fluid therapy and inotropic/vasopressor therapy
- Measures hemodynamic indices like:
  - CVP, PA Occlusion Pressure (PAOP)
  - PA pressure, PVR
  - PCWP, MVO_2
  - Intracardiac ECG
  - Right and left ventricular stroke work index
- Oxygenation variables like:
  - O_2 delivery
  - O_2 consumption
  - O_2 extraction
  - Mixed venous oxygen saturation (MvO_2)
- Used for intracardiac ECG monitoring
- Helps to measure thermodilution cardiac output
- Used to calculate lung water
- Helps to differentiate:
  - Cardiogenic and noncardiogenic pulmonary edema
  - Circulatory and respiratory failure

Types of PA Catheter

- Standard PA catheter
- Pacing PA catheter
- Continuous cardiac output PA catheter
- Continuous MvO_2 PAC
- RVEF PA catheter

Indications

Complex Fluid Management

- Shock
- Multiple organ failure
- Acute renal failure
- Massive trauma, acute burns
- Hemorrhagic pancreatitis

Specific Surgical Procedure

- Pericardiectomy
- Aortic cross-clamping (thoracic aortic aneurysm surgery)
- Sitting craniotomy
- Liver transplants, porto-systemic shunts

Cardiac Disease

- CAD with LV dysfunction/recent infarction
- Valvular heart disease/pulmonary HTN/pulmonary embolus
- Heart failure:
    - Cardiomyopathy
    - Cardiac tamponade
    - Cor pulmonale
- Those surgeries requiring CPB

Pulmonary Diseases

- Acute respiratory failure, ARDS
- Severe COPD
- Those requiring high levels of PEEP
- Differentiation of cardiogenic and noncardiogenic PE
- Aspiration of air emboli

High Risk Obstetrics

- Severe toxemia
- Placental abruption

Contraindications

Absolute Contraindications

- Tricuspid/pulmonary valve prosthesis
- Tricuspid/pulmonary endocarditis
- Right heart mass (thrombus/tumor)

Relative Contraindications

- Complete LBBB (due to risk of complete heart block)
- ***Wolff-Parkinson-White syndrome:***
    - Due to possibility of tachyarrhythmias
    - PAC with pacing capacity is better in WPW patients
- Ebsteins anomaly
- Septicemias as PAC may serve as nidus for injection
- Hypercoagulable states as thrombus may form

Description

- Typically multiple lumen catheter
- 5–7.5 French diameter
- 110 cm long with PVC body
- Extra connecting tubes for attachment to the pressure transducer
- Ports:
    - Tip: PA lumen/distal lumen
    - Port A:
        - Air channel for inflation of balloon
        - 1.5cc balloon is located just proximal to tip
    - Port B:
        - Used to measure temperature for calculation of cardiac output
        - Approximately 4 cm proximal to balloon is the thermistor
    - Port C:
        - Two additional lumens at 19 cm and 30 cm from tip
        - Proximal lumen at 30 cm from tip for:
            - Drug infusion
            - Cardiac output injection
            - Measurement of PA pressure
        - Distal lumen is ventricular port at 19 cm from tip for infusion of drugs
    - Port D: some PACs have connections for temporary pacing
    - Port E: some PACs are coated with heparin

PAC insertion technique: ***Seldinger technique:***

- After identifying major vein, instead of CV catheter, a dilator and sheets are threaded over guidewire
- Catheter placement is most commonly performed by observing the pressure waves as catheter is floated from CVP position through right heart chambers into PA
- Preparation of PA catheter:
    - PA catheter is first checked by inflating and deflating balloon
    - Irrigate all 3 intravascular lumens with heparinized saline
- Catheter is then threaded through the PA sheath
- Distal port connected to transducer and zeroed to patients midaxillary line
- At approximately 15 cm distal tip enters RA
- CVP tracing varying with respiration confirms an intrathoracic position
- Balloon is then inflated with 1.5 cc air to:
    - Protect endocardium from catheter tip
    - Allow right ventricles cardiac output to direct catheter forwards

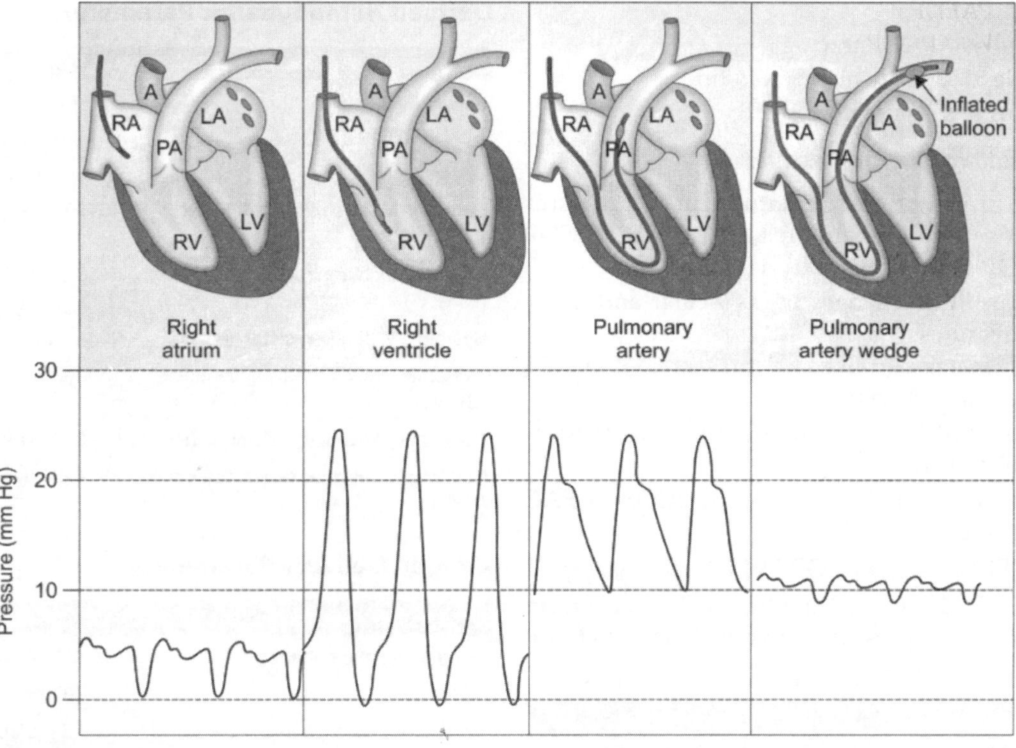

Fig. 17: PAC catheter insertion.

- Balloon is always deflated during withdrawal
- ECG monitoring done continuously at this stage
- A sudden increase in systolic pressure on distal tracing indicates RV location of catheter
- Sudden increase in diastolic pressure indicates PA entry which normally occurs at 40 cm
- Maneuvers to enhance catheter flotation in difficult cases:
  - Deep inhalation
  - Slight head up position
  - Right lateral tilt
  - Injecting iced saline through proximal lumen to stiffen catheter increases risk of RV perforation
  - Administer small dose of inotrope to increase CO

Access site	Distance to RV in cm
Right internal jugular vein	35
Right superior vena cava (subclavian vein)	35
Left internal jugular vein	45
Femoral vein	50
Right antecubital vein	60
Left antecubital vein	70

Prevention of PAC Infection

- Educate clinicians
- Use of maximal sterile barrier precautions:
  - Mask and cap,
  - Sterile gloves and gown
  - Large steri-drapes
- 2% chlorhexidine skin preparation
- Avoid routine change of CVP/PAC solely for reducing risk of injection

Factors Affecting Accuracy of PAC Monitoring

Pulmonary Vascular Resistance

- Increased PVR causes reduced pulmonary blood flow
- Causes of increased PVR:
  - Acute/chronic lung diseases
  - Pulmonary emboli
  - Alveolar hypoxia
  - Acidosis
  - Hypoxemia
  - Tachycardia
  - Vasoactive drugs

Alveolar Pulmonary Arterial Pressure Relationship

- Due to gravity dependant variation in pulmonary venous flow, directed PA catheter usually advances to gravity dependant areas of highest blood flow
- In zone III, $P_A > P_V > P_{ALV}$ meets the criteria for interrupted blood flow and continuous communication intracardiac pressure

- If PCOP > PAEDP:
  - Non-phasic PCOP tracing
  - Unable to aspirate blood from tip
  - Implies PAC is not in Zone III

Respiratory Pattern/Airway Pressures

- Changes in intrathoracic/intrapleural pressures affect transmural pressure, relation between PCOP and LVEDP
- Changes in PEEP changes intravascular and intrapleural pressures:
  - PEEP increases alveolar pressure: Zone III converted to zone II
  - Alters ventricular distensibility and reduces venous return
- If PEEP ≤ 10 cm H_2O, no effect in PCOP of PAC located in Zone III
- Higher PEEP changes PCOP-LVEDP relationship
- When PEEP > 10 cm H_2O, subtract 1–2 mm Hg from displayed wedge pressure for every 5 cm H_2O PEEP

Intracardiac shunts: PAWP waveform abnormalities:

Condition	Characteristics
Mitral regurgitation	Tall regurgitant C-V waveform
	Obliteration of X descent
Mitral stenosis	Tall a waves
	Attenuation of Y descent
Ventricular septal defect	Tall anterograde v waves
Myocardial infarction	Tall a waves
	Tall v waves

Reduced Ventricular Compliance

- Relationship between pressure and volume is not linear
- LV compliance is a dynamic factor
- Causes of reduced ventricular compliance:
  - MI, HTN
  - Restrictive myopathies
  - Right-left shunts
  - Aortic stenosis
  - Cardiac tamponade (***square pattern***)
  - Inotropic drugs

PAC Pressures

Pressures	Mean (mm Hg)	Range (mm Hg)
Right atrial pressure	5	1–10
RVESP/RVEDP	25/5	15–30/0–8
PA systolic/PA diastolic	23/9	15–30/5–15
Mean PA pressure	15	10–20
PCWP	10	5–15
LAP	8	4–12
LVEDP	8	4–12
LV systolic pressure	130	90–140

Derived Hemodynamic Parameters

Parameter	Normal value
Cardiac index (CI)	2.8–4.2 L/min/m^2
Stroke volume (SV)	50–110 ml/beat
Stroke index (SI)	30–65 ml/beat/m^2
Left ventricular stroke work index (LVSWI)	45–60 g.m/m^2
Right ventricular stroke work index (RVSWI)	5–10 g.m/m^2
Systemic vascular resistance (SVR)	900–1400 dyne sec cm^{-5}
Systemic vascular resistance index (SVRI)	1500–2400 dyne sec cm^{-5}/m^2
Pulmonary vascular resistance (PVR)	80–120 dyne sec cm^{-5}
Pulmonary vascular resistance index (PVRI)	250–400 dyne sec cm^{-5}/m^2

Oxygen Delivery Parameters

Parameter	Normal value
Arterial oxygen content	18–20 mL/dL
M_vO_2	13–16 mL/dL
Arteriovenous oxygen difference	4–5.5 mL/dL
Pulmonary capillary oxygen content	19–21 mL/dL
Pulmonary shunt fraction	2–8 %
Oxygen delivery	800–1100 mL/min
Oxygen consumption	150–300 mL/min

Complications

- Complication of central venous access:
  - Arterial puncture
  - Bleeding
  - Pneumothorax
  - Air embolism
- Complication of central venous catheterization:
  - Catheter shearing
  - Guidewire embolization
  - Arrhythmias:
    - Supraventricular tachycardia
    - Atrial fibrillation
    - Ventricular tachycardia/fibrillation
    - Right bundle branch block
    - Complete heart block
  - Air embolism
  - Arterial puncture
  - Postoperative pneumothorax
  - Minor increase in tricuspid regurgitation
  - RA rupture

- Complication of catheter residence: Late complication:
  - Mechanical problems:
    - Catheter entrapment
    - Catheter coiling/knotting/tip migration
    - Balloon rupture
    - Infection: Risk increases if catheter insitu for > 72 hours
    - Sepsis, endocarditis
    - Thrombosis, embolism
    - Pulmonary infarction
    - Valvular damage
  - Structural damage:
    - Delayed vascular injury/fistula
    - Cardiac perforation
    - TV/PV/endocardial damage
    - PA rupture/PA aneurysm:
      - More common in patients with:
        - Pulmonary HTN
        - Coagulopathy
        - Heparinization
        - Overwedging
      - Even trace hemoptysis not to be ignored as it heralds PA rupture
      - If suspected, place double lumen tube to maintain oxygenation of unaffected lung

PAC Modifications

- Mixed venous oxygen saturation:
  - Oximetric PAC uses *reflectance spectrophotometry*
  - Several wave lengths are transmitted through optical fibres embedded in PAC
  - The reflected intensity of light identifies saturation of blood surrounding tip of PAC
- Intermittent cardiac output monitoring:
  - Ice cold NS or 5% dextrose used for cardiac output measurement
  - Bolus of cooled fluid is injected into the PA
  - Thermistor at the tip of PAC records the reduction in temperature as bolus passes through PA
  - Factors which determine cardiac output:
    - Specific heat of blood and indicator
    - Volume of injectate
    - Catheter size
    - Specific gravity of blood and injectate
    - Area of blood-temperature curve
- Continuous cardiac output monitoring:
  - Pulsed thermodilution:
    - Uses coiled RV filament
    - Filament applies low power heating signal to RA and RV in cyclical manner
    - Thermistor at PAC tip detects changes in blood temperature
    - It sends major information to a computer
    - Computer uses stochastic analysis to create thermodilution curve
    - Cardiac output is calculated from thermodilution curve based on conservation of heat equation
  - Another technique:
    - Applies heat to a thermistor at PAC tip
    - RV out flow then cools the tip
    - The temperature changes registered are proportional to RV outflow
    - This determines the cardiac output
- RV ejection fraction:
  - Performed with special PA catheter which has a rapid response thermistor
  - Analyzes exponential decay of PA temperature over several cardiac cycles
  - Cardiac output calculated from the data
  - Ejection fraction = CO – mean residual fraction
  - RVEF useful in:
    - RV dysfunction
    - For assessment of RV preload
    - During liver transplantation
- Intracardiac pacing:
  - For bipolar ventricular/atrial/atrioventricular intracardiac pacing
  - PA catheter has 5 lumen
  - 2.4 French bipolar pacing electrode passed through additional lumen for pacing

Controversy of PAC Monitoring

- Perioperative outcomes reported as improved/worsened/unchanged by using PAC
- Errors in diagnosis and treatment are common as values are interpreted by health staff
- At present preponderance of studies have had difficulties in demonstrating outcome benefits

ICP MONITORING

Introduction

Normal ICP

- 10–15 mm Hg in adults and young children
- 3–7mm Hg for young children
- 1.5–6 mm Hg for preterm infants
- > 20 mm Hg: raised ICP

Lundberg's Classification

- 0–10 mm Hg – normal
- 15–20 mm Hg – mildly increased
- 20–40 mm Hg – moderately increased
- > 40 mm Hg – severely increased

Indications for ICP Monitoring

- Benign intracranial HTN
- Meningitis/encephalitis
- Encephalopathy:
  - Lead ingestion
  - Hypertensive crisis
  - Hepatic encephalopathy
- Post craniotomy cerebral edema
- Intracranial space occupying lesions
- Severe traumatic brain injury (GCS 3–8 with abnormal CT scan)
- Intracranial hemorrhage
- Post subarachnoid hemorrhage associated with hydrocephalus/coma
- Intracranial space occupying lesions (ICSOL):
  - Tumor, hematoma, abscess
  - AV malformation/aneurysm obstructing CSF
- Decompensated/normal pressure hydrocephaline
- Others:
  - Reyes syndrome
  - Venous sinus thrombosis

Contraindications

- Coagulopathy, anticoagulant therapy
- Prothrombin time > 13 seconds/INR > 1.3
- Scalp infection
- Severe midline shift causing ventricular displacement
- Cerebral edema causing ventricular collapse

Sites of Monitoring

Ventricular

- ***Gold standard***
- Most reliable

Subdural

- Hollow bolt inserted via burr hole
- Fiberoptic device/pressure transducer passed into subdural space by incising dura
- Hemorrhage and infection possible
- Underestimates ICP

Intraparenchymal

- Using silicone strain gauge monitor
- More accurate
- Can be inserted by non-neurosurgery staff

Extradural

- Using catheters in extradural space
- Not reliable and rarely used

Types of Monitoring Devices

- Fluid filled transduced ventriculostomy
- Fibreoptic sensors
- Microchips (internal strain gauge devices)
- Air pouch technologies

Locations of Monitoring Devices

- Ventricular
- Parenchymal
- Subdural

ICP Techniques

Invasive

Ventricular catheter:

- ***Gold standard***
- Most reliable, inexpensive, accurate and can be re-zeroed
- Consists of a catheter placed at level of foramen of Monroe/lateral ventricle
- Catheter attached to pressure resistant tubing filled with preservative free saline
- This catheter is attached to a non-flush strain gauge transducer
- Transducer is zeroed at external auditory meatus
- Maybe difficult if ventricles are narrow due to edema/ventriculitis
- Injury to basal ganglia, infection and blocked catheter can occur
- Antibiotic coated drains prevent infections

Fibreoptic transducers:

- Using fibreoptic catheter with flexible diaphragm
- Have fibreoptic probe which has a transducer at the tip which is inserted into brain
- Placed intraventricular/intraparenchymal
- Changes in light intensity reflected from diaphragm is calibrated as ICP
- Disadvantages:
  - High cost
  - Inability to zero device in situ
  - Can be broken if patient is restless
  - Has to replaced every 5 days to prevent infection

Implanted microchip Transducer:

- Solid state pressure transducer with piezoresistive strain gauze implanted at tip of nylon fibre (***Codman microsensor***)
- Pressure applied at the sensor tip generates electrical voltages
- Intraventricular/intraparenchymal/subdural/epidural
- Low infection and hemorrhage rates

Subarachnoid bolts:

- Metallic cylindrical instruments inserted such that their tip protrudes into subarachnoid space
- Most common device used: ***Richmond screw/Becker bolt***
- Easier to install but are less accurate

Continuous monitoring of intracranial compliance:

- ***Spiegelberg air pouch*** ICP/compliance monitor
- Balloon surrounding the end of a catheter is called airpouch
- Airpouch gets repeated inflated and deflated with 0.05–0.1 cc of air
- Pressure exerted on the balloon pouch is the pressure of the surrounding tissue
- Resultant pressure and volume changes calculates compliance and ICP
- ICP calculated in terms of PVI/VPR on a continuous basis
- PVI/VPR =Pressure volume index/volume pressure ratio)

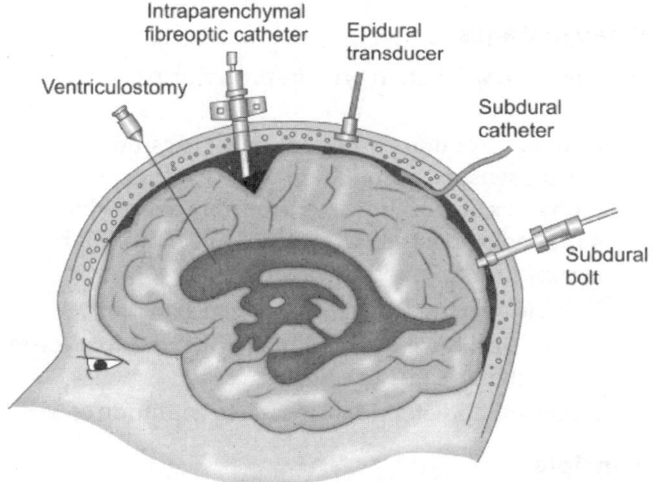

Fig. 18: ICP monitoring techniques.

Noninvasive

- Transcranial Doppler flow velocity to derive estimated CPP
- ***Rotterdam transfontanelle ICP transducer***
- USG guided Optic Nerve Sheath Diameter (ONSD)
- ONSD 5 mm = ICP > 20 mm Hg

ICP Waveforms

Normal Waveform

- Has two components
  - Baseline pressure
  - Variation of pressure (i.e., pressure waves)
- Variations due to small pulsations transmitted from systolic BP to intracranial cavity
- Blood pressure pulsations are superimposed on slower oscillations due to respiratory cycle

Pathological Waveforms

- Arterial pulses on ICP waveform become more prominent
- 3 types of pathological waveforms
- Lundberg A:
  - *Plateau waves*
  - ICP elevation > 50 mm Hg lasting 5–20 mins
- Lundberg B:
  - *Pressure pulses*
  - ICP elevations up to 50 mm Hg occurring every 30 sec-2 mins
- Lundberg C
  - Amplitude of 20 mm Hg
  - Frequency of 4–8/min

Complications

- Intraparenchymal/Intraventricular/Subdural hemorrhage
- Bacterial ventriculitis/meningitis
- CSF leakage
- Overdrainage causing ventricular collapse
- System malfunction- occlusion/opposition of catheter tip against ventricular wall

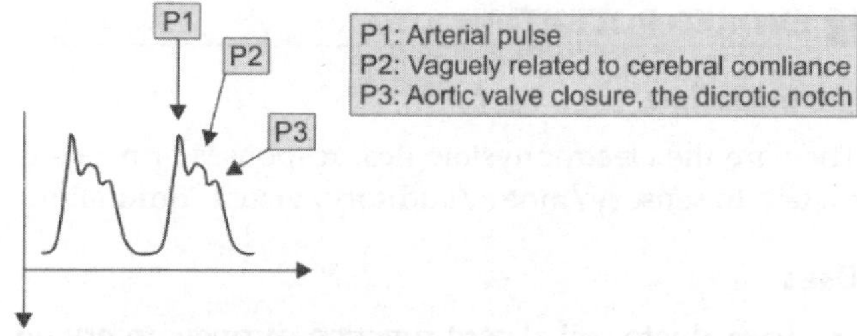

Fig. 19: Normal ICP waveform.

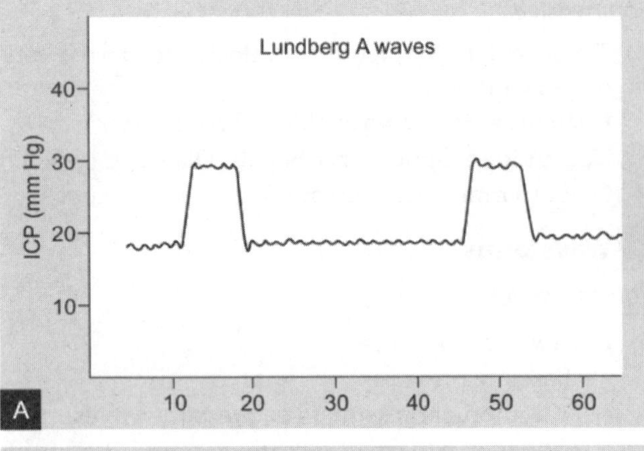

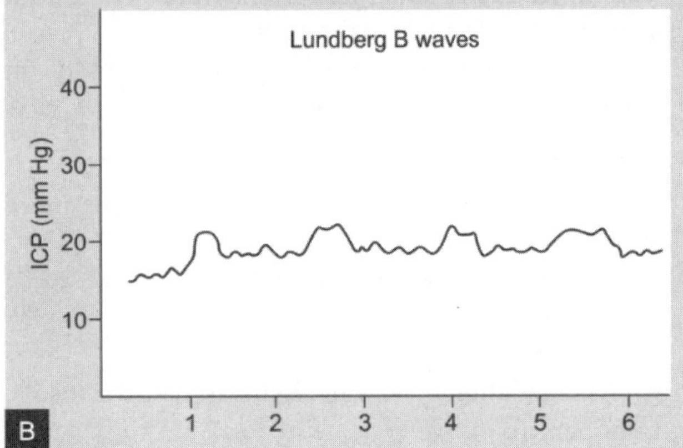

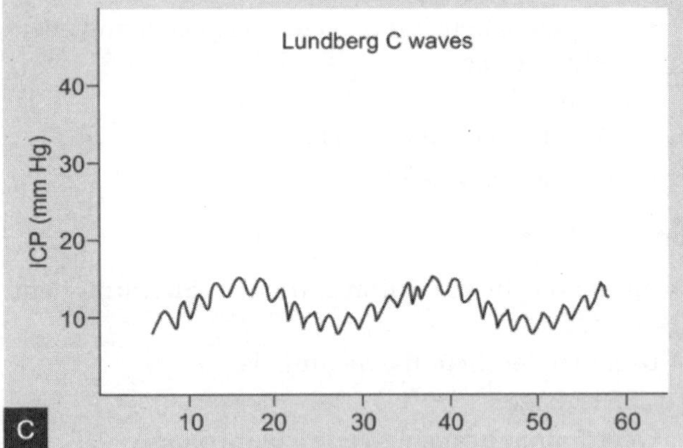

Figs. 20A to C: Lundberg waves.

EVOKED POTENTIAL

Introduction

They are the electrophysiological responses of nervous system to sensory/motor/auditory/visual stimulation.

Uses

- To evaluate spinal cord function during surgery on or near spinal cord
- Auditory nerve and brain stem function during surgery on pituitary tumors/optic N/optic chiasm

SOMATOSENSORY EVOKED POTENTIALS

Introduction

Somatosensory evoked potentials is a signal which is detectable on EEG, generated in response to a specific applied sensory input, by stimulating a peripheral sensory nerve.

Method

- Stimulus applied maybe electrical/mechanical/thermal/magnetic
- Stimulus is applied over:
  - Tibial nerve
  - Paroneal nerve
  - Median nerve
  - Ulnar nerve
  - Sometimes cranial nerves with sensory pathways
- Evoked potentials are recorded over sensory cortex

Indications

- During spine surgery when dorsal column is at risk
- During carotid surgery like:
  - Carotid endarterectomy
  - Aneurysm surgery
  - Embolization of AVM
- During streptokinase dissolution of occluding blood clot and to detect cerebral ischemia in SAH
- In comatose patients, the extent of CCT prolongation correlates with extent of injury Asymmetry between the 2 hemispheres is the most important criterion for recognizing the onset of cerebral ischemia

Disadvantages

- Detects dysfunction only in posterior part of spinal cord
- Cannot exclude anterior cord dysfunction as somatosensory stimulation follows dorsal column pathways of vibration and proprioception which are supplied by post spinal artery, while motor pathway is supplied by anterior spinal artery
- Volatile anesthetics produce depression of SSEP
- Opioids produce depression of SSEP, but to a lesser extent that volatile anesthetics
- Ketamine and etomidate increase amplitude of SSEP

Principle

- Low voltage electrical current which stimulates a peripheral nerve, is applied

- Resulting evoked potentials reflect integrity of sensory neural pathways from peripheral N to somatosensory cortex
- Due to presence of spontaneous EEG activity, a single peripheral stimulus which generates cortical activity of low amplitude would not be detectable amidst background noise
- Thus, summation followed by signal averaging of repetitive stimuli is necessary for meaningful signals

Results

- *Post stimulus latency*: Time from application of stimulus to occurrence of a peak/complex in evoked potential waveform
- *Peak amplitude*: Size of waveform is the peak amplitude
- *Polarity*: Direction of wave deflection (positive P or negative N)
- *Central conduction time and conduction velocity (CCT and CV)*: Derived from post stimulus latency

SSEPs are described in terms of polarity and latency, e.g. N 20 is SSEP generated by stimulation of median nerve which has a latency of 20 msec and a negative deflection.

Interpretation

Short Latency SSEPS

- <10–15 msec for BAEP
- <40 msec for SSEP
- Subcortical in origin and represent initial cortical activity
- Not affected by volatile anesthetics

Intermediate Latency SSEPS

- 40–120 msec
- They are near field potentials when recorded from scalp

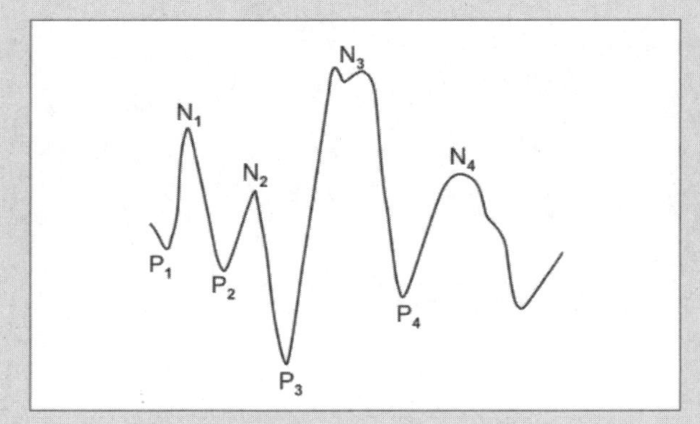

Fig. 21: Somatosensory evoked potentials.

- Have greater amplitude than short latency SSEPs
- Arise from primary sensory area of cerebral cortex
- Affected by volatile anesthetics but to a lesser extent than long latency SSEPs

Long Latency SSEPS

- 120–500 msec
- Depressed by volatile anesthetics
- Ischemia/mechanical disruption of nerve suggested by:
  - 50% reduction in signal amplitude
  - and 10% increase in latency

MOTOR EVOKED POTENTIALS

Introduction

Evoked potentials generated in response to stimulus applied over *motor cortex.*

Method

- Stimulus applied in a transcranial fashion over motor cortex
- Electromyographic deflection is detected by electrodes embedded in muscle belly
- Transcranial signal is applied as a rapid train of four or more stimuli
- Voltage of signal is adjusted to achieve adequate signals in upper and lower extremities
- Evoked potentials are detected at thenar eminence and abductor hallucis muscle
- Stimulus can also be applied to peripheral/cranial N/nerve roots/spinal cord

Disadvantages

- Recording MEPs require direct (epidural) or indirect (transosseus) stimulation of brain/spinal cord
- Extremely sensitive to volatile anesthetic: Use only TIVA
- Not possible to monitor MEPS if significant neuromuscular blockade present
- Stimulus can cause patient movement
- Obtain MEP only when slight patient movement is not problematic
- Bite block mandatory to prevent tongue injury

Uses

- Used during any spine/intracranial/cervical spine surgery
- Reflects integrity of motor pathway from peripheral to motor cortex
- Used to monitor anterior segment of spinal cord
- Obviates need for wakeup test during spine surgery

Interpretation

- Latency of signal is unreliable and not used to make clinical decisions
- Only amplitude is considered important
- 50% reduction in amplitude is considered significant

BRAINSTEM AUDITORY EVOKED POTENTIALS

Introduction

Instead of electrical stimulus applied to somatosensory nerve, a standardized sound (click) is applied to eighth cranial nerve via auditory apparatus.

Uses

- In comatose patients
- During surgery of cerebropontine angle and floor of IV ventricle
- During procedures close to CN V,VII or VIII
- Alternative to clinical assessment of sedation
- During acoustic neuroma surgery and any surgery around brainstem

Basis

- Arise from brainstem auditory pathways
- First 10–15 msec of AEPS is subcortical in origin and referred to as BAEP
- Volatile anesthetics produce depression of AEPs
- *Resistant to effects of anesthesia*

Interpretation

- Consists of series of positive and negative waves
- Latency of each peak has a significance with respect to integrity of various parts of auditory pathway
- Waves can be recorded in field far from vertex and ear or from vertex and non cephalic reference

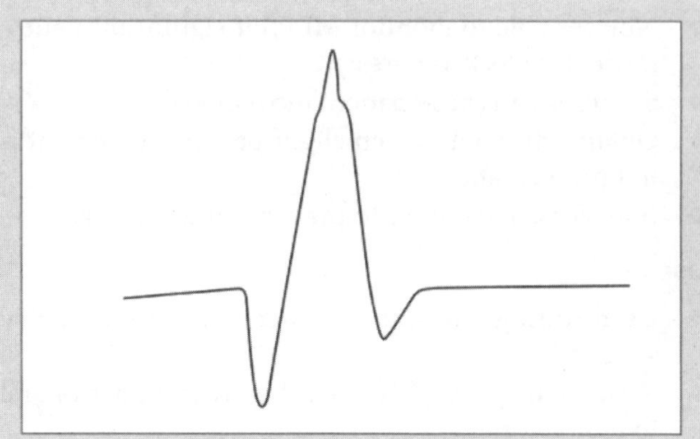

Fig. 22: Motor evoked potentials.

Peak	Generator
I	Acoustic nerve
II	Intracranial acoustic N/cochlear nucleus
III	Superior olive (pons)
IV	Lateral lemniscus (pons)
V	Inferior colliculus (mid brain)
VI	Medial geniculate body (thalamus)
VII	Thalamocortical radiation

Visual Evoked Potentials

- Produced by flashes from light emitting diodes which are mounted on goggles placed on patients closed eyes
- Evoked potentials over occipital cortex recorded
- Used during surgeries involving visual pathways
  - Transsphenoidal surgery
  - Anterior fossa surgery

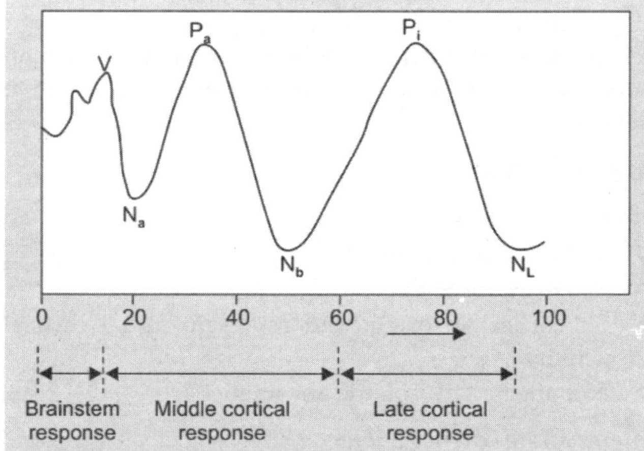

Fig. 23: Auditory evoked potentials.

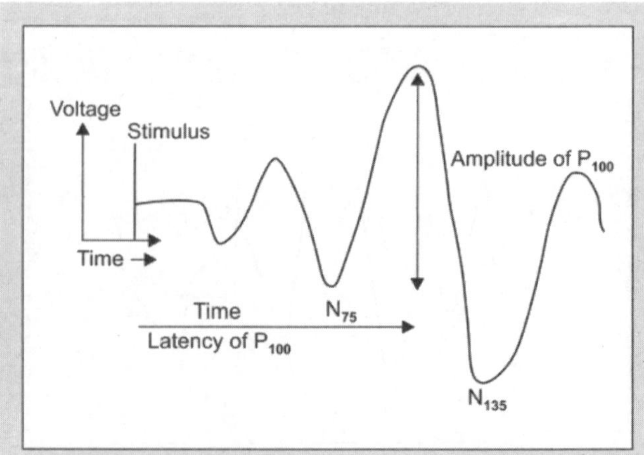

Fig. 24: Visual evoked potentials.

- Volatile anesthetics depress VEP, especially if MAC > 0.8
- Thus, signals are difficult to record during anesthesia
- Generated by light stimulation of retina

BISPECTRAL INDEX

Introduction

- Measure of level of consciousness by algorithmic analysis of patients EEG during general anesthesia
- Developed be ***Aspect Medical Systems***

Indications

- Patient factors:
  - Obesity
  - Geriatric
  - Pregnant
  - Critically ill
  - Opioid abuse
  - Previous history of awareness under GA
- Anesthetic technique:
  - TIVA
  - Low flow
  - Induced hypotension
  - Rapid sequence induction
- Surgery:
  - Cardiac surgery
  - Neurosurgery
  - Obstetric surgery

Working Principle

- 4 EEG electrodes are placed:
  - 2 inches above nose
  - Next to eyebrow
  - 2 electrodes in temple region
- Analysis of EEG data by 3 different approaches:
  - ***Fourier*** analysis
  - Bispectral analysis
  - Time – domain analysis
- Compares patients EEG data with that of EEG database
- Database has values of patients under GA since 1995
- BIS index displayed after analysis
- BIS index is a combination of 3 parameters derived from EEG analysis:
  - Burst Suppression Ratio
  - Relative β ratio
  - Sync Fast Slow
- BIS index is a dimensionless number on a scale from 0–100
- 0 represents cortical electrical silence
- 100 represents normal cortical activity

Interpretation

No.	BIS value	Correlation
1.	>93	Awake
		Intact memory
		Premedicated patient
2.	75–80	<10% event recall
3.	40–60	Recommended for GA maintenance
4.	65–85	Recommended for sedation
5.	<40	Deep sedation
		Burst suppression

Advantages

- Reduced risk of awareness
- Reduced use of narcotics and sedatives
- Reduced use of costly drugs like propofol
- Faster wake up time
- Shorter PACU stay
- Easy to use
- Inexpensive and noninvasive

Disadvantages

- Falsely elevated BIS index with:
  - Errors in electrode placement
  - EMG activity
  - Pacemakers
  - Patient warmers
- Does not predict movement in response to surgical stimulus as this occurs due to spinal reflexes
- BIS scores vary with type of BIS monitor
- Score based on adult population and cannot be extrapolated to children
- Poor correlation with sedation scores (***Ramsay*** scale) when used for ICU sedation
- Latency of 14–155 seconds
- Explicit recall occurred even with BIS value of 47

Clinical Applications

- Monitoring sedation and hypnosis
- Monitors awareness and recall during general anesthesia
- Guides optimal titration of anesthetics
- Predicts level of sedation in ICU

BIS Interactions

- ❖ Anesthetic doses of ketamine do not alter BIS values
- ❖ BIS not affected by even 75% N_2O producing unconsciousness
- ❖ Beta blockers may alter EEG response to stimuli and reduce BIS values
- ❖ Changes in body temperature can alter EEG signal and affect BIS index
- ❖ Greater with halothane than equipotent doses of isoflurane

Current Status

- ❖ ***Myles*** in a RCT of 2500 patients at high risk for intraoperative awareness found only 2 patients with *explicit recall* with use of BIS monitor
- ❖ Yet to be validated adequately by clinical trials

Recent Advances

- ❖ BIS-VISTA monitor
- ❖ Bilateral BIS monitor with:
  - 4 channel EEG
  - Asymmetry indicator (ASYM)
  - Density Spectral Array
- ❖ SYNCH-FAST SLOW subvariables:
  - Indicates quality of EEG overall
  - Determines effects of artifacts like EMG on BIS

DEPTH OF ANESTHESIA

Introduction

Measured indirectly as response to some form of stimulation.

Methods

I. Clinical signs:
- Blood pressure
- Heart rate
- Respiratory rate
- Pupillary response
- Perspiration
- Tearing
- Eyelash reflex
- Movement
- Response to command

II. Clinical scores
- ***EVANS*** or ***PRST*** score
- ***Modified Observer Assessment of Alertness and Sedation Score*** (MOAASS)

III. Clinical techniques
- Skin conductance
- Isolated forearm technique
- Surface electromyogram
- Facial electromyogram
- Lower esophageal contractility
- Heart rate variability

IV. Brain electrical activity monitoring:
- EEG
- Compressed Spectral Analysis (CSA)
- Cerebral Function Monitor (CFM)
- Bispectral Index
- Entropy
- Narcotrend
- Patient State Analyzer
- **SNAP** index

V. Evoked potential monitors:
- Motor Evoked Potentials
- Somatosensory Evoked Potentials
- Auditory Evoked Potentials
- Visual Evoked Potentials

CLINICAL SCORES

PRST Score/*Evans* Score

Introduction

Most commonly used system for depth of anesthesia monitoring.

No.	Index	Condition	Score
1.	Systolic BP	< Control +15	0
		< Control + 30	1
		>Control + 30	2
2.	Heart rate	<Control + 15	0
		<Control + 30	1
		>Control +30	2
3.	Sweating	Nil	0
		Moist skin	1
		Visible sweat beads	2
4.	Tears	No excess tears in open eyes	0
		Excess tears in open eyes	1
		Tears overflowing in closed eyes	2

Advantages

- ❖ Simple
- ❖ Does not require special instruments

Disadvantages

- ❖ Parameters nonspecific about anesthetic agents
- ❖ Tachycardia due to anticholinergic drugs may affect score

- Beta blockers opioids and regional anesthesia affect score
- Values widely variable among individuals

Modified Observer Assessment of Alertness and Sedation Score

Score	Description
5.	Responds readily to name spoken in normal tone
4.	Lethargic response to name spoken in normal tone
3.	Responds only after name called loudly/repeatedly
2.	Responds only after mild prodding/shaking
1.	Responds only after painful trapezius squeeze
0.	No response to painful trapezius squeeze

ISOLATED FOREARM TECHNIQUE

Technique

- Tourniquet applied to upper arm
- Tourniquet inflated to level above systolic BP before giving muscle relaxant
- Patient asked to move his hand
- Movement of arm either spontaneously or in response to command indicates awareness

Limitations

- Nonspecific response considered as awareness
- Level of anesthesia to prevent movement is higher than routinely used
- Tourniquet induced ischemia/complications possible

SPONTANEOUS SURFACE ELECTROMYOGRAM

Introduction

Electrical activity measured from the surface of various muscle groups in patients who are not completely paralyzed.

Rationale

- Frontalis muscle
- Less affected by neuromuscular blockade
- Innervated by facial N
- Stick acts as electrode and placed on frontalis muscle
- Levels falls during anesthesia
- Rises during awakening

LOWER ESOPHAGEAL CONTRACTILITY

Rationale: Non-striated fibres of lower half of esophagus retain activity even after complete skeletal muscle paralysis.

Types

I. Spontaneous Lower Esophageal Contractions

- Non responsive spontaneous contractions
- Detected by pressure transducers
- Under control of central esophageal contractility center
- Increased frequency of contractions occurs when:
  - Lightening of plane of anesthesia
  - Emotion and stress in awake patient

II. Provoked Lower Esophageal Contractions

- Due to sudden distention of esophagus by event such as arrival of bolus of food
- Induced by rapid inflation of balloon catheter in lower esophagus
- Smooth muscle contractions detected by distally placed pressure transducers

Interpretation

Esophageal contractility index = 70 * (SLOC rate + PLOC amplitude)

Current Status

- Limited role in measuring depth of anesthesia
- Easy to interprete
- Can be used with muscle relaxants
- Not a reliable method

HEART RATE VARIABILITY

Rationale

- Anesthetic agents first act on brainstem and then on cerebral cortex
- Measures brainstem mediated autonomic tone
- Not affected by any factor other than anesthetic depth

Components

- *Low frequency fluctuations:* Believed to be due to circadian rhythm
- *Medium frequency fluctuations*: Due to baroreceptor reflexes
- *High frequency fluctuations*: Coincides with frequency of ventilation
- Characterized by >10% variation in P waves of ECG over 5 mins

Limitations

- Depends on intact autonomic nervous system
- Depends on healthy myocardial conducting system

- Interference when:
  - Autonomic neuropathy
  - Beta blocker therapy
  - Sepsis
  - Conduction defects

COMPRESSED SPECTRAL ANALYSIS

Technique

- Superimposes linear plots of successive epochs of time on each other
- Generates 3 dimensional display of:
  - Amplitude – Y axis
  - Frequency – X axis
  - Time – Z axis

Limitations

- Patient variability
- Agent variability
- Confounded by hypoxia hypercarbia and hypotension
- Not reliable
- Can only provide a trend in conjunction with others

Parameters

- Total power
- *Spectral Edge Frequency*
- *Peak Power Frequency*

CEREBRAL FUNCTION MONITOR

Technique

- Uses single biparietal/bitemporal lead to obtain EEG signal
- Output is no longer a regular EEG signal
- It represents overall cortical background activity of brain
- Unreliable when using inhalational agents

ENTROPY

Introduction

Defined as amount of disorder in a system.

Rationale

- Describes irregularity complexity and unpredictability of a signal
- EEG signal most complex in awake patient
- Becomes more regular as anesthetic depth increases
- Entropy is high during awake state
- Entropy approaches zero (isoelectric EEG) with increasing anesthetic depth

Technique

- Based on processed EEG and frontalis muscle EMG signals
- Entropy algorithm used

Parameters

I. State Entropy

- Index from 0–97 (awake)
- Computed over frequency range 0.8–32 Hz
- Consists mostly of EEG activity

II. Response Entropy

- Index from 0–100 (awake)
- Computed over frequency range 0.8–47 Hz
- Consists mostly of EMG frontalis activity

III. Burst Suppression Ratio/Index

- Ratio of suppressed activity to total activity period in EEG in 1 minute

IV. Reproducible Hypnosis Index

- Used in neurosurgery for supratentorial lesions

Interpretation

- Target range for entropy – 40 to 60
- RE and SE around 40 indicate low probability of awareness
- Increasing EMG activity indicates impending arousal
- If SE is low and RE is high, consider:
  - Further analgesia
  - Further muscle relaxants

Current Status

- Correlates with BIS monitoring

NARCOTREND

Technique

- 2 electrodes placed on patients forehead
- 3rd electrode serves as reference
- Multivariate statistical algorithm transforms EEG data into 6 letter calculation of depth of anesthesia

Parameters

- *Narcotrend Index*
- *Signal Quality Index*
- EMG activity
- *Burst Suppression Ratio*
- *Narcotrend Stage Classification*

Narcotrend Stage

A= Awake
B= Sedated
C= Light anesthesia
D= General anesthesia
E= Deep hypnosis + general anesthesia
F= GA + burst suppression

Narcotrend Index

Similar to BIS score:

- 0 = Deeply anesthetized
- 100 = Fully awake

Current Status

- Reduces propofol consumption
- Reduces end tidal concentration of sevoflurane

PATIENT STATE INDEX

Rationale

- EEG in awake patient has occipital dominance
- EEG changes to frontal dominance on induction
- Returns to occipital dominance on awakening

Principle

- Uses 5 leads in frontotemporal region
- Uses time frequency and spatial information
- Uses collection of EEG databases for comparison and analysis
- Initially called ***PSA-400*** or ***Sedline monitor***
- Quantifies propofol/sufentanyl in ICU
- Patient State Index varies from 0–100

SNAP INDEX

Introduction

- Single channel device to monitor EEG

Technique

- Uses 3 SNAP electrodes:
  1. Centre of forehead
  2. Arch of eyebrow
  3. End of eyebrow line above temple

Current Status/Implications

- SNAP returns to baseline before awakening
- BIS remains below baseline after awakening
- SNAP more sensitive to unintentional awareness

MONITORS OF TISSUE OXYGENATION

Factors Affecting Tissue Oxygenation

- Hemoglobin concentration
- Percentage saturation of oxygen
- Oxygen consumption
- Hemoglobin affinity for oxygen (P_{50})
- Cardiac output

Methods

I. Clinical Signs

- Tachycardia
- Hypotension
- Oliguria
- Hypothermia

II. Surrogate Markers of Hypoperfusion

- pH
- Anion gap
- Base excess
- Serum lactate

III. Global Measures

- DO_2 and VO_2
- Blood lactate
- Mixed venous oxygen saturation
- Central venous oxygen saturation

IV. Regional Measures

- Brain tissue oxygen monitoring
- Jugular bulb oximetry
- Sublingual capnometry
- Gastric tonometry
  - Saline
  - Air
- Near infrared spectroscopy
  - Venous occlusion
  - Arterial occlusion
- Transcutaneous PO_2 and PCO_2

DO_2 AND VO_2

Introduction

Most commonly used methods of assessing global oxygen delivery.

Measurement

I. DO_2:

- Global measure of oxygen delivery

- DO_2 = cardiac output * arterial oxygen content
- $DO_2 = CO * [SaO_2 * Hb * 1.39 + (0.003 * PaO_2)]$

II. VO_2:

- $VO_2 = 10 * CO * (CaO_2\text{-}CvO_2)$
- CaO_2 = arterial oxygen content
- CvO_2 = venous oxygen content

III. OER:

- **Oxygen Extraction Ratio**
- VO_2/DO_2

Normal Values

- VO_2 = 250 mL/min if cardiac output = 5L/min (O_2 consumption)
- DO_2 = 1000 mL/min if cardiac output = 5L/min (O_2 delivery)
- OER = 25%

Significance

- Level of oxygen transport at which VO_2 begins to fall = ***Critical DO_2***
- Below critical DO_2, tissues start anaerobic glycolysis and cause lactic acidosis

SERUM LACTATE LEVELS

Introduction

Conventional measure of global oxygen demand supply balance.

Normal Values

- Normal value: 1 mmol/L
- In tissue hypoxia: >1.5 – 2 mmol/L

Physiology

- During shock, primary energy source is anerobic glycolysis
- Pyruvate converted to lactate instead of entering Tricarboxylic Acid cycle
- Pyruvate $\xrightarrow{\text{Lactate dehydrogenase}}$ Lactic acid + 2 ATP

Factors Affecting Lactate Levels

I. Elimination of Lactate

- Increased levels in liver dysfunction

II. Regional Blood Flow

- Complete obstruction to blood flow to limb/organ

III. Rate of Glucose Metabolism

- If glucose metabolism > oxidative capacity of mitochondria, lactate increases:
  - Inborn errors of metabolism
  - Catecholamine administration

Clinical Implications

- Follow changes in lactate levels rather than absolute values:
  - Continuous fall in level associated with survival
  - Persistent rise associated with continued ischemia
- Poor outcome levels if lactate levels do not reduce within 24 hrs

GASTRIC TONOMETRY

Introduction

Mostly widely studied technique of tissue capnometry.

Rationale

- Reduction in cardiac output elicits strong vasoconstriction response
- Also, during hypoperfusion, gut permeability increases
- Endotoxins and microorganisms enter systemic circulation
- Anerobic metabolism occurs in the gastric villi
- This increases gastric mucosal PCO_2 which is used as indicator

Physiology

- Vulnerability to hypoxia due to *countercurrent* mechanism of villi
- Most of oxygen diffuses directly out of arterioles into adjacent villi
- Tips of villi therefore have lower oxygen and higher CO_2 concentration
- Thus tips of villi are vulnerable to hypoxia

Indications

- Cardiac surgery
- Major vascular surgery
- Severe sepsis
- Trauma and burns patients
- Acute pancreatitis
- High risk surgical patients

Techniques

I. Saline Tonometry

- Gastric tube with gas permeable silicon balloon at tip placed in stomach
- Balloon filled with saline and left in situ for 60–90 minutes
- After 60–90 minutes saline aspirated and PCO_2 analyzed
- Intraluminal PCO_2 assumed to be equal to gastric Mucosal PCO_2
- Initial 1.2 mL saline discarded to avoid dead space sampling

Disadvantages

- Errors while sampling
- Loss of CO_2 during transport
- Underestimation by blood gas analyzer
- Long equilibration time: rapid changes not detected
- Only intermittent measurements possible

II. Air Tonometry

- Automated gas analyzer connected with gastric tonometer catheter
- 6 ml air pumped into balloon of catheter
- After predetermined time, monitor draws air from balloon
- Initial 1.2 ml discarded to avoid dead space sampling
- PCO_2 of rest of sample measured with infrared sensor
- Shorter equilibration time-can detect rapid changes in PCO_2

Variables Determined

I. Gastric Mucosal PCO_2 ($PgCO_2$)

- 3 variables determine $PgCO_2$:
  - Arterial oxygen content
  - Local blood flow
  - Tissue CO2 production
- If $PaCO_2$ constant, $PgCO_2$ determines local blood flow

II. Gastric Intramucosal pH

- Calculated using ***Henderson Hasselbach*** equation
- Assumes arterial HCO_3 to be equal to mucosal HCO_3
- Assumes that pH of fluid in hollow viscus equals that of surrounding tissue

III. CO_2-GAP

- $CO_2 - GAP = PgCO_2 - PaCO_2$
- Eliminates influence of ventilation on $PgCO_2$
- Increased CO_2 – GAP due to poor perfusion or increased demand

Current Status

- Most widely used technique of regional perfusion monitoring
- Useful to predict outcome in critically ill patients

Limitations

- Assumes gastric mucosal HCO_3 equals arterial HCO_3
- Respiratory acid base abnormality will affect pH calculation
- Enteral feeding can increase intraluminal CO_2 production

NEAR INFRA RED SPECTROSCOPY

Introduction

Method of continuous noninvasive bedside monitoring of global tissue oxygenation.

Principle

- Uses principle of light absorption and transmission
- Measures noninvasively:
  - Hb concentration
  - Percentage saturation of oxygen
  - Cytochrome aa_3
- Has greater tissue penetration than pulse oximetry
- 25 mm spacing between emission and detection probe
- 95 % of detected signal is from depth of 23 mm tissue penetration

Techniques

I. Venous Occlusion Method

- Pneumatic cuff inflated to 50 mm Hg
- Pressure blocks venous return but not arterial flow
- Venous blood volume and pressure increases
- This causes increase in total Hb and HbO_2
- This reflects change in regional blood flow and oxygen consumption

II. Arterial Occlusion Method

- Pneumatic cuff inflated to 30 mm Hg above SBP
- Pressure blocks venous and arterial flow
- Local available O_2 depleted
- This causes reduced HbO_2, increased Hb with constant total Hb
- After release of cuff, hyperemic response with increase in HbO_2 occurs

Parameters

- Fraction of oxyhemoglobin (HbO_2)
- Fraction of deoxyhemoglobin (Hb)
- Tissue Hb saturation (S_tO_2)
- Total tissue Hb (HbT)
- Absolute tissue Hb index (THI)
- Cytochrome aa_3 redox state:
  - Monitors changes in cytochrome aa_3 redox state
  - Measures adequacy of tissue oxidation
  - In reduced state, cyt aa_3 shows weak peak at 70 nm

Muscle Oxygen Tension

- NIRS measures muscle oxygenation
- Applied in superficial muscles like:
  - Brachioradialis
  - Tibialis anterior
  - Deltoids
- S_tO_2 maybe similar in severe sepsis/in normal volunteer

Limitations

- Represents average HbO_2 saturation in arterioles, venule and capillaries
- Relative contribution of arteriole/venule cannot be measured
- Does not measure microcirculatory blood flow
- Interpretation of StO_2 in terms of tissue oxygenation difficult
- Measurements influenced by adipose tissue thickness
- Thenar eminence most commonly used as adipose tissue is minimal
- No gold standard to which NIRS can be compared

TRANSCUTANEOUS PO_2 AND PCO_2

Principle

- Based on ***Polarography***
- Principle that at higher temperature, ability of skin to transport gases is increased
- Amperometric transducer used
- Rate of chemical reaction is detected by current drained through an electrode
- Sensor heats skin to 43–45 °C

Factors Affecting Transcutaneous Measurement

I. Skin Thickness

- Good in newborns due to thin epidermal layer
- Thick skin causes $PtCO_2$ to be lower than $PaCO_2$

II. Tissue Perfusion

- Low tissue perfusion causes reduced $PtCO_2$
- $PtCO_2$ does not reflect $PaCO_2$ in shock

III. Temperature

- Heating stratum corneum to >40°C causes:
  - Change in structure causing faster oxygen diffusion
  - Shift of ODC in heated dermal capillary bed
  - Dermal capillary hyperemia

Parameters

I. Transcutaneous O_2 Index (tc-index)

- Measures changes in $PtCO_2$ relative to changes in PaO_2
- With adequate blood flow, $PtCO_2 = PaO_2$ and tc-index = 1
- In shock, $PtCO_2$ drops and tc index falls
- Tc-index > 0.7 associated with hemodynamic stability
- Normally $PtCO_2$ is 70–80% of PaO_2 when circulation is normal

II. Transcutaneous CO_2 Partial Pressure

- Used as index of cutaneous blood flow
- Difference between $PaCO_2$ and $PtcCO_2$ occurs due to accumulation of CO_2 in skin due to hypoperfusion
- $PtcCO_2$ is less sensitive to changes in hemodynamics than $PtCO_2$

SUBLINGUAL CAPNOMETRY

Principle

- Sublingual mucosal PCO_2 used as a measure of tissue perfusion
- High $PslCO_2$ associated with impaired microcirculation

Method

- Uses ***Capnoprobe***
- Consists disposable $PslCO_2$ sensor which is CO_2 sensing optode
- Optode contains CO_2 permeable silicon capsule filled with fluorescent dye in a buffer solution at distal end of optical fibre
- Indicator excited by light travelling through optical fibre
- Changes in fluorescence causing changes in projected light is monitored by optical fiber
- Changes are due to formation of CO_2 and H_2CO_3 causing parallel changes in pH of solution
- Light signals are transferred via optical fibre and converted to numerical PCO_2 value

Current Status

- Reliable marker of tissue hypoperfusion
- $PsICO_2$ > 70 mm Hg predictive of circulatory failure
- Ps(I-a)CO_2 > 25 mm Hg indicates poor prognosis
- Capnoprobe not used anymore due to presence of bacteria in buffer solution

BRAIN TISSUE OXYGEN MONITORING

Introduction

- Allows continuous monitoring of cerebral oxygenation
- Oxygen sensor placed on white matter of brain
- Normal $PbrO_2$ = 25–35 mm Hg

Indications

I. *Traumatic brain injury*:
  - Low $PbrO_2$ during first 24 hrs after injury
  - Increased mortality associated with long duration of values <15 mm Hg
  - Currently $PbrO_2$ of 15 mm Hg is critical limit in TBI

II. *Subarachnoid hemorrhage*:
  - Low $PbrO_2$ values
  - Depth of tissue hypoxia related to severity of hemorrhage

III. Ischemic stroke

IV. Selection of critical perfusion pressure

Principle

- Based on ***Polarography principle***
- Employs ***Clark cell*** method to measure tissue oxygenation
- Clark cell is semipermeable membrane embracing set of bipolar electrodes
- One end has silver and other end has gold electrodes
- Dissolved oxygen permeates membrane into electrolyte solution
- Depolarization occurs at cathode which generates current
- Electrical current generated, is delivered to brain tissue O_2 monitor

Technique

- Small O_2 sensitive catheter introduced into white matter
- Position catheter in ischemic penumbra for information about parts of brain at risk
- Oxygenation measured by polarography technique
- Values reflect balance between O_2 demand and supply
- Catheter inserted through bolt inserted into skull

Types of Electrodes

I. Neurotrend
  - Requires larger burr hole
  - Measures $PbrO_2$, PCO_2 and pH

II. Licox
  - Measures only $PbrO_2$
  - 0.5 mm diameter and 5 mm long area

Factors Affecting $PbrO_2$:

I. PO_2 Values
  - $PbrO_2$ increases with increasing PaO_2 or FiO_2 values

II. PCO_2 Values
  - $PbrO_2$ decreases on hyperventilation

III. PEEP
  - Causes reduced ICP with no influence on oxygen delivery/consumption

IV. Cerebral perfusion pressure
  - When CPP < 60 mm Hg, $PbrO_2$ decreases by 6 mm Hg
  - When CPP > 60 mm Hg, effect on $PbrO_2$ is less significant
  - Thus, maintain CPP > 60 mm Hg

V. $SjvO_2$
  - If $SjvO_2$ < 55% it reflects drop in CPP and increased risk of ischemia

VI. Brain metabolic waste
  - When $PbtO_2$ < 10 it causes reduction in glutamate and aspartate
  - When glucose reduces, $PbtO_2$ also reduces
  - When glucose reduces, anaerobic respiration causes increased lactate

Complications

- Infection
- Cerebral hemorrhage
- Parenchymal laceration

Current Status

- Used in TBI to prevent *Secondary brain injury*

MIXED VENOUS OXYGEN TENSION

Introduction

- Direct measurement of reduced Hb percentage of blood in right ventricle, i.e., mixture of blood from SVC, IVC and coronary sinus

- Represents end result of both oxygen delivery and consumption at the tissue level

Procedure

- Continuous monitoring based on *Reflectance spectrometry*
- Light of selected wavelength transmitted down one fibreoptic filament to blood flowing past catheter tip
- Reflected light transmitted back via second filament to photodetector

Formula

- $SvO_2 = \frac{SaO_2 - VO_2 \, (mlO_2/min)}{Q * 13.9 * Hb \, (g/dL)}$

  SvO_2 = MvO_2 saturation
  SaO_2 = arterial O_2 saturation
  VO_2 = O_2 consumed
  CO = cardiac output
  Hb = Hemoglobin

Normal Values

- SvO_2 normally >75 %
- SvO_2 < 60 %: Imbalance between O_2 demand and supply causing the use of venous O_2 reservoir due to:
  Hypoxemia
  Low cardiac output
  High O_2 consumption

No.	SvO_2 levels	Consequences
1.	> 75%	Normal extraction
		O_2 supply > O_2 demand
2.	50 – 75%	Compensatory extraction
		Increasing O_2 demand/reducing O_2 supply
3.	30 – 50%	Exhaustion of extraction
		Beginning of lactic acidosis
		O_2 supply < O_2 demand
4.	25 – 30%	Severe lactic acidosis
5.	< 25%	Cellular death

Conditions Affecting SvO_2

No.	SvO_2	Conditions	Examples
1.	Increased > 75%	Increased O_2 delivery	Increased FiO_2
		Reduced O_2 demand	Sepsis
			Paralysed patient
			Post anesthesia
			Hypothermia
		Impaired O_2 utilization	Sepsis
			Cyanide poisoning
		Technical problems	Improper catheter wedging
2.	Decreased < 60%	Increased O_2 demand	Shivering
			Increased physical activity
			Seizures
			Pain
			Fever
			Raised BMR
		Poor O_2 supply	Hypoxic hypoxia (low FiO_2)
			Anemia
			Low cardiac output states
			Shock
			Hypovolemia
			Arrhythmias
			During suctioning
		Depletion of venous reservoir	Prolonged hypoxia

False Increase in SvO_2

- Wedging of catheter
- Improper PAC tip positioning
- Inaccurate calibration
- L to R shunting
- Sepsis
- Mitral regurgitation

Uses

- Reflects cardiac output and cardiac index status (normal value indicates adequate tissue perfusion)
- Reflects O_2 delivery and consumption
- To calculate ***oxygen extraction ratio*** **(OER)** = $\frac{SaO_2 - SvO_2}{SaO_2}$ (Normal 24–28)
- To determine optimum PEEP (that which increases SaO_2 without causing drop in SvO_2)

JUGULAR VENOUS OXIMETRY

Introduction

- Provides information about balance between global cerebral O_2 delivery and metabolic demand
- For non quantitative assessment of adequacy of cerebral blood flow
- Normal value 55 – 75 %

Principle

1. $SjvO_2$ catheter:
   - Based on unique light absorption spectrum of Hb
   - Uses 2 – 3 wavelengths of light for ***Reflectance photospectrometry***
   - Light directed into blood by one optical fibre and reflected back to a photosensor
   - Sensor measures absorption of reflected light at various wavelengths
   - Final $SjvO_2$ displayed as percentage of oxyHb to total Hb
2. Methods of monitoring:
   - Intermittent measurements with serial samples
   - Continuous monitoring with fibreoptic catheter

Procedure

Two methods:

- Direct puncture:
  - Direct puncture of jugular bulb
  - 1 cm below and 1 cm anterior to mastoid process
- Retrograde IJV catheterization:
  - IJV cannulation similar to Central venous cannulation procedure
  - Needle guidewire and catheter advanced in cephalad direction
  - J shaped guidewire to avoid injury to jugular bulb
  - Guidewire advanced only 2–3 cm beyond needle insertion
  - Position confirmed by lateral skull XRAY
  - Tip to be at level of and just medial to mastoid process

Site of Insertion

- Bilateral brain injury: In IJV on side of dominant drainage (usually right)
- *Focal brain injury*: In IJV ipsilateral to side of brain injury

Indications

- Head injury:
  - Provides early diagnosis of ischemia
  - Useful guide for hyperventilation therapy and fluid management
- Following SAH
- To diagnose cerebral vasospasm
- During AVM embolization (to determine adequacy of embolization)
- During aneurysmal surgery
- During cardiac surgery

Interpretation

I. **$SjvO_2$**: Percentage saturation of oxyhemoglobin
   - < 50%: Pathological
   - 50 – 55%: Critical
   - 55 – 75%: Normal
   - > 75 %: Hyperemic

II. **$AjvDO_2$**: Difference in O_2 content between arterial and jugular venous blood ($SaO_2 - SjvO_2$)
   - 4 – 8 mL O_2/100 ml blood => normal
   - < 4 mL O_2/100 ml blood => O_2 supply > demand (excess)
   - > 8 mLO_2/100 mL blood = > O_2 demand > supply (ischemia)

III. **OER**:
   - Oxygen extraction ratio
   - Normal 24 – 28 %

$$\frac{SaO_2 - SjvO_2}{SaO_2}$$

IV. **CEO_2**:
   - Normal: 24 – 40 %
   - Hyperemia: < 24%
   - Ischemia: > 40%

Factors Affecting $SjvO_2$:

I. Factors causing fall in $SjvO_2$:
   a. Fall in DO_2:
      - Hypocapnea
      - Hypotension
      - Vasospasm
      - Hypoxia
      - Anemia
      - Hemorrhage
      - Sepsis
      - Cardiorespiratory insufficiency

   b. Raise in VO_2:
      - Raised BMR
      - Seizures
      - Shivering
      - Pain
      - Light anesthesia

II. Factors causing raised $SjvO_2$:
   a. Raise in DO_2:
      - Hypercarbia
      - Drug induced vasodilation
      - Arterial HTN
      - AV malformation

   b. Fall in VO_2:
      - Coma
      - Hypothermia

- Sedatives
- Cerebral infarcts
- Brain death

Complications

- Infection
- Raised ICP
- Pneumothorax
- Arterial puncture
- Thrombosis

Limitations

- Poor correlation of $SjvO_2$ with cerebral oximeter
- Extracerebral contamination with blood from scalp /meninges possible
- False low reading if catheter tip abuts vessel wall
- Not sensitive to focal ischemia – measure of global cerebral oxygenation
- Hemodilution can alter $SjvO_2$
- Side of cannulation unclear in focal brain injury: ipsilateral/contralateral
- Frequent calibration required

Current Status

- Recommended in patients with head injury on hyperventilation therapy
- Benefits of $SjvO_2$ on long term cerebral function yet to be proven
- ***Best monitor*** at present for continuous monitoring of cerebral oxygenation

ANESTHESIA MACHINE CHECK LIST

Aims

- To ensure that the machine delivers the set percentage of oxygen
- To rule out leaks in the system
- To rule out obstructions
- Called ***Cock Pit Drill***

1993 FDA Recommendations

A. Check emergency ventilation equipment:
   - Verify back up ventilation equipment available and functioning

B. Check high pressure system:
   1. Check O_2 cylinder supply:
      - Cylinder should be shut off
      - Check cylinder by color coding and label
      - Ensure cylinder is connected to correct yoke
      - Verify O_2 cylinder is at least half full, i.e, 1000 PSIG
      - Open O_2 flow control valve, register flow of 4–5 L/min
      - Open N_2O flow control valve and note that no flow
      - Close flow meter and note bobbins fall to zero
      - Listen to O_2 pressure failure alarm if present
   2. Check pipeline supply:
      - Pipelines should be disconnected
      - Pipeline pressure should be between 50–60 PSIG
      - Check initial status of low pressure system (flow control knob to common gas outlet)
      - Close flow control valve and turn vaporizer off
      - Check fill level and tighten filler caps
   3. Check O_2 pressure fail safe mechanism:
      - Open N_2O cylinder, note pressure gauge shows any flow
      - Open N_2O flowmeter: should register no flow as O_2 line is not pressurized
      - Open O_2 cylinder and register flow in both $O_2$and N_2O flowmeters
      - Close O_2 cylinder and note flowmeter bobbins fall to zero and O_2 fail safe alarm is activated
      - Close both flow control valves

C. Check low pressure system:
   1. Check initial status:
      - Close flow control valves and turn off vaporizer
      - Check fill level of vaporizer and tighten filler caps
   2. Perform *Leak test of machine low pressure system*:
      - Verify flow control valves are closed and master switch off
      - Attach suction bulb to common gas outlet
      - Squeeze bulb repeatedly till fully collapsed
      - Verify it stays collapsed for at least 10 seconds
      - Open vaporizer one at a time and repeat suction test
      - Remove suction bulb and reconnect breathing system
   3. Test flowmeter:
      - Perform test flow of all gases through full range
      - Check smooth operation of floats
      - Check if proportionating device is working by creating hypoxic mixture and verifying correct changes in flow

D. Check breathing system:
  1. Calibrate oxygen analyzer:
     - Turn on master switch and all monitors
     - Remove analyzer and calibrate to read 21% at room air
     - Verify low O_2 alarm is enabled and functioning
     - Connect to common gas outlet
     - Flush with 100% oxygen
     - Verify that it reads > 90%
  2. Check initial status of breathing system:
     - Set selector switch to bag mode
     - Circuit should be complete, undamaged and unobstructed
     - Verify CO_2 absorbent is adequate
     - Install breathing circuit accessory equipment
       - Humidifier
       - Positive end respiratory pressure valve
  3. Perform *Leak test of breathing system*:
     - Check integrity of inner and outer tube of Bains circuit
     - Set all gas flows to zero or minimum
     - Close APL valve and occlude Y piece
     - Pressurize breathing system to 30 cm H_2O with O_2 flush
     - Ensure pressure remains fixed for at least 10 seconds
     - Open APL valve, ensure pressure decreases
  4. *Flow test*:
     - Checks integrity of unidirectional valves
     - Detects obstruction in circle system
     - Remove Y piece from circle system
     - Breathe through the two corrugated tubes individually
     - Valves should be present and move appropriately
     - Operator should be able to inhale but not exhale through inspiratory limb
     - Should be able to exhale but not inhale through expiratory limb

E. Check manual and automatic ventilation systems:
  1. Test ventilation system and unidirectional valves:
     - Place second breathing bag on Y piece
     - Set appropriate ventilatory parameters for next patient
     - Switch to ventilator mode
     - Turn ventilator on
     - Fill bellows and breathing bag with O_2 flush
     - Set O_2 flows to minimum, other gas flows to zero
     - Verify during inspiration that bellows deliver appropriate tidal volume
     - Verify during expiration that bellows fill completely
     - Set gas flows at 5 L/min
     - Verify bellows and simulated lungs fill and empty appropriately
     - Check for proper action of unidirectional valves
     - Exercise breathing circuit accessories and ensure proper function
     - Turn ventilator to bag mode
     - Ventilate manually and ensure inflation and deflation of artificial lungs
     - Remove second breathing bag from Y piece

F. Scavenging system:
  - Ensure proper connection between scavenging system, APL and ventilator relief valve
  - Adjust waste gas vacuum (if possible)
  - Fully open APL valve and occlude Y piece
  - With minimal O_2 flow, allow scavenger bag to distend fully
  - Verify absorber pressure gauge reads < 10 cm H_2O

G. Monitors:
  1. Check, calibrate and set alarm limits of all monitors:
     - Pulse oximeter
     - Capnometer
     - Oxygen anlayzer
     - Respiratory volume monitor (spirometer)
     - Pressure monitor with high and low airway pressure alarm

H. Others:
  - Laryngoscope
  - Blades
  - Ambu bag
  - Suction
  - Airways, masks
  - Other accessories for intubation

I. *Final position*: Check final status of machine:
  - Vaporizers off
  - APL valve open
  - Selector switch to bag
  - All flow meters to zero/minimum
  - Suction level adequate
  - Breathing system ready to use

Work Station Self Tests

- Present in many new anesthesia machines
- Comprehensiveness of these tests varies from model to another
- Checks for functioning of:

- Electronic components
- Mechanical components
- Pneumatic components
- ❖ Tested components are:
  - Gas supply system
  - Flow control valve
  - Circle system
  - Ventilator
  - Integrated vaporizers

Modifications in Boyle Mark IIIs

Gross

- ❖ Extra shelf on top of machine
- ❖ Bigger size and facility for extra cylinder

Circuits

- ❖ Simple lever movement changes open and close circuits
- ❖ Change of circuits at platform level
- ❖ Connections for jet ventilator
  - With preset valve pressure reduced to 60 PSIG
  - In older machines: 15–20 PSIG

Vaporizers

- ❖ Space present for another vaporizer
- ❖ No trilene lock

Flowmeters

- ❖ O_2 is made down stream
- ❖ O_2 flow control valve is touch and color coded
- ❖ *Master and slave regulator system, Link 25 system*
- ❖ Emergency O_2 button type
- ❖ Pressure gauge for N_2O
- ❖ Only 2 flow tubes with the flow:
  - Boyle mark IIIs: O_2 8L and N_2O 12L
  - Others: O_2 5L and N_2O 10L

SAFETY FEATURES OF ANESTHESIA MACHINE

Aims

Aims at avoiding:

- ❖ Delivery of hypoxic mixtures
- ❖ Delivery of excessive anesthetic concentrations
- ❖ Development of excessive machine pressures
- ❖ Administration of wrong agent
- ❖ ***Tipping***: high concentrating of volatile anesthetics delivered
- ❖ ***Overfilling:*** high, sometimes lethal concentrations delivered

Safety Features

1. To the OT personnel:
   - Antistatic rubber in anesthesia machine tubing, wheels and reservoir bags
   - Prevents generation of static electricity which can lead to fires
2. To the patient:
   A. To prevent delivery of hypoxic mixtures:
      i. Before flow control valves:
         - Pipelines
           - Non interchangeable quick couplers
           - Flexible pipelines
           - Color coding
           - ***Diameter index safety system (DISS)***
         - Cylinders
           - Color coding
           - Cracking of cylinders
           - ***Pin index safety system (PISS)***
         - Master switch
           - All alarms activated on turning on switch
         - Pressure regulators
         - Oxygen pressure failure safety devices
           - Pressure sensor shut off valve
           - Gas loaded regulator
      ii. At flow control valve level:
         - Oxygen ratio control devices
           - Oxygen ratio monitor
           - Oxygen ratio monitor
           - ***Link 25 system***
      iii. Beyond flow control valves:
         - Flow meter:
           - Touch and color coded knobs
           - Calibration
           - Flow meter sequence
         - Oxygen analyzer
         - *Vaporizer*: Use of only one vaporizer
   B. To prevent delivery of excess anesthetic:
      – Vaporizers constructed with back flow compensation
      – Locking device: prevents use of more than 1 vaporizer simultaneously
      – Back flow check valve: to prevent pumping effect
      – Trilene interlock (in older machines)
         - Prevents use of trilene vaporizer and closed circuit at same time
         - This prevents phosgene formation
   C. To prevent excess pressure on machine:
      – Reservoir bag
      – Adjustable pressure limiting (APL) valve
      – Pressure relief valve before common gas outlet
      – Pressure relief valve after pressure regulator

TO PREVENT DELIVERY OF HYPOXIC MIXTURE

A. Before Flow Control Valves

Pipelines

1. Non interchangeable quick couplers:
   - To tap gases at wall outlets
   - Each coupler contains pair of non-threading, gas specific, male and female component
   - Insertion into incorrect outlet prevented by using different shapes, space/combination of both for mating portions
   - Wall outlet and connector should be from same manufacturer
2. ***Diameter index safety system (DISS):***
   - Developed to provide non-interchangeable connections for pipelines
   - Consists of a body, nipple and nut combination
   - There are two concentric and specific shoulders on the nipple
   - Small bore mates small shoulder
   - Large bore mates large shoulder
   - Diameter of each port varies for specific gases
   - Color coding of outlets, noses and couplers are additional features
   - *Not followed in India*

CYLINDERS

1. Color Coding

- Different color of cylinders to help identify gas
- Top and shoulder of each cylinder painted with color assigned to the contained gas
- Coding also used on pipelines, connectors, knobs and gauges

Gas	Color
Oxygen	Black with white shoulder
Nitrous oxide	Blue
Nitrogen	Grey
Air	Grey body, white and black shoulder
Cyclopropane	Orange
Ethylene	Red
O_2-CO_2 (CO_2> 7.5%)	Predominant green
O_2-CO_2 (CO_2< 75)	Predominant green, rest grey
O_2-He (He < 80.5%)	Predominant brown
O_2-He (He > 80.5%)	Predominant brown, rest green
Entonox (N_2O 7.5%, O_2 52.5%)	Blue body, white shoulder

2. Cracking of Cylinders

- Cylinder valve to be opened slightly for a moment to clear outlet of dust which might enter the regulator
- Also helps to know if cylinder is full/empty
- Outlet to be painted away from operator and other personnel
- Performed before attaching cylinder to yoke

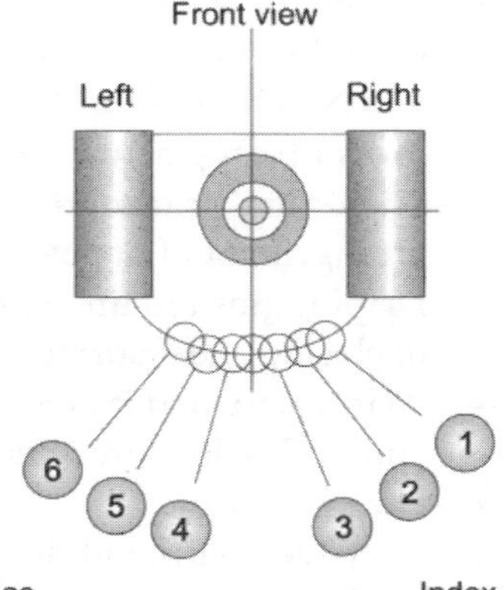

Gas	Index pins
Air	1 and 5
CO_2 mix (CO_2<7%)	2 and 6
CO_2 mix (CO_2>7%)	1 and 6
Cyclopropane	3 and 6
Ethylene	1 and 3
He-O_2 (<80%)	2 and 4
He-O_2 (>80%)	4 and 6
Nitrous oxide	3 and 5
Oxygen	2 and 5

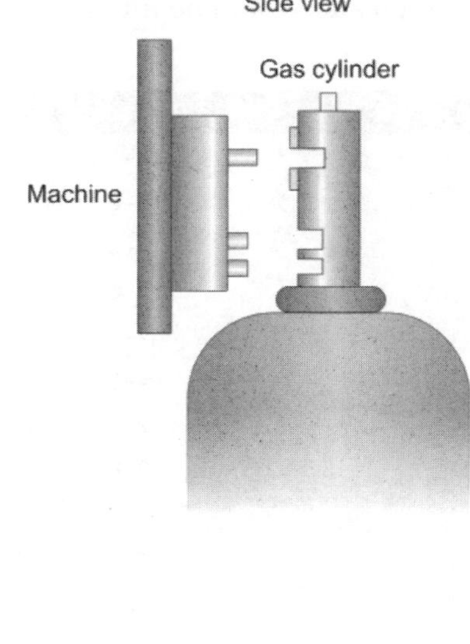

Fig. 25: Pin index safety system.

Pin Index Safety System

Introduction

- Consists of holes on cylinder valves positioned in an arc below the outlet port
- Pins on yoke/pressure regulator positioned to fit into these holes

Uses

- Prevents connection of wrong gas cylinder to machine
- Used in small cylinders (E type) to fit directly to machines

Components

- Contains two pins projecting from inner surface of yoke
- Two corresponding holes present in cylinder valve
- Seven hole locations present
- Holes are on circumference of a circle of 9/16 inch radius, centred in the port
- Two pins are assigned to each gas, one on either side of midline
- Pin are 4 mm in diameter and 6 mm long
- Except pin 7 which is slightly thicker

Disadvantages

- Problems arise when special gas mixtures used
- For e.g., 5% CO_2 mixture with O_2 has different pin index from 100% CO_2
- CO_2 mixtures of 7% or greater would be fitted with pin index for 100% CO_2

Gas	Piss score
Air	1–5
O_2	2–5
N_2O	3–5
O_2- CO_2 (CO_2> 7.5%)	1–6
O_2- CO_2 (CO_2<7.5%)	2–6
O_2-He (He > 80.5%)	4–6
O_2-He (He < 80.5%)	2–4
Cyclopropane	3–6
Ethylene	1–3
Nitrogen	1–4
Entonox(N_2O 7.5%, O_2 52.5%) (N_2O 7.5%, O_2 52.5%)	7

Master Switch

- Turning on master switch causes both pneumatic and electric functions to be activated
- All alarms and safety devices automatically activated before machine can be used
- There should be batteries for backup should main power fail

Pressure Regulators

- Reduces pressure and keeps it constant till the end
- Prevents damage to flow meters, vaporizers and ventilators

Oxygen Pressure Fail Safe Precautions

- Prevents delivery of 100% anesthetic when O_2 depletion goes unnoticed:
  - Cuts off supply of gases other than O_2
  - Gives audible/visible alarms
- Shuts off/proportionately reduces supply of N_2O and other gases
- Activated when O_2 pressure falls below critical level
- These devices are:
  - Pressure sensor shut off valve: Interrupts N_2O supply if O_2 pressure falls below threshold
  - Gas loaded regulator:
    - Where O_2 pressure regulator (primary regulator) controls secondary/slave regulators in N_2O line
    - If primary regulator fails, slave valve ensures only O_2 is delivered

At Flow Control Valves: *Proportionating Systems*

1. Oxygen ratio monitor (ORM)
   - Present in Drager machines
   - Contains linear resistors inserted between O_2 and N_2O flow control valves
   - Pressure drop across resistors monitored
   - These are transmitted via pilot line to an arrangement of opposing diaphragms
   - Diaphragms are linked together with a capacity of closing a leaf spring contact
   - Alarm activated if O_2% drops in a mixture of O_2 and N_2O below predetermined level
   - Drawbacks:
     - Gives alarm but does not control gas flow
     - No alarm activated when piping system contains gas other than O_2
2. Oxygen ratio monitor controller (ORMC)
   - Present in Drager machine
   - Design same as ORM
   - Salve regulator additionally present
   - This is controlled by a mechanism of opposing diaphragms which controls N_2O delivery pressure to N_2O control valve and thus N_2O flow

- Monitors ratio of O_2 flow and gives alarm when it falls < 30%
- Also reduces N_2O flow proportionally to maintain ratio
- Disadvantages:
  - Operator cannot override function of device when desired
  - Limits N_2O flow when O_2 falls only, unlike Link 25 also increases O_2 flow as N_2O flow is increased

3. *Link 25 control*

Introduction

Hypoxic safe guard/proportionating system which links N_2O flow control valve to O_2 flow control valve in order to maintain a minimum O_2 concentration of 25%.

Mechanism

- Present in Ohmeda and Boyle Ultima machines
- There is mechanical integration of N_2O and O_2 flow control valves
- Integration allows independent adjustment of either valve to maintain minimum O_2 concentration of 25%
- N_2O has a gear with 14 teeth fixed to the spindle
- O_2 has a gear with 29 teeth which is mounted on O_2 spindle which threads so that it can float over the spindle
- For every 2.07 rotation of N_2O spindle, O_2 gear will rotate once
- N_2O gear will engage O_2 spindle only when proportion of N_2O in mixture exceeds 75%
- Thread mounting of O_2 gear is such that it allows independent rotation of O_2 flow control valve
- Flows in flow meter are linked to rotation by regulating supply pressure of gases with secondary regulators situated just before flow meters, i.e. N_2O is supplied at 26 PSIG and O_2 at 14 PSIG

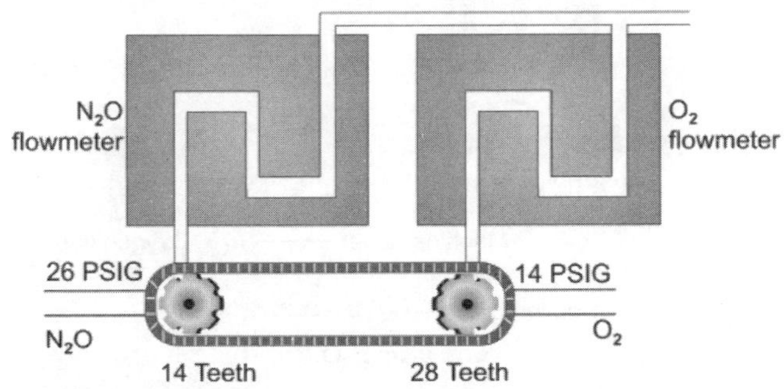

Fig. 26: Link 25 system.

- Ratio of O_2 to N_2O flow can never be <1:3
- When N_2O flow valve is turned through two revolutions/28 teeth, O_2 flow valve revolves once due to 2:1 gear ratio
- The final 3:1 flow ratio is because N_2O is supplied at 26 PSIG and O_2 is supplied at 14 PSIG
- Thus, combination of mechanical and pneumatic aspects of system yields final O_2 concentration

Advantages

- Prevents administration of FGF with $FiO_2 < 0.25$
- N_2O flow automatically lowered when O_2 flow decreased too much

Disadvantages

- 97% N_2O concentration can be delivered if chain is cut/broken
- Ratio of N_2O:O_2 other than 3:1 occurs if regulators are not precise
- Malfunctioning of spindle and gear if not properly aligned
- Malfunctioning possible if threads in spindle undergo wear and tear
- Leaks downstream like a broken O_2 flow tube can cause delivery of hypoxic mixture
- Device links only $N_2O$and O_2. So if third gas like air is induced in flow meter assembly, there is no assurance of 25% O_2 delivery in the mixture
- When using air and desflurane, it is possible to deliver < 21% O_2
- Does not detect if correct gas is actually flowing through its flow meters (whether gas is actually flowing in flow meter is really O_2)

Beyond Flow Control Valves

Flow Meters and Control Knobs

- Touch and color coded knobs
- O_2: white, fluted, larger and more projected
- N_2O: blue, not fluted and smaller
- Bar placed in front of knobs in some machines to prevent alteration in setting
- Float has radiolucent material, so it can be seen in dark
- Glass behind flow meter bank is radiolucent
- Use flow meters only to calibration: not possible to give less than calculated flows
- Flow meter sequence:
  - O_2 flow meter always downstream

- If O_2 is upstream and leak occurs through the flow meter not in use:
  - O_2 escapes through leak
  - N_2O is directed towards common gas outlet
  - This leads to delivery of hypoxic mixture

Oxygen Analyzer

- ***Only*** safety device which detects hypoxic mixture delivery
- Measures O_2% using fuel cell/by polarographic method
- Calibration done daily at room air to read 21%

FEATURES TO PREVENT EXCESS ANESTHETIC

- Back flow check valve at common gas outlet to prevent pumping effect
- Vaporizers constructed with back flow compensation
- Use of only one vaporizer at a time with locking device- ensures that only one vaporizer turned on at a time
- ***Keyed Index Safety System (KISS)*** to prevent filling of vaporizer different agent
- Trilene interlock as reaction of trilene and sodalime in closed circuit forms phosgene

FEATURES TO PREVENT EXCESS PRESSURE

- Safety blow off valves downstream of regulator to allow escape of gas if by accident, the regulators fail and allow high output pressures
- Pressure relief valve fitted to protect back bar which opens at 3–5 PSIG
- Barotrauma may occur if gases are flowing but breathing circuit is obstructed
- Whole back bar would be subjected to pressure of 60 PSIG and patient may be exposed to that pressure
- APL which opens at > 60 cm H_2O
- Reservoir bag: Made of compliant material but gives way when pressure > 50 cm H_2O

LEAK TEST

Introduction

- Checks integrity of machine from flow control valve to common gas outlet
- Evaluates machine which is downstream of all safety devices, except O_2 analyzer

Sites of Leaks

- Flow tube cracks/breaks
- Interface between flow tubes and manifold
- O ring junction between vaporizer and its manifold
- Loose filler caps on vaporizers

Complications of Leaks

- Hypoxia
- Patient awareness

Types of Leak Tests

- Oxygen flush test
- Common gas outlet occlusion test
- Traditional positive pressure leak test
- North American Drager positive pressure leak test
- Ohmeda 8000 interval positive pressure leak test
- Ohmeda negative pressure leak test
- *1993 FDA Universal negative pressure leak test*

Prequisites

- To be done daily/whenever vaporizer is changed
- Should be performed with machine switched off as minimum mandatory flow may reduce ability to detect small leaks
- Test repeated with each vaporizer turned on
- If this is not done, leaks associated with vaporizer or its mounting may not be found

Negative Pressure Leak Test

- Also called ***Universal leak test***
- Used for machines with check valves but also for those without valves
- Uses suction bulb attached to a tubing with 15 mm adaptor

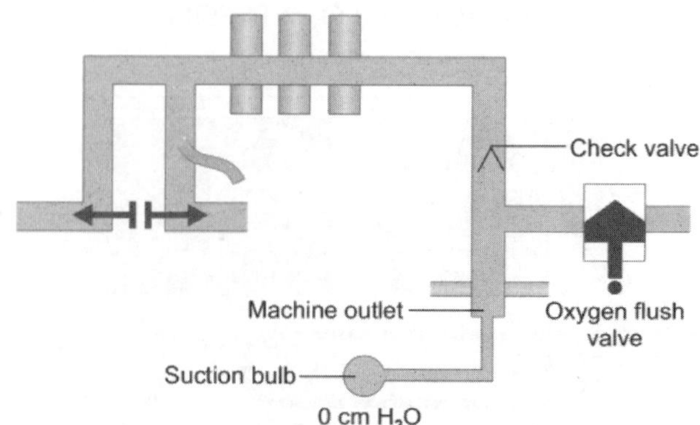

Fig. 27: Universal leak test.

- Suction bulb is fitted to the common gas outlet
- When leak is present in circuit, room air is entrained through the leak and suction bulb inflates
- In the absence of leak, suction bulb remains deflated
- Many newer machines not compatible with universal leak test

Procedure

- Verify flow control valve and master switch is off
- Attach suction bulb to common gas outlet
- Squeeze bulb repeatedly till fully collapsed
- Verify bulb stays collapsed for at least 10 sec
- Open vaporizer one at a time and repeat suction test
- Remove suction bulb and connect breathing system

Positive Pressure Leak Test

- Used for machines without an outlet check valve
- Detection of leak by pressurizing breathing circuit with O_2 flush valve

Disadvantages

- Dangerous if used in Ohmeda machines with check valves
- Inappropriate evaluation if leaking flush valve is present
- Positive pressure from breathing circuit results in closure of outlet check valve
- Valve on airway pressure gauge fails to decline
- System appears tight with the test but only circuit downstream of check valve is leak free
- Thus, vulnerable area exists from check valve back to flow control valves which is not tested by positive pressure test

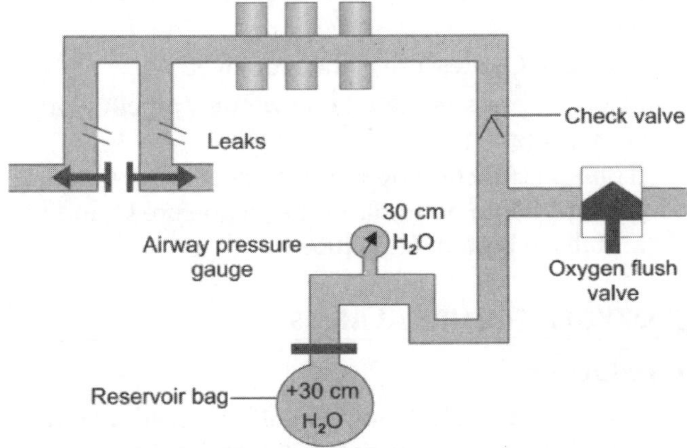

Fig. 28: Positive pressure leak test.

Types of Positive Pressure Leak Test

I. Pressure Gauge Test

- Pressure gauge attached to common gas outlet (CGO)
- Flow control valve slowly opened till pressure on gauge reaches 30 cm H_2O (22 mm Hg)
- Flow is lowered till that pressure is steady
- Flow rate then is equal to leak rate in machine
- Leak rate should be < 50 mL/min
- Cannot be performed if minimum mandatory flow present as this is around 200 mL/min

II. Fresh Gas Line Occlusion Test

- Flow of 50 ml/min set on flowmeter
- Fresh gas line is kinked
- Indicator on flowmeter should more downwards
- Can be used during case
- Cannot be used if minimum mandatory flow present

Combination Breathing System and Machine Leak Tests

I. Retrograde Fill Test

Procedure

- APL valve closed, patient port closed
- Master switch turned on
- O_2 flush used to fill reservoir bag
- As pressure on manometer rises, flow on flow meter adjusted to maintain 30 cm H_2O pressure in breathing system
- Flow to maintain steady flow should be < 350 mL/min

Advantages

- Checks breathing system and low pressure parts of machines
- Can be performed quickly
- Allows continuous airway pressure alarms to be checked

Disadvantages

- Insensitive to small leaks
- Does not localize leak

II. Squeeze Bulb Test

- Master switch and flow control valves switched off
- Occlude Y piece and close APL valve
- Suction bulb with 22 mm connector attached to reservoir bag mount

- Bulb squeezed till breathing system pressure gauge is > 50 cm H_2O
- If drop in pressure from 50 to 30 cm H_2O takes > 30 sec, leak rate is acceptable

III. In Use Test

- During machine use, leak can be quantified
- Lower fresh gas flows to as low as possible
- If ventilator bellows/reservoir bag continues to fill, leak rate is less than fresh gas flow

Identifying Site of Leak

- Systematic check of machine/breathing system
- Follow route of gas travel
- Apply alcohol on hands and move hands over components

OXYGEN FAILURE DEVICES

Introduction

On delivery of hypoxic mixture oxygen failure devices:

- Cuts off supply of gases other than O_2
- Gives an audible/visible alarm when O_2 pressure falls to a dangerous level

Types

- Oxygen failure safety device (OFSD)
- Oxygen failure alarm

OXYGEN FAILURE SAFETY DEVICES

Introduction

Safety devices which shuts off/proportionately reduces and ultimately stops supply of N_2O and other gases if O_2 supply pressure decreases.

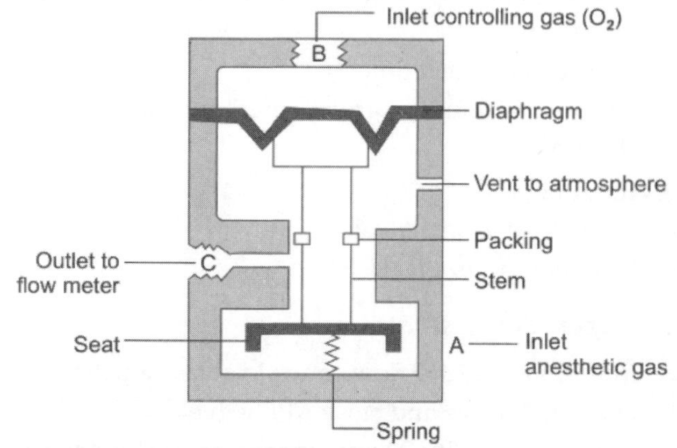

Fig. 29: Oxygen failure safety devices.

Mechanism

- Machine designed such that when O_2 supply pressure is reduced below normal, set O_2 concentration at common gas outlet does not fall below 19%
- Incorporated at level of pressure regulator
- O_2 pressure regulator works as primary regulator
- Output from this regulator controls secondary regulator located in N_2O line
- If O_2 pressure falls, N_2O flow will be automatically stopped
- O_2 failure safety valve closes the line at pressure between 15and 30 PSIG

Types

In Ohmeda machine:

- N_2O regulator totally out off when O_2 pressure falls below critical level (20–25 PSIG)

In Drager Narcomed:

- N_2O outlet pressure falls proportionate to fall is O_2 pressure
- But further decrease in O_2 pressure causes N_2O to fall and finally stop

Example

- When O_2 pressure is normal, diaphragm and stem pushed downwards, opening the valve
- The anesthetic gas flows is at A, around the stem and out at C
- When pressure falls, stem move upwards, closing the valve
- Middle chamber is vented to atmosphere to prevent mixing of anesthetic gas and O_2 if diaphragm ruptures or packing leaks

Checking OFSD

- Flows of O_2 and other gas (usually N_2O) are turned on
- Source of O_2 pressure is then removed
- Fall is O_2 pressure noted on cylinder/pipeline pressure gauge
- If OFSD is functioning properly, flow meter for other gas will fall to bottom of tube just before O_2 indicator falls to bottom of its tube

OXYGEN FAILURE ALARMS

Introduction

When O_2 pressure falls below 30 PSIG, at least a medium priority alarm to be enunciated within 5 seconds and it shall not be possible to disable this alarm.

Mechanism

- Pressurized canister is filled with O_2 during normal use
- When O_2 pressure falls, O_2 flows out from this canister through a whistle giving an audible alarm of 60 dB for 7–10 seconds
- End of whistle does not mean low pressure conditioner has been activated

Limitations

- Can permit hypoxic mixtures if:
  - Crossover in pipeline system cylinder with wrong gas
  - Accidentally closed/partially closed O_2 flow control
  - Low O_2 flow: Depleted cylinder/disconnected pipeline
- Does not offer total protection against hypoxic mixture as it does not prevent anesthetic gas from flowing if there is no O_2 flow
- Equipment problems like leaks/operator errors are not prevented

OXYGEN FLUSH VALVE

Introduction

Receives O_2 from pipeline inlet/cylinder and directs it to common gas outlet at high unmetered flows.

Mechanisms

- Flow rates will be 35–75 L/min
- Only O_2 flushed through this valve
- Consists of button and stem connected to a ball which is in contact with seat
- When button is depressed ball is forced away from seat and O_2 flows to common gas outlet
- Spring forces ball to close seat when button is not pressed

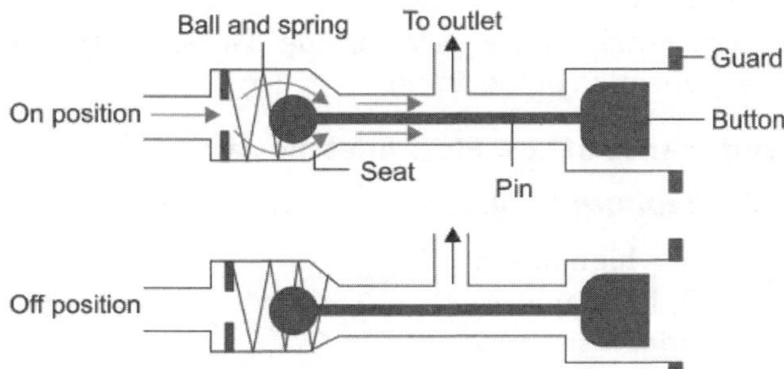

Fig. 30: Oxygen flush valve.

- Activation of flush may produce positive/negative pressure in machine which can be transmitted back to flow meter and vaporizer, causing reading to change

Hazards

- *Barotrauma*: Due to use during inspiration delivered by anesthesia ventilator
- Internal leakage:
  - O_2 enriched mixture delivery
  - Dilution of anesthetics in low flow (closed circuit)
- *Sticking of flush valve*: Obstruction of O_2 flow and anesthetic gas
- *Accidental activation*: Prevented by placing it in a collar

LOW FLOW ANESTHESIA

Definition

- Technique which uses fresh gas flows less than minute ventilation
- Technique in which at least 50% expired gases have been returned to lung after CO_2 absorption
- For most practical considerations FGF of 2 L/min is called low flow anesthesia

Bakers Classification

- Metabolic flow – 250 mL/min
- Minimal flow – 250–500 mL/min
- Low flow – 500–1000 mL/min
- Medium flow – 1–2 L/min

Equipment

- Circuit with CO_2 absorber to reutilize expired gases required
- Two circuits commonly used are:
  - To and fro circuit by ***Walters***
  - Closed circuit by ***Brain Sword***
- To and Fro Circuit:
  - Consists of a single channel for inspiration and expiration

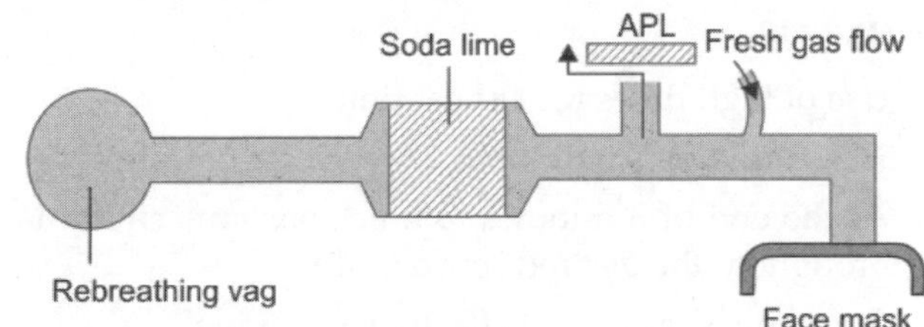

Fig. 31: To and fro circuit.

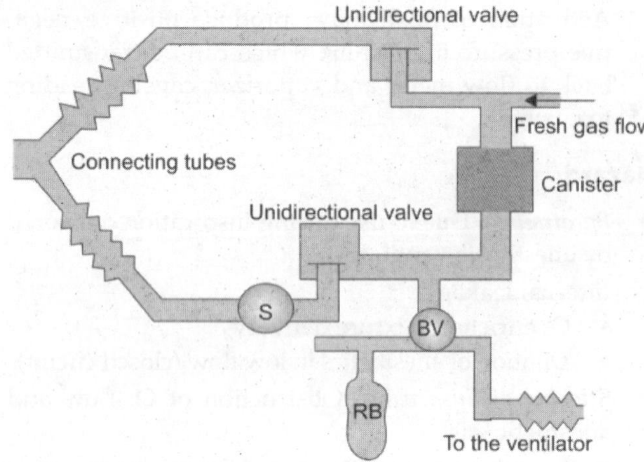

Fig. 32: Closed circuit.

- Advantages:
  - Simple and requires minimum breathing components
  - Resistance to spontaneous breathing is minimal
  - Easy to clean and sterilize
- Disadvantages:
  - Cumbersome and heavy near patients head end
  - Difficult to manage, especially the CO_2 absorber
  - Possibility of inhaling soda time dust
  - Increase in dead space of apparatus as soda lime is exhausted

Monitoring

- Inspired O_2 analyzer (when N_2O is being used)
- Monitoring of end tidal anesthetic concentration by:
  - Mass spectrometry
  - *Raman spectrometry*
  - *Riken gas indicator*
  - Photo acoustic surface absorption
  - Infra red absorption

Techniques of Low Flow Anesthesia

I. Loading

- Use of high flows for a short time
- 10 L/min flows with upto 2 MAC concentration
- At the end of 3 minutes/3 time constants circuit is brought to the desired concentration
- Commonest and most effective technique
- Disadvantages of high flows and OT pollution

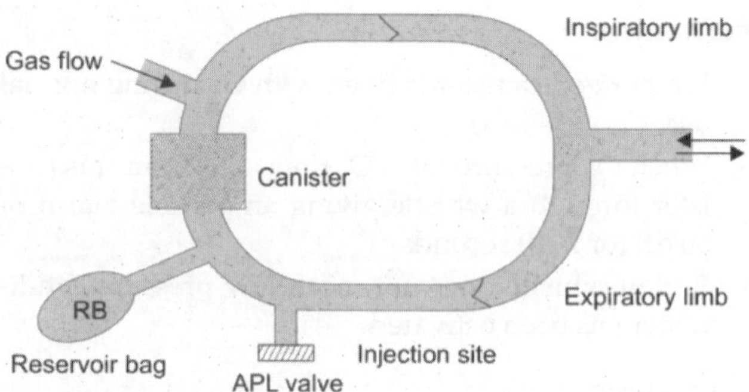

Fig. 33: Injection technique of low flow anesthesia.

II. Prefilled Circuit

- Use of 2 circuits
- Magills circuit used for preoxygenation
- Circle is fitted with test lung and entire circuit filled with gas mixture of desired concentration
- Following intubation circuit is connected to patient

III. Using Large Dose of Anesthetics

- Fresh gas flow started with metabolic flow of O_2 and large amount of N_2O (3–5 L/min)
- O_2 concentration which falls is continuously monitored and N_2O flow reduced once desired O_2 concentration is achieved(33–40 %)
- Seldom used as increased chances of hypoxia
- Setting in vaporizer brought to 0.5–0.8 % after 10 min

IV. Injection Technique

- Extremely reliable method
- Injection of agent directly into circuit
- 1 mL halothane gives 226 mL vapor at 20°C
- 1 mL isoflurane gives 196 mL vapor at 20°C
- Around 2 mL agent injected in graded aliquots into circuit
- Injection through self sealing rubber diaphragm covering one limb of metal T piece into either inspiratory /expiratory limb
- Wire mesh/gauze piece inside T-piece helps in vaporization of the liquid

Maintenance of Low Flow Anesthesia

*I. **Gothenburg** Technique*

- Initially high flows:
  - O_2 1.5 L/min and N_2O 3.5 L/min for 6 min after induction
  - Called *loading phase*
- Followed by O_2 4 mL /kg/min

- N_2O adjusted to maintain O_2 concentration around 40% in circuit
- This is detected by O_2 analyzer which is thus very important
- In the absence of O_2 analyzer:
  - Use 10 L/min for 3 mins
  - Followed by 400 mL/min O_2 and 600 mL/min N_2O for 20 mins
  - 500 mL O_2 and 500 mL N_2O thereafter
  - This maintains O_2 concentration between 33–40% at all times

*II. Injection Methods of **Kennedy and Lowe***

For halothane in a 50 kg patient:
- 0–5 min – 27 mL/hr
- 5–30 min – 5.5 mL/hr
- 30–60 min – 3.5 mL/hr
- 60–120 min – 2.5 mL/hr

Termination of Low Flow Anesthesia

I. High Flows

- At the end of surgery, open circuit
- Use high flows and let out agent
- Causes wastage of gas and OT pollution

II. Activated Charcoal

- Activated charcoal heated to 220°C adsorbs volatile anesthetics
- Charcoal containing canister with a bypass placed in circuit at the end of surgery
- Gas is directed through this canister

Advantages of Low Flow Anesthesia

- Economical
- Humidified gases are provided
- Maintains body temperature in long surgeries
- Less OT pollution

Disadvantages of Low Flow Anesthesia

- Accurate adjustment of fresh gas flows required
- Accumulation of trace gases
- Oxygen analyzer required
- Expired gas mixture analysis
- Risk of hypoxia if leaks/O_2 supply failure

Precautions

- Leaks should be sought during maintenance phase
- Most gas monitors sample gas at rate of 200 mL/min which may be more than half fresh gas flow
- Thus sample to be returned back to the circuit to maximize FGF utilization

Factors Affecting Low Flow Anesthesia

During Initiation

- Factors governing inhaled tension of anesthetic:
  - Volume of circle system (usually 6–7L)
  - FRC of lung to be de-nitrogenated (around 3 L)
  - Diffusion of anesthetic through rubber tubes
- Factors responsible for increase in alveolar tension of volatile anesthetics:
  - Concentration effect
  - Minute ventilation
- Factors responsible for uptake from lungs
  - Blood solubility of volatile agents (Blood-Gas Partition Coefficient)
  - Cardiac output
  - Alveolar-venous partial pressure gradient

During Maintenance

- Delivery of hypoxic mixture
- Steady alveolar anesthetic concentration to be maintained
- Two theories to explain volatile anesthetic uptake:
  - Exponential theory by ***Lowe***
  - Linear theory by ***C.Y Lin***

STERILIZATION AND DISINFECTION

Definition

- *Sterilization*: Process capable of removing/destroying all viable forms of microbial life, including bacterial spores, to an acceptable sterility assurance level (usually 10^{-6} implying that possibility of microorganism surviving on item is less than 1 in 1,000,000 or 1×10^{-6})
- *Disinfection*: Process capable of destroying most microorganisms but as ordinarily used, not bacterial spores

Levels of Disinfection: Centre for Disease Control

- High Level:
  - Kills all organisms
  - Except spores and species such as *Creutzfeldt-Jakob* Disease
  - Most high level disinfectants produce sterilization with sufficient contact time
- Intermediate level:
  - Kills vegetative bacteria; mycobacterium tuberculosis, fungi and viruses
  - Does not kill spores

- Low level:
  - Kills most vegetative bacteria but not mycobacterium TB
  - Kills some fungi and viruses, but not spores

Methods of Sterilization

1. Physical methods:
   A. Moist heat:
   - Around 100°C:
     - Boiling (100°C for 15 min)
     - Tyndallization
   - Below 100°C: Pasteurization, low pressure autoclaving
   - Above 100°C: Autoclaving

   B. Dry heat:
   - Hot air oven
   - Flames

Organisms	Germicidal level
Bacterial spores • B. subtilis • Cl. sporogenes	High level disinfection
Mycobacteria • M. bovis • M. tuberculosis	Intermediate level disinfection
Non lipid/small viruses • Polio virus • Rhino virus	Low level disinfection
Fungi • Cryptococcus • Candida	
Vegetative bacteria • Pseudomonas • Salmonella	
Lipid of medium sized viruses • Herpes simplex • Hepatitis B, HIV	

2. Chemical methods:
   - Glutaraldehyde
   - Orthophthaldehyde
   - Quaternary Ammonium compounds
   - Phenolic compounds
   - Alcohols
   - Chlorhexidene
   - Iodine
   - Chlorine compounds
   - Hydrogen peroxide
   - Formaldehyde
   - Ozone
   - Peracetic acid
3. Gas sterilization:
   - Ethylene oxide
   - Propylene oxide
4. Radiation:
   - Gamma rays
   - Ultraviolet rays
5. Filteration

CLEANING

Introduction

First and most important step in decontamination.

Method

- Prevent drying of blood/body fluids as devices
- Enzymatic foam sprays breakdown proteins and blood
- Stainless steel and other metals are not soaked in saline/sodium hypochlorite to prevent erosion
- Item is soaked in water and enzyme pre-soak, with or without detergent for > 3 mins
- Consult manufacturer instructors for each device

Steps

1. Remove tape and adhesive residue with solvent
2. Disassemble and water rinse with water temperature < 45 C for 15 mins
3. Thoroughly scrub with attention to corners, crevices and lumens
   - Immersible devices cleaned under water to prevent aerosolization of microorganisms
   - Non immersible items cleaned with cloth soaked in detergent
   - Cleaning accomplished by:
     - Manually
     - Washer-sterilizer
     - Ultrasonic cleaner
4. Rinsing to remove soil/residual detergent
5. Dry thoroughly as:
   - Humid environment increases growth of microorganisms
   - Water on item may dilute chemical agent
   - Ethylene oxide may form ethylene glycol with water which is toxic
   - Towel/air dried
6. Inspect for cleanliness and functionality

Area for Cleaning

- Designated location
- Separate from other parts of facility
- Entry only for authorized personnel
- Away from traffic, patients and clean storage

- Floor, wall, ceiling and work surface made of non-porous materials
- Air pressure to be negative relative to surrounding space
- This prevents air flowing out of space
- Minimum of 6–10 total air exchanges per hour with 100% fresh air
- Air to be exhausted outside without recirculation

PASTEURIZATION

Introduction

- Equipment immersed in water at elevated temperature (but <100°C) for a specific time
- Tyndallization: Steaming of object at around 100°C for 30 mins on consecutive days, only for heat sensitive culture media

Techniques

- 70°C for 30 minutes
- 80°C for 40 minutes
- Holder method: 60°C for 30 mins
- Flash modification: 71.1°C for 15 seconds

Mechanism of Action

- Moisture increases cellular permeability
- Heating coagulates proteins

Applications

- Breathing tubes, reservoir bags
- ETT, face mask, airway
- Laryngoscope blade, stylet, bite-blocks
- Elbows, adaptors, Y- connectors
- Ventilator Bellows

Advantages

- Low temperature is less damaging to equipment
- No toxic fumes/residues
- Simple, inexpensive, reliable

Disadvantages

- Treated equipment is wet
- Should be dried and packaged
- May get re-contaminated during packing
- Heat may damage some materials

AUTOCLAVING

Introduction

Utilizes saturated steam under pressure for sterilization.

Principle

- At sea level, water at 100°C
- When boiled in closed vessel and higher pressure, temperature at which it boils and that of the steam it forms, exceeds 100°C
- Increase in temperature depends on pressure within chamber
- Steams transfers heat to materials rapidly, on contact
- Moisture increases all permeability
- Heating coagulates proteins

Techniques

- 121°C for 15 mins
- 126°C for 10 mins
- 134°C for 3–5 mins at 32 PSIG pressure
- 150°C for few seconds
- Flash sterilization:
  - Items steam sterilized for immediate use
  - Usually items sterilized unwrapped

Design: Parts of autoclave machine:

1. Chamber/Pressure vessel:
   - Items to be sterilized placed here
   - Can withstand high pressure
   - Safety valve prevents excess pressure
2. Jacket:
   - Portion surrounding chamber
   - Maintains temperature of chamber
3. Doors:
   - 1 or 2 doors
   - Hinged/sliding
4. Shelf:
   - Items placed on shelf in chamber
   - Door closed and secured

Functioning: Phases of autoclaving:

1. Conditioning/heatup phase:
   - Air displaced from chamber
   - Incoming steam displaces air through port/drain at bottom of chamber
   - Chamber drain remains open till temperature in drain is same as temperature of steam entering chamber
   - This indicates that air has been removed
2. Sterilization/exposure phase:
   - Steam enters load to be sterilized and gives up latent heat
   - Sterilization time at intended temperature is set
   - Lowest temperature in sterilizer is 121°C
   - Cycles may be programmed at 134°C and 145°C

- Wrapped items sterilized for 30 mins at 121°C
- Unwrapped items for 20 mins at 121°C

3. Post-exposure/exhaust phase:
   - Items dried before being removed
   - Chamber exhausted to atmosphere
   - Filtered air circulated through chamber or deep vacuum is created within chamber

Monitors of Autoclaving

1. Mechanical indicators:
   - Indicates and records time, temperature and pressure
2. Biological indicators:
   - Standardized preparation of *Basillus subtilis*
   - Spores packed in strips/ampules
   - Placed in most difficult to sterilize location in load
   - Exposed to sterilization, retrieved, incubated and examined for growth
   - Rapid detection system gives fluorescence when it is exposed to UV light
3. Chemical indicators:
   - 5 classes of chemical indicators
   - Higher classes are more sensitive
     - Internal and External indicators
       - Indicates that item has been exposed to sterilization
       - Eg., autoclave tape/signaloc tape
       - Exhibit color change from white to black
     - ***Bowie Dick vacuum test***
       - Only assesses vacuum pump efficiency
     - Single parameter indicator
       - Test tube containing a chemical
       - Chemical melts on exposure to correct combination of sterilization parameters
     - Respond to one or more sterilization parameters
       - Contains ink which changes color on exposure to correct combination of sterilization parameters
     - Integrating indicators/integrators
       - Responds to all parameters of sterilization over a specified range of temperature

Sources of Error

1. Problems with steam:
   - Steam quality/saturation = percentage of liquid in steam
   - Steam quality to be > 97% (< 3% liquid water)
   - Low pressure:
     - Implies steam will be super heated
     - Steam is less able to transfer heat energy
   - High pressure:
     - Implies steam will change to liquid
     - Pack becomes wet
2. Air in chamber:
   - Impairs sterilization
   - Reduces steam penetration as poor conductor of heat
3. Equipment malfunction:
   - Out of calibration temperature/pressure gauges
   - Incorrect steam supply pressure
   - Faulty pressure control valves, vacuum pumps
4. Personnel errors:
   - Inadequate cleaning/packing
   - Poor loading techniques, overcrowding of items

Advantages

- Kills viruses and spores
- Economical, fast and good penetration
- Easy to use, reliable
- Absence of toxic products and residues
- Material pre-packaged and sterile until use
- Linen and rubber not destroyed

Disadvantages

- Equipment damage
- Metal corrosion, blunts, cutting edges
- Shortened life of electronic components
- Reduces light transmission in fibreoptic laryngoscope blades
- Inequality in level of disinfection at different sites

Low Pressure Autoclaving

- 73°C at 290 mm Hg for 2 hrs
- Pressure is sub-atmospheric (1/3rd atmospheric press)
- Steam is formed at 73°C
- Good for heat sensitive objects
- Also called *Low Temperature Steam (LTS)*
- If formaldehyde is added, spores are also killed (LTS-F)

DRY HEAT STERILIZATION

1. Hot air oven:

   Uses:
   - For items damaged by moist heat
   - Talc, glycerine, oils, petroleum jelly, waxes, powders

Advantages:
- Technique penetrates well
- Does not corrode metal

Disadvantages: Slow

Techniques:
- 170°C for 60 mins
- 160°C for 120 min
- 150°C for 150 min

2. Flames: Ophthalmic instrument heated directly on flames (1000°C)

CHEMICAL DISINFECTION

Introduction

- Involves immersing an item in a solution containing a disinfectant
- Also called ***Cold Sterilization***

Factors Influencing Chemical Disinfection

1. Concentration of chemical:
   - Higher concentration increases bactericidal activity (except alcohol)
   - Very high concentration damages item and skin of personnel
   - Water left on item dilutes active chemical
   - Equipment to be dried before chemical disinfection
2. Temperature: Higher temperature increases effectiveness of agent
3. Evaporation and light deactivation:
   - Evaporation occurs in uncovered container
   - If active agent more volatile than diluent, dilution occurs
   - Chlorine products are susceptible to evaporation
4. Bioburden: Higher the microbial load, longer the exposure time required
5. pH:
   - Increase in pH decreases the efficiency of phenols, iodine and hypochlorites
   - Increase in pH increases the efficacy of glutaraldehyde and quaternary ammonium compounds
6. Time:
   - For high level disinfection, minimum contact time of 20–30 min is recommended
7. Use pattern and use life:
   - Use pattern refers to how many times a solution can be used
   - Use life is time during which activated solution may be used once disinfectant solution is mixed

Area for Disinfection

- Designated areas
- Cleaning area separate to be from chemical storage area
- Area to be large enough to ensure vapor dilution
- Air exchange rate not less than 10 per hour
- Local exhaust ventilation to be installed
- Training to be given to each employee
- Personnel to wear protective gear for skin, eyes, clothing and gloves
- Minimize splashing, spilling and personnel exposure
- Chemical kept in closed container with tight fitting lid
- Small spills absorbed and neutralized with special mats
- Large spills treated with chemical spill kits with neutralizer/deactivator

Monitoring

- Standard biological preparations available only for sterilization
- Only way to assess is direct assay sterility test which is difficult and time consuming
- Physical monitors:
  - Exposure time
  - Temperature
  - Pressure

Advantages

- Economical, easy and fast
- Suitable for heat sensitive equipment

Disadvantages

- Equipment will be wet
- Pre-packaging not possible
- Risk of recontamination during drying/wrapping
- Cannot be used for all types of equipment
- More prone for error
- Impregnates rubber and plastic
- Irritating to skin, unpleasant odor
- Maybe harmful to patient
- Difficult to monitor efficacy
- Instruments have to be disassembled

1. Glutaraldehyde (2% solution with 0.3% Na_2CO_3)
   Advantages:
   - Excellent germicidal property
   - Acts in the presence of organic matter

- Non-corrosive equipment
- Long shelf life, around 30 days

Uses:

- Endoscopes
- ETT, breathing, equipment

Disadvantages:

- Dilution during use (≥ 1–1.5% recommended)
- Evaporates at room temperature
- Needs activation (made alkaline with Na_2CO_3) to become sporicidal
- pH kept between 7.5–8.5 to be sporicidal

Side effects:

- Headache, skin, eyes and mucous membrane irritation
- Asthma like symptoms
- Salivary gland enlargement in contaminated oral airways

Spectrum:

- Bacteria, fungi, viruses at room temperature within 15 mins
- High level disinfection requires 20–30 mins
- Sporicidal if between 3–10 hrs exposure

2. Orthophthaldehyde (OPA/Cidex OPA)

Spectrum:

- High level disinfection at room temperature after 12 mins
- Sporicidal with prolonged exposure

Advantages:

- Non corrosive, faster disinfection
- Minimal odor
- No need of activation/mixing
- Effective in presence of organic soil
- Can be discarded through drain

Disadvantages: Stains proteins

Side effects:

- Stinging, tearing and redness of eyes
- Dermatitis on repeated contact
- Lesions of skin, lip, mouth and esophagus if residues present

3. Quarternary ammonium compounds:

Spectrum:

- Low level disinfectant
- No sporicidal effects
- Bacteria, viruses and fungi at room temperature in 10 mins
- More active against gram positive than gram negative bacteria
- Inactivates HIV but some do not inactivate hepatitis
- Ineffective against mycobacterium TB
- Only chemical agent ineffective against TB

Advantages:

- Quick to act, nontoxic, non-caustic
- No noxious fumes

Disadvantages:

- Early generation Quotes affected by hard water, soap and preterm
- Inactivated by organic materials
- Deteriorates with age

4. Chlorhexidene:
   - 0.1% aqueous solution for 20 min for ETT decontamination
   - 0.5% in 50% ethyl alcohol for skin sterilization in 30 sec
   - Ideal hand scrub
   - Residual effect ensures prolonged disinfection
5. Alcohols: Ethyl/isopropyl alcohol (70–90% by volume)

Spectrum:

- Intermediate-low level disinfectants
- Effective against most viruses including HIV, Hepatitis B, bacteria, fungi and mycobacterium TB
- Inactive against spores

Advantages: Reduces bacterial count in hand rubs

Disadvantages:

- May not maintain contact time: Evaporates rapidly
- Inactivated by proteins
- Incorrect results while measuring anesthetic agents if it gets into gas sampling lines
- Hardens rubber and plastics on repeated use
- Inflammable- fire hazard

6. Phenols: 1.5% to clean surface of equipment

Spectrum:

- Bacteria, fungi, mycobacterium TB, most viruses
- Common respiratory viruses resistant to phenols
- Not sporicidal except at ≥ 100 °C
- Intermediate: low level disinfectant
- ***Disinfectant of choice*** for gross organic contamination

Advantages:

- Activate in presence of organic matter
- Active after mild heating, very stable
- Used mainly on environmental surfaces and non critical devices

Disadvantages:

- Bad odor
- Irritating to skin
- Absorbed by rubber
- Damage to skin and mucous membrane
- Difficult to rinse off most materials

7. Iodine:
   - 0.5–2% in alcohol used
   - *Iodophore* is combination of iodine and a solubilizing agent

   Spectrum:
   - Bacterial, virucidal, tuberculocidal
   - Prolonged contact for fungi and spores
   - Intermediate-low level disinfectant

   Advantages: Principally used as antiseptic

   Disadvantages:
   - Unstable in presence of hard water, heat and organic soil
   - Corrosion of metals
   - Staining of non-metallic objects
   - Tincture iodine irritates skin
8. Chlorine compounds:
   - Sodium and calcium hypochlorite (household bleach)
   - Chlorine dioxide and chloramine

   Spectrum:
   - 50–100 ppm for vegetative bacteria and fungi
   - 200 ppm for virus, Hepatitis B at 500 ppm
   - 1000 ppm for high level disinfection, not sporicidal

   Advantages: Inexpensive and fast acting

   Disadvantages:
   - Corrosive, irritating to personnel
   - Irritates eye and mucus membranes
   - Inactivated by organic matter
   - Not used for instruments, environmental disinfection agent
9. Hydrogen peroxide

   Spectrum:
   - Bacteria, viruses, fungi and spores
   - 3% hydrogen peroxide for work surfaces
   - 7.5% solution for 30 mins for high level disinfection

   Advantages: Not inactivated by organic matter

   Disadvantages:
   - Reduced effectiveness on exposure to heat and light
   - Damages rubber and plastic
   - Corrodes metal
   - Irritant to skin and eye
10. Formaldehyde

    Spectrum:
    - High level disinfectant
    - Bacteria, viruses, fungi, TB
    - Ineffective against spores

    Advantages:
    - Not corrosive
    - Not inactivated by organic matter

    Disadvantages:
    - Highly toxic, flammable gas
    - Pungent odor, irritates eyes and skin
    - Potential carcinogen
11. Ozone

    Advantages:
    - Compatible with plastic
    - Environment friendly, non-toxic residues
    - No exhaust ventilation required
    - Treated objects are dry
    - Less expensive compared gas plasma

    Disadvantages:
    - Corrodes metal
    - Unsuitable for natural rubber
    - Unsuitable for some metals (brass and copper)
12. Peracetic acid/***steris 20***

    Introduction: It is 36% peracetic acid with corrosion and degradation inhibitors contained in a single use container.

    Spectrum:
    - Bacteria, fungi, viruses
    - Spores at low temperature itself
    - Maybe effective against *prions*

    Advantages:
    - Effective in the presence of organic matter
    - Decomposition products not harmful (acetic acid, O_2, H_2O and H_2O_2)
    - Useful for heat sensitive items like endoscopes
    - Less damaging than autoclaving
    - Quick method, wrapping not necessary
    - Can be used on wet/dry items
    - Personnel are not exposed to toxins
    - No sterilant dilution necessary
    - Can be located in OT itself
    - Leaves no residues

    Disadvantages:
    - Can corrode metals
    - Can cause skin and eye damage
    - Can oxidize untreated metals
    - More costly
    - Only small number of items sterilized per cycle

    Procedure:
    - Equipment must be clean, need not be dry
    - Placed in special tray which is placed in processor
    - Each tray has holes for fluid entry and drainage
    - Continuous flow of sterilant on exposed surfaces occurs
    - Sealed package of sterilant concentrate placed in sterilizer
    - Lid closed and cycle is started

Sterilization cycle:
- Sterilized concentrate mixed with filtered sterile water
- Mixture heated to between 50–55 °C
- Diluted sterilant enters trays and covers instruments
- Circulation of sterilant continues for 12 minutes
- Sterilant is drained
- Instruments and chamber rinsed 4 times with sterile water
- Sterile air is pumped into chamber to displace water
- Cycle takes 20–45 minutes
- Printout confirming parameters were met is handed out at the end of cycle

GAS STERILIZATION

Chemistry

- Ethylene oxide is colorless, poisonous gas with sweet odor
- Inflammable in concentrations ≥ 3%

Preparation

- Available in high pressure tanks, ampoules and cartridges
- Mixed with CO_2 or CFCS or freon to reduce flammability
- 10% gas in CO_2 with humidity of 30–50% used
- Cylinder has aluminium color body with red shoulders
- Circular yellow band present below shoulders

Spectrum: Bacteria, fungi, viruses and spores

Physical Parameter of EOS

- Gas concentration: EOS between 450–750 mg/L recommended
- Temperature: Between 38–60 C
- Relative Humidity: Between 40–80 %
- Exposure time: Between 1.5– 6 hrs, upto 12 hrs

Design of Machine

- Pressure rated vessel with port for admitting air
- Vacuum pump for evacuating chamber gas components
- Jacket to heat vessel
- Steam source to humidify chamber and contents
- A means to inject sterilant
- Computer and monitors to document process

Uses

- Pump oxygenator
- ***Ruben valve***, plastic pump tubing
- Teflon prosthesis
- Grafts
- Catheters

Preparation of Instrument

- Item should be suitable for EOS
- Items disassembled, cleaned, dried and wrapped
- Caps, plugs, valves and stylets removed
- Equipment thoroughly cleaned and rinsed, dried with towel/air
- Wrap item in material permeable to EO gas and water vapor
- Devices sorted according to sterilization time
- Devices placed in wire baskets/metal carts which do not absorb EO
- Items loosely loaded to allow gas penetration
- Items not to be in contact with chamber walls

Sterilization Cycle

- Warming of chamber
- Evacuation of air
- Introduction of moisture and maintaining it for dwell period
- Introduction for ethylene oxide
- Raising of chamber pressure and temperature
- Exposure to EO for required time
- Releasing pressure in chamber
- Removal of EO mixture (***Purge cycle***)
- Introducing filtered air in chamber which re-establishes atmospheric pressure

Aeration Cycle

- Reduces retained EO on items to safe level
- Done by ambient aeration/mechanical aeration
- Takes long time

Indication of Gas Sterilization

1. Physical: Measures exposure time, temperature, humidity and pressure
2. Chemical:
    - Tapes/strips/cards/sheets
    - Changes color when sterilization parameters are met
3. Biological:
    - Used at least once a week
    - Placed in most inaccessible region of load

Complications

1. To patient:
   - Skin reaction
   - Respiratory tract inflammation
   - Hemolysis if blood is exposed to item
   - Sensitization and anaphylaxis
   - Increases risk of latex sensitization
2. Equipment alteration:
   - Leaches plastics, weakens integrity
   - ETT becomes soft and kinks easily
3. Personnel:

   Acute exposure:
   - Headache, eye irritation, coughing, metallic taste
   - Nausea, vomiting, diarrhea, fatigue ability
   - Memory loss, drowsiness, weakness, dizziness, CNS symptoms
   - Lack of coordination, convulsions
   - Upper respiratory tract irritation, dyspnea, respiratory paralysis

   Chronic exposure:
   - Corneal burns, cataract, keratitis
   - Skin reaction, respiratory infection
   - Affects CNS and PNS: reduces cognition
   - Anemia
   - Mutagenic, carcinogenic
   - Affects reproductive system

Advantages

- Reliable: Gas permeates crevices and narrow lumens
- Use on heat/moisture labile materials
- Minimal damage to equipment
- Items can be pre-packaged
- Can be stored sterile for long periods
- Eliminates risk of re-contamination
- Large load can be sterilized at a time

Disadvantages

- Fires and explosion hazard
- Long total processing time
- Costly and needs trained personnel
- Monitoring is required to reduce personnel exposure
- Some materials deteriorate after repeated EOS
- Petroleum based lubricants cannot be EO sterilized

GAS PLASMA STERILIZATION

Introduction

Called *fourth state of matter.*

Physics

- Contains cloud of reactive ions, electrons and neutral atomic and molecular particles
- Produced by applying energy to hydrogen peroxide
- Reactive species interact with intracellular molecules required for metabolism and reproduction

Advantages

- Effective, simple to operate
- Temperature during cycle does not exceed 50°C
- Useful for heat and moisture labile items
- Less corrosive than steam
- Used for hinged and non-hinged items
- Uses low concentration of agent
- No toxic residues: only O_2 and water, lack of personnel exposure
- Short processing time
- Sterilized product is dry and ready to use

Disadvantages

- Small size of sterilization chamber
- Cellulose, paper, linen, powders and implants cannot be processed
- Penetration not as good as EOS
- Items with collapsible surfaces like bags need a block to keep surfaces apart
- May require modification of wrapping and stacking techniques

Procedure: Has 5 phases:

1. Prepacking phase:
   - Item cleaned and dried
   - Can be unwrapped/kept in non-woven wrap
   - Hydrogen peroxide cassette placed inside sterilizer along with items
2. Preconditioning/Vacuum phase:
   - Door closed, chamber is evacuated
   - Vacuum is created in gas chamber
   - Filtered air reintroduced to restore atmosphere pressure
3. Diffusion phase:
   - Chamber evacuated again
   - Small volume of H_2O_2 is injected from cassette
   - H_2O_2 vaporizes and diffuses around items for a fixed time

4. Plasma phase:
    - Low temperature plasma is formed using radiofrequency energy
    - Temperature increases by around 5 °C during this phase
5. Vent phase:
    - Filtered air is introduced into chamber
    - Air displaces vapor from chamber
    - H_2O_2 vapor passes through device which decomposes it

RADIATION STERILIZATION

Principle: Uses electromagnetic waves produced during disintegration of radioactive elements.

Spectrum: Bacteria, viruses, spores, fungi

Advantages

- Items can be pre-packaged
- Item remains sterile until use
- Heat labile substances can be sterilized
- No risk from retained radioactivity

Disadvantages: Expensive, not practical for everyday use

Gamma Rays

- Derived from Co^{60} source
- Lethal dose for bacteria is 2.5 megarads
- ETT, catheters, plastic equipment can be sterilized
- Highly expensive
- Used for sterilizing disposable equipment after manufacturing

Ultraviolet Rays

- Special lights emitting UV rays fixed on roof at appropriate angles
- Whole OT and equipment to be exposed for 6 hrs or more
- Patients and personnel to be protected (especially skin and eyes)

CLASSIFICATION OF INSTRUMENTS

Introduction

Centre for Disease Control.
Instruments and other items classified by risk of infection involved to prevent nosocomial infection.

I. Critical items
    - Must be sterile
    - Present high risk of infection if contaminated
    - Vascular, regional block needles and catheters

II. Semi critical items
    - Do not pierce mucus membrane
    - Should be sterile/at least high level disinfected
    - Example:
        - Endoscope
        - Oral/nasal airways
        - Laryngoscope blades
        - Resuscitation bags
        - Temperature probes
        - Breathing tubes and connectors
        - Temperature probes
        - Breathing tubes and connectors
        - Facemask
        - Oxygen mask
        - Esophageal stethoscope
        - ETT

III. Non-critical items
    - Come in contact with intact skin
    - Require only cleaning followed by intermediate disinfection
    - Example:
        - Stethoscope
        - Head straps
        - BP cuff
        - Blood warmers
        - Pulse oximeter
        - CO_2 absorber assemblies
        - Arm board
        - Adaptors for O_2 sensors
        - ECG cable and electrode
        - Exterior of machine, ventilator
        - Humidifier
        - Scavenging system
        - IV fluid pump
        - Monitors
        - Equipment carts

IV. Environmental surfaces
    - Do not ordinarily come into direct contact with patient
    - If they do, it is only with intact skin
    - Can cause secondary cross contamination by health care workers
    - Adjustment knobs/handles, floors, walls, window sills

Sterilization of Individual Instruments

ET Tube, Airways, Suction Catheter

- Wash with soap and water, rinse
- Brush clean inner aspect of ETT and airway
- Soak for 30–60 mins in 0.1% chlorhexidine for sterilization
- Autoclaving is effective but must be replaced after six uses

- Gamma radiation effective
- Boiling effective but softens tubes

Facemask

- Wash with soap and water
- Do not boil
- Soak in water at 60–70°C for 20 minutes

Laryngoscope Blade

- Clean, wipe with 70% alcohol
- 0.1% chlorhexidine in 70% alcohol is alternative
- Boil/autoclave after cleaning (remove bulb)

Humidifier

- 60°C when in use keeps it pasteurized
- Pasteurization, Cu sponges
- Frequent and thorough washes

Syringes and Needles

- Gamma radiation ideal for disposable syringes and needles
- Glass syringes autoclaved
- If emergency, boil in distilled water for 5 mins

Ventilator

- Use bacterial filters at the time of usage
- Ethylene oxide/ultrasonic nebulization with H_2O_2/alcohol
- Internal irrigation with antiseptic
- Breathing units autoclaved/disposable breathing units used
- Formalin chambers
- Immerse breathing circuits in Cidex for 1 hour and then rinse

Machine Ventilator

- Outside of ventilator cleaned and disinfected with germicide
- Bellows and tubings sterilized with EOS
- Most parts of newer ventilators can be autoclaved
- Follow manufacturer recommendation

Machine

- Top surface supplied with clean cover for every case
- Cleaned between cases and end of day, then sprayed with germicide
- Do not get liquid in vaporizer filling tunnels
- Attention to frequently used knobs
- Drawers cleaned regularly after removing contents

Gas cylinder: Wash with soap, water, wipe and spray germicide.

Absorbers

- Effective filter, rarely contaminated
- Follow manufacturer instruction
- Autoclaving possible with newer absorbers
- Canister cleaned when absorbent is changed
- EOS/glutaraldehyde/gamma radiation

Maplesons Systems

- Disassembled and components cleaned
- Metal components are autoclaved
- Rubber and plastic sterilized with gas/plasma/glutaraldehyde
- Use disposable tubing
- Bain and Lack circuit sterilization difficult as central tubing is present

Pulse Oximeter Probe and Cable

- Cleaned with alcohol/recommended cleaning solution
- Cables sterilized by gas plasma
- Usually done at end of day/when visibly contaminated

BP Cuff, Tubing, Stethoscope

- Spray cuff with topical disinfectant
- Clean with detergent at end of day/when contaminated
- Gas sterilization/chemical/plasma sterilization (only for non-fabric cuffs)
- Stethoscope washed with water and wiped with alcohol
- Earplugs cleaned with alcohol applicator

Resuscitation Bags

- Valve disassembled and cleaned
- Disinfected after each use if possible
- Follow manufacturer instructions

Transesophageal Echo Probes

- Clean carefully, soak in disinfectant
- Automated reprocessor for ultrasound probes available
- Glutaraldehyde used

Reservoir Bag

- High level disinfection required
- Cleaned manually/washing machine

- EOS/pasteurization are preferred sterilization methods
- May result in gradual deterioration
- Chemical disinfection: Care to empty air pockets with disinfectants

Breathing Tubing

- Corrugated tubes to be periodically drained during use
- Water which has condensed may run into patient/absorber
- Subject to high level disinfection
- Soak in container with water and detergent to clean
- Remove Y tubing and pasteurize (intact Y tube loosens fit)
- Chemical disinfection, with care to exclude air pockets

STERILIZATION OF LARYNGEAL MASK AIRWAYS

Introduction

- 76% LMAS have occult blood
- Consult manufacturer recommendations
- Disposable device economical
- Class: Semi-critical device
- Warrants high level disinfection/sterilization

Cleaning

- Soak in 8–10% $NaHCO_3$ solution before cleaning to remove secretion
- Inflation valve not to be exposed to any fluid
- Clean with diluted (8–10%) Na HCO_3/detergent solution
- Pipe cleaner type brush inserted through distal aperture
- Ultrasonic cleaning more effective for proteinaceous material
- Supplementary potassium permanganate cleaning reduces protein content
- Rinsed with water and dried
- Packaged in cover

Sterilization Methods

- Autoclaving is the ***only recommended*** method
- Up to 134°C used: Higher temperature makes tube brittle
- Remove as much air as possible from cuff before autoclaving
- Residual air will expand in heat and damage cuff/valve/pilot balloon
- Use sterilizer without vacuum phase
- After sterilization, LMA left in package until prior to use
- Chemical/gas not used as pharyngitis and laryngitis possible
- Radiation sterilization for disposable LMAS

STERILIZATION OF FIBREOPTIC ENDOSCOPES

Introduction

- Semi-critical device
- Fragile, complex and heat sensitive
- Difficult to sterilize
- High level disinfection/sterilization recommended

Preparation

- Store in clean area with distal tip protected
- Best decontaminated in endoscopy unit
- Leak test performed before immersion to avoid damage which occurs during cleaning
- If leak occurs, remove unit from service and consult manufacturer

Cleaning

- Follow manufacturer recommendations as each solution is toxic to FOB
- Remove from patient and wipe exterior with disinfectant
- Flush all channels with water/enzymatic solution (diluted)
- Place FOB in enzymatic detergent solution
- Place water resistant cap over video connector before submersion
- All channels filled with solution and allowed to soak for 2–5 min
- Clean fibrescope with special cleaning devices for channels
- Short strokes used to introduce the brush
- If resistance felt, proceed from other direction
- Solution suctioned from all channels until free of debris
- Rinse with sterile water
- FOB hung vertically to drain any residual fluid
- Brush is inserted into suction port in anterograde fashion
- Retrograde introduction increases damage to internal lining of suction port

Methods of Sterilization

Chemical

- All lumens/channels to be filled with disinfectant
- After disinfection, wash with sterile water then 70% alcohol
- Agents used:
  - Glutaraldehyde (2% for 10 mins)
  - Hydrogen peroxide (for 20 mins)
  - Orthophthaldehyde
  - Steris-20

Gas/EO Sterilization

Automated Endoscope Reprocessors

- Have been implicated in infection
- Have filteration systems
- Change filters regularly
- FOB cooled for 5–7 mins after processing

HOSPITAL WASTE MANAGEMENT

Cat.	Name	Content	Disposal
I	Human anatomical waste	Human tissues, Organs	Incineration
		Body parts	Deep burial
II	Animal waste	Animal tissues, organs	Incineration
		Waste of veterinary hospital	Deep burial
III	Microbiology waste	From lab culture	Autoclaving
		Stocks/specimens	Microwaving
		Live/attenuated vaccines	Incineration
IV	Waste sharps	Needles	Disinfection (chemical)
		Syringes	Autoclaving, Microwave
		Scalpels/blades	Mutilation, Shredding
V	Discarded medicine	Outdated medicines	Incineration
			Drug disposal-secured landfills
VI	Solid waste	Blood contaminated items	Incineration
			Autoclaving
			Microwave
VII	Solid waste	Items other than waste sharps	Chemical treatment
		Tubings, catheter, IV sets	Autoclave, Microwave
IX	Incineration ash	Ash from incineration	Municipal landfill
X		Chemicals in disinfectants	Chemical treatment
			Discharge in drainage for liquids
			Secure landfills for solids

COLOR CODING OF HOSPITAL WASTE

Color	Container	Category	Treatment
Yellow	Plastic bag	I, II, III. VI	Incineration
			Deep burial
Red	Plastic bag Disinfected container	III, VI, VII	Autoclaving/ Microwave
			Chemical treatment
Blue/White translucent	Plastic bag Puncture proof container	IV, VII	Autoclave/Microwave
			Chemical treatment
			Shredding/Mutilation
Black	Plastic bag	V, IX, X (solids)	Secured landfill

ANESTHESIA CIRCUITS

Introduction

Breathing circuit is an interface which connects patients airway to anesthetic machine creating an artificial atmosphere from which the patient breathes.

Components

- Fresh gas entry port
- Reservoir for gas:
  - Bag
  - Corrugated tube
- Expiratory valve (APL), unidirectional valve, non-rebreathing valve
- CO_2 absorber
- Patient connections port
- Corrugated tubes connecting these components
- Filters: Bacterial HME filters

Requirements

Essential

- Deliver gases to alveoli in same concentration as set concentration
- Effectively eliminates CO_2
- Have minimal apparatus dead space
- Low resistance

Desirable

- Economy of fresh gas
- Conservation of heat
- Humidification of inspired gases
- Light weight
- Convenient
- Efficient during controlled and spontaneous ventilation
  - Efficient CO_2 elimination
  - Efficient fresh gas utilization

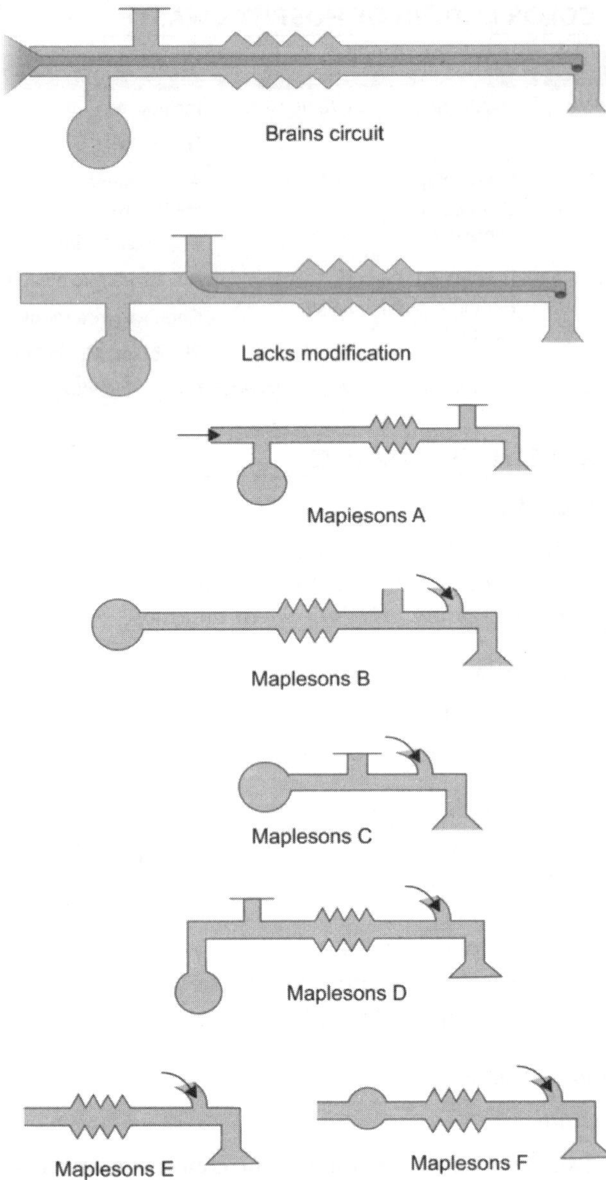

Fig. 34: Classification of anesthesia circuits.

- Adaptable for adults/children and ventilators
- Provision to reduce OT pollution

Classification Systems

- *McMohans* classification
- *Dripps* classification
- *Millers* classification
- *Moyers* classification
- *Collins* classification
- *Conway* classification
- ISO classification

McMohans classification:

Open circuit	No rebreathing
Semi closed circuit	Partial rebreathing
Closed circuit	Total rebreathing

Dripps classification:

Open	Inhales air + agent
	Exhales to atmosphere
	No reservoir bag
	No rebreathing
	Open drop, T piece
Semi-open	Inhales air + agent from machine
	Exhales to atmosphere
	Small reservoir
	Minimal rebreathing
	T piece with small reservoir (***Jackson-Rees***)
Semi-closed	Inhales from machine
	Exhales to atmosphere and machine
	Large reservoir bag
	Rebreathing possible
	Maplesons systems
Closed	Inhales from machine
	Exhales to machine
	Large reservoir bag
	Rebreathing present with CO_2 absorbent
	Brian Swords Circle system

Millers classification:

Systems without CO_2 absorbent	Systems with CO_2 absorbent
Unidirectional flow	
• Non-rebreathing system • Circle system	• Circle systems with absorber • Brian-Sword
Bidirectional flow	
1. Afferent reservoir system: – Mapleson A – Mapleson B – Mapleson C – Lacks system	***Ralf Waters*** To and Fro system
2. Efferent reservoir system: – Mapleson D – Mapleson E – Mapleson F – Bains system	
3. Enclosed afferent reservoir system: – Millers	
4. Combined system: – Humphrey ADE	

Advantages

- Simple inexpensive and rugged
- Variation in minute volume does not affect E_TCO_2 much
- In coaxial systems inspiratory limb is warmed by expiratory gases
- Low circuit resistance
- Easy to position conveniently
- Light weight and not bulky
- Compression and compliance volume losses from circuit is less
- No toxic compounds like compound A/Carbon monoxide

Disadvantages

- Requires high gas flows
- Inspired heat and humidity low due to high fresh gas flows
- Optimal FGF difficult to determine
- Difficult to scavenge Maplesons E and F
- Not suitable for patients with malignant hyperthermia as it is not possible to increase FGF enough to remove increased CO_2 load
- APL valve close to patients and inaccessible in Maplesons A,B and C

MAPLESON A/MAGILLS

Description

- ***Most efficient*** system for *spontaneous ventilation*
- ***Least efficient*** system for *controlled ventilation*
- FGF from machine end, near reservoir bag
- APL valve present near patient end
- Corrugated tube connecting bag and APL valve
- Sensor/E_TCO_2 monitor between APL valve and patient in adults
- Sensor present between APL valve and corrugated tube in paediatrics to decrease dead space
- Dead space at patient end and upto APL valve

Technique of Use

- For spontaneous ventilation, APL valve kept fully open

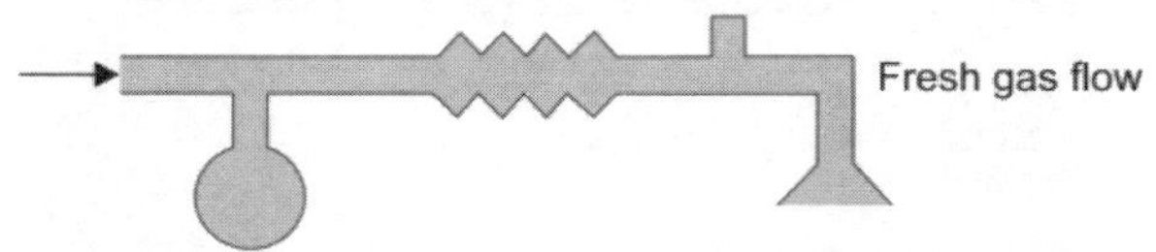

Fig. 35: Maplesons A circuit during 1st spontaneous inspirations.

- For controlled ventilation, APL valve partially closed
- APL valve opens during expiration in spontaneous and inspiration during controlled ventilation
- Ideally FGF rates around 60–80 mL/kg/min

Functional Analysis

Spontaneous Respiration

1. *Inspiration (1st)*: Fresh gas from prefilled circuit enters lung
2. Expiration
   - Dead space (first) and then alveolar gas flows into corrugated tube and bag
   - Fresh gas from inlet flows into reservoir bag
   - When reservoir bag fills, APL valve opens up
   - First, alveolar gas is vented out followed by alveolar gas in corrugated tube
   - During expiratory pause:
     - If FGF > MV, dead space gas pushed out
     - If FGF = MV, some dead space gas remains
     - If FGF < MV, more alveolar gas retained
3. Inspiration (2nd)
   - First gas inhaled is that present between patient and APL valve
   - Next gas will be alveolar gas/dead space gas/fresh gas depending on FGF rates

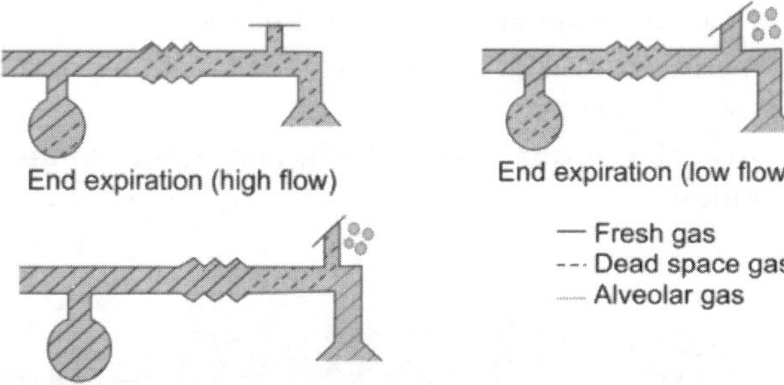

Fig. 36: Maplesons A circuit during 1st spontaneous expiration.

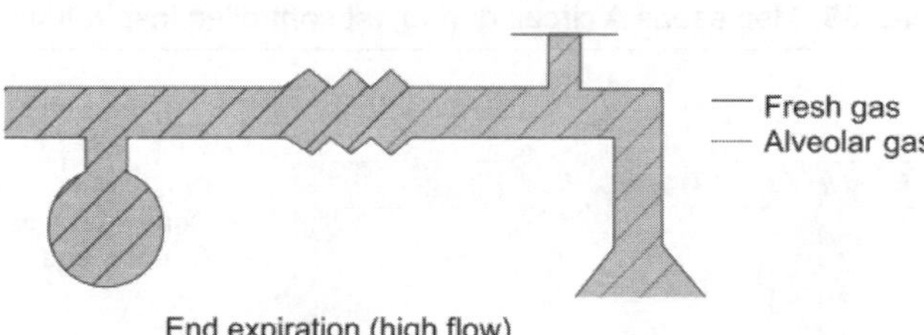

Fig. 37: Maplesons A circuit during 2nd spontaneous inspiration.

Controlled Ventilation

1. Inspiration (First inspiration)
   - Fresh gas from prefilled circuit alone is inhaled
   - APL valve opens during inspiration
2. Expiration
   - No gas escapes APL valve unless bag fills
   - Thus all exhaled gases remain within circuit
   - Alveolar and dead space gas enters corrugated tube
   - If tidal volume is large, alveolar gas may enter bag
3. Inspiration (Second inspiration)
   - Alveolar gas inhaled first
   - APL valve opens when pressure in the circuit increases
   - Gas flows to patient and exits APL valve too
   - When all exhaled gas is driven out of tube, fresh gas fills tubing
   - Some fresh gas enter patient while some is vented out
   - Rebreathing of alveolar gas and wastage of fresh gas occurs
   - ***Least efficient*** for controlled ventilation

Lacks Modification of Mapleson

- Added expiratory limbs, running from patient to APL valve
- APL valve at the machine end of system
- Easier to adjust APL valve
- Facilitates scavenging of excess gases
- Increased resistance and work of breathing due to coaxial tube
- Available as dual/parallel tube and coaxial configuration

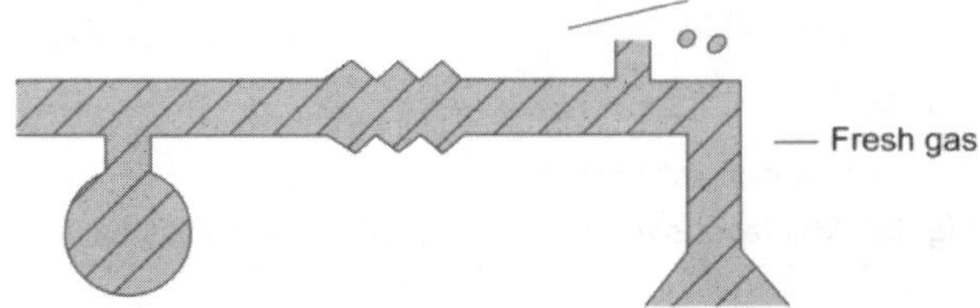

Fig. 38: Maplesons A circuit during 1st controlled inspiration.

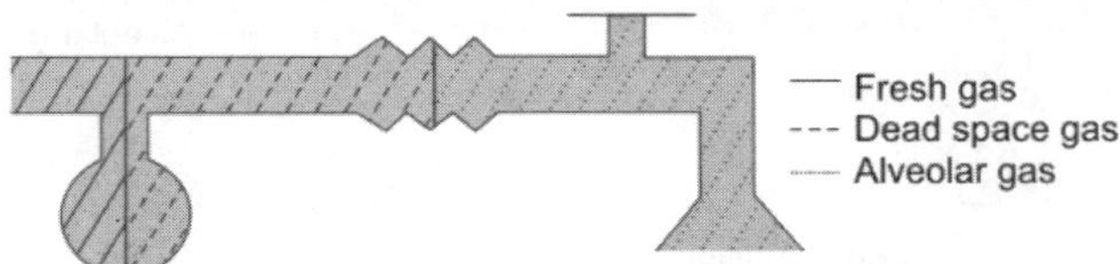

Fig. 39: Maplesons A circuit during 1st controlled expiration.

Preuse Check

- Positive pressure check by closing APL valve and patient port
- If coaxial system:
  - Attach tracheal tube to inner tube
  - Blow with APL valve closed
  - Reservoir bag will move if leak is present
  - Occlude both tubes at patient end
  - Open APL valve and pressure reservoir bag
  - If leak in inner tube is present, gas escapes APL valve

MAPLESON D

Description

- Has T-piece near patient end
- T-piece is 3 way tubular connector:
  - Patient connection port
  - Fresh gas port
  - Port with connected corrugated tubing
- Fresh gas flow (FGF) near patient end
- APL valve present near machine end, between reservoir and corrugated tube

Technique of Use

- ***Most efficient*** of Mapleson circuits for controlled ventilation
- For spontaneous ventilation, APL valve kept fully open
- Excess gas vented through APL during expiration in spontaneous ventilation

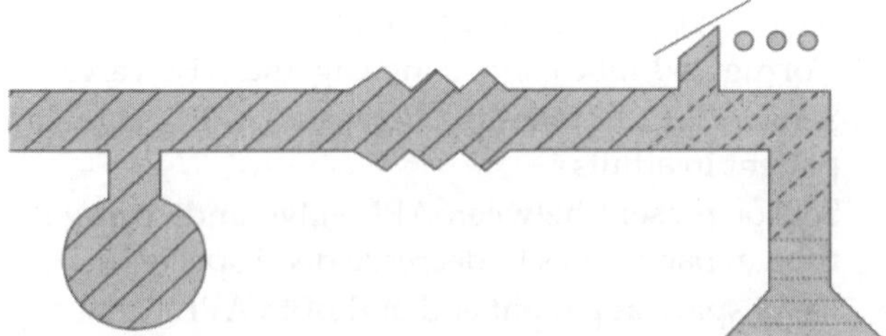

Fig. 40: Maplesons A circuit during second controlled inspiration.

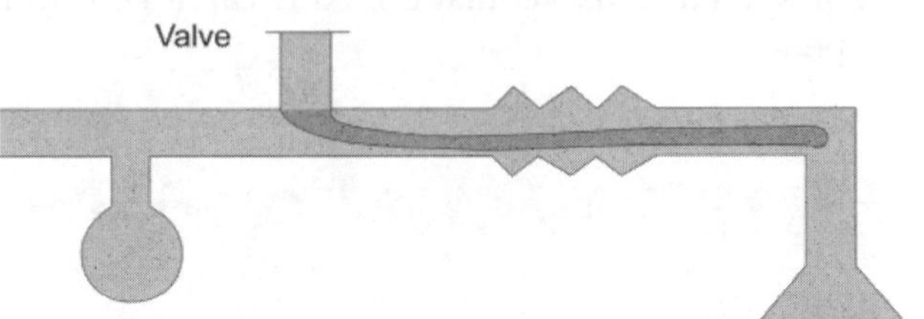

Fig. 41: Lacks modification of Maplesons A circuit.

- ❖ Excess gas vented through APL during inspiration in controlled ventilation
- ❖ FGF at 150–200 mL/kg/min (2–4 times minute volume)

Functional Analysis

Spontaneous Respiration

1. During Inspiration (first inspiration): FGF enters lungs
2. During Expiration:
   - Alveolar gas and dead space gas enters tube
   - FGF keeps mixing with alveolar gas
   - When reservoir bag fills, APL valve opens
   - During expiratory pause
     - If FGF > MV, corrugated tube filled with fresh gas
     - If FGF = MV, corrugated tube fills with some alveolar gas
     - If FGF < MV, most of corrugated tube fills with alveolar gas
3. During inspiration (second inspiration):
   - If FGF is high, all the gas drawn from corrugated tube will be FG
   - If FGF is low, some exhaled gas with CO_2 will be inhaled
   - E_TCO_2 increases and thus respiratory rate of patient will increase to compensate

Controlled Ventilation

1. Inspiration (first inspiration):
   - FGF flows into lung from prefilled circuit
   - APL valve opens
2. Expiration:
   - Gas exhaled, flows down corrugated tubing
   - Fresh gas enters at the same time
   - During expiratory pause, fresh gas pushes exhaled gas down the tubing
3. Inspiration (Second inspiration)
   - FGF and gas from tubing enters patient
   - If FGF is low, some exhaled gas is inhaled
   - If FGF is high, little rebreathing occurs

Preuse Check

- ❖ Occlude patient end, close APL valve and pressurize systems

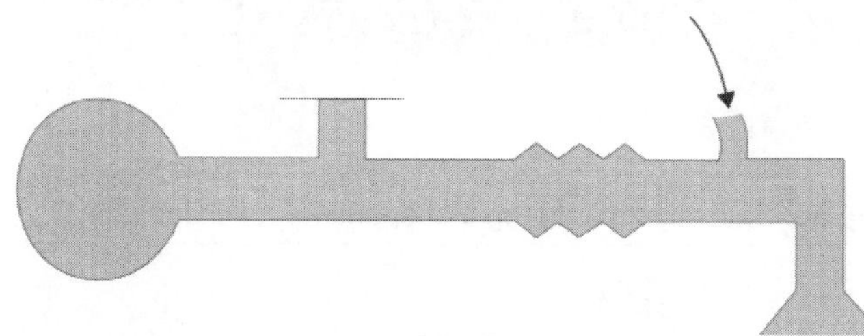

Fig. 42: Maplesons D system.

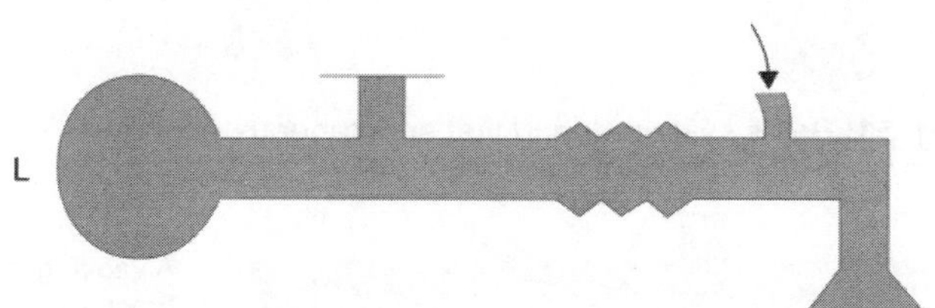

Fig. 43: Maplesons D during first spontaneous inspiration.

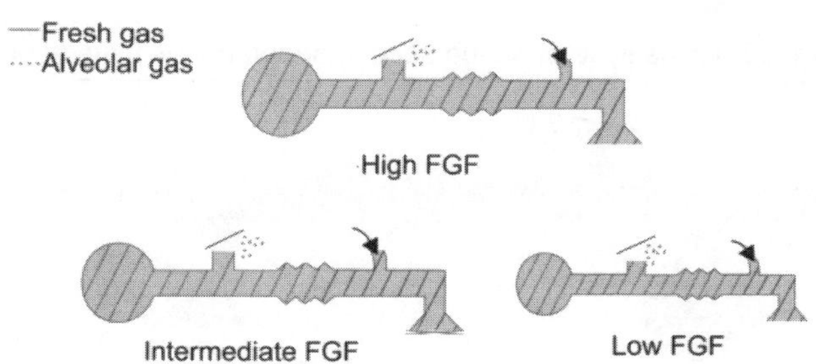

Fig. 44: Maplesons D during first spontaneous expiration.

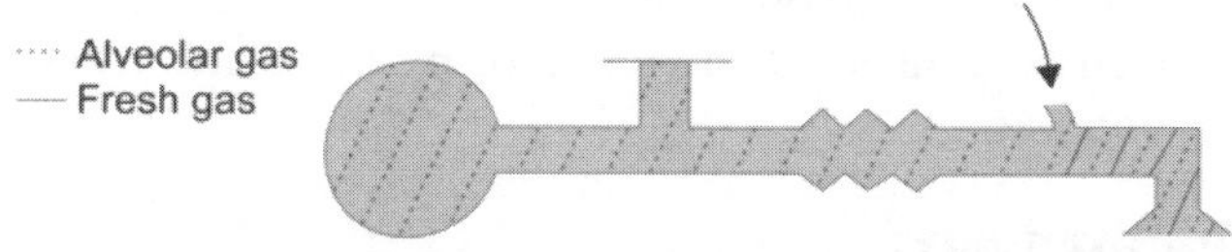

Fig. 45: Maplesons D during second spontaneous inspiration.

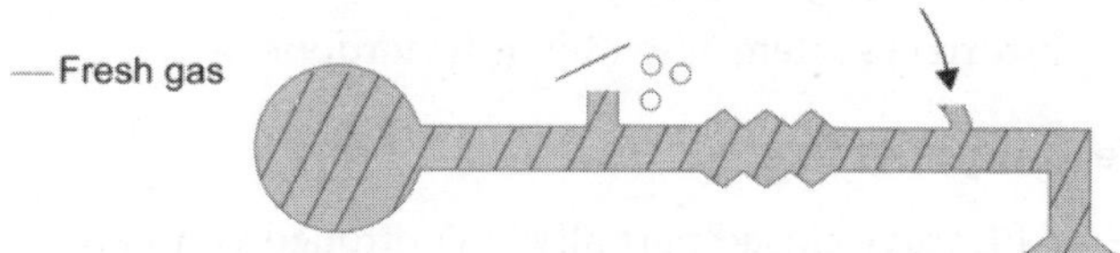

Fig. 46: Maplesons D during first controlled inspiration.

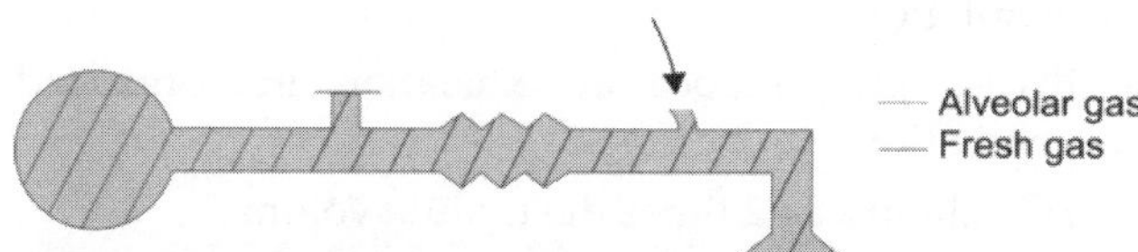

Fig. 47: Maplesons D during first controlled expiration.

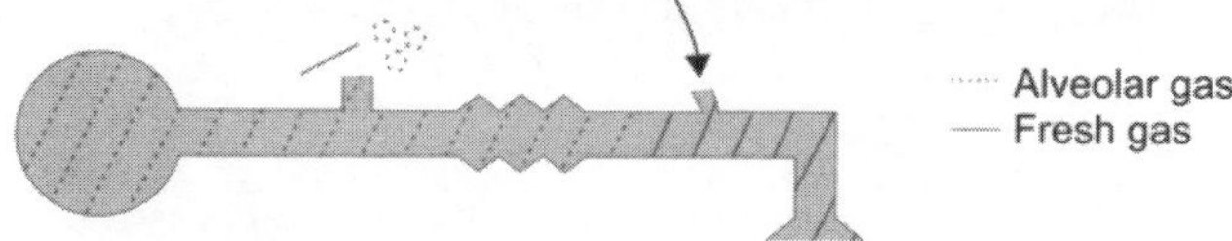

Fig. 48: Maplesons D during second controlled inspiration.

- Coaxial systems:
    - Flow meter test
    - Pethicks test

BAINS SYSTEM

Description

- Coaxial modification of Mapleson D
- FGF tube runs coaxially inside corrugated tubing
- FGF tube ends at point where FGF enters Mapleson D
- Traditionally, 1.8 metres long
- Length can be increased by adding additionally corrugated tube at machine end
- Outer tube is transparent to allow inner tube inspection

Advantages

- Light weight ,convenient
- Easily sterilized
- Reusable
- Facilitates scavenging from APL valve
- Exhaled gases in outer tube warms fresh gas
- Useful in remote location (MRI suite) by adding corrugated tube to machine end
- Can be connected to ventilator by removing reservoir bag

Disadvantages

- Kinking/leakage/disconnection of inner tube causing severe hypercarbia
- Incorrect system assembly is hazardous

Technique of Use

- APL valve closed partially in controlled ventilation
- Valve opened fully for spontaneous ventilation
- Excess gas escapes at exhalation in spontaneous ventilation
- Excess gas escapes at inhalation in controlled ventilation
- FGF should be 2 times the minute volume

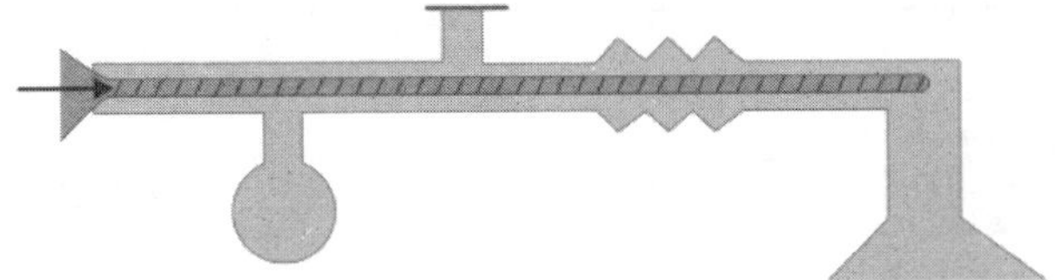

Fig. 49: Bains coaxial system

Functional Analysis: (Same as Mapleson D)

Spontaneous Ventilation

1. Inspiration (first inspiration): FG from machine flows into patient
2. Expiration:
    - Continuous FGF at patient end
    - Expired gas continuously mixed with FG at patient end
    - Expired gas flows back to corrugated tube and bag
    - APL valve opens when bag is full
    - During expiratory pause, FGF pushes exhaled gases more into reservation bag
3. Inspiration (Second inspiration):
    - Patient inhales FG as well as mixed gas from tube
    - Amount of mixed gas depends on FGF

Controlled Ventilation

1. Inspiration (First inspiration):
    - FG flows from prefilled circuit to patient
    - APL valve opens to allow FG escape

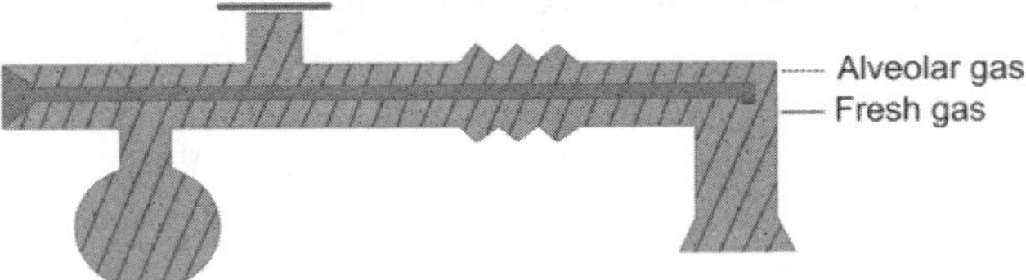

Fig. 50: Bains system during first spontaneous inspiration.

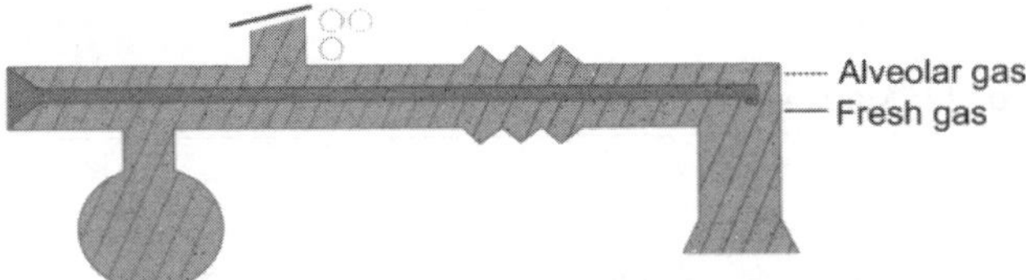

Fig. 51: Bains system during first spontaneous expiration.

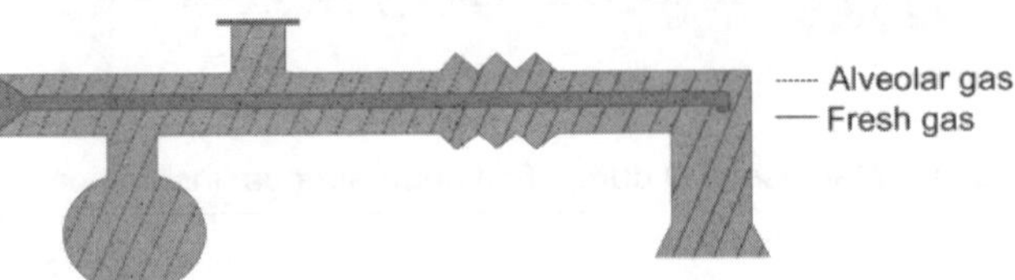

Fig. 52: Bains system during second spontaneous inspiration.

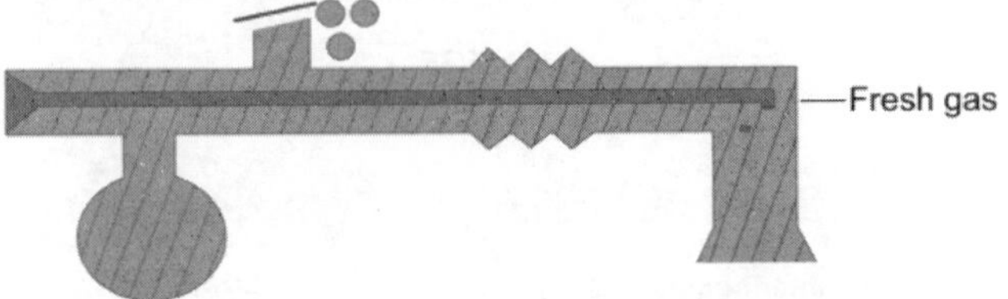

Fig. 53: Bains system during first controlled inspiration.

2. Expiration:
    - Continuous mixing of FG with expired gas
    - During expiratory pause FG pushes MG into reservoir bag
3. Inspiration (Second inspiration):
    - Patient ventilated with a mixture of gases
    - Mostly fresh gas if FGF is high
    - Some rebreathing occurs if FGF is low
    - APL valve opens and some mixed gas vented out

Preuse Test

A. Outer tube:
- Pressurize system with closed APL valve and patient end
- Bag inflates

B. Inner tube:

i. Set low flow on flowmeter
Occlude inner tube at patient end with finger
If flowmeter indicator falls, inner tube is intact

ii. ***Pethicks test***
- Activate O_2 flush and observe bag
- High flow at patient end creates negative pressure in outer tube
- Bag will collapse if inner tube is intact
- Bag will inflate if inner tube not intact

MAPLESON E

Design

- Length of tubing may be attached to T-piece to form a reservoir
- Does not have a bag
- Expiratory port may be enclosed in a chamber from which excess gas is evacuated

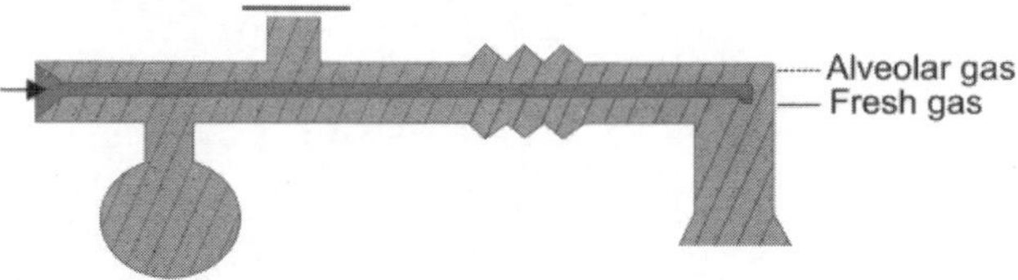

Fig. 54: Bains system during first controlled expiration.

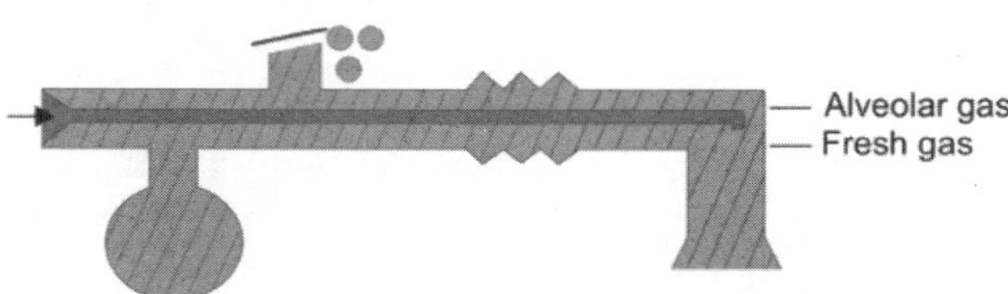

Fig. 55: Bains system during second controlled inspiration.

- E_TCO_2 placed between expiratory port and expiratory tubing
- Difficulty is scavenging: Rarely used
- Used for providing O_2 to spontaneously breathing patients

Technique of Use

- Expiratory limb open to atmosphere for spontaneous ventilation
- Controlled ventilation by occluding expiratory limb and allowing FG to inflate lung

Functional Analysis

- Similar to Mapleson D
- Rebreathing depends on:
    - FGF
    - Patients minute volume
    - Volume of exhalation limb
    - Respiratory pattern
    - Type of ventilation

Rebreathing

- If no expiratory limb is present, no rebreathing is possible
- If expiratory limb is present FGF kept at twice the MV to prevent rebreathing
- During controlled ventilation, no rebreathing as only FG inflates lung

Air Dilution

- Not possible during controlled ventilation
- During spontaneous ventilation, if no expiratory limb is present or volume of limb is less than patients tidal volume, air dilution prevented by providing FGF > PIFR (3–4 times MV)
- FGF of twice MV with reservoir of 1/3rd tidal volume prevents air dilution

Disadvantages

- Barotrauma during controlled ventilation
- Cannot assess lung compliance
- No APL valve to buffer pressure

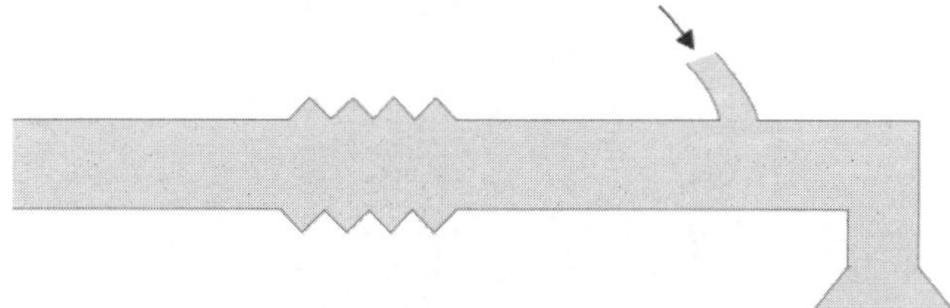

Fig. 56: Maplesons E system.

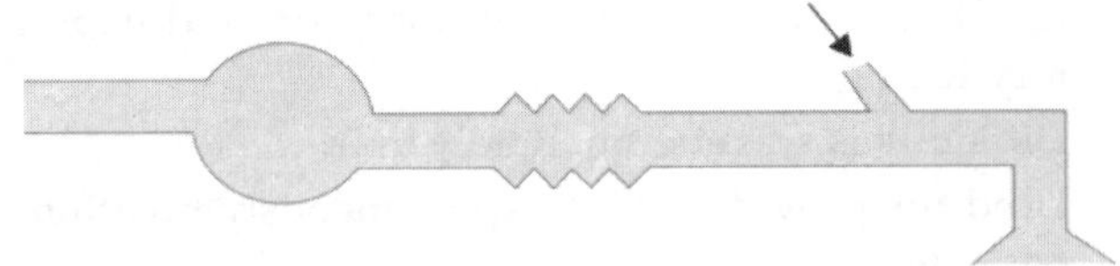

Fig. 57: Maplesons F system.

Modifications

- FGF inlet extending inside T-piece body towards patient connection
- Pressure limiting device addition

MAPLESON F

Description

- ***Jackson Rees modification of T-piece***
- Hole in tail/side of bag to vent gases
- Ventilator may be used instead of bag
- APL valve may be placed at patient end to protect against high pressure
- Scavenging by enclosing bag in chamber which is suctioned

Technique of Use

- Relief mechanism, i.e. the hole in tail, is left fully open during spontaneous ventilation
- Relief mechanism is occluded during controlled ventilation
- HME not preferred with spontaneous ventilation
- FGF to be more than twice the minute volume

Functional Analysis

- Similar to Mapleson D
- Decreased work of breathing than pediatric circle system
- If HME is added between patient and T-piece during inhalational induction, more of FGF will enter expiratory limb delaying induction as HME increase resistance

Hazards

- No APL valve present to buffer pressure
- If ventilators are used, disconnection at common gas outlet may not be detected by airway pressure monitor due to high resistance of FG tubing

SUGGESTED READING

1. Aitkenhead, A.K., Thompson, K., Rowbotham, D.J., Moppett, I. (2013). *Smith and Aitkenhead's Textbook of Anesthesia*. 6th ed. Philadelphia: Churchill Livingstone Elsevier.
2. Barash, P.G. (2017). *Clinical Anesthesia*. 8th ed. China: Wolters Kluwer.
3. Butterworth, J., Mackey, D., Wasnik, J. (2018). *Morgan and Mikhails Clinical Anesthesiology*. 6th ed. New York: McGraw-Hill Education/Medical.
4. Davey, A.J., Diba, A. (2012). *Wards Anesthetic equipment*. 6th ed. Philadelphia: Saunders Elsevier.
5. Davis, P.J., Cladis, F. (2017). *Smith's anesthesia for infants and children*. 9th ed. Philadelphia: Elsevier.
6. Dorsch, J.A., Dorsch, S.E. (2008). *Understanding Anesthesia Equipment*. 5th ed. Philadelphia: Wolters Kluwer/LWW.
7. Flood, P. (2015). *Stoeltings Pharmacology and Physiology in Anesthetic Practice*. 5th ed. China: Wolters Kluwer.
8. Gropper, M., Eriksson, L., Fleisher, L., Wiener-Kronish, J., Cohen, N., Leslie, K. (2020). *Millers Anesthesia*. 9th ed. Philadelphia: Elsevier Saunders.
9. Miller, R.D., Eriksson, L., Fleisher, L, Wiener-Kronish, J., Cohen, N., Young, W. (2014). *Millers Anesthesia* (8th edition ed.). New York: Elsevier Health.
10. Murray, M.J., et al. (2015). *Fausts Anesthesiology Review*. 4th ed. Philadelphia: Elsevier.

10 CHAPTER

Ophthalmic Anesthesia

INTRAOCULAR PRESSURE

Introduction

Intraocular pressure (IOP) is the pressure exerted by the intraocular contents on the layers of the eyeball.

Physiology

- Intraocular pressure is mainly generated by the presence of aqueous humor
- Aqueous humor is formed in the ciliary body, within the posterior chamber
- It is actively secreted by a sodium pump mechanism
- Ciliary body produces around 2.5 μL/minute of aqueous humor
- It drains over the lens and through the pupil, into the anterior chamber
- Here it bathes the inner corneal endothelium
- Thereafter, it drains via trabecular spaces of Fontana into Schlemm's canal
- Finally it is cleared by the episcleral venous system

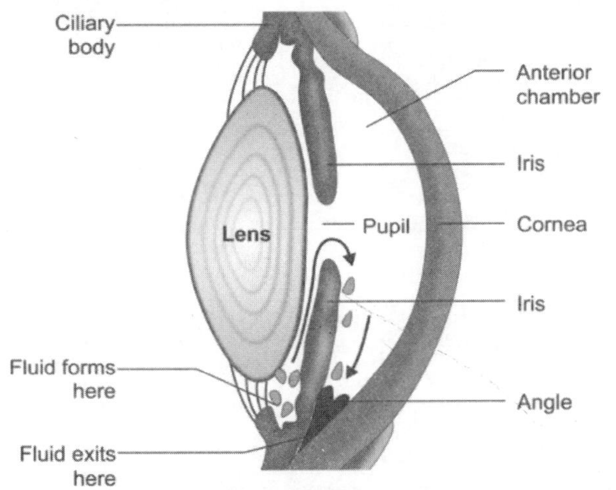

Fig. 1: Formation of acqueos humor.

Normal Values

- Normal volume of aqueous humor is 250 mL
- Normal IOP is between 10–20 mm Hg

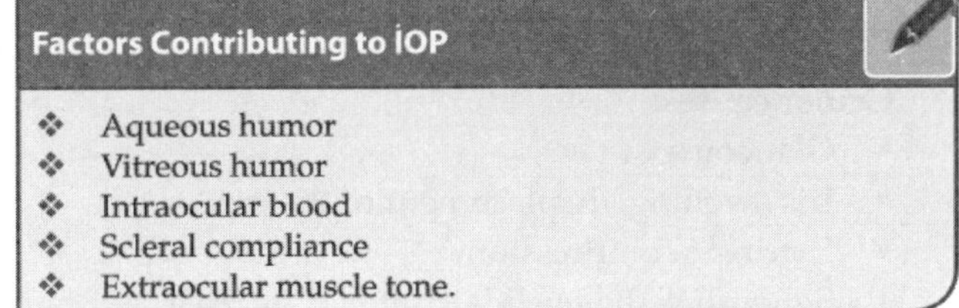

Factors Contributing to IOP

- Aqueous humor
- Vitreous humor
- Intraocular blood
- Scleral compliance
- Extraocular muscle tone.

Measurement

- IOP measurement is usually done with a tonometer
- IOP measurement is affected by corneal thickness and rigidity
- Types of tonometers:
  - Applanation tonometer:
    - Goldmann applanation tonometer
    - Perkins tonometer
    - Pneumatic tonometer
    - Non-contact (air puff) tonometer
  - Indentation tonometer: Schiotz tonometer.

Significance

- Intraocular perfusion pressure (IPP):
  - Intraocular perfusion pressure maintains the blood supply to retina and optic nerve
  - Intraocular perfusion pressure = MAP–IOP
  - Thus, increase in IOP causes a reduction in IPP
  - This impairs blood supply to retina and optic nerve
  - This eventually results in loss of optic nerve function, causing blindness
- Expulsion of intraocular contents:
  - This happens when the ocular integrity is breached, as in penetrating eye injuries
  - This results in the equalization of IOP and atmospheric pressures

- Thus, any increase in IOP thereafter will lead to leakage of intraocular contents
- This will lead to loss of intraocular contents and permanent visual loss

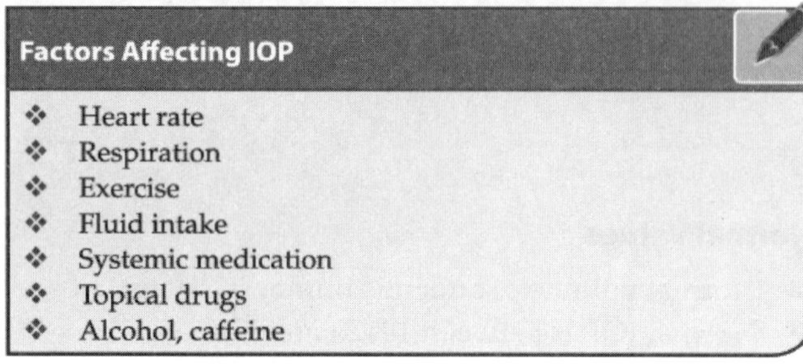

Factors Causing Raised IOP

- Ocular causes:
  - Glaucoma
  - Iris swelling, displacement of the iris
  - Extrinsic compression
  - Squeezing the eyelids shut can increase IOP up to 50 mm Hg
- Arterial pressure:
  - Arterial pressure regulates the choroidal blood volume (CBV)
  - Changes in choroidal blood volume causes changes in IOP
  - Rise in MAP may cause a detrimental increase in IOP, especially in open injuries
- External compression:
  - Facemasks and ETT tube ties may impede venous return if forcefully applied
  - This may cause a retrograde increase in the IOP
- Raised venous pressure: Can increase IOP to 30–40 mm Hg
  - Coughing, straining
  - Vomiting
- Hypoxia and hypercarbia:
  - This causes vasodilatation of blood vessels
  - This may in turn increase choroidal blood volume
  - Eventually IOP increases
- Drugs:
  - Succinylcholine: Raises IOP by 6–8 mm Hg
  - Ketamine
- Procedures:
  - Laryngoscopy and endotracheal intubation
  - Ryles tube insertion

Factors Causing Reduced IOP

- Reduced venous pressure:
  - Head up tilt reduces venous return
  - This reduced choroidal blood volume and thus the IOP
- Arterial pressure:
  - Lowering arterial blood pressure reduces IOP
  - Systolic BP less than 90 mm Hg is recommended to in open eye injuries
- Anesthetic drugs:
  - Propofol, thiopentone
  - Opioids do not affect IOP
  - Volatile anesthetics
  - Nondepolarizing muscle relaxants
  - Mannitol, acetazolamide

OCULOCARDIAC REFLEX

Introduction

- Oculocardiac reflex is a trigemino-vagal reflex response which results in bradycardia, junctional rhythm or asystole, secondary to traction on eye/extraocular muscle
- First described by ***Aschner and Dagnini*** in 1908

Prevalence

- 30–90% prevalence in ocular surgery
- More common in children and young adults undergoing strabismus surgery

Pathway

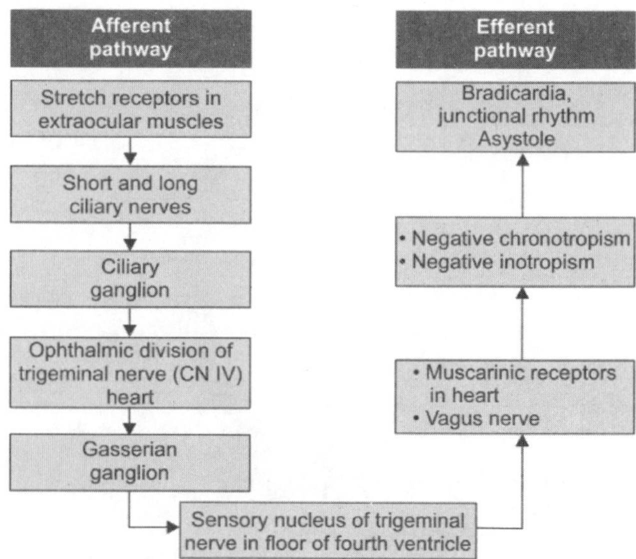

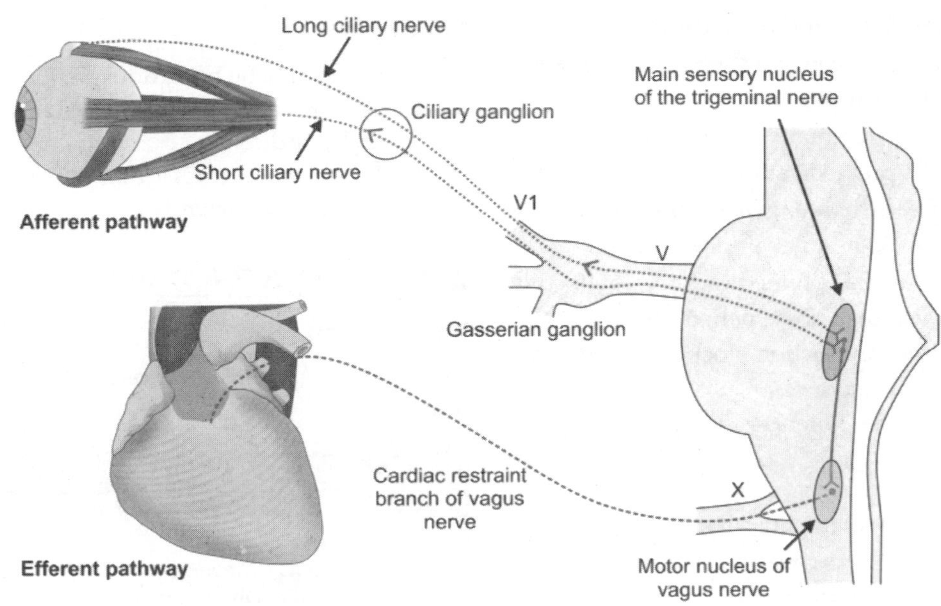

Fig. 2: Oculo cardiac reflex.

Triggers

- Pressure on eyeball
- Traction on extraocular muscles/conjunctiva/periosteum/any orbital structure
- Orbital trauma
- Orbital hematoma
- Manipulation of globe
- ***Forced duction test***
- Raised intraocular pressure
- During retrobulbar block

Aggravating Factors

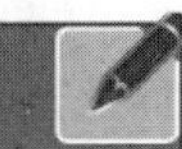

- Can occur in an empty orbit due to:
  - Extraocular muscle stimulation
  - Traction on orbital remnants following enucleation
- Hypoventilation, hypercarbia and acidosis augments the risk
- Light planes of anesthesia
- Anesthesia technique which includes fentanyl, remifentanyl and sufentanyl increases risk
- Reduced incidence of OCR with:
  - Sevoflurane, as compared with halothane
  - Pancuronium, as compared with other NDMR

Occurrence

- Common during
- Retrobulbar block:
  - Occurs due to retrobulbar hemorrhage
  - May occur up to 1.5 hours after surgery, as additional blood extravasates out
- Strabismus surgery (medical rectus is most sensitive to manipulation)
- Enucleation, cataract surgery
- Retinal detachment surgery (during giving retrobulbar block)
- Non-ocular surgery if pressure applied on eyeball
- Ocular trauma and pain
- Ocular manipulation

Manifestations

- *Most common in pediatric patients undergoing strabismus surgery*
- Triad of bradycardia, nausea and syncope
- Somnolence and nausea in awake patients
- *Sinus bradycardia most common manifestation*
- Nodal/junctional rhythm may manifest
- AV block, wandering pacemaker, asystole
- Ventricular trigeminy, multifocal VPCs, VT, VF

Prevention

- Retrobulbar block as it inhibits afferent links of reflex arc
- Gentle manipulation of ocular muscle

- Avoid hypoventilation and hypercarbia
- Communication between anesthetist and surgeon
- Deep planes of anesthesia
- Avoid fentanyl/remifentanyl/sufentanyl
- Intravenous (IV) premedication:
  - Done with IV atropine/glycopyrrolate
  - Given within 30 minutes prior to surgery
  - Intramuscular (IM) premedication is ineffective
  - Especially useful in those patients with:
    - History of conduction block
    - Vasovagal response
    - Currently on β-blocker therapy

Management

- Ask the surgeon to stop manipulation of muscle
- Ensure adequate oxygenation, ventilation and adequate depth of anesthesia
- Most often, heart rate and rhythm return to baseline within 20 seconds if these are done
- Deepen anesthetic plane and maintain normocarbia
- IV atropine:
  - 7 μg/kg increments is used
  - Given if conduction disturbance persists
  - To be given only once surgeon stops manipulation of extraocular muscles (EOM)
  - If it is given when OCR is still active, more dangerous arrhythmias may occur
- IV glycopyrrolate:
  - 10 μg/kg increments can also be used
  - It causes less tachycardia
  - Takes 3-4 minutes to act
- In recalcitrant episodes, infilterate rectus muscle with local anesthetics
- Repeated stimulation of EOM causes fatigue of the reflex arc at level of cardio-inhibitory center
- Cardiopulmonary resuscitation, if asystole, as it helps to circulate atropine

Postoperative Management

- Reflex may occur up to 1½ hours after uncomplicated retrobulbar block
- It may occur late due to:
  - Expanding retrobulbar hemorrhage
  - Persistent bleeding causing raised IOP
- Careful monitoring is therefore warranted
- Maintain adequate oxygenation and ventilation

Controversy

- Atropine may be hazardous as:
  - Elderly patients with CAD will not tolerate tachycardia
  - It may cause VPCs, LBBB, VT and VF if halothane is used concurrently

ANESTHESIA FOR STRABISMUS SURGERY

Introduction

Deviation of visual axis of one eye with respect to the other.

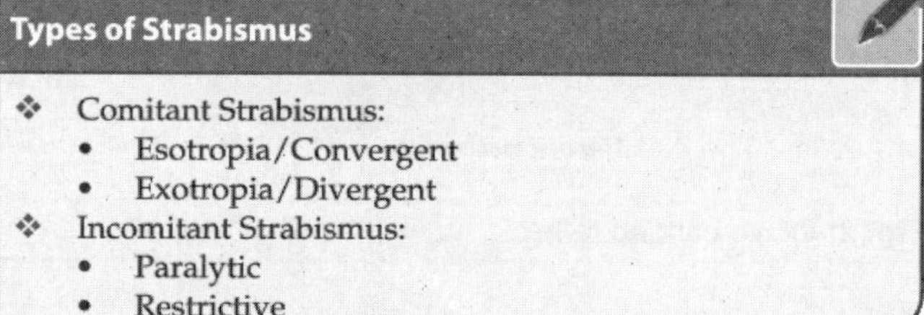

Types of Strabismus

- Comitant Strabismus:
  - Esotropia/Convergent
  - Exotropia/Divergent
- Incomitant Strabismus:
  - Paralytic
  - Restrictive

Comitant Strabismus

- Abnormal relation of eyes retained in all directions of gaze
- Attributed to abnormal afferent pathways/central mechanism
- Efferent pathways are usually normal
- Esotropia common in hypermetropes
- Exotropia common in myopes

Incomitant Strabismus

- Attributed to abnormal efferent pathways
- Afferent pathway and central pathways are, however, normal
- Paralytic incomitant strabismus occurs due to CN III trauma
- Restrictive incomitant strabismus occurs due to:
  - Muscular fibrosis
  - Local space occupying lesions of orbit

Timing of Surgery

- Visual maturation occurs by 5 years of age
- Thus strabismus has to be corrected by 4–5 years
- It is preferably done at 18 months of age
- In older children, it is done mostly for cosmesis

Anesthetic Considerations

- Remote airway
- Forced duction test
- Profound analgesia with minimal muscle relaxation
- Risk of malignant hyperthermia
- Risk of PONV—*Oculogastric* reflex
- *Oculocardiac* reflex
- Quiet emergence without coughing

Preoperative Assessment

- Assess for presence of:
  - URTI
  - Other assciated myopathies
- History of drug intake/eye drops, especially echothiophate as:
  - Echothiophate reduces plasma cholinesterase levels
  - This causes increased duration of action of succinylcholine
- Avoid excess preoperative sedation:
  - IV glycopyrrolate 10 µg/kg
  - PO midazolam 0.5 mg/kg half hour before surgery
  - Alternatively, IV midazolam can be given in the preoperative holding area

Monitors

- Pulse oximetry
- End tidal carbon dioxide
- ECG
- NIBP
- Temperature
- Neuromuscular monitoring

Induction

- Inhalational induction with halothane/sevoflurane in the absence of IV access
- IV induction with thiopentone 3–4 mg/kg + atracurium 0.5 mg/kg
- IV fentanyl 2 µg/kg can be used for analgesia
- Ketamine avoided due to nystagmus and blepharospasm
- IV droperidol 75 µg/kg 15 min before manipulation of EOM
- IV 0.15 mg/kg metaclopramide after induction to reduce postoperative nausea and vomiting (PONV)
- Dexamethasone or ondansetron 0.15 mg/kg IV can also be used
- Minimize subsequent opioid use

Maintenance

- O_2 + N_2O + sevoflurane can be used for maintenance of anesthesia
- Controlled ventilation with muscular paralysis preferred
- Atracurium boluses can be used to maintain paralysis
- If oculocardiac reflex develops during surgery:
  - Stop surgical stimulus immediately
  - Increase anesthetic depth
  - Assess ventilation
  - IV atropine if persistent bradycardia
- Warming blankets can be used to maintain the temperature of the patient

Extubation

- Smooth emergence mandatory
- IV neostigmine 0.05–0.06 mg/kg with glycopyrollate 0.01 mg/kg used for reversal
- Extubation in deep planes preferred to avoid coughing
- Extubation usually done in lateral position once spontaneous respiration is established

Postoperative Management

- Correct fluid deficits
- Delay ingestion of fluids to reduce chances of PONV
- Thin, clear juice can be attempted once fully awake
- Pain:
  - IV paracetamol 30 mg/kg PR at induction
  - IV ketorolac 0.75 mg/kg IV
- Do not arouse the patient forcefully

LMA FOR STRABISMUS SURGERY

Advantages

- Avoids the need for muscle relaxants
- Lighter planes can be used for tube tolerance
- Avoids hemodynamic changes at intubation and extubation
- Reduced straining/coughing on extubation compared with ETT
- Armoured laryngeal mask airway (LMA) is usually preferred

Disadvantages

- Increases risk of aspiration
- LMA displacement can occur intraoperatively due to proximity to surgical field
- Increased risk of oculocardiac reflex due to:
  - Maintenance in lighter planes
  - Spontaneously breathing patient

Forced Duction Test

- Done in incomitant strabismus
- Done to differentiate between paretic muscle and restrictive force preventing ocular motion
- Procedure:
  - Surgeon grasps sclera near corneal limbus
  - Moves eye in each field of gaze
  - Assesses tissue and elastic properties
  - This gives clues about site of mechanical restriction of EOM
- Test is valuable for :
  - Detection of paralysis of EOM
  - Patients with previous orbital trauma
  - History of previous strabismus surgery
- Anesthetic significance :
  - Test cannot be performed for 20 minutes after succinylcholine dose as:
    - Skeletal muscle paralysis following the dose lasts only less than 5 minutes
    - But force required to rotate globe remains high for 15–20 minutes
  - Can be performed immediately after intubation with nondepolarising agents
  - Increased chances of oculocardiac reflex during test
  - Can be done under deep inhalational anesthesia

ANESTHESIA FOR EYE INJURY

Introduction

Eye injuries demand urgent therapy, within the first few hours after presentation.

Types of Ocular Emergencies

- True emergencies:
  - Therapy should be started within minutes to first hours after presentation
  - Examples:
    - Chemical burns
    - Central retinal artery occlusion
- Urgent situations:
  - Therapy to be started in one- several hours
  - Examples:
    - Open-globe injuries
    - Corneal foreign body
    - Lid laceration
    - Endophthalmitis
    - Acute narrow angle glaucoma
    - Acute retinal detachment
  - Factors determining degree of urgency in eye injuries include:
    - Size of laceration
    - Risk of loss of ocular contents
    - Contamination of the wound
    - Risk of endophthalmitis and infection
- Semiurgent situations:
  - Therapy to be started within days
  - Examples:
    - Congenital cataract
    - Ocular tumors
    - Blowout fractures of the orbit
    - Chronic retinal detachment

Types of Eye Injuries

- Extraocular
- Ocular:
  - Blunt injuries
  - Penetrating injuries (open eye)
- Intraorbital
- Orbital fracture

Choice of Anesthetic Technique

- General anesthesia preferred for most cases
- Most patients are uncooperative and frightened to attempt local anesthesia
- Indications for general anesthesia include:
  - Uncooperative patients
  - Intoxicated patients
  - Children
- Disadvantages of local anesthesia:
  - Spread of LA is poor in those with infections
  - Peri or retrobulbar technique increases IOP and lead to vitreous loss
  - Ocular compression following administration of block is not possible

Anesthetic Requirements

- Akinesia
- Profound analgesia
- Minimal bleeding
- Avoidance of oculocardiac reflex
- Control of IOP
- Awareness of drug interactions
- Emergence without coughing, straining or vomiting

Anesthetic Considerations

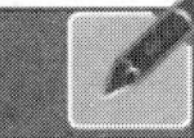

- Strategies to prevent increases in IOP:
  - Avoid direct pressure on the globe:
    - No retrobulbar or peribulbar injections
    - Careful facemask technique
  - Avoid increases in central venous pressure:
    - Avoid head down position
    - Prevent coughing during induction and intubation
    - Ensure adequate relaxation prior to laryngoscopy
    - Ensure deep anesthetic planes during the procedure
    - Extubate under deep plane of anesthesia
- Strategies to prevent aspiration pneumonia:
  - Premedication:
    - H_2 receptor antagonists
    - Non-particulate antacids
    - Metaclopramide
  - Rapid sequence induction:
    - Rapid induction agent
    - Cricoid pressure
    - Rapid acting muscle relaxant
    - Avoidance of positive pressure ventilation
    - Intubation as soon as possible

Preoperative Evaluation and Premedication

- Evaluate associated injuries, if polytrauma
- *Size of the perforation:* Small puncture have higher resistance to changes in IOP
- *Pulmonary status:* Decreased functional residual capacity become rapidly hypoxic
- NPO status:
  - Risk of pulmonary aspiration with inadequate NPO status
  - General NPO guidelines if visual prognosis is bad or minor degrees of injury:
    - 6 hours for solids
    - 2 hours for clear fluids
- Premedication:
  - IV metaclopramide 0.15 mg/kg to hasten gastric emptying
  - IV ranitidine 50 mg

Induction

- Adequate preoxygenation for 3–4 minutes
- Care to avoid exerting pressure on eyes with face mask during preoxygenation
- Rapid sequence induction preferred, if full-stomach status
- Propofol and fentanyl are preferred for induction
- High dose rocuronium with cricoid pressure preferred to succinylcholine
- Intubation after complete relaxation and deep planes to avoid coughing and bucking
- Care to be taken to prevent rise in IOP during laryngoscopy
- Methods used to prevent rise in IOP during laryngoscopy:
  - IV lidocaine 1.5 mg/kg 90 seconds prior to intubation
  - IV remifentanil 0.7 μg/kg 3–5 minutes prior to induction
  - Mild head up tilt at laryngoscopy helps to reduce IOP
- If ETT tube tie is used:
  - Ensure looseness around the neck to allow venous drainage
  - Tight ties limit venous drainage and cause retrograde rise in IOP

Monitors

- Pulse oximetry
- ECG
- End tidal CO_2
- NIBP
- Neuromuscular monitoring

Maintenance

- Balanced anesthesia technique preferred
- O_2 + air + sevoflurane or isoflurane can be used
- All volatile agents reduce IOP and can be used
- Maintain deep anesthetic planes to avoid movement of the patient
- Limit narcotic dose to minimize chances of PONV
- Paralysis maintained with vecuronium or atracurium based on the duration of surgery

Ventilation

- Slight head up tilt during ventilation preferred as it reduces IOP

❖ Mild hypocarbia (32–35 mm Hg) preferred as it reduces IOP

Hemodynamics

❖ Target systolic BP below 90 mm Hg to reduce IOP
❖ Avoid tachycardia as this increases IOP
❖ Judicious fluid loading to avoid acute increases in venous pressure
❖ Slight head up tilt maintained to control IOP

Extubation

❖ Extubation in deep planes for those who are at low risk of aspiration
❖ Patient should be fully reversed and breathing spontaneously
❖ Avoid bucking at extubation using:
  • IV lidocaine 1.5 mg/kg 90 seconds prior to extubation
  • IV remifentanyl 0.5 µg/kg 5 minutes prior to awakening
❖ Extubation done in lateral position to avoid coughing and straining

Postoperative

Management

❖ PONV can cause detrimental rise in IOP
❖ Multimodal approach used to prevent PONV
❖ Strategies to prevent PONV include:
  • Antiemetic agents:
    – Ondansetron
    – Metaclopramide
  • Anticholinergic agents
  • Dexamethasone

Monitors

❖ Pulse oximetry
❖ ECG
❖ NIBP.

Analgesia

❖ Multimodal analgesia used
❖ Satisfactory analgesia important as crying increases IOP and postoperative hemorrhage
❖ Subtenon block at the end of surgery is a useful technique
❖ Adequate analgesia is achieved most often using paracetamol and NSAIDs

RETROBULBAR BLOCK

Introduction

It is a type of regional anesthetic block, where LA is injected into the retrobulbar space.

Relevant Anatomy

❖ Retrobulbar space lies inside the extraocular cone, behind the globe
❖ Muscle cone:
  • Extraocular muscle form a cone around the globe
  • The base of this cone is formed by insertions of the muscles into the globe
  • Apex of the cone is formed by the optic foramen
❖ Motor innervation:
  • CN VI (abducens) innervates the lateral rectus muscle
  • CN IV (trochlear) innervates the superior oblique muscle
  • CN III (oculomotor) innervates all other extraocular muscles
  • CN III and VI pass within the cone to innervate their muscles
  • CN IV travels outside the muscle cone to innervate the superior oblique muscle
  • CN IV is affected in retrobulbar block by diffusion of the LA
❖ Sensory innervation:
  • Afferent fibers from the globe travel via long and short posterior ciliary nerves
  • These fibers pass through the intraconal ciliary ganglion
  • The fibers then join the nasociliary nerve, a branch of the trigeminal nerve

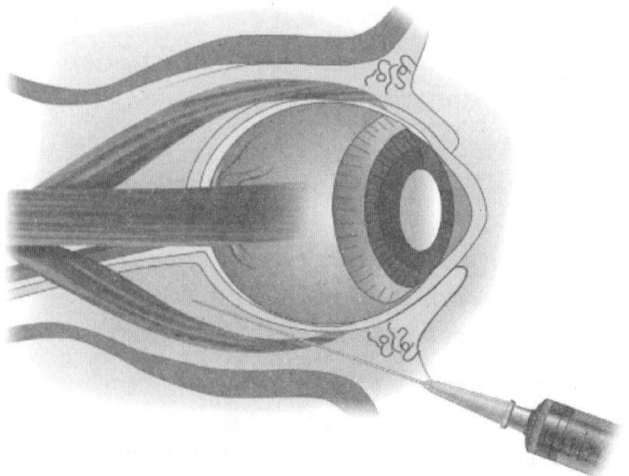

Fig. 3: Retrobulbar block.

Indications

- Intraocular procedures:
  - Cataract surgery
  - Vitrectomy
  - Tube shunt placement
- Cyclodestructive procedures
- Strabismus surgery
- Enucleation and evisceration

Contraindications

- Absolute contraindications:
  - Hypersensitivity to local anesthetics
  - Orbital infections
- Relative contraindications:
  - Increased axial length of the globe more than 25 mm length
  - Bleeding diathesis
  - Thyroid associated orbitopathy
  - Space occupying lesions of the orbit
  - Previous scleral buckling

Preparation

- Usually done with a retrobulbar needle, also called the ***Atkinson needle***
- The needle is 23–25 gauge and 1.5 inches (38 mm) long
- IV sedation:
  - Used to provide analgesia and amnesia
  - Improves patient cooperation
  - Midazolam and propofol are useful
- Ocular surface can be anesthetized with 1% tetracaine or other LA
- Position:
  - Patient placed in supine position
  - Patient should be staring straight at the ceiling
  - Globe is therefore fixed in primary gaze

Choice of Anesthetic Agents

- Lidocaine:
  - 2% lidocaine alone is adequate for short cases
  - 2% lidocaine used in a 1:1 mixture with 0.75% bupivacaine for longer cases
- Additives:
  - Epinephrine:
    - Used in 1: 200,000 dilution
    - Increases duration of action of lidocaine by causing local vasoconstriction
    - Effect is limited with bupivacaine use
    - Risk of retinal artery vasoconstriction
  - Sodium bicarbonate:
    - Neutralizes the pH of local anesthetics
    - Hastens the onset of action of bupivacaine
  - Hyaluronidase:
    - Used as 7.5 U/mL dilution
    - Facilitates spread of the anesthetic agent through muscle cone

Technique

- Lower eyelid is prepared with topical isopropyl alcohol
- Globe is placed in primary gaze
- Inferior orbital rim is palpated through the lower eyelid
- While palpating, the globe is elevated with the same finger with mild pressure
- Needle is oriented with the bevel facing up toward the globe
- Point of insertion of the needle is just superior to lateral third of the inferior orbital rim
- Temporal limbus is used as a guide to the point of entry
- Needle is advanced posteriorly, parallel to the orbital floor
- When 50% of the needle has passed, angle of insertion changed to medial and superior
- This allows the needle to enter the intraconal space
- No resistance or rotation of the globe should occur during the needle advancement
- This would suggest engagement of the sclera by the needle tip
- Syringe is aspirated to ensure no return of blood
- 3–4 mL of local anesthetic is slowly injected, observing proptosis of the globe
- Ocular compression is performed intermittently for 15 seconds till 2 minutes
- Degree of anesthesia and akinesia is assessed after 5 minutes

Complications

- Corneal abrasion
- Chemosis
- Retrobulbar hemorrhage—*most common* complication
- Ocular perforation: Risk is increased with myopic eyes

- Central retinal artery occlusion
- Optic nerve injury
- Subarachnoid or intradural injection
- Seizures, bradycardia
- Respiratory depression

Advantages

- Provides akinesia of EOM by blocking CN II, III and VI
- Provides sensory anesthesia of cornea, uvea and conjunctiva by blocking ciliary nerve
- Low volume injected
- Rapid onset
- Minimum anterior hemorrhage

Disadvantages

- Skill required
- Injection of LA is very close to the key structures in the apex
- Risk of major complications.

Differences from Peribulbar Block

- Uses lesser volume of local anesthetic
- Does not anesthetize CN VII (facial nerve)
- This allows the patient to close his eye with orbicularis oculi (CN VII)
- But patient will not be able to open his eye with levator superioris (CN III)

PERIBULBAR BLOCK

Introduction

Ocular anesthetic technique where LA is injected into the extraconal compartment of eye.

Relevant Anatomy

- Peribulbar space lies around the extraocular cone
- Thus, LA is deposited within the orbit, but does not enter the muscle cone
- Thus, this technique offers some safety, compared to retrobulbar block
- Muscle cone:
  - Extraocular muscle form a cone around the globe
  - The base of this cone is formed by insertions of the muscles into the globe
  - Apex of the cone is formed by the optic foramen
- Motor innervation:
  - CN VI (abducens) innervates the lateral rectus muscle
  - CN IV (trochlear) innervates the superior oblique muscle
  - CN III (oculomotor) innervates all other extraocular muscles
  - CN III and VI pass within the cone to innervate their muscles
  - CN IV travels outside the muscle cone to innervate the superior oblique muscle
- Sensory innervation:
  - Afferent fibers from the globe travel via long and short posterior ciliary nerves
  - These fibers pass through the intraconal ciliary ganglion
  - The fibers then join the nasociliary nerve, a branch of the trigeminal nerve

Indications

- Intraocular procedures:
  - Cataract surgery
  - Vitrectomy
  - Tube shunt placement
- Cyclodestructive procedures
- Strabismus surgery
- Enucleation and evisceration.

Contraindications

- Absolute contraindications:
  - Hypersensitivity to local anesthetics
  - Orbital infections
- Relative contraindications:
  - Increased axial length of the globe more than 25 mm length

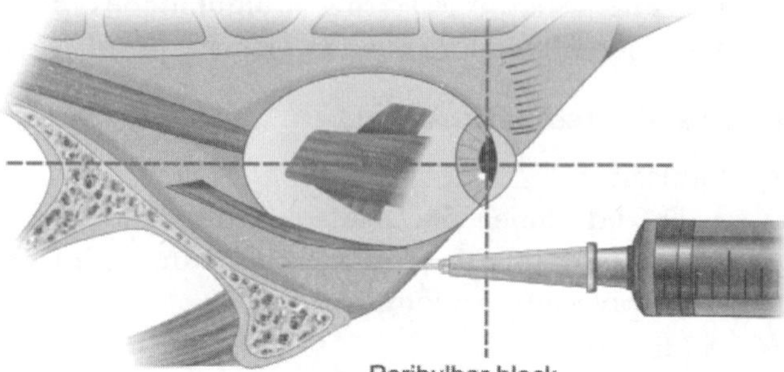

Fig. 4: Peribulbar block.

- Bleeding diathesis
- Thyroid associated orbitopathy
- Space occupying lesions of the orbit
- Previous scleral buckling

Preparation

- 0.75 inch 24–26 G needle is used for the block
- IV sedation:
  - Used to provide analgesia and amnesia
  - Improves patient cooperation
  - Midazolam and propofol are useful
- Ocular surface can be anesthetized with 1% tetracaine or other LA
- Position:
  - Patient placed in supine position
  - Patient should be staring straight at the ceiling
  - Globe is therefore fixed in primary gaze
- Mixture of 5 mL 0.5% bupivacaine along with 5 mL 2% lignocaine can be used

Technique

- Injections can be made through the conjunctival reflection or percutaneously
- 2 injections can be used in this block (superior and inferior)
- Inferior injection:
  - Point of insertion is at junction of outer 1/3rd and inner 2/3rd of lower orbital rim
  - Needle is directed vertically backwards, parallel to the floor of the orbit
  - If contact is made with the bone, needle is redirected slightly upwards
  - Syringe is aspirated and checked for the presence of blood
  - LA is injected after negative aspiration test
- Superior injection:
  - Point of insertion is just above the medial canthus
  - Needle is inserted and aimed tangentially away from the globe
  - Superior injection may be avoided till the time the inferior injection takes effect
  - If good akinesia occurs with the inferior injection, it maybe avoided

Advantages

- Reasonable akinesia
- Reliable anesthesia
- Less painful
- Need for facial block avoided
- Insignificant rise in IOP
- Injection away from key structures of the apex
- Minimum anterior hemorrhage
- Sight or life-threatening complications are rare

Disadvantages

- Skill required
- Akinesia of EOM may be less complete
- Greater volume of LA required
- More time required to achieve satisfactory block
- Chemosis may occur due to anterior spread of higher volume LA
- Multiple injections required as LA is injected outside the cone
- Significant rise in IOP and need for oculocompression

Complications

- Venous orbital hemorrhage
- Anterior orbital hemorrhage
- Spread of LA subcutaneously, to the opposite eye
- Periorbital echhymoses
- Ophthalmoplegia: Direct damage to the EOM or its nerve
- Globe perforation

SUGGESTED READING

1. Batterbury, M., Bowling, B., Murphy, C. (2004). *Ophthalmology*. 3rd ed. St. Louis: Mosby.
2. Butterworth, J., Mackey, D., and Wasnick, J. (2013). *Morgan and Mikhails Clinical Anesthesiology*. 6th ed. New York: McGraw Hill Education.
3. Hamilton RC. (1995). Techniques of orbital regional anesthesia. *British Journal of Anesthesia*, 75(1), 88–92.
4. Miller, R.D., Eriksson, L., Fleisher, L, Wiener-Kronish, J., Cohen, N., Young, W. (2018). *Millers Anesthesia*. 8th edition. Amsterdam: Elsevier Health.
5. Patil, B.B., Dowd, T.C. Ocular physiology. In: CM Kumar, C Dodds, GL Fanning, eds. 2002. *Ophthalmic Anaesthesia*. Lisse, Netherlands: Swets and Zeitlinger.
6. Shields, B. (1998). *Textbook of glaucoma*. 4th ed. Baltimore: Williams and Wilkins.
7. Stanek, G. (1908). *Wiener Klinische Wochenschrift*. New York: Springer Nature.
8. Wong, D.H. (2005). Regional anesthesia for intraocular surgery. *Continuing Education in Anesthesia, Critical Care and Pain*, 40(7), 93–7.

11 CHAPTER

Obstetric Anesthesia

UTEROPLACENTAL CIRCULATION

Introduction

- Placenta is the union of maternal and fetal tissues for purpose of:
  - Physiological exchange of nutrients
  - Respiration
  - Exchange of fetal metabolic waste
- The placenta is described as:
  - Discoid (in shape)
  - Hemo-choroidal (due to direct contact of chorion with maternal blood)
  - Deciduate (due to shedding of maternal tissue at parturition)

Placental Anatomy

- Placenta at term:
  - Weighs approximately 500 grams
  - Occupies 30% of uterine wall
- Grossly, it has 2 surfaces
  - Fetal surface:
    - Covered by smooth amnion
    - Umbilical cord is attached to the center
    - At term, about four-fifths of the placenta is from fetal origin
  - Maternal surface:
    - Rough and spongy
    - Maternal surface is dull red due to maternal blood
    - It is made up of 15–20 cotyledons, separated by fissures.
- Components of the placenta:
  - Placenta is composed of 2 plates:
    - Chorionic plate:
      - Lies towards the fetal side
      - Lined by amniotic membrane
      - Umbilical cord is attached to this plate
      - Consists of primary, secondary and tertiary villi
      - These villi are the functional unit of the placenta
      - Thus, they are responsible for feto-placental exchange
    - Basal plate:
      - Lies towards the maternal side
      - Perforated by the spiral branches of the uterine blood vessels
      - Blood from these spiral vessels enters the intervillous space
  - Intervillous space:
    - Lies in between the plates
    - This space is filled with maternal blood

Placental Circulation

- Consists of 2 independent circulation systems:
  - Uteroplacental circulation (maternal circulation)
  - Fetoplacental circulation
- Uteroplacental circulation (UPC):
  - Responsible for circulation of maternal blood through the intervillous space
  - Blood supply to the intervillous space is derived from 120–200 spiral arteries
  - These arteries funnel out as they pierce the intervillous space
  - This results in the formation of utero-placental arteries
  - Uteroplacental arteries supply blood to the IVS at low pressure (10–15 mm Hg)
  - Mature placenta has approximately 500 mL of blood:
    - 150 mL is present in the intervillous space
    - 350 mL is present in the system of villi
  - Blood in the intervillous space is completely replaced 3–5 times per minute

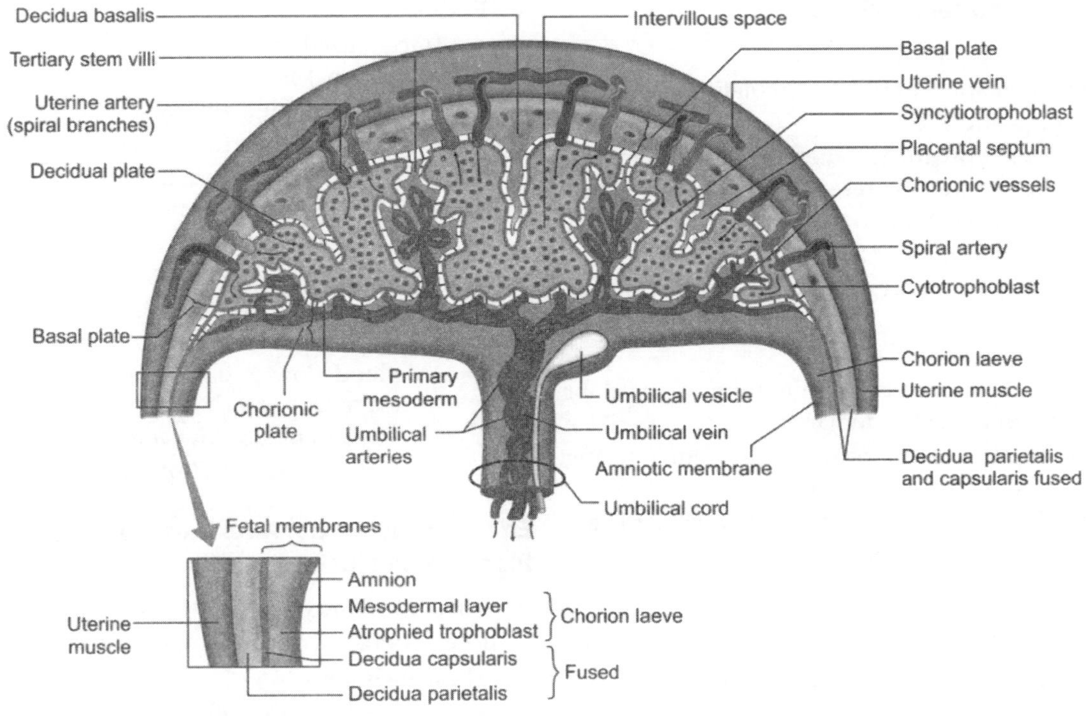

Fig. 1: Structure of the placenta.

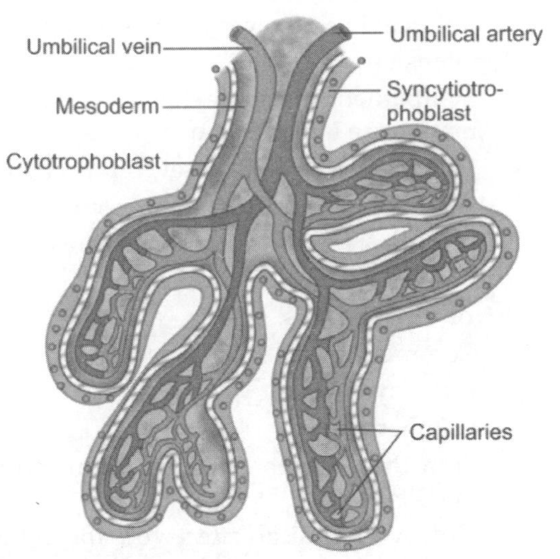

Fig. 2: Placental microanatomy.

- Fetoplacental circulation (FPC):
  - The 2 umbilical arteries carry impure blood from the fetus
  - They enter into the chorionic plate and break up into smaller branches
  - Each branch enters the chorionic villi dividing into smaller vessels
  - Blood flows into the venous network through terminal capillary networks
  - Ultimately, the umbilical vein carries oxygenated blood back to the fetus
- Maternal and fetal circulations therefore flow side-by-side in opposite directions
- This counter-current flow facilitates exchange of nutrients between the 2 circulations

Determinants of Uterine Blood Flow

- The uterine blood flow is dependent on:
  - Uterine perfusion pressure
  - Uterine venous pressure
- Uterine perfusion pressure is determined by:
  - Uterine arterial pressure
  - Uterine venous pressure
- Thus,

$$\text{Uterine blood flow} = \frac{(\text{Uterine arterial pressure}) - (\text{Uterine venous pressure})}{\text{Uterine vascular resistance}}$$

Uteroplacental Buffer Mechanisms

- Uterine autoregulation:
  - Non-pregnant uterine circulation exhibits autoregulation
  - However, pregnant uterine circulation is complicated due to presence of both:
    - Placental circulation
    - Non-placental circulations
  - Thus, uterine autoregulation during pregnancy may be suboptimal
- Luxury perfusion:
  - Uterine flow exceeds the minimum required for maintaining fetal O_2 demand
  - This buffer system protects the fetus during transient fluctuations in UPC
  - Also, the human placenta is a relatively inefficient oxygen exchanger normally
  - Thus, oxygen transfer is less affected by alterations in placental perfusion

Causes of Diminished Uterine Blood Flow

- Decreased perfusion pressure:
  - Decreased uterine arterial pressure:
    - Supine position
    - Hemorrhage
    - Hypovolemia
    - Drug-induced hypotension
    - Sympathetic blockade
  - Increased uterine venous pressure:
    - Vena caval compression
    - Uterine contractions
    - Seizures
    - Valsalva maneuver
- Increased uterine vascular resistance:
  - Endogenous vasoconstrictors:
    - Catecholamines
    - Vasopressin
  - Exogenous catecholamines:
    - Epinephrine
    - Phenylephrine> ephedrine

Methods of Measurement of Uteroplacental Flow

- Using Ficks principle:
  - Substances used include nitrous oxide and 4-amino-antipyrine
  - Not commonly used as it is error prone
- Radioactive tracers:
  - Tracers used include:
    - Xenon-133
    - Radiolabelled albumin
  - Uteroplacental perfusion is indicated by:
    - Decrease in radioactivity
    - Directly using scintigraphy
- Doppler ultrasonography:
  - Most commonly used technique
  - Uterine artery is identified using color Doppler
  - Blood flow is quantified using continuous-wave Doppler derived variables:
    - Mean blood flow velocity
    - Vessel cross sectional area

Effects of Neuraxial Anesthesia on Placental Perfusion

- Effect of neuraxial (NA) block on UPP depends on interactions between many factors
- These include:
  - Analgesia: Pain relief due to NA blockade increases uterine perfusion due to:
    - Reduced circulating catecholamines
    - Preventing hyperventilation
    - Reducing uterine vascular resistance
  - Hypotension:
    - Sympathetic blockade due to NA anesthesia may cause hypotension
    - This decreases UPP by several mechanisms:
      - Reduction in perfusion pressure
      - Reflex release of vasoconstrictors
      - Steal of blood to lower limbs
  - Use of vasopressors:
    - Commonly used vasopressors are:
      - Phenylephrine
      - Ephedrine
    - Both these drugs cause transient reduction in UPP
    - However, clinical effects on the fetus are minimal as suggested by:
      - Fetal blood pH
      - Base excess
  - Local anesthetic agents:
    - Local anesthetics do not produce clinically relevant reductions in UPP
    - However, UPP may be reduced due to inadvertent systemic injection

- Opioids:
  - Intrathecal opioids may result in increased uterine tone and reduced UPP
  - This causes fetal bradycardia commonly seen with intrathecal opioids
- Causes of increased uterine blood flow under neuraxial blockade:
  - Pain relief
  - Decreased sympathetic activity
  - Decreased maternal hyperventilation
- Causes of decreased uterine blood flow under neuraxial blockade:
  - Hypotension
  - Local anesthetic systemic toxicity
  - Systemically absorbed local anesthetic (minimal effect)

Effects of General Anesthesia on Placental Perfusion

- Induction agents:
  - Commonly used induction agents have no direct effects on UPP
  - However, indirect mechanisms altering UPP at induction include:
    - Systemic vasodilatation
    - Intubation response
- Inhalational agents:
  - Effects of inhalational agents on UPP depends upon the dose of administration
  - At MAC values 0.5–1.5, no clinically relevant change in UPP is produced
  - However, at MAC values >2, changes in UPP may be determined by:
    - Reduction in systemic BP causing reduced perfusion
    - Uterine relaxation improving UPP
- Ventilation:
  - Marked hypoxemia and hypoventilation reduce UPP by sympathetic activation
  - Effect of hyperventilation on UPP is controversial
  - Thus, maintenance of eucapnia or mild hypocapnia is recommended
- Anesthetic drugs which do not produce clinically relevant changes include:
  - Opioids
  - NMBAs

Methods of Optimizing Uteroplacental Perfusion

- Optimize maternal hemodynamics:
  - In the presence of maternal hypertension:
    - Decrease SVR:
      - Hydralazine
      - Alpha-methyl-dopa
    - Supplemental analgesia with opioids
    - Diuretics in the presence of hypervolemia
    - β-blockade with labetolol in the presence of hyperdynamic circulation
  - In the presence of maternal hypotension:
    - Restore intravascular volume status with crystalloids/colloids/blood
    - Left uterine displacement
    - Abdominal decompression if laparoscopic insufflation >16 mm Hg
    - Vasopressors if neuraxial block induced sympathectomy
- Low cardiac output syndrome:
  - Inotropes
  - Vasopressors
- Improve oxygenation:
  - Supplemental oxygen
  - Propped up positioning
  - Endotracheal intubation and mechanical ventilation
- Alteration of uterine tone:
  - Discontinuation of uterotonic agents:
    - Oxytocin
    - Prostaglandins
  - Initiation of tocolytic agents:
    - Beta-adrenergic agonists (terbutaline 0.25 mg IV)
    - Nitroglycerine

PLACENTAL TRANSFER OF DRUGS

Introduction

- Medications administered to pregnant women may cross the placenta
- This may have harmful effects on the fetus
- Placental permeability and pharmacokinetics determines fetal exposure to maternal drugs

Mechanisms of Transfer

I. *Simple Diffusion*

- Most drugs cross the placenta by simple diffusion
- Transfer of drugs occurs along concentration gradient
- Simple diffusion requires no carrier molecule/energy
- Transfer occurs through synctitiotrophoblast layer or through water channels

- Diffusion is governed by ***Ficks principle***
- Examples of drugs transferred by simple diffusion:
  - Midazolam
  - Paracetamol
- Formula for rate of diffusion:

  Rate of diffusion $Q/t = \frac{KA\,(C_m - C_f)}{D}$

  Q/t = rate of diffusion

  K = diffusion coefficient

  A = surface area of membrane available for exchange

  C_m-C_f = concentration gradient between maternal and fetal circulation

  D = thickness of membrane

II. *Facilitated Diffusion*

- It is a form of passive transport dependant on trans-membrane proteins
- It occurs *along* concentration gradient and requires a carrier molecule
- Proteins assist transport of polar molecules unable to passively cross a membrane
- The carrier molecules do not require energy but require a concentration gradient
- Examples of drugs transferred through facilitated diffusion:
  - Cephalosporins
  - Glucocorticoids

III. *Active Transport*

- Similar to facilitated diffusion as it requires a carrier molecule
- However, transport occurs *against* concentration gradient
- Requires carrier molecules and energy for transport across the membrane
- Examples of drugs transferred by active transport:
  - Norepinephrine
  - Dopamine

IV. *Pinocytosis*

- Molecules are engulfed by invagination of placental membrane
- These molecules are then transferred across the membrane to the opposite side
- Molecules are therefore transferred to fetal circulation
- These processes are very slow to have a significant impact on fetal drug concentration

Factors Governing Transfer

Drug Factors

- Molecular weight:
  - Low molecular weight molecules (< 1000 Da) cross placenta
  - Most drugs have molecular weight less than 500 Da
  - These molecules are easily transferred across the placenta
  - Drugs with molecular weight > 500 Da show incomplete transfer
- Lipid solubility:
  - Lipid soluble drugs cross placenta
  - Examples of lipid soluble drugs:
    - Thiopentone
    - Local anesthetics
    - Benzodiazepines
- Protein binding:
  - Protein binding determines the amount of free drug available to cross placenta
  - Drugs may be bound to albumin or α-1-acid glycoprotein (AAG)
  - Highly protein bound drugs do not cross placenta
- Degree of ionization:
  - Ionized drugs do not cross placenta
  - Examples of ionized drugs:
    - Glycopyrrolate
    - Heparin
    - Succinylcholine
    - Non-depolarizing NMBAs
- pKa: If pKa of drugs is close to physiological pH, more drug will be ionized and won't cross placenta

Maternal Factors

- Total dose and maternal drug concentration
- Addition of adjuvants like adrenaline reduces peak LA level
- Route of administration: injection into high vascular epidural space increases peak concentration of drug
- Maternal metabolism and excretion: hepatic/renal dysfunction increases toxicity
- Maternal protein binding: Increased protein binding reduces transfer
- Maternal pH alters extent of ionization and transfer

Placental Factors

- Placental blood flow:
  - Reduction in placental blood flow reduces the drug delivery to the membrane
  - This reduces the drug available for transfer
  - Factors reducing placental blood flow include:
    - Hypotension
    - Low cardiac output states
    - Aortocaval compression
    - Uterine contraction
    - Umbilical cord compression
- Placental ageing
- Placental area available for shunting:
  - The area available ranges from 3.4 m^2 at 28 weeks to 12.6 m^2 at term
  - Shunting of blood flow occurs in pre-eclampsia
  - This may present an increased barrier to transfer of molecules
  - Thus placental blood flow has to be adequate to ensure adequate transfer

Fetal Factors

- Solubility of drug in fetal blood
- Concentration of drug in fetal blood returning to placenta
- Uptake by fetal tissues
- Fetal hepatic metabolism and renal excretion
- Non placental routes of fetal drug exertion
- Fetal protein binding
- Fetal pH and adequacy of fetal circulation

Specific Drugs

I. *Drugs Which Readily Cross the Placenta*

- Anticholinergic agents:
  - Atropine
  - Scopolamine
- Benzodiazepines:
  - Diazepam
  - Midazolam
- Induction agents:
  - Propofol
  - Ketamine
  - Etomidate
  - Thiopentone
- Volatile anesthetics:
  - Halothane
  - Isoflurane
  - Sevoflurane
  - Desflurane
  - Nitrous oxide
- Opioids
- Local anesthetics
- Vasopressors: Ephedrine

II. *Drugs Which do Not Readily Cross the Placenta*

- Anticholinergic agents: glycopyrrolate
- Anticoagulants: heparin
- Muscle relaxants:
  - Depolarizing agents: succinylcholine
  - Nondepolarizing agents
- Vasopressor: phenylephrine

Types of Transfer

- Complete transfer (type 1):
  - These drugs cross the placenta rapidly
  - Concentrations equilibrate in maternal and fetal blood
  - Thus, F/M ratio of the drug is 1
  - Example: Thiopental
- Exceeding transfer (type 2):
  - These drugs cross the placenta rapidly
  - The concentration in fetal blood exceeds that in maternal blood
  - Thus, F/M ratio of the drug is greater than 1
  - Example: ketamine
- Incomplete transfer (type 3):
  - These drugs are unable to cross the placenta completely
  - Concentration in fetal blood is always lesser than that in maternal blood
  - Thus, F/M ratio of the drug is lesser than 1
  - Example: succinylcholine

Teratogenicity

Opioids

- Increased incidence of neonatal jaundice
- Neonatal depression if used during labor
- Withdrawal syndrome with chronic abuse

Nonopioids

- Paracetamol: safe
- Aspirin: IUGR, still birth
- Ibuprofen and ketorolac:
  - Increased maternal hemorrhage
  - Premature PDA closure
  - Prolonged labor

Warfarin

- ***Contradi syndrome***
- Stippled epiphysis, nasal and limb hypoplasia
- CNS effects
- Increased fetal hemorrhage
- Heparin and LMWH is safe during pregnancy

Anticonvulsants

- Phenytoin:
  - Fetal hydantoin syndrome
  - Growth and performance delays
- Carbameazepine:
  - Craniofacial defects
  - Developmental delay

Antiemetics

- Prochlorperazine: extrapyramidal effects
- Promethazine: fetal platelet aggregation
- Droperidol, metaclopramide, ondansetron: no risks
- Omeprazole and ranitidine: no risks

Antihypertensives

- ACE inhibitors: IUGR, neonatal renal failure
- β-blockers: IUGR, fetal bradycardia and hypoglycemia
- Calcium channel blockers, α_2 agonsists, methyldopa: no adverse effects

Benzodiazepines

- Cleft lip and palate
- ***Floppy infant syndrome***: hypotonia, lethargy, cyanosis, hypothermia

Hormones

- Antithyroid: fetal hypothyroidism and goitre
- Steroids:
  - Low birth weight
  - Congenital cataract
  - Cleft lip and palate

Antibiotics

- Aminoglycosides: ototoxicity, potentiate NMBAs
- Sulfonamides:
  - Hyperbilirubinemia
  - Anemia if maternal G6PD deficiency
- Tetracycline:
  - Teeth discoloration and hypoplasia
  - Skeletal growth restriction

Bronchodilators: No effects

PHYSIOLOGICAL CHANGES OF PREGNANCY

Introduction

- Successful anesthetic management of the pregnant woman depends on:
  - Recognition of anatomical and physiological changes
  - Appropriate adaptation of anesthetic techniques
- Physiological changes occur during pregnancy in major systems due to:
  - Hormones secreted by corpus luteum and placenta in first trimester
  - Mechanical effects and compression by enlarging uterus in 2nd and 3rd trimester

Central Nervous System

- Increase in cerebral blood flow
- Increased sensitivity to general anesthetics:
  - Reduced MAC of volatile anesthetics by up to 30% from non-pregnant state
  - More rapid uptake of volatile anesthetics due to reduced FRC
  - Altered pain threshold
  - Increased susceptibility to sedatives as progesterone has sedative effects
  - Increased sensitivity to benzodiazepines and propofol
- Increased sensitivity to local anesthetics:
  - Epidural venous engorgement resulting in:
    - Raised peak local anesthetic concentration
    - Increased incidence of bloody tap
  - Reduced volume of CSF due to:
    - Swelling of epidural veins
    - Increased epidural and CSF pressure:
      - This occurs due to raised intra-abdominal pressure
      - Epidural pressure is positive in term pregnant women
      - It is usually negative in 90% of non-pregnant women
      - Epidural pressure returns to non-pregnant level by 6–12 hours post-partum
  - Increased lumbar lordosis causing more cephalad spread of local anesthetic
  - 30% reduction in LA dose at term due to increased neuronal sensitivity to LA

Cardiovascular System

- Cardiovascular changes:
  - Blood volume increases by 45–50% at term
  - Heart rate increases by 15–20%, elevated by 10–20 bpm at term
  - Increased cardiac output by 40–50% by term:
    - Cardiac output increases from 5th week of gestation
    - Most of the increase occurs by 20 weeks of gestation
    - Cardiac output reaches maximum by 32 weeks
    - Approximately 1L of blood is contained in uterus and placenta
    - Initial increase in cardiac output is due to increase in heart rate
    - Thereafter, increased stroke volume causes increase in cardiac output
  - Contractility (variable) + 10%
  - Systemic vascular resistance reduced by 20%, causing a fall in diastolic BP
  - Systolic BP decreases in mid-trimester by up to 15 mm Hg
  - Diastolic BP reduces in mid trimester by 10–20 mm Hg
  - Central venous pressure and PCWP remains unchanged
  - PAP and PVR slightly decreased by 30%
  - Wide, loud and split S_1, S_3 and soft ejection systolic murmur
  - Left axis deviation, due to upward displacement of heart by uterus on ECG
  - Increased incidence of arrhythmias:
    - Sinus tachycardia
    - Ventricular ectopics
    - Paroxysmal supraventricular tachycardia
    - Paroxysmal atrial complexes
    - Ventricular arrhythmias
- Anesthetic implications of changes in cardiovascular system:
  - Venodilatation increases incidence of accidental epidural vein puncture
  - Healthy parturients tolerate up to 1500 mL blood loss
  - High hematocrit (> 42%) indicates low volume states and dehydration
  - Cardiac output remains high for first few hours post partum
  - Supine hypotension syndrome
    - IVC compression occurs by 13–16 weeks
    - Aortic compression occurs by 28–30 weeks

Respiratory System

- Anatomical changes:
  - Friable mucosa of nasopharynx due to estrogen-epistaxis
  - Capillary engorgement of mucosa, edema of oropharynx, larynx and trachea
  - Reduced airway resistance due to bronchiolar dilatation by progesterone
  - Vocal cord fatigue with decrease in maximum time of phonation
- Gas exchange:
  - Increase in minute ventilation by 45–50%
  - Increased oxygen demand and consumption by up to 35% due to:
    - Increased metabolic needs of:
      - Fetus
      - Uterus
      - Placenta
    - Increased respiratory work
    - Increased cardiac work
  - Increased requirement for CO_2 elimination
  - Increased work of breathing
  - Rightward shift of ODC facilitating oxygen delivery to fetus
  - PaO_2 increases to 100–106 mm Hg due to increased minute ventilation
  - $PaCO_2$ falls to 30 mm Hg by 12 weeks and remains at this level
- Mostly diaphragmatic pattern of breathing due to:
  - Limited thoracic cage movement
  - Pressure of gravid uterus
- Changes in pulmonary function tests:
  - Increased tidal volume by 45%, unchanged respiratory rate
  - Increased minute volume by 45%
  - Reduced FRC by 20% due to:
    - Increased intra-abdominal pressure
    - Upward displacement of diaphragm
  - Closing capacity unchanged
  - Reduced total lung capacity by 5%
  - Reduced expiratory reserve volume by 25%
  - Reduced residual volume by 15%
- Anesthetic implications of changes in respiratory system:

- Airway management is more challenging:
  - Breast engorgement may hinder laryngoscopy
  - Swollen, edematous mucosa which bleeds easily
  - Smaller size endotracheal tube preferred
- Greater risk of hypoxemia due to:
  - Decreased oxygen reserve due to reduced FRC
  - Increased oxygen consumption
  - Rapid airway obstruction

Gastrointestinal System

- Impaired esophageal and intestinal motility due to relaxant effect of progesterone
- Increased risk of aspiration and GERD due to:
  - Raised intragastric pressures (up to 40 cm H_2O at term)
  - Relaxation of lower esophageal sphinter: Reduced LES tone
  - Delayed gastric emptying
  - Shift in stomach position:
    - Enlarging uterus changes angle of GE junction and rotates the stomach
    - This removes *the pinch valve* effect at the point of entry in diaphragm
    - This increases the risk of aspiration
- Gastric and placental secretions:
  - Placental gastrin secretion increases volume and acidity of gastric secretions
  - Increased secretion of human placental lactogen:
    - This causes reduced glucose tolerance
    - This causes hyperglycemia and ketosis
- Anesthetic implications of changes in gastrointestinal system:
  - *Rapid sequence induction* with cricoid pressure for *> 12 weeks* gestation
  - Consumption of clear liquids promotes gastric emptying
  - Therefore, current ASA recommendations encourages clear liquid consumption by laboring patients

Renals

- Increased renal blood flow by 50–80%
- Kidneys enlarge by up to 30%
- GFR increases by 40–65% (from 100 mL/min to 150 mL/min) causing:
  - Raised creatinine clearance (from 120 mL/min to 150–200 mL/min)
  - Lower BUN and creatinine values (9 mg/dL and 0.5 mg/dL during pregnancy)
  - Glycosuria up to 1–10 g/day
  - Proteinuria up to 200–300 mg/day
- Dilatation of calyces, pelvis and ureters: urinary stasis causing frequent UTIs
- Anesthetic implications of changes in genitourinary system:
  - Gravid uterus may compress ureters and cause hydronephrosis
  - Urinary stasis results in increased risk of urinary infections
  - BUN and creatinine values which are normal for non-parturients indicate abnormal renal function during pregnancy
  - Glucosuria and mild proteinuria is normal during pregnancy

Hematological

- Blood volume:
  - Plasma volume increases by 45–50% by 34 weeks gestation
  - RBC volume on the other hand increases by only 30% at term
  - The increase in plasma volume exceeds the increase in RBC volume
  - This results in physiological anemia of pregnancy
  - Hemoglobin ranges from 9.5–15 g% and HCT from 28-40% in third trimester
  - Platelet count remains unchanged and may be increased in third trimester
- Increased oxygen transport:
  - Oxygen transport is increased in order to deliver more oxygen to fetus
  - This occurs due to:
    - Increased PaO_2 due to increased minute ventilation
    - Rightward shift of ODC facilitating easy delivery of oxygen
    - Increased cardiac output increasing uterine blood flow
- Plasma proteins:
  - Increased total protein levels
  - Reduced albumin levels and albumin: globulin ratio
  - Reduced plasma colloid oncotic pressure by up to 14%

- Raised levels of all clotting factors:
  - Factors VII, VIII, IX, X, XII
  - Fibrinogen
  - Plasminogen, prothrombin fragment
- Reduced anticoagulant activity:
  - Reduced protein C and S, antithrombin III
  - Impaired fibrinolysis
- Relative reduction in protein levels due to increased plasma volume: raised free drug fraction

❖ Changes in tests of coagulation:
- Prothrombin time shortened by 20%
- Partial thromboplastin time shortened by 20%
- Hypercoagulable trace on TEG
- No change or decreased platelet count
- Increased plasminogen and fibrin degradation products

❖ Anesthetic implications of hematological changes:
- Anemia of pregnancy occurs due to disproportionate raise in plasma volume
- Increase in blood volume prepares the parturient for blood loss during delivery
- Hemodynamic changes due to blood loss are not seen till it exceeds 1500 mL
- Due to alterations in coagulation system, risk of thromboembolism is increased

Implications of Pregnancy on Neuraxial Anesthesia

❖ Technical considerations:
- Increased lumbar lordosis:
  - Causes a reduction in vertebral interspinous gap
  - Results in difficulty in administering neuraxial anesthesia
- Apex of thoracic kyphosis at higher level
- Lateral position:
  - Head down tilt occurs when pregnant women lies in lateral position
  - This is due to a wider pelvis resulting in a downward tilt
  - This may result in rostral spread of local anesthetic when administered in lateral position

❖ Treatment of hypotension: relative resistance to vasopressors

❖ Local anesthetic dose requirements:
- Subarachnoid dose reduced by 25%
- Epidural dose is unaltered or slightly reduced

Implications of Pregnancy on General Anesthesia

❖ Drugs:
- Thiopentone:
  - Reduced induction dose
  - Prolonged elimination half life
- Propofol:
  - Reduced induction dose
  - Unaltered elimination half life
- Volatile anesthetic agents:
  - Minimum alveolar concentration decreased
  - Increased speed of induction
- Succinylcholine: unaltered duration of blockade
- Rocuronium: increased sensitivity
- Chronotropic agents and vasopressors: reduced sensitivity

❖ Tracheal intubation:
- Accelerated desaturation during apnea
- Smaller endotracheal tube required (6.5 or 7 mm ID)
- Increased risk of bleeding with nasal intubation

SUPINE HYPOTENSION SYNDROME

Introduction

❖ Term given to hypotension (reduction of SBP by at least 15–30 mm Hg) occurring when a parturient adopts supine position

❖ This occurs due to compression of abdominal aorta and IVC by the enlarging uteroplacental mass

❖ First reported in 1931

❖ Occurs in up to 15% of pregnant patients near term

❖ Also called ***Aortocaval syndrome***

Risk Factors

❖ Primigravida with tight skin around abdomen
❖ Obesity
❖ Multiple pregnancy
❖ Polyhydramnios
❖ Pregnancy induced hypertension
❖ Dehydration, bleeding, hypovolemia

Pathogenesis

❖ Syndrome has been clinically demonstrated from middle of second trimester onwards

❖ IVC compression:
- Occurs as early as 13–16 weeks gestation
- Causes 50% rise in femoral venous pressure in supine position at 16 weeks

- At term, femoral venous pressure increases to 2.5 times the normal value
- Aortic compression:
  - Aortic compression by gravid uterus occurs later by 28–30 weeks gestation
  - This results in lower femoral arterial pressures in supine position
- This causes a profound drop in venous return to the heart
- Cardiovascular system may not be able to compensate for the drop in venous return
- Compensatory mechanisms:

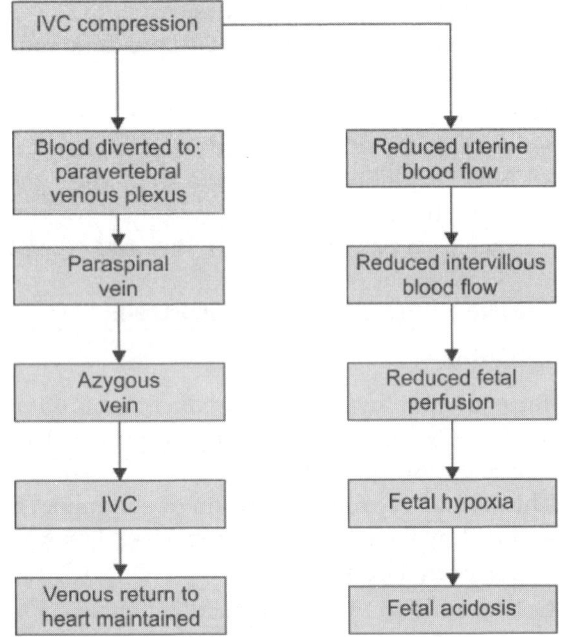

Types

- Concealed caval compression:
  - Occurs when compensatory mechanisms act to restore venous return to heart
  - No clinical symptoms
- Revealed caval compression:
  - When compensatory mechanisms are insufficient to maintain preload to heart
  - Occurs in 10% of patients causing serious reduction in venous return to heart
  - Clinical symptoms manifest

Clinical Features

- Usually occur within 3–10 minutes of assuming supine position
- Symptoms:
  - Faintness, giddiness, visual disturbances, numbness, paresthesias
  - Dyspnea, restlessness
  - Nausea, vomiting
  - Pallor, sweating, cold and clammy skin
  - On long standing:
    - Pooling of venous blood
    - Edema, varicose veins, thrombophlebitis
- Signs:
  - Hypotension
  - Tachycardia and narrow pulse pressure (*earliest sign*)
  - Reduced femoral artery pressures: ***Poseiro sign***
  - Placental abruption may occur due to transmission of raised venous pressures
  - Aggravated by:
    - Spinal anesthesia
    - Epidural anesthesia
    - Thiopentone
    - Halothane
- Fetal effects:
  - Fetal hypoxia
  - Slow irregular fetal heart rate

Prevention and Treatment

- Position:
  - Avoid supine position ***after 20 weeks*** gestation
  - Left lateral tilt of table to 15° by:
    - Tipping table
    - ***Crawford wedge***
    - Stationary ***Colon Morales left uterine displacers*** under right hip
    - Foam wedge
    - Folded sheets
  - Left lateral tilt to 30° indicated for:
    - Polyhydramnios
    - Twin pregnancy
    - During labor
  - Aortocaval compression exists even at 30° tilt, causing low cardiac output
  - However, steeper tilt of the table results in an insecure patient and is avoided
  - Inflatable bag may be used to elevate right buttock and back by 10–15 cm
- Fluid therapy:
  - 10–20 mL/kg IV fluids bolus before spinal anesthesia
  - Preloading done 15–20 minutes before giving spinal anesthesia
  - Large bore IV cannula preferred

- Vasopressors:
  - IV 5 mg ephedrine/phenylephrine 25–50 μg IV bolus
  - IV epinephrine infusion if hypotension associated with bradycardia
- Supplemental oxygen: 4 L/min oxygen supplementation by face mask
- Refractory severe hypotension:
  - Manual left uterine displacement (LUD):
    - Most effective way to prevent aortocaval compression
    - Advantages of manual LUD:
      - Can be done with patient in supine position
      - Allows airway management
      - Facilitates more effective CPR during maternal cardiac arrest
  - Trendelenburg position if severe
  - Immediate Cesarean section if patient is in shock

INTRAPARTUM FETAL EVALUATION

Introduction

- Intrapartum asphyxia is a major cause of perinatal morbidity and mortality
- This can result in still birth of the fetus or long-term neurological sequelae
- Fetal heart rate (FHR) acts as an indirect marker of fetal responses to changes in:
  - Oxygen delivery
  - Blood pressure
  - Blood gases
  - Acid-base status
- Intrapartum fetal monitoring enable early identification of fetal heart rate changes
- This plays a vital role in preventing perinatal complications

Advantages

- Associated with reduction in intrapartum fetal death
- Reduced incidence of neonatal seizures

Disadvantages

- Not proven to be clearly superior to intermittent auscultation
- High false positive rate
- Increases incidence of Cesarean sections and instrumental vaginal births
- No significant reduction in long-term neurological sequelae
- Low specificity as pre-existing neurological disease may cause changes in FHR

Predictive Criteria for Cerebral Palsy

- Essential criteria:
  - Evidence of cord blood metabolic acidosis at delivery:
    - pH < 7.0
    - Base deficit > 12 mmol/L
  - Early onset encephalopathy in preterm infants > 34 weeks gestational age
  - Neonatal spastic quadriplegic cerebral palsy
  - Neonatal dyskinetic cerebral palsy
  - Exclusion of other identifiable causes
- Criteria related to timing of hypoxic insult:
  - Sentinel hypoxic event immediately before or during delivery
  - Changes in FHR patterns at delivery:
    - Sudden, sustained fetal bradycardia lasting > 10 minutes
    - Absence of FHR variability with persistent late of variable deceleration
  - APGAR score of 0–3 beyond 5 minutes of delivery
  - Multisystem involvement within 72 hours of delivery
  - Early imaging signs of acute, non-focal cerebral abnormality

Techniques of Fetal Monitoring

- Fetal heart rate monitoring
- FHR response to stimulation
- Fetal scalp blood sampling
- Fetal pulse oximetry
- ST analysis

Indications 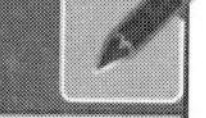

- Intermittent auscultatory monitoring is advised for low risk pregnancies
- FHR monitoring is advised for high risk pregnancies:
  - Preeclampsia
  - Suspected fetal growth restriction
  - Type I diabetes mellitus
  - Infective pathology:
    - Chorioamnionitis
    - Sepsis
    - Persistent fever > 38°C
  - Intrapartum use of oxytocin
  - Significant meconium
  - Antepartum hemorrhage

Techniques of Fetal Heart Rate Monitoring

Non-invasive (external) electronic fetal heart rate monitoring:

- Performed intermittently or continuously
- Done with a Doppler ultrasound device on maternal abdomen
- Motion of the heart is utilized by the device to create a complex waveform
- Peaks of successive waves are then used to calculate the R-R interval
- This estimates FHR, which closely correlates to FHR derived from fetal ECG
- Monica AN24 monitors:
  - Alternatively, several electrodes may be placed on maternal abdomen
  - Wireless monitors are used to enable FHR monitoring

❖ Intermittent auscultation:
- Done using Pinard or DeLee fetal stethoscope
- This technique is preferred for uncomplicated pregnancies

❖ Invasive (internal) fetal heart rate monitoring:
- This is done by obtaining fetal electrocardiogram tracings
- Electrodes used are:
  - Bipolar spiral electrode placed on fetal scalp transcervically
  - Reference electrode placed on the maternal thigh
- Reference electrode eliminates interference from maternal cardiac activity
- FHR is then calculated from the R-R interval

Frequency of Monitoring

❖ Labor admission test:
- Performed upon admission into the labor unit
- FHR patterns are assessed for a minimum of 20–30 minutes
- Aims to identify fetuses with an increased risk for abnormal FHR pattern
- In these patients, continuous rather than intermittent monitoring is continued

❖ For low risk pregnancies:
- FHR is continuously monitored
- FHR is reviewed:
  - At least every 30 minutes during active phase of first stage of labor
  - At least every 15 minutes in second stage

❖ In high risk pregnancies:
- FHR is continuously monitored
- FHR is reviewed:
  - At least every 15 minutes in active phase of first stage of labor
  - At least every 5 minutes in the second stage of labor

FHR Characteristics

Term	Definition
Baseline FHR	110–160 bpm, measured over > 2 min
Bradycardia	Baseline rate < 110 bpm for > 10 min
Tachycardia	Baseline rate > 160 bpm for > 10 min
Variability	Fluctuations in baseline FHR of > 2 cycles/min
Acceleration	Abrupt increase in FHR > 15 bpm above Baseline lasting > 15 sec and < 2 min
Prolonged acceleration	Acceleration > 2 min and < 10 min duration
Early deceleration	Gradual decrease in FHR below baseline, uniform shape, early onset
	Return to baseline associated with uterine contraction
	Nadir of deceleration at same time as peak of contraction
Late deceleration	Gradual decrease in FHR below baseline, uniform shape, early onset
	Return to baseline associated with uterine contraction
	Nadir of deceleration occurs after peak of contraction
Variable deceleration	Abrupt decrease in FHR below baseline
	Decrease is > 15 bpm, duration > 15 sec and < 2 min
	Variable shape
Prolonged deceleration	Abrupt prolonged decrease in FHR below baseline
	Decrease is > 15 bpm
	Duration >2 min but < 10 min

Significance of FHR Characteristics

❖ Normal baseline FHR:
- Reflects a normal cardiac conduction system
- This includes:
  - Intrinsic cardiac pacemakers:
  - Sinoatrial node
  - Atrioventricular node
  - Cardiac conduction pathways
- Also rules out extrinsic and intrinsic factors affecting FHR
- This includes:
  - Autonomic innervation
  - Humoral factors such as catecholamine
  - Maternal medications

❖ Baseline bradycardia:
- Fetal hypoxia
- Bradyarrhythmias (complete heart block)

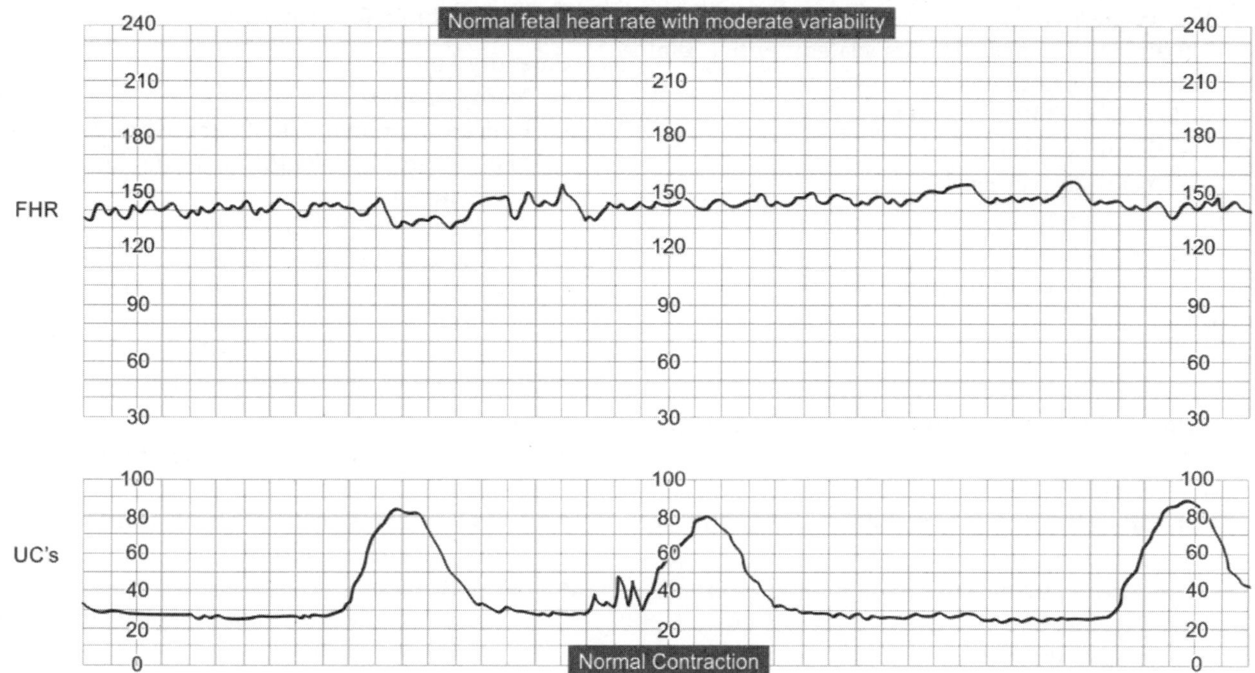

Fig. 3: Normal fetal heart rate pattern.

- Maternal β-blocker therapy
- Hypothermia
- Hypoglycemia
- Hypothyroidism

❖ Baseline tachycardia:
- Fetal causes:
  - Hypoxemia
  - Anemia
  - Tachyarrhythmias
  - Congenital cardiac anomalies
- Maternal causes:
  - Fever, dehydration
  - Hyperthyroidism
  - Elevated catecholamines

❖ FHR variability:
- Reflects interaction between fetal sympathetic and parasympathetic NS
- FHR variability has a high sensitivity to detect fetal hypoxia
- Thus, presence of FHR variability predicts normal fetal oxygenation
- However, specificity of FHR variability is low
- Thus, absence of FHR variability does not always indicate fetal hypoxia
- Other causes associated with low/absent FHR variability are:

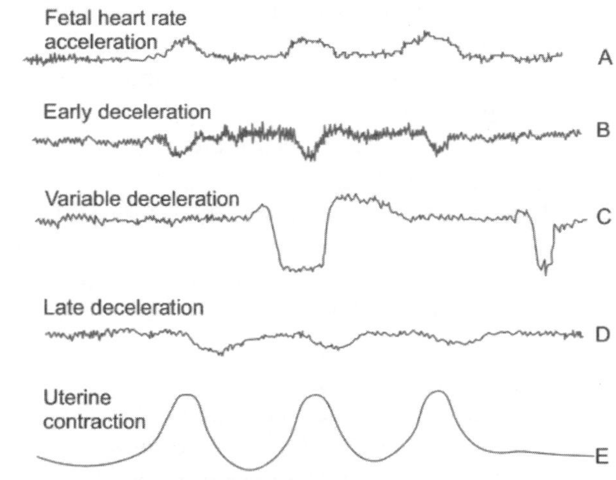

Fig. 4: Variations in fetal heart rate.

  - Fetal sleep cycle
  - Arrhythmias
  - Maternal medications
  - Extreme prematurity
  - Pre-existing neurological injury
- Increased FHR variability is seen in:
  - Normal fetuses due to exaggerated autonomic reflexes
  - Fetal hypoxia

- FHR acceleration:
  - FHR acceleration is associated with fetal movements normally
  - Absence of FHR acceleration suggests:
    - Fetal hypoxia
    - Fetal sleep cycle
    - Arrhythmias
    - Fetal anemia
    - Pre-existing neurological injury
- Early deceleration:
  - Clinically benign
  - *Not associated with fetal hypoxia*
  - Occurs due to increase in fetal ICP during uterine contraction
- Late deceleration:
  - Due to fetal response to transient hypoxia during uterine contraction
  - Can also occur due to severe pathological fetal hypoxia due to:
    - Maternal hypoxia
    - Maternal hypotension
    - Reduced fetal cardiac output
  - Pathological late decelerations are differentiated from reflex deceleration by:
    - Presence of baseline FHR variability in reflex deceleration
    - Recurrent late decelerations
- Variable decelerations:
  - Reflects a fetal reflex response to transient cord compression
  - However, recurrent variable decelerations suggest fetal hypoxia due to:
    - Maternal hypoxia
    - Maternal hypotension
    - Reduced fetal cardiac output
  - Recurrence is defined by occurrence with:
    - At least 50% of uterine contractions
    - Recorded over a 20-minute window
- Prolonged deceleration:
  - Caused by prolonged fetal hypoxia
  - Associated with absent or minimal FHR variability and no accelerations
- Sinusoidal pattern:
  - Smooth sine-like wave with undulating pattern in FHR baseline
  - Cycle frequency of 3-5 cycle per minute persisting for at least 20 minutes
  - Associated with severe fetal anemia

Classification of FHR Patterns

- Category I pattern:
  - Normal pattern
  - Indicates minimal risk of fetal hypoxia
  - FHR recordings ***should have all*** the following characteristics:
    - Baseline FHR of 110–160 bpm
    - Moderate FHR variability
    - Absence of late or variable FHR decelerations
    - Early decelerations maybe present
    - Accelerations maybe present
- Category II pattern:
  - Has an uncertain diagnostic significance
  - Tends to be prolonged with uncertain prognosis
  - Includes all FHR patterns which are not classified under categories I and III
  - These include:
    - Bradycardia not accompanied by absent baseline variability
    - Tachycardia
    - Minimal or excessive baseline FHR variability
    - Absent baseline variability not accompanied by recurrent decelerations
    - Absence of stimulated FHR accelerations
    - Recurrent variable decelerations with minimal baseline variability
    - Prolonged deceleration > 2 minutes but < 10 minutes
- Category III pattern:
  - Abnormal pattern
  - Associated with high risk of severe fetal hypoxia
  - FHR recordings ***should have at least one of***:
    - Absent FHR variability with recurrent late decelerations
    - Absent variability with recurrent variable decelerations
    - Absent variability with fetal bradycardia
    - Sinusoidal pattern
  - Necessitates prompt therapeutic action
  - This is because persistence of the pattern results in fetal demise

Causes of Monitoring Errors

- Fetal sleep cycle
- Technical factors:
  - Faulty electrodes
  - Faulty monitor setting
  - Faulty leg plate

- Maternal heart rate artefacts
- TENS signal artefacts
- Effect of drugs:
  - Opioids
  - Magnesium sulphate
  - Beta-blockers
  - Atropine
- Pre-existing fetal neurological injury

Ancilliary Tests

- FHR response to stimulation:
  - Scalp stimulation is performed in the absence of spontaneous accelerations
  - This is done by:
    - Manual stimulation trans-vaginally
    - Vibroacoustic stimulation on maternal abdominal wall
  - A positive response is indicated by:
    - Gestational age > 32 weeks:
      - FHR acceleration > 15 bpm above baseline
      - Lasting for > 15 seconds
    - Gestational age < 32 weeks:
      - FHR acceleration > 10 bpm above baseline
      - Lasting for > 10 seconds
  - Presence of stimulated-FHR-accelerations excludes ongoing hypoxia
- Fetal scalp blood sampling:
  - Assesses the fetal capillary blood for presence and degree of fetal acidosis
  - Technique:
    - Amnioscope with a light source is used to expose fetal scalp
    - Fetal scalp is cleaned and smeared with silicone gel
    - Scalp is punctured with a 2-mm blade to draw a droplet of blood
    - This is collected in long heparinized capillary tubes
    - The sample is analyzed for pH and lactate levels
    - However, test requires cervical dilatation of at least 2–3 cm
  - Contraindications:
    - Maternal HIV or hepatitis
    - Fetal coagulopathy
  - Associated with serious complications:
    - Fetal CNS infections
    - Leakage of fetal CSF
  - Not routinely performed due to:
    - Unproven diagnostic benefits
    - High sample failure rates
    - Patient discomfort
    - Serious complications

Latest Advances

- Fetal reflectance pulse oximetry:
  - Uses the Nellcor N-400 fetal pulse oximeter system
  - Used for term singleton neonates with vertex presentation
  - Probe is placed on the neonatal cheek or scalp with pressure from cervix
  - Reliable pulse oximeter signal may not be obtained due to:
    - Thick fetal hair
    - Fetal scalp congestion
    - Vernix caseosa
    - Movement artefacts
  - Thus, it is not routinely performed
  - Normal values:
    - Fetal SpO_2 50–70% during first stage of labor
    - Fetal SpO_2 45–65% during second stage of labor
  - Fetal SpO_2 < 30% for more than 10 minutes is associated with poor outcomes
- ST analysis:
  - Utilizes the STAN S31 fetal heart monitor
  - Monitors fetal electrocardiogram during labor
  - ST segment analysis is performed of ECG obtained from fetal scalp electrode
  - Not frequently used due to:
    - Interference with external electrical activity:
    - Maternal electrical signals
    - Transcutaneous electrical nerve stimulation signals
    - Poor correlation with fetal outcomes
- Other techniques include:
  - Proton MR spectroscopy
  - Transabdominal near infrared spectroscopy (NIRS)

APGAR SCORE

Introduction

- Score used to evaluate newborns immediately after birth
- This score is useful to identify depressed infants requiring resuscitation
- Useful in predicting short term mortality for low birth weight infants

❖ Developed by ***Dr. Virginia Apgar***, an anesthesiologist at Columbia University in 1952

Score

		0	1	2
Appearance	Color	Blue, pale	Pink body, blue limbs	Completely pink
Pulse	Heart rate	Absent	<100	>100
Grimace	Reflex Irritability	No response	Grimace	Cough, sneeze, cry
Activity	Muscle tone	Limp	Some flexion	Active motion
Respiration	Resp.effort	Absent	Slow, irregular	Good, crying

Technique

- ❖ Originally used to assess the need for intervention to establish breathing at 1 minute
- ❖ Usually performed by pediatrician/ individual not directly involved in care of mother
- ❖ Scoring usually done at 1 and 5 minutes after birth
- ❖ Each category is weighted evenly and assigned a value of 0, 1 or 2
- ❖ The components are then added together to yield the total score
- ❖ Repeated at 10, 15 and 20 minutes if the 5 minute score is less than 7
- ❖ Heart rate and respiratory effort are *most important* in identifying distressed new born
- ❖ Heart rate is assessed with the stethoscope rather than by palpation
- ❖ Color is of *least value*

Clinical Significance

- ❖ Resuscitation based on 1 minute score

Score	Category	Intervention
≥7	Normal	No ventilatory assistance
	Mild respiratory acidosis	
4-6	Moderately depressed	Oxygen via mask
	Respiratory acidosis	
0-3	Severe depression	Endotracheal intubation
	Combined respiratory and metabolic acidosis	Cardiac massage

Prognostic Value

- ❖ Low 1 min score:
  - Usually not predictive of adverse clinical outcome
  - Is not considered as evidence of intrapartum hypoxemic event
  - Most children with low 1 minute scores will have normal scores by 5 minutes

Contd...

Contd...

- ❖ Low 5 minute score:
  - Correlates with mortality at 1 year
  - These patients may have increased risk of cerebral palsy
  - This is especially so if low scores persist at later evaluations
  - Scores < 5 at 5 and 10 minutes correlate with increased risk of cerebral palsy
  - APGAR score 0 at 10 minutes indicates need for termination of resuscitation

Limitations

- ❖ Subjective score
- ❖ Observation only for very brief period
- ❖ Crude measurements: only looks at vital signs
- ❖ No agreement on how to score infants with a low gestational age
- ❖ Does not account for interventions taken during resuscitation
- ❖ Subtle effects of perinatal asphyxia/ maternal medication may be missed
- ❖ Little value when used to predict survival in any individual case
- ❖ Does not predict neurological outcomes
- ❖ Factors leading to errors in APGAR score:
  - Maternal sedation or anesthesia
  - Congenital malformations
  - Gestational age
  - Trauma
  - Inter-observer variability

Factors Affecting Apgar Score

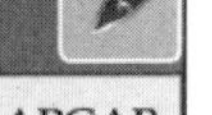

- ❖ False positive results: (absence of acidosis with low APGAR score)
  - Prematurity
  - Congenital myopathy
  - Congenital neuropathy
  - Acute cerebral trauma
  - Spinal cord trauma
  - Central nervous system anomalies
  - Precipitous delivery
  - Diaphragmatic hernias
  - Choanal atresia
  - Hemorrhage, hypovolemia
  - Drugs:
    - Analgesics, narcotics, sedatives
    - Magnesium sulphate
- ❖ False negative results: (acidosis with normal APGAR score)
  - Maternal acidosis
  - High fetal catecholamine levels

AAG/ACOG Policy Statement

- APGAR score should not be used to predict outcomes for individual infants
- APGAR score is not an appropriate method to diagnose asphyxia
- Umbilical artery samples are obtained for ABG when 5 minute APGAR score is < 5
- Expanded APGAR score reporting is more useful during resuscitative efforts

Modifications of the APGAR System

- Specified APGAR score:
  - Specifies the items of the APGAR score
  - Infants condition is scored regardless of gestational age and interventions
  - Thus, it calculates the APGAR score ignoring the extent of resuscitation
  - Maximal score which can be attained is 10 points
  - Accordingly, a full score of 10 points can be allocated to either:
    - A healthy term infant
    - Preterm infant without any problems postpartum
    - Infant receiving resuscitation with adequate response to interventions
- Expanded APGAR score:
  - Consists of basic interventions during resuscitation that are required to achieve optimal APGAR score
  - Components included along with the conventional APGAR score include:
    - Continuous positive airway pressure
    - Oxygen administration
    - Endotracheal intubation
    - Chest compressions
    - Epinephrine
  - Thus, maximal score which can be attained is 7
- Combined APGAR score:
  - Incorporates detailed interventions during resuscitation into the APGAR score
  - Combines both the Specified and Expanded APGAR scores
  - Thus, this score allows a more detailed assessment of the neonate
  - Has been found superior to conventional APGAR score in multiple studies
  - Components to be assessed along with conventional APGAR score include:
    - Continuous Positive Airway Pressure (C)
    - Oxygen administration (O)
    - Mask and Bag ventilation (M-B)
    - Intubation and ventilation (I)
    - Neonatal chest compressions (N)
    - Exogenous surfactant (E)
    - Drugs (D)
  - Maximal score that can be attained is 17 points

PHYSIOLOGICAL EFFECTS OF LABOR PAIN

Introduction

- Labor pain is ranked one of the highest on the pain rating scale
- However, very limited research exists on the mechanisms of labor pain

Stages of Labor

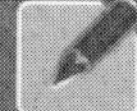

- First stage of labor:
  - Starts for onset of true labor pain
  - Ends with full dilatation of cervix
  - Also called cervical stage of labor
  - Average duration:
    - 12 hours in primigravida
    - 6 hours in multiparous women
- Second stage of labor:
  - Starts from full dilatation of the cervix (not from rupture of membranes)
  - Ends with expulsion of fetus from birth canal
  - Occurs in 2 phases:
    - Propulsive phase:
      - Starts from full dilatation of the cervix
      - Ends with descent of presenting part to pelvic floor
    - Expulsive part:
      - Starts with propulsive efforts to deliver baby
      - Ends with delivery of the baby
  - Average duration:
    - 2 hours in primigravidae
    - 30 minutes in multiparous women
- Third stage of labor:
  - Begins with expulsion of the fetus
  - Ends with expulsion of placenta and membrane
  - Average duration 15 minutes in primigravidae and multiparous women

Components of Labor Pain

- Visceral pain:
  - Occurs during early first stage and second stage of labor
  - Mainly due to dilatation of:

- Cervix
- Lower uterine segment

- Transmitted by small un-myelinated C-fibres
- Pain is dull in character and not easily localized
- Pain is referred to T_{10}-T_{12} dermatomoes such as:
  - Lower abdomen
  - Sacrum
  - Back
- Pain is not always sensitive to opioid therapy

❖ Somatic pain:
- Occurs during late first stage and second stage of labor
- Due to distention of:
  - Pelvic floor
  - Perineum
  - Vagina
- Transmitted by fine, myelinated A-delta fibres
- Pain is sharp in character and easily localized
- Occurs closer to delivery
- Radiates to adjacent T10-L1 dermatomes
- More resistant to opioids

Labor Pain Pathways

❖ Visceral pain:
- Transmitted via small un-myelinated C-fibres
- These travel along with the sympathetic fibres to:
  - Uterine plexus
  - Cervical plexus
  - Hypogastric plexus
- Fibres from sympathetic chain enter white rami communicantes with T_{10}-L_1
- They synapse in dorsal horn of spinal cord via posterior nerve roots
- Some fibres cross over at the dorsal horn level with multiple extensions
- This leads to poor localization of pain
- From dorsal horn cells, they are transmitted via spino-thalamic tract to brain
- Chemical mediators involved in this pathway include:
  - Bradykinin
  - Leukotrienes
  - Prostaglandins
  - Serotonin
  - Substance P
  - Lactic acid

❖ Somatic pain:
- Transmitted by fine, myelinated, rapidly transmitting A-delta fibres
- Transmission occurs to S_2-S_4 nerve roots via:
  - Pudendal nerves
  - Perineal branches of posterior cutaneous nerve of thigh
- Afferent fibres are also carried to L_1 and L_2 roots via:
  - Ilioinguinal nerve
  - Genitofemoral nerve
- From dorsal horn cells, they are transmitted via spino-thalamic tract to brain

Factors Affecting Severity of Labor Pain

❖ Parity:
- Severity of pain varies between nulliparous and multiparous women
- Nulliparous women experience more severe pain

❖ Prior education:
- Prior education about the process of labor reduces intensity of pain
- This may also explain cultural differences in perception of labor pain

❖ Severity of labor pain increases with progression of labor due to:
- Cervical distension (primarily)
- Increase in uterine pressure during contractions

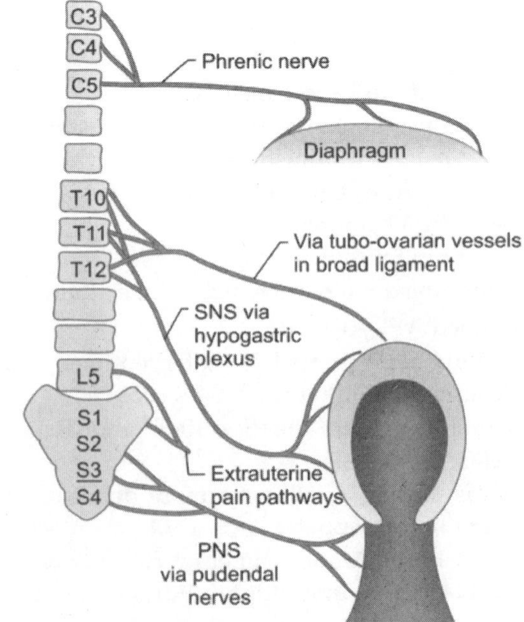

Fig. 5: Labor pain pathways.

Effects of Labor Pain on the Mother

- Obstetric course: Pain can affect the course of labor by several mechanisms:
  - Release of epinephrine causing tocolysis by β_2 adrenergic activity
  - *Fergusons reflex*:
    - Labor causes release of neural input from ascending spinal tracts to midbrain
    - This leads to an enhanced release of oxytocin
    - Oxytocin in turn stimulates uterine activity and contractility
  - Release of local mediators:
    - Pain results in the secretion of several substances with local actions
    - These include:
      - Substances which stimulate myometrial activity:
        - Substance P
        - Glutamate
        - Vasoactive intestinal peptide
    - Substances which inhibit myometrial activity:
      - Calcitonin gene related peptide (CGRP)
      - Nitric oxide
- Cardiorespiratory effects:
  - Reflex epinephrine secretion due to pain results in:
    - Increased cardiac output
    - Increased peripheral vascular resistance
    - Reduced uteroplacental circulation
  - Pain also stimulates the respiratory system
  - This leads to:
    - Intermittent hyperventilation during pain
    - Compensatory hypoventilation during the absence of pain
  - This may lead to fetal hypoxia during the hypoventilation phase
  - Also, hyperventilation causes respiratory alkalosis
  - This shifts maternal ODC curve to the left
  - This may reduce delivery of oxygen to the fetus
  - These changes may cause maternal or fetal decompensation in sick patients
- Gastrointestinal effects:
  - Labor pain causes increased release of gastrin
  - This causes increased acidity of gastric secretions
  - It also inhibits segmental and suprasegmental reflexes of GI motility
  - Thus, delayed gastric emptying results predisposing to aspiration
  - These changes are further aggravated by:
    - Recumbent position
    - Administration of opioids
- Metabolic effects:
  - Sympathetic response associated with pain increases metabolic rate
  - This may result in metabolic acidosis in decompensated patients
  - This may potentiate maternal hyperventilation as compensatory mechanism
  - This will shift the ODC curve to the left and prevent O_2 delivery to the fetus
  - Pain during labor causes cortisol release which is associated with:
    - Increase in protein catabolism
    - Hyperglycemia
    - Decrease in insulin secretion
    - Sodium and water retention
    - Increased ketone production
- Psychological effects:
  - Psychological effects of labor pain are greatly influenced by:
    - Psychosocial factors
    - Environmental factors
  - Severe labor pain can have adverse psychological effects on patients such as:
    - Post-partum depression
    - Psychotic reactions resembling post-traumatic stress disorder
- Post-labor pain:
  - Incidence of post-delivery pain:
    - Perineal pain 8-weeks post-partum is as high as 7%
    - Residual pain 6-months following cesarean section is 23%
  - Persistent post-delivery pain may lead to:
    - Post-partum depression
    - Chronic pain syndromes

Effects of Labor Pain on the Fetus

- There are no direct neural connections between mother and the fetus
- Thus, maternal labor pain has no direct effects on the fetus
- However, labor pain can cause fetal effects by altering uteroplacental circulation
- Uteroplacental circulation is altered by several mechanisms:
  - Altered uterine contractions by pain-induced release of:

- Oxytocin
- Adrenaline

• Uterine artery vasoconstriction by release of epinephrine
• Maternal desaturation during periods of hypoventilation

Beneficial Effects of Labor Analgesia

❖ Cardiovascular system:
  • Labor analgesia reduces circulating catecholamines
  • This results in:
    – Improved peripheral circulation
    – Better uteroplacental circulation

❖ Respiratory system:
  • Waxing and waning pattern of breathing due to labor pain is avoided
  • Thus, hyperventilation and respiratory alkalosis is not seen
  • This prevents leftward shift in maternal ODC curve
  • Thus oxygen delivery to fetus in increased

❖ Metabolic effects:
  • Glucose homeostasis normalises following relief of pain
  • Metabolic acidosis and ketosis are reversed

❖ Gastric emptying:
  • No significant direct change occurs
  • This is because most changes are due to physiological changes with pregnancy
  • However, avoidance of opioids may prevent gastric stasis

❖ Psychological effects:
  • Labor analgesia relieves the fear and anxiety associated with labou pain
  • This in turn may reduce the incidence of:
    – Elective cesarean sections during subsequent pregnancies
    – Post-traumatic stress disorder
    – Post-partum depression

INNERVATION OF FEMALE GENITAL TRACT

External Genitalia

❖ Antero-superior part:
  • Ilioinguinal nerve (L_1, L_2)
  • Genital branch of genitofemoral nerve (L_1, L_2)

❖ Posterior inferior part:
  • Pudendal branch from posterior cutaneous nerve of thigh (S_1-S_3)

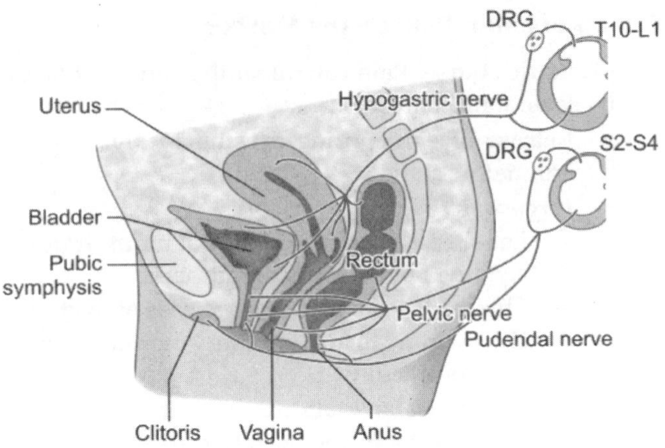

Fig. 6: Innervation of female genital tract.

❖ Vulva: Labia and perineal branch of pudendal nerve ($S_{2,3,4}$)

Internal Genitalia

❖ Vagina:
  • Sympathetic and parasympathetic from pelvic plexus
  • Lower part supplied by pudendal nerve

❖ Uterus:
  • Sympathetic:
    – T_{5-6} motor
    – T_{10} to L_1 sensory
    – Uterine pain is thus referred to that area of abdomen supplied by T_{10}-L_1
    – Uterus and cervix are insensitive to touch and handling
  • Parasympathetic: Pelvic nerve containing motor and sensory fibres from $S_{2,3,4}$

❖ Fallopian tubes:
  • Nerve supply is derived from uterine and ovarian nerves
  • Fallopian tube is very sensitive to handling

❖ Ovary:
  • Sympathetic supply via ovarian nerve (T_{10})
  • Nerve runs along the course of ovarian artery
  • Ovaries are sensitive to manual squeezing and handling

Pelvic Floor

❖ Inferior rectal nerve
❖ Perineal branch of pudendal nerve ($S_{2,3,4}$)
❖ 4th sacral nerve

Urinary Bladder

- Sympathetic:
  - Pelvic plexus
  - Conveys pain of over distension
- Parasympathetic:
  - Pelvic plexus from ***nervi erigentes*** ($S_{2,3,4}$)
  - Produces contraction of detrusor muscles and relaxation of internal sphincter
  - This is also called ***nerve of bladder evacuation***
- Urethra: pudendal nerve

Pelvic Ureter

- Sympathetic: Hypogastric and pelvic plexus
- Parasympathetic: Sacral plexus
- Urethra: Supplied by the pudendal nerve

Pain Pathway During Labor

- Source of pain:
  - Contraction of myometrium against cervical resistance
  - Progressive dilation of cervix and lower uterine segment
  - Stretching and compression of pelvic and perineal structures
- First stage of labor:
  - Visceral pain due to uterine contraction and cervical dilatation
  - Involves upto T_{10}–L_1 dermatomes
  - Primarily in lower abdomen, referred to lumbosacral/gluteal or thighs
  - Visceral afferents ⟶ sympathetic N ⟶ uterine and cervical plexus

    ↓

    Spinal cord (T_{10}–L_1) ⟵ hypogastric and aortic plexus
- Second stage of labor:
  - Perineal pain, due to compression of pelvic and perineal structures
  - Involves T_{10}-S_4 segments
  - Carried via pudendal N to spinal cord T_{10}–S_4 segments

LABOR ANALGESIA

Techniques

I. *Nonpharmacological*

- Low resource methods:
  - Psychoprophylaxis:
    - Education program
    - Strong focus of attention
    - Human support, soothing touch, hand holding
    - Relaxation techniques of voluntary muscles
    - Breathing techniques:
      - Slow breathing
      - Counting breaths
      - Reciting mantras in rhythm with breathing
  - Use of birth ball
  - Acupuncture
  - Application of hot or cold packs
  - Music and audioanalgesia
- Moderate resource methods:
  - Hypnosis
  - Yoga
  - Acupuncture
  - TENS
  - Sterile water injection
  - Biofeedback
  - Water immersion
  - ***The Bradley method***
  - ***Lamaze approach***
- High resource methods: Includes pharmacological interventions like opioids

II. *Pharmacological*

- Opioids:
  - Meperidine
  - Remifentanyl
  - Butorphanol
  - Fentanyl
  - Nalbuphine
  - Tramadol
- Sedative tranquilizers:
  - Benzodiazepines
  - Hydroxyzine
  - Barbiturates
  - Phenothiazines
- Others: Ketamine

III. *Inhalational Analgesia*

- Entonox
- Sevoflurane (0.8%)
- Isoflurane
- Enflurane (0.25%)
- Desflurane

IV. *Regional Analgesia*

- Epidural analgesia
- Subarachnoid block
- Combined spinal epidural analgesia

- Paracervical block
- Pudendal block
- Lumbar sympathetic block
- Caudal block

V. *Newer Advances*

- Patient controlled analgesia:
  - PCIVA: Patient Controlled IV Analgesia with remifentanyl
  - PCIA: Patient Controlled Inhalation Analgesia with sevoflurane
  - PCEA: Patient Controlled Epidural Analgesia
  - CI-PCEA: Computer Integrated PCEA
  - CI-AMB: Computer Integrated Automated Mandatory Boluses
- Acoustic Puncture Assisted Devices for identifying epidural space
- Ultrasound guided epidural anesthesia
- Transverse abdomen plane block (TAP block)
- EREM: Extended Release Epidural Morphine

Water Immersion

- Involves immersing the parturient in warm water deep enough to cover the abdomen
- This is thought to enhance relaxation and reduce labor pain
- Parturient may remain in the bath for a few minutes to hours during first stage of labor
- Water is kept at or slightly above the body temperature
- This is done to avoid increasing the mothers core temperature
- Analgesia is provided due to the warmth, influencing nociceptive input to brain
- Validation:
  - Water immersion may be offered during first stage of labor to:
    - Healthy parturients
    - Uncomplicated pregnancies
    - Between 37-41 weeks gestation
  - Hydrotherapy is usually safe, but used cautiously due to risk of infection

Hypnosis

- Technique aims at the attainment of an altered state of consciousness
- This prevents normal feelings such as pain from reaching the conscious mind
- Induction of altered state is through the patient herself or the partner
- Methods used to induce hypnosis include:
  - Guided imagery
  - Relaxation audio tapes
- Modulates pain via suppression of neural activity in the anterior cingulate gyrus
- This method is contraindicated in patients with previous history of psychosis
- Validation:
  - It can be used as an adjunct to pharmacological or epidural analgesia
  - Patients using hypnosis usually do not require pharmacological analgesia

Acupuncture

- Form of traditional medicine which deals with a specific type of energy, Qi
- Involves placement of needles at specific points on body, called acupuncture points
- Placement of these needles restores the harmony of Qi energy
- Placement of needles and type of stimulation depends on:
  - Degree and location of pain
  - Stage of labor
  - Level of maternal fatigue
- Validity:
  - Acupuncture was associated with superior pain relief
  - Acupuncture also reduces the requirement for pharmacological analgesia

Biofeedback

- Trains the patient to gain control over physiological responses
- This is done using electronic instruments
- This enables patient to consciously regulate both psychological and physical processes
- Validation:
  - Does not appear to be effective in reducing labor pain
  - Most patients treated with biofeedback require additional analgesia
  - Thus, it may be attempted as an analgesic adjuvant
  - At present, there is insufficient evidence that biofeedback is effective

Transcutaneous Electrical Nerve Stimulation (TENS)

- Involves transmission of low-voltage electrical impulses to skin via surface electrodes
- Impulses are generated with the help of a hand held battery powered generator
- Parturient is allowed to adjust the frequency, intensity and waveform of impulses
- Mechanism of action:
  - Relieves pain through gate-control theory
  - Nociceptive inhibition at presynaptic level in dorsal horn
  - Inhibits propagation of nociception along ummyelinated small fibres
  - Blocks impulses to target cells in substantia gelatinosa
  - Stimulates release of endorphins in the brain
- Method:
  - One pair of electrodes is placed paravertebrally between T_{10}-L_1
  - The second pair is placed at the level of S_2-S_4
  - The parturient controls the intensity of current using a dial
  - Continuous stimulation is self-applied during contractions
  - Intermittent, pulsing stimulation is used in between contractions
  - Stimulation causes a buzzing or pricking sensation
  - This reduces the awareness of contraction pain, thus providing analgesia
- Validity:
  - May provide analgesia during 1st stage of labor
  - Traditionally used as an analgesic adjuvant, not as sole analgesic
  - Found to have no benefit when used as an adjuvant to epidural analgesia

Lamaze Philosophy

- Developed by French obstetrician ***Dr. Fernand Lamaze***
- This is a technique of psychoprophylaxis
- Follows the philosophy that child-birth is a normal, natural and healthy process
- Breathing and relaxation techniques are employed by parturients
- Health practises adopted during labor include:
  - Labor is allowed to begin on its own
  - Walking, moving around and changing positions is recommended
  - Interventions that are not medically necessary are avoided
  - Rooming in of mother and baby is an important part of the Lamaze philosophy

The Bradley Method

- Described by Dr. Robert Bradley, an obstetrician in 1965
- Focuses on methods to achieve natural birth without the use of:
  - Surgery
  - Medication
  - Medical intervention
- Revolves around the principle that birth is a natural process
- Advocates that babies should be brought into the world in an ideal state
- Husbands play an important part in this technique
- Husbands are taught to coach their partner in:
  - Deep breathing and concentrated awareness during labor
  - Ensuring a distraction free environment during childbirth
- Does not support the use of labor analgesia or any other medications during labor

Pharmacological Analgesia

- Meperidine:
  - Most commonly used parenteral opioid
  - Dose:
    - Intermittent boluses:
      - 50–100 mg IM given Q4H
      - Onset of action 30–45 minutes
      - Duration of action 2–3 hours
    - IV-PCA:
      - Bolus dose 15 mg
      - Lockout interval 10 minutes
  - Clinical utility:
    - Less than 20% parturients experience effective analgesia
    - Other opioids may provide better relief compared with meperidine
    - Still remains the *most commonly used opioid* for labor analgesia worldwide
  - Associated with several significant maternal and fetal side effects:
    - Maternal side effects:
      - Seizures
      - Drug interactions

- Fetal side effects:
  - Associated with prolonged fetal side effects
  - This is due to generation of nor-meperidine
  - Greatest risk if meperidine is given 3-5 hours prior to delivery
  - Least risk if administered 1 hour before delivery
  - Side effects may be seen up to 72 hours after delivery
  - Fetal side effects include:
    - Low APGAR scores
    - Reduced fetal aortic flow
    - Reduced fetal muscular activity
    - Loss of beat-to-beat variability in FHR tracings

❖ Fentanyl:

- Analgesic efficacy:
  - 100 times that of morphine
  - 800 times that of meperidine
- Dosage:
  - Intermittent boluses:
    - 50–100 µg IV once every hour or 1 µg/kg
    - Onset of action 3–5 minutes
    - Duration of action 30–60 minutes
  - PCA regimen:
    - Loading dose of 50–100 µg
    - Patient controlled dose of 10–25 µg
    - Lockout interval of 10–12 minutes
- Can be given IV, SC, orally or transdermally
- Preferably used as PCIA due to:
  - Rapid onset
  - High potency
  - Good analgesia
  - Short duration of action
  - Absence of active metabolites
- Clinical utility:
  - Provides an attractive alternative due to pharmacokinetic profile
  - *Effectively used in IV-PCAs* for analgesia
  - Less effective when used as intermittent boluses
- Provides reasonable analgesia with:
  - Minimal neonatal depression
  - Minimal maternal sedation
  - Reduced vomiting

❖ Morphine:

- ***Twilight sleep:***
  - Refers to historical use of morphine with scopolamine during labor
  - Good analgesia is seen in the presence of maternal and fetal depression
  - Technique is associated with:
    - Delirium, extreme agitation
    - Sedation, amnesia
- Dosage:
  - 5–10 mg IM:
    - Time of onset 20–40 minutes
    - Duration of action 3–4 hours
  - 2–5 mg IV:
    - Time of onset 3–5 minutes
    - Duration of action 3–4 hours
- Clinical utility:
  - Good analgesia with morphine is usually obtained only at higher doses
  - There is a lack of analgesic efficacy seen at non-sedating doses
  - Therefore, *not very commonly used* for labor analgesia
- Morphine administration is associated with neonatal and maternal side effects
- Morphine is not routinely used as an infusion in PCAs for labor analgesia
- This is because of morphine-6-glucuronide accumulation
- M-6-G can in turn cause maternal and fetal respiratory depression

❖ Remifentanyl:

- Ultra short acting opioid with rapid onset and offset of action
- Rapid metabolism occurs by maternal non-specific esterases
- This accounts for the ultra short duration of action
- Mostly used in IV-PCA regimens
- Dose:
  - Bolus dose 15–50 µg (0.3–0.5 µg/kg)
  - Lockout interval of 3–5 minutes
  - Onset of action: 30–60 seconds
  - Peak action: 2.5 minutes
  - Context sensitive $T_{1/2}$ 3.5 minutes independent of duration of infusion
- Clinical utility:
  - Bolus dose is self administered at the beginning of one contraction

- Effect of this dose usually lasts during the subsequent contraction
- However, it remains an *inferior alternative to epidural analgesia*
- May be used in patients in whom epidural is contraindicated

- Side effects:
  - Major adverse effects are rare due to short duration of action
  - Respiratory depression is possible due to frequent boluses
  - Overall, fetal side effects are lesser as compared with meperidine

❖ Nalbuphine:
- Mixed agonist-antagonist opioid analgesic
- Agonist-antagonist:
  - Partial κ agonist
  - μ antagonist
  - Minimal affinity
- Analgesic potency of nalbuphine is comparable with morphine
- However, the respiratory depressant effect shows a ceiling effect
- Nalbuphine dose beyond 0.5 mg/kg fails to increase respiratory depression
- This is due to the mixed receptor affinity of nalbuphine
- Dosage:
  - Intermittent boluses:
    - 10–20 mg IV/ IM/ SC Q4-6H
    - Onset of action 2–3 minutes following IV injection
    - Onset of action 15 minutes following IM/ SC injection
    - Duration of action up to 3–6 hours
  - IV-PCA:
    - Bolus dose 1 mg
    - Lockout interval 6–10 minute
- Clinical utility:
  - Analgesia is comparable to that produced by meperidine
  - Associated with lesser nausea and vomiting, compared with meperidine
  - However, patients are more sedated when compared with meperidine
  - It is *not routinely used* for labor analgesia
  - Intermittent nalbuphine boluses is used when epidural and PCA are not options

❖ Butorphanol:
- Agonist: Antagonist:
  - Partial κ agonist
  - μ antagonist
  - Minimal α affinity
- Pharmacodynamic properties resemble that of nalbuphine
- Similar to nalbuphine, respiratory depressant action has ceiling effect
- Beyond a 2 mg dose, respiratory depression action of butorphanol plateaus
- Analgesic potency:
  - 5 times as potent as morphine
  - 40 times as potent as meperidine
- Dosage:
  - 1–2 mg IM/IV
  - Duration of action 4 hours
- Clinical utility:
  - Produces analgesic effect comparable to meperidine
  - However, adverse effects are fewer compared with meperidine
  - *Not routinely used* for labor analgesia

❖ Phenothiazines:
- Most commonly used phenothiazine is promethazine
- 25–50 mg IV/IM promethazine is used clinically
- This dose results in profound sedation and respiratory stimulation
- The respiratory stimulation is useful to counter opioid induced depression
- Clinical utility:
  - Rarely used nowadays as the sole analgesic
  - Used *most commonly in combination with opioids* for:
    - Additive sedation
    - Prevention of nausea and vomiting
    - Respiratory stimulation
- Disadvantages:
  - Produces profound maternal sedation
  - Can cause variation in FHR

❖ Ketamine:
- Potent analgesic which preserves airway reflexes
- However, increase in airway secretions may cause laryngospasm
- Dosage:
  - Intermittent boluses:
    - 0.2–0.5 mg/kg IV
    - Can be repeated every 2–5 minutes up to total of 1 mg/kg in 30 minutes

- Continuous infusion:
  - Bolus dose 0.1 mg/kg
  - Followed by infusion of 0.2 mg/kg/hour titrated to effect
- Clinical utility:
  - Rarely used as the sole analgesic agent
  - Usually used to supplement incomplete neuraxial block
  - Causes hypertension and psychomimetic effects
  - Therefore, it is not routinely used for labor analgesia

❖ Tramadol:
- It is an atypical weak synthetic opioid
- Has a low μ receptor affinity
- 10% as potent as morphine
- Dosage:
  - 1–2 mg/kg IV/IM
  - Onset of action within 10 minutes of IV administration
  - Duration of action 2–3 hours
- Clinical utility:
  - *Not very useful* for labor analgesia
  - Analgesic profile is inferior to meperidine
  - Causes more nausea and vomiting compared with meperidine
- Causes no clinically significant respiratory depression at normal doses

❖ Benzodiazepines:
- Clinical utility: *Not routinely used* as:
  - High incidence of maternal and fetal side effects
  - Non-preference for a sedated parturient in active labor
- Maternal side effects:
  - Sedation, hypnosis
  - Cyanosis and amnesia
- Fetal side effects:
  - Neonatal hypotonicity
  - Respiratory depression
  - Impaired thermoregulation

❖ Meptazinol:
- Mixed agonist-antagonist activity
- Partial opioid agonist at μ receptors
- Dosage:
  - 100 mg given IM
  - Onset of action 15 minutes after IM administration
  - Duration of action 2–3 hours
- Clinical utility:
  - Produces less neonatal depression compared with meperidine
  - Analgesic profile is also better than meperidine
  - However, it is neither widely available nor used for labor analgesia

Inhalational Analgesia

❖ Entonox:
- 50% $N_2O : O_2$ mixture
- Was used both as sole analgesic and as adjuvant earlier
- Maximal effect after 45–60 mins
- Important to use entonox at early onset of contraction
- Use discontinued after peak of contraction
- Causes nausea, dizziness, dysphoria, lack of cooperation
- OT pollution
- Not routinely used
- Used now as adjunct or when regional analgesia not possible

❖ Volatile anesthetics:
- Not routinely used
- Sevoflurane 0.8% most commonly used
- Isoflurane and enflurane (0.2–0.25%) and desflurane (0.2%)
- Causes more intense sedation, unpleasant smell, OT pollution
- Unconsciousness and loss of airway reflexes occur if accidental overdose
- PCIA uses sevoflurane and special vapourizes

Regional Anesthesia

I. *Epidural Analgesia*

❖ Indicated when patient is in active labor:
- Cervix 5–6 cm dilated in primigravida
- Cervix 3–4 cm in multigravida

❖ Required level of analgesia:
- $T_{10} - L_1$ level required for 1st stage of labor
- S_2-S_3 level required in 2nd stage of labor

❖ Advantages:
- Good analgesia
- Stable therapeutic analgesic level without fluctuations in pain relief
- Minimizes motor block: allows greater patient mobility

- Minimizes hypotensive episodes
- Reduces stress response
- Avoids parenteral drug therapy

❖ Disadvantages:
- Subarachnoid puncture or migration of catheter
- Longer time for onset of analgesia
- Catheter related infections

❖ Epidural analgesia regimen:
- Initial bolus:
  - 10–15 mL bupivacaine 0.0625–0.125% with 50–100 µg fentanyl
  - 10–15 mL ropivacaine 0.1-0.2 % with 50–100 µg fentanyl
- Maintenance dose:
  - Bupivacaine 0.0625–0.125% with fentanyl 1–2 µg/mL at 10–15 mL/hour
  - Alternatively, intermittent boluses may be injected as per requirement

❖ Patient Controlled Epidural Analgesia (PCEA) regimen:
- Initial bolus:
  - 10–15 mL bupivacaine 0.0625–0.125% with 50–100 µg fentanyl
  - 10–15 mL ropivacaine 0.1–0.2 % with 50–100 µg fentanyl
- Maintenance:
  - Basal infusion of 5–10 mL/hour 0.0625–0.125% bupivacaine
  - Demand bolus of 5–10 mL 0.0625–0.125% bupivacaine
  - Lockout interval of 5–15 minutes
  - Total 1 hour lockout of 20–25 mL 0.0625–0.125% bupivacaine

II. *Subarachnoid Block*

❖ Clinical utility:
- Useful as it provides immediate analgesia of a wider dermatome (T_{10}-S_5)
- Effective alternative when placement of epidural catheter is not feasible
- Single shot spinal analgesia is rarely indicated
- Continuous spinal analgesia is avoided due to high risk of complications
- Therefore, SAB is *rarely used outside the premise of operative delivery*

❖ Spinal analgesia is useful for:
- Multiparous women in rapidly progressing labor
- Primipara in advanced labor (fully dilated and significant pain)
- High likelihood of emergent operative delivery
- Following accidental dural puncture during epidural analgesia
- When epidural catheter placement is technically difficult:
  - Patients with abnormal anatomy
  - Post extensive spine surgery

❖ Saddle block (sacral-only anesthesia):
- Indications:
  - Forceps delivery
  - Repair of vaginal/rectal tears postpartum
  - Removal of placenta
- Regimen used for saddle block:
  - Hyperbaric bupivacaine 4–5 mg
  - Hyperbaric lidocaine 15–20 mg
  - Hyperbaric tetracaine 3 mg
  - Opioid additive can be used with the local anesthetic:
    - Fentanyl 10–25 µg or
    - Sufentanil 2.5–5 µg
- Injection of the drug is followed by the patient sitting up to establish block
- This allows accomplishment of sacral-only anesthesia

❖ Continuous spinal analgesia:
- Rarely used due to high incidence of complications
- Usually performed using 19–20 G epidural catheters
- The placement of these catheters requires 17–18 G spinal needles
- But the risk of PDPH is increased in this case due to larger dural rent
- 28–32 G microcatheters are rarely used due to risk of cauda equina syndrome
- Regimen:
  - Induction of analgesia is with hyperbaric bupivacaine 2.5–7.5 mg
  - Maintenance:
    - Intermittent boluses:
      - 0.5–1.5 mL 0.1–0.25% bupivacaine
      - 10–20 µg fentanyl may be added to the injection
    - Continuous infusion:
      - 0.0625–0.125% bupivacaine with 2 µg/mL fentanyl
      - Continuous infusion given at 1–5 mL/hour

- Advantages:
  - Provision of rapid analgesia
  - Allows flexibility in dosing
  - Limits degree of sympathectomy and hypotension
- Disadvantages:
  - Risk of PDPH as large needles are used for insertion of the catheter
  - Cauda equina syndrome: more common with:
    - Use of intrathecal lidocaine
    - Use of high concentrations of lidocaine
    - Use of finer gauge microcatheters (28–32 G)
    - Continuous infusions (rather than intermittent boluses)
    - This causes drug pooling around nerves of the cauda equina

III. *Combined Spinal Epidural*

- Includes intrathecal injection of drugs to initiate spinal analgesia
- This is followed by insertion of epidural catheter to allow:
  - Maintenance of analgesia
  - Conversion to surgical anesthesia
- CSE regimens commonly used:
  - Initial spinal injection:
    - 2.5–10 µg sufentanyl or 10–25 µg fentanyl alone or combined with 1–2.5 mg plain bupivacaine
    - This provides initial analgesia for approximately 60–90 minutes
  - Maintenance analgesia:
    - Usually 0.0625–0.125% bupivacaine with 2 µg/mL fentanyl is used
    - Alternatively 0.08–0.1% ropivacaine with 2 g/mL fentanyl can be used
    - 10–20 mL of this mixture can be injected to initiate the epidural
    - Alternatively, continuous infusion at 8–15 mL/hour can be used
- Indicated in:
  - Very early stage of labor when local anesthetics are avoided
  - Advanced stage when rapid analgesia required
  - Difficult epidural as it reduces failure rate of epidural
- Methods of CSE:
  - Epidural catheter followed by SAB at lower interspace
  - Epidural needle besides spinal needle at same interspace
  - Needle through needle technique at same interspace (preferred)
- Advantages:
  - Rapid onset of analgesia within 5 minutes
  - Duration of action of subarachnoid block 2–3 hours
  - Absence of significant motor block in most cases
  - Makes ambulation possible due to limited motor block
  - Reduces complications of epidural anesthesia:
    - Patchy block
    - Poor sacral spread
  - Reduces duration of 1st stage of labor
  - Same catheter can be used for operative anesthesia if required
- Disadvantages:
  - Potential for complications arising due to deliberate dural puncture
  - Risk of total spinal:
    - Epidural catheter remains untested at the time of insertion
    - This is because spinal injection during insertion precludes testing
    - Thus, subsequent epidural injection has to be done cautiously
  - Inadvertent spread of local anesthetic through dural rent into CSF fluid
  - Complications due to intrathecal administration of opioids
  - Increased risk of maternal respiratory depression
  - Increased incidence of fetal bradycardia

IV. *Caudal Anesthesia*

- Clinical utility:
  - *Rarely used,* unless lumbar epidural is contraindicated or technically difficult
  - However, it remains a useful option for analgesia once labor is established
- ***Double catheter technique***:
  - Used in the past
  - Lumbar epidural catheter was placed for early labor analgesia
  - Caudal epidural was placed to ensure analgesia at the time of delivery
  - This allowed higher dermatomal analgesia (T_{10}-L_1) during early labor

- During later stages caudal activation permits parturient to feel contractions
- At the same time, profound perineal analgesia is provided

❖ Regimen:
- 10–15 mL bupivacaine 0.0625–0.125% with 50–100 µg fentanyl
- 10–15 mL ropivacaine 0.1–0.2 % with 50–100 µg fentanyl
- 15–20 mL local anesthetic volume is required to ensure a block level upto T_{10}

❖ Advantages:
- Onset of perineal analgesia is more rapid, compared with lumbar epidural
- Allows parturient to feel uterine contractions
- At the same time it provides dense perineal analgesia

❖ Disadvantages:
- Associated with higher incidence of CNS toxicity
- Inadequate during early phases of labor

V. *Paracervical Block*

❖ Can be used as an alternative when neuraxial blockade contraindicated

❖ Technique:
- Local anesthetic injected submucosally into fornix for vagina. lateral to cervix

❖ Injections are carried out at 3 and 9 o'clock positions

❖ 5–10 mL of 1.5% chloroprocaine or 1% mepivacaine is used

❖ Bupivacaine is avoided due to high incidence of maternal systemic absorption

❖ Clinical utility:
- Blocks transmission through the paracervical ganglion
- This is also called ***Frankenhauser's ganglion***
- This ganglion carries visceral sensory nerve fibres from:
  - Uterus, cervix
  - Upper vagina
- Thus, it is very effective during the first stage of labor
- However, somatic sensory fibres from the perineum are not blocked
- Thus, it is ineffective during the second stage of labor
- *Rarely used nowadays* due to fetal bradycardia

❖ Advantages:
- Provides good analgesia during 1st stage of labor
- Simple to perform, does not affect progress of labor

❖ Disadvantages:
- No pain relief offered during 2nd stage of labor
- Close proximity of injection site to uterine artery makes it technically difficult
- Relatively high incidence of fetal bradycardia

❖ Complications:
- Profound fetal bradycardia
- Local anesthetic systemic toxicity (LAST)
- Postpartum neuropathy
- Infection

VI. *Pudendal Nerve Block*

❖ Clinical utility:
- Usually administered during second stage of labor
- Alleviates pain from lower vagina and perineum
- However, clinical efficacy is limited compared to neuraxial analgesia
- Thus, *rarely used for labor analgesia* nowadays
- However, it also causes motor blockade of:
  - Perineal muscles
  - External anal sphincter

❖ Technique:
- Through transvaginal approach in lithotomy position
- Ischial spine is palpated transvaginally/transrectally

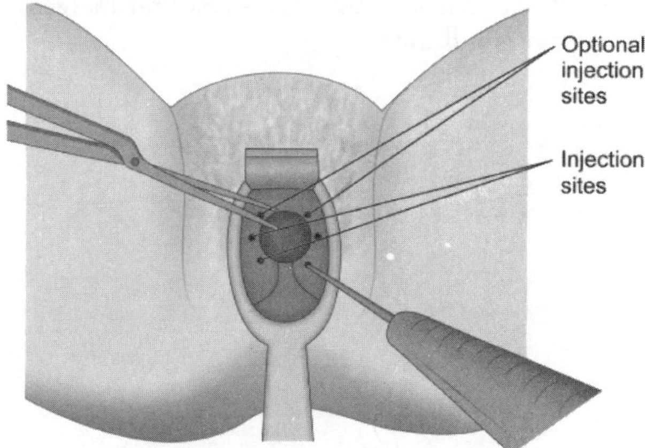

Fig. 7: Paracervical block.

- Needle guide (***Iowa trumpet***) is placed under ischial spine
- 20 G needle is passed through the guide until tip lies on the vaginal mucosa
- Needle is advanced 1–1.5 cm, piercing the sacrospinous ligament
- 10 mL of 1% lidocaine or mepivacaine, or 2% chloroprocaine is injected
- Local anesthetic is therefore deposited behind sacrospinous ligament
- The procedure is repeated on the opposite side

❖ Satisfactory analgesia for:
- Spontaneous vaginal delivery
- Outlet forceps delivery
- Vacuum delivery

❖ Not useful for:
- Mid-pelvic forceps delivery
- Repair of cervical or upper vaginal laceration
- Manual removal of retained placenta

❖ Complications:
- LAST
- Infection
- Hematoma
- Sciatic nerve block

VII. *Lumbar Sympathetic Block*

❖ Clinical utility:
- Bilateral lumbar sympathetic block may be used during first stage of labor
- This must be supplemented during second stage of labor with:
  - Pudendal nerve block
  - Spinal analgesia
- *Rarely used nowadays* unless epidural analgesia is contraindicated

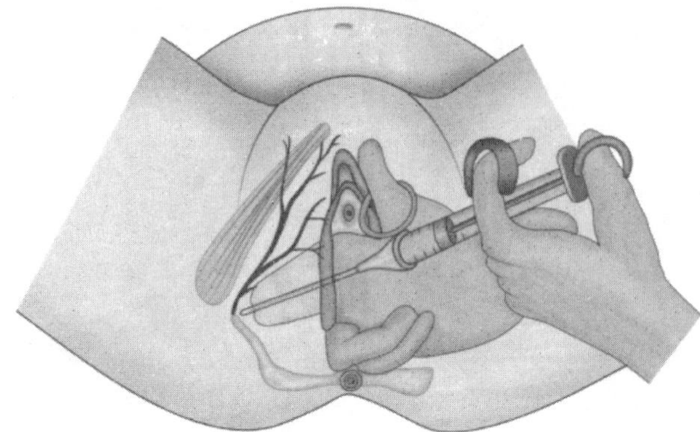

Fig. 8: Pudendal nerve block.

❖ Technique:
- Technically difficult to perform
- Performed at the level of L_2, using a 22 G, 10 cm needle
- Transverse spinous process is used as the landmark to guide needle placement
- Injection is performed anterior to medial attachment of psoas muscle
- Injection is performed on both sides
- Total of 20 mL 0.0625–0.125% bupivacaine is divided between the 2 sides

❖ Advantages:
- Fewer complications than paracervical block
- Useful when epidural analgesia has failed due to prior spine surgery

❖ Disadvantages:
- Technically more difficult to perform
- More painful needle placement
- Does not provide second stage analgesia
- Accelerates first stage of labor
- Thus, it should be used cautiously in rapidly progressive labor

PARACERVICAL BLOCK

Introduction

❖ Paracervical block is used to provide analgesia during the first stage of labor

❖ Can be used as an alternative when neuraxial blockade contraindicated

❖ Technically easy to perform and can be done by the obstetrician

Anatomy

❖ Upper vagina, cervix and lower uterus are innervated by the paracervical plexus

❖ This is also called ***Frankenhauser's plexus***

❖ This plexus contains fibres derived from:

❖ Inferior hypogastric plexus (T10-L1)

❖ Sacral nerve roots (S1-S4)

❖ This block however, does not affect the motor pathways

❖ Thus, progress of labor is not significantly affected

Indications

❖ Useful for procedures involving cervical dilatation or manipulation such as:
- Medical termination of pregnancy

- Hysteroscopy
- Cervical ablation or excision
- Intrauterine device placement

❖ First stage labor analgesia (not preferred nowadays due to fetal bradycardia)

Technique

❖ General preparation:
- Performed with the patient in lithotomy position
- Strict aseptic precautions are followed
- Vaginal speculum maybe used to provide exposure

❖ Approach:
- Local anesthetic injected submucosally into fornix for vagina, lateral to cervix
- Two point technique: Injections are given at 3 and 9 o'clock positions
- Four point technique: Injections are given at 2, 4, 8 and 10 o'clock positions
- Two point technique is preferred as:
  - It avoids multiple painful injections
  - Has similar efficacy to four point injection
- 5–10 mL of 1% lidocaine, 1.5% chloroprocaine or 1% mepivacaine is used
- Bupivacaine is avoided due to high incidence of maternal systemic absorption

Clinical Utility

❖ Blocks transmission through the paracervical ganglion

❖ This ganglion carries visceral sensory nerve fibres from:
- Uterus, cervix
- Upper vagina

❖ Thus, paracervical block is very effective during the first stage of labor

❖ However, somatic sensory fibres from the perineum are not blocked

❖ Thus, it is ineffective during the second stage of labor

❖ Onset of analgesia is rapid within 2–5 minutes of injection

❖ Duration of analgesia is dependent on the local anesthetic used

Advantages

❖ Provides good analgesia during 1st stage of labor

❖ Simple to perform, does not affect progress of labor

Disadvantages

❖ No pain relief offered during 2nd stage of labor

❖ Close proximity of injection site to uterine artery makes it technically dangerous

❖ Relatively high incidence of fetal bradycardia

Complications

❖ Profound fetal bradycardia

❖ Local anesthetic systemic toxicity (LAST)

❖ Cervical shock:
- Occurs due to failure of paracervical block
- Due to inadequate analgesia during gynecological procedures

❖ Postpartum neuropathy

❖ Infection

PUDENDAL NERVE BLOCK

Introduction

❖ Involves blocking the pudendal nerve which supplies lower vagina, perineum and vulva

❖ Typically performed by the obstetrician

Anatomy

❖ Pudendal nerve ($S_{2,3,4}$) supplies sensory and motor supply to:
- Lower vagina
- Vulva
- Perineum

❖ Nerve crosses posterior to sacrospinous ligament

❖ It lies in close relation to attachment of the ligament with ischial spine

❖ LA is injected around the trunk of pudendal nerve, posterior to sacrospinous ligament

Indications

❖ Minor procedures involving the perineum

❖ Spontaneous vaginal delivery

❖ Outlet forceps delivery

❖ Vacuum delivery

❖ Perineal repair following delivery

❖ Diagnosing and treating suspected pudendal neuralgia

Clinical Utility

❖ Ineffective for pain associated with uterine contractions in the first stage of labor

❖ Usually administered during the second stage of labor

- Effectively alleviates pain from lower vagina and perineum
- This was the preferred analgesic modality for second stage prior to adoption of neuraxial methods
- Within 5 minutes of performing the injection, analgesia is obtained
- Maximal analgesia is obtained after 10–20 minutes
- Average duration of lidocaine induced pudendal analgesia is 30–60 minutes
- Clinical efficacy is however, limited compared to neuraxial analgesia
- Pudendal nerve block is associated with motor blockade of:
  - Perineal muscles
  - External anal sphincter
- Clinical utility is limited for:
  - Mid-pelvic forceps delivery
  - Repair of cervical or upper vaginal laceration
  - Manual removal of retained placenta

Technique

- General preparation:
  - Performed with the patient in lithotomy position
  - Usually performed bilaterally
  - Ipsilateral blocks can be given when unilateral procedures are planned
  - Strict aseptic precautions are followed
- Approaches:
  - Can be performed through transvaginal/ transperineal approach
  - When fetal head has descended, transvaginal approach is not used
  - Transperineal approach is used in these circumstances
- Transvaginal approach:
  - Ischial spine is palpated along posterolateral vaginal sidewall
  - Needle guide (***Iowa trumpet***) is placed against the vaginal mucosa
  - Guide is positioned on sacrospinous ligament, 1 cm medial and inferior to ischial spine
  - 20 G needle is passed through the guide until tip lies on the vaginal mucosa
  - Needle is advanced 1–1.5 cm, piercing the sacrospinous ligament
  - 10 mL of 1% lidocaine or mepivacaine, or 2% chloroprocaine is injected
  - Local anesthetic is therefore deposited behind sacrospinous ligament
  - The procedure is repeated on the opposite side for bilateral blocks
- Transperineal approach:
  - Ischial spine is palpated through the rectum
  - The point of entry lies 2.5 cm posteromedial to ischial tuberosity
  - A 20 G needle is introduced at right angles to the skin
  - The needle is then advanced lateral to guiding finger
  - The needle is directed to the ischial spine transcutaneously
  - The sacrospinous ligament is then pierced by advancing the needle
  - 10 mL of 1% lidocaine or mepivacaine, or 2% chloroprocaine is injected
  - The procedure is repeated on the opposite side for bilateral blocks
  - The success rate is much lesser with the transperineal approach

Advantages

- Relatively easy to perform
- No effects on uterine contractions or progress of labor
- Minimal side effects on fetus

Disadvantages

- Limited utility during first stage of labor
- High rate of unilateral or bilateral block failure (10–50%)
- High rate of complications:
  - Accidental fetal injection through the fontanelle
  - LAST
  - Infection
  - Hematoma
  - Nerve injury: can cause sacral neuropathy

WALKING EPIDURAL

Introduction

- Term first used for low-dose combined spinal epidural technique using opioid, used for labor analgesia as motor function was maintained, which allowed maternal ambulation
- Currently used to describe any neuraxial technique which allows safe ambulation
- Also called ***minimal motor block epidural***

Indications

- Early in labor when local anesthetics are not preferred
- Late in labor when immediate analgesia required
- Difficult epidural as the initial intrathecal injection reduces failure rate of epidural
- Initial profound analgesia required but ongoing analgesia not required for sometime (e.g., Artificial Rupture of Membranes in anxious mother)
- Where rapid analgesia required and epidural catheter may be useful for later intervention (trial for forceps extraction where Cesarean section may follow)

Techniques

- Epidural catheter at higher space, SAB at one interspace lower
- Epidural catheter besides spinal needle in same space
- Needle through needle technique in same space (preferred technique)

Dosages

- For initial subarachnoid block:
  - Fentanyl 10–15 μg
  - Sufentanyl 5–10 μg
- For later epidural block:
  - 0.0625–0.125% bupivacaine at 8–15 mL/hour
  - 2 μg/mL fentanyl can be used as opioid adjuvant

Criteria for Ambulation

- Maternal criteria:
  - Maternal desire to ambulate
  - No obstetric or medical contraindications
  - Presence of second person to walk with patient
  - Ambulate only when spinal anesthesia given with only opioids
  - Avoid when spinal anesthesia is given with local anesthetics
  - Ability to sustain straight leg raising test > 10 seconds against resistance
  - Ability to perform partial knee bends at bedside using step stool
  - Stable orthostatic vital signs: asymptomatic and within 10% of baseline
- Fetal criteria:
  - Reassuring fetal status
  - Engagement of fetal presenting part
  - Intermittent fetal heart rate monitoring (every 15 minutes)

Advantages

Maternal

- Rapid onset of analgesia
- Reduces chances of patchy/unilateral block as with plain epidural
- Lesser amount of local anesthetic in systemic circulation
- Reduced motor block
- Better hemodynamic stability
- Ability to ambulate and void urine: avoids urinary catheterization
- Reduced residual urinary volume
- Analgesia can be prolonged using epidural catheter
- Same catheter can be used for operative analgesia
- Greater maternal satisfaction
- Feeling of self control

Obstetric

- Reduced duration of 1st stage of labor
- Enhanced rate of cervical dilation due to gravity
- Correct positioning of fetal head due to gravity
- Lesser need for augmentation
- Reduced need for assisted deliveries
- Improved APGAR scores

Side Effects

- Pruritus, nausea and vomiting, respiratory depression
- Urinary retention
- Hypotension, PDPH
- FHR abnormalities and fetal bradycardia
- Costly kits
- Epidural hematoma
- Broken catheter

Contraindications

- Coagulopathy
- Abruptio placentae
- Platelet count < 1,00,000/mm^3
- Hemodynamically unstable patient
- Non-reassuring fetal heart rate
- Patient refusal
- Medical/obstetric contraindications to ambulation
- Technique: As for continuous spinal epidural
- Monitoring: As for continuous spinal epidural

TOCOLYTICS

Introduction

- These are drugs which prevent preterm labor by suppressing uterine contraction
- Tocolytic drugs reduce the frequency and strength of uterine contractions
- Preterm labor is defined as:
  - Labor between 20–37 completed wks from 1st day of last menstrual period with:
    - Regular uterine contraction at least 30 seconds duration every 10 min
    - Cervical effacement/dilation
- Low Birth Weight (LBW) if birth weight < 2500 g
- Very Low Birth Weight (VLBW) if birth weight < 1500 g

Risk Factors for Preterm Labor

- History of previous preterm delivery
- Smoking, low socio-economic status
- Subclinical chorio-aminotis, genital infection, pyelonephritis
- Infection/thrombosis of placenta
- Placenta previa/abruption
- Pregnancy Induced Hypertension
- Antepartum Hemorrhage
- Cervical incompetence

Indications for Tocolytics

Prolonged Tocolysis

- Fetus < 2500 g
- 22–34 weeks gestational age
- Intact membrane
- Documented contraction
- Cervical effacement > 80%
- Cervical dilation 2–4 cm

Short-term Tocolysis

- Fetal distress: To prepare for immediate delivery
- In utero fetal surgery
- EXIT procedures
- Patient transfer to better setup
- Postoperative tocolysis

Contraindications for Tocolysis

- Fetal anomalies incompatible with life
- Non reassuring fetal status
- Intrauterine fetal demise
- Preeclampsia with severe features of eclampsia
- Maternal hemorrhage with hemodynamic instability
- Intra-amniotic infection
- Medical contraindications to the tocolytic drug

Goals of Tocolytic Therapy 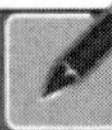

- To delay delivery by at least 48 hours to allow antenatal steroids to achieve maximal effects
- Provide for safe transport of mother to higher facility
- To prolong pregnancy in conditions which cause labor such as:
  - Acute pyelonephritis
  - Abdominal surgery
  - Recurrent preterm labor

Drugs Used for Tocolysis

- β_2 adrenergic agonists:
  - Ritodrine
  - Terbutaline
  - Salbutamol
- Calcium channel blockers: Nifedipine
- Oxytocin antagonists: Atosiban
- COX inhibitors:
  - Indomethacin
  - Sulindac
  - Aspirin
  - Ketorolac
- Nitric oxide donors: Nitroglycerine IV 30–50 µg bolus or 200–400 µg sublingually
- Magnesium sulphate

Calcium Channel Blockers

- Introduction:
  - Nifedipine is most commonly used and extensively studied
  - CCBs have a low incidence of significant maternal and fetal side effects
  - Thus, they are slowly becoming the first line of therapy for tocolysis
- Mechanism of action:
  - Block calcium selective aqueous voltage dependant cell membrane channels
  - CCBs also prevent release of calcium from the sarcoplasmic reticulum
  - This results in a reduction in the intracellular calcium levels
  - This reduces the intracellular actin-myosin interaction
  - This causes relaxation of uterine smooth muscle
- Dose (nifedipine):
  - Induction dose: 20–30 mg PO
  - Maintenance dose: 10–20 mg Q4-6H PO

- Side effects:
  - Has fewer side effects compared with beta blockers
  - Hypotension is most common side effect
  - Most other side effects are mild
  - These include:
    - Headache, flushing
    - Dizziness, nausea
  - Safe side effect profile makes it tocolytic agent of choice

Cycloxygenase Inhibitors

- Introduction:
  - Indomethacin is the prototype COX inhibitor used for tocolysis
  - Sulindac and ketorolac are also effective tocolytic agents
- Mechanism of action:
  - Inhibit COX enzyme, thus preventing synthesis of prostaglandins
  - PGE_2 and $PGF_2\alpha$ are important precipitants of uterine contractions
  - Thus, by inhibiting prostaglandin synthesis, tocolysis is ensured
- Dose:
  - Indomethacin:
    - Induction dose: 50–100 mg PO/ PR
    - Maintenance dose: 25–50 mg Q4H
  - Ketorolac:
    - Induction dose: 60 mg IM
    - Maintenance dose: 30 mg PO Q6H
  - Sulindac:
    - Induction dose: 200 mg PO
    - Maintenance dose: 200 mg PO Q12H
- Side effects:
  - Maternal side effects are minimal
  - Transient inhibition of platelet aggregation may result
  - Premature closure of ductus arteriosus in-utero is possible
  - Other fetal complications include:
    - Oligohydramnios, reduced fetal urine output
    - Intraventricular hemorrhage, necrotizing enterocolitis

Beta Adrenergic Agonists

- Introduction:
  - Ritodrine and terbutaline were used extensively in the past
  - However, maternal side effects have substantially reduced their usage
- Mechanism of action:
  - These drugs act on β_2 receptors present on uterine smooth muscle
  - Stimulation of these receptors results in relaxation of uterine smooth muscle
  - This is responsible for the tocolytic action of β_2 agonists
- Dose (terbutaline):
  - Induction dose: 0.25 mg subcutaneously
  - Maintenance dose: 0.25 mg subcutaneously Q2-3 H
- Maternal side effects:
  - Hypotension, tachycardia
  - Pulmonary edema
  - Hyperglycemia, hypokalemia

Magnesium Sulphate

- Mechanism of action:
  - Functions as an antagonist of calcium at the motor end-plate and cell membrane
  - This reduces calcium influx into the myocyte
  - Mg^{2+} also competes with Ca^{2+} for binding sites on sarcoplasmic reticulum
  - This prevents the rise in free intracellular calcium concentration
  - Magnesium decreases release of acetylcholine at the neuromuscular junction
  - The sensitivity of motor end plate to acetylcholine is also reduced
  - Thus, magnesium has a multi-pronged action causing tocolysis
- Dose:
  - Induction dose: 4–6 g IV bolus over 20 minutes
  - Maintenance: 2–4 g/Hr IV as continuous infusion
- Side effects:
  - Causes less frequent and less severe side effects, compared with β-agonists
  - Palpitations, nausea, blurred vision
  - Transient hypotension, pulmonary edema
  - Should be used with caution in patients with renal dysfunction

Oxytocin Antagonists

- Atosiban is a competitive oxytocin antagonist
- It binds to both decidual and myometrial receptors
- However, it does not alter the subsequent sensitivity of myometrium to oxytocin
- This is important as it reduces the risk of post-partum uterine atony and hemorrhage
- Phase II and III trial have shown it to be an effective tocolytic agent

- It has few maternal side effects and undergoes minimal placental transfer
- Atosiban has a tocolytic efficacy similar to CCBs and β blockers
- This drug has not yet been approved by the FDA due to risk of perinatal deaths
- However, it is extensively used in Europe

Anesthetic Considerations of Tocolytic Drug Co-Therapy

- β_2 AGONISTS:
  - Tachycardia:
    - Delay anesthetic induction after discontinuation of β-agonist therapy
    - This allows time for tachycardia to subside
    - A delay of 15 minutes is warranted to allow the heart rate to settle
    - Depth of anesthesia becomes difficult to assess due to tachycardia
    - This may result in over administration of sedative agents
    - Avoid co-therapy with drugs which cause tachycardia such as:
      - Atropine
      - Glycopyrrolate
      - Pancuronium
    - Avoid halothane as it sensitizes myocardium to catecholamine-induced arrhythmias
    - Ectopics and atrial fibrillation is possible with β_2 agonist therapy
  - Fluid therapy:
    - Tachycardia should not be misconstrued as a sign of hypovolemia
    - Avoid aggressive hydration preoperatively
    - This may precipitate pulmonary edema
    - Risk of fluid overload is high due to increased ADH activity
  - Avoid hyperventilation:
    - Hyperventilation exacerbates hypokalemia
    - This may potentiate hyperpolarization of the cell membrane
- Calcium channel blockers:
  - Co-administration of volatile agents with CCBs may result in:
    - Hypotension
    - Vasodilatation
    - Myocardial depression
    - Conduction defects
  - Increased postpartum hemorrhage may result from CCBs due to uterine atony
  - These drugs potentiate neuromuscular blocking agents
  - When co-administered with $MgSO_4$, they may *cause* neuromuscular blockade
- COX inhibitors:
  - Effects of indomethacin therapy on platelet function are transient
  - Epidural anesthesia in patients receiving low dose COX inhibitors is safe
  - Increased chances of post partum hemorrhage however exists
- Magnesium sulphate:
  - Magnesium therapy has to be discontinued prior to induction
  - This is because it causes hypotension due to generalized vasodilatation
  - Hypotension may be profound following administration of SAB
  - Magnesium also increases sensitivity to NMBAs as:
    - It attenuates the release of ACH at NMJ
    - Reduces sensitivity of motor end plate to ACH
    - Decreases excitability of muscle membrane
  - This sensitization occurs with both depolarizing and non-depolarizing agents
  - Magnesium therapy also reduces postoperative analgesic requirement
  - Magnesium increases PPH due to increased uterine blood flow

Choice of Tocolytic Agents 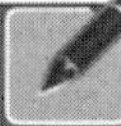

- 24–32 weeks gestational age:
  - Indomethacin is preferred as first line therapy
  - However, indomethacin is not used for more than 72 hours
  - This is due to fear of premature closure of fetal ductus arteriosus
  - In patients with medical contraindications to indomethacin, nifedipine is used
  - Nifedipine is used as second line therapy in case of failure of first line therapy
- 32–34 weeks gestational age:
  - Nifedipine is used as first line therapy between 32-34 weeks gestational age
  - Terbutaline is used as second line therapy in case of failure of first line therapy
  - However, first line therapy is stopped prior to initiation of second line drugs
  - This is because of:
    - Absence of evidence of efficacy of concurrent therapy
    - Increased risk of side effects

Drug	Contraindications	Maternal side effects	Fetal side effects
CCBs	Cardiac disease	Transient hypotension	None
	Renal disease	Flushing, headache	
	Maternal hypotension	Nausea, dizziness	
Beta blockers	Arrhythmias	Arrhythmias, hypotension	Tachycardia
	Poorly controlled thyroid	Pulmonary edema	Myocardial hypertrophy
	Uncontrolled DM	Hyperglycemia, hypokalemia	Myocardial ischemia
		Tremors, palpitations	Hyperglycemia
		Altered thyroid function	
Magnesium sulphate	Myasthenia gravis	Flushing, lethargy, headache	Lethargy, hypotonia
	Myotonic dystrophy	Weakness, diplopia, dry mouth	Respiratory depression
			Demineralization

Efficacy of Tocolytic Agents

- Tocolytic drugs are effective for delaying delivery for 48 hours, upto 7 days
- However, they may not be effective for delaying delivery to 37 weeks
- Also, tocolytic therapy does not alter other important clinical outcomes such as:
  - Neonatal respiratory distress
  - Neonatal survival

ANTICOAGULATION IN PREGNANCY

Introduction

- Pregnancy is a hypercoagulable prothrombotic state
- There is almost a five-fold increase in risk of VTE during pregnancy
- This risk remains elevated until 12 weeks post-partum
- However, multiple risks are associated with anticoagulation during pregnancy:
  - Teratogenic effects on the fetus
  - Hemorrhage during labor
- Thus, anticoagulation during pregnancy should be carefully titrated to minimize maternal and fetal risk

Indications

- Prophylaxis for DVT and pulmonary embolism
- Therapy for DVT and pulmonary embolism
- Inherited thrombophilia
- Sickle cell disease
- Atrial fibrillation
- Prosthetic heart valves
- Antiphospholipid antibody syndrome

Choice of Anticoagulants

- Warfarin:
  - Warfarin crosses placenta and can cause fetal anticoagulation
  - Associated with teratogenicity ***(Contradi syndrome/Warfarin Embryopathy)***
  - Warfarin administration during pregnancy is associated with:
    - Teratogenic effects in first trimester
    - Fetal bleeding and intracranial hemorrhage at later stages of pregnancy
  - Thus, it is generally not used during pregnancy
  - It may be used in mechanical valve recipients with a high risk of thrombosis
  - Does not cross over into breast milk
  - Not contraindicated during postpartum period
  - Can be restarted 7 days after delivery
  - Warfarin is indicated throughout pregnancy only for patients with:
    - Mechanical valve with past history of clot
    - Older generation prosthetic valve
- Low molecular weight heparin:
  - LMWH are preferred over UFH except during the peri-partum period
  - This is because:
    - LMWH heparin produces a more predictable response
    - Thus, it does not require frequent monitoring
    - Also associated with lower incidence of HIT

- LMWH does not cross the placenta and cause fetal anticoagulation
- Can cause significant maternal hemorrhage and osteoporosis rarely

❖ Unfractionated heparin:
- Preferred over LMWH in patients with severe renal dysfunction
- This is due to combined renal and hepatic elimination of UFH
- LMWH on the other hand have exclusive renal elimination
- Does not cross placenta to cause fetal anticoagulation
- Can cause maternal hemorrhage/osteoporosis/HIT
- Relative heparin resistance occurs in pregnancy
- Reversal of anticoagulation before delivery makes it preferred choice
- UFH does not cross into breast milk and is safe during breast feeding

❖ Fondaparinux:
- Factor Xa inhibitor
- Limited information on fetal effects exists
- Preferred alternative in HIT when heparin is contraindicated

❖ Danaparoid:
- Heparinoid anticoagulant
- Limited information on fetal effects exists
- Can be used as an alternative in HIT when heparin is contraindicated

❖ Argatroban:
- Direct thrombin inhibitor
- Evidence exists that it may cross the placenta
- Thus, it is less preferred to fondaparinux in the presence of HIT

❖ Direct oral anticoagulants (DOAC):
- Drugs include:
  - Dabigatran
  - Direct factor Xα inhibitors:
    - Rivaroxaban
    - Apixaban
    - Edoxaban
- They are avoided during pregnancy and lactation due to lack of adequate studies
- Evidence of teratogenicity has been found in animal studies

Initiation of Anticoagulation during Pregnancy: ASH 2018 Guidelines

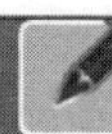

❖ Patients on chronic anticoagulation:
- Warfarin therapy:
  - Teratogenicity of warfarin is maximal between 6-12 weeks of gestation
  - Thus, LMWH substitution should be initiated:
    - During attempted conception or
    - Immediately after becoming pregnant
- DOACS:
  - Human teratogenic effects of DOACs are not known
  - However, LMWH substitution should be initiated:
    - During attempted conception or
    - Immediately after becoming pregnant
- Direct thrombin inhibitors: switch to LMWH on confirmation of pregnancy

❖ Patients not on chronic anticoagulation:
- LMWH is initiated on confirmation of pregnancy
- Absence of vaginal bleeding is ensured prior to initiation of therapy

Monitoring

❖ Baseline tests to be performed prior to initiation of anticoagulation are:
- Platelet count: Used as a baseline value to diagnose HIT
- Creatinine levels: For determining appropriate dose

❖ The lab tests are repeated 3–4 weeks after initiation of therapy and include:
- Platelet count
- Hemoglobin
- Hematocrit

❖ Stable platelet count rules out HIT and warrants no drug alterations

❖ Patients with stable platelet counts do not require subsequent monitoring

❖ Platelet counts may be repeated on occurrence of thrombosis during LMWH therapy

Antepartum Dosage

Drug	Dose level	Dosage
LMWH	Prophylactic	Enoxaparin 40 mg SC OD
		Dalteparin 5000 IU SC OD
	Therapeutic	Enoxaparin 1 mg/kg SC Q12H
		Dalteparin 100 IU/kg SC Q12H
Unfractionated heparin	Prophylactic	5000 IU SC Q12H
	Therapeutic	As continuous infusion or SC Q12H
		Titrated to therapeutic aPTT levels
Fondaparinux	Therapeutic	5–10 mg PO OD

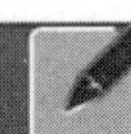

Anticoagulation During Labor and Delivery: ASH 2018 Guidelines

- Anticoagulation is avoided during labor except in very high risk patients
- LMWH is substituted with UFH at 36-37 weeks gestation
- This minimizes risk of persistent anticoagulation during labor due to LMWH
- Replacement with UFH is done earlier in patients at high risk for preterm delivery
- In case of scheduled delivery:
  - LMWH is discontinued 24 hours prior to:
    - Cesarean section
    - Induction of labor
  - UFH is discontinued
    - 12 hours prior to intervention for prophylactic doses
    - 24 hours prior to intervention for therapeutic doses
- Patients who may require continued anticoagulation during delivery include:
  - Prosthetic heart valve
  - Atrial fibrillation with LA thrombus
  - Recent pulmonary embolism
- Therapy is individualized in these patients
- Timing of neuraxial anesthesia during delivery:
  - Neuraxial block given at least 12 hours after last dose of prophylactic LMWH
  - Neuaraxial block given at least 24 hours after last dose of therapeutic LMWH
  - Neuraxial block given after normalization of aPTT for UFH:
    - Usually within 6 hours for IV administration of UFH
    - Upto 24 hours for SC administration of UFH

Postpartum Resumption of Anticoagulation

- Acute VTE requiring therapeutic dosing:
  - Initiation of anticoagulation is begun:
    - 4-6 hours after vaginal delivery
    - 6-12 hours after cesarean section
  - Indications for delayed resumption of anticoagulation:
    - Traumatic epidural puncture
    - Active bleeding
    - High risk PPH patients
  - Therapeutic dose of LMWH or UFH is continued for at least 5 days post-partum
  - Slow transition to oral anticoagulants is recommended with:
    - Warfarin
    - Fondaparinux
    - Danaparoid
  - DOACs are avoided in breast feeding patients
  - Bridging to oral anticoagulants is titrated with close monitoring of INR
  - Duration of oral anticoagulation therapy is individualized according to patient
  - Most patients require 3-6 months of anticoagulation post-partum
- Patients receiving prophylaxis for VTE
  - Urgency of resuming anticoagulant therapy following delivery is less
  - Thus, initiation of anticoagulation is begun:
    - 6-12 hours after vaginal delivery
    - 12-24 hours after cesarean section
  - Slow transition to oral anticoagulants is recommended with:
    - Warfarin
    - Fondaparinux
    - Danaparoid
  - DOACs are avoided in breast feeding patients
  - Bridging to oral anticoagulants is titrated with close monitoring of INR
  - Oral anticoagulation prophylaxis is continued for at least 6 weeks post-partum

Complications

- Bleeding:
  - Due to UFH therapy:
    - Can be rapidly reversed with protamine administration
    - Indications for protamine therapy:
      - Severe bleeding unrelated to pregnancy
      - Imminent cesarean section or delivery in high-risk patients
      - Antepartum complications:
        - Placental abruption
        - Placenta previa
  - Due to LMWH:
    - Not completely reversed by protamine
    - Anticoagulation has to withheld till the bleeding subsides
    - However, for severe bleeding protamine reversal may be used
- Heparin induced thrombocytopenia:
  - Incidence of HIT in pregnancy is very low
  - It is more commonly seen with UFH than LMWH
  - Diagnosis of HIT should immediately prompt:
    - Laboratory tests for PF_4 antibody testing
    - Discontinuation of heparin therapy
    - Substitution with alternative anticoagulant
- Osteoporosis:
  - Osteoporosis is a known complication of prolonged heparin therapy
  - Incidence is more with UFH compared to LMWH

PERIPARTUM CARDIOMYOPATHY

Introduction

- Dilated cardiomyopathy occurring between 36 weeks of gestation and 5 months postpartum
- Peripartum cardiomyopathy is also called:
  - ***Toxic post-partum heart failure***
  - ***Postpartum heart disease***
  - ***Cardiomyopathy of pregnancy***
  - ***Puerperal cardiomyopathy***
  - ***Meadows syndrome***
  - ***Zaria syndrome***
- It is a diagnosis of exclusion, when no other cause of heart failure is found
- Heart failure presenting before the last month of pregnancy is called:
  - Pregnancy-associated cardiomyopathy or
  - Early pregnancy-associated cardiomyopathy

Definition: ESC 2011 Guidelines

- Development of heart failure:
  - Towards the end of pregnancy or
  - Within 5 months post-partum
- Absence of another identifiable cause of heart failure
- LV systolic dysfunction
- LVEF < 45%

Incidence

- 1 in 300 to 1 in 4000 pregnancies worldwide
- High in Nigeria:
  - Due to the tradition of ingesting ***Kanwa*** (dried lake salt)
  - Ingested while lying on heated mud beds twice a day for 40 days post partum
  - High salt intake causes volume overload and hypertension
  - This leads to post partum cardiomyopathy
- Mortality ranges from 18–56%
- 90% occur within first 2 months post-partum
- Only 10% develop in last months of pregnancy

Etiology: Various Theories to Explain Occurrence

- Accelerated HTN reported in 30% cases
- Maternal immunological response to fetal antigen:
  - Fetal cells escaping into maternal circulation are not rejected due to:
    - Suppressed immune system in pregnancy
    - Weak immunogenicity of fetal antigen
  - These fetal cells lodge into the cardiac tissue during pregnancy
  - After delivery, maternal immune competency is restored
  - Fetal cells are then recognized as nonself
  - An autoimmune response may subsequently be triggered
  - This can lead to dilated cardiomyopathy
- Fragmentation of tropocollagen:
  - Fast involution of uterus after delivery causes fragmentation of tropocollagen
  - This causes release of actin, myosin and metabolites
  - Antibodies against actin cross react with myocardial tissue
  - Patient acquires cardiomyopathy
- Beri Beri:
  - Onset of lactation associated with increased BP and nutritional requirements
  - This may reduce vitamin B_1 levels: Wet beri beri and CCF

Predisposing Factors

- Black race:
  - High BP and increase in incidence of sickle cell anemia
  - This can cause CCF due to longstanding anemia
- Old age > 30 years old
- Multiparous women
- Twin pregnancies
- Obesity > 30 BMI
- Diabetes
- Smoking
- Preeclampsia
- Chronic HTN > 140/90 mm Hg
- Prolonged tocolytic therapy with β agonists:
  - Terbutaline and ritodrine
  - β agonist activity: Tachycardia, arrhythmias, MI, sodium retention, hypertension
- Family history
- Malnutrition:
  - Reduced selenium levels
  - Wet beri beri
  - Nutritional anemia
  - Hypoproteinemia: Causes edema

Pathology

- Dilatation of heart
- Increased weight of heart (double the normal weight of 300–350 grams)

- Hypertrophy and mural thrombi on LV
- Loss of myocardial fibers with interstitial edema

Pathophysiology

- Patients with significant myocardial damage remain asymptomatic when at rest
- Physiological stress like pregnancy increases cardiac work
- Pregnancy causes:
  - Increase in preload associated with uterine contraction or surgery
  - Increase in cardiac demand:
    - Heart rate
    - Stroke volume
    - Increased contractility
  - This causes increased stress on myocardial function
- With progressive ventricular failure:
  - End diastolic volume increases, reducing subendocardial blood flow
  - Cardiac output reduces, reducing coronary perfusion further
  - Myocardial O_2 demand–supply imbalance ensues
  - This causes further ventricular compromise

Clinical Features

Symptoms

- *Most commonly* present during first month post-partum
- Gradual/insidious onset/sometimes acute onset dyspnea and pulmonary edema
- Edema, dyspnea on exertion, orthopnea, fatigue, PND, cough, hemoptysis

Signs

- Signs of LVF:
  - Crackles
  - Cyanosis
  - Tachycardia
  - Cold extremities
  - Diaphoresis
  - LV thrust
  - Narrow pulse pressure
  - S_3 gallops at apex and radiating to axilla
  - Audible S_4
- Signs of RVF:
  - Raised JVP
  - Hepatojugular reflex
  - Anasarca
  - Hepatomegaly
  - RV heave
- Systemic embolization of mural thrombi:
  - LV thrombus formation can occur in patients with LVEF < 35%
  - Especially to kidneys causing pyelonephritis
  - Cerebral embolization, pulmonary embolization and infarction
- Signs of valve regurgitation:
  - Mitral regurgitation
  - Tricuspid regurgitation (functional)
- Arrhythmias:
  - Supraventricular tachycardia
  - Atrial fibrillation
  - Ventricular tachycardia/fibrillation

Investigations

- Chest X-ray:
  - Taken only after first trimester
  - Findings:
    - Cardiomegaly, pulmonary vascular congestion
    - Patchy infiltrates and intestitial congestion in lower lung fields
    - Pleural effusion
- CT scan lungs for pulmonary emboli
- ECG: Non-specific changes:
  - Non-specific ST-T changes
  - Ectopics, sinus tachycardia
  - Rarely atrial fibrillation
  - LV hypertrophy: High voltage complexes
  - P pulmonale in lead V_1
  - First degree heart block, bundle branch block patterns
- Echocardiography:
  - LV enlargement
  - Global systolic dysfunction with or without LVH
  - Objective indices:
    - LVEF < 45%
    - Fractional shortening < 30%
    - LV end-diastolic dimension >2.7 cm/m^2 BSA
  - Elevated filling pressures
  - Intracardiac thrombi
- Cardiac catheterization is rarely required
- Endomyocardial biopsy if condition does not improve after 2 weeks therapy for CCF
- Routine blood with: D-dimers, factor V, anticardiolipin Abs for differentiating DIC

- ❖ Viral serological tests:
  - Viral HIV
  - Rickettsial
  - Toxoplasmosis
  - Syphilis
  - Chagas disease (trypanosomiasis)
  - Diphtheria
- ❖ Nuclear study/angiography with fetal shield after first trimester

Diagnostic Criteria: NHLBI/NIH 2000 Recommendations

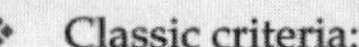

- ❖ Classic criteria:
  - Onset of heart failure between 36 weeks of pregnancy to 5 months post partum
  - No evidence of heart disease prepartum
  - No other causes of heart failure
- ❖ Additional criteria:
  - LVEF < 45%
  - LV fractional shortening < 30%
  - LV end-diastolic diameter > 2.7 cm/m^2

Differential Diagnosis

- ❖ Toxic: Cocaine, alcoholic cardiomyopathy
- ❖ Infective:
  - HIV
  - Rickettsial
  - Toxoplasmosis
  - Syphilis
  - Chagas disease (trypanosomiasis)
  - Diphtheria
- ❖ Collagen vascular disease: Sarcoidosis
- ❖ Endocrine: Thyrotoxicosis, pheochromocytoma
- ❖ Previous heart ailment: Valvular, ischemic, myopathic

Goals of Anesthesia

- ❖ Rate: Maintain high-normal
- ❖ Rhythm: Maintain sinus rhythm
- ❖ Preload: Reduce or maintain preload
- ❖ Afterload: Reduce afterload
- ❖ SVR: Reduce SVR
- ❖ PVR: Reduce PVR
- ❖ Contractility: Maintain/increase contractility
- ❖ Maintain uteroplacental adequacy

Choice of Anesthesic Technique

- ❖ Regional anesthesia:
  - Used for:
    - Labor analgesia (*technique of choice*)
    - Non-emergent Cesarean section
  - Advantages:
    - Early administration of labor analgesia reduces cardiac stress
    - Continuous epidural offers better hemodynamic control
    - RA causes sympathectomy induced reduction in afterload
    - This improves myocardial performance
    - If fixed cardiac output state exists, RA with only opioids may be used
  - Guidelines for regional anesthesia:
    - Continuous FHR monitoring required
    - Preloading and prophylactic ephedrine not used
- ❖ General Anesthesia:
  - Used for:
    - Fetal distress
    - Moderately symptomatic parturients
    - Acute maternal decompensation
  - Complications:
    - Hypotension
    - Pulmonary edema
    - Hypoxemia
    - MI and dysrhythmias
  - Slow maternal circulating time causes:
    - Late onset of action of drugs
    - This may be presumed to be insufficient dosage
    - This may lead to additional dosage administration and overdosage

Technique of General Anesthesia

Premedication

- ❖ Supplemental oxygen administration
- ❖ Bed rest not recommended due to increased risk of DVT
- ❖ Left uterine displacement to avoid supine hypotension syndrome
- ❖ Premedication is essential to avoid anxiety induced increase in SVR
- ❖ Premedication with IV midazolam can be used
- ❖ Anti-aspiration prophylaxis
- ❖ Anticoagulation in case of:
  - Markedly enlarged heart
  - History of embolization
  - History of atrial fibrillation
  - Significantly reduced cardiac output
- ❖ Stop ACE inhibitors and angiotensin II antagonists on day of surgery
- ❖ Diuretics and digoxin continued on morning of surgery

Monitoring

- BP: invasive BP monitoring preferred in case of elective procedures
- Pulse oximetry
- ECG
- Urine output
- Pulmonary artery catheter for management of hemodynamic status
- Cardiac output monitoring
- FHR monitoring

Induction

- Preoxygenation important as maternal oxygen demand increases by 20% at birth
- Opioid induction preferred with neonatologist to manage neonatal depression
- Etomidate + fentanyl + vecuronium can be used for induction
- Induction takes longer time as circulation is slow due to heart failure
- Adequate time should be given for induction drugs to act
- This is because in the presence of cardiac failure, circulation time is prolonged
- Deep anesthetic plane is preferred during intubation

Maintenance

- Balanced anesthesia with O_2 + air + 1 MAC isoflurane
- Avoid anesthetics associated with myocardial depressant effects like halothane
- Graded doses of anesthetic drugs to avoid postoperative depression
- N_2O avoided if pulmonary hypertension
- Prevent tachycardia at the time of incision
- PEEP to reduce pulmonary congestion and increase forward output

Hemodynamics

- Avoid fluid overload: judicious use of colloids
- NTG/SNP for preload and afterload reduction if cardiac decompensation occurs
- Inotropes:
  - Dobutamine/ milrinone can be used for persistent hypotension
  - Levosimendan may be a useful inodilator to maintain cardiac output
- If condition does not improve with standard medical therapy, consider:
  - Pacemaker placement
  - Intra Aortic Balloon Pump (IABP)
  - Left Ventricular Assist Devices (LVAD)
  - Cardiac transplantation
- Non-anesthetic drugs:
  - Ergometrine is avoided as it increases SVR
  - Oxytocin should be given slowly, to avoid tachycardia seen with rapid boluses
  - Avoid β blockers and calcium channel blockers
  - Furosemide may be used to counter autotransfusion occurring during delivery
- CO increases 65% after delivery due to:
  - Release of IVC compression
  - Autotransfusion of blood back into maternal circulation

Extubation: Fully awake extubation in left lateral position to avoid aspiration

Intraop Complications

- Hypotension
- Pulmonary edema
- Hypoxemia
- MI
- Arrhythmias
- Delayed awakening

Postoperative

- ACE inhibitor and angiotensin II inhibitor in postpartum period (not during pregnancy)
- Captopril avoided as it crosses placenta and causes renal failure in neonate
- Hydralazine with NTG/amlodipine are alternatives to decrease preload and after load
- Blood gases to be taken every 6th hourly for 24 hours postoperatively

Prognosis

- Mortality rate 10% in 2 years
- Common causes of death in PPCM:
  - Progressive pump failure
  - SVT (AF and atrial flutter)
  - Thromboembolic events
- Poor prognosticators include:
  - Black race

- Multiparity
- Age > 35 years
- Poor NYHA status at presentation
- LVEF < 25%

❖ Predictors of persistent LV dysfunction postoperatively:
- Black race
- Diagnosis during pregnancy
- LVEF < 30%
- FS < 20%
- LV end-diastolic diameter > 6 cm
- Elevated cardiac troponin T

GESTATIONAL DIABETES MELLITUS

Introduction

Gestational diabetes mellitus is defined as diabetes with onset or first recognition during the second or third trimester of pregnancy that was not clearly overt diabetes prior to gestation.

Definition of Diabetes Mellitus: ADA 2012 Guidelines

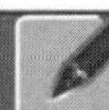

❖ Diagnosis requires that two or more glucose threshold values must be exceeded

❖ Fasting blood sugar:
- FBS > 126 mg/dL or 7 mmoL/L
- Fasting is defined as no caloric intake for at least 8 hours

❖ 2 hour post-prandial sugar (PPBS):
- PPBS > 200 mg/dL or 11.1 mmoL/L
- Test is performed after a 75 g anhydrous glucose load dissolved in water

❖ Random blood sugar (RBS):
- RBS > 200 mg/dL or 11.1 mmoL/L in the presence of hyperglycemic symptoms
- Random is defined as any time during the day, without regard to last meal
- Hyperglycemic symptoms include:
  - Polyuria
  - Polydipsia
  - Unexplained weight loss

Incidence

❖ GDM complicates approximately 2-9% of pregnancies

❖ An additional 1% of pregnancies are complicated by pregestational or preexisting DM

❖ Prevalence has been increasing over time due to increasing obesity

Modified White Classification

Gestational diabetes				
Class	Age of onset	Duration	Vascular disease	Insulin required
A_1	Any age	Any duration	None	No
A_2	Any age	Any duration	None	Yes
Pregestational diabetes				
Class	Age of onset	Duration	Vascular disease	Insulin required
B	> 20 yrs	< 10 yrs	None	Yes
C	10-19 yrs	10-19 yrs	None	Yes
D	< 10 yrs	> 20 yrs	Benign retinopathy	Yes
F	Any age	Any duration	Nephropathy	Yes
R	Any age	Any duration	Proliferative retinopathy	Yes
H	Any age	Any duration	Heart	Yes

Risk Factors

❖ Age > 30 years

❖ Obesity

❖ Asian race

❖ Family history of diabetes mellitus

❖ Glucose intolerance with previous pregnancy

❖ Previous birth of overweight baby > 4 kgs

❖ Polyhydramnios

❖ Recurrent vaginal candidiasis

❖ Persistent glucosuria

Maternal Hazards

❖ Acute complications:
- Diabetic ketoacidosis
- Hyperosmolar non-ketotic hyperglycemic coma
- Dehydration

❖ Chronic complications:
- Coronary artery disease
- Diabetic retinopathy
- Diabetic nephropathy
- Autonomic neuropathy

❖ Peripartum complications:
- Preeclampsia, gestational hypertension
- Abortion, preterm labor, prolonged labor
- Polyhydramnios, perineal injuries due to large baby, risk of operative delivery
- Postpartum hemorrhage
- Puerperal sepsis
- Lactation failure

Fetal Hazards

- Hazards during in-utero development:
  - Hydramnios
  - Large-for-gestational-age fetus
  - Small-for-gestational-age fetus
  - Macrosomia
- Hazards during labor:
  - Preterm delivery
  - Shoulder dystocia
  - Brachial plexus injury
  - Clavicular fracture
  - Risk of operative delivery
- Neonatal complications:
  - Hypoglycemia
  - Hyperbilirubinemia
  - RDS
  - Hypocalcemia
  - Acidosis
  - Hypertrophic cardiomyopathy
- Birth defects:
  - Nervous system:
    - Caudal regression
    - Neural tube defects, spina bifida
    - Meningomyelocele
    - Anencephaly, microcephaly, hydrocephaly
    - Holoprosencephaly
  - Cardiopulmonary system:
    - VSD, ASD
    - Coarctation of aorta
    - TGA, situs inversus
    - Hypoplastic left heart syndrome
    - Pulmonary hypoplasia
  - Renal system:
    - Renal agenesis
    - Hydronephrosis
    - Multicystic dysplasia
    - Duplex ureter
  - Gastrointestinal system:
    - Duodenal/anorectal atresia
    - Small left colon
  - Others:
    - Single umbilical artery
    - Lower 2, 3 DPG concentration causing polycythemia
    - Decreased buffering capacity to acid load
- Neonatal pathological syndrome: (acute complications)
  - Neonatal respiratory distress syndrome
  - Organomegaly
  - Hypertrophic cardiomyopathy
- Long term complications:
  - Adolescent obesity
  - Impaired glucose tolerance
  - Inheritance of diabetes mellitus

Anesthetic Considerations 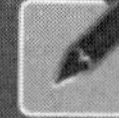

- Difficult intubation due to:
  - Stiff joint syndrome
  - Pregnancy induced changes
- Risk of aspiration due to:
  - Diabetic gastroparesis
  - Pregnancy induced changes
- In the presence of autonomic neuropathy:
  - Increased risk of hypothermia
  - Poor response to atropine/catecholamines
  - Precipitous hypotension on neuraxial blockade
  - Increased risk of nerve injury
  - Increased risk of silent MI
- Reduced oxygen saturation and transport
- Reduced sympathetic response to hypoglycemia under GA
- Perioperative complications:
  - Congestive cardiac failure
  - Renal failure
  - Infections

Choice of Technique

- For labor analgesia:
  - Small dose systemic opioids for mild-moderate pain
  - Epidural analgesia may be used for severe pain
- For cesarean section:
  - Both epidural and subarachnoid block are safe
  - However, in severe diabetics, epidural anesthesia may be preferred
  - This is because of slower onset of sympatholysis with epidural anesthesia
- General anesthesia is used in case of operative emergencies or coagulopathy

Anesthetic Technique

- Preoperative assessment:
  - Assess for areas of increased risk:
    - Hypertension, pre-eclampsia
    - Difficult airway: ***prayer sign***
    - Sepsis
    - Renal dysfunction
  - Evaluation of end-organ damage: autonomic neuropathy

- Management of blood glucose levels:
  - Insulin dose is withheld on the morning of surgery
  - Intravenous normal saline infusion is begun prior to surgery
  - If blood glucose level is < 70 mg/dL, 5% dextrose at 100-150 mL/hr is started
  - Goal of management is to maintain blood glucose levels around 100 mg/dL
  - Short-acting regular insulin at 1.25 IU/hr is begun if RBS > 100 mg/dL
  - Insulin infusion is subsequently titrated to maintain blood glucose levels
  - Hourly measurement of blood sugar is required to prevent hypoglycemia
  - Half-hourly blood sugar measurement is indicated in patients undergoing general anesthesia
- Preoperative optimization:
  - Anti-aspiration prophylaxis:
    - Non-particulate antacid immediately before surgery
    - IV metaclopramide 10 mg 30-40 minutes prior to induction
  - Positioning:
    - Routine left uterine displacement during positioning
    - Gradual positional changes to avoid hypotension
    - Padding of extremities to avoid peripheral nerve injuries
  - Two separate intravenous cannulae to be secured prior to induction:
    - One cannula is used for perioperative fluid therapy
    - The other is used for administration of perioperative glucose control regimen
- Monitors:
  - Routine ASA monitors are indicated in diabetic parturients
  - Fetal monitoring is mandatory in all cases
  - Invasive hemodynamic monitoring required in cases of:
    - Severe preeclampsia
    - Severe gestational hypertension
    - Diabetic nephropathy
- Induction:
  - Adequate preoxygenation is essential
  - *Rapid sequence induction* with cricoid pressure for GA
  - Induction is begun after surgical preparation and draping of the patient
  - Difficult airway cart with *polio blade* and short handle is kept ready
  - Hypotension promptly treated with IV ephedrine to prevent fetal acidosis
- Maintenance:
  - O_2+ 1 MAC isoflurane may be used for maintenance of balanced anesthesia
  - IV fentanyl 1 g/kg may be administered following delivery
  - Compression stockings may be applied for DVT prophylaxis
- Hemodynamics:
  - Judicious fluid administration as diabetics are prone for pulmonary edema
  - This is because renal protein wasting results in low colloid osmotic pressure
  - Hypotension is aggressively treated with ephedrine boluses
- Postoperative:
  - Monitor mother and neonate for postoperative hypoglycemia
  - Maternal insulin requirements decrease in the early postpartum period
  - Adequate analgesia is important to prevent catecholamine and glucose swings
  - Intravenous/ intrathecal morphine and NSAIDs can be used to ensure analgesia
  - Early resumption of enteral nutrition
- Specific precautions in patients with proliferative retinopathy:
  - Valsalva manuver during 2nd stage of labor is contraindicated
  - Vitreous hemorrhage may occur during Valsalva manuver due to retinopathy

ANEMIA IN PREGNANCY

Introduction

- Hb concentration of < 11g% or HCT < 33% in 1stand 3rd trimester
- Hb concentration < 10.5 g% in 2nd trimester
- Hb concentration < 10g% at any time in pregnancy

Classification

I. *Physiological Anemia in Pregnancy:*

- Hb < 10 g%
- RBC count 3.2 million/mm^3
- PCV 30%
- Normal RBC morphology with central pallor on peripheral smear

II. *Pathological Anemia in Pregnancy*

- Nutritional:
  - Iron
  - Vitamin B_{12}
  - Folate
  - Proteins
- Hemorrhagic:
  - Acute: Antepartum hemorrhage
  - Chronic: Hookworm, hemorrhoids
- Bone marrow insufficiency:
  - Aplastic anemia
  - Radiation
  - Infection with parvovirus B_{12}
  - Drugs (aspirin, indomethacin)
- Anemia of chronic disease:
  - Chronic renal failure
  - Neoplasms
- Infections:
  - Malaria
  - Hookworm
  - Tuberculosis

III. *Hereditary Anemia*

- Sickle cell disease
- Thalassemia
- Other hemoglobinopathies
- Hereditary hemolytic anemia: spherocytosis

Compensatory Mechanisms

- Increased cardiac output
- Reduced blood viscosity
- Increased 2,3 DPG in RBC
- Rightward shift of Oxygen Dissociation Curve (ODC)
- Increased production of erythropoietin

Severity of Anemia

- Mild anemia: 10-10.9 g/dL
- Moderate anemia: 7-9.9 g/dL
- Severe anemia: < 7g/dL

Complications

Maternal Complications

- Heart failure at 30-32 wks
- Uterine atony, APH
- PPH
- Preeclampsia
- Preterm labor
- Infection
- Puerperal sepsis
- Uterine subinvolution
- Pulmonary embolism
- Puerperal venous thrombosis

Fetal Complications

- Low birth weight
- Intrauterine death
- Fetal acidosis

Preoperative Assessment

- History of tiredness, fatigueability, breathlessness, palpitation, angina
- Tachycardia, wide pulse pressure, ejection systolic murmur, pallor, crepts
- Investigations:
  - Complete hemogram, reticulocyte count
  - Stool and urine analysis, ESR, serum creatinine, BUN, bilirubin
  - Serum proteins, iron, B_{12} and folate levels, TIBC, Hb electrophoresis
  - ECG for evidence of MI
  - MCHC, MCV, MCH

Goals of Anesthesia

- Minimize factors affecting O_2 delivery
- Prevent increase in O_2 consumption
- Optimize PaO_2 in arterial blood

Choice of Anesthesia

- Regional anesthesia preferred (SAB/CSE) as:
  - Good analgesia
  - Ability to provide supplemental O_2
  - Reduce blood loss
  - Reduce DVT
- Disadvantages of regional anesthesia:
  - Hypotension and hemodilution
  - Chance of pulmonary edema due to overload
- Avoided in B_{12} deficiency with CNS symptoms as it worsens subacute degeneration of cord

Monitoring

- ECG, SpO_2, NIBP, E_TCO_2, temperature, urine output
- IBP, CVP in unstable patients
- PA catheter and mixed venous oxygen saturation helpful

- Serial Hb and HCT when major blood loss anticipated

Anesthetic Considerations

- Avoidance of hypoxia:
  - Preoxygenate with 100% O_2 for 3-5 mins or 4 vital capacity breaths
  - High FiO_2 (40-50%) intraoperatively
  - Spontaneous ventilation used only for short surgeries
  - Difficult airway anticipation
  - Avoid conditions increasing O_2 consumption:
    - Shivering
    - Fever
    - Acute blood loss
    - Pain
    - Light planes
- Minimize anesthesia induced oxygenation changes:
  - N_2O used cautiously in B_{12} and folate deficiency
  - Avoid hypoventilation to minimize alkalosis
  - Avoid hypoventilation to avoid acidosis
  - Titrate induction agents to prevent hypotension
  - Careful and slow positioning to avoid hypotension
  - Left lateral tilt beyond 28 weeks
  - Avoid hypothermia
- Blood transfusion:
  - Hb > 10 g%: Rarely indicated
  - Hb < 6 g%: Always indicated
  - Hb 7–9 g%: Decision based on:
    - Ongoing blood loss
    - Coexisting disease
    - Threat of bleeding

Sickle Cell Disease

- Complications:
  - Increased preterm labor
  - Abruption, placenta previa
  - Pregnancy Induced Hypertension
- GA/RA acceptable
- Avoid factors predisposing sickling
  - Hypoxemia
  - Hypovolemia
  - Hypotension
  - Acidosis
  - Hypoventilation
  - Hypothermia
  - Light planes

Thalassemia

- Chronic anemia causes tissue hypoxia
- Multiple transfusion: Hemosiderosis and heart failure
- Concomitant difficult airway due to abnormal facies

AMNIOTIC FLUID EMBOLISM

Introduction

- Catastrophic condition which occurs when amniotic fluid enters maternal circulation
- AF embolism, though rare, is a condition with a mortality rate of 80–100%
- First reported by Meyer in 1926
- First described by Steiner and Lushbaugh in a case series of 8 women in 1941
- Also called ***obstetric shock*** or ***anaphylactic syndrome of pregnancy***

Incidence

- Incidence of AFE is rare
- Ranges from 1.9-6.1 cases per 1,00,000 deliveries
- Responsible for 10% of all maternal deaths
- Maternal mortality rate is high (reduced from 86% in 1979 to 37% in 2005)
- 25% of patients die within the first hour of initial symptoms
- Neonatal mortality rate is as high as 20–25%
- Only 50% of neonatal survivors remain neurologically intact

Components of Amniotic Fluid

- Volume of amniotic fluid increases from 50 mL at 12 weeks to 1000 mL at term
- It is hypotonic due to dilution with fetal urine
- The damage to the lungs is irreversible because of contents of amniotic fluid
- pH = 6.9 – 7.15
- Suspended particles:
  - Lanugo fetal squames fetal gut mucin
  - Hair meconium trophoblasts
  - Vernix caseosa
- Nitrogenous products:
  - Amino acids uric acid proteins
  - Urea creatinine
- Others:
  - Glucose enzymes hormones
  - Vitamins steroids lipids
- Electrolytes:
  - Na Mg Fe Cl Mn
  - K Ca PO_4 S Zn
- Biochemical mediators:
  - Surfactant — IL_1 prostaglandin E_1, E_2, F_{1x} F_{2z}
  - Endothelin — TNFα arachidonic acid
  - Leukotriene C_4 and D_4 — TxA_2 thromboplastin
  - Collagen — TF3 phospholipase A_2

- PF3 (TF Tissue factor, PF= platelet factor)
- PG F2α is the *most significant* for causing syndrome

Predisposing Factors

- Elderly and multiparous
- Multiple pregnancy
- Polyhydramnios
- Macrosomia
- Intrauterine death
- Term pregnancy in the presence of IUCD

Precipitating Factors

- Artificial rupture of membranes, use of oxytocics, tumultuous labor
- 1st trimester curettage abortion
- 2nd trimester abortion using saline, glucose, PG, urea, hysterotomy
- Abdominal trauma, placenta rupture, uterine rupture
- Amniocentesis, intrauterine fetal monitoring
- During LSCS
- When uterine/decidual blood vessels are abnormally opened:
  - Placenta accreta
  - Ruptured uterus
  - Retained placenta
  - Trauma from intrauterine manipulation:
    - Rupturing membrane
    - Inserting catheter for pressure recording
  - Endocervical venous laceration/lower uterine tear during normal labor

Pathogenesis

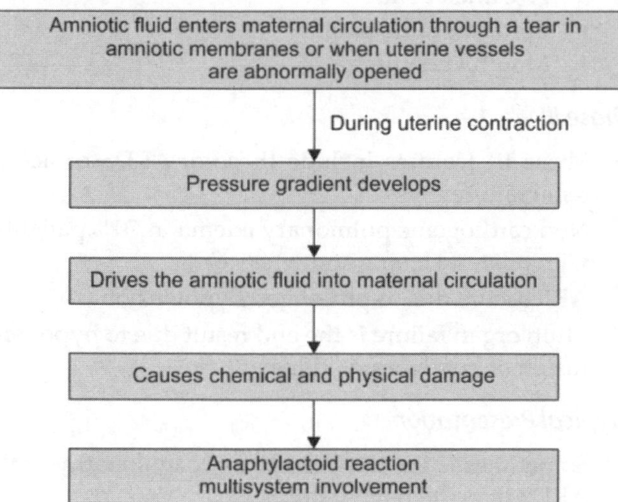

Pathogenetic Theories of AFE

Anaphylactic Shock Theory

- Fetal contents of amniotic fluid produce a reaction similar to anaphylactic shock
- Hallmark symptoms of cutaneous flare, bronchospasm and airway edema
- Controversial as:
  - Symptoms not due to histamine: histamine usually absent in amniotic fluid
  - Symptoms not due to antigenic reexposure: AFE seen in both prime and multigravida

Pulmonary Vascular Obstruction Theory

- Physical plugging of pulmonary capillaries due to:
  - Abnormal volume of amniotic fluid entering maternal circulation
  - Abnormal substances present in amniotic fluid like lanugo

Alveolar Capillary Leak Theory

- Alveolar capillary leak occurs secondary to acute micro vascular emboli
- ARDS and pulmonary edema due to alveolar capillary leakage
- Increase in ECF volume and decreased colloid osmotic press contribute

LV Dysfunction Theory

- Biphasic pattern of hemodynamic disturbances seen in AFE
- Initially pulmonary vasospasm due to amniotic fluid present in pulmonary vasculature
- This causes pulmonary hypertension and hypoxia
- Secondary phase of LVF with secondary elevation of pulmonary arterial pressure
- LV dysfunction may be due to:
  - Hypoxic LV injury
  - Direct depressant effect of amniotic fluid on myocardium
  - Myocardial ischemia due to coronary vasospasm: by endothelin present in AF

Bleeding Diathesis Theory

- Amniotic fluid assists in post partum hemostasis
- Entry into maternal circulation produces intravascular clotting

- This consumes fibrinogen producing increased bleeding
- AF also has thromboplastin like effect and contains plasmin proactivator and factor X activator
- This causes intravascular coagulation and multisystem damage

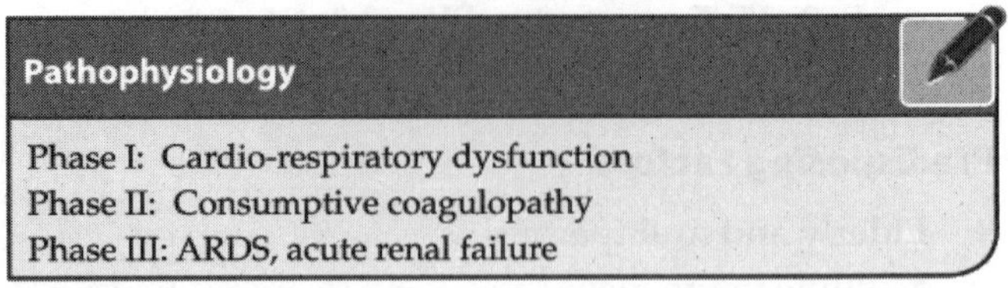

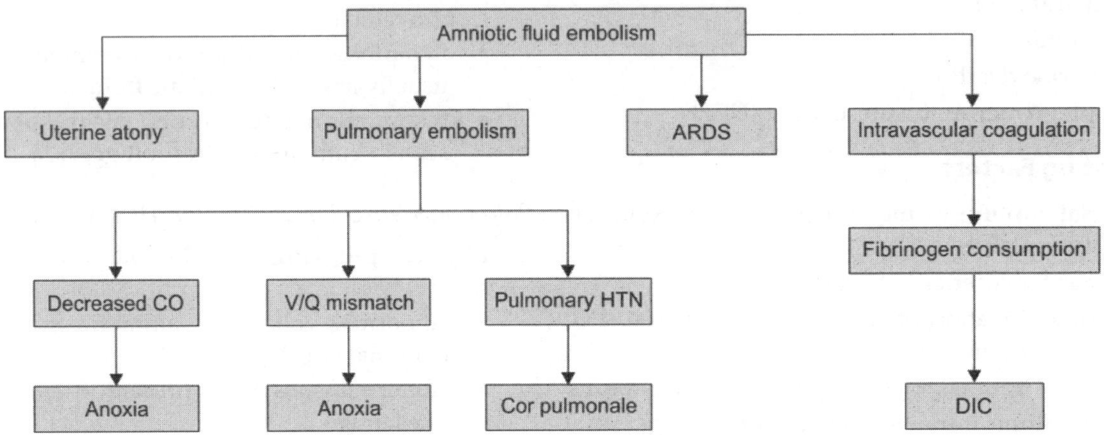

Clinical Features

- Approximately 70% of cases occur before delivery
- The remaining 30% of cases can occur up to 48 hours post-partum
- AFE can occur during:
  - Abdominal trauma
  - After first trimester abortion
  - Second trimester
  - Labor and normal delivery
  - Cesarean section
  - Post-partum period
- Prodromal symptoms such as chills and vomiting are rare
- Patient usually goes into cardiac arrest soon after prodromal symptoms

Phase I

- Phase I symptoms include respiratory and cardiovascular dysfunction
- Classical presentation of:
  - Sudden onset dyspnea and hypotension
  - Hypoxia with altered mental state
  - Followed soon by cardiorespiratory arrest
- Hypotension and shock is the first clinical presentation in most cases
- GTCS occurs in 50% cases of AFE
- If meconium stained AF, shorter time from initial symptoms to arrest
- Cardiac arrest and DIC may occur simultaneously

Phase II

- Phase II features include features of coagulopathy
- This may present as postpartum hemorrhage, uterine atony or frank DIC
- Isolated coagulopathy may present as bleeding from
  - Per vagina
  - From incision site
  - IV catheter site
  - Epidural catheter site
  - Mouth and gums

Phase III

- Phase III features include those of ARDS or acute renal failure
- Non cardiogenic pulmonary edema in 70% patients with bilateral crepts and wheeze
- ARF occurs due to prolonged hypotension
- Multi organ failure is the end result due to hypoperfusion of heart, brain, kidneys

Atypical Presentation

- Sometimes, AFE can present as coagulopathy with ARDS or acute renal failure

- This happens without the initial phase of cardiorespiratory dysfunction
- This results in an atypical presentation without the 3 classic phases of AFE

Clinical Features Under GA

- Hypotension, arrhythmias
- Pulmonary edema
- Generalized bleeding

Diagnosis

Clinical Tests

- Decreased O_2 saturation in pulse oximetry
- Decreased E_TCO_2 with increased $[PaCO_2–E_TCO_2]$ gradient
- ECG: Arrhythmias, MI, asystole
- Chest X-ray: Normal/effusion/cardiomegaly/pulmonary edema
- ABG: Reduced $PO_2$and SO_2, reduced gradient between alveolar and arterial PO_2
- TEE: Long axis 4 chamber view:
  - Acute RVF
  - Suprasystemic right sided pressures
  - Bulging of interatrial septum
  - LV dysfunction
- PA catheter:
  - Increased PCWP
  - Reduced LV stroke work index
  - Reduced SVR
  - Increased PA pressure
  - Increased pulmonary vascular resistance

Confirmatory Tests

- Pulmonary artery catheter/CVP aspirate:
  - For pulmonary microvascular cytology
  - Only used for confirmation, not for early diagnosis and treatment
  - PAC/CVP blood used:
    - Blood is stained for fetal squames/mucin with:
      - *Nile Blue A*
      - *Papanicola Oil Red O*
      - *Acid mucopolysaccharides*
    - Fetal squames: Not sensitive/specific (not confirmatory)
    - Fetal mucin: More sensitive indicator
  - Newer technique using monoclonal antibodies:
    - Uses TKH 2 antibodies
    - Measures maternal serum zinc coproporphyrin I
    - This is characteristic of meconium
- Autopsy:
  - Section from all parts of lungs are examined for:
    - Squames (fetal skin)
    - Bile containing meconium
    - Lanugo
    - Fat from vermix caseosa
    - Mucin from fetal gut
  - Finding AF elements in lungs is confirmatory

Diagnostic Criteria

- AFE is a clinical diagnosis based upon:
  - Presence of certain characteristic clinical findings
  - Exclusion of other potential causes
- AFE is suspected in pregnant or recent postpartum women with cardiovascular collapse
- Presence of amniotic fluid debris in maternal lung tissue is not diagnostic of AFE
- Amniotic fluid debris can be found in maternal lung in the absence of AFE as well
- A diagnostic score has been suggested based on four criteria
- All four diagnostic criteria must be present to establish a diagnosis of AFE:
  1. Clinical onset during labor or within 30 minutes of placental delivery
  2. Sudden onset cardio-respiratory arrest or hypotension (SBP< 90 mm Hg) with evidence of respiratory compromise (dyspnea, cyanosis, SpO_2 < 90%)
  3. Absence of fever (>38°C) during labor
  4. Documentation of over DIC using ISTH score
- ISTH score for diagnosis of overt DIC: (score >3 implies overt DIC)

	0 Points	1 Point	2 Points
Platelet count	> 1,00,000/mL	50,000-1,00,000/mL	< 50,000/mL
Prolonged PT/INR	< 25% increase	25-50% increase	> 50% increase
Fibrinogen level	> 200 mg/L	< 200 mg/L	

Differential Diagnosis

- Acid aspiration
- Pulmonary thromboembolism
- Air embolism
- Acute LV failure
- Hemorrhagic/septic shock/anaphylactic shock

- Abruptio placentae/uterine/hepatic rupture
- Acute MI/peripartum cardiomyopathy
- Eclampsia (if convulsion present)
- Local anesthetic drug reaction
- Total spinal anesthesia
- Cerebrovascular accident

Management

Objectives

- Maintain oxygenation
- Restore normal BP and cardiac output for vital organ perfusion
- Correct coagulopathy
- **Cardiopulmonary resuscitation**: In case of cardiac arrest:
  - In left lateral position
  - Continuous cricoid pressure during positive pressure ventilation
  - Higher level of DC shock (above midpoint of sternum)
  - Removal fetal and maternal monitors before shocking
  - Reduced tidal volume breaths

Airway and Breathing

- 100% oxygen
- If unconscious intubate with 0.5-1 mm smaller ETT
- Prevent traumatic intubation
- High FiO_2 to maintain $SpO_2 > 90\%$
- PEEP may help to improve oxygenation

Circulation

- IV access, prevent bleeding from IV site
- Fluid administration guided by CVP monitoring
- Rapid volume infusion to optimize preload
- After correction of hypotension, fluid therapy at maintenance levels to avoid pulmonary edema
- Inotropes: Dopamine, dobutamine or norepinephrine
- Foleys catheter with urine output > 0.5 mL/kg/hr
- Diuretics only to mobilize excess fluids
- Relieve uterine compression of IVC in left lateral position

Coagulopathy

- FFP, fresh blood, platelet concentrate and cryoprecipitate
- Cryoprecipitate helpful as it is rich in both fibrinogen and fibronectin

Uterine Atony

- Oxytocin, methylergometrine, $PGF_2\alpha$ and manual massage
- Oxytocics may cause increased pulmonary vascular resistance
- If persistent bleeding, uterine exploration for tears and retained placenta

Prophylatic Antibiotics

Steroids

- 500 mg (high dose) hydrocortisone IV Q 6H
- May be helpful but not tested

Cardiopulmonary Bypass

Open pulmonary artery thromboembolectomy in moribund patients with AFE.

Care of Fetus

- Fetal monitoring
- Delivery to be done within 5 mins of maternal cardiac arrest
- This gives best chance of fetal survival at > 24 wks gestational age
- Delivery may increase likelihood of success of CPR in cardiac arrest

Treatment of Complications

- Hemodialysis for acute renal failure
- Anticonvulsants for seizures
- Industrial surfactant-***pluronic F68***, antiprostaglandins

Prevention

- Prophylactic measures difficult
- Avoid uterine trauma during amniotomy
- Placental incision during cesarean section avoided
- Avoid trauma at IV catheter insertion site during labor
- Do not strip membranes from cervix in labor
- Avoid Intra Uterine Death
- Care with syntocinon in prolonged labor
- Do early termination with curettage

Prognosis

- Neurological morbidity rates are high and few patients are without consequences
- If amniotic fluid is meconium stained, no mother survived without neurodeficits
- Rapid death within 1 hour of onset of symptoms common

St George's Hospital Recommendations

- Blood grouping, cross matching and screening for antibodies in all patients at ANC
- Anticipate those at risk: Previous PPH
- Ergometrine to be avoided, prefer oxytocin
- Control source of bleeding
- IV fluids–RL, hestarch, gelatin, albumin, dextran
- FFP/cryoprecipitate/platelet concentrate
- 2 large bore IV lines
- Monitoring: BP, SPO_2, ECG
- Assess blood loss
- Maintain input/output
- Prompt surgical intervention
- Warming of blood
- Inotropic support
- Consult hematologist, anesthetist

PULMONARY ASPIRATION

Introduction

- Leading cause of maternal anesthetic deaths
- All pregnant patients are to be considered full stomach regardless of NPO status

Incidence

- One of the leading causes of maternal anesthetic deaths
- Incidence is 1 in 661 pregnancies undergoing cesarean section
- Incidence is 0.4% in patients undergoing cesarean section under GA
- Mortality due to pulmonary aspiration has reduced significantly due to:
  - Alterations in anesthetic technique
  - Strict NPO guidelines
  - Use of routine anti-aspiration prophylaxis
- Mortality from aspiration pneumonia can range from 5-15%

Effects of Pregnancy on Gastric Function

- LES function and tone is altered during pregnancy due to:
  - Altered anatomical relationship of esophagus to stomach and diaphragm
  - Progesterone induced relaxation of LES tone from 35 to 24 cm H_2O
  - Increased gastric volume
- This results in higher incidence of GERD in pregnant mothers
- The physiological changes return to normal within 48 hours of delivery
- Gastric emptying:
  - Pregnancy does not significantly delay gastric emptying
  - Gross obesity may be associated with hiatus hernia delaying gastric emptying
  - Gastric emptying is progressively delayed as labor progresses
  - This may be due to:
    - Physiological responses to pain
    - Opioid analgesic administration
- Changes in nature of gastric fluid:
  - Almost all pregnant women have gastric fluid pH < 2.5
  - 60% of pregnant women have gastric volume > 25 mL
  - Hypersecretion of gastric acid occurs due to gastrin release in pregnancy

Determinants of Severity

- Morbidity and mortality from aspiration depend on 3 major risk factors:
  - Chemical nature of the aspirate
  - Physical nature of the aspirate
  - Volume of aspirate
- Volume of aspirate:
  - Higher volumes of aspirate increase severity of manifestations
  - Threshold volumes for aspiration pneumonitis are:
    - 0.4 mL/ kg of non-particulate gastric fluid
    - This amounts to approximately 25 mL
- Chemical nature of aspirate:
  - pH of the liquid aspirated is an important determinant of aspiration pneumonia
  - pH < 2.5 causes pulmonary granulocytic reaction
  - Thus, pH< 2.5 is the threshold for causing aspiration pneumoia
- Physical nature of aspirate:
  - Solid aspirates are more likely to cause asphyxia due to airway obstruction
  - Liquid aspirates cause more severe clinical manifestations

Risk Factors for Aspiration Pneumonia

- Patient related risk factors:
  - Gastroesophageal reflux
  - Abdominal muscle weakness

- Associated gastrointestinal pathology
- Hiatus hernia
- Maternal obesity
- Polyhydramnios
- Twin pregnancy
- Supine hypotension syndrome causing increased nausea

❖ Anesthesia related risk factors:
- General anesthesia:
  - General anesthetia itself increases risk of aspiration
  - Inadequate depth of anesthesia at intubation
  - Difficult airway/intubation with multiple attempts at intubation
- Neuraxial anesthesia:
  - Concomitant opioid administration due to delayed gastric emptying
  - Deep sedation with un-secured airway
  - Local anesthetic systemic toxicity (LAST) causing seizures

❖ Surgery related risk factors:
- Emergency surgery
- Lithotomy position
- Trendelenburg position

Determinants of Aspiration Pneumonia During General Anesthesia

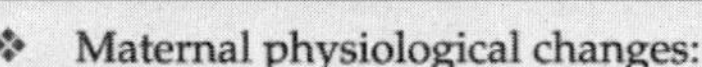

❖ Maternal physiological changes:
- Maternal GERD
- Increased gastric volumes > 25 mL
- Reduced gastric pH < 2.5

❖ Anesthetic drugs aggravating maternal GERD:
- Opioids
- Glycopyrrolate

❖ Difficult intubation due to:
- Pharyngeal and laryngeal mucosal edema
- Enlarged breasts impairing laryngoscopic introduction
- Enlarged tongue causing difficult mask ventilation

Types of Pulmonary Aspiration

❖ Chemical pneumonitis/acid aspiration syndrome
- Materials with pH < 2.5

❖ Solid/particulate matter

❖ Fecal/bacterial contaminated material (rare):
- Intestinal obstruction
- Perforation
- Bowel infract

Prevention of Aspiration Under General Anesthesia

❖ Avoid loss of consciousness:
- Avoid GA when other alternatives are present
- Avoid over sedation when regional anesthesia is used
- Avoid LA systemic toxicity induced seizures
- Avoid hypotension of regional anesthesia
- Avoid supine hypotension syndrome
- Appropriate GA techniques:
- Assume all second trimester patients are at increased risk of aspiration
- Intubate all second trimester patients receiving GA
- Avoid GA techniques with LMA
- During intubation:
  - *Rapid sequence induction* with succinylcholine
  - Trained assistant for induction *mandatory*
  - De-fasiculation with NDMR unnecessary
  - Cricoid pressure from before loss of consciousness, to cuff inflation
  - Use of cuffed ETT
- During extubation:
  - Extubate only when fully awake
  - Inflate lungs and during inflation, cuff of ETT deflated
  - Positive pressure is maintained as ETT is removed

❖ Appropriate positioning:
- During induction:
  - Head up position increases risk of aspiration if vomiting occurs
  - Head up position also makes laryngoscopy difficult
  - Supine with right hip elevation by 10–15° is ideal during intubation
  - Support head on small pillow in sniffing position
- During extubation: lateral, head down position

Options for Antiaspiration Prophylaxis

❖ Oral antacid therapy:
- Particulate antacids are not used as when aspirated they cause:
- Intra-pulmonary shunting
- Severe hypoxia
- Non-particulate antacids reduce severity of pneumonitis if aspiration occurs

- Sodium citrate:
  - 0.3 M non-particulate sodium citrate is used
  - 30 mL sodium citrate neutralizes 255 mL of gastric acid with pH of 1
  - 15–30 mL dose given to those scheduled for Cesarean section
  - Should be given within 20 minutes of induction of GA
  - Action lasts for 40 minutes – 1 hour
  - Side effects: metabolic alkalosis, laxative effect, bad taste
- Sodium bicarbonate:
  - 8.4% dilute $NaHCO_3$ 20 mL
  - Not very effective
  - Can release about 0.4 L of intragastric gas

❖ H_2 antagonists:
- Cimetidine:
  - Given in doses of 200-400 mg IV
  - Reduces gastric acidity within 60-90 minutes
  - Largely replaced by other H_2 antagonists as:
    - Causes arrhythmias and cardiac arrest on rapid injection
    - Interferes with cytochrome P-450 clearance of local anesthetics
- Ranitidine:
  - Oral dose 150 mg ranitidine
  - IV dose 50-100 mg
  - Onset of action within 30 minutes
  - Peak action within 60-90 minutes
  - Duration of action 8 hours
  - Does not interfere with LA metabolism or cause cardiac arrest
- Other less commonly used alternatives:
  - Nizatidine:
    - Dose 150–300 mg PO
    - Duration of action 10 hours
  - Famotidine:
  - Dose 20–40 mg IV or PO
  - Duration of action 10 hours
  - Does not interfere with LA metabolism or cause cardiac arrest

❖ Proton pump inhibitors:
- Omeprazole 20-40 mg PO
- Lansoprazole 10-30 mg PO
- Inhibits proton pump of oxyntic cells
- Advantages:
  - Longer duration of action
  - Reduced incidence of adverse reactions
  - Lower fetal concentration
- Ranitidine is more effective than PPI in reducing gastric volume and pH

❖ Metoclopramide:
- Dose 10 mg which can be given PO/IM/IV:
  - One hour before surgery for oral and IM dose
  - 1-3 mins before induction for IV dose
- Reduces gastric volume below 25 mL within 15 minutes
- Can cause extrapyramidal symptoms
- Crosses the placenta, but with no major fetal side effects

❖ Anticholinergic therapy:
- Glycopyrrolate/ atropine/scopolamine
- Reduces volume of gastric secretions and amount of acid secreted
- May reduce lower esophageal sphincter tone and increase GERD risk
- Not routinely recommended during pregnancy
- Reserved for specific medical/anesthetic indications

❖ Nasogastric tube: used to decompress stomach if distended, before extubation

❖ Role of routine anti-aspiration prophylaxis:
- Anti-aspiration prophylaxis not recommended routinely as:
  - Most patients will not require GA
  - Not cost effective
- Routine prophylaxis causes:
  - Increased pH of stomach
  - This increases intragastric bacterial growth
  - If aspiration occurs, aspiration of colonized gastric content occurs

Recommendations for Antiaspiration Prophylaxis: ASA 2016 Guidelines

❖ Fasting guidelines:
- Clear fluids:
  - Oral intake may be allowed upto 2 hours before induction of anesthesia
  - Examples of clear fluids:
    - Water
    - Fruit juice without pulp
    - Carbonated beverages
    - Clear tea
    - Black coffee
    - Sports drinks

- Volume is less important compared to presence of particulate matter
- Moderate amounts are allowed for:
  - Uncomplicated laboring patients
  - Uncomplicated patients undergoing cesarean section
- Complicated patients requiring further oral restriction include:
  - Obesity
  - Difficult airway
  - Increased risk of emergency cesarean section
  - Non reassuring fetal heart rate pattern on NST

- Solids:
  - Oral intake is allowed upto 6-8 hours before induction of anesthesia
  - Duration depends upon type of solid food (fatty foods)
  - Complicated patients requiring further restriction include:
    - Obesity
    - Difficult airway
    - Increased risk of emergency cesarean section
    - Non reassuring fetal heart rate pattern on NST
    - Avoid solid foods in actively laboring patients

❖ Elective cesarean section:
- Oral antacid not given prior to elective cesarean sections
- H_2 receptor blockers and PPIs:
  - Drugs used:
    - Ranitidine 150 mg
    - Famotidine 20 mg
    - Omeprazole 20 mg
  - Timing of administration:
    - Night before planned surgery
    - Repeated 2 hours before induction of anesthesia
- Metoclopramide:
  - 10 mg PO on the night before surgery
  - 10 mg PO 2 hours prior to induction of anesthesia or
  - 10 mg IV at least 15 minutes prior to induction

❖ Emergency cesarean section:
- 30 mL non-particulate sodium citrate within 15 minutes of induction
- This is important as sodium citrate has a short duration of action
- Ranitidine 50 mg IV at least 30 minutes prior to induction
- Metoclopramide 10 mg IV at least 30 minutes prior to induction

❖ High risk labor:
- Oral antacids and metoclopramide are not recommended
- Ranitidine 150 mg given Q6H during labor

Clinical Presentation

❖ Usually present within first 2 hours of aspiration
❖ Latency period may be upto 6–8 hours

Clinical Staging

Stage I	Profound dyspnea Tachycardia Bronchospasm with normal X-ray
Stage II	Increasing cyanosis and hypoxemia Minor X-ray findings
Stage III	Profound hypoxemia with wide (A-a) DO_2 Reduced compliance Diffuse bilateral infilterates on X-ray
Stage IV	ARDS

Investigations

❖ Gastric aspirate analysis
❖ ABG for PaO_2, alveolar – arterial gradient, hypercarbia
❖ CVP and urine output for fluid therapy
❖ Chest X-ray:
- Right lower lobe most commonly involved
- Bilateral lung involvement may be seen in upright-position aspiration
- Soft, mottled densities in peripheral and dependant lung areas characteristic
- Occurs 12–24 hrs after aspiration
- ***Snow storm*** appearance

Differential Diagnosis

❖ Foreign body aspiration
❖ Barium aspiration
❖ Lipoid pneumonia
❖ Bronchitis
❖ Viral pneumonia
❖ Necrotizing pneumonia

Treatment

- Rigid bronchoscopy:
  - Procedures done prior to rigid bronchoscopy include:
    - Suctioning of upper airway followed by tracheal intubation
    - Suction of primary bronchi through endotracheal tube
  - RB is useful for removing large food particle causing airway obstruction
- Flexible bronchoscopy:
  - Useful for clearing aspirates from distal airway
  - Also useful for obtaining BAL samples
  - Lung lavage:
    - Previously done using sodium bicarbonate and saline
    - Not recommended currently as:
      - Not associated with clinical benefit
      - Increases hypoxemia
- Antibiotics:
  - Prophylactic antibiotics are not useful for preventing aspiration pneumonia
  - Indications for prophylactic antibiotic therapy include:
    - Fever
    - Worsening infiltrates on chest X-ray
    - Leucocytosis
    - Clinical deterioration
    - Failure to resolve within 48 hours
  - BAL/protected specimen brush may be used to obtain culture samples
  - Specific antibiotic therapy can be initiated once pathogen is identified
- Treatment of hypoxemia:
  - Supplemental oxygen is given as required
  - Clinical deterioration may warrant endotracheal intubation
  - Ventilatory strategy should be lung-protective with:
    - Limitation of inspiratory plateau pressures < 30 cm H_2O
    - Minimal tidal volumes (6 mL/kg)
    - High PEEP values
- Fluid therapy:
  - Restrictive fluid strategy is preferred in severe aspiration pneumonia
  - Fluid therapy may be guided by CVP or PCWP
- Corticosteroid therapy:
  - No longer routinely recommended for aspiration pneumonia
  - Indications include:
    - Severe bronchospasm
    - Steroid replacement therapy

HYPERTENSIVE DISORDERS OF PREGNANCY

Introduction

- Most common medical disorder of pregnancy
- Associated with significant maternal and fetal morbidity and mortality

Incidence

- Affects 6-10% of pregnancies
- One of the leading causes of maternal morbidity and mortality
- Maternal morbidity and mortality is lower in developed countries
- Incidence of preeclampsia is 4.6% of all pregnancies

Classification of Hypertensive Disorders in Pregnancy

- Gestational HTN
- Preeclampsia:
  - Preeclampsia without severe features
  - Severe preeclampsia
- Eclampsia
- Chronic HTN
- Chronic HTN with superimposed preeclampsia

Diagnostic Criteria: ACOG 2019 Guidelines

- Gestational HTN:
  - Gestation:
    - Occurs after 20 weeks of gestation
    - Regresses soon after delivery
  - HTN:
    - Sustained elevation of BP on 2 separate occasions at least 4 hours apart:
      - SBP > 140 mm Hg
      - DBP > 90 mm Hg
    - Single occasion of high BP recording:
      - SBP > 160 mm Hg
      - DBP > 110 mm Hg
- Preeclampsia without severe features:
  - Gestation:
    - Occurs after 20 weeks of gestation
    - Regresses within 3 months postpartum

- HTN: sustained elevation of BP on 2 separate occasions at least 4 hours apart:
  - SBP > 140 mm Hg
  - DBP > 90 mm Hg
- Proteinuria:
  - More than 300 mg in 24 hours
  - Protein: creatinine ratio > 0.3
  - Two clear catch midstream urine samples 4 hours apart with:
    - More than +1 on dipstick assay
- Protein concentration > 30 mg/dL
- Edema: not essential for diagnosis

❖ Preeclampsia with severe features:
- Hypertension:
  - Sustained elevation of BP on at least 2 occasions 4 hours apart:
    - SBP > 140 mm Hg
    - DBP > 90 mm Hg
  - Single occasion of high BP recording:
    - SBP > 160 mm Hg
    - DBP > 110 mm Hg
- New onset of at least one of the following:
  - Pulmonary edema
  - Hepatocellular dysfunction:
    - Raised ALT more than twice the normal levels
    - Raised AST more than twice the normal levels
  - Thrombocytopenia < 1,00,000 cells/ µL
  - Raised serum creatinine:
    - Serum creatinine > 1.1 mg/dL
    - Serum creatinine > 2 times baseline serum creatinine levels
  - New onset cerebral or visual symptoms:
    - Visual disturbances:
      - Blurred vision
      - Flashing lights
      - Scotomata
    - Persistent headache:
      - Not explained by other diagnosis
      - Unresponsive to usual analgesics

❖ Eclampsia: new onset tonic-clonic, focal or multifocal seizures in the absence of other causes

❖ Chronic hypertension:
- Pre-pregnancy SBP > 140 mm Hg
- Pre-pregnancy DBP > 90 mm Hg
- Elevated BP which fails to resolve after delivery

Feature	Preeclampsia	Gestational HTN	Chronic HTN
Onset of HTN	> 20 weeks gestation	> 20 weeks gestation	Pregestation
Resolution	3 months post-partum	3 months post-partum	Does not resolve
Severity of HTN	Mild-severe	Mild	Mild-severe
Proteinuria	Present	Absent	Absent
Serum uric acid > 5.5 mg/dL	Present	Absent	Rare
Hemoconcentration	In severe disease	Absent	Absent
Thrombocytopenia	In severe disease	Absent	Absent
Hepatic dysfunction	In severe disease	Absent	Absent

Adverse Effects in Hypertensive Disorders of Pregnancy

❖ Maternal complications:
- Intracerebral hemorrhage
- Hypertensive encephalopathy
- Pulmonary edema
- Eclampsia
- Abruptio placentae
- Disseminated intravascular coagulation
- Renal failure
- Liver failure

❖ Fetal-neonatal complications:
- Oligohydramnios
- Severe IUGR
- Preterm delivery
- Hypoxia-acidosis
- Neurological injury
- Intrauterine death

PREECLAMPSIA

Definition: ACOG 2019 Guidelines

❖ Preeclampsia without severe features:
- Gestation:
  - Occurs after 20 weeks of gestation
  - Regresses within 3 months postpartum

- HTN: Sustained elevation of BP on 2 separate occasions at least 4 hours apart:
  - SBP > 140 mm Hg
  - DBP > 90 mm Hg
- Proteinuria:
  - More than 300 mg in 24 hours
  - Protein: creatinine ratio > 0.3
  - Two clear catch midstream urine samples 4 hours apart with:
    - More than +1 on dipstick assay
    - Protein concentration > 30 mg/dL
- Edema: Not essential for diagnosis

❖ Preeclampsia with severe features:
- Hypertension:
  - Sustained elevation of BP on at least 2 occasions 4 hours apart:
    - SBP > 140 mm Hg
    - DBP > 90 mm Hg
  - Single occasion of high BP recording:
    - SBP > 160 mm Hg
    - DBP > 110 mm Hg
- New onset of at least one of the following:
  - Pulmonary edema
  - Hepatocellular dysfunction:
    - Raised ALT more than twice the normal levels
    - Raised AST more than twice the normal levels
  - Thrombocytopenia < 1,00,000 cells/ μL
  - Raised serum creatinine:
    - Serum creatinine > 1.1 mg/dL
    - Serum creatinine > 2 times baseline serum creatinine levels
  - New onset cerebral or visual symptoms:
    - Visual disturbances:
      - Blurred vision
      - Flashing lights
      - Scotomata
    - Persistent headache:
      - Not explained by other diagnosis
      - Unresponsive to usual analgesics

Types of Preeclampsia

❖ Early preeclampsia:
- Symptom onset before 34 weeks gestation
- High rate of recurrence
- Strong genetic predisposition

❖ Late preeclampsia:
- Symptom onset beyond 34 weeks gestation
- Strong metabolic predisposition

Feature	Early onset	Late onset
Onset of symptoms	< 34 weeks gestation	> 34 weeks gestation
Relative frequency	Rare, 20% incidence	80% incidence
Placental morphology	Abnormal	Normal
Risk for adverse outcomes	High	Negligible
Associated IUGR	Present	Absent
Genetic predisposition	Present	Absent
Etiology	Primarily placental	Primarily maternal
Risk factors	Family history	Diabetes
		Multiple pregnancy Increased BMI Maternal age > 35 years Cardiovascular disorders

Risk Factors for Preeclampsia

❖ Demographic factors:
- Advanced maternal age > 35 years
- Afro-americans, Black race
- Hispanic ethnicity
- Cigarette smoking (associated with risk reduction)

❖ Hypertensive disease:
- History of chronic HTN
- Family history of HTN during pregnancy
- History of preeclampsia in previous pregnancy
- History of systolic HTN during early pregnancy

❖ Associated diseases:
- Pregestational diabetes
- Gestational diabetes
- Thrombophilia
- Obesity with BMI > 30
- Obstructive sleep apnea
- Chronic kidney disease
- Systemic lupus erythematosus
- Circulating anticardiolipin antibodies
- Protein S deficiency
- Protein C resistance
- APLA syndrome

❖ Obstetric factors:
- Nulliparity
- Multifetal gestation, twin pregnancy
- Large for gestational age baby
- Polyhydramnios
- Unexplained fetal growth restriction
- Hydatidiform mole
- Assisted reproduction techniques

Pathogenesis

❖ Genetic factors:
- Maternal genetic factors play an important role
- But no single genetic variant has been found with a strong predisposition

- Polygenic inheritance pattern is seen in preeclampsia involving:
  - Altered expression of angiotensinogen T235
  - Endothelial nitric oxide synthase (eNOS)

❖ Immunological factors:
- Immunological intolerance between mother and fetus contribute to preeclampsia
- Abnormal HLA antigens:
  - Extravillous trophoblasts cells express unusual HLA class I antigens:
    - HLA-C
    - HLA-E
    - HLA-G
  - These may be recognized by natural killer cells (NK-cells)
  - The NK-cell response causes abnormal placental implantation
  - This in turn causes preeclampsia
- Role of dendritic cells:
  - Dendritic cells initiate antigen-specific T-cell responses to decidual tissue
  - This leads to abnormal placental implantation

❖ Inflammation:
- Maternal inflammatory response is important in preeclampsia
- Inflammatory response is seen towards:
  - Circulating synctitio-trophoblast debris
  - Cell-free DNA released due to placental hypoxia
  - Maternal infections

❖ Complement activation:
- This is an important mechanism in patients with connective tissue disorders
- Activation of both classical and alternative complement pathways occurs

❖ Environmental factors:
- Low calcium intake:
  - Low calcium intake alters the effects of calcium regulatory hormones
  - This may contribute to preeclampsia
- Obesity:
  - Obesity predisposes to preeclampsia by inducing:
    - Chronic inflammation
    - Endothelial cell dysfunction
  - This may result in the alteration of placental angiogenic factors
  - The resulting microangiopathy causes preeclampsia

❖ Abnormal placental development:
- Abnormal remodelling of spiral arteries:
  - Spiral A are terminal branches of uterine artery supplying placenta
  - Normally placental cytotrophoblasts invade tunica media of spiral A
  - Due to this, spiral arteries undergo morphological transformation
  - They transform into large capacitance vessels of low resistance
  - In preeclampsia, trophoblasts fail to invade the tunica media
  - Thus, spiral A remain as narrow, high resistance muscular arterioles
  - This results in preeclampsia
- Defective trophoblast differentiation:
  - Normal trophoblasts express adhesion molecules of epithelial cells
  - During endothelial invasion trophoblasts undergo differentiation
  - Adhesion molecules are altered into those of endothelial cells
  - This process is known as pseudo-vasculogenesis
  - Preeclamptic trophoblasts do not show pseudo-vasculogenesis
- Placental hypoperfusion:
  - Placental hypoperfusion causes abnormal placental development
  - Placental hypoperfusion results in release of several factors into circulation
  - These alter maternal endothelial cell function causing preeclampsia

❖ Endothelial dysfunction:
- Imbalance between angiogenetic factors results in endothelial dysfunction
- These factors include:
  - Proangiogenic factors:
    - VEGF (vascular endothelial growth factor)
    - PlGF (placental growth factor)
  - Antiangiogenic factors: sFlt-1
- Endothelial dysfunction results in various clinical features of preeclampsia:
  - HTN due to altered endothelial control of vascular tone
  - Coagulopathy due to altered expression of procoagulants
  - Endothelial dysfunction in target organs causing:
    - Brain: Headache, seizures
    - Liver: Epigastric pain
    - Placenta: Fetal growth retardation

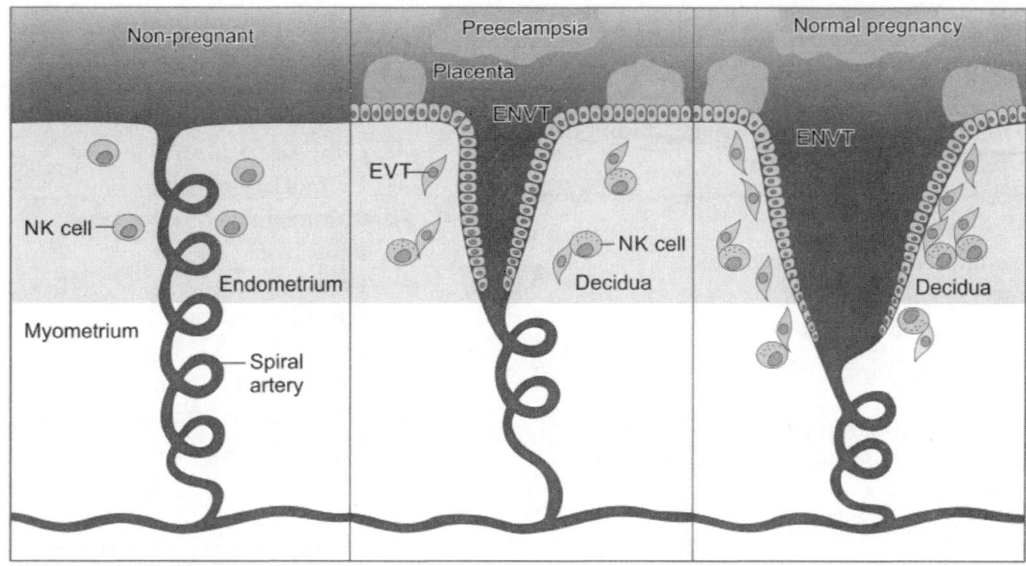

Fig. 9: Pathogenesis of preeclampsia.

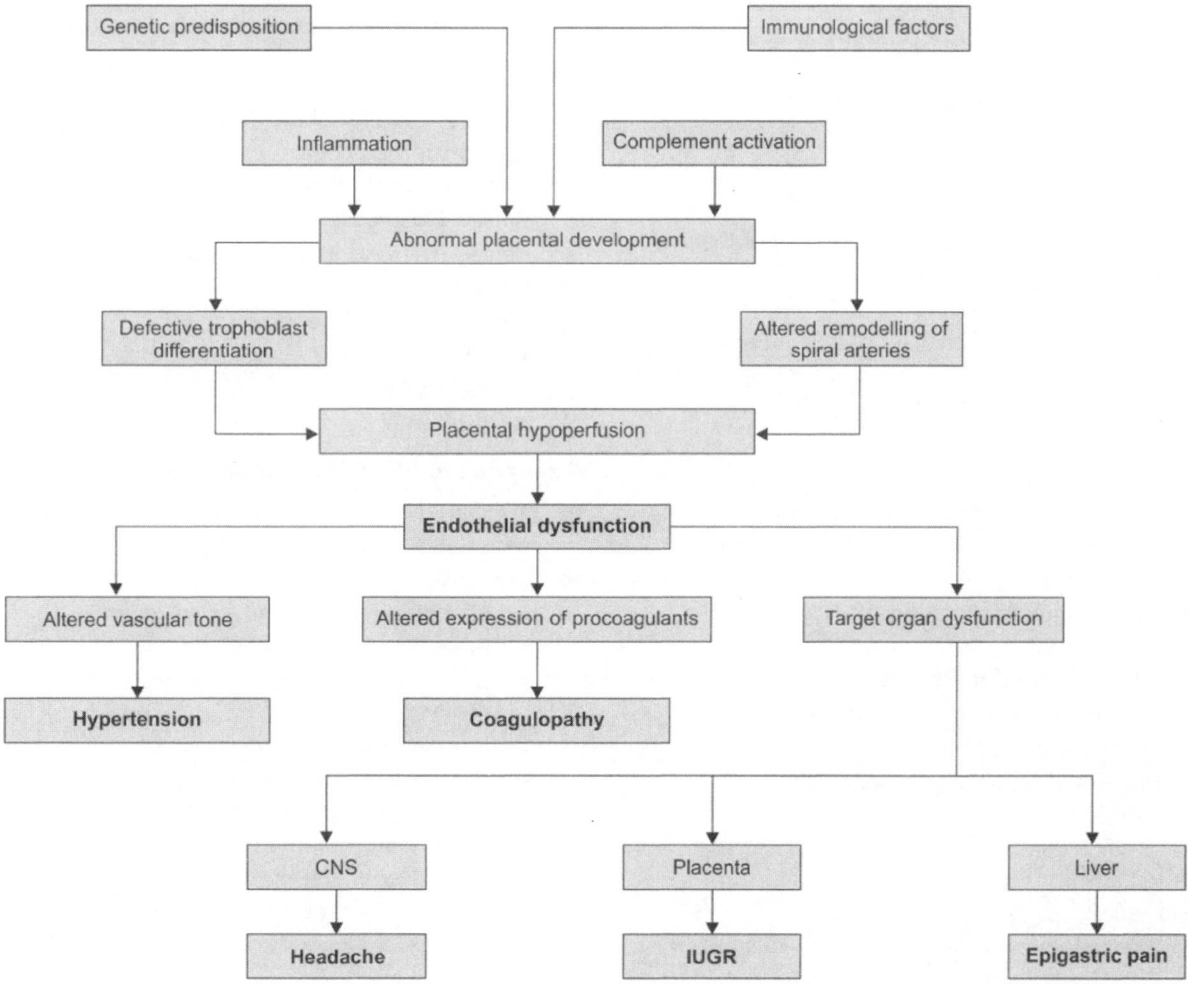

Genetic predisposition → Abnormal placental development

Immunological factors → Abnormal placental development

Inflammation → Abnormal placental development

Complement activation → Abnormal placental development

Abnormal placental development → Defective trophoblast differentiation → Placental hypoperfusion

Abnormal placental development → Altered remodelling of spiral arteries → Placental hypoperfusion

Placental hypoperfusion → **Endothelial dysfunction**

Endothelial dysfunction → Altered vascular tone → **Hypertension**

Endothelial dysfunction → Altered expression of procoagulants → **Coagulopathy**

Endothelial dysfunction → Target organ dysfunction

Target organ dysfunction → CNS → **Headache**

Target organ dysfunction → Placenta → **IUGR**

Target organ dysfunction → Liver → **Epigastric pain**

Pathophysiology

- Central nervous system:
  - Cerebral edema
  - Micro infarcts, punctate hemorrhage, thrombosis
  - Hyperreflexia, hyperreactivity
  - Headache, visual disturbances, vertigo, convulsions
- Cardiovascular:
  - Renin angiotensin axis stimulation
  - Increased systolic BP
  - Increased cardiac output
  - Reduced intravascular volume: sensitive to fluid overload
  - Reduced colloid osmotic pressure
  - Reduced blood volume: hemoconcentration
- Respiratory:
  - Edema of upper airways due to:
    - Increased capillary permeability
    - Reduced colloid osmotic pressure
  - Mild ventilation perfusion mismatch
  - Increased chances of pulmonary edema
- Hepatic:
  - Periportal necrosis
  - Subcapsular hemorrhage
  - Fibrin deposits in sinusoids
  - Impairment in function
  - Hepatomegaly, fatty liver, rupture of liver
- Coagulation:
  - Thrombocytopenia
  - Consumption, increased platelet activation
  - DIC
  - Altered factor VIII: vWF levels
- Renals:
  - Reduced GFR
  - Decreased renal flow, vasospasm
  - Increased BUN, serum creatinine and uric acid levels
  - Acute renal failure, oliguria, azotemia
- Uteroplacental:
  - Placental modular infarcts
  - Reduced intervillous blood flow
  - Hyperactive uterus
  - Increased sensitivity to oxytocin
  - IUGR

Complications

- Maternal:
  - Neurological complications:
    - Convulsions, eclampsia
    - Cerebrovascular accidents
    - Cerebral edema
    - Intracranial hemorrhage
  - Cardiovascular complications:
    - Congestive cardiac failure
    - Pulmonary edema
  - Gastrointestinal complications:
    - Fatty liver
    - Liver rupture
    - HELLP syndrome
  - Others:
    - Acute renal failure
    - DIC, post-partum hemorrhage, abruption
    - Septic shock
- Fetal:
  - Preterm labor
  - IUGR, small for gestational age
  - Respiratory distress syndrome
  - Meconium aspiration
  - Intracranial/ intraventricular hemorrhage

Early Predictors

- Rollover test: HTN on turning patient from left lateral to supine position
- Angiotensin II infusion test
- Raised plasma fibronectin
- Raised uric acid levels > 5.9 mg/dL
- Hypocalciuria
- Raised placental peptides
  - CRH
  - Activin A
  - Inhibin B

Prevention: ACOG 2019 Guidelines

- Till date no intervention has been proven to eliminate the risk of preeclampsia
- Low dose aspirin prophylaxis:
  - 60-150 mg aspirin PO given daily
  - Started before 16 weeks of gestation
  - Recommended in the presence of:
    - More than one high risk factors:
      - History of preeclampsia
      - Multifetal gestation
      - Chronic hypertension
      - Diabetes mellitus
      - Renal disease
      - Autoimmune disorders:
        - SLE
        - APLA

- More than two moderate risk factors:
  - Nulliparity
  - Obesity with BMI > 30
  - Family history of preeclampsia
  - Personal history factors:
    - Age > 35 years
    - Maternal LBW or small for gestational age at birth
    - Previous adverse outcome during pregnancy
    - More than 10-year pregnancy interval

- Common interventions with insufficient evidence:
  - Dietary modification:
    - Garlic supplementation
    - Sodium restriction
    - Fish oil supplements
  - Folic acid supplementation
  - Antioxidants: vitamin C and E
- Newer interventions under investigation:
  - Metformin
  - Sildenafil
  - Statins

Obstetric Management of Severe PE

- Expedited delivery if:
  - Maternal indicators:
    - Severe uncontrolled HTN
    - Persistant CNS symptoms, eclampsia
    - Pulmonary edema
    - AST or ALT > twice normal range with abdominal tenderness
    - Thrombocytopenia < 1,00,000/mm^3
    - Acute renal failure
  - Fetal indicators:
    - Fetal distress in NST
    - Amniotic fluid index < 2
    - USG determined fetal weight < 5th percentile
    - Retrograde umbilical artery end diastolic flow
- Conservative management if:
  - Maternal indicators:
    - Controlled HTN
    - AST and ALT increased but no abdominal tenderness
    - Oliguria < 0.5 mL/kg/hr which improves with rest/fluids
    - Proteinuria < 5 g/day
  - Fetal indicators:
    - BPP > 6
    - Amniotic Fluid Index > 2
    - USG estimated fetal weight > 5th percentile

Preoperative Evaluation

- Clinical evaluation:
  - Duration and severity of preeclampsia
  - Compliance with therapy
  - Time and dose of last drug intake: $MgSO_4$/β blockers
  - Assessment of other organ involvement
  - Coexistent diseases
  - History of last food intake
  - Airway assessment
  - Intravascular volume status assessment
- Investigations:
  - Complete blood count: Hemoconcentration
  - Peripheral blood smear: Schistocytes, Burr cells, Mexican hat cells
  - Blood urea, serum creatinine, uric acid
  - Liver function tests: AST, ALT, LDH, serum albumin
  - Coagulation studies: BT, CT, PT, INR, FDP, D-dimer, TEG
  - Urine analysis:
    - Microscopy
    - 24 hours sample for albuminuria
  - Baseline ultrasound for fetal growth
  - NST weekly from time of diagnosis

Choice of Anesthetic Technique

Labor Analgesia

- Conventional epidural analgesia:
  - Continuous epidural is *technique of choice*
  - Early placement of neuraxial block is recommended:
    - Reduces the requirement of general anesthesia
    - Optimizes timing of catheter placement
    - Optimizes utero-placental circulation early
  - Level of analgesia:
    - Epidural catheter is placed through the L_2-L_3 level
    - T_{10} – L_1 level required for 1st stage of labor
    - S_2 – S_3 level required for 2nd stage of labor
    - Allows verification of catheter function within 15–20 minutes

- Epidural analgesia regimen:
  - Initial bolus:
    - 10-15 mL bupivacaine 0.0625-0.125% with 50-100 μg fentanyl
    - 10-15 mL ropivacaine 0.1-0.2 % with 50-100 μg fentanyl
  - Maintenance dose:
    - Bupivacaine 0.0625-0.125% with fentanyl 1-2 μg/mL at 10-15 mL/hour
    - Alternatively, intermittent boluses may be injected as required
- Advantages:
  - Provides excellent analgesia
  - Prevents hypertensive response to pain
  - Analgesia provided for both 1st and 2nd stage of labor
  - Reduces circulating levels of catecholamines
  - Increases intervillous blood flow
  - Able to produce relaxation if forceps delivery/vacuum
  - Can be converted to surgical anesthesia if cesarean section is planned
- Disadvantages:
  - Time consuming with delayed onset
  - Hypotension, infection, catheter breakage
  - Hematoma if coagulopathy present
  - Nerve injury due to fat needle
  - Increased risk of bloody tap due to fat needle

❖ Other regional anesthesia alternatives:
- Continuous spinal epidural anesthesia:
  - Less preferred to sole continuous epidural anesthesia
  - This is because of coadministration of intrathecal anesthesia
  - Thus, epidural efficacy cannot be evaluated until intrathecal resolution
- Quadratus lumborum block
- Patient controlled epidural anesthesia

❖ Other less commonly used alternatives:
- Paracervical block
- Pudendal nerve block with:
  - Entonox
  - Local perineal infiltration if forceps application or vacuum extraction
- Patient controlled opioid analgesia

Anesthesia for Cesarean Section

❖ Combined spinal-epidural anesthesia (CSE):
- *Technique of choice* for planned cesarean sections in preeclamptic patients
- Spinal anesthesia is activated with combination of:
  - Hyperbaric bupivacaine 75 mg
  - Fentanyl 25 μg
- Epidural anesthesia is activated if duration of surgery exceeds spinal block
- Advantages:
  - Avoidance of GA:
    - No intubation and extubation response
    - Reduced risk of aspiration
    - Reduced risk of failed intubation
    - Awake patient: Easy assessment of CNS status
  - CSE advantages:
    - Immediate onset of action due to intrathecal injection
    - More intense block compared with conventional epidural
    - This enables a much better surgical exposure
    - Produces profound analgesia
    - Epidural catheter can be used for postoperative analgesia
    - Maintains utero-placental perfusion
    - Improves intervillous blood flow
    - Reduces stress response to surgery and catecholamine levels
- Disadvantages:
  - Epidural efficacy cannot be evaluated until intrathecal block resolves
  - No airway control
  - Risk of total spinal/ high spinal
  - Risk of IV infusion of LA if bloody tap-LAST
  - Epidural hematoma if associated coagulopathy
  - Time consuming procedure: not useful in the presence of fetal distress

❖ Conventional epidural anesthesia:
- Advantages:
  - Avoidance of GA:
    - No intubation and extubation response
    - Reduced risk of aspiration
    - Reduced risk of failed intubation
    - Awake patient: Easy assessment of CNS status
  - Epidural advantages:
    - Better hemodynamic stability compared with CSE/ GA
    - Maintains utero-placental perfusion

  - Improves intervillous blood flow
  - Effective pain relief
  - Can be used for postoperative analgesia
  - Reduces stress response to surgery and catecholamine levels
  - Stable cardiac output
- Disadvantages:
  - Slow onset of action in 15-20 minutes is the primary disadvantage
  - Less intense block compared to CSE, compromising surgical exposure
  - No airway control
  - Risk of total spinal/high spinal
  - Risk of IV infusion of LA if bloody tap-LAST
  - Hematoma if associated coagulopathy
  - Time consuming procedure: Not useful if fetal distress

❖ Spinal anesthesia:
- Traditionally contraindicated in the presence of severe preeclampsia
- However, recent data suggests that SAB is appropriate in severe preeclampsia
- Advantages:
  - Causes quick onset of anesthesia
  - Avoids risks associated with GA:
    - No intubation and extubation response
    - Reduced risk of aspiration
    - Reduced risk of failed intubation
    - Awake patient: Easy assessment of CNS status
- Disadvantages:
  - Profound hypotension due to:
    - Sympathetic blockade
    - Pre-existing intravascular volume depletion
    - Concomitant $MgSO_4$ and β-blocker therapy

❖ General anesthesia:
- Less desirable compared with neuraxial techniques due to:
  - Possibility of difficult airway in pregnant patients
  - Exacerbation of HTN during intubation
- Indications for GA:
  - Ongoing maternal hemorrhage
  - Sustained fetal bradycardia
  - Severe thrombocytopenia precluding neuraxial techniques
  - Coagulopathy precluding neuraxial techniques
- Advantages:
  - Controlled airway
  - Faster onset < 5 mins
  - Better hemodynamic stability
  - Avoids spinal hematoma
- Disadvantages:
  - Difficult airway
  - Increased risk of airway trauma and bleeding
  - Intubation response
  - Interaction between $MgSO_4$ and NDMR: delayed awakening
  - Increased chances of aspiration

Preoperative Optimization

❖ Goals:
- To minimize vasospasm
- Improve intravascular volume
- Improve circulation especially to uterus, placenta and kidneys
- To correct fluid and electrolyte imbalance
- Seizures prophylaxis
- Prevent and treatment of coagulation abnormalities

❖ Optimization:
- General:
  - Bed rest
  - Nurse in left lateral position
  - Diuretics if pulmonary edema
  - Keep grouped and cross matched blood ready
  - Continuous fetal monitoring
  - Secure two IV lines (large bore)
- Intravascular volume resuscitation:
  - IV fluids at 60-125 ml/hr of RL/NS
  - Goals of volume resuscitation:
    - Urine output > 1ml/kg/hr
    - CVP around 4-5 mm Hg
    - 5-10 mm Hg of PCWP
- Treatment of acute severe hypertension:
  - Goals:
    - Systolic BP: 120-160 mm Hg
    - Diastolic BP: 80-105 mm Hg
- Drugs used:
  - Labetalol:
    - *First line agent*
    - Onset of action within 5-10 minutes

  - 10–20 mg IV stat dose
  - 40–80 mg increments every 10 minutes
  - Restrict total dose to a maximum of 220 mg
- Hydralazine:
  - Second line agent
  - Onset of action within 10-20 minutes
  - 5 mg IV stat dose
  - Followed by 5 mg increments every 20 minutes
  - Restrict total dose to a maximum of 20 mg IV
- Nifedipine:
  - Used when labetolol and hydralazine are contraindicated
  - Onset of action 10-20 minutes
  - 10 mg PO stat dose
  - Dose is repeated every 20 minutes
  - Restrict total dose to maximum of 50 mg
- Nicardipine:
  - Onset of action 10-15 minutes
  - Initial IV infusion 5 mg/hour
  - Increased by 2.5 mg/hour every 5 minutes
  - Restrict maximum rate of infusion to 15 mg/hour
- Sodium nitroprusside:
  - Onset of action 30 seconds-1 minute
  - 0.25 – 2 µg/kg/min IV infusion
  - Doses above 2 µg/kg/min may result in fetal side effects
  - Less commonly used alternatives:
    - NTG-0.5-5 µg/kg/min IV or 50-100 µg/min or 400 µg sublingual
    - α-methyl dopa: 250 mg PO TID upto maximum 3g/day
    - Trimethaphan: 1–4 mg IV bolus followed by 1 mg/ml infusion
    - Clonidine: 4 µg/kg PO
    - Prazosin

- Seizure prophylaxis:
  - Magnesium sulphate:
  - Drug of choice for seizure prophylaxis in severe preeclampsia
  - Insufficient data to justify use in PE without severe features
  - Therapy is initiated once decision regarding delivery is made
  - Infusion is continued for 24 hours postpartum
  - $MgSO_4$ IV regimen:
    - 4–6 g IV over 20–30 minutes
    - This is followed by 1–2 g/hour infusion
  - Diazepam 5–10 mg followed by 30 mg in 500 ml NS titrated to effect
  - Phenytoin:
    - 10 mg/kg loading dose
    - This is followed by 5 mg/kg at 2 hrs
    - This is followed by 200 mg TID for 5 days
  - Thiopentone 75–100 mg IV for immediate control of ongoing seizures
- Corticosteroid administration:
  - Used to accelerate fetal lung maturation
  - Indicated in parturients between 24–34 weeks gestation
- Anti-aspiration prophylaxis:
  - 15 mL of 0.3 M sodium citrate
  - 1 mg/ kg IV ranitidine
  - 0.15 mg/kg IV metoclopramide
- Prevention and treatment of coagulopathy:
  - Maintain platelet count > 1,00,000/mm^3
  - Use whole blood, FFP, platelet concentrates and cryoprecipitate

Monitoring

- SpO_2, NIBP, ECG
- Capnography and neuromuscular monitoring if GA is planned
- Foleys catheter, hourly intake – output chart
- Hourly deep tendon reflexes
- Maternal muscle strength and $MgSO_4$ levels
- Uterine contraction monitor – tocodynamometer
- Fetal heart rate monitoring
- Indications for invasive BP in preeclampsia:
  - Need for continuous monitoring of BP in severe preeclampsia
  - Poorly controlled maternal blood pressure
  - Planned use of rapid acting vasodilator therapy
  - Need for frequent ABGs as in pre-existing pulmonary edema
  - Use of systolic pressure variation to estimate intravascular volume status
- CVP catheter:
  - Presence of severe preeclampsia alone is not an indication for CVP placement
  - This is because time taken to placement may delay definitive management

- Indications in preeclampsia:
  - Prior to surgery:
    - Preoperative pulmonary edema
    - Difficulties in vascular access
  - Post-surgical indications:
    - Assessment of refractory preoperative oliguria
    - Guide for fluid therapy
    - Assessment of fluid responsiveness
    - Administration of vasoactive inotropes
- PA catheter is used only in the presence of coexisting severe cardiac disease

Conduct of Cesarean Section Under Epidural Anesthesia

- Anti-aspiration prophylaxis
- Large bore IV cannula (16 G) secured for unexpected intraoperative fluid shifts
- *Crystalloid preloading prior to neuraxial techniques is no longer recommended*
- O_2 is administered by face mask
- Appropriate monitors are connected
- Epidural catheter under strict asepsis in L_2-L_3 or L_3 L_4 levels
- Level of analgesia preferred for cesarean section is T_4
- Local anesthetic preparations with adrenaline are avoided in preeclamptic patients:
  - May result in unreliable response due to cotherapy with beta-blockers
  - Causes severe HTN if inadvertent intravascular injection
- For combined spinal epidural anesthesia:
  - Spinal anesthesia is activated with combination of:
    - Hyperbaric bupivacaine 75 mg
    - Fentanyl 25 μg
  - Epidural anesthesia is activated if duration of surgery exceeds spinal block
- For conventional epidural anesthesia:
  - Confirmation using LA-adrenaline mixture is not used in preeclampsia
  - Alternative methods of confirming epidural catheter position have to be used
  - Upon confirmation of epidural catheter location:
    - 0.5% bupivacaine is given in incremental doses till T_4 level is reached
    - If additional perineal relaxation required, 2% lidocaine 5–10 mL given
    - Followed by 0.125% bupivacaine and 2 μg/mL fentanyl at 10 mL/hr
- Treat hypotension with:
  - IV phenylephrine 25–50 μg bolus is the agent of choice
  - IV ephedrine 2.5–5 mg as alternative
  - Left uterine displacement
  - Additional IV fluids
- Uterotonic medications:
  - Administered following delivery of fetus
  - Oxytocin is the first line agent used
  - Misoprostol or carboprost can be used for refractory hemorrhage
  - Ergometrin is contraindicated due to risk of severe HTN
- Postoperative monitoring of platelet count prior to removal of catheter

Conduct of General Anesthesia

Preoperative Preparation

- 2 large bore IV cannula
- IV fluids at 60–100 ml/hr NS/RL
- Informed consent taken
- Antiaspiration prophylaxis 30–60 minutes prior to anesthetic induction
- Antihypertensive therapy
- Seizure prophylaxis
- Keep adequate blood ready

Anesthetic Considerations 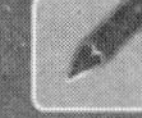

- Difficult airway due to edema
- Exaggerated hypertensive response to intubation and extubation
- Increased risk of aspiration
- Drug interaction with $MgSO_4$:
  - Increased sensitivity to NDMR
  - Increased duration of action of NDMR
  - Reduced BP: profound hypotension with RA
  - Hypotension refractory to therapy
  - Platelet aggregation: increased bleeding
  - Neonatal hyporeflexia and respiratory depression
  - Reduced beat to beat variability in FHR
  - Increased post-partum hemorrhage (PPH) due to:
    - Tocolysis
    - Increased uterine blood flow

OT Preparation

- Emergency drugs
- Facemask (transparent), airways
- ETT – 7, 6.5, 6 and 5.5 size
- Different laryngoscopy blade sizes, gum elastic bougie

- Anesthetic drugs
- Skilled assistant for rapid sequence induction
- Working suction kept ready

Induction

- Adequate preoxygenation with 100% O_2 and tight-fitting face mask:
  - 3 minutes of tidal volume breathing or
  - 8 vital capacity breaths
- Labetolol may be administered to titrate BP to < 140/90 mm Hg
- Rapid sequence induction technique is used
- Induction agent used is IV propofol 2 mg/kg
- Ketamine is avoided due to exaggerated sympathomimetic response
- IV succinylcholine IV 1-1.5 mg/kg for neuromuscular paralysis
- Dose adjustment for succinylcholine due to magnesium therapy is not required
- Topical anesthesia of airway may be used to reduce intubation response
- Intubation is carried out with smaller sized ETT
- Intubation response may be controlled with:
  - IV lidocaine 1.5 mg/kg
  - IV labetalol 10 mg bolus
  - IV esmolol 0.5-1 mg/kg bolus
  - IV NTG infusion
- Awake intubation preferred in the presence of preoperative:
  - Dyspnea
  - Stridor
  - Dysphonia

Maintenance

- 100% O_2 + 0.5 MAC isoflurane used to maintain balanced anesthesia
- 2/3rd MAC of volatile anesthetics used
- Give titrated small doses of cisatracurium/atracurium for NMB
- Neuromuscular monitoring mandatory due to concomitant magnesium therapy
- $MgSO_4$ therapy is continued intraoperatively
- Restrictive IV fluid regimen is preferred to prevent fluid overload
- Following delivery of fetus:
  - Volatile anesthetic dose is reduced to prevent uterine atony
  - Nitrous oxide or propofol infusion may be used to prevent awareness
  - IV fentanyl 1–2 µg/kg is given after delivery of fetus
  - Uterotonic therapy is administered:
    - Oxytocin 20–40 IU in 1000 mL RL is given over 4–8 hours
    - If uterine atony unresponsive to oxytocin:
      - Carboprost 0.25 mg IM Q 15–60 mins as required
      - Misoprostol 800-1000 mg PO/PR/PV Q2H
    - Avoid ergot alkaloids like methergine due to risk of hypertensive crisis

Extubation

- Fully awake, fully reversed
- IV xylocard/esmolol to decrease extubation response

Postoperative

Monitors

- Urine output and intake output chart hourly till post-partum diuresis occurs
- Monitor CNS status, convulsions
- Monitor for neuromuscular weakness
- Monitor for 12–24 hrs

Analgesia

- Multimodal analgesia
- NSAIDs:
  - May potentiate PPH and postpartum HTN
  - Thus they are generally avoided when HTN persists beyond the first POD
  - Agents commonly used are:
    - Ketorolac 30 mg IV Q6H
    - Ibuprofen 600–800 mg PO Q6H
- IV/ IM/neuraxial opioids /PCA/ PCEA
- Epidural/CSE

Management

- Fluids at < 80 ml/hr
- $MgSO_4$ is continued for 24 hours after last seizure episode
- Change from IV to oral antihypertensives
- May require antihypertensives for 3 months
- Advise about risk of preeclampsia in later pregnancies

ECLAMPSIA

Introduction

- New onset seizures or coma in preeclamptic patients with:
  - No pre-existing neurological disorder
  - No other known cause of seizures

- Onset of eclampsia may occur:
  - Antepartum (50%)
  - Intrapartum (25%)
  - Postpartum (25%)

Incidence

- Major cause of maternal morbidity and mortality
- Incidence ranges from 0.1-5.9 per 10000 pregnancies
- Maternal mortality rate is approximately 4.2%
- Perinatal mortality rate ranges from 13-30%

Pathogenesis

- Precise mechanism of eclamptic seizures is not known
- Two mechanisms have been proposed
- Breakdown of cerebral autoregulation:
  - Severe HTN causes breakdown of cerebral autoregulation
  - This leads to hyperperfusion and endothelial dysfunction
  - This ultimately results in vasogenic and cytotoxic edema
- Activation of cerebral autoregulation:
  - Severe HTN causes activation of autoregulatory mechanisms
  - This results in cerebral vasoconstriction and hypoperfusion
  - Localized ischemia results, causing endothelial dysfunction
  - This ultimately results in vasogenic and cytotoxic edema

Clinical Features

- Can occur before, during or after labor
- Premonitory symptoms:
  - Most often seizures are preceded by premonitory symptoms
  - These include:
    - Hypertension most commonly (75%)
    - Headache (66%):
      - Persistent frontal or occipital headache
      - Thunderclap headaches
    - Visual disturbances (27%):
      - Scotomata
      - Loss of vision due to cortical blindness
      - Blurred vision
      - Visual field defects: Homonymous hemianopia
      - Photophobia
    - Right upper quadrant or epigastric pain (25%)
    - Other rarely associated symptoms:
      - Vertigo, vomiting
      - Sudden onset severe edema with oliguria
- Premonitory signs:
  - Hyperreflexia with clonus
  - Visual perception deficits
  - Visual perception deficits
  - Altered mental status
  - Memory deficits
  - Cranial nerve deficits
- Onset of GTCS of variable duration:
  - Tonic phase: 15-20 seconds
    - Sudden loss of consciousness
    - Loss of posture with self-injury
    - Brief flexion of arms, deviation of eyes
    - Extension of back, neck and arms
    - Involuntary cry due to contraction of respiratory muscles
    - Shallow breathing
    - Ends with tremors to merge with clonic phase
  - Clonic phase: 60-90 seconds
    - Brief violent generalized flexor contractions
    - Muscle relaxation is progressively prolonged
    - Cyanosis
    - Tongue and cheek biting
    - Frothy salivation
    - Loss of bowel and bladder control
    - Ends with deep inspiration, sustained muscle relaxation
  - Post-ictal phase: several hours
    - Most patients recover consciousness within 10-20 minutes of clonic phase
    - Headache, mild confusion
    - Myalgia
    - Fatigue
- Fetal response to eclampsia:
  - Fetal bradycardia lasting for 3-5 minutes occurs during seizure activity
  - Resolution of maternal seizures is associated with:
    - Fetal tachycardia
    - Loss of fetal heart rate variability
  - Persistent fetal heart rate changes are associated with post-eclamptic abruption

- Associated with:
  - Respiratory arrest and cyanosis during convulsions
  - Postictal hemiparesis due to intracranial hemorrhage

Complications

- Cerebral edema
- Raised ICP
- Status epilepticus
- Cerebral hemorrhage
- Pulmonary edema due to:
  - Aspiration
  - Cardiac failure
- Acute renal failure
- Liver rupture
- Placental abruption
- Respiratory failure
- Death

Differential Diagnosis

- Seizures without neurological deficits:
  - Metabolic anomalies:
    - Hypocalcemia
    - Hyponatremia
    - Hypoglycemia
  - Toxins:
    - Drug intoxication
    - Alcohol withdrawal
  - Infections:
    - Meningitis
    - Encephalitis
    - Sepsis
  - Others:
    - Thrombotic thrombocytopenic purpura
    - Hemolytic uremic syndrome
- Seizures with neurological deficits:
  - Stroke
  - Intracranial hemorrhage
  - Mass lesion
  - Metabolic encephalopathy
  - CNS infections

Treatment

- Supportive therapy:
  - Maternal oxygenation and protection:
    - Nurse in eclampsia unit
    - *Nurse in left lateral position*
    - Supplemental O_2 administered at 8-10 L/min via non-rebreathing mask
    - Reduce light and sound stimulation
    - Protect head and body from injury
    - Oral airway is avoided until resolution of seizure
    - Raised, padded bed rails may be used to prevent injury
  - Maintain patent airway in patients with altered consciousness:
    - Suction airway to remove secretions
    - Apply jaw thrust and head tilt
    - Attempt ventilation using bag and mask with 100% FiO_2
    - Soft, lubricated nasal airway may be used to maintain airway patency
  - Circulation:
    - Secure two large bore IV lines
    - Restrict IV fluids to 75 -100 mL/hour to minimize cerebral edema
    - Foleys catheter with intake output monitor
    - CVP and IBP placement
    - Monitor BP and ECG continuously
- Antihypertensive therapy:
  - Indications:
    - Persistent elevation for > 30 minutes:
      - SBP > 200 mm Hg
      - DBP > 120 mm Hg
      - MAP > 140 mm Hg
    - Persistent elevation for > 1 hour:
      - SBP > 160 mm Hg
      - DBP > 110 mm Hg
      - MAP > 130 mm Hg
    - Hypertension with pre-existing thrombocytopenia or CCF:
      - SBP > 155 mm Hg
      - DBP > 105 mm Hg
      - MAP > 125 mm Hg
  - Drugs used:
    - Labetalol:
      - *First line agent*
      - Onset of action within 5-10 minutes
      - 10-20 mg IV stat dose
      - 40-80 mg increments every 10 minutes
      - Restrict total dose to a maximum of 220 mg

- Hydralazine:
  - Second line agent
  - Onset of action within 10-20 minutes
  - 5 mg IV stat dose
  - Followed by 5 mg increments every 20 minutes
  - Restrict total dose to a maximum of 20 mg IV
- Nifedipine:
  - Used when labetolol and hydralazine are contraindicated
  - Onset of action 10-20 minutes
  - 10 mg PO stat dose
  - Dose is repeated every 20 minutes
  - Restrict total dose to maximum of 50 mg
- Nicardipine:
  - Onset of action 10-15 minutes
  - Initial IV infusion 5 mg/hour
  - Increased by 2.5 mg/hour every 5 minutes
  - Restrict maximum rate of infusion to 15 mg/hour
- Sodium nitroprusside:
  - Onset of action 30 seconds-1 minute
  - 0.25 – 2 μg/kg/min IV infusion
  - Doses above 2 μg/kg/min may result in fetal side effects

❖ Anticonvulsant therapy:

- Magnesium sulphate therapy:
  - Magnesium sulphate is the anticonvulsant of choice
  - Therapeutic range of 4.8-8.4 mg/dL is recommended
  - Therapeutic regimen:
    - Loading dose of 4-6 grams over 20-30 minutes
    - Followed by 1-2 g/hour maintenance infusion
    - For seizure recurrence additional bolus dose of 2-4 grams IV
  - Previous regimens used:
    - ***Pitchards*** regimen:
      - Loading dose 4 grams $MgSO_4$ IV over 5 minutes
      - Followed by 5 grams IM in each buttock (total 10 gram)
      - Subsequently 5 gram IM in alternate buttock Q4H
    - ***Zuspan*** regimen:
      - 4 grams $MgSO_4$ IV loading dose over 5-10 minutes
      - Followed by 1-2 gram/ hour infusion
    - ***Sibai*** regimen:
      - 6 grams $MgSO_4$ IV loading dose over 15-20 minutes
      - Followed by 2 gram/ hour infusion
- Other anticonvulsant regimens used:
  - ***Lytic cocktail*** regimen/***Menon*** regimen:
    - Loading dose:
      - 25 mg chlorpromazine + 100 mg pethidine IV
      - 50 mg chlorpromazine + 25 mg promethazine IM
    - 100 mg pethidine in 1L 20% dextrose over 24 hours
    - IV promethazine 25 mg Q4H
    - IV chlorpromazine 50 mg Q8H
  - ***Lean*** regimen:
    - Diazepam 10 mg IV every 2 minutes to maximum 40 mg
    - Followed by 40 mg in 500 mL normal saline over 24 hours
  - Thiopentone used for magnesium sulphate refractory seizures
  - Phenytoin:
    - Used for magnesium sulphate refractory seizures
    - 1.25 grams IV bolus at rate of 50 mg/minute

❖ Obstetric management:

- Eclampsia is considered as an absolute contraindication for expectant therapy
- Thus, delivery of the fetus is the only definitive management
- Trial of labor with inducing agents may be attempted in:
  - Gestational age > 34 weeks
  - Favourable Bishops score
- Cesarean section is preferred for:
  - Gestational age < 34 weeks
  - Unfavorable cervix

❖ Postpartum management:

- Seizures always resolve following delivery
- Diuresis (> 4 L/day) is the most accurate clinical indicator of resolution
- Absence of seizure activity is confirmed prior to stopping anticonvulsants
- Magnesium sulphate therapy is continued for 24 hours postpartum

- For post-partum eclampsia magnesium sulphate is continued for 24-48 hours
- Antihypertensive therapy is continued post-partum to prevent stroke
- Transition to oral medications is considered in those with persistent HTN

Complications

- Cerebral edema: mannitol/hypertonic saline, hyperventilation
- Pulmonary edema: diuretics, IPPV
- Acute renal failure: diuretics, RRT
- Liver rupture: IV fluids, surgical repair
- DIC: FFP, cryoprecipitate

ANESTHESIA FOR ECLAMPSIA PATIENTS

Preoperative Preparation

- 2 large bore IV cannula
- *IV fluids restricted to 75-100 mL/hour to minimize cerebral edema*
- Informed consent taken
- Antiaspiration prophylaxis 30-60 minutes prior to anesthetic induction
- Antihypertensive therapy for:
  - SBP > 160 mm Hg
  - DBP > 110 mm Hg
- Seizure prophylaxis should be continued intra-operatively
- Keep adequate blood ready

Anesthestic Considerations

- *Difficult airway due to:*
  - *Airway edema*
  - *Swollen tongue due to injury during seizure activity*
- Exaggerated hypertensive response to intubation and extubation
- Increased risk of aspiration
- Presence of pre-existing neurological deficits should be recorded
- *Raised ICP predisposing to intracranial hemorrhage at induction*
- Drug interaction with $MgSO_4$:
  - Increased sensitivity to NDMR
  - Increased duration of action of NDMR
  - Reduced BP: Profound hypotension with RA
  - Hypotension refractory to therapy
  - Platelet aggregation: Increased bleeding
  - Neonatal hyporeflexia and respiratory depression
  - Reduced beat to beat variability in FHR
  - Increased post-partum hemorrhage (PPH) due to:
    - Tocolysis
    - Increased uterine blood flow

OT Preparation

- Emergency drugs
- Facemask (transparent), airways
- ETT – 7, 6.5, 6 and 5.5 size
- Different laryngoscopy blade sizes, gum elastic bougie
- Anesthetic drugs
- Skilled assistant for rapid sequence induction
- Working suction kept ready

Monitoring

- SpO_2, NIBP, ECG
- Capnography and neuromuscular monitoring if GA is planned
- Foleys catheter, hourly intake – output chart
- Hourly deep tendon reflexes
- Maternal muscle strength and $MgSO_4$ levels
- Fetal heart rate monitoring
- Indications for invasive BP in eclampsia:
  - Need for continuous monitoring of BP
  - Poorly controlled maternal blood pressure
  - Planned use of rapid acting vasodilator therapy
  - Need for frequent ABGs as in pre-existing pulmonary edema
  - Use of systolic pressure variation to estimate intravascular volume status
- CVP catheter:
  - Presence of eclampsia alone is not an indication for CVP placement
  - This is because time taken to placement may delay definitive management
  - Indications in eclampsia:
    - Prior to surgery:
      - Preoperative pulmonary edema
      - Difficulties in vascular access
    - Post-surgical indications:
      - Assessment of refractory preoperative oliguria
      - Guide for fluid therapy
      - Assessment of fluid responsiveness
      - Administration of vasoactive inotropes
- PA catheter is used only in the presence of coexisting severe cardiac disease

Conduct of Cesarean Section Under Epidural Anesthesia

- *Neuraxial anesthesia may be used in patients with:*
  - *Well controlled seizures*
  - *No evidence of raised ICP*
  - *Normal coagulation parameters*

- Anti-aspiration prophylaxis
- Large bore IV cannula (16 G) secured for unexpected intraoperative fluid shifts
- *Crystalloid preloading prior to neuraxial techniques is no longer recommended*
- O_2 is administered by face mask
- Appropriate monitors are connected
- Epidural catheter under strict asepsis in L_2-L_3 or L_3 L_4 levels
- Level of analgesia preferred for cesarean section is T_4
- Local anesthetic preparations with adrenaline are avoided in eclamptic patients:
    - May result in unreliable response due to co-therapy with beta-blockers
    - Causes severe HTN if inadvertent intravascular injection
- For combined spinal epidural anesthesia:
    - Spinal anesthesia is activated with combination of:
        - Hyperbaric bupivacaine 75 mg
        - Fentanyl 25 μg
    - Epidural anesthesia is activated if duration of surgery exceeds spinal block
- For conventional epidural anesthesia:
    - Confirmation using LA-adrenaline mixture is not used in eclampsia
    - Alternative methods of confirming epidural catheter position have to be used
    - Upon confirmation of epidural catheter location:
        - 0.5% bupivacaine is given in incremental doses till T_4 level is reached
        - If additional perineal relaxation required, 2% lidocaine 5-10 mL given
        - Followed by 0.125% bupivacaine and 2 μg/mL fentanyl at 10 mL/hr
- Treat hypotension with:
    - IV phenylephrine 25-50 μg bolus is the agent of choice
    - IV ephedrine 2.5-5 mg as alternative
    - Left uterine displacement
    - Additional IV fluids
- Uterotonic medications:
    - Administered following delivery of fetus
    - Oxytocin is the first line agent used
    - Misoprostol or carboprost can be used for refractory hemorrhage
    - Methergine is contraindicated due to risk of severe HTN
- Postoperative monitoring of platelet count prior to removal of catheter

Induction

- Adequate preoxygenation with 100% O_2 and tight-fitting face mask:
    - 3 minutes of tidal volume breathing or
    - 8 vital capacity breaths
- Labetolol may be administered to titrate BP to < 140/90 mm Hg
- Rapid sequence induction technique is used
- Induction agent used is IV propofol 2 mg/kg
- *Ketamine is avoided due to:*
    - *Exaggerated sympathomimetic response*
    - *Increase in ICP*
- IV succinylcholine IV 1-1.5 mg/kg for neuromuscular paralysis
- Dose adjustment for succinylcholine due to magnesium therapy is not required
- Topical anesthesia of airway may be used to reduce intubation response
- *Deep plane of anesthesia is preferred at intubation to prevent increase in ICP*
- Intubation is carried out with smaller sized ETT
- Intubation response may be controlled with:
    - IV lidocaine 1.5 mg/kg
    - IV labetalol 10 mg bolus
    - IV esmolol 0.5-1 mg/kg bolus
    - IV NTG infusion

Maintenance

- 100% O_2 + 0.5 MAC isoflurane used to maintain balanced anesthesia
- 2/3rd MAC of volatile anesthetics used
- Give titrated small doses of cisatracurium/atracurium for NMB
- Neuromuscular monitoring mandatory due to concomitant magnesium therapy
- $MgSO_4$ therapy is continued intraoperatively
- Restrictive IV fluid regimen is preferred to prevent fluid overload
- Hyperventilation is avoided as it reduces CBF without reducing $CMRO_2$
- *Hypoventilation is also avoided as it reduces seizure threshold*
- *Eucapneic ventilation is preferred (E_TCO_2 35-45 mm Hg)*
- Following delivery of fetus:

- Volatile anesthetic dose is reduced to prevent uterine atony
- Nitrous oxide or propofol infusion may be used to prevent awareness
- IV fentanyl 1-2 μg/kg is given after delivery of fetus
- Uterotonic therapy is administered:
  - Oxytocin 20-40 IU in 1000 mL RL is given over 4-8 hours
  - If uterine atony unresponsive to oxytocin:
    - Carboprost 0.25 mg IM Q 15-60 mins as required
    - Misoprostol 800-1000 mg PO/PR/PV Q2H
  - Avoid ergot alkaloids like methergine due to risk of hypertensive crisis

Extubation

- Fully awake, fully reversed with absence of seizure activity
- Patients with inadequate neurological recovery require postoperative ventilation
- IV xylocard/ esmolol may be used to decrease extubation response

Postoperative Management

Monitors

- Urine output and intake output chart hourly till post-partum diuresis occurs
- Monitor CNS status, convulsions
- Monitor for neuromuscular weakness
- Monitor for 12-24 hrs

Analgesia

- Multimodal analgesia
- NSAIDs:
  - May potentiate PPH and postpartum HTN
  - Thus they are generally avoided when HTN persists beyond the first POD
  - Agents commonly used are:
    - Ketorolac 30 mg IV Q6H
    - Ibuprofen 600-800 mg PO Q6H
- IV/IM/neuraxial opioids /PCA/PCEA
- Epidural/CSE

Management

- Seizures always resolve following delivery
- Diuresis (> 4 L/day) is the most accurate clinical indicator of resolution
- Absence of seizure activity is confirmed prior to stopping anticonvulsants
- Magnesium sulphate therapy is continued for 24 hours postpartum
- For post-partum eclampsia magnesium sulphate is continued for 24-48 hours
- Antihypertensive therapy is continued post-partum to prevent stroke
- Transition to oral medications is considered in those with persistent HTN

HELLP SYNDROME

Introduction

- HELLP syndrome is one of the most serious complications of severe preeclampsia
- Formerly known as edema-proteinuria-hypertension gestosis type B
- Renamed as HELLP syndrome by ***Louis Weinstein*** in 1982
- The syndrome can occur in pregnant and postpartum women
- It is characterized by specific abnormalities:
  - Hemolysis with a microangiopathic blood smear
  - Elevated liver enzymes
  - Low platelet count

Incidence

- Occurs in 0.1-1% of all pregnancies
- Complicates 4-12% of preeclampsia cases
- Most patients stabilize within 24-48 hours
- Maternal mortality rate of 1-3%
- Perinatal mortality rate of 35%
- Recurrence rate of 2-27% in subsequent pregnancies
- More commonly seen in multiparous, white females

SIBAIS Diagnostic Criteria

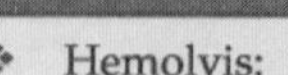

- Hemolyis:
  - Bilirubin > 1.2 mg/dL
  - Abnormal peripheral smear
  - Reduced serum haptoglobulin
- Elevated liver enzymes:
  - AST/SGOT > 70 IU/L
  - LDH > 600 IU/L or twice the upper limit of normal
- Low platelets < 1,00,000 cells/mm^3

Risk Factors

- Previous history of preeclampsia/HELLP syndrome
- Genetic factors:
  - Membrane cofactor protein
  - Complement factor-I
- Multiparity

Pathophysiology

- Placental ischemia theory:
  - Postulates that mechanisms of HELLP and preeclampsia are similar
  - Defective placental development occurs due to abnormalities in spiral artery
  - This results in the release of various factors such as:
    - Placental growth factors
    - Vascular endothelial growth factor
  - This results in endothelial cell dysfunction and HELLP syndrome
- Immune rejection theory:
  - HELLP arises due to maternal immune response to fetal antigens
  - This in turn results in endothelial dysfunction and multiorgan damage
  - Fetal genetic variants associated with long-chain 3-hydroxyacyl CoA dehydrogenase (LCHAD) are commonly responsible
- Inborn errors of fatty acid metabolism:
  - Medium-long chain fatty acid mutations result in defective metabolism
  - This results in insufficient mitochondrial oxidation of fatty acids
  - This causes hepatocellular damage seen in HELLP syndrome
- Complement dysregulation theory:
  - Abnormal placentation results in complement dysregulation
  - Dysregulation of complement cascade results in multisystem dysfunction

Pathogenesis

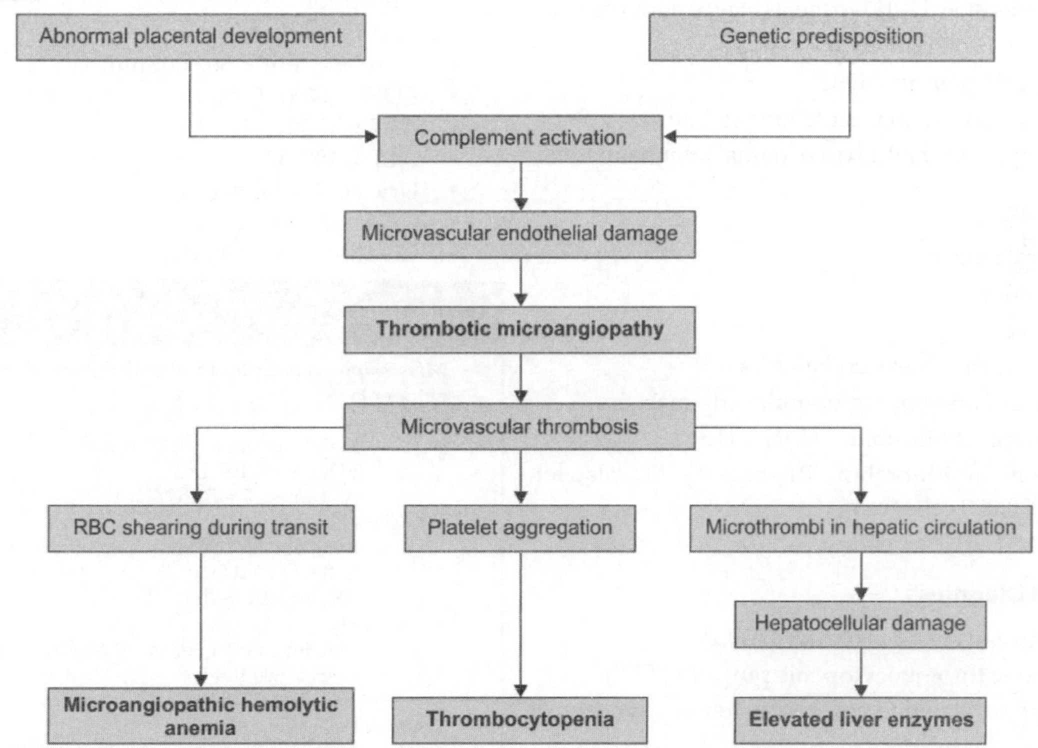

Clinical Features

- Onset of HELLP syndrome:
  - Antepartum presentation:
    - Occurs antepartum in 70% of cases
    - Typically develops between 28-36 weeks of gestation
  - Postpartum presentation:
    - Occurs post-partum in 30% of cases
    - Mostly present within 48 hours of delivery
    - May occur upto 7 days post-partum
- Symptoms:
  - Clinical presentation is varied

- Common symptoms include:
  - Abdominal pain: (40-90% patients)
    - Most common symptom
    - Pain localized to:
      - Mid-epigastrium
      - Right upper quadrant
      - Below the sternum
  - Nausea, vomiting and malaise (29-84% patients)
  - Uncommon symptoms:
    - Headache (33-68% patients)
    - Visual disturbances (10-20% patients)
    - Thrombocytopenia related bleeding:
      - Mucosal hematuria
      - Petechial hemorrhage
      - Ecchymosis
      - Retinal hemorrhage

❖ Signs:
- Hypertension: 12–18% patients may be normotensive
- Edema, proteinuria
- Abruptio placenta, DIC
- Pulmonary edema, acute kidney injury
- Subcapsular of intraparenchymal liver hematoma

Investigations

❖ Peripheral smear:
- Schistocytes
- Burr cells
- Spherocytes, Mexican hat cells

❖ Raised LDH and haptoglobulin: early markers

❖ Raised indirect bilirubin, reduced Hb

❖ FDP and antithrombin III activity if platelet count < 50,000 cells/mm^3

❖ Raised AST, ALT levels

Differential Diagnosis

❖ Acute fatty liver of pregnancy (AFLP)

❖ Thrombotic thrombocytopenic purpura (TTP)

❖ Pregnancy related hemolytic uremic syndrome (HUS)

❖ Preeclampsia with severe features

❖ Other disorders:
- Lupus flare
- Hepatitis
- Cholecystitis
- Appendicitis
- Pancreatitis

Feature	HELLP	TTP/HUS	AFLP
Hypertension	Present	±	±
Anemia	±	Severe	Normal
Thrombocytopenia	Present	Severe	±
Proteinuria	Present	±	±
Antithrombin III	±	Normal	Decreased
AST	Elevated	Normal	Elevated
Bilirubin	Elevated, indirect	Elevated	Elevated, direct
Creatinine	±	Elevated	Elevated
Fibrinogen	Normal	Normal	Decreased
Glucose	Normal	Normal	Decreased
Ammonia	Normal	Normal	Elevated
LDH	Elevated	Grossly elevated	Elevated

Risk Factors Increasing Morbidity

❖ Clinical factors:
- Epigastric pain
- Nausea, vomiting
- Eclampsia
- Severe HTN
- Abruption

❖ Laboratory factors:
- Platelet count < 50,000/mm^3
- LDH > 1400 IU/L
- AST > 150 IU/L
- ALT > 100 IU/L
- Uric acid > 7.8 mg/dL
- CPK > 200 IU/L
- Creatinine > 1 mg/dL

Classification

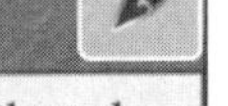

❖ ***Mississippi*** classification: Based on severity of thrombocytopenia
- Class I:
  - Platelet count < 50,000/ mm3
  - LDH > 600 IU/L
  - AST or ALT > 70 IU/L
- Class II:
  - Platelet count 50,000 – 1,00,000/mm^3
  - LDH > 600 IU/L
  - AST or ALT > 70 IU/L
- Class III:
  - Platelet count 1,00,000 – 1,50,000/ mm^3
  - LDH > 600 IU/L
  - AST or ALT > 40 IU/L

❖ *Tennessee* classification:
- Complete HELLP: When more than 2 criteria are present:
  - Severe anemia unrelated to blood loss
  - Platelet count < ₹1,00,000/mm^3
  - LDH > 600 IU/L or more than twice upper limit of normal
  - AST > 70 IU/L or more than twice upper limit of normal
  - Serum bilirubin > 1.2 mg/dL
  - Peripheral smear with schistocytes and burr cells
- Incomplete HELLP: Only 1 or 2 of the above

Management

- Definitive therapy:
  - In general, there is no role for expectant management in HELLP syndrome
  - Only definitive therapy is immediate delivery via Cesarean section under GA
  - If gestational age is below 34 weeks:
    - Delivery may be delayed for 24-48 hours
    - This is done to accelerate fetal lung maturation with corticosteroids
    - However, maternal and fetal condition must be stable
    - Continuous monitoring of mother and fetus is essential
    - Expectant management beyond 48 hours is not recommended
    - This is because risk of serious complications is high
  - Trial of labor with inducing agents may be attempted in:
    - Gestational age > 34 weeks
    - Favourable Bishops score
  - Cesarean section is preferred for:
    - Gestational age < 34 weeks
    - Unfavorable cervix
- Supportive therapy:
  - *Nurse in left lateral position*
  - Supplemental O_2 administered at 8-10 L/min via non-rebreathing mask
  - Reduce light and sound stimulation
  - Secure two large bore IV lines
  - Restrict IV fluids to 75 -100 mL/hour
  - Platelet transfusion therapy:
    - Indications:
      - Significant bleeding
      - Platelet count < 20,000 cells/mm^3 in all pregnant patients
      - Platelet count < 40,000 cells/mm^3 for cesarean section
    - Dose:
      - 6-10 units of random donor platelets
      - 2 units of single donor platelets
  - Packed cells are transfused when hemoglobin falls below 7 g/dL
  - Foleys catheter with intake output monitor
  - CVP and IBP placement
  - Monitor BP and ECG continuously
  - Complete counts are repeated 24 hours after steroid therapy
- Antihypertensive therapy:
  - Goals:
    - Systolic BP < 160 mm Hg
    - Diastolic BP < 110 mm Hg
  - Drugs used:
    - Labetalol:
      - *First line agent*
      - Onset of action within 5-10 minutes
      - 10-20 mg IV stat dose
      - 40-80 mg increments every 10 minutes
      - Restrict total dose to a maximum of 220 mg
    - Hydralazine:
      - Second line agent
      - Onset of action within 10-20 minutes
      - 5 mg IV stat dose
      - Followed by 5 mg increments every 20 minutes
      - Restrict total dose to a maximum of 20 mg IV
    - Nifedipine:
      - Used when labetolol and hydralazine are contraindicated
      - Onset of action 10-20 minutes
      - 10 mg PO stat dose
      - Dose is repeated every 20 minutes
      - Restrict total dose to maximum of 50 mg
    - Nicardipine:
      - Onset of action 10-15 minutes
      - Initial IV infusion 5 mg/hour
      - Increased by 2.5 mg/hour every 5 minutes
      - Restrict maximum rate of infusion to 15 mg/hour
    - Sodium nitroprusside:
      - Onset of action 30 seconds-1 minute
      - 0.25–2 μg/kg/min IV infusion
      - Doses above 2 μg/kg/min may result in fetal side effects
- Anticonvulsant therapy with magnesium sulphate:
  - Magnesium sulphate is the anticonvulsant of choice
  - Therapeutic range of 4.8-8.4 mg/dL is recommended
  - Therapeutic regimen:
    - Loading dose of 4-6 grams over 20-30 minutes
    - Followed by 1-2 g/hour maintenance infusion
    - For seizure recurrence additional bolus dose of 2-4 grams IV
- Postpartum care:
  - Supportive care is continued postoperatively
  - Laboratory values worsen during first 48 hours following delivery

- Laboratory testing every 12 hours is recommended following delivery
- In most patients, laboratory values return to normal within 7 days
- Magnesium sulphate therapy is continued for 24 hours post-partum
- Antihypertensive therapy is continued to prevent intracranial hemorrhage
- Transition to oral antihypertensive is considered for persistent HTN

❖ Dexamethasone rescue therapy:
- Currently obsolete as it does not improve maternal outcomes
- Was used for both antepartum and post-partum therapy
- Regimens used:
  - High risk patients: 20 mg IV Q6H for 24 hours
  - Mild-moderate risk patients:
    - 10 mg IV Q6H 2 doses
    - Followed by 6 mg IV Q6H for 2 doses

Complications

❖ Maternal complications:
- Intracranial hemorrhage, cerebral venous thrombosis, retinal detachment
- Myocardial infarction, pulmonary edema, pulmonary embolism
- Subcapsular liver hematoma and infarction, liver failure
- DIC, abruption, GI bleed, retinal detachment
- Acute renal failure
- ARDS, sepsis, stroke

❖ Fetal complications:
- Prematurity
- IUGR
- Thrombocytopenia

Anesthetic Implications

❖ Impaired drug metabolism due to hepatic involvement

❖ Hepatic rupture possible-care during positioning changes

❖ Invasive hemodynamic monitoring

❖ Large bore IV cannula, central venous access

❖ Blood readily available for massive blood transfusion

❖ Epidural is safe if:
- Platelet count > 80,000 cells/mm^3
- Normal bleeding time
- Normal PT, aPTT and fibrinogen levels

❖ GA preferred if:
- Platelet counts < 50, 000 cells/mm^3
- Abruption, subcapsular hematomas
- Hemodynamically unstable
- Non reassuring FHR

❖ Rapid sequence induction technique

❖ Perioperative availability of vascular surgeons in addition to obstetricians

❖ Avoidance of IM injections

❖ Massive blood transfusion protocol:
- Aims to maintain FFP: PC: PLT = 1:1:1
- Packed cells 6 units
- FFP 6 units
- Platelets 1 SDP or 6 RDP
- Cryoprecipitate 5 units (1 pooled unit)

ANTEPARTUM HEMORRAGE

Introduction

❖ Obstetric hemorrhage defined as that which occurs during pregnancy and includes:
- Antepartum hemorrhage
- Peripartum hemorrhage
- Postpartum hemorrhage

❖ APH is hemorrhage from or into genital tract occurring before delivery

Incidence

❖ Incidence of upto 25% amongst hospital deliveries

❖ Most common cause of maternal morbidity and mortality

❖ Associated with mortality rates of 2.3% and 12% for placenta previa and abruptio

Etiology

❖ Abnormal placentation:
- Placenta previa
- Placenta accreta
- Abruption
- Vasa previa
- Hydatiform mole
- Circumvallate placenta

❖ Uterine atony:
- Over distended uterus
- Halogenated anesthetics
- Polyhydramnios
- Previous uterine atony
- Multiple gestation

❖ Trauma during labor:
- Uterine rupture
- Cesarean section
- Complicated vaginal delivery
- Hysterectomy

❖ Coagulopathies:
- Abruption
- Massive transfusion
- Amniotic fluid embolism

- Congenital/acquired coagulopathy
- Severe preeclampsia, HELLP syndrome: sepsis
- Retention of dead fetus
- Others:
  - Vaginal/vulvar varicosities
  - Ectopic pregnancy
  - Cervical polyp/malignancy

Types of APH

- Early antepartum hemorrhage:
  - Occurs before 20 weeks gestation
  - Most commonly due to:
    - Threatened abortion
    - Ectopic pregnancy
- Late antepartum hemorrhage:
  - Occurs after 20 weeks gestation
  - Most commonly due to:
    - Placental abruption
    - Placenta previa

PLACENTA PREVIA

Introduction

- Refers to the abnormal implantation of placenta in lower uterine segment
- The term previa (in front of) refers to position of placenta relative to presenting part

Incidence

- Incidence of 4 per 1000 pregnancies
- Accounts for one-third of the case of antepartum hemorrhage
- Reported perinatal mortality rate is 2.3%
- Prevalence is much higher at 20 weeks than at term
- This is because most placenta previas resolve before delivery

Risk Factors

- Previous uterine trauma:
  - Occurs commonly in patients with history of cesarean section
  - Also seen in other surgeries causing uterine scarring such as myomectomy
  - The placenta may implant in the scarred area
  - Typically includes lower uterine segment
- Advanced maternal age > 35 years
- Multiparity
- Smoking
- Male fetus
- Prior placenta previa

Etiology

- Dropping down theory:
  - This postulates that decidual reaction in the upper uterine segment is weak
  - Thus, fertilized ovum drops down and is implanted in the lower uterine segment
  - Failure of zona pellucida to disappear in time may be a possibility
  - This results in central placenta previa
- Persistence of chorionic activity theory:
  - Chorionic activity persists in the decidua capsularis
  - This subsequently develops into capsular placenta
  - The placenta comes into contact with decidua vera of lower uterine segment
  - This may be responsible for lesser degrees of placenta previa
- Defective decidua theory:
  - Postulates that defective decidua causes spreading of chorionic villi
  - This spread occurs over a wide area of uterine wall to get nourishment
  - During this process, spread into the lower uterine segment occurs
  - This results in placenta previa

Types of Placenta Previa

- Type I: low lying placenta previa:
  - Major portion of placenta is attached to the upper segment of uterus
  - Only lower margin of placenta encroaches onto lower segment
  - Lower margin however, does not reach the cervical OS
- Type II (marginal placenta previa):
  - Major portion of placenta is within the lower segment
  - Placenta lies within 2 cm of cervical os, without covering it
- Type III (incomplete or partial central placenta previa):
  - Placenta covers the internal os partially
  - This results in uncovering of internal os when it is fully dilated
- Type IV (complete placenta previa):
  - Placenta completely covers the cervical os
  - Even full dilatation does not uncover the cervical os

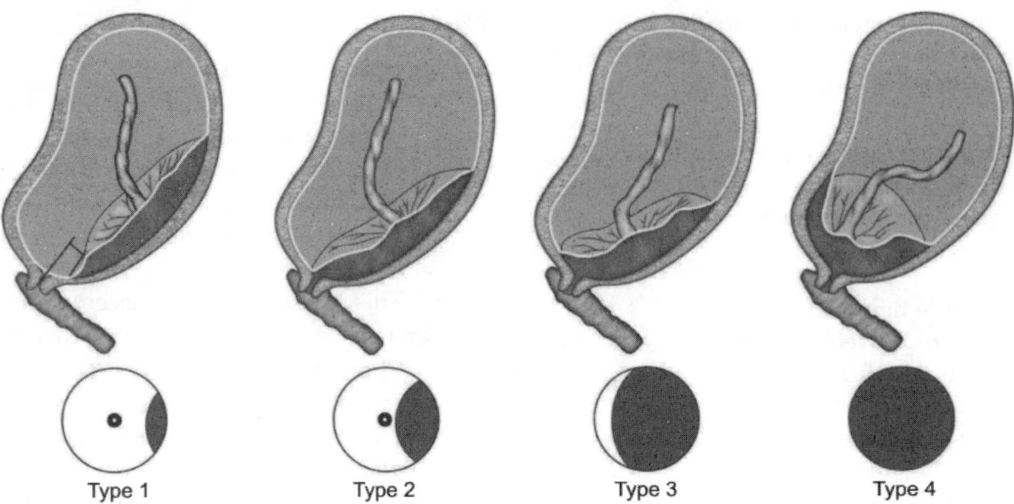

Fig. 10: Types of placenta previa.

Grades of Placenta Previa

- Mild placenta previa: Includes type I and type II anterior placenta previa
- Major placenta previa:
  - Includes:
    - Type II posterior placenta previa
    - Types III and IV placenta previa
  - Dangerous placenta previa:
    - Name given to type II posterior placenta previa
    - This is because in this type, the placenta overlies sacral promontory
    - Since birth canal is curved this narrows the A-P diameter of the inlet
    - This prevents engagement of the presenting part
    - Also, during vaginal delivery, compression of the placenta may occur
    - This may result in fetal anoxia and death

Classification

- Placenta accrete:
  - Placenta is attached onto myometrium
  - Anchoring placental villi attach onto the myometrium rather than the decidua
- Placenta increta:
  - Placenta is attached into myometrium
  - Anchoring placental villi penetrate into the myocardium
- Placenta percreta:
  - Penetration through full thickness of myometrium
  - Also penetrates through uterine serosa onto adjacent organs
  - Implanted on bowel/bladder/pelvic organs

Diagnosis

- Transabdominal ultrasonography:
  - Accuracy after 30 weeks gestation is 98%
  - Poor imaging can result from:
    - Maternal obesity
    - Posteriorly situated placenta due to:
      - Acoustic shadow from fetal presenting part
      - Absence of anatomical landmark to define presence in lower segment
  - False positive results may occur due to:
    - Full bladder
    - Myometrial contractions
- Transvaginal ultrasonography:
  - It is currently the gold standard for diagnosis
  - Transducer is inserted into the vagina without touching the cervix
  - Higher frequency transducers may be used to attain better resolution
  - Distance from placental edge to the internal os is measured
  - This predicts the possibility of APH and need for cesarean section
  - Advantages:
    - Does not require full bladder
    - More accurate than transabdominal ultrasound
- Double setup examination:
  - Examination is performed in the operating room
  - Vaginal examination is done with all personnel ready for cesarean section
  - Preparation for double setup examination includes:
    - Application of all monitors
    - Two wide-bore intravenous cannulae

    - Administration of non-particulate antacid
    - Sterile preparation and draping of abdomen
  - Palpation of the placenta in the lower segment confirms the diagnosis
  - It also helps in identifying the degree of placenta previa
  - This has become almost obsolete nowadays
- MRI:
  - Non invasive method with no risk of ionizing radiation
  - More sensitive than ultrasound for diagnosis of:
    - Posterior placenta previa
    - Placenta previa accrete
  - Disadvantages:
    - Time consuming
    - Lack of portability
  - Thus, use of MRI is not practical although it is a very useful modality

Obstetric Management

- Obstetric management is based on:
  - Severity of vaginal bleeding
  - Maturity and status of the fetus
- Patients with persistent bleeding and non-reassuring fetal status:
    - Immediate delivery is recommended
    - Techniques:
      - Cesarean section: When placenta is within 2 cm of internal os
      - Vaginal delivery: When placenta is 2-3 cms away from the cervical os
- Patients with controlled bleeding:
  - Expectant management in the hospital:
    - Aims to continue pregnancy without compromising maternal health
    - This is done to enable full attainment of fetal maturity
    - Prolongs pregnancy by at least 4 weeks after initial bleeding episode
    - Components:
    - Complete bed rest
    - Supplementary hematinics
    - Blood transfusion for severe anemia
    - During this time, periodic assessments are made of:
      - Maternal vital signs and hemoglobin concentration
      - Fetal evaluation with NST or biophysical profile
      - Fetal lung maturity studies as indicated
    - Tocolytic therapy:
      - Indicated when gestational age < 32 weeks
      - Tocolysis is used to decrease preterm contractions
      - Ritodrine is the commonly used agent
    - Rh immunoglobulin is given to all Rh-negative patients
    - Betamethasone:
      - Given for patients between 24-34 weeks of gestation
      - Steroids are used to accelerate lung maturity
  - OPD management: reserved for:
    - Stable patients without bleeding in previous 48 hours
    - Should have quick transport facility to the hospital

ABRUPTIO PLACENTA

Introduction

- Refers to the premature separation of a normally implanted placenta
- Occurs anytime between 20 weeks to term
- Results in fetal compromise due to loss of placental surface area
- This adversely impacts maternal-fetal exchange of oxygen and nutrients

Incidence

- Abruption is seen in 0.4-1% of pregnancies
- Overall incidence is:
  - 5.9-6.5 per 1000 singleton births
  - 12.2 per 1000 twin births
- Incidence is increasing particularly in patients with:
  - History of respiratory illness
  - Advancing gestational age:
    - 20% before 34 weeks
    - 40% between 34 and 37 weeks
    - 40% bewong 37 weeks
- Perinatal mortality rate has dropped from 80% in the past to almost 12% currently

Risk Factors

- Obstetric factors:
  - Preeclampsia (most common risk factor associated with 50% of all abruptions)

- Multiparity
- Advanced maternal age
- Premature rupture of membranes
- Chorioamnionitis

❖ Maternal comorbidities:
- Hypertension
- Acute or chronic respiratory illness
- Substance abuse
- Maternal cocaine use
- Maternal or paternal tobacco use

❖ Trauma:
- Blunt abdominal trauma
- Acceleration/ deceleration injury

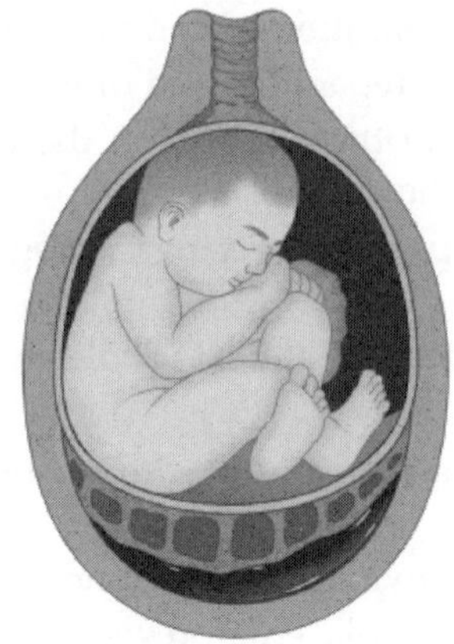

Fig. 11: Abruptio placenta.

Pathophysiology

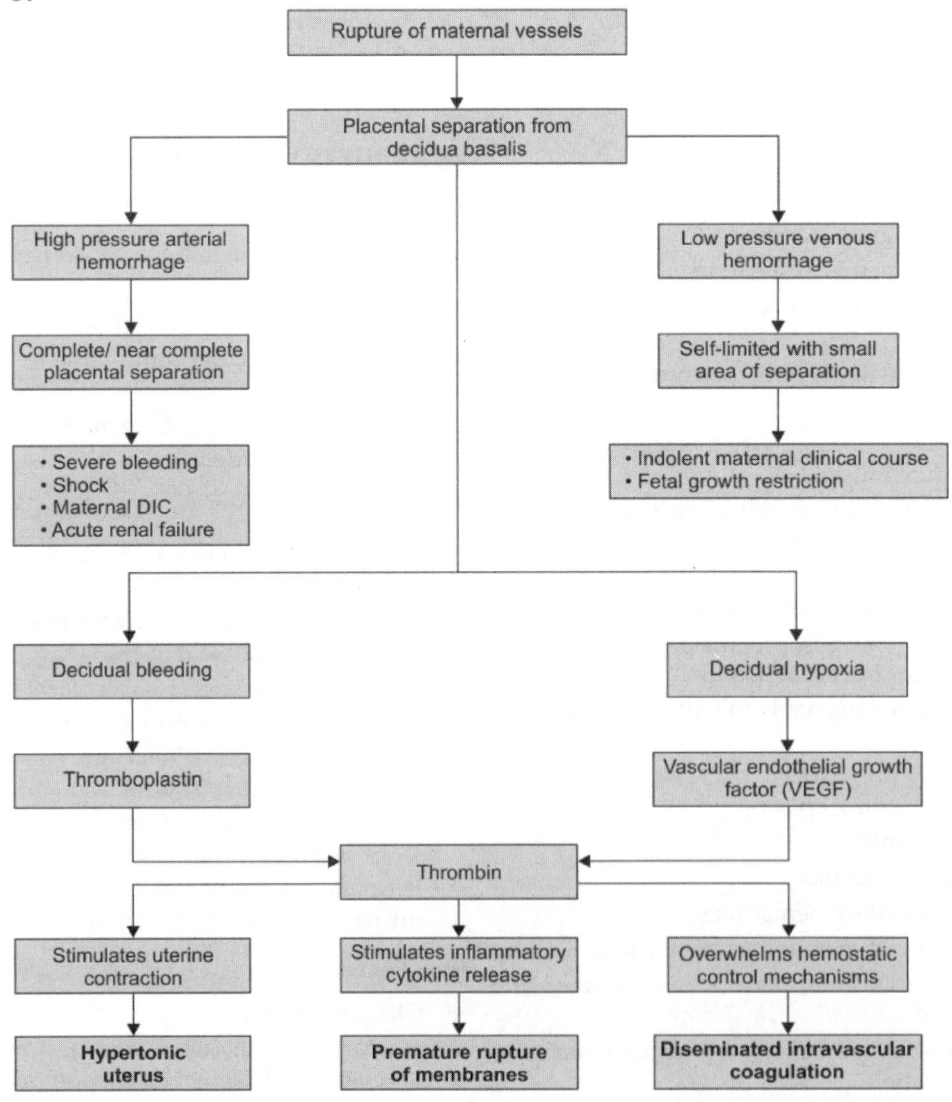

Types of Abruption

- Concealed abruption:
  - Blood collects behind the separated placenta and is not visible outside
  - Collected blood is prevented from exteriorizing by the fetal presenting part
  - This is because the presenting part compresses on the lower segment
  - This effectively seals the uterine exit
  - Blood may also percolate into amniotic sac after rupturing the membranes
  - Associated with multiple maternal complications:
    - Shock
    - Anuria
    - Coagulopathy
    - Postpartum hemorrhage
    - Puerperal sepsis
  - Risk of fetal death is high (50–100%)
  - This type is rarely seen
- Revealed abruption:
  - Following separation, blood insinuates downwards between the membranes and decidua
  - Blood eventually exits the cervical canal to be visible externally
  - Risk of fetal death is comparatively lower (25–30%)
  - This is the most common type of abruption
- Mixed abruption:
  - This is a mixture of both concealed and revealed types
  - Usually one variety predominates over the other
  - Second most common type of abruption

Grades of Abruption

- Grade 0:
  - Absent clinical features
  - No vaginal bleeding or abdominal tenderness
  - Diagnosis made after inspection of placenta following delivery
- Grade 1 (40%):
  - Slight vaginal bleeding is present
  - Uterus is irritable with minimal abdominal tenderness
  - Normal heart rate and BP
  - Fibrinogen levels are unaffected
  - Normal coagulation profile
  - Fetal heart sounds are unaffected
- Grade 2 (45%):
  - Mild-moderate vaginal bleeding
  - Always associated with uterine tenderness
  - Maternal tachycardia with orthostatic hypotension
  - Mild hypofibrinogenemia (> 150 mg/dL)
  - Mild abnormality in coagulation profile
  - Fetal distress or fetal death may be result
- Grade 3 (15%):
  - Moderate-severe bleeding or may be concealed
  - Associated with severe uterine tenderness
  - Hypovolemic shock:
    - Tachycardia with heart rate > 120 bpm
    - Systolic BP < 80 mm Hg
  - Almost always associated with fetal death
  - Maybe associated with other maternal complications:
    - Coagulopathy
    - Acute renal failure and anuria

Obstetric Management

- Obstetric management is based on:
  - Severity of vaginal bleeding
  - Grade of abruption
  - Maturity and status of the fetus
- Patients with persistent bleeding and non-reassuring fetal status:
  - Immediate delivery is recommended
  - Cesarean section is the rule for viable fetuses
  - Vaginal delivery: Used for intrauterine fetal demise
- Patients with controlled bleeding and minimal abruption:
  - Term or near-term gestation: Urgent delivery
  - Pre-term:
    - Complete bed rest
    - Supplementary hematinics
    - Blood transfusion for severe anemia
    - During this time, periodic assessments are made of:
      - Maternal vital signs and hemoglobin concentration

  - Fetal evaluation with NST or biophysical profile
  - Fetal lung maturity studies as indicated
- Tocolytic therapy:
  - Indicated when gestational age < 32 weeks
  - Tocolysis is used to decrease preterm contractions
  - Ritodrine is the commonly used agent
- Rh immunoglobulin is given to all Rh-negative patients
- Betamethasone:
  - Given for patients between 24-34 weeks of gestation
  - Steroids are used to accelerate lung maturity

UTERINE RUPTURE

Risk Factors

- History of previous scar
- Weak myometrium due to multiple gestation
- Polyhydramnios
- Trauma
- History of prolonged labor under influence of oxytocin

Presentation of APH

- Profuse vaginal bleeding
- Hypovolemic shock with no bleeding if concealed hemorrhage
- Abnormal uterine tone
- Pain and uterine tenderness in abruptio
- Painless bleeding in placenta previa
- Retroplacental hematoma in USG

Anesthetic Considerations

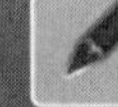

- Inadequate preoperative preparation due to emergency surgery
- Estimate volume of blood loss
- Profuse bleeding perioperatively:
  - Preoperative hypotension and fetal distress
  - Requirement of large amount of blood intraoperatively
  - Gross underestimation of blood loss due to concealed hemorrhage
  - Increased chances of post-partum hemorrhage
- Possibility of extended surgery for:
  - Emergency hysterectomy
  - Uterine/internal iliac artery ligation

Feature	Class I	Class 2	Class 3	Class 4
Blood loss (%)	< 15	15-30	30-40	> 40
Heart rate (bpm)	< 100	> 100	> 120	> 140
Systolic BP (mm Hg)	Normal	Normal	Decreased	Decreased
Pulse pressure	Normal/ high	Decreased	Decreased	Decreased
Respiratory rate (breaths/min)	14–20	20–30	30–40	> 35
Mental state	Slight anxiety	Slight anxiety	Anxious, confused	Lethargic

OT Preparation

- Small sized ETT (upto 6 size)
- Laryngoscope blade: Polio blade with short handle
- Airways, facemask, bougie, LMA, cricothyrotomy set
- Anesthetic drugs preloaded, emergency drugs, atropine, adrenaline
- Suction apparatus
- CVP and IBP transducer systems
- Fluid warmer, rapid fluid infusion devices, hand inflated pressure bags
- Adequate amount of crystalloids and colloids
- Cross matched blood (at least 4–6 units)

Patient Preparation

- For expectant management patients:
  - Intravenous access:
    - Only one peripheral line is maintained during stay in the hospital
    - Alternatively, PICC lines may be used for drug administration
    - Other veins are preserved for emergencies requiring large bore venous access
  - Investigations:
    - Blood typing and cross matching should be done every 3 days
    - This is due to risk of developing new allo-antibodies during pregnancy
  - DVT prophylaxis:
    - DVT prophylaxis with pneumatic compression device is recommended
    - Pharmacological prophylaxis is not recommended due to bleeding risk
- Coagulation profile with:
  - PA, aPTT, INR
  - Serum fibrinogen levels, TEG
  - Emergency coagulation profile with ***clot coagulation test***:

- Done as a bedside test
- 5 mL of blood is withdrawn in a clean glass tube
- In normal patients, blood clots within 6–7 minutes of sample collection
- The formed clot breaks down within 60 minutes
- Coagulopathy is suspected if:
  - No clot formation occurs within 6 minutes
  - Clot lysis begins after 1 hour
- Suspect hypofibrinogenemia if no clot forms in 30 minutes

- Two large bore 14-16 G IV access
- Oxygen via face mask 6-8 L/min
- Volume resuscitation:
  - Non dextrose containing crystalloid (lactated ringers, plasmalyte)
  - Colloids upto 1.5 litres may be given in 24 hours
  - Cross matched blood (4-6 units)
  - O^{-ve} blood if cross matched blood is unavailable
- Anti-aspiration prophylaxis:
  - 0.3 M sodium citrate 30 mL
  - IV ranitidine 1 mg/kg
  - IV metoclopramide 0.15 mg/kg
- Stop $MgSO_4$ and $CaCl_2$ therapy
- ***Double setup examination*** may be done if placenta previa suspected

Monitors

- Pulse oximetry, E_TCO_2
- NIBP, ECG
- Invasive blood pressure:
  - May be indicated in:
    - Hemodynamically unstable patients
    - Ongoing blood loss
    - Massive concealed abruptions
  - May be used for:
    - Beat-to-beat hemodynamic monitoring
    - Frequent arterial samples for ABG and hemoglobin levels
- Central venous pressure in unstable patients to guide fluid therapy
- Urine output, temperature
- BIS monitoring for intraoperative awareness

Choice of Anesthetic Technique

- Neuraxial anesthesia:
  - Abruptio placentae:
    - Indicated for vaginal delivery and cesarean section in stable patients
    - Options for neuraxial anesthesia include:
      - Spinal anesthesia
      - Combined spinal-epidural anesthesia
      - Epidural anesthesia
    - Catheter based techniques are preferred
    - This is to allow extension of anesthesia for unexpected hysterectomy
    - Neuraxial anesthesia is safe provided:
      - Mild to moderate abruption
      - Minimal bleeding
      - No hypovolemia
      - No coagulopathy
      - No uteroplacental insufficiency
  - Placenta previa:
    - Preferred in patients with:
      - No active bleeding
      - Hemodynamic stability
      - Pre-existing volume deficit
      - No history of placenta accreta
    - Not preferred in patients with active bleeding
    - This is because risk of intraoperative bleeding is high in these patients
    - Options for neuraxial anesthesia include:
      - Spinal anesthesia
      - Combined spinal-epidural anesthesia
      - Epidural anesthesia
    - Catheter based techniques are preferred
    - This is to allow extension of anesthesia for unexpected hysterectomy
    - Advantages of epidural anesthesia for placenta previa patients include:
      - Stable blood pressure after delivery
      - Lower intraoperative transfusion rates
      - Lower intraoperative transfusion volumes
      - Comparable neonatal outcomes with general anesthesia
- General anesthesia preferred if:
  - Uncontrolled hemorrhage
  - Coagulopathy
  - Maternal hemodynamic instability
  - Fetal distress
  - Patient refusal

Induction

- Adequate preoxygenation
- Induction is carried out following painting and draping of the patient
- Ketamine 0.75-1 mg/kg or etomidate 0.3 mg/kg are the *induction agents of choice*
- Thiopentone and propofol are avoided as risk of cardiovascular collapse is high
- *Rapid sequence induction* with cricoid pressure and left uterine displacement

Maintenance

- Balanced anesthesia with low dose volatile agents if controlled bleeding
- 50% O_2 + 50% N_2O + 0.5-1% isoflurane depending on maternal tolerance
- Volatile anesthetics are avoided in severe maternal hemorrhage or fetal compromise
- TIVA with IV infusion of ketamine may be used in these cases
- In case of increase in severity of hemorrhage following delivery:
  - Discontinuation of volatile agent
  - IV ketamine or midazolam may be used to ensure amnesia
- NDMR:
  - Pancuronium used if shock
  - Atracurium if acute renal failure
  - Vecuronium for uncomplicated cases
- Following delivery of the baby:
  - Uterotonic agents are administered to reduce bleeding:
    - IV oxytocin
    - IM methylergonovine
    - Rectal misoprostol
  - IV fentanyl 1 µg/kg may be administered for analgesia
- For uterine relaxation during dilatation and curettage:
  - IV NTG 50-100 µg bolus o
  - Increased concentration of volatile anesthetic

Hemodynamics

- Aggressive resuscitation of intravascular volume is important
- Either crystalloids or colloids may be used
- Choice of fluids is less important compared to adequacy of restoration
- Correct coagulopathy:
  - FFP/ cryoprecipitate
  - Platelet concentrate
  - Factor VII 60-120 µg/kg if no DIC
- Cryoprecipitate is used for suspected hypofibrinogenemia
- Blood is transfused to maintain Hb > 7 g/dL
- Massive transfusion may be required for patients with placenta accreta

Control of Bleeding

- Uterotonic therapy:
  - Oxytocin 20-40 IU in 1000 mL RL over 4-8 hours
  - Methergine 0.2 mg IM Q2-4 H as required
  - Carboprost 0.25 mg IM Q 15-60 mins as required
  - Misoprostol 800-1000 mg PO/PR/PV Q2H
  - Dinoprostone 20 mg PO Q2H
  - Intra-myometrial PGE_2 0.5 mg or PGF 2 α 0.2 mg
- Medical management:
  - Estimated blood loss replacement:
    - Crystalloids are administered in a 3:1 ratio to estimated blood loss
    - This allows initial resuscitation until blood products are arranged
    - Blood component therapy may be started following initial resuscitation
    - Improved outcomes have been reported when PRBC: FFP: PLT : 1:1:1
    - Platelets transfused to maintain counts > 50,000/mm^3
    - Cryoprecipitate may be transfused to maintain fibrinogen > 150 mg%
    - Early replacement of fibrinogen minimizes coagulopathy
  - Prothrombin concentrates: Needs further clinical trials
  - Tranexemic acid:
    - 1 g slow IV bolus over 5 minutes
    - Repeated once within 30-60 minutes if bleeding continues
  - Aprotinin/ methotrexate
  - Uterine massage
- Surgical management:
  - Uterine tamponade with:
    - ***Sengstaken – Blackmore esophageal catheter***
    - Bimanual compression
    - Uterine packing
  - Compression sutures ***(B-Lynch)***

- Selective radiological embolization with:
  - Gelatin sponge
  - Polyurethane foam
  - Polyvinyl methyl alcohol particle
- Arterial ligation:
  - U/L or B/L uterine artery
  - U/L internal iliac artery
  - U/L or B/L ovarian artery
- Emergency hysterectomy
- Exploration and repair if trauma/retained products

Extubation

- Fully conscious, awake, reversed
- Hemodynamically stable with controlled bleeding
- Extubated in lateral position

Complications

- Hemorrhagic shock
- Postpartum hemorrhage
- Coagulopathy, DIC
- Couvelaire uterus: Extravasated blood dissects between myometrial fibres
- Sheehans syndrome: Anterior pituitary necrosis
- Intrauterine death of fetus
- Acute renal failure

POSTPARTUM HEMORRHAGE

Introduction: ACOG 2017 Practice Bulletin

- Postpartum hemorrhage is an obstetric emergency
- It is commonly defined as cumulative blood loss:
  - Exceeding 500 mL for vaginal delivery within 24 hours
  - Exceeding 1000 mL for cesarean section within 24 hours of birth
  - Associated with:
    - Symptoms of hypovolemia
    - 10% reduction in hematocrit after delivery
    - Requirement of blood product transfusion

Incidence

- Incidence varies widely as multiple definitions have been used to define PPH
- Estimated to be 1-5% of deliveries
- Leading cause of maternal morbidity and mortality worldwide
- Death from PPH occurs in approximately 1 in 1000 deliveries
- Incidence is increasing as a result of increasing incidence of:
  - Postpartum uterine atony
  - Abnormal placentation
  - Obstetric interventions such as induction of labor
  - Obesity and multiple gestations

Etiology

- Primary causes:
  - Uterine atony
  - Uterine inversion
  - Genital lacerations:
    - Upper genital tract: broad ligament
    - Lower genital tract:
      - Perineal, periclitoral, vaginal
      - Cervical, periurethral
  - Retained products of conception (placenta, membranes)
  - Abnormal placentation:
    - Placenta accreta
    - Placenta increta
    - Placenta percreta
  - Uterine rupture
  - Amniotic fluid embolism
  - Coagulopathy
- Secondary causes:
  - Uterine infection
  - Retained products of conception
  - Placental site subinvolution
  - Anticoagulation

Risk Factors

- Patient related factors:
  - Previous history of PPH
  - Abnormal placentation:
    - Placental previa
    - Placenta accreta
    - Placental abruption
  - Acquired coagulopathy:
    - Severe preeclampsia
    - Preoperative anticoagulation
    - Amniotic fluid embolism
    - Intrauterine fetal demise
  - Advanced age
  - Uterine overdistension:
    - Multiparity
    - Obesity
    - Polyhydramnios

- Chorioamnionitis
- Fibroids

❖ Procedure related:
- Prolonged labor due to failure to progress in second stage
- Lacerations during instrumental delivery
- Prolonged use of oxytocin

Types

❖ Primary or early PPH:
- Occurring within 24 hours of delivery
- Most commonly occurs within 2 hours following delivery
- Primary PPH is of 2 types:
  - Third stage hemorrhage: occurring before expulsion of placenta
  - True PPH: Occurs subsequent to placental expulsion (more common)

❖ Secondary or late PPH: Occurring between 24 hours to 6 weeks of delivery

Pathogenesis

❖ Uterine atony:
- Refers to inability of myometrium to contract effectively
- It is the *most common cause of PPH*
- Accounts for almost 80% of all cases of PPH
- At term, myometrial fibres contract around spiral arterioles
- This acts as a tourniquet and helps to control bleeding
- Inadequate contraction leads to uterine atony and PPH
- Risk factors for uterine atony:
  - Factors related to obstetric condition:
    - Uterine overdistension due to:
      - Multiple gestation
      - Polyhydramnios
      - Fetal macrosomia
    - Prolonged labor
    - Chorioamnionitis
  - Factors related to obstetric management:
    - Cesarean delivery
    - Induced labor
    - Augmented labor
  - Factors related to maternal comorbidities:
    - Advanced maternal age
    - Hypertension
    - Diabetes
  - Others:
    - Prolonged oxytocin use
    - Prolonged tocolytic therapy
    - High concentration of volatile agents

❖ Genitourinary tract trauma:
- Second most common cause of PPH
- May result in:
  - Genitourinary tract hematoma:
    - Vaginal, vulvar hematomas
    - Vulvovaginal, retroperitoneal hematomas
  - Genitourinary tract lacerations
- Causes of lacerations:
  - Operative delivery
  - Fetal malpresentation
  - Fetal macrosomia
  - Episiotomy
  - Precipitous delivery
  - Shoulder dystocia

❖ Retained products of conception:
- Defined as failure to expel placenta completely within 30 minutes of delivery
- Retained products inhibit adequate uterine contractions
- Occurs in approximately 3% of vaginal deliveries
- Most commonly retained products:
  - Placental tissue
  - Amniotic membrane
- Risk factors for retained products:
  - History of retained placenta
  - Preterm delivery
  - Oxytocin use during labor
  - Chorioamnionitis
  - Accessory placental lobes

❖ Uterine rupture:
- Rare in occurrence
- Risk factors for uterine rupture:
  - Previous cesarean section
  - Multiparity
  - Fetal malpresentation
  - Obstructed labor
  - Prior uterine interventions:
    - Hysterotomy
    - Myomectomy

❖ Uterine inversion:
- Rare in occurrence
- Occurs due to fundal placentation with excessive cord traction
- Risk factors:
  - Short umbilical cord
  - Uterine anomalies
  - Excessive cord traction
  - Inappropriate fundal pressure
- Types of uterine inversion:
  - Complete uterine inversion:
    - Internal lining of fundus crosses cervical os
    - Fundus forms a rounded mass in the vagina
    - No palpable fundus in the abdomen
  - Incomplete uterine inversion:
    - Partial extrusion of fundus into the cervix
    - Fundus does not cross the cervical os

❖ Coagulopathy:
- May be due to congenital or acquired causes
- Acquired causes:
  - Anticoagulant administration
  - Intrauterine fetal death
  - Placental abruption
  - Sepsis
  - Amniotic fluid embolism

Clinical Features

Feature	Class I	Class 2	Class 3	Class 4
Blood loss (%)	< 15	15-30	30-40	> 40
Heart rate (bpm)	< 100	> 100	> 120	> 140
Systolic BP (mm Hg)	Normal	Normal	Decreased	Decreased
Pulse pressure	Normal/ high	Decreased	Decreased	Decreased
Respiratory rate (breaths/min)	14-20	20-30	30-40	> 35
Mental state	Slight anxiety	Slight anxiety	Anxious, confused	Lethargic

Pathophysiology

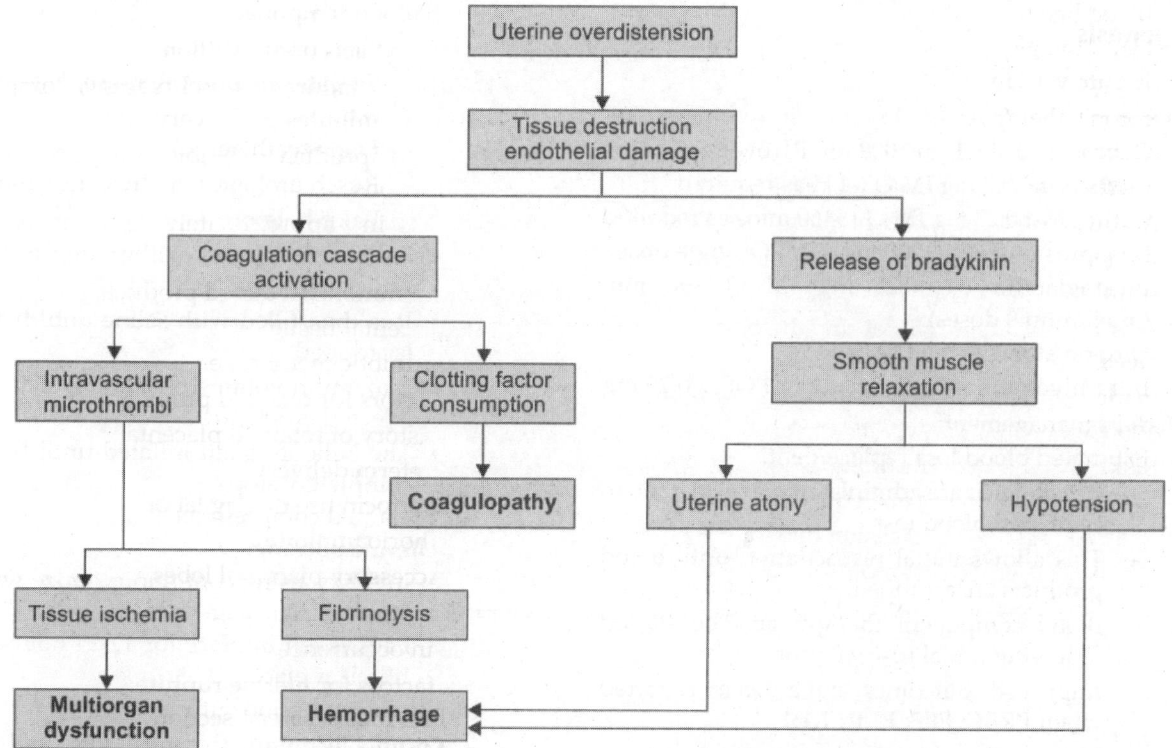

Prevention

❖ Uterotonic agents:
- Oxytocin:
  - Preoperative infusion is continued for at least 1 hour post delivery
  - Oxytocin 5 IU slow IV is given within 1 minute of birth of baby

- Misoprostol:
  - More stable compared with oxytocin
  - Can be given by oral, sublingual and per-rectal routes
  - 600 μg PO/SL if oxytocin unavailable
- Active management of third stage labor:
  - Reduces the incidence of PPH by 60%
  - Controlled cord traction by skilled assistant
  - Uterine massage after delivery of placenta

Management

- Treatment goals:
  - Restore adequate circulatory volume to prevent hypoperfusion
  - Restore tissue oxygenation
  - Reverse or prevent coagulopathy
  - Eliminate cause of PPH
- Multidisciplinary team approach to treatment:
  - Obstetrician
  - Anesthetist
  - Blood bank
  - Hematologist
  - ICU physician
- Uterotonic therapy:
  - Oxytocin 10–80 IU in 1000 mL RL over 4–8 hours
  - Methergine 0.2 mg IM Q2-4 H as required
  - Carboprost 0.25 mg IM Q 15–60 mins as required
  - Misoprostolol 600–1000 mg PR/PO single dose
  - Prostaglandin $F_2\alpha$ 0.25 mg IM Q15-90 min (maximum 8 doses)
  - Dinoprostone 20 mg PO Q2H
  - Intra-myometrial PGE_2 0.5 mg or $PGF_2\alpha$ 0.25 mg
- Medical management:
  - Estimated blood loss replacement:
    - Crystalloids are administered in a 3:1 ratio to estimated blood loss
    - This allows initial resuscitation until blood products are arranged
    - Blood component therapy may be started following initial resuscitation
    - Improved outcomes have been reported when PRBC: FFP: PLT : 1:1:1
    - Platelets transfused to maintain counts ≥ 50,000/mm^3
    - Cryoprecipitate may be transfused to maintain fibrinogen > 150 mg%
    - Early replacement of fibrinogen minimizes coagulopathy
  - Recombinant factor VIIa:
    - Given as *Novoseven* 60-100 μg/kg slow IV
    - Has rapid onset of action and achieves hemostasis within 10-40 minutes
    - Duration of action is short (2 hours)
    - Thus, repeat dosing may be required
  - Other blood-based products:
    - Fibrinogen concentrates (RiaSTAP)
    - Prothrombin concentrates: Needs further clinical trials
    - Fibrin sealant (Tisseal)
    - Hemostatic matrix (Floseal)
  - Tranexemic acid:
    - 1 g slow IV bolus over 5 min
    - Repeated once within 30-60 mins if bleeding continues
  - Aprotinin/ methotrexate
  - Uterine massage
- Surgical management:
  - Uterine tamponade with:
    - Balloon tamponade:
      - Devices used include:
        - ***Sengstaken–Blackmore esophageal catheter***
        - Foleys catheter
        - Rusch urological hydrostatic balloon
        - Bakri balloon
      - Balloon is placed within uterine cavity under USG guidance
      - It is then filled with saline until bleeding is stopped
      - Maximum volume of saline which can be injected is 500 mL
      - The balloon is left inflated until bleeding completely stops
    - Bimanual compression
    - Uterine packing:
      - Involves using continuous gauze within a sterile plastic bag
      - Pack is left in place for 12-24 hours while EBL is replaced
  - Uterine compression sutures:
    - Simple technique to control PPH and avoiding hysterectomy
    - Best used for uterine atony controlled by bimanual massage
    - Sutures used include:
      - B-Lynch suture

- Hayman vertical suture
- Pereira transverse and vertical suture
- Selective radiological embolization:
  - Pelvic angiography is done to visualize bleeding vessels
  - Pledgets of different materials may then be placed for vessel occlusion
  - Advantages:
    - Selectivity
    - Preservation of uterus
    - Success rate of 95%
  - Disadvantages:
    - Post-procedure infections
    - Postembolization fever
    - Tissue necrosis
  - Materials used for embolization include:
    - Gelatin sponge
    - Polyurethane foam
    - Polyvinyl methyl alcohol particle
- Systematic pelvic devascularization:
  - Involves laparotomy with stepwise devascularization
  - Sequential arterial ligation of:
    - Ipsilateral or B/L uterine artery
    - Ipsilateral or B/L ovarian artery
    - Ipsilateral internal iliac artery
  - Iliac artery ligation usually controls bleeding from any genital source
  - Reported success rate varies between 40-100%
  - However, it is technically difficult and risks injury to surrounding organ
- Emergency cesarean hysterectomy:
  - Reserved as the final option in the management of PPH
  - Should not be delayed in PPH refractory to conventional methods
  - Subtotal hysterectomy is not preferred as it is ineffective for:
    - Bleeding in lower segment
    - Bleeding from cervix or vaginal fornices
- Exploration and repair-curettage if trauma/retained products:
  - Done in the presence of retained products of conception
  - Banjo curette is used with gentle traction to avoid uterine perforation
  - Transabdominal USG is used to guide removal of retained products

Special Situations

- $MgSO_4$ therapy: Stop $MgSO_4$ infusion and IV Ca gluconate given
- Uterine inversion:
  - Manual replacement
  - Hydrostatic pressure to revert uterus
- Placental adherence:
  - Hysterectomy
  - Embolization if massive hemorrhage

Anesthesia for PPH Patients

OT Preparation

- Small sized ETT (upto 6 size)
- Laryngoscope blade: Polio blade with short handle
- Airways, facemask, bougie, LMA, cricothyrotomy set
- Anesthetic drugs preloaded, emergency drugs, atropine, adrenaline
- Suction apparatus
- CVP and IBP transducer systems
- Fluid warmer, rapid fluid infusion devices, hand inflated pressure bags
- Adequate amount of crystalloids and colloids
- Cross matched blood (at least 4-6 units)

Patient Preparation

- Coagulation profile with:
  - PA, aPTT, INR
  - Serum fibrinogen levels, TEG
  - Emergency coagulation profile with ***clot coagulation test***:
    - Done as a bedside test
    - 5 mL of blood is withdrawn in a clean glass tube
    - In normal patients, blood clots within 6-7 minutes of sample collection
    - The formed clot breaks down within 60 minutes
    - Coagulopathy is suspected if:
      - No clot formation occurs within 6 minutes
      - Clot lysis begins after 1 hour
    - Suspect hypofibrinogenemia if no clot forms in 30 minutes
- Two large bore 14-16 G IV access
- Oxygen via face mask 6-8 L/min
- Volume resuscitation:
  - Non dextrose containing crystalloid (lactated ringers, plasmalyte)

- Colloids upto 1.5 litres may be given in 24 hours
- Cross matched blood (4-6 units)
- O^{-ve} blood if cross matched blood is unavailable

❖ Anti-aspiration prophylaxis:
- 0.3 M sodium citrate 30 mL
- IV ranitidine 1 mg/kg
- IV metoclopramide 0.15 mg/kg

Monitors

❖ Pulse oximetry, E_TCO_2

❖ NIBP, ECG

❖ Invasive blood pressure:
- May be indicated in:
  - Hemodynamically unstable patients
  - Ongoing blood loss
  - Massive concealed abruptions
- May be used for:
  - Beat-to-beat hemodynamic monitoring
  - Frequent arterial samples for ABG and hemoglobin levels

❖ Central venous pressure in unstable patients to guide fluid therapy

❖ Urine output, temperature

❖ BIS monitoring for intraoperative awareness

Induction

❖ Adequate preoxygenation

❖ Induction is carried out following painting and draping of the patient

❖ Ketamine 0.75-1 mg/kg or etomidate 0.3 mg/kg are the *induction agents of choice*

❖ Thiopentone and propofol are avoided as risk of cardiovascular collapse is high

❖ *Rapid sequence induction* with cricoid pressure and left uterine displacement

❖ ETT is downsized as rapid fluid resuscitation causes airway edema

Maintenance

❖ Balanced anesthesia with low dose volatile agents to prevent awareness

❖ 50% O_2 + 50% N_2O + 0.5-75% isoflurane may be used

❖ Volatile anesthetics are avoided in the presence of:
- Severe maternal hemorrhage
- Fetal compromise

❖ TIVA with IV infusion of ketamine may be used in these cases

❖ NDMR:
- Pancuronium used if shock
- Atracurium if acute renal failure
- Vecuronium for uncomplicated cases

Hemodynamics

❖ Aggressive resuscitation of intravascular volume is important

❖ Either crystalloids or colloids may be used

❖ Choice of fluids is less important compared to adequacy of restoration

❖ Correct coagulopathy:
- FFP/ cryoprecipitate
- Platelet concentrate

❖ Cryoprecipitate is used for suspected hypofibrinogenemia

❖ Blood is transfused to maintain Hb > 7 g/dL

Extubation

❖ Usually extubated late due to massive intraoperative fluid shifts

❖ Extubated when:
- Fully awake, reversed
- Hemodynamically stable with controlled bleeding

❖ Extubated in lateral position

Complications

❖ DIC, TRALI, ARDS, MODS

❖ Acute tubular necrosis, ARF

❖ Venous thromboembolism

❖ ***Sheehans syndrome***

❖ Surgical complications:
- Urinary tract/bowel/vascular injury
- Genitourinary fistula, genitointestinal fistula
- Uterine synechiae: ***Ashermans syndrome***
- Pelvic hematoma and sepsis

POST-PARTUM STERILIZATION

Introduction

❖ It is the most popular technique of terminal sterilization all over the world

❖ It is also one of the most commonly performed surgeries

Types

❖ Post-partum sterilization:
- Done at the time of child birth or in the early post-partum period

- Advantages:
  - Fallopian tubes easily accessible:
    - Uterine fundus remains near umbilicus for several days postpartum
    - This allows easier access in immediate post-partum period
  - Simpler surgical procedure
  - Reduced incidence of bowel vessel injury
  - Reduced incidence of bowel laceration
  - Eliminates need for re-hospitalization
  - Reduced length of hospital-stay
- Disadvantages of immediate sterilization:
  - Increased risk of uterine atony:
    - Causes post-partum hemorrhage
    - Risk reduces 12 hours post-partum
  - Sterilization is performed before complete assessment of the newborn

❖ Interval sterilization:
- Done when complete involution of uterus occurs: 3 months after delivery
- Ideal time of operation is following menstrual period in the proliferative phase
- Done laparoscopically usually
- Indications: Complicated pregnancy/associated medical conditions

Methods

❖ Tubal ligation using conventional laparotomy:
- ***Madleners technique:***
  - Easiest technique
  - Loop of fallopian tube is crushed with an artery forceps
  - Crushed area is tied with silk suture
  - Loop is not excised
  - Failure rate is very high (1.5–7%)
  - Abandoned in preference to Pomeroys technique
- ***Irving technique:***
  - Fallopian tube is ligated on either side
  - The mid-portion of the tube is excised
  - Free medial end is turned backwards and buried in posterior uterine wall
- ***Pomeroys technique:***
  - A loop is made of the fallopian tube using Allis forceps
  - Loop consists of:
    - Mainly isthmus
    - Part of the ampullary portion of the tube
  - Through a vascular area in mesosalpinx, catgut suture is passed
  - Both the limbs of the loop are tied together
  - About 1.5 cm of the tube distal to the ligature is excised
  - Excised segment is sent for histopathological examination
  - The same procedure is repeated on the opposite side
  - Cut ends become independently sealed off due to absorbable sutures
  - This is the most commonly used technique for tubectomy
  - Advantages:
    - Easy, safe and effective
    - Low failure rate of 0.1–0.6%
- ***Uchidas technique:***
  - Saline solution is injected sub-serosally in mid-portion of the tube
  - The serous coat is incised to expose the muscular tube
  - Tube is then ligated on either side
  - 3–5 cm of the tube is then resected off
  - The proximal stump is allowed to retract under the serous coat
  - The serous coat is then closed such that:
    - Proximal stump is buried
    - Distal stump is open to peritoneal cavity
  - No failure has been observed so far

❖ Mini-laparotomy (MINI-LAP):
- Small abdominal incision is used
- Performed using specialized equipment
- Tubectomy is performed using one of above techniques followed by closure

❖ Laparoscopic sterilization:
- Most commonly used method of sterilization
- Mostly done under local anesthesia
- Failure rate of 0.1%
- Tubectomy is performed using:
  - Silastic rings (silicone rubber with 5% barium sulfate)
  - Filshie clip made of titanium lined with silicone rubber
  - Hulka-Clemens spring clip
  - Electrosurgical methods which desiccates tubal tissue using heat

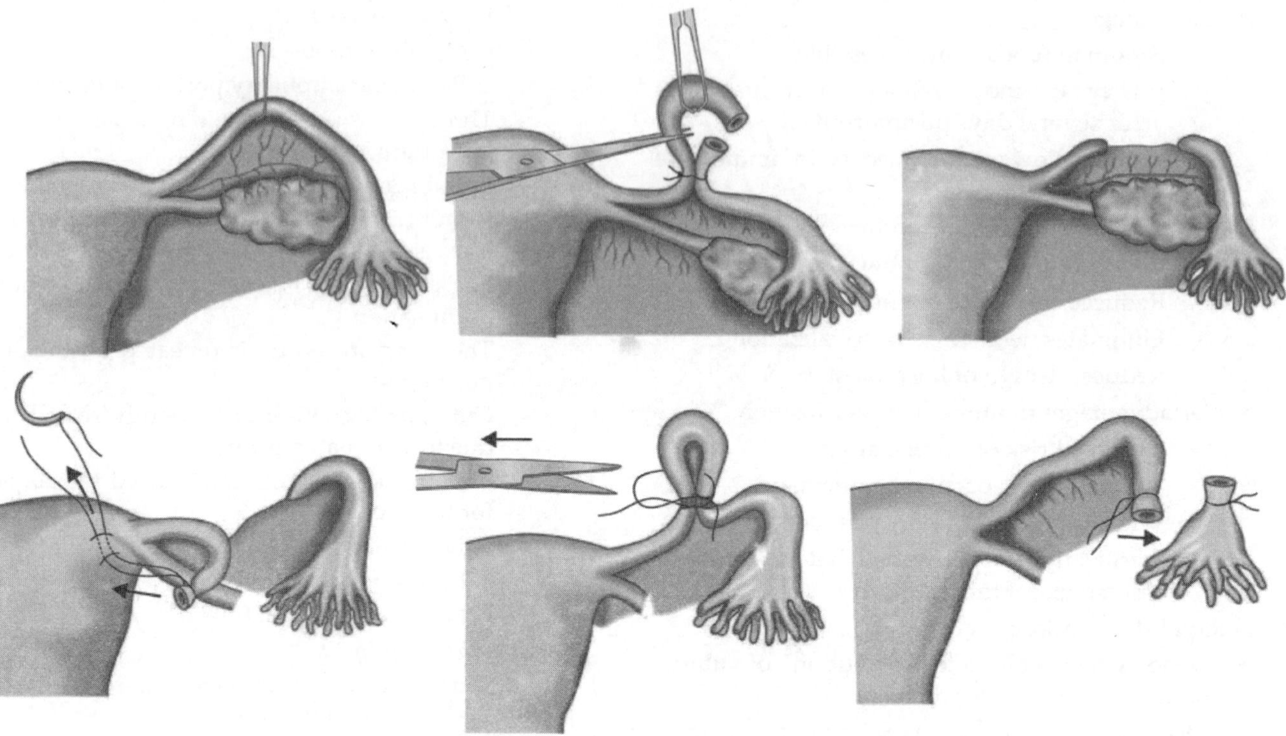

Fig. 12: Techniques of tubal ligation for post-partum sterilization.

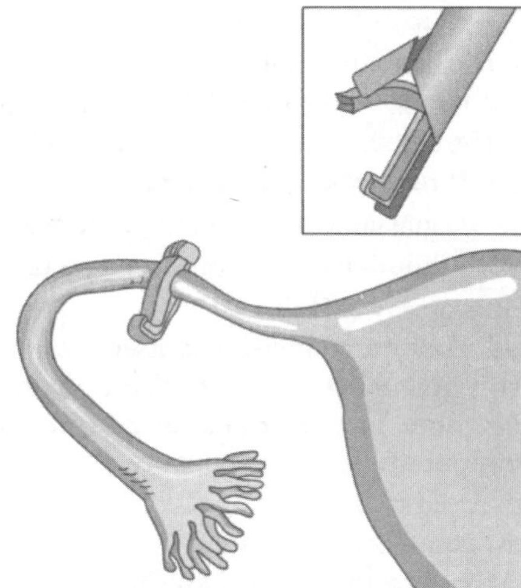

Fig. 13: Laparoscopic sterilization using Filshie clip.

Preoperative Evaluation

- Requires thorough re-evaluation even if in the immediate post-partum period
- This is because many diseases may present in the post-partum period:
  - Preeclampsia
  - Eclampsia
  - HELLP syndrome
- Patient should be evaluated for:
  - Volume status:
    - Blood loss may be under-estimated during cesarean section
    - Evaluation should include:
      - Orthostatic changes in blood pressure and heart rate
      - Hematocrit for sterilization performed > 8 hours post-partum
  - Fever:
    - May occur due to:
      - Endometritis
      - Urinary tract infections
    - Postponement of surgery is advised to facilitate antibiotic therapy
  - Condition of the neonate to exclude problems incompatible with life
  - Adequacy of epidural anesthesia during labor/ cesarean section

- Risk of aspiration:
  - Time of last oral intake
  - Type of last oral intake
  - Administration of opioids by any route

Preoperative Fasting

- Aspiration is a major risk associated with anesthesia for post-partum tubal ligation
- This is due to:
  - Delayed gastric emptying:
    - Occurs due to:
      - Physiological changes occurring during labor
      - Opioids administered for labor analgesia
    - Gastric emptying however is not delayed for clear fluids unless opioids have been given
  - Gastroesophageal reflux:
    - LES sphincter tones reduces during third trimester of pregnancy
    - This change lasts till the second day post-partum
    - Thus, patients undergoing early post-partal tubal ligation may be at increased risk of GER
- Thus, preventive measures for aspiration pneumonia are essential
- These include:
  - Fasting interval of 6-8 hours depending upon the nature of intake
  - Anti-aspiration prophylaxis given at least 1 hour prior to induction:
    - 0.3 M sodium citrate 30 mL
    - IV ranitidine 1 mg/kg
    - IV metoclopramide 0.15 mg/kg

Techniques of Anesthesia

- Local anesthesia with IV sedation:
  - Technique:
    - Maternal IV sedation with:
      - Midazolam 1-2 mg IV
      - Fentanyl 50-100 µg IV
    - This is followed by infiltration with 100 mg lidocaine of:
      - Skin
      - Subcutaneous tissue
    - Intraperitoneal instillation of 400 mg lidocaine is then used
    - This is administered into peritoneal cavity as 80 mL of 0.5% solution
    - For laparoscopic tubal ligation:
      - Maternal sedation with:
        - Midazolam 1-2 mg IV
        - Fentanyl 50-100 µg IV
      - Skin infiltration is performed with 10 mL of 0.5% bupivacaine
      - This was followed by:
        - Surgical exposure of the fallopian tubes
        - Local spraying of 5 mL 0.5% bupivacaine on each tube
        - Tubal ligation is carried out after 5 minutes of spraying
  - Advantages:
    - Rapid onset and recovery
    - Ease of administration
    - No nausea and vomiting
    - Reduced postoperative complications
- Neuraxial anesthesia:
  - Spinal/epidural anesthesia may be used
  - Sensory level of T_4 required to block visceral pain due to tubal manipulation
  - Spinal anesthesia:
    - Local anesthetic dose:
      - LA requirement reduces to pre-pregnant levels 12-36 hours after delivery
      - 0.75% hyperbaric bupivacaine 10–12 mg is commonly used
      - Fentanyl 10-25 µg may be added to the intrathecal injection
      - Hyperbaric lidocaine:
        - Provides short-acting anesthesia
        - It is avoided due to risk of cauda equina syndrome
    - Intrathecal pethidine:
      - Used as an alternative to local anesthetics
      - 1 mg/kg of prepartum weight preservative-free pethidine used
      - Onset time: 3-5 minutes
      - Duration of action: 30-60 mminutes
    - Hypotension:
      - Risk of hypotension due to SAB is reduced following delivery
      - Thus hypotension during post-partal tubal ligation is rare
      - This is because of auto-transfusion of blood during delivery
    - Advantages:
      - Immediate onset of action
      - Provides dense block

- Avoids reactivation of dormant epidural catheter
- Reduces risk of LAST

- Epidural anesthesia:
  - Catheter used for labor analgesia/ cesarean section may be used
  - However, failure rate is high if activated more than 10 hrs post-partum
  - Epidural test dose is important to rule out intrathecal catheter migration
  - 2% lidocaine with 1:2,00,000 adrenaline may be an ideal agent
  - Epidural fentanyl 50-100 µg may be given for postoperative analgesia
  - Disadvantages:
    - Delayed onset of action
    - Onset of action may exceed duration of surgery
    - Risk of epidural failure in delayed tubal ligation
    - Risk of total spinal and LAST due to catheter migration

❖ General anesthesia:
- Associated with higher morbidity and mortality
- Used for immediate postpartum laparoscopy
- Trendelenburgs position is used
- Induction:
  - Rapid sequence induction with cricoid pressure to avoid aspiration
  - Induction agents preferred are thiopentone and propofol
- Maintenance:
  - Volatile anesthetic requirement is reduced during pregnancy
  - This takes 12-36 hours to return to pre-gestational values
  - Thus, high concentration volatile agents are avoided (> 1 MAC)
  - Use of high concentration VA cause uterine relaxation
  - This may predispose the patient to post-partum hemorrhage
  - TIVA may be used as an alternative in patients at high risk for PPH
  - Cisatracurium may be used for subsequent doses of NMBAs
  - Neuromuscular monitoring is recommended due to:
    - Varied response of NDMR in post-partum period
    - NMBA potentiation by drugs such as metaclopramide
  - Prevent light anesthesia during manipulation of fallopian tube
  - Light anesthesia predisposes the patient to bradycardia
  - This occurs due to vagal stimulation
  - Drugs used to treat bradycardia include:
    - Glycopyrrolate
    - Atropine

Postoperative Analgesia

❖ Post-partum tubal ligation is associated with short-duration modest pain

❖ Thus, single dose of opioid may be sufficient in the postoperative period

❖ This is followed by oral analgesic supplementation

❖ Oral analgesics are begun before resolution of neuraxial block

❖ NSAIDs used are:
- Ketorolac (compatible with breast feeding and ductal patency)
- Ibuprofen

❖ Other options include:
- Infiltration of skin and mesosalpinx with bupivacaine
- Epidural analgesia

Complications

❖ Immediate complications:
- Wound infections
- Peritonitis (rare)

❖ Delayed complications:
- Chronic pelvic pain
- Congestive dysmenorrhea
- Menstrual abnormalities:
  - Menorrhagia
  - Dysmenorrhea
  - Hypomenorrhea
- ***Post-ligation syndrome*** comprising of:
  - Pelvic pain
  - Menorrhagia
  - Cystic ovaries

- Psychological complications
- Incisional hernia
- Failure of sterilization:
  - Occurs due to:
    - Fistula formation
    - Spontaneous re-anastomosis
  - Overall failure rate is 0.7%
  - Pomeroys technique has the lowest failure rate 0.1–0.6%
  - Madleners technique has highest failure rate of 1.5–7%
  - Failure rate is higher if performed:
    - Hysterotomy
    - Cesarean section

ANESTHESIA FOR FETAL SURGERY

Introduction

- Fetal surgery is performed for congenital lesions with poor neonatal outcomes
- Correction of fetal anomalies in-utero prevents irreversible organ damage
- This results in healthier neonates with better perinatal outcomes
- First procedure performed was fetal blood transfusion in 1963 by Sir William Liley

Advantages

- In-utero environment supports rapid post-operative healing
- Umbilical circulation meets nutritional and respiratory needs without outside assistance

Prerequisites

- Prerequisites for fetal surgery include:
  - Accurate diagnosis of the lesion
  - Accurate assessment of severity of the lesion
  - Absence of contraindications to the planned intervention
  - Risk of maternal morbidity low
  - Fetal surgical outcome should be better than neonatal surgical outcome
- Fetal surgery should be performed only for fetal anomalies which:
  - Can progress in utero
  - Cause harm to fetus before fetal lungs are mature

Indications 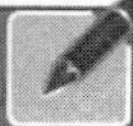

- Minimally invasive fetal surgical procedures:
  - Spina bifida: fetoscopic closure of the malformation
  - Aortic and pulmonary stenosis: valvuloplasty
  - Cyanotic congenital heart disease: balloon atrial septostomy
  - Twin twin transfusion syndrome: Laser ablation of blood vessels
  - Twin reversed arterial perfusion: Radiofrequency ablation
  - Congenital diaphragmatic hernia: Tracheal balloon occlusion
  - Obstructive uropathy:
    - Shunt insertion
    - Valve ablation
- Open fetal surgery:
  - Meningomyelocele repair
  - Sacrococcygeal teratoma excision
  - Resection of intrathoracic masses
  - Congenital diaphragmatic hernia: Temporary tracheal occlusion
  - Congenital cystic adenoid malformation: Excision

Types of Surgical Interventions

- Open surgical procedures:
  - Involve both maternal laparotomy and hysterotomy
  - Performed during pregnancy at mid-gestation
  - Pregnancy is allowed to continue to term after the procedure
  - Tocolytic agents are used to maintain uterine relaxation
  - Open surgical procedures done include:
    - Repair of fetal meningomyelocele
    - Resection of congenital pulmonary airway abnormalities
    - Debulking of sacrococcygeal teratomas
  - Associated with higher maternal and fetal risk
  - Complications include:
    - Premature rupture of membranes (PROM)
    - Preterm labor
    - Uterine dehiscence
    - Oligohydramnios
    - Hemorrhage, pulmonary edema
    - Fetal mortality
- Minimally invasive procedures:
  - Include both endoscopic and percutaneous procedures
  - Generally done with ultrasound guidance at mid-gestation

- Pregnancy is allowed to continue to term following the procedure
- Minimally invasive procedures performed include:
  - Intrauterine fetal blood transfusion
  - Fetoscopic laser coagulation for twin-twin-transfusion syndrome (TTS)
  - Aspiration of:
    - Thoracic cysts
    - Pleural effusions
    - Ascites
  - Biopsy of fetal skin/muscle/liver
- Associated with significantly lower risk of preterm labor and delivery

❖ Intrapartum procedures:
- Performed on fetuses at term, just prior to delivery
- Involves modification of cesarean delivery to allow intrapartum fetal therapy
- During this procedure, fetus remains supported by placental gas exchange
- These are also called EXIT procedures (ex-utero intrapartum therapy)
- EXIT procedures are commonly performed for:
  - Cystic hygroma
  - Lymphangioma
  - Cervical teratoma
  - Cardiopulmonary diseases as a bridge to ECMO

Fetal Effects of Anesthesia

❖ Teratogenic effects:
- Anesthetic agents produce harmful effects on fetal cells:
  - Decreased cell motility
  - Prolongation of DNA synthesis
  - Inhibition of cell cleavage
- The teratogenic effects of anesthetic agents on the fetus depends upon:
  - Timing of exposure to the drug
  - Dose of anesthetic drug
- However most anesthetic drugs are devoid of teratogenic effects
- These include:
  - Opioids
  - Benzodiazepines
  - Induction agents
  - Neuromuscular blockers
  - Inhalational agents
- Nitrous oxide has been found to be teratogenic in animal studies

❖ Direct fetal effects of anesthetic agents;
- Volatile anesthetic agents:
  - These cause direct depressant actions on fetal cardiovascular system
  - Effect is more pronounced at high doses (>1.5 MAC)
- Induction agents and opioids:
  - Produce fetal anesthesia
  - Reduce fetal heart rate variability

❖ Neuroplasticity:
- Anesthetic drugs may hamper neurological development in the fetus
- This may result from:
  - Accelerated neuro-apoptosis
  - Inhibitory effects on synaptogenesis
  - Decreased neurogenesis
- Clinical implications of fetal exposure on neuroplasticity has to be determined

❖ Indirect effects:
- Intrauterine asphyxia:
  - This may occur due to maternal hypoxia
  - Mild hypoxia is tolerated due to high O_2 affinity of fetal hemoglobin
  - Prolonged maternal hypoxia may lead to fetal hypoxia and death
- Fetal acidosis:
  - Maternal hypoventilation may cause maternal hypercapnia
  - This may in turn lead to fetal acidosis
- Compromised uteroplacental circulation:
  - Maternal hyperventilation:
    - This may result in hypocapnia and umbilical A vasoconstriction
    - This decreases uteroplacental circulation
  - Maternal hypotension reduces utero-placental circulation

Fetal Sentience

❖ Ability of the fetus to experience pain is termed as fetal sentience

❖ Maturation of pain pathways:
- Pain pathways should be fully functional for fetal sentience
- Peripheral pain receptors are completely developed by 20 weeks of gestation
- Spinothalamic connections are also fully developed by this time

- Pain transmission is therefore:
  - Possible from 16 weeks gestational age
  - Completed by 26 weeks gestational age
- Due to inability to communicate, objective measurement of pain is not possible
- Subjective methods using hypothalamo-pituitary-adrenal (HPA) axis response is used
- Activation of the HPA axis is the surrogate indicator of fetal pain
- This axis is completed and fully functional from 20 weeks gestational age
- Methods of studying fetal sentience:
  - Hormonal responses:
    - Fetal interventions causes alterations in stress hormones:
      - Noradrenaline
      - Cortisol
      - B-endorphin
      - Corticotrophin
    - These hormonal responses can be prevented by fetal analgesia
  - Hemodynamic responses:
    - Painful stimuli to fetus cause significant hemodynamic responses
    - This stress response causes redistribution of blood flow to the brain
    - This phenomenon is evaluated using Doppler USG techniques

Anesthetic Considerations

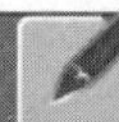

- Maternal considerations:
  - Avoid maternal hypotension as it causes fetal acidosis and asphyxia
  - Reduce material anxiety: can be due to:
    - Concerns about fetal safety
    - Fear of pain and complication due to procedure
  - Risk of preterm labor:
    - Uterine stimulation during interventions may cause uterine contraction
    - This can lead to preterm labor
    - Stimulation reduces uterine blood flow and causes placental separation
    - This is more likely at GA > 27 weeks as uterus is more irritable
    - Less likely when gestational age < 20 weeks.
  - Risk of aspiration
  - Avoidance of supine hypotension syndrome
  - Adequate maternal analgesia to be ensured:
    - Pain may stimulate uterine contractions
    - This in turn may precipitate preterm labor

Contd...

Contd...

- Fetal considerations:
  - Fetal analgesia to be ensures to avoid fetal sentience
  - Blood loss:
    - Blood volume in the fetus is low (approximately 50 mL)
    - Further, immature coagulation cascade predisposes to bleeding
    - Blood transfusion may be required with minimal blood loss (10 mL)
  - Hypothermia:
    - Fetal skin is thin, offering little barrier to evaporative heat losses
    - This may predispose the fetus to hypothermia
    - This can be prevented by:
      - Limiting surgical duration
      - Warm uterine irrigation system
  - Avoid fetal hypoxia:
    - Avoid maternal hypoxia (hyperoxia is not a problem)
    - Avoid maternal hyperventilation:
      - Alkalosis shifts oxyhemoglobin dissociation curve to left
      - Reduces delivery to fetus
    - Avoid maternal hypoventilation as it causes fetal acidosis

Anesthetic Techniques

- Maternal local anesthesia with fetal paralysis:
  - Indications:
    - For percutaneous needle aspiration/catheter insertions
    - For fetal umbilical vein sampling
    - Fetoscopic procedures
  - Maternal local anesthesia with 0.5 mL of 1% lidocaine as field block
  - Narcotics like remifentanil as supplement 0.1-0.2 µg/kg/min
  - Fetal anesthesia through IM injection with:
    - Fentanyl 10 µg/kg
    - Pancuronium 0.3 mg/kg IV
    - Atropine 20 µg/kg
  - Alternatively fetal anesthesia may be provided through umbilical V injection
  - Advantages:
    - Minimal parenteral analgesia to mother
    - Minimal risk to maternal airway
    - No risk of maternal neuromuscular blockade
    - Fetal drugs do not cross placental barrier in retrograde fashion
    - Loss of fetal movements for 2-4 hours
  - Disadvantages:
    - If emergency delivery is required, fetus would be paralysed

  - Fetus would require respiratory assistance after delivery
- Disadvantages
  - Increased chances of hypoxia
  - Unprotected airway: Increased risk of aspiration
  - Persistence of fetal movements
  - Does not block peritoneal/uterine pain
  - Monitoring required for 3-4 hrs for ventilation and hemodynamics

❖ Regional anesthesia:
- Used for major procedures
- Fetal anesthesia through IM injection with:
  - Fentanyl 10 μg/kg
  - Pancuronium 0.3 mg/kg IV
  - Atropine 20 μg/kg
- Advantages:
  - Excellent analgesia and good relaxation of abdomen
  - Avoids problems associated with intubation
  - Keeps mother awake: safe airway
- Disadvantages:
  - Can cause maternal hypotension
  - Avoided when fetal status is compromised

❖ General anesthesia:
- Useful for major open procedures
- Fetal anesthesia through IM injection with:
  - Fentanyl 10 μg/kg
  - Pancuronium 0.3 mg/kg IV
  - Atropine 20 μg/kg
- Advantages:
  - Excellent analgesia
  - Excess fetal movements reduced with direct muscle relaxant injection
  - Safe airway and reduces risk of aspiration
- Disadvantages:
  - Problems associated with intubation
  - Halogenated agents may cause fetal hypotension and acidosis

Surgery	Maternal anesthesia	Fetal anesthesia
Open surgery	GA with epidural anesthesia	Direct fetal IM injection
Fetoscopic fetal surgery	LA or regional anesthesia	Direct fetal IM injection Umbilical cord injections
Fetoscopic cord surgeries	LA or regional anesthesia	Maternal opioids
EXIT procedures	GA or RA	Fetal IM injection

ANESTHESIA FOR OPEN FETAL PROCEDURES

Preoperative Evaluation

❖ Maternal evaluation:
- USG for evaluating placental size and abnormalities
- Placentomegaly should be evaluated as it may:
- Alter pharmacokinetics of administered drugs
- May be injured during hysterotomy causing massive hemorrhage
- History of smoking to be ascertained as it impairs uteroplacental perfusion
- ***Mirror syndrome*** to be ruled out:
  - Also called ***Ballantynes syndrome***
  - Syndrome seen in mothers of hydrops fetalis babies
  - Characterized by:
    - Generalized edema
    - Proteinuria
    - Hypertension
  - The mother clinically mirrors the features seen in the fetus
  - Associated with high perinatal mortality and mortality
  - Thus, it is a contraindication for fetal surgery

❖ Fetal evaluation:
- Fetal imaging is performed preoperatively to identify alterations in physiology
- Detailed USG to confirm diagnosis and rule out other congenital anomalies
- Fetal echocardiogram to rule out congenital heart defects
- Amniocentesis or umbilical blood sampling for fetal karyotyping

❖ Only healthy parturients are approved for surgery (between 24-29 weeks)

❖ Family counselling about fetal benefits, maternal risks and alternatives

❖ Family to be warned that current and all subsequent pregnancies will be C-section

Premedication

❖ Parturient is nursed in:
- Quiet room to avoid maternal stress
- Thermoneutral environment to avoid fetal stress response

❖ Separate consent for per-rectal tocolytic suppository

❖ O negative, CMV negative irradiated blood cross matched for fetal transfusion

- Maternal sedation with 0.05 mg/kg midazolam IV
- Avoid heavy sedation to prevent aspiration and maternal hypoxia
- Anti-aspiration prophylaxis with:
  - 30 mL of non-particulate antacid like sodium citrate
  - H_2 receptor antagonist: 50 mg ranitidine IV
  - Antiemetics: 8 mg ondansetron IV/ 10 mg metaclopramide IV
- Shift to operation theatre in left lateral position: avoid supine hypotension syndrome
- Pneumatic compression devices are placed due to prolonged postoperative bed rest
- Epidural catheter is placed and tested preoperatively
- Epidural anesthesia is not used intraoperatively due to risk of hypotension
- Per-rectal indomethacin suppository 50 mg is placed to ensure tocolysis

Monitoring

- Maternal monitoring
  - Invasive BP monitoring for close regulation of blood pressure
  - Pulse oximetry
  - E_TCO_2, ECG
  - Temperature, urine output
  - BIS monitoring to prevent awareness
  - Neuromuscular monitoring as magnesium therapy may prolong NMBA action
  - Tocodynamometer especially in the postoperative period
- Fetal monitoring
  - Important to monitor for fetal asphyxia/ distress
  - Blood gas: pH and electrolytes
  - Blood glucose
  - Fetal pulse oximetry:
    - Indications:
      - Resection of large fetal masses
      - Moderate degree of fetal exposure
      - High risk of fetal cardiovascular depression
    - Monitored with separate sterile probe placed on fetal extremity
    - Normal fetal oxygen saturation ranges from 50–70%
    - Fetal SpO_2 < 50% indicates:
      - Maternal hypotension
      - Umbilical cord compression
    - Difficulty in probe placement may arise due to wet skin of the fetus
    - The skin is wiped dry repetitively to circumvent the problem
    - Placement of aluminium foils over the probe is useful as:
      - Prevents probe dislodgement
      - Prevents interference from ambient light
  - Fetal ECG
  - Fetal BP and umbilical blood flow
  - Transvaginal ultrasonography for fetal cardiac contractility
  - Continuous fetal echocardiography:
    - Requires the presence of fetal cardiologist
    - May not be practical for routine use
    - Echocardiography is begun at the beginning of fetal exposure
    - Continued till the time of uterine closure

Induction and Intubation

- 100% oxygen with tight fitting mask to adequately preoxygenate patient:
  - 3 minutes of tidal volume breathing or
  - 8 vital capacity breaths
- ***Rapid sequence induction*** with cricoid pressure
- Thiopentone 3 mg/kg, succinylcholine 1 mg/kg IV is used for induction
- Small sized ETT is used to secure the airway
- Immediately following induction other invasive monitors are placed:
  - Ryles tube
  - Radial arterial catheter
  - Other large bore IV access
  - Urinary catheter
- Surgical antibiotic prophylaxis is given
- Per-rectal indomethacin suppository 50 mg is placed if not done already
- Ultrasonography is performed prior to incision to:
  - Confirm fetal parameters
  - Placental position prior to surgical incision
- Type O-negative irradiated blood in 50 mL aliquots is kept ready for fetal transfusion
- Position: Supine with left uterine tilt.

Maintenance

- Balanced anesthesia with volatile agents is the preferred technique

- Sevoflurane or isoflurane may be used
- Desflurane is avoided due to higher incidence of fetal bradycardia
- Sevoflurane is preferred as it enables expeditious recovery following surgery
- 100% O_2 with 1 MAC sevoflurane may be used until surgical incision
- Volatile agent concentration is increased to 2-3 MAC just prior to incision
- This ensures uterine muscle relaxation and are agents of choice for open fetal surgery
- IV nitroglycerine may be used in case of inadequate uterine relaxation
- IV atracurium in low doses (2 mg) may be supplemented for muscle relaxation
- Doses are carefully titrated as magnesium is used for tocolysis during uterine closure
- Tocolytic therapy is initiated at the time of uterine closure:
  - Loading dose of 4–6 g given IV
  - Followed by 2–4 g/hour continuous infusion
- Fentanyl 1 µg/kg may be given to ensure analgesia at the time of uterine closure
- Epidural analgesia may be activated at the time of closure to augment analgesia
- Volatile anesthetic dose is subsequently reduced to 1 MAC
- Alternatively, volatile agents may be stopped during closure to facilitate recovery
- Propofol and nitrous oxide may be used to prevent awareness in the absence of VA

Hemodynamics

- Blood pressure is maintained to within 10% of baseline perioperatively
- Maintenance of BP is important as fetal distress can occur with hypotension
- Patient in lateral position or tilting table to left to avoid supine hypotension syndrome
- Restrictive fluid strategy is preferred due to risk of perioperative pulmonary edema
- Risk of perioperative pulmonary edema is high due to:
  - Fluid absorption from continuous uterine irrigation
  - Magnesium sulphate therapy
- Total intraoperative IV crystalloid infusion is restricted to 500 mL to 1L
- Hypotension is treated with:
  - IV fluid boluses
  - IV ephedrine 2.5-5 mg bolus
  - IV phenylephrine 10-25 µg bolus
  - Phenylephrine is not associated with decreased uteroplacental flow
- Special staplers available for vascular hemostasis to reduce hemorrhage

Fetal Anesthesia

- Following adequate hysterotomy and uterine exposure, the specific fetal part is exposed
- Supplemental fetal anesthesia is provided with intramuscular injections
- Drug cocktail is usually injected comprising of:
  - Fentanyl 5–10 µg/kg
  - Pancuronium 0.1-0.2 mg/kg
  - Atropine 20 µg/kg
- The drug cocktail is injected into either of:
  - Deltoid muscle
  - Gluteal region
  - Thigh of the fetus
- Following this, appropriate fetal monitors and vascular access catheters are secured
- Intraosseous routes and umbilical cord may be used in the presence of difficult access
- Prevention of fetal hypothermia:
  - Operating room to be maintained at 25–30°C
  - Rapid infusion system:
    - Warm fluid may be continuously infused into the uterine cavity
    - Fluid most commonly used for uterine irrigation is lactated ringers
    - This is delivered into the uterus via a sterile tubing system
    - Upto 10 L of fluid may be required to maintain irrigation
    - Uterine irrigation has multiple beneficial effects:
      - Replaces lost amniotic fluid
      - Maintains uterine volume
      - Prevents placental separation and fetal expulsion
      - Keeps the fetus warm
      - Prevents compression of umbilical cord

Extubation

- Awake extubation to reduce risk of aspiration
- Avoid coughing/straining as it can jeopardize integrity of uterine closure

Postoperative Management

Monitoring

- SpO_2, ABG
- BP, FHR
- Urine output and temperature
- Tocodynamometer to monitor uterine activity
- Periodic ultrasonography for:
  - Fetal monitoring
  - Patency of ductus arteriosus especially with indomethacin therapy

Management

- Tocolysis is continued with indomethacin therapy 50 mg Q4-6H
- Magnesium sulphate therapy is continued for 48–72 hours postoperatively
- Additional tocolytic therapy may be required:
  - Terbutaline
  - Calcium channel blockers

Complications

- Preterm labor
- Pain
- Pulmonary edema
- Aspiration
- Respiratory depression: Fetal distress

Analgesia

- Plays a vital role in preventing preterm labor
- Inadequate analgesia stimulates placental estrogen production and uterine activity
- Epidural analgesia with 0.05% bupivacaine and 10 µg/ mL fentanyl
- Patient controlled epidural analgesia
- NSAIDs are avoided due to risk of failure of ductal patency
- Fentanyl 1 µg/kg

EXIT PROCEDURE

Introduction

- Method of delivery utilizing placental support while surgery is performed to secure the fetal airway
- This allows continuing placental perfusion of the fetus while airway is established
- *Also called:*
  - ***Ex-utero Intrapartum Treatment***
  - ***Operation On Placental Support (OOPS)***

Indications 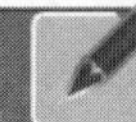

- Fetal cervical masses:
  - Lymphangioma
  - Teratoma
  - Hemangioma
  - Neuroblastoma
  - Goiter
- Fetal lung masses:
  - Congenital cystic adenomatoid malformations
  - Bronchopulmonary sequestration
- Fetal mediastinal masses:
  - Teratoma
  - Lymphangioma
- Congenital high airway obstruction (CHAOS) syndrome:
  - Tracheal atresia
  - Laryngeal atresia
- As a bridge to ECMO:
  - Hypoplastic left heart syndrome
  - Aortic stenosis

Fetal Procedures Performed during Exit

- Laryngoscopy
- Bronchoscopy
- Tracheostomy
- Tumor decompression or resection
- ECMO cannulation

Differences between Exit and Cesarean Section

Feature	Cesarean	Exit
Goal for uterine tone	Minimal hypotonia	Maximal hypotonia
Preferred anesthetic	Regional anesthesia	General anesthesia
Anesthetic plane	Minimal to avoid fetal depression	Deep planes
Warm uterine irrigation	Not required	Required
Anesthesiologists required	1	2 (for mother and fetus)

Anesthetic Considerations

- Maternal considerations:
  - Avoid maternal hypotension as it causes fetal acidosis and asphyxia
  - Reduce material anxiety: Can be due to:
    - Concerns about fetal safety
    - Fear of pain and complication due to procedure
  - Risk of aspiration due to general anesthesia
  - Avoidance of supine hypotension syndrome

- Minimal uterine relaxation is sufficient
- Uterotonic drugs following cord clamping to reduce maternal blood loss
- Deep anesthetic planes:
  - Deep anesthetic plane is preferred
  - This is because the fetus remains intubated postoperatively
  - Thus, opioids can be administered to the mother during the surgery

❖ Fetal considerations:
- Fetal analgesia to be ensured to avoid fetal sentience
- Blood loss:
  - Blood volume in the fetus is low (approximately 50 mL)
  - Further, immature coagulation cascade predisposes to bleeding
  - Blood transfusion may be required with minimal blood loss (10 mL)
  - O^{-ve} irradiated blood should be readily available
- Hypothermia:
  - Fetal skin is thin, offering little barrier to evaporative heat losses
  - This may predispose fetus to hypothermia especially with long surgery
  - This can be prevented by:
    - Limiting surgical duration
    - Overhead warming lamps
    - Uterine irrigation with warm fluids
- Avoid fetal hypoxia:
  - Avoid maternal hypoxia (hyperoxia is not a problem)
  - Avoid maternal hyperventilation:
    - Alkalosis shifts oxyhemoglobin dissociation curve to left
    - Reduces delivery to fetus
  - Avoid maternal hypoventilation as it causes fetal acidosis

❖ Technical considerations:
- Requires 2 operation theatres (for mother and fetus post-separation)
- Requires 2 teams of anesthesiologists (for mother and fetus)
- Requires 2 sets of monitoring equipment (for mother and fetus)
- Involves sterile manipulations: sterile anesthetist team is required
- Perinatal cardiologist for continuous fetal monitoring
- Perfusion team in case ECMO is planned

Preoperative Evaluation

❖ Maternal evaluation:
- USG for evaluating placental size and abnormalities
- Placentomegaly should be evaluated as it may:
  - Alter pharmacokinetics of administered drugs
  - May be injured during hysterotomy causing massive hemorrhage
- History of smoking to be ascertained as it impairs uteroplacental perfusion
- Gross polyhydramnios may be present in mother
- This may necessitate volume-reduction amniocentesis to:
  - Enable preoperative examination
  - Improve intraoperative visualization

❖ Fetal evaluation:
- Fetal imaging is performed preoperatively to:
  - Identify alterations in physiology
  - Determine weight of fetus for administration of medications
- Detailed USG to confirm diagnosis and rule out other congenital anomalies
- Fetal echocardiogram to rule out congenital heart defects
- Amniocentesis or umbilical blood sampling for fetal karyotyping

❖ Family counselling about:
- Fetal and maternal risks involving complex surgery
- Possibility of fetal blood transfusion

Preoperative OT Preparation

❖ Maternal equipment:
- Small sized ETT (upto 6 size)
- Laryngoscope blade: Polio blade with short handle
- Airways, facemask, bougie, LMA, cricothyrotomy set
- Anesthetic drugs preloaded, emergency drugs, atropine, adrenaline
- Suction apparatus
- IBP transducer systems
- Fluid warmer, rapid fluid infusion devices, hand inflated pressure bags
- Adequate amount of crystalloids and colloids
- Cross matched blood (at least 4-6 units)

❖ Fetal equipment: (to be maintained sterile)
- Fetal pulse oximeter
- Fetal E_TCO_2 monitor
- Intravenous catheters 24 G

- Saline flush with extensions for connection to IV cannula
- Sterile tourniquet for IV catheter placement
- Aluminium foil to:
  - Secure IV cannula
  - Protect pulse oximeter from ambient light
- Resuscitation medications:
  - Preloaded adrenaline syringes (1 µg/kg)
  - Preloaded calcium gluconate syringes (30 mg/kg)
- Preloaded fetal anesthesia syringe for intramuscular injection
- Appropriate size ETT (2.5, 3, 3.5 cm)
- Sterile ventilation bag with separate oxygen source
- Sterile stethoscope
- Type O-ve irradiated cross matched blood (50 mL aliquots)
- CPB pump if ECMO is planned

Choice of Anesthetic Technique

- General anesthesia is the preferred technique
- EXIT surgery is usually avoided in the presence of contraindications to GA
- Epidural anesthesia may be used as an alternative when required
- IV NTG 0.5-1.5 µg/kg/min may be used to improve uterine relaxation

Premedication

- Informed consent to be taken
- Maternal counselling regarding fetal separation in contrast with cesarean section
- Maternal sedation with 0.05 mg/kg midazolam IV
- Avoid heavy sedation to prevent aspiration and maternal hypoxia
- Anti-aspiration prophylaxis with:
  - 30 mL of non-particulate antacid like sodium citrate
  - H_2 receptor antagonist: 50 mg ranitidine IV
  - Antiemetics: 10 mg metaclopramide IV
- Shift to operation theatre in left lateral position: avoid supine hypotension syndrome
- Pneumatic compression devices are placed due to prolonged postoperative bed rest
- Epidural catheter is placed and tested preoperatively
- Epidural anesthesia is not used intraoperatively due to risk of hypotension

Monitoring

- Maternal monitoring
  - Invasive BP monitoring for close regulation of blood pressure
  - Pulse oximetry
  - E_TCO_2, ECG
  - Temperature, urine output
  - BIS monitoring to prevent awareness
  - Neuromuscular monitoring
- Fetal monitoring
  - Important to monitor for fetal asphyxia/distress
  - Blood gas and blood glucose
  - Fetal pulse oximetry:
    - Monitored with separate sterile probe placed on fetal extremity
    - Intra-EXIT normal fetal oxygen saturation ranges from 50-70%
    - Fetal SpO_2 < 50% indicates:
      - Maternal hypotension
      - Umbilical cord compression
    - Fetal saturation increases to 90% following fetal lung ventilation
    - Difficulty in probe placement may arise due to wet skin of the fetus
    - The skin is wiped dry repetitively to circumvent the problem
    - Placement of aluminium foils over the probe is useful as:
      - Prevents probe dislodgement
      - Prevents interference from ambient light
  - Fetal ECG, fetal BP, temperature
  - E_TCO_2 following fetal intubation
  - Continuous fetal echocardiography:
    - Requires the presence of fetal cardiologist
    - Especially important during resection of large lung masses

Induction and Intubation

- 100% oxygen with tight fitting mask to adequately preoxygenate patient:
  - 3 minutes of tidal volume breathing or
  - 8 vital capacity breaths
- ***Rapid sequence induction*** with cricoid pressure
- Thiopentone 3 mg/kg, succinylcholine 1 mg/kg IV is used for induction
- Small sized ETT is used to secure the airway
- Immediately following induction other invasive monitors are placed:
  - Ryles tube
  - Radial arterial catheter
  - Other large bore IV access
  - Urinary catheter

- Surgical antibiotic prophylaxis is given
- Ultrasonography is performed prior to incision to:
    - Confirm fetal parameters
    - Placental position prior to surgical incision
- Opioids may be administered following intubation as fetus is usually ventilated postoperatively
- Position: Supine with left uterine tilt

Maintenance

- Balanced anesthesia with volatile agents is the preferred technique
- Sevoflurane or isoflurane may be used
- Desflurane is avoided due to higher incidence of fetal bradycardia
- Sevoflurane is preferred as it enables expeditious recovery following surgery
- 100% O_2 with 1 MAC sevoflurane may be used until surgical incision
- Volatile agent concentration is increased to 2–3 MAC just prior to incision
- This ensures uterine muscle relaxation
- IV nitroglycerine may be used in case of inadequate uterine relaxation
- Volatile anesthetic dose is reduced to 1 MAC following umbilical cord clamping
- Alternatively, volatile agents may be stopped altogether to facilitate recovery
- Propofol and nitrous oxide may be used to prevent awareness in the absence of VA
- IV atracurium (10 mg) may be supplemented for intraoperative muscle relaxation
- Epidural analgesia may be activated during uterine closure to augment analgesia
- Uterotonic therapy:
    - Communication with the surgeon about timing of administration is vital
    - Administration is begun just prior to division of the cord
        - Oxytocin:
            - Most commonly used uterotonic agent
            - 20–40 IU in 1000 mL RL over 4–8 hours
        - Other agents used include:
            - Methergine 0.2 mg IM Q2-4 H as required
            - Carboprost 0.25 mg IM Q 15–60 mins as required
            - Misoprostol 800–1000 mg PO/PR/PV Q2H
            - Dinoprostone 20 mg PO Q2H
            - Intra-myometrial PGE_2 0.5 mg or PGF 2 α 0.2 mg

Hemodynamics

- Blood pressure is maintained to within 10% of baseline perioperatively
- Maintenance of BP is important as fetal distress can occur with hypotension
- Patient in lateral position or tilting table to left to avoid supine hypotension syndrome
- Restrictive fluid strategy is preferred due to risk of perioperative pulmonary edema-
- Total intraoperative IV crystalloid infusion is restricted to 500 mL to 1L
- Hypotension is treated with:
    - IV fluid boluses
    - IV ephedrine 2.5–5 mg bolus
    - IV phenylephrine 10–25 µg bolus
    - Phenylephrine is not associated with decreased uteroplacental flow
- Special staplers available for vascular hemostasis to reduce hemorrhage

Fetal Anesthesia

- A separate OR may be required for extensive post-EXIT fetal procedures
- Anesthetic management of the fetus is performed by a separate sterile anesthesia team
- Following adequate hysterotomy and uterine exposure, fetal limb is exposed
- Supplemental fetal anesthesia is provided with intramuscular injections
- Drug cocktail is usually injected comprising of:
    - Fentanyl 5–10 µg/kg
    - Pancuronium 0.1–0.2 mg/kg
    - Atropine 20 µg/kg
- The drug cocktail is injected into either of:
    - Deltoid muscle
    - Gluteal region
    - Thigh of the fetus
- Following this, appropriate fetal monitors and vascular access catheters are secured
- Intraosseous routes and umbilical cord may be used in the presence of difficult access
- IV fluid boluses (RL or blood) may be administered to maintain intravascular volume
- Fluid status and ventricular filling is constantly monitored by the cardiologist
- Continuous fetal echocardiographic monitoring is important to assess:
    - Ventricular filling
    - Myocardial contractility

- Securing the fetal airway:
  - Usually done once complete/adequate resection of the mass is performed
  - Following intubation ETT position is confirmed by:
    - Bilateral auscultation with sterile stethoscope
    - E_TCO_2 monitoring
  - Endotracheal tube position is then secured by suturing it to the gums
- Intra-EXIT normal fetal oxygen saturation ranges from 50–70%
- Fetal saturation increases to 90% following fetal lung ventilation
- Prevention of fetal hypothermia:
  - Pre-EXIT procedure:
    - Operating room to be maintained at 25–30 °C
    - Rapid infusion system:
      - Warm fluid may be continuously infused into the uterine cavity
      - Fluid most commonly used for irrigation is lactated ringers
      - This is delivered into the uterus via a sterile tubing system
      - Upto 10 L of fluid may be required to maintain irrigation
      - Uterine irrigation has multiple beneficial effects:
  - Keeps the fetus warm
  - Prevents inadvertent compression of umbilical cord
  - Maintains uterine volume
  - Prevents placental separation
  - This ensures placental integrity during the procedure
  - Post-EXIT procedure:
    - Operating room to be maintained at 25–30 °C
    - Forced air warmers
    - Multiple pre-warmed towels
- Following clamping of the cord and delivery of the baby:
  - Umbilical catheters may be placed for vascular access
  - Lung/mass resection is completed in a separate operation theatre

Extubation

- Awake extubation to reduce risk of aspiration
- Avoid coughing/straining as it can jeopardize integrity of uterine closure.

Postoperative Management

Monitoring

- SpO_2, ABG
- BP, FHR
- Urine output and temperature

Management

- Foleys catheter and NGT are removed when the patient is:
  - Fully awake
  - Hemodynamically stable
  - Voiding adequately
- Supplemental O_2 as per requirement
- Ondansetron or metoclopramide can be used to reduce PONV incidence

Complications

- Blood loss is the most common complication
- Pain
- Pulmonary edema
- Aspiration
- Intraoperative respiratory depression: fetal distress

Analgesia

- Analgesic requirements are similar to that for cesarean section
- Epidural analgesia with 0.05% bupivacaine and 10 µg/mL fentanyl
- Patient controlled epidural analgesia
- NSAIDs
- Fentanyl 1 µg/kg

NON-OBSTETRIC SURGERY IN PREGNANCY

Introduction

- Frequency of non-obstetric surgeries during pregnancy ranges from 0.3–2.2%
- Non-obstetric surgery may be required at any stage of pregnancy:
  - First trimester 42%
  - Second trimester 35%
  - Third trimester 23%
- Most commonly performed surgeries include:
  - Laparoscopic gynecological surgeries during first trimester
  - Appendicectomy during other stages of pregnancy

Types of Non-obstetric Surgery during Pregnancy

- Pregnant patients should never be denied medically necessary non-obstetric surgery
- Elective surgery:
  - Surgery which does not involve a medical emergency
  - Can be delayed without increasing risk of permanent disability
- Semi emergency surgery:
  - Surgery which is necessary
  - Can be delayed without increasing risk of permanent disability
- Emergency surgery:
  - Surgery which is necessary
  - If delayed can cause maternal morbidity and mortality

Indications for Non-obstetric Surgery during Pregnancy: ACOG 2019 Guidelines

- Pregnancy related surgeries:
  - Cervical incompetence
  - Presence of ovarian cysts
  - Fetal surgeries
- Non-pregnancy related surgeries:
  - Acute abdomen:
    - Appendicitis
    - Cholecystitis
  - Cancer surgeries
  - Trauma surgery

Risks Associated with Nonobstetric Surgeries: ACOG 2019 Guidelines

- Maternal risks:
  - Associated with non-obstetric surgery:
    - Infection
    - Reoperation
    - Respiratory complications
    - Blood transfusion
  - Associated with pregnancy:
    - Venous thromboembolism
    - Aspiration penumonia
    - Risk of preterm delivery
    - Risk of PPH in the event of cesarean section due to tocolytic therapy
- Fetal risks:
  - Teratogeneicity to non-anesthetic medications
  - None of the anesthetic agents have been found to be teratogenic
  - Fetal hypoxia due to alterations in utero-placental circulation
  - Preterm delivery

Timing of Surgery

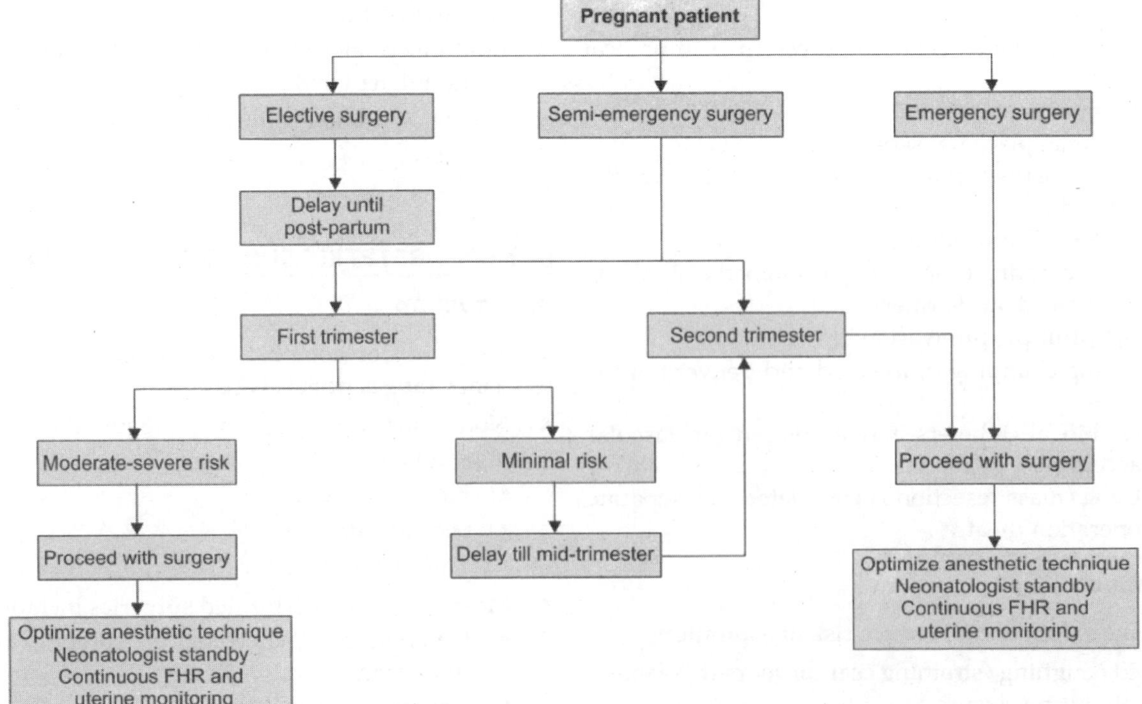

Preoperative Evaluation and Optimization

- Medical and obstetric history
- Anesthesia directed physical examination:
  - Airway assessment
  - Screening for VTE risk
- Laboratory investigations:
  - As per the medical condition
  - Additional testing is not warranted in uncomplicated pregnancies
- VTE prophylaxis should be initiated in indicated patients
- Counselling about risk of preterm labor should be explained
- Consent taken should include cesarean section due to fetal indications

Anesthetic Considerations

- Maternal considerations:
  - Maintenance of mild physiological alkalosis during ventilation
  - Difficult intubation due to:
    - Soft tissue edema
    - Enlarged breasts
  - Difficult mask ventilation due to swollen tongue
  - Aspiration prophylaxis
  - Avoidance of supine hypotension syndrome
  - Reduced anesthetic requirements during pregnancy:
    - Induction agents
    - Volatile anesthetics
  - Reduced NMBA requirement due to enhanced sensitivity to NMBAs
  - Avoidance of preterm labor: use of perioperative tocolytics
  - VTE prophylaxis as high risk of thromboembolism during pregnancy
- Fetal considerations:
  - Avoidance of non-anesthetic teratogenic agents:
    - Hyperthermia
    - Ionizing radiation
    - Iodinated contrast media
  - Drugs:
    - Captopril, enalapril
    - Phenytoin, valproic acid
  - Availability of qualified personnel for FHR monitoring
  - Avoidance of preterm labor

Choice of Anesthetic Technique

- Choice of anesthetic technique should be guided by:
  - Nature of surgery
  - Maternal indications
- Local and regional anesthesia:
  - Advantages:
    - Avoids airway instrumentation
    - Minimizes alterations in utero-placental flow
    - Minimizes risk of aspiration
  - Disadvantages:
    - SAB may cause precipitous hypotension and fetal distress
    - High block can cause paralysis and hypotension
    - Difficulty in controlling ventilation and maintaining $PaCO_2$
    - Inadvertent intrathecal/intravascular injection of local anesthetic
- General anesthesia:
  - Useful for emergencies
  - Secures the airway

Preoperative Preparation and Premedication

- Informed consent
- NPO guidelines:
  - NPO for 6–8 hours with non-fatty solids
  - NPO for 2 hours for clear liquids
- Nursing with 15° left-lateral tilt to avoid supine hypotension beyond 20 weeks GA
- Placement of large bore IV cannula as surgically appropriate
- Anti-aspiration prophylaxis:
  - 10 mg metoclopramide at least 30 minutes prior to induction
  - 50 mg ranitidine IV at least 30 minutes prior to induction
- Thromboprophylaxis:
  - Mechanical thromboprophylaxis for procedures less than 45 minutes
  - LMWH for procedures lasting more than 45 minutes
- Per-rectal indomethacin for prophylactic tocolysis 50–100 mg
- Sedative premedication:
  - Sedative premedication is usually avoided
  - In anxious patients, IV midazolam 1 mg may be administered

Monitors

- Maternal monitors:
  - As indicated by the type of surgery
  - No additional maternal monitors are required
  - Pulse oximetry, E_TCO_2

- ECG, temperature monitoring
- Neuromuscular monitoring and BIS
- Tocodynamometer for uterine contraction

❖ Fetal monitoring:
- All patients should have documented FHR pre and postoperatively
- Need for continuous intraoperative FHR monitoring should be individualized
- Continuous FHR monitoring is indicated when:
  - Fetus is viable
  - Fetus is previable to facilitate positioning and oxygenation interventions
  - Anatomically possible
- Simultaneous FHR monitoring and uterine contraction monitoring

Induction

❖ Adequate preoxygenation

❖ General anesthesia with LMA may be used in appropriate cases upto 18 weeks GA

❖ Endotracheal intubation is preferred beyond 18 weeks of gestation

❖ Rapid sequence intubation is indicated for pregnancy beyond 18 weeks GA

❖ Propofol, ketamine and etomidate may be used for induction

❖ Succinylcholine may be used to ensure neuromuscular paralysis

❖ Fentanyl is preferred to ensure analgesia and limit intubation response

❖ Nasogastric tube may be inserted to prevent aspiration post-extubation

Position

❖ Supine with left uterine displacement beyond 20 weeks gestation

❖ 15° left lateral tilt is used to prevent aorto-caval compression

Maintenance

❖ Balanced anesthesia with 50% O_2 + 50% nitrous oxide + 0.5 MAC volatile anesthetic

❖ Inhaled nitrous oxide has no effect on:
- Uterine tone
- Maternal hemodynamics
- FHR variability

❖ Thus, < 50% N_2O may be used safely beyond 6 weeks pregnancy

❖ Pregnant patients are more sensitive to the effects of NMBAs

❖ Also concurrent magnesium sulphate therapy reduces NMBA requirements

❖ Neuromuscular monitoring must be used to guide dosing of NMBAs

❖ Short acting NMBAs such as atracurium (5–10 mg) are preferred

❖ Titrated fentanyl boluses may be used (1 µg/kg) to prevent delayed recovery

❖ Intraoperative tocolysis:
- Should not be used prophylactically
- Should be considered when high risk of preterm labor is present
- When indicated, magnesium sulphate is preferred for intraoperative tocolysis:
  - IV 2–4 grams over 20 minutes
  - 1–2 grams/hour infusion thereafter

Hemodynamics

❖ Maternal hemodynamics:
- Maternal BP is the most important determinant of utero-placental perfusion
- Thus, systolic blood pressure is maintained:
  - Above 100 mm Hg
  - With 20% variation from baseline BP
- Drugs used to treat hypotension:
  - Both phenylephrine and ephedrine may be used
  - Phenylephrine is associated with reflex bradycardia

❖ Fetal hemodynamics:
- Anesthesia usually results in changes in the FHR patterns:
  - Reduced FHR variability
  - Low-normal baseline FHR
- Treatment to optimize utero-placental circulation is warranted when:
  - Persistent fetal bradycardia
  - Persistent fetal tachycardia
  - Repetitive decelerations
  - Prolonged decelerations
- Techniques to optimize uteroplacental perfusion include:
  - Left uterine displacement
  - Increasing maternal blood pressure
  - Increased delivered FiO_2
  - Maintenance of normocarbia

Ventilation

- Minimum FiO_2 of 50% is recommended during anesthesia
- Ventilation is adjusted to maintain normal physiological alkalosis of pregnancy
- Vigorous hyperventilation and hypoventilation have to be avoided
- E_TCO_2 is maintained between 30-32 mm Hg

Extubation

- Patient is extubated once fully awake and fully reversed
- Postoperative ventilation should be considered for:
  - Prolonged surgeries
  - Excessive blood loss

Postoperative Management

Management

- Nursing is done with LUD position
- Early resumption of oral feeds and ambulation is recommended
- Mechanical VTE prophylaxis is continued in postoperative period until ambulation
- Tocolysis continued in the postoperative period for 24 hours:
  - Indomethacin 25-50 mg Q4H
  - Magnesium sulphate 1-2 g/hour

Monitors

- Maternal monitoring:
  - Pulse oximetry
  - ECG, NIBP
  - Tocodynamometer
  - ABG
- Fetal monitoring:
  - FHR should be documented postoperatively in all cases
  - Continuous FHR is recommended in high-risk patients

Analgesia

- Multimodal analgesia preferred
- Local anesthetic infiltration
- Regional anesthesia techniques
- Opioids
- NSAIDs:
  - Single dose NSAIDs may be safe
  - Repeated doses should be avoided especially during first and third trimesters
  - This is due to potential fetal ductal-closure side effects of NSAIDs

APPENDICITIS IN PREGNANCY

Introduction

Most common nonobstetric surgical emergency in pregnancy.

Clinical Features

Most common in 1st and 2nd trimester.

Symptoms

- Abdominal pain variable in position due to growing uterus
- Anorexia nausea vomiting
- Diarrhea/constipation, dysuria

Signs

- Fever 37–38°C
- Tachycardia > 100 bpm
- Abdominal guarding and rigidity
- Tenderness:
  - Right iliac fossa
  - Right upper quadrant
  - Mid epigastric
  - Diffuse
- Rectal tenderness
- ***Rebound pain***
- Reduced bowel sounds
- ***Psoas test:***
  - Indicates inflammation of iliopsoas group of muscles
  - Occurs in retrocecal appendicitis
  - Actively flex thigh at hip joint
  - Alternately passive extension of thigh with patient lying on the side
  - Abdominal pain indicates positive psoas test
- ***Obdurator test:***
  - Indicates inflammation of obdurator internus
  - Patient lies on back
  - Knees and hips flexed to 90°
  - Flexion and internal rotation of hip causes pain
- ***Rovsings sign***:
  - Palpation of left lower quadrant increases pain in right lower quadrant of abdomen
  - Not useful in pregnancy

- *Alders sign:*
  - To differentiate uterine and appendiceal pain
  - Pain localized with patient supine
  - Patient turned to her left side
  - If pain shifts to the left , it is assumed to be uterine

Differential Diagnosis

Obstetric

- Preterm labor
- Salpingitis
- Abruption
- Degenerating myoma
- Chorioamnionitis
- Tuboovarian abscess
- Ovarian cyst tortion
- Threatened abortion

Nonobstetric

- Glomerulonephritis
- Pyelonephritis
- Cholecystitis
- Pancreatitis
- Renal calculus
- Sickle cell crisis
- Porphyria
- Pneumonia
- Intestinal obstruction
- Mesenteric adenitis

Anesthetic Goals

- Delay elective surgery till second trimester if possible
- Preserve maternal life in emergency surgery
- Optimize maternal physiological function
- Avoid teratogenicity
- Avoid oxytocic effects on myometrium
- Optimize uteroplacental blood flow
- Use regional anesthesia where possible
- Avoid awareness under general anesthesia

Anesthetic Considerations

- Avoidance of teratogenic agents:
  - Category D: Diazepam
  - Category C:
    - Thiopentone
    - Etomidate
    - Sufentanyl
    - Chloroprocaine
    - Ketamine
    - Morphine
    - Bupivacaine
    - Halothane
- Prevention of supine hypotension syndrome
- Maintenance of fetal oxygenation:
  - Maintain PaO_2, $PaCO_2$, BP
  - Avoid hyperventilation – alkalotic shift of ODC
  - Avoid high MAC of volatile anesthetics
  - Avoid excess airway pressures–hypotension
  - Use regional anesthesia where possible
- Prevention of preterm labor:
  - β2 agonists
  - magnesium sulphate
  - indomethacin
  - Atosiban
  - NTG
  - Nifedipine

Preoperative Preparation

- Large bore IV access
- Preload with 10–20 mL/kg crystalloid
- Nurse in 15° left lateral tilted position if > 16–20 weeks gestation
- Premedication avoided
- Avoid NSAIDs to avoid premature closure of ductus arteriosus
- Benzodiazepines for sedation if required
- IV glycopyrrolate 10 μ/kg
- Antiaspiration prophylaxis after 16 weeks gestation
  - Non particulate 0.3 M sodium citrate 30 mL 30 min before surgery
  - IV ranitidine 1 mg/kg
  - IV metaclopramide 0.15 mg/kg
- Prophylactic tocolysis if indicated

Choice of Anesthesia

- Regional anesthesia is *technique of choice*
- Spinal preferred as:
  - Lower doses of LA reduces chances of fetal LA toxicity
  - Accidental injection of LA intravascularly avoided
- Epidural anesthesia with graded doses alternative
- GA with ETT and IPPV if patient hemodynamically unstable

Advantages of Regional Anesthesia

- Minimizes fetal drug exposure
- Airway management simplified
- Decreased blood loss

Effects of Surgery on Fetus

- Hypovolemia
- Hypotension
- Hypoxemia
- Intrauterine fetal asphyxia
- Fetal acidosis
- Preterm labor
- Teratogenicity

General Anesthesia

Monitors

- Pulse oximetry
- Temperature
- NIBP
- IBP/CVP if hemodynamically unstable
- ECG
- Cardiotocometer
- End tidal CO_2
- Tocodynamometer
- Urine output
- entropy
- FHR monitoring feasible after 18 weeks when fetus becomes viable

Induction

- 3–5 mins preoxygenation with 100% oxygen
- ***Rapid sequence induction*** with ***Sellicks maneuver***
- Thiopentone succinycholine for induction
- Avoid ketamine in early pregnancy as it increases uterine tone
- Intubation with 6.5 or 7 mm ETT
- Left lateral position tilt

Maintenance

- O_2 air (50:50) morphine/pethidine NDMR isoflurane 0.5–1 MAC
- Avoid teratogenic agents
- Avoid N_2O in early pregnancy as:
  - it inhibits methionine synthetase
  - inhibits DNA synthesis
  - reduces placental blood flow

Ventilation

- Maintain E_TCO_2 within normal limits of pregnancy
- Avoid maternal hypercarbia as it causes fetal acidosis
- Avoid PEEP as it may aggravate hypotension

Hemodynamics

- Hypotension aggressively treated to avoid uteroplacental insufficiency
- Judicious fluid boluses as increased chances of pulmonary edema
- Ephedrine used to treat hypotension unresponsive to fluid boluses
- Phenylephrine and metaraminol alternatives

Extubation

- Fully awake and fully reversed
- Return of protective airway reflexes
- Extubate in left lateral position

Postoperative

- Routine administration of tocolytics controversial
- Thromboprophylaxis with heparin essential to avoid risk of DVT
- Multimodal analgesia essential
- Pain increases risk of preterm labor
- Regional analgesia techniques important to reduce dosage of opioids
- Avoid NSAIDs to reduce risk of premature closure of ductus arteriosus
- Postoperative analgesia may mask awareness of early contractions
- Tocometry important monitor for preterm labor
- Monitor tocodynamometer and fetal heart rate

Complications

- Preterm labor
- Perforation of viscera
- Abortion
- Peritonitis
- Maternal and fetal mortality epidural hematoma
- Pulmonary edema (very common)

LAPAROSCOPIC SURGERY IN PREGNANCY

Introduction

- Laparoscopy was avoided during pregnancy due to concerns of fetal complications
- However, pregnancy is no longer considered a contraindication to laparoscopy

Concerns

- Rise in intra-abdominal pressure during pneumoperitoneum causing:
  - Reduced utero-placental blood flow
  - Fetal hypoxia
  - Fetal acidosis
- Absorption of carbon dioxide by the fetus resulting in fetal acidosis
- Mechanical injury to the fetus by trocar or Veress needle
- Uterine perforation causing PROM and preterm delivery

Advantages

- Lesser risk with laparoscopy, compared to laparotomy
- Earlier ambulation and return to routine activity reduces chances of DVT
- Earlier return of GI function
- Reduced operative time and hospital stay duration
- Reduced infection and reduced postop incisional hernia
- Lesser bleeding
- Lesser pain: reduces narcotic use
- Lesser manipulation of uterus while obtaining adequate exposure:
  - Reduces chances of preterm labor
  - Reduces premature delivery
  - Reduced likelihood of spontaneous abortion
- Avoidance of a large abdominal scar with an enlarging uterus
- Better visualization due to optical magnification

Disadvantages

- Increases chances of hypoxia, hypercapnea and hypotension
- Increased postoperative nausea and vomiting (PONV)
- Narrow field of vision during surgery
- Harmful effects of CO_2:
  - Fetal tachycardia and HTN
  - Severe maternal acidosis
  - Severe fetal acidosis

Indications

- Diagnostic:
  - For acute abdomen in pregnancy
  - Diagnosis of ectopic pregnancy
- Therapeutic:
  - Laparoscopic appendicectomy
  - Laparoscopic cholecystectomy
  - Linear salpingotomy for unruptured ectopic pregnancy
  - Laparoscopic fundoplication and hernia repair
  - Other rare procedures:
    - Radical nephrectomy
    - Retroperitoneal lymphadenectomy
    - Adrenalectomy

Contraindications

- Hemodynamic instability
- Large ovarian mass
- Multiple prior surgeries
- History of adhesive disease

Timing of Surgery: SAGES 2017 Guidelines

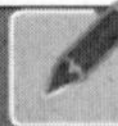

- Laparoscopic surgery can be performed safely during any trimester of pregnancy (Level II, Grade B)
- Limitations of Ist trimester:
  - Risk of teratogenicity
  - 12% miscarriage rate
- Limitations of IIIrd trimester:
  - 30% risk of preterm labor which increases with gestational age
  - Gravid uterus prevents proper visualization of surgical field
  - Laparoscopic surgery has been successfully performed up to 34 weeks
- IInd trimester:
  - 0% miscarriage rate, 8% preterm labor
  - No risk of teratogenicity
  - Gravid uterus does not cause obstruction
  - *Safest* trimester to perform surgery
  - Ideally done at < 23 weeks gestational age

Modifications of Surgical Technique: SAGES 2017 Guidelines

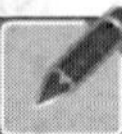

- Trocar placement:
  - All patients undergoing laparoscopy are at risk for trocar injury
  - Hassens (open) or Verres needle (closed) techniques can be used safely
  - Gravid uterus causes difficult trocar insertion and increases risk of:
    - Risk of bowel perforation
    - Uterine perforation
    - Preterm labor
  - Thus, the port is placed at least 6 cm above the uterine fundus
  - Alternative techniques to lift abdominal wall are:
    - Use of abdominal wall lifting devices (gasless laparoscopy)
    - Optical trocar which allows visualization at the time of trocar insertion
- Pneumoperitoneum:
  - Maintenance of a low IAP is mandatory
  - IAP is usually maintained between 8-12 mm Hg
  - IAP should not exceed 15 mm Hg

Anesthetic Technique

1. Regional anesthesia

- Disadvantages:
  - May cause precipitous hypotension and fetal distress
  - High block can cause paralysis and hypotension

- Difficulty in controlling ventilation and maintaining $PaCO_2$
- Inadvertent intrathecal/intravascular injection of local anesthetic
- Increased incidence of shoulder tip pain
- Nasogastric tube is usually not well tolerated in an awake patient

❖ Advantageous as awake mother prevents aspiration
❖ Therefore, regional anesthesia is usually not preferred for laparoscopic surgery
❖ When used, epidural anesthesia is preferred over spinal anesthesia

2. General anesthesia: ***Technique of choice*** as:

❖ Avoids patient anxiety
❖ Respiratory compromise and dyspnea possible in awake patient
❖ Nasogastric tube may be uncomfortable in awake patient
❖ Allows control of ventilation to adjust hyperapnea

Preoperative Management

❖ NPO orders:
- 6 hours solids
- 2 hours clear fluids

❖ Preoperative antibiotics
❖ Premedication: Midazolam 0.05 mg/kg IV
❖ Anti-aspiration prophylaxis for gestation > 16 weeks: (Wong CA, 2007)
- 30 mL of non-particulate sodium citrate
- IV ranitidine 50 mg
- IV metoclopramide 10 mg or ondansetron 8 mg

❖ Antisialogogue:
- IV glycopyrrolate 0.01 mg/kg
- Also combats reflex vagal activity from peritoneal stretching

❖ *Prophylactic* glucocorticoids and tocolytic agents: not recommended
❖ Mechanical DVT prophylaxis
❖ Preoperative fetal heart rate monitoring
❖ Parturient is shifted to OT in left lateral position

Intraoperative Management

Induction and Intubation

❖ Adequate preoxygenation with 100% oxygen as desaturation is rapid
❖ ***Rapid sequence induction*** with cricoid pressure is ***technique of choice***
❖ Thiopentone 3 mg/kg + succinylcholine 1 mg/kg + O_2 + isoflurane 1 MAC
❖ Smaller sized ETT is used to secure the airway
❖ Nasogastric tube is inserted to:
- Prevent perforation of distended stomach
- Reduce risk of aspiration

Monitoring

Maternal Monitors

❖ Monitors:
- Pulse oximetry
- NIBP/ IBP
- ECG
- E_TCO_2
- Nasopharyngeal temperature
- Nerve stimulator
- Peak airway pressure
- Minute ventilation
- Serial ABG for $PaCO_2 - E_TCO_2$ difference
- Intra-abdominal pressure

❖ Clinical assessment:
- Skin color, turgor, capillary refill
- Cornea and conjunctiva for edema in prolonged Trendelenburg position
- Upper chest for subcutaneous emphysema
- Urine output as oliguria is possible especially when IAP > 15 mm Hg

Fetal Monitors

❖ Done pre and postoperatively during urgent abdominal surgery (Level III, Grade B)
❖ Monitors used include:
- FHR: Cardio tachometer
- Uterine activity: Tocodynamometer
- Transvaginal ultrasonography

Position

❖ Trendelenburg position with left sided tilt used in most cases
❖ All parturients are placed with a slight leftward tilt after 16 weeks of gestation
❖ Amount of Trendelenburg position that the parturient tolerates depends on:
- Patients habitus
- Co-morbid risk factors
- Gestational age of pregnancy

❖ Left sided tilt up to 30 degrees improves visualization of appendix and gall bladder\
❖ Initiate al positional alterations slowly

Maintenance

- Propofol infusion used for maintenance in TIVA (reduces PONV incidence)
- Fentanyl 1 µg/ kg and vecuronium 0.1 mg/kg IV boluses for maintenance
- O_2 + 1 MAC isoflurane used to maintain balanced anesthesia
- Halothane avoided as it can cause arrhythmias in the presence of CO_2
- N_2O avoided as:
  - It causes bowel distention
  - It increases risk of PONV
  - It reduces the delivered FiO_2
- E_TCO_2 maintained between 32-34 mm Hg
- Intermittent NGT suctioning required as CO_2 diffuses into stomach and distends it
- Table is tilted to left and Trendelenburg restricted to 10°
- Thromboprophylaxis:
  - Mechanical thromboprophylaxis for procedures less than 45 minutes
  - LMWH for procedures lasting more than 45 minutes
- Tocolytic agents: (Level I, Grade A)
  - Should not be used prophylactically
  - Should be considered when signs of preterm labor are present

Hemodynamics

- Strict maintenance of BP with fluid boluses and vasopressors
- 2.5-4 mL/kg/hour of Ringers Lactate through 16-18 G IV cannula
- Third space and insensible fluid loss is negligible
- Restrictive fluid strategy is used for maintenance of intravascular volume status
- Volume of retained intraperitoneal saline is added to the total volume of fluid infused
- Volume of retained intraperitoneal saline = (Volume of fluid used for irrigation)– (Volume of fluid in suction container)

Extubation

- Fully awake in lateral and head down position to reduce risk of aspiration
- Shifted to PACU in left lateral position

Postoperative

Management

- Foleys catheter and NGT are removed when the patient is:
  - Fully awake
  - Hemodynamically stable
  - Voiding adequately
- Supplemental O_2 mandatory as O_2 demand increases following laparoscopic surgery
- Ondansetron or metoclopramide can be used to reduce PONV incidence

Complications

- Air leak syndromes:
  - Subcutaneous emphysema
  - Pneumothorax
  - Pneumopericardium
  - Pneumomediastinum
- Gas embolism usually when laparoscopy is associated with hysteroscopy
- PONV:
  - Main complication post laparoscopic surgery
  - May be severe
  - Steps to reduce PONV:
    - Preoperative nasogastric tube drainage
    - Propofol based anesthesia
    - Intraoperative administration of ondansetron /metaclopramide
- Aspiration pneumonia
- Postoperative pulmonary dysfunction:
  - Lesser in pelvic surgery compared with upper abdominal surgery
  - FRC returns to baseline values within 72 hours
- Pulmonary edema: excess fluid administration (chasing low urine output intraoperatively)
- Pain:
  - More of visceral nature
  - Lesser compared with open laparotomy

Monitoring

- Pulse oximetry
- ECG
- BP-as hemodynamic changes outlast duration of pneumoperitoneum
- Urine output
- ABG

Postoperative Analgesia

- Topical anesthesia and infiltration reduces postoperative pain
- Intraperitoneal instillation of 0.5% lidocaine 80 mL or 0.125% bupivacaine with epinephrine in right subdiaphragmatic area reduces shoulder tip pain
- NSAIDs:
  - Are avoided for postoperative analgesia especially after 32 weeks gestation
  - This is due to the risk of ductus arteriosus closure
- Opioids and clonidine can also be used

SUGGESTED READING

1. AAP Committee on Fetus and Newborn. (2015). The APGAR score. *Pediatrics*, 117(4), 819–22.
2. Abalos, E., Cuesta, C., Grosso, A.L., Chou, D., Say, L. (2013). Global and regional estimates of preeclampsia and eclampsia: a systematic review. *European Journal of Obstetrics, Gynecology and Reproductive Biology*, 170(1), 1–7.
3. Abildgaard, U., Heimdal, K. (2012). Pathogenesis of syndrome of hemolysis, elevated liver enzymes, and low platelet count (HELLP): a review. *European Journal of Obstetrics, Gynecology and Reproductive Biology*, 116(2), 117–23.
4. ACOG. (2019). ACOG practice bulletin no. 202: gestational HTN and preeclampsia. *Obstetrics and Gynecology*, 133(1), e1–e25.
5. ACOG. (2019). Non-obstetric surgery during pregnancy. *Obstetrics and Gynecology*, e285–e286.
6. Akamatsu, T.J., Bonica, J.J., Rehmet, R., Eng, M., Ueland, K. (1974). Experiences with the use of ketamine for parturition as primary anesthetic for vaginal delivery. *Anesthesia Analgesia*, 52(6), 284–7.
7. Alfirevic, Z., Devane, D., Gyte, G.M. (2017). Continuous cardiotocography as a form of electronic fetal monitoring for fetal assessment during labour. *Cochrane Database of Systematic Reviews*.
8. Alshawabkeh, L., Economy, K.E., Valente, A.M. (2016). Anticoagulation during pregnancy: evolving strategies with a focus on mechanical valves. *Journal of American College of Cardiology*, 68(16), 1804–13.
9. American College of Obstetricians and Gynecologists. (1996). Pulmonary disease in pregnancy. *International Journal of Gynecology and Obstetrics*, 54(2), 187–96.
10. American College of Obstetricians and Gynecologists. (2009). ACOG practice bulletin: intrapartum FHR monitoring: nomenclature, interpretation and general management principles. *Obstetrics and Gynecology*, 114(1), 192–202.
11. American College of Obstetricians and Gynecologists. (2016). Practice bulletin: management of preterm labor. *Obstetrics and Gynecology*, e155–164.
12. American College of Obstetricians and Gynecologists' Committee on Obstetric Practice. (2016). Committee opinion no.679- immersion in water during labor and delivery. *Obstetrics and Gynecology*, 128(5), e231–e236.
13. American College of Surgeons. (2008). *Advanced Trauma Life Support for Doctors*. Chicago: AAS.
14. American Diabetes Association. (2012). Diagnosis and classification of diabetes mellitus. *Diabetes Care*, 33(Suppl 1), S64–S71.
15. American Diabetes Association. (2019). Classification and diagnosis of diabetes: standards of medical care in diabetes. *Diabetes Care*, 43(Suppl 1), S13–S28.
16. American Society of Anesthesiologists. (2007). Practise guidelines for obstetric anesthesia. *Anesthesiology*, 124(2), 843–63.
17. American Society of Anesthesiologists. (2016). Practice guidelines for obstetric anesthesia: an updated report be the ASA task force on obstetric anesthesia and Society for Obstetric Anesthesia and Perinatology. *Anesthesiology*, 124(2), 270–300.
18. Amin SM, Amr, Y.M., Fathy, S.M., Alzeftawy, A.E. (2011). Maternal and neonatal effects of nalbuphine given immediately before induction of general anesthesia for elective cesarean section. *Saudi Journal of Anesthesia*, 5(4), 371–5.
19. Anderson, D. (2014). Pudendal nerve block for vaginal birth. *Journal of Midwifery and Womens Health*, 59(6), 651-9.
20. Antonucci, R., et al. (2012). Use of NSAIDs in pregnancy: impact on the fetus and newborn. *Current Drug Metabolism*, 13(4), 474–90.
21. Babenco, H.D., Conard, P.F., Gross, J.B.. (2000). The pharmacodynamic effect of a remifentanil bolus on ventilatory control. *Anesthesiology*, 92, 393–8.
22. Bach, V., et al. (1989). A randomized comparison between midazolam and thiopental for elective cesarean section anesthesia. *Anesthesia Analgesia*, 68(3), 234–7.
23. Bakker, J.J., et al. (2013). Internal vs external tocodynamometry during induced or augmented labour. *Cochrane Database of Systematic Reviews*.
24. Barragan Loayza, I.M., Solà, I., Juandó Prats, C. (2011). Biofeedback for pain management during labor. *Cochrane Database Systematic Review*.
25. Barton, J.R., Sibai, B.M. (2004). Diagnosis and management of hemolysis, elevated liver enzymes & low platelets syndrome. *Clinical Pernatology*, 31(4), 807-33.
26. Bates, S.M., et al. (2018). ASH 2018 guidelines for management of VTE in the context of pregnancy. *Blood Advances*, 2(22), 3317–59.
27. Bradley, R.A., Hathaway, M., Hathaway, J. (1965). *Husband- Coached Childbirth*. New York: Harper & Row.
28. Cantwell, R., et al. (2011). Saving mothers lives: reviewing maternal deaths to make motherhood safer. *British Journal of Obstetrics and Gynecology*, 118 (Suppl 1), 1–203.
29. Cefalo, R.C., Bowes, W.A. (1998). Managing labor: never walk alone. *New England Journal of Medicine*, 117–8.
30. Chandraharan, E. (2014). Fetal scalp blood sampling during labour: is it a useful diagnostic test or a historical test that no longer has a place in modern clinical obstetrics. *British Journal of Obstetrics and Gynecology*, 121(9), 1056–62.

31. Chen, L.K., et al. (2006). The effects of continuous epidural analgesia on doppler velocimetry of uterine arteries during different periods of labour analgesia. *British Journal of Anesthesia*, 96(2), 226–30.
32. Chestnut, D.H. (2019). *Chestnuts Obstetric Anesthesia: Principles and Practice*. 6th ed. Philadelphia: Elsevier Saunders.
33. Cicinelli, E., Einer-Jensen, N., Galantino, P., Alfonso, R., Nicoletti, R. (2004). The vascular cast of the human uterus: from anatomy to physiology. *Annals of New York Academy of Science*, 19–26.
34. Clark, K., Lam, L.T., Gibson, S., Currow, D. (2009). The effect of ranitidine versus proton pump inhibitors on gastric secretions: a meta-analysis of RCTs. *Anesthesia*, 64(6), 652–7.
35. Clark, R.B. (1983). Systemic modification during labor and delivery. *Obstetrics and Gynecology*, 165–97.
36. Clark, S.L., et al. (2016). Proposed diagnostic criteria for the case definition of amniotic fluid embolism in research studies. *American Journal of Obstetrics and Gynecology*, 215(4), 408–12.
37. Committee on Practice Bulletins-Obstetrics. (2017). Practice bulletin no. 183: postpartum hemorrhage. *Obstetrics and Gynecology*,;130(4):e168–e186.
38. Committee on Practice Bulletins—Obstetrics. (2017). Practise bulletin 177: obstetric analgesia and anesthesia. *Obstetrics and Gynecology*, 129(4), e73–e89.
39. Conron, R.W. Abbruzzi, K., Cochrane, S.O., Sarno, A.J., Cochrane, P.J. (1999). Laparoscopic procedures in pregnancy. *The American Surgeon*, 65(3), 259–63.
40. Cresswell, J.A., Ronsmans, C., Calvert, C., Filippi, V. (2013). Prevalence of placenta previa by world region: a systematic review and meta-analysis. *Tropical Medicine and International Health*, 18(6), 712–24.
41. Cyna, A.M., McAuliffe, G.L., Andrew, M.I. (2004). Hypnosis for pain relief in labour and childbirth: a systematic review. *British Journal of Anesthesia*, 93(4), 505–11.
42. DC Dutta, Konar, H. (2015). *DC Duttas Textbook of Obstetrics*. 8th ed. Kolkata: Jaypee Brothers Medical Publishers (P) Ltd.
43. De-Giorgio, F., Grassi, V.M., Vetrugno, G., d'Aloja, E., Pascali, V.L., Arena, V. (2012). Supine hypotensive syndrome as the probable cause of both maternal and fetal death. *Journal of Forensic Sciences*, 57(6), 1646–9.
44. De Buck F., Deprest J., Van de Velde M. (2008). Anesthesia for fetal surgery. *Current Opinion in Anesthesiology*, 21(3), 293–7.
45. Ditisheim, A., Sibai, B.M. (2017). Diagnosis and management of HELLP syndrome complicated by liver hematoma. *Clinical Obstetrics and Gynecology*, 60(1), 190–7.
46. Dodd, J.M., Crowther, C.A., Antoniou, G., Baghurst, P., Robinson, J.S. (2007). Screening of GDM: the effect of varying blood glucose definitions in the prediction of adverse maternal and infant health outcomes. *Australian and New Zealand Journal of Obstetrics and Gynecology*, 47(4), 307–12.
47. Dowswell, T., Bedwell, C., Lavender, T., Neilson, J.P. (2009). Transcutaneous electrical nerve stimulation (TENS) for pain relief in labour. *Cochrane Database Systematic Reviews*.
48. Duley, L., Gulmezoglu, A.M. (2010). Magnesium sulphate versus lytic cocktail for eclampsia. *Cochrane Database of Systematic Reviews*.
49. European Society of Gynecology. (2011). ESC guidelines for the management of cardiovascular diseases during pregnancy: the task force on the management of cardiovascular diseases during pregnancy of the ESC. *European Heart Journal*, 32(24), 3147–97.
50. Fang, C., Richards, A., Liszewski, M., Kavanagh, D., Atkinson, J.P. (2008). Advances in understanding of pathogenesis of aHUS and HELLP. *British Journal of Hematology*, 143(3), 336–48.
51. Foley, M.R., Strong, T., Graite, T. (2018). *Obstetric Intensive Care Manual*. 5th ed. Arizona: McGraw-Hill Education.
52. Fonseca, J.E., Méndez, F., Cataño, C., Arias, F. (2005). Dexamethasone treatment does not improve outcome in women with HELLP syndrome: a double blind placebo controlled RCT. *American Journal of Obstetrics and Gynecology*, 193(5), 1587–90.
53. Gad, C. (1967). Paracervical block. *Acta Obstetricia et Gynecologica Scandinavica*, 7–18.
54. Gandhi, A., Malhotra, N., Malhotra, J., Gupta, N., Bora, N. (2016). *Principles of Critical Care in Obstetrics*. 1st ed. Agra: Springer India.
55. George, L.M., Gatt, S.P., Lowe, S. (1997). Peripartum cardiomyopathy: four case histories and a commentary on anesthetic management. *Anesthesia and Intensive Care*, 25(3), 292–6.
56. Gibbs, C.P., Krischer, J., Peckham, B.M., Sharp, H., Kirschbaum, T.H. (1986). Obstetric anesthesia: a national survey. *Anesthesiology*, 65(3), 298–306.
57. Gist, R.S., Stafford, I.P., Leibowitz, A.B., Beilin, Y. (2009). Amniotic fluid embolism. *Anesthesia Analgesia*, 1808(5), 1599–602.
58. Gleicher, N. (2007). Why much of the pathophysiology of preeclampsia- eclampsia must be of autoimmune nature. *American Journal of Obstetrics and Gynecology*, 196(1), 5.e1–7.
59. Goldszmidt, E. (2008). Principles and practices of obstetric airway management. *Anesthesiology Cllinics*, 26(1), 109–25.
60. Greer, I.A., Nelson-Piercy, C. (2005). LMWH for thromboprophylaxis and treatment of VTE in pregnancy: a systematic review of safety and efficacy. *Blood*, 106(2), 401–7.
61. Guyatt, G.H., et al. (2012). Executive summary: antithrombotic therapy and prevention of thrombosis, ACCP evidence based clinical practise guidelines. *Chest*, 141(2 Suppl), S7–S47.
62. Gyte, G.M., Richens, Y. (2006). Routine prophylactic drugs in normal labour for reducing gastric aspiration and its effects. *Cochrane Database of Systematic Reviews*.
63. Haas, D.M., Imperiale, T.F., Kirkpatrick. P.R., Klein, R.W., Zollinger, T.W., Golichowski, A.M. (2009). Tocolytic therapy: a meta analysis and decision analysis. *Obstetrics and Gynecology*, 113(3), 585–94.
64. Hall, J.E. (2016). *Guyton and Hall Textbook of Medical Physiology*. 13th ed. Philadelphia: Elsevier.

65. Harms, K., Rath, W., Herting, E., Kuhn, W. (1995). Maternal hemolysis, elevated liver enzymes, low platelet count and neonatal outcome. *American Journal of Perinatology*, 12(1), 1–6.
66. Hedderson, M.M., Gunderson, E.P., Ferrara, A. (2010). Gestational weight gain and risk of gestational diabetes mellitus. *Obstetrics and Gynecology*, 115(3), 597–604.
67. Hemmings, H.C. Jr, Egan, T. (2013). *Pharmacology and physiology for anesthesia: foundations and clinical application*. Philadelphia: Elsevier Saunders.
68. Hibbard, J.U., Lindheimer, M., Lang, R.M. (1999). A modified definition of PPCM and prognosis based on echocardiography. *Obstetrics and Gynecology*, 94(2), 311–6.
69. Hoefnagel, A., Yu, A., Kaminski, A. (2016). Anesthetic complications in pregnancy. *Critical Care Clinics*, 32(1), 1–28.
70. Horlocker, T.T., Vandermeulen, E., Kopp, S.L., Gogarten, W., Leffert, L.R., Benzon, H.T. (2010). Regional anesthesia in the patient receiving antithrombotic or thrombolytic therapy: American Society of Regional Anesthesia and Pain Medicine evidence-based guidelines. *Regional Anesthesia and Pain Medicine*, 43(3), 64–101.
71. Hughey, M.J., McElin, T.W., Young, T. (1978). Maternal and fetal outcome of Lamaze prepared patients. *Obstetrics Gynecology*, 51(6), 643–7.
72. Jauniaux, E., Bunce, C., Grønbeck, L., Langhoff-Roos, J. (2019). Prevalence and main outcomes of placenta accreta spectrum: a systematic review and meta-analysis. *American Journal of Obstetrics and Gynecology*, 221(3): 208–18.
73. Keskin, H.L., Keskin, A.E., Avsar, A.F., Tabuk, M., Caglar, G.S. (2003). Pethidine versus tramadol for pain relief during labor. *International Journal of Gynaecology and Obstetrics*, 82(1), 11–6.
74. Kinesella, S.M. (2003). Lateral tilt for pregnant women: why 15 degrees? *Anesthesia*, 58(9), 835–7.
75. Kinsella, S.M., Lohmann, G. (1994). Supine hypotensive syndrome. *Obstetrics and Gynecology*, 83(5 Pt 1), 774–88.
76. Knight, M., et al. (2010). Incidence and risk factors for amniotic fluid embolism. *Obstetrics and Gynecology*, 115(5), 910–7.
77. Knight, M., et al. (2012). Amniotic fluid embolism incidence, risk factors and outcomes: a review and recommendations. *BMC Pregnancy and Childbirth*, 1–7.
78. Kodali, B.S., Bharadwaj, S. (2018). Fetal surgery: anesthetic implications and strategic management. *Indian Journal of Anesthesia*, 62(9), 717–23.
79. Labor, S. Maguire, S. (2008). The pain of labour. *Reviews in Pain*, 2(2), 15–9.
80. Lachmeijer, A.M., Dekker, G.A., Pals, G., Aarnoudse, J.G., ten Kate, G.P., Arngrímsson, R. (2002). Searching for preeclampsia genes: the current position. *European Journal of Obstetrics Gynecology and Reproductive Biology*, 105(2):94–113.
81. Landon, M.B. (1992). Diabetes mellitus and pregnancy. *Obstetrics Gynecology Clinics of North America*, 633–54.
82. Macones, G.A., Hankins, G.D., Spong, C.Y., Hauth, J., Moore, T. (2008). The 2008 National Institute of Child Health and Human Development workshop report on electronic fetal monitoring update on definitions, interpretation, and research guidelines. *Obstetrics and Gynecology*, 112(3), 661–6.
83. Madden, K., Middleton, P., Cyna, A.M., Matthewson, M., Jones, L. (2016). Hypnosis for pain management during labor and childbirth. *Cochrane Database Systematic Review*.
84. Marik, P.E. (2011). Pulmonary aspiration syndromes. *Current Opinion in Pulmonary Medicine*, 17(3), 148–54.
85. Marin, J.J., Briz, O., Serrano, M.A. (2004). A review on the molecular mechanisms involved in the placental barrier for drugs. *Current Drug Delivery*, 1(3), 275–89.
86. Marra, A., Vargas, M., Striano, P., Del Guercio, L., Buonanno, P., Servillo, G. (2014). Posterior reversible encephalopathy syndrome: the endothelial hypotheses. *Medical Hypotheses*, 82(5), 619–22.
87. Martin, J.N., Magann, E.F. (1996). HELLP syndrome current principles and recommended practice. *Current Obstetric Medicine*, 129–75.
88. Martin JN Jr, Rose, C.H., Briery, C.M. (2006). Understanding and managing HELLP syndrome: the integral role of aggressive glucocorticoids for mother and child. *American Journal of Obstetrics and Gynecology*, 195(4), 914–34.
89. May, A., Elton, C.D. (1998). The effects of pain and its management on mother and fetus. *Baillieres Clinical Obstetrics and Gynecology*, 12(3), 423–41.
90. Metzfer, B.E., et al. (2012). Hyperglycemia and adverse pregnancy outcomes (HAPO). *Diabetes Care*, 358(19), 574–80.
91. Miyakoshi, K., et al. (2013). Perinatal outcomes: intravenous patient controlled fentanyl versus no analgesia in labor. *Journal of Obstetrics and Gynaecology Research*, 39(4), 783–9.
92. Morrison, C.E., Dutton, D., Howie, H., Gilmour, H. (1987). Pethidine compared with meperidine during labour. *Anesthesia*, 42(1), 7–14.
93. Murali, S., Baldisseri, M.R. (2005). Peripartum cardiomyopathy. Critical Care Medicine, 33(10 Suppl), s340–s346.
94. Myers, L.B., Cohen D, Galinkin, J., Gaiser, R., Kurth, C.D. (2002). Anesthesia for fetal surgery. *Pediatric Anesthesia*, 12(7), 569–78.
95. Nair, A., Bharuka, A., Rayani, B.K. (2018). The reliability of surgical APGAR score in predicting immediate and late postoperative morbidity and mortality: a narrative review. *Rambam Maimonides Medical Journal*, 9(1), 1–4.
96. NICE (UK). (2014). Intrapartum care for healthy women and babies. *NICE guidelines*.
97. Nonnenmacher, A., Hopp, H., Dudenhausen, J. (2010). Predictive value of pulse oximetry for the development of fetal acidosis. *Journal of Perinatal Medicine*, 38(1), 83-6.
98. Novikova, N., Cluver, C. (2012). Local anesthetic nerve block for pain management in labor. *Cochrane Database Systematic Reviews*.
99. Osol, G., Mandala, M. (2009). Maternal uterine vascular remodelling during pregnancy. *Physiology*, 58-71.
100. O'Rourke, N., Kodali, B.S. (2006). Laparoscopic surgery during pregnancy. *Current Opinion in Anesthesiology*, 19(3), 254–9.
101. Pacifici GM, Nottoli, R. (1995). Placental transfer of drugs administered to the mother. *Clinical Pharmacokinetics*, 28(3), 235–69.
102. Palmer, C.M. (2010). Continuous spinal anesthesia and analgesia in obstetrics. *Anesthesia Analgesia*, 111(6), 1476–9.
103. Papile, L.A., P. (2001). The APGAR score in the 21st century. *New England Journal of Medicine*, 344(7), 519–20.

104. Pearl, J.P., Price, R.R., Tonkin, A.E., Richardson, W.S., Stefanidis, D. (2017). SAGES guidelines for the use of laparoscopy during pregnancy. *Surgical Endoscopy*, 31(10), 3767–82.
105. Pearson, G.D., et al. (2000). Peripartum cardiomyopathy. *Journal of American Medical Association*, 283(9), 1183–8.
106. Pijnenborg, R., Vercruysse, L., Hanssens, M. (2006). The uterine spiral arteries in human pregnancy: facts and controversies. *Placenta*, 27(9-10,)939–58.
107. Preston, R. (2010). Walking epidurals for labour analgesia: do they benefit anyone? *Canadian Journal of Anesthesia*, 103–6.
108. Ramachandran, R., Rewari V, Trikha A. (2011). Anesthetic management of patients with peripartum cardiomyopathy. *Journal of Obstetric Anesthesia and Critical Care*, 5–12.
109. Redman, C.W., Sargent, I.L. (2005). Latest advances in understanding preeclampsia. *Science*. 308(5728):1592–4.
110. Renner, R.M., Edelman, A.B., Nichols, M.D., Jensen, J.T., Lim, J.Y., Bednarek, P.H. (2016). Refining paracervical block techniques for pain control in first trimester surgical abortion: a randomized controlled non-inferiority trial. *Contraception*, 94(5), 461–6.
111. Rüdiger, M., et al. (2012). Newborn assessment in the delivery room. *Neoreviews*.
112. Salmon, J.E., et al. (2011). Mutations in complement regulatory proteins predispose to preeclampsia: a genetic analysis of the PROMISSE cohort. *PLOS Medicine*. 8(3), e1001013.
113. Saloheimo, A.M. (1968). Paracervical block anesthesia in labor. *Acta Obstetricia et Gynecologica Scandinavica*, 47(5), 1–21.
114. Schierup, L., Schmidt, J.F., Jensen, A.T., Rye, B.A. (1988). Pudendal block in vaginal deliveries: mepivacaine with and without epinephrine. *Acta Obstetricia et Gynecologica Scandinavica*, 195–7.
115. Schnider, S.M., Levinson, G., Rosen, M.A. (2013). *Schnider and Levinsons Anesthesia for Obstetrics*. 5th ed. Baltimore: Lippincott Williams & Wilkins.
116. Sen, G., et al. (2002). Laparoscopic cholecystectomy in third trimester of pregnancy. *Journal of Obstetrics and Gynecology*.
117. Shah, A.K., Rajamani, K., Whitty, J.E. (2008). Eclampsia: a neurological perspective. *Journal of Neurological Sciences*, 271(1-2), 158–67.
118. Sheiner, E., Sarid, L., Levy, A., Seidman, D.S., Hallak, M. (2005). Obstetric risk factors and outcome of pregnancies complicated with early postpartum hemorrhage: a population based study. *Journal of Maternal and Fetal Neonatal Medicine*, 18(3):149–54.
119. Simhan, H.N., Caritis, S.N. (2007). Prevention of preterm delivery. *New England Journal of Medicine*, 357(5), 477–87.
120. Simkin, P.P., O'Hara, M. (2002). Nonpharmacological relief of pain during labor: systematic reviews of five methods. *American Journal of Obstetrics and Gynecology*, 186(5), S131–159.
121. Simons, S.H., Tibboel, D. (2006). Pain perception development and maturation. *Seminars in Fetal and Neonatal Medicine*, 11(4), 227–31.
122. Singh, S., Behera, A. (2010). Eclampsia in Eastern India: incidence, demographic profile and response to 3 different anticonvulsant regimens of magnesium sulphate. *The Internet Journal of Gynecology and Obstetrics*, 15(2), 1–7.
123. Skupski, D.W., Rosenberg, C.R., Eglinton, G.S. (2002). Intrapartum fetal stimulation tests: a meta-analysis. *Obstetrics and Gynecology*, 99(1), 129–34.
124. Sliwa, K., et al. (2017). Clinical characteristics of patients from the worldwide registry on PPCM. *European Journal of Heart Failure, 19(9)*, 1131–41.
125. Smith, C.A., Collins, C.T., Crowther, C.A., Levett, K.M. (2011). Acupuncture or acupressure for pain management in labor. *Cochrane Database Systematic Reviews*.
126. Stepp, K., Falcon, T. (2004). Laparoscopy in the second trimester of pregnancy. *Obstetrics and Gynecology Clinics of North America*, 485–96.
127. Toyoda, K. (2013). Antithrombotic therapy for pregnant women. *Neurologia Medico Chirurgica*, 53(8), 526–30.
128. Tukur, J. (2009). The use of magnesium sulphate for the treatment of severe pre-eclampsia and eclampsia. *Annals of African Medicine*, 8(2), 76–80.
129. Ullman, R., Dowswell, T., Smith, L., Burns, E. (2010). Parenteral opioids for maternal pain relief in labour. *Cochrane Database Systematic Review*.
130. Upadhyay, A., Stanten, S., Kazantsev, G., Horoupian, R., Stanten, A. (2007). Laparoscopic management of a non-obstetric emergency in the third trimester of pregnancy. *Surgical Endoscopy*, 21(8), 1344–48.
131. Van de Velde, M., De Buck, F. (2012). Fetal and maternal analgesia/anesthesia for fetal procedures. *Fetal Diagnosis and Therapy*, 201–9.
132. Vayssiere, C., Haberstich, R., Sebahoun, V., David, E., Roth, E., Langer, B. (2007). Fetal ECG ST-segment analysis and prediction of neonatal acidosis. *International Journal of Gynecology and Obstetrics*, 97(2), 110–4.
133. Vogel. J.P., Nardin, J.M., Dowswell, T., West, H.M., Oladapo, O.T. (2014). Combination of tocolytic agents for inhibiting preterm labour. *Cochrane Database Systematic Reviews*.
134. Vohra, A., Kumar, S., Charlton, A.J., Olukoga, A.O., Boulton, A.J., McLeod, D. (1993). Effect of diabetes mellitus on the cardiovascular responses to induction of anesthesia and tracheal intubation. *British Journal of Anesthesia*, 71(2), 258–61.
135. WOMAN Trial Collaborators. (2017). Effect of early tranexamic acid administration on mortality, hysterectomy and other morbidities in women with PPH (WOMAN): an international randomized double blind placebo-controlled trial. *Lancet*, 389(10084), 2105–16.
136. Wong, C.A., McCarthy, R.J., Fitzgerald, P.C., Raikoff, K., Avram, M.J. (2007). Gastric emptying in obese pregnant women at term. *Anesthesia Analgesia*, 105(3), 751–5.
137. Wright, W.L. (2017). Neurological complications in critically ill pregnant patients. *Handbook of Clinical Neurology*, 657–74.
138. Yentis, S., Malhotra, S. (2013). *Analgesia, Anaesthesia and Pregnancy*. 3rd ed. New York: Cambridge University Press.
139. Zador, G., Lindmark, G., Nilsson, B.A. (1974). Pudendal block in normal vaginal deliveries. clinical efficacy, lidocaine concentrations in maternal and fetal blood, fetal and maternal acid-base values and influence on uterine activity. *Acta Obstetricia et Gynecologica Scandinavica*, 51–64.
140. Zera, C.A., Seely, E.W., Wilkins-Haug, L.E., Lim, K., Parry, S.T., McElrath, T.F. (2014). The association of BMI with serum angiogenic markers in normal & abnormal pregnancies. *American Journal of Obstetrics andGynecology*, 221(3), e1–e7.

12 CHAPTER

Miscellaneous Topics

AMERICAN SOCIETY OF ANESTHESIOLOGISTS FUNCTIONAL STATUS CLASSIFICATION

Introduction

- American Society of Anesthesiologists (ASA) classification is a system designed for assessing fitness of patients before surgery
- Originally consisted of six categories which described the physical status of the patient
- This was revised in 1961 ***by Dripps*** to 5 classes

Classification

- Category I:
  - Healthy patient
  - No comorbidities
  - Mortality 0.05%
- Category II:
  - Mild systemic disease with no functional limitation
  - Examples: Bronchial asthma or well controlled hypertension
  - Mortality 0.4%
- Category III:
  - Severe systemic disease with functional limitation
  - Examples: Chronic renal failure on dialysis, class II CCF
  - Mortality 4.5%
- Category IV:
  - Severe systemic disease which constantly threatens survival
  - Examples: Acute MI, respiratory failure requiring mechanical ventilation
  - Mortality 25%
- Category V:
  - Moribund disease
  - Not expected to survive more than 24 hours with or without surgery
  - Mortality 50%
- Category VI:
  - Currently it has been removed
  - Declared brain dead patient whose organs are being removed for donor purposes
- Category E:
  - Additional code for emergency surgery
  - Called as emergency if delay in treatment would significantly increase threat to patients life or body part

Uses

- Used to indicate patient's overall physical health/ sickness preoperatively
- Regarded by lawyers and hospitals as a scale to predict risk and decide if a patient should have had an operation
- Used to predict operative risk, planning anesthetic management and monitoring technique
- As the ASA grade increases, mortality risk also rises

Trial of Ratings Modification

- Class Ia: Normal healthy individual
- Class Ib:
  - Mild systemic disease or,
  - Healthy individual with operative or anesthetic risk
- Class IIa:
  - Moderate systemic disease or,
  - Mild systemic disease with anesthetic/operative risk
- Class IIb:
  - Moderate-severe systemic disease with no functional impairment
  - Moderate systemic disease with operative/ anesthetic risk
- Class III: Severe systemic disease with functional limitation
- Class IV: Severe systemic disease which constantly threatens survival
- Class V: Moribund disease, not expected to survive more than 24 hours with or without surgery

Limitations

- Subjective score:
  - Physical status classification is a rating conferred by the practitioner
  - So individual variation existed i.e. it was subjective score rather than objective
- There exists no class for diseases which are moderate (only mild and severe are mentioned)
- Class of a patient suffering simultaneously from more than two diseases is not clear
- The word systemic creates a lot of confusion as:
  - MI, although grave, is a local disease with poor postsurgery survival rates
  - However it does not fit in any category of ASA classification, being a local disease
- The classification assumes that age has no relation to physical fitness which is not true as neonates and elderly even in the absence of any systemic disease tolerate similar anesthetics poorly compared to young adults
- Classification ignores malignancy entirely
- Does not consider age, sex, pregnancy status, operative/difficult airway risk

Other Health Grading Systems

- *APACHE II score, Goldman index*
- *APGAR score, Malinas score*
- *Barnes akathisia score*
- *Blantyre Coma Scale*
- *Glasgow Coma Scale*

DRUG ERRORS IN ANESTHESIA

Introduction

Leading cause of morbidity and mortality in hospitalized patients.

Types

- Omission—drug not given
- Repetition—extra dose
- Substitution—incorrect drug/drug swap
- Insertion—unintended drug use
- Incorrect dose—wrong dose
- Incorrect route—wrong route of administration

Risk Factors

- Inadequate experience
- Inadequate familiarity with equipment
- Carelessness, haste
- Lack of staff
- Odd working hours
- Fatigue
- Poor communication
- Failure to perform routine check
- Inadequate familiarity with surgery
- Teaching activity underway

Mechanisms

- Slips: Due to attention failures
- Lapses: Due to memory failure
- Rule based errors: Lack of expertise
- Fixation errors: Misapplication of knowledge due to fixed ideas
- Violation: Deliberate deviation from standard instructions

Drugs Involved

- Induction agents:
  - Ketamine
  - Thiopentone
- Muscle relaxants
- Narcotics
- Anticholinergics
- Local anesthetics

Error Reduction in OT: APSF Recommendations

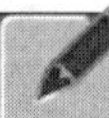

- Color coding
- Drug labels
- Checking labels with second observer
- Double checking before labeling syringe and before administration of drug
- Pre filled syringes
- Bar codes with audible readers on syringes
- Smart pumps
- Preparation of IV medication in pharmacy rather than at point of care
- Standardization of preparation procedures
- Standardization of preparation syringes
- Standardization of infusion concentrations and units
- Standardization of drug workspace layout
- Radiofrequency identification (RFID)
- Computerized order entry (CPOE)
- Avoid storing hazardous concentrated solutions like KCl in syringes

Error Reduction in ICU

- Reduce physician work hours
- Computerized devices
- Computerized physician order entry

ASTM Label Standards

1.	Induction agents	Yellow
2.	Tranquilizers	Orange
3.	Relaxants	Fluorescent red
4.	Narcotics	Blue
5.	Relaxant antagonists	Fluorescent red/white stripes
6.	Narcotic antagonists	Blue/white stripes
7.	Anticholinergics	Green
8.	Local anesthetics	Gray
9.	Hypotensive agents	Violet/white stripes
10.	Vasopressors	Violet
11.	Narcotic/tranquilizer combination	Blue/salmon
12.	Major tranquilizers	Salmon

EVIDENCE BASED MEDICINE

Introduction

Optimal integration of the best research evidence with clinical expertise and patient preferences to aid in clinical decision making.

Advantages

- ❖ Minimizes errors in patient care
- ❖ Reduces cost of treatment
- ❖ Optimizes quality of patient care
- ❖ Clinicians updated on latest developments

Disadvantages

- ❖ RCTS do not guarantee absence of publication bias-more likelihood of positive trials being published than negative trials
- ❖ Difficult to practice clinically
- ❖ Suppresses clinical freedom
- ❖ Not useful in many clinical situations

Grading Systems

- ❖ Hierarchy of study types
- ❖ SIGN methodology
- ❖ GRADE methodology.

Hierarchy of Study Types

- ❖ Systematic reviews and meta-analyses of randomized controlled trials (RCTs)
- ❖ Randomized controlled trials
- ❖ Nonrandomized intervention studies—case control studies
- ❖ Observational studies—case series/reports
- ❖ Nonexperimental studies
- ❖ Expert opinion, pathophysiological inference

Grade Methodology

- ❖ Quality of evidence: Extent to which one can be confident that an estimate of effect is correct
- ❖ Strength of recommendation: Extent to which one can be confident that adherence to the recommendation will do more good than harm

Strength of Recommendations

Factors Affecting Strength of Recommendations

- ❖ Quality of evidence
- ❖ Specificity: Should be specific to patient groups
- ❖ Trade offs: Involves compromises between benefits and risks

No.	Class	Benefit	Recommendation
1.	I	Benefit >>> Risk	General consensus—treatment is useful
			Procedure should be performed
2.	IIa	Benefit >> Risk	Weight of evidence favoring usefulness
			Additional studies with focused objectives needed
			Reasonable to administer treatment
3.	IIb	Benefit ≥ Risk	Usefulness less well established by evidence
			Additional studies with broad objective required
			Treatment may be considered
4.	III	Risk ≥ Benefit	Evidence exists that treatment not useful/may be harmful
			No additional studies required
			Procedure/Treatment should not be performed

Levels of Evidence

Factors Affecting Levels of Evidence

- ❖ Study design: Should minimize bias
- ❖ Study quality: Should use appropriate randomization blinding methods
- ❖ Consistency: Indicates similarity of effect in different studies
- ❖ Directness: Extent to which patients and interventions are similar to those of population of interest

LOE	Description
A (High)	Multiple (3–5) population risk strata evaluated
	Sufficient evidence from multiple RCTS/meta analyses
	General consistency of direction and magnitude of effect
B (Low)	Limited (2–3) population risk strata evaluated
	Limited evidence from single RCT/nonrandomized studies
C (V Low)	Very limited population risk strata evaluated
	Only expert opinion/case studies

Clinical Use

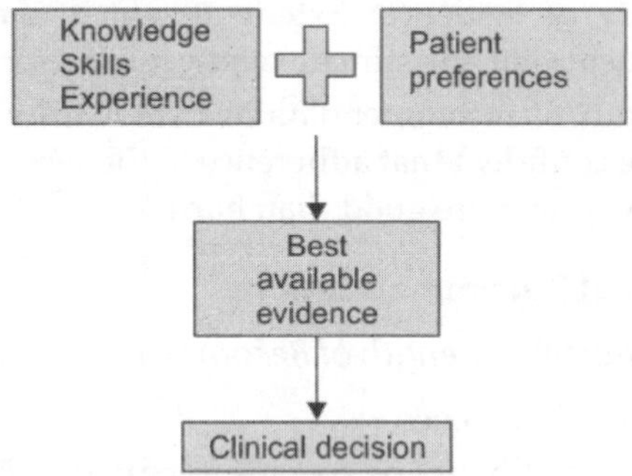

HYPERBARIC OXYGEN THERAPY

Introduction

Refers to administration of oxygen at higher than atmospheric pressure.

Indications: ***Undersea and Hyperbaric Medical Society*** guidelines:

- Global hypoxia:
  - Carbon monoxide poisoning
  - Cyanide poisoning
  - Severe anemia
  - During therapeutic lung lavage
- Regional hypoxia:
  - Crush/thermal injuries
  - Non healing wounds/ulcers
  - ***Meleneys*** ulcer
  - Acute peripheral vascular insufficiency
  - Compromised surgical graft
  - Flap osteonecrosis
  - ***Osteoradionecrosis***
  - Radiation cystitis
- Infections:
  - ***Gas gangrene***/clostridial myonecrosis
  - Necrotizing fasciitis
  - ***Fournier's*** gangrene
  - Refractory osteomyelitis
  - Mucormycosis
- Gas lesions:
  - Gas embolism
  - Decompression sickness/***Caissons*** disease
- Others:
  - Septic shock
  - ARDS
  - Plastic surgery
  - Cancer therapy
  - Congenital cardiac anomalies
  - Disseminated sclerosis
  - Acute cerebral edema

Physiological Effects of Hyperbarism

- Trapped air pockets:
  - Contract on compression and expand on decompression
  - Middle ear, paranasal sinuses, intestinal gas, pneumothorax have air pockets
- Altered temperature:
  - Increased heat production and increased chamber temperature during compression
  - Cooling and reduced chamber temperature during decompression
- Elevation of absolute pressure:
  - Causes ***High Pressure Nervous Syndrome***
- Elevated partial pressure of oxygen (PaO_2):
  - Raised PaO_2
  - Raised blood oxygen content
  - Vasoconstriction
  - Antibacterial action especially against anaerobes
- Elevated inert gas pressure:
  - Elevated nitrogen pressure
  - Associated with narcosis—nitrogen narcosis
  - Causes euphoria, memory loss, unconsciousness
- Reversal of anesthesia:
  - Both intravenous and inhalational anesthetics reversed
  - Insignificant at clinically used pressures

Mechanism of Action

I. In global hypoxia:
  - Competes with CO molecules for Hb and eliminates CO
  - Increases dissolved oxygen in plasma
  - Shifts oxygen dissociation curve to right

II. In regional hypoxia:
  - Increases oxygen gradient at tissue level by increasing PaO_2
  - Increases oxygen delivery to tissues
  - Stimulates angiogenesis due to improved fibroblast function

III. Infections:
  - Inhibits clostridial alpha toxins
  - Improves osteoclast function
  - Leukocyte oxidative killing when O_2 tension > 130 mm Hg
  - Inhibits growth of microorganism:
    - *Clostridium* welchii
    - *Clostridium tetani*
    - *Staphylococcus aureus*
    - *Pseudomonas* pyocyanea

IV. Gas lesions:
- Reduces volume of embolus
- Increases arterial hydrostatic pressure
- Improves oxygen delivery to tissues downstream of emboli
- Maximizes gradient for removal of gas from emboli

V. Others:
- Increases sensitivity of cells to radiotherapy
- Improves collateral flow in grafts—reduces area of ischemia

Rationale

❖ Increases PIO_2 and thus improves PAO_2
❖ Increases oxygen carried in plasma
❖ O_2 dissolved in plasma at 3 atm pressure is 6 mL/100 mL blood (0.3 mL/100 mL blood at 1 atm pressure)
❖ Tissues oxygenated even if blood flow reduced by half
❖ DO_2 can be increased without using O_2 bound to Hb
❖ Tissues can survive anoxia for longer time

Methods of Administration

❖ Single person chamber:
- Made of transparent acrylic
- Only patient is subject to compression
- Staff remains outside

❖ Multiperson chamber:
- Made of steel/aluminium
- Can be used for surgery
- Staff breathes compressed air
- Patient breathes 100% O_2 at pressure from mask/ETT
- Used for critically ill patients

Technique

❖ For decompression sickness:
- 2.8 atm followed by slow decompression to 1.9 atm
- Periods of oxygen breathing interspersed with 5–15 minutes periods of breathing room air
- Technique reduces oxygen toxicity

Limitations

❖ Contraindicated if pulmonary blebs/bullae
❖ Factors limiting dose and duration of therapy:
- Oxygen toxicity
- Decompression sickness of accompanying staff
- Difficulty with monitoring
- Patient discomfort

Side Effects

❖ Decompression sickness:
- Gaseous emboli
- Rupture of tympanic membrane
- Can be reduced by reducing decompression rate
- Reduced by O_2 inhalation before decompression

❖ Oxygen toxicity:
- CNS—reduced cerebral blood flow, convulsions
- RS—pulmonary edema, CO_2 narcosis, absorption atelectasis
- Retrolental fibroplasia
- Testicular damage

❖ Barotrauma:
- Pneumothorax
- Pneumomediastinum
- Gas embolism

❖ Visual disturbances:
- High pressure myopia: Effect of high pressure on lens shape/refractory index
- Retrolental fibroplasia
- Cataract

❖ High pressure nervous syndrome:
- Nausea, vomiting, vertigo, tinnitus, paresthesia, anxiety
- Involuntary muscle movement
- Occurs at > 15–20 atm pressure

Anesthesia Under Hyperbaric Oxygen Therapy

Indications

❖ Carotid endarterectomy
❖ Therapeutic bronchoalveolar lavage
❖ Emergency surgery in a saturation dive
❖ Injured divers
❖ Open heart surgery
❖ Radiation therapy for cancer

Evaluation

❖ Ability to vent middle ear—eustachian tube patency on Valsalva maneuver
❖ Chest X-ray for blebs/bullae
❖ Visual acuity checks for hyperbaric myopia
❖ Anxiolytic therapy initiated if claustrophobic

Machines

❖ Standard machines used in chamber
❖ Cylinders and reducing valves function normally
❖ Gases piped from outside should be at higher pressure (>60 PSIG)

- Flow meters show high value due to increased gas density
- Flow meters calibrated to higher pressure levels
- Expired gases absorbed and vented outside

Monitors

- Most instruments left outside chamber
- View oscillometric measurements through glass port in chamber
  - Blood pressure:
    - Ordinary/fluid filled BP cuffs
    - Finger plethysmography/intra-arterial catheter
    - Aneroid manometer preferred to mercury manometer
  - ECG and EEG:
    - Standard equipment
    - Recording apparatus placed outside
  - Blood gas:
    - Machine placed in adjacent lab
    - Polarographic microelectrodes recommended
  - Respiratory function: With normal instruments

Technique of Anesthesia

- Regional anesthesia:
  - Safe and effective
  - Avoids need for mechanical ventilation
  - Extreme aseptic precautions as increased bacterial growth in warm and humid chamber
- General anesthesia: Less preferred

Inhaled Anesthetics

- Can pollute chamber
- Effect of volatile agents proportional to partial pressure of anesthetic and not alveolar concentration
- Effect of 1% halothane at 1 atm equivalent to 0.5% at 2 atm
- Prefer nonexplosive agents
- Standardized vaporizers used
- Recalibrate vaporizers within chamber

Nitrous Oxide

- May be used as sole anesthetic
- Induction rapid (<60s)
- Increased atm pressure allows MAC to be exceeded
- Induction with nitrous oxide associated with HTN, tachycardia, tachypnea
- Rapid emergence but severe postoperative nausea and vomiting (PONV)
- May cause embolism during decompression
- Dilutional hypoxia possible

Intravenous Anesthetics

- Behavior unaffected by pressure
- No pharmacokinetic alteration up to 6 atm pressure

Intravenous Fluids

- Air volume in drip chamber shrinks during compression and expands during decompression
- Exclude glass bottles to avoid risk of explosion during decompression
- Use plastic infusion bottles
- Infusion pumps to be capable of handling pressure differential

Tubes

- ETT cuff inflated with water to avoid volume changes during compression/decompression
- Intragastric tube left open
- Bladder catheters filled with saline
- Repressure pressure bags during compression and vent out during decompression
- PA balloon ports left open to chamber during compression and decompression

Ventilation

- Pressure controlled/volume controlled used
- Pressure controlled ventilation needs frequent adjustment of PC level
- Risk of fire hazard due to O_2 build up in ventilator case
- ETT cuff inflated in chamber and released before decompression

HIGH ALTITUDE

Introduction

No.	Level	Height
1.	Baseline	3,000 m above sea level
2.	Mild high altitude	3,000–3,600 m
3.	Moderate high altitude	4,200–4,800 m
4.	Extreme high altitude	>4,800 m

Pathophysiological Changes

I. *Central nervous system*

- Vasodilatation causing:
  - Raised ICP
  - Increased cerebral blood flow
  - Altered behavior
  - Drowsiness, incoordination
  - Lack of judgment
  - Sleep—speech disturbances
  - Unconsciousness, seizures

II. *Cardiovascular:*
- Tachycardia
- Hypertension
- Increased blood volume by 30%
- Increased erythropoiesis
- Hematocrit increases from 40 to 65%
- Local vasodilation due to tissue hypoxia
- Pulmonary HTN due to hypoxic pulmonary vasoconstriction

III. *Hypothermia*:
- Causes:
  - Arrhythmias
  - AV block
  - Hypotension
  - Negative inotropism

IV. *Respiratory system (RS)*:
- Reduced PIO_2
- Reduced ambient pressure
- Reduced gas density
- Increased diffusion capacity (normal 2.1 mL/mm Hg/min)
- Reduced oxygen gradient leading to ventilation perfusion mismatch
- Hypoxia induced hyperapnea: Leftward shift of ODC
- Pulmonary edema due to:
  - Increased hydrostatic pressure
  - Increased pulmonary vascular permeability
  - Coagulation defect
  - Increased oxygen free radicals
  - Increased autonomic activity causing neurogenic pulmonary edema

Anesthetic Considerations

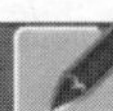

- Remote site:
  - Suboptimal equipment
  - Increased risk of infection and pollution—lack of properly built OT
  - Risk of fire hazard and explosion
- Risk of perioperative hypoxia—supplemental oxygen therapy very important
- Hypothermia common—maintain OT temperature between 21 and 24°C
- Warm intravenous fluids essential
- Judicious fluid doses to avoid pulmonary edema
- Increased bleeding tendency due to:
  - Raised venous pressure
  - Increased capillary density
  - Venodilation
  - Raised blood volume
  - Coagulopathies
- Increased risk of aspiration

Preoperative Preparation

- NPO 6 hours
- Informed consent
- Opioid/benzodiazepine premedication
- Antisialogogues—glycopyrrolate/atropine
- Antibiotic prophylaxis
- Antiaspiration prophylaxis
- DVT prophylaxis

Machine

- Boyles type F with Goldman vaporizer for halothane
- Spirometers used to calibrate flowmeters
- Flowmeters show low reading at high flows due to low gas density
- Hazardous if low flow anesthesia used with high nitrous oxide concentration
- Oxygen analyzers show false low reading unless calibrated
- Oxygen analyzer essential if low flow used
- Venturi devices deliver higher O_2 than at sea level
- Venturi mask delivering 35% at sea level delivers 41% at 10,000 feet
- Reduce fire hazard by:
  - Avoiding ether
  - Use battery operated lights in OT
  - Reduced overall fire risk as PIO_2 is low

Regional Anesthesia

- Increased incidence of bowel and bladder distension after subacromial bursal block (SAB)
- Increased incidence of postdural puncture headache due to:
  - Chronically increased CSF pressure
  - Dehydration
- Duration of action of local anesthetics shortened
- Prevent Phrenic N palsy during:
  - Interscalene block
  - Supraclavicular block
  - Stellate ganglion block

Induction

- All patients at risk of aspiration due to delayed gastric emptying
- Rapid sequence induction (RSI) preferred
- Thiopentone has slower onset due to prolonged brain arm circulation time at high altitude
- Propofol, etomidate, benzodiazepines safe

- Larger amounts of propofol required
- Ether induction slow and requires high concentration
- Gas volume in ETT cuff and PAC balloon expands
- Periodic checking of blood glucose levels as high altitude increases glucose consumption

Inhalational Agents

- Potency proportional to partial pressure and not percentage in mixture of O_2
- Nitrous oxide potency reduced as barometric pressure reduces
- Nitrous oxide to be given at 50% to be effective
- Fixed concentration of volatile anesthetics have reduced potency
- Halothane can be used:
  - Ideal for rapid induction and recovery
  - High potency
  - Non inflammable
  - Reduced incidence of laryngospasm
- Delivery of halothane increased at high altitude though partial pressure remains constant
- Isoflurane also suitable

Neuromuscular Blockade

- Succinylcholine safe for short duration surgery
- NDMR action prolonged in hypothermic patients
- Continue assisted ventilation till patient regains complete consciousness
- Complete reversal mandatory as patients are dependent on hyperventilation for oxygenation
- Maintain PaO_2 and $PaCO_2$ at baseline levels rather than normal values

Ventilation

- High oxygen concentration to be given due to:
  - Anesthetic deprived compensatory mechanisms
  - Reduced PIO_2 and PAO_2 at high altitude
  - Hypoxic brain damage at lower PaO_2
  - Reduced compensation for acidosis at high altitude
- Ventilation at high altitude dependant on hypoxic drive
- Administration of narcotics blunts hypoxic drive and precipitates hypoxia

Temperature

- Warm OT and warm IV fluids mandatory
- Warming blankets
- Humidified inspired gases
- Heated peritoneal/bladder/colonic lavage

Fluid Balance

- Challenging due to preexisting hypovolemia and hypoosmolarity
- Fluid bolus prior to induction in hypovolemic patients
- Avoid aggressive fluid challenges in patients at high risk *for High Altitude Pulmonary Edema*
- Titrate to maintain renal perfusion
- Clear IV lines of air bubbles as development of R to L shunts through *Patent Foramen Ovale* common in high altitude

Deep Vein Thrombosis

- Common due to:
  - Hypercoagulability
  - Polycythemia
- Increased risk of postoperative stroke/TIA/DVT

Dissociative Anesthesia

- Advantageous as:
  - Minimally suppresses ventilation
  - Reduces dose of opioids
- Ketamine 1–6 mg/kg total dose + atropine 20 µ/kg + midazolam 0.05 mg/kg for TIVA useful
- Useful if supplemental O_2 not available for use

ANESTHESIA IN SPACE

Physiological Changes in Space

- Cardiovascular changes:
  - Increase in LV end diastolic volume
  - Paradoxical reduction in CVP due to microgravity
  - Reduced LV mass due to cardiac atrophy/injury
  - Central redistribution of blood
  - Facial edema
  - Diuresis with plasma volume depletion (≥20%)
- Autonomic dysfunction:
  - Especially on return to earth
  - Occurs due to:
    - Cardiovascular deconditioning
    - Reduced intravascular volume
    - Increased NO expression
    - Downregulation of α-adrenergic receptors
    - Ventricular atrophy
    - Changes in arterial stiffness
- G forces:
  - Increase in gravitational forces during launch as space craft accelerates to orbital speed
  - Absence of gravitational stress (microgravity) during the period in space
- Neuromuscular changes: Skeletal muscle atrophy even after short missions

Technical Challenges

Airway

- Difficult intubation due to facial edema
- Both intubator and patient to be secured
- Intubator to stabilize head of patient by holding it between knees
- Use smaller size ETT if vocal cord edema is present
- LMA, intubating LMA, cuffed oropharyngeal airway used alternatively

Fluid Therapy

- Hypovolemia may not be adequately treatable due to reduced quantity of supplies
- Air fluid interface in IV fluids generate bubbles as fluids and gases do not separate on basis of differing densities due to lack of gravity
- Air bubbles do not rise up but remain mixed in solution
- IV bag to be degassed before flight/removed by in-line filteration as IV fluid bags contain fluids akin to foam

Neuromuscular Blockade

- Succinylcholine to be avoided as it may cause cardiovascular collapse
- Disuse and skeletal muscle atrophy due to immobilization causes proliferation of extra-junctional receptors causing hyperstimulation and cardiac arrest on SCH use
- Resistance to NDMR may occur

Subarachnoid block: Increased risk of cardiovascular collapse due to autonomic dysfunction

Vaporizers

- Devices which depend on gravity induced separation of fluids and gases malfunction
- This is because vaporizers require gravity to confine liquids to bottom of reservoir

Closed Environment

- Safe use of anesthetic gases difficult in space craft
- Drugs used in flight should not be capable of reaching crew through the closed cabinet atmosphere
- Dumping of exhaust O_2 into cabin atmosphere avoided to prevent fire hazard
- Minimum flow system for xenon may be useful

Complications

Nephrolithiasis and Osteoporosis

- Due to gravitational unloading
- This causes loss of calcium from bones along with hypercalciuria

Space Motion Sickness

- GERD may occur during flight and after landing
- Dizziness, drowsiness, nausea, and vomiting
- Increased risk of aspiration

Hemorrhage and Hypovolemia

- Reduced chances of bleeding
- This is because due to high surface tension of blood, it will remain on surface of wound
- Chances of arterial bleeds spilling out still remains
- Hypotension may be increased by preexisting volume loss and increased G forces during reentry

Ebullism

- Cabin pressure in space craft is 760 mm Hg
- That of extra-vehicular activity (EVA) space suits is 222 mm Hg
- This reduced pressure in EVA suit increases risk of decompression sickness
- If the suit is disrupted during EVA, astronauts ambient pressure quickly drops to zero
- This causes generalized bubble formation called ebullism
- Body fluid boils due to ambient pressure being lower than saturated water vapor pressure

Hypoxia

- Astronauts breathe 100% oxygen in EVA suits
- Disruption of the suit causes hypoxia

Electrolyte disturbances: Hypokalemia and hypomagnesemia common due to reduced dietary intake

Other Advantages

- On board diagnostic tools like remotely guided USG examination
- Remote robotic surgery substituted for on-board surgeon

INTRAOPERATIVE ANAPHYLAXIS

Introduction

Rapid systemic reaction, with potentially life threatening consequences, to a substance to which the individual is already sensitized.

Types

- Allergic anaphylaxis:
    - Type I IgE mediated release of inflammatory mediators
    - Involves mast cells and basophils

- Anaphylactoid reaction:
    - Direct non-immune mediated release of inflammatory mediators
    - Direct complement activation contributory

Risk Factors

- Female gender
- Old age
- History of pulmonary/cardiovascular disease
- History of atopy
- Food allergy
- Latex allergy
- Intravenous drug administration

Etiology

- Muscle relaxants: *Most common*
    - Succinylcholine
    - Rocuronium
    - Atracurium
- Natural rubber:
    - Latex gloves
    - Tourniquets
    - Foleys catheter
- Antibiotics:
    - Penicillins
    - Betalactams
    - Bacitracin
    - Vancomycin
    - Polymyxins
    - Amphotericin
- Hypnotics:
    - Thiopentone
    - Propofol
- Opioids:
    - Morphine
    - Meperidine
- Colloids:
    - Dextran
    - Gelatin
    - Mannitol
- Drugs affecting coagulation:
    - Aprotinin
    - Heparin
    - Protamine
- Others:
    - Bupivacaine
    - Ester local anesthetics
    - β-blockers
    - Radiocontrast allergy
    - Povidone iodine

Mechanism

- Initial exposure to antigens causes IgE release
- IgE binds to mast cells and basophils
- Reexposure to multimeric antigen causes cross linking of IgE receptors
- Degranulation of mast cells and basophils
- Release of inflammatory mediators:
    - Histamine
    - Prostaglandins
    - Serotonin
    - Tryptase
    - Kinins
    - Leukotrienes

Symptoms

- Flushing
- Urticaria
- Dyspnea
- Periorbital/perioral edema
- Wheezing
- Generalized rashes
- Localized edema

Signs

- Hypotension
- Bronchospasm
- Cardiovascular collapse
- Arrhythmias
- Laryngeal edema
- Tachycardia
- Angioedema
- Pulmonary HTN
- Acute tubular necrosis
- Pulmonary edema

Signs Under Anesthesia

- Increased peak inspiratory pressure
- Increased end tidal carbon dioxide
- Decreased oxygen saturation
- Decreased urine output
- Disseminated intravascular coagulation

Severity: Ring and Meissner scale

No.	Severity	Description
1.	Grade I	Erythema, pruritis
		Angioedema, urticaria
2.	Grade II	Urticaria, erythema
		Hypotension, tachycardia, presyncope
		Dyspnea, wheezing, bronchospasm
		Nausea, vomiting, diarrhea
3.	Grade III	Profound hypotension, arrhythmias
		Bradycardia, cardiovascular collapse
		Laryngeal edema, bronchospasm, hypoxia
		Confusion, unconsciousness
4.	Grade IV	Pulseless electrical activity
		Cardiac arrest

Investigations

I. *General*:

- Carboxypeptidase levels
- Complement C3 and C4 levels elevated at 30 minutes, 1 and 4 hours post episode
- Tryptase estimation:
  - Blood sample taken 30 minutes after onset of reaction
  - Values > 20 ng/mL suggestive of anaphylaxis
  - Half life of tryptase 2 hours
  - Serum levels decrease over time
  - Repeat sample at 6 and 24 hours after reaction for tryptase levels
  - Does not differentiate anaphylaxis and anaphylactoid reaction
  - May be absent in the presence of anaphylaxis

II. *Invivo tests*:

- Skin prick testing:
  - Done 4–6 weeks after anaphylactic episode due to mast cell depletion
  - Test with suspected agents and positive and negative controls
  - Freshly prepared diluted drugs used
  - Skin pricked with needle containing small quantity of allergen
  - On front of forearm/back of trunk
- Intradermal skin testing:
  - Done 4–6 weeks after anaphylactic episode due to mast cell depletion
  - Done only if skin prick test is negative
  - Drug concentration of prick test diluted by 1:10
  - 0.2–0.3 mL introduced intradermally with hypodermic needle
  - Slightly greater risk of systemic reaction
- Scratch test: Deep dermal scratch done with blunt bottom of lancet
- Patch test: Patch containing allergen applied to skin
- Bronchial challenge test:
  - In cases of strong suspicion
  - Patient inhales nebulized histamine or methacholine
  - Degree of airway obstruction measured with spirometry
  - Patients with airway hyperreactivity respond to lower dose of drug
  - Post bronchodilator may be used to differentiate asthma from COPD
  - Done only with availability of full resuscitation facilities

III. *Invitro tests*:

- Radioallergosorbent test (RAST):
  - Measures presence of specific IgE antibodies in serum
  - Insoluble disk coupled with specific drug added to patients serum
  - Radiolabeled anti-human antibody added to mixture
  - Radiolabeled anti-human antibody binds to IgE antibodies already bound to antigen
  - Unbound IgE antibodies washed away
  - Amount of radioactivity proportional to serum IgE for allergen

Management

General

- Stop administration of offending drug
- Terminate or rapidly complete surgery
- IV fluids:
  - Loss of 40–50% IV volume
  - Rapid administration to compensate for peripheral vasodilatation
  - 1–2 liters boluses of balanced salt solution
  - Titrate to maintain SBP > 90 mm Hg

Airway

- Administer 100% oxygen
- Endotracheal intubation:
  - Secure airway early
  - Those with apnea, coma, increasing hypercapnea, exhaustion
  - *Rapid sequence intubation*
  - Largest sized ETT used if no airway edema to minimize resistance
  - Ventilatory strategy:
    - Small tidal volume (6–8 mL/kg)
    - Slower respiratory rate
    - Shorter inspiratory time
    - Longer expiratory time (I:E = 1:4 or 1:5)
    - Permissive hypercapnea
  - Delay extubation as airway edema may continue for 24 hours

Bronchodilators

- Ipratropium bromide 0.03%—500 µg in 2.5 mL NS nebulization
- Albuterol 0.3% 2.5–5 mg in 3 mL NS nebulization
- Albuterol 100–200 µg IV bolus
- Terbutaline 250–500 µg subcutaneously repeated every 20 minutes for 3 doses
- Aminophylline 5 mg/kg IV over 20–30 minutes

Epinephrine

- *Drug of choice* as α_1 supports blood pressure while β_2 supports bronchodilation
- Highest peak blood levels with intramuscular administration in anterolateral thigh
- Subcutaneous injection provides uncertain and delayed absorption
- 0.2–0.5 mg IM (1:1,000) repeat every 5–15 minutes if no improvement (*Class I, LOE C*)
- 50–100 μg IV boluses if anaphylactic shock (*Class I, LOE B*)
- 5–15 μg/min infusion to maintain blood pressure in shock (*Class IIa, LOE C*)
- 2–2.5 mg in 10 mL instilled endotracheally

Antihistaminics

- Diphenhydramine (H_1 blocker)—0.5–1 mg/kg IV
- Ranitidine (H_2 blocker)—1 mg/kg IV

Corticosteroids

- Methylprednisolone 0.5–1 mg/kg bolus followed by 0.8 mg/kg Q4–6H
- Hydrocortisone 1–5 mg/kg IV bolus followed by 2.5 mg/kg Q4–6H
- Decrease airway edema and reduce recurrence
- Hydrocortisone preferred due to fast onset

Vasopressors

- Other vasopressors useful in those cases unresponsive to epinephrine (*Class IIb, LOE C*)
- Dopamine 2–20 μg/kg/min infusion
- Norepinephrine 0.05 μg/kg/min infusion
- Vasopressin:
  - 1–2 IU IV for hypotension
  - 40 IU IV for cardiac arrest
- Methoxamine and metaraminol other alternatives

Others

- Ketamine: May be useful if intubation planned
- Heliox:
  - Mixture of 70% helium and 30% oxygen
  - Reduces turbulence in airflow
  - Not useful if >30% oxygen required
- Volatile anesthetics:
  - Isoflurane/sevoflurane in refractory bronchospasm
  - Increases ease of mechanical ventilation
- Glucagon:
  - 20–30 μg/kg or 1–5 mg bolus followed by 5–15 μg/min infusion
- Magnesium sulfate:
  - 40–60 mg/kg or 2 g IV bolus
  - Used for refractory bronchospasm

Extracorporeal Life Support

- Cardiopulmonary bypass for anaphylaxis followed by cardiac arrest (*Class IIb, LOE C*)
- Requires equipment and expertise

Differential Diagnosis

- Pulmonary embolism
- Acute myocardial infarction
- Aspiration
- Vasovagal reaction

ELECTRICAL SAFETY IN OPERATING ROOM

Introduction

- Operating theater is at a high risk for fire hazards as:
  - Variety of electrical equipment are close to each other
  - Unconscious patient who cannot protect himself

Predisposing Factors

- Confined space
- Electrical items
- Electrically sensitive persons:
  - Patient with breaks in skin—abrasions
  - Wet dressings
  - Implanted pacemakers
  - Monitoring lines connected to transducer
- Inflammable materials:
  - Oxygen
  - Ether
  - Bowel gas

Risk Factors

I. *Circumstantial*:
  - Non uniformity of electrical fixtures
  - Poorly designed electrical distribution system
  - Poor maintenance

II. *Human*:
  - Unskilled electrician
  - Non adherence to regulations
  - Overloaded cables
  - Excessive fuse sizes
  - Inadequate earthing

III. *Environmental*:
  - Heat
  - Humidity
  - Animals: Rats and rodents

Types of Electrical Hazard

- Shock—when person becomes final component that closes electrical circuit
- Electrocution—when amount or path of flow of current through person becomes lethal
- Burns
- Fires
- Explosions
- Failure of equipment

Classes of Electrical Equipment

Describes method of electrical protection.

Class I

- Any conducting part of equipment is earthed
- Fuses present at wall socket, live and neutral sides of equipment
- Any electrical leakage channeled to earth and breaks circuit

Class II

- Accessible conducting parts have doubly reinforced insulation
- This prevents possibility of accessible part becoming live
- Earthing wire not required

Class III

- Uses voltages not higher than Safety Extra Low Voltage (SELV)
- Usually less than 25 V for AC and 60 V for DC
- Unlikely for electrocution at such low voltages
- Equipment which uses either batteries or SELV transformers
- Can cause microshock
- Does not meet current standards as limitation of voltage alone not sufficient to ensure patient safety

Electrocution

Mechanisms

I. *Resistive coupling*:
   - Person touches faulty wire or equipment while in contact with earth
   - Body becomes part of an electrical circuit
   - Leakage current passes through the body to the earth

II. *Capacitative coupling*:
   - Occurs in presence of high frequency current
   - Equipment attached behaves like one of the plates of the capacitor
   - Body becomes part of an electrical circuit
   - Current passes through the body

Factors Affecting Severity

- Type of current—AC current more dangerous
- Size of current—50–60 Hz frequency most dangerous
- Electrical path (especially current density through the heart)
- Duration of current flow
- Timing in relation to ECG

No.	Strength of current	Injury
1.	<1 mA	Nil
2.	1 mA	Tingling
3.	5 mA	Pain
4.	15 mA	Muscular tetany, pain, asphyxia
5.	50 mA	Expiratory respiratory arrest
6.	75 mA	Arrhythmias
7.	100 mA	Ventricular fibrillation
		Cardiac arrest
8.	>5 Amp	Sustained asystole
		Contact burns

Injuries Caused

- Functional disruption of tissues
- Burns
- Respiratory failure
- Ventricular fibrillation
- Blunt trauma

Types of Shocks

Macroshock

- *Most common*
- 100–300 mA current, as low as 50 mA
- Electrical charge occurs through intact skin
- Travels to heart and out again
- Current distributed somewhat evenly through body parts
- Examples:
  - Contact with faulty class I equipment
  - Defibrillator use

Microshock

- Very low level shocks which go undetected
- Usually <1 mA current
- Charge directly delivered to heart muscle
- Examples:
  - Shock delivered via central line/pacemaker wire

Precautions

I. *Technical measures*:
- Polarities to be correctly identified
- Prevent interruption of neutral conductor
- Earth connections on all socket outlets in an area to be interconnected by a low resistance conductor
- Exposed metal objects to be interconnected to a good earth
- Earth leakage trip device
- Regular testing and maintenance
- International standard theater electrical equipment
- Do not block access to electrical panels with carts/equipment

II. *Cautery measures*:
- Keep cautery forceps in protective quiver
- Use of buzzer which is activated on depression of foot switch
- Proper plugging in of cautery plate
- Use of bipolar cautery in the presence of pacemakers

III. *Utilization measures*:
- Plug equipment into wall receptacles with power switches in off position
- Do not unplug equipment by grasping cord
- Check for frayed or exposed wiring on equipment cords
- Do not drape cord over hot/sharp objects
- Do not plug in equipment with wet hands
- Do not plug in equipment when cord is wet
- Ensure patient is not in contact with earthed objects
- Wear antistatic shoes

IV. *Appropriate selection of equipment*

Types of Electrical Equipment

Describes degree of protection of medical equipment.

Type B

- Equipment may be class I, II or III
- Maximum leakage current not to exceed 100 μA
- Not suitable for direct connection to heart

Type BF

- Equipment may be class I, II or III
- Maximum leakage current not to exceed 100 μA
- Uses *floating/isolated circuit*

Type CF

- Provides highest degree of protection
- Have maximum leakage current <10 μA
- Suitable for direct cardiac connection
- Examples:
  - ECG leads
  - Pressure transducers

TOTAL INTRAVENOUS ANESTHESIA

Introduction

Method of inducing and maintaining general anesthesia by drugs administered exclusively by intravenous route in the absence of all inhalational agents including nitrous oxide.

Ideal Intravenous Anesthetic

- Rapid onset of action
- Rapid offset of action
- Noncumulative
- Nonactive metabolites
- Nontoxic metabolite

Aims

- Achieve smooth general anesthesia
  - Smooth induction
  - Reliable and titratable maintenance of anesthesia
  - Rapid emergence on termination of infusion
- Avoid undesirable clinical effects
- Avoid under or overdosing
- Allow rapid and smooth emergence

Indications

- Previous history of PONV
- High risk of PONV: Orchidopexy, strabismus
- Scoliosis surgery: Intraoperative wake-up test
- History of malignant hyperthermia/malignant hyperthermia susceptible
- Airway procedures
- Neurosurgery—endoscopic neurosurgeries for hypotensive anesthesia
- Thyroid surgeries for recurrent laryngeal nerve monitoring

Advantages

- Avoids the peaks and troughs of repeated bolus dosing
- Better hemodynamic control—controlled hypotension
- Reduced stress response
- Reduced bleeding
- Reduced intraocular pressure
- Improved V/Q matching
- Increases maximum attainable FiO_2
- Reduces OT pollution
- Smooth emergence

- Lesser hangover
- Reduced bowel distention
- Reduced PONV

Disadvantages

- Delay to peak effect (equivalent of four to five drug elimination $T_{1/2}$)
- Decrease in plasma concentration at transition from loading dose to maintenance dose
- No single intravenous anesthetic provides all components of anesthesia
- Combination of drugs necessary
- Early or late respiratory depression
- Opioid side effects—muscle rigidity, gastroparesis, pruritus
- Adverse effects if IV line disrupted
- Risk of awareness

Modes of Delivery

- Simple intravenous boluses
- Variable rate continuous infusion

Instruments Used

- Controllers
  - Drops (***Exadrop***)
  - Volumetric (***Dosifix***)
- Pumps
  - Syringes (***Intrafusor***)
  - Volumetric (***Infusomat***)
  - Peristaltic drops (***Digifusa***)

TIVA Alarms

- Occlusion
- Empty syringe
- Absent syringe
- Wrong syringe position
- Low battery
- Bolus delivery
- Setting changes

Monitoring During TIVA

- ASA minimum monitoring standards:
  - Pulse oximetry
  - Electrocardiogram
  - Noninvasive blood pressure (NIBP)
  - Capnography
- Depth of anesthesia:
  - Bispectral Index (BIS)
  - Auditory evoked potential
  - Entropy

Drugs Used

- Hypnotic agents:
  - Propofol
  - Benzodiazepines
  - Ketamine
  - Barbiturates
- Analgesic agents:
  - Remifentanyl
  - Alfentanil
  - Fentanyl
  - Morphine
- Muscle relaxants:
  - Vecuronium
  - Atracurium
  - Rocuronium

Drug Dosages

Opioids

- Fentanyl 2 µg/kg bolus followed by 0.2 µg/kg/min infusion
- Alfentanil 20 µg/kg bolus followed by 0.25 µg/kg/min infusion
- Sufentanil 0.15 µg/kg bolus followed by 0.003 µg/kg/min infusion
- Remifentanil 1 µg/kg bolus followed by 0.02 µg/kg/min

Hypnotics

Propofol 1.5–2 mg/kg induction followed by:

- 100–150 µg/kg/min first 10 minutes
- 90–140 µg/kg/min from 10 minutes to 2 hours
- 75–125 µg/kg/min beyond 2 hours
- Turn off propofol 5–10 minutes prior to desired time of emergence

Ketamine

- No initial bolus
- Infusion started at 1 mg/min, maintained up to 1 hour
- 1–4 hours: 0.6 mg/min
- >4 hours: 0.4 mg/min
- Turned off 15–30 minutes prior to end of surgery

Infusion Schemes

- BET infusion scheme:
  - B = Loading dose
  - E = Terminal elimination
  - T = Transfer to peripheral compartment
- Open loop system:
  - Blood or brain drug concentration chosen
  - Microprocessor of pump adjusts rate of infusion

- Microprocessor maintains effect site drug concentration
- No feedback signal of output

❖ Closed loop system:
- Future technology
- Feedback signal of effect site concentration built into delivery system

TIVA Models

❖ ***Roberts*** manual infusion regimen
❖ ***Marsh*** weight based regimen
❖ ***Schnider*** model
❖ ***Kataria, Paedfusor*** pediatric models

Recent Advances

❖ Newer hypnotics:
- ***Remimazolam***
  - Sedation with 6 mg initial loading dose
  - Followed by 3 mg doses at >2 minutes intervals
  - Recovery within 16 minutes for 90% patients
- Dexmedetomidine
- S+ketamine enantiomer
- Propofol prodrug

❖ Closed loop anesthesia
❖ Target controlled infusion (TCI)
❖ Noninvasive monitoring of propofol concentration

TARGET CONTROLLED INFUSIONS

Introduction

Target controlled infusion is an infusion controlled in such a manner as to attempt to achieve a user defined drug concentration at the effect site.

Goals

❖ Avoid over-dosage
❖ Ensure constant concentration
❖ Allow accurate titration
❖ Account for patient covariates

Advantages

❖ Improves stability and titration
❖ Minimal workload—convenient to use
❖ Displays calculated blood concentration
❖ Good control of depth of anesthesia
❖ Optimizes drug properties
❖ Cardiovascular stability—lower heart rate, less stress hormones
❖ Improved ciliary function postoperatively
❖ Reduced intracranial pressures (ICP)
❖ Quickens recovery
❖ Helps anticipating recovery—predicts patient waking time
❖ Avoids OT pollution
❖ Less incidence of PONV

Disadvantages

❖ Concentration calculation errors
❖ Possibility of awareness when used with muscle relaxants
❖ Requires dedicated IV cannula for administration
❖ IV access needs constant check for occlusion

Components

❖ User interface for patient details
❖ Software with pharmacokinetic model validated for specific drug
❖ Infusion device—capable of infusion rates up to 1,200 mL/hr with precision of 0.1 mL/hr
❖ Communication between control unit and pump hardware

Functions of TCI Pump

❖ Bolus: Ability to rapidly increase plasma concentration
❖ Flow rate: Accurate function at low flow rates
❖ Alarms: Facilitates identification of improper positioning of syringe in pump
❖ Tight syringe fitting: Prevents syringe from moving when pump is in action
❖ Battery indicator

Target Controlled Infusion (TCI) Pharmacokinetic Models 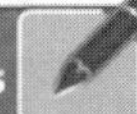

❖ ***Marsh*** model used by Diprifusor for propofol
- Assumes that central compartment volume proportional to weight alone
- Age is entered but not used in calculations

❖ ***Schuttler and White-Kenny*** models for propofol
❖ ***Schnider*** model for propofol
- Incorporated in newer generation TCI pumps
- Follows a three compartment model
- Age, height and weight are entered into the system
- Calculated lean body mass used to calculate infusion rates

❖ ***Kataria*** model for children
- Minimum age of 3 years and body weight 15 kg

❖ ***Paedfusor*** model for children
- Minimum age limit is 1 year and lowest body weight permissible is 5 kg

❖ ***Minto*** model for remifentanil
- Uses three compartment model
- Covariates age, weight, height, and gender considered for calculation of dose
- Questionable efficacy owing to fixed context sensitive half life of remifentanil
- May producer higher concentrations in elderly or sick patients

Rationale

- End result always a variation of bolus, elimination and transfer scheme
- Pharmacokinetic model used in reverse
- Desired effect site concentration chosen
- Computer calculates rate of administration using pharmacokinetic model
- Calculations done to keep desired concentration in target compartment constant every 10 seconds
- Infusion pump changes infusion rate depending upon target concentration

Usage

- Initial programming of pump based on patients age, height, weight and sex
- Initial induction blood propofol levels of 6–8 μg/mL
- Caution in elderly and those with cardiovascular disease
- Reassessment of dosage during airway manipulation
- Target concentration adjusted subsequently based on response to surgical stimulus
- Coadministration of benzodiazepines and opioids necessitate dose adjustments
- Target concentration reduced towards end of case to promote rapid recovery
- Infusion stopped once final sutures applied
- Time to awakening displayed by machine, usually at propofol concentration of 1 μg/mL

Precautions

- High concentration of drugs that run at slow speeds avoided
- Syringe pump connected closer to patient
- Vasoactive drugs should not be combined with primary drug
- Pump should not be placed above level of patient
- Use separate IV access for TCI infusion

Validation

- Median prediction error (MDPE): Median of procentual difference, positive or negative
- Median absolute prediction error (MDAPE): Median of procentual difference between measured and predicted concentration in absolute value
- Divergence: Slope of linear regression analysis of evolution in time of MDAPE
- Wobble: Median of variability in individual patients

MONITORED ANESTHESIA CARE

Introduction

"Refers to instances in which an anesthesiologist has been called upon to provide specific anesthesia services to a patient undergoing a planned procedure and is in control of the patients nonsurgical or nonobstetrical medical care (including monitoring patients vital signs, and is available to administer anesthetics or provide medical care as appropriate)".

Requirements

- Performance of preanesthetic examination and evaluation
- Prescription of anesthetic care
- Personal participation in, or medical direction of entire plan of care
- Continuous physical presence of anesthesiologist
- Proximate presence of anesthesiologist for diagnosis and management of emergencies

Goals

- To maintain patient safety and sense of well being
- To alleviate pain and minimize discomfort
- Administration of sedatives, hypnotics, anesthetic agents and other medications
- To minimize psychological response: Anxiolysis, analgesia and amnesia
- To control behavior
- Support of vital functions
- Diagnosis and treatment of clinical problems which occur during the procedure
- Provision of other medical services as needed to complete the procedure safely
- To return patient to preprocedural state

End Points

- Providing patient comfort
- Maintaining cardiorespiratory stability
- Improving operative conditions
- Prevent recall of unpleasant perioperative events

Contraindications

- Severe comorbidity (ASA III, IV)
- Morbid obesity
- Documented history of sleep apnea
- Increased risk of airway obstruction:
  - Sleep apnea/stridor
  - Dysmorphic facies

- Oral abnormalities: Macroglossia
- Neck abnormalities: Neck mass
- Jaw abnormalities: Micrognathia

- Inability to follow simple commands:
  - Cognitive dysfunction
  - Intoxication
  - Psychological problems
  - Acutely agitated
  - Uncooperative patients
- Medical problems associated with alcohol/drug abuse
- Patients of extreme age: Younger than 18 years, older than 70 years
- History of intolerance to standard sedatives:
  - Chronic opioid use
  - Chronic benzodiazepine use
- Spasticity or movement disorders
- Pregnancy
- Prolonged procedures requiring deep sedation

Preoperative Assessment

- Similar to preanesthetic evaluation of other patients
- Patient's ability to lie motionless and actively cooperate is assessed
- Ability to verbally communicate with the patient assessed as it:
  - Is a means of reassuring the patient?
  - Allows requests for active participation by the patient
  - Assists in monitoring level of sedation and cardiorespiratory function

Monitoring

- Visual, tactile, and auditory assessment:
  - Response to verbal stimulation evaluated for effective titration of sedation
  - Rate, depth, and pattern of breathing
  - Peripheral perfusion and capillary refill
  - Diaphoresis, shivering, cyanosis, and changes in neurological status
- Auscultation: Precordial stethoscope
- Pulse oximetry
- Capnography
- ECG
- BP recorded at least every 5 minutes
- Temperature: For prolonged procedures

Drugs Used

- Benzodiazepines
- Midazolam 1–2 mg IV before propofol/remifentanil infusion
- Diazepam 2.5–5 mg IV

Opioids

- Alfentanyl 5–20 μg/kg IV bolus 2 minutes before stimulus
- Fentanyl 0.5–2 μg/kg IV bolus 2 minutes before stimulus
- Remifentanyl 0.1 μg/kg/min infusion 5 minutes before stimulus, 0.05 μg/kg IV maintenance as tolerated

Others

- Propofol 250–500 μg/kg bolus, 25–75 μg/kg/min infusion
- Ketamine 0.25–1 mg/kg IV bolus
- Dexmedetomidine 0.5–1 μg/kg loading dose over 10 minutes, 0.2–0.7 μg/kg/hr infusion

ANESTHESIA FOR DAYCARE SURGERY

Introduction

An operation or procedure, an office or outpatient operation/procedure, where the patient is discharged on the same working day—***International Association of Ambulatory Surgery (IAAS).***

Advantages

- Reduced dependence on availability of hospital beds
- Greater flexibility in scheduling surgeries
- Shorter surgical waiting lists
- Lower overall procedural costs
- Lower requirements of nursing and medical supervision
- Greater turnover of patients
- Minimal psychological disturbances, especially children
- Less incidence of hospital acquired infections
- Lesser incidence of respiratory complications
- Reduced incidence of venous thromboembolism

Procedure Requirements

- Minimal risk of postoperative hemorrhage
- Minimal risk of postoperative airway compromise
- Rapid return to normal fluid and food intake
- Postoperative pain controllable by outpatient management techniques
- Postoperative care managed by patient/responsible adult

Patient Requirements

- ASA I and ASA II patients
- ASA III patients whose disease is well controlled preoperatively

- Should have understanding of the process and be able to follow discharge instructions
- Patients place of residence to be within easy access to surgical facilities
- Normal term infants of over 6 weeks age
- Ex-premature infants more than 52 weeks post-conceptual age

Common Daycare Surgeries

General Surgery

- Herniorraphy
- Hemorrhoidectomy
- Herniotomy
- Upper and lower gastrointestinal tract endoscopy/ biopsy
- Lymph node excision biopsy
- Laparoscopic procedures

Plastic Surgery

- Otoplasty
- Excision skin lesions
- Scar revision

Gynaecology

- D and C
- Hysteroscopy
- Vaginal hysterectomy
- Tubal ligation

Orthopedics

- Implant removal
- Arthroscopy
- Closed reduction procedures

Urology

- Circumcision
- Cystoscopy
- Lithotripsy
- Prostate surgery
- Orchidectomy/orchidopexy

Otolaryngology

- Myringotomy
- Mastoidectomy
- Tympanoplasty
- Adenoidectomy
- Tonsillectomy
- Polypectomy

Ophthalmology

- Examination under anesthesia
- Lacrimal duct probing
- Strabismus correction

Contraindications

- Serious life threatening diseases
- Morbid obesity complicated by cyclic vomiting syndrome (CVS) and RS symptoms
- Chronic use of centrally acting drugs
- Extremely premature infants (<60 weeks postconceptional age)
- Lack of responsible adult at home to take care of patient postdischarge
- Surgical procedures involving:
  - Major fluid shifts
  - Significant blood loss
  - Significant postoperative pain
  - Significant PONV

Preoperative Evaluation

- Detailed history with specific focus on comorbidities
- Identify difficult airway
- Recording of vital signs
- Preoperative counseling to allay fear and anxiety
- Written and verbal communication regarding arrival time and fasting guidelines
- Need for a responsible adult to accompany patient specified
- Investigations:

Age	Male	Female
<40 yrs	Nil	Hematocrit
		Pregnancy test
40–49 yrs	ECG	Hematocrit
		Pregnancy test
50–64 yrs	ECG	Hematocrit
		ECG
65–74 yrs	Hematocrit	Hematocrit
	ECG	ECG
	BUN	BUN
	Glucose	Glucose
>75 yrs	Hematocrit	Hematocrit
	ECG	ECG
	BUN	BUN
	Glucose	Glucose
	Chest X-ray	Chest X-ray

Anesthetic Goals

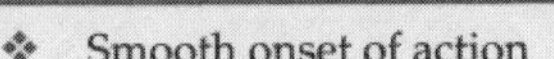

- Smooth onset of action
- Adequate intraoperative analgesia and amnesia
- Good surgical conditions
- Rapid recovery
- Minimal adverse effects

Choice of Anesthetic Technique

- General anesthesia most commonly preferred
- Central neuraxial blockade not encouraged as persistant motor block delays discharge
- Local nerve and plexus blocks are good options for peripheral surgeries

Choice of Drugs

Induction Agents

- Propofol
- Ketamine

Analgesics

- Fentanyl
- Alfentanil
- Sufentanil
- Remifentanil

Maintenance

- Nitrous oxide along with sevoflurane, desflurane or propofol

Muscle Relaxants

- Succinylcholine
- Atracurium, cisatracurium
- Mivacurium

Regional Anesthesia

- Short acting drugs like lignocaine and procaine desirable for central NAB
- Bupivacaine used if anticipated duration of surgery >2 hours
- Intrathecal fentanyl and sufentanil prolong sensory blockade without affecting motor block
- Low spinal is recommended

CRITERIA FOR DISCHARGE FROM POSTANESTHESIA CARE UNIT

Introduction

Minimum mandatory stay in postanesthesia care unit (PACU) is not required and patients must be observed until:

- They are no longer at risk for ventilatory depression
- Their mental status is clear/has returned to baseline
- They are hemodynamically stable

Recommendations for Discharge

- Minimum mandatory stay not required
- Vital signs stable and within acceptable limits
- Patient should be alert, oriented/mental status returned to baseline
- Discharge after patient meets certain criteria
- Scoring system used to document fitness for discharge
- Requirements to urinate and retain clear fluids are *not part of routine criteria*
- Outpatients discharged with responsible adults who will accompany their home
- Written instructions regarding postprocedure diet, medications and emergency phone number provided

Scoring Systems

Modified Aldrete Scoring System

Respiration	
Able to take deep breath and cough	2
Dyspnea/shallow breathing	1
Apnea	0
Oxygen saturation	
Maintains SpO_2 > 92 on room air	2
Needs oxygen to maintain SpO_2 > 90%	1
SpO_2 < 90% even with supplemental oxygen	0
Consciousness	
Fully awake	2
Arousable on calling	1
Not responding	0
Circulation	
BP + 20 mm Hg preoperatively	2
BP + 20–50 mm Hg preoperatively	1
BP + 50 mm Hg preoperatively	0
Activity	
Able to move four extremities voluntary/on command	2
Able to move two extremities	1
Unable to move extremities	0
Score more than 9 required for discharge	

Postanesthesia Discharge Scoring System

Vital signs	
BP and pulse within 20% preoperative level	2
BP and pulse within 20–40% preoperative level	1
BP and pulse more than 40% preoperative level	0
Activity	
Steady gait, no dizziness, meets preoperative level	2

Contd...

Contd...

Requires assistance	1
Unable to ambulate	0
Nausea and vomiting	
Minimal/treated with oral medications	2
Moderate/treated with parenteral medications	1
Severe/continues despite therapy	0
Pain	
Controlled with oral analgesics and acceptable to patient:	
Yes	2
No	1
Surgical bleeding	
Minimal/no dressing changes	2
Moderate/up to two dressing changes required	1
Severe/more than three dressing changes required	0
Score more than 9 required for discharge	

Discharge after Regional Anesthesia

- Must meet same criteria as patients recovering from general anesthesia
- Additional criteria present, to ensure safe ambulation if neuraxial block or major lower limb nerve block has been administered
- Before ambulation, patients with neuraxial must have:
  - Return of normal sensation, muscle strength, proprioception and sympathetic function
  - Normal perianal sensation (S_4 and S_5)
  - Ability to plantar flex toes
  - Proprioception of big toe
  - Advisable to void before discharge

CLINICAL TESTS FOR CORRECT PLACEMENT OF ENDOTRACHEAL TUBE

Introduction

Detection of esophageal intubation is significant as it contributes to 15% of major anesthetic catastrophies.

Clinical Tests

- Direct visualization of tube passing through larynx
- Observation of chest movement
- Observation of abdominal movements
- Observation of moisture condensation in ETT: *Tracheal mist*
- Auscultation of breath sounds
- Auscultation of epigastrium
- Movement of reservoir bag in unparalysed patients

Diagnostic Aids

- Exhaled carbon dioxide (CO_2):
  - Exhaled CO_2 waveform observed for *a minimum of 3 cycles*
  - False positives occur when:
    - Alveolar gas forced into stomach during mash ventilation
    - Ingestion of carbonated soft drinks preoperatively
- Esophageal detector device (EDD):
  - Is a 60 mL catheter tip syringe fitted with one end of 15 mm tracheal tube
  - Works on principle that esophagus is a fibromuscular tube with no intrinsic structure to maintain patency
  - Trachea is kept patent by C-shaped cartilaginous rings
  - Withdrawal of plunger of EDD will aspirate gases from lung if ETT is in trachea with minimal resistance
  - However, if ETT is in esophagus, withdrawal of plunger will cause opposition of esophageal walls around syringe
  - This occludes lumen causing increased resistance when plunger is pulled back
  - Inflated stomach may give false positive result: EDD to be applied before starting ventilation through the tube
- ***Ellicks evacuator bulb***: Modification of EDD
- Transtracheal illumination:
  - Lighted stylet placed inside ETT just proximal to the cuff, with cricoid pressure and overhead light dimmed
  - When stylet was introduced into esophagus, no transesophageal illumination can be demonstrated
  - Disadvantages: Cannot be used in midline neck masses and red rubber ETT
- Fiberoptic scope:
  - *Best method* of confirming tracheal intubation
  - Visualization of carina and tracheal rings
  - Impractical for routine use but mandatory for doubtful cases and difficult intubation

VICARIOUS LIABILITY

Introduction

An employer is responsible not only for his own negligence but also for the negligence of his employees, if such acts occur in the course of employment and within its scope, by the *principle of respondent superior (let the master answer)*.

Explanation: Employees are liable under the law principle *"qui facit per alium facit per se"*, i.e., one who acts through another, acts in his or her own interests.

Prerequisites: Three conditions must be satisfied to prove vicarious liability:

- There must be an employer-employee relationship
- The employees conduct must occur within the scope of his employment
- While on the job

Determination of negligence: Fourfold test to determine negligence:

- It must be established that there is a duty of care (between a doctor and patient, this can be taken for granted)
- It must be shown that duty of care has been breached, using ***Bolam*** test, as falling below the standard of a responsible body of medical men means the doctor may be considered negligent
- Should be shown that there was a *causal link* between the breach of duty and harm
- It must be shown that the harm was not too remote

Implications in Medicine

- The principal doctor becomes responsible for any negligence of the assistant. Both may be sued by the patient even though the principal has not been professionally concerned. The same applies where the principal employs nonmedical servants.
- When two doctors practice as partners, each is liable for the negligence of the other, even though one may have no part in the negligent act.
- When two or more independent doctors are attending to a patient, each may be held liable for the negligence of others that he observes, or in the ordinary course should have observed and allows it to continue without objection.

PREOPERATIVE EVALUATION CLINIC

Introduction

The preoperative evaluation clinic was developed with the goal of focusing all preoperative clinical services into hospital location to establish a center of visibility competitiveness and efficiency.

Operative Goals

- Provide a centralized site for preoperative evaluation
- Avoid logistic shuffling of patients to multiple hospital sites
- Provide anesthesia consultation for evaluation of medically complex patients
- Establish rapport with patients and reduce anxiety
- Improve patient care by provide personalized care, comfort and convenience
- Improved education of patients and families about their surgical procedure and proposed anesthesia care, including postoperative pain control options
- Educate patients about what to expect regarding postoperative feeding and discharge needs
- Ensure cost effective ordering of preoperative laboratory and diagnostic studies
- Reduce number of cancellation and delays in operative procedures on the day of surgery
- Ensure availability of medical records at the time of preoperative evaluation
- Ensure patients and surgeon satisfaction

Components: Preoperative evaluation clinic is a visible collaboration between departments of surgery, anesthesia, nursing, and hospital administration

Requisite Facilities

- Registration and reception area
- Adequate number of examination rooms
- Patient and family education room
- Phlebotomy and ECG room
- Area for admitting, financial, and insurance services
- Computer support room and rest rooms

Importance

- Prostate artery embolization (PAE) clinic aims at evaluating patient for potential risks during surgery and postoperative period
- Patients should be screened and triaged to determine patients current health status
- Standardization of preoperative process done in preanaesthetic clinic (PAC). This is useful as:
  - Allows for development and implementation of clinical algorithms to optimize preoperative medical management and reduce complications
  - This can reduce cost of admission and length of stay
  - Allows more accurate data collection
  - Minimize complications caused by communication errors

Prostate Artery Embolization Clinic Activities

- Surgeon office schedules PAC appointment. Flexibility in scheduling appointment is required to accommodate patients with urgent surgical requirements
- Anesthetist interviews and examines patient, obtains relevant medical information and determines appropriate diagnostic, laboratory, ECG and other evaluation requirements

- Phlebotomy/ECG and hospital admitting and insurance registration are available at the clinic
- Patients ECG is assessed during the visit and lab results evaluated at the end of each clinic day. Thus, significant abnormalities can be addressed immediately and cases cancelled the day before surgery
- A nurse educator trained in perioperative teaching discusses the surgery and hospital process with each patient and family member to increase patient awareness and comfort thus reducing fear and anxiety

Role of Anesthetist

- The anesthetist is the only specialist who can decide on whether the patient is appropriate for anesthesia and stable to proceed
- The anesthetist should develop leadership and management position in the preanesthetic evaluation program

ANESTHETIC CONSIDERATIONS OF PRONE POSITION

Introduction

- In the classic prone position, face, chest, abdomen, front of thighs, knees, toes and some surface of hands and arms all touch the supporting surface
- Also called *concorde position or face down position*

Modifications

- *Jack-knife position*:
  - Used for anorectal surgeries
  - Patient lies flexed on table with pelvis at flexion point
- *Knee-chest position:*
  - Exaggeration of jack-knife position
  - Knee and chest are supported
- ***Buie position***:
  - For proctological work
  - Patient kneels on a padded shelf, places chest on table proper
  - Table is tilted to head down position
- ***Georgia position***: For perineal and rectal work
- ***Overholt position***:
  - Used for thoracic problems
  - To prevent drainage of infected material and blood from the involved lung into the other lung
- ***Sellor-Brown position***:
  - Lower part of body in one plane
  - Chest neck and head are on a lower plane
  - Used to drain blood and infected material from the uninvolved lung
- Crouching or Carpenters rule position:
  - Knees and hips are flexed maximally
  - Patients weight rests on back of legs
  - Abdomen rests on front of thigh
  - Associated with:
    - Knee injury
    - Femoral venous obstruction
    - Abdominal wall restriction

Indications

- Posterior cervical and occipital surgeries
- Spine surgeries: Laminectomy, spinal fusion, scoliosis
- Thoracotomy by posterior approach
- Adrenal exploration, renal biopsies, percutaneous nephro-lithototripsy, PCN
- Surgeries on back of leg, e.g. varicose vein stripping, tendon repair
- Prone ventilation for ARDS
- Anorectal surgery in jack-knife position

Contraindications

- Crush injury to chest, flail chest
- Contusion of heart
- Severe *pectus excavatum*

Problems

- Care must be taken in keeping head safe in relation to rest of body
- Body weight against abdominal wall leads to:
  - Reduced diaphragmatic movement: Reduced FRC
  - Reduced tidal volume
- Increased intra-abdominal pressure causes reduced venous return
- Pressure on body prominences and toes: Pressure injuries

Physiological Effects

- Cardiovascular system:
  - Blood supply to brain must be protected:
    - Avoid severe twisting or neck extension
    - This may impede flow through vertebral artery
  - Venous return from head may get occluded:
    - Eyelid edema, swollen and engorged eye vessels
    - Headache, subglottic edema can occur macroglossia
  - Pressure on carotid sinus may cause severe arrhythmias

- Pressure on inferior vena cava and femoral vein:
  - Causes reduced venous return
  - This leads to hypotension
  - This is compounded by sympathetic block associated with SAB/GA
- Venous air embolism
- Increased bleeding from abdominal pressure due to epidural venous engorgement

❖ Respiratory system:
- Less airway pressure is required to ventilate patient in prone position
- This is because weight of chest and abdominal wall does not have to be lifted
- Patients thorax and pelvis should be raised by support
- A hand should be able to pass between abdomen and bed
- Body weight against abdominal wall leads to reduced diaphragmatic movement and tidal volume

Complications

Neurological Complications

❖ Ophthalmological:
- Corneal abrasions: Eyes may be injured during:
  - Turning patient
  - Protracted pressure in prone position during long duration surgeries
- *Anterior ischemic optic neuropathy (AION)*
- *Posterior ischemic optic neuropathy (PION)*
- *Central retinal artery occlusion (CRAO)*
- Cortical blindness

❖ Facial nerve injury in infra-parotid region

❖ Brachial plexus injuries due to:
- Neck rotation: Stretching of nerve roots
- Compression of plexus between ribs and clavicle
- Injury to neurovascular bundle from head of humerus
- Compression of ulnar nerve before, within or after the cubital tunnel
- Lateral compression of radial nerve proximal to elbow

❖ Ulnar nerve: At risk against sharp edges of supporting devices when arms are positioned above the head

❖ Spine injury if hips and shoulder not in same plane always

❖ Jack-knife position:
- Can injure femoral nerve
- Lateral cutaneous nerve of thigh injury causing ***meralgia paresthetica***

❖ Injury to nerves and tendons of dorsum of foot

Other Injuries

❖ Orbital compression can cause retinal ischemia and blindness

❖ Nasotracheal tubes:
- To be positioned carefully
- Avoid pressure on nasal cartilage in anterior margin

❖ Pressure necrosis of maxilla and forehead in prolonged procedures

❖ In cervical and posterior fossa procedures:
- Flexion of neck causes reduced anteroposterior diameter of hypopharynx
- This leads to compression ischemia of base of tongue and macroglossia
- This causes unexpected postextubation airway obstruction

❖ Ear cartilage damage if folded over

❖ Turning an extended neck causes:
- Neck muscle spasm and headache postoperatively
- This is due to pressure on C_2 between atlas and axis vertebrae

❖ Chest support devices may block venous return from neck

❖ In females:
- Breasts may get injured along sternal border
- Common if breast prosthesis is present
- Thus, medial and cephalad displacement of breast should be done

❖ Male genitals: Electrocautery grounding plate should not touch them

❖ Skin overlying iliac crest should be protected

❖ Compartment syndrome in prolonged kneeling position

❖ Toes should be protected using pillows under ankles

❖ Air embolism is a risk when operating field is higher than the heart

Accidental extubation: In prone position there is:

❖ Poor access to airway

❖ Traction from head movements and circuit

❖ Loosening of adhesive tapes due to sweating/saliva

ANESTHETIC CONSIDERATIONS OF LITHOTOMY POSITION

Introduction

It is the position in which the patient is on his back with the legs and thighs flexed to right angles.

Modification

- For combined vaginal-abdominal approach to pelvic viscera:
  - Leg elevation is less
  - Flexion of thigh to abduction is less than 90°
- ***Walcher's position*** for obstetrics: Thighs pressed firmly onto trunk and legs left dangling
- ***Blandy's position*** for TURP where legs are supported in such a way that thighs create an obtuse rather than acute angle with the body

Types of Lithotomy Position

- Low lithotomy position:
  - Used for most urological procedures
  - Degree of thigh elevation is only 35–40°
  - Reduces perfusion gradients and improves perineal access
- High lithotomy position:
  - Thigh flexed to 90° or more on trunk
  - Legs are almost fully extended on thighs by suspending patients feet from high poles
  - Significant uphill perfusion gradient exists
  - Poorly tolerated in less mobile patients
  - Complications:
    - Sciatic nerve stretching
    - Compression of contents of femoral canal
- Exaggerated lithotomy position:
  - For transperineal approach to retropubic area
  - Patient's pelvis is flexed ventrally on the spine
  - Thighs are flexed on trunk with lower legs aimed skywards
  - Significant uphill perfusion gradient exists for feet perfusion
  - Restricted ventilation: Controlled ventilation necessary
  - Avoided in preexisting lumbar spine diseases
  - High frequency of compartment syndrome of lower limbs
- Tilted lithotomy position:
  - Lithotomy position with head down tilt
  - Patient may slide cephalad and have head injuries
  - Cranial vascular compression and raised ICP
  - Use of shoulder brace to prevent cephalad displacement:
    - This may compress neurovascular bundle in neck
    - May also compress subclavian neurovascular bundle between clavicle and first rib
  - Weight of abdominal viscera on the diaphragm limits ventilation
  - It also causes gravitational accumulation of blood in the poorly ventilated lung apices
  - During controlled ventilation higher airway pressures are required to expand the lung

Indications

- Perineal and rectal surgeries
- Vaginal surgery
- Urological operations: Transurethral resection of the prostate (TURP), cystoscopy, retrograde pyelography, etc.

Contraindications

- Painful lumbar spine diseases
- Obese patients: Relative contraindication
- Decompensated CCF
- Raised ICP: Tilted lithotomy position contraindicated

Physiological Changes

- Respiratory system:
  - Vital capacity reduces by 18%
  - Thus is due to:
    - Restriction of diaphragmatic movement
    - Reduced volumetric expansion of lung due to pulmonary vascular congestion
  - Tidal volume reduces by 3%
  - FEV_1 increases by 9% due to:
    - Weight of abdominal viscera acts as a belt
    - This improves resting position of diaphragm
    - This increases inspiratory reserve
    - This adds force to maximum expiratory effort
  - Increase in postoperative respiratory complications due to paralysis of abdominal muscles with resultant inability to cough following SAB/epidural anesthesia
- Cardiovascular system:
  - Sudden elevation of lower limb causes increased venous return to right heart and precipitates CCF
  - Sudden lowering of lower limb may cause significant hypotension

Complications

- Venous stasis: Any patient placed in lithotomy position for more than 15 minutes should have legs protected by elastic stockings
- Damage to hip and knee especially of elderly women
- Injury to hand and fingers when caudal portion of table is lowered

- Sudden hypotension, congestive cardiac failure
- Compartment syndrome in high and exaggerated lithotomy position
- Peripheral nerve injuries:
  - Obdurator nerve ($L_{2,3,4}$):
    - Due to acute flexion of thigh on groin
    - Causes paralysis of thigh adductors
  - Femoral nerve:
    - Due to acute thigh flexion with angulation against underlying surface of pubic ramus
    - Causes abnormal gait and numbness
  - Saphenous nerve:
    - Compression of leg to knee brace medially
    - Causes loss of sensation on medial aspect of leg
  - Common peroneal nerve (L_4–S_2):
    - Due to pressure on head of fibula
    - Causes foot drop due to tibialis anterior palsy
  - Stretching of sciatic nerve: foot drop
  - Compression of popliteal neurovascular bundle by edges of holder
  - Improper technique of lowering legs may cause torsion stress on lumbar spine
  - ***Transient neurological symptoms (TNS):***
    - Especially common with 5% lidocaine and 1% tetracaine
    - Neuronal damage due to:
      - Increased release of glutamate causing increased intracellular calcium levels
      - This causes vacuolation and central chromatolysis of neurons in ***Obersteiner-Redlich zone***
    - More common when:
      - 5% lidocaine used for spinal anesthesia
      - In lithotomy position due to stretching of nerve fibers

NEURONAL TRANSMISSION

Definitions

- Action potential: Brief localized spikes of positive charge/depolarization on the cell membrane caused by rapid influx of Na^+ ions down its electrochemical gradient
- Threshold potential: The point at which the rate of depolarization abruptly increases

Types of Impulses

- Local, nonpropagated disturbances in potential: *Synaptic potential*
- Propagated disturbances in potential: *Action potential*
- Measurement of electrical events in living tissue is done with *cathode ray oscilloscope*

All or None Law

- Whether or not an impulse is conducted across the nerve fiber is determined by all or none law
- Once the threshold intensity is reached, a full fledged action potential is fired
- Further increase in intensity of stimulus produce no increment or change in action potential
- If the stimulus is subthreshold in magnitude, action potential fails to occur
- Thus, action potential is ***all or none*** in character

Electrogenesis of Action Potential

- Two factors contribute to electrical potential in cells:
  - Concentration gradient of ions across membrane
  - Selective permeation of ions through membrane
- Electrogenic Na^+K^+ATPase complex:
  - Transports 3 Na^+ ions out of the cell, for every 2 K^+ ions it moves into the cell
  - This creates a concentration gradient which favors movement of extracellular Na^+ into the cell and intracellular K^+ out of the cell
  - This gradient thus produces forces which tend to move the ions
- At rest:
  - The membrane is more permeable to K^+ than Na^+
  - Thus, a relative excess of negatively charged ions (anions) accumulates intracellularly
  - This accounts for the resting membrane potential (RMP) (–70 mv)
  - This RMP is close to the MP of K^+ (–80 mv)
- On application of a mechanical/chemical/electrical stimulus:
  - Depolarization occurs which fires an action potential when it exceeds the threshold potential (–55 mv)
  - This occurs as depolarization causes opening of VGSC (*voltage gated sodium channels*)
  - This causes influx of Na^+ ions and thus, a progressive reduction of negative polarity
- When the membrane potential reaches + 35 mv:
  - A sudden inactivation of Na^+ channels causes a drop in Na^+ permeability
  - This occurs along with an increased conductance of K^+ out of the cell
  - This returns the membrane to its resting potential
  - After reaching baseline, persistent K^+ efflux causes *after-hyperpolarization*

- After hyperpolarization:
  - Minor changes in the Na^+ and K^+ concentrations occur during this process
  - Baseline concentrations are then established using Na^+K^+ ATPase

Impulse Conduction

- Inward current entering the axon during depolarization flows within axoplasm and spreads to adjacent inactive regions
- These regions are rapidly depolarized by this local circuit current to levels far in excess of threshold potential, thus generating its own inward current
- Depending on presence of myelin, three types of conduction occur:
  - ***Saltatory conduction***:
    - Occurs in myelinated axons where depolarization jumps from one ***node of Ranvier*** to the next
    - Thus, myelinated axons conduct up to 50 times faster than unmyelinated fibers
  - ***Orthodromic conduction***: Conduction of impulses in one direction from synaptic junction along axons to their termination
  - ***Antidromic conduction***: Conduction in opposite direction

Factors Affecting Neuronal Responsiveness

- pH: Alkalosis increases excitability (seizures common in hyperventilated patients)
- Hypoxia: Total inexcitability of neurons within 3–5 seconds
- Inhaled anesthetics increase threshold for excitation and thus, reduce activity

Synaptic fatigue: Refers to a reduction in number of discharges by postsynaptic membrane, when synapses are repetitively and rapidly stimulated.

Post-tetanic Facilitation

- Increased responsiveness of postsynaptic neuron to stimulation after a rest period which was preceded by repetitive stimulation of an excitatory synapse
- This occurs due to increased release of neurotransmitters due to increased permeability to Ca^{2+}
- This may be responsible for mechanism ***of short term memory***

CONCENTRATION EFFECT

Definition

- Increasing inspired concentration of an anesthetic agent not only increases alveolar concentration but also the rate of rise of alveolar concentration (i.e.; F_A/F_I ratio)
- Predominantly seen for N_2O as it has low blood gas partition coefficient (0.47)

Factors Causing Concentration Effect

- *Concentrating effect*:
  - When a certain amount of gas is taken up by the blood (i.e. uptake), the alveolar size reduces
  - This reduction in alveolar size concentrates the gas remaining in the lung
  - The magnitude of this effect is influenced by concentration of gas within the lung
  - For example:
    - When the lung is filled with 1 part N_2O and 99 parts of O_2:
      - If one half of N_2O is taken, 0.5 parts N_2O and 99 parts of O_2 remains
      - Thus N_2O concentration is 0.5% (0.5/99.5)
    - If the same lung is filled with 80 parts of N_2O and 20 parts of O_2:
      - If one half of N_2O is taken, 40 parts of N_2O and 20 parts O_2 remain
      - Thus, concentration of N_2O remaining is 67% (40/60)
    - When inspired gas contains 100% of N_2O:
      - If 50% of N_2O is taken up, 50 parts of N_2O is present in 50 parts of alveolar gas
      - Thus, concentration remains 100%
- *Augmented inflow effect*:
  - When N_2O is taken up by blood, the alveolar volume reduces
  - To prevent alveolar collapse, additional inflow of gas occurs due to negative pressure and gas is drawn from trachea
  - This fresh inflow of gas replaces the volume of N_2O lost by uptake in blood
  - Thus, increased alveolar ventilation makes alveolar gas more like inspired gas
  - This reduces F_I/F_A concentration difference
  - For example:
    - If one half of N_2O is taken from an 80 parts N_2O and 20 parts O_2 mixture
    - 40 parts of N_2O and 20 parts of O_2 remain
    - N_2O concentration will be 67%

- The remaining 40 parts of gas is again filled by an 80% N_2O and 20% O_2 mixture, i.e.; by 32 parts of N_2O (80% of 40 parts) and 8 parts of O_2 (20% of 40 parts)
- Thus, total volume is now made by 72 parts of N_2O (40+32) and 28 (20+8) parts of O_2
- Thus, N_2O concentration becomes 72%

SECOND GAS EFFECT

Definition

Uptake of a large volume of first or primary gas (usually N_2O) from alveoli, increases rate of rise in alveolar concentration of a second gas given concomitantly.

Factors Causing Second Gas Effect

- *Concentrating effect*:
  - Uptake of large volume of N_2O causes a reduction in alveolar volume
  - Thus, concentration of all remnant gases in alveolus increases, including that of inhaled anesthetics
  - This is especially important for less soluble agents as their uptake into blood is less
- *Augmented inflow effect*:
  - The loss of volume of alveoli when large volume of N_2O is taken up by blood is replaced by fresh gas inflow with more inhaled anesthetic
  - This also increases alveolar concentration of inhaled anesthetic
  - This is especially important for more soluble agents as their uptake into blood is larger

Clinical importance: Since uptake of large volume of N_2O is limited to first 5–10 minutes of induction, these effects are important only during this period.

Controversy: ***Sun-X 1999 anesthesia analogue*** demonstrated that N_2O did not effect alveolar/blood concentration of enflurane under controlled ventilation.

DIFFUSION HYPOXIA/FINK EFFECT

Definition

Desaturation of a patient on termination of anesthetic which includes nitrous oxide within 5–10 minutes

Etiology

- As N_2O has low BGPC (0.47), large volume of N_2O diffuses from blood into alveoli upon termination of N_2O administration
- This occurs within 5–10 minutes of termination
- This has a twofold effect to cause hypoxia:
  - Displacement of alveolar oxygen:
    - N_2O diffusing into alveolus displaces alveolar O_2
    - If only room air is being administered during this time, fraction of alveolar O_2 can fall below 0.21 and cause hypoxia
  - Displacement of alveolar CO_2:
    - N_2O also displaces CO_2
    - If this causes the fraction of alveolar CO_2 to fall below the level needed to maintain $PaCO_2$ sufficient to drive ventilation, hypoventilation results
    - This causes further hypoxia
    - This is more important when residual narcotics are present or in patients with COPD
    - Diffusion hypoxia is prevented by administration of 100% O_2 for 5–10 minutes on termination of N_2O

PRINCIPLES AND USE OF ULTRASOUND IN ANESTHESIA

Introduction

- Ultrasound is a form of mechanical sound energy which travels through a conducting medium (e.g. body tissue) as a longitudinal wave producing compressions (high pressure) and rarefactions (low pressure)
- Human hearing range is 20–20,000 Hz
- Frequency of ultrasound wave is ≥ 20,000 Hz
- Medical ultrasound commonly is 2.5–15 mHz range

Generation of Ultrasound Wave

- An ultrasound wave is generated when a strong electrical field is applied to an array of piezoelectric crystals located on the transducer surface
- Electrical stimulation causes distortion of these crystals which then start vibrating
- This results in production of sound waves and is called ***converse piezoelectric effect***
- Each crystal generates an ultrasound wave
- The summation of all these waves produces an ultrasound beam
- The waves are generated in intermittent trains called pulses
- *Pulse length* is the distance travelled by one pulse
- Pulse repetition frequency (RPF):
  - Refers to the rate at which pulses are generated by the transducer (number of pulses per unit time)
  - This is important as ultrasound pulses must be spaced with enough time between pulses to permit the waves to reach the target, and return to the transducer before the next pulse is generated

Attenuation

- As the ultrasound beam travels through tissue layers, the amplitude of the original signal reduces and depth of penetration increases
- This is due to:
  - Absorption (conversion of acoustic energy to heat)
  - Reflection
  - Scattering at interfaces
- The attenuation caused by each tissue is represented by its *attenuation coefficient*
- Thus tissues like bone have a high attenuation coefficient and severely limits beam transmission
- Attenuation also varies with frequency of the ultrasound wave
- High frequency waves are more attenuated and thus have lesser tissue penetration and vice versa

Generation of Image

- The transducer waits to receive the returning wave (echo) after each pulsed wave
- The transducer then converts the echo (mechanical energy) into an electrical signal which is displayed on screen
- This is called ***piezoelectric effect***

Components of Ultrasound Scanner

- Pulser: Applies high amplitude voltage to energize crystals
- Transducer: Converts mechanical to electrical energy and vice versa
- Receiver: Receives and amplifies weak signals
- Memory: Stores video display
- Display: Displays ultrasound signals in a variety of modes

Modes of Display

- Amplitude (A) mode
- Brightness (B) mode
- Motion (M) mode
- B-modes is most often used for regional blocks

Echogenecity

- When an echo returns to the transducer, its amplitude is represented by the degree of brightness of a dot on display (***echogenicity***)
- Strong specular reflection produce bright dots (*hyperechoic shadows*):
  - Diaphragm
  - Pericardium
  - Bone
  - Gall and bladder stones
- Weaker diffuse reflections produce grey dots (*hypoechoic shadows*), e.g. solid organs
- No reflection produces dark dots (*anechoic shadows*), e.g. blood and fluid filled structure as the beam passes through without any reflection
- Nerves exhibit the phenomenon of ***anisotropy***:
  - Phenomenon where the echogenecity of the nerve varies with angle of insonation
  - Thus at 90°, reflection from the scanned nerve is maximal and image is best

Resolution

- Spatial resolution determines the degree of image clarity
- Resolution refers to the ability of ultrasound machine to distinguish two structures that are close together as separate
- Spatial resolution is influenced by axial and lateral resolution
- Axial resolution refers to the ability of to distinguish two structures which lie along the axis of ultrasound beam as separate and distinct
- Lateral resolution refers to resolution of objects lying side by side, i.e., perpendicular to beam axis

Imaging Plane and Approaches

- Nerves can be imaged in either short (transverse) axis or long (longitudinal) axis
- Blocks are usually performed in short axis (SAX) view
- With this view, identification of nerve fibers as modular structures is easy with good resolution
- Circumferential spread of LA on injection is also viewable

Color Doppler

- Instrument used to characterize blood flow and useful in identifying blood vessels in close proximity to nerves
- ***Doppler effect:***
  - Occurs when there is a moving source (RBCs) and a stationary listener (USG transducer)
  - There is an apparent change in frequency of returning echoes due to relative motion between sound source and receiver
  - RBCs moving towards transducer are perceived as higher frequency (red)
  - RBCs moving away from transducer are perceived as lower frequency (blue)

Uses of Ultrasound in Anesthesia

- First used by ***La Grange*** in 1978 for supraclavicular block
- In 1994 detailed paper on the same published by ***Stephen Kapral***
- Ultrasound guided nerve blocks:
  - Regional anesthesia
  - Chronic pain
- Ultrasound guidance for vascular access
- Diagnostic modality:
  - Pleural/pericardial effusion
  - Intra-abdominal hemorrhage
  - Perforated hollow viscus
  - Trauma patients
- Monitoring:
  - Transesophageal echocardiography
  - Cardiac output monitoring
  - Transthoracic echocardiography

Advantages of Ultrasound Guided Nerve Blocks

- Higher rate of success with failure rate 20% with paresthesia technique
- Reveals nerve localization and surrounding vascular structures
- Real time imaging guidance during needle advancement
- Images local anesthetic spread pattern during injection (***Doughnut sign***)
- Improves quality of sensory block, onset time and success rate compared to nerve stimulator technique
- Reduces number of needle attempts and the risk of nerve injury
- Prevents intravascular and intraneural injection

Ultrasound Guided Vascular Access

- Advantages:
  - High success rate
  - Less number of punctures: Reduces skin transfer of pathogens
  - Reduced incidence of complications
- Limitations:
  - Impractical: USG probes/sterile scanner manipulation
  - Unavailability of equipment
  - Lack of trained personnel

RAPID SEQUENCE INDUCTION

Introduction

- Rapid intravenous induction and muscle relaxation to aid endotracheal intubation, combined with cricoid pressure to reduce risk of pulmonary aspiration
- Virtually simultaneous administration of sedative hypnotic and neuromuscular blocking agent to render a patient rapidly unconscious in order to facilitate emergency tracheal intubation (*within 60–90 seconds*) and to minimize risk of aspiration by applying ***Sellicks maneuver***

Indications: Full stomach patients:

- Pregnancy
- Intestinal obstruction
- Preoperative gastroesophageal reflux, esophageal dilatation
- Hiatus hernia, strangulated hernia
- Inadequate NPO status:
  - Less than 6 hours for solids
  - Less than 4 hours for breast milk
  - Less than 2 hours for clear fluids
- Trauma, head injury, burns
- Maxillofacial trauma
- Autonomic neuropathy, associated with delayed gastric emptying

Principles for Rapid Sequence Induction

- Adequate preoxygenation must be performed (3–5 minutes)
- Sufficient dose of IV drugs to be given to ensure patient is adequately anesthetized
- Intubation within 60–90 seconds is considered acceptable
- Cricoid pressure:
  - Applied subsequent to injection of induction agent
  - Removed after checking position of ETT and inflating cuff

Preparation for Rapid Sequence Induction

- Trained assistant
- Working suction
- Tilting trolley
- Tested cuffed endotracheal tube
- Two functioning laryngoscopes, gum elastic bougie
- Routine monitoring, IV cannula
- Drawn up predefined dose of induction agent and succinylcholine
- Emergency drugs
- Plan for failed rapid sequence induction (RSI)

Conduct of RSI

- Check equipment
- Take baseline BP, heart rate, SPO_2 on room air

- Switch on suction and place within easy reach
- Preoxygenate with at least tidal volume breathing with tight fitting face mask for:
  - At least 3 minutes
  - Or, until ETO_2 reaches 90%
- Thiopentone 3–5 mg/kg administered IV
- Cricoid pressure at 30 N/3 kg force (9.8 N = 1 kg)
- Succinylcholine 1.5 mg/kg
- Intubate, inflate cuff, check position of ETT in sniffing position
- Remove cricoid pressure and continue anesthesia
- Nasogastric tube inserted to deflate stomach
- Awake extubation in lateral position

Other Methods of Rapid Muscle Relaxation

- Priming technique:
  - 10% of intubating dose of NMBA, administered 2–4 minutes before intubation dose
  - This accelerates onset of action of NMBA by 30–60 seconds
  - But, intubating condition not very good
  - Also, associated with aspiration and difficulty in swallowing
- High dose neuromuscular blocking agents:
  - Useful with rocuronium
  - Increasing dose of rocuronium from 0.6 mg/kg IV to 1.2 mg/kg IV reduces onset of action from 90 to 60 seconds
- Combination of NMBAs:
  - Mivacurium and rocuronium used in combination often
  - Does not have consistent effect

Adverse Effects of RSI

- Hemodynamic instability:
  - Due to excessive dose of induction agent
  - Hypertension, tachycardia and awareness if inadequate anesthesia
- Problems with cricoid pressure:
  - BURP (backwards, upwards, rightwards pressure) improves view but increases chances of airway obstruction
  - Impedes laryngoscopy and distorts view
  - May cause esophageal rupture
  - Cricoid cartilage fracture, especially if patient is on steroids.

Failed RSI Regimen after Succinylcholine

- Announce failed intubation and call for help
- Maintain cricoid pressure
- Insert oral airway
- Ventilate with face mask and 100% oxygen
- Try four handed bag and mask ventilation with extra person
- Insert laryngeal mask airway (LMA): Release cricoid force temporarily as LMA is swept into place
- Reapply cricoid force and attempt ventilation
- Release cricoid force and attempt ventilation
- If ventilation not possible, emergency cricothyrotomy if patient is not waking up or spontaneously breathing

Other Techniques to Prevent Aspiration

- *Newcastle technique*:
  - Based on assumption that patient cannot hyperventilate and vomit simultaneously
  - Uses hyperventilation with N_2O, O_2 and ether
- 20° head down tilt in lateral position
- 40° head up tilt:
  - Maneuver raises larynx by 19 cm above lower esophageal sphincter
  - It prevents passive reflux, but increases likelihood of aspiration if vomiting occurs

Special Situations

- Myasthenia gravis:
  - May be resistant to succinylcholine
  - Use 1.5 mg/kg succinylcholine with vecuronium 0.01 mg/kg IV
- Pediatric patients:
  - May not cooperate for preoxygenation
  - Desaturation occurs faster
  - Force for cricoid pressure not yet established
  - Gentle face mask ventilation after induction
  - If uncuffed tube used, put throat pack to prevent intraoperative aspiration
  - Succinylcholine is preceded by atropine to prevent bradycardia
  - Nasogastric tube inserted after intubation

CRICOID PRESSURE

Introduction

- Temporary occlusion of upper end of esophagus by backward pressure on cricoid cartilage against body of C5/C6 vertebra
- Also called ***Sellicks maneuver***

Indications

- ❖ Pregnancy
- ❖ Intestinal obstruction
- ❖ Preoperative gastroesophageal reflux, esophageal dilatation
- ❖ Hiatus hernia, strangulated hernia
- ❖ Inadequate NPO status:
  - Less than 6 hours for solids
  - Less than 4 hours for breast milk
  - Less than 2 hours for clear fluids
- ❖ Trauma, head injury, burns
- ❖ Maxillofacial trauma
- ❖ Autonomic neuropathy, associated with delayed gastric emptying

Contraindications

- ❖ Suspected cricotracheal injury
- ❖ Active vomiting
- ❖ Unstable cervical spine injury
- ❖ May be difficult in patients with history difficult intubation

Mode of Application

- ❖ Position:
  - Tonsillectomy position/sniffing position
  - Extension on neck, cervical spine flexed on thorax
- ❖ Timing:
  - Upon initiation of induction
  - Incremental forces:
    - 20 N while patient is conscious
    - 30 N upon loss of consciousness
- ❖ Methods of application:
  - Single handed cricoid pressure:
    - Thumb and middle finger placed on cricoid cartilage
    - Index finger placed above, to prevent lateral movement of cricoid cartilage
  - Double handed cricoid pressure:
    - Counter pressure with hand placed beneath cervical vertebrae to support neck
    - One hand placed under hyperextended neck
    - Other hand applies cricoid pressure
    - Better in cervical spine pathology
- ❖ Cricoid yoke:
  - Hand held device with foam contact cushion molded to fit over cricoid cartilage
  - Applies pressure set at predetermined values
- ❖ Nasogastric tube (NGT):
  - NGT must be left open to atmosphere to vent air/liquid
  - This limits rise in intragastric pressure during induction
  - Presence of NGT may reduce incidence of aspiration
  - Chances of passive regurgitation may be higher
  - If NGT already present, empty stomach before induction

Withdrawal of cricoid pressure: After tube position is checked and ETT cuff is inflated.

Complications of Cricoid Pressure

- ❖ Insufficient pressure may allow aspiration
- ❖ Excessive pressure (more than 40 N):
  - Completely occludes laryngeal lumen, especially in young females
  - Difficulty in laryngoscopy and intubation
  - Difficulty with fall mask ventilation
  - Difficulty with LMA insertion
  - Esophageal rupture
  - Cricoid cartilage fracture, especially if patient is on long term steroids (asthmatics)

VENTURI PRINCIPLE

Introduction

- ❖ It is a reduction in fluid pressure which results when a fluid flows through a constricted section of pipe
- ❖ *Coanda effect*: If such a constriction occurs at a bifurcation, due to increase in velocity and decrease in pressure, fluid (air, blood) tends to stick to one side of the branch causing maldistribution

Explanation

- ❖ Any apparatus containing a tube with a constriction and an opening at the constriction will suck in air/fluid due to low pressure at that site (***Bernoulli's principle***). Such an apparatus is called Venturi apparatus
- ❖ When a gas passes through a tube with a narrowed diameter, its pressure is reduced
- ❖ So as to keep the energy constant, velocity of the gas increases.

Applications

Clinical Signs

- ❖ Obstructive sleep apnea syndrome: Collapse of airway occurs due to turbulent flow through obstructed airways
- ❖ Mucus plug present at branching of tracheobronchial tree may cause maldistribution of gases.
- ❖ *Pulsus bisferiens* in aortic regurgitation
- ❖ Unequal flow may occur due to plaques in vascular tree (*coronary steal* due to Coanda effect)

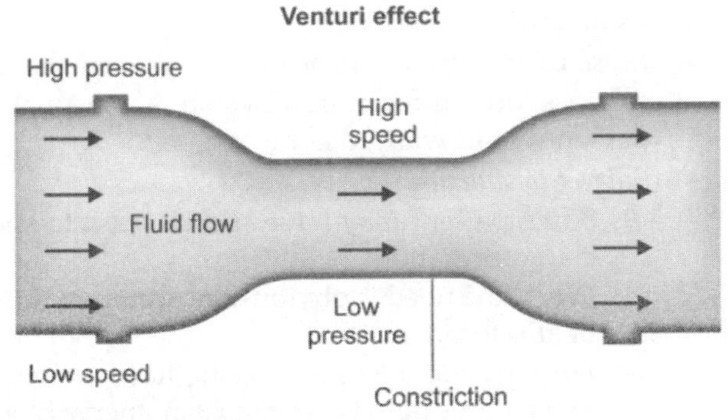

Fig. 1: Venturi principle.

Venturi Devices

- Venturi mask:
  - Color coding:
    - Color of the mask's aperture determines the FiO_2
    - FiO_2 delivered by blue mask 24%
    - FiO_2 delivered by white mask is 28%
    - FiO_2 delivered by yellow mask is 35%
    - FiO_2 delivered by red mask is 40%
    - FiO_2 delivered by green mask is 60%
  - Working principle:
    - Oxygen mask having different diameter ports at the distal end
    - It thus entrains air into oxygen flow
    - At point A, 100% oxygen flows into wider point B via narrow orifice
    - Due to narrowing, oxygen speeds up and pressure drops at that point is below atmospheric pressure
    - Thus, room air is drawn to this point, diluting the 100% oxygen to a calibrated value set by the colored nozzle
    - The nozzle has a varying aperture open to room air, which sets the entrapment ratio and thus the FiO_2 given to the patient
- Oxygen tents
- ***Pethick's test*** for checking Bains circuit
- Nebulizer:
  - Oxygen passes through the liquid present in reservoir containing medication
  - Water droplets containing medication is generated which is inhaled
- Vaporizers, humidifier
- Jet ventilation:
  - High-frequency jet ventilation (HFJV) through a small catheter in trachea
  - Oxygen flow through catheter entrains air
- ***Saunders injector*** in Venturi ventilation for bronchography:
  - Two 16 gauge cannulae are attached to proximal end of bronchoscope
  - A jet of oxygen blows through the cannula
  - This will generate sufficient force to draw in room air and deliver air at substantial positive pressure
- PEEP valve
- For driving gases in a ventilator
- Suction apparatus
- Use of helium for treating laryngospasm:
  - Helium is a gas of low density and hence reduces turbulent flow
  - This reduces velocity of gas flow through the narrow laryngeal orifice
  - Therefore, laryngeal obstruction is relieved

INFORMED CONSENT

Introduction

Legal and moral imperatives for informed consent are based on ethical principle of respect for patient autonomy, i.e., ability to choose without controlling interference by others and without personal limitations which prevent meaningful choices.

Components

- Name and purpose of diagnostic test or procedure
- Most significant risks of test/procedure
- Benefits of intervention, including chances of success if pertinent
- Probable outcome of intervention/refusal of proposed plan
- Possible alternatives and procedure
- Patient must be free from concerns

Definition

- Consent requires an active communication between doctor and patient wherein the physician educates the patient explaining the nature and purpose of the proposed procedure or therapy, along with the attendant risks and benefits
- In the Indian context, informed consent was nonexistent till Consumer Protection Act was made applicable to medical profession

Documentation of Consent

- Hand written note:
  - Is the best evidence of discussion and consent?
  - Time consumed in the process however, is unacceptable

- Separate anesthesia consent form required, with common risks detailed in separate form
- Reliance on surgical consent is not very reliable

Ethical Aspects of Consent

- Ethical obligation to respect patients autonomy
- Obligation to respect patients right to be involved in decisions which affect them
- Patient must be supplied adequate information to make a balanced decision free from coercion
- Need to respect autonomy may conflict with other obligations like *principles of beneficence (doing good)*
- For example, patient may decline life saving therapy and this may have to be respected

Legal Aspects of Consent

- Touching a patient without consent may lead to chain of battery or assault
- Treating doctor is responsible for ensuring that patient has consent for treatment
- Consent is valid if given voluntarily by appropriately informed patient who has capacity to exercise a choice
- Patient without capacity to consent, may be treated without consent, if it is in their best interest/consent is taken from guardian
- Pain, illness, premedication does not necessarily render a patient incompetent to consent

Informed Refusal

- Informed consent is meaningless if patient cannot also refuse medical treatment
- For example:
  - Request to withdraw life support and care in ICU
  - Do not resuscitate (DNR) orders in operation theater
  - Jehovahs witness patients who refuse blood transfusion
  - Patient refusing preoperative testing like HIV and pregnancy test

Disclosure

- Informed consent requires honest disclosure of medical information to patient
- Therapeutic privilege cited if stress of discussing risk can harm patient psychologically/physically
- Physician must discuss therapy, its alternatives and no therapy
- He should also disclose the common and serious risks
- Two standards of disclosure:
  - *Reasonable person standard*: Physician must disclose any information which a reasonable person would want to know
  - *Subject to standard*:
    - Some patient may have special need to special information
    - When the need is obvious, information must be disclosed
    - For e.g.: Violinist has specific need to know about nerve damage from axillary nerve block

Outcome

- Patient will have sufficient knowledge to make an educated decision whether or not to undergo the proposed therapeutic intervention
- Physicians have ethical obligation to avoid exploiting their influence on patients and to coerce or manipulate than into decision by threats/misinterpreting information

COMPUTERS IN ANESTHESIA

Introduction

Various applications of computers in anesthesia are:

- Hospital information systems
- Electronic health record
- Computerized order entry
- Decision support system/artificial intelligence
- Telemedicine
- Computer integrated private cloud appliance (PCA) devices
- Target control infusion

Hospital Information System

- Network of interfaced subsystems, both hardware and software, which coexist to serve the multiple computing requirements of a hospital including:
  - Admission and discharge
  - Transfer
  - Billing
  - Laboratory, radiology
- Component elements:
  - Administrators
  - Clinical documentation
  - Billing systems
  - Business systems

Electronic Health Record

- It is a computerized record of patient care
- It includes:
  - ICU record

- Out patient record
- Emergency department record
- Nursing home electronic record
- Dialysis electronic record

❖ Core function (benefits) includes:
- Management of patients health information and data
- Presentation of results acquired from patients testing
- Computerized order entry
- Decision support: Autogenerated reminder to inform the behavior of clinician

❖ Patient support tools such as discharge directions generated automatic billing management, insurance validation

❖ Internal and external reporting requirements simplified

Computerized Ordered Entry

❖ It is a computer based ordering system, designed to automate the ordering process

❖ Example, for drugs, pathology/radiology tests

❖ Benefits of computerized order entry:
- Identification of prescribers
- Standardized legible orders
- Link to adverse drug reporting system
- Cost management
- Reduce confusion of drug name
- Improved order turn around

Decision Support System/Artificial Intelligence

❖ Provides immediate access to current medical knowledge, institutional best practices, billing compliance information, administrative function and facilitates cost control

❖ Acts in three ways:
- Passive system: Responds when information is asked
- Semiactive system: Provides alarms only when certain condition are met
- Active/autonomous system: Generates order and manages medical process automatically

❖ For example: Automated weaning of mechanical ventilator

Telemedicine

❖ Application of healthcare server across space, time, social and cultural barriers

❖ Useful in underserved areas and providing access to specialist in remote areas

❖ Allowing patients to receive medical attention at home when physical contact is not a critical element

❖ New technologies like teleimmersion, telepresence, telesurgery are coming up

ANESTHESIA FOR SCOLIOSIS CORRECTION

Introduction

Deformity characterized by coronal, sagittal and horizontal plane deviation of spine associated with rotation of vertebrae.

Classification

I. Nonstructural/Mobile Scoliosis

❖ Sciatica

❖ Leg length discrepancy

❖ Hip contracture causing pelvic tilt

II. Structural Scoliosis

❖ Idiopathic:
- Infantile < 3 yrs
- Juvenile 3–10 yrs
- Adolescent >10 yrs

❖ Congenital:
- Hemivertebrae
- Spinal dysmorphism
- Fused ribs

❖ Syndromes:
- *VATER anomaly*
- *Von-Recklinghausen's*/neurofibromatosis
- *Marfan syndrome*
- Rheumatoid arthritis
- *Ehlers Danlos syndrome*

❖ Post-trauma:
- Vertebral fracture
- Postsurgery
- Post-thoracoplasty
- Postradiation
- Postburns contracture

❖ Neuromuscular:

Neuropathic:
- Cerebral palsy
- Polio myelitis
- Spinal cord injury
- *Freidrich's ataxia*
- Meningomyelocele

Myopathic:
- *Duchenne muscular dystrophy*
- Myotonic dystrophy

Pathophysiology

- Pulmonary:
  - Reduced vital capacity
  - Reduced total lung volume
  - Reduced functional residual capacity
  - Ventilation perfusion mismatch
  - Hypoxia, hypercarbia
  - Respiratory failure
- Cardiovascular:
  - Pulmonary HTN
  - RV hypertrophy and failure
  - Associated defects:
    - Mitral valve prolapse
    - Coarctation of aorta
    - Mitral regurgitation
    - Cyanotic heart disease
    - Aortic regurgitation

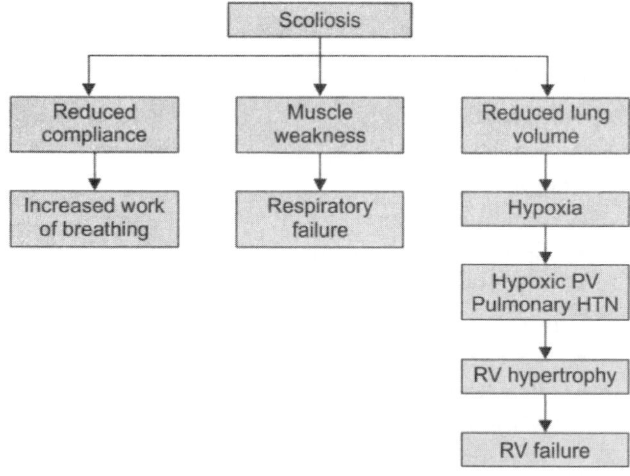

(PV: pressure-volume; HTN: hypertension; RV: right ventricular)

Assessment of Severity

Severity increases with:

- Greater number of vertebrae involved
- More cephalad location of curve
- Loss of normal thoracic kyphosis
- Increased Cobb's angle

Cobb's Angle

Measurement

- Perpendicular drawn from bottom of lowest vertebrae whose bottom tilts towards concavity of curve
- Perpendicular from top of highest vertebra whose top tilts towards concavity
- Angle at which perpediculars intersect is Cobb's angle

No.	Angle	Implication
1.	<20°	Benign
		Monitored every 4 months by X-ray
		No surgery required
2.	>40°	Cardiorespiratory impairment present
		Restrictive lung disease
3.	>100°	Severe cardiorespiratory involvement
		Severe impairment of gaseous exchange

Indications for Surgery

- Cobb's angle > 50°
- Neurological involvement
- Pain
- Cosmetic purposes

Surgical Technique

- Posterior spinal fusion with:
  - ***Herrington rod***
  - ***Cotrel Dubousset instrumentation***
- Anterior approach
  - Thoracotomy
  - Transdiaphragmatic
  - Transabdominal
- Combined posteroanterior approach

Preoperative Evaluation

- Cardiovascular, respiratory and neuromuscular status
- Cobb's angle
- Associated congenital anomalies
- Neurological deficits especially on neck rotation

Investigations

- Complete blood count—increased HCT due to chronic hypoxia
- Coagulation profile—PT and INR on day of surgery
- ECG for cor pulmonale
- Pulmonary function tests:
  - Reduced vital capacity, TLC, FRC, IC, ERV
  - Normal FEV_1/FVC
- PEFR as bedside test to assess severity
- 2D ECHO as mitral valvce prolapse MR, AR, and cardiomyopathy possible
- ABG—baseline values noted: Reduced PaO_2 with normal $PaCO_2$ and pH
- X-ray spine, CT thorax, preoperative myelogram/MRI for cysts/lipomas/teratomas

Preoperative Preparation

- Preoperative teaching of incentive spirometry and coughing

- Aggressive pulmonary toilet
- Bronchodilator therapy if COPD
- If intraoperative wake-up test planned:
  - Rehearse the test
  - Reassure patient about lack of pain
- Discuss with the patient:
  - Autologous transfusion
  - Awake intubation/tracheostomy
  - Postoperative ventilation
  - Postoperative pain management
  - Sleep apnea syndrome
  - Prone position and inability to lie flat

Premedication

- Sedatives avoided if neuromuscular disease/pulmonary HTN
- Antisialogogues—glycopyrrolate
- Antibiotics before catheterization/laryngoscopy
- Steroids if any neurodeficits
- DVT prophylaxis

Monitors

- General:
  - Pulse oximeter: IBP for hypotensive anesthesia
  - End tidal CO_2: CVP/PA catheter for pulmonary HTN
  - ECG: Urine output
  - Temperature: Esophageal stethoscope
  - Thromboelastography: Neuromuscular monitoring
- Spinal cord monitoring:
  - Intraoperative wake-up test
  - Somatosensory evoked potentials (SSEPS-posterior column)
  - Motor evoked potentials (MEPS-anterolateral tracts)

Anesthetic Considerations

- Long duration surgery
- Blood loss:
  - Blood conservation strategies
  - Hypotensive anesthesia
- Hypothermia due to large surgical field exposure
- ***Difficult airway***
- ***Remote airway***
- Difficult regional anesthesia technique
- One lung ventilation if anterior approach
- Restrictive lung defect:
  - Increased risk of postoperative respiratory insufficiency
  - Retention of secretions
  - Postoperative respiratory failure
  - Right ventricular failure and pulmonary HTN postoperative
- Increased risk of ***Malignant hyperthermia***

Induction

- On trolley with all monitors
- Thiopentone/etomidate/propofol as induction agents
- Fentanyl and nondepolarizing neuromuscular blocking agents
- Succinylcholine avoided in muscular dystrophy
- Intubate with fiberoptic bronchoscopy
- Sometimes tracheostomy done
- Fix tube properly as remote airway
- Armoured tube to avoid kinking
- DLT/bronchial blocker with one lung ventilation if anterior approach
- Nasogastric tube as ***postoperative ileus*** common

Maintenance

$O_2 + N_2O$ + volatile agents + fentanyl + vecuronium

OR

TIVA with propofol and remifentanyl infusion

Position

- Prone position:
  - If posterior approach
  - Prevent neck extension—to minimize venous pressure and blood loss
  - Abdomen should be free to avoid IVC compression
  - Protect pressure points
  - Eye protection
  - ***Wilson frame/Jackson table*** to free chest and abdomen
- Lateral position:
  - If anterior approach
  - Pad pressure points adequately

Ventilation

Avoid hypoxia hypercarbia and acidosis.

Hemodynamics

- Deliberate hypotension:
  - MAP between 60 and 70 mm Hg to maintain spinal cord perfusion
  - NTG/SNP/esmolol/propranolol used
- Maintain normothermia/normocarbia
- Warming devices for patients and fluids
- Moderate third space losses: Replace with BSS at 5–7 mL/kg/hr

Blood Conservation

- Preoperative optimization of Hb
- Modest hypotension

- Coagulation control
- *Cell salvage*
- Antifibrinolytic agents
- Autologous blood transfusion
- *Isovolemic hemodilution*
- Reduce intra-abdominal pressure:
  - NMBAs to avoid increased abdominal wall tension
  - Careful positioning
  - Deep plane of anesthesia

Extubation

- Most need elective postop ventilation
- Extubate patients with mild-to-moderate PFT abnormalities
- Extubation parameters:
  - Vital capacity > 10 mL/kg
  - Tidal volume > 5 mL/kg
  - Spontaneous respiratory rate < 30/min
  - Negative inspiratory force > –30 cm H_2O
- Postoperative ventilation if:
  - Severe restrictive lung defects
  - Vital capacity < 30% predicted
  - CO_2 retention
  - *Duchenne muscular dystrophy*
  - Cerebral palsy

Postoperative

I. Complications

- Pneumothorax, hemothorax/pleural effusion
- Atelectasis, hypoxia
- Ventilation perfusion mismatch
- Disseminated intravascular coagulation
- SIADH
- Infections
- Paralytic ileus
- Spinal cord injury
- Thoracic duct injury: *Chylothorax*
- Thromboembolism

II. Monitoring

- Pulse oximetry
- ABG
- Blood urea nitrogen
- PT INR
- Platelet count
- Blood pressure
- X-ray
- Serum creatinine
- Urine output
- Serum electrolytes Q12H for 24 hours

III. Pain

- Epidural analgesia
- Patient controlled analgesia
- Intravenous opioids
- Intrathecal opioids
- Paravertebral blocks
- Extrapleural catheters
- *Multimodal analgesia*

IV. Management

- Aggressive chest physiotherapy
- Incentive spirometry
  - Deep breathing
  - Coughing
  - Bronchodilator therapy
- Maintain urine output > 0.5 mL/kg/hr
- Avoid hypotonic fluids for 1st 24–36 hours postoperative
- Compression stockings/pneumatic leg pumps for DVT prophylaxis

WAKE-UP TEST

Introduction

- Intraoperative awakening of patient after completion of spinal instrumentation to assess integrity of spinal motor pathways
- Described first by ***Vauzelle***

Preparation

- 1–2 assistants to be available in the event of excessive movement
- Discontinue propofol and muscle relaxants 30–45 minutes before test
- Discontinue volatile agents 20 minutes before test
- Continue opioid infusion to allow patient to tolerate pain
- Patients usually respond within 5 minutes
- Avoid naloxone as it causes pain and patient may become agitated
- If necessary naloxone 0.3–0.5 μg/kg boluses every 2–3 minutes
- Reversal of NM blockade unnecessary if 3 twitches are present on TOF
- Excessive movement rare if nitrous – narcotic – relaxant technique used

Procedure

- Patient instructed to squeeze anesthetists hand—confirms responsiveness

- Then asked to move feet and toes
- If patient moves hands but unable to move feet reduce amount of distraction and repeat test
- Once patient moves feet deepen plane of anesthesia with benzodiazepines, thiopentone and muscle relaxant

Interpretation

- Patient moves hands and feet—correct screw placement
- Patient moves hands but not feet—screws need realignment
- Patient does not move hands/feet—patient not awake

Disadvantages

- Only one time indicator
- Cannot be done in children/mentally retarded
- Rarely may be false negative—patient can have neurodeficit at the end of surgery
- Replaced largely by SSEP/MEP

Complications

- Prone position extubation
- Intraoperative awareness
- Self injury
- Dislodgement of instruments
- Air embolus from open venous sinus if patient inhales vigorously
- Myocardial infarction

OBESITY

Introduction

Disease characterized by abnormally high percentage of body weight as fat.

Pathological Changes

- Respiratory system:
  - Pulmonary function tests:
    - Reduced FRC, VC, TLC, ERV
    - Normal FEV_1, FVC
  - Obstructive sleep apnea
  - Obesity hypoventilation syndrome: ***Pickwickian syndrome***:
    - Obesity (BMI > 30 kg/m^2)
    - Awake arterial hypercapnea ($PaCO_2$ >45 mm Hg)
  - Small airway obstruction, asthma
  - Pulmonary HTN, cor pulmonale
- Cardiovascular system:
  - Increased total blood volume
  - Increased cardiac output: Up to 20–30 mL per kg of excess fat
  - Left ventricular hypertrophy, reduced ventricular compliance
  - Increased left ventricular filling pressures, diastolic dysfunction
  - Pulmonary edema, biventricular failure
  - Dormant CAD
  - Cardiac arrhythmias due to:
    - Fatty infilteration of conduction system
    - CAD, myocardial hypertrophy
    - Hypoxia and hypercapnea, OSAS
    - Electrolyte imbalance
    - Increased circulating catecholamines
  - ECG changes:
    - Low voltage QRS complexes
    - LVH, left atrial enlargement, left axis deviation
    - T wave inversion in inferior and lateral leads
  - Hypertension:
    - SBP increases by 3–4 mm Hg with every 10 kg weight gained
    - DBP increases by 2 mm Hg with every 10 kg weight gained
    - Occurs due to RAS stimulation causing sodium retention and HTN
- Gastrointestinal tract:
  - Predisposed to aspiration:
    - Gastric volumes > 25 mL
    - Gastric pH > 2.5 causes increased pneumonitis if aspiration occurs
    - Delayed gastric emptying
    - GERD, acid peptic disease, hiatus hernia
  - Colonic carcinoma, cholelithiasis
  - Nonalcoholic Fatty Liver Disease (NAFLD)
  - Nonalcoholic Steatohepatitis (NASH)
- Genitourinary system:
  - ESRD
  - Macrosomia
  - Prostatic carcinoma
  - Urinary incontinence
  - Menorrhagia, ecclampsia, preeclampsia
- Endocrine system:
  - Type II diabetes mellitus
  - Dyslipidemia
  - Hypothyroidism
  - ***Insulin resistance, metabolic syndrome***
- Central nervous system:
  - Carpal tunnel syndrome
  - ***Pseudotumor cerebri***

- Stroke
- Endogenous depression

❖ Blood:
- Hypercoagulability: Increased factor VII, vWF, PAI-I
- Relative polycythemia

❖ Musculoskeletal system:
- ***Acanthosis nigricans***
- Gout
- Osteoarthritis
- Rheumatoid arthritis

Anesthetic Considerations

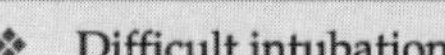

❖ Difficult intubation
❖ Difficult IV access
❖ Difficult monitoring
❖ Difficult positioning
❖ Increased dosage of anesthetic agents
❖ Judicious fluid administration as CCF may be precipitated
❖ Increased chances of nerve injuries
❖ Difficult regional anesthetic technique

Regional Anesthesia

❖ Useful alternative to GA

❖ Technically difficult as:
- Difficult to identify bony landmarks
- Higher regional block failure rates
- Easier in lumbar region as less fat in this area

❖ Longer needles, sitting position, USG and fluoroscopy used to make procedure easier

❖ Dose requirement for epidural analgesia may be reduced due to:
- Vascular engorgement
- Fatty infilteration which reduces volume of the space

❖ Subarachnoid block:
- Not as difficult as epidural
- Height of block is difficult to control causing fast upward spread of the LA
- Continuous catheter SAB is better

❖ Combination of epidural and GA:
- Allows use of larger oxygen concentration
- Provides optimal muscle relaxation
- Provides option for postoperative analgesia

Ambulatory Anesthesia

❖ Done in obese individuals with stable concomitant diseases

❖ Morbidly obese patient with unstable comorbidities and no patient escort are unsuitable

❖ Individual evaluation and proper selection is important

❖ Use of regional blocks where feasible, rapidly dissipating anesthetic agents and appropriate sized equipment should be combined

❖ Technically challenging as dose titration is required

Preoperative Evaluation

❖ Respiratory system:
- Pulmonary function tests: Reduced ERV is the *most sensitive* indicator for pulmonary impairment
- Sleep study: May be necessary in patients with OSA/OHS

❖ Cardiovascular system:
- ECG: RVH, RAD, RV strain: Pulmonary HTN
- ECHO: Tricuspid regurgitation is confirmatory for pulmonary HTN
- Stress test:
  - Patients lead a sedentary lifestyle
  - These patients may have a dormant CAD without symptoms
  - Thus, stress test may be necessary

❖ Blood tests:
- Serum glucose and thyroid hormone status
- Serum electrolytes especially important in a setting of chronic hypercapnea
- Serum creatinine
- Serum vitamin B_{12}, folate, iron, and calcium levels: ***Acute postgastric reduction surgery polyneuropathy***
- Arterial blood gas
- Liver function tests (LFTs):
  - Raised alanine aminotransferase *most commonly* seen
  - Clearance is usually preserved even in the presence of abnormal LFTs

❖ Airway: Difficult airway due to:
- Short, thick neck
- Excessive tissue folds in the mouth and pharynx
- Thick suprasternal, presternal, submental fat pads
- Limited movement of atlanto-occipital joints by low cervical fat pads: Causes reduced thyromental distance

❖ Neck circumference:
- *Neck circumference > 40 cm* indicates increased incidence of OSA
- This is *single biggest predictor* of difficult intubation in these patients

❖ Difficult venous access: CVP may be necessary for venous access

Preoperative Medications

- All medications to be continued on morning of surgery except insulin and OHAs
- Anxiolysis with benzodiazepines
- Antiaspiration prophylaxis:
  - 30 mL of nonparticulate sodium citrate
  - 50 mg ranitidine IV
  - 10 mg metoclopramide or 8 mg ondansetron IV
- DVT prophylaxis:
  - S/C heparin 5,000 IU before surgery and every 12 hours after surgery till fully mobile
  - S/C enoxaparin 40 mg Q12H

Intraoperative Care

Position

- Specially designed ***Hercules table*** available
- Particular care of pressure points as increased chances of:
  - Nerve injuries
  - Rhabdomyolysis
  - Pressure sores
- ***Walters Henderson maneuver*** for shifting patient on and off table
- Supine position:
  - IVC and aortic compression
  - Reduced FRC and oxygenation
  - Worsened in head down position
- Prone position: Reduced lung compliance and ventilation
- Lateral decubitus position: *Best preferred* as better diaphragmatic movement
- Position at intubation:
  - Stacking with towels or pillows to bring chin above the level of chest
  - ***Head ELevated Laryngoscopy Position (HELLP):***
    - Done with *troop elevation pillows*
    - Brings external auditory meatus in line with sternal angle

Monitors

- Pulse oximetry, E_TCO_2
- ECG, precordial stethoscope
- NIBP cuff size may be small for arm circumference
- Invasive arterial BP monitoring required as spuriously high BP values may result from small cuffs
- PA catheter inserted if pulmonary hypertension present
- Temperature, neuromuscular monitoring, urine output

Pharmacological Considerations

- Increased blood volume in obese patients reduces the plasma concentration of drugs injected
- Fat has low blood flow and thus, calculating the dose based on TBW may cause excess plasma concentration
- Calculating initial dose based on LBW with subsequent doses based on pharmacological response is best approach
- LBW in obese persons calculated by adding 20–30% to the ideal body weight (IBW)
- $IBW = 22 \times height^2$
- IBW = height (cm) – x, where:
  x = 100 in males
  x = 105 in females
- Repeated injection accumulates in fat and causes prolonged response

Induction

- Difficult mask ventilation: Gather fat pads in cheek around the mask for better fit
- Preoxygenation:
  - Preoxygenate adequately as rapid desaturation occurs due to reduced FRC
  - Four vital capacity breaths with 100% oxygen within 30 seconds *recommended*
- Induction agents:
  - Larger doses are required
  - Dose of all agents except succinylcholine is calculated according to LBW
  - Dosage of succinylcholine is according to TBW as the pseudocholinesterase increases proportionately to TBW
- Intubation:
  - Difficult intubation anticipated
  - LMA, gum elastic bougie kept ready
  - Use *polio blade with short handle*
  - Awake fiberoptic intubation preferred
  - Sedation with dexmedetomidine useful
  - Head ELevated Laryngoscopy Position
  - Xylocard 1.5 mg/kg IV given prior to intubation if hypertensive
  - Intubation attempted when expired oxygen ≥ 90%

Maintenance

- TIVA or balanced anesthesia with inhalation agents can be used
- Nitrous oxide:
  - May be a good choice
  - Avoid if pulmonary HTN present

- High oxygen demand limits its use
- Also causes abdominal distention reducing FRC further

❖ Desflurane may be preferred due to better hemodynamic stability

❖ Halothane avoided as:
- Increased sensitization to catecholamines
- Increased chances of halothane hepatitis

❖ Short acting opioids facilitate rapid and smooth emergence

❖ Cisatracurium, vecuronium and rocuronium useful

❖ Dexmedetomidine may be a useful sedative and analgesic

Ventilation

❖ Pressure control mode very useful

❖ Tidal volumes > 10 mL/kg offer no added advantages

❖ Maintain minute volume of around 5 liters

❖ PEEP:
- Improves lung compliance and oxygenation
- Prevents V-Q mismatch
- Detrimental if pulmonary HTN present

Hemodynamics

❖ Judicious fluid administration as CCF may be precipitated

❖ Adipose tissue masks tissue perfusion: fluid balance may be difficult to assess

❖ Blood loss is greater due to more extensive dissection to reach the surgical site

❖ Early colloid and blood product infusion required as these patients are less able to compensate for blood loss

Postoperative Care

Extubation

❖ Prompt extubation necessitated as patient may become ventilator dependant

❖ Extubated in semi-recumbent position as this has lesser adverse effect on respiration

❖ Reversal:
- Prompt and early reversal but slow full recovery seen with neostigmine induced reversal of vecuronium
- Neostigmine dosed according to TBW

❖ Sugammadex:
- Modified cyclodextrin derivative
- Encapsulates rocuronium
- Causes rapid and complete reversal of rocuronium induced neuromuscular blockade

Management

❖ Walter Henderson maneuver with patient transfer device to safely transfer patient

❖ Nursed in semirecumbent position

❖ Respiratory care:
- Adequate analgesia
- Use of elastic binder
- Early ambulation
- Deep breathing exercises
- Incentive spirometry
- CPAP or bilevel positive airway pressure initiated for those with OSAS

Monitors

❖ Pulse oximetry

❖ IBP, ECG, temperature

❖ Blood sugar, arterial blood gas monitoring.

Postoperative Analgesia

❖ Epidural analgesia:
- Useful analgesia with opioids and local anesthetics
- Allows early ambulation and prevents DVT

❖ Patient controlled analgesia:
- Done with morphine-PCA
- Nausea and pruritus is also reduced

❖ Local infilteration of wound with bupivacaine

❖ Multimodal analgesia:
- Combines PCA and local infilteration
- Better analgesia than either techniques done alone

OBSTRUCTIVE SLEEP APNEA

Definition

❖ Obstructive sleep apnea:
- Complete cessation of airflow
- Lasting 10 seconds or longer
- Despite maintaining ventilatory effort
- Occurring ≥ 5 times per hour of sleep
- Reduction of at least 4% in SaO_2

❖ Obstructive sleep hypopnea:
- Partial cessation of airflow (≥ 50%)
- Lasting ≥ 10 seconds
- Despite maintaining ventilatory efforts
- Occurring ≥ 15 times per hour of sleep
- Reduction of at least 4% in SaO_2

- Obesity hypoventilation (Pickwickian) syndrome:
  - Obesity (BMI > 30 kg/m^2)
  - Awake arterial hypercapnea ($PaCO_2$ > 45 mm Hg)
  - Absence of other causes of hypoventilation

Grading

- Done using the ***apnea-hypopnea index (AHI)*** which is derived from polysomnography
- $$AHI = \frac{\text{Number of episodes of apnea/hypopnea}}{\text{Total sleep time in hours}}$$
- Normal limit of AHI = 5–10 events per hour
- Grading of OSAS:
  - Mild disease = 5–15 events/hr
  - Moderate disease = 16–30 events/hr
  - Severe disease = ≥ 30 events/hr
- ***Total arousal index (TAI)*** = total no of arousals/hr
- ***Respiratory disturbance index*** = AHI + TAI

Pathophysiology: Sleep apnea causes hypoxia and hypercapnea which results in:

- Systemic HTN due to systemic vasoconstriction
- Acute carbon dioxide retention due to chronic hypoventilation
- Polycythemia due to increased levels of TNF-α, IL_1, ICAM, VCAM
- Excessive daytime somnolence and intellectual deterioration due to:
  - Cerebral dysfunction
  - Sleep fragmentation
  - Loss of deep sleep
  - Excessive motor activity
- Left heart failure due to:
  - Reduced pleural pressure
  - Reduced intrathoracic pressure
  - Increased cardiac afterload
- Sudden cardiac death due to:
  - Vagal bradycardia
  - Ventricular arrhythmias
- Pulmonary HTN and cor pulmonale due to hypoxic pulmonary vasoconstriction

Preoperative Screening

- History of:
  - Heavy snoring with sudden awakening with choking
  - Daytime somnolence, headaches
- On examination:
  - Nasal obstruction, tonsillar hypertrophy
  - Retrognathia, crowding of pharynx, macroglossia
  - Obesity, GERD
  - Pulmonary HTN, systemic HTN, intracranial HTN
  - IHD, right and left heart failure, arrhythmias
- Investigations:
  - Blood urea and serum creatinine
  - Blood glucose and thyroid function tests
  - Serum electrolytes and ABG especially for chronic hypercapnea
  - Raised LFTS: Especially alanine aminotransferase
  - Cardiovascular:
    - Echocardiogram and ECG
    - Stress tests: As these patients may have dormant CAD due to sedentary life style
  - Respiratory:
    - Sleep study or polysomnography
    - *Gold standard* for diagnosis
    - Monitors:
      - Electroencephalography
      - Electrocardiography
      - Electrooculography
      - Electromyography
      - Nasal/oral airflow, pulse oximetry, capnography
      - BP and esophageal pressure for GERD
      - Room noise
    - Results expressed as AHI
    - Costly test
  - Nasopharyngoscopy for assessing surgical benefits like uvulopharyngoplasty for obstruction
  - Overnight recording of SaO_2 by pulse oximetry can be used for diagnosis

Choice of Anesthesia

- Regional anesthesia preferred as respiratory drive is not affected
- Difficult to establish land marks
- Should be ready for airway management if inadvertent respiratory paralysis
- If GA, intubation with controlled ventilation preferred

Preoperative Preparation

- NPO orders
- Informed consent
- Preoperative sedation:
  - Usually with benzodiazepines
  - Sedation may increase airway obstruction
  - If sedation is given, SpO_2 should be monitored or patient should be placed on CPAP
- Antiaspiration prophylaxis

- ❖ DVT prophylaxis
- ❖ Continue all preoperative medications except OHAs and insulin
- ❖ Difficult venous access if patient is obese: Central line may be only venous access
- ❖ Facilitate ventilation:
  - CPAP is required in moderate-to-severe OSAS
  - If refractory to CPAP, noninvasive positive pressure ventilation is given (NIPPV)

Monitors

- ❖ Pulse oximetry, capnography, ECG
- ❖ Temperature, urine output
- ❖ Precordial stethoscope, neuromuscular monitoring
- ❖ Invasive arterial BP measurement preferred over NIBP as NIBP becomes unreliable due to cuff size
- ❖ PA catheter inserted and monitored if pulmonary HTN present

Induction

- ❖ Preoxygenate with FiO_2 of 100% with APL value set to deliver 5–15 cm H_2O of CPAP for 3 minutes
- ❖ Difficult mask ventilation: Gather fat pads in cheek around mask for better seal
- ❖ Avoid large doses of drugs and longer acting drugs
- ❖ All drugs given according to lean body weight except for succinylcholine and neostigmine (according to TBW)
- ❖ *Rapid sequence induction* for emergencies with cricoid pressure and succinylcholine
- ❖ Difficult airway equipment and gum elastic bougie kept ready
- ❖ ***McCoy laryngoscope***, LMA kept standby
- ❖ Awake intubation and extubation preferred in difficult airway
- ❖ *Awake fiberoptic intubation* preferred for elective cases
- ❖ Oxygen insufflation with nasopharyngeal catheter during intubation delays desaturation
- ❖ Cricothyrotomy set and ENT surgeon standby for can't ventilate can't intubate situation

Maintenance

- ❖ TIVA or balanced anesthesia with inhalation agents can be used
- ❖ Nitrous oxide:
  - May be a good choice
  - Avoid if pulmonary HTN present
  - High oxygen demand limits its use
  - Also causes abdominal distention reducing FRC further
- ❖ Desflurane may be preferred due to better hemodynamic stability
- ❖ Halothane avoided as:
  - Increased sensitization to catecholamines
  - Increased chances of halothane hepatitis
- ❖ Short acting opioids facilitate rapid and smooth emergence
- ❖ Cisatracurium, vecuronium, and rocuronium useful
- ❖ Dexmedetomidine may be a useful sedative and analgesic

Ventilation

- ❖ Tidal volumes > 10 mL/kg offer no added advantages
- ❖ Maintain minute volume of around 5 liters
- ❖ PEEP:
  - Improves lung compliance and oxygenation
  - Prevents V-Q mismatch
  - Detrimental if pulmonary HTN present

Hemodynamics

- ❖ Judicious fluid administration as CCF may be precipitated
- ❖ Early colloid and blood product infusion required as these patients are less able to compensate for blood loss

Extubation

- ❖ Consider short period of postoperative mechanical ventilation if:
  - Duration of surgery is longer
  - Upper airway surgeries where serious compromise of upper airway is expected
- ❖ Fully awake extubation with patient is sitting or reverse Trendelenburg position
- ❖ Adequate suctioning and cricoid pressure during extubation may prevent aspiration

Postoperative Care

Position

- ❖ Head elevated to 30° to increase upper airway stability
- ❖ Lateral posture relieves upper airway obstruction

Complications

- ❖ Respiratory: Hypercapnea, desaturation (episodic)
- ❖ Cardiovascular: HTN, MI, arrhythmias

Management

- ❖ Nursed in high dependency unit for few days if:
  - Severe BMI/OSAS
  - Severe cardiovascular disease

- Severe intraoperative complication
- High postoperative opioid requirement
- Maintenance of CPAP:
  - Insert NG tube before initiation of therapy to prevent distension of stomach
  - Even if NG tube is present, CPAP can be used but leakage may be present
  - 2–4 L/min of oxygen via side port on CPAP mask achieves adequate FiO_2
- Advantages of CPAP:
  - CPAP reduces risk of complication
  - Sedative analgesic drugs can be used safely
  - After nasal surgery, surgeon may use nasopharyngeal airway with packing around it
  - CPAP is very useful in this scenario to prevent dangerous desaturation

Postoperative Analgesia

- Multimodal analgesia is best
- Opioids:
  - Patient controlled analgesia useful
  - Basal rate set at zero and dosing is restricted
  - Morphine is preferred opioid
- Local infilteration of incision site
- Epidural analgesia:
  - Allows early ambulation
  - Reduces risk of DVT
  - NSAIDs can be used

POLYSOMNOGRAPHY

Introduction

- Comprehensive recording of the biophysical changes which occur during of sleep
- Usually done at night except for patients with Circadian rhythm sleep disorders

Indications

- Narcolepsy, parasomnias
- Restless leg syndrome
- REM behavioral disorder
- Obstructive sleep apnea syndrome
- Circadian rhythm sleep disorder
- Congenital central hypoventilation syndrome (***Ondine's curse***)

Monitors

- Electroencephalography
- Electrooculography
- Electromyography
- Electrocardiography
- Nasal and oral airflow
- Jaw and chin movements
- Abdominal and chest wall movements
- Pulse oximetry

Interpretation

- Sleep latency: Time taken to fall asleep from the time lights were switched off (normally < 20 min)
- Sleep efficiency:
  - Calculated as:
    - Number of minutes of sleep
    - Number of minutes in bed
  - Normally > 85–90%
- Sleep stages:
  - REM sleep and NREM sleep (stages I–IV)
  - 20–25% of sleep is REM sleep
  - Majority of sleep is stage II sleep
- Breathing irregularities:
  - Obstructive sleep apnea:
    - Complete cessation of air flow
    - Lasting more than 10 seconds
    - Despite maintaining ventilatory effort
    - Occurs more than 5 times per hour of sleep
    - Reduction of at least 4% in SaO_2
  - Obstructive sleep hypopnea:
    - Partial cessation of airflow
    - Lasting more than 10 seconds
    - Despite maintaining ventilatory efforts
    - Occurs more than 15 times per hour of sleep
    - Reduction of at least 4% in SaO_2
- Arousals: Sudden shifts in brain wave activity due to leg movements, environmental noise, etc.
- Cardiac rhythm abnormalities
- Leg movements
- Body position during sleep
- Oxygen saturation during sleep

CPAP Titration Study

- Polysomnography done for an OSAS patient after CPAP mask is applied
- This is done to determine:
  - Correct CPAP mask size
  - Correct amount of pressure
  - Tolerance to treatment
- When CPAP titration and diagnostic polysomnography are done on the same night the study is called ***split night study***

- Minimum of 2 hours of polysomnography required to diagnose OSAS before a CPAP mask is applied in a split night study

Alternatives

- Nowadays polysomnography is replaced by ***actigraphy*** which is used to measure gross motor activity
- Usually measured by an actigraph unit at the wrist

PHYSIOLOGICAL CHANGES DURING LAPAROSCOPY

Introduction

Three major forces alter the patients physiology during laparoscopic surgery:

- Increase in intra-abdominal pressure and volume, which are transmitted to the thorax
- Patient position
- Carbon dioxide insufflation

Effects of Carbon Dioxide Insufflation

- Procedure:
  - Gas is insufflated via a midline percutaneous puncture
  - Rate of insufflation 2–3 L/min
  - Insufflation occurs through a Veress needle
  - Laparoscope is passed into the expanded peritoneal cavity through a subumbilical incision
  - Once pneumoperitoneum is established gas flow is reduced to 200–300 mL/min
  - IAP is maintained at 14–20 mm Hg
- Effects of carbon dioxide pneumoperitoneum:
  - Effects on RS:
    - $PaCO_2$ rises during first 15–30 minutes of insufflation to reach a plateau
    - In an apneic patient $PaCO_2$ rises at the rate of 3–6 mm Hg/min
    - Rise in $PaCO_2$ during pneumoperitoneum occurs due to:
      - Absorption of CO_2 from peritoneal cavity due to raised IAP
      - Impairment of pulmonary ventilation
      - Due to patient position
    - Hypercarbia and acidosis stimulate respiratory center
    - As a compensatory mechanism, minute volume increases
    - Each mm Hg rise in $PaCO_2$ increases ventilation by 2–3 L/min
    - Increase in respiratory rate is higher than increase in tidal volume
    - $PaCO_2$–E_TCO_2 gradient does not change significantly in normal patients
    - In ASA II and III patients $PaCO_2$ increases more than E_TCO_2
    - $PaCO_2$ between 35 and 45 mm Hg desirable
  - Effects on cardiovascular system:
    - Direct effects of carbon dioxide:
      - Direct myocardial depression causing:
        - Negative chronotropism
        - Increased bathmotropism
        - Stimulates myocardial irritability and arrhythmias
        - Mainly occurs due to acidosis
      - Vasodilatation:
        - Hypercarbia directly causes vasodilation of all blood vessels, except pulmonary blood vessels
        - Hypercarbia also reduces responsiveness to catecholamines
        - In pulmonary blood vessels hypercarbia causes vasoconstriction
    - Indirect effects of hypercarbia:
      - Occurs secondary to CNS and sympathoadrenal stimulation
      - Results in:
        - Increased cardiac output and heart rate
        - Increased force of contraction, BP, and CVP
        - Reduced peripheral vascular resistance
  - Effects on central nervous system:
    - CO_2 first used as an anesthetic by Hickman in 1824
    - CO_2 causes nitrous oxide like narcosis at 90–120 mm Hg
    - Slight elevation of $PaCO_2$ causes:
      - Direct cortical depression
      - Increased seizure threshold
    - Further elevation causes cortical and subcortical depression
    - Carbon dioxide is the most important factor in regulating of cerebral blood flow:
      - Hypercarbia increases CBF and ICP
      - Each 1 mm Hg rise in $PaCO_2$ increases cerebral blood flow (CBF) by 1.8 mL/100 g/min
  - Effects on regional hemodynamics:
    - Urine output, renal plasma flow and GFR reduce to less than 50% of baseline values
    - Causes bicarbonate retention and compensatory metabolic alkalosis
    - Reduces splanchnic and hepatic blood flow: Reduces drug metabolism
    - Increases cerebral blood flow velocity

- Neuroendocrine effects: Increases levels of:
  - Epinephrine, norepinephrine
  - Renin, cortisol
  - Antidiuretic hormone, atrial natriuretic peptide

Effects of Raised Intra-abdominal Pressure

- Effects on RS:
  - Reduces thoracopulmonary compliance by 30–50%
  - Reduces FRC and aids development of atelectasis due to diaphragmatic displacement
  - Increases airway pressures and causes V-Q mismatch
  - Increases risk of aspiration by reducing esophageal sphincter tone
  - Can cause various complications:
    - Subcutaneous emphysema
    - Pneumothorax
    - Capnothorax
    - Carbon dioxide air embolism
    - Endobronchial intubation
- Effects on cardiovascular system:
  - Causes reduced cardiac output due to:
    - Reduction in venous return occurring due to:
      - Pooling of blood in lower limbs
      - Inferior vena cava compression
      - Increased venous resistance
    - Direct negative inotropism
    - Increase in systemic vascular resistance occurring due to:
      - Raised intrathoracic pressure
      - Stimulation of peritoneal stretch receptors
      - Increased vascular resistance of intra-abdominal organs
  - Increases propensity for arrhythmias:
    - Occurs due to sudden stretching of peritoneum during insufflations
    - This causes increased vagal tone
    - This may result in sinus bradycardia and even asystole
- Effects on central nervous system:
  - Raised IAP reduces venous return from the upper body
  - This causing venous engorgement
  - This may result in raised ICP and IOP

Effects of Patient Position

- Usually Trendelenburg position with head down tilt preferred
- Effects on RS:
  - Reduction in FRC, TLV, pulmonary compliance
  - Favors development of atelectasis
- Effects on cardiovascular system:
  - Increase in CVP, cardiac output and BP: May precipitate CCF
  - Sudden hypotension on lowering limbs
- Effects on central nervous system:
  - Causes raised ICP, CBF, and IOP
  - Increased incidence of nerve injuries:
    - Brachial plexus
    - Obdurator nerve
    - Femoral nerve
    - Common peroneal nerve

LAPAROSCOPIC SURGERY

Introduction

Laparoscopy (or peritoneoscopy) is a minimally invasive procedure allowing endoscopic access to the peritoneal cavity after insufflation of a gas (CO_2) to create a space between anterior abdominal wall and viscera.

Advantages

- Better cosmesis: Smaller nonmuscle splitting incision
- Reduced blood loss intraoperatively
- Lesser incidence of postoperative complications:
  - Pain, respiratory muscle dysfunction
  - Ileus, infection
  - Dehiscence of wound
- Shorter hospitalization and convalescence
- Lower cost
- Lesser incidence of incisional hernia
- Reduced levels of C-reactive protein and IL_6
- Lesser incidence of hyperglycemia and leukocytosis postoperatively

Disadvantages

- Narrowed two dimensional visual field
- Need for longer duration of general anesthesia
- Longer learning curve for surgeons
- Increased incidence of PONV:
  - Occurs in 40–75% patients
  - PONV can be reduced with:
    - Propofol based anesthesia
    - Intraoperative gastric emptying: Nasogastric tube
    - IV fluid administration perioperatively
    - Droperidol, ondansetron, palanosetron administration intraoperatively

- Postoperative pain:
  - More of visceral pain:
    - Biliary colic
    - Pelvic spasm
  - Referred shoulder tip pain common: Occurs due to intrapleural carbonic acid formation
  - Reduced with preoperative administration of NSAIDs and COX II inhibitors
  - Dexamethasone is effective

Choice of Gas for Pneumoperitoneum

- Carbon dioxide:
  - Insufflating agent of choice
  - Advantages:
    - Odourless, nontoxic, noncombustible
    - Readily available
    - 20 times more soluble in blood than air
    - *Blood gas partition coefficient (BGPC)* of 0.8
  - Disadvantages:
    - Causes hypercapnea
    - Gas embolism possible: Least risk amongst other gases
    - Shoulder pain due to formation of carbonic acid intrapleurally
- Nitrous oxide:
  - Advantages:
    - Less irritating to peritoneum
    - Lower potential for embolism compared to air/oxygen
    - Reduced risk of arrhythmias and shoulder pain
  - Disadvantages: Supports combustion
- Oxygen:
  - Causes explosion while using cautery
  - Possibility of gas embolism
  - It was used in 1993
- Air:
  - Originally used to produce pneumovulgaris
  - High risk of causing air embolism
  - Delayed absorption causes shoulder pain
- Inert gases:
  - Helium, argon, and xenon used
  - Nonflammable but high risk of embolism
  - Avoids hyperoxia and hyperventilation
  - Not safe if gas embolism occurs as less soluble

Gasless Laparoscopy

- Peritoneal cavity expanded using abdominal wall lift using a fan retractor
- Advantages:
  - Avoids hemodynamic and respiratory consequences of raised IAP and hypercarbia
  - Renal and splanchnic perfusion not altered
  - Incidence of port site metastasis after laparoscopic surgery is reduced
  - Good for patients with severe cardiopulmonary disease
- Disadvantages:
  - Compromises surgical exposure
  - Increases technical difficulty
  - Combining gasless laparoscopy with low pressure CO_2 pneumothorax (<5 mm Hg) may improve surgical condition

Indications

- Urological:
  - Uncomplicated adrenelectomy
  - Nephrectomy
- General surgery:
  - Cholecystectomy
  - Hernia repair, antireflux surgery
  - Splenectomy, appendicectomy
  - Bowel surgery
- Gynecological:
  - Tubal surgeries, cystectomy
  - Hysterectomy, endometrial ablation
- Thoracoscopic and neurosurgery without gas insufflations: Recent advances
- Lumbar discectomies and spine surgeries using anterior approach

Contraindications

- Raised ICT, intracranial space occupying lesions (ICSOL)
- Ventriculoperitoneal shunt:
  - Continuous ICP monitoring and ventricular drainage may be required
  - Patients are at increased risk of:
    - Gas emboli
    - Shunt obstruction
    - Raised ICT
- Severe cardiopulmonary disease (including bullae)
- Gastrointestinal disorders:
  - History of previously extensive surgery with adhesions
  - Large intra-abdominal/abdominal wall tumor
  - Obesity, peritonitis
  - Diaphragmatic hernia

- Coagulopathy, sickle cell disease: As acidosis precipitates crisis
- Hypovolemia, patient on β-blockers
- Patient refusal, inexperienced surgeon
- Pregnancy: Was considered contraindication as:
  - Increased risk of damaging gravid uterus
  - Carbon dioxide pneumoperitoneum may cause fetal acidosis
  - May cause miscarriage/premature labor

Laparoscopy in Pregnancy

- Should be done during second trimester
- Ideally done at *less than 23 weeks* to:
  - Minimize risk of preterm labor
  - Maintain adequate surgical field
- Tocolytics used intraoperatively, to arrest preterm labor
- Avoid blind/closed technique using ***Veress needle***
- Use open laparoscopy for abdominal access using ***Hasson cannula*** to avoid damaging uterus
- Continuous fetal monitoring using transvaginal USG
- Mechanical ventilation adjusted to maintain material physiological alkalosis

Choice of Anesthesia

- General anesthesia with ETT and CMV: Best as:
  - Duration of surgery may be long
  - Patient may be anxious
  - Dyspnea common in awake patient in Trendelenburg position
  - NGT/OGT may be uncomfortable in awake patient
  - Most importantly muscle paralysis essential as:
    - Raised IAP makes spontaneous breathing difficult
    - Provides quieter surgical field and better exposure
    - Bucking causes increased risk of pneumothorax and gas dissection
    - Coughing increases IAP: Hollow viscus perforation
    - Necessary to control ventilation to adjust for hypercarbia and acidosis
- Role of GA with LMA:
  - Advantages:
    - Fewer cases of sore throat
    - Useful for short cases
  - Disadvantages:
    - Does not protect airway against aspiration
    - Limits ability to apply positive pressure
    - Interferes with use of OGT
- Role of local anesthesia:
  - Advantages:
    - Quicker recovery
    - Fewer cardiovascular changes
    - Reduced incidence of PONV
    - Allows early diagnosis of complications in awake patient
  - Disadvantages:
    - Carbon dioxide may irritate peritoneum
    - OGT in awake patient is uncomfortable
    - Disadvantages if conversion to open laparotomy
- Regional anesthesia:
  - May require high level sensory block (T4): Results in dyspnea
  - OGT not tolerated
  - Hyperventilation causes excessive movement in surgical field
  - Sympathetic denervation results in hypotension and reduced cardiac output
  - Shoulder tip pain: Alleviated with opioids/clonidine

Anesthetic Management

Preoperative Evaluation

- Examination:
  - Look for dyspnea, kyphoscoliosis, body weight distribution, URTI
  - Cardiac function evaluated in patients with heart disease
  - Patients with severe valvular disease and CCF are more prone for cardiac complications than patients with IHD
  - Patients with renal failure:
    - Optimize hemodynamics
    - Avoid nephrotoxic agents
  - In patients with respiratory diseases, laparoscopy preferable
- Investigations:
  - CBC, urinalysis, CT, BT, ECG, blood grouping and typing
  - Baseline electrolytes, ABGs, pulse oximetry and pulmonary function tests
  - BUN and SC: As possibility of oliguria during long surgery
  - Baseline CXR:
    - To rule out active disease: Bulla on X-ray contraindicates laparoscopy
    - Postoperative comparison of acute changes such as:
      - Emphysema

- Pneumothorax
- Pulmonary edema

Preoperative Preparation

- Informed consent:
  - Inform about general complications of surgery
  - Explain about:
    - Specific complications of laparoscopic surgery
    - Postoperative referred pain
  - Inform and obtain consent for possible laparotomy
- NPO orders:
  - 6 hours solids
  - 2 hours clear fluids
- Premedication:
  - Preoperative sedation with midazolam/morphine
  - Preoperative NSAIDs: Reduce postoperative pain and opioid requirements
  - Clonidine and dexmedetomidine:
    - Reduce intraoperative stress response
    - Improves hemodynamic stability
- Preoperative antibiotic prophylaxis as per hospital protocol
- DVT prophylaxis if long duration surgery
- Antiaspiration prophylaxis if delayed gastric emptying
- Complete bowel preparation preoperatively

Monitors

- Mechanical monitors:
  - BP measurement
  - ECG with ST segment trending
  - Pulse oximetry: Watch for sudden bradycardia and SAN arrest during insufflation
  - Capnography mandatory:
    - E_TCO_2 stabilizes after 15–30 minutes of insufflation
    - If E_TCO_2 increases after 30 minutes suspect:
      - Subcutaneous emphysema
      - Pneumothorax
  - Nerve stimulator, indicators of FiO_2
  - Monitor minute volume and peak airway pressure
  - Temperature monitoring with esophageal probe
  - Arterial line for long surgeries/ASA III patients
  - TEE/Doppler/CVP for hemodynamically unstable patients
  - Serial ABGs to monitor $PaCO_2$-E_TCO_2 difference
- Clinical monitors:
  - Skin:
    - Monitor color turgor and capillary refill
    - Head, neck, and upper chest may become purplish in dependent position
    - Suggestive of hypercarbia
  - Cornea and conjunctiva:
    - Monitor for edema
    - Important in:
      - Trendelenburg position
      - When oliguria occurs as it may indicate fluid overload
  - Upper chest wall: Monitor for subcutaneous emphysema
  - Pulse: For volume and rhythm
  - Urine output:
    - Oliguria may occur despite adequate hydration
    - Common when IAP > 15 mm Hg
    - Also monitor color and concentration of urine

Position

- Trendelenburg position used for urology
- Dorsolithotomy position used for gynecology
- Head-up position used for upper GI and biliary tract surgeries
- Lateral decubitus used for thoracoscopy, nephrectomy and adrenelectomy
- Precautions:
  - Adequate padding to protect from nerve compression
  - Shoulder braces used in Trendelenburg position
  - Patient tilt limited to 15–20°
  - Tilting to be slow and progressive to avoid sudden cardiovascular changes
  - Position of ETT to be checked after any change in position
  - Endobronchial intubation possible in obese patient with Trendelenburg position

Induction

- Adequate preoxygentaion
- Induction with thiopentone + fentanyl + muscle relaxant like vecuronium
- Rapid sequence induction if delayed gastric emptying present
- Lidocaine 1.5 mg/kg IV 90 seconds before intubation to prevent intubation response
- Insert orogastric/NG tube for:
  - Deflating stomach of air entry during mask ventilation
  - Prevention of regurgitation

- During pneumoperitoneum, CO_2 continuously inflates stomach
- ❖ Foleys catheter inserted to empty urinary bladder

Maintenance

- ❖ Mixture of oxygen + air + isoflurane used
- ❖ Use of air + O_2 + inhalation agent mandates use of higher MAC of inhalation anesthetic
- ❖ Intermittent fentanyl and vecuronium boluses may be used to maintain balanced anesthesia
- ❖ Careful dosing as closure of laparoscopy procedure may be abrupt
- ❖ Avoid halothane as it can cause arrhythmias in the presence of hypercarbia
- ❖ TIVA:
  - Propofol maintenance results in fewer postoperative side effects
  - Propofol avoided in fertility procedures as it causes lower pregnancy rates
- ❖ Nitrous oxide:
  - Avoided as:
    - It distends bowel and disrupts surgical field
    - May cause increased incidence of PONV
  - If used, N_2O limited to 50% of inspired mixture
- ❖ Maintain deep planes: Bucking causes hollow viscus/blood vessel perforation by trocar
- ❖ Intermittent suctioning of OGT as CO_2 continues to diffuse into stomach and distend it
- ❖ Intermittent sequential compression stocking to be applied if long surgery
- ❖ Maintain intra-abdominal pressure < 15 mm Hg
- ❖ Adjuvants:
  - Vagolytic drugs:
    - To be available as bradycardia and sinoatrial arrest possible
    - Usually occurs during sudden peritoneal distension by gas
- ❖ Vasodilating drugs:
  - Nicardipine, α_2 blockers, remifentanyl useful
  - Improve hemodynamic stability
- ❖ Antiemetics:
  - Droperidol: Sedative, long acting and α-inhibitory action
  - 5 HT_3 blockers: Ondansetron and palanosetron

Ventilation

- ❖ Positive pressure ventilation preferred
- ❖ Maintain $ETCO_2$ between 35 and 40 mm Hg
- ❖ This requires a 15–25% increase in minute volume
- ❖ Increase in respiratory rate rather than tidal volume preferable in patients with COPD/spontaneous pneumothorax

Hemodynamics

- ❖ Large bore angiocatheter placed due to possibility of major hemorrhage
- ❖ Minimal third space loss, blood loss and insensible water loss
- ❖ Maintenance fluids:
  - 2.5–4 mL/kg/hr of lactated Ringers ideal
  - Despite adequate hydration oliguria common
  - Volume of fluids infused may be mistakenly increased
  - This may lead to postoperative pulmonary edema
  - Thus restrict fluids to 2.5–4 mL/kg/hr as after deflating abdomen diuresis occurs
- ❖ *Retained intraperitoneal saline*:
  - Volume of retained intraperitoneal saline should be added to maintenance fluids
  - Calculated as (Volume of fluids for irrigation–volume of fluid in suction containers)
- ❖ Vasodilators:
  - Nicardipine, α_2 blockers, remifentanil useful
  - These reduce cardiovascular changes of pneumoperitoneum
- ❖ Bradycardia common at the time of peritoneal distension

Extubation

- ❖ Extubation might be delayed as high concentration of inhalation agents must be used
- ❖ Delayed extubation if patient has:
  - Edema
  - Venous congestion
  - Duskiness of head and neck
  - Tongue, conjunctival, and lid edema: Keep head end up till edema subsides
  - Oliguria: Wait till diuresis has begun

Postoperative Care

Monitors

- ❖ Monitor SpO_2: Supplemental oxygen mandatory even in healthy patients as O_2 demand increases after laparoscopy
- ❖ Monitor BP as hemodynamic changes induced by pneumoperitoneum outlast duration of pneumoperitoneum
- ❖ Temperature, urine output, ABG monitoring

Management

- PONV:
  - 40–75% incidence
  - Treated with 5 HT_3 inhibitors, scopolamine and droperidol
- Chest X-ray: Immediate chest X-ray taken if:
  - Respiratory distress
  - Subcutaneous emphysema
  - Suspected pneumothorax
  - Pulmonary edema
  - History of cardiac disease
- Remove Foleys catheters and OGT if patient fully awake, stable and voiding adequately

Analgesia

- Multimodal analgesia with opioids and NSAIDs
- Intraoperative peritoneal LA administration useful
- Wound site infilteration reduces incisional pain
- Shoulder pain: Opioids, clonidine

Complications

- Postoperative nausea and vomiting
- Shoulder tip pain
- Injuries from instruments:
  - Abdominal wall bleeding
  - Blood vessel/hollow viscus perforation, peritonitis
  - Subcutaneous emphysema, wound infection, hernia at trocar site
  - Hemorrhage
  - Staples and clips can causes nerve entrapment
  - Thermal injury from cautery/laser
- Complications of pneumoperitoneum:
  - Raised IAP:
    - Bowel ischemia
    - Omental/bowel herniation
    - Gastric regurgitation
    - IVC compression
  - Reduced venous return:
    - Hypotension
    - Raised intrathoracic pressure
  - Airleak syndromes:
    - Mediastinal emphysema
    - Subcutaneous emphysema
    - Capnothorax
    - Pneumothorax
  - Air embolism
  - PONV
  - Bradycardia, shoulder tip pain
  - Endobronchial intubation
- Complications of hypercarbia:
  - Acidosis
  - HTN, tachycardia
  - Arrhythmias
  - Precipitation of sickle cell crisis
  - Raised ICT
- Complications of Trendelenburg position:
  - Raised ICP, IOP, glaucoma
  - Corneal and conjunctival edema
  - Retinal hemorrhagge, retinal detachment
  - Upper airway edema
  - Hypoxemia, ventilation perfusion mismatch
  - Brachial plexus injury
  - Endobronchial intubation
  - Femoral and obdurator N injuries
- Late complications:
  - Bowel obstruction due to injury, cautery, burns
  - Incisional hernia
  - Adhesions, DVT
  - Nerve injuries
  - Bowel necrosis
  - Cutaneous metastasis at port site

PHEOCHROMOCYTOMA

Introduction

- These are functional catecholamine secreting tumors of chromaffin tissue derived from neural crest
- Tumors are called *pheochromocytoma* when they are present in adrenal medulla
- When tumors are located extra-adrenally, they are called *paraganglionomas*

Incidence

- Account for 0.1–1% of all cases of hypertension
- In adults 55–60% occur in females
- In children 70% occur in boys

Syndromic association: Can occur as part of:

- ***MEN 2A syndrome (Sipples syndrome)***:
  - Parathyroid adenomas
  - Medullary carcinoma of thyroid
  - Pheochromocytoma
- ***MEN 2B syndrome (Gordon's syndrome):***
  - Medullary carcinoma of thyroid
  - Pheochromocytoma
  - Marfanoid habitus, muscosal neuroma
  - ***Von-Hippel-Lindau syndrome***
  - Hemangioblastoma of retina, cerebellum
  - Pheochromocytoma

- ***Neurofibromatosis type I (Von-Recklinghausen's disease):***
  - Neurofibromatosis
  - Pheochromocytoma
- ***Familial paraganglionoma syndrome***
- Nonsyndromic familial pheochromocytoma

Location

- Pheochromocytomas:
  - Adrenal medulla
  - Sympathetic ganglia
- Paraganglionomas:
  - Thorax, right atrium
  - Urinary bladder, spleen, broad ligament of ovary
  - ***Organs of Zuckerkandl*** at aortic bifurcation

Rule of Ten

- 10% of tumors occur in children
- 10% familial
- 10% malignant
- 10% extradrenal
- 10% bilateral

Pathophysiology

- Pheochromocytomas predominantly secrete epinephrine and norepinephrine
- Malignant pheochromocytomas may secrete dopamine also

Dopaminergic Pathway

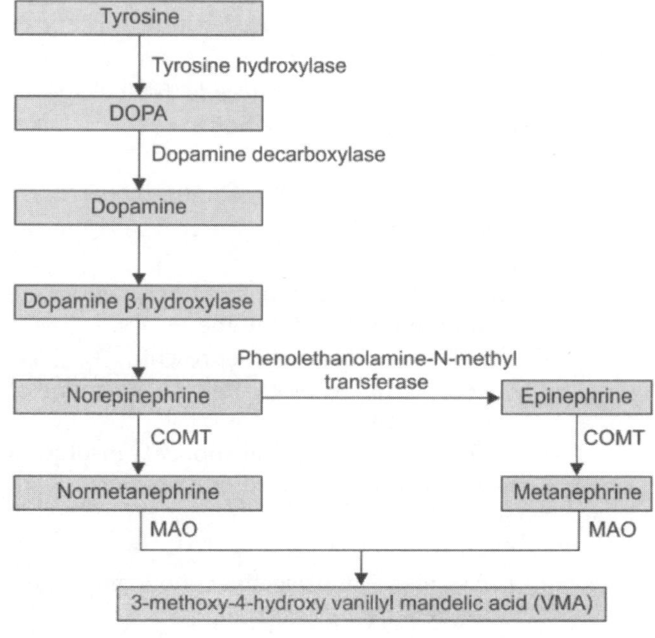

Clinical Features

- Most commonly occur in young to mid-adult life
- In adults it is more common in females
- Considered greatest mimic due to varied clinical presentation
- Hypertension:
  - 5–15% cases are normotensive
  - Seen in 90% cases, intermittent or continuous
  - HTN with narrow pulse pressure and reflex bradycardia if norepinephrine secreting tumor
  - HTN with raised SBP, low DBP and tachycardia if epinephrine secreting tumor
- ***Paroxysms/pheochromocytoma crisis***:
  - Presents with classical triad of headache, palpitation and sweating
  - Symptoms:
    - Fever due to raised BMR
    - HTN or orthostatic hypotension
    - Hyperglycemia, polyuria, polydipsia
    - Headache, palpitation, dyspnea, weakness
    - Panic attacks, blurred vision, weight loss
    - Atypical manifestations like:
      - Acute abdomen secondary to hemorrhagic rupture
      - ***Catecholamine cardiomyopathy***:
        - Congestive cardiac failure, LVF
        - Myocardial infarction, acute pulmonary edema, arrythmias
- Symptoms precipitated by:
  - Palpation of abdomen
  - Uterine contraction during labor
  - Defecation, changes in posture
  - Micturition (if tumor present in bladder)
  - Drugs:
    - Tricyclic antidepressants
    - MAO inhibitors
    - Phenothiazines, droperidol
    - *Metaclopramide*, naloxone
- Complications:
  - Patients are at high risk for cerebrovascular accidents
  - Rhabdomyolysis due to muscle ischemia from vasoconstricted state

Indicators of Suspicion

- Family history of MEN/pheochromocytoma
- Paroxysmal headache/sweating and palpitation
- HTN at an early age (<20 yr) or if resistant to therapy
- Unexplained grade III/IV retinopathy

- Orthostatic hypotension in patients who are not on antihypertensive therapy
- Incidentaloma in adrenal gland
- ***Carneys triad***: Coexistence of three types of neoplasms in young women:
  - Gastric stromal tumor
  - Pulmonary chondromas
  - Extra-adrenal paraganglionomas

Differential Diagnosis

- Thyrotoxic crisis
- Malignant hyperthermia
- Acute anxiety neurosis
- Toxemia of pregnancy

Diagnosis

- Nonspecific investigations:
  - Raised hematocrit due to reduced intravascular volume and hemoconcentration
  - Hypercalcemia due to ectopic parathyroid related protein
  - Uncontrolled hyperglycemia
  - Raised BUN and serum creatinine due to myoglobinuric renal failure
  - ECG:
    - LVH, LBBB/RBBB
    - T wave changes, MI
    - Tachyarrythmias
  - Chest X-ray: Cardiomegaly
  - Echocardiography: LVH, catecholamine cardiomyopathy
- Specific investigations:
  - Urine 24 hours assay of adrenal hormones:
    - Considered as better screening test
    - Stat samples may have normal values as catecholamine secretion is paroxysmal
    - Urinary metanephrine is *most specific*
    - Normal values:
      - Catecholamines: Less than 100–150 µg/day
      - Metanephrine: Less than 1.3 mg/day
      - Vanillyl mandelic acid less than 7 mg/day
    - In pheochromocytoma:
      - Catecholamines: More than 250 µg/day
      - Metanephrine: More than 1.3 mg/day
      - Vanillylmandelic acid: More than 14 mg/day
  - Plasma catecholamines: Stat sample:
    - Normal value: Less than 1 µg/mL
    - Pheochromocytoma: More than 1 µg/mL
  - Pharmacological tests:
    - Provocative test:
      - No longer used
      - Glucagon, histamine, tyramine
    - Suppression test:
      - With clonidine and pentolinium
      - Used when other tests are negative but very strong clinical suspicion exists
    - Tumor localization:
      - CT scan: Identities 90% tumors > 1 cm diameter
      - MRI: Useful in pregnancy as less radiation
      - Selective venous catheterization:
        - Useful in locating multiple extra-adrenal tumors
        - Blood samples taken from vein draining tumor
        - Catecholamine levels are measured in these samples
      - Arteriography: Rarely used as contrast releases catecholamines
      - MIBG scintigraphy:
        - With meta-iodo-benzyl-guanethidine
        - To diagnose ectopic and multiple tumors
        - Guanethidine taken up by chromaffin granules
        - Tumor is then visualized with gamma camera
      - PET scan: For extra-adrenal tumors
      - Ultrasonography and IV pyelography: Insensitive

Preoperative Preparation

- Have to be adequately prepared before surgery to resolve volume contracted state
- α-blockade should always precede β-blockage to avoid unopposed vasoconstriction
- α-adrenergic blockage:
  - Aim: To restore blood volume status by reversing vasoconstriction
  - Duration:
    - At least 2 weeks before surgery for complete restoration of blood volume
    - If ST-T wave changes are present:
      - Long-term α-blockade (1–6 months) recommended
      - This produces clinical and ECG resolution of catecholamine cardiomyopathy
  - Drugs used:
    - Phenoxybenzamine:
      - Provides nonselective noncompetitive irreversible α-blockade

- Start with 10 mg bid/tid
- Increase 10–20 mg every 3 days until maximum of 80–250 mg/day
- Longer duration of action:
  - Facilities BID dosing
  - α-blockade may persist in postoperative period causing hypotension
- Somnolence, headache, stuffy nose are side effects

- Prazosin:
  - Started at 1 mg Q8H
  - Gradually increases dose till maximum of 8–12 mg/day
  - ***First dose phenomenon***, so given at bed time
- Doxazosin, terazosin
- Doxazosin allows once daily dosing
- $MgSO_4$, dexmedetomidine, calcium channel blockers, clonidine also used

❖ β adrenergic blockade:
- Commenced only after α-blockade has started
- Only used if persistent tachycardia (>100 bpm) or arrhythmias
- β-blockade may precipitate CCF in catecholamine cardiomyopathy

❖ Rapid IV α-blockade:
- Done over at least 3 days
- Day 1:
  - Phenoxybenzamine 1 mg/kg in 500 mL 5% dextrose
  - Given over 2 hours
  - Oral propranolol given if heart rate increases beyond 120 bpm
- Day 2:
  - Phenoxybenzamine 1–1.5 mg/kg in 500 mL of 5% dextrose
  - Given over 2 hours
  - Oral propranolol given if heart rate increases beyond 100 bpm
- Day 3:
  - Phenoxybenzamine 1.5–2 mg/kg in 500 mL 5% dextrose
  - Given over 2 hours
  - Oral propranolol given if heart rate increases beyond 100 bpm

❖ α-methyl tyrosine:
- Inhibits tyrosine hydroxylase which is rate limiting step in catecholamine biosynthesis
- Reduces catecholamine production and secretion
- Reserved for patients with metastatic disease or in whom surgery is contraindicated
- Dose: 0.5–4 g/day

Roizens Criteria: Used for assessment of adequacy of preparation

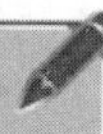

❖ No in-hospital BP reading more than 160/90 mm Hg for 24 hours prior to surgery
❖ Orthostatic hypotension with standing BP > 80/45 mm Hg
❖ ECG free of ST-T changes for 1 week prior to surgery
❖ No more than 1 ectopic beat every 5 minutes
❖ Other indicators: Serial hematocrit, RBS control, improved psychological status

Premedication

❖ NPO orders
❖ Informed consent
❖ Sedatives/anxiolytics: Useful as they prevent catecholamine release
❖ Avoid use of:
- Morphine and pethidine as they cause histamine release
- Metoclopramide and droperidol as they cause catecholamine release
- Atropine as parasympathetic block causes unimposed sympathetic NS activity

❖ Steroid supplementation if bilateral adrenelectomy planned
❖ *Adequate volume expansion*: Careful in patients with cardiomyopathy
❖ Drug to be avoided:
- Morphine, pethidine, curare, atracurium: Histamine releasers
- Succinylcholine: Catecholamine release
- Pancuronium: Sympathomimetic effect
- Droperidol, metaclopramide: Inhibits catecholamine reuptake and potentiates their action
- Halothane: Sensitizes myocardium to catecholamines

Induction

❖ Adequate preoxygenation
❖ Induction with etomidate/benzodiazepine/thiopentone/propofol
❖ Fentanyl as opioid and vecuronium as muscle relaxant
❖ Adequate depth of anesthesia before intubation is very important
❖ Intubation response:
- IV lidocaine 1–1.5 mg/kg IV
- Nitroglycerine infusion as alternative
- Might be more severe as more catecholamine stores present in N terminals due to reuptake of already increased catecholamines

- Avoid use of:
  - Morphine pethidine, atracurium: Histamine release
  - Pancuronium: Sympathomimetic effect
  - Succinylcholine:
    - Releases catecholamines by increasing intra-abdominal pressure
    - Also has direct effect on sympathetic ganglia

Maintenance

- Maintenance with O_2 with N_2O and isoflurane for balanced anesthesia
- Opioids (fentanyl/alfentanyl) with vecuronium as intermittent boluses
- Inhalational agents:
  - Isoflurane/sevoflurane preferred
  - Desflurane use is controversial
  - Avoid halothane as it sensitizes myocardium to catecholamines
- Avoid use of:
  - Pancuronium, metoclopramide, droperidol
  - Ketamine, ephedrine
- Avoid hypoventilation as it causes sympathetic nervous system stimulation
- Handling of tumor may cause life threatening hypertensive crisis
- Hypotension may occur following ligation of venous supply to tumor

Monitoring

- E_TCO_2, pulse oximetry, ECG monitoring
- IBP monitoring is *mandatory*
- Urinary catheter, temperature probe may be used
- Urinary output measurement hourly ($\geq$ 0.5 mL/kg/hr)
- CVP and pulmonary wedge pressure in patients with cardiomyopathy
- Echocardiography may be done
- Arterial blood gases, blood sugar: Done second hourly

Hemodynamics

- Hypertensive crisis:
  - Occurs during:
    - Intubation
    - Tumor manipulation for tumor removal
    - Also due to hypocalcemia, hypercarbia
    - If SBP $\geq$ 200 mm Hg for more than 1 minute, treat HTN
  - Drugs used:
    - SNP: 0.5–10 µg/kg/min as infusion
    - NTG: 0.5–10 µg/kg/min as infusion
    - Phentolamine 2–5 mg IV bolus or as infusion
- Control of hypotension:
  - Occurs following ligation of venous drainage of tumor
  - Prevented by preoperative preparation
  - Treated by volume expansion and vasopressors like dopamine and phenylephrine
- Laparoscopic surgery increases IAP and hypercarbia which cause catecholamine release
- Control of tachyarrhythmias:
  - β-blockers:
    - Propranolol 1 mg increments
    - Atenolol, labetolol
    - Esmolol: Preferred as half life of 9 minutes
  - Amiodarone: Supraventricular arrhythmias especially with CCF
  - Lidocaine: For ventricular arrhythmias

Postoperative Care

Monitor

- Pulse oximetry
- BP for hypotension/hypertension: HTN more common
- Blood sugar levels
- Urinary output, ABG

Analgesia

- Multimodal approach safest
- Epidural analgesia useful
- NSAIDs can be used as adjuvants
- Opioids: Lower doses preferred as patients will be somnolent

Complications

- Hypertension:
  - Common usually up to 3 days postoperatively
  - If it persists more than 2 weeks postoperatively, measure urinary plasma catecholamine levels
  - Done to rule out residual disease
  - Usually, catecholamine levels reduce to normal within 72 hours
  - Other causes of HTN:
    - Pain, urinary retention
    - Hypoxia, hypercarbia
- Hypotension: Occurs due to:
  - Sudden catecholamine withdrawal post surgery
  - Persistent α-blockade
  - If acute, it may indicate intra-abdominal hemorrhage

- Hypoglycemia:
  - Occurs due to disappearance of inhibition of β-cell function by catecholamines
  - This causes increased insulin secretion
- Somnolence:
  - Most common occurs for up to 48 hours postoperatively
  - Occurs due to catecholamine withdrawal post-surgery
  - Normal opioid doses may cause respiratory depression

Role of Regional Anesthesia

- Epidural preferred over spinal anesthesia as:
  - Sudden drop in SVR with hypotension avoided
  - Level of block can be extended
  - Duration can be prolonged
  - Epidural anesthesia reduces catecholamine release
- Epidural preferred over GA for hemodynamic benefits as:
  - Deep GA must be given to prevent tachycardia and HTN
  - This can cause myocardial depression
  - Vasopressors more effective during epidural rather than GA

Pheochromocytoma in Pregnancy

- Investigations:
  - Difficult to localize the tumor with radiological studies due to risk of fetal radiation exposure
  - MRI is safest modality
- Supine hypotension syndrome:
  - Aortocaval compression effects may be aggravated by volume constricted state
  - Also, left lateral tilt might stimulate catecholamine release by uterine compression of the tumor
- Preoperative preparation:
  - α-blockers considered safe
  - α-blockade commenced before β-blocker therapy
  - β-blockers might cross placenta and cause fetal bradycardia and hypotension
- Cesarean section:
  - *Vaginal delivery absolutely contraindicated*
  - Surgery for pheochromocytoma done during 1st trimester/3rd trimester at the time of cesarean section
  - Epidural anesthesia preferred over GA/SAB
- Uterotonics:
  - Following delivery syntocinon given safely
  - Ergonovin/prostaglandin avoided as may precipitate hypertensive crisis
- Magnesium sulphate:
  - Can be used to maintain cardiovascular stability
  - Hypomagnesemia occurs during pregnancy as increased utilization of magnesium occurs
  - Treated with 40–60 mg/kg IV bolus followed by 2 g/hr IV infusion
  - Magnesium not deleterious to fetus

CLEFT LIP AND PALATE

Introduction

Most common occurring anomaly due to defective embryological development of the lip and palate.

Incidence

- Occurs in 1:300–600 live births
- Isolated cleft palate: 1:2,000 live births
- Cleft present in both lip and palate in 50% cases
- Cleft lip with or without palate: 1:1,000 births (more common in boys)
- Isolated cleft palate more common in Asian girls

Development

- Congenital clefts of upper lip occur due to failure of fusion of maxillary with medial and lateral nasal processes
- Face develops between 4 and 7 weeks of fetal life
- Palate development completed at 12 weeks
- Anatomy:
  - Cleft palate is divided into prepalatal and postpalatal clefts
  - The incisive foramen marks the boundary between the two
  - Prepalatal cleft involves anterior palate, alveolus, lip, nostril floor and ala nasi
  - Postpalatal cleft may extend from soft and hard palate to incisive foramen
- *Most common* cleft of palate is left complete cleft of pre and palatal structures
- Second most common is midline cleft of all soft palate and part of hard palate without a cleft is prepalatal area

Pathophysiology

- Pharynx communicates more extensively with nasal fossae and oral cavity
- Thus, complex mechanisms of swallowing, breathing, hearing and speech are impaired
- Difficulty in feeding:
  - Presence of cleft lip and palate in neonates causes feeding difficulty

- Presence of cleft makes creation of negative pressure difficult
- Thus, baby cannot suck
- Breast feeding is improbable and bottle feeding difficult

❖ Chronic middle ear effusion/infection:
- Abnormal anatomy of nasopharynx effects Eustachian tube function
- Palatopharyngeus muscle function is impaired owing to the cleft palate
- ASOM, SOM occur commonly
- These cause conductive hearing loss

❖ Abnormal speech:
- Nasal septation between food and air is absent
- Secondary defects in growth of ala nasi and velopharyngeal function can occur
- This causes rhinolalea aperta
- Speech of these children is typically nasal
- Usually unable to pronounce *plosives (p, k, d, t) and fricatives (s, f)*

Conditions Associated with Cleft Lip and Palate

❖ Limb and ear deformities
❖ Club foot
❖ ***Pierre-Robins syndrome***: Micrognathia, cleft palate, respiratory, and digestive disorders
❖ ***Downs syndrome***
❖ ***Velocardiofacial syndrome***
❖ ***Goldenhaar syndrome (facio-auriculo-vertebral syndrome)***
❖ ***Treacher-Collins syndrome:***
- Antimongoloid slant of eyes
- Eyelid colobomas (outer part of lower lid)
- Pointed nasal prominence
- Small oral cavity with normal sized tongue
- Dental malocclusion
- High arched palate/cleft palate
- Increased anterior facial height
- Hypoplastic cheeks, zygomatic arch, mandible
- Microtia with possible hearing loss

Indication and Timing of Closure

❖ Cleft lip:
- Usually done at 3 months
- Repaired early to improve scar and assist maternal bonding

❖ Cleft palate:
- Closure of soft palate at 6–9 months
- Secondary closure of residual hard palate at 15–18 months of age

❖ This repair provides total palatal closure before speech evolves
❖ If soft palate is repaired at the time of lip repair, additional anesthetic avoided

Rule of ten: Operate child when:
❖ Age less than 10 weeks
❖ Weight approximately 10 pounds
❖ Hemoglobin: 10 g/dL or more
❖ WBC count ≤ 10,000/μL

Preoperative Evaluation

❖ History of:
- Repeated droplet infection:
  - Respiratory, ear, gastrointestinal infections
  - Treat with antibiotics
- Feeding problems: Low body weight, anemia
- Previous surgery or anesthetic exposure
- Previous history of aspiration
- Immunization and development milestones

❖ Investigations:
- Complete blood count, blood grouping and cross matching
- Bleeding time, clotting time
- X-ray mandible, X-ray chest
- Echocardiography if congenital heart disease suspected

Preoperative Preparation

❖ NPO orders:
- Clear fluids 2 hours
- Breast milk 4 hours
- Cow's milk and solids 6 hours

❖ Informed consent
❖ Specific consent to be taken for suppository use
❖ 10% glucose solution started to avoid hypoglycemia at 4 mL/kg/hr
❖ Premedication:
- Syrup phenergan 0.3 mL/kg 90 minutes prior to surgery
- Syrup diazepam 0.2 mg/kg 1 hour prior to surgery
- Oral midazolam 0.25–0.5 mg/kg 30 minutes prior to surgery as alternative
- Atropine 20 μg/kg IM 30 minutes before surgery

Induction

❖ Two techniques of induction: Inhalational induction or IV induction
❖ Inhalation induction:
- Used when difficult airway suspected or when IV access is absent

- Preoxygenate for 3–5 minutes
- $O_2 + N_2O$ + halothane/sevoflurane used
- Concentration is slowly increased
- Once limb is relaxed, IV line taken with 22 G cannula

❖ Intravenous induction:
  - Used when IV access is available
  - Preoxygenate for 3–5 minutes
  - IV ketamine 1–2 mg/kg or
  - IV thiopentone 4–5 mg/kg double diluted given slow intravenously
  - Succinylcholine 1–1.5 mg/kg or vecuronium 0.1 mg/kg IV as muscle relaxants

Intubation

❖ Timing of intubation:
  - Deep intubation with child breathing spontaneously or
  - Intubation following muscle relaxation

❖ Laryngoscopy:
  - Straight forward in patients with cleft lip
  - In patients with cleft palate, insert gauze pack in cleft before laryngoscopy
  - Intubation done with a small, Miller laryngoscope
  - ***Retromolar intubation:***
    - Done if left sided cleft palate or bilateral cleft with protruding premaxilla
    - In such cases slant laryngoscope from incisor, support on left molar
    - ET tube inserted through right cleft (retromolar intubation)

❖ Endotracheal tube:
  - RAE tube (***Ring-Adeyer-Ellwyn tube***)
  - Reinforced tube used, which resists compression
  - ET tube secured in midline after confirming air entry to avoid distortion and maintain symmetry

❖ Throat is packed and eyes are protected

❖ NG tube inserted after intubation to empty stomach of gas and secretions which are removed before preparation of surgical field

Position

❖ Slight head up: Reduces risk of aspiration

❖ Neck extended: Reduces bleeding

❖ Shoulder support: For better exposure

Monitoring

❖ Heart rate, pulse oximetry, E_TCO_2

❖ Precordial stethoscope

❖ ECG, temperature, urine output

❖ Blood loss: Lesser compared with other surgeries

Maintenance

❖ $O_2 + N_2O$ + sevoflurane/isoflurane + fentanyl (1 μg/kg) + NDMR

❖ Clonidine and ketamine can be used as opioid sparing techniques

❖ Adrenaline infilteration of 1:200,000 used to control bleeding

❖ Thus, halothane use is not advised as it sensitizes heart to arrhythmias

❖ ***Dingmans gag*** used by surgeon causes tongue swelling postoperatively

❖ Dexamethasone 0.1 mg/kg given to avoid postoperative tongue swelling

❖ IV fluid management using 4:2:1 rate (***Halliday formula***)

Extubation

❖ Reversal of NDMR with 0.02 mg/kg atropine and 0.06 mg/kg neostigmine IV

❖ Extubation after early/deep and proper suctioning (done gently)

❖ Fully awake extubation in head down and lateral decubitus position

❖ Nasal stents to maintain airway patency

Postoperative Care

Monitoring

❖ Pulse oximetry and apnea alarm

❖ Blood pressure

❖ Urine output

❖ ABG with blood sugar levels

Postoperative Management

❖ Elbow restraints for some days to prevent child from taking his hands to operation site

❖ Feeding started as soon as child is fully awake with clear water and half diluted milk

❖ ***Logan's bow***:
  - Traction suture placed through tongue and tied loosely
  - Traction on the suture stimulates respiration
  - Done to prevent child from going into deep sleep and apnea
  - The suture is removed when child leaves PACU

Analgesia

- LA infilteration by surgeon
- Regional blocks:
  - Infraorbital/palatine/nasopalatine block
  - Consider infraortbital nerve block for cleft lip repair
  - Nasopalatine with palatine block done for palatal surgery
- NSAIDs: Paracetamol suppository/ketorolac (0.5 mg/kg IV up to maximum 30 mg)
- Opioid analgesics fentanyl (1 µg/kg IV) or morphine (0.1 mg/kg IV)

Complications

- Laryngeal edema/spasm (1 mm laryngeal edema causes 60% narrowing)
- Delayed recovery
- Respiratory depression
- Airway obstruction due to:
  - Closed palate
  - Small mandible pushing tongue into pharynx
  - Edema
  - Blood and residual anesthesia
- Bleeding
- Hypothermia
- Abbe-Estlander flap:
  - Taken from lower lip to upper lip
  - Done to make up for tissue loss in bilateral cleft lip
  - Thus, problems of closed mouth is common like vomiting and aspiration

ANESTHESIA FOR TONSILLECTOMY

Introduction

Tonsillitis is infection of tonsil which are aggregates of lymphoid tissue, present on both sides of throat.

Anatomy: ***Waldeyer's ring*** is formed by:

- Tubal tonsils
- Palatine tonsils
- Lingual tonsils
- Adenoid

Indications

- Infections:
  - Chronic tonsillitis
  - Recurrent acute tonsillitis (more than 3 episodes of tonsils/adenoids per year)
  - Peritonsillar abscess unresponsive to medical therapy
  - Recurrent chronic otitis media/SOM
  - Chronic tonsillitis with streptococcal carrier state unresponsive to antibiotics with valvular heart disease
- Obstruction:
  - OSAS, severe dysphagia
  - Sleep disorder
  - Cardiopulmonary complications due to hypertrophy
  - Dental malocclusion/affecting facial growth
- Others:
  - Malignancy of tonsils for biopsy/resection
  - Persistent halitosis unresponsive to therapy due to chronic tonsillitis
  - Chronic nasal obstruction with rhinorrhea and obligate mouth breathing

Contraindications

- Acute tonsillitis, abnormal coagulation people
- Uncorrected partial/complete cleft palate as adenoids help fill retropharyngeal gap and facilitate speech

Methods for Tonsillectomy

- Conventional ***cold steel*** tonsillectomy:
  - Tonsillar snare used as dissector
  - More intraoperative bleeding
  - Less postoperative pain and post-tonsillectomy bleeding
- Hot surgical techniques:
  - Bipolar radio frequency
  - Electrocautery, ultrasonic dissection
  - Laser powered microdebrider:
    - Less intraoperative bleeding
    - Increased postoperative pain and bleeding

Clinical Features

- Pain in throat, fever, tachycardia
- Dysphagia/odynophagia, failure to thrive
- Mouth breathing, inflamed tonsil with discharge
- Cervical lymphadenopathy
- Cor pulmonale:
  - If long standing hypoxia and hypercapnea due to airway resistance
  - Cardiac enlargement is reversible with digitalis and tonsillectomy
- Two most common levels of obstruction during sleep are at soft palate and base of tongue
- Long standing hypoxia and hypercapnea:
  - This leads to increased airway resistance

- This causes pulmonary artery constriction and pulmonary HTN
- Ultimately right heart failure and cor pulmonale results

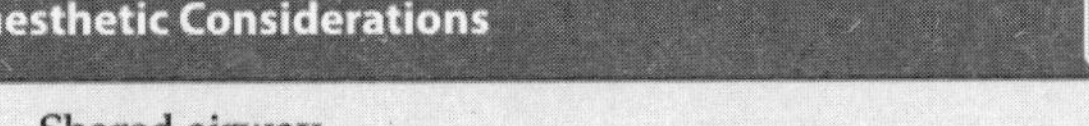

Anesthetic Considerations

- Shared airway
- Difficult airway if enlarged lymphoid tissue
- Obstruction of ETT/LMA by ***Boyle-Davies*** gag used by surgeons
- Maintain deep planes of anesthesia with rapid recovery of consciousness and reflexes

Preoperative Assessment

- History:
  - History of fever, pain, dysphagia: Defer surgery
  - Bleeding disorders: Easy bruising/bleeding gums/epistaxis
  - Family history of bleeding disorders/intake of aspirin/NSAIDs
  - History of allergy/GERD sinusitis
  - History of rhinorrhea/postnasal drip
  - History of anemia/sickle cell disease
  - History of antibiotics/anti-histaminics/NSAIDs/previous surgeries
- Examination:
  - Wheezing/rales for LRTI
  - Inspiratory stridor/prolonged expiration: Partial airway occlusion
  - Loose/missing teeth: Care during mouth gag application
  - Enlarged and tender lymph nodes (≥2 cm)
  - Tonsillar/pharyngeal exudate
  - Thorough airway assessment
  - ***Adenoid facies:***
    - Long face, flat midface, open mouth
    - Retrognathia, high arched palate, hyponasal speech

Investigations

- Complete blood count, blood grouping and typing
- Clotting profile, chest X-ray
- ECG if recent URTI/pneumonia/bronchitis/cor pulmonale

Premedication

- Avoid sedation if history of OSAS/airway obstruction
- In older children/adults, 0.05 mg/kg midazolam PO if age ≥2 years
- IV access taken after EMLA cream application
- 0.02 mg/kg glycopyrollate given IV
- IV fluids if dehydrated due to odynophagia
- Antibiotics before surgery if acute tonsillitis present
- Consent for rectal analgesia

Technique of Anesthesia

- Local anesthesia:
  - Rarely done under local anesthesia
  - Used with GA for postoperative analgesia and bleeding
  - No single nerve block is adequate as multiple areas of nerve supply to tonsils
  - Following topical anesthesia of mucus membrane, three LA injections into:
    - Region of upper pole
    - In anterior pillar
    - In lower pole (between capsule and pharyngeal wall)
  - Care to prevent injection into blood vessel as it is a very vascular area
  - If local anesthetic spreads to glossopharyngeal nerve, airway reflexes may lost
- GA with ETT: Most commonly used
- GA with LMA: Flexible LMA can be used
  - Advantages:
    - Avoids muscle relaxants
    - Reduces aspirations of blood
    - Reduces laryngospasm/bronchospasm/desaturation
    - Requires light plane of anesthesia: Faster recovery
  - Disadvantages:
    - Difficult to control situation if airway is lost during surgery
    - May get compressed on opening mouth gag
    - Access to inferior pole is difficult
    - Maneuvers to aid insertion:
      - Head extension
      - Lateral insertion of LMA
      - Pressure on tip of LMA with index finger
      - Anterior displacement of tongue
      - Use of laryngoscope

Monitors

- Pulse oximetry, E_TCO_2
- NIBP, ECG
- Precordial stethoscope
- Urine output, temperature

Induction

- Intravenous: Propofol + fentanyl with or without short acting NDMR
- Inhalational:
  - In uncooperative children with poor venous access
  - Difficult/slow in significant OSAS: Also may cause hypoxia
- Intubation:
  - South facing ETT (nasal ETT used in some adults)
  - Intubate under deep inhalation/after administering muscle relaxants
  - Nasotracheal intubation may be used in adults as adenoids is absent
  - Secure ETT in midline and ensure that it lies correctly in Boyle-Davis gag
  - Pack throat with petroleum gauze to prevent aspiration
  - Limit cuff pressure to avoid postextubation croup

Position

- Eyes protected especially if gag is used
- Head extended and held by a sand bag/bolster kept under shoulder
- Mouth kept open by Boyle-Davis gag
- Advantages:
  - Direct view of tonsils
  - Posterior pharynx forms sump into which blood drains

Maintenance

- Oxygen + N_2O + isoflurane 1 MAC
- Fentanyl is given in intermittent boluses
- Maintain adequate depth to prevent reflex induced HTN, tachycardia and bucking/straining during surgery
- Intraoperative dexamethasone 0.15 mg/kg IV to reduce edema
- Spontaneous ventilation/CMV with muscle relaxants can be used
- Care to prevent accidental extubation/aspiration of blood and secretions if throat pack displaced
- LA + adrenaline injected in tonsillar fossa:
  - Gives bloodless field
  - But, increases postoperative pain
  - If large volume is used, respiratory obstruction/aspiration can occur due to bilateral glossopharyngeal nerve block

Hemodynamics

- Instrumentation of postnasal space may cause bradycardia
- Blood loss difficult to assess
- IV fluids like RL/DNS to maintain volume status
- Blood transfusion may be required in some cases

Extubation

- No difference in rate of complications between extubating in deep/awake planes
- Fully awake plane with complete return of reflexes preferred
- Head down tilt with lateral position
- Avoid blind suctioning of pharynx to avoid trauma
- Suction done under vision after removal of throat pack: ***Coroners clot*** may result otherwise
- Antiemetic like ondansetron 0.15 mg/kg IV
- Neostigmine 0.05 mg/kg + atropine 0.01 mg/kg IV
- Remove LMA when patient opens eyes to command
- Transfer to recovery room in tonsillar position with oxygen inhalation

Postoperative Care

Pain

- Moderate-to-severe pain present after tonsillectomy
- Oral syrup/rectal paracetamol and NSAIDs (do not increase bleeding)
- LA infilteration into tonsillar bed
- Opioids
- Avoid aspirin to prevent risk of bleeding
- Increased pain if laser or electrocautery used
- Pain is less in those who have had sharp surgical dissection and ligation of blood vessels

Management

- IV fluid administration as swallowing may be reduced due to pain
- IV cannula kept in-situ in case of postoperative bleeding
- Dexamethasone 0.05–0.15 mg/kg to reduce PONV, pain and increase oral feed tolerance
- Continue antibiotics
- Metoclopramide 0.15 mg/kg IV to reduce PONV

Complications

- Post-tonsillectomy bleeding: *Most common*
- Airway obstruction:
  - Due to upper airway edema, blood, secretions, and laryngospasm

- Greater incidence following ETT than LMA use
- Avoided by giving topical anesthesia to upper airway

❖ PONV:
- During first 24 hours, incidence 30–65%
- Due to pharyngeal irritation from surgery and swallowed blood
- Decompress stomach with OGT
- Ondansetron 0.1 mg/kg given IV
- May cause dehydration: Start IV fluids

❖ Pain and sore throat may last for 3–4 days

❖ *Creutzfeldt–Jakob* disease:
- Transmission due to contamination of instruments with lymphoid tissue
- Use disposable surgical and anesthesia equipment between December and January to reduce transmission
- Single use ETT, laryngoscope blades, tongues and LMAs preferred

❖ Pulmonary edema:
- Due to increased pulmonary hydrostatic pressure from rapid relief of airway obstruction
- Most cases resolve within 24 hours
- Treat with ETT, PPV, and PEEP application, diuretic therapy

POST-TONSILLECTOMY BLEEDING

Introduction

❖ Most common complication following tonsillectomy

❖ It is an emergency procedure involving a hypovolemic, tachycardic child on full stomach

❖ Usually bleeding is venous in origin

Incidence

❖ 0.1–8.1% incidence

❖ More common in older children (above 11 years age at 69% incidence)

❖ More common in chronic tonsillitis

❖ Most common in first 6–8 hours postoperatively and may occur till sixth day

❖ 67% of bleeds originate from tonsillar fossa

❖ 26% originate in nasopharynx and 7% from both tonsillar fossa and nasopharynx

Types

❖ Primary hemorrhage: Occurs during surgery

❖ Reactionary hemorrhage:
- Approximately 75% occurs in first 6 hours postsurgery
- Remaining 25% occurs within 24 hours
- Occurs due to:
  - Slippage of ligature from bleeding vessels
  - Dislodgement of clots due to retching/vomiting
  - Bleeding from adenoid bed common in first 4 hours

❖ Secondary hemorrhage:
- From 24 hours to 5–10 days postsurgery
- Due to secondary infection with sloughing of tissues

Blood Supply to Tonsil

❖ Superior pole of tonsil:
- Ascending pharyngeal artery
- Lesser palatine artery

❖ Inferior pole:
- Facial artery branches
- Dorsal lingual artery
- Ascending palatine artery

Venous Return

❖ Plexus around tonsillar capsule

❖ Lingual vein

❖ Pharyngeal plexus

Anesthetic Considerations 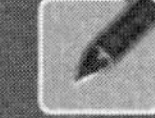

❖ Hypovolemia: Needs urgent fluid resuscitation

❖ Full stomach: Due to ingested food and swallowed blood

❖ Difficult intubation:
- Active bleeding in airway
- Formed clots obstructing airway access
- Edema from previous instrumentation and surgery

❖ Residual narcotic effects: Due to previous anesthesia

❖ Shared airway

Preoperative Evaluation

❖ History:
- Elicited from the mother
- History of frequent swallowing
- Vomiting with coffee brown vomitus

❖ Previous anesthesia record:
- Difficult intubation
- Anesthetic agents used

❖ Examination:
- General:
  - Assess level of consciousness and look for signs of restlessness
  - Pallor and dehydration
  - Stridor and intercostal retractions: Suggests difficult intubation

- Blood loss is difficult to assess as most of blood is swallowed
- Cardiovascular:
  - Hypotension (occurs late), tachycardia
  - Capillary refill time more than 2 seconds
  - Bradycardia in late stages
- Respiratory: Tachypnea, stridor, accessory muscle use
- Others: Oliguria, cold extremities, metabolic acidosis

Treatment

- If history of intermittent bleeding with no active bleed:
  - Observe
  - IV fluids
  - Coagulation parameters
  - If coagulation study abnormal, hematology consult
  - Complete blood count and hematocrit as baseline
- If active minor bleeding:
  - IV fluid resuscitation
  - Ice water gargling and packing
  - If persistent and patient is uncooperative, reexploration is done

Preoperative Preparation and Resuscitation

- Secure large bore IV access
- Resuscitation with crystalloids/blood/plasma:
  - 20 mL/kg repeated depending on clinical signs
  - Up to 40–60 mL/kg may be required
  - Avoid hypotonic fluids: 5% dextrose, 0.45% saline, 2.5% dextrose
- Send blood for hematocrit, cross-matching and coagulation profile
- Avoid preoperative sedation
- Antisialogogues: Glycopyrrolate 0.02 mg/kg IV
- Anti-aspiration prophylaxis:
  - IV metoclopramide 0.15 mg/kg
  - IV ranitidine 1 mg/kg
- Check blood pressure in erect and supine position for orthostatic changes

OT Preparation

- Machine check, AMBU bag, masks
- Variety of ETT and laryngoscope blades
- Variety of large bore suction catheters as blood in airway may plug the catheter/ETT
- Tilting table
- Emergency drugs: Atropine, adrenaline
- Anesthetic agents

Monitors

- Pulse oximetry, E_TCO_2
- NIBP, urine output
- ECG, precordial stethoscope
- Temperature

Induction: Two techniques can be used:

- Inhalational induction with sevoflurane/halothane:
  - Disadvantages:
    - Challenging as position of patient is lateral to avoid aspiration
    - Can be slow
    - Blood may be inhaled and precipitate laryngospasm
    - Tracheal intubation in lateral position is difficult
    - Halothane may cause cardiac arrest
  - Advantages:
    - Oxygenation is well maintained in spontaneous ventilation
    - Lateral position helps in draining blood
    - Clots can be easily suctioned
- Rapid sequence IV induction with cricoid pressure:
  - *Preferred method*
  - Ketamine 2 mg/kg + succinylcholine 1 mg/kg + fentanyl 1 µg/kg used
  - Etomidate 0.2–0.4 mg/kg IV used as alternative
  - Avoid thiopentone and propofol due to risk of precipitous hypotension
  - Advantages:
    - Supine position with cricoid pressure reduces risk of aspiration
    - Less stressful to child
  - Disadvantages:
    - Preoxygenating a bleeding child may be difficult
    - Face mask ventilation following succinylcholine may inflate stomach
    - Risk of hypoxia if difficult intubation with paralyzed patient
- Technique:
  - Adequate preoxygenation with 100% oxygen for 3–5 minutes
  - Rapid sequence induction with cricoid pressure
  - Head down tilt to keep blood away from larynx
  - 0.5–1 mm smaller than appropriate sized ETT as airway edema will be present

- Decompress stomach with Ryles tube after intubation
- Dexamethasone 0.1 mg/kg IV to reduce airway edema
- Ondansetron 0.1 mg/kg IV to prevent vomiting
- Suction to be readily available

Maintenance

- O_2 + N_2O + isoflurane 1 MAC used for maintaining balanced anesthesia
- Fentanyl and vecuronium given in intermittent boluses
- Intermittent positive pressure ventilation

Hemodynamics

- Continue volume resuscitation throughout surgery
- IV fluids and blood as per clinical signs and hematocrit
- Maintain temperature

Extubation

- Head down lateral position
- Extubate when fully awake with normal cough and gag reflex, and stable hemodynamics
- Neostigmine 0.05 mg/kg + glycopyrollate 0.02 mg/kg IV for reversal of NM blockade
- Avoid coughing during extubation to prevent reactionary hemorrhage due to slippage of ligature

Postoperative Care

Management

- Nurse in tonsil position/***Fowlers position***
- Tonsil position: Pillow under chest so that head falls below chest level and fluids drain from mouth
- May require midazolam/opioids to tolerate postnasal packs
- Oxygen administration till fully awake
- Maintain normal temperature
- Continue IV fluids and blood as per hematocrit

Analgesia

- Adequate analgesia to prevent restlessness
- Opioids/NSAIDs used in combination

Monitors

- Pulse oximetry, ECG, NIBP
- Temperature, urine output
- Serial hematocrit
- Monitor for further bleeding

PHYSIOLOGICAL CHANGES WITH AGEING

Introduction

- Progressive, universally prevalent physiological process producing measurable changes in the structure and decremental alteration in function of tissues and organs
- Generally, patients more than 65 years are called geriatric
- 65–74 years: Elderly
- 75–84 years: Aged
- More than 85 years: Very old

Central Nervous System Changes

- Reduction in brain mass, starts at 50 years
- 10% reduction in brain weight occurs at 80 years
- Atherosclerosis of cerebral blood vessels
- Reduced cerebral blood flow
- Reduced neurotransmitters: Dopamine, serotonin, GABA, acetylcholine
- Increased incidence of postoperative delirium and cognitive decline

Cardiovascular System Changes

- Cardiac output:
  - Cardiac output is stroke volume dependant as heart rate is low
  - Reduced maximal cardiac output
  - Output is volume dependant but volume intolerance
- Structural changes:
  - Stiffening of myocardium, arteries and veins causing:
    - Slow diastolic filling
    - Postural hypotension with mild hypovolemia
  - Increased capillary permeability: Increased chances of pulmonary edema
- Conduction system:
  - Fibrosis of conduction system
  - Loss of sinoatrial node cells
  - Atrial fibrillation common, sick sinus syndrome, complete heart block
- Blood pressure:
  - Old age represents a volume contracted state
  - Increased sympathetic nervous system activity and reduced parasympathetic activity
  - Labile blood pressure during anesthesia
  - Reduced PNS activity may limit increase in heart rate in response to administration of atropine

- Reduced arterial compliance: Systolic HTN and widened pulse pressure
- ❖ Defective ischemic preconditioning as protective effect of angina is absent

Respiratory System Changes

- ❖ Structure:
  - More upper airway obstruction
  - Stiffening of chest wall, barrel shaped chest
  - Increased elasticity of lung parenchyma
  - Reduced alveolar surface area: Reduced resting PaO_2
  - Less effective cough: Increased chances of aspiration
  - Flattened diaphragm and loss of muscle mass: Increased dyspnea
- ❖ Physiology:
  - Increased anatomical and physiological dead space
  - Ventilation-perfusion mismatch
  - Increased closing capacity
  - Closing capacity exceeds FRC in mid 60s
  - 50% reduction in ventilatory response to hypoxia and hypercarbia: Increased risk of postoperative apnea
  - PaO_2 falls steadily [$PaO_2 = \frac{(100 - \text{age})}{4}$]
  - Reduced minute volume requirements as O_2 consumption and CO_2 production reduces
  - Patients tolerate longer periods of apnea
  - Edentulous patient: Maintenance of patent airway and face mask seal difficult

Endocrine System Changes

- ❖ Insulin resistance
- ❖ Insulin secretion reduces in response to glucose load
- ❖ Reduced estrogen, testosterone and GH production
- ❖ Subclinical hypothyroidism in females

Hepatocellular Changes

- ❖ Reduced liver mass, 20–40% reduction in liver blood flow
- ❖ Size of liver reduces to 40% by 80 years
- ❖ Reduced hepatic function
- ❖ Reduced phase I metabolism and bile secretion with age
- ❖ Reduced plasma cholinesterase in men

Renal Changes

- ❖ Reduced renal cortical mass by 20–25%
- ❖ Loss of up to half the glomeruli by 80 years
- ❖ Reduction in GFR by 1 mL/min/yr after 40 years age
- ❖ Increased risk of acute renal failure perioperatively

Body Composition and Fluid Homeostasis

- ❖ Gradual loss of skeletal muscle and body fat
- ❖ Reduced total body water and plasma albumin
- ❖ Low responsiveness to ADH
- ❖ Reduced aldosterone secretion: Altered Na^+ homeostasis
- ❖ Reduced ability to conserve Na^+ and concentrate urine
- ❖ Reduced basal metabolism

Thermoregulation

- ❖ Prone to hypothermia as:
  - Reduced subcutaneous fat insulation
  - Reduced BMR: Reduced heat production
- ❖ Ineffective shivering and vasoconstriction
- ❖ Vasoconstriction not activated till temperature falls by more than 4°C

Hematology

- ❖ Hypercoagulability and DVT
- ❖ Anemia more common
- ❖ Reduced immune response: Increased infection

Musculoskeletal

- ❖ Reduced muscle mass fragile skin
- ❖ Osteoporosis: Positional fractures and dislocations
- ❖ Osteoarthritis/rheumatoid arthritis deformities: Difficult IV line
- ❖ Increased chances of nerve injuries: pad pressure points
- ❖ Osteoporosis, ligament laxity and calcification causes difficult spinal

Drug Pharmacology

- ❖ Reduced body mass
- ❖ Reduced total body water
- ❖ Relative reduction in fat
- ❖ Reduced albumin
- ❖ Increased acid glycoprotein
- ❖ Reduced cardiac output
- ❖ Mildly contracted blood volume
- ❖ Reduction in hepatic and renal clearance
- ❖ Also altered drug responses as in:
  - Drugs have more pronounced effect

- Bolus doses take longer time to act
- Increased drug interactions
- Target organs more sensitive to drug level
- Increased context sensitive half life

❖ Examples:
- Use meperidine only for shivering
- Fentanyl, sufentanyl, remifentanyl, alfentanyl and morphine: 50% reduction in dosage
- Thiopentone and propofol warrant 20% reduction in dose
- Midazolam requires modest reduction in dose at 60 years and 75% reduction in dose at 90 years
- Vecuronium, rocuronium, cisatracurium and succinylcholine:
  - Have slower onset of action
  - Increased incidence of residual paralysis especially if multiple doses used
- Residual paralysis occurs due to drug accumulation
- Neostigmine dose increases with age in some studies
- Decrease in MAC value of volatile anesthetics with age
- Reduced sensitivity to β-agonists, antagonists and digoxin with age
- Increased chances of renal failure and GI bleed with NSAIDs
- Increased hypotension with CCBs, nitrates and diuretics due to volume contracted state

ANESTHETIC MANAGEMENT OF GERIATRIC PATIENT

Introduction

With geriatric population on the rise, anesthetist is bound to encounter more number of elder patients in the near future.

Preoperative Evaluation

❖ Preoperative risk factors:
- Emergency surgery
- ASA class ≥ 3
- Low functional status
- Clinical evidence of CCF

❖ Coexisting diseases:
- History of cardiac (MI/CCF), respiratory (COPD), renal/hepatic diseases
- History of RA/OA deformities:
  - Difficult IV access
  - Cervical instability
- Polypharmacy and drug interactions are common
- Dehydration, malnutrition are very common: *Anorexia of ageing*

❖ History and evaluation:
- History of previous illness, medication history
- Current functional status of all organ systems
- Assessment of level of physical activity for CVS and RS status is limited due to bone and joint disease
- Mental status examination important
- Low albumin levels associated with increased morbidity and motality

❖ Preoperative management:
- Continue all medication except OHAs
- Avoid sedatives, especially benzodiazepines and pethidine
- Perioperative β-blockade considered
- Care towards *Do not resuscitate orders*
- Optimize preoperative medical status
- Postpone elective surgery until concurrent illnesses are optimized

Regional Anesthesia

❖ Use wherever possible

❖ Most common used for TURP, herniorrhaphy, gynecological surgeries, hip fractures

❖ Requires alert and cooperative patient

❖ Advantages:
- Reduced chances of DVT, early mobilization
- Low incidence of postoperative cognitive decline
- Rapid recognition of CNS changes and onset of angina pectoris

❖ Spinal anesthesia:
- Difficult spinal due to ligament calcification and laxity
- Prolonged duration of action due to reduced vascular absorption of LA due to atherosclerosis
- Profound hypotension on induction due to volume contracted state
- T_8-T_{10} level acceptable for most cases

❖ Epidural anesthesia:
- More gradual onset of hypotension than spinal anesthesia
- Dose required to produce sensory block lesser as progressive occlusion of intervertebral foramina with connective tissue occurs

Conduct of General Anesthesia

Monitoring

❖ Pulse oximetry, capnography

❖ NIBP, ECG

- Temperature, urine output
- BP/CVP considered in cardiac patients
- Neuromuscular monitoring (residual palsy)

Positioning

- Osteoporosis increases chances of positional injuries
- Intermittently relieve pressure points in long duration surgeries
- Positional changes should be gradual as defectives baroreceptor function

Induction

- Smaller induction doses used
- Difficult IV access due to thin veins and bony deformities
- Onset of IV induction delayed due to longer brain-arm circulation time
- Significant hypotension with induction
- Difficult mask ventilation in edentulous patients
- Precautions to prevent aspiration as:
  - Blunted airway reflexes
  - Increased incidence of hiatus hernias in elderly
- ET tube to be used where possible

Maintenance

- Reduced MAC value of volatile anesthetics
- Reduced doses of intravenous drugs
- Reduced fentanyl, sufentanyl, alfentanyl, remifentanyl and morphine requirements by 50%
- Reduce doses of muscle relaxants as high incidence of residual muscular paralysis
- Forced air warmers to prevent hypothermia

Ventilation

- Mechanical ventilation with supplemental oxygen preferred to spontaneous ventilation
- High tidal volume with PEEP used to prevent atelectasis
- Avoid hyperventilation if patient receiving digoxin to prevent hypokalemia

Postoperative Care

Monitors

- Pulse oximetry, NIBP
- ECG, urine output
- Temperature
- Neuromuscular monitoring
- ABG, fluid balance

Management

- Early establishment of nasogastric tube feeding
- Early mobilization, physiotherapy and thromboprophylaxis, elastic support stockings
- Maintain hemoglobin level at 9–10 g% if cardiac disease present
- Continue oxygen for 24 hours except in minor surgeries
- Monitor fluid balance and fluid overload

Postoperative Analgesia

- May be more tolerant of acute pain
- Delirium and cognitive decline hinder pain reporting by patient
- More difficulty with visual analog scale rather than verbal/numerical scales
- Epidural analgesia superior, it also reduces opioid requirements
- NSAIDs used with caution and reduces opioid requirement

Complications

- Pain causing:
  - Sleep deprivation
  - Gastric ileus
  - Suboptimal mobilization
  - Insulin resistance
  - Tachycardia, perioperative MI
- Cardiovascular system:
  - Myocardial infarction, cardiac arrest
  - Arrhythmias
- Respiratory system:
  - Pneumonia: If more than 48 hours on ventilator
  - Reintubation
  - Atelectasis
- Central nervous system:
  - Stroke: Usually occurs more than 7 days postoperatively
  - Delirium, cognitive decline

ANESTHESIA FOR TOTAL HIP REPLACEMENT

Introduction

Performed commonly in geriatric patients who usually have associated comorbidities.

Preoperative Evaluation

History

- Underlying medical illness and review of organ systems

- Drug history: For *polypharmacy*
- Surgical history and anesthetic history

Examination

- Deafness, dementia and cognitive dysfunction common
- Vital parameters: BP, heart rate, rhythm, respiratory rate
- CVS, RS, CNS, abdominal examination
- Difficult IV access in rheumatoid arthritis if small joints of wrist and foot are involved
- Check if patient can tolerate lying flat after spinal (orthopnea may limit lying flat)

Investigations

- Routine blood, urea, creatinine, clotting profile
- *Chest X-ray*: Pleural effusion, interstitial fibrosis
- Echocardiography for LV function, RWMA, valve abnormality
- Dobutamine stress test:
    - Exercise tolerance is limited by hip disease
    - Hence, cardiovascular reserve may be difficult to assess
- Lung function tests, ABG and SpO_2 on room air
- Renal function tests may be impaired due to chronic NSAID use

Airway Assessment

- In rheumatoid arthritis, cervical spine and temporomandibular joint (TMJ) may be involved
- Atlanto-axial subluxation occurs in 25% patients with severe rheumatoid arthritis
- Treat as unstable spine: Use manual in line stabilization maneuver
- TMJ involvement may cause restricted mouth opening

Preoperative Preparation

- NPO orders
- Informed consent
- Optimize comorbidities
- Two units of cross matched blood to be available
- Antibiotic prophylaxis
- 16–18 G large bore IV cannula in nondependant arm for laterally positioned patients
- Time DVT prophylaxis as per ASRA guidelines for regional anesthetic techniques
- Invasive monitors if severe disease/large blood loss is anticipated
- ACE inhibitors stopped to avoid sudden hypotension
- Continue other antihypertensives
- Stop morning dose of hypoglycemic agents
- Avoid NSAIDs, especially if neuraxial block planned

Anesthetic Considerations

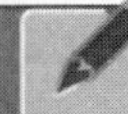

- Anesthetic consideration of lateral position
- Hypotensive anesthetic technique may be preferred
- Keep patient warm: OT may be set at 18–20°C
- OT temperature usually set at 18–20°C to prevent premature cement setting
- Ensure adequate volume filling prior to cementing
- Watch for ***bone cement implantation syndrome***
- Patient warming device and warm fluids should be used where possible
- Blood loss may be around 300–500 mL
- Strategies to avoid blood transfusion:
    - Avoid HTN and tachycardia
    - Regional anesthesia technique
    - Hypotensive anesthesia
    - Acute normovolemic hemodilution
    - Intraoperative and postoperative blood salvage
- Anterior restraints used in lateral position may prevent chest expansion

Choice of Anesthetic Technique

- Regional anesthesia:
    - Advantages:
        - Reduces blood loss intraoperatively
        - Reduced need for blood transfusion
        - Improved cement bonding due reduced bleeding
        - Reduced incidence of DVT and PE
        - Avoids effects of GA on pulmonary function
        - Good postoperative analgesia
        - Low cost
    - Conduct of anesthesia:
        - Monitors: NIBP, SpO_2, ECG, urine output
        - Preload with IV fluid 10 mL/kg
        - Subarachnoid block with 0.5% heavy bupivacaine
        - Phenylephrine better for treating hypotension
        - Protect pressure points with gel pads, cotton pads and gamgee rolls
        - Patient warming devices connected
        - Tranexemic acid 500 mg in NS given over 30 minutes pre-incision and postoperatively
        - Sedate with midazolam and fentanyl combination
        - Oxygen by face mask at 4–6 L/min

- 10° head down tilt with normal to slight hypervolemia when hypotensive anesthesia planned
- Basal BP restored after cementing is complete

- Epidural anesthesia:
  - For longer and more complex surgery
  - Also for postoperative analgesia
  - Insert urinary catheter if epidural anesthesia given
  - Time removal of catheter with DVT prophylaxis
- Peripheral nerve blocks for THR:
  - No single peripheral nerve block is sufficient for THR
  - Lumbar plexus block gives effective analgesia
  - 3 in 1 femoral block is easier to perform but less effective
- General anesthesia:
  - Advantages:
    - Better in patients unable to the flat
    - Safer in patients with fixed cardiac output states like aortic stenosis
    - Patients comfortable
    - Less likely to require urinary catheterization
  - Expect:
    - Late recovery from GA
    - Reduced MAC values
    - Increased benzodiazepine requirements
    - Increased LA concentration as albumin levels are lower in blood

Anesthetic Problems

Preoperative Problems

- Deafness, dementia, and cognitive impairment: Difficult to communicate
- Difficult to assess cardiac status: Stress dobutamine test
- Volume contracted state if hypertensive: Judicious preloading
- Associated comorbities: DM, HTN, polypharmacy, ARF, NSAID nephropathy
- May have reduced FRC and V-Q ratio: Pulmonary function test done
- Anemia of chronic disease
- Antiaspiration prophylaxis as reduced LES tone and airway reflexes
- DVT prophylaxis as prolonged immobilization

Intraoperative Problems

- Lateral position:
  - Might decrease FRC more
  - May be dangerous in patients prone for pathological fractures
  - Padding to prevent brachial plexus injuries
- Blood loss of around 500 mL: Use blood conservation strategies
- Bone cement implantation syndrome
- Fat embolism syndrome from femur reaming
- Judicious fluid management to prevent fluid overload
- Prone for hypothermia as thermoregulatory center impaired
- Profound fall in BP after SAB if isolated systolic HTN exists preoperatively
- If general anesthesia chosen:
  - Prolonged and late recovery as although weight is less, fat proportion is increased
  - Difficulty airway: Atlanto-axial joint and TMJ involvement
  - Unstable cervical spine: Use MILS maneuver

Postoperative Care

Position: Supine with legs abducted using pillow.

Ventilations

- Oxygen therapy for 24 hours postoperatively
- Given for 72 hours postoperatively in those at high risk for M1

Monitors

- NIBP, SpO_2
- ECG, urine output
- Drains
- Hemoglobin 24 hours postoperatively

Postoperative Analgesia

- Less severe compared with TKR
- Multimodal analgesia preferred
- Patient controlled analgesia may be used
- Use NSAIDs with caution as renal impairment may occur in elderly
- Epidural analgesia very useful
- Time the removal of catheter with DVT prophylaxis regimen
- Epidural infusion of 0.125% bupivacaine and fentanyl 2–4 μg/mL for 48 hrs at 6–10 mL/hr started around 2 hours after SAB

ARTERIAL TOURNIQUET

Introduction

Use of arterial tourniquet greatly facilitates bloodless field during upper and lower limb orthopedic surgeries.

Indications

- For intravenous regional anesthesia or Biers block
- To provide bloodless field for surgery:
  - For better identification of structures
  - Reduced operative time
  - Reduced surgical complications
  - Reduced need for blood transfusion

Guidelines for Use

- Position: Point of overlap of tourniquet to be placed 180° from neurovascular bundle as there is some area of reduced compression at overlap point
- Cuff width:
  - Width of inflated cuff to be more than half the limb diameter
  - To be more than 7 cm, especially for leg, to minimize drainage to skin
- Tourniquet time:
  - Minimum time for IVRA is 30 minutes
  - Maximum duration of inflation:
    - 2 hours as increased risk of rhabdomyolysis and nerve palsy if longer duration
    - 5 minutes of intermittent perfusion allowed beyond 2 hours inflation
    - This is followed by repeat exsanguination through elevation and compression of limb
    - This may allow prolonged use of tourniquet
- Tourniquet pressure:
  - Systolic BP + 150 mm Hg for IVRA
  - Systolic BP + 100 mm Hg for lower limb surgeries
  - Systolic BP + 50 mm Hg for upper limb surgeries

Changes on Cuff Deflation

- Mild systemic metabolic acidosis (preinflation pH of 7.4 reduces to 6.9, 2 hours after deflation)
- Increased $PaCO_2$ (1–8 mm Hg)
- Raised lactate levels
- Increased K+ levels (5–10% increase)
- Transient rise in $ETCO_2$ levels
- Transient fall in systolic BP: 14–19 mm Hg
- Transient fall in heart rate: 6–12 bpm
- Transient fall in temperature by 0.7°C
- All these changes are due to release of toxic metabolites from the occluded limb, such as carbon dioxide, lactic acid, and potassium

Contraindications

- Peripheral vascular disease (*Raynaud's disease*)
- Deep vein thrombosis
- AV fistula/arterial calcific disease
- Peripheral neuropathy/CNS disorder
- Severely injured/traumatized limb
- Severe infection in limb
- Bone abscess
- Sickle cell disease: Use is controversial as sickling is promoted by hypoxia/acidosis

Complications

Tourniquet Pain

- Occurs in 66% cases 30–60 minutes after giving RA
- Due to faster recovery of unmyelinated C fibers from SAB as the block wanes, as compared to A fibers
- Bupivacaine is associated with reduced tourniquet pain as it blocks C unmyelinated fibers in a better way
- Likelihood of pain varies with anesthetic technique:
  - IVRA > epidural > SAB > GA
  - Hyperbaric tetracaine > isobaric bupivacaine
- Clinical features:
  - Dull, deep, burning, and poorly localized pain
  - Hypertension, tachycardia, diaphoresis
- Treatment:
  - Definitive treatment is cuff deflation
  - Sedatives, IV opioids
  - Double cuff application
  - EMLA cream application under cuff
  - TENS/vibratory massages: Not useful

Hemodynamic Changes

- Exsanguination:
  - Results in movement of blood from peripheral to central circulation
  - Causes increased SVR and preload to heart
- 10–15% increase in heart rate and HTN on cuff inflation
- Cardiac arrest, LV failure
- Deflation of cuff:
  - Causes reduced SVR
  - This causes acute blood loss which may continue for 24 hours
  - Also causes release of metabolites: May require cardiac support with inotropes

Tourniquet Hypertension

- Occurs due to tourniquet pain
- Begins three-fourths to 1 hour after cuff inflation

Pulmonary Embolism

- Pulmonary embolism possible following exsanguinations/cuff deflation in TKR
- Silent DVT may be the cause and high index of suspicion is required

Metabolic Changes

- Increased $PaCO_2$ (1–8 mm Hg), reduced pH, increased lactate and K^+ levels
- Only increase in $PaCO_2$, in head injury patients may cause increased CBF and raised ICP
- Body temperature increases in pediatric patients during tourniquet inflation

Postoperative Edema

- Due to return of exsanguinated blood and post-ischemic reactive hyperemia
- Can be due to arterial flow with no venous return during cuff inflation
- Post-tourniquet syndrome: Pale and swollen limb for 1–6 weeks postoperatively
- Cold compression of limb is useful

Bleeding

- Bleeding during tourniquet inflation:
    - More commonly due to intramedullary blood flow in long bones
    - Particularly common in skeletally immature patients
    - Also due to small arteries between two long bones in distal limb
- Post-tourniquet release, bleeding may continue for 24 hours

Tourniquet Failure

Occurs due to:

- Inadequate pressure and exsanguination
- Calcified arteries

Delayed Return of Blood Flow After Tourniquet Release

Causes are:

- Arterial injury
- Compartment syndrome
- Reperfusion injury due to formation of lipid peroxides which is reduced by propofol (which inhibits superoxide formation)

Trauma

- Skin trauma:
    - Due to improper placement of padding under cuff
    - Causes bruising, abrasions, and blistering
- Arterial trauma: Causes arterial spasm, arterial thrombus
- Venous trauma: Venous thrombus due to stagnant blood
- Muscle rhabdomyolysis: If inflation time more than 2 hours
- Nerve injury:
    - Called ***tourniquet palsy***
    - Paroneal and tibial nerve palsy common following TKA with tourniquet inflation ≥ 2 hours

BONE CEMENT

Introduction

Bone cement consists of polymethyl-methacrylate which interdigitates with interstices of cancellous bone and strongly binds prosthetic device to patients bone during TKR/THR.

Components

- Components of ampule:
    - Methylmethacrylate monomer
    - N,N–dimethyl paratoluidene
    - Hydroquinone
- Components of powder:
    - Methylmethacrylate styrene copolymer
    - $BaSO_4$
- Hydroquinone prevents premature polymerization which occurs due to exposure to light or elevated temperatures
- N,N dimethylparatoluidene promotes cold curing of finished therapeutic compound
- $BaSO_4$ for contrast for X-ray examination

Indications

- Fixation of prosthesis to living bone:
    - Osteoarthritis
    - Rheumatoid arthritis
    - Traumatic arthritis
    - Avascular necrosis
    - Sickle cell anemia
    - Collagen vascular diseases
- Fixation of pathological fractures where loss of bone substance/recalcitrance of fracture renders conventional measures ineffective

Contraindications

- Allergy to any of the components
- Infective arthritis/active joint infection/history of such injection
- Where loss of musculature/neuromuscular compromise in affected limb would render procedure unjustifiable

Pathophysiological Changes

- Polymerization of methylmethacrylate:
    - Is an exothermic reaction
    - *Temperatures can reach up to 110°C*
    - This can cause RBC and bone narrow lysis

- Methacrylic acid:
  - Residual methylmethacrylate monomers gets hydrolysed to methacrylic acid
  - Significant fraction of circulating methacrylate is in the form of free acid and rather than methylester
  - This can cause vasodilation and reduced systemic vascular resistance
- Femoral reaming and prosthetic implantation can cause embolization of fat, bone marrow and air into femoral venous channels due to intramedullary hypertension (≥ 500 mm Hg)
- Release of tissue thromboplastin may trigger platelet aggregation and microthrombus formation in lungs

Complications

- Most frequent complications:
  - Exothermic reaction: Red cell and bone marrow lysis
  - Transient hypotension:
    - Occurs primarily in:
      - Patients with increased or high normal BP
      - Patients with hypovolemia
      - Those with preexisting cardiovascular abnormalities
    - Onset of hypotension is within 10–165 seconds
    - Hypotension lasts for 30 seconds to 5–6 minutes
  - Thrombophlebitis
  - Surgical wound infection, deep wound infection
  - Trochanteric bursitis, trochanteric separation
  - Hemorrhage and hematoma
  - Loosening and displacement of prosthesis
- Most serious complications:
  - Cardiac arrest due to:
    - Direct embolization
    - Secondary to hypoxia due to pulmonary embolism
    - Myocardial infarction
  - Cerebrovascular accidents
- Other complications:
  - Heterotopic bone formation
  - Short-term cardiac conduction abnormalities

Bone Cement Implantation Syndrome

Components

- Hypoxia (increased pulmonary shunting)
- Hypotension
- Dysrhythmias including heart block and sinus arrest
- Pulmonary hypertension (increased pulmonary vascular resistance)
- Reduced cardiac output
- Fat embolization syndrome (FES)
- Cardiac arrest

Risk Factors for Syndrome

- Revision surgery
- Long stem femoral prosthesis
- THA/TKA for pathological fractures
- Quantity of cement used

Strategies to Minimize Embolization

- Increase FiO_2 prior to cementing: Prevents hypoxia
- Maintain euvolemia by monitoring CVP: Prevents hypotension
- Create vent hole in distal femur to relieve intramedullary pressure
- Perform high pressure lavage of femoral shaft to remove debris: Potential microemboli
- Use cement-less prosthesis
- Discontinue N_2O several minutes prior to bone cement application

FAT EMBOLISM

Introduction

- Fat embolism can be defined as the presence of fat in peripheral circulation
- Fat embolism syndrome (FES) can be defined as the physiological response to fat within systemic circulation
- Seen in almost all patients who sustain a pelvic/femur fractures, but incidence of FES is < 1%

Etiology

- Long bone/pelvic fractures
- Hip/knee replacement (during implantation of femoral prosthesis/during reaming)
- Following CPR, bone marrow transplant
- Lipid emulsion therapy or lipid infusion in parental feeding
- Liposuction
- Acute pancreatitis, acute fatty liver
- Acute sickle cell crisis: Bone marrow crisis

Pathogenesis

- Two theories to explain FES: Mechanical theory and biochemical theory
- Mechanical theory:
  - Fat globules are released by disruption of fat cells in the fractured bone
  - These enter circulation through tears in medullary blood vessels

- Biochemical theory: Two mechanisms:
  - Toxic mechanism:
    - Free fatty acids released due to trauma
    - These directly affect pneumocytes in lung and cause ARDS
    - This is increased by trauma mediated release of catecholamines
    - Catecholamines increase mobilization of free fatty acids
  - Obstructive mechanism:
    - Unspecified chemical event occurs at site of fracture
    - This causes release of mediators
    - These mediators affect lipid solubility, resulting in coalescence of lipids
    - Consequently, fat embolization occurs
- Other predisposing factors such as shock, hypovolemia, sepsis or DIC may be required to convert fat emboli to FES
- ARDS:
  - Increased fatty acid levels can have a toxic effect on capillary alveolar membrane
  - This leads to the release of vasoactive amines and prostaglandins
  - This causes development of SIRS/ARDS due to damage to pulmonary endothelium
- Neurological manifestations are due to capillary damage to cerebral circulation and cerebral edema

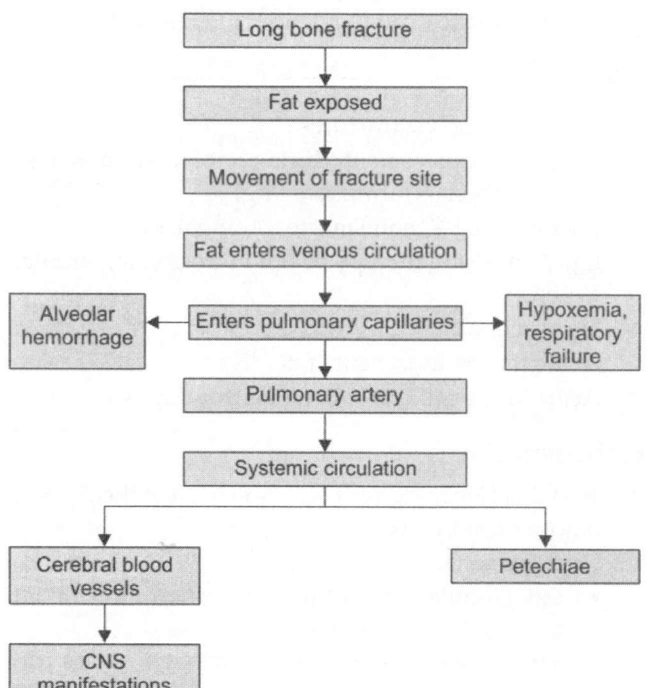

Risk Factors for Fat Embolism Syndrome

- Male gender
- Age 20–30 years
- Hypovolemic shock
- Intramedullary instrumentation
- Total hip arthroplasty using cementing femoral stems
- Bilateral total knee arthroplasty

Incidence

- Incidence of FES in isolated long bone fractures is 3–4%
- Mortatility rate associated with FES is 10–20%
- Self limiting condition with adequate supportive therapy

Types

Subclinical FES

- Occurs in 50% patients with long bone fractures
- Can occur up to 3 days after injury
- Associated with mild hypoxemia and hematological abnormalities

Non-fulminant FES

- Occurs in 1–5% cases of major trauma
- Develops within 12–72 hours gradually
- Severe hypoxia, respiratory depression, rashes fever, tachycardia, CNS symptoms

Fulminant FES

- Rapid onset occurring within few hours
- Severe form associated with RVF, cardiac arrest, fat particles in systemic circulation, DIC
- Can occur during surgery causing fatal outcome

Clinical Features

- Classically presents within 72 hours following long bone fractures
- Males 20–30 years of age affected more often
- Dermatological manifestations:
  - Petechiae over axilla, neck, conjunctiva face *pathognomonic*
  - Occurs due to rupture of small blood vessels by fat globules
- Respiratory manifestations:
  - Hypoxemia, tachypnea, dyspnea
  - Initial chest X-ray is normal, 10% have fluffy appearance

- Less than 10% cases progress to frank ARDS
- Inspiratory crackles due to RV failure

❖ Central nervous system:
- Drowsiness, confusion, coma, seizures
- Can occur in the absence of respiratory complications
- This may be due to passage of fat across ASD/ other AV shunts

❖ Others:
- Pyrexia, tachycardia
- ECG: RV strain pattern

❖ Renals: Oliguria, lipiduria, hematuria, proteinuria

Signs During General Anesthesia

❖ Hypotension, tachycardia, rashes

❖ Reduction in E_TCO_2 and SpO_2 with increase in E_TCO_2-$PaCO_2$ gradient

❖ Reduced alveolar-arterial gradient

❖ Raised pulmonary arterial pressure, reduced cardiac index

❖ ECG: ST elevation, right ventricular strain pattern

❖ Transesophageal echocardiography

❖ Delayed awakening following GA

Investigations

❖ Blood: Thrombocytopenia (< 1.5 lakh/mm^3), anemia (unexplained cause)

❖ Fat globules in blood/urine/retina (***cotton wall spots***)

❖ Increased clotting time, hypocalcemia due to affinity of calcium to FFA

❖ Increased serum lipase may be present

❖ Increased levels of free fatty acids and triglycerides in blood

❖ ECG: RV strain pattern, ST elevation

❖ Transesophageal echocardiography, pulmonary artery catheter: For pulmonary HTN

❖ MRI/CT scan

❖ Broncho-alveolar lavage: Macrophages with fat

Gurds Diagnostic Criteria for Fat Embolism Syndrome

❖ Major features:
- Respiratory insufficiency, tachypnea > 30 cycles/ min
- Cerebral involvement
- Petechial rashes

❖ Minor features:
- Pyrexia > 38°C
- Tachycardia
- Jaundice
- Retinal changes: Retinal fat globules
- Renal changes: Urinary fat globules

❖ Lab findings:
- Fat microglobulinemia: Essential
- Anemia, thrombocytopenia, raised ESR

❖ *One major and four minor criteria with evidence of fat microglobulinemia required*

Schonfeld Fat Embolism Syndrome Index

Sign	Score
Petechial rash	5
Diffuse alveolar infilterates	4
Hypoxemia, PaO_2 <70, FiO_2 100%	3
Confusion	1
Fever >38°C (>100.4°F)	1
Heart rate >120 bpm	1
Respiratory rate >30/min	1

❖ Ranks/score given according to incidence of presentation

❖ Score > 5 required for diagnosis of FES

Management

Prophylactic

❖ Early stabilization of fracture

❖ Reduce intramedullary instrumentation and manipulation

❖ Use of cemented prosthesis

❖ Change in surgery such as converting IM nailing to external fixator application

❖ Reversal of possible risk factors such as hypovolemia

Supportive

❖ Monitor pulse oximetry, ECG, capnography

❖ Oxygen therapy:
- Continuous positive pressure ventilation may be required
- If SpO_2 < 90% tracheal intubation and mechanical ventilation
- Ventilation with FiO_2 100% and respiratory rate > 35 breaths/min
- Ventilation to be instituted before onset of respiratory failure
- Only 10% cases require mechanical ventilation as symptoms resolve within 3–7 days

❖ Correct hypovolemia, cardiac support with inotropes

- Heparin: Useful as it increases lipase action and clears FFAs from blood
- Alcohol and dextran bind FFA: Unproven role, results may be disappointing
- Corticosteroids: Beneficial especially if cerebral edema present
- Aspirin as prophylactic agent as it inhibits TXA_2 production

PALLIATIVE CARE

Introduction

- Palliative care is defined as care which aims at mitigating the sufferings of the patient, not to affect a cure
- Hospice refers to the philosophy of care that seeks to support dignified dying or a good death experience for those with terminal illness

Definition (WHO 2002 Definition)

Defined as an approach that improves the quality of life of patients and their families facing problems associated with life-threatening illness, through the prevention of suffering by means of early identification and impeccable assessment and treatment of pain and other problems, physical, psychosocial and spiritual.

Roles of Palliative Care [National Council for Palliative Care (NCPC) 2002]

- Providing relief from pain and other symptoms
- Integrates psychological and spiritual aspects of patient care
- Offers a support system to help patients live as actively as possible until death
- Offers a support system to help the family cope with the patients illness

AIMS of Palliative Care (Canadian Palliative Care Association Guidelines 2001)

- Access is foundational: Care should be available to all those who require it
- Care is patient focused: Strives to meet physical, psychological and spiritual needs
- Care should be sensitive to patient's cultural and religious values
- Patient should be ready to deal with the dying process
- Right to choice: Each patient should have right to choose best possible treatment option
- Palliative care never intentionally hastens death or provides physician assisted death
- Care choices are guided by quality of life as defined by the patient

Indications of Palliative Care 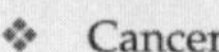

- Cancer
- Chronic obstructive pulmonary disease
- Chronic renal failure
- Chronic heart failure
- Parkinsonism
- Progressive neurological conditions
- HIV/AIDS

Timing of Palliative Care

- To be instituted within 8 weeks of newly diagnosed advanced cancer
- Should be started soon after a known cancer patient's disease becomes advanced

Components of Palliative Care

- Build rapport with patients and family caregivers
- Exploration of patient's understanding and education about illness and prognosis
- Manage symptoms, distress, and functional status
- Clarification of treatment goals
- Assistance with medical decision making
- Assessment and provision of dignity therapy
- Coordination with other care providers
- Provision of referral to other care providers

Services Provided by Palliative Care

- Interdisciplinary healthcare:
  - Healthcare
  - Nursing services
  - Medical, social, pastoral counseling
  - Home health aide
- Bereavement counseling
- Dietary counseling
- Physical therapy
- Occupational therapy
- Speech therapy
- Investigations and drugs
- Durable medical equipments and supplies

Drugs used in Palliative Care

- Analgesics:
  - Non-opioids:
    - Paracetamol
    - NSAIDs
  - Opioids:
    - Codeine, dihydrocodeine
    - Morphine, methadone
    - Oxycodone, hydromorphone

- ❖ Corticosteroids:
  - Prednisolone
  - Dexamethasone
- ❖ Laxatives:
  - Senna, sodium docusate
  - Lactulose, mineral oil
  - Magnesium hydroxide
- ❖ Diarrhea:
  - Loperamide
  - Codeine phosphate
- ❖ Antidepressants:
  - Diazepam, lorazepam
  - Chlorpromazine, haloperidol
  - Phenytoin, sodium valproate
- ❖ GI drugs:
  - Hyoscine butylbromide
  - Metaclopramide, dimenhydrinate

Model of Palliative Care

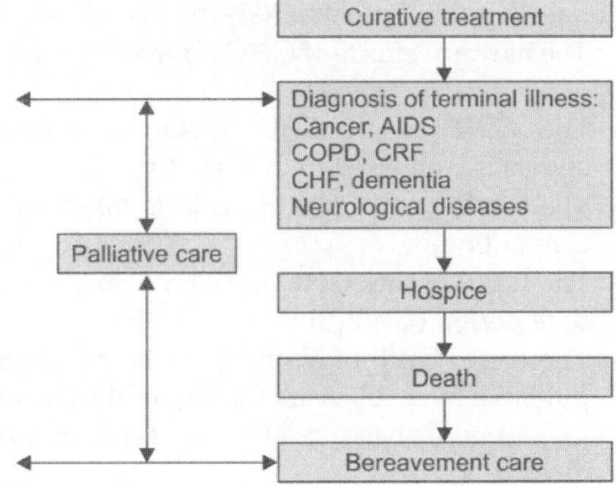

Cancer Pain

- ❖ Choice of analgesics: ESMO 2018 guidelines:
  - Mild pain:
    - NPS score 1–3
    - Acetaminophen
    - NSAIDs
  - Mild-moderate pain:
    - NPS score 4–6
    - Weak opioids preferred in combination with NSAIDs
    - Tramadol
    - Codeine
    - Dihydrocodeine
  - Moderate-severe pain:
    - NPS score 7–10
    - Strong opioids preferred
    - Oral morphine
    - Oral hydromorphone
    - Oxycodone
- ❖ Choice of route of administration:
  - Oral route preferred for chronic pain
  - Parenteral administration preferred for:
    - Acute exacerbations and breakthrough pain
    - Inability to receive oral opioids
  - Transdermal buprenorphine and fentanyl used for:
    - Inability to swallow
    - Poor oral compliance
    - Poor tolerance of oral morphine

End of life care: ***National Consensus Project for Quality Palliative Care 2018 Guidelines***:

- ❖ Involves an interdisciplinary team (IDT)
- ❖ End of life care involves:
  - Assessment of patient and family needs
  - Development of a treatment plan
  - Bereavement care plan
- ❖ Assessment: End of life care includes thorough assessment by the IDT of:
  - Physical, social, and spiritual needs of the patient
  - Patient and family preferences regarding setting of care
  - Patient and family wishes during and immediately following death
- ❖ Development of treatment plan:
  - Comprehensive plan is developed in consultation with the patient and family members
  - Plan aims to anticipate, prevent and treat physical, psychological and spiritual symptoms
  - Aims to provide treatment in a culturally appropriate manner
- ❖ Bereavement care plan:
  - Patient and family needs are respected and supported during the dying process
  - Post-death care is provided in a manner which honors the patients and family's cultural beliefs
  - Bereavement care plan is activated after the death of the patient
  - This plan addresses immediate needs of the patient and long term needs of the family

Advantages of Palliative Care

- ❖ Reducing transfer to acute care setting by skill upgrading of care personnel
- ❖ Reducing distress to patient and family caused by transfer to acute care setting
- ❖ Increasing familial involvement in decision making about patient care

- Encourages open and early discussion on death
- Allows for advance care planning
- Provides opportunity for improved control of pain

Barriers in Palliative Care

- Delays in decision making
- Prohibitive costs
- Limited availability of essential drugs like morphine
- Social and cultural issues
- Limited number of palliative care centers
- Long time for development of trust between staff and family members

GREEN ANESTHESIA

Introduction

- Volatile anesthetic agents are aggressive greenhouse gases
- Use of these agents results in addition of greenhouse gases to the earths atmosphere
- This in turn leads to ozone layer depletion and global warming
- The global warming potential of a halogenated anesthetic is up to 2,000 times that of CO_2
- Green anesthesia refers to the measures taken to reduce the effects of these agents on the atmosphere

Atmospheric Structure

- Components of earths atmosphere:
- Troposphere:
  - Extends up to 10 km above the earths surface
  - Comprises 80% of the atmospheric mass
  - Contains almost all of the atmospheric water vapor
- Tropopause:
  - Represents the boundary between the troposphere and stratosphere
  - Height of the tropopause is defined by the change in temperature with altitude
- Stratosphere: Extends from 10 to 50 km from earths surface
- Mesosphere: Beyond 50 km from earths surface
- Ozone layer:
  - Eighty percent of atmospheric ozone is in the ozone layer
  - This belt is in the stratosphere between 20 and 30 km
  - Ozone layer limits the earthward bound transmission of ultraviolet radiation (280–315 nm)

The Greenhouse Effect

- To be energy neutral, incoming solar radiation should equal outgoing reflected radiation
- Greenhouse gases (GHG) absorb outgoing infrared radiations (IR)
- These gases then re-emit the radiation back to the earths surface
- This results in a positive energy balance and net energy gain
- Volatile anesthetic agents are halogenated fluorocarbons and potent GHG
- Other greenhouse gases include:
  - Water vapor
  - Carbon dioxide
  - Methane
  - Nitrous oxide
  - Halogenated fluorocarbons (HCFCs)
  - Ozone (O_3)
  - Perfluorinated carbons (PFCs)
  - Hydrofluorocarbons (HFCs)
- Global Warming Potential (GWP):
  - The harmful effects of GHG is measured in terms of GWP
  - The GWP of all GHG, including anesthetic agents is compared to that of CO_2
  - The GWP_{100} of carbon dioxide is taken as 1 by convention
  - The GWP of any GHG is taken over a 100 year time period (GWP_{100})
  - Therefore, GWP of a substance is the warming potential over 100 years for 1 kg of the substance in gaseous phase, relative to 1 kg of carbon dioxide
  - GWP of a GHG is dependent on:
    - Radiative efficiency
    - Atmospheric lifetime
- Carbon footprint is the total GHG emission caused by the product, event or organization

Greenhouse Effect of Anesthetic Gases

- Most anesthetic gases are chlorine containing compounds
- Less than 5% of anesthetic vapors are metabolized by the patient
- These are predominantly exhaled unchanged via the circuit, into the AGSS
- Therefore, all vapor in the anesthetic circuit eventually ends up in the atmosphere
- Chlorine containing compounds photolyse in the atmosphere and liberate chlorine atoms

- Each chlorine atom has the propensity to destroy 100,000 molecules of ozone
- This in turn leads to global warming
- Sevoflurane has the smallest GWP_{100}, while desflurane has the greatest GWP_{100}
- 1 bottle of desflurane when vaporized has the same global warming potential as 886 kg of CO_2

Characteristic	Isoflurane	Sevoflurane	Desflurane
Atmospheric lifetime	3.2 years	1.1 years	14 years
GWP_{100}	510	130	2,540
IR absorption range	7.5–9.5 µm	7–10 µm	7.5–9.5 µm

Green Anesthetic Strategies Greenhouse Gas Protocol

Modification of Anesthetic Equipment

- Use of Anesthetic Gas Scavenging System (AGSS)
- Preference of closed or circle system over open or semiclosed systems
- Ensuring good seals with airway devices
- Use of low flow anesthetic techniques
- Use of cuffed endotracheal tubes in pediatrics
- Minimize disconnections between anesthetic circuit and the machine
- Use of reusable anesthetic equipment compared with disposable items:
    - Laryngoscope blades
    - LMAs
    - Operating room gowns
    - Operating room drapes
- Turn off ventilation, AGSS and equipment lighting when not in use

Modification of Anesthetic Technique

- Choice of volatile anesthetic:
    - Minimize desflurane usage
    - Prefer isoflurane and sevoflurane instead of desflurane
    - Limit use of nitrous oxide
    - Encourage xenon anesthesia
- Vapor capture condensation:
    - Condensation of exhaled gases from the AGSS prevents atmospheric release
    - Fractional distillation separates the exhaled gases and salvages anesthetic gases
    - This salvaged anesthetic agent can then be reused for delivering anesthetic care
    - Devices have been developed for salvaging exhaled anesthetic agents
    - ***Deltasorb***: *Blue zone technologies*:
        - Zeolite, when placed in the scavenging line absorbs the exhaled anesthetic
        - This has been developed as zeolite canisters placed in the scavenging line
        - Zeolite adsorbs the exhaled gas and prevents release into the environment
        - Trapped agents are processed by steam extraction and fractional distillation
        - This reduces the volatile agent released into the atmosphere by 40–75%
        - However, FDA approval is still pending for implementation into practice
- TIVA:
    - Use of TIVA avoids the use of inhaled agents altogether
    - TIVA with propofol emits 4 time lesser GHG than anesthesia with desflurane
- Regional anesthesia techniques:
    - Regional anesthesia techniques plays a major role in ensuring green anesthesia
    - Preference of epidural analgesia techniques, over N_2O for labor analgesia
- Green disposal:
    - Minimize wastage, including that of drugs
    - Discard unused propofol along with sharps to be incinerated
    - Avoid environmental contamination with toxic drugs that persist and accumulate

ENHANCED RECOVERY AFTER SURGERY

Introduction

- Refers to evidence based protocols to minimize surgical stress response, postoperative pain, expedite recovery following elective procedures and decrease length of stay in the hospital
- First introduced by ***Henrik Kehlet***, a gastrointestinal surgeon in 1997
- Originally described in colorectal surgery, but includes other surgical specialities now

Principles

- Preoperative principles:
    - Preoperative optimization of patients comorbidities
    - Prehabilitation and counseling for postoperative patient participation
    - Selective bowel preparation
    - Reduced preoperative fasting intervals
    - Carbohydrate rich drink in immediate preoperative period
    - Avoidance of long acting sedatives as premedication

- Intraoperative principles:
  - Preference of minimally invasive techniques
  - Reliance on nerve blocks for opioid sparing analgesia
  - Zero-balance fluid therapy
  - Maintenance of normothermia
  - Multimodal PONV prophylaxis
  - Protocol driven anesthetic techniques
  - Avoidance of tubes, drains and lines
- Postoperative principles:
  - Immediate resumption of alimentation
  - Ileus prophylaxis
  - Heplock flushing of vascular access lines
  - Accelerated mobilization
  - Avoidance of Foleys catheter
  - Removal of drains and tubes on postoperative day 1
  - Multimodal analgesia

Anesthetic Goals

- Minimize stress response to surgery
- Provide optimal operating conditions
- Select most appropriate surgical approach:
  - Minimally invasive techniques are essential to Enhanced Recovery After Surgery (ERAS) protocols
  - Advantages of minimally invasive techniques include:
    - Decreased inflammatory mediator release
    - Improved pulmonary function
    - Expeditious return of bowel function
    - Reduced length of hospital stay
- Multimodal analgesia as opioid-sparing strategy:
  - Fundamental to ERAS protocols is minimizing opioid dosage
  - Analgesia aims at preventing pain at time of rest postoperatively
  - However, analgesia should be judicious so as to facilitate early ambulation
- Restrictive perioperative fluid therapy:
  - Intraoperative fluid therapy for ERAS aims at maintaining euvolemia
  - Zero-balance approach is preferred by replacing only the fluid lost during surgery
- Avoidance of nasogastric tube:
  - Nasogastric tubes are associated with patient discomfort and delays oral intake
  - Thus, NG tubes are avoided in ERAS protocols for elective surgeries
- Maintenance of normothermia:
  - Maintenance of normothermia plays a key role in early, enhanced recovery
  - Deleterious effects of hypothermia include:
    - Coagulopathy
    - Adverse cardiac events
    - Surgical wound infections
- Rapid recovery of physical functions:
  - Early ambulation
  - Early oral intake
- Rapid recovery of cognitive function
- PONV prophylaxis
- Avoidance and early removal of drains and catheters:
  - Peritoneal drains are usually omitted from ERAS protocols
  - Drains do not reduce perioperative mortality and morbidity
  - Drains also do not ameliorate the effect of anastomotic leakage in bowel surgeries
  - Therefore, insertion of drains is avoided in ERAS protocols
  - When inserted, these drains are removed as soon as possible after surgery

Preoperative Evaluation and Preparation

- Identification of comorbidities and optimization of comorbidities
- Avoid preoperative hyperosmotic bowel preparation
- Mechanical bowel preparation and oral antibiotics for bowel preparation may be used
- Minimize fasting interval
- Maintain adequate hydration during fasting period
- Clear carbohydrate drink is advised in appropriate volumes 2 hours prior to surgery
- Preoperative planning for postoperative analgesia
- Educate patient about importance of self involvement in postoperative recovery

Premedication

- PO paracetamol 1.5 g given 2 hours prior to surgery
- PO celecoxib (or any COX_2 inhibitor) 400 mg 2 hours prior to surgery
- PO gabapentin 300–600 mg given 2 hours preoperatively
- S/C heparin 5,000 IU for thromboprophylaxis given 1 hour prior to surgery
- Bilateral sequential compression devices placed for mechanical thromboprophylaxis
- Routine benzodiazepine premedication avoided to prevent:
  - Delayed extubation

- Postoperative amnesia, drowsiness
- Cognitive dysfunction in postoperative period
- Postoperative pharyngeal dysfunction
- Postoperative discoordinated breathing and swallowing

Monitors

- ❖ Pulse oximetry
- ❖ ECG
- ❖ NIBP
- ❖ Capnography
- ❖ Temperature monitoring
- ❖ Neuromuscular monitoring
- ❖ BIS is useful to monitor awareness as all drugs are used in minimal doses
- ❖ Invasive hemodynamic monitoring depending on complexity of surgery

Induction

- ❖ Adequate preoxygenation for 3–5 minutes
- ❖ IV propofol 1–1.5 mg/kg is induction agent of choice due to:
  - Rapid recovery
  - Anti-emetic actions
  - Clear headed recovery
- ❖ IV fentanyl 1 μg/kg can be used at induction for intraoperative analgesia
- ❖ IV vecuronium 0.1 mg/kg for neuromuscular paralysis to facilitate intubation
- ❖ Antibiotic prophylaxis administered 30–60 minutes prior to skin incision
- ❖ Induction agents and technique can be modified depending upon:
  - Hemodynamic stability
  - Risk of aspiration
  - Anticipation of difficult airway

Maintenance

- ❖ Balanced anesthesia techniques or TIVA can be used for maintenance of anesthesia
- ❖ Balanced anesthesia:
  - Balanced anesthetic techniques has added advantages such as:
    - Small degree of muscle relaxation
    - Ease of titration
    - Rapid recovery
  - O_2 + air + 1 MAC sevoflurane or desflurane used for balanced anesthesia
  - Opioid doses are minimized (1 μg/kg/hr) to avoid opioid related adverse effects
  - Small doses of IV fentanyl 25–50 μg used to supplement intraoperative analgesia
  - Neuromuscular blockade is titrated to a TOF count of 2–3 in intraoperative period
- ❖ TIVA:
  - TIVA can be used in patients at high risk of PONV
  - IV propofol at 75–150 μg/kg/min titrated according to BIS is used for TIVA
  - IV remifentanil infusion is used with propofol in TIVA regimens
- ❖ Multimodal antiemetic prophylaxis is used to prevent PONV:
  - IV dexamethasone 8 mg after induction of anesthesia
  - IV ondansetron 4 mg at end of surgical procedure

Ventilation

- ❖ Lung protective ventilation preferred to reduce postoperative pulmonary complications
- ❖ Typical initial ventilator settings include:
  - Tidal volume 6–8 mL/kg
  - FiO_2 50%
  - Respiratory rate 10–12 breath/min titrated to maintain $ETCO_2$ 40–42 mm Hg
  - PEEP 5 cm H_2O
  - Performance of recruitment maneuvers when indicated

Hemodynamics

- ❖ Restrictive fluid therapy (RFT) and zero-balance strategy is used to minimize fluid administration
- ❖ RFT has been found equivalent to goal directed therapy (GDT)
- ❖ GDT and liberal fluid therapy is unwarranted in the setting of early alimentation
- ❖ Thus, preloading prior to neuraxial blockade is not practiced
- ❖ Also, administration of hourly maintenance fluid is restricted by avoiding replacement of:
  - Urine output
  - Calculated insensible losses
  - Third space losses
- ❖ Warming devices are used to maintain core body temperature and normothermia:
  - Forced air warming devices
  - Insulation water mattresses
  - IV fluid warmers
- ❖ Perioperative glycemic control is targeted to maintain glucose levels between 140 and 200 mg/dL

Extubation

- Extubation strategy depends on type of surgery and duration of anesthetic exposure
- Early extubation forms a key role in most ERAS protocols

Postoperative Management

Management

- PONV prophylaxis is essential to hasten recovery
- Fluid therapy:
  - Restricted fluid administration of balanced salt solution at 50 mL/hr
  - Fluid administration may be titrated to hemodynamic benefit
  - Fluid administration is discontinued once oral fluid intake is tolerated
- Diet:
  - Resumption of diet within few hours of surgery is important
  - Bowel sounds are not associated with tolerance of oral intake
  - High calorie drinks are used to minimize negative protein balance postsurgery
  - Early removal of catheters and drains is an important principle in ERAS
  - Alvimopan:
    - Peripherally acting μ-opioid receptor antagonist
    - Has limited ability to cross blood brain barrier
    - Reduces prolonged ileus after bowel surgery, when given preoperatively
- Early ambulation:
  - Early ambulation improves quality of surgical care
  - This forms a key component of ERAS protocols
  - Early ambulation prevents:
    - Postoperative pneumonia
    - Venous thromboembolism

Monitors

- Pulse oximetry
- ECG
- NIBP
- Adequacy of ventilation
- Urine output

Analgesia

- Multimodal analgesia practiced for pain relief
- Goal is to minimize pain at rest and facilitate early ambulation
- Useful opioid adjuncts include:
  - Paracetamol (if not administered at beginning of surgery)
  - IV ketorolac 15–30 mg at the end of surgical procedure
  - Local anesthetic techniques may be used to supplement analgesia

ISOMERISM IN ANESTHESIA

Introduction

- Isomerism is the phenomenon by which two molecules with the same atomic formulae have different structural composition
- The constituent atoms of the molecule are the same, but they are arranged in a different configuration

Types of Isomerism

- Structural isomerism
- Stereoisomerism:
  - Enantiomers:
    - Levo isomer [(−) or λ-isomer]
    - Dextro isomer [(+) or δ-isomer]
  - Diastereoisomers

Structural Isomerism

- They have identical atomic components and molecular formula
- However, their inter-atomic bonds are arranged differently
- Thus, they can be completely different molecules with different physical properties
- Examples of structural isomers:
  - Molecules with similar actions: Isoflurane and enflurane:
    - Both agents have the same molecular formula $C_3H_2ClF_5O$
    - Both volatile agents with similar profile
  - Molecules with different actions:
    - Prednisolone and aldosterone:
      - Both drugs have a molecular formula $C_{21}H_{28}O_5$
      - Prednisolone has both glucocorticoid and mineralocorticoid actions
      - Aldosterone has predominantly mineralocorticoid action
    - Isoprenaline and methoxamine:
      - Both drugs have a molecular formula $C_{11}H_{17}NO_3$
      - Isoprenaline acts predominantly on β-adrenoceptors
      - Methoxamine acts on α-adrenoceptors

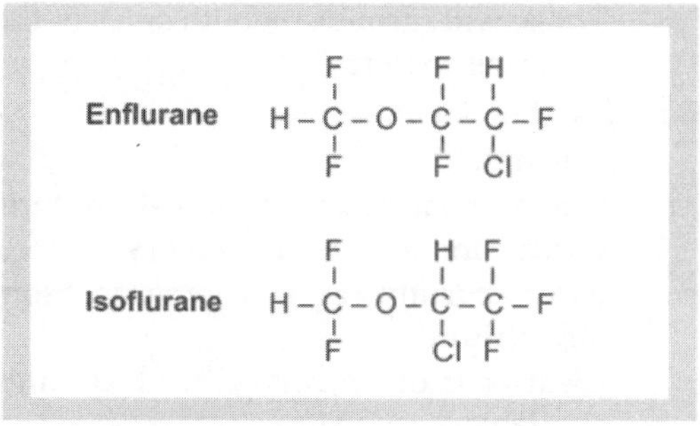

Enflurane H–C(F)(F)–O–C(F)(F)–C(H)(Cl)–F

Isoflurane H–C(F)(F)–O–C(H)(Cl)–C(F)(F)–F

Fig. 2: Structural isomerism.

- Dobutamine and dihydrocodeine:
  - Both drugs have a molecular formula $C_{18}H_{23}NO_3$
  - Dobutamine is an inotropic agent
  - Dihydrocodeine is an opioid.

Tautomerism

- Refers to the dynamic interchange between 2 forms of a molecule, with a change in physical environment
- Example:
  - Midazolam is ionized in solution at a pH of 4
  - At pH of 7.4, it changes into a 7—membered unionized ring structure
  - This renders it lipid soluble and rapidly acting at physiological pH 7.4

Steroisomerism

- They have identical components and interatomic bonds
- However, their three dimensional configuration is different
- Almost 60% of anesthetic drugs are stereoisomers
- Stereoisomers are of two types:
  - Enantiomers
  - Diastereoisomers

Enantiomers

- Enantiomers are nonsuperimposable mirror images of each other
- These are akin to the right and left hands, which are mirror images of each other
- Thus, they cannot be superimposed on each other with palms facing in the same direction
- It is for this reason that enantiomers are also called chiral (*chiros* in Greek means hand)
- In such molecules, the therapeutic activity resides mainly in one enantiomer
- This enantiomer with therapeutic activity is called ***eutomer***

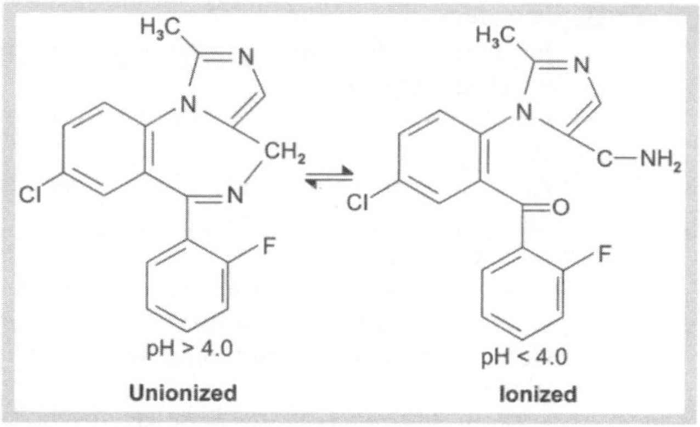

Fig. 3: Tautomerism of midazolam.

- The other enantiomer can have:
  - Undesirable properties
  - Different therapeutic properties
  - Inert pharmacological properties
- This isomer with undesirable properties is called the ***distomer or isomeric ballast***
- The physicochemical properties of enantiomers are very similar
- They differ only in their ability to rotate plane-polarized light in opposite directions
- Therefore, enantiomers are also called optical isomers
- Depending on the direction in which they rotate light, they are of two type
- An enantiomer rotating polarized light to the right is called dextro isomer
- An enantiomer rotating polarized light to the left is called levo isomer
- A racemic mixture is an equal mixture of two enantiomers, with no optical activity
- Almost all chiral drugs were being administered as racemic mixtures
- However, recent advances in technology allows synthesizing drugs as single isomers
- Advantages of single isomer drugs include:
  - Selective pharmacodynamic profile of the drug
  - Specific pharmacokinetic profile of the drug
  - Predictable concentration-response relationships
  - Improved therapeutic index
  - Decreased propensity for drug-drug interactions
- Examples of enantiomers:
  - Isoflurane:
    - Optical isomers of isoflurane exhibit stereoselectivity in their effects
    - Thus, (+) isoflurane is twofold more effective as (–) isoflurane

- Bupivacaine:
  - Bupivacaine has two optical isomers with varying properties
  - Levobupivacaine is longer acting than racemic bupivacaine
  - Also, cardiotoxicity with levobupivacaine is lesser
- Dexmedetomidine:
  - It is the pharmacologically active dextro-enantiomer of medetomidine
  - Compared to medetomidine, dexmedetomidine is:
    - More selective receptor agonist
    - More potent sedative and analgesic
- Levosimendan:
  - Levosimendan binds stereoselectively to cardiac troponin C
  - It is 47 times as potent as its stereoisomer dextrosimendan

Diastereoisomers

- Diastereoisomers are nonenantiomeric stereoisomers (do not demonstrate handedness)
- They are compounds that are not nonsuperimposable mirror images of each other
- Diastereoisomers differ in their physico-chemical properties and are easily separated
- Diastereoisomerism can be due to:
  - Presence of more than one chiral center
  - Geometric isomerism:
    - Occurs when two groups are attached to adjacent atoms by a rigid bond
    - Such isomers typically contain a double bond, which cannot rotate
    - Cis-trans isomerism is an example of geometric isomerism
    - Isomers with groups on the same side of the bond are cisisomers
    - Those with groups on both sides of the bond are transisomers
- Examples of diastereoisomers:
  - Atracurium:
    - Commercial atracurium is a mixture of 10 optical and geometric isomers
    - Cisatracurium is a geometric isomer of atracurium
    - Cisatracurium forms 15% of commercially available atracurium
    - Ciastracurium has been isolated and synthesized separately

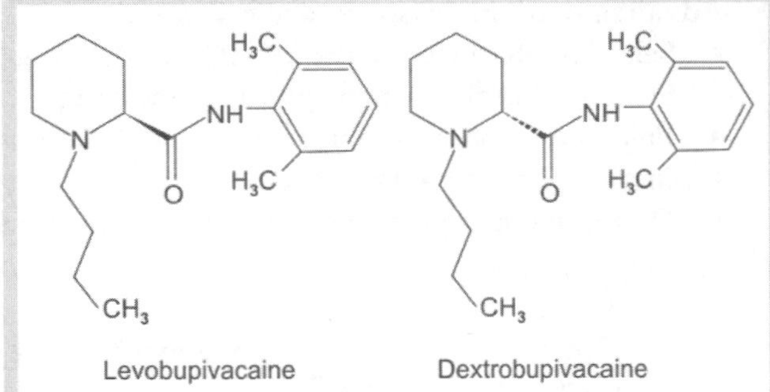

Fig. 4: Bupivacaine enantiomers.

Clinical Significance of Isomerism

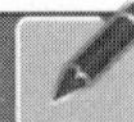

- Stereospecific biological interactions:
  - Interaction of molecules with biological systems is highly stereospecific
  - This followed the glove-to-the-hand hypothesis by ***Easson and Stedman***
  - Thus, enantiomers differ in receptor affinity due to different 3-D configuration
- Stereospecific pharmacokinetics:
  - Pharmacokinetic properties may vary widely among enantiomers
  - This can affect:
    - Absorption:
      - Due to change in lipophilicity at physiological pH
      - Tautomerism in midazolam is an example
    - Protein binding:
      - Isomers may have different affinity to plasma proteins
      - S(–) and R(+) isomers of warfarin have different albumin affinity
    - Metabolism: Due to competition between isomers for metabolic pathways

Chiral Switch

- Drugs previously sold as racemates, are being redeveloped as single enantiomers
- This process is referred to as chiral switch
- This leads to pharmacologically superior old drugs with better side effect profiles
- Examples:
  - Bupivacaine and levobupivacaine
  - Atracurium and cisatracurium

Methods of Enantioselective Synthesis of Drugs

- Chromatography:
  - Uses the countercurrent chromatographic process with the simulated moving bed
  - Tramadol is synthesized using this technology
- Crystallization:
  - Chiral salt of the drug is placed under specific conditions

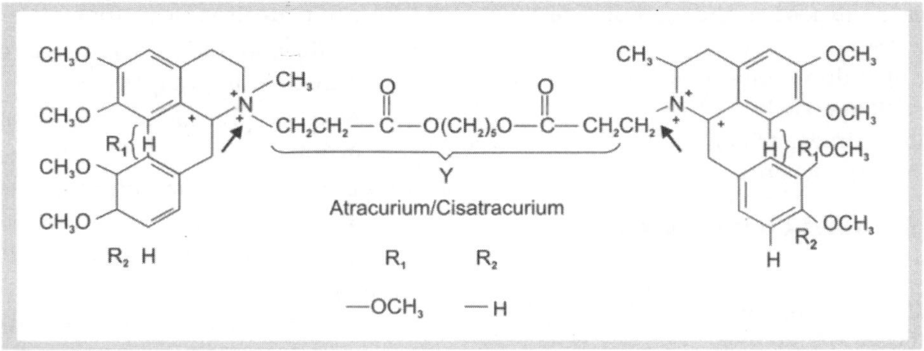

Fig. 5: Atracurium diastereoisomers.

- This yields the isomer in crystal form
- Used in the synthesis of methadone

❖ Enzymatic resolution:
- Uses the principle that certain enzymes react only with one isomer of a molecule
- This method has been used in the synthesis of benzodiazepines

NEUROTOXICITY, NEUROPLASTICITY, AND ANESTHESIA

Introduction

❖ Exposure to anesthetic agents and sedatives can cause neurodegeneration and neuroapoptosis

❖ Thus, they are potentially damaging to neuronal cells and can contribute to neurotoxicity

Physiology

❖ Neurodevelopment:
- Neuroplasticity refers to the ability of the brain to form synaptic connections in response to learning, experience or following injury
- Synaptogenesis involves formation of synaptic contacts between neurons
- This enables formation of neuronal circuitry, pathways and meaningful maps
- Synaptogenesis is based on activity dependant remodeling
- Thus, synapses undergo constant remodeling where:
  - New synapses are being formed
  - Old synapses are being pruned away
- New synapses are formed along pathways of constant neural stimulation
- Old synapses along dysfunctional neural pathways undergo apoptosis
- Two neurotransmitters (GABA and NMDA) control all aspects of neurodevelopment:
  - Neuronal migration
  - Differentiation
  - Maturation
  - Synaptogenesis

❖ Phases of neurodevelopment:
- Neurodevelopment occurs mainly during:
  - Last trimester of in-utero life
  - First 3 years of postnatal life
- The brain weighs 335 g at birth and almost triples its weight by 12 months age
- This time period is called the *brain growth spurt period or period of synaptogenesis*
- During this time period, trillions of synaptic connections are being formed
- Thus, general anesthetic exposure during this period can be particularly harmful

❖ Effect of anesthetic agents:
- Anesthetic agents act via these two receptors and turn off neuronal communication
- This ensures adequate anesthetic planes with:
  - Amnesia
  - Analgesia
  - Hypnosis
- Therefore, since general anesthetics act via the same receptors which are essential for neurodevelopment, they have a potential for causing neurotoxicity
- Two critical factors determine anesthetic neurotoxicity:
  - Stage of brain development at the time of anesthetic exposure:
    - Risk of toxicity increases at extremes of age in human beings
    - Humans are vulnerable to injury from 2nd trimester to 3 years age

- Degree of exposure and cumulative anesthetic dose:
  - Use of multiple anesthetic agents increases the risk of toxicity
  - Also, maintenance of anesthesia for more than 3 hours increases risk

Mechanisms of Anesthetic Neurotoxicity

- Apoptosis:
  - This is an energy consuming process wherein unwanted cells are removed
  - Apoptotic process involves:
    - Chromatin aggregation
    - Condensation of cellular organelles
    - Development of apoptotic bodies
    - Phagocytosis
  - Anesthetic agents may cause apoptosis and cause neurotoxicity
- Effects on synaptogenesis:
  - Anesthetic exposure can lead to a reduction in the number of synapses
  - During the brain growth spurt period, GABA acts as an excitatory neurotransmitter
  - At this stage, GABA stimulation leads to depolarization and excitatory synaptogenesis
  - Exposure to anesthetic agents at this stage potentiates GABA excitatory transmission
  - This causes a rise in intracellular calcium concentration and neuronal injury
- Effects on neurogenesis:
  - Exposure to isoflurane in young non-human mammals causes loss of stem cells
  - Also, there was a decline in the production of new neurons
  - This may lead to impaired memory and learning at a later stage, causing neurotoxicity
- Role of neurotrophic factors:
  - Isoflurane and propofol use causes significant reduction in synaptic density
  - Neurotrophic factors may be responsible for this action
  - Brain derived neurotrophic factor (BDNF) plays an important role in this process
- Reactive oxygen species and mitochondrial injury:
  - GABA activation in developing brain causes raised intracellular calcium
  - This leads to disturbances in mitochondrial membrane potential
  - This eventually leads to neuronal cell death
  - Also, increased production of reactive oxygen species occurs with:
    - Isoflurane
    - Sevoflurane
    - Propofol
  - This can lead to increased neuronal lipid peroxidation and neuronal deletion
- Complement activation:
  - Complement pathways play an important role in modification of synaptic connections
  - Isoflurane activates complement cascade via modulation of C1q and C3 complement
  - This could lead to deleterious effects during synaptogenesis
- Nitrous oxide neurotoxicity:
  - Nitrous oxide causes massive swelling of neuronal organelles
  - Mitochondria and endoplasmic reticulum swell and can cause neuronal damage
  - This may lead to short and long term neurocognitive dysfunction

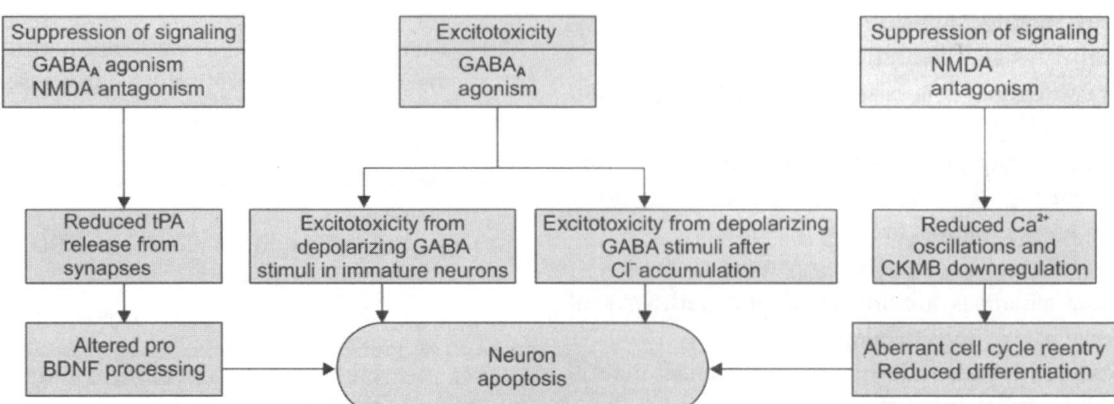

Neurotoxicity of Individual Anesthetic Agents

- Ketamine:
  - Dose dependant neuroapoptosis
  - Oligodendrocyte apoptosis
  - Synergistic neurotoxicity when co-administered with propofol
- Propofol:
  - Neurotoxic in subanesthetic doses
  - Oligodendrocyte apoptosis
  - Synergistic neurotoxicity when co-administered with ketamine
- Nitrous oxide:
  - Toxic effects in cell organelles
  - Potentiates neurotoxic effects of volatile agents
- Volatile anesthetics:
  - Neurotoxic at sub-MAC levels
  - Oligodendrocyte apoptosis
  - Sevoflurane < isoflurane < desflurane
- Benzodiazepines:
  - Toxic effects on neuronal differentiation
  - Causes neuroapoptosis on prolonged administration
- Barbiturates:
  - Induces dose-dependant neuroapoptosis
  - Less neurotoxic compared with propofol
  - Potentiates ketamine neurotoxicity

Types of Anesthesia Induced Neurotoxicity

- Anesthesia induced developmental neurotoxicity (AIDN)
- Postoperative cognitive decline (POCD)

Prevention of Anesthesia Induced Neurotoxicity

- Alpha 2 adrenoceptor agonists:
  - α_2 adrenoceptor signaling plays a trophic role during neurodevelopment
  - Dexmedetomidine reduces expression of apoptotic enzymes
  - Other neuroprotective mechanisms include:
    - Inhibition of calcium entry
    - Scavenging of glutamate
    - Reduction in NMDA receptor activation
- Xenon:
  - Xenon inhibits both intrinsic and common apoptotic pathways
  - Thereby, neuronal cell death can be prevented by using xenon
- Anesthetic preconditioning:
  - Prior exposure to low dose or short duration of anesthetic attenuates injury
  - Preconditioning with isoflurane and propofol protects against neurotoxicity
- Vitamins:
  - Nicotinamide attenuates ketamine induced neuronal cell loss in rats
  - Other vitamins which show neuroprotective effect are:
    - Vitamin D_3 (enhances trophic factors)
    - Vitamin C (antioxidant effect)
- Erythropoietin:
  - Has a direct neurotrophic and neuroprotective effect
  - Anesthetic agents may inhibit release of erythropoietin
  - Thus, supplementation with erythropoietin may afford some neuroprotection
- Other agents which are being investigated are:
  - Lithium
  - Melatonin
  - Acetyl-L-carnitine
  - Activity dependant neuroprotective protein
  - Bumetanide
  - Cyclosporin A

Validation

- General Anesthesia compared to Spinal anesthesia trial (***GAS trial***):
  - Randomized infants undergoing inguinal hernia repair
  - Received either awake-regional technique or general anesthetic
  - Secondary outcomes measured at 2 years of age
  - Showed no risk of adverse neurodevelopment in children exposed to general anesthetic
- Pediatric anesthesia and neurodevelopment assessment study (***PANDA study***):
  - Aims to reduce genetic contributions to cognitive performance
  - Compared children undergoing inguinal hernia repair with general anesthesia below 3 years age with unexposed siblings
  - No difference in IQ was found between exposed and unexposed siblings

SUGGESTED READING

1. Aitkenhead, A.K., Thompson, K., Rowbotham, D.J., Moppett, I. (2013). *Smith and Aitkenheads Textbook of Anesthesia.* 6th ed. Philadelphia: Churchill Livingstone Elsevier.
2. Barash, P.G. (2017). *Clinical Anesthesia.* 8th ed. China: Wolters Kluwer.

3. Butterworth, J., Mackey, D., Wasnik, J. (2018). *Morgan and Mikhails Clinical Anesthesiology*. 6th ed. New York: McGraw-Hill Education/Medical.
4. Chang, D.W. (2014). *Clinical Application of Mechanical Ventilation*. 4th ed. Noida: Delmar Cengage Learning.
5. Davis, P.J., Cladis, F. (2017). *Smiths anesthesia for infants and children*. 9th ed. Philadelphia: Elsevier.
6. Flood, P. (2015). *Stoeltings Pharmacology and Physiology in Anesthetic Practice*. 5th ed. China: Wolters Kluwer.
7. Gropper, M., Eriksson, L., Fleisher, L., Wiener-Kronish, J., Cohen, N., Leslie, K. (2020). *Millers Anesthesia*. 9th ed. Philadelphia: Elsevier Saunders.
8. Marino, P.L. (2017). *The little ICU book of facts and formulas*. 2nd ed. China: Wolters Kluwer.
9. Marschall, K., Hines, R.L. (2017). *Stoeltings Anesthesia and Coexisting Disease*. 7th ed. New York: Elsevier.
10. Miller, R.D., Eriksson, L., Fleisher, L, Wiener-Kronish, J., Cohen, N., Young, W. (2014). *Millers Anesthesia*. 8th ed. New York: Elsevier Health.
11. Miller, T., Myles, P.S. (2019). Perioperative fluid therapy for major surgery. *Anesthesiology*, 130(5), 825-32.
12. Murray, M.J., et al. (2015). *Fausts Anesthesiology Review*. 4th ed. Philadelphia: Elsevier.

13

CHAPTER

Pediatric Anesthesia

DIFFERENCES IN ADULT AND PEDIATRIC AIRWAY

Feature	Pediatric	Adult
1. Supraglottic		
Nares	Narrow	Wide
Angle of jaw	Obtuse	Acute
Tongue size	Larger	Smaller
Palate	Non-ossified	Ossified
Epiglottis	Large, floppy, Ω shaped, more cephalad	Thinner
Position of larynx	Newborn—C3	C5–6
	At 6 years—C4–5	
Description of larynx	More anterior and cephalad	Lower
Vocal cords	Anterior slanting	Not so
Aryepiglottic folds	Thicker—difficult to fix laryngoscope blade	Thinner
Submucosal tissue	More—increased chance of edema	Less
2. Subglottic		
Cartilages	Soft, collapse easily—reduce cricoid pressure	Harder, stable
Lumen	Narrow, circular—uncuffed tube	Wide, elliptical
Subglottis	Funneled	No funneling
Cricoid	Narrow before puberty	Wide
Narrowest part	Subglottis	Vocal cord
Tracheal length	Reduced (4 cm)	More
Angulation of bronchi	More horizontal	Less
Diaphragm	Higher	Lower
Ribs	Horizontal	Slanted
Alveoli	Lesser (20–50 million)	More (300 million)

PHYSIOLOGICAL DIFFERENCES IN NEONATE

System	Features	Anesthetic implications
CNS	Small brain (10% of body weight)	Lowers MAC values by 25%
	Poorly developed blood brain barrier	Increased drug toxicity
	Immature neuromuscular junction	Increased sensitivity to d-TC
	Spinal cord ends at L2L3	SAB given at lower level
	Increased CSF volume (4 mL/kg)	Increased drug dose in SAB
	Thin unmyelinated neurons	Faster onset of neuraxial blocks
	Increased body surface area: weight ratio	More hypothermia
	Less insulating tissue	More hypothermia
	Shivering nonexistent	Non-shivering thermogenesis for temperature regulation
	Increased chances of intraventricular hemorrhage	Avoid drastic BP changes

Contd...

Contd...

System	Features	Anesthetic implications
Cardiovascular	Myocardium has 30% less contractile tissue	Fixed stroke volume Cardiac output depends more on HR
	Right ventricular muscle thicker than left ventricle till 3–6 months	ECG axis +180° Normalizes to +90° at 3–6 months
	Patent shunts—PDA, PFO	Avoid air bubbles in IV lines
	BP lower (50–65 mm Hg at birth)	Systolic BP good indicator of blood volume
	Higher heart rate 100–170 bpm	< 80 bpm indicates cardiac arrest
	Higher cardiac output (350–400 mL/kg @ birth)	70 mL/kg in adults
	Volume dependent but volume intolerant	Avoid fluid overload
	Blood volume more: 100 mL/kg preterm 90 mL/kg term 75 mL/kg school age	
	Hemoglobin drops during first 3 months	Physiological anemia
	Inactive baroreceptor reflexes	Difficult to maintain if hypovolemic Replace fluid deficits promptly
	Immature sympathetic nervous system	Vagal predominance Bradycardia common
Respiratory	Obligate nose breathers	Care while passing nasogastric tube
	Increased airway resistance	Position head carefully Minimize apparatus resistance
	Increased dead space	Use circuits with low dead space Rendall-Baker-Soucek mask
	Surfactant appears at 28 weeks	RDS babies < 28 weeks
	Lecithin-sphingomyelin ratio	>2 is normal
	Narrow caliber of airway	Increased work of breathing
	Narrowest area is subglottis	Increased subglottic area
	Cartilages are soft	Gentle cricoid pressure
	Thick aryepiglottic folds	Laryngoscope blade difficult to fix
	Circular cricoid cartilage	No need of cuffed ETT
	Reduced FRC and lung volumes	Accelerated desaturation
	Increased basal metabolic rate	Mandatory adequate preoxygenation
	Poorly developed lung elastic tissue	Airway closure during tidal ventilation due to low compliance
	Less compliance Lesser number of alveoli	High respiratory rate to maintain ventilation as fixed tidal volume
	Poor respiratory mechanics	Small tidal volume
	More horizontal ribs	No bucket handle movement Only piston movement
	Increased basal metabolic rate	Alveolar ventilation 100 mL/kg/min
	Increased alveolar ventilation	Rapid emergence from volatile anesthetics
	Increased closing volume	Air trapping more common
	O_2 and N_2O almost completely absorbed	Air O_2 mixture below 3 months age to prevent absorption atelectasis
	Immature respiratory center	Very sensitive to depressants
	CO_2 dissociation curve shifts to left	Hyperventilation at lower CO_2 levels
	Lower PO_2	50 mm Hg term neonate 75 mm Hg after 1 week
Renals	Reduced GFR and tubular reabsorption	Judicious fluid therapy
	Obligatory salt losers	Hyponatremia in postoperative period
	Reduced drug elimination	Increased drug toxicity and DOA

Contd...

Contd...

System	Features	Anesthetic implications
Liver	Immature enzyme systems	Increased duration of action of drugs
	Lack of fats and proteins	Reduced gluconeogenesis Increased hypoglycemia
Blood	Fetal Hb normalizes by 3–6 months	Shift of ODC to left
	Reduced 2, 3-DPG	Shift of ODC to left
	Parenchymal shunt due to atelectasis	Low PO_2
	Cardiac shunts—PFO and PDA	
	Anatomical AV shunts	
	Increased chances of hypocalcemia in 1st 48 hours	Supplement after birth
	Increased hypoglycemia chances in LBW babies	Supplement after birth
	Water retention postoperatively	Reduce maintenance fluids by 1/3rd in postoperative period
	Hyperglycemia causes osmotic diuresis and IVH	Use dextrose containing fluids only in VLBW and endocrinopathies

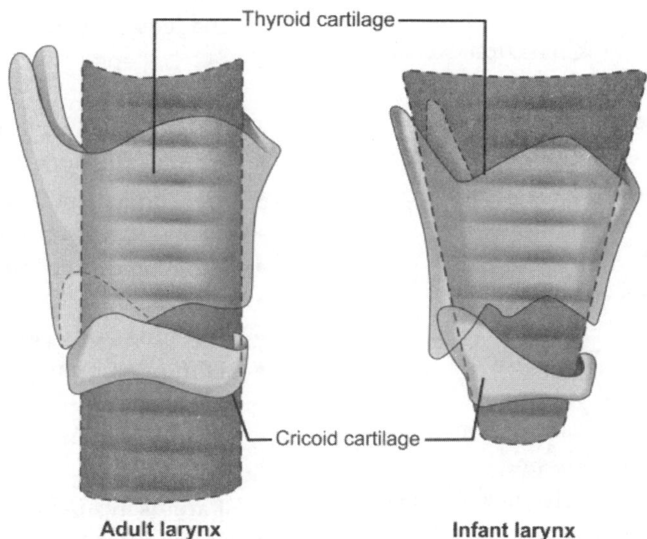

Fig. 1: Adult vs pediatric larynx.

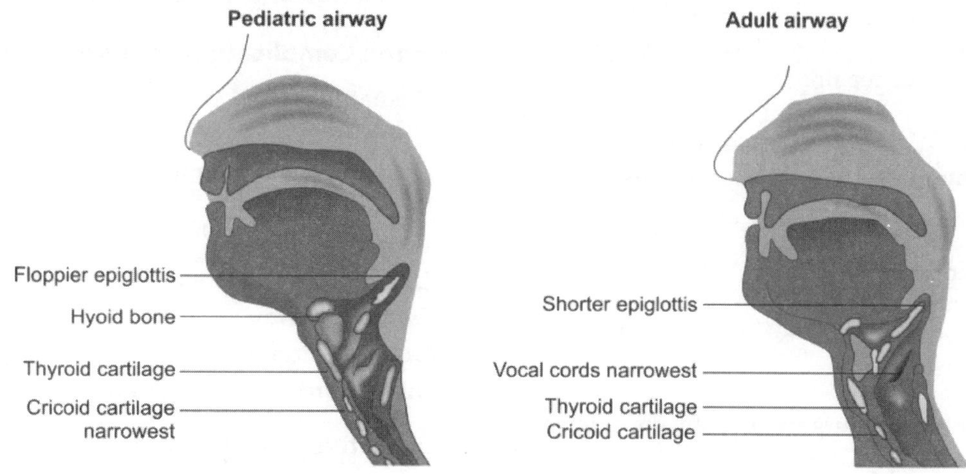

Fig. 2: Adult vs pediatric airway.

PEDIATRIC DAY CARE SURGERY

Introduction

- Day care surgery was first reported in 1909
- Outpatient anesthesia was recognized as a separate entity only in 1984

Challenges in Day care Anesthesia

- Anesthesia at remote locations
- Ensure minimal perioperative complexity
- Management of pain
- Complex comorbidities

Indications

- Ophthalmology:
  - Examination under anesthesia
  - Trabeculectomy
  - Strabismus surgery
  - Chalazion excision
- ENT:
  - Adenoidectomy (>4 years age)
  - Frenulectomy
  - Tonsillectomy (>4 years age)
  - Laryngoscopy
  - Myringotomy
  - Foreign body removal
  - Endoscopic sinus surgery
- Dental procedures:
  - Extraction
  - Restoration
- General surgery:
  - Hernia repair
  - Cyst excision
  - I and D abscess
  - Dressing
  - Endoscopy
  - Excision of skin lesions
  - Suture of lacerations
  - Removal of sutures
- Urology:
  - Circumcision
  - Meatotomy
  - Cystoscopy
  - Hydrocelectomy
  - Orchiopexy
  - Testicular biopsy
  - Hypospadiasis repair
- Plastic surgery:
  - Otoplasty
  - Scar revision
  - Septorhinoplasty
  - Cleft lip surgery
- Orthopedics:
  - Closed reduction of fractures
  - Arthroscopy
  - Cast change
  - Implant removals
  - Percutaneous tenotomies
  - Manipulation

Prerequisites

- Limited duration of surgery (usually considered as 4 hours)
- Low risk of anesthetic and surgical complications
- Minimal blood loss
- Minimal physiological derangements
- Minimal postoperative pain
- Pain should be easily treatable with oral analgesics
- Ability to resume oral feeds in the immediate post-operative period

Selection Criteria

- ASA I-II physical status patients are preferred
- ASA III children considered, if systemic disease is well controlled
- Good preoperative evaluation is a prerequisite

Exclusion Criteria for Day care Surgery

- Age and medical exclusions:
  - Ex-preterm infants < 60 weeks post-conceptual age
  - Inadequately controlled systemic disease:
    - Epilepsy
    - Asthma
  - Active viral/bacterial infections
  - Complex congenital heart disease
- Surgical and anesthetic exclusions:
  - Inexperienced surgeon or anesthetist
  - Prolonged procedure (>4 hours)
  - Significant risk of perioperative hemorrhage
  - Opening body cavity (excluding laparoscopy)
  - Difficult airway
  - Sleep apnea
  - Severe pain unrelieved by oral medications
- Social exclusions
  - Parents incapable of taking care for child at home
  - Inadequate housing conditions
  - Unsupported parent with numerous children
  - Inadequate postoperative transport arrangements

Common Complicating Comorbidities

- Prematurity
- Upper respiratory tract infections
- Obstructive sleep apnea
- Obesity
- Bronchial asthma
- Uncorrected congenital heart disease
- Difficult airway
- Downs syndrome
- Inborn errors of metabolism

Preoperative Evaluation

- Preoperative evaluation should be done well in advance of planned procedure

- Assess feasibility of day care surgery by evaluating:
  - Time required for surgery <4 hours
  - Complexity of surgery
  - Severe complicating comorbidities
  - Blood loss
- Upper respiratory tract infections (URTIs):
  - Benign recurrent viral illnesses usually do not necessitate delay in surgery
  - However, infections increase airway inflammation which can persist up to 6 weeks
  - Recent or active URTI increases risk of perioperative complications like:
    - Atelectasis
    - Hypoxemia
    - Laryngospasm
    - Bronchospasm
  - Surgery should be postponed for 4 weeks in the presence of:
    - Fever
    - Productive cough
    - Purulent secretions
    - Lethargy
    - Pulmonary involvement

Preoperative Preparation

- Ensure shortest time between admission and anesthetic induction to prevent orientation
- Informed consent to be taken
- Ensure NPO status
- Anxiolysis:
  - Midazolam:
    - Midazolam 0.25–0.5 mg/kg PO given 30 minutes prior is *most commonly* used
    - Midazolam 0.2 mg/kg nasal can be used as alternative to oral route
  - Oral ketamine:
    - 5 mg/kg ketamine is given orally as an alternative to benzodiazepines
    - However, it is associated with prolonged recovery
  - IM ketamine:
    - Used in exceptionally uncooperative patients
    - 3–4 mg/kg ketamine IM in combination with midazolam and glycopyrrolate
    - Avoided in strabismus and intraocular surgeries
  - Oral fentanyl:
    - 15–20 µg/kg fentanyl is preferred dose
    - However, it is associated with PONV and pruritus
  - Sufentanyl 1.5–3 µg/kg intranasal
- Continue other medications as appropriate
- Parental presence preferable at the time of induction

Anesthetic goals

- Rapid induction
- Prompt recovery
- Early discharge
- Minimal side effects
- Minimal pain

Ideal Anesthetic Agent for Ambulatory Surgery

- Smooth and rapid induction
- Prompt recovery
- Should have analgesic properties
- Should have minimal side effects
- Be free of postoperative nausea and vomiting

Induction

- Intravenous and inhalational techniques are suitable in pediatric patients
- Technique used in the absence of IV access is inhalational induction
- Intravenous agents:
  - Thiopentone 5–6 mg/kg
  - Ketamine 2 mg/kg
  - Propofol 2–2.5 mg/kg
- IM Induction:
  - Ketamine 5 mg/kg
- Inhalational induction:
  - Sevoflurane
  - Halothane
- Rectal:
  - Ketamine 6 mg/kg
  - Midazolam 0.4 mg/kg
- Muscle relaxants:
  - Atracurium 0.5 mg/kg
  - Vecuronium 0.1 mg/kg
  - Rocuronium 0.6–0.9 mg/kg

Airway Management

- Face mask; LMA; COPA preferred as airway interfaces
- ETT avoided to prevent risk of:
  - Post-extubation stridor
  - Use of neuromuscular blocking agents

Maintenance

- O_2+ air + sevoflurane 1 MAC most commonly used for maintenance of anesthesia
- Short acting narcotics may be used for maintenance of analgesia:
  - Fentanyl
  - Remifentanyl
  - Sufentanyl
- TIVA is a useful alternative in patients undergoing strabismus surgery

Hemodynamics

- Day care surgery is usually not associated with major fluid loss
- Fluids given according to type of surgery and weight

Extubation

- Lesser respiratory complications seen when extubated in deeper planes
- However, full reversal and adequate core temperature to be ensured prior to extubation

Postoperative Care

- Analgesia:
  - Ketorolac
  - Paracetamol:
    - Most commonly used agent
    - 10–15 mg/kg given Q4H
    - Maximum dose is:
      - 4 g in adolescents
      - 75 mg/kg in infants and children
  - *Ibuprofen*: 10 mg/kg given Q6H
  - Diclofenac:
    - 1 mg/kg can be given Q8H
    - Can be given in the same dose through PO, IV or PR route
- Treat PONV

Complications

- Pain
- PONV
- Sore throat (LMA)
- Croup (ETT)
- Fever
- Headache

Advantages

- Reduces separation anxiety when parents are allowed to be present at induction
- Increased parental involvement
- Reduces postoperative behavioral problems in children
- Reduces risk of nosocomial infections
- Reduced morbidity and mortality
- Greater efficiency
- Reduced waiting list
- Reduced hospital stay
- More economical

Disadvantages

- Multiple trips to be done by the patient for preoperative preparation
- Skilled anesthetist required
- Good postoperative care mandatory

Regional Anesthesia

- Useful for orthopedic and urological day care procedures
- Peripheral nerve blocks can provide analgesia lasting 8–12 hours, up to 24 hours
- Neuraxial blocks performed with low concentration local anesthetics to avoid:
  - Motor blockade
  - Urinary retention
- Caudal anesthesia most popular
- Spinal less popular

Criteria for Discharge to Ward

Steward recovery scale:

Sign	Criterion	Score
Consciousness	Awake	2
	Responds to stimuli	1
	Not responding	0
Airway	Coughing/crying on command	2
	Maintaining good airway	1
	Airway requiring maintenance	0
Movement	Purposeful movement	2
	Non-purposeful movement	1
	Not moving	0

- Score of 0 indicated needs for securing the airway
- Score of 6 indicates a fully awake patient, ready for discharge
- Criteria for discharge to ward does not mandate tolerance of oral feeds and voiding of urine

Criteria for Discharge to Home

- Able to tolerate oral feeds with minimal PONV
- Caregivers to be able to provide basic postoperative care

- Caregivers should have adequate understanding of discharge instructions
- In those who have received neuraxial anesthesia:
  - Should be able to transfer with assistance
  - Should be able to void urine within 6 hours of surgery
  - Should call for further assistance if unable to void after 6 hours of surgery

PERIOPERATIVE FLUID THERAPY IN PEDIATRICS

Introduction

- Meticulous fluid management is required in pediatrics due to limited margin of error
- Main objective of perioperative fluid therapy is to ensure adequate tissue perfusion

Goals of Fluid Therapy in Pediatrics

- Ensure adequate intravascular volume
- Ensure good cardiac output and stable hemodynamics
- Ensure adequate tissue perfusion
- Prevent electrolyte disturbances and hypoglycemia
- Correction of fluid deficits
- Replace ongoing losses
- Compensate for autonomic changes under anesthesia
- Prevent volume overload

Challenges in Pediatric Fluid Therapy

- Increased basal metabolic rate
- Small surface area—volume ratio
- Immature homeostasis
- Immature renals
- Reduced GFR
- Reduced glomerular surface area
- Differences in total body water:
  - Preterm infants: 90% of body weight
  - Term infants: 75–80% of body weight
  - Adults: 60% of body weight
- Increased circulating blood volume:
  - Preterm neonate: 100 mL/kg
  - Full term neonate: 85–90 mL/kg
  - Infants: 75–80 mL/kg
  - Older infants- adolescents: 75–80 mL/kg
  - Adults: 65–70 mL/kg

Effects of Anesthesia on Fluid Status

- Preoperative fasting increases deficit
- Reduced basal metabolic rate under GA
- Reduced sympathetic tone
- Increased venous capacitance and peripheral pooling
- Blunted baroreceptor reflexes
- Reduced cardiac output with use of:
  - Halothane
  - Sevoflurane
  - Thiopentone
  - Propofol
- Reduction in venous return due to IPPV and CPAP
- Surgery induced third spacing due to capillary leak and tissue edema

Types of Perioperative Fluid Requirements

Deficit fluids:

- Fluid deficit is dependent on the duration of fasting prior to surgery
- Fluid deficit = (Maintenance fluid per hour   Number of hours of fasting)
- Causes of fluid deficits:
  - Reduced oral intake and fasting
  - Increased fluid losses:
    - Diarrhea
    - Vomiting
    - Polyuria
    - Hemorrhage
    - Burns
    - Fever
  - Maldistribution
  - Third space loss
  - Hypoalbuminemia—cirrhosis, CCF
  - Other illnesses

Maintenance Fluids

- Maintenance fluids replaces losses from physiological processes like:
  - Urine
  - Sweat
  - Respiration
  - Stools
- Causes of maintenance losses:
  - Insensible losses:
    - Refers to loss which is not perceived by the individual
    - This loss usually cannot be measured
    - Causes of insensible loss:
      - Cutaneous loss:
        - Accounts for 2/3rd of insensible losses
        - 30 mL per 100 kcal spent is lost via sweating

- Respiratory loss:
  - Occurs due to humidification and warming of inspired air
  - Accounts for 1/3rd of insensible losses
  - Approximately 15 mL per 100 kcal is lost via respiration
- Sensible losses:
  - Refers to loss which can be sensed by the individual
  - This loss can be measured
  - Causes of sensible loss:
    - Urine
    - Feces

Ongoing Losses

- Ongoing losses accounts for fluid losses occurring during surgery
- Estimation of loss requires constant supervision of fluid and blood loss
- Causes of ongoing losses:
  - Drainage of ascitic fluid or cystic fluid
  - Fluid sequesterated in gastrointestinal tract
  - Evaporation from exposed surgical field
  - Bleeding

Assessment of Preoperative Dehydration

No.	Signs	Level of dehydration		
		Mild	Moderate	Severe
1.	Weight loss (%)	5	10	15
2.	Fluid deficit (mL/kg)	50	100	150
3.	Pulse	Normal	Increased, weak	Increased, feeble
4.	Blood pressure	Normal	Normal or low	Low, orthostatic
5.	Skin turgor	Normal	Decreased	Greatly decreased
6.	Anterior fontanelle	Normal	Sunken	Markedly depressed
7.	Mucous membranes	Moist	Dry	Very dry
8.	Eyes	Normal	Sunken	Markedly sunken
9.	Urine rate (mL/kg/hr)	<2	<1	<0.5
10.	Urine specific gravity	1.02	1.020–1.030	> 1.030

Calculation of Intraoperative Fluid Requirements

- *Maintenance fluids*: ***Holliday and Segar formula***:
  - Formula used to calculate hourly maintenance fluid requirement:
    - *0–10 kg*: 4 mL/kg/hr up to first 10 kg
    - *10–20 kg*: 40 mL + 2 mL/kg/hr above 10 kg
    - *More than 20 kg*: 60 mL + 1 mL/kg/hr above 20 kg
- *Deficit fluids*:
  - Deficit = (Number of NPO hours) × (Maintenance requirement per hour)
  - 50% of calculated deficit is given during 1st hour
  - Remaining 50% of the calculated deficit is given over next 2 hours
  - Consider fever, prematurity and renal concentrating ability at time of calculation
- *Third space losses*:
  - Refers to the sequestration of fluid to a non-functional extracellular space
  - 1 mL/kg/hr for minor surgeries like hernia repair
  - 15–20 mL/kg/hr for major abdominal and thoracic surgeries
  - 50 mL/kg/hr for necrotizing enterocolitis surgery
- *Blood loss*:
  - Estimated using gravimetric method
  - Replaced in 1:1 ratio with blood or colloid
  - Can be replaced in 3:1 ratio with crystalloids: blood as a temporizing measure

Composition of Commonly Used Fluids

Fluid	pH	OSM	Tone	Na	Cl	K	Ca	Others
0.9% NS	5.5	308	Iso	154	154	0	0	–
RL	6.5	275	Iso	130	109	4	3	Lactate 28 mEq/L
D5	4.5	285	Hypo	0	0	0	0	–
DNS	4	308	Hypo	154	154	0	0	–
1/2 DNS	4	405	Hypo	77	77	0	0	–
Plasmalyte A	7.4	294	Iso	140	98	5	0	Mg 3 mEq/L, acetate 27 mEq/L, gluconate 23 mEq/L

Choice of Intraoperative Fluids

- Role of dextrose containing fluids:
  - Perioperative fluid therapy aims at preventing hypoglycemia and hyperglycemia
  - Currently, predominantly non-dextrose containing isotonic fluids are used
  - Dextrose is given only in those children at risk for hypoglycemia
  - This is because:
    - Preoperative fasting duration has reduced drastically
    - Hypoglycemia occurs only in 0.2–2.5% patients
    - Also, dextrose administration is associated with risk of hyponatremia
  - Glucose infused at 120–300 mg/kg/hr is enough to maintain blood sugar
  - Routine dextrose administration in perioperative period is no longer advised, even in neonates
- Choice of fluids:
  - Isotonic crystalloids with sodium in range 131–154 mmol/L preferred
  - Fluids restricted to 50–80% of routine maintenance needs if suspicion of SIADH
  - Plasma electrolytes are measured when starting maintenance fluids
  - Plasma electrolytes have to be measured every 24 hours thereafter
- Maintenance:
  - Isotonic crystalloids
  - 0.9% NS or RL used most often
- Third space:
  - Isotonic crystalloids
  - 0.9% NS or RL used most often
- Deficit:
  - Isotonic crystalloids
  - 0.9%NS or RL used most often
- Blood loss:
  - 1 mL blood replaced with 1 mL blood
  - 1 mL blood replaced with 1 mL colloid
  - 1 mL blood with 3 mL crystalloid

Postoperative Fluid Therapy

- Timing of fluid therapy:
  - Usually kept NPO during the first 3 postoperative hours
  - If intake delayed for more than 3 hours, administration of fluids required
  - Consider:
    - Maintenance requirements to provide basic metabolic requirements
    - Additional requirements:
  - GI losses from gastric suctioning
  - Additional losses from fever
  - Fluid for drug dilution
- Choice of fluids:
  - Maintenance fluids should be isotonic with appropriate amounts of:
    - Potassium chloride
    - Dextrose
  - 0.9% NS or RL preferred fluids
  - 0.9% NS with 5% dextrose may be used if prolonged fasting expected
  - 5% dextrose and hypotonic fluids increase chances of hyponatremia
- SIADH:
  - SIADH is common in the postoperative period in pediatric population
  - This is due to non-osmotic stimulation of ADH release
  - SIADH results in diminished free water excretion and hyponatremia
  - Causes of postoperative SIADH:
    - Pain
    - Nausea and vomiting
    - Narcotic administration
    - Inhalational agents
    - Positive pressure ventilation
  - Thus, maintenance fluid is reduced to 1/3rd the calculated dose

Complications of Fluid Therapy

- Fluid overload:
  - Anasarca
  - Pulmonary edema
  - Bowel swelling
  - Laryngeal edema
- Hyperchloremic metabolic acidosis from excess use of normal saline
- Hyponatremia if large amounts of ringers lactate
- Coagulopathy if colloids like dextran

NPO GUIDELINES

For Pediatric Age

Age	Fasting time	
	Milk and solids (hours)	Clear fluids (hours)
< 6 months	4	2
6 months–3 years	6	3
>3 years	8	3

For all Ages

Ingested material	Fasting time
Clear fluids	2 hours
Breast milk	4 hours
Infant formula	6 hours
Non human milk	6 hours
Light meal (toast with clear fluids)	6 hours

Clear Fluids

- Water
- Clear tea
- Fruit juice without pulp
- Carbonated beverages
- Black coffee

Advantages of Liberal NPO Guidelines

- Improved patient comfort
- Reduced dehydration
- Reduced hypovolemia at induction
- Reduced chances of hypoglycemia
- Clear fluids 2 hours preoperative stimulates peristalsis, reduces gastric volume and pH

Administration of Drugs

- To be given 60–90 minutes before arrival to OT
- Can be ingested with up to 150 mL water

CHILD WITH RECENT UPPER RESPIRATORY INFECTION

Introduction

- Upper respiratory infection is the most common infection in childhood
- Administration of anesthesia for children with recent URTI increases risk of perioperative respiratory adverse events (PRAE)

Etiology

- Gram positive bacteria:
  - *Staphylococcus*
  - Pneumococcus
  - *Streptococcus*
  - Hemophilus
- Gram negative bacteria:
  - *Pseudomonas*
  - *E. coli*
  - *Klebsiella*
- Viruses:
  - Myxovirus
  - Paramyxovirus
  - Rhinovirus
  - Coronavirus
  - Adenovirus
  - Picornavirus

Types of Respiratory Infections

- URTI:
  - Pharyngitis
  - Laryngitis
  - Croup
  - Epiglottitis
  - Otitis media
  - Tonsillitis
  - Sinusitis
- LRTI
  - Pneumonia
  - Bronchiolitis
  - Bronchiectasis
  - Cystic fibrosis

Implications of Concomitant URTI

- Increased secretions
- Breath holding
- Increased risk of apnea, stridor, coughing
- Seeding of lower respiratory tract causing nosocomial pneumonia

Perioperative Respiratory Adverse Events

- Anesthetizing children with recent URTI increases risk of PRAE
- This is mostly due to persistent airway hyperreactivity following URTI
- Respiratory events are the 2nd most common cause of perioperative cardiac arrest in children
- PRAE includes:
  - Hypoxia
  - Airway obstruction
  - Breath-holding
  - Atelectasis
  - Laryngospasm
  - Bronchospasm

Risk Factors for Nosocomial Pneumonia

- Preoperative antibiotic therapy
- Existence of active URTI
- Presence of tracheostomy tube
- Increased duration of intubation
- Presence of azotemia
- Increased gastric pH

Risk Predictors of PRAE

- Patient related:
  - Young age, infancy
  - Active URTI:
    - Increased airway reactivity can last up to 4 weeks after URTI
    - But incidence of PRAE decreases considerably 2–4 weeks after URTI
    - Thus, anesthesia in patients with URTI < 2 weeks poses increased risk
  - Passive or active smoking
  - Reactive airway disease:
    - Recurrent wheezing
    - Wheezing during exercise
    - Hay fever
    - Past or current eczema
  - Airway anomalies:
    - Subglottic stenosis
    - Cleft palate
    - Pierre-Robin syndrome
    - Laryngomalacia
  - Inadequate fasting status
  - Previous history of apnea
  - Obstructive sleep apnea
  - Down's syndrome
  - Anemia with hematocrit less than 30%
- Surgery related:
  - Shared airway procedures:
    - ENT procedures
    - Dental procedures
    - Respiratory procedures
  - Sudden surgical stimulation
  - Blood or secretions in upper airway
  - Emergency procedures
- Anesthesia related:
  - Inhalational induction of anesthesia
  - Desflurane administration
  - Administration of NMBAs
  - High opioid administration
  - Choice of airway device:
    - Increased airway stimulation increases risk of PRAE
    - Thus, ETT have highest risk of PRAE
    - Risk of PRAE associated with airway device is ETT > LMA > face mask

Prediction of PRAE: The COLDS Score

- Decision making tool which identifies risk of PRAE
- Incorporates most risk factors for PRAE in a child with URTI

Characteristic	1 point	2 points	5 points
Current signs	None	Mild	Moderate-severe
Onset	>4 weeks ago	2–4 weeks ago	<2 weeks ago
Lung disease	None	Mild	Moderate-severe
Device planned	None or face mask	SGAD	ETT
Surgery planned	Non-airway	Minor airway	Major airway
		Flexible bronchoscopy	Rigid bronchoscopy
		Dental extractions	Cleft palate

Preoperative Evaluation

- Assess for obvious signs of URTI:
  - Nasal discharge
  - Repeated coughing
  - Fever
- Auscultation for:
  - Signs of lower respiratory tract infections
  - Wheeze
  - Crackles
- Child with active RTI for elective procedures: Postpone for 2–4 weeks
- Child with active RTI for emergency procedures: Take adequate precautions and continue

Preoperative Optimization and Premedication

- Glucocorticoids:
  - Corticosteroids if taken should be continued
  - Perioperative steroid cover is started in patients with poorly controlled asthma
- β_2 agonists:
  - Inhaled Short Acting Beta Agonists (SABA) used for children with rhonchi
  - SABA is repeated 20–30 minutes prior to induction of anesthesia:
    - Albuterol 2.5 mg via nebulization preferred when < 20 kg weight
    - Albuterol 5 mg via nebulization when weight > 20 kg
  - If on β_2 agonists, monitor theophylline levels between 10 and 20 µg/mL
- Antisialagogue:
  - Glycopyrrolate 4 µg/kg administered intravenously
  - This helps to minimize secretions and decrease chances of laryngospasm
- Nasal decongestant:
  - Topical decongestant spray can be used for older patients prior to induction

- This helps in reducing tracheal irritation from secretions
- Decongestant sprays are avoided in infants

- Premedication:
  - Benzodiazepines are avoided as they increase risk of respiratory complications
  - Distraction techniques and parental presence is preferred

Induction

- Preoxygenate for 3–5 minutes
- Use transparent face mask for induction
- IV induction preferred over inhalational induction
- IV propofol is the preferred induction agent to minimize airway reactivity
- IV lidocaine 1–2 mg/kg can be used to reduce airway reactivity
- Maintain deep anesthetic planes at intubation
- Airway instrumentation is minimized to reduce risk of laryngospasm
- LMA preferred over ETT as reduced risk of laryngospasm.
- Suction can be done following ETT placement in deep planes

Ventilation

- Ventilatory strategy aims at minimizing atelectasis
- Lung protective ventilator strategy preferred:
  - Low tidal volumes
  - High respiratory rates
  - Positive end expiratory pressure
  - Prolonged I:E ratio

Emergence and Extubation

- Avoid extubation in light planes
- Extubation in deep planes preferred as it reduces incidence of PRAE
- Contraindications to deep planes of extubation:
  - Blood or secretions in airway
  - Previous difficult mask ventilation
  - Difficult airway

Postoperative Management

- Nebulization with ipratropium or humidified air following extubation
- Humidification of delivered gases to reduce inspissation of secretions
- Usually uneventful postoperative course as laryngospasm is mostly an intraoperative event
- Complications:
  - Desaturation and hypoxia
  - Bronchospasm
  - Persistent cough

HYPERTROPHIC PYLORIC STENOSIS

Introduction

- First described by Hirschsprung in 1888
- Hypertrophic pyloric stenosis is a medical emergency but not a true surgical emergency
- Condition characterized by hypertrophy of muscularis propria of the pylorus
- Results in functional obstruction of the gastric outlet

Incidence

- Incidence ranges from 2 to 4 per 1,000 live births
- Male:Female = 4:1
- Presents early in life, between 3 and 5 weeks age

Etiology

- Familial inheritance:
  - Common in monozygotic twins
  - Genetic loci which may be responsible IHPS1
  - Causes deficient production of neuronal nitric oxide synthase
  - This causes impaired relaxation of pyloric smooth muscle
  - Common associations:
    - Turners' syndrome
    - Edwards' syndrome
    - Esophageal atresia
- Hyperacidity:
  - Occurs due to high gastric parietal cell mass
  - This results in impaired gastrin control and duodenal hyperacidity
  - This causes repeated contraction of the pylorus, causing IHPS
- Other suspected factors:
  - Abnormal myenteric plexus innervations
  - Cow's milk protein allergy
  - Exposure to macrolide antibiotics

Clinical Features

- Classical presentation is at 4–8 weeks old
- Vomiting:
  - Non-bilious vomitus
  - Vomiting intensity increases until pathognomonic projectile vomiting ensues
  - Projectile vomiting occurring immediately after feeds

- Signs of dehydration:
  - Occur in cases where diagnosis is delayed
  - Sunken fontanelle, dry mucous membrane
  - Poor skin turgor, lethargy
  - Malnutrition, poor weight gain
- Jaundice:
  - Seen as a result of starvation and caloric deprivation
  - This causes deficiency of hepatic glucuronyl transferase
  - This results in jaundice
- Palpable mass:
  - Mass palpable on lateral edge of rectus abdominis
  - *Olive* in right upper quadrant of abdomen in 60–80% infants
  - Best time to appreciate is immediately after a feed
  - *Visible peristalsis* may be appreciable

Lab Findings

- *Hypochloremic metabolic alkalosis*:
  - Classical picture is hypochloremic metabolic alkalosis
  - Occurs due to repeated vomiting
  - This causes loss of hydrochloric acid in the vomitus
- Dyselectrolytemias:
  - Hypokalemia:
    - Hypokalemia may arise due to renal compensation for alkalosis
    - Kidney excretes K^+ ions in order to retain H^+ ions
    - This compensates for alkalosis, while causing hypokalemia
  - Hypo/hypernatremia may occur due to persistent vomiting
- Ultrasound:
  - *Diagnostic test of choice*
  - High sensitivity (90–99%), high specificity (97–100%)
  - Diagnostic features:
    - Pyloric muscle thickness > 4 mm
    - Pyloric muscle length > 14–20 mm
    - Pyloric diameter > 10–14 mm
- Barium studies:
  - Only used in cases where USG is inconclusive, to avoid radiation
  - Elongated pyloric canal (***string sign***)
  - Thickened pyloric mucosa (***double-track sign***)
  - Removal of any residual barium from the stomach after the study is important
  - This is done, to prevent aspiration

Management

- Resuscitation:
  - Airway, breathing, circulation supported
  - Serial electrolytes, acid-base and blood glucose measurements are made
  - Nasogastric tube inserted to decompress the stomach
  - Cimetidine rapidly normalizes the metabolic alkalosis in IHPS
- Fluid therapy:
  - If dehydrated, 20 mL/kg of 0.9% saline bolus used
  - Maintenance fluid started to maintain hydration
  - Focus is on preventing hypoglycemia and hypernatremia
  - 5% $D_{1/2}$NS or DNS may be used as maintenance fluid
  - KCl 2–4 mEq per 100 mL fluid can be added, in the absence of renal insufficiency
  - $D_{1/2}$NS with 40 mmol/L of K^+ infused at 3 L/m^2/day can be used as maintenance
  - Hourly intake-output chart is essential
  - Fluid and electrolyte status can be normalized within 24 hours in most infants
- Conservative management:
  - Reserved for those in whom surgery is contraindicated
  - Nasoduodenal feeding continued for several months
- Surgical management:
  - *Considered only after fluid and electrolyte status have been normalized*
  - Risk of postoperative apnea, if metabolic alkalosis is uncorrected
  - Ramstedt pyloromyotomy:
    - First described in 1907
    - Longitudinal incision of the pylorus
    - Approach is via right upper quadrant transverse incision
    - Blunt dissection performed to the level of the submucosa
    - Associated with minimal morbidity and mortality
    - May be performed laparoscopically

- Endoscopic balloon dilatation:
  - Not as successful as surgery
  - Reserved for those in whom surgery is a definite risk

Anesthetic Considerations

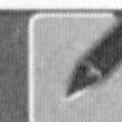

- ❖ Surgery usually performed in infancy
- ❖ Malnourished, dehydrated infant—difficult venous access
- ❖ Gastric outlet obstruction—full stomach considerations
- ❖ Severe preoperative electrolyte disturbances
- ❖ Chances of postoperative respiratory depression

Preoperative Preparation

- ❖ Fluid and electrolyte status:
  - Optimize fluid and electrolyte status prior to induction
  - Surgery deferred until:
    - Sodium level 130 mEq/L
    - Potassium level 3 mEq/L
    - Chloride level 85 mEq/L
    - Urine output 1 mL/kg/hr
- ❖ Nasogastric tube:
  - Aspiration of nasogastric tube essential to avoid aspiration
  - Large multi-orifice orogastric catheter preferable
  - This however does not guarantee evacuation of gastric fluid
  - Volume of gastric contents is often significant (>100 mL)
  - Suctioning NGT in lateral position may be useful
  - *4-quadrant aspiration:*
    - Performed in some centers
    - Infant turned through full rotation
    - Stomach is aspirated at each quarter turn
- ❖ Since most surgeries are done in early infancy, premedication is usually not required

Induction

- ❖ Nasogastric tube inserted prior to induction and suctioned
- ❖ Adequate preoxygenation with 100% oxygen
- ❖ Awake intubation is not superior to modified RSI in IHPS
- ❖ Inhalational induction with sevoflurane or halothane if no IV access
- ❖ Rapid sequence induction with propofol or thiopentone if IV access is present
- ❖ IV succinylcholine 1–2 mg/kg is used to ensure muscle paralysis
- ❖ Classic RSI not possible in infants as child will desaturate with cricoids pressure
- ❖ Role of classic RSI with cricoids pressure is therefore controversial
- ❖ Modified RSI with gentle PPV is useful
- ❖ Atropine may be used to treat bradycardia during laryngoscopy
- ❖ IV co-amoxiclav 30 mg/kg or cefuroxime 50 mg/kg for antibiotic prophylaxis

Monitors

- ❖ Pulse oximetry
- ❖ NIBP
- ❖ ECG
- ❖ Capnography
- ❖ Temperature
- ❖ Neuromuscular monitoring
- ❖ Urine output

Maintenance

- ❖ O_2 + air + sevoflurane used for maintenance
- ❖ Nitrous oxide avoided in laparoscopic surgery
- ❖ Sevoflurane or desflurane preferred due to risk of postoperative apnea
- ❖ Air may be injected through NGT at the end of the procedure to ensure pyloric patency
- ❖ Narcotic dose is minimized to ensure fully awake child at the end of surgery
- ❖ Intraoperative analgesia may be achieved with IV fentanyl 1 µg/kg
- ❖ Muscle relaxation maintained with small doses of atracurium (0.05–0.1 mg/kg)
- ❖ Wound infilteration at end of procedure with 0.25% bupivacaine 0.8 mL/kg useful

Ventilation

- ❖ Increased risk of postoperative apnea and respiratory depression
- ❖ Deliberate hypoventilation in order to combat CNS alkalosis may be prudent

Hemodynamics

- ❖ Active warming with warming blankets to ensure euthermia
- ❖ 10 mL/kg boluses of NS may be used to restore circulating blood volume
- ❖ Glucose containing maintenance solutions should not be used for fluid boluses

- Ensure normoglycemia if glucose containing fluids are not used introperatively
- Bradycardia and hypotension can result from celiac reflex due to traction on pylorus

Extubation

- Child can be extubated once fully reversed and awake
- Extubation usually performed in left lateral position

Postoperative

Management

- Nasogastric tube usually removed at the end of the procedure
- Oral feeds usually initiated 6–8 hours postsurgery
- Feeding sometimes commenced as soon as 4 hours postprocedure
- Maintenance fluids continued until feeds have been fully established
- Graded feeds initiated starting with pedialyte and progressing to full-strength formula
- Resumption of full feeds usually takes 2–3 days
- Persistent vomiting resolves within 1–2 days post surgery
- Respiratory depression:
  - Apnea may occur postoperatively, if alkalosis was uncorrected prior to surgery
  - This may occur up to 7 hours postsurgery
  - This is due to delayed correction of CNS alkalosis, affecting the pH of the CSF

Monitors

- Pulse oximetry
- NIBP
- ECG
- Urine output
- Respiratory rate

Analgesia

- Multimodal analgesia preferred
- Paracetamol and NSAIDs useful to augment analgesia
- IV Ibuprofen 5 mg/kg useful for severe pain

Complications

- Duodenal perforation
- *Incomplete myotomy*: Recurrent vomiting
- Wound dehiscence
- Hernia

GASTROSCHISIS AND OMPHALOCELE

Introduction

- Gastroschisis and omphalocele are fetal abdominal wall defects causing herniation of abdominal contents
- Failure of gut to return to abdominal cavity during fetal development causes persistent herniation of abdominal contents without a covering sac
- Gastroschisis:
  - It is a full thickness abdominal wall defect
  - It is usually associated with evisceration of bowel and other abdominal organs
  - This causes protrusion of the contents through a defect close to base of umbilicus
  - No sac is present to cover the abdominal contents
  - Contents may be thickened, matted together or edematous
- Omphalocele:
  - It is a midline abdominal wall defect
  - Abdominal contents are covered by amnion and peritoneum
  - Thus, contents are covered by a 2-layered sac

Omphalocele

- Occurs in 10th week of fetal life
- Also called exomphalos
- Occurs due to non-return of bowel from extra-embryonic coelom
- Thus, the gut fails to return to abdominal cavity and undergo the obligatory 270° rotation
- Thus, omphalocele is considered a rotational anomaly
- It is covered by an outer membrane called amnion and inner layer of peritoneum
- Differentiating features from gastroschisis:
  - Intestinal contents are commonly in the midline
  - Umbilical cord is inserted into umbilical sac
  - Umbilical cord is present at the apex of sac
  - Presence of extracorporeal liver
  - Bowel is completely covered with peritoneum
  - Thus, usually not associated with infections and dyselectrolytemias
  - Not considered a surgical emergency (requires urgent surgery though)
  - Higher rate of associated defects (80%) like:
    - Mental retardation
    - Cloacal/bladder dystrophy
    - Metabolic defects
    - Cardiac defects (tetralogy of Fallot)

- Associated syndromes:
  - ***Beckwith—Wiedemann syndrome***
  - ***Pentalogy of Cantrell***

❖ Types:
- Exomphalos minor: Small defect (2–5 cm diameter)
- Exomphalos major: Large defect (>10 cm diameter) involving liver and spleen

❖ Risk factors associated with development of omphalocele include:
- Extremes of maternal reproductive age
- Maternal selective serotonin reuptake inhibitor (SSRI) exposure
- Maternal obesity
- Black race

Gastroschisis

❖ Occurs earlier (6–8 weeks) of fetal life

❖ Several hypotheses to explain the pathogenesis:
- Failure of formation of mesoderm in the abdominal wall
- Rupture of amnion surrounding the umbilical ring
- Abnormal involution of right umbilical vein
- Disruption of right vitelline artery:
  - This causes ischemia and atrophy of anterior abdominal wall
  - Thus, the bowel is uncovered and exposed
  - This causes a defect in the lateral abdominal wall

❖ Thus, gastroschisis is a true abdominal wall defect

❖ Differentiating features are:
- Generally less than 5 cm diameter
- Intestinal contents are usually towards one side (commonly right side)
- Umbilical cord insertion is para-umbilical
- Umbilical cord is present towards one side of the wall (not at the apex)
- Absence of extracorporeal liver
- Bowel is not encased in peritoneum:
  - Therefore, it is prone to getting infected
  - Appears thickened, edematous and covered by fibrin peel
  - Also associated with fluid and electrolyte abnormalities
- Considered a surgical emergency
- Lower rate of associated defects (32%)

❖ Risk factors for gastroschisis:
- Low maternal age (less than 20 years)
- Maternal smoking
- Maternal alcohol consumption
- Maternal intake of drugs such as:
  - Pseudoephedrine
  - Aspirin
  - Ibuprofen
  - Acetaminophen
- High agricultural chemical content in surface water

No.	Character	Gastroschisis	Omphalocele
1.	Incidence	1: 3000	1: 5,000
2.	Maternal age	<20 years	>40 years
3.	Location of defect	Lateral to umbilicus	Through center of umbilicus
4.	Covering sac	Absent	Present
5.	Condition of bowel	Thick, edematous	Normal
6.	Size of defect	Usually small	Usually large
7.	Contents	Only small, large bowel	Liver
8.	Infections	Common	Rare
9.	Associated anomalies	Rare	Common
10.	Surgical emergency	Emergent surgery	Urgent surgery

Incidence

❖ Gastroschisis and omphalocele are the most common abdominal wall defects

❖ Prevalence of these defects is:
- 1 per 5,386 live births for omphalocele
- 1 per 2,229 live births for gastroschisis

Differential Diagnosis

❖ Ectopia cordis

❖ Limb-body wall complex

❖ Cloacal exstrophy

❖ Urachal cyst

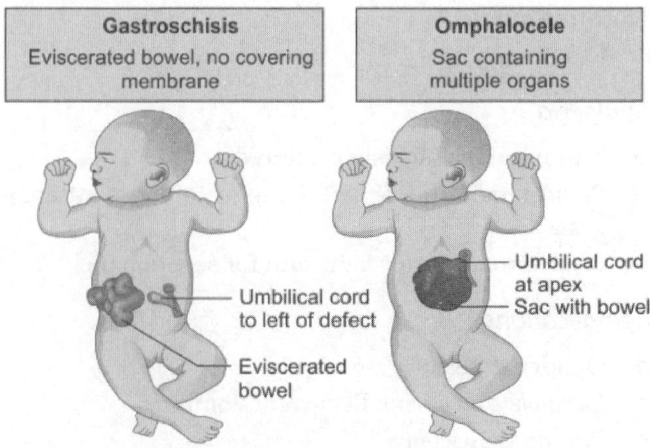

Fig. 3: Gastroschisis and omphalocele.

Treatment

- Primary closure:
  - Done within few hours of birth if the defect is small
  - Successful in 70% of the cases
  - Criteria for safe primary closure:
    - Intragastric pressure < 20 cm H_2O
    - Intravesical pressure < 20 cm H_2O
    - $ETCO_2$ < 50 mm Hg
    - Peak airway pressure < 30 cm H_2O
  - Small bowel is decompressed by aspirating stomach contents
  - Large bowel is evacuated through the rectum
  - Size of the defect is increased by 1–2 cm during reduction of contents
  - This is in order to prevent intestinal injury at the time of reduction
  - Abdominal wall is stretched and bowel contents are replaced
- Staged closure:
  - Indications:
    - For smaller abdominal wall defects
    - Distended intestinal loops
  - Done using Dacron reinforced silastic silo
  - Silo acts as temporary housing for bowel
  - Silo is secured at the edges of the defect
  - Size is gradually reduced over 3–7 days
  - Allows abdominal cavity to accommodate contents gradually
  - This avoids compromising perfusion or ventilation

Anesthetic Considerations

- Prevention of infection and sepsis especially in gastroschisis
- Fluid balance:
  - Correction of hypovolemia and electrolyte imbalance preoperatively
  - Anticipation of massive fluid losses intraoperatively
- Prevention of hypothermia:
  - Anticipation of massive heat loss intraoperatively
  - Aggressive prevention of hypothermia preoperatively and intraoperatively
- Rapid sequence induction in view of associated intestinal obstruction
- Difficult ventilation postoperatively due to reduced FRC

Preoperative Preparation

- Informed consent
- Maintenance of temperature during transport:
  - Should be nursed in incubator at all times to prevent hypothermia
  - Overhead radiant heaters
  - Intravenous fluid warmers
  - Humidified, warm anesthetic gases
- IV access:
  - IV line in preferred in upper limb
  - Increased abdominal pressure limits venous return from lower limb
  - 2 large bore IV cannulae preferred
  - Central venous access preferred if postoperative parenteral nutrition is planned
  - Umbilical vessel catheterization is contraindicated
- Fluid resuscitation with isotonic crystalloids (6–10 mL/kg/hr) and albumin if hypovolemic
- Antibiotic prophylaxis especially if gastroschisis
- NGT is inserted to decompress stomach contents
- Handling the viscera:
  - Defect is covered with a warm sterile saline-soaked gauze piece
  - This is further wrapped in a sterile plastic wrap to prevent heat loss
  - Viscera is physically supported to ensure no twisting occurs at the herniation site
- Nursing position:
  - Gastroschisis
    - Children with gastroschisis are nursed in the right lateral position
    - This is to enhance venous return from the gut and avoid vascular compromise
  - Large omphalocele:
    - Nursed in left lateral position
    - This is because the viscera and liver may compress the IVC in supine position

Monitors

- Pulse oximetry
- Capnography
- ECG
- NIBP
- Temperature
- Urine output
- Invasive BP
- Precordial stethoscope
- Pulse oximeter and NIBP to be secured in lower limb
- This is in order to check for reduced venous return following abdominal closure

Induction

- Preoxygenation to maintain SpO_2 between 85 and 95% to prevent retinopathy of prematurity
- Nasogastric or progastric tube inserted prior to induction

- Awake intubation with video laryngoscopy or fiberoptic intubation if difficult airway
- Rapid sequence induction with gentle cricoid pressure
- Difficult airway with large tongue is anticipated in Beckwith-Wiedemann syndrome
- Epidural via thoracic or caudal tip at T_4–T_8
- Central line placement if postoperative parenteral nutrition is planned

Maintenance

- Avoid nitrous oxide for maintenance of anesthesia
- Balanced anesthesia with O_2 + air + 1 MAC isoflurane may be used
- Increased dose of relaxants is used to facilitate primary closure
- IV 5–10 µg/kg fentanyl or epidural infusion can be used for analgesia
- Ventilatory requirements increase once bowels are placed in the abdomen
- Hand-ventilation may be necessary to maintain gas exchange

Hemodynamics

- Massive fluid losses occur during surgery due to:
  - Exposed visceral surfaces
  - Third space losses due to partial bowel obstruction
- Dextrose containing fluids used for maintenance in order to avoid hypoglycemia
- 6–10 mL/kg RL along with 5% albumin can be used for volume resuscitation
- Prevent hypothermia
  - Cover head of baby
  - Warm IV fluids
  - Warm theater
  - Adequate blankets
- Watch for aortocaval compression and hypotension
- This can occur during tight primary closure causing reduced venous return
- If hypotension occurs following wound closure:
  - Notify the surgeon
  - Reopen wound
  - Aggressive hydration
  - Inotropic support

Complications

- Postoperative ileus
- Intestinal obstruction
- Aortocaval compression
- Hepatic vein compression, liver damage
- Compression of renal vessels
- Reduced organ perfusion
- Intestinal perforation
- Peritonitis, necrotizing enterocolitis, sepsis
- Lower lobe atelectasis due to diaphragmatic splinting
- Abdominal compartment syndrome

Postoperative Care

- Postoperative ventilation preferred
- Mechanical ventilation is required for 24–48 hours due to deterioration in lung function
- Opioid requirements are lesser as hepatic function is reduced
- Head up position is preferred while nursing
- TAP block or caudal epidural can be used for postoperative analgesia

TRACHEOESOPHAGEAL FISTULA

Introduction

- Represents an abnormal connection between esophagus and trachea
- First described by Thomas Gibson in 1697
- First successful primary repair was performed in 1941 by Cameron Haight
- Current survival rates in healthy infants undergoing surgery approach 100%

Incidence

- This is the most common type of airway fistula
- Incidence of 1 in 3,500–4,500 live births
- Acquired TEFs occur in approximately 0.5% patients undergoing tracheostomy
- Incidence of malignant TEF:
  - 4.5% for primary esophageal tumors
  - 0.3% for primary lung tumors

Etiology

- Congenital: Associated with trisomy 13, 18, and 21
- Acquired:
  - Blunt trauma/avulsion injury of neck
  - Postintubation/tracheostomy complication:
    - Traumatic intubation
    - Prolonged intubation
    - Abrasive tube
    - Cuff pressure > 30 mm Hg
  - Esophageal carcinoma
  - Postradiation therapy
  - Esophageal stents causing persistent pressure on esophageal wall
  - Impacted dentures

Classification

Gross classification	Vogt classification	Description
– (not included)	Type 1	Esophageal agenesis, no fistula present No fistula is present Not included in Gross classification
Type A	Type 2	Proximal and distal esophageal stumps Missing mid segment No fistula present
Type B	Type 3A	Proximal esophagus meets lower trachea Distal esophageal stump
Type C	Type 3B	Proximal esophageal atresia Esophagus ends in blind loop superior to sternal angle Distal esophagus arises from lower trachea or carina
Type D	Type 3C	Proximal esophagus terminates on lower trachea or carina Distal esophagus arises from carina
Type E or type H		Type D variant Esophagus is continuous Presence of fistula appears like the letter H
Type F		Esophageal stenosis

Associated Anomalies

- Vater:
  - Vertebral defects
  - Anal atresia
  - Tracheoesophageal fistula
  - Esophageal atresia
  - Radial aplasia
  - Renal anomalies
- Vacterl:
  - Vertebral defect
  - Anal malformation
  - Cardiac defects
  - Tracheoesophageal fistula
  - Esophageal anomalies
  - Radial aplasia
  - Renal anomalies
  - Limb defects
- Musculoskeletal
  - Hemivertebrae
  - Syndactyly
  - Radial aplasia
  - Rib anomalies
  - Polydactyly
  - Scoliosis
- Cardiac:
  - VSD
  - TOF
  - COA
  - PDA
  - Right sided aortic arch
  - ASD
- Gastrointestinal:
  - Imperforate anus
  - Meckels diverticulum

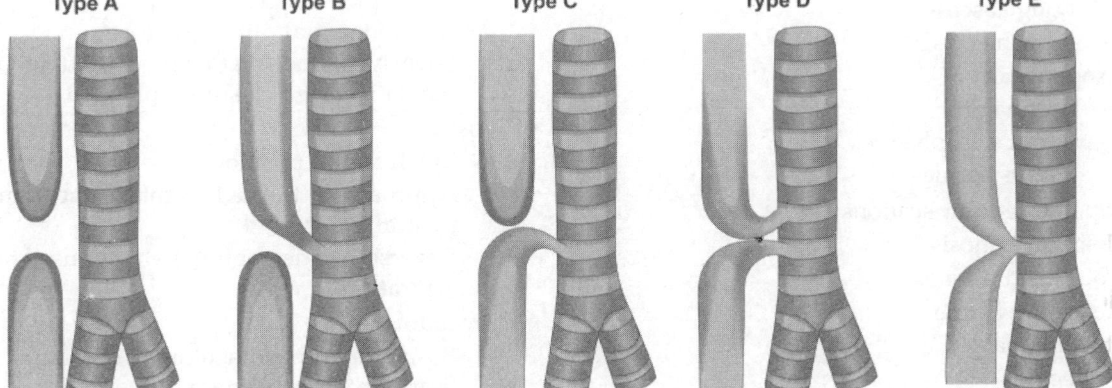

Fig. 4: Types of tracheoesophageal fistula.

- Duodenal atresia
- Annular pancreas
- Malrotation

❖ Genitourinary:
- Renal agenesis
- Hypospadiasis
- Horseshoe kidney
- Polycystic kidney disease

Clinical Features

❖ History:
- Polyhydramnios in mother is suggestive of TEF with esophageal atresia
- Presence of fundic gas shadow on prenatal USG is another indication of TEF
- Classically presents with copious fine white frothy mucus in mouth of neonates
- Secretions recur in spite of suctioning
- Choking, coughing and cyanosis occur with first feed due to aspiration of saliva
- Frequent LRTI

❖ On examination:
- Signs of dehydration
- Scaphoid abdomen in the absence of fistula
- If fistula present, abdominal distension due to build up of air in stomach
- Inability to pass 8–10 Fr feeding tube beyond 10–15 cm suggests TEF
- Normal distance to infant's gastric cardia is 17 cm

Complications

❖ Preoperative complications:
- Pulmonary:
  - Recurrent pneumonia
  - Acute lung injury
  - ARDS
  - Lung abscess
  - Bronchiectasis
- Esophageal:
  - Esophagitis
  - Barret's esophagus
  - Hiatus hernias

❖ Postoperative complications:
- Tracheal stenosis
- Vocal cord paralysis
- Recurrent fistula
- Pneumonia
- Atelectasis
- Pneumothorax
- Gastroesophageal reflux disease

Investigations

❖ Chest X-ray:
- Pulmonary infilterates, aspiration pneumonia
- Coiled NGT in proximal esophageal pouch
- Right aortic arch
- Rib anomalies

❖ Abdomen X-ray:
- Skeletal anomalies
- Intestinal malrotation
- Intestinal obstruction

❖ Contrast upper GI X-ray:
- Usually not required as it increases risk of aspiration
- Useful in case of uncertain diagnosis or suspicion of proximal TEF

❖ Esophageal endoscopy and bronchoscopy:
- May be useful to diagnose TEF
- Methylene blue may be used as contrast material
- Methylene blue is injected into the trachea
- Appearance of contrast in the esophagus confirms diagnosis of TEF

❖ Multi-detector row CT scans may be useful to confirm diagnosis

❖ Echocardiography: To diagnose associated defects

❖ Renal USG

❖ Prenatal USG:
- Polyhydramnios
- Air in stomach confirms presence of fistula

Procedure

❖ Timing of surgery:
- Primary closure is always preferably done as an emergency procedure
- Staged repair several weeks after birth is preferred in:
  - Premature babies
  - Severe respiratory distress syndrome
  - Aspiration pneumonia
  - Congenital cardiac disease
- Fogarty balloon catheter is used to obliterate fistula if staged closure is planned

❖ Position:
- In left lateral position
- Approach is through right thoracotomy, extra-pleurally
- Reverse Trendelenburg is always used to prevent aspiration

❖ Procedure:
- Posterolateral thoracotomy incision is made in fourth intercostal space
- Retropleural exposure is obtained and vagus nerve identified

- Fistula usually present where azygous vein crosses trachea to enter SVC
- Azygous vein is divided and fistula is then isolated and divided
- Tracheal end of the fistula is sutured and repaired
- Tracheal suture line may be covered with a flap of mediastinal pleura
- Esophageal end is identified and dissected to assess length for primary anastomosis
- Anastomosis is then completed if the length is sufficient

❖ If length of esophagus is inadequate for primary repair:
- Gastrostomy is created for feeding
- Esophagostomy is created for drainage of saliva
- Gastrostomy feeding, upper pouch suction done till 1 year age
- Colonic interposition for esophagus or gastric pull up is done at 1 year age

Prognostication

❖ *Waterston classification*:
- Group A:
  - Birth weight more than 2,500 g
  - No other problems
  - Associated with lowest mortality
  - Can undergo surgery
- Group B:
  - Birth weight 1,800–2,500 grams
  - Associated with moderate pneumonia or other congenital problems
  - Need stabilizing treatment prior to surgery
  - Associated with 32% mortality
- Group C:
  - Birth weight less than 1,800 g
  - Associated with severe pneumonia or other severe congenital problems
  - 94% mortality
  - Requires staged repair

❖ *Spitz classification*:
- Group I:
  - Birth weight more than 1,500 g
  - No major cardiac anomaly
  - Survival rate of 98.5%
- Group II:
  - Birth weight less than 1,500 g *or* major cardiac anomaly
  - Survival rate of 82%
- Group III:
  - Birth weight less than 1,500 g *and* major cardiac anomaly
  - Survival rate of 50%

Anesthetic Considerations

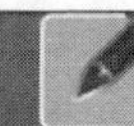

❖ Pediatric patients
❖ Difficult IV access
❖ Shared airway
❖ Difficult airway—difficult placement of ETT
❖ Preoperative dehydration
❖ Preoperative respiratory distress/aspiration pneumonia
❖ Perioperative hypothermia
❖ Associated anomalies (cardiac anomalies are most commonly associated with mortality)

Preoperative Preparation

❖ Prevent and treat aspiration pneumonia:
- Nurse in semi-upright position with head end up
- Low pressure suction to upper esophageal pouch using 8Fr ***Replogle sump tube***
- Oral feeding contraindicated
- Preoperative antibiotic therapy with chest physiotherapy

❖ Note down baseline SpO_2 values and start supplemental O_2 therapy

❖ Dextrose containing fluids started at 4 mL/kg/hr as these children are usually NPO

❖ Cover extremities, head with gumgee pads/aluminium foil

❖ Shift with thermal protection

OT Preparation

❖ Provide thermoneutral environment:
- Air conditioner is switched off
- OT table can be prewarmed with heating mattress
- All fluids and blood to be prewarmed
- Warmed and humidified gases to be used

❖ Include manometer in circuit

❖ Suction

❖ Oxygen source

❖ Airway equipment

❖ *Pharmacy*: Anesthetic drugs

❖ Monitors checked and calibrated

❖ Emergency drugs

Monitors

❖ Pulse oximetry ❖ End tidal carbon dioxide

❖ ECG ❖ Temperature

❖ Urine output ❖ Airway pressure

❖ Invasive arterial pressure monitoring, especially in the presence of cardiac disease

❖ Central venous access usually not required unless:
- Difficult peripheral access
- Postoperative TPN planned

Induction

- Awake intubation:
  - *Traditionally used* but traumatic and associated with IVH in preterm neonates
  - Done rarely nowadays if:
    - Severe airway problems
    - Sick gasping infant
    - In emergencies
  - Disadvantages:
    - Technically difficult
    - Increases arterial and venous pressure
    - Increased ICP and increased incidence of intracranial hemorrhage
    - Increased incidence of hypoxemia
- Intravenous induction:
  - Preferred over awake intubation
  - 22/24 G cannula is inserted with EMLA cream
  - IV thiopentone 3–4 mg/kg or ketamine 2 mg/kg can be given for induction
  - Endotracheal tube in inserted and position is confirmed
  - Muscle relaxants are avoided till ventilation is assured
  - Avoid positive pressure ventilation to avoid stomach distension
- Inhalational induction:
  - Useful if IV access is absent
  - Sevoflurane, oxygen and air are used for induction
  - Avoid prolonged use of high sevoflurane concentrations
  - Watch for apnea, breath holding and bradycardia

Intubation

- Ideal ETT position is between carina and TEF, lying just above carina
- The tip of the ETT should ideally lie just distal to the TEF
- Position of patient:
  - Sniffing position
  - Pillow avoided
  - Flat shoulders
  - Head in doughnut to stabilize
- Straight/curved blade can be used
- 2.5–3.5 mm ID ETT
- Correct ETT size is that which has leak at 30 cm H_2O airway pressure
- Two techniques of intubation:
  - Routine intubation with tip of ETT positioned above the carina
  - Intentional endobronchial intubation:
    - ETT is passed through the cords and beyond the carina
    - This ensures endobronchial intubation
    - The ETT is then withdrawn till breath sounds are just heard on both sides
    - Position of the tube is confirmed by flexible fiber-optic bronchoscopy
- Confirmation of ETT position:
  - Feel for ETT tip at suprasternal notch
  - Auscultation of breath sounds is done with neck flexed
  - Auscultate stomach to ensure no distension occurs through TEF
  - Flexible fiber-optic bronchoscopy is technique of choice
- Following bronchoscopy, Fogarty catheter can be positioned into the TEF
- This helps to isolate esophagus from trachea and aid intraoperative ventilation

Maintenance

- O_2 + air + isoflurane is used for maintenance of balanced anesthesia
- Atracurium is *drug of choice* for muscle paralysis
- Epidural analgesia:
  - Used to supplement analgesia
  - Epidural injection can be given via thoracic/caudal approach
  - Tip of epidural catheter should lie at T_{6-7} level to ensure adequate analgesia
  - 0.1–0.2 mL/kg/hr infusion of 0.125% bupivacaine can be used

Ventilation

- Aims at ventilating the lungs without ventilating the fistula
- Inflation pressures are kept minimal until gastrostomy is opened or fistula is controlled
- Typical ventilatory settings:
  - Tidal volume 7–10 mL/kg
  - Respiratory rate 35–40 breaths/min
  - Titrate FiO_2 to maintain SpO_2 between 95 and 98%
- Hand ventilation is preferred during lung retraction
- Increase FiO_2 if hypoxemia occurs during lung retraction
- Suction blood and secretions from ETT intermittently
- ETT may get blocked by blood clot leading to sudden crisis scenarios
- Thus, regular suctioning of ETT is vital to safe conduct of anesthesia

- Monitor for problems associated with shared airway:
  - ETT kinking
  - Accidental extubation

Hemodynamics

- Maintain hematocrit >35%
- Choice of fluids:
  - $D_{1/2}$ NS can be used as replacement fluid
  - Maintenance with isotonic crystalloids
- Warming blanket, warm IV fluids

Extubation

- Patients can be extubated at the end of surgery
- Deep planes are preferred at extubation
- This is because an awake, retching patient affects the anastomotic site

Postoperative Management

- Postoperative ventilation considered if:
  - Aspiration pneumonia
  - Associated cardiac anomalies
  - Low birth weight less than 2,000 g
  - Premature infant
  - Respiratory distress syndrome
- Nurse in lateral and supine position
- Prolonged intubation may be required if tracheomalacia/bronchomalacia is associated
- Multimodal analgesia is usually preferred for postoperative pain relief

CONGENITAL DIAPHRAGMATIC HERNIA

Introduction

- Failure of closure of diaphragm allows abdominal contents to herniate into the thorax
- This characterizes congenital diaphragmatic hernia
- As a result of this herniation, normal development of the lungs is hampered
- First successful operative repair accomplished by ***Heidenhain*** in Germany in 1905
- Progress in the techniques of management of CDH has been exceedingly slow

Incidence

- Six times more common on the left than the right hemithorax
- Incidence of 1 in 2,200–3,500 live births
- Mortality rate is generally high (30–45%)
- If ECMO has been employed as a treatment strategy, mortality rises to 50%
- Bilateral defects are usually fatal

Classification

- Absent diaphragm
- Diaphragmatic hernia
  - ***Bochdalek's*** posterolateral hernia (70–75%):
    - Left sided hernia (85%)
    - Right sided hernia (13%)
    - Bilateral hernia (2%)
  - ***Morgagnis*** anterior hernia (23–28%)
  - Central hernias (2–7%)
- Eventration

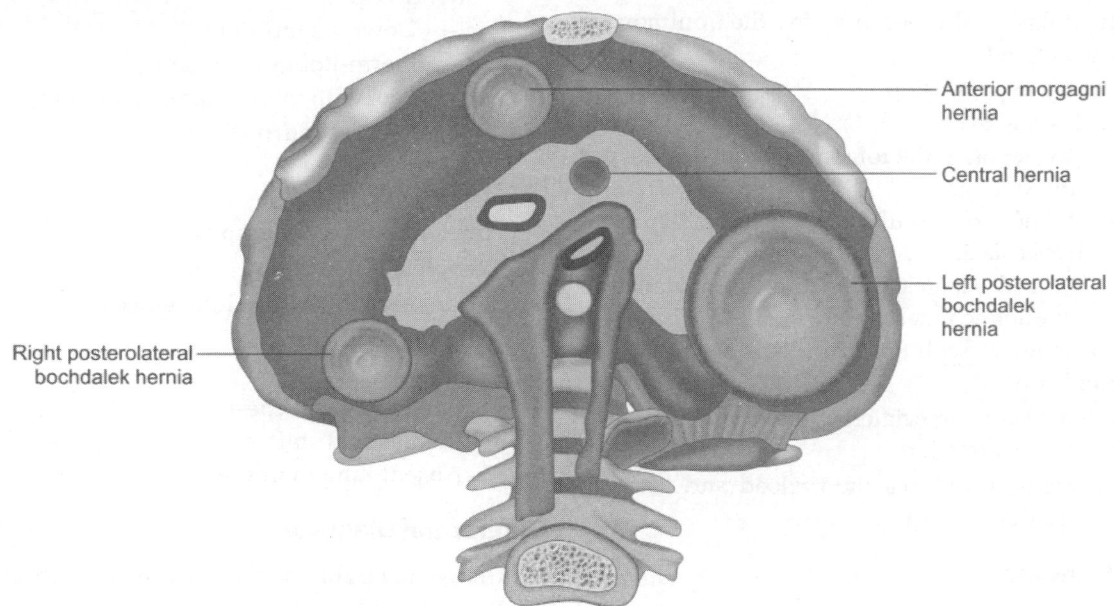

Fig. 5: Types of congenital diaphragmatic hernia.

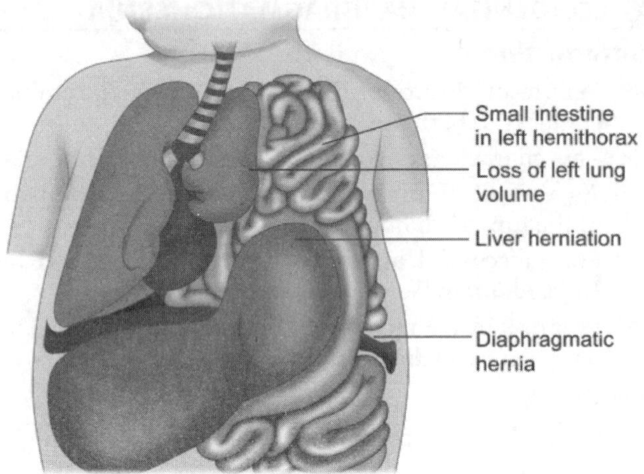

Fig. 6: Congenital diaphragmatic hernia.

Pathophysiology

- Pulmonary hypoplasia and pulmonary HTN are critical derangements in CDH
- Pulmonary hypoplasia:
  - Hypoplasia occurs due to:
    - Compression by bowel
    - Global embryopathy
  - Usually occurs on the ipsilateral side of the hernia
  - Contralateral side may be involved to a variable extent
  - Results in reduced lung volume and impaired alveolarization
  - Hypoplasia also occurs in the pulmonary vascular bed
- Pulmonary hypertension:
  - Occurs due to:
    - Reduction in the total number of vessels per unit of lung
    - Pulmonary vascular remodeling with medial hyperplasia
    - Altered vasoreactivity due to imbalance in autonomic innervation
  - This together with RVH results in severe PPHN after birth
- CDH may also be associated with varying degree of ventricular dysfunction
- IVC obstruction reduces the preload and leads to reduced cardiac output

Clinical Features

- Routine prenatal screening may identify CDH at a mean gestational age of 24 weeks
- Classical triad:
  - Dyspnea and respiratory distress at birth
  - Cyanosis
  - Apparent dextrocardia
- Degree of distress is dependent on:
  - Severity of lung hypoplasia
  - Presence of persistent pulmonary HTN of the newborn (PPHN)
- Physical findings:
  - Most CDH usually occur in the left hemithorax
  - Right sided CDH (15%) and bilateral herniation (1–2%) are rare
  - Pulmonary complications are less commonly seen with right sided CDH
  - This is because the liver prevents translocation of bowel loops
  - Child usually has a scaphoid abdomen with barrel-shaped chest
  - Reduced air entry in chest
  - Bowel sounds audible in chest
  - Displaced heart sounds
  - Hypoxia, acidosis
- Associated anomalies:
  - Adrenal insufficiency
  - Congenital heart disease:
    - ASD
    - VSD
    - TOF
    - Hypoplastic left heart
  - Neural tube defects
  - Syndromes:
    - Down's syndrome
    - Pierre-Robin syndrome
    - Beckwith-Wiedemann syndrome
    - Fryn's syndrome

Investigations

- Antenatal ultrasonography
- Complete blood count
- Serum electrolytes, calcium, glucose
- Arterial blood gas
- Chest X-ray:
  - Bowel loops in chest
  - Mediastinal shift
  - Absent lung markings

Differential Diagnosis

- Congenital pulmonary airway malformation (CPAM)
- Bronchogenic cyst
- Eventration

Medical Management

- Antenatal management:
  - Antenatal steroids given to mother may help improve lung maturation
  - Delivery of the fetus is usually targeted after completion of 39 weeks of gestation
  - This avoids complications associated with prematurity
- Initial medical management followed by surgical correction improves survival
- Goals of medical management:
  - Avoid bag and mask ventilation
  - Immediate intubation and gastric suction after birth
  - Central or peripheral venous access for administration of fluids
  - Placement of preductal arterial line in right upper limb
  - Hemodynamic goals:
    - Volume boluses/inotropes can be used
    - Maintain mean BP > 35 mm Hg
    - Urine output > 1 mL/kg/h
    - Arterial pH > 7.2
    - Lactate levels < 3–5 mmoL/L
  - Titration of FiO_2 to maintain preductal saturation of more than 85%
  - Surfactant therapy:
    - Has poor results unless given prophylactically before first breath
    - Exosurf 5 mL/kg Q12H (3 doses given)
    - Further prospective trials are required to establish benefit in CDH
  - Other drugs which can be used are:
    - Sildenafil
    - Bosentan
    - Milrinone
    - Prostaglandin (PGE_1)
    - Prostacyclin (PGI_2)
  - Inhaled nitric oxide therapy:
    - Used in a dose of 5–20 ppm
    - Indicated when the oxygen saturation index (OI) reduces below 25 ± 9
    - Has not been found to be useful in reducing the need for ECMO
    - Plays an important role in treating exacerbations of pulmonary HTN

Modes of Ventilation

- Conventional ventilation:
  - Gentle ventilation with low peak inspiratory pressures preferred
  - Ideally not to involve use of muscle relaxants and paralysis
  - Prevent over distension of alveoli and barotrauma
  - Initial settings:
    - Peak inspiratory pressure < 25 cm H_2O
    - PEEP 3–5 cm H_2O
    - Respiratory rate 40–60 cycles/min
  - Prevent hypoxia, excess hypercarbia and acidosis
  - Permissive hypercapnea up to 60 mm Hg may be acceptable
  - Dobutamine or tolazoline tried if persistent hypoxemia
- High frequency oscillatory ventilation
  - Considered when PIP > 25 cm H_2O is required to maintain $PaCO_2$ < 60 mm Hg
  - Target eight rib expansion on contralateral side on HFOV
  - Initial HFOV settings:
    - Mean airway pressure 2–3 cm H_2O above that used in conventional ventilation
    - Amplitude/ΔP 1.5–2 times the MAP
    - Inspiratory time 33%
    - Frequency 10 Hz
  - Reduces need for ECMO
  - Yet to be proven to have positive impact on survival
  - Found to have no added benefits over conventional ventilation
- ECMO:
  - Indications:
    - Maximal ventilatory support fails to maintain:
      - Preductal SpO_2 > 85%
      - Postductal SpO_2 > 70%
    - Respiratory acidosis with pH > 7.15
    - Requirement of PIP > 28 cm H_2O
    - Requirement of MAP > 17 cm H_2O
    - Inadequate oxygen delivery with metabolic acidosis
    - Consistently elevated OI > 40
  - Used when CDH is unresponsive to conventional therapy with:
    - Age > 34 weeks gestation
    - Weight > 2 kg
    - No associated major lethal anomalies
  - Veno-arterial (VA) ECMO is used in the presence of hemodynamic instability
  - Mortality rate increases when duration of ECMO therapy exceeds 2 weeks
  - Surgical closure is planned once patient status has optimized:

- Maintenance of age appropriate arterial pressures for > 12–24 hours
- Preductal SpO_2 > 85% with FiO_2 < 50%
- Absence of acidosis
- Urine output > 1–2 mL/kg/hr
- Surgical closure is planned following ECMO decannulation in sick patients

Surgical Management

- Techniques of surgical closure:
  - Conventional open approach:
    - Surgical repair is usually preferred 48–72 hours after birth
    - Can be via thoracic or abdominal approach
    - Bowel contents are replaced into the abdomen
    - Diaphragmatic defect is then closed
    - Small defects can be closed primarily and have low recurrence rates
    - Larger defects may need placement of a patch for closure of the defect
    - Goretex graft or autologous muscle flaps may be used for closure
  - VATS:
    - Associated with longer operative times and higher recurrence rates
    - Not found to be particularly advantageous over open technique
    - Persistent pulmonary hypertension contra-indicates thoracoscopic approach
  - ***FETO (Fetoscopic endotracheal occlusion)***:
    - This is a prenatal intrauterine surgery
    - In this technique, fetal trachea is occluded with the ***Fetendo*** clip
    - Tracheal occlusion prevents outward movement of lung fluid
    - This promoted fluid retention and improves lung expansion
    - This may also promote reduction of viscera into abdominal cavity
    - Large multicentric trials are needed to demonstrate benefits of FETO

Anesthetic Considerations

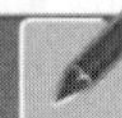

- Full stomach patient: avoid bag and mask ventilation
- Potential hypoxia and hypotension at induction
- Difficult IV access
- Difficult intubation
- Avoid precipitating pulmonary hypertensive crisis:
  - Deep anesthetic planes
  - Avoid hypoxia, hypercarbia and acidosis
  - Hypothermia

Preoperative Preparation

- Informed consent
- Nasogastric tube to reduce abdominal distension
- Venous access preferred in upper limbs
- Prevent hypothermia
- Lateral nursing of neonate with hernia side down

OT Preparation

- Suction
- Oxygen source
- Airway equipment
- *Pharmacy*: Anesthetic drugs
- Monitors calibrated and ready
- Emergency drugs

Anesthetic Management

Monitors

- Pulse oximeter
- End tidal carbon dioxide
- ECG
- Temperature
- Airway pressure
- Esophageal stethoscope
- Urine output
- Invasive BP
- Precordial stethoscope right axilla
- Two pulse oximeters used for preductal and postductal measurements
- Lower limb congestion should be monitored at the end of surgery (IVC compression)
- Central venous access is useful to:
  - Measure central venous pressure
  - Administer inotropes
  - Administer postoperative TPN

Induction

- Adequate preoxygenation followed by rapid sequence induction
- High dose fentanyl 2–5 μg/kg is used to reduce pulmonary HTN
- Avoid positive pressure ventilation or mask ventilation
- Nasogastric tube is inserted to decompress stomach (if not already inserted)
- Avoid lower limb IV access as raised intra-abdominal pressure reduces venous return
- Maintain both preoperative umbilical venous and arterial catheter during surgery
- In sick neonates, repair may be required with HFOV or ECMO support
- In these patients TIVA is used as the anesthetic plan

Maintenance

- Balanced anesthesia with O_2 + air + isoflurane + fentanyl boluses + NDMR
- 100% oxygen may be used in the presence of inadequate oxygenation
- Vecuronium or rocuronium are appropriate NDMRs
- Pancuronium is avoided due to its sympathomimetic properties
- Avoid N_2O to avoid abdominal distension (difficult closure)
- Maintain deep planes to avoid precipitating pulmonary hypertensive crisis
- Vasopressors required to increase SVR and reduce shunt fraction
- Avoid increasing R-L shunt:
  - Hypoxia
  - Acidosis
  - Hypercarbia
  - Hypothermia
- Surgical access may cause compression of blood vessels and hypotension
- Forced air warmers may be used to prevent hypothermia
- Replace significant blood loss

Ventilation

- Adjust FiO_2 to maintain:
  - Preoperative PaO_2 and $PaCO_2$ levels
  - In the absence of preoperative reference ranges, maintain $SpO_2 > 85\%$
- Small tidal volume and rapid respiratory rate is used to maintain:
  - Airway pressure < 20–30 cm H_2O
  - $PaCO_2 > 30$ mm Hg
  - Peak airway pressures < 25 cm H_2O
  - PEEP 2–4 cm H_2O
- Avoid recruitment maneuvers at the end of the procedure to expand ipsilateral lung

Complications

- *"Honeymoon phenomenon"*
  - Characterized by good early oxygenation followed by sudden desaturation
  - Smooth early recovery followed by sudden pulmonary hypertensive crisis
  - Postoperative ventilation is therefore beneficial
  - Weaning is attempted slowly over 48–72 hours once clinical stability attained
  - Occurs due to:
    - Impaired visceral perfusion
    - Reduced diaphragmatic excursion
    - Worsened pulmonary compliance
    - Raised intra-abdominal pressure
- Persistent pulmonary hypoplasia
- Contralateral pneumothorax
- Abdominal compartment syndrome
- IVC compression, hypotension
- Cardiac arrest

Postoperative Management

- Most patients are ventilated postoperatively
- Postoperative ventilatory goals:
  - $PaO_2 > 70–80$ mm Hg
  - $SpO_2 > 95\%$
  - $PaCO_2$ 35–40 mm Hg
  - Peak inspiratory pressures < 25 cm H_2O
- Opioid infusion may be used to maintain sedation and analgesia
- Judicious fluid management with prompt correction of any acidosis
- Maintain normothermia
- Management of pulmonary hypertensive crisis:
  - Hyperventilate with 100% oxygen
  - Maintain alkalosis
  - Pulmonary vasodilators:
    - Milrinone
    - Dobutamine
    - Inhaled nitric oxide
  - ECMO

HERNIA REPAIR

Introduction

- Protrusion of part or whole of a viscus from its normal position through an opening in the wall of its containing cavity
- Inguinal hernias result from presence of intestinal contents in the patent process vaginalis (PPV)
- An incarcerated hernia is an irreducible hernia which does not slide back into the abdominal cavity
- When vascular supply of the bowel is disrupted due to bowel entrapment, the hernia is called strangulated

Types

- Inguinal
- Femoral
- Epigastric
- Umbilical
- Paraumbilical
- Obdurator
- Spigelian
- Lumbar
- Gluteal
- Perineal
- Sciatic
- Diaphragmatic
- Incisional
- Hiatus

Preoperative Assessment

- Most herniorrhaphies are planned as day-care surgery
- History:
  - Chronic cough
  - Constipation
  - Obesity with concurrent diseases
  - Undescended testes
- If bowel obstruction:
  - Vomiting
  - Dehydration
  - Fluid and electrolyte balance
  - Hypovolemia
- Investigations:
  - Complete blood count
  - ECG
  - Chest X-ray
  - Arterial blood gases
  - Pulmonary function tests

Timing of Surgery

- Inguinal hernias do not heal spontaneously
- Incarcerated hernias can usually be manually reduced
- Following manual reduction, hernia repair is usually performed within 24–48 hours
- Strangulated hernias require immediate surgical correction
- Previously exploration of the contralateral side was performed to rule out PPV
- This however risks damage to the vas deferens and infertility
- Current consensus is therefore to avoid exploration of the contralateral side

Surgical Techniques

- Can be done laparoscopically or via open repair
- Laparoscopic surgery has similar efficacy and complication rate compared to open surgery
- However, large scale randomized trials are required to form a consensus
- Open repair can be performed under awake regional or general anesthesia
- However, laparoscopic surgery requires administration of general anesthesia

Anesthetic Techniques

- Awake regional anesthesia:
  - Can be used in older children undergoing open repair
  - Advantages of regional anesthesia:
    - Less hypotension
    - Less hypoxemia
    - Better analgesia
  - However, incidence of long term cognitive decline is similar to general anesthesia
  - Alternatives for regional anesthesia include:
    - Spinal anesthesia: for bilateral hernias
    - Epidural anesthesia: for bilateral hernias
    - Caudal anesthesia: for bilateral hernias
    - Ilioinguinal/iliohypogastric nerve block: For unilateral hernias
- GA with ETT:
  - For large abdominal wall hernias which need muscle relaxation
  - Obstructed/strangulated hernias
  - Hernias with increased aspiration risk
  - Laparoscopic approach
  - Hemodynamically unstable patients
- GA with LMA:
  - Anxious patients
  - Children
  - Inguinal/femoral hernia (minimal risk of aspiration)

Premedication

- Informed consent
- NPO guidelines
- Anti-aspiration prophylaxis:
  - Ranitidine 1 mg/kg IV
  - Metaclopramide 0.15 mg/kg
- IV fluids if vomiting/dehydration
- Midazolam 0.05–0.15 mg/kg IV for anxiolysis
- Glycopyrrolate 10 µg/kg IV
- Sedation is avoided if increased risk of aspiration
- Preoperative antibiotic prophylaxis

Monitor

- Pulse oximetry
- NIBP
- ECG
- End tidal CO_2
- Invasive BP if hemodynamically unstable patient

Induction

- NGT if strangulated

- *Rapid sequence induction* with gentle cricoid pressure if strangulated/obstructed hernia
- Epidural insertion if large laparotomy wound

Maintenance

- O_2 + air + isoflurane used for maintenance
- Avoid N_2O in view of bowel distention
- Adequate muscle relaxation is required for reduction if large abdominal hernias
- Depth of anesthesia is increased at the time of manipulation of spermatic cord
- Inadequate depth of anesthesia may result in laryngospasm or bradycardia
- Prevent hypothermia if the surgical field of exposure is large
- Multimodal intraoperative analgesia can be used to reduce opioid dose
- Extubation in deep planes with minimal coughing to protect hernia repair

Postoperative Management

- Multimodal analgesia with:
  - Opioids
  - NSAIDs
  - Wound infilteration with local anesthetic agents
  - Single shot caudal anesthesia
  - Diclofenac/paracetamol PR or PO

ILIOINGUINAL/ILIOHYPOGASTRIC BLOCKS

Introduction

- Ilioinguinal/ iliohypogastric blocks provide ipsilateral analgesia in the inguinal area

Anatomy

- Nerves arise from T_{12}–L_1 and pass over the quadratus lumborum
- They then pierce the internal oblique muscle just medial to anterior superior iliac spine
- The nerves then become subcutaneous by piercing external oblique aponeurosis
- This occurs 2–3 cm superior to superficial inguinal ring
- These nerves can be found in the transverse abdominis plane
- These nerves control the sensory and motor supply to inguinal region and perineum

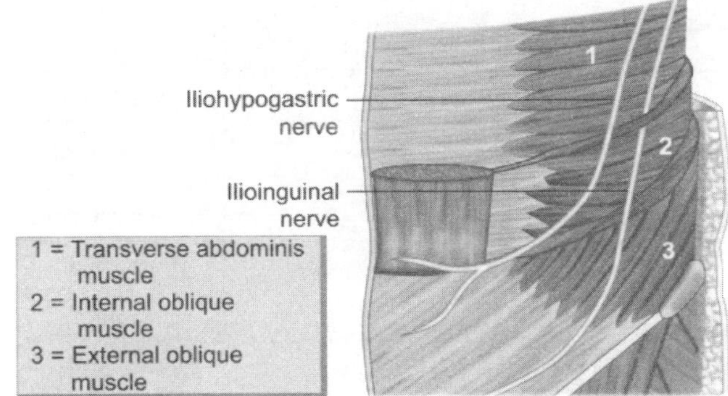

Fig. 7: Ilioinguinal nerve block anatomy.

- Areas supplied include:
  - Skin of lower abdominal wall
  - Upper thigh
  - Lateral hip

Indications

- Inguinal herniorrhaphy
- Orchiopexy
- Hydrocele surgery

Drugs Used

- Drugs used:
  - 0.25% bupivacaine
  - 0.2% ropivacaine
- 0.4–0.5 mL/kg of local anesthetic volume is used, depending on size of patient

Technique

- 24–26 G 40–50 mm short bevel needle is used for puncture
- Line is drawn from Anterior Superior Iliac Spine (ASIS) to umbilicus
- Point of insertion is on this line, 3–4 mm away from ASIS
- Needle is inserted at this point, perpendicular to the skin
- Needle is advanced till LOR is felt as it pierces external oblique aponeurosis
- 0.3 mL/kg of local anesthetic is injected in a fan shaped manner
- Advance further till it pierces internal oblique muscle and LOR felt
- 0.1–0.2 mL/kg LA injected between internal oblique and transverse abdominis muscles
- Gently massage the area to spread the LA

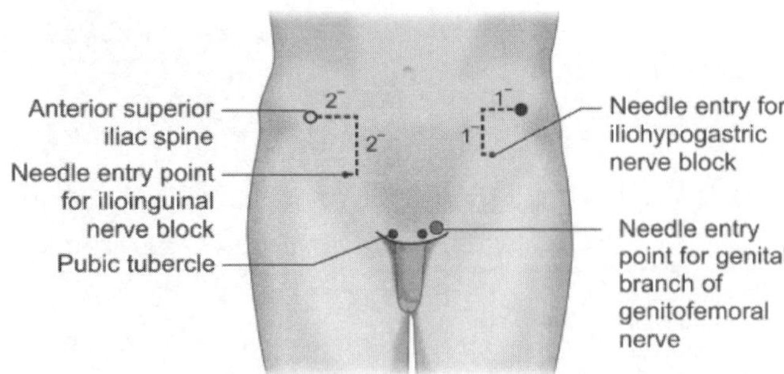

Fig. 8: Ilioinguinal and iliohypogastric nerve block technique.

- Block genital branch of genitofemoral nerve if required with 1–2 mL LA

Complications

- Intravascular injection: Local anesthetic systemic toxicity (LAST)
- Intraperitoneal injection
- Hepatic laceration
- Bowel perforation
- Femoral nerve block

PEDIATRIC SPINAL ANESTHESIA

Introduction

- First spinal anesthesia in pediatric patient was given by August Bier in 1898
- Interest in pediatric spinals waned subsequently into the 20th century
- Subsequently, it was shown to be effective in ex-preterms in preventing postoperative apnea
- Since then (1980s), it has become a standard of care in moribund neonates
- Its safety has been established as an alternative to GA

Anatomical Differences

- Spinal cord and meninges:
  - Spinal cord ends as the conus medullaris at L_2–L_3 level (L_1–L_2 in adults)
  - Conus medullaris reaches the adult level (L_1–L_2) at one year age
  - Dura ends at S_3 (S_2 in adults)
  - Pia mater:
    - It is highly vascular in children
    - This causes rapid re-absorption of local anesthetic
    - This leads to a shorter duration of spinal block in children
  - Myelination:
    - In children, endoneurium is loose
    - This presents little barrier to drug diffusion
    - Therefore, onset and offset of the block is relatively faster
- Dural sac:
  - Subarachnoid space is narrow (6–8 mm)
  - CSF volume is more:
    - 10 mL/kg in neonates
    - 4 mL/kg in infants and toddlers
    - 2 mL/kg in adults
    - Thus, higher dose of local anesthetic is required
  - CSF pressure is lesser
- Surface landmarks:
  - Smaller pelvis and sacrum
  - Spinal laminae are cartilaginous—avoid paramedian approach
  - ***Tuffiers*** line at L_4 spinous process
  - Lower approach commonly used to avoid spinal cord injury (L_{4-5} or L_5–S_1)
- Ligaments:
  - Ligaments are thinner and less densely packed
  - Thus, they are easy to penetrate
  - Also, it is difficult to feel the fascial planes during penetration
  - Therefore, it is more difficult to feel loss of resistance
- Level of block:
  - Normal thoracic kyphosis is limited due to increased spinal flexibility
  - This facilitates cephalad spread of the local anesthetic
  - This results in higher level of sensory block
  - This has deleterious effects on respiratory system:
    - Reduced outward movement of ribcage
    - Decreased intercostal muscle activity
- Hemodynamic response:
  - Peripheral blood pool is lesser in children
  - Thus, the vascular response is less marked compared with adults
  - Immature sympathetic system contributes to better hemodynamic stability
  - Hence, preloading is not necessary prior to spinal anesthesia in children

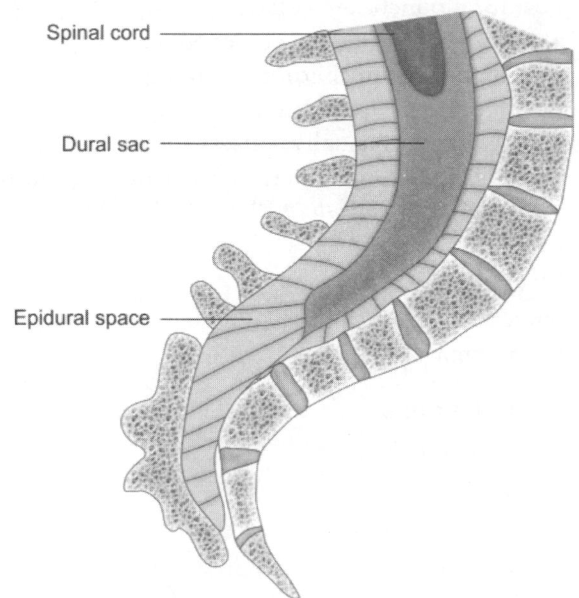

Fig. 9: Anatomy spinal cord—adults.

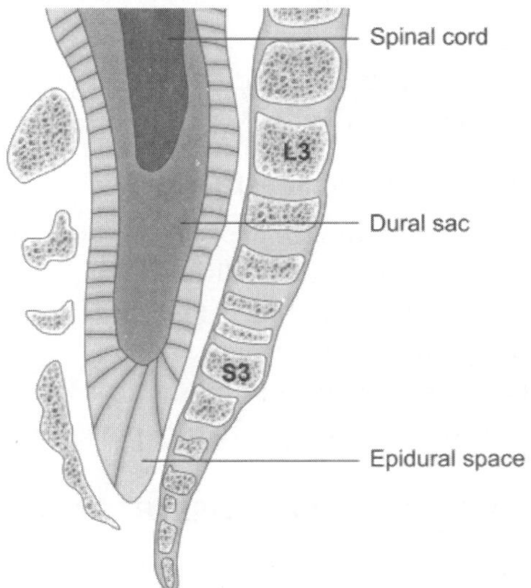

Fig. 10: Anatomy spinal cord—at birth.

Differences in Technique

- Test dose of local anesthetic essential for allergy
- Performed at lower level as spinal cord reaches L_3 in infants
- Requires sedation/GA to ensure patient cooperation
- Rarely causes hypotension in children less than 10 years age
- Crystalloid preloading not required
- Dose of local anesthetic higher as CSF volume is twice that in adults (4 mL/kg)
- Block duration shorter than in adults

Indications

- General surgery:
  - Hernia
  - Lower abdomen surgery
  - Colostomy
  - Anoplasty
  - Rectal biopsy
  - Perineoplasty
  - Appendicectomy
- Orthopedic surgery:
  - Clubfoot tendon lengthening
  - Closed reduction of fracture hip
  - Incision and drainage of abscess
  - Amputations of lower limb
- Urological surgery:
  - Circumcision
  - Vesicostomy
  - Orchidotomy
  - Orchiopexy
  - Varicocelectomy
  - Hydrocelectomy
  - Hypospadiasis repair
  - Meatoplasty
  - Urethroplasty
  - Ureteral reimplant
  - Ectopia vesicae

Advantages

- Patient is awake and breathing spontaneously
- Provides all components of balanced anesthesia
- Minimal physiological alterations
- Avoids general anesthesia complications:
  - Respiratory depression
  - Postoperative apnea
  - Cardiovascular instability
  - Airway manipulation
  - Reduced total anesthetic requirements
  - Hastens wake up time
  - Smooth recovery
  - Reduced PONV as no opioids are used
  - Reduced postoperative pulmonary complications
- Avoids airway manipulation in high risk patients:
  - Subglottic stenosis
  - Laryngo-tracheomalacia
  - Difficult airway
  - Muscular dystrophy
  - Hyper-reactive airways
- Anesthetic method of choice in malignant hyperthermia

- Excellent postoperative analgesia
- Reduced stress response to surgery
- Reduced bleeding intraoperatively
- Facilitates limb immobilization after nerve repair/skin graft
- Reduces cost:
  - Rapid recovery
  - Early ambulation
  - Rapid return of appetite
  - Shorter hospital stay

Disadvantages

- Requires expertise
- Requires GA/sedation for patient cooperation
- Limited duration of action—unsuitable for long surgeries
- Increased risk of inadvertent complications

Technique

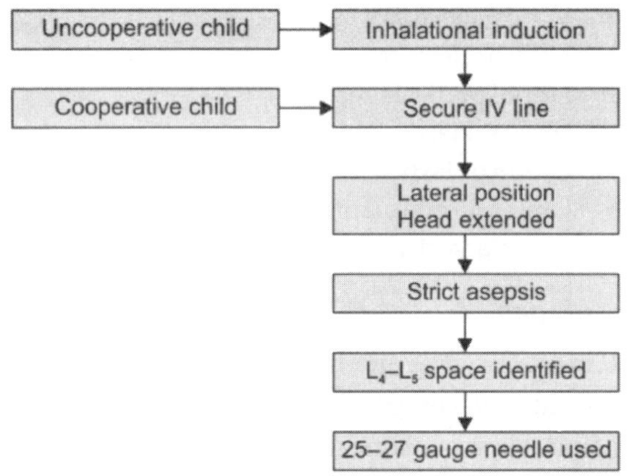

Dosage

Bupivacaine (0.5%)	0–5 kg	5–15 kg	> 15 kg
Amount (mg/kg)	0.5–0.6	0.4	0.3
Volume (mL/kg)	0.1–0.12	0.08	0.06
Duration (minutes)	65–75	70–80	75–85

Complications

- High spinal:
  - Can result with:
    - High doses of local anesthetic
    - Lifting of legs postadministration of spinal anesthetic
  - Causes cardiorespiratory insufficiency
  - This results in hypotension and desaturation
  - Bronchospasm has been reported with higher block
- Postdural puncture headache:
  - Incidence of PDPH is independent of age
  - Can be seen in children as young as 2 years age
  - Severe symptoms are usually rare
  - Treatment is usually conservative
  - Epidural blood patch (0.2–0.3 mL/kg) recommended in persistent PDPH (> 1 week)
- Backache
- Meningitis
- Shivering
- Hematoma

Contraindications

- Local site infection
- Sepsis
- Meningomyelocele
- Spina bifida
- Hydrocephalus
- Coagulopathy
- Convulsive disorder
- VP shunt
- Vertebral implants
- Progressive neuromuscular disorders

Limitations of Spinal Anesthesia

- Provides short duration of anesthesia (70–80 minutes) in the absence of additives
- Requires administration of sedation and GA to ensure patient cooperation
- Failure rates as high as 5–15%
- Lack of availability of pediatric spinal needles

PEDIATRIC EPIDURAL ANESTHESIA

Introduction

- Routine use of thoracic and lumbar epidural catheters in infants is uncommon
- Less commonly performed due to:
  - Technical difficulties
  - Risk of spinal cord trauma
  - Unavailability of instruments
- Caudal approach to epidural space is therefore preferred to direct approach

Anatomical Differences

- Epidural space:
  - Space itself is more superficial
  - Shallower epidural space: Spread of local anesthetic is more even

- Shorter skin—epidural distance:
  - 1.5 mm/kg till 1 year
  - 1 mm/kg thereafter
- Thinner ligaments:
  - Easy to penetrate
  - Difficult to feel fascial planes and loss of resistance
- More rapid onset of action due to:
  - Thinner nerve fibers
  - Less densely packed epidural fat facilitating faster spread of local anesthetic
- Local anesthetic absorption:
  - Incomplete myelination of spinal cord: Block achieved at lower LA concentration
  - Higher cardiac output in children: Systemic absorption occurs faster
- Increased chances of catheter coiling which can be avoided by:
  - Use of 21 G catheters
  - Increasing cephalad angulation of epidural needle
  - Use of introducer
  - Injection of saline to open up epidural space

Technical Differences

- Test dose local anesthetic essential for LA allergy
- Hanging drop method not done due to short skin-space distance
- Needle continuously advanced with continuous loss of resistance monitoring
- Saline preferred for LOR as air can cause air embolism
- Catheter passes easily in space; can even reach cervical cord level

Determination of Catheter Position

- Measurement of depth of epidural space from skin:
  - Epidural space usually encountered at 2.2–2.5 cm
  - Depth of insertion of needle (cm) = 1 + (0.15 × age in years)
- The *Tsui test*:
  - Uses stimulating epidural catheters
  - Nerve stimulator is connected with an insulated Tuohy needle
  - Stimulator is then stimulated while watching for muscular jerks in the dermatome
  - Jerk indicates position of needle tip in the corresponding dermatomal segment
  - Threshold current for an insulated needle is usually 6–17 mA
  - Epidural catheters require lower threshold currents (1–10 mA)
  - Allows placement of catheter tip within 1–2 cm of the nerve root
- Ultrasound guidance:
  - Less challenging in young children as ossification is less developed
  - Spinal cord fibers, dura mater and CSF are easily visualized
  - Thus, epidural space can be readily identified using linear high-frequency probes
- Radiography:
  - Radio-opaque dyes like iohexol can be used for epidurography
  - Fluoroscopy can be used for real time monitoring of catheter placement
  - X-ray imaging with contrast to identify tip of catheter

Dosages

- Local anesthetic:
  - Higher concentration (0.5%) of bupivacaine and ropivacaine avoided
  - 0.2% bupivacaine or ropivacaine can be used
  - 0.3–0.5 mL/kg is adequate for thoracolumbar epidural
  - As infusion:
    - 0.125% bupivacaine:
      - 0.2 mg/kg/hr for neonates
      - 0.4 mg/kg/hr for older children
    - 0.1% ropivacaine:
      - 0.2 mg/kg/hr for neonates
      - 0.4 mg/kg/hr for older children
- Additives:
  - Fentanyl:
    - Commonly used additive
    - Dose of 1–2 µg/mL for postoperative continuous epidural infusion
  - Ketamine:
    - Dose of 0.25–0.3 mg/kg
    - Ketamine has unpredictable duration of action and hallucination
  - Buprenorphine 1–2 µ/kg
  - Preservative free morphine 30–50 µg/kg
  - Clonidine 0.5–1 µg/kg
  - Buprenorphine
    - Acts for 24–30 hours
    - Less respiratory depression
    - Causes nausea and vomiting

Advantages

- Patient awake and breathing spontaneously
- Complete analgesia
- Minimal hemodynamic alterations owing to:
  - Low resting sympathetic tone in children
  - Reduced blood in lower extremities
- Avoids complications of general anesthesia:
  - Respiratory depression
  - Postoperative apnea
  - Cardiovascular instability
  - Airway manipulation
  - Reduced total anesthetic requirements
  - Hastens wake up time
  - Smooth recovery
  - Reduced PONV as opioids are not used
- Reduced postoperative pulmonary complication
- Excellent postoperative analgesia for 48–72 hours
- Reduced stress response to surgery
- Reduced bleeding intraoperatively

Disadvantages

- Uncertain depth of epidural space
- Risk of dural puncture as epidural space is narrow
- Difficult to feel loss of resistance as under GA, ligaments are lax

Technique

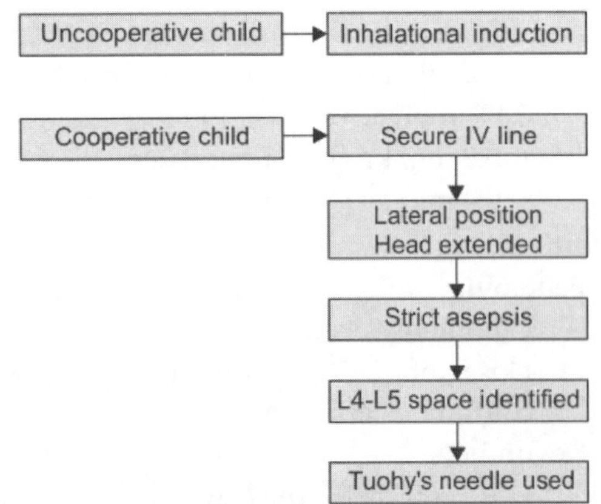

- Typically done in an anesthetized child in lateral position with knees flexed
- Depth of epidural space is calculated using the formula
- Under strict aseptic precautions with draping, needle is placed in midline position
- Paramedian approach is less commonly preferred
- A 5 cm 20 G Tuohy needle with a 21–24 G catheter is used in children less than 2 years age
- A 5 cm 18 G Tuohy needle with a 20 G epidural catheter is used in older children
- Saline and less commonly air (<1 mL total) is used for loss of resistance technique
- Air is usually avoided in view of venous air embolism
- On identification of the space, direct LA injection or catheter insertion is carried out
- Test dose of local anesthetic is always given to verify correct placement

Modified Bromage Scale: >2 Years Age

Score	Description
1	Complete motor block
2	Patient able to move feet, almost complete motor block
3	Partial motor block, patient able to move knees
4	Weakness of hip flexion, able to raise leg but unable to keep it raised
5	No detectable weakness of hip flexion, able to keep leg raised > 10 seconds
6	No weakness at all, able to perform partial knee bend when supine

Complications

- Dural puncture, total spinal, postdural puncture headache
- Backache
- Infections
- Meningitis
- Epidural abscess
- Epidural hematoma
- Intravascular injection—LAST

Adverse Effects

- Itching
- Nausea and vomiting
- Ileus, bowel dysfunction
- Urinary retention

Contraindications

- Local site infection
- Sepsis
- Meningomyelocele
- Spina bifida
- Hydrocephalus
- Coagulopathy
- Convulsive disorder
- VP shunt

- Vertebral implants
- Progressive neuromuscular disorders

CAUDAL ANESTHESIA

Introduction

Local anesthetic injection into epidural space via sacral canal through sacral hiatus.

Anatomy

- Sacral hiatus is formed by failure of union of S_4 and S_5 vertebra in the midline
- Bony defect is covered by posterior sacrococcygeal ligament
- Remnants of S_5 articular process is called sacral cornua
- This contains:
  - Terminal part of dural sac terminating at S_3
  - Cauda equina formed by S_1–S_5 and coccygeal nerve
  - Valveless venous plexus
  - Areolar tissue
  - Lymphatics

Indications

- Pediatric anesthesia:
  - General surgery:
    - Rectal
    - Inguinal
    - Urogenital
    - Circumcision
    - Orchidectomy
    - Orchidotomy
  - Orthopedic surgery:
    - Clubfoot
    - Fracture reduction
    - I and D of abscess
- Adult anesthesia:
  - Vaginal hysterectomy
  - Inguinal herniorrhaphy
  - Hemorrhoidectomy
  - Anal dilation
  - Lower limb surgeries
- Obstetric analgesia
- Postoperative analgesia:
  - Circumcision
  - Hemorrhoidectomy
  - Anal dilation
- Chronic pain: Lower back pain

Technique

- Done under sedation
- Lateral Sim's position
- Strict asepsis
- Posterior superior iliac spine is identified
- Injection is carried out in the midline
- Tip of coccyx is palpated
- Sacral hiatus is palpated proximally
- The epidural needle is then inserted perpendicular to skin
- Once sacral surface is hit, the needle is slightly withdrawn
- It is then redirected and advanced at 45° angle
- Needle is advanced till sudden "POP" is felt
- Check aspiration is done for blood or CSF
- The local anesthetic is injected in graded aliquots

Dose of Local Anesthetic

- Armitage formula:
  - 0.5 mL/kg of 0.25% bupivacaine:
    - Anal surgery
    - Circumcision
  - 1 mL/kg of 0.25% bupivacaine: Lower thoracic level
  - 1.25 mL/kg of 0.25% bupivacaine: Mid thoracic level:
    - Herniorrhaphy
    - Orchidectomy
- Additives:
  - Morphine 50–70 µg/kg
  - Clonidine 1 µg/kg
  - Butadol 5–25 µg/kg

Continuous Caudal Epidural

- Done using a catheter threaded into caudal space
- Position of catheter tip confirmed with fluoroscopy or a nerve stimulator

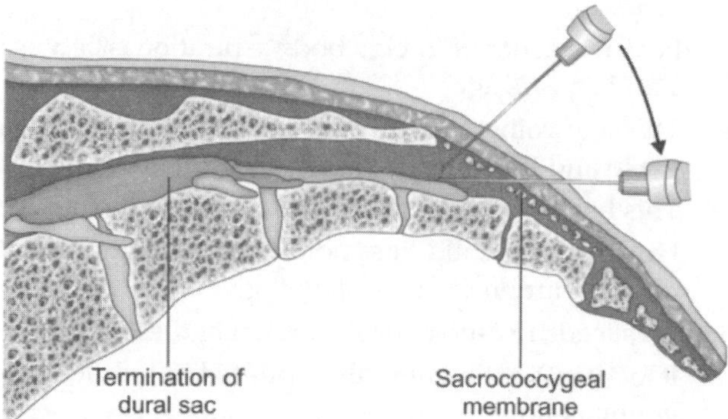

Fig. 11: Caudal anesthesia technique.

- Catheter can be threaded up to thoracic epidural to achieve T_2–T_4 block
- Dose of LA is the same as bolus dose with frequent top ups

Complications

- Absent/patchy block
- IV or IO placement: LAST
- Dural puncture
- Injection into fetal scalp when used for obstetric anesthesia
- Excessive spread
- Pain at injection site
- Periosteal hematoma
- Urinary retention
- Infection
- Permanent neurodeficits

Contraindications

- Local pathology:
  - Pilonidal sinus
  - Sacrococcygeal teratomas
  - Sepsis
- Fixed cardiac ouput state:
  - Aortic stenosis
  - Mitral stenosis

FOREIGN BODY ASPIRATION

Introduction

- Foreign body aspiration is a leading cause of mortality and morbidity in young children
- Tracheobronchial foreign body aspiration (FBA) is a potentially life-threatening event

Epidemiology

- Common cause of mortality in children below 2 years age
- Peak incidence of foreign body aspiration is between 1 and 2 years age
- This age coincides with the development of pincer grasp and fine motor skills
- This bestows the ability to put objects in the mouth
- However, the child does not have adequately developed dentition to allow chewing
- This leads to aspiration of foreign bodies
- Food items are commonly aspirated in toddlers and young children
- In older children, non-edible item aspiration is more common

Types of Foreign Body

- Organic:
  - Peanuts
  - Tamarind seeds
  - Jelly beans
  - Custard apple
  - Popcorn
- Inorganic:
  - Beads
  - Coins
  - Pins
  - Buttons
  - Small toys

Sites of Foreign Body

- Larynx 3%
- Trachea/carina: 13%
- Right lung 60%
- Left lung 23%
- Bilateral lung fields 2%

Phases of Aspiration

- Immediate phase:
  - Choking
  - Gagging
  - Coughing
  - Wheezing
  - Stridor
- Asymptomatic second phase:
  - Few minutes to months after first phase
  - Depends on location, degree of obstruction and type of foreign body
- Renewed symptomatic phase:
  - Airway infection and inflammation
  - Repeated coughing bouts, sputum, wheezing, fever, hemoptysis

Clinical Features

- History:
  - Foreign body aspiration
  - Coughing, choking, stridor on feeding
  - Voice changes, barking cough: Suggestive of laryngeal edema
  - Stridor, aphonia, hoarseness: Indicates presence of foreign body in trachea/larynx
- Examination:
  - Chest retraction: Upper airway obstruction
  - Unilateral diminished breath sounds
  - Bilateral reduced breath sounds: Tracheal foreign body
- Investigations:
  - Chest X-ray:
    - More than 90% foreign bodies are radiolucent

- Mediastinal shift
- Ipsilateral atelectasis
- Contralateral hyperinflation
- Absence of mediastinal shift on lateral decubitus film
- CT scan: For symptomatic children with normal chest X-rays

Differential Diagnosis

- Asthma
- Croup
- Pneumonia
- Bronchitis
- Tracheomalacia
- Bronchomalacia
- Vocal cord dysfunction
- Psychogenic cough

Complications

- Acute:
  - Organic foreign body: Foreign body swells up and causes airway edema
  - Oil containing seeds: Chemical inflammation
  - Vegetable seeds swell and fragment, causing distal airway obstruction
- Chronic:
  - Tracheal/bronchial stenosis
  - Bronchiectasis
  - Lung abscess
  - Tissue erosion
  - Pneumomediastinum
  - Pneumothorax

Management

- Emergency out of hospital management:
  - If complete obstruction:
    - Back blows, chest thrust is used in infants
    - ***Heimleichs*** maneuver, abdominal thrust in children
    - Never use blind finger sweeps
    - CPR initiated if the child has a cardiorespiratory arrest
  - If incomplete obstruction:
    - Encourage coughing and spontaneous respiration
    - Shift to hospital
- In hospital management:
  - Phase I presentation:
    - Rigid bronchoscopy is *treatment of choice*
    - Flexible fiber-optic bronchoscope may be used in specialized centers
    - Thoracotomy in indicated when the FB is not accessible via bronchoscope
  - Phase II presentation:
    - Bronchodilators
    - Antibiotics
    - Steroids
    - Chest physiotherapy
    - Rigid bronchoscopy

Anesthetic Considerations

- Pediatric patient
- Shared airway
- Absence of a secure airway
- Avoidance of muscle paralysis
- Requirement of deep anesthetic planes

Preoperative Preparation

- Informed consent
- Stable children can be fasted as the airway is not secure during rigid bronchoscopy
- NPO guidelines in non-emergency cases:
  - 6 hours solids
  - 2 hours clear fluids
- Antibiotics coverage
- Steroids and bronchodilator therapy
- IV midazolam 0.05–0.15 mg/kg as most children are very anxious
- Anti-aspiration prophylaxis:
  - Metaclopramide 0.15 mg/kg IV
  - Ranitidine 1 mg/kg IV

OT Preparation

- Suction
- Oxygen source: Pipeline/cylinder
- Airway equipment: Prepare for emergency airway rescue
- Pharmacy: Anesthetic drugs preloaded
- Monitors
- Emergency drugs: Especially atropine

Monitors

- Pulse oximetry: Has a lag phase before detecting desaturation
- NIBP
- ECG
- End tidal CO_2 not reliable as most expired gases escape around the bronchoscope

Induction

- Spontaneous ventilation postinduction is preferred in children with proximal FBA
- Use of positive pressure ventilation may dislodge the foreign body
- This can move the FB distally and convert a partial obstruction to complete obstruction
- Avoidance of positive pressure ventilation is less important in the presence of a distal FB
- Thus, the bronchoscopist should be consulted prior to administration of NMBA
- IV induction:
  - IV propofol/thiopentone used for induction
  - Propofol is preferred as it is stable in the presence of a reactive airway
  - Muscle relaxants are avoided till location of foreign body is determined
  - This is followed by the application of cricoid pressure
  - Early cricoid pressure can cause coughing and laryngospasm
  - However, forceful cricoid pressure causes airway obstruction
  - ETT may dislodge highly placed foreign body at the time of insertion
- Inhalational induction:
  - Less preferred and done only in the absence of IV access
  - Induction may be delayed if foreign body is highly placed
  - 100% oxygen with sevoflurane is used for inhalational induction
  - N_2O avoided as it may cause distal lung expansion
  - Topical spray with 10% lidocaine is used to reduce coughing during laryngoscopy
- Rigid bronchoscopy is carried out when adequate depth of anesthesia is attained

Maintenance

- Adequate depth of anesthesia cannot be maintained with inhalational agents alone
- This is due to intermittent interruption of ventilation and leak around the bronchoscope
- Thus, TIVA allows for maintenance of a continuous depth of anesthesia
- Thus, TIVA anesthesia for rigid bronchoscopy is maintained with:
  - Propofol (boluses or infusion)
  - Dexmedetomidine infusion
  - Neuromuscular blocking agents
- Avoidance of NMB causes:
  - Increased mocement
  - Breath holding
  - Laryngospasm

Ventilation

- Spontaneous ventilation avoids dislodgement of the foreign body distally
- However, positive pressure ventilation allows for controlled ventilation
- This reduces incidence of hypoxemia and desaturation during the procedure
- Thus, once the distal location of the foreign body has been confirmed, NMB is advisable
- Ventilation may be achieved through the ventilation port of ventilating bronchoscope
- Regular suction is required during bronchoscopy to prevent airway obstruction

Technique

- Using ventilating bronchoscope
- 2.5–6 mm ID sizes available, ED is 2 mm larger
- This bronchoscope enables visualization of airway and ventilation simultaneously
- Whole airway and subglottic area is visualized first
- Foreign body is removed with forceps
- Tracheobronchial tree is then visualized for any remnants and airway inflammation
- Vigorous irrigation and suction is done to remove secretions

Extubation and Emergence

- Vigorous suction in deep anesthetic planes is required to clear the airway of secretions
- This is important to prevent laryngospasm post-procedure
- Emergence of the child is then allowed usually without airway instrumentation
- Intubation may however be required in the presence of airway edema

Postoperative

Management

- Steroids, bronchodilators and antibiotics
- Nebulized racemic epinephrine
- Humidified oxygen
- Monitor for airway obstruction

Complications

- Trauma to airway and teeth
- Dislodgement of foreign body
- Complete airway obstruction
- Barotrauma
- Hypoxia and hypercarbia:
  - Frequently remove telescope
  - Withdraw bronchoscope to midtrachea and ventilate
- Bronchospasm: Bronchodilators, albuterol nebulization
- Pneumothorax, pneumomediastinum
- Iatrogenic tracheoesophageal fistula

Modes of Ventilation

- Spontaneous ventilation:
  - Advantages:
    - Reduced risk of foreign body dislodgement
    - Allows continuous ventilation during bronchoscopy
    - Rapid airway assessment is possible once foreign body is removed
  - Disadvantages:
    - Requires deep planes at bronchoscopy
    - May cause hypoventilation
    - May cause arrhythmias
    - Requires assistance and additional manpower
- Controlled ventilation:
  - Advantages:
    - Airway immobilized
    - Good exposure
    - Less volatile anesthetic doses required
    - Reduced atelectasis
    - Better oxygenation
  - Disadvantages:
    - May be difficult if not airtight
    - May be impossible during suction/instrumentation
    - May dislodge foreign body distally
- Jet ventilation:
  - Causes barotrauma
  - Dislodges foreign body distally

CIRCUMCISION

Introduction

- Circumcision involves the excision of prepuce or foreskin around the penis
- It is the most commonly performed surgical procedure in the world

Indications

- Persistent phimosis
- Balanitis xerotica obliterans
- Recurrent balanoposthitis
- Recurrent UTIs
- Paraphimosis
- Cultural and religious reasons
- Not routinely recommended in healthy boys

Contraindications

- Local infection
- Penile congenital anomalies
- Hypospadiasis

Preoperative Assessment and Preparation

- When possible, circumcision is delayed till child is older than 1 year age
- Rule out active URTI
- Rule out bleeding diathesis/previous anesthesia
- No investigations required unless clinically indicated
- NPO orders
- Informed consent for local anesthesia and rectal suppository
- Topical EMLA applied at IV access site 60–90 minutes before surgery

Premedication

- If less than 2 years age:
  - Paracetamol 15 mg/kg PO
  - Paracetamol 30 mg/kg PR
- If above 2 years age:
  - Diclofenac 1 mg/kg PO
  - Diclofenac 1 mg/kg PR
  - Midazolam 0.5 mg/kg 45 minutes before
  - IV glycopyrrolate 10 μg/kg

Anesthetic Technique

- GA with LMA and regional block for postoperative analgesia is most commonly used
- Penile block or caudal anesthesia are options for regional analgesia
- Caudal anesthesia is a more efficacious analgesic technique
- There is lesser need for rescue analgesia when caudal anesthesia is used for circumcision
- However, caudal anesthesia not preferred as:
  - More time spent performing the block
  - Larger volume of local anesthetic injection

Monitoring

- Pulse oximetry
- NIBP
- ECG
- E_TCO_2

Induction

- IV/inhalational induction techniques can be used depending on the presence of IV line
- IV propofol and fentanyl can be used for induction
- Spontaneous ventilation is usually preferred
- Atracurium can be used for paralysis if controlled ventilation is required
- Opioid requirement is usually less as regional analgesia is used for supplementation

Maintenance

- O_2 + air + 1 MAC isoflurane may be used for maintenance of anesthesia
- Atracurium boluses may be used to maintain paralysis
- However, opioid requirement will be low with regional analgesia supplementation

Extubation

- Thorough suction to be done prior to extubation
- Deep extubation preferred to reduce the risk of laryngospasm

Postoperative

- Circumcision is a very painful procedure
- Good postoperative analgesia is essential
- Multimodal analgesic strategy is useful
- Topical lidocaine gel can be applied frequently
- Lidocaine gel should contact suture lines for it to be effective
- PO paracetamol can be given 15 mg/kg TID to supplement analgesia

Complications

- Urinary retention which may be due to:
  - Inadequate analgesia
  - Persistent caudal block
- Bleeding, infection
- Nausea and vomiting
- Residual redundant skin
- Meatal stenosis
- Skin bridges

PENILE BLOCK

Introduction

- Penile block is used for procedures of the distal penis such as circumcision
- This block can be achieved via:
  - Subcutaneous ring block
  - Dorsal nerve block
  - Subpubic block

Anatomy

- Distal two thirds of the penis is supplied by:
  - Right and left dorsal nerve of penis (branches of pudendal nerve)
  - The nerve passes under pubic bone and crosses subpubic space from back to front
  - Enters suspensory ligament and then penis
  - Runs along inner side of ***Bucks*** fascia accompanied by artery and vein
- Proximal one third of the penis is supplied by branches from:
  - Perineal nerve
  - Ilioinguinal nerve
  - Genitofemoral nerve
- Suspensory ligament divides subpubic space into two separate compartments
- Subpubic space is filled with areolar tissue
- Covered with membranous layer of superficial fascia or *SCARPAS* fascia which continues as *BUCKS* fascia

Indications

- Circumcision
- Hypospadiasis repair
- Surgery for phimosis and paraphimosis
- Preputioplasty

Drugs

- Drugs used:
  - Bupivacaine 0.25%
  - Ropivacaine 0.2%
- 0.1 mL/kg volume of local anesthetic is used for each side
- Up to 10 mL can be used for adolescent
- Total dose of bupivacaine/ropivacaine not to exceed 1.5 mg/kg
- ***Adrenaline is not used*** as an additive for penile block
- This is because it can cause spasm of the dorsal artery of the penis
- This can in turn lead to ischemia and necrosis of the glans

Technique

- Procedure is performed under complete aseptic precautions
- 21 G 30 mm long regional block needle can be used for puncture

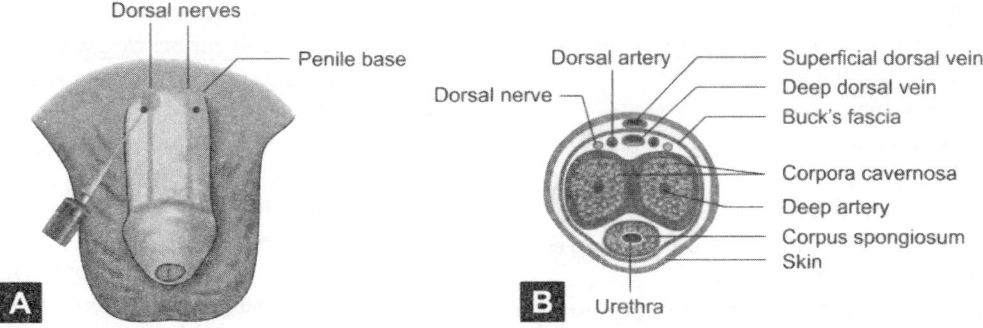

Figs. 12A and B: Penile block. (A) Injection sites; (B) Section through penis.

- Superficial ring block:
  - Local anesthetic is injected circumferentially around the base of penis
  - Injections are directed superficial to the Bucks fascia
- Dorsal nerve block:
  - Palpate lower border of pubic symphysis with index finger and retract penis
  - Insert needle perpendicular to skin between fingers and pubic arch
  - Advance till bone is struck or slight loss of resistance felt
  - If bone is struck, walk the needle inferiorly until it becomes free
  - Depth of insertion correlates with age:
    - 8 mm for newborn
    - 30 mm for young adult
  - Once loss of resistance is felt, inject:
    - Half the volume of local anesthetic at 11 O' clock position
    - Remaining half volume of local anesthetic at 1 O' clock position
    - Final 1 mL of local anesthetic on underside of penis
  - *Repeat the procedure on the other side*
- Subpubic block:
  - Penis is pulled downward and needle is inserted perpendicular to the skin
  - Point of insertion is 0.5–1 cm lateral to midline and caudal to pubic symphysis
  - Needle is directed medially and caudally until fascia scarpa is pierced
  - On appreciation of loss of resistance, local anesthetic is injected

Complications

- IV injection: Local anesthetic systemic toxicity (LAST)
- Damage to dorsal nerve of penis: Necrosis of glans penis
- Damage to dorsal artery of penis especially with midline punctures
- Compressive hematomas
- Penile necrosis due to inadvertent adrenaline use

PEDIATRIC POSTOPERATIVE ANALGESIA

Introduction

- Pain is defined as an unpleasant sensory and emotional experience associated with actual or potential tissue damage or described in terms of such damage
- Components required for pain perception are fully developed by 25 weeks of gestation
- Descending inhibitory pathways remain underdeveloped till mid infancy
- Pain is often undertreated in children due to:
  - Difficulty in assessment as most common symptom is crying which is nonspecific
  - Fear of side effects of medications

Assessment of Pain

- Neonates and infants:
  - ***Premature Infant Pain Profile:***
    - It is an observational- behavioral tool
    - Relies on:
      - Gestational age
      - Heart rate
      - Oxygen saturation
      - Facial actions
    - Clinical utility is well established
  - *CRIES* postoperative pain scale:
    - It is an observational- behavioral tool
    - 10 point toll similar to APGAR scoring system
    - Acronym which stands for:

  - Crying
  - Requirement of oxygen supplementation
  - Increased vital signs
  - Expression
  - Sleeplessness
- *FLACC* scale:
  - It is an observational- behavioral tool
  - Used to assess pain in children between 2 months and 7 years of age
  - Useful in children unable to communicate their pain

❖ Toddler age group:
- FLACC scale
- COMFORT-Behavior scale:
  - It is an observational-behavioral tool
  - The scale relies on:
    - Alertness
    - Calmness
    - Respiratory response or crying
    - Body movements
    - Facial tension
    - Muscle tone
  - Pain is scored between 6 and 30 points
  - Intervention is required when the score exceeds 17

❖ Children between 3 and 8 years:
- ***Poker chip scale***:
  - It is a self report measure
  - Also called the Pieces of Hurt tool
  - Allows children to quantify pain using four poker chips
  - The poker chips represent the amount of pain felt by the child
  - Selection of more poker chips by the toddler indicates severe pain
- ***Wong baker faces scale:***
  - It is a self report measure
  - Created for children older than 3 years age
  - Scored as 0, 2, 4, 6, 8, 10 with increasing intensity of pain
  - Shows series of faces ranging from happy face at 0 to crying face at 10
  - Appropriate for children who do not know how to count
- ***Faces pain scale***:
  - It is a self report measure
  - Requires selecting a picture of a face that represents pain intensity
  - These pictures can be drawings or photographs
  - Scored 0, 2, 4, 6, 8, 10 with increasing severity
- ***Manchester pain scale:***
  - It is a self report measure
  - Uses panda bear faces on a scale to represent intensity of pain
  - Removes ethnic bias associated with scales using photographs
  - Validated in emergency department setting
- ***CHEOPS scale:***
  - It is an observational-behavioral measure
  - Analogue for children's hospital of eastern ontario pain scale
  - Lengthy scoring system with inconsistent scoring among categories
  - Cumbersome and used extensively in research settings
- ***Oucher scale:***
  - It is a self report measure
  - There are two scales on the oucher poster:
    - A number scale for older children
    - A photographic scale for younger children
  - Allows children to match pain intensity with photos of other children
  - Photographs depict faces with increasing levels of pain

❖ Children more than 8 years of age:
- ***Visual analogue scale:***
  - Requires selecting a point on a line representing pain intensity
  - Scale shows good sensitivity for children above 8 years of age
- ***Colored analo scale***:
  - Similar to VAS but uses a mechanical slider to indicate pain intensity
  - Good sensitivity like VAS, but requires purchase of the tool
- ***Numerical rating scale***:
  - Requires child to rate the severity of pain between numbers 0 and 10
  - Convenient as it requires no additional equipment
  - Not very well researched with children

❖ Pain assessment in cognitively impaired children:
- The Non-Communicating Children's Pain Checklist (NCCPC-PV):
  - Tool comprises a checklist of 27 pain behaviors across 6 categories
  - Each behavior is scored on a 0–3 point scale after a 10 min observation
  - Good correlations have been achieved with the VAS score
  - It may be time consuming and cumbersome for frequent assessments

- The University of Wisconsin Pain Scale for Preverbal and Nonverbal children:
  - Scale consists of five behavior categories with 4 descriptors for each
  - Scoring is more subjective and precision is therefore limited
  - Unclear reliability owing to subjective scoring and lack of reproducibility
- The Pain Indicator for Communicatively Impaired Children:
  - Six core pain indicators are scored on a 4 point scale
  - Provides a simple method of pain assessment
  - Can be used in the out-of-hospital setting

CRIES scale:

Indicator	Score		
	0	1	2
Crying	No	High pitched, consolable	Inconsolable
Requires oxygen for $SpO_2 > 95\%$	No	$FiO_2 < 30\%$	$FiO_2 > 30\%$
Increased vital signs	No	HR or BP increased < 20%	HR or BP increased > 20%
Expression	No	Grimace	Grimace and grunt
Sleepless	No	Wakes often	Constantly awake
Score < 4	Initiate non-pharmacological methods		
Score > 4	Initiate pharmacological and non-pharmacological methods		

FLACC behavioural pain score:

Categories	Score		
	0	1	2
Face	No particular expression or smiling	Occasional grimace	Quivering chin, clenched jaw
Legs	Normal position or relaxed	Uneasy, restless	Kicking, legs drawn up
Activity	Lying quietly, moves easily	Squirming, tense	Arched, rigid or jerking
Cry	No cry (awake/ asleep)	Moans or whimpers	Crying steadily, screaming
Consolability	Content, relaxed	Reassured by touch	Difficult to console

Strategies for Pain Management

- ❖ Behavioral methods:
  - Hypnosis
  - Biofeedback
  - Relaxation
  - Behavioral pain therapy
- ❖ Physical methods:
  - Rest and limb elevation.
  - Cold application
  - TENS
- ❖ Pharmacological methods:
  - NSAIDs
  - Opioids
  - Local anesthetics.
- ❖ Regional blocks
- ❖ Recent advances:
  - EMLA cream
  - Ethylchloride vapocoolant spray
  - Iontophoresis with fentanyl
  - Liposomal lidocaine

Rationale

- ❖ Multimodal analgesia used, which targets multiple sites along pain pathway:
  - Peripheral level:
    - Local anesthetics
    - Peripheral nerve blockade
    - NSAIDs
    - Antihistamines
    - Opioids
  - Spinal level:
    - Local anesthetics
    - Neuraxial opioids
    - α_2 adrenoceptor agonists
    - NMDA receptor antagonists
  - Cortical level:
    - Systemic opioids
    - α_2 adrenoceptor agonists
    - Voltage gated calcium channel proteins
- ❖ Choose drugs with synergistic effect and different side effect profile
- ❖ Timing of analgesic medications:
  - Pain is most severe in first 24–72 hours
  - Thus analgesic requirement is highest during the first 72 hours
  - Round the clock coverage is required for first 24 hours
  - Analgesic medications are then prescribed as required

Considerations for Analgesic Plan

- ❖ Surgical considerations:
  - Analgesic regimen should be tailored to the surgical procedure
  - This is especially important in the event of a planned regional block
  - Considerations at the time of placement of a regional block include:
    - Site of placement of the regional block catheter
    - LA solution to be used

- Correct placement of epidural catheters improves diaphragmatic function

❖ Age and cognitive ability:
  - Neonates and young infants:
    - Children in this age group possess an impaired respiratory drive
    - Thus, opioid sparing techniques such as regional blocks are preferred
    - Care should be taken to avoid local anesthetic toxicity
  - Toddlers:
    - May be treated with oral opioids when pain is severe
    - Analgesic therapy can be supplemented or reduced with:
      - Non-pharmacological interventions
      - Parental presence in the postoperative period
  - Preschool and school going children:
    - Have a better understanding of the postoperative experience
    - Patient-controlled analgesia is helpful in this age group
    - Regional techniques are excellent for opioid sparing in all age groups

❖ Previous pain experience:
  - In case of previous analgesic exposure, history should be obtained regarding:
    - Analgesic history
    - Previous analgesic regimens
    - Response to treatment
    - Adverse effects from analgesic medications
  - Opioid naïve children require smaller opioid doses
  - This is in contrast to those with prior opioid exposure who require higher doses

Drug Dosages

Paracetamol

❖ 7.5 mg/kg IV for neonates
❖ 15 mg/kg IV older children
❖ 30 mg/kg PR followed by 20 mg/kg TID
❖ Total daily dose:
  - Less than 100 mg/kg in children
  - Less than 75 mg/kg in infants
  - Less than 50 mg/kg in neonates

NSAIDs

❖ Diclofenac 1 mg/kg IM Q8H
❖ Ibuprofen 6–10 mg/kg Q6H
❖ Ketorolac 0.5 mg/kg Q8H

Opioids

❖ Tramadol 1–2 mg/kg Q6H
❖ Morphine 50–100 μg/kg or 10–40 μg/kg/hr infusion
❖ Fentanyl 0.5–1 μg/kg or 0.1–0.2 μg/kg/min infusion
❖ Remifentanyl 0.1–0.5 μg/kg or 0.05–5 μg/kg/min infusion
❖ Alfentanyl 5–10 μg/kg or 1–4 μg/kg/min infusion
❖ Sufentanyl 0.5–5 μg/kg or 0.01–0.05 μg/kg/min infusion

Local Anesthetics: Ropivacaine/Bupivacaine

❖ 2 mg/kg bolus
❖ 0.4 mg/kg/hr is maximum allowable dose

Others

❖ Ketamine 0.5 mg/kg followed by 10–20 μg/kg/min infusion
❖ Dexmedetomidine 0.5–1 μg/kg over 10 minutes followed by 0.2–0.3 μg/kg/min infusion

Regional Blocks

❖ Local infilteration
❖ Ilioinguinal—iliohypogastric block for herniorrhaphy
❖ Penile block for circumcision
❖ Fascia iliaca block for lower limb
❖ Intercostal block for thoracic/upper abdominal surgeries
❖ Subarachnoid, caudal, epidural-perineal and lower limb surgeries

ANESTHESIA FOR CONJOINED TWIN

Introduction

❖ Conjoined twins are identical twins whose bodies are joined in-utero
❖ They are monozygotic, monochorionic twins who develop from a single placenta
❖ Incomplete splitting of monozygotic twins occurs after day 12 of embryogenesis
❖ This results in the fetuses being physically joined at some anatomical location

Incidence

❖ Rare phenomenon
❖ Incidence ranges from 1: 50,000 to 1: 200,000 live births
❖ Both twins are always of the same sex
❖ Higher incidence in:
  - Females (ratio 3:1)
  - Southwest Asia and Africa
❖ Overall survival rate of 20%

Etiology

- Theory of fission:
  - This is the older theory
  - Fertilized ovum splits incompletely, resulting in conjoined twins
- Theory of fusion:
  - This is the current generally accepted theory
  - Fertilized ovum separates completely
  - However, stem cells in both twins search for similar cells
  - Fusion of these cells with like- stem cells in the twin results in fusion of the twins

Classification

- Classified according to the site of conjunction
- Craniopagus:
  - Incidence 1–2%
  - Have fused skulls but separate bodies
  - Can be joined at:
    - Front of head
    - Side of the head
    - Back of the head
  - Usually not joined at the face or base of skull
  - Brains may be separate or fused
  - Variable amounts of shared brain tissue, CSF spaces and blood vessels
  - Separation surgery depends on amount of shared brain tissue
- Thoracopagus:
  - *Most common* type
  - Incidence 35–40%
  - Involves fusion of anterior upper thorax
  - Usually have conjoined hearts, liver and upper GI tract
  - Separation surgery depends on cardiac anatomy
- Omphalopagus:
  - Second most common type of conjoined twins
  - Incidence 30–33%
  - Joined at lower chest or upper abdomen with a conjoined liver
  - However, conjoined heart is not present
  - Separation rate is highest for this subset of conjoined twins
- Pyopagus:
  - Incidence 18–19%
  - Twins are joined at the sacrum
  - Separation is possible with a high success rate
- Ischiopagus:
  - Incidence 6%
  - Joined at the pelvis causing anterior union of lower half of body
  - Usually involves genitourinary tract
  - Separation is possible with a high success rate

Timing of Surgery

- Timing of separation surgery depends on several factors, including associated conditions
- Usually twin separation surgery is best performed at 9–12 months of age
- Ideally combined weight of the twins by this time should be at least 8 kg
- This weight will provide for greater skin surface area and blood volume
- Indications for emergency twin separation:
  - Damage to the connecting bridge at the time of delivery (omphalopagus)
  - Condition of one twin threatens survival of the other:
    - Complex congenital heart disease
    - Cardiomyopathy
    - Sepsis
  - Condition of one twin is incompatible with life:
    - Anencephaly
    - Acardia
    - Still born
    - Complex congenital heart disease

Investigations

- Routine blood tests, urinalysis
- 3-D CT imaging
- MRI scan, angiography
- Cerebral angiography
- CT angiographic reconstruction
- Electroencephalogram
- SSEPs, VEPs, MEPs

Anesthetic Considerations

- Informed consent: should include explanation of:
  - Procedural steps
  - Risks associated with procedure
  - Risk of losing one or both babies
- Large logistical requirements:
  - Requirement of large operating room to accommodate multidisciplinary staff
  - Requirement of two operating theatre tables
  - Requirement of two separate monitors with separate equipment
  - Requirement of two anesthetic teams, one for each twin

- Each twin has to be treated as a separate entity and anesthetized separately
- Inter-twin cross circulation:
  - Possibility of varying degrees of cross circulation amongst twins exists
  - This may account for varying pharmacokinetics of the drugs administered
  - However, cross circulation may not be adequate to justify drug administration in a single twin
  - The extent of cross circulation has to be determined prior to induction
- Difficult airway especially in thoraco-omphalopagus patients due to:
  - Opisthotonus
  - Hyperextension of neck
  - Inability to position each twin supine
  - Difficult access to mouth as the twins faces are close to each other
  - Angulation of trachea may make ETT placement difficult
- Hypothermia:
  - Difficult to maintain temperature of the patient
  - This is because of the large surface area exposed at the surgical field
- Massive blood loss:
  - Seen especially in pyopagus and ischiopagus
  - Concealed blood loss occurs commonly following twin separation
- Abnormal positioning of the patient especially in thoracopagus
- Determination of weight:
  - Weight of each twin has to be determined prior to induction
  - If both twins appear equal in size, combined weight may be divided in half
  - If both twins differ in size, weight may be determined by ratio of size difference

Monitors

- Each twin needs its own set of monitors
- Pulse oximetry
- NIBP
- E_TCO_2
- ECG
- Nasopharyngeal temperature
- Invasive blood pressure monitoring for each twin
- CVP monitoring in each twin as surgery involves massive fluid shifts
- Frequent ABG analysis to assess hemoglobin and electrolyte status
- SSEP and MEP in case neurological disruption is likely

Preoperative Preparation

- Adequate NPO status
- Placement of invasive vascular access in both twins on the day prior to surgery
- Central venous access may be difficult as:
  - Usual landmarks are usually unreliable
  - Difficult positioning of patient
- Calculation of approximate weight of each twin for drug administration
- Avoid injection of air bubbles as septal defects may coexist, causing systemic embolism
- Determination of extent of cross circulation:
  - Glycopyrollate is administered to one twin
  - Heart rate response is noted in the other twin
  - This determines the extent of cross circulation between twins

Induction

- Each twin should be anesthetized individually, one after the other
- Sequential induction is preferred over simultaneous induction of both twins
- Administration of double induction dose to one twin will not anesthetize the other
- Small amount of induction dose administered to one twin crosses over to the other twin
- However, this amount is not adequate to anesthetize the other twin
- Administration of muscle relaxants however produces muscle weakness in the other twin
- Ketamine and fentanyl are used as induction agents for both the twins
- First twin is intubated without the administration of muscle relaxants
- This is done in order to prevent subclinical paralysis in the second twin
- Positional changes at the time of intubation may lead to hypotension in the second twin
- Fixation of ETT may be challenging in craiopagus patients

Maintenance

- Balanced anesthesia with O_2+ air + sevoflurane preferred
- Intermittent boluses of fentanyl and atracurium may be used to maintain anesthetic plane
- Lung compliance may be low when the chest wall is involved (thoraco-omphalopagus)
- This may necessitate higher ventilation pressures
- Color coding may be useful to differentiate drugs and blood products of both twins

Hemodynamics

- Massive third space losses may occur due to large incision and long operative times
- Goal directed fluid therapy may be used to maintain euvolemia
- Crystalloid replacement may reach levels up to 15 mL/kg/hr
- In such a scenario, colloids such as 5% albumin may be used in place of crystalloids
- Blood sugars should be monitored frequently in view of prolonged duration of surgery
- Blood loss and transfusion:
  - It may be difficult to determine the source of bleeding (i.e., which twin is bleeding)
  - Transfusion trigger is usually accepted as a hematocrit of 30%
  - Blood transfused to one twin will not reach the other twin
  - Thus, blood and component therapy should be individualized to each twin
- Vasopressors may be used to support circulation when fluid therapy has been optimized
- Maintain normothermia:
  - Fluid warmer
  - Forced air warmer
  - Warming lights
  - Warm blankets
  - Control of ambient OR temperature
- Intertwin steal phenomenon:
  - Vasodilatation in one twin may cause steal phenomenon in the other twin
  - This may lead to precipitous hypotension in both twins

Postoperative Care

Monitors

- Pulse oximetry
- ECG
- NIBP/IBP
- CVP
- Continuing blood loss
- ABGs for hypoxia, hypercarbia and acidosis

Management

- Fluid management may be challenging owing to massive fluid shifts
- Diaphragmatic dysfunction and sterna/chest wall insufficiency may complicate extubation

Analgesia

- Multimodal analgesia is key
- Good analgesia is essential to facilitate adequate ventilation

ANESTHESIA FOR DENTAL PROCEDURES

Introduction

- Anesthetic requirements for pediatric dental procedures may vary from MAC to administration of GA
- First demonstrated by Dr. Horace Wells for wisdom tooth extraction, when he used nitrous oxide to anesthetize himself

Indications for General Anesthesia

- Extensive dental restoration:
  - Multiple amalgam
  - Resin based composite restorations
  - Pulpal therapy
  - Impacted wisdom tooth extraction
- Children with orofacial trauma
- Neurological disorders:
  - Atheroid cerebral palsy
  - Poorly controlled seizures
  - Post-encephalitic children
  - Hyperactive children
- Communication disorders:
  - Mental retardation
  - Autism
- Local anesthetic allergy

Pediatric Dental Procedures

- Stainless steel crowns
- Pulp treatments
- Tooth extractions
- Operative restorations
- Orthognathic plates for cleft palate

Anesthetic Considerations

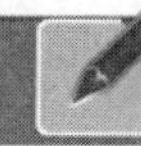

- Surgery related:
  - Remote anesthesia
  - Shared airway
  - Arrhythmias due to trigeminal nerve stimulation
- Patient related:
  - Pediatric patient
  - May be associated with adenotonsillar hypertrophy
  - Difficult airway in cases of cleft palate
  - High risk of aspiration owing to semi-erect position
  - High risk of laryngospasm due to pooled secretions

Types of Anesthesia

- Local anesthesia
- Conscious sedation:
  - Oral sedation
  - IV sedation
  - Inhalational sedation with nitrous oxide
- General anesthesia

Local Anesthesia

- Types of local anesthesia for dental procedures:
  - Intrapulpal anesthesia
  - Intraligamental anesthesia
  - Topical anesthesia
  - Nerve block
  - Intraosseus anesthesia
  - Submucosal injections
- Drugs used include:
  - 2% lidocaine 4–5 mg/kg
  - 2% lidocaine with 1:80,000 epinephrine up to 7 mg/kg
  - 3% prilocaine with felypressin up to 6 mg/kg
  - 4% articaine with 1:100,000 epinephrine up to 7 mg/kg
  - 0.25–0.5% bupivacaine up to 2 mg/kg

Oral Sedation

- Peroral midazolam:
  - Oral midazolam is usually used to achieve sedation via oral route
  - 0.4–0.6 mg PO given 30 minutes prior to procedure up to maximum of 10 mg
- Other drugs used are:
  - Chloral hydrate and trichlofos
  - Promethazine
  - Ketamine
  - Clonidine
- Disadvantages:
  - Delayed onset of action
  - Variable absorption in GI tract
  - Bitter taste of drug

Intravenous Sedation

- Usually achieved with titrated doses of benzodiazepines
- Target controlled infusion of propofol may also be used to maintain anesthesia
- Facilities to secure the airway on an urgent basis should be available

Nitrous Oxide Sedation

- Useful in slightly older children
- Nitrous oxide is administered with a nasal mask/hood
- The child is asked to breathe through the nose with mouth closed
- 100% oxygen is delivered to the child at 4–6 L/min for 2–3 minutes
- Nitrous oxide is then introduced at 10–20% and slowly increased to reach the desired plane
- The jaw is thrust upwards to prevent tongue fall, while the hood is supported with thumb
- Local anesthetic is then injected to ensure adequate analgesia
- The concentration of nitrous oxide can then be gradually reduced
- Recovery is achieved by reverse titration (inhaling 100% oxygen for 5 minutes)

General Anesthesia

Preoperative Preparation

- Adequate NPO orders
- Informed consent
- Premedication is rarely required
- Short acting benzodiazepines like midazolam may be used in very anxious patients
- EMLA cream may be useful to secure IV access prior to induction

Monitors

- Minimum monitoring standards
- NIBP
- Pulse oximetry
- E_TCO_2
- ECG

Position

- Usually in semi-upright position
- This position is preferred as:
  - It helps to prevent aspiration of secretions
  - It facilitates surgical access

Induction

- Adequate preoxygenation
- Induction:
  - Intravenous induction with propofol is the technique of choice
  - In the absence of an IV line, inhalational induction with sevoflurane is preferred

- Inhalational induction with halothane is associated with risk of arrhythmias
- Succinylcholine is avoided, especially if early discharge is planned
- Succinylcholine may cause body pain, which may preclude early discharge
- NMB is achieved with non-depolarizing NMBA of appropriate duration of action
- NMBA may be avoided in select cases by intubating the patient in deep planes

❖ Intubation:
- Laryngeal mask or endotracheal tube may be used to secure airway
- Endotracheal intubation may be required in patients undergoing extensive surgery
- LMAs may be moved and displaced during surgical field exposure
- Nasotracheal ETT is preferred as it prevents interference with the surgical field
- Orally inserted ETT it may be manipulated during surgery to aid field exposure

❖ Throat packs:
- Throat packs may be placed to prevent aspiration of blood or debris
- Bite blocks may be used on the side opposite to extraction to open the mouth
- These have to be removed without fail at the end of surgery

Maintenance

❖ Maintenance of anesthesia may be achieved via TIVA or balanced anesthesia

❖ Balanced anesthesia is maintained with O_2 + air + sevoflurane

❖ Target controlled infusions of propofol may be used as an alternative to provide TIVA

❖ This helps prevent OT pollution, especially in the backdrop of shared airway

Emergence

❖ Pharyngeal packs should be removed prior to extubation

❖ Thorough suctioning to clear all pooled secretions and debris is very important

❖ Extubation is preferred in fully awake planes with the patient able to protect his airway

❖ Lateral position with Trendelenburg tilt is the preferred position at extubation

❖ Paracetamol, NSAIDs and dexamethasone may be used for postoperative analgesia

SUGGESTED READING

1. Abajian, J.C., Mellish, R.W., Browne, A.F., Perkins, F.M., Lambert, D.H., J Mazuzan, J.E., Jr. (1984). Spinal anesthesia for surgery in the high risk infant. *Anesthesia Analgesia*, 63(3), 359–62.
2. American Academy of Pediatric Dentistry. (2004). Guidelines for elective use of conscious sedation, deep sedation and general anesthesia in pediatric dental patients. *AAPD Reference Manual*, 27(7 Suppl), 74–80.
3. Andrews, K., Fitzgerald, M. (1999). Cutaneous flexion reflex in human neonates: a quantitative study of threshold and stimulus-response characteristics after single and repeated stimuli. *Developmental Medicine and Child Neurology*, 41(10), 696–703.
4. Bailey, A.G., McNaull, P.P., Jooste, E., Tuchman, J.B. (2010). Perioperative crystalloid and colloid fluid management in children: where are we and how did we get there. *Anesthesia Analgesia*, 110(2), 375–90.
5. Beck with, J.B. (2003). Conjoined twins: developmental malformations and clinical implications. *Pediatric Developmental Pathology*, 6(4), 361–4.
6. Bhananker, S.M., et al. (2007). Anesthesia related cardiac arrest in children: update from the Pediatric Perioperative Cardiac Arrest Registry. *Anesthesia Analgesia*, 105(2), 344-50.
7. Cantlay, K., Williamson, S., Hawkings, J. (2005). Anesthesia for dentistry. *Continuiung Education in Anesthesia Critical Care and Pain*, 5(3), 71–5.
8. Chen, L.H., Zhang, X., Li, S., Liu, Y., Zhang, T., Wu, J. (2009). The risk factors for hypoxemia in children younger than 5 years old undergoing rigid bronchoscopy for foreign body removal. *Anesthesia Analgesia*, 109(4), 1079–84.
9. Davis, P., Cladis, F. (2017). *Smiths anesthesia for infants and children*. 9th ed. Philadelphia: Elsevier.
10. Dhayagude, H.S., Dave, N.M. (2017). *Principles and Practise of Pediatric Anesthesia*. 1st ed. New Delhi: Jaypee Brothers Medical Publishers.
11. Dohi, S., Seino, H. (1986). Spinal anesthesia in premature infants: Dosage and effects of sympathectomy. *Anesthesiology*, 65(5), 559–61.
12. Downey, P., Middlesworth, W., Bacchetta, M., Sonett, J. (2017). Recurrent and congenital tracheoesophageal fistula in adults. *European Journal of Cardiothoracic Surgery*, 52(6), 1218–22.
13. Downward, C.D., et al. (2003). Analysis of an improved survival rate for congenital diaphragmatic hernia. *Journal of Pediatric Surgery*, 38(5), 729–32.
14. Drake Brockman, T.F., Ramgolam, A., Zhang, G., Hall, G.L., von Ungern-Sternberg, B.S. (2017). The effect of endotracheal tubes versus LMAs on perioperative respiratory adverse events in infants: a randomized controlled trial. *Lancet*.
15. Duhamel, B. (1963). Embryology of exomphalos and allied malformations. *Archives of Disease in Childhood*, 38(198), 142–7.
16. Eren, S., Balci, A.E., Dikici, B., Doblan, M., Eren, M.N. (2003). Foreign body aspiration in children: experience of 1160 cases. *Annals of Tropical Paediatrics*, 23(1), 31–7.

17. Feld, L.G., et al. (2018). Clinical practice guideline: maintenance intravenous fluids in children. *Pediatrics*, 142(6), e20183083.
18. Feldkamp, M.L., Carey, J.C., Sadler, T.W. (2007). Development of gastroschisis: review of hypothesis, a novel hypothesis, and implications for research. *American Journal of Medical Genetics Part A*, 143(7), 639–52.
19. Furman, E., Roman, D.G., Lemmer, L.A., Hairabet, J., Jasinska, M., Laver, M.B. (1975). Specific therapy in water, electrolyte and blood volume replacement during pediatric surgery. *Anesthesiology*, 42(2), 187–93.
20. Gander, J.W., et al. (2011). Early recurrence of congenital diaphragmatic hernia is higher after thoracoscopic than open repair: A single institutional study. *Journal of Pediatric Surgery*, 46(7), 1303–8.
21. Greer, J.J. (2013). Current concepts on the pathogenesis and etiology of CDH. *Respiratory Physiology and Neurobiology*, 189(2), 232–40.
22. Gregory, G.A., Andropoulos, D.B. (2012). *Gregory's Pediatric Anesthesia*. 5th ed. West Sussex, United Kingdom: Wiley-Blackwell.
23. Habre, W., et al. (2017). Incidence of severe critical events in pediatric anesthesia: a prospective multicentre observational study in 261 hospitals in Europe. *Lancet Respiratory Medicine*, 5(5), 412–25.
24. Hanson, J.W. (1975). Incidence of conjoined twins. *Lancet*, 2(7947), 1257.
25. Hicks, C.L., von Baeyer, C.L., Spafford, P.A., van Korlaar, I., Goodenough, B. (2001). The Faces Pain Scale-revised: towards a common metric in pediatric pain management. *Pain*, 93(2), 173–83.
26. Holder, T.M., Ashcraft, K.W., Sharp, R.J., Amoury, R.A. (1987). Care of infants with esophageal atresia, Tracheoesophageal Fistula and associated anomalies. *Journal of Thoracic and Cardiovascular Surgery*, 94(6), 828–35.
27. Holliday, M.A., Segar, W. (1957). The maintenance need for water in parenteral fluid therapy. *Pediatrics*, 19(5), 823–32.
28. Imbelloni, L.E., Vieira, E.M., Sperni, F., Guizellini, R.H., Tolentino, A.P. (2006). Spinal anesthesia in children with isobaric local anesthetics: Report on 307 patients under 13 years of age. *Paediatric Anesthesia*, 16(1), 43–8.
29. Ke, M., Wu, X., Zeng, J. (2015). The treatment strategy for tracheoesophageal fistula. *Journal of Thoracic Disease*, 7(Suppl 4), S389–S397.
30. Kirby, R.S. (2017). The prevalence of selected major birth defects in the United States. *Seminars in Perinatology*, 41(6), 338–44.
31. Kokki, H. (2012). Spinal blocks. *Pediatric Anesthesia*, 22(1), 56–64.
32. Kokki, H., Salonvaara, M., Herrgård, E., Onen, P. (1999). Postdural puncture headache is not an age related symptom in children: a prospective, open-randomized, parallel group study comparing a 22-G Quincke with a 22-G Whitacre needle. *Pediatric Anesthesia*, 9(5), 429–34.
33. Lee, B.J., August, D. (2014). COLDS: a heuristic preanesthetic risk score for children with upper respiratory tract infection. *Pediatric Anesthesia*, 24(3), 349–50.
34. Lopez, T., Sánchez, F.J., Garzón, J.C., Muriel, C. (2012). Spinal anesthesia in pediatric patients. *Minerva Anesthesiologica*, 78(1), 78–87.
35. Lupo, P.J., et al. (2017). Population based birth defects data inthe United States 2010-2014: a focus on gastrointestinal defects. *Birth Defects Research*, 109(8), 1504–14.
36. Macksey, L.F. (2017). *Pediatric Anesthesia and Emergency Drug Guide*. United States of America: Jones and Bartlett Learning.
37. McCann, M.E., Greco, C., Matthes, K. (2018). *Essentials of Anesthesia for Infants and Neonates*. Cambridge: Cambridge University Press.
38. McGrath, P.A., Seifert, C.E., Speechley, K.E., Booth, J.C., Stitt, L., Gibson, M.C. (1996). A new analogue scale for assessing childrens pain: an initial validation study. *Pain*, 64(3), 435–43.
39. Murat, I., Dubois, M. (2008). Perioperative fluid therapy in pediatrics. *Pediatric Anesthesia*, 18(5), 363–70.
40. Neilson, J. (2015). Intravenous fluid therapy in children and young people: summary of NICE guidance. *British Medical Journal*.
41. New York School of Regional Anesthesia Guidelines. (2009). Pediatric epidural and caudal analgesia and anesthesia in children. New York: NYSORA.
42. Pascucci, R.C., Hershenson, M.B., Sethna, N.F., Loring, S.H., Stark, A.R. (1985). Chest wall motion of infants during spinal anesthesia. *Journal of Applied Physiology*, 2087–91.
43. Perro, M., Thébaud, B. (2014). Understanding and treating pulmonary hypertension in CDH. *Seminars in Fetal and Neonatal Medicine*, 19(6), 357–63.
44. Pretorius, D.H., Drose, J.A., Dennis, M.A., Manchester, D.K., Manco-Johnson, M.L. (1987). Tracheoesophageal Fistula in utero: twenty two cases. *Journal of Ultrasound Medicine*, 6(9), 509–13.
45. Pullerits, J., Holzman, R.S. (1993). Pediatric neuraxial blockade. *Journal of Clinical Anesthesia*, 5(4), 342–54.
46. Rea, C., Escalona, M., Churion, J., Pastrana, R. (2000). First 300 cases of peditraic regional anesthesia in Venezuela (caudal, spinal and peridural). *Internet Journal of Anesthesiology*, 4(4), 1–5.
47. Sharma, V., Berkelhamer, S., Lakshminrusimha, S. (2015). Persistent pulmonary hypertension of the newborn. *Maternal Health Neonatology Perinatology*, 14.
48. Skarsgard, E.D. (2016). Management of gastroschisis. *Current Opinion in Pediatrics*, 28(9), 363–9.
49. Smith, N. (2014). Esophageal atresia and tracheoesophageal fistul. *Early Human Development*, 947–50.
50. Snaith, R., Peutrell, J., Ellis, D. (2008). An audit of intravenous fluid prescribing and plasma electrolyte monitoring; a comparison with guidelines from the NPSA. *Pediatric Anesthesia*, 18(10), 940–6.
51. Snoek, K.G., et al. (2010). Standardized postnatal management of infants with CDH in Europe: the CDH EURO consortium consensus. *Neonatology*, 110(1), 354-64.
52. Snoek, K.G., et al. (2016). Conventional Mechanical Ventilation Versus High-frequency Oscillatory Ventilation for Congenital Diaphragmatic Hernia: A Randomized Clinical Trial (The VICI-trial). *Annals of Surgery*, 263(5), 867–74.
53. Soodan, A., Pawar, D., Subramanium, R. (2004). Anesthesia for removal of inhaled foreign bodies in children. *Pediatric Anesthesia*, 14(11), 947–52.

54. Spitz, L., Kiely, E. (2003). Conjoined twins. *Journal of American Medical Association, 289(10), 1307–10.*
55. Spitz, L., Kiely, E.M., Morecroft, J.A., Drake, D.P. (1994). Esophageal atresia: at risk groups for the 1990s. *Journal of Pediatric Surgery*, 29(6), 723–5.
56. Srinivas, J., Visram, A. (2002). Survey of pediatric epidural practise in the UK. *Pediatric Anesthesia*, 12(9), 820.
57. Steward, D.J. (1975). A simplified scoring system for the postoperative recovery room. *Canadian Anesthesia Society Journal*, 22(1), 111-3.
58. Tan, H.K., Brown, K., McGill, T., Kenna, M.A., Lund, D.P., Healy, G.B. (2000). Airway foreign bodies: a 10 year review. *International Journal of Pediatric Otorhinolaryngology*, 56(2), 91–9.
59. Tusi, B.C. (2006). Innovative approaches to neuraxial blockade in children: the introduction of epidural nerve root stimulation and ultrasound guidance for epidural catheter placement. *Pain Research and Management*, 11(3), 173–80.
60. VanderWall, K.J., Skarsgard, E.D., Filly, R.A., Eckert, J., Harrison, M.R. (1997). Fetendo clip: a fetal endoscopic tracheal clip procedure in a human fetus. *Journal of Pediatric Surgery*, 32(7), 970–2.
61. van Dijk, M., Peters, J.W., van Deventer, P., Tibboel, D. (2005). Pain control-The COMFORT Behavior scale: a tool for assessing pain and sedation in infants. *American Journal of Nursing*, 105(1), 33–6.
62. Varughese, A., McCullock, D., Lewis, M., Stokes, M. (1994). Removal of LMA in children-awake or asleep? *Anesthesiology*, 81, A1321.
63. Voepel-Lewis, T, Zanotti, J, Dammeyer, J.A., Merkel, S. (2010). Reliability and validity of FLACC behavioural tool in assessing acute pain in critically ill patients. *American Journal of Critical Care*, 19(1), 55–61.
64. von Ungern-Sternberg, B.S., et al. (2010). Risk assessment for respiratory complications in pediatric anesthesia: a prospective cohort study. *Lancet*, 376(9743), 773–83.
65. von Ungern-Sternberg, B.S., Habre, W., Erb, T.O., Heaney, M. (2009). Salbutamol premedication in children with a recent respiratory tract infection. *Pediatric Anesthesia*, 19(11), 1064–9.
66. Waterston, D.J., Carter, R.E., Aberdeen, E. (1962). Esophageal atresia: tracheoesophageal fistula. a study or survival in 218 infants. *Lancet*, 1(7234), 819–22.
67. Williams, D.G., Howard, R. (2003). Epidural analgesia in children: a survey of current opinions and practices amongst UK pediatric anesthetists. *Pediatric Anesthesia*, 13(9), 769–76.
68. Wong, D.L., Winkelstein, M.L. (1997). *Whaley and Wongs Essentials of pediatric nursing*. 5th ed. St. Louis: Mosby.
69. Worthington, L.M., Flynn., P.J., Strunin, L. (1998). Death in the dental chair: an avoidable catastrophe? *British Journal of Anesthesia*, 80(2), 131–2.

14

CHAPTER

ICU and Mechanical Ventilation

HYPONATREMIA

Introduction

- Hyponatremia is the condition of excess water relative to sodium
- It is defined as serum sodium levels < 138 mEq/L
- Symptomatic hyponatremia rarely occurs until serum sodium falls below 135 mEq/L

Etiology

- Pseudohyponatremia:
  - Occurs when there is marked increase in lipid or protein levels
  - In pseudohyponatremia, low sodium level is a result of laboratory artefact
  - This is because high lipids or proteins in plasma causes an increase in volume
  - This results in sample dilution before measurements
  - In this situation, measured plasma sodium may be considerably lower
  - Types of pseudohyponatremia:
    - Hyponatremia with normal plasma osmolality:
      - Hyperlipidemia (chylomicronemia)
      - Hyperproteinemia
      - Marked glycine absorption during TURP surgery
    - Hyponatremia with increased plasma osmolality:
      - Hyperglycemia
      - Mannitol
- Hyper-osmolar hyponatremia: (P_{osm} > 295 mOsm/kg H_2O):
  - Hyperglycemia
  - Mannitol administration
  - Glycerol administration
  - Maltose administration
- Hypo-osmolar hyponatremia: (P_{osm} < 275 mOsm/kg H_2O):
  - With increased total body sodium:
    - CCF
    - Nephrotic syndrome
    - Cirrhosis
  - With low total body sodium:
    - Renal wasting:
      - Thiazide diuretics
      - Mineralocorticoid deficiency
      - Salt losing nephropathies
      - Osmotic diuretics:
        - Mannitol
        - Hyperglycemia
      - Renal tubular acidosis
      - ***Cerebral salt wasting syndrome***
    - Extra-renal losses:
      - Vomiting, diarrhea
      - Integumentary loss:
        - Sweating
        - Burns
      - Third spacing
  - With normal total body sodium:
    - Primary polydipsia
    - SIADH
    - Drug induced:
      - Chlorpropamide
      - Cyclophosphamide
    - Fluid overload due to CRF
    - Glucocorticoid deficiency
    - Hypothyroidism
- Iso-osmolar hyponatremia: (P_{osm} 275–295 mOsm/kg H_2O):
  - γ-globulins
  - Lithium
  - THAM
- Causes as related to volume status:
  - Hypovolemic hyponatremia:
    - Hemorrhage
    - Burn wound edema

  - Peritonitis
  - Cerebral salt wasting syndrome
- Hypervolemic hyponatremia:
  - CCF, nephrotic syndrome
  - Cirrhosis, TURP syndrome
- Euvolemic hyponatremia:
  - SIADH
  - Pseudohyponatremia
  - Iatrogenic administration of vasopressin
  - Increased AVP secretion from:
    - Small cell carcinoma of lung
    - Duodenal and pancreatic carcinoma

Cerebral Salt Wasting Syndrome

- Severe salt wasting diathesis due to secretion of brain natriuretic peptide
- In this condition, ADH levels are normal unlike in SIADH
- Predisposing factors:
  - Cerebral lesions due to trauma
  - Subarachnoid hemorrhage
  - Tumors, infections
- Hydrocortisone 1200 mg/day prevents cerebral salt wasting syndrome

Pathophysiology

- Acute hyponatremia:
  - Rapid reduction in plasma sodium occurs during acute hyponatremia
  - The blood brain barrier is more permeable to water than sodium
  - Rapid reduction in plasma sodium increases both ECF and ICF brain water
  - Fall in plasma sodium levels causes hypo-osmolality
  - *Hypoosmolality* (not hypoNa^+) causes symptoms due to cerebral edema
- Chronic hyponatremia:
  - Gradual compensatory loss of intracellular solutes occurs
  - Gradual rate of loss restores cell volume to normal
  - Thus, edema is absent even though hyponatremia occurs

Pathogenesis

- Hyponatremia with low total body sodium (TBN):
  - Occurs due to the loss of both sodium and water
  - This leads to extracellular volume depletion
  - But the loss of sodium is more than that of water
  - As intravascular deficit reaches 10% non-osmotic ADH secretion is activated
  - This occurs through:
    - Atrial stretch receptors
    - Carotid baroreceptors from preoptic muscles in hypothalamus
  - This causes decreased renal free water elimination resulting in hyponatremia
  - In hyponatremia due to vomiting:
    - Chloride is lost from the gastrointestinal tract
    - Kidney starts bicarbonaturia as a compensatory mechanism
    - Thus sodium is also lost along with bicarbonate ions
    - Hence, urinary sodium is usually more than 20 mEq/L
- Hyponatremia with increased total body sodium (TBN):
  - Edematous disorders are associated with hyponatremia and an increased TBN
  - When the increase in water exceeds that of sodium, hyponatremia results
  - HypoNa^+ results from progressive impairment of renal free water clearance
  - Aquaporin is therefore upregulated in CCF, cirrhosis and CRF
  - Progressive impairment of renal free water excretion occurs due to:
    - Non-osmotic ADH release
    - Decreased delivery of fluid to distal diluting segment in nephrons
- Hyponatremia with normal TBN:
  - Occurs in:
    - Glucocorticoid insufficiency
    - Hypothyroidism
    - Drugs:
      - Chlorpropamide
      - Cyclophosphamide
    - SIADH

Clinical Features

- Mild to moderate hyponatremia ($Na^+ > 130$ mEq/L) are frequently asymptomatic
- Severe hyponatremia (< 120 mEq/L) causes symptoms of cerebral edema
- Hyponatremia primarily results in neurological manifestations

- Nausea and malaise are the *earliest symptoms*
- Severity depends on rate of development of extracellular hypoosmolality
- Acute hyponatremia:
  - Neurological manifestations:
    - Cerebral edema occurs when:
      - Serum Na^+ < 123 mEq/L
      - Rapid reduction in serum sodium in less than 24 hours
    - Apathy, lethargy
    - Agitation, altered consciousness
    - Headache, obtundation
    - Disordered reflexes and thermoregulation
    - Muscle twitching, seizures, coma
    - Hyponatremic encephalopathy has a poor prognosis (33% mortality)
  - Cardiovascular manifestations:
    Symptoms usually seen serum Na+ <100 mEq/L
    - Vasoconstriction and increased PVR causing HTN
    - Bradycardia
    - Increased blood flow to liver and kidneys
    - Decreased blood flow to skin and muscles
  - Musculoskeletal:
    - Muscle cramps
    - Weakness during strenuous exercise
  - Renal:
    - Dilute urine
    - Urine Na^+ < 10 mEq/L indicates extra-renal losses with intact renal sodium handling
    - Urine Na^+ > 20 mEq/L indicates intrinsic renal tubular damage
  - Gastrointestinal:
    - Usually occurs early and first
    - Anorexia, nausea, vomiting
- Chronic hyponatremia:
  - Focal weakness, hemiparesis
  - Weakness, ataxia
  - Positive Babinski sign

HYPONATREMIA SEVERITY

Serum levels	ECG	CNS	CNS
120 mEq/L	Wide QRS complex	Hypotension	Restlessness
		Bradycardia	Confusion
115 mEq/L	Wide QRS complex	Cardiac depression	Nausea
	ST elevation		Somnolence
	Ectopics		
110 mEq/L	VT	CCF	Seizures
	VF		Coma

Diagnostic Approach to Hyponatremia

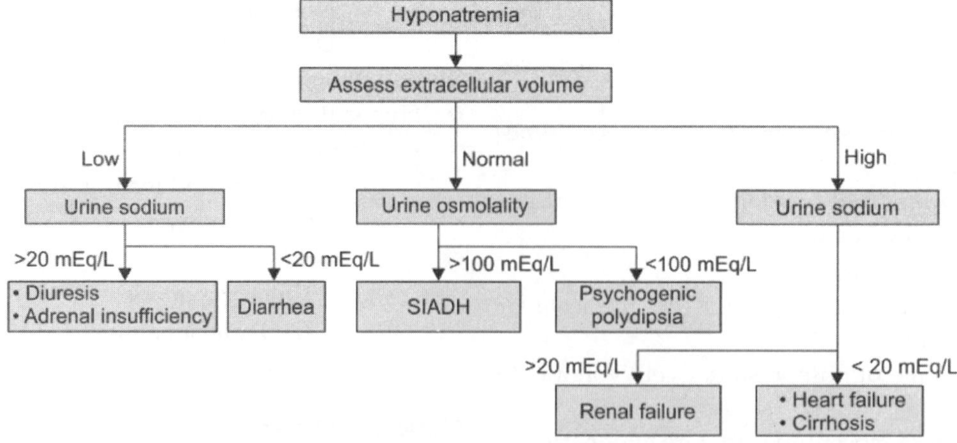

Treatment

- Treatment of cause:
  - Treat underlying disease
  - Remove offending drugs
  - Hyponatremia with normal or high serum osmolality: Remove non-sodium solute:
    - Glucose
    - Mannitol
    - Urea

- Hyponatremia with low serum osmolality:
  - High total body sodium:
    - Restrict salt and water
    - Improve renal perfusion:
      - Increase cardiac output:
      - Inotropes
      - Vasodilators
    - Increase renal blood flow:
      - Dopamine
      - Diuresis
      - Dialysis
  - Low total body sodium:
    - Restore blood volume: saline
    - Eliminate sodium losses
    - Treat adrenal insufficiency
    - Cortisol
  - Normal total body sodium:
    - Restrict water
    - Loop diuretic
    - Urinary sodium replacement with 0.9% or 3% saline
    - Lithium, demeclocycline
    - Thyroid replacement, hemodialysis
    - V_2 receptor antagonists:
      - Conivaptan
      - Tolvaptan

❖ Replacement of sodium:
- Choice of fluid:
  - Hypertonic saline given if:
    - Seizures
    - Severely symptomatic
    - Serum $Na^+ < 110$ mEq/L
    - Rapid development of hyponatremia
    - More than 0.5 mEq/L/hr reduction in sodium levels
  - Isotonic saline: fluid of choice in mild-moderate cases
- Rate of correction:
  - Not to exceed 0.6-1 mEq/L/hour for acute hyponatremia
  - For chronic hyponatremia, rate of correction not to exceed:
    - 6 mEq/ 24 hours in high-risk patients
    - 12 mEq/24 hours in low-risk patients
  - Hypertonic saline is usually administered at 1-2 mL/kg/hour
  - Rate can be reduced or stopped once symptoms improve
  - Once Na^+ levels reach 125 mEq/L, water restriction alone is sufficient
  - Serum sodium levels are checked at least every 2 hours
- Amount to be administered:
  - Na^+ deficit = TBW × [(desired Na^+) – (present Na^+)]
  - Free water excess =
    $$\text{TBW} \times \frac{125}{(\text{Measured plasma Na}^+)}$$
  - Urine volume for diuresis =
    $$\text{FWE} \times \frac{[1\text{- urine Na}^+]}{154}$$
- Duration of administration:
  - First half of deficit given over 8 hours
  - Next half is given over 1–3 days if symptoms persist
- Monitoring:
  - Serial serum Na^+ levels (every 2 hours)
  - Sodium levels are used to prevent correction at more than:
    - 1–2 mEq/L/hour
    - 8 mEq/L in 24 hours
- Recovery:
  - CNS signs and symptoms usually improve within 24 hours
  - It may require 4 days for complete recovery

❖ Newer modalities: Urea administration is under investigation

❖ Complications of therapy:
- Delayed correction causes neurological injury
- Cerebral hemorrhage/CCF if rapid rates of correction
- Complications of using hypertonic saline:
  - Pulmonary edema
  - Hypokalemia
  - Hyperchloremic metabolic acidosis
  - Transient hypotension
  - Coagulation defects: raised PT and aPTT
- ***Central pontine demyelination/osmotic demyelination***:
  - Lesion occurring due to correction of sodium levels at a rate faster than brain can adapt to higher osmolality
  - Pathophysiology:
    - Rapid correction causes abrupt brain dehydration
    - This causes neuronal crenation
    - This results in permanent neurological sequelae
  - Risk factors: More likely if:
    - Hyponatremia has persisted for longer than 48 hours
    - Correction rates:
      - More than 20 mEq/L/day
      - More than 0.6 mEq/L/hr

    - Associated alcoholism, poor nutritional status
    - Liver disease, burns, hypokalemia
  - Clinical features:
    - Fluctuating levels of consciousness
    - Behavioural disturbances, dysarthria, dysphagia
    - Convulsions, pseudobulbar palsy, quadriplegia
  - Prognosis:
    - Improvement may occur after several weeks
    - Some patients may be permanently impaired

Treatment Algorithm for Symptomatic Hyponatremia (ERA-EDTA Guidelines, 2014)

- Step I:
  - Indication for 3% hypertonic saline is assessed
  - Regardless of whether acute/chronic onset, 3% saline is indicated for acute life- threatening hyponatremia
- Step II: 100 mL of 3% hypertonic saline is infused over 10–15 minutes
- Step III: Serum sodium level is measured after each 3% saline infusion
- Step IV: Infusion of hypertonic saline is stopped when there is:
  - Improvement in symptoms
  - Increase in 4–6 mEq/L serum sodium concentration
- Step V: 100 mL bolus of 3% hypertonic saline may be repeated up to 3 total doses
- Step VI:
  - IV line is kept patent with minimal volume of 0.9% normal saline
  - Increase in sodium level is limited to below 8 mEq/L for the first 24 hours

Anesthetic Considerations of Hyponatremia

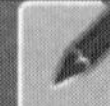

- Safe serum sodium levels for anesthetic fitness is 130 mEq/L
- For all elective procedures, serum sodium levels have to be corrected to 130 mEq/L
- Failure to do so may result in intraoperative cerebral edema causing:
  - Decreased MAC values of volatile agents
  - Agitation, confusion
  - Delayed postoperative recovery.

HYPERNATREMIA

Introduction

- Refers to the condition where:
  - Serum $Na^+ > 145$ mEq/L
  - Serum osmolality > 295 mOsm/L
- Usually seen in association with severe systemic diseases
- Thus, it is associated with mortality rates as high as 70%

Etiology

- Hypernatremia with low total body sodium: hypotonic fluid loss:
  - These patients lose both sodium and water
  - However, the volume of water lost is excess to that of sodium
  - The loss can either be renal or extra-renal (GIT/sweat)
  - Renal losses are associated with urinary sodium levels greater than 20 mEq/L
  - Extra-renal losses are associated with urinary sodium level below 10 mEq/L
  - Causes of hypernatremia with low TBN include:
    - GI losses: vomiting, diarrhea, intestinal fistula
    - Skin loss: Burns, sweating
    - Impaired renal concentrating ability:
      - Osmotic diuresis, hypercalcemia
      - Prolonged water intake, reduced protein intake
      - Sickle cell disease, multiple myeloma
- Hypernatremia with normal total body sodium:
  - These patients manifest signs of water loss without overt hypovolemia
  - The total body sodium content is usually normal
  - Causes of hypernatremia with normal total body sodium include:
    - Intracellular movement of water due to:
      - Exercise
      - Seizures
      - Rhabdomyolysis
    - Central diabetes insipidus
    - Nephrogenic diabetes insipidus
- Hypernatremia with high total body sodium:
  - Iatrogenic:
    - $NaHCO_3$ (contains 1000 mEq/L of sodium)
    - 3% hypertonic saline (contains 514 mEq/L of sodium)

- Deliberate/ accidental ingestion:
  - Substitution of sugar with salt in infant feeds
  - Sea water ingestion/ drowning
- Mineralocorticoid/ glucocorticoid excess:
  - Primary hyperaldosteronism
  - Cushings syndrome
  - Ectopic ACTH production
- Peritoneal dialysis

PATHOPHYSIOLOGY OF ACUTE HYPERNATREMIA

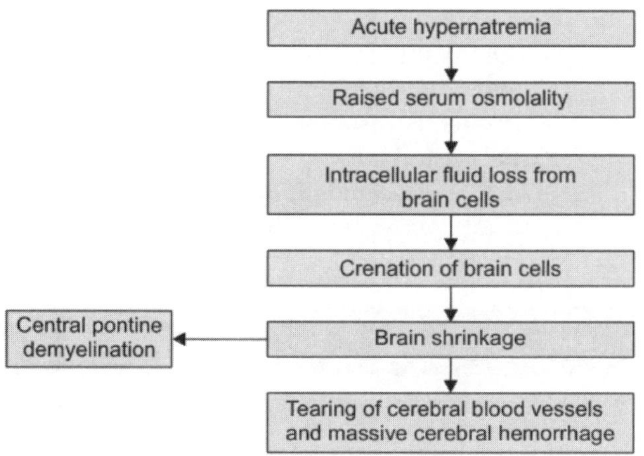

PATHOPHYSIOLOGY OF CHRONIC HYPERNATREMIA

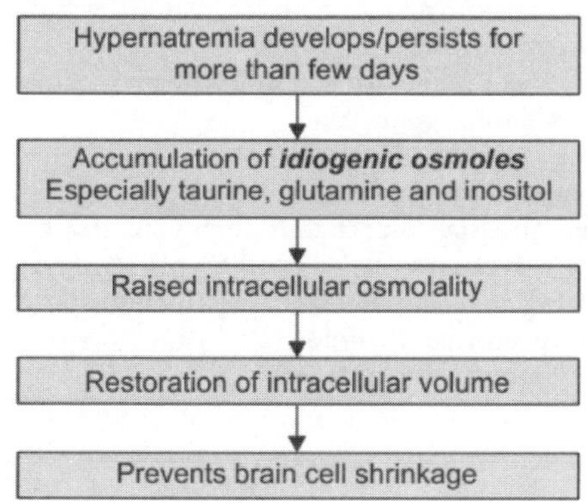

Clinical Features

- Neurological symptoms predominate in patients with hypernatremia
- Hypernatremia is associated with a history of:
  - Nausea and vomiting
  - Lethargy and weakness
  - Increased thirst with low water intake
  - Excess salt intake
  - Polyuria more than 3000 mL of urine in 24 hours
  - Drugs:
    - Demeclocycline causing diabetes insipidus
    - Lithium
    - Loop diuretics
    - Lactulose
- Common in:
  - Debilitated patients who cannot drink
  - Very old/young patients
  - Patients with altered consciousness
- Each liter of water deficit raises serum Na^+ by 3–5 mEq/L
- Acute symptoms occur once $Na^+ > 150$ mEq/L although rate of change of Na^+ is important
- Associated hypocalcemia may contribute to brain damage
- Fever can be a contributing cause/a result of hypernatremic dehydration
- Neurological symptoms predominant

Osmolarity (mOsm/kg)	Manifestations
350–375 mOsm/kg	Restlessness, irritability
375–400 mOsm/kg	Tremulousness, ataxia
400–430 mOsm/kg	Hyper-reflexia, spasticity, twitching
> 430 mOsm/kg (serum Na^+ > 158 mEq/L)	Seizures, death

COMPLICATIONS

- Massive/multiple small parenchymal hemorrhages
- Subdural/subarachnoid hemorrhage
- Cortical venous thrombosis
- Renal insufficiency and ARF
- Polyuria causing hydronephrosis and bladder distension

EVALUATION

- Hypovolemic hypernatremia:
  - Non-renal losses:
    - U_{Na} less than 10–15 mEq/L
    - U_{OSM} more than 400 mOsm/kg
  - Renal water losses:
    - U_{Na} more than 20 mEq/L
    - U_{OSM} less than 300 mOsm/kg
- Euvolemic hypernatremia:
  - Non-renal water losses:
    - U_{Na} variable
    - U_{OSM} more than 400 mOsm/kg
  - Renal water losses:
    - U_{Na} variable
    - U_{OSM} less than 290 mOsm/kg

- Hypervolemic hypernatremia:
  - Iatrogenic
  - Mineralocorticoid excess:
    - U_{Na} more than 20 mEq/L
    - U_{OSM} more than 300 mOsm/kg

Treatment

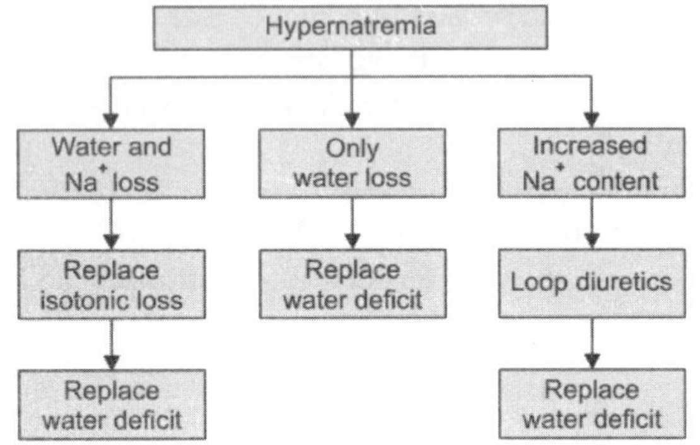

- Cornerstone of treatment is volume replacement and restoring plasma osmolality
- Calculation of free water deficit:

  Free water deficit (L) =

$$TBW \times \frac{(\text{Measured } Na^+ - \text{Normal } Na^+)}{\text{Normal } Na^+}$$

- Rate of correction:
  - Not more than 1–2 mEq/L/hour
  - In chronic cases especially, correction of Na^+ deficit should be gradual
  - Rapid correction can cause brain cells to swell and cause edema
  - In acute cases, correction can be more rapid as ***idiogenic osmoles*** are absent
- Choice of fluids:
  - Hypernatremia with low total body sodium:
    - Isotonic saline/fluids initially, for correction of hypernatremia
    - Hypotonic solution given later, for correction of TBW deficit
  - Hypernatremia with high total body sodium: treated with D_5W
  - Hypernatremia with normal total body sodium: treated with D_5W
- Role of normal saline: NS can be used even in hypernatremia as:
  - Na^+ in solution, will be less than patients serum Na^+
  - In most hypernatremia situations, there is total body sodium deficit
  - Use of NS allows more gradual reduction in serum Na^+ levels
- Duration of therapy:
  - Serial sodium levels and osmolality to be obtained
  - Plasma expanding fluids continued till tissue perfusion is restored
  - Urine output should be more than 0.5 mL/kg/hour
  - This is done with 0.45 NS or hypotonic solutions
- Treat diabetes insipidus:
  - Nephrogenic DI:
    - Salt and water restriction
    - Thiazide diuretics
  - Central DI:
    - DDAVP 1–4 µg S/C or 5–20 µg intranasally every 12–24 hours
    - Aqueous vasopressin can be used
  - Partial central DI:
    - Chlorpropamide (potentiates vasopressin)
    - Carbamazepine (increases vasopressin secretion)

Anesthetic Implications 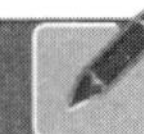

- Postpone elective surgery if serum sodium > 150 mEq/L until corrected
- Both water and isotonic fluid deficits have to be corrected completely prior to surgery
- Hypernatremia increases MAC value of volatile anesthetics
- Thus, increased utilization of volatile agents is seen in hypernatremia due to:
  - Increased MAC values causing increased use of volatile agents
  - Reduction in cardiac output causing increased uptake of volatile agents
- On the other hand, for IV anesthetics, a reduction in V_d necessitates dose reduction
- Hypernatremia associated hypovolemia and cardiac depression causes:
  - Precipitous hypotension on induction due to anesthetic induced vasodilatation
  - Hypoperfusion of tissues.

Prognosis

When plasma osmolality > 350 mOsm/kg, mortality of 40–55%

Example: 70 kg man with serum sodium level of 160 mEq/L:

- Normal TBW × 140 = present TBW × present Na^+
- (70 × 0.6) × 140 = present TBW × 160
- Thus, present TBW = 36.7 L
- Water deficit = Normal TBW – Present TBW = 42–36.7 = 5.3 L
- This volume has to be replaced over 48 hours

- Thus, 110 mL/hr of D_5W has to be given over 48 hours for correction of sodium levels

HYPOKALEMIA

Introduction

- Normal potassium levels are 3.5–5 mEq/L
- Hypokalemia is defined as plasma K^+ levels <3.5 mEq/L
- Plasma potassium levels correlate poorly with the total potassium deficit

Etiology

There are 2 main causes of hypokalemia:

- Transcellular K^+ shifts from ECF to ICF:
  - Iatrogenic causes:
    - Insulin therapy
    - Lithium therapy
    - Vitamin B_{12} therapy
    - Barium ingestion
    - Exogenous catecholamines:
      - Isoproterenol, epinephrine
      - Ritodrine, terbutaline
  - Stress related catecholamine release
  - Acute alkalosis
  - Hypothermia
  - Hypokalemic periodic paralysis
  - Thyrotoxicosis (rarely)
- Potassium depletion:
  - Insufficient intake:
    - Anorexia nervosa, geophagia
    - Starvation, primary aldosteronism
    - Alcoholism, secondary aldosteronism
  - Increased losses:
    - GI losses:
      - Vomiting, malabsorption
      - NG suction
      - Diarrhea (especially secretory diarrhea)
      - Ureterosigmoidostomy
      - Villous adenomas
      - Enteric fistulas
    - Renal losses:
      - Primary hyperaldosteronism (Conns syndrome)
      - Bartters syndrome
      - Liddles syndrome
      - Chronic metabolic acidosis
      - Renal tubular acidosis
      - Renovascular hypertension
      - Licorice ingestion
      - Excessive use of chewing tobacco
      - Drugs:
        - Carbenicillin
        - Gentamicin
        - Amphotericin B
        - Levodopa
        - Lithium
        - Theophylline
        - Chloroquine
    - Sweat losses:
      - Heat stroke
      - Heavy exercise
      - Fever

Pathophysiology

- K^+ is the principle intracellular cation
- 98% of K^+ in body is intracellular
- Extracellular K^+ is found mainly in muscles
- Hypokalemia results in a reduction of the extracellular potassium levels
- Reduction in ECF K^+ leads to a reduction in the resting membrane potential (RMP)
- This causes reduced responsiveness to sodium shifts into the cell
- Therefore, cellular excitability reduces
- Chronic K^+ loss causes ratio of ICF: ECF K^+ to remain stable
- Acute K^+ loss causes redistribution from ECF to ICF, causing changes in RMP
- This causes hyperpolarization of cardiac cell resulting in:
  - Ventricular premature ectopics
  - Re-entrant phenomenon
  - Ectopic tachycardias

Clinical Features

- Cardiovascular system:
  - Hypertension
  - Autonomic neuropathy
  - Orthostatic hypotension
  - ECG changes:
    - U waves
    - T wave inversion
    - ST depression
    - QT shortening
  - *Dysrhythmias*: ventricular ectopics and AF most commonly
  - Potentiation of digitalis toxicity
  - Myocardial dysfunction
- Neuromuscular:
  - Malaise, fatigue
  - Skeletal muscle weakness, hyporeflexia

- Cramps, paralysis, tetany
- Paresthesias, rhabdomyolysis

❖ Gastrointestinal:
- Nausea, vomiting
- Abdominal distension
- Paralytic ileus

❖ Renal:
- Metabolic alkalosis
- Paradoxical aciduria
- Nephrogenic diabetes insipidus
- Increased ammonia production
- Low GFR, chronic intestitial damage

❖ Metabolic:
- Negative nitrogen balance
- Encephalopathy in patients with liver disease

❖ Endocrine:
- Glucose intolerance due to decreased insulin secretion
- Decreased aldosterone secretion

Diagnostic Approach to Hypokalemia

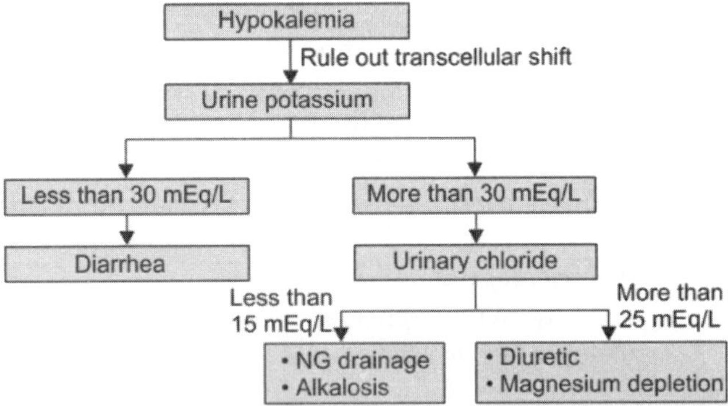

ECG Changes

❖ ECG changes do not correlate with the severity of hypokalemia

❖ Changes include:
- Narrow QRS complexes
- ST depression > 0.5 mm
- QT_c prolongation
- T wave inversion and flattening
- U wave amplitude > 1 mm
- U wave amplitude greater than T wave amplitude in the same lead

❖ These patients are predisposed to serious ventricular arrhythmias such as:
- Ventricular tachycardia
- Torsades de-pointes
- Ventricular fibrillation.

Treatment

❖ Treat any condition that promotes transcellular K^+ shifts:
- Correct alkalosis
- Stop β_2 agonist /insulin therapy
- Warm the patient

❖ Correcting potassium deficit: 1 mEq/L reduction in serum K^+ level represents 10% loss of total body K^+ stores (100–200 mEq of K^+)
- Oral replacement:
  - In stable patients with mild hypokalemia (> 3 mEq/L)
  - Should be able to tolerate oral intake
  - 20 mEq/L K^+ given every hour until optimum levels are achieved
  - Salt substitutes and K^+ supplements are commonly used
- Monitoring:
  - Blood pressure
  - Pulse oximetry
  - ECG
  - Bedside K^+ levels
- Foods rich in K^+:
  - Oranges, tomatoes
  - Grapes, banana
  - Coconuts water, raisin
  - Dried fruits
- Intravenous replacements:
  - Indications:
    - Severe hypokalemia < 2.5 mEq/L
    - Symptomatic patients with moderate hypo K^+ 2.5–3 mEq/L
    - Prolonged QT_c
    - Cardiac arrhythmias
    - When oral replacement is not feasible
  - Solutions used:
    - KCL:
      - 1 and 2 mEq/mL available
      - Packed as 10–40 mEq per ampule
      - Extremely hyperosmolar with osmolality 4000 mOsm/L
      - Preferred solution, especially in presence of alkalosis
    - K phosphate:
      - 4.5 mEq K^+ and 3 mmol phosphate per mL
      - Solutions should be diluted due to high osmolality
      - Especially used for DKA when phosphate levels are low

- Infusion rate and method:
  - KCL required in mL = $\frac{(\text{Body weight}) \times (\text{Potassium deficit})}{2} \times \frac{1}{3}$
  - Maximum rate is 0.5 mEq/kg/hr or 250 mEq/day
  - 20 mEq K^+ is added to 100 mL of NS and infused over 1 hour
  - Maximum rate of infusion is usually set at 20 mEq/hr
  - Rate of infusion may be increased to 40 mEq/hour K^+ if:
    - Serum K^+ level < 1.5 mEq/L
    - Serious arrhythmias
  - Continuous ECG monitoring required for infusion at 40 mEq/hr
- Choice of vein:
  - Rate of infusion via peripheral line should not exceed 8 mEq/h
  - This is due to the irritant nature of KCl to the endothelium
  - Rate of infusion via central line should not exceed 20 mEq/h
  - This is due to risk of developing right atrial hyperkalemia
  - This in turn can lead to cardiac standstill and arrest in diastole
  - If higher rates of administration are required, it can be administered via a second peripheral line

❖ Correct cause of K^+ depletion:
- Treat fever, diarrhea and vomiting adequately
- Stop use of diuretics
- Consider change if antibiotics

❖ Refractory hypokalemia:
- Could be due to hypomagnesemia
- Check serum magnesium levels and correct if low

Anesthetic Implications

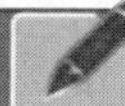

❖ Following factors have to be considered before cancelling surgery
- Urgency of surgery
- Concomitant medications given (digitalis toxicity with serum K^+ < 4 mEq/L)
- Acid base balance
- Suddenness of development of hypokalemia

❖ Postponement of surgery:
- All patients undergoing elective surgery to have normal K^+ levels

Contd...

Contd...

- Postponement of surgery not required if K^+ > 3 mEq/L
- K^+ < 3.5 mEq/L in cardiac surgery is associated with increased perioperative arrhythmias

❖ Preoperative considerations:
- Patients with ESRD should undergo dialysis except during emergency surgery
- Plasma K^+ levels measured 1–3 days before surgery:
  - Is 0.2-0.8 mEq/L higher than if measured immediately before surgery
  - Beta blockers like propranolol can be used to prevent this effect
- Prevent hypokalemia from anxiety induced hyperventilation by premedication with dexmedetomidine/clonidine

❖ Intraoperative considerations:
- Glucose free intravenous fluids are used
- No change in anesthetic requirements immediately perioperatively
- Avoid hyperventilation as it aggravates hypokalemia by causing respiratory alkalosis
- Increased sensitivity to NMBAs may be seen
- This may necessitate:
  - Reduction in dosage of NMBAs
  - Monitoring with nerve stimulator
- Prolonged NMB action expected post-surgery: delayed recovery.

HYPERKALEMIA

Introduction

❖ Defined as serum potassium levels above 5.5 mEq/L
❖ Hyperkalemia rarely occurs in normal individuals
❖ This is owing to the kidneys ability to excrete large potassium loads
❖ The kidneys can excrete up to 500 mEq or potassium per day

Etiology

❖ Pseudohyperkalemia:
- Tourniquet use
- In vitro hemolysis
- Marked leucocytosis
- Marked thrombocytosis

❖ Transcellular potassium shift:
- Acidosis
- Hypertonicity
- Heavy exercise
- Drugs:
  - Beta blockade
  - Succinylcholine
  - Digitalis intoxication

- Insulin deficiency
- Hyperkalemic periodic paralysis
- ❖ Potassium overload:
  - Potassium supplementation:
    - Potassium-rich foods
    - Intravenous potassium
    - Potassium containing drugs
  - Transfusion of aged blood
  - GI bleeding
  - Cell destruction after chemotherapy
  - Rhabdomyolysis/ crush injury
  - Hemolysis (in-vitro)
  - Extensive tissue necrosis
- ❖ Decreased potassium excretion:
  - Renal failure
  - Aldosterone deficiency
  - Selective defect in renal potassium excretion:
    - Obstructive uropathy
    - Renal transplantation
    - Type IV renal tubular acidosis
    - Systemic lupus erythematosus
    - Sickle cell disease
- ❖ Enhanced chloride reabsorption:
  - Gordons syndrome
  - Cyclosporine
- ❖ Drugs:
  - Potassium sparing diuretics: spironolactone, triamterene, amiloride
  - NSAIDs: inhibit prostaglandin mediated renin release
  - ACE inhibitors and AT-II antagonists:
    - Interfere with AT-II mediated aldosterone release
    - Especially common:
      - In CCF patients
      - When combined with K+ sparing diuretics
  - Trimethoprim, pentamidine
  - Heparin: interferes with aldosterone secretion
  - Mannitol, cyclosporine

PSEUDOHYPERKALEMIA

- ❖ Refers to conditions in which hyperkalemia is due to the technique of blood sampling
- ❖ Causes:
  - Sample lysis in vitro
  - Tourniquet use
  - Marked leucocytosis
  - Marked thrombocytosis
  - Abnormal red cell morphology (stomatocytosis)
- ❖ Sample lysis in vitro:
  - This can occur due to various causes:
    - Mechanical trauma during venepuncture
    - Potassium extrusion from the cell during fist clenching:
      - Potassium moves out of the muscle cells with exercise
      - Fist clenching during sampling raises serum K^+ by 1–2 mEq/L
    - Potassium extrusion during delayed sample processing:
      - Clotted blood has more K^+ than heparinized sample by 0.5 mEq/L
      - This is because K^+ gets extruded from RBCs during clotting
- ❖ Tourniquet use:
  - Tourniquet use may result in spurious hyperkalemia due to RBC lysis
  - Thus, while sampling in the presence of tourniquet:
    - Tourniquet is released after needle enters the vein
    - This is followed by a wait of 1–2 minutes
    - Blood samples are drawn after 2 minutes of tourniquet release
- ❖ Marked thrombocytosis:
  - Marked thrombocytosis may result in spurious hyperkalemia
  - This is because potassium moves out of platelets once clotting has occurred
  - Thus, serum K^+ levels exceed plasma K^+ levels by 0.1–0.5 mEq/L
  - K^+ levels increase 0.15 mEq/L for every 1,00,000/μL increase in platelet count
- ❖ Marked leucocytosis:
  - Marked leucocytosis as in chronic leukemia can lead to spurious hyperkalemia
  - This is due to increased cellular fragility of WBCs
  - Unlike hyperkalemia seen with thrombocytosis, high K+ is present in serum and plasma samples
- ❖ Abnormal red cell morphology (stomatocytosis):
  - Causes a hereditary form of pseudohyperkalemia
  - This is caused by an increase in passive potassium permeability of RBCs
  - Pseudohyperkalemia may be the only manifestation of this disorder

EFFECT OF SUCCINYLCHOLINE ON POTASSIUM LEVELS

- Succinylcholine in a normal patient raises serum K^+ by 0.5 mEq/L
- This is because being a depolarizing agent, it causes Na^+ uptake into the cell
- In exchange, K^+ is thrown out of the cell, causing hyperkalemia
- Hyperkalemia with succinylcholine occurs in:
  - Metabolic acidosis and hypovolemia
  - Severe abdominal infections
  - Closed head injury
  - After massive trauma: patients are susceptible for at least 60 days
  - Conditions causing proliferation of extra-junctional ACH receptors:
    - Guillain-Barre syndrome
    - Cerebrovascular accidents with hemiplegia
    - Muscular dystrophy

Pathophysiology

- Manifestations of hyperkalemia are due to impaired neuromuscular transmission
- Skeletal muscle weakness occurs due to:
  - Sustained depolarization
  - Inactivation of Na^+ channels of muscle membrane
- Hyperkalemia causes:
  - Reduction in RMP of cardiac cells
  - Reduction in duration of myocardial action potential
  - Reduction in upstroke velocity
- *Sine wave pattern*:
  - Hyperkalemia reduces rate of ventricular depolarization
  - This coincides with beginning of repolarization in some areas of myocardium
  - Other areas of the myocardium are still undergoing depolarization
  - This causes a progressive widening of QRS complexes
  - These merge with T waves, to yield *sine wave pattern*
- Hyperkalemic cardiotoxicity is enhanced by hyponatremia and hypocalcemia

CLINICAL FEATURES

- Mainly skeletal muscle and cardiac manifestations
- Neuromuscular manifestations:
  - Neuromuscular weakness (with serum K^+ levels above 8 mEq/L)
  - Areflexia, ascending paralysis
  - Paresthesias, muscle weakness and flaccid paralysis
  - Inability to phonate and respiratory arrest in severe cases
- Gastrointestinal: nausea, vomiting and diarrhea
- Cardiovascular:
  - Cardiac effects are negligible when K^+ is less than 6 mEq/L
  - Death occurs due to diastolic arrest or ventricular fibrillation

ECG Changes in Hyperkalemia

- Hyperkalemia is associated with a variety of changes on the ECG
- However, it is an insensitive and nonspecific method of detecting hyperkalemia
- ECG changes may be the first indicator of hyper-kalemia
- Usually the first ECG changes to occur are:
  - Tall symmetrical peaked T waves (*pinched at the base* appearance of T waves)
  - Shortened Q_T interval
- ***Hyperkalemic Brugada sign:***
  - Seen in critically ill patients with significant hyperkalemia (> 7 mEq/L)
  - ECG changes seen include:
    - Pseudo-right bundle branch block
    - Persistent coved ST segment elevation in at least 2 precordial leads
- ECG stages of hyperkalemia:
  - Mild hyperkalemia: 5.5–6.5 mEq/L:
    - Increased PR interval
    - Tall, peaked T waves
  - Moderate hyperkalemia: 6.5–8 mEq/L:
    - Loss of P wave
    - Prolonged QRS complex
    - ST-elevation
    - Ectopic beats
    - Escape rhythms
  - Severe hyperkalemia: more than 8 mEq/L:
    - Progressive QRS widening
    - Cardiac arrhythmias:
      - Sine wave ventricular flutter
      - Ventricular tachycardia
      - Ventricular fibrillation
      - Sinus bradycardia
      - Sinus arrest
      - Asystole
    - Conduction abnormalities:
      - Right bundle branch block

- Left bundle branch blocks
- Bifascicular blocks
- Advanced atrioventricular block

Treatment

- General measures:
  - Confirm hyperkalemia by repeat blood sample, if no cardiac derangements
  - Monitor ECG and serum potassium levels
  - Stop further K^+ administration
- Treatment of causes:
  - Aldosterone agonists: 9-fludrocortisone 0.025–0.10 mg/day
  - Digitalis intoxication:
    - Resistant to treatment
    - Attempts to shift K^+ into the cell are ineffective
    - Consider digoxin specific antibodies
- Drugs contributing to hyperkalemia are stopped
- Physiological antagonism:
  - Calcium:
    - Mechanism of action:
      - Stabilizes myocardium
      - Reverses membrane excitability
    - Dosage:
      - Calcium chloride:
        - Contains 13.6 mEq in 10 mL of 10% solution
        - Thus, calcium chloride is irritant to peripheral veins
        - Hence, central or deep veins are preferred
        - 0.5–1 g calcium chloride is given IV over 3–5 minutes
      - Calcium gluconate:
        - Contains 4.6 mEq in 10 mL of a 10% solution
        - 1 g calcium gluconate given over 10 minutes
        - 2–3 g can be given over 5 minutes in emergencies
    - Onset of action: 1–3 minutes
    - Duration of action: 30–60 minutes
    - Repeat dosage:
      - Calcium administration may be repeated every 30–60 minutes
      - Serum calcium levels have to be checked on repeated administration
- Shift potassium back into the cell:
  - Insulin with glucose:
    - Mechanism of action:
      - Through Na^+–H^+ antiporter
      - Insulin administration causes Na^+ entry into the cell
      - When Na^+ enters the cell, H^+ is extruded from it
      - This is done to maintain electrical neutrality
      - K^+ must therefore enter the cell, for the same purpose
      - This reduces ECF potassium levels
    - Dosage:
      - 5–10 IU regular insulin given IV as a bolus dose
      - Given along with 25 grams glucose (50 mL of 50% dextrose)
      - Insulin is given alone if blood glucose > 250 mg/dL
      - Alternatively, 2 ampoules of 50 mL 50% dextrose can be given
      - 0.15 IU/kg insulin with 1 mL/kg of 50% dextrose is alternative
    - Onset of action: 10–20 minutes
    - Peak action: 30–60 minutes
    - Duration of action: 4–6 hours
    - Repeat dosing:
      - Bolus doses may be repeated every 2–3 hours
      - Serial monitoring of blood glucose levels is necessary
      - Continuous infusion of insulin with glucose is an alternative
  - Sodium bicarbonate:
    - Mechanism of action:
      - Increases extracellular fluid pH
      - This causes H^+ ion release from the cells as part of buffering
      - This increases K^+ influx into the cell to maintain neutrality
      - It is not useful when used alone however
      - Thus, not recommended as a sole agent for hyperkalemia
    - Dosage:
      - 50–150 mEq given over 5–10 minutes
      - Alternatively, 1 mEq/kg IV
    - Onset of action: 5–10 minutes
    - Duration of action: 1–2 hours
  - β-agonists:
    - Mechanism of action:
      - Increases Na^+-K^+ ATPase activity:
        - Bind to cell surface of receptors and upregulate cAMP
        - Increase potassium influx in skeletal muscle

- Also act by activating the Na^{+}–K^{+}–$2Cl^{-}$ cotransporter
- Dosage:
  - 10–20 mg albuterol in 4 mL NS over 10 minutes
  - This is four times the dose used for bronchodilatation
  - This is administered via nebulization
- Onset of action: 15–30 minutes
- Duration of action: 2–4 hours
- Effectiveness: may lower serum K^{+} concentration by 0.5–1.5 mEq/L

- Hyperventilation:
  - Mechanism of action:
    - Promotes respiratory alkalosis
    - K^{+} is therefore shifted intracellularly, in exchange for H^{+} ions
    - Each 0.1 change in pH changes K^{+} by 0.4–1.5 mEq in opposite direction
  - Dosage: Maintain $PaCO_2$ around 25–35 mm Hg

❖ Eliminate potassium from the body:

- Sodium polysterone sulphonate:
  - Mechanism of action: exchanges K+ for Na+ in GIT
  - Dosage:
    - Oral administration:
      - 15–30 grams with 20% sorbitol given orally
      - Dose can be repeated every 4–6 hours as necessary
    - Per rectal administration:
      - 50 g diluted in 150 mL tap water (not sorbitol)
      - This solution is given PR as enema via a rubber tube
      - Rubber tube is positioned with the tip in sigmoid colon
  - Onset of action: 1–2 hours
  - Duration of action: 4–6 hours
  - Contraindications: (due to risk of intestinal necrosis)
    - Ileus
    - Large/ small bowel obstruction
    - Ulcerative colitis
- Diuretics:
  - Mechanism of action: promotes kaliuresis
  - Dosage: 40–80 mg furosemide given IV
  - Onset of action variable
  - Duration of action variable
- Dialysis:
  - Mechanism of action:
    - Exchange of K^{+} with hypokalemic dialysate
    - This reduces extracellular K^{+} levels
  - Effectiveness:
    - Hemodialysis is more effective than peritoneal dialysis
    - Hemodialysis removes 25–50 mEq/hour of potassium
    - Peritoneal dialysis removes 10–15 mEq/hour of potassium
  - Onset of action: Within minutes
  - Duration of action: Variable

Anesthetic Considerations

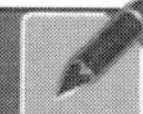

❖ All patients undergoing elective surgery to have normal K^{+} levels
❖ Delaying surgery not recommended if K^{+} level is less than 5.9 mEq/L
❖ Stress during surgery itself causes serum K^{+} to fall by 0.2–0.8 mEq/L
❖ Patients on ESRD should undergo dialysis except in emergencies
❖ Factors to consider before cancelling surgery:
- Urgency of surgery
- Degree of hyperkalemia
- Medications given
- Acid base balance
- Suddenness of electrolyte imbalance

❖ Careful perioperative ECG monitoring is mandatory
❖ Neuromuscular function is monitored as hyperkalemia potentiates effects of NMBAs
❖ Succinylcholine is contraindicated
❖ K^{+} containing solutions like RL contraindicated
❖ Avoid respiratory and metabolic acidosis
❖ Mild hyperventilation is desirable.

HYPOCALCEMIA

Introduction

❖ Hypocalcemia is diagnosed on the basis of plasma *ionized calcium* concentration

❖ Hypocalcemia is defined as plasma ionized Ca^{+} less than:
- 4 mg/dL
- 1.1 mmol/L
- 2 mEq/L

❖ Hypocalcemia is called true hypocalcemia when free Ca^{2+} levels are low

INCIDENCE

- Hypocalcemia occurs in 88% of critically ill patients
- Occurs in 66% of less severely ill ICU patients
- Multiple trauma and post-CPB patients are at higher risk for hypocalcemia

Causes

- Low albumin level is *most common* cause
- Hypoparathyroidism:
  - Following parathyroidectomy: due to ***hungry bones*** post-surgery
  - Suppression of PTH by:
    - Severe hypo/hypermagnesemia
    - Burns, sepsis
    - Pancreatitis, I^{131} therapy
    - Hemosiderosis, hemochromatosis
    - Idiopathic causes
  - As a part of multiple endocrine defects (most commonly adrenal insufficiency)
- ***Pseudohypoparathyroidism:***
  - Refers to the group of disorders defined by target organ resistance to PTH
  - Occurs due to abnormalities in G-protein function
  - Characterized by:
    - Short stature, obesity
    - Round face and short metacarpals
    - Hypocalcemia and hyperphosphatemia
    - Elevated PTH concentration
  - Causes:
    - Familial unresponsiveness of PTH
    - Vitamin D dependant rickets type II
- Vitamin D deficiency:
  - Nutritional, inadequate sunlight exposure
  - Malabsorption: post-surgical (post-gastrectomy), IBD
  - Altered Vitamin D metabolism:
    - Anti-convulsant therapy
    - Vitamin-D dependant rickets type I
- Hyperphosphatemia:
  - Overzealous phosphate therapy
  - Tumor lysis secondary to chemotherapy
  - Rhabdomyolysis, chronic renal failure
  - ***Osteitis fibrosa cystica*** following parathyroidectomy
- Calcium chelation:
  - Pancreatitis:
    - Causes precipitation of calcium with fats (soaps)
    - This occurs following release of lipolytic enzymes and fat necrosis
  - Rhabdomyolysis, fat embolism
  - Multiple transfusions > 5 PRBCs or > 1.5 mL/kg/min
  - Rapid infusion of large volumes of albumin and isotonic saline
- Alkalosis:
  - Acute hyperventilation
  - Sodium bicarbonate therapy
  - Post-CPB patients
  - Nasogastric suctioning, diuresis
  - Occurs due to more calcium binding to albumin with rising pH
- Miscellaneous and rare causes:
  - Calcitonin secreting medullary carcinoma of thyroid
  - Osteoblastic neoplastic disease (breast and prostate)
- Drugs:
  - Phosphates (enema, laxatives)
  - Phenytoin, phenobarbital
  - Gentamycin, tobramycin, actinomycin
  - Heparin, protamine
  - Theophylline, $MgSO_4$
  - Diuretics (loop), citrate
  - Glucagon, glucocorticoids
  - Sodium nitroprusside

Clinical Features

- General:
  - Weakness, fatigue are usually the *first symptoms*
  - Parasthesia also occurs commonly
  - Hypocalcemia becomes symptomatic when serum ionized Ca^{2+} falls below 0.7 mmol/L
  - *Hallmark* of hypocalcemia is tetany, characterized by neuromuscular irritability
- Neurological:
  - Increased neuronal membrane irritability
  - Muscle spasm, circumoral and digital paresthesias
  - Tetany, Chvostek sign, Trousseaus sign
  - Seizures, abdominal cramps, biliary colic, urinary frequency
  - Papilledema

- Seizures:
  - May be focal/jacksonian/petitmal/grand-mal/cerebral tetany
  - *Cerebral tetany*:
    - Generalized tetany followed by tonic spasms
    - Treatment with standard anti-convulsants is ineffective
- Extrapyramidal disturbances, Parkinsonism

❖ Psychiatric:
- Anxiety, depression
- Dementia, hallucination, confusion, psychosis

❖ Cardiovascular system:
- Dysrhythmias
- Digitalis insensitivity, congestive cardiac failure
- Hypotension
- ECG:
  - Prolonged QTc
  - Long and flattened ST segment
  - Heart block

❖ Respiratory:
- Laryngeal spasm
- Bronchospasm
- Apnea, respiratory arrest

❖ Skeletal:
- Osteodystrophy
- Rickets, osteomalacia

❖ Dermatological:
- Dry scaly skin, brittle nails
- Coarse hair, metastatic soft tissue calcification

❖ Miscellaneous:
- Cataract, dental hypoplasia
- Reduced insulin secretion

❖ Tests for latent hypocalcemia:
- ***Chvostek sign*** (masseteric spasm):
  - Tapping on facial nerve, at angle of mandible, just anterior to the ear
  - This causes ipsilateral facial muscle spasm/masseteric spasm
  - The response to tapping depends on the severity of hypocalcemia:
    - Twitching of the lip in mild cases
    - Hemifacial spasm in severe cases
  - But this sign is *nonspecific* as it can occur in 10% normal individuals
- ***Trousseaus sign*** (carpopedal spasm):
  - Sphygmomanometer cuff is inflated for 3 min to 20 mm Hg above SBP
  - This produces the characteristic carpopedal spasm
  - Occurs due to the increased muscle irritability caused by hypocalcemia
  - On inflation of the BP cuff, ischemia of radial and ulnar nerves occurs
  - This increases the excitability of the nerve trunk under the cuff
  - Excitability is maximal at 3 minutes following cuff inflation
  - Excitability returns to normal even if ischemia is prolonged
  - Characteristics of carpopedal spasm:
    - Adduction of the thumb
    - Extension at inter-phalangeal joints
    - Flexion at metacarpophalangeal joints
    - Flexion at the wrist joint
    - Pronated forearm
    - Clinically, it is *more specific* than Chvosteks sign

INVESTIGATIONS

❖ ECG manifestations:
- Severity of ECG manifestations do not correlate with degree of hypocalcemia
- ECG changes usually occur at serum calcium less than 6 mg/dL
- Heart block:
  - Hypocalcemia prolongs plateau phase of action potential
  - This causes a delay in ventricular repolarization
  - Thus, ventricles do to respond to next electrical impulse from SA node
  - This results in a 2:1 type of heart block
- Prolonged QT_C (more than 44 msec)- *most characteristic ECG sign*
- Long, flat ST segment, heart block

❖ X-ray features:
- Metastatic soft tissue calcification occurs
- Calcium deposits in and around blood vessels of basal ganglia
- This may cause extrapyramidal effects

TREATMENT

❖ Treatment of cause:
- Improve overall nutrition in critically ill patients with low albumin levels
- Remove offending drugs
- Repletion of magnesium if hypomagnesemia present

- Removal of phosphate if hyperphosphatemia
- Correct potassium disturbances:
  - Hyperkalemia with hypocalcemia:
    - Hyperkalemia potentiates hypocalcemia induced arrhythmias
    - Thus, in this setting, *correct hypocalcemia first*
  - Hypokalemia with hypocalcemia:
    - Hypokalemia protects against hypocalcemic tetany
    - Thus, correction of hypokalemia first may provoke tetany
    - Thus, even in this setting, *correct hypocalcemia first*

❖ Replacement of calcium:
- Administration of calcium: ***Rules of '10's***
  - Intravenous regimen:
    - Indications:
      - Symptomatic hypocalcemia
      - Severe hypocalcemia with ionized calcium below:
        - » 1.9 mEq/L
        - » 0.95 mmol/L
    - Calcium chloride:
      - Contains 13.6 mEq in 10 mL of 10% solution
      - This amounts to 272 mg of elemental calcium
      - Thus, calcium chloride is irritant to peripheral veins
      - Hence, central or deep veins are preferred
      - On extravasation $CaCl_2$ causes ***calcinosis cutis***
      - 1 g 10% calcium chloride is given IV over 10–20 min
      - Maintenance dose regimens can include:
        - » 1 g IV repeated hourly until symptoms resolve
        - » Continuous infusion at 0.02–0.08 mL/kg/hr
    - Calcium gluconate:
      - Contains 4.6 mEq in 10 mL of a 10% solution
      - This amounts to 93 mg of elemental calcium
      - Calcium gluconate is less irritant to veins
      - Thus, it is preferred over calcium chloride
      - 1–3 g 10% calcium gluconate given over 10–20 min
    - Followed by elemental Ca^{2+} 0.3–2 mg/kg/hr infusion
  - Oral regimen:
    - 500–1000 mg elemental calcium Q6H
    - Available as:
      - Calcium lactate
      - Calcium glubionate
      - Calcium carbonate
      - Calcium ascorbate
      - Calcium gluconate
    - IV Ca^{2+} is given till ionized calcium is between 4–5 mg/dL
    - Once ionized Ca^{2+} is 4–5 mg/dL, oral therapy is started
- Administration of Vitamin D:
  - Indications:
    - If calcium supplementation fails to maintain serum Ca^{2+} levels
    - If hypercalciuria develops
  - Preparations:
    - Ergocalciferol 1200 μg/day ($T_{1/2}$: 30 days)
    - Dihydrotachysterol 200–400 μg/day ($T_{1/2}$: 7 days)
    - 1,25 dihydrocholecalciferol 0.25–1 μg / day ($T_{1/2}$: 1 day)

❖ Monitors:
- ECG: heart block, ventricular fibrillation
- Serum calcium, potassium, magnesium, phosphate and creatinine levels
- Urinary calcium: to prevent hypercalciuria (> 5 mg/kg/day)

❖ Mode of administration:
- Choose larger peripheral vein to prevent irritation and thrombosis
- Calcium to be diluted in 50–100 mL D_5W to reduce irritation and thrombosis
- Extravasated $CaCl_2$ causes severe tissue destruction and calcinosis cutis
- Thus, *calcium gluconate is considered safer*
- Not to be mixed with phosphate or bicarbonate to prevent precipitation
- Given with caution in digitalized patients as calcium increases digoxin toxicity
- Dosage adjusted to keep serum calcium in low normal range

❖ Adverse effects of therapy:
- Hypercalcemia
- Hypercalciuria
- Renal stones

Anesthetic Considerations

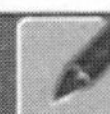

- Preoperative preparation:
  - Hypocalcemia to be corrected preoperatively:
    - 10–20 mL calcium gluconate given at 5 mL/min
    - 10 mL/min 10% Ca gluconate in 500 mL D_5W over 6 hours
  - Maintain serum ionized calcium in lower half of normal range in patients with chronic hypoparathyroidism
  - Normalize serum magnesium and phosphate levels also
- Monitors:
  - Serial ionized calcium measurements to be done intraoperatively
  - Preoperative ECG useful to maintain QT_C levels
- Intraoperatively:
  - Hypocalcemia potentiates negative inotropic effects of:
    - Barbiturates
    - Volatile anesthetics
  - NMBA blockade requires close monitoring with nerve stimulator
  - Avoid hyperventilation and alkalosis to prevent further decrease in serum Ca^{2+}
  - IV calcium to be given following rapid transfusion of:
    - Blood products
    - Albumin solutions.

HYPERCALCEMIA

Introduction

- Hypercalcemia refers to:
  - Total serum calcium more than 10.5 mg/dL
  - Ionized calcium levels above 2.7 mEq/L
- Primary hyperparathyroidism and malignancy account for more than 90% of cases

Etiology

- Endocrinopathies
  - Hyperparathyroidism:
    - Primary hyperparathyroidism:
      - Parathyroid secretion increases independent of serum Ca^{2+}level
      - Occurs due to adenomas secreting PTH
    - Secondary hyperparathyroidism:
      - Parathyroid secretion increases due to chronic hypocalcemia
      - Occurs in chronic renal failure
    - Tertiary hyperparathyroidism:
      - Autonomous PTH secretion
      - Occurs following prolonged secondary hyperparathyroidism
    - MEN II syndrome
  - Hyperthyroidism, pheochromocytoma
  - Adrenal insufficiency, acromegaly
- Malignancy: ***Humoral hypercalcemia of malignancy:***
  - Squamous cell carcinoma of lung
  - Breast carcinoma:
    - *Most common malignancy*
    - Causes 25–50% of malignancy associated hypercalcemia
  - Renal cell carcinoma, leukemias
  - Multiple myeloma: hypercalcemia occurs due to:
    - Bone destruction
    - Derangement of RANK-L/osteoprogenerin system
    - Secretion of hormones:
      - PTH-like peptide
      - Prostaglandins, cytokines
      - $IL_{1\alpha}$ and $IL_{1\beta}$ and also TNF which stimulates osteoclast activity
- Drugs:
  - Hypervitaminosis D and A
  - Thiazide diuretics, lithium
  - Hormonal therapy for breast cancer
- Granulomatous diseases:
  - Sarcoidosis, histoplasmosis
  - Tuberculosis, coccidioidomycosis
  - Hypercalcemia occurs due to conversion of calcidiol to calcitriol by granulomatous tissue
- Miscellaneous:
  - Acidosis, post-renal transplantation
  - Immobilization, ***Pagets disease of bone***
  - Recovery from acute renal failure, phosphate depletion syndrome
  - Hypocalciuric hypercalcemia, ***milk alkali syndrome***
  - ***Idiopathic hypercalcemia of infancy,*** aluminium intoxication

Severity

- Mild hypercalemia:
  - Serum levels 10.5-11.9 mg/dL
  - Usually asymptomatic
- Moderate hypercalcemia:
  - Serum levels 12–13.9 mg/dL
  - Lethargy, anorexia, nausea, polyuria

Contd...

Contd...

- ❖ Severe hypercalcemia:
  - Serum levels more than 14 mg/dL
  - Muscle weakness, depression
  - Impaired memory, emotional lability
  - Lethargy, stupor, coma
- ❖ Serum levels more than 20 mg/dL causes cardiac arrest.

Clinical Features

- ❖ General:
  - Malaise, polydipsia
  - Weakness, dehydration
- ❖ Central nervous system:
  - Confusion, proximal muscle weakness
  - Impaired memory, muscular dystrophy
  - Headache, irritability
  - Ataxia, hypotonia
  - Mental retardation in infants
- ❖ Psychiatric:
  - Apathy, anxiety, depression
  - Stupor, hallucinations
- ❖ Cardiovascular:
  - Hypertension
  - Arrhythmias (heart block)
  - Metastatic calcification of:
    - Heart valves
    - Coronary arteries
    - Myocardium
  - Cardiomyopathy
  - Increased digitalis sensitivity
  - ECG changes:
    - QT_c shortening
    - Coving of ST segment
    - Normal or increased QRS duration
    - Widening of T wave
- ❖ Gastrointestinal:
  - Anorexia, weight loss
  - Nausea, vomiting
  - Constipation, abdominal pain
  - Peptic ulcer disease due to increased gastrin production
  - Pancreatitis due to:
    - Deposition of calcium in pancreatic duct
    - Calcium activation of trypsinogen within pancreatic parenchyma
- ❖ Genitourinary:
  - Nephrogenic diabetes insipidus
  - Nephrolithiasis
  - Renal insufficiency
  - Type I renal tubular acidosis
- ❖ Skeletal:
  - Pathological fractures, osteopenia, osteoporosis
  - Bony pain especially along anterior margin of tibia
  - Osteitis fibrosa cystica
- ❖ Metastatic calcification:
  - ***Band keratopathy***, conjunctivitis, pruritus
  - Brain, kidney, blood vessels, myocardium

INVESTIGATIONS

- ❖ ECG changes:
  - ST segment shortening and depression
  - Widening of QRS complex and T waves
  - Reduction of QT_c interval
  - Arrhythmias (uncommon):
    - Bundle branch block
    - Complete heart block
- ❖ Double antibody PTH assay:
  - Differentiates between malignancy/hyperparathyroidism induced hypercalcemia
  - Serum PTH levels are low in malignancy but high in hyperparathyroidism
- ❖ Radio immunoassay for PTH: Most useful confirmatory test of hyperparathyroidism

TREATMENT

Mild-Moderate Hypercalcemia

- ❖ Does not require immediate therapy
- ❖ Warrants only supportive therapy to avoid factors aggravating hypercalcemia

Severe Hypercalcemia

- ❖ Supportive therapy:
  - Ensure adequate hydration:
    - At least 6–8 glasses of water per day
    - This is necessary to minimize the risk of nephrolithiasis
  - Correct associated abnormalities
  - Remove offending drugs:
    - Thiazide diuretics
    - Lithium carbonate therapy
  - Dietary calcium restriction (< 1000 mg/day)
  - Increase physical activity
  - Monitors:
    - ECG, cardiovascular status
    - Serum calcium, magnesium and potassium levels
    - Total serum calcium more than 14 mg/dL is treated as a medical emergency

- Calciuresis:
  - Saline hydration:
    - Normal saline dilutes serum calcium and promotes calciuresis
    - Rate of administration depends on:
      - Severity of hypercalcemia
      - Age of the patient
      - Presence of cardiac/renal comorbidities
    - Volume expansion done with:
      - Normal saline at 200–300 mL/hour
      - Rate adjusted to maintain adequate urine output
    - Reduces serum calcium by 1.5–3 mg/dL
    - Saline hydration is continued for 2–4 hours as tolerated by the patient
    - Duration of repletion:
      - 3–4 L of normal saline is administered during first 24 hours
      - This is followed by saline volumes of 2–3 L/day
      - Therapy is continued until a urine output of 2 L/day is achieved
    - Volume repletion is aimed to re-establish euvolemia
    - Onset of action: immediate
    - Duration of action: during therapy
  - Diuretics:
    - Furosemide increases calcium excretion by increasing tubular secretion
    - Can achieve net calcium excretion rate of 2000–4000 mg/day
    - Initial dose 20–40 mg furosemide given IV Q2–4H
    - Dose may be increased in the presence of suboptimal response
    - Dose is titrated to maintain a urine output of 150–200 mL/hour
    - Other dyselectrolytemias have to be treated prior to diuresis:
      - Hypokalemia
      - Hypomagnesemia
    - Diuretics, if given before saline hydration may aggravate hypercalcemia by causing additional volume depletion
    - Onset of action: 1–2 hours
    - Duration of action: during therapy
- Reduce calcium resorption:
  - Increased physical activity
  - Bisphosphates:
    - First line therapy for acute hypercalcemia
    - Inhibits osteoclast function and viability
    - Drugs used:
      - Zoledronate:
        - Most commonly used
        - 4 mg given IV over 15 minutes
        - Most rapid onset of action
        - Long acting drug which worsens ARF
        - Preferred over palmidronate for malignant hyper Ca^{2+}
      - Pamidronate:
        - Used when zoledronate is not available
        - 60–90 mg given IV over 2 hours
        - Is avoided if serum creatinine > 2.5 mg/dL
      - Other bisphosphonates used:
        - Ibandronate:
          - Used for treating hypercalcemia of malignancy
          - 2 mg IV given over 2 hours
          - As effective as palmidronate
        - Alendronate:
          - Third generation bisphosphonate
          - Gastrointestinal side effects present
          - Not used for treatment of hypercalcemia
        - Risedronate:
          - Third generation bisphosphonate
          - Less gastrointestinal side effects
          - Not used for treatment of hypercalcemia
        - Clodronate
        - Etidronate
    - Onset of action: 24–72 hours
    - Duration of action: 2–4 weeks
  - ***Salmon calcitonin***:
    - Second line therapy for acute hypercalcemia
    - Mechanism of action:
      - Inhibits bone resorption by interfering with osteoclast function
      - Increasing renal calcium excretion
    - Dosage:
      - 2–8 IU/kg calcitonin is given subcutaneously or IM
      - This dose is repeated every 6–12 hours up to 48 hours
      - Tachyphylaxis develops after 48 hrs and therefore limits its use
    - Efficacy:
      - Reduces serum calcium by a maximum of 1–2 mg/dL

    - Most beneficial when used in patients with $Ca^{2+} > 14$ mg/dL
    - 25% patients may not respond to therapy
  - Onset of action: 4–6 hours
  - Duration of action: 48 hours
- Steroids:
  - Mechanism of action:
    - Reduces intestinal calcium absorption
    - Inhibits osteoclast activity
    - Thus, it limits calcium mobilization from the bone
  - Indications:
    - Addisons disease
    - Steroid responsive malignancies
  - Drugs used:
    - Prednisolone 1–2 mg/kg PO
    - Hydrocortisone 200–300 mg IV bolus
  - Onset of action: 2–5 days
  - Duration of action: days- weeks
- Denosumab:
  - Indications:
    - Patients in whom bisphosphonates are contraindicated
    - Bisphosphonate resistant hypercalcemia
  - Dose:
    - 120 mg subcutaneously given once a week
    - Therapy is continued weekly for 4 weeks
    - This is followed by once a month dosing
  - Can be used in CRF patients as it has extra-renal clearance
- Phosphates:
  - Reduce serum calcium by deposition of calcium in bone and soft tissue
  - Rarely used and given oral if used
  - IV route not preferred due to risk of metastatic calcification
  - IV route only used if life threatening hypercalcemia
- Hemodialysis:
  - Generally used when all other therapeutic options are exhausted
  - Can remove up to 6000 mg/day
  - Indications:
    - Severe malignancy associated hypercalcemia
    - Congestive cardiac failure
    - Renal failure
- Mithramycin:
  - This is an antibiotic-antineoplastic agent
  - Used earlier for treating hypercalcemia associated with malignancy
  - 15–25 μg/kg/day given IV over 4–6 hours for 3–4 days
  - This regimen may be repeated every week until desired response is attained

❖ Treatment of cause:
- Parathyroidectomy:
  - Treatment of choice for primary hyperparathyroidism
  - Indications:
    - Age less than 50 years
    - Serum calcium more than 11.5 mg/dL
    - More than 30% reduction in GFR
    - Severe bone demineralization
- Calcimetics:
  - Used for primary, secondary and tertiary hyperparathyroidism
  - Also reduces inorganic phosphorus levels
  - Indicated if patient refuses surgery or is medically unfit for surgery
  - Sensitizes PTH calcium receptor to calcium
  - Thus, it is also useful in tertiary hyperparathyroidism
  - Cinacalcet is the only calcimimetic currently available
- Secondary hyperparathyroidism:
  - Calcium supplementation
  - Phosphate binders, Vitamin D analogues
  - Calcimetics

Anesthetic Considerations

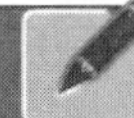

❖ Preoperative measures:
- Hypercalcemia is a medical emergency
- 200–400 mL/hour normal saline given preoperatively
- Careful monitoring to avoid fluid overload
- Correct hypercalcemia if possible before anesthetic administration

❖ Monitors:
- Ionized calcium, magnesium, potassium levels and ECG
- Neuromuscular function with nerve stimulator
- CVP and PA catheter advisable for patients with reduced cardiac reserve

❖ Controlled ventilation to avoid:
- Acidosis: worsens hypercalcemia
- Alkalosis:
  - Reduces plasma K^+ levels
  - This causes unopposed hypercalcemia resulting in tetany

❖ Avoid thiazides, maintain hydration and urine output with sodium containing fluids

❖ Reduce dose of NMBA in those with muscle weakness.

HYPOMAGNESEMIA

Introduction

- Normal serum magnesium levels range from 1.6–2.4 mg/dL
- Hypomagnesemia is defined as serum Mg^{2+} level less than 1.6 mg/dL or 0.66 mmol/L
- Clinical signs are usually not seen until the levels fall below 1.2 mg/dL or 0.5 mmol/L

Incidence

- Seen in up to 12% of hospitalized patients
- Incidence ranges from 15–60% in ICU patients
- In ICUs, it is most commonly associated with liver transplants and cardiac surgeries

Etiology

- Slight hypomagnesemia in:
  - Athletes
  - Hypermetabolic states (pregnancy)
  - Cold weather
  - Use of β-agonists
- Inadequate GI intake: rare
  - Alcoholics (30% are hypomagnesemic)
  - Malnutrition
  - Total parenteral nutrition
  - Refeeding syndrome
- Inadequate GI absorption: most common cause:
  - Malabsorption syndrome
  - Severe, prolonged vomiting or diarrhea
  - Prolonged nasogastric suction
  - Pancreatitis
  - Chronic laxative abuse
- Extra-renal losses:
  - Small bowel/biliary fistulas
  - Intestinal drains
  - Lactation Profuse sweating, burns
- Increased renal losses:
  - Polyuria due to:
    - Diuretics
    - Alcoholism
    - Volume expansion (saline diuresis)
  - Advanced renal disease, following renal transplant
  - Recovery phase of acute tubular necrosis
  - Drugs:
    - Loop and thiazide diuretics
    - Aminoglycosides
    - Amphotericin B
    - Proton pump inhibitors
    - Cisplatin, cardiac glycosides
    - Cyclosporin
    - Theophylline, pentamidine
    - Colony stimulating factor therapy
- Endocrine disorders:
  - Hyperaldosteronism
  - Hyperparathyroidism
  - Hyperthyroidism
  - SIADH
  - Diabetic ketoacidosis
- Metabolic disorders:
  - Hypercalcemia
  - Hypophosphatemia
  - Hypoalbuminemia
- Others:
  - Post- CPB
  - Post CRRT

Predisposing Conditions

- Alcoholism due to malnutrition and chronic diarrhea
- Diuretic therapy due to urinary magnesium loss
- Antibiotic therapy due to inhibition of renal reabsorption
- Secretory diarrhea due to loss of Mg^{2+} rich lower GI secretions
- Diabetes mellitus due to glycosuric magnesium loss
- Acute myocardial infarction due to intracellular Mg^{2+} from excess catecholamines

Pathophysiology

- Hypomagnesemia is commonly associated with hypokalemia and hypocalcemia
- Thus, clinical consequences of isolated hypomagnesemia are difficult to determine
- ECG changes seen in hypomagnesemia are similar to those seen with hypokalemia
- This may be due to hypomagnesemia altering the cardiac intracellular K^+ content
- Hypomagnesemia also increases myocardial sensitivity to digitalis
- This is because both inhibit the Na^+–K^+ exchange pump on cell membranes
- Hypomagnesemia depresses the CNS by causing presynaptic inhibition
- It also decreases the seizure threshold by competitively inhibiting NMDA receptors

Clinical Features

- Neurological:
  - Irritability, weakness, confusion
  - Apathy, depression
  - Fasciculations, tetany, seizures
  - Chvostek sign, Trousseaus sign
  - Ataxia, nystagmus, vertigo, hyper-reflexia
  - Obtundation, coma
- Cardiovascular:
  - Electrical irritability
  - Dysrhythmias:
    - Prolongation of QT_c interval
    - Can provoke *torsades de pointes* (characteristic)
    - Atrial fibrillation
  - Heart failure, hypotension
  - Potentiates digoxin toxicity
  - ECG changes:
    - Prolonged PR interval
    - Prolonged QT_C
    - Atrial fibrillation
- Gastrointestinal:
  - Anorexia, dysphagia
  - Nausea, vomiting
- Other dyselectrolytemias:
  - Hypocalcemia (due to reduced PTH secretion)
  - Hypokalemia (due to renal K^+ wasting)
  - Hyponatremia
  - Hypophosphatemia

Severity

Severity	Serum level	Clinical features
Moderate hypomagnesemia	1.2–1.6 mg/dL	• Neuromuscular irritability • Hypocalcemia • Hypokalemia
Severe hypomagnesemia	< 1.2 mg/dL	• Tetany • Arrhythmias • Seizures

ECG Changes

- Low P-wave voltage
- Prolonged PR internal
- Wide QRS complexes
- Increased QT_c interval
- ST segment depression
- Flat/inverted T-waves especially in precordial leads
- Prominent U-waves
- Predisposed to AF, torsades de pointes, long QT Syndrome.

Investigations

- Peripheral lymphocyte magnesium concentration:
  - Correlates with skeletal and cardiac magnesium content
  - Serum magnesium may not reflect intracellular Mg^{2+} content
  - Thus, serum magnesium is an insensitive marker for Mg^{2+} depletion
- Magnesium retention test:
  - Based on principle that renal reabsorption of Mg^{2+} is close to maximum rate
  - Thus, normally, most of the infused Mg^{2+} load will be excreted in the urine
  - However, when Mg^{2+} stores are deficient, it is reabsorbed in the renal tubules
  - Thus, a smaller fraction of injected Mg^{2+} is excreted in the urine
  - Procedure:
    - 24 mmol of magnesium is added to 250 mL of isotonic saline
    - This saline is infused over 1 hour
    - Urine is collected for 24 hours, beginning at the onset of the infusion
  - Results:
    - Urinary Mg^{2+} < 50% of infused Mg^{2+}, implies hypoMg^{2+} is likely
    - Urinary Mg^{2+} > 80% of infused Mg^{2+}, implies hypoMg^{2+} is unlikely

Treatment

- Magnesium preparations:
  - Oral preparations:
    - Magnesium chloride tablets containing 64 mg elemental magnesium
    - Magnesium oxide tablets 400 mg containing 241 mg elemental Mg^{2+}
    - Magnesium oxide tablets 140 mg containing 85 mg elemental Mg^{2+}
    - Magnesium gluconate tablets 500 mg with 27 mg elemental Mg^{2+}
  - Parenteral preparations:
    - Magnesium sulphate (50%) containing 500 mg/dL elemental Mg^{2+}
    - Magnesium sulphate 12.5% containing 120 mg/dL elemental Mg^{2+}
    - Magnesium chloride containing 1 mmol/mL Mg^{2+}

- Administration:
  - The 50% $MgSO_4$ preparation contains 500 mg magnesium per mL
  - This preparation has an osmolality of 4000 mOsm/L
  - Thus, it has to be diluted to 10% or 20% solution for IV use
  - Saline solutions should be used for dilution of the preparation
  - This is because calcium is present in Ringers lactate
  - This calcium will counteract the actions of magnesium
- Replacement protocols:
  - Mild deficiency:
    - 1 mEq/kg is replaced for the first 24 hours
    - This is followed by 0.5 mEq/kg daily for the next 3–5 days
    - Oral 60–90 mEq/day of MgO or $MgSO_4$ heptahydrate can be used
    - HypoCa^{2+} and hypoMg^{2+} patients should receive Mg^{2+} as $MgCl_2$
    - This is because $MgSO_4$ can chelate calcium and aggravate hypocalcemia
  - Moderate deficiency:
    - Loading dose:
      - 6 g $MgSO_4$ added to 250–500 mL isotonic saline
      - This is infused over 3–4 hours
    - Maintenance dose:
      - 5 g $MgSO_4$ added to 250–500 mL isotonic saline
      - This is infused over the next 6 hours
      - This dose is repeated every 12 hours for 5 days
  - Severe deficiency (< 1 mg/dL) or life-threatening hypomagnesemia:
    - Loading dose: 1–2 g $MgSO_4$ given IV over 2–5 minutes
    - Maintenance dose:
      - 5 g $MgSO_4$ added to 250–500 mL isotonic saline
      - This is infused over the next 6 hours
      - This dose is repeated every 12 hours for the next 5 days
- Monitors:
  - Serum Mg^{2+}, Ca^{2+}, K^+ levels
  - BP and cardiac output and ECG
  - Patellar reflexes: withhold magnesium if decreased reflexes
  - Caution if renal failure present
- Treat associated conditions as isolated hypomagnesemia is rare:
  - Hypokalemia
  - Hypocalcemia
  - Hypophosphatemia

Anesthetic Considerations 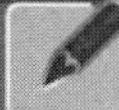

- No specific anesthetic interactions due to hypomagnesemia have been described
- But, associated dyelectrolytemias such as hypo K^+ cause perioperative interactions
- Thus, hypokalemia, hypocalcemia and hypophosphatemia are corrected prior to surgery
- Isolated hypoMg^{2+} is associated with an increased risk of perioperative arrhythmias
- Hence hypomagnesemia has to be corrected prior to elective surgery
- Hypomagnesemia is also associated with:
  - Prolonged action of neuromuscular blockers
  - Increased incidence of respiratory depression with sedation
- Elective postoperative ventilation is therefore preferred.

HYPERMAGNESEMIA

Introduction

- Hypermagnesemia is defined as serum Mg^{2+} levels more than 2.4 mg/dL or 1 mmol/L
- Rarely encountered as kidneys can increase fractional Mg^{2+} excretion up to 100%

Incidence

- Occurs in approximately 10–15% of hospitalized patients with renal failure
- Patients with cardiovascular disease usually have higher serum magnesium levels
- High serum magnesium levels are associated with higher in-hospital mortality rates

Etiology

- Increased magnesium load:
  - Treatment of pre-eclampsia/eclampsia
  - Magnesium containing laxatives/antacids/enemas
  - Untreated diabetic ketoacidosis
  - Tumor lysis
  - Rhabdomyolysis

- Increased renal magnesium absorption:
  - Hyperparathyroidism
  - Hypothyroidism
  - Adrenal insufficiency
  - Mineralocorticoid deficiency
  - Familial hypocalciuric hypercalcemia
  - *HELIX* syndrome:
    - *H*ypohidrosis
    - *E*lectrolyte imbalance:
      - Hypocalciuria
      - Hypokalemic metabolic alkalosis
    - *L*acrimal gland dysfunction
    - *X*erostomia

Predisposing Factors

- Pre-eclampsia, eclampsia
- Chronic renal failure
- Laxative abuse
- Lithium ingestion

Pathophysiology

- Magnesium decreases the transmission of neuromuscular signals
- Thus, it acts as a CNS depressant and decreases neuromuscular activity
- It also antagonizes the release and effect of ACH at the neuromuscular junction
- Effects on the neuromuscular junction include:
  - Depressed skeletal muscle function
  - Potentiation of neuromuscular blockade

Clinical Features

- Hypermagnesemia rarely produces clinical symptoms at serum levels < 4 mg/dL
- When seen, effects are most commonly neuromuscular and cardiovascular
- Neuromuscular effects:
  - These are the most consistently observed complications of hypermagnesemia
  - Increasing magnesium levels inhibits neuromuscular transmission
  - This produces a curare like effect of the neuromuscular junction
  - This eventually results in respiratory paralysis and flaccid quadriplegia
- Cardiovascular effects:
  - Magnesium is an effective intracellular and extracellular Ca^{2+} channel blocker
  - In addition, magnesium blocks several cardiac potassium channels
  - This results in delayed cardiac conduction and brady-arrhythmias
  - However, cardiac contractility and vascular tone remain unaffected

Severity of Hypermagnesemia

Serum levels	Clinical features
2.4–5 mg/dL	• Decreased cardiac conduction, nausea • Wide QRS complexes • Increased PR interval
5–7.2 mg/dL	• Sedation • Hypoventilation • *Decreased deep tendon reflexes* • Muscle weakness
7–12 mg/dL	• Hypotension • Bradycardia • Diffuse venous dilation • *Loss of deep tendon reflexes*
More than 12 mg/dL	• *Areflexia, flaccid quadriplegia* • Respiratory paralysis, paralytic ileus • Coma • Cardiac arrest, complete heart block

ECG Changes

- Prolonged PR internal
- Widening of QRS complexes
- Elevated T waves
- Atrioventricular/intraventricular conduction disturbances
- Cardiac arrest can occur if serum levels exceed 12 mEq/L.

Treatment

- Stop all magnesium containing preparations (antacids)
- Antagonize effects of magnesium:
  - Ca^{2+} administration reverts the calcium channel blockade provoked by Mg^{2+}
  - 10 mL of 10% calcium chloride IV is given over 2–3 minutes
  - Further infusion of 40–60 mL during the next 24 hours may be given
  - However, the effects are transient and should not delay hemodialysis
- Eliminate magnesium:
  - Extracellular volume expansion:
    - Half normal saline with 5% dextrose is used
    - In most cases, impaired renal function restricts fluid resuscitation
    - Thus, fluid resuscitation is used only if renal function is preserved

- Diuresis with 40–80 mg furosemide IV following fluid resuscitation
- Hemodialysis done with low magnesium bath is the *treatment of choice*
- Diuresis with normal saline is not recommended as:
  - This reduces the likelihood of iatrogenic hypocalcemia
  - Hypocalcemia potentiates effects of hypermagnesemia

Anesthetic Considerations 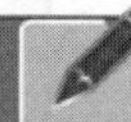

- ❖ Monitor ECG, BP and neuromuscular function, serial Ca^{2+} and Mg^{2+} levels
- ❖ Effects of hypermagnesemia include:
  - Potentiation of local anesthetic action
  - Potentiation of NMBA action by causing presynaptic NM blockade
- ❖ Thus, dose of NDMR used intra-operatively is reduced by 25–50%
- ❖ Hypermagnesemia can precipitate severe weakness in:
  - Patients with Eaton-Lambert syndrome
  - Myasthenic patients
  - Patients treated with small doses of defasciculating agonist
- ❖ Effects of hypermagnesemia on action of succinylcholine:
  - Prolongs action of succinylcholine
  - Also, it prevents succinylcholine provoked K^+ release
- ❖ Hyper Mg^{2+} potentiates vasodilatation and negative inotropic action of anesthetics
- ❖ Hypermagnesemia also aggravates hypotension seen with spinal anesthesia
- ❖ Urinary catheter can be used to monitor output if diuretics are used.

HYPOPHOSPHATEMIA

Introduction

Hypophosphatemia refers to inorganic phosphorus level less than 2.5 mg/dL.

Causes

- ❖ Intracellular shift of phosphorous:
  - During treatment of DKA:
    - Occurs due to insulin induced cellular uptake of phosphorous
    - Occurs 12–24 hours after initial therapy
  - Hyper-alimentation
  - ***Nutritional recovery syndrome***
  - Carbohydrate induced hypophosphatemia: ***refeeding syndrome***
  - Change from catabolic state to anabolic state
  - Respiratory alkalosis:
    - Increases rate of glycolysis
    - This in turn increases intracellular consumption of phosphorous
    - Effects of hyperventilation progress even after cessation of hyperventilation
  - Therapeutic hyperthermia
  - Acute correction of acidosis
  - Gram-negative sepsis and salicylate poisoning due to respiratory alkalosis
  - ***Neuroleptic malignant syndrome***
- ❖ Excessive renal losses:
  - Hyper-parathyroidism
  - Chronic alcoholics and alcohol withdrawal: *most common cause*
  - Diuretic therapy
  - Renal tubular defects, acute renal failure, following renal transplantation
  - Severe hypo-magnesemia
- ❖ Excessive GI losses:
  - Phosphorus binding antacids
  - Malabsorption syndrome

Pathophysiology

Hypophosphatemia results in:

- ❖ Low levels of ATP
- ❖ Low levels of 2,3–DPG
- ❖ Membrane phospholipid dysfunction: results in:
  - Defective phagocytosis
  - Defective chemotaxis
  - Reduced bactericidal activity

Clinical Features

- ❖ Severe life threatening organ dysfunction when serum P_i levels < 1 mg/dL
- ❖ Central nervous system:
  - Circumoral and finger tip paresthesias
  - Myopathy, reduced deep tendon reflexes, malaise
  - Encephalopathy, seizures, delirium, coma
- ❖ Cardiovascular:
  - Impaired myocardial function
  - Low cardiac output, hypotension
- ❖ Hematological:
  - Dysfunction of WBC, RBC and platelets
  - Reduced chemotaxis, phagocytosis, bactericidal activity
  - Immune dysfunction

- Reduced survival of WBC, RBC, platelets: spherocytosis
- Tissue hypoxia due to low 2, 3-DPG levels
- Metabolic acidosis
- Miscellaneous:
  - Respiratory failure
  - Rhabdomyolysis if severe hypophosphatemia

Investigations

Urinary phosphorus:

- If urinary P_i <100 mg/day: Suggests extra-renal causes
- If urinary P_i > 100 mg/day: implies renal loss of P_i

Treatment

- Calculation of P_i deficit:
  - P_i deficit = V_d {(desired P_i level) – (current P_i level)}
  - V_d = 400 mL/kg
  - The calculated deficit to be given at not more than 0.25 mmol/kg over 4–6 hours
- Phosphorous repletion:
  - Severe or symptomatic hypo-phosphatemia
    - 0.2–0.68 mmol/kg or 5–16 mg/kg elemental phosphorus
    - Rate of infusion < 0.25 mmol/kg over 4–6 hours to avoid hypocalcemia
  - Moderate hypo-phosphatemia: 15 mmol boluses (465 mg) with 100 mL NS over 2 hours
  - Mild hypo-phosphatemia:
    - Oral phosphorus < 30 mmol/day (1 g/day) as higher doses cause diarrhea
    - Available as sodium or potassium phosphate
    - Milk (contains 100 mg/dL or 33 mmol/L of phosphorus)
- Choice of fluid and duration of therapy:
  - Potassium phosphate: 93 mg/dL of phosphorus
  - Sodium phosphate: 93 mg/dL of phosphorus
  - Oral phosphorus started once serum P_i > 2 mg/dL
  - P_i supplements continued for 5–10 days to replenish body stores
- Monitors: Phosphorus and other electrolytes after 6 hours of initiating therapy
- Precautions:
  - Administer cautiously in hypo-calcemic patients: risk of precipitating severe hypocalcemia
  - If hyper-calcemia present, P_i administration may cause metastatic calcification
  - Use with caution if renal failure present and avoid hyper-phosphatemia

Anesthetic Considerations 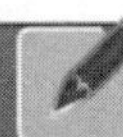

- Hyperglycemia and respiratory alkalosis have to be avoided
- Avoid DNS and dextrose containing fluids
- Neuromuscular blockade monitoring
- Postoperative ventilation may be required if severe hypophosphatemia.

HYPERPHOSPHATEMIA

Introduction

Hyper-phosphatemia refers to serum inorganic P_i levels more than 5 mg/dL.

Etiology

- Increased intestinal absorption:
  - Phosphorus containing cathartics
  - Granulomatous diseases
  - Vitamin-D therapy
- Parenteral administration:
  - IV phosphate salts
  - IV lipid infusions
- Internal redistribution:
  - Acute metabolic/respiratory acidosis
  - Reduced insulin levels
  - Clonidine administration
- Binding to serum proteins:
  - Plasma cell dyscrasias
  - Liver failure
- Cellular release:
  - Rhabdomyolysis
  - Tumor lysis as in:
    - ***Burkitts lymphoma***
    - Lymphoblastic lymphomas
  - Sepsis
- Decreased renal excretion:
  - Renal insufficiency when GFR < 25 mL/min
  - Hypo-parathyroidism, pseudo-hypoparathyroidism
  - Tumoral calcinosis
  - ***Pseudoxanthoma elasticum***
  - ***Infantile hypo-phosphatasia***
  - Hypo-parathyroidism, hyperthyroidism, adrenal insufficiency
  - Bisphosphonate therapy

Clinical Features

Those of:

- Hypocalcemia
- Hypomagnesemia
- Renal failure

- Risk of metastatic calcification if: Calcium x-phosphorus product > 70 mg^2/dL^2

Investigations

- Normal renal function with P_i excretion more than 1500 mg/day suggests excessive P_i supply
- Abnormal renal function with low GFR suggests reduced renal P_i excretion
- Normal function and P_i excretion less than 1500 mg/day suggests P_i reabsorption

Treatment

- Eliminate cause
- Correct hyperphosphatemia:
  - Restrict intake of calcium phosphate to less than 200 mg/day
  - Increase renal elimination:
    - 1–2 L of normal saline over 4–6 hours
    - Acetazolamide 500 mg QID
  - Increase GIT losses:
    - Enteric aluminium hydroxide 30–45 mg Q6H
    - Sucralfate, calcium citrate, calcium carbonate
  - Calcimetics: useful in patients with renal failure
  - Phosphorus binders use with caution in patients with ARF:
    - ***Sevelamer hydrochloride:*** binds bile acids
    - ***Lanthanum carbonate***
  - Hemodialysis and peritoneal dialysis
- Correct hypocalcemia: Give calcium supplements only when serum P_i < 2 mmol/L or 6 mg/dL

Anesthetic Considerations

- Monitor renal functions, serum P_i and Ca^{2+} levels
- Secondary hypo-calcemia to be excluded
- Neuromuscular monitoring
- Avoid hypoventilation and acidosis.

PARACETAMOL/ACETAMINOPHEN POISONING

Introduction

- Analgesic-antipyretic which is used very commonly
- It is one of the most common drugs causing Drug-Induced Liver Injury (DILI)

Prevalence

- Considered safe when taken at the usual therapeutic doses up to 4000 mg/24 hours
- Even slightly higher doses can be hepatotoxic in susceptible patients like alcoholics
- Considered to be the most common cause of acute liver failure in the United States
- Paracetamol poisoning accounts for approximately 50% of acute liver failure cases
- If overdose is identified early, mortality rates are extremely low
- However, once acute liver failure has developed, mortality rate approaches 28%

Mechanism of Toxicity

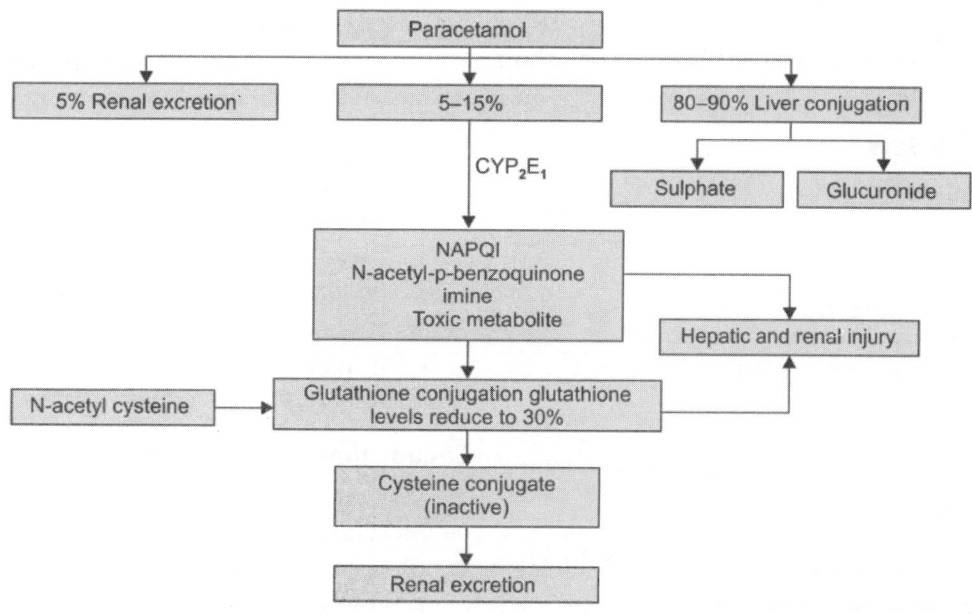

- Where there is ingestion of high levels of paracetamol, excessive amount of NABQI is formed
- This overwhelms the hepatic glutathione conjugation capacity
- When the glutathione stores are depleted to 30%, NABQI precipitates proteins in the liver and kidney by oxidant injury
- This causes liver failure, centrilobular hepatic necrosis and acuter tubular necrosis
- Centrilobular necrosis seen as CYP_2E_1, which produces NABQI is maximally concentrated around the central veins and minimally around the portal triad

Factors Influencing Biochemical Toxicity

- Excessive intake of paracetamol
- Excessive cytochrome P450 activity
- Decreased capacity for glucuronidation or sulfation
- Depletion of glutathione stores

Toxic Dose

- Maximum recommended daily dose of paracetamol is:
  - 80 mg/kg in children
  - 4 g in adults
- Toxicity results from:
  - Single ingestion of > 200 mg/kg in children or > 10 g in adults
  - 24–hour ingestion of > 200 mg/kg in children or > 10 g in adults
  - 150 mg/kg in children or > 6 g in adults per day for 2 consecutive days
- Single dose ingestion of more than 350 mg/kg results in severe hepatotoxicity
- 5–6 g/day for a few days in alcoholics (as alcohol induces CYP_2E_1)

Fatal Period: 3–5 days

Clinical Presentation

Four stages of toxicity:

- Stage I:
  - Between 0–24 hours
  - Symptoms are absent or non-specific
  - If present, symptoms include:
    - Anorexia, malaise
    - Nausea, vomiting
  - No clinical/laboratory evidence of hepatic injury except hypokalemia
- Stage II:
  - Between 24–72 hours
  - Minimal clinical manifestations
  - Usually there will be improvement in symptoms present during the first stage
  - Symptoms if present during this stage include:
    - Generalized abdominal pain
    - Hepatic tenderness
    - No other clinical evidence of hepatic injury
  - Laboratory abnormalities:
    - Lab evidence of hepatic injury begins to appear at this stage
    - Elevated levels of AST: *most sensitive*
    - Raised ALT, serum bilirubin
    - Prolonged prothrombin time if severe toxicity
- Stage III:
  - Between 72–96 hours
  - Recurrence of stage I symptoms such as anorexia, nausea and vomiting
  - Clinical evidence of hepatic and renal injury appear and include:
    - Jaundice, hypoglycemia
    - Coagulopathy, encephalopathy
    - Flapping tremors
    - Anuria
  - Laboratory abnormalities at this stage include:
    - Peaking of AST levels
    - Frank hepatic failure
    - Metabolic acidosis
    - Coagulopathy
    - Renal failure
    - Pancreatitis
- Stage IV:
  - Presents beyond 96 hours
  - Can progress to either:
    - Clinical improvement and recovery
    - Deterioration to multiorgan failure and death
  - Features consist of:
    - Hemorrhagic pancreatitis, DIC
    - Cardiac arrhythmias
    - Confusion, coma
  - Death occurs within 3–5 days of onset of stage IV symptoms
  - If patient survives hepatic failure, complete resolution with recovery occurs

Circumstances of Poisoning

- Very rarely suicidal
- Most often due to accidental overdose
- Especially common in children due to inadequate glucuronide conjugating ability

Clinical Factors Affecting Toxicity

- Age:
  - Older patients are at a higher risk of developing paracetamol toxicity
  - Adults above 40 years are at a higher risk of:
    - Hepatic failure
    - Liver transplantation
- Nutritional status:
  - Malnutrition and prolonged fasting predispose to paracetamol toxicity
  - Hepatic glucuronidation is dependent upon carbohydrate reserves
  - In malnourished patients, carbohydrates reserves are minimal or absent
  - Thus, hepatic glucuronidation in impaired in these patients
  - This leads to enhanced microsomal metabolism and NABQI production
- Acute alcohol ingestion:
  - Alcohol is a substrate for CYP_2E_1 enzyme
  - Thus, alcohol may compete with paracetamol for CYP_2E_1 binding sites
  - Therefore, concomitant alcohol ingestion may reduce NABQI formation
  - Acute alcohol ingestion may therefore prevent hepatotoxicity
  - Incidence of hepatotoxicity is lesser in those who overdose PCT with alcohol
- Chronic alcohol ingestion:
  - Not associated with increased risk of toxicity following a single overdose
  - However, risk is increased following multiple sub-therapeutic doses of PCT
  - This is because chronic alcohol abuse induces CYP_2E_1 enzyme
  - This results in enhanced generation of NABQI causing hepatotoxicity
- Chronic liver disease:
  - Not associated with an increased risk of hepatotoxicity
  - This is because the levels of CYP_{450} enzyme is lesser in this population
  - This may offer some degree of hepatoprotection following overdose
  - However, elimination $T_{1/2}$ of PCT is prolonged in these patients by 2–2.5 hours
  - Thus, the daily dose of paracetamol should be restricted to 2000 mg/day
- Tobacco use:
  - Tobacco smoke contains CYP_2A_1 inducers and increases oxidative metabolism
  - Thus, tobacco consumption increases the risk of mortality following overdose
- Other medications:
  - Concomitant use of medicines which induce CYP_2E_1 enhances risk of toxicity
  - These drugs include:
    - Anticonvulsants:
      - Carbamazepine
      - Phenobarbital
      - Phenytoin
    - Antituberculosis drugs:
      - Isoniazid
      - Rifampicin
- Herbal products:
  - Simultaneous use of herbal products which induce CYP_{450} increases toxicity
  - These include:
    - St. Johns wort
    - Garlic, germander

Diagnosis

- Routine blood investigations:
  - Complete blood count
  - ESR, hemoglobin
  - Bleeding time, clotting time: Coagulopathy common
- Liver function tests
- Renal function tests
- Plasma drug levels:
  - Plasma acetaminophen levels are obtained within 4–24 hours following overdose
  - This value is plotted on a ***Rumack-Matthew*** nomogram
  - This nomogram was derived from retrospective analysis of PCT overdose patients
  - The nomogram separates possible toxicity from unlikely toxicity
  - The nomogram applies only to:
    - A single sample
    - Obtained after a single ingestion
    - Within the window period (4–24 hours)
  - The nomogram cannot be used to predict outcomes if:
    - Recurrent/ chronic PCT exposures
    - Samples obtained outside the window period
  - Obtaining multiple samples following acute overdose is not indicated
  - Useful to predict the risk of hepatotoxicity
  - If the plasma level falls above the nomogram line:
    - Risk of hepatotoxicity (ALT > 1000 IU/mL) is 60%
    - Risk of renal failure is 1%
    - Risk of mortality is 5%
    - This necessitates antidote therapy

- If plasma levels are below the nomogram line:
  - Risk of hepatotoxicity is only 1%
  - Antidote therapy is not required
  - All patients usually recover without complications

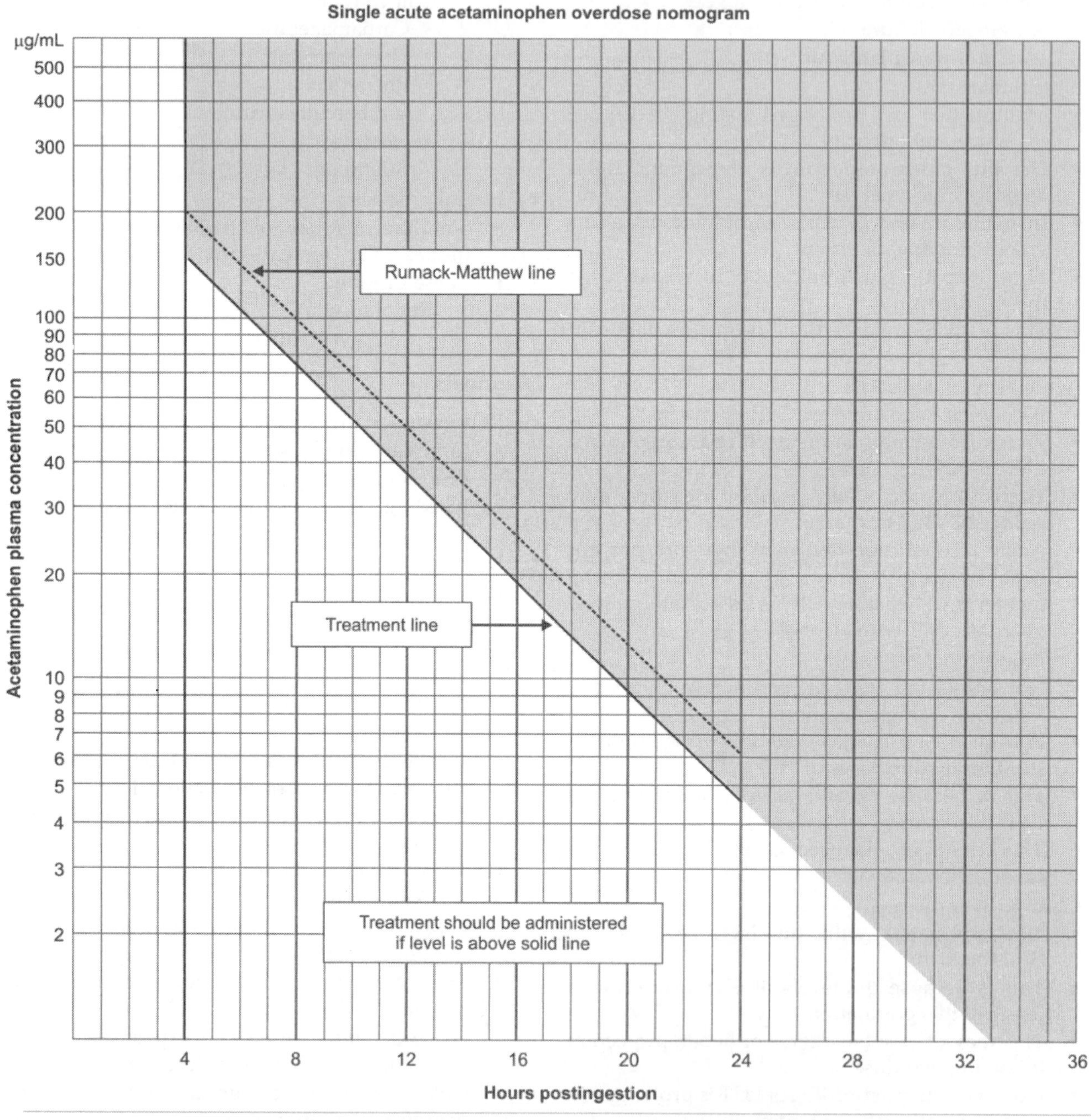

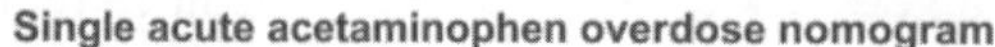

Nomogram: acetaminophen plasma concentration vs time after acetaminophen ingestion (adapted with permission from Rumack and Matthew. *Pediatrics*. 1975;55:871-875). The nomogram has been developed to estimate the probability of whether a plasma acetaminophen concentration in relation to the interval postingestion will result in hepatotoxicity and, therefore, whether acetylcysteine therapy should be administered.

Caitions for use of the chart:

1. Time coordinates refer to time postingestion.
2. Graph relates only to plasma concentrations following a single, acute overdose ingestion.
3. The treatment line is plotted 25% below the Rumack-Matthew line to allow for potential errors in plasma acetaminophen assays and estimated time from ingestion of an overdose (Rumack et al. *Arch Intern Med*. 1981;141 (suppl):380-385).

Fig. 1: Rumack Matthew nomogram.

Treatment

- Monitor:
  - BT, CT to check for coagulopathies
  - Prothrombin time helpful to predict course of liver disease
  - FDPs and D-dimer assay to diagnose DIC
  - Plasma levels of PCT
  - Serum amylase levels to detect pancreatitis
  - Fractional excretion of sodium, blood urea and creatinine to detect ATN
  - Strict intake output chart maintenance
- Non-specific measures:
  - Airway:
    - Check if airway is patent
    - Use head tilt, chin lift and jaw thrust maneuver
  - Breathing:
    - Check if spontaneous breathing is present
    - Mechanical ventilation may be required if efforts are inadequate
  - Circulation:
    - Check for pressure of carotid pulse
    - Secure IV lines and start IV fluids
    - Avoid IM injections to prevent hematomas due to coagulopathy
  - Gastric decontamination:
    - Gastric decontamination maneuvers include:
      - Induced vomiting with syrup ipecac
      - Activated charcoal therapy
      - Gastric lavage
      - Whole bowel irrigation
    - Not recommended nowadays due to high success with NAC therapy
    - The only maneuver recommended is activated charcoal therapy
  - Activated charcoal (AC):
    - 1 g/kg orally is recommended within first 4 hours after overdose
    - This is because PCT is completely absorbed from GIT within 4 hours
    - Thus, AC is not used in those who present beyond 4 hours of ingestion
    - Maximum dose of activated charcoal recommended is 50 grams
    - Administration of AC is reduces the incidence of hepatotoxicity
    - However, it should be withheld in:
      - Sedated patients
      - Those who are unable to protect the airway
- Specific measures:
  - Goal of therapy is to replenish glutathione levels in liver
  - N-acetyl cysteine (NAC):
    - In early PCT poisoning (< 8 hrs after ingestion):
      - Prevents binding of NABQI to hepatic macromolecules
      - This is done by:
        - Acting as a glutathione precursor/ substitute
        - Acting as a sulphate precursor
        - Directly reducing NABQI back to PCT
    - In established PCT toxicity (> 24 hrs after ingestion):
      - NAC reduces hepatic necrosis by:
        - Acting as an antioxidant
        - Reducing neutrophil infiltration
        - Increasing microcirculatory blood flow
        - Increasing tissue oxygen delivery and extraction
    - Effectiveness:
      - Serious hepatotoxicity is rare if NAC is administered within 8 hours
      - Key to effective treatment is to start therapy before onset of hepatotoxicity
    - NAC regimens:
      - Both IV and oral regimens are available for PCT poisoning
      - However, both regimens are effective with minimal differences
    - IV regimen:
      - Indicated in:
        - Vomiting
        - Pancreatitis
        - Bowel ileus
        - Bowel injury
        - Hepatic failure
      - Follows a 20–hour protocol
      - 20% NAC (200 mg/ml) is used
      - Loading dose:
        - 150 mg/kg in 200 mL of 5% dextrose
        - Given over 15– 60 minutes

- First maintenance dose:
  - 50 mg/kg in 500 mL of 5% dextrose
  - Given over the next 4 hours (12.5 mg/kg/hour)
- Second maintenance dose:
  - 100 mg/kg in 1000 mL of 5% dextrose
  - Given over 16 hours (6.25 mg/kg/hour)

– Oral regimen:
  - Follows a 72–hour protocol
  - 10 and 20% solutions of NAC are available
  - These are diluted to 5% solution for oral administration
  - Loading dose: 140 mg/kg
  - Maintenance dose: 70 mg/kg every 4 hours for 17 doses

- Methionine therapy:
  – Less effective than NAC
  – 2.5 mg orally Q4H up to a total of 10 grams

❖ Complication management:
- Protein restriction, lactulose and oral neomycin for hepatic encephalopathy
- FFP and heparin for DIC
- Antibiotic prophylaxis
- Liver transplant: Early transplant beneficial
- Fulminant hepatic failure:
  – NAC therapy continued past standard regimen until:
    - Patient recovers
    - Receives transplant/dies
  – Correct coagulopathy and acidosis
- Hemodialysis: may be required in severe cases with high plasma levels of PCT
- Monitor and aggressively treat cerebral edema

Complications of Therapy

❖ Anaphylactic reactions with IV regimen

❖ Rotten egg taste with oral NAC regimen (due to –SH group)

❖ Nausea and vomiting with oral NAC regimens:
- Avoided by diluting the 10–20% NAC solutions to 5% using chilled beverages
- Odour can be minimized by using NG tube to administer the solution
- Persistent nausea and vomiting may require metoclopramide 0.1 mg/kg IV

❖ NG tube administration of NAC may be required to prevent vomiting

❖ Dose dependent diarrhea with oral NAC regimens (resolves on continual therapy)

Treatment Algorithm for PCT Poisoning

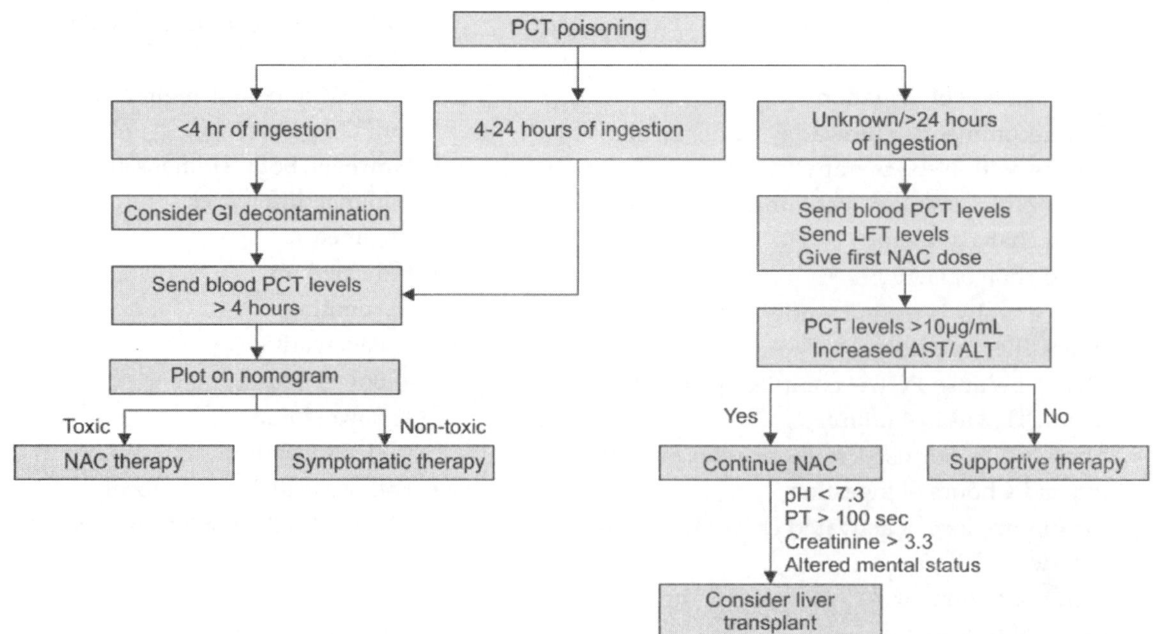

Poor Prognosticators

- Metabolic acidosis, pH < 7.3 despite fluid resuscitation
- Combination of coagulopathy (PT > 100)
- Renal insufficiency (creatinine > 3.3 mg/dL)
- Grade III/IV hepatic encephalopathy.

ORGANOPHOSPHORUS POISONING

Introduction

- These compounds are derivates of phosphoric acid, used mainly as insecticides
- They are potent cholinesterase inhibitors causing cholinergic toxicity
- Use of organophosphates has declined due to development of carbamate insecticides
- Incidence of toxic organophosphate exposure is 30,00,000 persons per year
- Incidence of fatalities from organophosphate exposure is 3,00,000 persons per year

Classification of Organophosphate Compounds

- Alkyl phosphates:
  - HETP, OMPA
  - TEPP, malathion
  - Trichlorfon
- Aryl phosphates:
  - Parathiol (follidol), chlorothion
  - Paraoxon, diazion (TIK–20)
  - Methylparathion

Routes of Absorption

- GI tract
- Transconjunctival
- Transdermal
- Mucous membrane
- Inhalation

Fatal Dose

- Parathion: 80 mg IM/ 175 mg orally
- Malathion and diazinon: 1 g orally

Fatal Period

- Less than 24 hours in untreated cases
- Complete recovery in 10 days if treated early

Causes of Death

- Respiratory muscle paralysis
- Respiratory arrest due to failure of respiratory centre
- Intense broncho-constriction
- Cardiovascular collapse due to vasodilatation

Pathophysiology

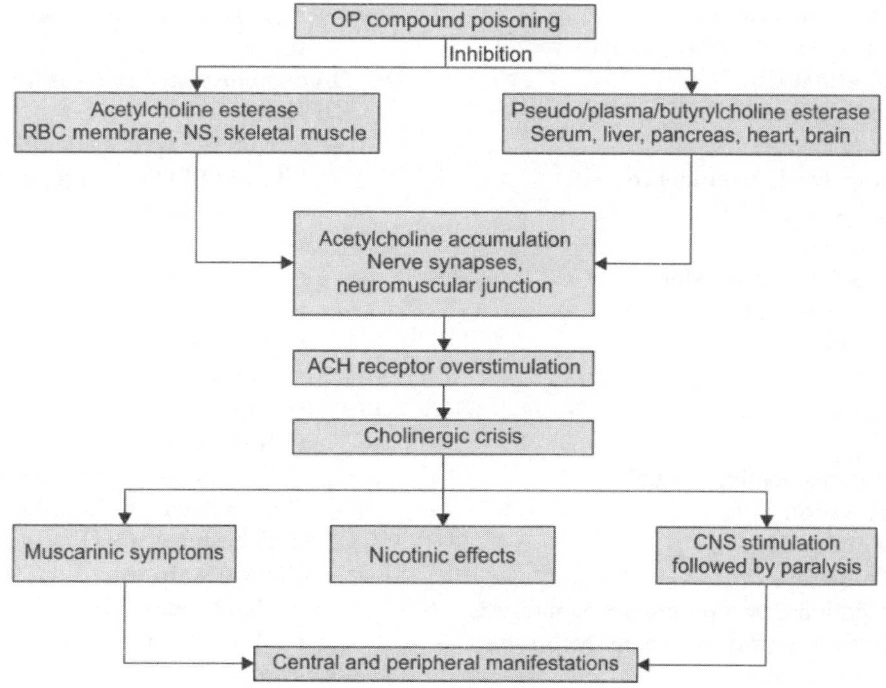

Clinical Features

- Immediate sequelae:
  - Onset of symptoms:
    - Most rapid following inhalational exposure
    - Slowest following transdermal absorption
    - Oral exposure causes symptoms within 3 hours
    - Transdermal absorption may result in symptoms after 12 hours
    - Manifests maximally in 24 hours
    - Lipophilic agents:
      - Examples:
        - Fenthion
        - Malathion
      - Associated with delay in onset of symptoms up to 5 days
      - Manifestations are also more prolonged (greater than 30 days)
  - RS/GI symptoms are more marked depending on route of entry
  - Hydrocarbon/garlic like odour from patient
  - Muscarinic manifestations:
    - S: Salivation
    - L: Lacrimation
    - U: Urination
    - D: Defecation
    - G: GI pain/ distress
    - E: Emesis
    - Respiratory:
      - Bronchoconstriction, dyspnea
      - Bronchorrhea, cyanosis
      - Persistent reactive airway disease rarely
    - Gastrointestinal:
      - Anorexia, cramps
      - Nausea, diarrhea
      - Vomiting, fecal incontinence
      - Tenesmus
    - Cardiovascular:
      - Bradycardia, hypotension
      - Pulmonary edema
      - Arrhythmias:
  - Heart block
  - QT_c prolongation
    - Pupils:
      - Miosis occasionally unequal
      - Blurred vision
  - Nicotinic manifestations:
    - Striated muscle:
      - Fasciculations, cramps, areflexia, paralysis
      - Respiratory paralysis, acute respiratory failure and death
    - Sympathetic ganglia: hypertension, tachycardia, pallor, mydriasis
    - Neurological:
      - Restlessness, drowsiness, emotional lability, slurred speech
      - Headache, ataxia, tremors, weakness
      - Confusion, coma, convulsions
    - ***Chromolacryorrhea:***
      - Formation of red tears
      - Occurs due to porphyrin accumulation in lacrimal glands
- Delayed sequelae:
  - ***Intermediate syndrome (IMS):***
    - Seen in 10–40% of patients
    - Occurs 1–4 days after exposure and resolution of cholinergic excess
    - Most patients have complete resolution within 2–3 weeks
    - Risk factors for IMS:
      - Exposure to highly fat-soluble OP agent
      - Inadequate doses of oximes
      - Rare following carbamate poisoning
    - Clinical features:
      - Characteristic neurological findings
      - Paralysis of neck flexors causing neck flexion weakness
      - Cranial nerves abnormalities
      - Proximal muscle weakness
      - Decreased deep tendon reflexes
      - Respiratory insufficiency
    - Aggressive antidote therapy and respiratory support
  - ***Organophosphate induced delayed neuropathy (OPIDN):***
    - Occurs 1–3 weeks after exposure
    - Risk of OPIDN is independent of severity of acute manifestations
    - Drugs causing OPIDN:
      - Chlorpyrifos
      - Leptophos
      - Malathion
      - Merphos
      - Mipafox
      - Trichlorfon
      - Triorthocresylphosphate (TOCP)
    - Occurs due to inhibition of neuropathy target esterase (NTE)
    - Clinical features:
      - Mixed sensori-motor syndrome
      - May resemble Guillain-Barre syndrome
      - Begins with stocking-glove paresthesias

- Followed by symmetrical flaccid paralysis of lower extremities
- Ascends to involve upper extremities
- Antidotal therapy does not help
- Prognosis:
  - Most cases of mild delayed neurotoxicity improve with time
  - In severe cases spasticity of lower limbs causes permanent disability
- Irreversible neuropsychiatric deficits may occur such as:
  - Decreased memory
  - Parkinsonism

Diagnosis

- Mainly clinical diagnosis
- Symptoms, signs and garlicky odour from patient
- Atropine test:
  - 2 mg atropine given IV/6 mg given IM
  - Normal persons will have marked atropinization
  - In OP poisoning, symptoms are relieved and secretions decrease
- RBC and plasma acetylcholinesterase levels:
  - Measurement of RBC cholinesterase activity indicates the degree of toxicity
  - Cholinesterase levels reduce to less than 50% of baseline values
  - RBC cholinesterase is a more accurate indicator of synaptic cholinesterase
  - Plasma cholinesterase levels, however are more readily available
  - Sequential measurements help in determining effectiveness of oxime therapy
- Non-specific indicators:
  - Leucocytosis
  - Hypo/hyperglycemia
  - Abnormal LFTs
  - Raised serum amylase: pancreatitis like findings
  - Pulmonary edema on chest X-ray
  - ECG:
    - Heart block, prolonged QT_c
    - Idioventricular rhythm
    - VF/torsades-de-pointes
- Electromyography:
  - Helps identify OP poisoning
  - Quantifies ACHE at the neuromuscular junction

Treatment

- Decontamination:
  - Personnel protection:
    - Personnel must wear protective clothing
    - Neoprene/nitrile gloves are used instead of latex for better protection
  - Dermal decontamination:
    - All contaminated clothing must be removed
    - Exposed areas are washed with soap, water and alkaline solution
    - A second wash with diluted ethanol may be done
    - Thorough irrigation should be performed of:
      - Conjunctival recesses
      - Skin folds
      - Fingernails
      - Scalp and hair
  - Gastric decontamination:
    - Useful if given within 1 hour of ingestion
    - Single dose activated charcoal 1 g/kg (50 g in adults) can be used
    - Gastric lavage may be given prior to charcoal therapy
    - However, it is associated with increased risk of pulmonary aspiration
    - Thus, gastric lavage is limited to intubated patients
    - Forced emesis is currently contraindicated
- Airway:
  - *Provide 100% oxygen via facemask*
  - Keep airway patent: head tilt, chin lift, jaw thrust
  - Gentle suctioning to remove secretions
  - *Early intubation* is often needed due to nicotinic respiratory paralysis
  - Intubation/tracheostomy if:
    - Coma, bronchospasm
    - Respiratory failure, excess secretions, seizures
    - Depressed mental status
  - Succinylcholine may cause prolonged paralysis and is avoided
  - On the other hand, NDMR may be less effective at standard doses
- Antimuscarinic therapy
  - Atropine:
    - *First line* of treatment for OP poisoning
    - 2-4 mg IV is given as the initial dose in adults
    - 0.05 mg/kg is given as the initial dose in children
    - Dose is *doubled* every 5–10 mins until signs of atropinization occur
    - Characteristics of full atropinization:
      - Dry skin and mucous membranes
      - Tachycardia > 110 bpm
      - Hypertension
      - Reduced secretions
      - Decreased/ absent bowel sounds
      - Dilated pupils
      - Absence of bronchospasm

- Full atropinization has to be maintained for at least 24 hours
- IV infusion can be used to maintain full atropinization:
  - Initiated at 10–20% of the total loading dose per hour
  - Maximum dose of 2 mg/hour
- Atropine does not block the nicotinic receptors
- Thus, it does not address the muscular manifestations of OP poisoning
- Oxygen therapy has to be initiated preferably prior to atropinization
- This is because of the risk of inducing ventricular tachyarrhythmias
- However, in the absence of oxygen, there is no need to delay therapy

- Glycopyrrolate:
  - Glycopyrrolate has similar actions to atropine
  - However, it does not cross the blood-brain barrier
  - Thus, it does not reverse the CNS manifestations of OP poisoning
  - However, it can be used in combination with atropine therapy
  - This is done when atropine causes CNS toxicity with inadequate reversal of peripheral muscarinic manifestations
  - The usual dose of glycopyrrolate used is *1–2 mg IV*
  - This dose can be repeated as required until symptoms subside

❖ Cholinesterase reactivators:

- Agents used:
  - *Pralidoxime* (2–pyridine aldoxime methiodide)
  - *Diacetyl monoxime* (DAM)
  - *Obidoxime*
- Rationale:
  - Restores ACHE activity by regenerating phosphorylated ACHE
  - Reactivators have to be started as early as possible after OP poisoning
  - This is due to aging of ACHE enzyme (usually within 24 hours)
  - These are continued till the patient is clinically well
  - Therefore, these agents treat nicotinic, muscarinic and CNS symptoms
  - However, pralidoxime should not be used without concurrent atropine
  - This is because transient oxime-induced ACHE inhibition may worsen symptoms
- Indications:
  - Signs of cholinergic toxicity
  - Those with neuromuscular dysfunction
  - Exposure to OP compounds known to cause OIDN:
    - Chlorpyrifos
    - Leptophos
    - Malathion
    - Merphos
    - Mipafox
    - Trichlorfon
    - Triorthocresylphosphate
- Dosage:
  - 1–2 g (30 mg/Kg) given slow IV as 5% solution over 30 minutes
  - In children 25–50 mg/kg may be given IV
  - The drug has to be administered slowly due to risk of cardiac arrest
  - This can be repeated at 6–12 hour intervals for 24–48 hours
  - Alternatively, therapy can be continued as IV infusion:
    - 8 mg/kg/hour in adults
    - 10–20 mg/kg/hour in children
- Maximum dose: less than 12 g in 24 hours
- Not to be administered in:
  - Asymptomatic patients
  - Patients with carbamate poisoning and minimal symptoms

❖ Treatment of complications:

- Convulsions:
  - Treated with benzodiazepines and antidote therapy
  - Preferred agents:
    - Midazolam
    - Lorazepam
    - Diazepam
  - Prophylactic diazepam also reduces incidence of cognitive dysfunction
  - Currently, there is no evidence for anticonvulsants such as phenytoin
- Hypotension:
  - IV line is secured and baseline blood sample taken for ACHE levels
  - Large fluid boluses of normal saline can be given

- Bradycardia:
  - Usually secondary to bronchospasm
  - Atropine can be used to treat bradycardia
- Pulmonary edema and bronchospasm: Oxygen, intubate, CPPV, atropine
- Cardiac arrest: resuscitate as per ACLS guidelines

❖ Avoid agents which potentiate poisoning such as:
- Succinylcholine
- Ester anesthetics
- Beta blockers

CARBON MONOXIDE POISONING

Introduction

❖ Carbon monoxide is a gas formed by incomplete combustion of hydrocarbons
❖ It is a common cause of occupational poisoning causing mortality and morbidity
❖ This is due to difficulty in environmental detection even with high concentrations
❖ It is associated with increased risk of delayed sequelae despite adequate acute therapy

Prevalence

❖ Fire related smoke inhalation causes most cases of CO poisoning
❖ Non-fire related CO poisoning accounts for up to 1200 mortalities per year
❖ Thus, it is one of the most common causes of poisoning related deaths
❖ It most commonly occurs during winter season in cold climates

Physiological Characteristics of Carbon Monoxide

❖ Colorless, odourless and tasteless gas
- Molecular weight: 28.01 Da
- Density: 0.968 (air is 1)

❖ Blood carboxyhemoglobin levels:
- Non-smokers: 0–5%
- Smokers: 5–10%

❖ TLV– TWA: 50 ppm (Threshold Limit Value- Time Weighted Average)

Circumstances of Poisoning

❖ Closed space burns
❖ Fires and natural disasters
❖ Underground mine explosions
❖ Faulty furnaces
❖ Motor vehicle exhaust
❖ Hookah smoking

Sources of Carbon Monoxide

❖ Anesthetic adsorbents
❖ Banked blood
❖ Boats
❖ Camp stoves and lanterns
❖ Charcoal grills
❖ Gasoline powered equipment such as generators
❖ Natural combustion furnaces
❖ Methylene bromide (industrial solvent)
❖ Methylene chloride (paint remover)

Pathophysiology

❖ Hemotoxicity:
- CO binds to hemoglobin, rendering it incapable of delivering oxygen to tissues
- Thus, arterial O_2 content is low despite adequate partial pressures of oxygen
- CO also causes a leftward shift in the oxyhemoglobin dissociation curve
- This decreases the offloading of oxygen from hemoglobin to tissues
- The net result is a reduced ability of oxygen delivery by hemoglobin to the tissues

❖ Cardiotoxicity:
- Myoglobin has 60 times greater affinity for CO than oxygen
- Almost 15% of the total body store of CO is extravascular, bound to myoglobin
- The myocardial myoglobin bound CO is responsible for myocardial dysfunction

❖ Neurotoxicity:
- CO exposure causes inactivation of cytochrome oxidase
- This in turn causes endothelial damage and destroys microvasculature
- On reperfusion, platelets adhere to these regions of compromised vasculature
- This eventually results in ischemia-reperfusion injury
- CO also causes peroxidation of lipids and damage to the brain
- Another factor contributing to neurotoxicity is neuronal apoptosis

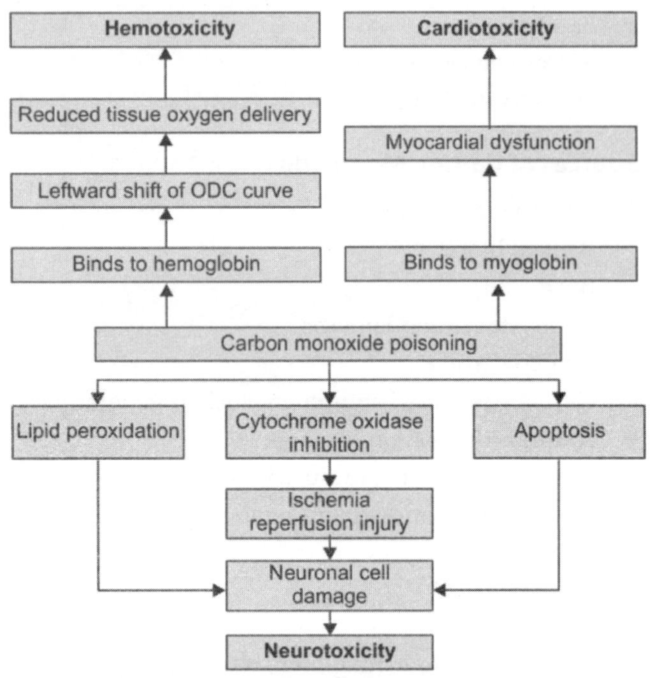

Toxicokinetics

- CO is readily absorbed after inhalation
- After absorption, CO is carried in the blood primarily bound to hemoglobin
- Hemoglobin has 200–250 times greater affinity for CO than oxygen
- Thus, CO is mainly confined to the intravascular compartment
- However, over time, it binds to myoglobin and is transported into the tissues
- The ***Coburn-Forster-Kane*** equation is used to calculate the concentration of COHb
- This equation assumes that the patient weighs 70 kgs and is not anemic

$$\text{COHb (\%)} = \frac{100}{1 + (643/\text{ppm CO})}$$

- The half-life of CO ranges between 249–320 minutes on room air
- With 100% oxygen, the half-life reduces to 47-80 minutes.

Clinical Features

- Symptoms:
  - Largely non-specific symptoms at presentation
  - Most common symptom is headache
  - Others include:
    - Malaise, nausea, vomiting
    - Loss of consciousness
- Signs:
  - *Cherry red* appearance of lips and skin (not very sensitive)
  - Cutaneous bullae after severe exposures (rare)
  - Neurological:
    - Most sensitive organ to CO poisoning is the CNS
    - Altered mental status
    - Seizures, syncope, coma
    - Ataxia
    - Retinal hemorrhages
  - Cardiovascular:
    - Myocardial ischemia (in up to one-third of the patients)
    - Transient myocardial stunning in prolonged exposures (lasts < 24 hours)
    - Ventricular arrhythmias
  - *Delayed neuropsychiatric syndrome (DNPS):*
    - Occurs in up to 40% of patients with significant CO exposure
    - Can occur anywhere between 3–240 days after apparent recovery
    - Incidence of DNPS correlates poorly with COHb levels
    - Manifestations include:
      - Varying degrees of cognitive deficits
      - Personality changes:
        - Psychosis
        - Dementia
      - Movement disorders like:
        - Parkinsonism
        - Chorea
      - Focal neurological deficits
      - Amnestic syndromes
      - Cortical blindness
      - Apraxia, agnosia and incontinence

Diagnosis

- Diagnosis is made based on history, physical examination and cooximetric COHb levels
- Pulse oximetry:
  - Cannot be used to screen for carbon monoxide poisoning
  - Usually normal as carboxy-hemoglobin is interpreted as oxy-hemoglobin
  - This is due to the similar extinction coefficients of COHb and oxyHb
  - Thus, pulse-oximetry is mostly normal even in the setting of severe poisoning

- Carboxy-hemoglobin levels:
  - Technique of measurement:
    - Usually done using a co-oximeter
    - This device reads the% of total hemoglobin saturated with CO
    - Arterial or venous blood can be used for measurements
    - This is because CO extraction across the capillary bed is very low
    - Thus, values obtained from arterial and venous blood usually correlate
  - Levels of carboxyhemoglobin:
    - 5% in normal individuals
    - Up to 8% in neonates due to fetal hemoglobin
    - Up to 10% in smokers
- Direct blood CO levels using infrared spectrophotometry
- ABG analysis:
  - Blood PO_2 levels tend to be normal
  - This is because PO_2 reflects O_2 dissolved in blood which is not affected by CO
  - Shows severe lactic acidosis
- ECG shows features of ischemia
- Cardiac enzymes (creatinine phosphokinase) may be elevated
- CT scan
- MRI
- Assessment of regional cerebral perfusion:
  - Positron emission tomography (PET)
  - Single photon emission CT (SPECT)

Treatment

- Oxygen:
  - CO is removed almost exclusively in the pulmonary circulation
  - This occurs through competitive binding of hemoglobin to oxygen
  - The half-life of CO ranges between 249-320 minutes on room air
  - With 100% oxygen, the half-life reduces to 47-80 minutes
  - Thus, high flow O_2 via non-rebreathing mask is the most important intervention
  - Oxygen therapy is continued till COHb < 5% in those who do not require HBO
  - Patients with altered sensorium should be intubated and ventilated with FiO_2 of 1
  - Concomitant cyanide toxicity should be considered in smoke inhalation
- Hyperbaric oxygen therapy:
  - Rationale:
    - Exposes patient to 100% oxygen under supra-atmospheric conditions
    - This results in a decrease in the half-life of COHb to 30 minutes
    - The dissolved oxygen in blood also increases with HBO
    - This increases the delivery of non-Hb bound oxygen to the tissues
  - Indications:
    - Age > 36 years
    - Prolonged CO exposure > 24 hours (even if intermittent)
    - CO level > 25%
    - Loss of consciousness
    - Coma, seizures
    - Altered mental status (GCS < 15), confusion
    - Abnormal cerebellar function
    - Evidence of end organ ischemia:
      - ECG changes
      - Chest pain
    - Severe metabolic acidosis (pH < 7.1)
    - Fetal distress in pregnancy
    - Use of HBO in low risk patients is not recommended
  - Timing of therapy:
    - Benefit of HBO is greatest if started early (ideally within 6 hours)
    - Benefit in patients treated more than 12 hours after exposure is unproven
  - Efficacy:
    - Patients treated with HBO had lower mortality
    - This benefit extends for up to 4 years after poisoning
    - It may also be beneficial in preventing DNPS in these patients
- Isocapnic hyperpnea:
  - This is a technique used in mechanically ventilated patients
  - It is based on the fact that elimination $T_{1/2}$ of COHb depends on minute volume
  - These patients are hyperventilated with a mixture of oxygen and carbon dioxide
  - The technique aims to maintain a $PaCO_2$ of 40 mm Hg in spite of hyperventilation
  - Respiratory acidosis can occur in the absence of adequate hyperventilation

- This technique is much less expensive compared with HBO therapy
- Airway burns:
  - Intubation
  - Humidified 100% oxygen
  - Bronchoalveolar lavage
  - Chest physiotherapy
  - Bronchodilator therapy
  - Nebulization with heparin 10000 IU in 4 mL saline
  - N-acetyl cysteine nebulization

CYANIDE POISONING

Introduction

- Cyanide is a chemical molecule consisting of:
  - One atom of carbon
  - One atom of nitrogen
  - Bound by three molecular bonds
- Cyanide is a mitochondrial and is one of the most rapidly lethal poisons

Prevalence

- Incidence of exposures to cyanide was 1148 from 2007 to 2011
- Majority of reported cases of cyanide poisoning are accidental
- Mortality rate is 8.3% for intentional overdose patients
- Incidence of cardiac arrest was 9% amongst the survivors

Physiological Properties of Cyanide

- Low molecular weight: 26.02 Da
- Whole blood < 1 µg/mL
- Concentration in air:
  - Immediately fatal: 270 ppm
  - Life threatening: 110 ppm for more than 30 minutes

Circumstances of Poisoning

- Smoke inhalation
- Domestic fires
- Occupational poisoning:
  - Laboratory mishaps
  - Industrial accidents
  - Fumigation
  - Photographic development
  - Jewellers
- Suicidal attempts
- Homicidal activity
- *Iatrogenic cyanide poisoning:*
  - Occurs during the use of nitroprusside for hypertension
  - Occurs even at therapeutic doses (2–10 µg/kg/min) in malnourished patients

Sources of Cyanide

- Inorganic cyanides (cyanide salts):
  - Sodium cyanide
  - Potassium cyanide
- Gaseous cyanides:
  - Hydrogen cyanide
  - Cyanogen gas
  - Cyanogen chloride
- Organic cyanides:
  - Cassava
  - Apricots, bitter almond
  - Cherry, peaches
- Combustion of materials such as:
  - Wool, silk
  - Synthetic rubber
  - Polyurethane
- Ingestion of cyanogenic chemicals:
  - Acetonitrile
  - Acrylonitrile
  - Proprionitrile

Routes of Poisoning

- Inhalation
- Ingestion
- Transdermal
- Parenteral

Toxicodynamics

- Toxic dose of cyanide depends upon:
  - Form of cyanide
  - Route of exposure:
    - Inhalational:
      - 100 ppm for 30 minutes
      - 270 ppm for 5 minutes
    - Oral toxic dose: 1.52 mg/kg
    - Dermal toxic dose: 100 mg/kg
    - Intravenous toxic dose: 5–10 µg/kg/min for 3–10 hours
  - Duration of exposure
- For potassium cyanide, adult lethal dose is 200 mg

- For hydrogen cyanide:
  - Airborne concentration of 270 µg/mL may be immediately fatal
  - Exposures of more than 110 ppm for more than 30 minutes is life threatening
  - Permissible Exposure Limit (PEL) is 10 ppm at an 8-hour Time-Weighted Average (TWA)
  - Immediate Dangerous to Life or Health (IDLH) value is 50 ppm
- HCN readily crosses biological membranes because:
  - It has a low molecular weight
  - It is unionized
- After absorption, it exists in equilibrium as:
  - Cyanide anion (CN^-)
  - Undissociated HCN
- Being a weak acid with a pKa of 9.21, it exists primarily as HCN at physiological pH
- Thus, rapid lethality associated with inhalation is due to:
  - Rapid diffusion across biological membranes
  - Rapid and direct diffusion to target organs

Toxicokinetics

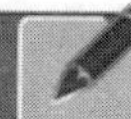

- Volume of distribution for cyanide anion varies between 0.075–1.5 L/kg
- Approximately 60% is plasma protein bound
- Cyanide is eliminated from the body by multiple pathways
- Cyanide is detoxified by enzymatic conversion to thiocyanate via:
  - Rhodanese:
    - Most important mechanism
    - Catalyses transfer of sulfane sulfur from thiosulphate to cyanide
    - This results in formation of thiocyanate, which is eliminated in urine
    - Highest concentration in the liver
  - β- mercaptopyruvate- cyanide sulfurtransferase
- Elimination of cyanide follows first order kinetics (range 1.2–66 hours)
- Small amounts are also excreted via urine, sweat and expiration.

Pathophysiology

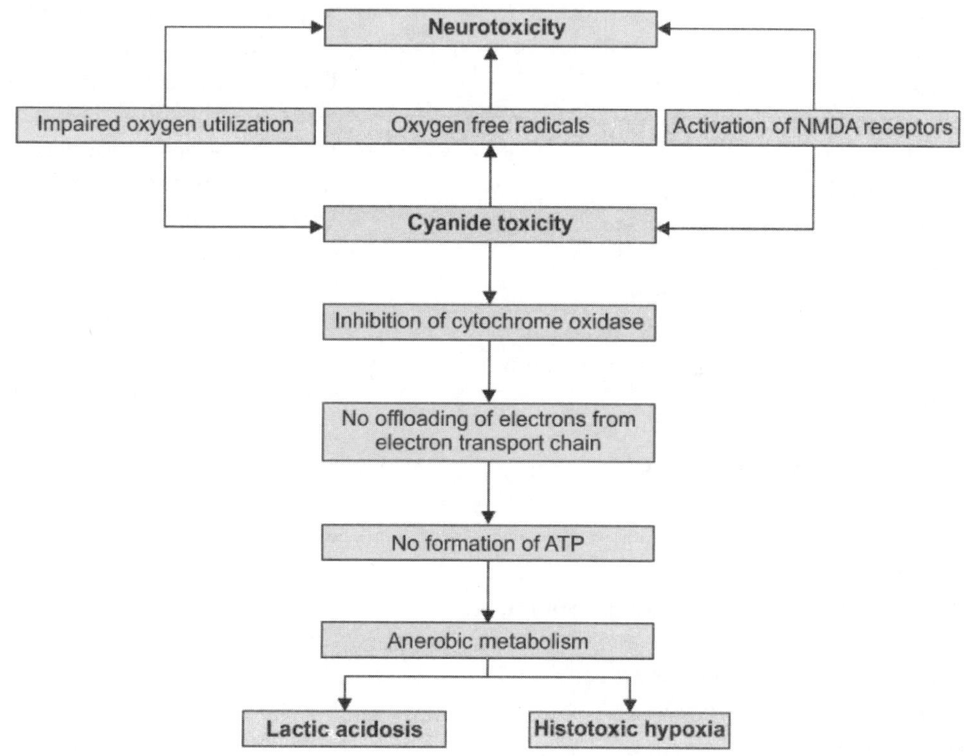

Clinical Features

- Acute poisoning:
  - Neurological:
    - Headache, anxiety
    - Confusion, vertigo
    - Loss of consciousness, seizures
  - Cardiovascular:
    - Tachycardia and HTN initially
    - Bradycardia and hypotension
    - Dysrhythmias
  - Respiratory:
    - Tachypnea followed by bradypnea
    - Pulmonary edema
  - Gastrointestinal:
    - Vomiting
    - Abdominal pain
  - Skin:
    - Cherry red color:
      - Occurs due to flushing
      - Cyanide impairs the utilization of oxygen by the tissues
      - Thus, venous oxyhemoglobin concentration is high
      - This imparts a cherry red color to the skin
      - However, it is not a very specific sign
      - It is seen only in 11% of cyanide toxicity patients
    - Cyanosis occurs more commonly than cherry red color
    - Irritant dermatitis
  - Renal failure
  - Hepatocellular necrosis
  - Others:
    - Rhabdomyolysis
    - Bitter almond or unusual odour
- Delayed sequelae:
  - Occurs in survivors of acute exposure
  - Basal ganglia is very sensitive to cyanide toxicity
  - Thus, it manifests predominantly as movement disorders like Parkinsonism
- Chronic exposure:
  - Non-specific manifestations such as:
    - Headache, dysgeusia
    - Vomiting, chest pain
    - Abdominal pain, anxiety
  - Manifestations specific to cyanide poisoning include:
    - *Tropical Ataxic Neuropathy (TAN)*
    - *Lebers hereditary optic neuropathy*
    - *Tobacco amblyopia*

Diagnosis

- Requires a high index of suspicion as it is a rare toxin
- Non-specific tests include:
  - Blood glucose estimation to rule out hypoglycemia
  - Salicylate levels
  - ECG for prolongation of QRS or QT_c intervals
  - In suspected carbon monoxide poisoning:
    - Carboxyhemoglobin levels
    - Methemoglobin levels
- Specific tests:
  - ABG analysis:
    - Reveals high anion gap metabolic acidosis
    - Metabolic acidosis is usually severe
    - This is usually because of:
      - Cyanide poisoning causing anerobic metabolism
      - Secondary manifestations such as seizures
  - Blood lactate levels:
    - High blood lactate levels are usually seen in cyanide poisoning
    - Lactate levels correlate with the severity of cyanide toxicity
    - Also, serial lactate levels can be used to monitor progress of treatment
  - Central venous blood gas:
    - Narrow venous-arterial PO_2 gradient is seen in cyanide poisoning
    - This is because cyanide inhibits cellular oxidative phosphorylation
    - This decreases peripheral tissue oxygen extraction from the blood
    - This results in venous hyperoxia and cherry red skin color
    - However, venous hyperoxia is a nonspecific sign and can be seen in:
      - Carbon monoxide poisoning
      - Hydrogen sulphide poisoning
      - Azide poisoning
  - Cyanide concentration:
    - Blood cyanide levels may not correlate with toxicity
    - Also, results are rarely available on time to guide therapy
    - Results of direct testing may be unreliable due to:
      - Improper storage conditions of the sample
      - Delay in processing samples

- Symptomatic correlation with levels of blood cyanide:
  - 12–23 μmol/L: tachycardia and flushing
  - 23–58 μmol/L: obtundation
  - 58–69 μmol/L: coma
  - 69 μmol/L: death

Treatment

- Evaluation:
  - Careful evaluation is essential as cyanide poisoning is rapidly lethal
  - High index of suspicion should be maintained, especially in smoke inhalation
  - Cyanide poisoning must be considered in all smoke inhalation patients with:
    - Carbonaceous material in oropharynx
    - Neurological dysfunction
    - Severe metabolic acidosis
    - Serum lactate levels > 8 mmol/L
- Initial resuscitation:
  - Airway and breathing:
    - Airway should be secured as per the clinical condition
    - 100% O_2 should be given irrespective of the pulse oximetric saturation
  - Circulation:
    - Large bore IV access is secured rapidly
    - Hypotension is treated with fluids and vasopressors as required
    - CPR should be provided as per ACLS protocol
    - *Rescue breaths are contraindicated* in cyanide poisoning
    - This is due to the risk of exposure of the CPR provider to cyanide
- Decontamination:
  - Personnel protection:
    - Personnel must wear protective clothing
    - Neoprene/nitrile gloves are used instead of latex for better protection
    - Respirators are worn until proper decontamination is completed
  - Dermal decontamination:
    - All contaminated clothing must be removed and discarded safely
    - Exposed areas are washed with soap and water solution
    - Thorough irrigation should be performed of:
      - Conjunctival recesses
      - Skin folds
      - Fingernails
      - Scalp and hair
  - Gastric decontamination:
    - Must be performed quickly as cyanide is absorbed rapidly
    - Single dose activated charcoal 1 g/kg (50 g in adults) can be used
    - However, cyanide is poorly absorbed by activated charcoal
    - Thus, administration of activated charcoal is of questionable benefit
    - Gastric lavage is generally not recommended unless ingestion is recent
- Antidotal treatment: consists of three modalities:
  - Direct cyanide binding:
    - Hydroxocobalamin:
      - It is considered as the *first line therapy* in cyanide poisoning
      - This is a precursor of vitamin B_{12}
      - It contains a cobalt moiety which binds to intracellular cyanide
      - This results in the formation of cyancobalamin
      - This molecule is readily excreted in the urine
      - Hydroxocobalamin may be used in combination with sodium thiosulfate
      - Dose:
        - IV 70 mg/kg for children
        - Typical adult dose is IV 5 g
        - A second dose may be repeated depending on response
        - This is usually given at half the initial dose
      - Disadvantages:
        - Causes reddish discoloration of:
          » Skin and mucous membranes
          » Urine
        - These changes last for 2–3 days
        - Therefore, it may affect other blood and urine tests
        - May interfere with cooximetric measurements
    - Dicobalt edetate:
      - It is an intravenous chelator of cyanide
      - Used rarely as an antidote for cyanide poisoning
      - Dose used is 20 mL of a 1.5% solution
      - This is given IV rapidly over 5 minutes
      - It is use can be associated with serious side effects such as:
        - Anaphylaxis
        - Seizures
        - Hypotension and cardiac dysrhythmias

- Induction of methemoglobinemia:
  - Formation of methemoglobin oxidizes Fe^{2+} moiety in heme to Fe^{3+}
  - This provides an alternative binding site for cyanide
  - Thus, methemoglobin acts as a competitor for cytochrome oxidase
  - Binding of cyanide results in formation of cyan-methemoglobin
  - This is relatively less toxic
  - Induction of methemoglobinemia is accomplished using:
    - Amyl nitrite:
      - Available as volatile liquid in ampules
      - Ampules are broken and inhaled by the patient
      - In ventilated patients, vapour is introduced into the ETT
      - This is done for 30 seconds every minute
      - The remaining 30 sec is used to oxygenate the patient
      - Amyl nitrite induces only a 5% methemoglobinemia
      - Thus, it is only a temporizing measure
      - Used in emergencies in the absence of an IV access
    - Sodium nitrite:
      - Administered IV 300 mg
      - This induces a 15–20% methemoglobinemia
      - Thus, it is more effective than amyl nitrite
      - Dose should be reduced in children and anemic patients
    - Dimethylaminophenol:
      - Used infrequently to induce methemoglobinemia
      - Dose of 5 mL of 5% solution IV
      - This is given rapidly within 1 minute
- Use of sulfur donors: (AP, 2005)
  - Sulfur donors act by maximizing the substrate for rhodanese enzyme
  - This enables formation of thiocyanate and cyanide detoxification
  - The agent usually used is sodium thiosulphate
  - Given in a dose of 50 mL of a 25% solution or 12.5 g IV

❖ Hyperbaric oxygen therapy:
- Effective when used in combination with antidotal therapy
- Advantages of HBO therapy include:
  - Transfer of cyanide from tissues to blood, thus hastening elimination
  - Improved respiratory status
  - Decrease brain lactate levels
- Currently however, data for the use of HBO in cyanide poisoning is limited

METHEMOGLOBINEMIA

Introduction

❖ Methemoglobin is formed by the oxidation of ferrous atom in heme to ferric moiety

❖ Normally, less than 2% of circulating hemoglobin exists as methemoglobin

❖ Methemoglobin *levels above* 2% is called as methemoglobinemia

Etiology

❖ Congenital methemoglobinemia:
- Cytochrome b_5 reductase deficiency
- Hemoglobin M disease
- Cytochrome b_5 deficiency

❖ Acquired methemoglobinemia:
- Analgesics:
  - Phenacetin
  - Phenazopyridine
- Antimicrobials:
  - Antimalarials:
    - Chloroquin
    - Primaquine
  - Dapsone
- Local anesthetics:
  - Benzocaine
  - Lidocaine
  - Prilocaine
  - Dibucaine
- Nitrates/ nitrites:
  - Amyl nitrite
  - Isobutyl nitrite
  - Butyl nitrite
  - Sodium nitrite
  - Ammonium nitrate
  - Silver nitrate
  - ***Nitroglycerin***
  - ***Nitroprusside***
  - Nitric oxide
- Sulfonamides:
  - Sulfanilamide
  - Sulfathiazide

- Sulfapyridine
- Sulfamethoxazole

Circumstances of Poisoning

- Use of xenobiotic compounds such as:
  - Topical anesthetics especially benzocaine
  - Dapsone
  - Nitric oxide
- Consumption of nitrate-contaminated well water
- Drug abuse with contaminated heroin/cocaine
- Fires, automobile exhaust fume poisoning

Toxicodynamics

- In normal homeostasis auto-oxidation of hemoglobin occurs spontaneously and slowly
- This results in conversion of 0.5–3% of hemoglobin to methemoglobin every hour
- This auto-oxidation is paralleled with continuous reduction of methemoglobin
- This helps in maintaining a constant level of methemoglobin below 2%
- The methemoglobin homeostatic mechanism is shown below

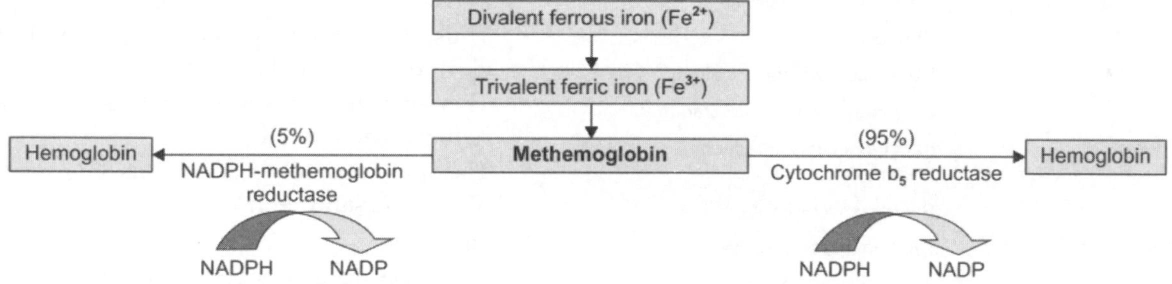

Pathophysiology

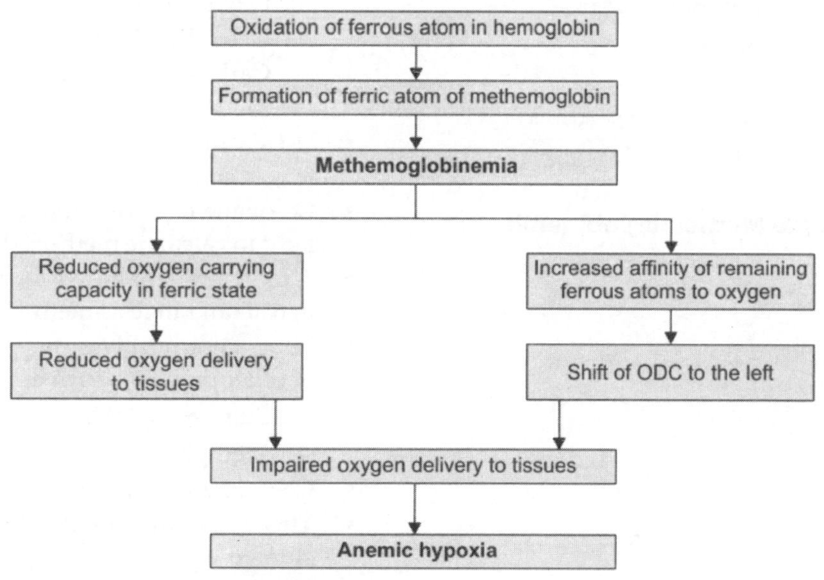

Toxicokinetics

- Methemoglobin enzyme systems are immature until approximately 4 months of age
- Thus, even genetically normal infants are more susceptible to methemoglobinemia
- Half-life of methemoglobin formed due to exposure to oxidants is between 1-3 hours
- With continued exposure to the oxidant, half-life is prolonged

Clinical Features

- Signs and symptoms occur due to acute impairment in oxygen delivery to tissues
- The severity of signs and symptoms depends on the level of methemoglobin
- Cyanosis is clinically detected when absolute concentration of meth-Hb is > 1.5 g/dL
- This is equivalent to meth-Hb concentration above 8–12% in the absence of anemia

- In anemic patients, cyanosis occurs at higher concentrations of meth-Hb
- This is because cyanosis detection is dependant on the absolute level of meth-Hb
- It does not depend on the percentage concentration of meth-Hb

No.	Methemoglobin level	Features
1.	1–3%	Asymptomatic
2.	3–15%	Possibly none
		Low SpO_2 on pulse oximeter
		Slate gray cutaneous coloration
3.	15–20%	Chocolate brown blood
		Cyanosis
4.	20–50%	Dizziness, syncope
		Dyspnea, exercise intolerance
		Fatigue, anxiety, headache, weakness
		Sinus tachycardia
5.	50–70%	CNS depression, coma
		Myocardial ischemia, dysrhythmias
		Metabolic acidosis
		Seizures
		Tachypnea
6.	> 70%	Grave hypoxic symptoms
		Death

Factors Predisposing to Methemoglobinemia

- Advanced age
- Age < 36 months
- Diarrhea
- Anemia
- Hospitalization
- Acidosis
- Renal failure
- Malnutrition
- Sepsis

Investigations

- Meth-Hb should be considered in:
  - Sudden onset cyanosis after intake of oxidative agent
  - Any cyanosis unresponsive to supplemental oxygen
  - Abnormal color of blood observed at phlebotomy
  - Clinical cyanosis in the presence of normal arterial PaO_2
- Pulse oximetry:
  - Is *inaccurate* for monitoring oxygen saturation in meth-Hb
  - Standard pulse oximeter uses 2 wavelengths of light:
    - 660 nm
    - 940 nm
  - The percentage of oxyhemoglobin is calculated using both these wavelengths
  - Meth-Hb also absorbs light at both the pulse oximeter's wavelengths
  - Therefore, meth-Hb will also be falsely reported as oxy-Hb
  - Thus, the pulse oximeter will report falsely elevated values of SpO_2
  - This leads to errors in estimating percentage of reduced and oxy-Hb
  - The SpO_2 is usually displayed as 85%, regardless of the true saturation
- Cooximetry:
  - It is a spectrophotometric method which is used to differentiate between:
    - Oxyhemoglobin
    - Deoxyhemoglobin
    - Carboxyhemoglobin
    - Methemoglobin
  - Uses a micro-processor controlled, fixed wavelength co-oximeter
  - Co-oximeters use additional wavelengths of light to calculate meth-Hb levels
  - This instrument how-ever measures all readings in 630 nm range as meth-Hb
  - Thus, false positives may occur in the presence of other pigments such as:
    - Sulf-hemoglobin
    - Methylene blue
  - Co-oximetry requires fresh blood samples
  - This is because meth-Hb levels increase with storage

Treatment

- Lesser degrees of methemoglobinemia (< 20%):
  - Do not require specific antidotal therapy
  - Discontinuation of offending agent is usually sufficient
- Symptomatic/severe methemoglobinemia (> 20%):
  - General considerations:
    - Do not require gastric decontamination as meth-Hb presents late

  - By the time of presentation, the entire toxic load is already absorbed
  - 100% oxygen supplementation
  - Secure airway, breathing and circulation
  - This may require use of mechanical ventilation and inotropes
- Methylene blue (MB):
  - Indications:
    - Severely symptomatic patients
    - Methemoglobin level >20%
  - Dose:
    - 1–2 mg/kg given slow IV over 5 minutes
    - This is because rapid injections are painful
    - Response is usually rapid
    - Dose can be repeated every 60 minutes
    - Avoid doses above 7 mg/kg as it can cause hemolysis
  - Mechanism of action:
    - Converted to leucomethylene blue by NADPH
    - Leucomethylene blue reduces methHb to Hb
  - Efficacy:
    - Considered as drug of choice
    - Rapidly reduces meth-Hb levels to non-toxic levels (< 10%)
    - This action is usually completed within 10–60 minutes
  - Contraindications:
    - G6PD deficiency
    - Serotonergic medications such as SSRIs
  - Causes of MB treatment failure:
    - Ongoing oxidant stress
    - NADPH methemoglobin reductase deficiency
    - Sulfhemoglobinemia
- Ascorbic acid:
  - Treatment with ascorbic acid requires multiple doses
  - Reduction of meth-Hb to non-toxic levels require up to 24 hours
  - Thus, it may not be the ideal drug in emergency scenarios
  - It is useful in situations where MB is contraindicated
  - Only few case reports exist of ascorbic acid for methemoglobinemia
  - Doses vary from 1–10 g IV Q6H until clinical improvement
- Blood transfusion:
  - May be useful in:
    - Patients in shock
    - Contraindications to methylene blue (e.g., G6PD deficiency)
    - Unavailability of methylene blue
  - However, the clinical response is usually less marked than with MB
- Hyperbaric oxygen therapy: May be used in severe cases

ABDOMINAL COMPARTMENT SYNDROME

Introduction

- For most critically ill patients, IAP of 5–7 mm Hg is considered normal
- Intra-abdominal HTN is defined as a sustained elevation of IAP above 12 mm Hg
- Intra-abdominal HTN (IAH) is classified into 4 grades based on the IAP:
  - Grade I: 12–15 mm Hg
  - Grade II: 16–20 mm Hg
  - Grade III: 21–25 mm Hg
  - Grade IV: above 25 mm Hg
- Abdominal compartment syndrome (ACS) is defined as sustained IAP >20 mm Hg associated with attributable organ dysfunction

Incidence

- Incidence of ACS is low (approximately 1%)
- ACS occurs most frequently in critically ill patients
- Incidence in patients undergoing laparotomy varies from 2–36%
- 35% of mechanically ventilated patients can have intra-abdominal HTN or ACS

Classification 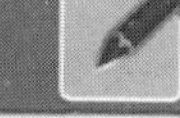

- Primary ACS:
  - Associated with injuries/ diseases of abdominopelvic region
  - Etiology:
    - Abdominal trauma
    - Hemoperitoneum
    - Pancreatitis
  - Surgical or radiological intervention of the primary cause is required
- Secondary ACS:
  - Results from conditions that do not originate in the abdominopelvic region
  - Typically related to the need for and the extent of volume resuscitation
  - Etiology:
    - Massive fluid resuscitation
    - Sepsis
    - Burns

Contd...

Contd...

- Tertiary or recurrent ACS:
  - Occurs in lieu of prior medical or surgical therapy for ACS
  - Typically seen in patients with:
    - Recurrent hemorrhage
    - Persistent accumulation of ascites.

Predisposing Factors

- Medical factors:
  - Massive fluid resuscitation (> 5 L in 24 hours)
  - Intra-abdominal infections
  - Sepsis
  - Ileus
  - Pneumonia
- Surgical factors:
  - Blunt/penetrating abdominal trauma
  - Open abdomen
  - Pelvic fractures
  - Retroperitoneal bleeding
  - Recent abdominal surgery
  - Abdominal packing after temporary abdominal closure for:
    - Multiple trauma
    - Liver transplantation

Etiology

- Increased abdominal contents:
  - Intestinal obstruction
  - Large abdominal tumor
  - Pregnancy
  - Abdominal aortic aneurysm
  - Ascites
  - Hemoperitoneum
  - Pneumoperitoneum
  - Large pelvic/ retroperitoneal hematoma
  - Abdominal packs
  - Peritonitis
  - Retroperitoneal edema (pancreatitis)
- Capillary leak:
  - Acidosis
  - Hypotension
  - Hypothermia
  - Massive fluid resuscitation
  - Polytransfusion
  - Coagulopathy
  - Oliguria
  - Sepsis
  - Major trauma
  - Burns
- Decreased abdominal wall compliance:
  - Abdominal surgery with tight primary closure
  - Prone positioning
  - Central obesity
- Decreased abdominal volume:
  - Reduction of large, long-standing hernia
  - Direct closure of large, chronic abdominal wall defect
  - Retroperitoneal edema (pancreatitis)
  - Large pelvic and retroperitoneal hematoma

Pathophysiology

- The volume of the abdominal compartment is limited by the abdominal fascia
- Once IAP is > 20 mm Hg, small changes in volume can cause drastic increases in IAP
- The increase in IAP can in turn affect multiple organ systems
- Central nervous system:
  - Increase in IAP forces the diaphragm cephalad
  - This increases the intrathoracic pressure and impedes venous return from brain
  - As a result, the ICP increases and cerebral blood flow decreases
  - The elevated ICP is sustained as long as the IAP remains elevated
  - This can result in progressive cerebral ischemia
- Cardiovascular system:
  - Increase in IAP causes:
    - A reduction in venous return to the heart (preload)
    - Increase in systemic vascular resistance (afterload to left heart)
    - Increase in pulmonary vascular resistance and right ventricular afterload
  - These changes lead to:
    - Leftward displacement of the ventricular septum
    - Impairment of LV filling
    - Reduction in cardiac output and cardiac index
- Respiratory function:
  - Raised IAP results in a cephalad displacement of the diaphragm

- This results in:
  - Reduced spontaneous tidal volumes
  - Arterial hypoxemia and hypercarbia
  - Reduced the thoracic compliance
  - Increased peak and mean airway pressures
- Thus, increased airway pressures are required during mechanical ventilation
- This can result in alveolar barotrauma

❖ Renal function:
- Increased IAP results in:
  - Direct compression of the renal parenchyma
  - Decreased perfusion of the kidneys
  - Na^+ and water retention due to activation of the renin angiotensin axis
- This results in progressive reduction in glomerular perfusion and oliguria

❖ Gastrointestinal:
- The gut is one of the most sensitive organs to increases in IAP
- Increased IAP results in a reduction in abdominal perfusion pressure (APP)
- APP is defined as the difference between mean arterial pressure and IAP
- Thus, APP = MAP – IAP
- Any increase in the IAP can therefore adversely affect APP
- Hypoperfusion of the gut may incite loss of the mucosal barrier
- This results in bacterial translocation and sepsis
- Thus, resuscitation in ACS should target improvement in APP rather than IAP

❖ Peripheral perfusion:
- The increase in IAP causes:
  - Excessive femoral venous pressure
  - Increased peripheral vascular resistance
  - Decreased femoral artery blood flow (by as much as 65%)
- This leads to peripheral limb edema and increases risk of DVT

Systemic Effects of Abdominal Compartment Syndrome

❖ Central nervous system:
- Raised ICP
- Reduced cerebral perfusion pressure

❖ Cardiovascular system:
- Reduced cardiac output
- Reduced venous return
- Increased PCWP and CVP
- Raised SVR

❖ Respiratory system:
- Raised intra-thoracic pressure
- Raised peak inspiratory pressure
- Reduced compliance
- Increased shunt fraction

❖ Gastrointestinal:
- Reduced celiac blood flow
- Reduced SMA blood flow
- Reduced mucosal blood flow
- Reduced portal blood flow
- Reduced lactate clearance

❖ Renal:
- Reduced glomerular blood flow
- Reduced GFR and oliguria

Clinical Features

❖ Most patients are critically ill with a tensely distended abdomen

❖ In the ICU, ACS most commonly presents as oliguria and increased ventilatory requirements

❖ Other clinical findings include:
- Hypotension, tachycardia
- Raised JVP
- Peripheral edema
- Abdominal tenderness
- Acute pulmonary decompensation

Evaluation

❖ Imaging:
- Helps in localizing the cause of elevated abdominal pressure
- However, they do not make a specific diagnosis of ACS
- Chest X-ray shows:
  - Reduced lung volumes
  - Atelectasis
  - Elevated hemi-diaphragms
- CT scan may show:
  - Dense infiltration of retroperitoneum
  - Extrinsic compression of IVC
  - Massive abdominal distension
  - Direct renal compression
  - Bowel wall thickening
  - Bilateral inguinal herniation

❖ Measurement of IAP:
- Is the *most accurate* method of diagnosing ACS

- Methods of measurement of IAP include:
  - Intragastric pressure
  - Intracolonic pressure
  - Intravesical pressure
  - Inferior vena cava catheters
- Intravesical pressure (IVP):
  - Simplest *and most accurate* method of measuring IAP
  - Technique:
    - IVP changes with alterations in head and body position
    - Thus, consistent position is important during measurements
    - Drainage tube of the Foleys catheter is clamped
    - 25–50 mL of sterile saline is instilled into the Foleys catheter
    - An 18-G needle is inserted into the aspiration port
    - The other end of the needle is attached to a pressure transducer
    - The transducer is zeroed at the level of mid-axillary line
    - IVP is usually measured 30-60 seconds after saline instillation
    - Abdominal contractions must be absent during measurement
    - Thus, IVP is measured at end expiration in supine position
    - IVP correlates closely with the IAP
  - IVP does not correlate with the IAP in:
    - Intraperitoneal adhesions
    - Pelvic hematomas
    - Pelvic fractures
    - Abdominal packs
    - Neurogenic bladder

Differential Diagnosis

- Mesenteric ischemia
- Ruptured abdominal aortic aneurysm
- Toxic megacolon
- Acute appendicitis
- Acute diverticulitis

Treatment

- Supportive measures:
  - Ventilation:
    - High peak airway pressures are required to maintain tidal volumes
    - Thus, ventilatory strategy should be modified to include:
      - Pressure limited volume guaranteed ventilation mode
      - Low tidal volumes
      - PEEP to reduce V/Q mismatch and improve hypoxia
      - Permissive hypercapnia
  - Hemodynamic support:
    - Mean arterial pressures must be titrated to maintain APP
    - Volume administration may temporarily improve cardiac output
    - Colloids may be used to reduce the volume of fluids administered
    - However, the type of fluid usually does not matter
    - This is because definitive treatment is abdominal decompression
- Non-surgical options:
  - Positioning:
    - Elevation of head end of the bed >20° increases the IAP
    - Patient should therefore be nursed only in the supine position
  - Prokinetic agents:
    - Metoclopramide and erythromycin ethyl succinate most commonly used
    - Efficacy of these agents is controversial
    - Therefore, they are not universally recommended
  - Gastric decompression:
    - Done using nasogastric suction
    - Useful for gaseous or liquid distention
    - Evacuation of luminal contents provides modest reduction in IAP
  - Rectal decompression:
    - Useful for fecal impaction
    - Can be done using:
      - Enemas
      - Rectal drainage catheter/tube
  - Sedation and neuromuscular blockade:
    - Abdominal wall compliance may be improved with adequate analgesia
    - Thus, sedation helps to maintain APP in the presence of elevated IAP
    - Paralysing agents prevent coughing and bucking which increases IAP
  - Paracentesis:
    - May be used as a temporizing measure for:
      - Recurrent ascites
      - Hemoperitoneum

- Retroperitoneal hematoma
- Intra-abdominal abscess
- Percutaneous drainage may prevent open abdominal decompression

❖ Surgical options:
- Abdominal decompression:
  - Remains the primary recommended intervention
  - Usually done when IAP exceeds 25 mm Hg
  - Done by opening the midline fascia along its full length via laparotomy
  - Offers immediate relief of hypotension and respiratory compromise
  - However, an open abdomen does not ensure low IAP
  - Thus, continuous monitoring of IAP is necessary
  - Temporary abdominal wall fascia closure may be done using:
    - Meshes
    - Zippers
    - Vacs
  - Fascia can be approximated after 5–7 days once IAP has normalized
  - Advantages of temporary abdominal wall closure include:
    - Bridging of fascial edges
    - Allowance of abdominal organ edema
    - Prevention of evisceration
    - Preservation of fascia for later closure
    - Retention of fluids and temperature
- Percutaneous decompression (PCD):
  - PCD is a less invasive and effective technique for decompression
  - Useful in the presence of free intraperitoneal fluid
  - Intraperitoneal fluid is detected by ultrasonography
  - Large volume USG- guided paracentesis is then done to reduce IAP
  - Causes of failure of PCD:
    - Catheter kinking
    - Catheter malposition
    - Secondary infections
    - Perforation of bowel
  - Indicators of failure of percutaneous drainage are:
    - Failure to drain > 1000 mL of fluid in first 4 hours
    - Failure to decrease IAP by 9 mm Hg in first 4 hours

Anesthetic Considerations for Abdominal Decompression

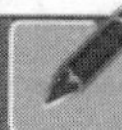

❖ Altered pharmacokinetics:
- Patients with ACS are sensitive to cardiac depression by induction agents
- This is due to:
  - Associated liver dysfunction
  - Altered volume of distribution of drugs
  - Hypovolemia
  - Altered drug metabolism
- Therefore, slow induction with titrated dose of anesthetic agents is required

❖ Sudden decrease in intra-thoracic pressure (ITP):
- Once abdomen is open, the ITP equilibrates with atmospheric pressure
- This results in a reduction in intrathoracic pressures
- Thus, a sudden increase in lung compliance may occur
- This in turn leads to barotrauma and volutrauma
- Thus, appropriate adjustments have to be made once abdomen is open

❖ Sudden decrease in SVR:
- Upon opening the abdomen, external pressure on blood vessels is relieved
- This results in a sudden fall in afterload and SVR
- This can lead to profound drop in the cardiac output and arterial pressures
- Cardiac output is maintained by:
  - Fluid resuscitation
  - Vasopressor therapy

❖ Reperfusion injury:
- Perfusion of previously ischemic bowel areas causes reperfusion injury
- This can result in myocardial depression, arrhythmias and cardiac arrest.

DROWNING

Introduction

❖ Defined as respiratory impairment resulting from submersion/immersion in liquid (***Utstein definition***)

❖ Any submersion or immersion without respiratory impairment is called water rescue

Incidence

❖ Common cause of accidental death worldwide

❖ Important cause of childhood fatalities worldwide

❖ Leading cause of death among children below 15 years age

❖ Incidence of drowning peaks in 3 groups:
- Highest in children < 5 years old
- Second peak in those aged 15-24 years
- Third peak in elderly

Risk Factors for Drowning

❖ Inadequate adult supervision

❖ Altered sensorium due to:
- Alcohol or other intoxication
- Hypoglycemia

- CNS disorders:
  - Syncope (e.g., due to hyperventilation prior to underwater diving)
  - Seizures
  - Dementia
  - Developmental disorders in children
- Concomitant spinal cord injuries due to:
  - Diving into shallow water
  - Significant fall from heights
  - Boating mishaps
- Intentional drowning:
  - Suicide
  - Homicide
  - Child abuse
  - Child neglect
- Cardiac conditions:
  - Dysrhythmias (Brugadas syndrome)
  - Ischemic heart disease

Pathophysiology

- Initial period following submersion is associated with:
  - Panic
  - Loss of normal breathing pattern
  - Breath holding
  - Air hunger
  - Struggle by the victim to stay above water
- Eventually reflex inspiratory efforts occur leading to hypoxemia due to:
  - Aspiration of liquid media
  - Laryngospasm when water contacts lower respiratory tract
- This in turn leads to hypoxic ischemia injury
- Drowning can also be associated with:
  - Cerebral hypoxia
  - Hypothermia
  - Respiratory distress
  - Aspiration of:
  - Foreign material
  - Particulate matter
  - Vomitus
  - Chemical irritants
  - Transient dyselectrolytemias
- Diving reflex:
  - Strongest in infants below 6 months age
  - Thought to be due to parasympathetic stimulation on submersion
  - Comprises of:
    - Apnea
    - Bradycardia
    - Peripheral vasoconstriction
    - Central shunting of blood flow
  - This provides transient protection against hypoxic brain injury during submersion
  - Diving reflex is however absent in adults
  - This is because diving is associated with sympathetic and parasympathetic stimulation
  - Thus, this reflex is not protective in adults

Types of Drowning

- Formerly, different types of drowning were recognized:
  - Dry drowning
  - Near drowning
  - Salt water drowning
  - Fresh water drowning
- Dry drowning:
  - Term used for drowning associated with absence of aspiration
  - Usually occurs when submersion is associated with laryngospasm
  - This prevents aspiration of fluid content
  - This may also be due to death of the patient prior to submersion
  - Term is no longer in use currently
- Near drowning:
  - Implies the patient almost died from submersion in liquid medium
  - Presently called non- fatal drowning
- Secondary drowning:
  - Term used to describe changes occurring due to aspiration of fluid content
  - This can cause interstitial or pulmonary edema
  - Can present up to 3 days after the initial submersion
  - Terminology is no longer used
- Salt water drowning:
  - Salt water is hypertonic
  - Aspiration of salt water causes massive exodus of fluid into pulmonary intestitium
  - This causes flash pulmonary edema with a hypertonic serum
- Fresh water drowning:
  - On the other hand, fresh water is hypotonic
  - Thus, on aspiration of fresh water, the fluid enters circulatory system
  - This causes massive fluid overload, hypervolemia, hemolysis and hyperkalemia
- Current concepts:
  - These distinctions and definitions are not used any longer
  - The Utstein definition is currently the only standard definition to avoid confusion
  - Distinction between salt and fresh water drowning:
    - No longer considered important

- This is because large volume aspiration is required to cause these changes
- More than 11 mL/kg fluid aspiration is required
- In reality, non-fatal drowning patients aspirate less than 3–4 mL/kg
- Thus, aspirated volumes seldom reach such levels to cause distinctions

Clinical Features

- Central nervous system:
  - Primary brain injury due to:
    - Hypoxia
    - Cerebral edema
  - Secondary brain injury due to:
    - Reperfusion
    - Sustained acidosis
    - Hyperglycemia
    - Cerebral edema
    - Seizures
    - Hypotension
- Respiratory system:
  - Fluid induced bronchospasm
  - Aspiration pneumonia
  - Chemical pneumonitis
  - Destruction of surfactant causing:
    - Atelectasis
    - Decreased compliance
    - Marked ventilation-perfusion mismatch
    - Non-cardiogenic pulmonary edema
  - Negative pressure pulmonary edema due to laryngospasm
  - Acute respiratory distress syndrome
- Cardiovascular system:
  - Arrhythmias:
    - Occur due to:
      - Hypothermia
      - Hypoxemia
    - Types of arrhythmias:
      - Sinus tachycardia
      - Sinus bradycardia
      - Atrial fibrillation
      - Ventricular arrhythmias
  - Pulmonary hypertension
  - Myocardial dysfunction
  - Myocardial infarction due to:
    - Takatsubo cardiomyopathy
    - Coronary artery spasm
    - Hypothermia
    - Cardiogenic pulmonary edema
- Dyselectrolytemias:
  - Transient dyselectrolytemias
  - Metabolic/ respiratory acidosis
- Renal system: acute tubular necrosis due to:
  - Hypoxemia
  - Shock
  - Hemoglobinuria
  - Myoglobinuria due to rhabdomyolysis
- Coagulopathy
- Rare and severe infections such as:
  - Pseudallescheria boydii complex
  - Naegleria
  - Burkholderia
  - Aeromonas

Injuries Associated with Drowning

- Spinal cord injuries due to shallow water diving
- Hypothermia
- Aspiration
- Respiratory failure

Investigations

- Complete blood counts, electrolyte levels, coagulation profile
- Arterial blood gas for hypoxemia, dyselectrolytemias, acidosis
- Co-oximetry for methemoglobinemia and carboxyhemoglobinemia
- Blood sugar levels
- Liver function tests: elevated AST, ALT
- Renal function tests for acute renal impairment
- Chest X-ray for:
  - Pulmonary edema
  - Aspiration
  - Atelectasis
- CT scan for spine injuries
- Cardiac troponin I for prognostication

Management

- Out of hospital care: modifications of BLS protocol:
  - CPR sequence:
    - Rescuer should pay attention to his own safety during rescue process
    - CPR for drowning victims should follow the traditional ABC approach
    - CAB approach is not used for resuscitation
    - This is because of the hypoxic nature of the cardiac arrest
    - Prompt initiation of rescue breathing increases chances of survival

- Rescue breathing begins as soon as the rescuer reaches a stable surface
- Cervical spine stabilization: (Class III, LOE B)
  - Incidence of cervical spine injury is rare in non-fatal drowning
  - Unnecessary cervical spine immobilization impedes airway manipulation
  - Routine spine stabilization is not recommended
  - Cervical spine stabilization used only if high suspicion of spine injury:
    - Facial or head injury
    - Unable to give adequate history
    - Diving accidents
- Airway clearance: (Class II, LOE C)
  - Only modest amount of water is aspirated by majority of victims
  - Most of the water aspirated is rapidly absorbed into central circulation
  - Removal of water by means other than suction is not recommended
  - These attempts include:
    - Abdominal thrusts
    - Heimlich maneuver
  - Routine use of these maneuvers is not recommended
  - These maneuvers may be potentially harmful
- Chest compressions and ACLS:
  - Initiated after confirmation of absent central pulse on delivery of two rescue breaths
  - Chest compressions are continued as per BLS guidelines
  - Defibrillation with AED is attempted in the presence of shockable rhythm
  - It is necessary to dry the area prior to application of defibrillation paddles
- Vomiting:
  - Most patients vomit while receiving CPR
  - In the presence of vomiting, turn the victim to the side
  - Vomitus can be removed with a cloth, suction or finger-sweep maneuver

❖ Emergency department management:
- Airway:
  - Securing the airway early is important
  - Indications for intubation include:
    - GCS score <13
    - Signs of neurological deterioration
    - Inability to protect airway
    - Inability to maintain oxygenation with high flow supplemental O_2:
      - $PaO_2 < 60$ mm Hg in adults
      - $PaO_2 < 80$ mm Hg in children
      - $SpO_2 < 90\%$
    - $PaCO_2 > 50$ mm Hg
  - In patients who do not require intubation:
    - Supplemental oxygen is titrated to maintain $SpO_2 > 94\%$
    - Non-invasive ventilation may be used to reduce V/Q mismatch
  - Orogastric tube is used to decompress stomach and relieve gastric distention
- Monitoring:
  - Pulse oximetry
  - ECG
  - End tidal CO_2
  - Invasive arterial BP and CVP in unstable patients
- Other measures:
  - Wet clothing is removed and warming initiated in hypothermic patients
  - Cervical spine stabilization used only if high suspicion of spine injury

❖ Inpatient management:
- Nervous system:
  - Head end elevated nursing to reduce ICP
  - Diuretics in the presence of cerebral edema
  - In the presence of imminent herniation, hyperventilation is used to reduce ICP
  - Prolonged hyperventilation should be avoided
  - Non-sedating anticonvulsants may be used to prevent seizure activity
  - Neuromuscular blocking agents are avoided
  - Euglycemia is maintained to optimize CNS status
  - Use of therapeutic hypothermia in drowning patients is controversial
- Respiratory system:
  - Inhaled beta- agonists are used to treat bronchospasm
  - Antibiotics are used only in the presence of:
    - Clinical pulmonary infection
    - Drowning in grossly contaminated water
  - No evidence to support routine use to glucocorticoids in drowning patients
  - Lung protective ventilator strategy used for ventilation
  - Higher ventilation pressures may be required due to poor lung compliance
  - PEEP is useful to prevent atelectasis and V/Q mismatch

- ECMO may be used when:
  - Inability to ventilate with:
    - Conventional mechanical ventilation
    - High frequency ventilation
  - Intact neurological function
- Surfactant therapy may be used (lack of evidence to support routine use)

- Cardiovascular system:
  - Hypovolemia and hypotension may occur due to cold diuresis
  - Volume repletion with isotonic crystalloids or colloids may be required
  - Myocardial dysfunction warrants:
    - Optimal fluid load
    - Inotropic support (dopamine, dobutamine)
- Others:
  - Dyselectrolytemias may occur due to cold diuresis and have to be treated
  - Bronchoscopy may be required in case of foreign body aspiration
  - Renal replacement therapy may be required in acute tubular necrosis

Prognostication

Orlowski score	
Category	*Score*
Age less than 3 years	1
Maximum estimated submersion time more than 5 minutes	1
Resuscitation no attempted for at least 10 minutes after rescue	1
Patient in coma on admission to hospital	1
Arterial blood pH less than 7.1	1

- 90% chance of complete functional recovery when score < 2
- 5% probability of survival in patients with a score > 3
- In general, poor prognostic factors following drowning include:
  - Unwitnessed event
  - Delayed resuscitation
  - Need for out of hospital CPR
  - Need for continued CPR in emergency department
  - Prolonged coma

THERAPEUTIC HYPOTHERMIA

Introduction

- Induced hypothermia has been shown to improve neurological outcome post cardiac arrest
- Maintaining a core body temperature 32–34°C for 24 hours after ROSC dramatically improves survival
- Therapeutic hypothermia refers to maintenance of temperature between 32–34°C
- ***Targeted Temperature Management*** refers to maintenance of temperature no higher than 36°C

Inclusion Criteria

- Pulse ROSC with GCS motor score < 6
- No other reason for coma
- No DNR/ DNI status
- Adult, age > 17 years

Exclusion Criteria

- Awake, alert after cardiac arrest
- Arrest of traumatic etiology
- Arrest associated with significant non-compressible bleeding
- Cerebral performance score 4–5 prior to arrest
- Pregnancy
- DNR/ DNI status

Monitoring during Therapeutic Hypothermia

- Pulse oximetry
- Capnometry
- Continuous cardiac monitoring
- Central venous pressure (maintain CVP 8–12 mm Hg)
- Invasive arterial pressure (maintain MAP > 60 mm Hg)
- Urine output (hypothermia associated cold-diuresis)
- Core body temperature:
  - Esophageal temperature is most accurate
  - Bladder temperature is not used as diuresis causes false readings
  - Rectal temperature lags behind acute temperature changes by 1.5°C
- Arterial blood gases and electrolytes Q4H:
  - Solubility of gases increases with a reduction in body temperature
  - Thus, with hypothermia, $PaCO_2$ reduces
  - But, blood gas machines interprete values assuming temperature as 37°C usually
  - Thus, the actual $PaCO_2$ may be slightly lower than the $PaCO_2$ measured at 37°C
  - This may lead to a source of error and hyperventilation during hypothermia
  - Thus, mild hyperventilation with higher $PaCO_2$ is targeted during hypothermia
  - Also, repeated electrolyte measurement is essential during cold-diuresis phase

Goals of Therapeutic Hypothermia

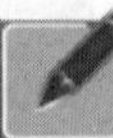

- Targeted temperature management (36°C):
  - Uncomplicated patients with moderate coma (some motor response)
  - Absence of cerebral edema on CT-scan
  - Absence of malignant EEG patterns
  - Those with concerns of non-compressible bleeding
- Therapeutic hypothermia (32–34°C):
  - Deep coma (loss of motor response or brainstem reflexes)
  - Malignant (epileptiform) EEG patterns
  - Cerebral edema on early CT scans.

Technique

- Cooling is begun as soon as possible post ROSC (but within 4–6 hours)
- Core body temperature is reduced to 32–34°C (below 36°C for TTM)
- Methods of cooling include:
  - Surface cooling:
    - Useful in patients with:
      - Heart failure
      - Pulmonary edema
      - Renal dysfunction
    - Reduce core temperature at 0.5–1°C per hour
    - Options for surface cooling include:
      - Chilled saline or ice packs in axillae, neck, groin
      - Cooling blankets, vests and leg wraps
      - Cooling helmet
      - Fans
  - Intravascular cooling:
    - 25–30 mL/kg isotonic fluids can be infused over 30 minutes
    - Temperature of the fluid at infusion is around 4°C
    - This reduces core temperature by > 2°C per hour
  - Thermostatically controlled cooling devices ***(Arctic Sun)***:
    - Provide precise temperature regulation
    - Useful as they allow avoidance of extreme temperatures
- Intubation and mechanical ventilation:
  - Essential to protect airway during induction of hypothermia
  - Sedation should be titrated to avoid shivering, rather than any sedation scale
  - Continuous infusion of propofol with fentanyl is usually used:
    - Propofol 20–50 µg/kg/min
    - Fentanyl 25–100 µg/hour
  - Midazolam infusion may be used in unstable patients (2–5 mg/hour)
  - Muscle paralysis may be required to treat hypothermia associated shivering
  - Muscular paralysis however masks seizures and is avoided in epileptic patients
- Avoid drop in temperature below 32°C
- Hypothermia is maintained for at least 24-48 hours post ROSC
- Avoidance of hyperthermia for at least 48–72 hours is mandatory for good outcome
- Gradual rewarming should be practiced at a rate < 0.25°C/hour

Complications

- More common:
  - Bradycardia:
    - Very common
    - Heart rate < 50 bpm is common with induction of hypothermia
    - However, bradycardia rarely requires treatment
  - Prolongation of QT interval
  - Coagulopathy with PTT prolongation
  - Cold diuresis:
    - Hypovolemia
    - Hypokalemia
    - Hypomagnesemia
    - Hypophosphatemia
  - Hyperkalemia during rewarming
  - Shivering
- Less common:
  - Arrhythmias:
    - Prolongation of QT interval
    - Tachydysrhythmias are uncommon unless core temperature drops < 32°C
    - Commonly seen tacharrhythmias are:
      - Atrial fibrillation
      - Non- sustained VT
  - Significant bleeding (< 5% cases)
  - Skin injury/ulceration

Validation

- Pediatric population:
  - TH after pediatric cardiac arrest has not been well established
  - However, it may be beneficial in neonates with hypoxic ischemic encephalopathy
  - Therefore, no supportive RCT exists for use in children after sudden cardiac arrest

- HACA study: (Hypothermia After Cardiac Arrest study group, 2002)
  - Hypothermia after Cardiac Arrest study:
  - Included 274 patients from 9 centers in 5 European countries
  - Mild cooling to 32–34°C was implemented following ROSC
  - Study found:
    - Improvement in functional recovery in hypothermia group (55% vs 39%)
    - Lower 6-month mortality in those patients who were cooled (41% vs 55%)

POSTCARDIAC ARREST SYNDROME

Introduction

It refers to the unique and complex combination of pathophysiological processes which occur after ROSC following a sudden cardiac arrest

Epidemiology

- In-hospital mortality rates are as high as 67% for sudden cardiac arrest survivors
- Amongst survivors of SCA, CNS injury is seen in up to 50% patients
- Less than 15% patients recover fully if coma persists > 6 hours after ROSC
- This number dwindles to less than 10% if the coma persists for > 24 hours
- GCS score < 5, 72 hours after ROSC indicate little or no chance of neurological recovery

Phases of Post Cardiac Arrest Syndrome

- Immediate post cardiac arrest phase: First 20 minutes after ROSC
- Early post cardiac arrest phase: 20 minutes to 12 hours after ROSC
- Intermediate phase: 12 hours to 72 hours after ROSC
- Recovery phase: Beyond 72 hours after ROSC

Components of Post Cardiac Arrest Syndrome

- Post cardiac arrest brain injury
- Post cardiac arrest myocardial dysfunction
- Systemic ischemia- reperfusion response
- Persistent precipitating pathology

Pathophysiology and Clinical Features

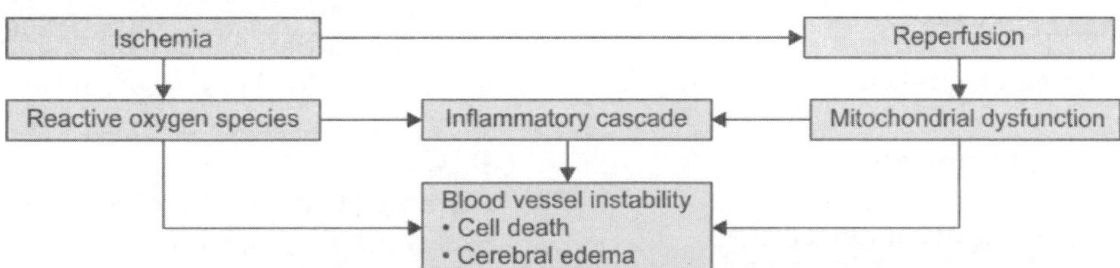

No.	Syndrome	Pathophysiology	Manifestations
1.	PCA-brain injury	Impaired cerebral autoregulation Cerebral edema Postischemic neurodegeneration	Coma, vegetative state Seizures, myoclonus Cognitive dysfunction Stroke Secondary Parkinsonism Brain death
2.	PCA- myocardial dysfunction	Myocardial stunning Global hypokinesia Low cardiac output syndrome ACS	Hypotension Dysrhythmias Cardiovascular collapse
3.	Systemic reperfusion response	SIRS Impaired vasoregulation Impaired coagulation Adrenal suppression Impaired tissue oxygenation Immunosuppression	Hypotension Cardiovascular collapse Pyrexia, lactic acidosis Hyperglycemia Multiorgan failure Infection
4.	Persistent precipitating pathology	AMI, cardiomyopathy COPD, asthma Cerbrovascular accidents Pulmonary embolism Poisoning, drug overdose Sepsis, pneumonia Hemorrhage, dehydration	Etiology specific

Diagnosis

- Neuroprognostication following sudden cardiac arrest is essential for planning treatment
- Earliest time for prognostication of poor neurological outcome is 72 hours after ROSC
- Head CT scan:
  - Has to be performed as soon as clinically possible
  - Useful to identify:
    - Subarachnoid hemorrhage
    - Epidural, subdural hematomas
    - Cerebral edema- usually peaks several days after resuscitation
- Nerve- specific enolase:
  - Is a very sensitive test for severe neurological injury
  - Levels > 33 μg/ L is a marker for poor neurological prognosis
- Continuous EEG:
  - Useful for assessment of electrical convulsive activity
  - Presence of seizures indicates poor prognosis usually
- BIS monitoring and SSEP may be simple alternatives to predict neurological outcome

Cerebral Performance Score

- Used to predict neurological outcome after ROSC
- Score 1:
  - Good cerebral performance
  - Conscious, alert
  - Able to work and lead a normal life
  - May have:
    - Minor psychological or neurological deficits
    - Mild dysphasia
    - Non-incapacitating hemiparesis
    - Minor cranial nerve abnormalities
- Score 2:
  - Moderate cerebral disability
  - Conscious with sufficient function for part time work
  - May have:
    - Hemiplegia, seizures
    - Ataxia, dysarthria
    - Dysphasia
    - Permanent memory or mental changes
- Score 3:
  - Severe cerebral disability
  - Conscious, but depends on others for daily support
  - Has at least limited cognition
  - Includes wide range of patients:
  - Ambulatory with severe memory disturbances
  - Dementia precluding independent existence
  - Locked in syndrome
- Score 4:
  - Coma or vegetative state
  - Unconscious, unaware of surroundings
  - No cognition
  - No verbal or psychological interaction with the environment
  - Score > 4 predicts poor quality of life (sensitivity 55.6%, specificity 96.8%)
- Score 5: Certified brain dead or dead by traditional criteria

Score	Description
1.	Awake, alert and can work
2.	Awake and alert, cannot work but can perform independent daily activities
3.	Conscious, but dependant on others
4.	Coma or vegetative state
5.	Brain death

Monitoring

- General intensive care monitoring:
  - Arterial catheter
  - Oxygen saturation by pulse oximetry
  - Continuous ECG
  - CVP, mixed venous oxygen saturation
  - Temperature
  - Urine output
  - Arterial blood gases, serum lactate
  - Blood glucose, electrolytes, CBC
  - Chest X-ray
- Advanced hemodynamic monitoring:
  - Echocardiography
  - Cardiac output monitoring
- Cerebral monitoring:
  - Continuous EEG
  - CT scan
  - BIS, SSEP

Goals of Therapy

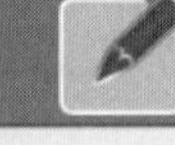

- Determining and treating the cause of cardiac arrest
- Minimizing brain injury
- Managing myocardial dysfunction and stunning
- Managing ischemia- reperfusion related complications.

Prevention

- Temperature:
  - Avoid fever for 48 hours post ROSC
  - Induced mild hypothermia 32–34°C for 12–24 hours
  - Rewarm slowly (< 0.25°C/hour)
- Cardiovascular:
  - Maintain MAP 65–90 mm Hg
  - Suppress dysrhythmias

- Reperfusion therapy
- Medical management of ACS (antiplatelets, anticoagulation)

❖ Pulmonary:
- Mechanical ventilation
- Avoid hyperventilation
- Avoid hypoxia and hyperoxia

❖ Gastrointestinal: Consider early refeeding after hypothermia

❖ Fluids:
- Monitor CVP and urine output
- Monitor potassium, glucose and electrolytes during temperature changes
- Maintain serum $K^+ > 3.5$ mEq/L
- Avoid hyperglycemia > 180 mg/dL

❖ Infections:
- Prophylactic antibiotics are of unproven benefit
- Antipyretics are reasonable

❖ Neurological:
- CT scan to exclude intracranial lesions
- Sedation and muscle relaxation, especially if neuro-monitoring is indicated
- Monitor for seizures with EEG

Therapeutic Targets

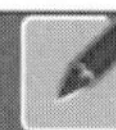

❖ Systolic blood pressure more than 90 mm Hg (Class IIb)
❖ Mean arterial pressure between 65–90 mm Hg (Class IIb)
❖ CVP 8-12 mm Hg
❖ Arterial oxygen saturation 94–96% (Class IIa)
❖ PaO_2 more than 60 mm Hg is desired, more than 100 mm Hg is optimal
❖ Avoid prolonged hyperoxia (> 300 mm Hg)
❖ Maintain temperature corrected normocarbia (Class IIb)
❖ Mixed venous oxygen saturation > 70%
❖ Hematocrit > 30% or Hb > 8 g/dL
❖ Lactates < 2 mmol/L
❖ Urine output > 0.5 mL/kg/hour
❖ Oxygen delivery index > 600 mL/min/m^2

Treatment

❖ Post-cardiac arrest brain injury:
- Therapeutic hypothermia:
  - Mild therapeutic hypothermia is effective for post-cardiac arrest syndrome
  - Cooling to 32–34°C for 24 hours is effective for neuro-protection
- Early hemodynamic optimization: According to the goals of therapy
- Airway protection and mechanical ventilation: (McKenzie N, 2017)
  - Indicated if inadequate signs of awakening > 5 mins after ROSC
  - Controlled reoxygenation targeting SpO_2 94–96%
  - Avoid hyperventilation
  - Ventilation adjusted to maintain normocarbia (35–45 mm Hg)
  - Lung protective ventilation:
    - Tidal volume 6–8 mL/kg
    - Plateau pressure < 30 cm H_2O
- Seizure control:
  - Prolonged seizures should be treated with anticonvulsant therapy
  - Maintenance therapy should be started after first event
  - Precipitating causes are excluded prior to starting maintenance therapy
  - Anticonvulsants which can be used are:
    - Benzodiazepines
    - Phenytoin
    - Sodium valproate
    - Propofol or barbiturates
- Supportive care:
  - Sedation and paralysis especially when initiating therapeutic hypothermia
  - Renal replacement therapy as indicated in other critically ill patients
  - Routine use of steroids is not indicated
  - Pressure sore prophylaxis

❖ Post- cardiac arrest myocardial dysfunction
- Early hemodynamic optimization: according to goals of therapy
- Intravenous fluids to optimize preload:
  - Avoid hypotonic fluids
  - Isotonic fluids at 4°C and 20–30 mL/kg maybe used to simultaneously:
    - Induce hypothermia
    - Optimize preload
- Inotropic optimization:
  - Useful to treat myocardial stunning, commonly seen after ROSC
  - Used when MAP < 80 mm Hg inspite of an adequate CVP (8–12 mm Hg)
- Coronary revascularization:
  - Emergency PCI recommended in all patients in whom ACS is suspected
  - Thrombolytic therapy may be used in the absence of PCI
- Mechanical circulatory support:
  - Used for circulatory support unresponsive to conventional measures
  - Typically used during 1st 24–48 hours when cardiac dysfunction is severe
  - Options to support circulation are:
    - IABP
    - ECMO
    - LVAD

- Systemic ischemia- reperfusion response:
  - Early hemodynamic optimization: According to goals of therapy
  - Intravenous fluids, vasopressors
  - High volume hemofiltration
  - Temperature control
  - Glucose control
  - Antibiotics only for documented infections
- Persistent precipitating pathology: Disease specific interventions:
  - Hypovolemia
  - Hypo/hyperkalemia
  - Metabolic disorders
  - Accidental hypothermia
  - Tension pneumothorax, cardiac tamponade

Adult Immediate Post-Cardiac Arrest Care Algorithm

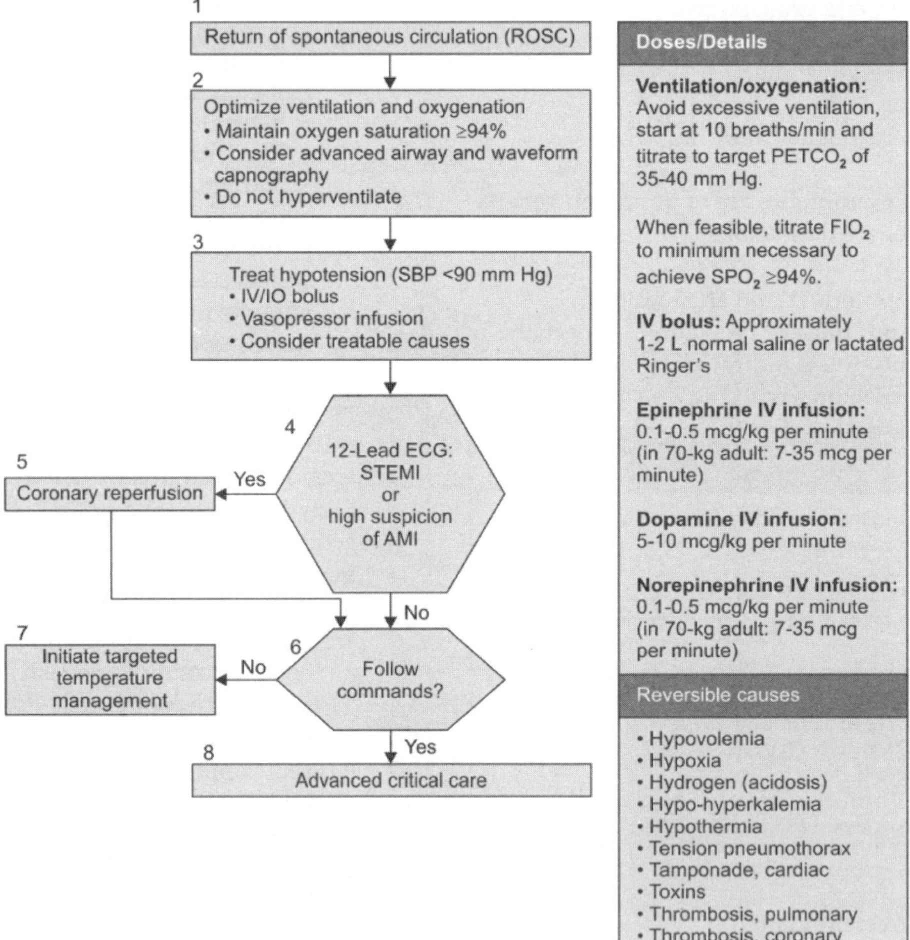

MULTIPLE ORGAN DYSFUNCTION SYNDROME

Introduction

- Development of potentially reversible physiological derangement involving more than 2 organ systems, not involved in the disorder resulted in ICU admission is called multiple organ dysfunction syndrome
- Earlier called:
  - Sequential organ failure
  - Progressive systems failure
  - Multiple organ failure
  - Multisystem organ failure (MSOF)

Incidence

- Estimating the exact incidence of sepsis is difficult
- Incidence of sepsis in the USA is greater than 5,00,000 cases per year
- Prevalence of SIRS in septic patients ranges from 20–60%
- Approximately 40% of patients with sepsis develop septic shock
- Mortality from MODS remains high and ranges from 40–90%
- Poor prognostic factors include:
  - Impaired host immune status

- Infection with a resistant organism
- Advanced age
- Poor prior functional status

Risk Factors for Mods

- Iatrogenic factors:
  - Blood transfusion
  - Mechanical ventilation
  - Iatrogenic intraabdominal HTN
- Infection:
  - Peritonitis, intra-abdominal infections
  - Pneumonia
  - Necrotizing soft tissue infections
  - Tropical infections
  - Pancreatitis
- Ischemia:
  - Ruptured aortic aneurysm
  - Hypovolemic shock
  - Mesenteric ischemia
- Immune reactions:
  - Autoimmune disease
  - Reactive hemophagocytic syndrome
  - Antiphospholipid antibody syndrome
  - Transplant rejection
  - Graft vs host disease
- Intoxications:
  - Ecstasy, cocaine
  - Salicylates, acetaminophen
- Endocrine risk factors:
  - Adrenal crisis
  - Pheochromocytoma
  - Thyroid storm
  - Myxedema coma

Etiology

- Sepsis
- Multiple trauma
- Burns
- Pancreatitis
- Pulmonary aspiration of gastric contents
- Massive hemorrhage
- Massive transfusions
- Ischemia reperfusion
- Ischemic necrosis
- Microvascular thrombosis
- Multiple sequential physiological insults

Pathogenesis

- Gut hypothesis:
  - Proposes that the gut serves as the motor of MODS in critically ill patients
  - MODS occurs primarily due to splanchnic hypoperfusion and mucosal ischemia
  - This increases the gut permeability and causes translocation of bacteria
  - Tissue injury subsequently occurs due to immune response
- Endotoxin macrophage hypothesis:
  - Gram-negative infections are common in patients with MODS
  - This theory proposes that endotoxins are principal mediators in MODS
  - Pro-inflammatory mediators include:
    - TNF- α
    - IL-1, IL-6
    - TXA_2, PAF, NO
- Tissue hypoxia-microvascular hypothesis:
  - Primarily occurs due to macro and microvascular changes
  - This results in insufficient supply of oxygen to the tissues
  - Hypoxemia results in cell death and organ dysfunction
- Integrated hypothesis: Combination of other 3 hypothesis
- Altered metabolism:
  - Extreme protein catabolism causes ***auto-cannibalism***
  - Ketone body ratio (Aceto-acetate: β-hydroxy butyrate) less than 0.4 is *characteristic* of MODS

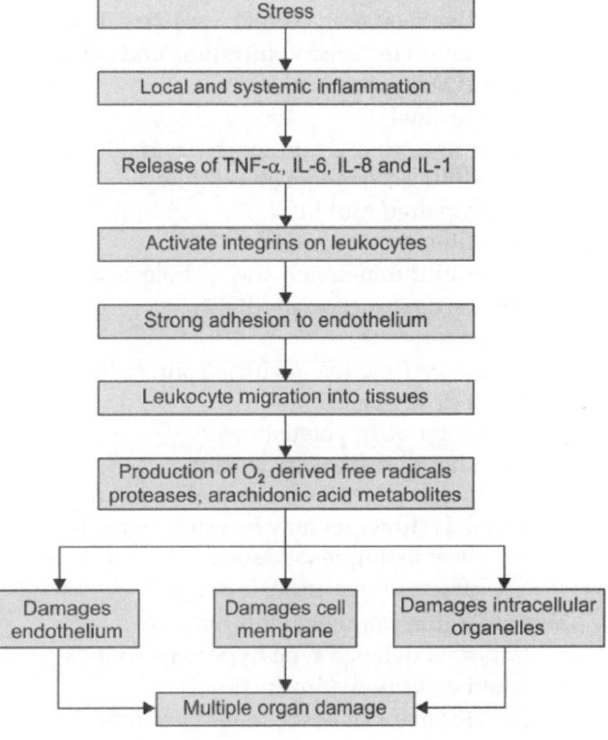

Pathophysiology

- Neurological:
  - Characteristic features of MODS include:
    - Reduced GCS score
    - Altered level of consciousness
  - Causes of neurological dysfunction in MODS include:
    - Subclinical cerebral edema
    - Metabolic derangements
    - Reduced cerebral perfusion pressure
    - Micro-abscesses in the brain
    - Iatrogenic sedatives and analgesics
- Cardiovascular: Five principal cardiovascular derangements occur:
  - Reduced peripheral vascular tone due to nitric oxide
  - Increased capillary permeability producing capillary leak
  - Alteration in regional blood flow to specific organ beds
  - Microvascular occlusion and stasis due to plugging by rigid RBCs and WBCs
  - Myocardial depression affecting right heart
- Respiratory:
  - Failure of normal gas exchange and arterial hypoxemia is characteristic
  - Ventilation-perfusion mismatch due to:
    - Atelectasis
    - Intravascular thrombosis
    - Altered regional blood flow
    - Alveolar edema due to capillary leak
  - Ventilation induced volutrauma and barotrauma aggravate lung injury
- Gastrointestinal:
  - Gastrointestinal dysfunction occurs due to:
    - Reduced regional blood flow
    - Impaired motility
    - Altered microbial flora
  - Hyperbilirubinemia and cholestasis reflect hepatic dysfunction in MODS
- Genitourinary:
  - Renal dysfunction results from reduced renal blood flow due to:
    - Systemic hypotension
    - Altered regional perfusion
    - Increased intra-abdominal pressure
  - Renal dysfunction may be exacerbated by:
    - Pre-existing renal deficit
    - Effects of nephrotoxic drugs
- Hematological derangements include:
  - Impaired delayed type hypersensitivity
  - Altered antibody production
  - Development of nosocomial infections

Clinical Features

- General:
  - Fever, tachycardia, tachypnea, leucocytosis
  - Rapid reduction in muscle mass, marked protein catabolism
- Neurological:
  - Encephalopathies, myopathy
  - Heterogenous neuropathies
  - ***Critical illness neuropathy***
  - Coma
- Cardiovascular:
  - Hypotension, tachycardia
  - Reduced cardiac output and SVR
  - Diffuse capillary leak and anasarca
  - LV and RV dysfunction, low output failure
  - Supraventricular arrhythmias
- Respiratory:
  - Hypoxemia and respiratory distress
  - Atelectasis, wasted ventilation, V/Q mismatch
  - ALI develops in 24-72 hours: *most common manifestation*
  - Acute respiratory failure
- Gastrointestinal:
  - Splanchnic ischemia
  - Upper GI bleeding and stress ulceration
  - Intolerance of enteral feeds: ileus
  - Abdominal distension and diarrhea
  - Hyperbilirubinemia and cholestasis, liver failure
  - Pancreatitis, hepatitis
- Genitourinary:
  - Prerenal/renal azotemia
  - Oliguric acute renal failure
  - Fluid and electrolyte derangement
- Endocrine:
  - Hyperglycemia and insulin resistance
  - Side euthyroid syndrome
  - Relative adrenal insufficiency
- Metabolic:
  - Hyperglycemia due to increased gluconeogenesis and decreased glucose clearance
  - Lipolysis, hypertriglyceridemia
  - Low ketone levels
  - Increased oxygen consumption
  - Increased energy expenditure
- Hematological:
  - Leukocytes, mild anemia due to bone marrow suppression
  - Thrombocytopenia and DIC
  - Nosocomial infections: gram negative infections are common

Clinical Staging

- Stage I:
  - Increased volume requirement
  - Mild respiratory alkalosis
  - Associated with oliguria, hyperglycemia, increased insulin requirement
- Stage II:
  - Tachypnea, hypocapnea, hypoxemia
  - Moderate liver dysfunction
  - Possible hematological abnormalities
- Stage III:
  - Shock with azotemia
  - Acid-base disturbances
  - Significant coagulation abnormalities
- Stage IV:
  - Patient is vasopressor dependant
  - Oliguric/anuric
  - Ischemic colitis/lactic acidosis.

Treatment

- Resuscitation:
  - Aimed at maintaining gastric intramucosal pH above 7.35
  - Hyperdynamic state is maintained to decrease oxygen debt/perfusion deficit
  - Volume loading > 40 mL/kg may be required in first hour in pediatric patients
  - Colloids or crystalloids may be used for volume expansion
  - Blood transfusion however, is not very beneficial
  - Effect of inotropes on splanchnic perfusion is unpredictable
- Control precipitating factors:
  - Appropriate antibiotics to be used if infection
  - Bleeding should be controlled early if trauma is the cause
  - Avoid delays in surgical therapy
  - Early fracture fixation
  - Early burn excision
- Supportive therapy:
  - Cardiovascular:
    - Inotropes and vasopressors used to maintain optimal cardiac output
    - Adequate perfusion pressure and DO_2 has to be maintained to cells
  - Respiratory:
    - Endotracheal intubation and ventilation
    - High intrathoracic pressure is avoided
  - Renals:
    - Renal perfusion is maintained with fluid therapy and inotropes
    - Renal dose dopamine may be detrimental
    - Renal replacement therapy should be initiated early
  - Hematological support if DIC manifests
- Metabolic:
  - Goal is to obtain nitrogen equilibrium
  - Early enteral nutrition helps to stimulate blood flow to gut
  - Vitamin-E, zinc, omega-3 fatty acids, glutamine and arginine are under investigation
  - Growth hormone can improve nitrogen balance
- Reduce stress response:
  - Sedation and analgesia
  - Prevent hypothermia
  - Residual foci of inflammation should be removed
  - Secondary catheter-related sepsis is avoided
- Experimental therapy:
  - Anti-inflammatory and anti-cytokine therapy
  - Monoclonal anti-TNF-α therapy
  - Platelet activating factor and phospholipase A_2 antagonists
  - Antioxidants:
    - N-acetyl-cysteine
    - ATP-$MgCl_2$
    - Inhibitors of NO synthase

Prevention

System	Preventive strategies
Cardiovascular	Restrict transfusion above Hb 7g%
Respiratory	Pressure/volume limited ventilation
Gastrointestinal	Stress ulcer prophylaxis with H_2 blockers
	Enteral nutrition
	Selective decontamination of digestive tract
Renals	Avoid nephrotoxins
Endocrines	
Hematology	DVT prophylaxis

Prognosis: *MODS score*

Characteristic	Score				
	0	1	2	3	4
GCS score	15	13–14	10–12	7–9	<6
Pressure adjusted heart rate	<10	10.1–15	15.1–20	20.1–30	>30
PaO_2/FiO_2	>300	226–300	151–225	76–150	<75
Serum bilirubin (μmol/L)	<20	21–60	61–120	121–240	>240

Characteristic	Score				
	0	1	2	3	4
Serum creatinine (μmol/L)	<100	101-200	201-350	351-500	>500
Platelet count	>120000	81000–120000	51000–80000	21000–50000	<20000

Pressure adjusted heart rate =

$$\frac{(\text{Heart rate}) \times (\text{Right atrial pressure})}{\text{Mean arterial pressure}}$$

Number of failing systems	Mortality
0	<10%
1	0–30%
2	20–50%
3	40–80%
4	60–100%
>5	>80%

NON-INVASIVE VENTILATION

Introduction

Technique of providing ventilation without the use of an artificial airway, using a mask or similar device.

Mechanism of Action

- Reduces inspiratory muscle work
- Reduces work of breathing
- Reduction in pressure-time product (PTP) of inspiratory muscles
- Also causes recruitment of alveoli
- Increases FRC
- Increases V/Q ratio

Types of NIPPV

Type	Term	Description
NPPV	Non invasive positive press vent	May be used as CPAP or BIPAP
CPAP	Continuous positive airway pressure	Positive pressure during spontaneous breathing
		No mechanical breaths given
		Active when IPAP = EPAP
PEEP	Positive end-expiratory pressure	Positive pressure applied at end-expiratory phase
		Applied during mechanical breaths
Bilevel PAP	Bilevel positive airway pressure	Provides IPAP and EPAP
		Also known as BIPAP
IPAP	Inspiratory PAP	Controls peak inspiratory pressure
EPAP	Expiratory PAP	Controls end expiratory pressure
		Used as PEEP when IPAP > EPAP
		Used as CPAP when IPAP = EPAP

Indications: *British Thoracic Society (BTS) 2002 Guidelines*

- Level I evidence: Using RCTs:
  - Acute hypercapneic respiratory failure due to COPD exacerbation
  - Facilitating weaning/extubation in patients with COPD
  - Cardiogenic pulmonary edema
  - Immunosuppressed patients with hypoxemic respiratory failure
- Level II evidence: Individual cohort studies:
  - Do not intubate status
  - End stage patients as palliative measure
  - Extubation failure (COPD/CCF: as a preventive measure)
  - Community acquired pneumonia in COPD
  - Post-operative respiratory failure (prevention and therapy)
  - Prevention of acute respiratory failure in asthma
- Level III evidence: Case control studies:
  - Neuromuscular diseases/kyphoscoliosis
  - Treatment of respiratory failure in asthma
  - Thoracic trauma
  - Partial upper airway obstruction
  - For ventilation in post-operative patients
- Level IV evidence: Case series:
  - Very old age > 75 yrs
  - Cystic fibrosis
  - *Obesity hypoventilation syndrome*

Patient Selection Criteria

- Patient criteria:
  - COPD
  - Cardiogenic pulmonary edema
  - Decompensated OSAS
  - Chest wall deformity
  - Neuromuscular disorders
- Clinical criteria:
  - Sick, but not moribund
  - Conscious and cooperate
  - Able to protect airway
  - No excessive respiratory secretions
  - Hemodynamically stable
  - Few comorbidities
- Blood gas criteria:
  - Respiratory acidosis with:
    - $PaCO_2 > 45$ mm Hg
    - pH < 7.35
    - $H^+ > 45$ nmol/L
  - Low P(A-a) O_2 gradient

Goals of NIPPV

- Short term goals:
  - Relieve symptoms
  - Reduce work of breathing
  - Improve gas exchange
  - Optimize patient comfort
  - Good patient-ventilator asynchrony
  - Minimize risk
  - Avoid intubation
- Long term goals:
  - Improve sleep duration and quality if OSAS
  - Maximize quality of life
  - Enhance functional status
  - Prolong survival

Monitoring during NIPPV

- Subjective responses: Assessment of:
  - Patient comfort level and consciousness
  - Respiratory rate and heart rate
  - Chest wall motion
  - Accessory muscle recruitment
  - Coordination with ventilator
- Physical responses:
  - Reduction in respiratory rate in first or second hour is most consistent sign
  - Reduced sternocleidomastoid activity
  - Abdominal paradox and heart rate reduces
  - Patient breathes in synchrony with ventilator
- Gaseous exchange:
  - Pulse oximetry
  - E_TCO_2
  - ABG after 4-6 hrs of initiating therapy and Q1-2H thereafter
  - Spirometry before discharge

Interfaces for NIPPV

- Nasal mask:
  - *Most commonly* used interface:
  - Cannot be used in dyspneic patients as they are mouth breathers: increases gas leak chances
  - Advantages:
    - Comfortable
    - Increased patient compliance
  - Disadvantages:
    - Gas leaks through mouth
    - Nasal dryness/drainage
    - Less effective at reducing $PaCO_2$
- Facial mask:
  - Advantages: Good seal possible
  - Disadvantages:
    - Claustrophobia
    - Non-compliance with therapy
    - Regurgitation and aspiration
    - Asphyxiation in cases of power/gas failure
    - Alarms and monitors may be necessary
  - In acute setting, use facemask initially and change to nasal mask after 24 hrs as patient improves
- Nasal pillows:
  - Resembles nasal mask but is smaller in size
  - Contains two cushions which fit under nose
  - Has pressure range of 3-20 cm H_2O
  - Used for CPAP
  - More comfortable, but gas leaks possible
- CPAP helmet

Problems with Interfaces

- Gas leaks
- Pressure points sores/dry eyes
- Nasal congestion/discharge
- Nasal airway drying
- Skin breakdown/irritation
- Sensitive front teeth

Initiating NIPPV

- Done in appropriate location and with appropriate monitors
- Patient in bed/chair, sitting at 30° angle
- Select and fit interface, select ventilator
- Apply headgear, avoid excessive strap tension: 1–2 fingers under strap
- Encourage patient to hold mask
- Connect interface to ventilator tubing and turn on ventilator
- Start with low pressure/volume in spontaneously triggered mode:
  - IPAP: 8–12 cm H_2O
  - EPAP: 3–5 cm H_2O
  - Tidal volume 10 mL/kg
- Gradually change the settings:
  - Increase IPAP to 10–20 cm H_2O
  - Increase tidal volume to 10–15 mL/kg as tolerated, as indicated by:
    - Alleviation of dyspnea
    - Reduced respiratory rate
    - Increased tidal volume
    - Good patient-ventilator synchrony
- Provide oxygen supplementation, keep $SpO_2 > 90\%$

- Check for air leaks, readjust straps
- Add humidifier as needed
- Consider mild sedation (IV lorazepam 0.5 mg) in agitated patients
- Encourage, reassure, frequently check and make adjustments
- Monitor ABGs every 1–2 hours

Weaning from NIPPV

- Criteria for weaning:
  - Respiratory rate < 24 breaths/min
  - SpO_2 > 90% on FiO_2 < 40%
  - Compensated pH > 7.35
  - Heart rate < 110 bpm
- Breaks can be made for drugs/meals, etc
- Ventilate as much as possible during first 24 hrs/ until patient improves

Contraindications to NIPPV

- Absolute contraindications:
  - Respiratory arrest
  - Cardiac arrest
  - Improperly fitting mask
- Relative contraindications:
  - General:
    - Agitated and uncooperative
    - Cannot protect airway
    - Clinically unstable patients
  - Local:
    - Facial trauma
    - Burns
    - Deformity
  - Upper airway:
    - Upper airway obstruction
    - Recent upper airway/GI/facial surgery
    - Increased secretions
    - Increased risk of aspiration/vomiting
  - Systemic:
    - Severe comorbidity
    - Focal consolidation on chest X-ray
    - Undrained pneumothorax
    - Life threatening hypoxemia
    - Hemodynamic instability
    - Bowel obstruction
    - Non-respiratory organ failure:
      - Encephalopathy
      - Severe upper GI bleed

Advantages of NIPPV

- No neuromuscular paralysis
- Reduced work of breathing
- Reduced intubation complications: injury to teeth, vocal cords and larynx
- Preserves airway defense mechanisms
- Allows patients to eat, drink and verbalize
- Reduces infectious complications: VAP, sinusitis
- Can be administered outside ICU settings
- Reduces hospital stay
- Reduces cost

Complications

- Mask related:
  - Discomfort
  - Claustrophobia
  - Facial skin erythema
  - Nasal bridge ulceration
  - Acneform rashes
- Air pressure/flow related:
  - Nasal congestion
  - Eye irritation
  - Sinus/ear pain
  - Gastric insufflation
  - Nasal/oral dryness
  - Air leaks
- Major complications:
  - Aspiration pneumonia
  - Hypotension
  - Pneumothorax

WEANING FROM MECHANICAL VENTILATION

Introduction

- Weaning refers to the process of gradually withdrawing ventilatory support
- Weaning success refers to the absence of ventilatory support 48 hrs after extubation
- Weaning failure refers to either:
  - Failure of the spontaneous breathing trial
  - Need for reintubation within 48 hours of extubation

Criteria for Weaning Readiness

Category	Examples	Values
Ventilatory criteria	Spontaneous breathing trial	Tolerates 20- 30 minutes of SBT
	$PaCO_2$	< 50 mm Hg with normal pH
	pH	7.35–7.45
	Spontaneous tidal volume	> 5 mL/kg

Contd...

Contd...

Category	Examples	Values
	Spontaneous respiratory rate	< 35 breaths/min
	Minute volume	< 10 L/min with satisfactory ABG
	Vital capacity	> 10 mL/kg
Oxygenation criteria	PaO_2 without PEEP	> 60 mm Hg at FiO_2 < 40%
	PaO_2 with PEEP (< 8 cm H_2O)	> 100 mm Hg at FiO_2 < 40%
	PaO_2/FiO_2	> 150 mm Hg
	SaO_2	> 90% at FiO_2 < 40%
	Intrapulmonary shunt (Qs/Qt)	< 20%
	P(A-a) O_2	< 350 mm Hg at FiO_2 100%
Pulmonary reserve	Maximum voluntary ventilation	Twice the minute volume at FiO_2 40%
	Maximum inspiratory pressure	> -30 cm H_2O in 20 seconds
Pulmonary measurements	Static compliance	> 30 mL/cmH_2O
	Airway resistance	Stable or improving
	V_D/V_T	< 60% while intubated
Combined weaning indices	***RSBI***	< 105 breaths/min/L
	Simplified weaning index	< 9 /min
	CROP index	> 13 mL/breath/min

Weaning Parameters

- Maximal inspiratory pressure (MIP):
  - Also called negative inspiratory force
  - Defined as the amount of negative pressure a patient can generate in 20 seconds when inspiring against an occluded measuring device
  - Normal values:
    - Healthy males: –120 cm H_2O
    - Healthy females: –90 cm H_2O
    - Intubated patients: –30 cm H_2O
- Forced vital capacity:
  - In normal subjects, FVC is 70–80 mL/kg
  - In intubated patients, FVC of 10–15 mL/kg is considered sufficient for weaning
- Airway resistance:
  - $\text{Airway resistance} = \dfrac{\text{PIP- } P_P}{\text{Constant inspiratory flow rate}}$
  - No critical weaning value has been established for airway resistance
  - Higher airway resistance causes greater work of breathing
- Intrapulmonary shunt fraction:
  - Shunt fraction $\dfrac{Q_s}{Q_T} = \dfrac{CcO_2 - CaO_2}{CcO_2 - CvO_2}$
  - Where:
    - Q_s/Q_T = Shunt percent
    - CcO_2 = End capillary O_2 content in volume%
    - CaO_2 = Arterial O_2 content in volume%
    - CvO_2 = Mixed venous O_2 content in volume%
  - Interpretation:
    - 10–20% = Mild physiological shunt
    - 20–30% = Moderate physiological shunt
    - 30% = Severe physiological shunt

Weaning Indices

- ***Simplified weaning index***:
  - Simplified Weaning Index = $\dfrac{F_{mv}\,(\text{PIP-PEEP})}{\text{MIP}} \times \dfrac{PaCO_{2mv}}{40}$
  - Where,
    - F_{mv} = ventilator frequency
    - PIP = peak inspiratory pressure
    - MIP= maximal inspiratory pressure
    - $PaCO_{2mv}$ = arterial CO_2 tension while on ventilator
  - SWI evaluates patients ventilatory endurance and efficiency of gas exchange
  - SWI <9/min suggests 93% chances of weaning success
  - SWI >11/min suggests 95% chances of weaning failure
- ***Compliance Rate Oxygenation and Pressure Index (CROP index)***
  - CROP index = $\dfrac{(C_{DYN} \times \text{MIP} \times PaO_2/PAO_2)}{f}$
  - Where:
    - C_{DYN} = Dynamic compliance
    - MIP = Maximum inspiratory pressure
    - PaO_2 = Arterial oxygen tension
    - P_AO_2 = Alveolar oxygen tension
    - f = Spontaneous respiratory rate per min
  - Useful for evaluation of:
    - Patients gas exchange
    - Balance between respiratory demand and neuromuscular reserve

- CROP index > 13 mL/breath/min indicates likelihood of weaning success

❖ ***Rapid shallow breathing index (RSBI)***:

- Introduction:
  - Determines ratio of spontaneous respiratory rate to tidal volume
  - Also called ***Tobin Index***
- Calculation:
  - $\text{RSBI} = \dfrac{\text{f (number of breaths/min)}}{\text{Tidal volume (in liters)}}$
  - $\text{RSBI rate} = \dfrac{(\text{RSBI}_2 - \text{RSBI}_1)}{\text{RSBI}_1} \times 100$
- Significance:
  - RSBI > 105 suggests potential weaning failure
  - RSBI 80–105 suggests weaning may or may not be successful
  - RSBI < 80 implies weaning may be successful
  - RSBI rate < 20% indicates chances of successful weaning trial
- Measurement:
  - Explain procedure to patient
  - Ensure ventilator sensitivity is appropriately set
  - Patient is taken off the ventilator and allowed to breath spontaneously
  - Alternatively, RSBI can be measured on:
    - CPAP of 5 cm H_2O with
    - Pressure support 5 cm H_2O for 5 minutes
  - Measurements are ideally taken:
    - Using hand held spirometer attached to endotracheal tube
    - With the patient breathing room air
  - Measurements are taken for 1 minute on room air
  - Measurements taken include:
    - Respiratory rate for 1 minute (f)
    - Minute expired volume (V_E)
  - V_T is then calculated by dividing V_E by f
  - Divide f by V_T to obtain RSBI
- Basis:
  - Better compliance is associated with adequate gas exchange and lower respiratory rate
  - Thus, greater is probability of sustaining spontaneous ventilation
  - Hence weaning is more likely to be successful if:
    - Respiratory rate is lower and
    - Tidal volume is higher
- Advantages:
  - Non-invasive measure
  - Can be obtained at bedside with portable device (ventilator)
  - Easily reproducible
  - Can be performed in short period of time
  - No need for laboratory data
- Limitations: RSBI has limited use in:
  - Patients with COPD
  - Neurosurgical patients
  - Pediatric patients
- Factors causing false elevation in RSBI:
  - Narrow endotracheal tube
  - Female gender
  - Sepsis, fever
  - Supine position
  - Suctioning
  - Restrictive lung disease
- Modifications of RSBI:
  - Serial RSBI:
    - Breathing pattern may deteriorate over time during SBT
    - This deterioration is ascribed to:
- Poor respiratory muscle endurance
- Worsening of pulmonary mechanics
    - This forms the basis of measurement of serial RSBI
    - Thus, serial RSBI is more useful to predict weaning failure
  - RSBI rate:
    - Refers to rate of change of RSBI during serial measurements
    - SBT is given for a 2-hour interval and serial RSBIs are measured
    - The RSBI rate is then calculated as:
    - $\text{RSBI rate} = \dfrac{(\text{RSBI}_2 - \text{RSBI}_1)}{\text{RSBI}_1} \times 100$
    - While predicting success of weaning, RSBI rate <20% has:
      - Sensitivity of 90%
      - Specificity of 100%
- Current status:
  - Predicts weaning failure more accurately than weaning success
  - Advantages of RSBI include:
    - Decreasing duration of ventilation
    - Elimination of delay in extubation of patients

Risk Factors for Weaning Failure

- Pathophysiological conditions:
  - Infections
  - Sepsis
  - Renal failure
  - Delirium
- Cardiovascular conditions:
  - Hypotension/hypertension
  - Low cardiac output
  - Arrhythmias
  - Fluid imbalance
  - Anemia
- Metabolic disturbances:
  - Acid-base imbalances
  - Dyselectrolytemias
  - Nutritional/caloric deficit

Signs of Weaning Failure

- Early signs:
  - Tachypnea, diaphoresis, delirium
  - Use of accessory muscles of respiration
  - Chest- abdomen asynchrony
  - Paradoxical abdominal movements
- Blood gases:
  - Progressive hypercapnia ($PaCO_2$ > 50 mm Hg)
  - Progressive respiratory acidosis
  - Progressive hypoxemia (PaO_2 < 60 mm Hg)
  - Decreasing PaO_2/ FiO_2 ratio (< 150 mm Hg)
- Vital signs:
  - Alteration in BP:
    - 20 mm Hg or systolic BP
    - 10 mm Hg for diastolic BP
  - Progressive tachycardia (> 110 b/min)
  - Arrhythmias
- Respiratory parameters:
  - Decreasing tidal volume (< 250 mL)
  - Progressive tachypnea (> 30/min)
  - Decreasing static compliance (< 30 mL/ cm H_2O)
  - Increasing V_D/V_T > 60%

SPONTANEOUS BREATHING TRIAL

Introduction

- Spontaneous breathing trial is a trial of unassisted breathing during which patient is observed for signs of respiratory failure
- Usually done for period of 30 minutes: ***Grade A, LOE I** Critical Care 2000*
- Can be carried out for upto 2 hours

Methods

- Using T piece
- Using pressure support and PEEP (minimal support with PS 5 cm H_2O and PEEP 5 cm H_2O)
- Using CPAP alone

Criteria to Assess Readiness for SBT: *Wean Screen*

Criteria	Value
Reversal of respiratory failure	Evidence of some reversal of underlying cause of respiratory failure
	f/V_T <105
Adequate oxygenation	$PaO_2/FiO_2 \geq$ 150–200
	PEEP ≤ 5–8 cm H_2O
	$FiO_2 \geq$ 40–50%
	pH ≤ 7.25
Hemodynamic stability	Absence of MI
	Absence of significant hypotension
	Minimal vasopressors
	Dopamine/dobutamine ≤ 5 μg/kg/min
Respiratory drive	Able to initiate inspiratory effort

Procedure

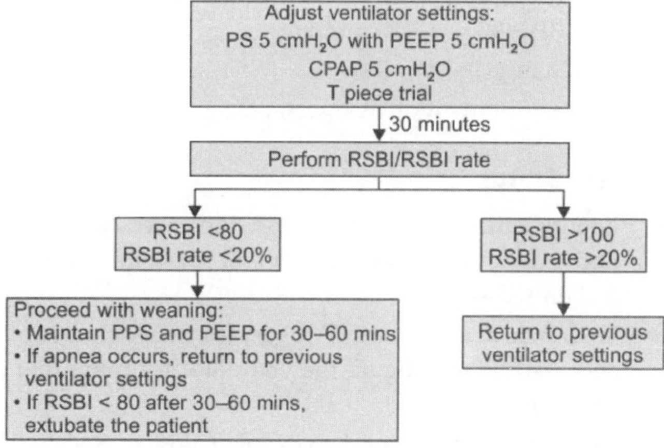

T Piece Trial

- May use new aerosol setup or existing ventilator circuit
- Let patient breathe spontaneously for up to 5 minutes every 30–180 minutes
- Return patient to mechanical ventilation after 5 minutes
- Increase duration of spontaneou breathing gradually for upto 2 hours at a time
- If patient tolerates trial with good ABG and stable vital sings, extubate the patient

Termination Criteria

- Change in mental status:
  - Coma
  - Agitation
  - Anxiety
  - Somnolence
- Signs of increased work of breathing:
  - Nasal flaring
  - Paradoxical breathing movement
  - Use of accessory respiratory muscles
  - Onset of worsening discomfort/diaphoresis
- Unstable ventilatory/respiratory pattern:
  - Respiratory rate > 30 breaths/minute
  - Change in respiratory rate of > 50%
- Inadequate gaseous exchange:
  - SpO_2 < 85–90%
  - PaO_2 < 60 mm Hg
  - pH < 7.32
  - Rise in $PaCO_2$ > 10 mm Hg
- Hemodynamic instability:
  - Heart rate > 140 bpm
  - Sustained change in heart rate > 20%
  - SBP < 90 or > 180 mm Hg
  - Change in BP > 20%
  - Requirement of vasopressors

Current Status

- Led to superior outcome and increased weaning and extubation success in several randomized controlled trials
- Tolerance of a 2 hour SBT suggests an 85% chance of successfully staying off the ventilator for more than 48 hours
- Currently, controversies exist regarding:
  - CPAP vs T-piece use for 1 hour
  - T-piece vs plain pressure support 7 cm H_2O for 1 hour
  - Duration of SBT 30 minutes vs 120 minutes

PERCUTANEOUS TRACHEOSTOMY

Introduction

PDT is a procedure in which placement of a tracheostomy tube is achieved after establishing a tracheal stoma through dilatation rather than surgical creation of a stoma.

Indications

- Need for prolonged mechanical ventilation *>7 days*:
  - Pneumonia refractory to treatment
  - Severe COPD
  - ARDS
  - MODS
  - Severe brain injury
- Airway protection against aspiration: Laryngeal incompetence due to:
  - Critical illness
  - Polyneuropathy
  - Bulbar palsy
- Upper airway obstruction:
  - Inflammatory diseases
  - Benign laryngeal pathology (web/cysts/papilla)
  - Malignant laryngeal tumors
  - Bilateral recurrent laryngeal nerve palsy
  - Laryngeal trauma/stenosis
  - Tracheal stenosis
- Facilitation of pulmonary toilet
- Facilitation of weaning in patients with COPD
- Obstructive sleep apnea syndrome

Timing

Tracheostomy indicated if artificial airway is anticipated for > 7 days.

Contraindications

- *Age < 15 years*
- Emergency airway access
- Known or suspected difficult intubation
- Local infection
- Unstable fractures of cervical spine
- Gross distortion of neck anatomy:
  - Hematoma/tumor
  - Thyromegaly
  - High innominate artery
  - Scars from previous surgery
  - Previous radiotherapy to neck
- Bleeding diathesis:
  - PT/APTT > 1.5 times reference
  - Platelet count < 50,000 /µL
  - Bleeding time > 10 minutes
- Need for PEEP > 15 cm H_2O

Advantages of Translaryngeal Intubation

- Ease and rapidity of insertion
- Avoids acute surgical complications
- Lower cost
- Avoids late surgical complications (stenosis, infection, RLN palsy)
- Reduces risk of VAP

Advantages of Tracheostomy

- Improved patient comfort
- Reduced need for sedation and analgesia
- Effective airway suctioning
- Reduced airway resistance
- Reduced work of breathing
- Reduced tube dead space
- Increased ease for speech
- Able to eat orally
- More secure airway: reduced risk of extubation
- Easy tube reinsertion
- Improved oral, nasal, facial hygiene
- Facilitates oral communication and speech
- Improves patient appearance
- Improves patient mobility
- Facilitates nursing care of airway
- Facilitates more rapid weaning off ventilator

Advantages of Percutaneous Tracheostomy

- Time required is shorter compared to surgical tracheostomy
- Avoids transport of critically ill patients to operation theatre
- Less expensive

Techniques

All have similar success rates:

- ***Sheldons trocar***
- ***Ciaglias percutaneous dilation tracheostomy*** (PDT) 1985:
  - Needle guide wire airway access
  - Serial dilation with sequentially large dilators
- ***Schachners Rapitrach technique*** 1989:
  - Contains dilating forceps device with beveled metal cones
  - Advanced forcibly over a wire into airway
- ***Griggs guidewire dilating forceps (GDWF) technique*** 1990:
  - Similar to Rapitrach forceps
  - Forceps has no cutting edge on tip of instrument
- ***Fantoni's translaryngeal technique:***
  - Initial puncture of the trachea is carried out with the needle directed cranially
  - Tracheal cannula inserted with a pull-through technique along the orotracheal route in a retrograde fashion
  - Cannula is then rotated downward using a plastic obturator
  - Advantages:
    - Minimal amount of skin incision required
    - Minimal bleeding observed
  - Disadvantages:
    - Procedure can only be carried out under endoscopic guidance
    - Rotating the tracheal cannula downward may pose a problem

Equipment

- PDT kit:
  - # 22 needle, syringe
  - 11 F short punch dilator
  - Guide wire
  - 8 F guiding catheter
  - 18 F, 21 F, 24 F, 28 F, 36 F, 38 F dilators
  - ***Shiley*** 8 size tracheostomy tube
  - Fibreoptic bronchoscope
- Rapitrach kit:
  - # 12 needle and syringe
  - Guidewire, scalpel
  - Rapitrach PCT dilator
  - Standard portex # 8 tracheostomy tube with curved obturator
  - Fibreoptic bronchoscope
- GWDF kit:
  - # 14 needles and syringe
  - Guide wire (J tipped Seldinger type)
  - Scalpel
  - ***Howard Kelly*** forceps
  - Shiley 8 # double cannula tracheostomy tube with curved obturator
  - Fibreoptic bronchoscope

Types of Tracheostomy Tubes

- Depending on cuff:
  - Cuffed tubes:
    High volume low pressure cuffs preferred
    Cuff pressure not to exceed 25 cm H_2O
    Higher pressures can cause tracheal mucosal ischemia

- Uncuffed metallic tubes:
  - ***Jacksons 3 cannula***
  - ***Fullers tube***
- Depending on number of cannula:
  - Single cannula tube
  - Double cannula tube:
    - If cannula gets blocked, inner cannula is removed and cleaned everyday
    - Outer cannula is not removed on 1st 3 days to allow track formation
- Depending on fenestration:
  - Fenestrated tubes
  - Unfenestrated tubes:
    - Fenestrated has opening in posterior part of outer tube
    - If tube is cuffed, fenestration lies above cuff
    - Deflation of cuff allows air to pass through tracheostomy lumen and fenestration
    - Maximal airflow then occurs through upper airways
    - This aids in speech

Investigations

- Complete blood count: platelets > 50000 /µL
- PT/APTT > 1.5 reference
- Bleeding time < 10 minutes
- Blood urea nitrogen < 40 mg/dL, creatinine < 4 mg/dL
- Chest X-ray for tracheal air column (AP and lateral view)

Preparation for Tracheostomy

- NPO orders
- Induce with 50-100 µg fentanyl and 1–2 mg/kg ketamine IV
- 5 mg morphine, 10 mg atracurium IV
- Patient kept on FiO_2 1 from at least 15 minutes before surgery
- Withdraw ETT under FOB vision to place cuff just under vocal cords
- Monitor ECG, NIBP, SpO_2, E_TCO_2

Position

- Patient kept supine
- Sand bag under neck and shoulder to hyperextend neck
- Head placed in neutral position
- Surface marking done for thyroid, cricoid cartilage and suprasternal notch marked

Technique

GRIGGS

- Intensivist stands at head end of patient
- ETT cuff deflated and tidal volume increased to twice desired volume with increase in peak inspiratory pressure limit
- Cleanse and drape neck below cricoid cartilage and upper chest
- Infiltrate skin and subcutaneous tissue with 2% xylocaine with 1:100000 adrenaline
- Identify puncture site by applying pressure between 2nd and 3rd tracheal rings
- ETT withdrawn from puncture site
- Pass FOB through ETT
- 1.5 to 2 cm midline transverse incision made between T_2 and T_3
- Pass needle (14# IV cannula with syringe attached) through tracheal wall and pass guidewire through it when air drawn into syringe
- Visualize entry of needle with FOB
- Remove needle as soon as air bubbles into syringe and advance sheath till it enters trachea
- Thread conical dilator to dilate soft tissue and enter trachea with continuous gentle pressure, verify with FOB
- Remove dilator, dilate trachea with both hands
- Suction out bleeding
- Thread TT over guide wire under FOB vision

Ciaglia

- Uses rhinos for dilation
- Technique is similar to Griggs otherwise
- Rhinos become smooth when placed in water
- With rhinos, dilation of trachea is more controlled
- In Griggs, dilation is done with forceps and force to be applied to place tube has to be learnt by trial and error

Postoperative Care

- Airway entry checked by auscultation and respiratory plethysmography
- Chest X-ray taken to confirm position
- Provide humidified gases:
  - ***Trach mask/mist collar***
  - Heat and moisture exchanger
  - Suction blood and secretions
- *Antiseptic wound and stoma care everyday*

- Monitor tube position to prevent dislodgement
- Suction tracheostomy tube when:
  - Audible rales or mucus rattling
  - Patient unable to generate effective cough
  - Visible secretions in airway
  - Increased respiratory rate or work of breathing
  - During cuff deflation
  - Before feeds
- Avoid frequent suctions to prevent build up of secretions
- Feeding with tracheostomy:
  - Suction tracheostomy tube before feeding
  - Encourage fluid intake which helps in loosening secretions
  - *Deflate cuff to enable swallowing*
  - *Use speaking valve, if present to make swallowing easier*
  - Monitor for vomiting and aspiration
- *Deflate balloon for 15 mins every hour for 1st 24 hours and then leave balloon inflated*
- *Clean inner cannula once every 8 hours*
- Tracheostomy tube exchange
  - *Done every 2 weeks if single lumen TT*
  - *Done every month if double cannula TT*
- Tube exchange to prevent obstruction and also formation of granulation tissue around tube

Decannulation

- The patient is decannulated when:
  - Able to obey commands in non-neurologically compromised patients
  - Cough reflex is sufficient
  - Suctioning is rarely needed
  - Mechanical ventilation has not been needed for more than 24 hours
  - FiO_2 is reasonably low
  - Airway is spontaneously patent
  - No new infilterates on chest X-ray
  - Tolerates cuff deflation for more than 24 hours
  - Tolerates speaking valve for more than 12 hours
  - Tolerates decannulation cap for upto 4 hours
- At discharge from ICU to the ward with a tracheal cannula in place:
  - Tracheal cannula should be without cuff (to avoid risk of total airway occlusion)
  - An individual plan for decannulation should be presented

Complications

Perioperative Complications (< 24 hours Postoperatively)

- Hemorrhage
- Hypoxia
- False passage:
  - Most common with short and thick neck
  - Paratracheal insertion
- Posterior tracheal wall perforation:
  - Due to guiding catheter/guidewire instability
  - Can cause pneumothorax/subcutaneous emphysema
- Subcutaneous emphysema:
  - False tracheostomy tube placement
  - Tracheal wall trauma
- Tension pneumothorax
- Accidental extubation
- Death

Postoperative Complications (> 24 hours Postoperatively)

- Hemorrhage: common if:
  - Multisystem disease
  - Sepsis
  - Coagulopathies
  - Renal failure
  - Tracheoarterial fistula
  - Stomal granulation
- Granulation tissue: Due to perichondritis of cricoid/tracheal cartilages
- Tracheoarterial fistula:
  - Tip of tube erodes into posterior branch of brachiocephalic artery
  - Risk is minimized if TT puncture is between 2-3 tracheal rings
- Stomal infections
- Tracheoesophageal fistula

Late Complications (> 6 months Postoperatively)

- Voice change
- Scar formation
- Tracheal stenosis:
  - Symptomatic if > 75% lumen obstructed
  - Incidence reduced by using properly sized TT
  - High volume, low pressure cuff preferred
  - Flexible connecting tube between TT and ventilator reduces traction on TT and pressure on trachea
  - Place TT between T_2 and T_3 or T_1 and T_2 to reduce risk of cricoid cartilage injury

- Tracheocutaneous fistula:
  - Due to excessive granulation tissue and chronic infection of stoma
  - Usually stoma closes within 2–5 days of decannulation

VENTILATION IN ARDS

Definition

- Acute onset arterial hypoxemia within 1 week
- Bilateral opacities consistent with pulmonary edema on chest X-ray or CT scan
- PaO_2/FiO_2 ratio < 300 mm Hg with a minimum of 5 cm H_2O PEEP
- No evidence of left atrial HTN/CCF
- PCWP < 18 mm Hg

ARDS Score

No.	Component	Value	Score
1.	Chest X-ray score:		
	No alveolar consolidation	—	0
	Consolidation confined to one compartment	—	1
	Consolidation confined to two quadrants	—	2
	Consolidation confined to three quadrants	—	3
	Consolidation in all four quadrants	—	4
2.	Hypoxemia score:		
	PaO_2/FiO_2	> 300	0
	PaO_2/FiO_2	225–299	1
	PaO_2/FiO_2	175–224	2
	PaO_2/FiO_2	100–174	3
	PaO_2/FiO_2	< 100	4
3.	PEEP Score:		
	PEEP	< 5 cm H_2O	0
	PEEP	6–8 cm H_2O	1
	PEEP	9–11 cm H_2O	2
	PEEP	12–14 cm H_2O	3
	PEEP	> 15 cm H_2O	4

$$\text{Final value} = \frac{\text{Aggregate sum}}{\text{Number of components used}}$$

Category	Score
No lung injury	0
Mild-moderate lung injury (ALI)	0.1– 2.5
Severe lung injury (ARDS)	≥ 2.5

Risks of Ventilation in ARDS

- Ventilation may cause *ventilator induced lung injury (VILI)* by:
  - Atelectrauma
  - Barotrauma
  - Volutrauma
  - Biotrauma
- Oxygen toxicity if high FiO_2:
  - Retrolental fibroplasia
  - Reduced surfactant

Goals of Ventilation: *ARDS Network Protocol*

- Oxygenation:
  - PaO_2 55–80 mm Hg or SpO_2 88–94%
  - SpO_2 > 94% if concomitant pregnancy/stroke/intracranial HTN
- Tidal volume 4–6 mL/kg of Ideal Body Weight
- Plateau pressure < 30 cm H_2O
- Respiratory rate < 35 breaths/min
- pH between 7.30–7.45

Ventilation Strategies

Lung Protective Strategies

- Open collapsed lung units with recruitment maneuvers
- Keep recruited units open with appropriate PEEP
- Prevent alveolar over-distension:
  - Limit plateau pressure < 30 cm H_2O
  - Limit tidal volume to 4–6 mL/kg of IBW
- Permissive hypercapnea

Other Ventilatory Strategies

- ***Prone ventilation***
- ***Liquid ventilation***
- ***Airway pressure release ventilation (APRV)***
- ***Inverse ratio ventilation***
- Tracheal gas insufflation
- ECMO
- High frequency ventilation

Newer Strategies

- Continuous Lateral Rotation Therapy
- ***NAVA***
- ***Upright ventilation***
- ***Negative pressure ventilation***

RECRUITMENT MANEUVER

Introduction

- Refers to the brief application of a CPAP maneuver with the goal of opening as many collapsed alveoli as possible

Mechanism: Three Steps to Open Lung Alveoli

- Overcome critical opening pressure during inspiration
- Maintain opening pressure for sufficient time
- Use auto-PEEP/apply high PEEP at expiration to prevent collapse
- ***Hysteresis***: for a given inflation pressure, lung volume is larger during exhalation than inhalation

Indications

- ARDS/ ALI:
  - Insufficient evidence to support routine use in ARDS
  - May be used in severe hypoxemia despite lung protective ventilation strategies
- Atelectasis during general anesthesia
- De-recruitment atelectasis following disconnection from ventilator
- After ETT suctioning

Contraindications

- Raised ICP
- Hemodynamic instability
- Existing barotrauma
- Predisposition to barotrauma:
  - Apical bullous lung disease
  - Focal lung pathology (lobar pneumonias)

Factors Affecting Recruitment

- Type of lung injury, pulmonary or extra-pulmonary origin
- Differences in the severity of lung injury
- The transpulmonary pressures reached during recruitment maneuvers
- The type of recruitment maneuver applied
- The PEEP levels used to stabilize the lungs after the recruitment maneuver
- Differences in patient positioning (prone position more favourable)
- Use of vasoactive drugs:
  - These affect the distribution of pulmonary blood flow
  - Thus gas-exchange may be modified due to alterations in V/Q matching

Consequences of Recruitment Maneuver

- Raised ICP
- Increased oxygenation
- ***Stretch reflex*** of alveoli stimulated: increased surfactant secretion
- Increased intrapulmonary shunt
- Barotrauma
- Increased pulmonary arterial pressure
- Decreased cardiac output

Types of Recruitment Maneuvers (RM)

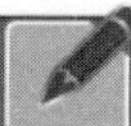

- Sustained inflation maneuvers
- Pressure controlled ventilation (PC-CMV) applied with escalating PEEP level
- Recruitment and decremental PEEP
- Extended sigh maneuvers (eSigh)
- *RAMP maneuver*: Long slow increase in inspiratory pressure upto 40 cm H_2O.

Timing of Recruitment Maneuver (RM)

- Most centres perform recruitment maneuvers early in the course of ARDS
- This is during the early exudative phase of ARDS (first 7–10 days)
- RM may not be effective if performed once ARDS enters the fibroproliferative phase

Procedure

- Sustained inflation maneuver:
  - Prior to beginning the maneuver:
    - FiO_2 is increased to 1.0
    - Ventilator is set to CPAP mode with mandatory rate 0
    - Patient is sedated to tolerate high airway pressures
  - 30–40 cm H_2O PEEP is applied for 40 seconds during the first RM
  - Most of the alveolar recruitment occurs during first 10 seconds of the RM
  - The results of first recruitment maneuver are then assessed
  - If the response is inadequate, RM is repeated in 15–20 minutes
  - Second maneuver can be done at a higher PEEP (35–40 cm H_2O)

- If RM is successful, PaO_2/FiO_2 ratio becomes > 300 mm Hg
- High PEEP value is maintained post RM to prevent *de-recruitment* of alveoli

❖ PC-CMV with escalating PEEP level:
- PC-CMV mode is selected with:
  - Pressure control set 20 cm H_2O above the PEEP value
  - Mandatory rate 10–12 breaths/min
- PEEP is then increased incrementally till the PIP is at least 40 cm H_2O
- This high PIP is sustained for 40–60 seconds
- The PEEP is then reduced to an appropriate level to prevent derecruitment
- Ventilation is then continued PC-CMV mode

❖ PC-CMV with increased PEEP levels:
- Uses PC-CMV with PEEP increments in 5 cm H_2O
- Each increment in PEEP is sustained for 2–5 minutes
- All other ventilatory parameters are held constant during the RM
- Continuous monitoring of the lung compliance is mandatory
- Following full inflation, PEEP levels are reduced in 5 cm H_2O decrements
- PEEP levels are reduced till there is a sudden drop in lung compliance
- This represents the upper inflection point of the lungs
- The lung is then reinflated to allow opening of lung units
- The PEEP is now set at 2–4 cm H_2O above the upper inflection point

❖ Recruitment and decremental PEEP:
- This technique can be used to determine optimal PEEP for lung recruitment
- Following full inflation of lungs, PEEP is progressively decreased
- This is done in 5 cm H_2O increments until compliance of the lungs decreases
- This PEEP value represents the upper inflection point (UIP) for the lungs
- Following this, lungs are reinflated with PEEP set 2–4 cm H_2O above the UIP

❖ Extended sigh maneuvers:
- Sigh breaths were used in 1960s to prevent low tidal volume atelectasis
- The use of sighs was eventually abandoned due to use of higher tidal volumes
- However, in ARDS, lung protective ventilation with low V_T is used
- This has renewed interest in sigh breaths
- Different techniques of sigh breaths include:
  - 3 consecutive breaths at a $P_{plateau}$ of 45 cm H_2O
  - Twice the tidal volume every 25 breaths with optimal PEEP

Monitoring during Recruitment Maneuver

❖ RM is considered successful if PaO_2/FiO_2 ratio increases by 20–50%

❖ RM is discontinued if:
- SpO_2 decreases by 5%
- Systolic BP falls by 30 mm Hg
- Heart rate decreases by 20 bpm
- Occurrence of arrhythmias

Advantages

❖ Effective in reducing lung atelectasis

❖ Improves oxygenation and respiratory mechanics

❖ Prevents endotracheal suctioning-induced alveolar derecruitment

Disadvantages

❖ Effects are short-lived (3–6 hours)

❖ Associated with circulatory impairment

❖ Increased risk of barotrauma/volutrauma

❖ Reduces net alveolar fluid clearance

Complications

❖ Hypotension:
- RM is associated with sustained increase in the transthoracic pressure
- This results in a reduced venous return to the heart
- Thus, hypotension may occur due to a reduction in the preload to the heart

❖ Desaturation

❖ Barotrauma:
- Not commonly reported following RM
- However, RM can rarely result in pneumothorax and subcutaneous emphysema

❖ Cardiac arrest (during prolonged recruitment maneuvers)

Current Status 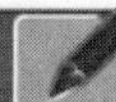

- Most studies of recruitment maneuvers report improvement in oxygenation
- However, meta-analyses do not report convincing benefits on key outcomes such as:
  - Mortality
  - Duration of hospital stay
  - Incidence of barotrauma
- Thus, clinical benefit is uncertain and it is not routinely recommended in ARDS
- Further trials are required to confirm the benefit from lung recruitment in ARDS.

POSITIVE END EXPIRATORY PRESSURE

Introduction

- Positive end expiratory pressure (PEEP) is the alveolar pressure above atmospheric pressure which exists at end expiration
- This is used as ventilatory strategy to treat refractory hypoxemia (extrinsic PEEP)

Indications

- Refractory hypoxemia, (PaO_2 < 60 mm Hg with FiO_2 of > 50%)
- During routine ventilation:
  - Low levels of PEEP are required for most ventilated patients
  - This is to prevent end-expiratory alveolar collapse
  - This reduces the incidence of VILI
- ARDS/ALI:
  - Remains the prime indication for application of PEEP
  - ARDS patients usually require > 5 cm H_2O PEEP
  - The major benefit in this population is an improvement in oxygenation
- Cardiogenic pulmonary edema
- Other indications:
  - Bilateral infiltrates on chest radiograph
  - Recurrent atelectasis with low FRC
  - Reduced lung compliance

Contraindications

- Absolute contraindications:
  - Untreated pneumothorax
  - Tension pneumothorax
- Relative contraindications:
  - Recent lung surgery
  - Emphysema
  - Bronchopleural fistula
  - Hypovolemia
  - Hemodynamic instability
  - Raised ICP
  - Right heart failure/pulmonary HTN
  - Post cardiac surgeries like ***Glenns/Fontans*** shunt

Physiology

- PEEP re-inflates collapsed alveoli and maintains alveolar inflation during expiration
- Normally alveolar end expiratory pressure equals atmosphere pressure
- Average pleural pressure is around –5 cm H_2O
- Thus, alveolar distending pressure (i.e., alveolar – pleural pressure) is +5 cm H_2O
- This alveolar distending pressure overcomes elastic recoil of alveolar wall
- Thus, PEEP of 5 cm H_2O is sufficient to maintain end expiratory alveolar volume

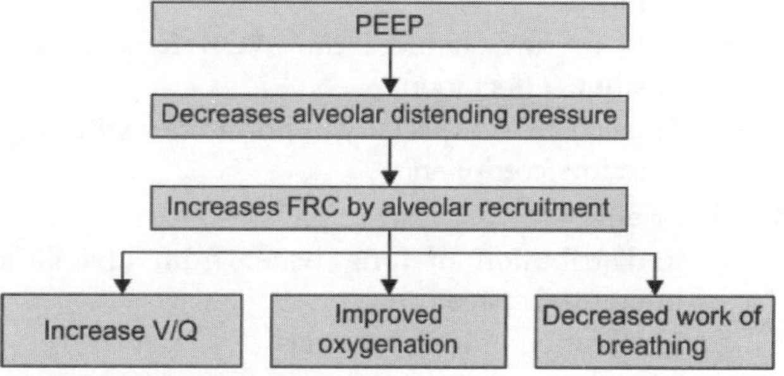

Mechanisms of PEEP

- Recruitment of atelectatic alveoli:
  - Use of extrinsic PEEP causes recruitment of atelectatic alveoli
  - This causes reinflation of previously collapsed alveoli
  - Thus, intrapulmonary shunting across atelectatic alveoli is reduced
  - This improves ventilation- perfusion mismatch
- Increase in dissolved arterial oxygen content:
  - Application of PEEP increases partial pressure of oxygen in the alveoli
  - By Henrys law, solubility of gas in a liquid is directly proportional to pressure of the gas above the surface of the solution
  - Increase in partial pressure of alveolar oxygen causes:
    - Increased gas exchange across the alveolar-capillary membrane
    - Increased solubility of oxygen in blood

- Thus, the dissolved oxygen content of blood increases

❖ Increasing surface area of alveolar basement membrane:
- Application of PEEP causes a re-expansion of collapsed alveoli
- This results in an increase in the surface area of alveolar basement membrane
- This creates more areas for gaseous exchange to occur

❖ Decrease in work of breathing (WOB):
- Use of extrinsic PEEP significantly reduces the work of breathing
- The WOB can be as high as 30% in intubated patients with low compliance
- This can cause an increase in the CO_2 production and lactate levels
- By decreasing the WOB, lactate and CO_2 production is reduced
- Thus, the need for high minute ventilation is reduced
- This in turn reduces the WOB further, in a positive- effect loop
- Thus, PEEP is especially important for stiff lungs with low compliance

❖ Other effects:
- Redistribution of lung water from alveoli to interstitial space
- Restoration of lung volumes

Goals of PEEP and CPAP

❖ To maintain PaO_2 > 60 mm Hg and SpO_2 > 90% with an acceptable pH

❖ To recruit alveoli and maintain them in an aerated state

❖ To restore functional residual capacity

❖ To enhance tissue oxygenation

Types of PEEP

❖ Extrinsic PEEP: PEEP which is provided by a mechanical ventilator

❖ Intrinsic PEEP: PEEP which occurs secondary to incomplete expiration

Optimal PEEP

❖ Term coined by Suter et al. in 1975

❖ Optimal PEEP is defined as the level of PEEP that maximizes clinical benefit with:
- Increased delivery of oxygen
- Improved FRC
- Improved static compliance (C_s)
- Decreased shunt fraction (Q_S/Q_T

❖ PEEP is said to be optimal when:
- FiO_2 is the lowest possible
- Adequate oxygenation is attained:
  - PaO_2 greater than 60 mm Hg
  - SaO_2 greater than 90%
- Optimal oxygen transport (> 1000 mL/minute of oxygen)
- PaO_2/FiO_2 ratio > 300
- Optimal mixed venous oxygen saturation
- Static lung compliance is maximal
- Intrapulmonary shunt fraction is reduced to less than 15%
- Absence of any cardiovascular adverse effects induced by PEEP:
  - Adequate systemic BP
  - Decrease of less than 20% in cardiac output
  - Stable pulmonary vascular pressures

The Optimal PEEP Study

❖ Oxygen delivery titrated PEEP study:
- In this study, PEEP values are titrated to oxygen delivery
- Oxygen delivery is calculated as:
  O_2 delivery (DO_2) = {Cardiac output (Q_T)) × {Oxygen content (CaO_2)}
- For optimal PEEP level, PEEP is increased in 2 cm H_2O increments
- Clinical parameters are continuously monitored
- PEEP is incrementally increased until there is a reduction in DO_2
- This is the point at which optimal PEEP has been exceeded
- PEEP is then ramped down to the previous level, called optimal PEEP

❖ Compliance titrated PEEP study:
- In this study, PEEP values are titrated to the static compliance
- Static compliance is calculated as:
- Static compliance C_s =

$$\frac{\text{Tidal volume delivered (mL)}}{P_{PLAT} - P_{BASELINE}}$$

- For optimal PEEP level, PEEP is increased in 2 cm H_2O increments
- As the PEEP increases, static compliance also increases
- Once optimal PEEP has been exceeded, there is a sudden fall in C_s

- PEEP in incrementally increased until there is a reduction in compliance
- PEEP is then ramped down to the previous level, called optimal PEEP

Weaning from PEEP

- Baseline ABG is reviewed to determine improvement in ventilatory indications
- Criteria for weaning from PEEP therapy should be met:
  - PaO_2 > 90 mm Hg on an FiO_2 < 0.40
  - Hemodynamically stable
  - Absence of septic picture
  - Improvement in lung compliance (C_s > 25 mL/cm H_2O)
  - PaO_2/FiO_2 ratio > 250
- PEEP value is initially reduced by 5 cm H_2O
- Clinical parameters are continuously monitored
- PEEP is returned to previous levels if there is:
  - Reduction in SpO_2 by > 20% from previous PEEP level
  - Reduction in PaO_2 by > 20% from previous PEEP level
- In the absence of these criteria, further weaning of PEEP levels may be considered
- Further reductions in PEEP levels are done at 1 to 6-hour intervals
- The duration of weaning depends on the clinical scenario
- Once the PEEP has been weaned to 5 cm H_2O, additional evaluation is necessary
- If reduction of PEEP to 0 worsens the condition, PEEP is continued at 5 cm H_2O
- This is done until criteria for extubation are met

Beneficial Effects of PEEP

- Improves oxygenation
- Recruits and stabilizes alveoli
- Improves lung compliance
- Improves FRC and prevents end expiratory collapse
- Minimizes potential for VILI

Complications

- Decreased venous return:
  - Pleural pressure becomes more positive with application of PEEP
  - This decreases pressure gradient between RA and central venous drainage
  - This decreases venous return to the right atrium
  - This causes decreased cardiac output and hypotension
- Barotrauma:
  - Increased risk of barotrauma if:
    - PEEP > 10 cm H_2O
    - Mean Airway Pressure > 30 cm H_2O
    - Peak inspiratory pressure > 50 cm H_2O
  - Causes of barotrauma:
    - Pneumothorax
    - Tension pneumothorax
    - Pneumomediastinum
    - Pneumopericardium
    - Pneumoperitoneum
    - Subcutaneous emphysema
- Raised ICP:
  - More common in patients with normally compliant lungs
  - Raised intrathoracic pressure impedes venous return from superior vena cava
  - This causes venous congestion and retrograde increase in ICP
  - Increase in ICP is rare in patients with ARDS/non-compliant lungs
  - Excessive pressure due to PEEP is not transmitted to SVC in ARDS
  - Thus, there is no increase in ICP in ARDS patients
- Renal function:
  - PEEP reduces perfusion to glomeruli
  - Glomerular filtration is less effective and reduced urine output results
- Others:
  - Decreased cardiac output
  - Increased pulmonary vascular resistance; right ventricular failure
  - Decreased cerebral perfusion pressure
  - Septal shift to left

AUTO PEEP

Introduction

- Intrinsic or auto-PEEP is a complication of mechanically ventilated patients
- This is the PEEP generated as a result of incomplete expiration

Mechanism

- Passive exhalation permits complete emptying of the air in the lungs
- Air is expelled until alveolar pressure equalizes atmospheric pressure

- However, when the lung fails to deflated completely, air is trapped at end expiration
- This generates a positive pressure at end expiration, called auto-PEEP

Etiology

- High minute ventilation:
  - A high minute ventilation can be caused by:
    - Large tidal volumes
    - High respiratory rates
  - Large tidal volume (TV):
    - High TV increases volume of air to be exhaled before the next breath
    - Thus, with high TV, some air may be retained at the end of the breath
    - This can result in the generation of auto-PEEP
  - High respiratory rates:
    - High respiratory rates decrease the duration of expiration
    - This results in inadequate time for complete expulsion of air
    - This results in air trapping and generation of auto-PEEP
- Expiratory flow limitation:
  - Expiratory flow may be limited by:
    - Bronchospasm
    - Bronchomalacia
  - This causes incomplete expulsion of air during expiration
  - Expiratory flow limitation is seen in most patients with COPD
  - Thus, auto-PEEP may be generated during mechanical ventilation
  - Flow limitation is higher in supine position compared with semi-recumbent
- Expiratory resistance:
  - Refers to expiratory flow limitation due to causes unrelated to airways
  - These include:
    - Narrow diameter endotracheal tube
    - Kinked ETT
    - Inspissated secretions
    - Exhalation/ PEEP valves
    - Patient- ventilator asynchrony

Factors Contributing to Auto-PEEP

- Airway inflammation and mucus plugging:
  - This results in the generation of dynamic airflow obstruction
  - Mucus plugging occludes the airway distal to the location of the plug
  - This causes expiratory airflow obstruction and air trapping in distal airways
  - During forced expiratory efforts, pressure around the airway increases
  - This is due to trapping of air in the alveoli that are dependent on that airway
  - This results in the generation of auto-PEEP
- High lung compliance:
  - The airways lack a scaffolding to stay open during forced expiration
  - This leads to dynamic airway collapse and air trapping
  - This ultimately results in the generation of auto-PEEP
- Slow inspiratory flow:
  - This may generate a higher inspiratory to expiratory time ratio
  - Thus, time taken for expiration may be very short
  - This can result in air trapping and the generation of auto-PEEP

Sequelae of Auto-PEEP

- Increase in intrathoracic pressure
- Decreased venous return
- Decreased cardiac output
- Alveolar overdistension and barotrauma
- Ventilator associated lung injury

Evaluation of Auto PEEP

- Flow versus time graphs:
  - With auto-PEEP, exhalation will be ongoing when next inspiratory cycle starts
  - Thus, inspiratory flow upstroke begins before expiratory tracing reaches zero
  - This can be detected on the flow vs time graphs on the ventilator display
- Palpation and auscultation:
  - With auto-PEEP, exhalation will be ongoing when next inspiratory cycle starts
  - Thus, inspiratory flow will be heard before the expiratory flow ceases
- Quantification of auto-PEEP:
  - Auto PEEP can be calculated from the end-expiratory alveolar pressure

Auto-PEEP = (end expiratory alveolar pressure) – (extrinsic PEEP)

- Measurement of end-expiratory alveolar pressure:
  - End-expiratory breath hold is applied by the ventilator
  - Airway pressure is read directly from the ventilator during breath hold

❖ Other signs:
- Increasing plateau pressures on the ventilator
- Active exhalation shown by the use of accessory muscles of expiration
- Hypotension
- Long expiratory times

Treatment of Auto PEEP

❖ Ensuring adequate exhalation time:
- Decreasing the tidal volume
- Decreasing respiratory rate
- Decreasing I:E ratio to 1:3 to 1:5
- Increasing inspiratory flow rate to 60-100 L/min

❖ Decreasing work of breathing:
- Minimize work of breathing by sedation and paralysis
- Control of fever and pain
- Optimal treatment of sepsis

❖ Minimize expiratory flow obstruction:
- Bronchodilators
- Steroids
- Suctioning of mucus plugs

❖ Minimize expiratory resistance:
- ETT suctioning
- Replace ETT
- Replace ventilatory circuits

❖ Disconnecting patient from ventilator and allowing enough time for exhalation

PERMISSIVE HYPERCAPNEA

Introduction

❖ Permissive hypercapnia (PHY) is a strategy used to minimize the incidence of VILI

❖ This is a central component of protective lung ventilatory strategy

❖ Refers to:
- Intentional hypoventilation of patient
- Acceptance of hypercapnia
- Continuation of the hypoventilation strategy

❖ This does not include patients with chronic hypercapnia whose baseline $PaCO_2$ levels are targeted during mechanical ventilation

Mechanism of Action

❖ Reduced tidal volume allowing permissive hypercapnea causes:
- Reduced peak inspiratory pressures:
- Reduced mean airway pressure
- Reduced likelihood of barotrauma

❖ Attenuation of inflammatory response of ALI:
- Interferes with coordination of immune response by reducing cytokine signalling
- Inhibits the release of TNF-α and IL-1
- Modulates neutrophil expression of selectins and intercellular adhesion molecules

❖ Effects on free radical generation and activity:
- Attenuates free radical production
- Modulates free radical induced tissue damage
- Production of superoxide by stimulated neutrophils is decreased at acidic pH
- Reduces free radical tissue injury following pulmonary ischemia/reperfusion

Effects of Hypercarbia

❖ Central nervous system:
- For each 1 mm Hg increase in CO_2, CBF increases by 1.8 mL/100 g/ min
- Increased $PaCO_2$ causes:
  - Raised pH of CSF
  - Cerebral vasodilatation
- This increases the intracranial pressure
- $PaCO_2$ > 90 mm Hg causes decreased seizure threshold

❖ Respiratory system:
- Hypercarbia increases pulmonary vascular resistance
- Increases hypoxic pulmonary vasoconstriction (HPV)
- Maximal HPV occurs when $PaCO_2$ is around 100 mm Hg

❖ Cardiovascular system:
- Increased plasma epinephrine and norepinephrine
- Increases heart rate and BP
- Very high $PaCO_2$ levels cause hypotension and bradycardia

- GIT and renals:
  - Increases hepatic and portal venous blood flow
  - Retention of HCO_3^- in renal tubules
  - Metabolic alkalosis (compensatory)

Metabolic Effects of Permissive Hypercarbia

$PaCO_2$	pH
80	7.15
70	7.22
60	7.28
50	7.34
40	7.40
35	7.45
30	7.50
25	7.55
20	7.60

Indications

- Acute respiratory distress syndrome (ARDS) managed with low tidal volumes
- Acute lung injury (ALI)
- Status asthmaticus
- COPD

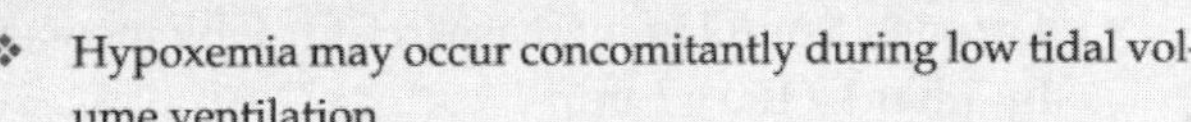

Recommendations

- Hypoxemia may occur concomitantly during low tidal volume ventilation
- Thus, higher FiO_2 is recommended during ventilation
- No acceptable lower limit of pH has been defined
- pH values above 7.25 are usually accepted
- Patients may tolerate pH values up to 7.10 in the absence of renal problems
- Actual $PaCO_2$ is of less importance as up to 150 mm Hg can be tolerated
- High $PaCO_2$ levels however increase the drive to breathe
- Thus, adequate sedation and neuromuscular paralysis must be ensured
- Limit carbon dioxide production during permissive hypercapnia by:
  - Antipyretics
  - External cooling.

Protocol for Implementation of Permissive Hypercapnea

- Hypercapnia must be implemented progressively in increments of 10 mm Hg
- Hypercapnia can be increased up to a maximum of 80 mm Hg/day
- Once hypercapnia exceeds 80 mm Hg, progress should be made more slowly
- FiO_2 is adjusted to maintain SpO_2 at 85-90%
- This may require intermittent use of 100% FiO_2
- Weaning from PHY:
  - When PHY has been used for less than 24 hours:
    - $PaCO_2$ is allowed to decrease by 10–20 mm Hg/hour
    - When the $PaCO_2$ levels are closer to normal, reductions are slower
  - When PHY has been used for > 24 hours, it is discontinued over 1–3 days

Ventilation During Permissive Hypercapnia

- Tidal volume is maintained in the range of 4–7 mL/kg
- Plateau airway pressure (PAP) more than 35 cm H_2O is avoided
- If PAP < 30 cm H_2O despite tidal volume of 10 mL/kg, PHY not likely to be needed
- Higher PAP may be accepted if chest wall compliance is decreased as in:
  - Tense ascites
  - Morbid obesity
  - Chest wall trauma
- $PaCO_2$ is allowed to increase and pH is allowed to drop
- Ventilatory settings are maintained constant as the pH falls
- CO_2 production is reduced by using:
  - Paralytic agents
  - Cooling the patient
  - Restricting glucose intake
- Buffering agents are administered to maintain pH above 7.25
- Buffering agents used include:
  - Sodium bicarbonate
  - Tromethamine (THAM)
  - Carbicarb (mixture of sodium carbonate and bicarbonate)

Contraindications

- Acute cerebral disease:
  - Cerebral hemorrhage
  - Mass lesions
  - Head injury
  - Cerebral edema
  - Known seizure disorder
- Cardiovascular diseases:
  - Active coronary artery disease
  - Heart failure

- Pulmonary HTN and right heart dysfunction
- Arrhythmias
- Hemodynamically unstable patients
- Hypovolemia

Advantages

- Reduced peak airway pressures
- Minimizes occurrence of VILI/VALI
- May exert direct protective effects in ALI states by attenuating inflammatory process
- Achieves faster weaning and improves survival rates
- Decreases incidence of chronic lung diseases
- Improved long term neurological outcome

Disadvantages

- Potential for hypercarbia and carbon dioxide retention
- May cause hyperventilation due to stimulation of respiratory center
- Respiratory acidosis, CNS dysfunction
- Intracranial HTN, neuromuscular weakness
- Cardiovascular impairment and increased pulmonary vascular resistance

Adverse Effects

- Cardiovascular:
  - Causes tachycardia and hypertension
  - Arrhythmias
  - Exacerbation of right heart dysfunction
  - Coronary artery steal
- Neurological:
  - Raised ICP
  - Agitation or CO_2 narcosis
  - Decreased seizure threshold
  - Cerebral artery steal
  - Interventricular hemorrhage
- Others:
  - Worsening of hypoxemia
  - Intracellular acidosis
  - Inhibition of cell division
  - Decreased glycolysis

Conclusion

- Data that suggest benefits from PHY are indirect
- These are derived from trials that examined the effect of low TV ventilation in ARDS
- This data shows improved patient outcomes from PHY due to low TV ventilation
- Thus, data are confounded by inability to differentiate benefits from PHY and low TV ventilation
- Further trials are required to establish clinical efficacy of PHY

LIQUID VENTILATION

Introduction

- Alternative mode of ventilation in ARDS
- Lung is insufflated with oxygenated PFC liquid rather than O_2- containing gas
- First attempted by ***Clark and Gollan*** for ventilating small mammals such as mice
- First used in humans in 1989 by ***Greenspan*** for ventilating a 28-week preterm baby

Rationale for Use

- ARDS is associated with loss of surfactant
- This causes increased surface tension
- Increased surface tension leads to alveolar collapse
- Filling lung with liquid removes air-liquid interface
- This supports alveoli and decreases chances of collapse
- Thus, liquid ventilation (LV) improves compliance of lungs

Indications

- Neonatal applications:
  - Hyaline membrane disease
  - Meconium aspiration syndrome
  - Persistent pulmonary HTN of the newborn
  - Congenital diaphragmatic hernia
- Adult applications:
  - Acute respiratory distress syndrome
  - Pneumonia for lavage
  - Pulmonary interstitial emphysema
- Experimental uses:
  - Drug delivery:
    - Exogenous surfactant
    - Bronchodilators
    - Antibiotics
    - Mucolytics
    - Antioxidants
  - Pulmonary contusion
  - Cystic fibrosis
  - Pulmonary alveolar proteinosis

- Lung protection during CPB
- Donor lung protection during organ donation

Mechanism of Action

- Decreases surface tension
- Alveolar recruitment and selective distribution to dependant lung regions
- Increases surfactant synthesis and secretion
- Improves arterial oxygenation as liquid used has PFC
- Anti-inflammatory property:
  - Indirect: by mitigation of VILI
  - Direct: decreases release of TNF-α, IL-1, IL-8

Properties of Ideal Fluid for Liquid Ventilation

- Non toxic
- Chemically stable
- Low surface tension to improve lung compliance
- High solubility for oxygen and carbon dioxide to maintain gas exchange
- Greater density compared to body fluids so it can descend to dependant lung regions
- Minimal systemic absorption
- Volatile to allow elimination in acceptable time

Choice of Fluid

- Perfluoro carbons are used most commonly for liquid ventilation
- PFCs are compounds where carbon-bound H^+ atoms are replaced with F^- atoms
- Perflubron (PFB) is the only medical grade PFC approved for use in human trials
- It is commercially called ***LiquiVent***
- Perflubron contains a long, linear fluorinated hydrocarbon chain with 1 bromide atom
- Perfluorocarbons are used as they:
  - Non- toxic and minimally absorbed
  - Easily eliminated by evaporation from lungs
  - Chemically inert
  - Eliminate air-liquid interface
  - Lower surface tension
  - Dissolve oxygen and carbon dioxide
  - Fill collapsed alveoli to prevent closure
  - Accumulate in dependant areas of lung as they are heavier than water

Physical Properties of PFCS

- Clear, colorless, odourless and inert liquids
- Stable, insoluble in water and can be stored indefinitely at room temperature
- They are non-biotransformable and can be autoclaved
- Have a very high solubility for oxygen, carbon dioxide and other gases
- Dissolve almost 15 times the volume of oxygen per given volume of plasma

Pharmacokinetics of PFCs

- Small amounts of PFCs may diffuse into the pulmonary circulation
- Uptake into the blood depends upon:
  - PFC vapour pressure
  - Permeability coefficient of the blood vessels
  - Solubility of the particular PFC used
  - Degree of ventilation-perfusion mismatch
- The absorbed PFCs are scavenged by macrophages
- Routes of elimination:
  - Through the skin via transpiration
  - Through lungs via volatilization
- PFB blood concentrations persist for > 8 days following the last dose of perflubron

Types of Liquid Ventilation

- Total liquid ventilation:
  - This technique uses PFCs instead of gas to obtain gas exchange
  - In this technique, the entire lung is initially filled with PFC fluid
  - LV is accomplished by delivery of tidal volumes of oxygenated PFC fluid
  - Thus, the entire lung volume is filled with oxygenated PFC liquid
  - This constitutes the entire FRC of the patient (almost 30 mL/kg)
  - Along with this, tidal volume of PFC is actively pumped in and out of lungs
  - Liquid tidal volume of PFC is therefore actively pumped in and out of the lungs
  - Thus, this technique requires a special ventilator
  - The ventilator delivers and removes the dense and viscous PFC liquid
  - Usually applied after a short period of partial liquid ventilation
  - Optimal ventilation depends upon:
    - Adequate minute volume
    - Adequate time for diffusion of respiratory gases
  - Typical ventilator settings include:
    - Tidal volumes of 15–20 mL/kg
    - Tidal volume is adjusted based upon blood gases

- Low respiratory rate (4-6 breaths per minute)
- I:E ratio of 1:2 to 1:3

- This allows a sufficient dwell time for the PFC fluid
- Thus, more effective diffusion of gases occurs across the basement membrane
- TLV is weaned off when sufficient clinical improvement has occurred
- Specific weaning parameters and techniques have not yet been established
- Return to gas ventilation may be accomplished by a transition to partial LV
- PFC fluid is removed at the end of expiratory phase once weaning is planned
- Gas ventilation is begun and the PFC fluid is not replaced as it evaporates
- Thus, elimination of PFC fluid occurs by passive evaporation from the lung
- This usually requires 7–10 days for complete clearance from the lung
- However, this technique is difficult and expensive
- Thus, it is less preferred, compared to partial liquid ventilation

❖ Partial liquid ventilation:
- Also called ***PFC Associated Gas Exchange (PAGE)***
- This technique uses tracheal insufflation of PFC with gas ventilation
- PFC is instilled into the lungs during continuous positive pressure ventilation
- The lungs are slowly filled with a volume of PFC equivalent to the FRC
- This amounts to approximately 20–30 mL/kg of PFC fluid
- The insufflation is done using a syringe pump over 15 mins- 1 hour
- FRC is reached when a fluid meniscus is seen in the ETT at end-expiration
- The PFC within the lung is then oxygenated by a conventional gas ventilator
- Tidal volumes are delivered with a conventional volume regulated ventilator
- Typically, pressure control ventilation is used to deliver gas ventilation
- FiO_2 and PEEP are adjusted based upon gas exchange and pulmonary mechanics
- As PFC fluid evaporates, it is replaced with additional PFC at 2–8 mL/kg/hour
- This maintains the total liquid volume close to the FRC

Character	TLV	PLV
Ventilator	Liquid ventilator	Conventional ventilator
Tidal volume delivered	Oxygenated PFC	Gas
Lungs are filled	Completely by PFC	Filled till FRC by PFC
Feasibility	Experimental	Yes

Procedure

❖ Total liquid ventilation:
- Liquid ventilation is initiated after sedation and skeletal muscle paralysis
- Conventional mechanical ventilation is stopped
- The lungs are gradually filled with warmed oxygenated PFC
- 30 mL/kg of PFC is introduced initially using a gravity assisted device
- Further quantities are administered until the lung has been completely filled
- Once air has been completely expelled, the special ventilator is connected
- Tidal volume is subsequently set at 15–20 mL/kg
- Respiratory rate is regulated to 4–6 breaths per minute
- The maximum inspiratory pressure is 30 cm H_2O
- Pressure of between 15 and 20 cm H_2O is usually sufficient
- The negative pressure required for expiration ranges from –15 to –30 cm H_2O
- At the end of the treatment conventional artificial ventilation is started
- Ventilation is continued till the PFC has evaporated from the lungs (7–10 days)

❖ Partial liquid ventilation:
- A volume of 20–30 mL/kg of PFC is introduced via ETT over 15 minutes
- This dose is repeated till:
  - A sustained meniscus is seen in the ETT at end expiration
  - Or till the infused volume reaches a maximum of 30 mL/kg
- This replaces the functional residual capacity
- PFC is then infused at 2–8 mL/kg/hour to replace the evaporative losses
- The PFC is re-dosed daily for 5–7 days until clinical improvement occurs

Adjuncts to Liquid Ventilation

Additive effect of PLV occurs in combination with:

❖ Nitric oxide

❖ Exogenous surfactant

- ❖ Conventional PEEP
- ❖ High frequency oscillatory ventilation (HFOV)
- ❖ Prone ventilation

Advantages of Liquid Ventilation

- ❖ Improves lung compliance:
  - Alveoli are recruited due to the hydraulic forces provided during LV
  - Alveolar expansion at lower pressures reduces the risk of barotrauma
  - This results in an improvement in oxygenation and lung compliance
- ❖ Better V/Q matching:
  - On insufflation, PFCs accumulate in the dependant areas of lung
  - In these areas, ARDS is typically more severe
  - Presence of PFCs improves gas exchange across alveolar basement membrane
  - Thus, intrapulmonary right-left shunt eventually reduces
  - This results in better ventilation-perfusion matching
- ❖ Lavage:
  - PFCs are heavier than body fluids
  - Thus, they mobilize purulent secretions from lungs
  - LV facilitates the removal of this exudative material from the lung
  - Thus, liquid ventilation is useful in lung diseases with secretions
  - LV also allows oxygenation during therapeutic lavage
- ❖ Anti-inflammatory effects:
  - PFCs also have anti-inflammatory properties
  - Anti-inflammatory properties are due to:
    - Inhibition of neutrophil function
    - Inhibition of macrophage function
    - Inhibition of cytokine expression
    - Attenuation of ICAM-1 expression in injured alveolar cells

Disadvantages

- ❖ Pneumothorax due to overdistension during gas ventilation in PLV
- ❖ Hypotension and low cardiac output due to raised pulmonary arterial pressure
- ❖ Lactic acidosis due to redistribution of blood flow
- ❖ Mucus plugging of airway and ETT blockade
- ❖ Hypercarbia due to ineffective elimination by high viscosity PFCs
- ❖ Interference with radiography due to radio-opaque nature of some PFCs

Current Status 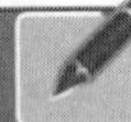

- ❖ Primary applications of LV techniques till date remains:
  - Potential to treat lung disease with less risk of barotrauma
  - Complement existing forms of respiratory therapy such as:
    - Surfactant therapy
    - ECMO
    - HFOV
    - Inhaled NO
- ❖ Several problems which are associated with LV remain to be solved:
  - Safety of liquid ventilation over prolonged periods of time
  - Return to conventional gas ventilation from liquid ventilation
  - Hemodynamic effects in the presence of pulmonary hypertension
  - Significant degree of lactic acidosis
  - Increase in hypoxemia in inhomogeneous lung pathology
  - The metabolism of PFC with regard to damage from long term persistence
- ❖ Thus, PLV is not routinely recommended in ARDS patients.

INVERSE RATIO VENTILATION

Introduction

- ❖ IRV is a strategy for mechanical ventilation that reverses the classic I:E ratio
- ❖ IRV is mechanical ventilation with inspiratory-expiratory time ratio more than 1
- ❖ I:E ratio typically ranges from 2:1 to 4:1
- ❖ This ensures improved oxygenation by increasing the mean airway pressure

Mechanism of Action

Improves oxygenation by:

- ❖ Increasing mean airway pressure
- ❖ Causing recruitment of alveoli
- ❖ Decreasing intrapulmonary shunt
- ❖ Improvement of V/Q matching
- ❖ Decreasing dead space ventilation

- Generation of auto PEEP by incomplete emptying of lungs

Physiological Changes

Increased	Decreased	No Change
Mean airway pressure	PEEP requirement	FiO_2
Central venous pressure	Peak airway pressure	Intrinsic PEEP
Pulmonary arterial pressure	Cardiac output	Blood pressure
PaO_2		$PaCO_2$

Physiological Basis

- Mean airway pressure (MAP):
  - MAP is calculated using airway pressures averaged over the respiratory cycle
    MAP = [(Fraction of cycle in inspiration) × PIP] + [(Fraction of cycle in expiration) × PEEP]
  - Where:
    PIP = peak inspiratory pressure
    PEEP = positive end expiratory pressure
  - Peak inspiratory pressure is always higher than PEEP
  - IRV increases the time spent in inspiration
  - Thus, it increases the time spent in the higher-pressure portion of the cycle
  - This results in an increase in the MAP without increasing the pressure itself
  - Higher MAP recruits alveoli without generating high PAP
  - This reduces shunting and improves oxygenation
- Auto-PEEP:
  - In conventional ventilation, E time is usually twice the I time
  - This allows expiration more time to be completed as it occurs passively
  - During IRV, time for expiration is shorter than the inspiratory time
  - This results in breath stacking due to incomplete lung emptying
  - This results in an increased end expiratory pressure causing auto-PEEP
  - Presence of auto-PEEP reduces shunting and improves oxygenation

Indications

- Primary indication is in the management of refractory hypoxemia in ARDS
- IRV is used as a rescue therapy when all other methods have been maximized

Contraindications

- Hypovolemia
- Vasodilatory shock
- COPD
- Bronchial asthma

Types

- Volume Controlled-IRV:
  - Inspiratory time extended with slow inspiratory flow
  - End expiratory pause/decelerating inspiratory flow also other features
  - Any ventilator can be adjusted to deliver VC-IRV
  - Allows control of minute volume and inspiratory flow
  - Requires careful monitoring of airway and alveolar pressure
- Pressure controlled-IRV:
  - *More commonly used*
  - Constant pressure is applied for the duration of inspiration
  - Causes decelerating gas flow into lungs
  - Permits exact adjustment of airway pressure
  - May cause variation in tidal and minute volume
  - Requires special ventilators

Adverse Effects

- Although PIP remains unchanged, average pressure in lungs is increased during IRV
- Increased of chances of barotrauma due to:
  - Increased mean airway pressure
  - Dynamic hyperinflation in the presence of auto-PEEP
  - Increased mean alveolar pressure and volume
- May cause a reduction in cardiac output
- Increased rate of transvascular fluid flow/ flooding due to increased alveolar pressure
- May worsen pre-existing pulmonary disease
- Requires sedation and NMBA as patients are often agitated

Current Status

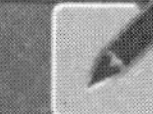

- IRV has not shown to improve objective clinical outcome measures such as:
  - Mortality
  - Length of mechanical ventilation
  - Length of ICU stay
- It has been shown to modestly improve oxygenation, although inconsistently

Contd...

Contd...

- I:E ratios above 2:1 are usually avoided due to adverse hemodynamic effects
- Currently, more data is required to evaluate the possible benefit of IRV.

PRONE VENTILATION

Introduction

- Prone ventilation is ventilation delivered with the patient lying in prone position
- It is used as a strategy to improve oxygenation in ARDS when traditional methods fail
- Proning has been reported to:
  - Increase PaO_2 by > 20%
  - Decrease intrapulmonary shunting by 10–12%

Physiological Effects on Oxygenation

- Reducing ventral-dorsal transmural pressure difference:
  - The transmural pressure (P_{TM}) differs between ventral and dorsal lung in supine posture
    Transmural pressure (P_{TM}) = {Alveolar pressure (P_{ALV})} – {Pleural pressure (P_{PL})}
  - In supine position, the dorsal P_{PL} is higher than the ventral P_{PL}
  - Thus, the transmural pressure is higher in the ventral lung regions
  - This effect is exaggerated in ARDS due to the increase in lung weight
  - Thus, in supine ARDS patients, there is a tendency towards:
    - Over-inflation of the ventral alveoli
    - Atelectasis of the dorsal alveoli
  - This difference between dorsal and ventral P_{TM} is reduced by proning the patient
  - Thus, prone position makes ventilation more uniform and prevents:
    - Ventral alveolar over-inflation
    - Dorsal alveolar collapse
  - This results in improved ventilation and oxygenation in ARDS patients
- Improved lung perfusion:
  - When supine, the blood flow is maximal in dependant (dorsal) lung regions
  - However, in ARDS, alveolar collapse is also maximal in the dorsal lung
  - Once the patient is placed in prone position, alveoli in these regions expand
  - However, blood flow patterns change only modestly upon proning
  - Thus, majority of the blood flow is still directed towards the dorsal lung
  - This results in an improvement in V/Q match and better oxygenation
- Reduced lung compression:
  - In supine ARDS patients:
    - Heart compresses the medial posterior lung parenchyma
    - Diaphragm compresses the posterior caudal lung parenchyma (abdominal pressure)
  - This exacerbates V/Q mismatch caused by posterior alveolar collapse in ARDS
  - In prone ARDS patients:
    - Heart becomes dependant and lies on the sternum
    - Diaphragm is displaced caudally (provided abdomen is unsupported)
  - This decreases the compression of posterior lung regions
  - This results in an improvement of ventilation and oxygenation
- Other beneficial effects:
  - Increased FRC
  - Improved cardiac output
  - Better drainage of secretions
  - Improved lymphatic drainage

Indications

- Severe ARDS unresponsive to protective ventilation with permissive hypercapnia
- As a bridge to ECMO
- Limited use in:
  - Mild-moderate ARDS
  - Non- ARDS patients

Patient Selection Criteria

- PaO_2/FiO_2 < 150 mm Hg with an FiO_2 > 0.6 and PEEP > 5 cm H_2O
- SAPS II score > 49
- High tidal volume > 12 mL/kg
- Oxygenation index > 30%

Contraindications

- Absolute contraindications:
  - Shock (MAP persistently below 65 mm Hg)
  - Acute bleeding:
    - Hemorrhagic shock
    - Massive hemoptysis
  - Unstable spine injuries

- Patients at risk for spinal instability (rheumatoid arthritis)
- Multiple fractures/ trauma: pelvis, femur, face
- Pregnancy
- Raised ICP > 30 mm Hg
- Cerebral perfusion pressure < 60 mm Hg
- Tracheal surgery/ sternotomy within 2 weeks
- Central cannulation for VA ECMO or BIVAD support

❖ Relative contraindications:
- Morbid obesity
- Severe burns
- Recent DVT
- Recent tracheostomy < 24 hours
- Anterior chest tubes with air leaks
- Recent pacemaker implantation
- Major abdominal surgery
- Lung transplant recipient

Duration of Therapy

❖ Useful in patients with ARDS and suboptimal oxygenation lasting > 12- 24 hours

❖ This is because prone ventilation is most beneficial when initiated early

❖ The optimal duration of prone positioning is not known

❖ Proning is usually done once a day for a duration ranging 2-20 hours/day

❖ Lower mortality rates have been reported with > 12 hours proning per day

❖ The frequency of turning severely ill patients should be minimized

❖ Thus, prone ventilation may be maintained for 18-20 hours/day

❖ Cessation of prone ventilation is appropriate when:
- Continued improvement in oxygenation:
  - PaO_2: FiO_2 > 150 mm Hg
  - FiO_2 < 0.6
  - PEEP < 10 cm H_2O
- For acute emergencies
- Prolonged interventions
- Surgical procedures

Preparation for Prone Positioning

❖ General:
- Assess daily hygiene such as:
  - Mouthcare
  - Dressings
  - Change of stoma bags
- Ventilator is repositioned to remain:
  - As close to the patient as possible
  - On the appropriate side
- Patient is positioned at one side of the bed towards the ventilator

❖ Sedation:
- Ensure adequate sedation of the patients
- Deep sedation is usually preferred (RASS score –5)
- Consider bolus dose muscle relaxants

❖ Airway and breathing:
- Difficult airway trolley kept ready
- Secure ETT tape and remove any anchor fast device
- *Suction oropharynx and airway prior to procedure*
- Ensure availability of closed-circuit suctioning
- Preoxygenation with 100% oxygen

❖ Note down:
- All vital signs
- Previous laryngoscopy grade
- Length of ETT at the lips
- Ventilator settings
- Inspiratory pressure
- Pre-proning ABG

❖ Invasive lines:
- Ensure all lines are sutured and secured
- Discontinue all non-essential infusions
- Ensure patient is hemodynamically stable
- Ensure adequate volume of all vasopressors/ inotropes
- This is in order to avoid changing connections in prone position

❖ Other tubes:
- NG feeds should be stopped and NGT aspirated
- Ideally, NGT aspiration has to be done 1 hour prior to position change
- Document NGT tube length
- Chest drains need to be well secured and below the patient
- Tube should be preferably clamped at the time of change in position
- Ensure adequate length of tubes and cables running above or below the patient
- Urinary catheter should be spigotted and taped to the side of the leg

❖ Skin/eyes:
- Monitor skin integrity prior to position change
- Eyes should be cleaned, lubricated and taped shut to avoid ulceration
- Ideally eyes should be protected with a gel pad

Positioning the Patient

- The procedure requires at least four health care providers:
  - One member to protect the ETT and turn the head
  - One member to turn the trunk
  - One member to turn the legs
  - One member to control and move arterial line, venous lines and catheters
- A Log roll may be used to aid positioning
- Once positioned, all lines and catheters should be checked for displacement
- Head should be turned towards the direction of the ventilator
- Head requires frequent turning to avoid facial edema
- Hands should be held in swimmers position:
  - Abducted at the shoulder
  - Flexed to 90° at the elbow
- Protective cushions should be placed under:
  - Shoulders
  - Hips
  - Ankles
- Immediately following prone positioning, there may be a brief period of:
  - Hemodynamic instability
  - Oxygen desaturation
- However, this usually improves over a period of time

Positioning AIDS

- Circular electric bed
- Manual two step, light weight, portable support frame
- ***Vollmans prone positioner***

Ventilatory Strategies in Prone Position

- Ventilation in prone position employs protective lung ventilation strategy
- Benefits are maximal when tidal volume is restricted to below 8 mL/kg
- Peak and plateau pressures may increase transiently after proning
- This phenomenon occurs due to:
  - Mobilization of secretions
  - Decrease in chest wall compliance
- However, these changes decline over a period of time due to alveolar recruitment
- Prone position is rarely combined with other modes such as high frequency ventilation

Assessment of Response

- Response to proning is assessed 1 hour after change in position
- Positive response:
  - Sustained improvement in gas exchange:

$PaO_2 > 10$ mm Hg

Increase in oxygenation index > 20% from baseline

  - Evidence of alveolar recruitment:
    - Increase in lung compliance
    - Decrease in plateau pressure
- Failure of therapy:
  - No change in gas exchange or lung mechanics
  - Worsening of gas exchange
  - Worsening hemodynamics

Complications

- Nerve compression: brachial plexus injury
- Crush injury
- Venous stasis
- Dislodgement of:
  - Endotracheal tube
  - Vascular catheters
  - Drains
- Diaphragmatic limitation
- Pressure sores (head)
- Retinal damage
- Transient fall in arterial oxygen saturation
- Vomiting
- Transient arrhythmias

Clinical Evidence

- Clinical evidence shows that proning reduces the risk of VILI
- However, it is difficult to prove that prone position alone reduces VILI
- This is because most trials utilize lung protective ventilation strategies concomitantly
- Proning may also provide an additional mortality benefit at 28 days and 90 days
- However, there is no evidence that prone ventilation prevents other organ dysfunction
- Thus, although the benefit has been proven, the clinical effect of prone position has not been firmly established and requires further trials

TRACHEAL GAS INSUFFLATION

Introduction

TGI is an adjunct to mechanical ventilation where trachea is filled with a stream of fresh gas at the end of exhalation.

Rationale

- Without TGI, trachea is filled with alveolar gas at end of exhalation
- This CO_2 rich air is forced back into alveoli at next inspiration
- With TGI a stream of fresh gas at 4–8 L/min is insufflated through a small catheter or channel into walls of ETT in lower trachea
- This flushes carbon dioxide from upper airways, prior to next inspiration
- Provides gas flow near carina thus washing carbon dioxide out of large airways

Mechanism of Action

- Reduces dead space
- Useful to decrease carbon dioxide and acidosis due to small tidal volume ventilation
- Enhanced gas mixing distal to TGI catheter tip due to turbulence at high gas flows through TGI catheter

Procedure

- TGI catheter passed to position through the ETT lumen using sidearm adaptor
- Fresh gas flow 4-8 L/minute used
- TGI may be selectively timed during expiration: also called Expiratory Wash Out or EWO
- EWO can be used to offset increases in Tv and airway pressure, seen with continuous TGI

Side Effects

- Desiccation of secretions
- Airway mucosal injury
- TGI catheter may be nidus for accumulation of secretions
- May causes auto-PEEP and increase airway pressure from expiratory flow
- May cause increased tidal volume delivery

Current Status

Ravenscraft found $PaCO_2$ decreased from 53 to 45 mm Hg when catheter was at 1 cm from carina and FGF at 6L/min

AIRWAY PRESSURE RELEASE VENTILATION

Introduction

Bilevel form of ventilation with sudden and short releases in pressure to rapidly reduce FRC and permit ventilation.

Indications

- ALI/ARDS
- Refractory hypoxemia
- Massive atelectasis

Components

- Contains CPAP circuit
- Release valve is expiratory limb of CPAP circuit to accomplish rapid release of CPAP

Principle

- A ventilatory mode which sets a level of CPAP which intermittently time cycles to a lower airway pressure to maintain alveolar recruitment throughout respiratory cycle
- Provides two levels of CPAP
- Allows spontaneous breathing at both levels when spontaneous effort is present
- Can work in apneic/spontaneously breathing patients
- Contains CPAP circuit which maintains baseline airway pressure above ambient
- Augmentation of alveolar ventilation determined by APRV rate and tidal volume
- If APRV release frequency and tidal volume are sufficient to reduce $PaCO_2$ below apneic threshold, controlled ventilation results
- Weaning from APRV done by lowering release frequency until patient is breathing with CPAP without any APRV

Mechanism

- Provides two levels of airway pressure P_{high} and P_{low}, during two set time periods T_{high} and T_{low}
- APRV strategy is for long T_{high} and short T_{low}
- Accomplished by setting P_{high} well above closing pressure of recruitable alveoli
- The set T_{high} generally maintains this pressure and alveolar recruitment for several seconds
- Set T_{low} is of duration adequate to assist in carbon dioxide removal

Advantages

- Augmented alveolar ventilation with low peak airway pressure
- Prevents over-distension of lung parenchyma
- Improves patient ventilator synchrony
- Improves mean airway pressure
- Reduces physiological dead space
- May be used with mask in patients already receiving NI-CPAP
- Reduces peak airway pressure, mean airway pressure and mean intra-thoracic pressure
- Decreases incidence of VILI
- Allows IRV with or without spontaneous breathing

Disadvantages

- Variable tidal volume delivered
- Could be harmful in COPD/asthma patients
- Auto-PEEP usually present
- Asynchrony if spontaneous breaths are out of sync with release time
- Requires presence of active exhalation valve
- Caution in hemodynamically unstable patients

HIGH FREQUENCY VENTILATION

Introduction

Ventilation with supra-physiological respiratory rates and tidal volumes equal to or less than dead space (usually 60-3000 breaths/minute).

Methods

- Small tidal volume rapid respiratory rate with conventional mechanical ventilator
- High frequency percussive ventilation
- Various forms of external chest oscillation
- High frequency positive pressure ventilation (HFPPV)
- High frequency jet ventilation (HFJV)
- High frequency oscillatory ventilation (HFOV)

Mode	Rate	Tidal volume	Exhalation	Gas
HFPPV	60–100 cycles/min	3–5 mL/kg	Passive	None
HFJV	100–150 cycles/min	2–5 mL/kg	Passive	Yes
HFOV	Upto 2400 cycles/min	< 3 mL/kg	Active	Yes

Advantages

- Reduced peak airway pressure: decreases barotrauma
- Reduced tidal volume: less volutrauma
- Alveolar recruitment maintained:
  - Increases oxygenation
  - Decreases oxygen toxicity
- More efficient carbon dioxide removal
- Avoids cyclical expansion and collapse of alveoli: decreases lung damage
- Decreased need for surfactant therapy
- Prevents bronchopulmonary dysplasias
- Decreased need for ECMO

Theories of Gas Transport in HFOV

i. *Direct alveolar ventilation theory:* Some proximal alveoli receive bulk gas flow

ii. *Inter-regional gas mixing theory:*
  - Called ***Pendelluft***
  - Alveoli with short time constants fill early in inspiration
  - These may empty into alveoli with longer time constants which are still filling

iii. *Corrective streaming theory:*
  - Air in the center of airway moves faster than air in contact with airway walls during inspiration
  - In expiration all gases move slowly
  - Thus gas flows rapidly into central alveoli while it flows away from alveoli, along the walls

iv. *Augmented dispersion theory:* ***Taylor***
  - Gas flowing through has a parabolic front
  - This increases dispersion of gas across the front of moving column (*Axial diffusion*)
  - This also causes molecular dispersion of gas along concentration gradients occurring laterally (*Radial diffusion*)

v. *Cardiogenic mixing theory:* Due to heartbeat induced oscillations in airway

vi. *Molecular diffusion theory:* Due to simple diffusion across alveolar capillary membrane along a concentration gradient

Indications

- Pulmonary:
  - Neonatal RDS/Hyaline membrane disease
  - Adult respiratory distress syndrome (ARDS)
  - Air-leak syndromes:
    - Pneumothorax
    - Bronchopleural fistula
  - *Oxygenation index* more than 13

- Persistant pulmonary HTN:
  - Meconium aspiration
  - Neonatal asphyxia
  - Congenital diaphragmatic hernia
  - Congenital heart defects with pulmonary HTN
- Ventilation during procedures: HFJV and HFPPV:
  - Direct laryngoscopy , bronchoscopy
  - Endoscopic laser surgery
  - Upper airway and tracheal surgeries
  - One lung ventilation
- Difficult airway algorithm: Percutaneous tracheal HFJV
- Others:
  - Ventilation in hemodynamically unstable patients
  - During weaning

Determinants of Gas Exchange

- FiO_2
- Mean airway pressure (P_{aw}):
  - Increased P_{aw} will improve oxygenation
  - P_{aw} used in HFOV is higher than that used in conventional ventilation
  - P_{aw} upto 35-40 cm H_2O is used in HFOV
- Amplitude (Power/ P):
  - Determines displacement of piston
  - Increasing amplitude/power of pressure wave increases tidal volume
  - This causes increased CO_2 elimination
  - Power adjusted till chest movement is optimal (***Chest wiggle***)
- Rate/frequency:
  - Increasing frequency shortens inspiratory and expiratory times
  - Thus, tidal volume decreases
  - Thus, in HFOV, increasing frequency reduces MV and increases carbon dioxide levels
  - Frequency adjusted between 3–15 Hz (180–900 breaths/min)
  - Also increased frequency increases barotrauma
- Bias flow:
  - Maintains P_{aw} and washes carbon dioxide out
  - Bias flow can be increased to 40–60 L/min
- I and E TIME: Inspiratory time usually fixed at 33%

Complications

- Cardiovascular depression
- Decreased venous return and cardiac output in initial stages
- Barotrauma and air-leak syndromes due to dynamic hyperinflation
- Necrotizing tracheobronchitis
- Inspissated airway secretions
- Slow movement of airway columns: may take upto 45 minutes for ABG changes to occur

Contraindications

- No absolute contraindications
- Obstructive airway disease:
  - As HFV devices have very short expiratory time
  - Asthma and bronchiolitis
  - Combination of active recruitment, high pressure and short expiratory time can cause barotrauma
- Hemodynamically unstable patients
- Severe acidosis
- Pregnancy

HIGH FREQUENCY POSITIVE PRESSURE VENTILATION

Introduction

- Use of conventional ventilator to deliver tidal volumes of 3-4 mL/kg at frequency of 1–2 Hz through a flow interrupter
- Also called ***High Frequency Flow Interrupter***

Example

Infrasonics Infant Star Ventilator.

Working Principle

- Essentially IPPV with increased respiratory rate and reduced tidal volume
- Breaths may be PC/VC with gas flow directed through insufflation catheter placed in airway or through side arm of pneumatic valve attached to an ETT or bronchoscope
- Requires ventilator with:
  - Low internal and circuit compliance
  - Negligible compressible volume
- Tidal volume 3–4 mL/kg
- Respiratory rate 60-100 breaths/min
- Inspiration: Expiration < 0.3
- Frequency of 1–2 Hz

Current Status

- Not gained widespread use
- Studies showed no difference in mortality

HIGH FREQUENCY JET VENTILATION

Introduction

Intermittent high pressure jet of gas delivered at high frequency (100–200 Hz) through small bore cannula built along sides of modified ETT.

Example: ***Bunnel Life Pulse Jet Ventilator***

Working Principle

- Frequency of 4–11 Hz
- Total volume 3–4.5 mL/kg
- Respiratory rate 100–150 breaths/min
- 1:E = 0.1 to 0.5
- Expiration is *passive*
- Driving pressure = 10–40 PSI

Mechanism

- High pressure jet entrains stream from conventional ventilator
- Thus, due to Venturi effect, actual tidal volume delivered is higher than volume of gas delivered from jet catheter, as entrainment of additional ambient gas occurs
- Has synergistic effect when used with recruitment maneuvers

Procedure

- Small 14–16 G cannula placed within specially designed ETT
- Less commonly, catheter is placed directly into trachea
- Ancillary circuit providing continuous humified gas flow is directed via side port into ETT
- Humidification by coaxial flow of saline in front of jet cannula
- Saline is nebulized by jet flow and humidifies air
- Tidal volume is adjusted by altering inspiratory time/driving pressure

High Frequency Flow Interruption

- Variation of HFJV
- High pressure source of gas is interrupted by valve
- Pulsatile flow is delivered to patients airway
- *Emerson rotating ball* used to interrupt flow.

Current Status

- Safe, but not superior to CMV in neonatal RDS
- Requires reintubation with special ETT in unstable patients
- Role is yet to be defined and thus, it has not found widespread use

HIGH FREQUENCY OSCILLATORY VENTILATION

Introduction

Uses continuous flow of gas and piston/loud speaker diaphragm to generate high frequency sinusoidal waves in this column of gas.

Example

- ***Sensormedics 3100 A*** (for patients' weighing less than 45 kg)
- ***Sensormedics 3100 B*** (for patients weighing more than 90 kg)

Working Principle

- Tidal volume 1-3 mL/kg
- Frequency between 3-15 Hz
- Respiratory rate up to 2400 breaths/min
- Expiration is *active*

Physics

- Back and forth motion of piston creates active expiratory phase which is unique to HFOV
- Mean airway pressure is constant
- Peak pressure gradually falls from proximal to distal airway
- Small tidal volume provides for relatively higher mean airway pressure
- This higher MAP may recruit lung more effectively than PEEP

Mechanism

- A bias flow of fresh, heated, humidified gas is provided at proximal ETT
- Bias flow is typically 20-40 L/min
- P_{aw} at proximal ETT is set at high level (25-35 cm H_2O)
- Oscillating piston vibrates the flowing gas
- P_{aw} modified by adjusting bias flow rate/back pressure

Inspiration

- Is an *active* process
- HFOV device placed in line with ETT
- Gas source placed perpendicular to ETT
- Fresh Gas Flow (FGF) is driven into ETT by waves from oscillator

Expiration

- Is also an *active* process
- Expiratory limb placed perpendicular to ETT but opposite to FGF
- Expiratory limb has high impendence to oscillations but low impendence to steady gas flow
- Rigid interconnecting tubes used to ensure proper transmission of oscillatory waves

Care of Patient

- Change in posture Q6H
- Encourage oral feeds
- DVT prophylaxis
- Consider weaning to conventional ventilation within 24 hours

Weaning Criteria

- Mean airway pressure < 25 cm H_2O in adults
- Mean airway pressure < 20 cm H_2O in children
- Frequency < 5 Hz

Current Status

- Proven by randomized controlled trial to be safe and effective in children with severe lung disease
- Not yet shown to improve outcome

VENTILATOR INDUCED LUNG INJURY

Introduction

- Ventilator induced lung injury is an acute lung injury affecting the airways and parenchyma that is caused by or exacerbated by mechanical ventilation
- It is mostly seen in patients ventilated for ARDS

Incidence

- More in earlier days with conventional tidal volumes of 12–15 mL/kg (up to 50%)
- Presently incidence has reduced (3% in all mechanically ventilated patients)
- Incidence is higher in ARDS patients (5–10%) due to a reduced lung compliance
- Associated with a high mortality rate of 40–60%

Mechanisms of VILI

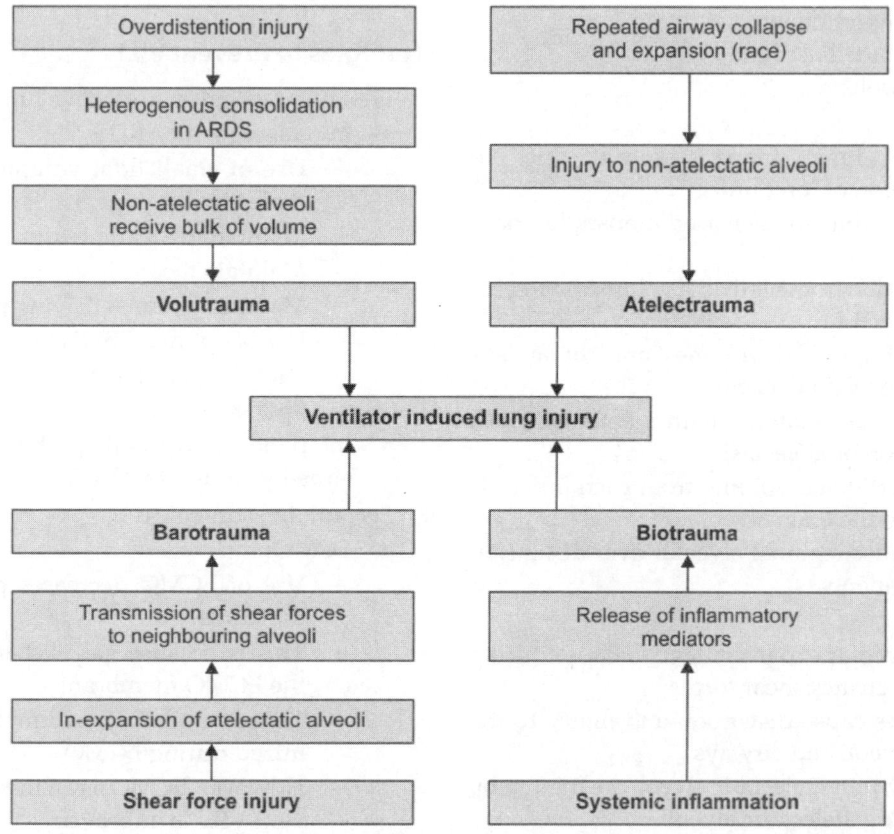

Pathophysiology

- Altered gene expression and cellular metabolism
- Upregulated inflammatory response
- Translocation of bacteria from lungs to systemic circulation
- *Mechanotransduction*: transduction of mechanical stimuli (like cell deformation) into biochemical alteration
- Alterations in surfactant

Types of VILI

- Barotrauma:
  - Mechanical ventilation initially equilibrates pressures in adjacent alveoli
  - However, alveolar pressures eventually increase
  - This creates pressure gradient between alveoli and adjacent perivascular sheath
  - The gradient may result in the rupture of alveoli adjacent to the sheath
  - This results in the entry of air into the perivascular sheath
  - This results in pulmonary interstitial emphysema (PIE)
  - Other manifestations include:
    - Pneumothorax
    - Pneumoperitoneum
    - Pneumomediastinum
    - Air embolism
- Volutrauma:
  - Represents lung injury caused due to overdistention of lung units
  - This occurs due to increased transpulmonary pressures
  - Overdistention from high tidal volumes increases the risk for VILI
  - However, high tidal volumes are not always necessary for VILI to occur
  - ARDS is associated with heterogeneous consolidation or atelectasis
  - A disproportionate volume from each breath is delivered to the open alveoli
  - This can cause regional alveolar over distension in ARDS patients
- Atelectrauma:
  - Cyclical alveolar expansion and collapse during ventilation creates shear forces
  - These forces cause distention and injury to the adjacent alveoli and airways
  - Specifically, non-atelectatic alveoli are injured by neighbouring atelectatic alveoli
  - This is due to the impact of cyclical opening and closing during tidal breathing
  - This process is referred to as cyclical atelectasis or atelectrauma
- Biotrauma:
  - This is characterized by ventilator induced release of inflammatory mediators
  - This can occur as a result of both atelectrauma and volutrauma
  - Biotrauma is associated with an increase in inflammatory mediators such as:
    - Tumor necrosis factor
    - IL-6 and IL-8
    - Metalloproteinase- 9

Clinical Features and Evaluation

- Tachypnea, tachycardia
- Worsening hypoxemia or requirement of higher FiO_2 to maintain PaO_2
- New/ increased bilateral interstitial or alveolar opacities
- CT scan shows:
  - Heterogenous consolidation/ atelectasis
  - Focal hyperlucent areas which represent over distended lung

Strategies to Prevent VILI

- First line strategies: protective lung ventilation:
  - In patients with ARDS:
    - Use of small tidal volumes (6 mL/kg predicted body weight)
    - Maintain plateau pressure below 30 cm H_2O
    - Maintain mean airway pressure < 40 cm H_2O
    - Maintain optimal driving pressure
    - Use of optimal PEEP to prevent atelectrauma
    - PaO_2 55-80 mm Hg
    - SpO_2 88-95%
  - In patients without ARDS: protective lung strategy similar to ARDS
- Second line strategies:
  - ECMO:
    - Use of ECMO decreases physical stress on the lungs
    - This is because gas exchange occurs across the ECMO membrane
    - Thus, ventilatory parameters can be minimized during ECMO
    - However, ECMO as an initial strategy to prevent VILI is unproven

- Sedation and paralysis:
  - Neuromuscular paralysis may be required when sedation is inadequate
  - Especially useful in clinical scenarios predisposing to auto-PEEP
  - However, no additional benefit has been proven with routine use of NMBAs in ARDS
- Prone positioning may be beneficial in refractory cases

❖ Other ventilatory strategies:
- Continuous lateral rotation therapy:
  - Therapy used to mechanically rotate patients continuously in bed
  - Advantages:
    - Promotes early mobilization
    - Mobilizes pulmonary secretions
    - Improves alveolar gas exchange
    - Causes redistribution of weight of edematous lung
    - Permits recruitment
  - Has been shown to reduce duration of ventilation and ICU stay
- Semi- upright mechanical ventilation:
  - This position is associated with:
    - Significant increase in oxygen saturation
    - Significant decrease in end-tidal CO_2
  - Advantages:
    - Decreases intrapulmonary shunting
    - Permits better alveolar recruitment
    - Increases FRC
    - Improves gastric emptying
    - Causes faster recovery of diaphragmatic function
  - Effects not proven in any trials
- Airway pressure release ventilation:
  - Best if spontaneous ventilation is present
  - Better recruitment of alveoli
- Neurally Adjusted Ventilatory Assist (NAVA):
  - Uses diaphragmatic electric activity to trigger inspiration
  - Less trigger delay and better patient-ventilator synchrony
  - Reduced work of breathing
  - Ventilatory assistance increases with diaphragmatic contraction

❖ Investigational therapies for preventing VILI:
- Aspirin
- Inhaled corticosteroids

❖ Investigational therapies for treating VILI:
- GM-CSF
- Stem cells
- Macrolide antibiotics
- Anti- inflammatory agents:
  - Tissue factor antibodies
  - Sevoflurane
- Lung transplantation

VENTILATOR ASSOCIATED PNEUMONIA

Introduction

Pneumonia occurring > 48 hours after endotracheal intubation with no clinical evidence suggesting presence of pneumonia at the time of initial intubation.

Definitions

❖ Ventilator associated conditions (VACs):
- At least 2 calendar days of stable or decreasing daily minimum PEEP or FiO_2
- This is followed by a sustained change for > 2 days comprising at least 1 of:
  - Rise in PEEP of at least 3 cm H_2O
  - Rise in FiO_2 of at least 20 points

❖ Infection-related ventilator associated complications (IVACs): VAC criteria with:
- Temperature < 36 °C or more than 38 °C OR
- WBC count more than 12,000 cells/mm^3 AND
- At least 1 new antibiotic continued for > 4 days within 2 days of VAC onset
- This excludes the first 2 days on ventilator

❖ Possible VAP: IVAC criteria along with one of the 3 criteria:
- Criterion 1: Positive culture meeting specific quantitative or semi-quantitative threshold
- Criterion 2: Purulent respiratory secretions and identification of organisms NOT meeting the quantitative or semi-quantitative thresholds
- Criterion 3: Organisms identified within 2 days of VAC onset (excluding 1st 2 days on MV) from:
  - Pleural fluid
  - Positive lung histopathology
  - Positive diagnostic test for legionella species
  - Positive diagnostic test for selected respiratory viruses

❖ Ventilator associated pneumonia (VAP):
- Radiographic criteria: New or progressive and persistent:
  - Infiltrates
  - Consolidation
  - Cavitation

- Systemic criteria:
  - Temperature < 36 °C or > 38 °C OR
- WBC count < 4000 cells/mm³ or > 12000 cells/mm³ Pulmonary criteria: at least 1 of:
  - Worsening gas exchange
  - New onset or increase of purulent aspirates

❖ Ventilator associated tracheobronchitis (VAT): criteria for VAP without radiographic criteria

Types of VAP

❖ *Early onset VAP:* Pneumonia occurring within first 96 hours of ventilation

❖ *Late onset VAP:* Pneumonia occurring more than 96 hours of ventilation.

Incidence

❖ VAP is the *second most common* nosocomial infection

❖ Likelihood of developing VAP increases with the duration of mechanical ventilation

❖ Incidence of VAP ranges from 2–16 episodes per 1000 ventilator-days

❖ Incidence of ranges from 8–28% for all ventilated patients

❖ The risk of developing VAP varies from:
- 3% per day during first 5 days of MV
- 2% per day during the next 5 days (days 5–10)
- 1% per day thereafter

❖ Late onset VAP has a higher mortality rate than early- onset VAP

❖ This is because early onset VAP is usually due to antibiotic sensitive bacteria

❖ Late onset VAP is commonly associated with MDR pathogens

Etiology

❖ Gram negative bacteria:
- Klebsiella, E. coli
- Pseudomonas, Acinetobacter
- Enterobacter, Serratia marcescens
- Proteus, Hemophilus

❖ Gram positive bacteria:
- Staphylococcus aureus (*most commonly* isolated organism)
- Streptococcus pneumoniae
- Legionella pneumophila
- Hemophilus influenza
- Pneumococcus

❖ Gram negative anerobes:
- Bacteroides fragilis
- Rare, usually occurs following aspiration in non-intubated patients

❖ Fungal:
- Candida
- Aspergillus fumigatus

❖ Viral:
- Influenza A
- Severe acute respiratory syndrome virus

❖ Usually, early onset VAP is caused by:
- Hemophilus influenza
- Staphylococcus aureus
- Pneumococcus

❖ Late onset pneumonia caused by:
- Methicillin resistant staphylococcus aureus
- Pseudomonas
- Acinetobacter

Pathogenesis

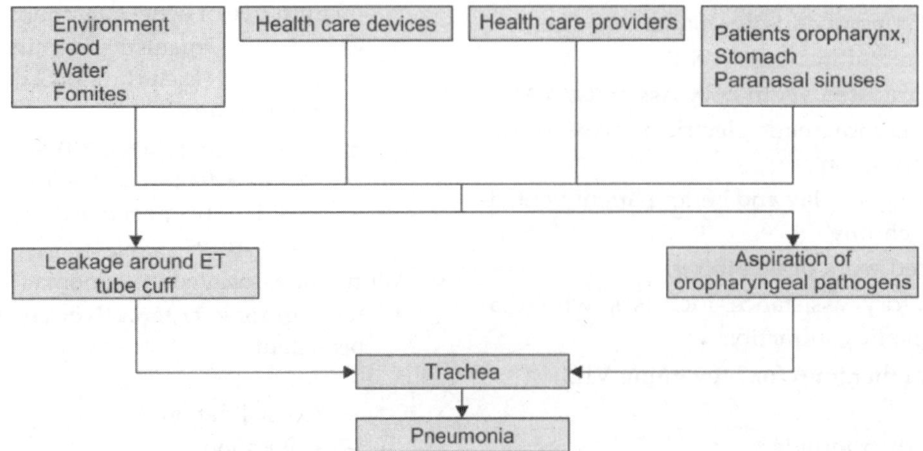

Risk Factors

- Host related risk factors:
  - Male gender
  - Extreme age
  - Prior CNS disorder
  - Immunocompromised individuals
  - Acute underlying diseases
  - Surgeries:
    - Emergent surgery
    - Neurosurgery
    - Thoracic surgery
    - Cardiac surgery
  - Burns
  - Re-intervention
  - Acute renal failure
  - Acute respiratory distress syndrome
  - ECMO
- Intervention related risk factors:
  - Peri-operative blood transfusion
  - Increased duration of mechanical ventilation
  - Re-intubation
  - Frequent ventilator circuit changes
  - Intracuff ETT pressure less than 20 cm H_2O
  - Tracheostomy tubes
  - Nasogastric tubes
  - Enteral nutrition
  - Absence of subglottic secretion drainage

Risk Factors for Multi-Drug Resistant VAP

- Antimicrobial therapy in preceding 90 days
- Current hospitalization for 5 or more days
- High frequency of antibiotic resistance in the hospital unit
- Hospitalization for > 2 days in the preceding 90 days
- Chronic dialysis within 30 days
- Immuno-suppressive disease/ therapy
- Home infusion therapy (including antibiotics)
- Home wound care

Diagnosis

Clinical pulmonary infection score (CPIS score):

Variable	0	1	2
Temperature	≥ 36.1, ≤ 38.4	38.5 - 38.9	≥ 39 to ≤ 36
Tracheal secretion	Absent	Non-purulent	Purulent
Leucocytosis	4000–11000	< 4000 or > 11000	< 4000 or > 11000 with > 500 band forms
PaO_2/FiO_2	> 240, ARDS	-	≤ 240, absence of ARDS
X-ray infiltrates	Absent	Patchy/ diffuse	Localized
Microbiology	Negative	Moderate-heavy growth	Moderate-heavy growth and
			Pathogen consistent with Gram stain
CPIS score > 6 is considered as evidence of the presence of VAP			

Prevention

- Mechanical ventilatory strategies:
  - Care of endotracheal tube:
    - Use of silver coated cuffed endotracheal tube
    - Incidence reduced by maintaining cuff pressure above 20 cm H_2O
    - Use of oropharyngeal ETT and orogastric tube reduces incidence
    - Use of nasopharyngeal and nasogastric tubes increases incidence
    - Thus, *oral intubation reduces incidence of VAP and is preferred*
    - Appropriate circuit changes when grossly contaminated
    - Use of heat and moisture exchangers when possible
  - ***Continuous Aspiration of Subglottic Secretions*** (CASS)
  - Other techniques:
    - Preference of non-invasive ventilation
    - Use of closed suction catheters and sterile suction technique
    - Adoption of a weaning protocol and daily assessment foe extubation
    - Avoiding contamination with ventilator circuit condensate
    - Careful use of in-line small-volume nebulizers
    - Use of expiratory line gas traps or filters
    - Single patient use of:
      - Monitors
      - Oxygen analyzers
      - Resuscitation bags
- Pharmacological methods:
  - Limiting the use of sedatives and paralytic agents

- ***Selective decontamination of digestive track (SDD):***
  - Involves application of a poorly absorbable mixture of:
    - Polymyxin
    - Amphotericin B
    - Aminoglycoside
  - Avoid use of systematic antibiotics for SDD
- ***Selective decontamination of oral cavity (SDO):***
  - Chlorhexidine mouth wash used to decontaminate oral cavity
  - Advantages: prevents antibiotic resistance
- Alternatives: Use mixture of:
  - 2% gentamicin
  - 2% colistin
  - 2% vancomycin
  - Applied as paste Q6H to oral cavity
- Stress ulcer prophylaxis:
  - PPI and H_2 blockers are avoided
  - Reducing gastric acidity enhances colonization of stomach
  - *Sucralfate* is the drug of choice for stress ulcer prophylaxis

❖ Improve host immunity:
- Maintain nutritional status
- Avoid agents which impair pulmonary defences:
  - Aminophylline
  - Anesthetic agents, sedatives
  - Corticosteroids
  - Anti-neoplastic agents
- Minimize use of invasive procedures when possible
- Remove/treat disease states which affect host defences:
  - Acidosis
  - Dehydration
  - Hypoxemia
  - Ethanol intoxication
  - Acid aspiration
  - Thermal injury
  - Diabetic ketoacidosis
  - Renal failure
  - Heart failure
  - Liver failure

❖ Blood products:
- Avoid unnecessary blood transfusions
- Transfusion trigger of 7 g% rather than 9 g% reduces risk of VAP

❖ Nursing considerations:
- Semi-recumbent position nursing: Position head of bed 30° above horizontal
- Oscillating beds reduce risk of VAP
- Staff education
- Strict adherence to
  - Hand washing
  - Use of accepted infection-control procedures/ practices
- Feeding:
  - Late administration of enteral foods (beyond 5 days of intubation)
  - Practice post-pyloric feeding
  - Immuno-nutrition (parenteral/enteral): Comprises of:
    - Selenium
    - Vitamin C, Vitamin E
    - Arginine, glutamine
    - Omega-3 fatty acids
- Prophylactic immunization in patients with neutropenia for:
  - Influenza
  - Pneumococcus
- ***FAST-HUG approach:***
  - F- Feeding
  - A-Analgesia
  - S-Sedation
  - T-Thrombopropylaxis
  - H-Head end elevation 30-40°
  - U-Ulcer prophylaxis
  - G-Glycemic control

Management

❖ Criteria for admission to ICU: 1 major OR 3 minor criteria required of:
- Minor criteria:
  - Respiratory rate more than 30 cycles/ min
  - Leucopenia (total count less than 4000 cells/ mm^3)
  - Thrombocytopenia (less than 100000 cells/ dL)
  - Confusion/ disorientation
  - Hypotesion requiring rapid fluid administration
  - Uremia (BUN > 20 mg/dL)
  - X-ray infilterates
  - Hypothermia (< 36 °C)
  - PaO_2/ FiO_2 < 250
- Minor criteria:
  - Invasive mechanical ventilation
  - Septic shock with need for vasopressors

- ❖ Antibiotic therapy:
  - Empirical therapy:
    - – For early onset VAP with no risk factors for MDR pathogens:
      - ▪ Ceftriaxone OR
      - ▪ Levofloxacin, monifloxacin, ciprofloxacin OR
      - ▪ Ampicillin/ sulbactam or ertapenem
    - – For late onset VAP with risk factors for MDR pathogens:
      - ▪ Antipseudomonal cephalosporins:
        - - Cefepime
        - - Ceftazidime
      - ▪ Antipseudomonal carbapenem:
        - - Imipenem
        - - Meropenem
      - ▪ Beta lactam piperacillin- tazobactam with antipseudomonal FQ:
        - - Ciprofloxacin
        - - Levofloxacin
      - ▪ Aminoglycoside with linezolid or vancomycin
    - – If MRSA, add vancomycin/ linezolid
  - Monotherapy vs combination therapy:
    - – Combination therapy is associated with higher rates of:
      - ▪ Therapy failure
      - ▪ Nephrotoxicity
    - – It also fails to prevent resistance
    - – Combination therapy used only if MDR or pseudomonas is suspected
  - Continuous vs intermittent infusion: continuous infusion maintains drug concentration above the MIC for longer duration
  - Aerosolized antibiotics:
    - – Polymyxin or aminoglycosides for MDR gram negative bacteria
    - – Especially useful in patients not improving with systemic therapy
  - *Antibiotic rotation/holiday*: may reduce incidence of resistance
  - Duration of therapy:
    - – Shorten duration from 14-21 to 8 days, provided organism is not pseudomonas
    - – If low suspicion of VAP (CPIS of < 6), stop after 3 days
- ❖ Supportive therapy:
  - Chest physiotherapy
  - Postural drainage
  - Humidification, aerosolization with bronchodilators

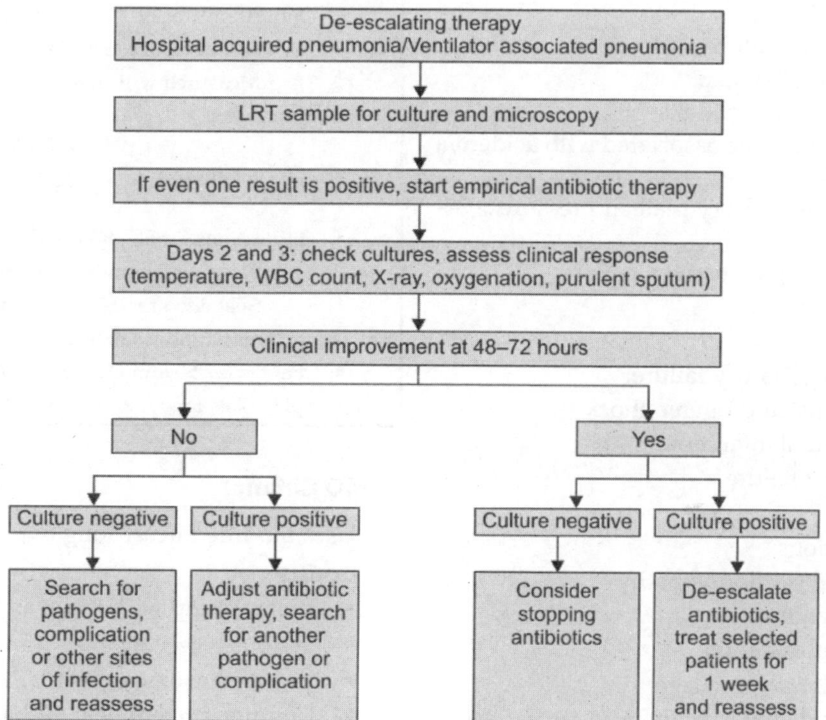

EXTRA-CORPOREAL MEMBRANE OXYGENATION

Introduction

- Refers to oxygenation of blood outside the body using a membrane oxygenator
- It is a form of mechanical cardiopulmonary support, delivered in a prolonged fashion
- First used in the clinical setting for respiratory failure in 1971

Indications in Pediatrics

- Primary pulmonary HTN of newborn (PPHN):
  - Idiopathic PPHN
  - Meconium aspiration syndrome
  - Respiratory distress syndrome
  - Asphyxia
  - Group-B streptococcal sepsis
- Pulmonary vaso-reactive crisis following repair of congenital heart defect
- Congenital Diaphragmatic Hernia
- *Low Cardiac Output Syndrome* due to:
  - Right/ left/ biventricular failure
  - Following repair of congenital heart defect
- As a bridge to cardiac surgery in patients with severe end organ damage
- As a bridge to cardiac transplant

Indications in Adults

- ECMO in respiratory failure:
  - Severe adult ARDS when:
    - PaO_2/ FiO_2 ratio < 50-80
    - Severe hypercarbia associated with acidemia (pH < 7.15)
    - High end-inspiratory plateau pressure > 35-45 cm H_2O
    - Failed proning maneuver
  - Lung transplantation
  - COPD
- ECMO in cardiorespiratory failure:
  - Post-cardiotomy cardiogenic shock
  - Acute myocardial infarction
  - End stage heart failure
  - Myocarditis
- Emerging indications:
  - Sepsis induced cardiomyopathy
  - Toxic shock syndrome
  - Severe drug intoxication
  - Diffuse alveolar hemorrhage
  - Following accidental hypothermic cardiac arrest

Patient Selection Criteria

- General criteria:
  - Gestational age > 34 weeks
  - Birth weight > 2000 grams
  - Failure of maximal medical therapy
  - If risk of mortality is > 80% with conventional ventilation
- Ventilation criteria:
  - Reversible lung injury
  - On mechanical ventilation for less than 14 days
  - Results are better when ECMO is instituted within 7 days of intubation
- Systemic criteria:
  - No intracranial hemorrhage
  - No significant coagulopathy/uncontrolled bleeding
  - No lethal malformation

ECMO Criteria

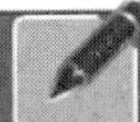

- These are qualifying criteria which apply only when:
  - Infant has reached maximum ventilatory support of 100% FiO_2
  - With peak inspiratory pressure > 35 cm H_2O
- ***Alveolar –Arterial oxygen pressure gradient {P(A-a) O_2}:***
  - Calculated with patient on 100% O_2
  - P(A-a) O_2 = Barometric pressure – 47 – $PaCO_2$ - PaO_2
  - Indications for ECMO therapy:
    - P(A-a) O_2 of 605–620 mm Hg
    - Measured with 100% FiO_2 for 4–12 hours
- ***Oxygen Index:***
  - Oxygen index = $\frac{mP_{aw} \times FiO_2}{PaO_2}$
  - Indications for ECMO therapy:
    - Oxygenation index of 0.35–0.6
    - Sustained for 0.5–6 hours with mP_{aw} > 20 cm H_2O
- Acute deterioration: Taken as:
  - PaO_2 < 35–50 mm Hg for 2–12 hours
  - pH < 7.25 for > 2 hours with hypotension.

ECMO Circuit

- Uses modified heart-lung bypass machine
- Consists of:
  - Roller pump with raceway tubing
  - Venous reservoir
  - Membrane oxygenator
  - Counter-current heat exchanger

- Blood pump can be either:
  - Single roller pump
  - Vortex centrifugal pump
- Oxygenators can be either:
  - Bubble oxygenator
  - Membrane oxygenator
  - Hollow fiber oxygenator

Safety Devices and Monitors

- Air bubble detectors
- Arterial line filters to trap air, thrombi and other emboli
- Pressure monitors
- Continuous venous O_2 saturation monitor
- Temperature monitors

Types

- Venoarterial (VA) ECMO:
  - Blood drawn from RA via IJV
  - Oxygenated blood back into aortic arch via right common carotid artery
  - Oxygenates blood and support cardiac function as blood flow to aorta is supported by ECMO
  - Most common route for ECMO
- Venovenous (VV) ECMO:
  - Blood drawn from RA via right IJV
  - Oxygenated blood back to RA via femoral vein
  - Only oxygenates blood, does not support cardiac output
  - Blood flow from right heart to left heart remains sole function of the heart

Venoarterial ECMO	Venovenous ECMO
Requires arterial cannula	Requires only venous cannula
Provides cardiac support to assist systemic circulation	Does not provide cardiac support
Bypasses pulmonary circulation	Maintains pulmonary blood flow
Reduces pulmonary arterial pressure	Elevates mixed venous PO_2
Lower perfusion rates needed	Higher perfusion rates needed
Higher PaO_2 achieved	Lower PaO_2 achieved

Technique

- Initiation:
  - Once ECMO revival has been decided, patient is anticoagulated with heparin
  - Cannulation sites and techniques are then decided
  - Types of cannulation:
    - Percutaneous cannulation:
      - Percutaneous VV ECMO:
        - Femoro-femoral approach: Using bilateral femoral veins
        - Femoro-jugular approach: Using femoral and jugular vein
      - Percutaneous VA ECMO: Using femoral artery and vein
    - Surgical cannulation:
      - Intra-thoracic cannulation: Using right atrium and ascending aorta
      - Peripheral cannulation:
        - Using femoral artery and vein
        - Using axillary artery and femoral vein:
          - Uses right axillary artery as ECMO inflow limb
          - Indicated in:
            - Post-cardiotomy patients
            - Peripheral vascular disease:
              - Aortoiliac aneurysms
              - Aorto-iliac occlusive disease
              - Femoral vessel atherosclerosis
- Titration:
  - The ECMO circuit is primed with the freshest available blood
  - Cannulae are connected to the appropriate limbs of the ECMO circuit
  - Venoarterial/venovenous bypass is then established
  - Flow is increased till respiratory and hemodynamic parameters are satisfactory
  - Once these goals have been achieved, blood flow is maintained at that rate

Maintenance

- General care:
  - Cultures from the circuit are obtained at least once a week
  - Strict aseptic precautions
  - Minimum sedation with fentanyl/ morphine/ midazolam after stabilization
  - Doses of other inotropes may be reduced once patient is on ECMO
  - Antacids and H_2 blockers
- Central nervous system:
  - Avoid paralytic agents
  - Frequent CNS assessment
  - Phenobarbital for seizures

- Respiratory management:
  - Pressure control modes of ventilation are usually preferred
  - Goals of ventilatory management:
    - $FiO_2 < 50\%$
    - PIP < 25 cm H_2O
    - Rate 10–20 breaths/min
    - PEEP 3–5 cm H_2O
    - Plateau airway pressures < 20 cm H_2O
    - $PaO_2 > 50$ mm Hg
    - $SpO_2 > 85\%$
  - ETT suction has to be done regularly
  - Daily chest X-ray
- Cardiovascular management:
  - ECMO flow rates should be high enough to maintain:
    - Adequate perfusion pressure
    - Adequate venous oxy-hemoglobin saturation
  - However, being a closed circuit, flow rates should be low enough to:
    - Maintain sufficient preload to left heart
    - To prevent air embolism
  - Systemic perfusion and intravascular volume have to be maintained
  - Typically, ECMO flow rates are maintained around 5 L/min in adults
  - Inotropes may be used to increase cardiac output
- Renals:
  - Most patients are fluid overloaded at the initiation of ECMO therapy
  - Aggressive diuretic therapy is recommended once patient is stable on ECMO
  - Oliguria and ATN are common during the first 24–48 hours
  - Diuretic phase, beginning within 48 hours is one of earliest signs of recovery
  - Ultrafiltration may be added to the ECMO circuit if oliguria persists
- Fluid balance:
  - Hyperalimentation for catabolic states
  - Fluid retention occurs in first 1–3 days

Anticoagulation during ECMO

- Anticoagulation is most commonly sustained with a continuous infusion of UFH
- Dose is titrated to maintain an ACT of 180–210 seconds
- Plasma PTT can also be used to titrate heparin dose
- This measures the intrinsic and common coagulation pathways
- Heparin dose can be titrated to maintain an aPTT 1.5 times the normal (50–70 sec)
- Patients with suspected HIT can be managed with direct thrombin inhibitors (DTI)
- DTI therapy is titrated to maintain aPTT values between 50- 70 seconds
- Hematological goals during ECMO include:
  - Hemoglobin > 7–8 g/dL
  - Platelet count > 40–50,000 cells/ mm^3
  - INR < 1.6–1.7
  - Fibrinogen > 100 mg/dL

Contraindications

- Absolute contraindications: conditions which are incompatible with recovery:
  - Severe neurological injury
  - End stage malignancy
- Relative contraindications:
  - Gestational age < 34 weeks due to risk of intracranial hemorrhage (ICH)
  - Weight < 2000 grams due to risk of intracranial hemorrhage (ICH)
  - Patient with pre-existing ICH as patients are anticoagulated during ECMO
  - Coagulopathies
  - Duration of mechanical ventilation for > 2 weeks before initiation of ECMO:
    - This is due to risk of development of chronic lung disease
    - ECMO cannot reverse chronic lung disease
    - Hence it is contraindicated as the primary disease is irreversible

Weaning Criteria

- For patients with respiratory failure:
  - Improvement in radiographic appearance
  - Improvement in pulmonary compliance
  - Improvement in arterial oxy-hemoglobin saturation
- For patients with cardiorespiratory failure:
  - Enhanced aortic pulsatility
  - Improved left ventricular output
- Temporary trials of weaning should be performed prior to permanent discontinuation
- Weaning of VV ECMO:
  - Countercurrent sweep gas flowing through the oxygenator is eliminated

- Extracorporeal blood flow remains constant, in the absence of gas transfer
- Ventilator settings are adjusted to maintain adequate gas exchange
- Patients are maintained off ECMO for several hours
- This helps to determine the feasibility of permanent weaning off ECMO

❖ Weaning off VA ECMO:
- Requires temporary clamping of both drainage and infusion lines
- ECMO circuit circulates through a bridge between arterial and venous limbs
- This prevents thrombosis of stagnant blood within the ECMO circuit
- VA ECMO weaning trials are shorter than VV ECMO trails
- This is due to the higher risk of thrombus formation with VA ECMO

Complications

❖ Mechanical complications:
- Failure of pump
- Airlock due to air in circuit
- Rupture of tubing
- Oxygenator failure
- Hypothermia due to heat exchanger malfunction
- Clots in ECMO circuit
- Damage to IJV with mediastinal bleeding during cannulation

❖ Physiological complications:
- Bleeding due to increased heparin
- Intracranial hemorrhage or infarcts due to:
  - Carotid artery ligation
  - Systemic heparinization
  - Thrombocytopenia
  - Coagulopathies
- Seizures
- Pulmonary hemorrhage
- Cardiovascular complications:
  - Hypovolemia/hypervolemia
  - Hypo/hypertension
  - Arrhythmias
  - Pericardial tamponade
  - Symptomatic PDA
  - Altered renin-angiotensin-aldosterone cycle due to non-pulsatile perfusion
- Blood:
  - Anemia
  - Thrombocytopenia
  - Leukopenia
  - Increased chances of infection
- GIT complications:
  - Gut hemorrhage
  - Biliary calculi
  - Direct hyperbilirubinemia

❖ Metabolic complications:
- Acidosis/alkalosis
- Hyper/hyponatremia
- Hypo/hyperkalemia
- Hyper/hypocalcemia
- Hypo/hyperglycemia

ECMO Prognositication: *The RESP score:*

❖ The score is a tool for predicting survival in ECMO initiated for respiratory failure

❖ The score was developed and validated on a specific ARDS population

❖ This may be a barrier to widespread use of this score with other diagnoses

❖ Immunocompromised status is defined as:
- Hematological malignancies
- Solid tumors
- Solid organ transplantation
- Human immunodeficiency virus
- Cirrhosis

❖ CNS dysfunction is defined as:
- Neurotrauma
- Stroke
- Encephalopathy
- Cerebral embolism
- Seizures
- Epileptic syndrome

Parameter	Score
Age (years)	
• 18–49	0
• 50–59	–2
• > 60	–3
Immunocompromised status	–2
Mechanical ventilation prior to ECMO initiation	
• Less than 48 hours	3
• 48 hours–7 days	1
• More than 7 days	0
Acute respiratory diagnosis group	
• Viral pneumonia	3
• Bacterial pneumonia	3
• Asthma	11

Contd...

Contd...

Parameter	Score
• Trauma and burns	3
• Aspiration pneumonia	5
• Other acute respiratory diagnoses	1
• Non-respiratory and chronic respiratory diagnoses	0
Central nervous system dysfunction	–7
Acute associated (non-pulmonary) infection	–3
Neuromuscular blockade agents before ECMO	1
Nitric oxide use before ECMO	–1
Bicarbonate infusion before ECMO	–2
Cardiac arrest before ECMO	–2
$PaCO_2$ (mm Hg)	
• < 75	0
• ≥ 75	–1
Peak inspiratory pressure (cm H_2O)	
• < 42	0
• ≥ 42	–1
Total	–22 to 15

Risk Category	Total RESP score	Survival
I	≥ 6	92%
II	3 to 5	76%
III	–1 to 2	57%
IV	–5 to –2	33%
V	≤ –6	18%

APACHE SCORE II

Introduction

- The *acute physiological assessment and chronic health evaluation (APACHE) score* is a widely used method for assessing severity of illness in acutely ill patients in ICUs, taking into account a variety of routine physiological parameters
- Outlined by ***Knauss*** in 1985
- Scores ranged from 0.71 with higher scores indicating greater severity of illness and increased risk of death

Applications

- Lower age for application is not specified but a good limit is to use the score only for patients above 15 years of age
- Some procedures and medicines are only given to patients with a certain Apache II score
- Apache II score can be used to describe mortality of a patient when comparing the outcome with other patients
- Predicted mortalities are averaged for groups of patients in order to specify the groups mortality

Calculation

- A point score is calculated from 12 routine physiological measurements during first 24 hours after admission
- Information about previous health status also is obtained at admission
- The resulting score is interpreted in relation to the illness of the patient
- After initial score has been determined within 24 hours of admission, no new score can be calculated during the hospital stay
- If a patient is discharged from ICU and readmitted, a new score can be calculated
- Using the patients Apache score and principle diagnosis at admission the predicted mortality can be calculated

Parameter	Range	Score
Age in years	Less than 44 years	0
	45–54 years	2
	55–64 years	3
	65–74 years	5
	More than 75 years	6
Severe organ insufficiency	Yes, non-operative/emergency postop patient	5
Immunocompromised status	Yes, elective postop patient	2
	No	0
Rectal temperature	More than 40.9 °C	4
	39–40.9 °C	3
	38.5–38.9 °C	1
	36–38.4 °C	0
	34–35.9 °C	1
	32–33.9 °C	2
	30–31.9 °C	3
	Less than 30 °C	4
Heart rate	More than 179 bpm	4
	140–179 bpm	3
	110–139 bpm	2
	70–109 bpm	0
	55–69 bpm	2
	40–54 bpm	3

Contd...

Contd…

Parameter	Range	Score
	Less than 40 bpm	4
Respiratory rate	More than 49 /min	4
Non-ventilated or ventilated	35–49 /min	3
	25–34 /min	1
	12–24 /min	0
	10–11 /min	1
	6–9 /min	2
	Less than 6 /min	4
Mean arterial pressure	More than 159 mm Hg	4
	130–159 mm Hg	3
	110–129 bpm	2
	70–109 bpm	0
	50–69 bpm	2
	Less than 50 bpm	4
Oxygenation	A-a gradient >499	4
Use PaO_2 if FiO_2 < 50%	A-a gradient 350–499	3
Else, use alveolar-arterial gradient	A-a gradient 200–349	2
	A-a gradient <200 if FiO_2 >49 or PaO_2 >70	0
	If FiO_2 less than 50%	
	PaO_2 61–70	1
	PaO_2 55–60	3
	PaO_2 less than 55	4
Arterial pH	More than 7.69	4
	7.6–7.69	3
	7.5–7.59	1
	7.33–7.49	0
	7.25–7.32	2
	7.15–7.24	3
	Less than 7.15	4
Serum sodium levels	More than 179 mmol/L	4
	160–179 mmol/L	3
	155–159 mmol/L	2
	150–154 mmol/L	1
	130–149 mmol/L	0
	120–129 mmol/L	2
	111–119 mmol/L	3
	Less than 111 mmol/L	4

Contd…

Contd…

Parameter	Range	Score
Serum potassium levels	More than 6.9 mmol/L	4
	6–6.9 mmol/L	3
	5.5–5.9 mmol/L	1
	3.5–5.4 mmol/L	0
	3–3.4 mmol/L	1
	2.5–2.9 mmol/L	2
	Less than 2.5 mmol/L	4
Serum creatinine	More than 3.4 mg/dL and ARF	8
	2–3.4 mg/dL and ARF	6
	1.5–1.9 mg/dL and ARF	4
	More than 3.4 mg/dL and CRF	4
	2–3.4 mg/dL and CRF	3
	1.5–1.9 mg/dL and CRF	2
	0.6–1.4 mg/dL	0
	Less than 0.6 mg/dL	2
Hematocrit	More than 59.9%	4
	50–59.9%	2
	46–49.9%	1
	30–45.9%	0
	20–29.9%	2
	Less than 20%	4
WBC count	More than 39000 /mm^3	4
	20000–38900 /mm^3	2
	15000–19900 /mm^3	1
	3000–14900 /mm^3	0
	1000–2900 /mm^3	2
	Less than 1000 /mm^3	4

Mortality Prediction

Total of all points Apache score is then calculated:

Apache score	Mortality rate
0–4	4%
5–9	8%
10–14	15%
15–19	25%
20–24	40%
25–29	55%
30–34	75%
More than 35	85%

DELIRIUM IN ICU

Introduction

- Delirium is an acute confusional state characterized by an alteration of consciousness with reduced ability to focus, sustain or shift attention
- ICU delirium is a non-specific, potentially preventable and often reversible disorder of impaired cognition seen in ICU patients
- Characteristic features of ICU delirium include:
  - Development over a short period of time
  - Fluctuating course
  - Disorientation
  - Impaired short-term memory
  - Impaired attention

Incidence

- Incidence of ICU delirium reported varies from 45–87%
- The incidence is highest in mechanically ventilated patients
- The risk of ICU delirium in decreasing frequency are:
  - Neurosurgical patients (highest risk)
  - Trauma patients
  - Medical ICU patients
  - Surgical patients (lowest risk)
- Delirium is the *most common* cause of acute brain dysfunction in the ICU
- Prolonged delirium following critical care illness is associated with:
  - 2.5- fold increased risk of short-term mortality
  - 3.2- fold increased risk of 6-month mortality

Risk Factors for ICU Delirium

- Modifiable risk factors:
  - Benzodiazepine use
  - Blood transfusions
  - Alcohol abuse, tobacco use
- Non-modifiable risk factors:
  - Advanced age > 70 years
  - HTN
  - Dementia
  - APOE4 polymorphism

Contd...

Contd...

  - Vision/hearing impairment
  - Prior coma
  - Pre-ICU emergency surgery or trauma
  - Increasing severity of illness scores.

Drugs Associated with ICU Delirium

- Benzodiazepines
- Opioids
- Anticholinergics
- Antihistaminics
- H2 blockers
- Antibiotics
- Corticosteroids
- Metoclopramide

Precipitating Factors

- Metabolic disturbances
- Hypotension
- Sepsis
- Poor pain control
- Mechanical ventilation
- Sleep disturbances
- Benzodiazepines
- Opioids (meperidine, morphine)
- Anticholinergics
- Steroids

Prediction of Delirium

- Predictive models including delirium risk factors are capable of predicting delirium
- Prediction of delirium in ICU (***PRE-DELIRIC***) model is most commonly used
- The 10 predictors include:
  - Age
  - APACHE-II score
  - Admission group
  - Urgent admission
  - Infection
  - Coma
  - Sedation
  - Morphine use
  - Urea level
  - Metabolic acidosis

Pathophysiology

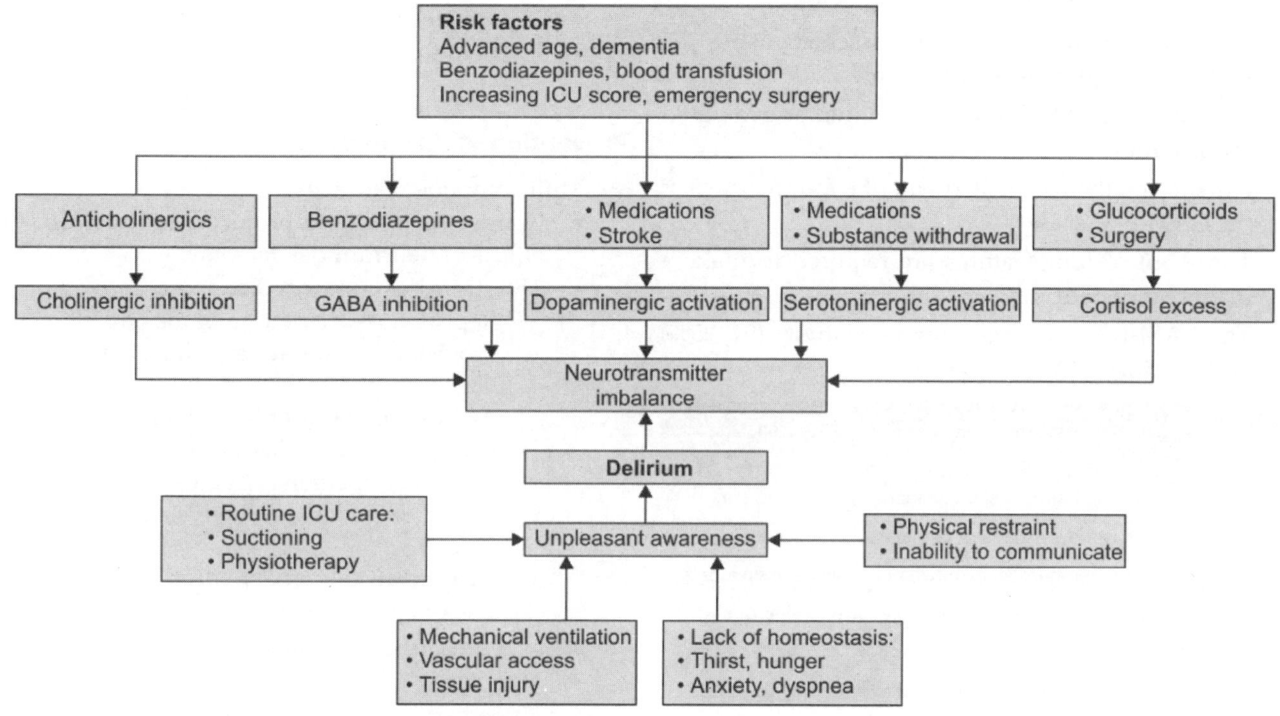

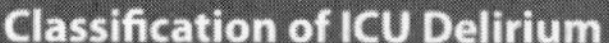

Classification of ICU Delirium

- Hyperactive delirium:
  - Characterized by:
    - Restlessness, agitation
    - Rapid mood changes
    - Hallucinations, refusal to cooperate with care
  - Most easily recognizable subtype
- Hypoactive delirium:
  - Characterized by:
    - Inactivity, reduced motor activity
    - Sluggishness, abnormal drowsiness
    - Occurs in older patients
    - Has a worse prognosis
    - Associated with:
    - Greater requirement of mechanical ventilation
    - Prolonged length of ICU stay
    - Higher 6-month mortality (approaches 32%)
    - 6- month mortality seen with other types is 8.7%
- Mixed delirium: includes both signs of hyperactive and hypoactive delirium.

Clinical Features

- Manifests as a constellation of symptoms with an acute onset and fluctuating course
- Common cognitive symptoms include:
  - Disorientation, inability to sustain attention
  - Impaired short-term memory
  - Impaired visuo-spatial ability
  - Reduced level of consciousness
- Common behavioural symptoms include:
  - Disturbances in sleep-wake cycle
  - Irritability, hallucinations, delusions
- Manifestations can range from somnolence and comatose to disruptive or combative
- Manifestations also depend on the precipitating factors:
  - Patients with sepsis present with encephalopathy and hypoactive delirium
  - Patients with alcohol withdrawal present with hyperactive delirium

Adverse Outcomes of Delirium

- Self extubation
- Removal of catheters
- Prolonged hospital stay
- Increased short term mortality
- Increased 6-month mortality
- Long term cognitive dysfunction

Evaluation of Delirium

- Done using the CAM-ICU scale in 2 steps
- Level of consciousness is first assessed using the Richmond Agitation Sedation Scale
- Patients with RASS scores > - 3 should be evaluated for delirium
- Patients are then evaluated with the four features of the CAM-ICU scale
- Three out of four features are required to make a diagnosis of delirium
- The CAM-ICU scale has a high sensitivity (91–95%) and specificity (98%)

RASS Score	
Score	*Description*
+ 4	Overtly combative, violent, immediate danger to staff
+ 3	Pulls or removes tubes or catheters, aggressive
+ 2	Frequent non-purposeful movements, fights ventilator
+ 1	Anxious but movements not aggressive or vigorous
0	Alert and calm
– 1	Not fully alert, but has sustained eye opening to voice (>10 seconds)
– 2	Briefly awakens with eye contact to voice (< 10 seconds)
– 3	Movement or eye opening to voice, but no eye contact
– 4	No response to voice, but movement or eye opening to physical stimulation
– 5	No response to voice or physical stimulation

CAM ICU Scale

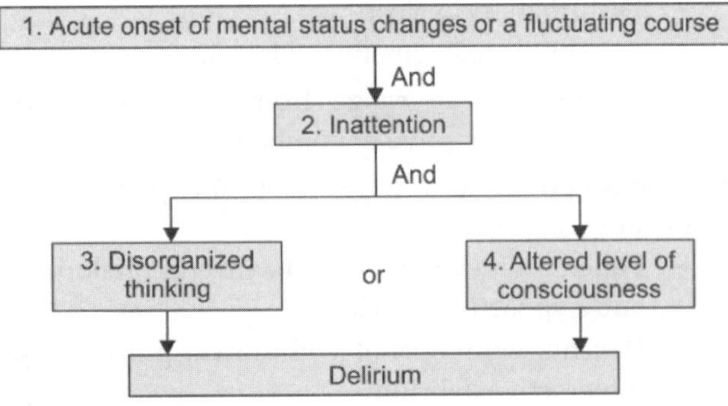

Biomarkers of Delirium

- S100B protein: Shown to be elevated in patients with delirium
- Procalcitonin: Higher baseline level is associated with more days of delirium
- C-reactive protein: Higher baseline level is associated with more days of delirium
- Additional serum biomarkers include:
    - Brain-derived neurotrophic factor
    - Neuron-specific enolase
    - Interleukins
    - Cortisol

Prevention of ICU Delirium

- Multicomponent strategy:
    - Consists of multiple protocols to minimize the effects of delirium risk factors
    - The strategies comprised of:
        - Repeated re-orientation of the patient
        - Provision of cognitively stimulating activities
        - Avoidance of bright light therapy
        - Non-pharmacological sleep protocol
        - Early mobilization activities
        - Timely removal of catheters and physical restraints
        - Early correction of dehydration
        - Use of eyeglasses and hearing aids
- Management of critical illnesses leading to delirium:
    - Hypoxia
    - Hypercarbia
    - Hypoglycemia
    - Shock
- Pharmacological strategies:
    - Reduced benzodiazepine use
    - Ensure adequate analgesia
    - Haloperidol, dexmedetomidine or ketamine are not used to prevent delirium

Treatment

- Non-pharmacological therapies:
    - Specifically devised to prevent the occurrence of delirium
    - These strategies may reduce the incidence of delirium by up to 40%
    - Strategies include:
        - Minimization of noise:
            - Use of ear plugs within 48 hours of admission
            - Discontinuation of unnecessary monitors
            - Avoidance of telephones in close vicinity of patient
            - Adjusting alarm limits to safest minimum levels
        - Other methods:
            - Reduce the frequency of room changes
            - Encouragement of family support
            - Avoidance of mechanical restraints

- Providence of clock and reading glasses
- Avoid interventions during sleeping hours
- Music therapy

❖ Delirium prevention bundles:
- ABCDE bundle for liberation and animation:
  - This is a critical care bundle which encourages weaning from MV
  - This bundle should be adopted for patients on a daily basis
  - Liberation refers to the use of:
    - Target based sedation protocols
    - Spontaneous awakening trials
    - Proper choice of sedatives
  - Animation refers to early mobilization of patients following extubation
  - Advantages of this bundle:
    - Minimizes delirium
    - Improves long-term cognitive outcomes
- Pain, agitation and delirium (PAD) care bundle:
  - The key recommendation of this bundle is the *analgesia-first strategy*
  - This strategy minimizes the use of sedation
  - Emphasizes on the treatment of pain prior to administration of sedation
  - This allows patient interaction with their environment without agitation
  - The PAD care bundle also integrates:
    - Spontaneous awakening trials
    - Spontaneous breathing trials
    - Early mobility
    - Sleep hygiene programs

❖ Pharmacological therapy:
- Haloperidol:
  - Most frequently used antipsychotic and is the *first line of treatment*
  - It is a butyrophenone antipsychotic
  - It is also a cortical dopamine (D_2) antagonist
  - Routine use of antipsychotics to treat delirium should be discouraged
  - Antipsychotics are used only in patients with significant distress:
    - Significant agitation, anxiety, delusions
    - Risk of physical harm to others
  - Commonly used dose is IV 2–10 mg Q6H
- Atypical antipsychotics:
  - These are alternatives to haloperidol and include:
    - Olanzapine
    - Risperidone
    - Haloperidol
    - Aripiprazole
  - Efficacy of haloperidol and atypical antipsychotics are comparable
- Cholinesterase inhibitors:
  - Use of anticholinergic drugs accentuates drug-associated ICU delirium
  - Thus, cholinesterase inhibitors may be effective in treating delirium
- Alpha 2 agonists:
  - Shown to be effective in decreasing the incidence of delirium
  - Intravenous alpha 2 agonists are associated with:
    - Reduced severity of delirium
    - Enhanced respiratory function
    - Reduced duration of weaning
    - Shorter overall ICU stay
  - α_2 agonists are more efficacious than BZDs in preventing delirium
  - Dexmedetomidine is useful in ventilated patients where agitation precludes weaning
- Benzodiazepines (BZDs):
  - Use of BZDs is associated with:
    - Suppressed level III or IV REM sleep
    - Higher incidence of ICU delirium
    - Prolonged ventilation
    - Prolonged ICU stay
  - BZD should be used to treat delirium only in alcoholics
- Other agents: lack of evidence precludes use of:
  - High dose HMG- CoA reductase inhibitors
  - Ketamine infusion

SUGGESTED READING

1. Abedin, Z. and Conner, R. (2008). *ECG Interpretation—The Self-Assessment Approach.* 2nd edition. Massachusetts: Wiley-Blackwell.
2. Abou-Donia, M. B. (2003). Organophosphorous ester induced chronic neurotoxicity. *Archives of Environmental and Occupational Health*, 58(8), 484–97.
3. Ahee, P. and Crowe, A.V. (2000). The management of hyperkalemia in the emergency department. *Journal of Accident and Emergency Medicine*, 17(3), 188–91.
4. Algaba, Á. and Nin, N. (2013). Alveolar recruitment maneuvers in respiratory distress syndrome. *Medicina Intensiva*, 37(5), 355–62.
5. Allon, M. and Shanklin, N. (1996). Effect of bicarbonate administration on plasma potassium in dialysis patients: interactions with insulin and albuterol. *American Journal of Kidney Disease*, 28(4), 508–14.
6. Alvisi, V., Romanello, A., Badet, M., Gaillard, S., Philit, F. and Guérin, C. (2003). Time course of expiratory flow limitation in COPD patients during acute respiratory failure requiring mechanical ventilation. *Chest*, 123(5), 1625–32.

7. American Thoracic Society; Infectious Diseases Society of America. (2005). Guidelines for the management of adults with hospital-acquired, ventilator associated & healthcare associated pneumonia. *American Journal of Respiratory and Critical Care Medicine*, 171(4), 388–416.
8. Anzueto, A. et al., (2004). Incidence, risk factors and outcome of barotrauma in mechanically ventilated patients. *Intensive Care Medicine*, 30(4), 612–9.
9. Armaganidis, A., Stavrakaki-Kallergi, K., Koutsoukou, A., Lymberis, A., Milic-Emili, J. and Roussos, C. (2000). Intrinsic positive end-expiratory pressure in mechanically ventilated patients with and without tidal expiratory flow limitation. *Critical Care Medicine*, 28(12), 3837–42.
10. Arumugam, S. et al., (2017). Delirium in the intensive care unit. *Journal of Emergencies, Trauma and Shock*, 10(1), 37-46.
11. Barbier, F., Andremont, A., Wolff, M. and Bouadma, L. (2013). Hospital acquired pneumonia and ventilator associated pneumonia: recent advances in epidemiology and management. *Current Opinions in Pulmonary Medicine*, 19(3), 216–28.
12. Beberta, V. S., Pitotti, R.L., Borys, D. J. and Morgan, D. L. (2011). Seven years of cyanide ingestions in the USA: critically ill patients are common, but antidote use is not. *Emergency Medicine Journal*, 28(2), 155–8.
13. Beitler, J.R. et al., (2014). Prone positioning reduces mortality from ARDS in the low tidal volume era. *Intensive Care Medicine*, 40(3), 332–41.
14. Benson, G.D., Koff, R.S. and Tolman, K. G. (2005). The therapeutic use of acetaminophen in patients with liver disease. *American Journal of Therapeutics*, 12(2), 133–41.
15. Berenson, J. R. (2002). Treatment of hypercalcemia of malignancy with bisphosphonates. *Seminars in Oncology*, 29(6 Suppl 21), 12–8.
16. Berry, N. and Fletcher, S. (2012). Abdominal compartment syndrome. *Continuing Education in Anesthesia Critical Care and Pain*, 12(3), 110–7.
17. Bersten, A. D. and Handy, J. M. (2019). *OHs Intensive Care Manual*. 8th edition. London: Elsevier.
18. Bilezikian, J. P. (1993). Clinical review 51: management of hypercalcemia. *The Journal of Clinical Endocrinology and Metabolism*, 77(6), 1445–9.
19. Blanch, L., Bernabé, F. and Lucangelo, U. (2005). Measurement of air-trapping, intrinsic positive end-expiratory pressure, and dynamic hyperinflation in mechanically ventilated patients. *Respiratory Care*, 50(1), 110–23.
20. Body, J. J. (2004). Hypercalcemia of malignancy. *Seminars in Nephrology*, 24(1), 48–54.
21. Bunchorntavakul, C. and Reddy, K. R. (2013). Acetaminophen related hepatotoxicity. *Clinical Liver Disease*, 17(4), 587–607, viii.
22. Butterworth, J. F., Mackey, D. C. and Wasnick, J. D. (2018). *Morgan and Mikhail's Clinical Anesthesiology*. 6th edition. United States: Lange.
23. Cairo, J. (2016). *Pilbeams Mechanical Ventilation: Physiological and Clinical Applications*. 6th edition. St. Louis: Elsevier.
24. Cavallazi, R., Saad, M. and Marik, P. E. (2012). Delirium in the ICU: an overview. *Annals of Intensive Care*, 2(1), 49.
25. Chang, D. W. (2014). *Clinical Application of Mechanical Ventilation*. 4th edition. New York: Delmar Cengage Learning.
26. Chastre, J. and Fagon, J. Y. (2002). Ventilator-associated pneumonia. *American Journal of Respiratory and Critical Care Medicine*, 165(7), 867–903.
27. Chiew, A.L., Gluud, C., Brok, J. and Buckley, N. A. (2018). Interventions for paracetamol (acetaminophen) overdose. *Cochrane Database of Systematic Reviews*.
28. Clark, R., Fisher, J. E., Sketris, I. S. and Johnston, G. M. (2012). Population prevalence of high dose paracetamol in dispensed paracetamol/opioid prescription combinations: an observational study. *BMC Clinical Pharmacology*, 12, 11.
29. Combes, A. et al., (2018). Extracorporeal membrane oxygenation for severe acute respiratory distress syndrome. *New England Journal of Medicine*, 378, 1965–75.
30. Constantin, J. M., Godet, T., Jabaudon, M., Bazin, J. E. and Futier, E. (2017). Recruitment maneuvers in acute respiratory distress syndrome. *Annals of Translational Medicine*, 5(14), 290.
31. Cooper, M. S. and Gittoes, N. J. L. (2008). Diagnosis and management of hypocalcemia. *British Medical Journal*, 336(7656), 1298–302.
32. Cox, C. A., Wolfson, M. R. and Shaffer, T. H. (1996). Liquid ventilation: a comprehensive overview. *Neonatal Network*, 15(3), 31–43.
33. Dart, R. C. et al., (2006). Acetaminophen poisoning: an evidence-based consensus guideline for out-of-hospital management. *Clinical Toxicology (Philadelphia)*, 44(1), 1–18.
34. Degraeuwe, P.L. J., de Vos, G. and Blanco, C. E. (1995). Perfluorochemical liquid ventilation: from the animal laboratory to the intensive care unit. *International Journal of Artificial Organs*.
35. Desai, N. R., Myers, L. and Simeone, F. (2012). Comparison of 3 different methods used to measure the rapid shallow breathing index. *Journal of Critical Care*, 27(4), 418, e1–6.
36. Devlin, J. W. et al., (2018). Clinical practice guidelines for the prevention and management of pain, agitation/sedation, delirium, immobility and sleep disruption in adult patients in the ICU. *Critical Care Medicine*, 46(9), e825–73.
37. Dietzek, A., Connelly, K., Cotugno, M., Bartel, S. and McDonnell, A. M. (2015). Denosumab in hypercalcemia of malignancy: a case series. *Journal of Oncology Pharmacy Practice*, 21(2), 143–7.
38. Eddelston, M. et al., (2005). Differences between organophosphorous insecticides in human self poisoning: a prospective cohort study. *Lancet*, 366(9495), 1452–9.
39. Eddleston, M. and Phillips, M. R. (2004). Self-poisoning with pesticides. *British Medical Journal*, 328(7430), 42–4.
40. Eddlestone, M., Roberts, D. and Buckley, N. (2002). Management of severe organophosphorous pesticide poisoning. *Critical Care*, 6, 259.
41. Ernst, A. and Zibrak, J.D. (1998). Carbon monoxide poisoning. *New England Journal of Medicine*, 339(22), 1603–8.
42. Fan, E. et al., (2017). An Official American Thoracic Society/European Society of Intensive Care Medicine/

Society of Critical Care Medicine clinical practice guideline: mechanical ventilation in adult patients with ARDS. *American Journal of Respiratory and Critical Care Medicine*, 195(9), 1253–63.

43. Feihl, F. and Perret, C. (1994). Permissive hypercapnea: how permissive should we be? *American Journal of Respiratory and Critical Care Medicine*, 150(6 Pt 1), 1722–37.
44. Felsenfeld, A. J., Levine, B. S. and Rodriguez, M. (2015). Pathophysiology of calcium, phosphorous and magnesium dysregulation in chronic kidney disease. *Seminars in Dialysis*, 28(6), 564–77.
45. Fielden, N. M., Lewicki, L. J., Meyer, K. H., Wollens, C. and Arroliga, A. C. (2007). The effects of continuous lateral rotation therapy. *Chest*, 132(4), 575A.
46. Fuhrman, B. P., Paczan, P. R. and DeFrancisis, M. (1991). Perfluorocarbon-associated gas exchange. *Critical Care Medicine*, 19(5), 712–22.
47. Garnacho-Montero, J., Escoresca-Ortega, A. and Fernández-Delgado, E. (2015). Antibiotic de-escalation in the ICU: how best is it done? *Current Opinion in Infective Diseases*, 28(2), 193–8.
48. Girard, T. D., Pandharipande, P. P. and Ely, E. W. (2008). Delirium in the intensive care unit. *Critical Care*, 12(Suppl 3), S3.
49. Glérant, J. Ch., Leleu, O., Rose, D., Mayeux, I. and Jounieaux, V. (2005). Oxygen consumption and PEEPe in ventilated COPD patients. *Respiratory Physiology and Neurobiology*, 146 (2–3), 117–24.
50. Goldfrank, L. R., Howland, M. A., Lewin, N., Nelson, L. and Goldfrank, L. (2015). *Goldfranks Toxicologic Emergencies*. 10th edition. New York: McGraw-Hill Education.
51. Goligher, E. C. et al., (2017). Lung recruitment maneuvers for adult patients with ARDS—a systematic review and meta-analysis. *Annals of American Thoracic Society*, 14(Suppl 4), S304–11.
52. Graber, M., Subramani, K., Corish, D. and Schwab, A. (1988). Thrombocytosis elevates serum potassium. *American Journal of Kidney Diseases*, 12(2), 116–20.
53. Guérin, C. et al., (2013). Prone positioning in severe acute respiratory distress syndrome: PROSEVA study.. *New England Journal of Medicine*, 368, 2159–68.
54. Hampson, N. B. (2016). US mortality due to carbon monoxide poisoning, 1994–2014: accidental and intentional deaths. *Annals of Americcan Thoracic Society*, 13(10), 1768–74.
55. Hayhurst, C. J., Pandharipande, P. P. and Hughes, C. G. (2016). Intensive Care Unit delirium: a review of diagnosis, prevention, and treatment. *Anesthesiology*, 125(6), 1229–41.
56. Haymond, S., Cariappa, R., Eby, C. S. and Scott, M. G. (2005). Laboratory assessment of oxygenation in methemoglobinemia. *Clinical Chemistry*, 51(2), 434–44.
57. Hess, D. R. (2011). Approaches to conventional mechanical ventilation of the patient with acute respiratory distress syndrome. *Respiratory Care*, 56(10), 1555–72.
58. Hodgson, C. et al., (2009). Recruitment maneuvers for adults with acute lung injuryreceiving mechanical ventilation. *Cochrane Database of Systematic Reviews*, (2), CD006667.
59. Holzheimer, R. G. and Mannick, J. A. (2002). *Surgical treatment: Evidence-based and problem-oriented*. Munich: Zuckschwerdt Publishers.
60. Hong, J. J., Cohn, S. M., Perej, J. M., Dolich, M. O., Brown, M. and McKenney, M. G. (2002). Prospective study of the incidence and outcome of intra-abdominal hypertension and the abdominal compartment syndrome. *British Journal of Surgery*, 89(5), 591–6.
61. Hshieh, T. T. et al., (2015). Effectiveness of multicomponent nonpharmacological delirium interventions: a meta-analysis. *JAMA Internal Medicine*, 175(4), 512–20.
62. Huang, C. C. et al., (2017). Hyperbaric oxygen therapy is associated with lower short- and long-term mortality in patients with carbon monoxide poisoning. *Chest*, 152(5), 943–53.
63. Hughes, K. T. and Beasley, M. B. (2017). Pulmonary manifestations of acute lung injury: more than just diffuse alveolar damage. *Archives of Pathology and Laboratory Medicine*, 141(7), 916–22.
64. Ichai, C., Hervé, Q. and Jean-Christophe, O. (2012). *Metabolic disorders and critically ill patients*. Switzerland: Springer International Publishing.
65. Indira, M., Andrews, M. A. and Rakesh, T. P. (2013). Incidence, predictors and outcome of intermediate syndrome in cholinergic insecticide poisoning: a prospective observational cohort study. *Clinical Toxicology*, 51(9), 838–45.
66. (1999). International consensus conferences in intensive care medicine: Ventilator-associated Lung Injury in ARDS. *American Journal of Respiratory and Critical Care Medicine*, 160(6), 2118–24.
67. Inzucchi, S. E. (2004). Understanding hypercalcemia: its metabolic basis, signs and symptoms. *Journal of Postgraduate Medicine*, 115(4), 69–70, 73–6.
68. Irwin, R. S. and Rippe, J. M. (2005). *Irwin and Rippes Intensive Care Medicine*. Philadelphia: Lippincott Williams and Wilkins.
69. Kacmarek, R., Stoller, J. and Heuer, A. (2017). *Egans Fundamentals of Respiratory Care*. 11th edition. St Louis: Elsevier.
70. Kaisers, U., Kelly, K. P. and Busch, T. (2003). Liquid ventilation. *British Journal of Anesthesia*, 91(1), 143–51.
71. Kao, L. W. and Nañagas, K. A. (2004). Carbon monoxide poisoning. *Emergency Medicine Clinics of North America*, 22(4), 985–1018.
72. Kavanagh, B.P. and Laffey, J. G. (2006). Hypercapnia: permissive and therapeutic. *Minerva Anesthesiologica*, 72(6), 567–76.
73. Khemani, R. G., Parvathaneni, K., Yehya, N., Bhalla, A. K., Thomas, N. J. and Newth, C. J. L. (2018). Positive end-expiratory pressure lower than the ARDS netweok protocol is associated with higher pediatric acute respiratory distress syndrome mortality. *American Journal of Respiratory and Critical Care Medicine*, 198(1), 77–89.
74. Kim, H. J. and Han, S. W. (2002). Therapeutic approach to hyperkalemia. *Nephron*, 92(Suppl 1), 33–40.
75. Kotani, T., Katayama, S., Fukuda, S., Miyazaki, Y. and Sato, Y. (2016). Pressure-controlled inverse ratio ventilation as a rescue therapy for severe acute respiratory distress syndrome.. *Springerplus*, 5(1), 716.

76. Kreit, J. W. (2018). *Mechanical Ventilation: Physiology and Practice*. 2nd edition. Oxford: Oxford University Press.
77. Larson, A. M. et al., (2005). Acetaminophen-induced acute liver failure: results of a United States multicenter, prospective study. *Hepatology*, 42(6), 1364–72.
78. Lee, H. K., Brough, T. J., Curtis, M. B., Polito, F. A. and Yeo, K. T. J. (2008). Pseudohyperkalemia—is serum or whole blood a better specimen type than plasma. *Clinica Chimica Acta*, 396(1–2), 95–6.
79. Lee, W. M. (2003). Drug-induced hepatotoxicity. *New England Journal of Medicine*, 349(5), 474–85.
80. Lin, S. M. et al. (2004). The impact of delirium on the survival of mechanically ventilated patients. *Critical Care Medicine*, 32, 2254–9.
81. Maerz, L. and Kaplan, L. J. (2008). Abdominal compartment syndrome. *Critical Care Medicine*, 36(4 Suppl), S212–5.
82. Makin, A. J., Wendon, J. and Williams, R. (1995). A 7-year experience of severe acetaminophen-induced hepatotoxicity. *Gastroenterology*, 109(6), 1907-16.
83. Malbrain, M. L. N. G. (2004). Different techniques to measure intra-abdominal pressure (IAP): time for a critical re-appraisal. *Intensive Care Medicine*, 30(3), 357–71.
84. Manzano, F. F. et al., (2008). Positive-end expiratory pressure reduces incidence of ventilator-associated pneumonia in non-hypoxemic patients. *Critical Care Medicine*, 36(8), 2225–31.
85. Marini, J. J. and Dries, D. J. (2019). *Critical Care Medicine: The essentials and more*. 5th edition. Philadelphia: Lippincott Williams & Wilkins.
86. Marino, P. L. (2017). *The little ICU book of facts and formulas*. 2nd edition. China: Wolters Kluwer.
87. Marrs, T. C. and Thompson, J. P. (2016). The efficacy and adverse effects of dicobalt edetate in cyanide poisoning. *Clinical Toxicology*, 54(8), 609–14.
88. Martin, C. M. et al., (2009). A prospective observational registry of patients with severe sepsis: the Canadian Sepsis Treatment and Response Registry. *Critical Care Medicine*, 37(1), 81–8.
89. Miller, R. D., Eriksson, L., Fleisher, L., Wiener-Kronish, J., Cohen, N. and Young, W. (2015). *Millers Anesthesia*. 8th edition. Philadelphia: Elsevier Saunders.
90. Mistry, M., Shea, A., Giguère, P. and Nguyen, M. L. (2016). Evaluation of sodium polystyrene sulfonate dosing strategies in the inpatient management of hyperkalemia. *Annals of Pharmacotherapy*, 50(6), 455–62.
91. Morocco, A. P. (2005). Cyanides. *Critical Care Clinics*, 21(4), 691–705, vi.
92. Mount, D. B. (2015). *Brenner and Recotr's The Kidney*. 10th edition. Philadelphia: WB Saunders.
93. Mughal, M. M., Culver, D. A., Minai, O. A. and Arroliga, A. C. (2005). Auto-positive end-expiratory pressure: mechanisms and treatment. *Cleveland Clinics Journal of Medicine*, 72(9), 801–9.
94. Munshi, L. et al., (2017). Prone position for acute respiratory distress syndrome. a systematic review and meta-analysis. *Annals of American Thoracic Society*, 14(Suppl 4): S280–8.
95. Neuville, M., Mourvillier, B., Bouadma, L. and Timsit, J. F. (2017). Bundle of care decreased ventilator-associated events—implications for ventilator-associated pneumonia prevention. *Journal of Thoracic Disease*, 9(3), 430–3.
96. Olson, K. R. et al., (2018). *Poisoning and drug overdose*. 7th edition. New York: McGraw Hill Education.
97. Ouimet, S., Kavanagh, B. P., Gottfried, S. B. and Skrobik, Y. (2007). Incidence, risk factors and consequences of ICU delirium. *Intensive Care Medicine*, 33(1), 66–73.
98. Owens, W. (2018). *The Ventilator Book*. 2nd edition. Columbia: First Draught Press.
99. Parker-Cote, J. L., Rizer, J., Vakkalanka, J. P., Rege, S. V. and Holstege, C. P. (2018). Challenges in the diagnosis of acute cyanide poisoning. *Clinical Toxicology*, 56(7), 609–17.
100. Pawar, K. S., Bhoite, R. R., Pillay, C. P., Chavan, S. C., Malshikare, D. S. and Garad, S. G. (2006). Continuous pralidoxime infusion versus repeated bolus injection to treat organophosphorus pesticide poisoning: a randomized controlled trial. *Lancet*, 368(9553), 2136–41.
101. Pelosi, P., de Abreu, M. G. and Rocco, P. R. M. (2010). New and conventional strategies for lung recruitment in acute respiratory distress syndrome. *Critical Care*, 14, 210.
102. Pham, P. C. T., Pham, P. A. T., Pham, S. V., Pham,P. T. T., Pham, P. M. T. and Pham, P. T. T. (2014). Hypomagnesemia: a clinical perspective. *International Journal of Nephrology and Renovascular Disease*, 7, 219–30.
103. Porzecanski, I. and Bowton, D. L. (2006). Diagnosis and treatment of ventilator-associated pneumonia. *Chest*, 130(2), 597–604.
104. Reade, M. C. and Finfer, S. (2014). Sedation and delirium in the intensive care unit. *New England Journal of Medicine*, 370(5), 444–54.
105. Reickert, C. et al., (2001). The pulmonary and systemic distribution and elimination of perflubron from adult patients treated with partial liquid ventilation. *Chest*, 119(2), 515–22.
106. Rello, J., Kollef, M., Diaz, E. and Rodriguez, A. (2007). *Infectious Diseases in Critical Care*. 2nd edition. Berlin: Springer.
107. Roberts, B. et al., (2005). Muticenter study of delirium in ICU patients using a simple screening tool. *Australian Critical Care*, 18(1), 6, 8–9, 11–4 passim.
108. Rose, B. D. and Post, T. W. (2001). *Clinical Physiology of Acid Base and Electrolyte Disorders*. 5th edition. New York: McGraw Hill Education.
109. Rumack, B.H. (2002). Acetaminophen hepatotoxicity: the first 35 years. *Journal of Toxicology: Clinical Toxicology*, 40(1), 3–20.
110. Sangalli, F., Patroniti, N. and Pesenti, A. (2014). *ECMO-Extracorporeal Life Support in Adults*. New York: Springer-Verlag Mailand, XII, 489.
111. Sauer, S. W. and Keim, M. E. (2001). Hydroxocobalamin: improved public health readiness for cyanide disasters. *Annals of Emergency Medicine*, 37(6), 635–41.
112. Schiødt, F. V., Lee, W. M., Bondesen, S., Ott, P. and Christensen, E. (2002). Influence of acute and chronic alcohol intake on the clinical course and outcome in acetaminophen overdose. *Alimentary Pharmacology and Therapeutics*, 16(4), 707–15.
113. Schmidt, L. E., Dalhoff, K. and Poulsen, H. E. (2002). Acute versus chronic alcohol consumption in acetaminophen induced hepatotoxicity. *Hepatology*, 35(4), 876–82.

114. Schmidt, M. et al., (2014). Predicting survival after extracorporeal membrane oxygenation for severe acute respiratory failure: the respiratory extracorporeal membrane oxygenation survival prediction score. *American Journal of Respiratory and Critical Care Medicine*, 189(11), 1374–82.
115. Segal, L. N. et al., (2008). Evolution of pattern of breathing during a spontaneous breathing trialpredicts successful weaning. *Intensive Care Medicine*, 36(3), 487–95.
116. Seo, K. W., Park, M., Kim, J. G., Kim, T. W. and Kim, H. J. (2000). Effects of benzothiazole on the xenobiotic metabolizing enzymes and metabolism of acetaminophen. *Journal of Applied Toxicology*, 20(6), 427–30.
117. Sklar, M. C., Sy, E., Lequier, L., Fan, E. and Kanji, H. D. (2016). Anticoagulation practices during venovenous extracorporeal membrane oxygenation for respiratory failure: a systematic review. *Annals of American Thoracic Society*, 13(12), 2242–50.
118. Smellie, W. S. A. (2007). Spurious hyperkalemia. *British Medical Journal*, 334(7595), 693–5.
119. Spasovski, G. et al., (2014). Clinical practice guideline on diagnosis and treatment of hyponatremia. *Nephrology Dialysis Transplant*, 29(Suppl 2), i1–i39.
120. Surawicz, B. and Knilans, T. (2008). *Chou's Electrocardiography in Clinical practice.* 6th edition. Philadelphia: Saunders.
121. Takeuchi, A. et al., (2000). A simple "new" method to accelerate clearance of carbon monoxide. *American Journal of Critical Care Medicine, 161(6), 1816–9.*
122. Teixeira, C., Zimermann Teixeira, P. J., Hohër, J. A., de Leon, P. P., Monteiro Brodt, S. F. and da Siva Moreira, J. (2008). Serial measurements of f/VT can predict extubation failure in patients with f/VT less than or equal to 105. *Journal of Critical Care*, 23(4), 572–6.
123. Thompson, J. P. and Marrs, T. C. (2012). Hydroxocobalamin in cyanide poisoning. *Clinical Toxicology*, 50(10), 875–85.
124. Tintinalli, J., Stapczynski, J., John Ma, O., Yealy, D., Meckler, G. and Cline, D. (2016). *Tintinallis Emergency Medicine.* 8th edition. New York: McGraw Hill Education, 2176.
125. Tonetti, T. et al., (2017). Driving pressure and mechanical power: new target for VILI prevention. *Annals of Translational Medicine*, 5(14), 286.
126. Valls i Soler, A. and Wauer, R. R. (2001). 2nd European symposium on liquid ventilation. *European Journal of Medical Research*, 6(3), 115–38.
127. Van Beers, F. and Vos, P. (2014). Semi-upright position improves ventilation and oxygenation in mechanically ventilated intensive care patients. *Critical Care*, 18(Suppl 1), 258.
128. Van den Boogaard, P. P. et al., (2012). Development and validation of the PRE-DELIRIC (PREdiction of DELIRium in ICu Patients) delirium prediction model for intensive care patients: observational multi-centre study. *British Medical Journal*, 344, e420.
129. Vincent, J. L., Moore, F. and Fink, M. (2017). *Textbook of Critical Care.* 7th edition. London: Elsevier.
130. Vuylsteke, A., Brodie, D., Combes, A., Fowles, J. a. and Peek, G. (2017). *ECMO in the Adult Patient: Core Critical Care.* Cambridge: Cambridge University Press.
131. Weaver, L. K., Howe, S., Snow, G. L. and Deru, K. (2008). UHMS guidelines: Hyperbaric oxygen: Indications and results. *The hyperbaric oxygen comittee report: Underwater and Hyperbaric Medical Society*, 35, 333–87.
132. Yoon, E., Babar, A., Choudhary, M., Kutner, M. and Pyrsopoulos, N. (2016). Acetaminophen-induced hepatotoxicity: a comprehensive update. *Journal of Clinical and Translational Hepatology*, 4(2), 131–42.

15 CHAPTER Perioperative Fluid Therapy and Blood Transfusion

PERIOPERATIVE FLUID THERAPY

Introduction

- Perioperative fluid therapy is a major factor which optimizes postoperative outcomes
- Fluid therapy is one of the most controversial aspects of perioperative care

Goals of Perioperative Fluid Therapy

- To maintain tissue perfusion
- To maintain adequate oxygen delivery to the tissues
- To avoid complications associated with hypovolemia:
  - Hypotension
  - Low cardiac output
  - Decreased tissue perfusion
  - Hypovolemic shock
  - Multiorgan failure
- To avoid complications associated with hypervolemia:
  - Central nervous system complications:
    - Cerebral edema
    - Impaired cognition
    - Postoperative delirium
    - Raised ICP
    - Reduced cerebral perfusion pressure
  - Cardiovascular complications:
    - Myocardial edema
    - Impaired contractility
    - Myocardial depression
    - Conduction disturbances
    - Pericardial effusion
  - Respiratory complications:
    - Pneumonia
    - Postoperative respiratory failure
    - Pulmonary edema
    - Pleural effusion
    - Increased extravascular lung water
    - Prolonged ventilation
  - Gastrointestinal complications:
    - Gut edema and ascites
    - Reduced abdominal perfusion pressure
    - Decreased gastric motility and ileus
    - Tension at bowel anastomotic site and anastomotic dehiscence
  - Renal system:
    - Renal interstitial edema
    - Increased renal venous pressure
    - Renal compartment syndrome
    - Reduced renal blood flow
    - Reduced GFR
    - Salt and water retention
  - Other complications:
    - Dilutional anemia
    - Dilutional coagulopathy
    - Impaired wound healing

Causes of Perioperative Volume Derangements

- Preoperative factors:
  - Fasting causing preoperative dehydration
  - Associated conditions:
    - Bowel obstruction
    - Pancreatitis
  - Mechanical bowel preparation
  - Preoperative bleeding
  - Other causes:
    - Fever
    - Diuresis
    - Vomiting
    - Diarrhea
- Anesthesia related factors:
  - General anesthetic induction causing vasodilatation and myocardial depression

- Sympathetic blockade due to neuraxial anesthesia
- Mechanical ventilation causing reduced preload due to:
  - Large tidal volume
  - High PEEP levels
  - Recruitment maneuvers
- Coagulopathy (causing hemorrhage) due to:
  - Hypothermia
  - Hemodilution

❖ Surgery related factors:
- Hemorrhage
- Decreased venous return due to:
  - Abdominal insufflation for laparoscopic procedures
  - Direct compression of IVC and other major veins
- Prolonged surgery causing bowel edema and fluid sequestration

Monitors of Intravascular Volume Status

❖ Static indices:
- Traditionally used for assessment of intravascular fluid status
- Sole reliance on these parameters is not recommended
- Examples:
  - Clinical parameters:
    - Blood pressure and heart rate:
      - Response to changes in intravascular volume is unpredictable
      - Responses may be blunted by:
        - » General anesthesia
        - » Neuraxial anesthesia
        - » Beta-blocker therapy
    - Orthostatic response
  - Central venous pressure and PCWP:
    - Inaccurate measures of cardiac preload
    - Poor predictors of fluid responsiveness
  - Urine output:
    - Inaccurate indicator of intravascular volume status
    - Oliguria < 0.5 mL/kg/hour does not predict AKI
    - Indicators of postoperative AKI are:
      - » Oliguria with urine output <0.3 mL/kg/hour
      - » Oliguria lasting more than 2 hours
  - Mixed venous oxygen saturation:
    - Not an accurate indicator of intravascular fluid status
    - This is because MvO_2 is also altered by:
      - Hemoglobin
      - Tissue oxygen extraction

❖ Dynamic indices:
- Useful in patients undergoing major surgery
- Provide superior assessment of volume responsiveness
- Indices based on respirophasic variation:
  - Physiological basis:
    - Based on changes in preload during respiratory cycle
    - During mechanical ventilation:
      - Inspiratory phase:
        - » Causes positive intrathoracic pressure
        - » Reduces venous return and preload
      - Expiratory phase:
        - » Reduction in intrathoracic pressure
        - » Increased venous return and preload
    - These changes result in alteration of:
      - Right ventricular filling volume
      - Stroke volume
      - Pulse pressure
      - Systolic blood pressure
  - Significance:
    - Normal physiological variation in these indices is below 10%
    - Variation exceeding 10% indicates hypovolemia
  - Limitations: not useful during:
    - Open chest procedures
    - Low tidal volume ventilation (< 8 mL/kg)
    - High PEEP levels (> 15 cm H_2O)
    - High intra-abdominal pressure
    - Cardiac arrhythmias
  - Examples:
    - Pulse pressure variation (PPV)
    - Stroke volume variation (SVV)
    - Systolic pressure variation (SPV)
    - Change in distensibility index
- Transesophageal echocardiography derived indices:
  - Useful in:
    - Major invasive surgeries

- High risk patients with high anticipated blood loss
- Major surgery in patients with myocardial dysfunction
- Useful when indices based on respirophasic variation cannot be used
- Disadvantages:
  - More invasive
  - Needs technical expertise
- Examples:
  - Stroke volume index
  - Cardiac output
  - Cardiac index
  - LV end diastolic diameter

- Laboratory derived indices:
  - Fractional excretion of sodium
  - Blood lactate levels
- Less commonly used indices: Prone to error:
  - Pulse contour analysis
  - Thoracic electrical bioimpedance
  - Bioreactance

Choice of Fluid Therapy

- Crystalloids:
  - Balanced salt solutions:
    - Have an electrolyte concentration similar to plasma
    - Preferred as maintenance fluids
    - Can be used for replacement of intraoperative blood loss
    - Resuscitation ratio:
      - 3 mL crystalloid for 1 mL blood lost in liberal strategy
      - 1.5 mL crystalloid for 1 mL blood lost in restrictive strategy
    - Include ringers lactate and plasmalyte A
  - Preferred crystalloids:
    - Ringers lactate
    - Plasmalyte A
  - Crystalloids not preferred:
    - Dextrose containing solutions: Due to adverse effects of hyperglycemia
    - Normal saline: due to risk of hyperchloremic metabolic acidosis
- Colloids:
  - Commonly used to replace volume lost by massive intraoperative hemorrhage
  - Administered in a ratio 1 mL colloid for 1 mL blood lost perioperatively
  - Use of colloids over crystalloids is associated with:
    - No additional survival benefit
    - No reduction in risk of complications
  - Thus, preference of colloids over crystalloids offers no added benefit
  - Examples:
    - Hydroxyethyl starch:
      - Produces 100% volume expansion
      - Avoided due to perioperative AKI and coagulopathy
    - Albumin:
      - Produces 90% volume expansion
      - Most commonly used colloid, especially in children
      - Routine use precluded by cost
    - Gelatins:
      - Produce 70–80% volume expansion which is short lived
      - Not commonly used due to:
        - More common association with anaphylaxis
        - Short lived action (2–3 hours)
      - Examples:
        - Hemaccel
        - Gelofusine
- Blood: Used when specific transfusion triggers are reached:
  - Perioperative anemia:
    - Rarely required when Hb > 10 gm%
    - Almost always indicated when Hb < 6 gm%
    - The decision to transfuse between 6–10 g% depends on:
      - Cardiopulmonary risk factors
      - Ongoing blood loss
      - Clinical judgement
    - Restrictive transfusion strategy (Hb <8 g/dL) should be used
  - Acute blood loss:
    - > 1500 mL in adults
    - > 40 mL/kg in children
- Plasma derivatives:
  - Used to correct perioperative coagulopathies
  - Use is guided by laboratory evaluation of hemostasis

Intraoperative Fluid Therapy Strategies

- Liberal fluid strategy:
  - Uses the traditional Holliday Segar formula
  - Term is used when perioperative fluid administration exceeds 5 liters
  - Fluid replacement includes:
    - Preoperative fluid deficits
    - Maintenance fluid therapy
    - Replacement of third space loss& insensible losses
    - Intraoperative blood and urine loss
  - Grosslyover-estimatesperioperativefluidrequirements
  - Strategy is inappropriate as third space does not exist
  - Crystalloid replaced: Blood lost ratio is very high (3:1)
  - This strategy is usually avoided due to increased incidence of:
    - Tissue edema
    - Postoperative adverse outcomes
  - Current status:
    - Not preferred usually for any surgery
    - May be used for very specific indications:
      - Renal transplantation (goal directed liberal fluid therapy)
      - Palliative procedures for TOF (modified BT shunt)
      - Single ventricle physiology:
        - Post BD Glenn shunt
        - Post Fontan surgery
- Restrictive fluid strategy:
  - Also called zero-balance strategy
  - Fluid replacement is this strategy includes:
    - Maintenance fluid therapy at 1–3 mL/kg/hour
    - Intraoperative blood and urine loss is replaced with:
      - Crystalloid or colloid when Hb > 8 grams/dL
      - Blood when transfusion trigger is reached
    - Replacement of third space loss and insensible losses is avoided
    - Vasopressors are preferred to treat hypotension
    - Preloading is avoided prior to:
      - Neuraxial blockade
      - Induction of general anesthesia
    - Zero-fluid balance is targeted at the end of surgery
  - Crystalloid replaced: Blood lost ratio is lesser (1.5:1)
  - Advantages:
    - Associated with better outcomes than liberal fluid strategy
    - Improved clinical outcomes
    - Lower risk of mortality
    - Reduced incidence of pneumonia and AKI
    - Reduced incidence of wound infections
    - Shorter duration of hospital stay
  - Current status:
    - Superior to liberal fluid strategy
    - May be associated with slightly higher risk of AKI
    - Preferred for:
      - Mild-moderate risk surgeries
      - All major surgeries with:
        - Expected blood loss < 500 mL
        - Limited hemodynamic monitors
- Goal directed fluid therapy:
  - Titrated perioperative fluid therapy to specific hemodynamic goals
  - Fluid therapy in this strategy includes:
    - Maintenance fluid therapy at 1–3 mL/kg/hour
    - Fluid boluses are used when specific hemodynamic goals are exceeded
    - Role of Trendelenburg position:
      - Used to assess fluid responsiveness
      - Done prior to administration of fluid boluses
      - Hemodynamic improvement suggests fluid responsiveness
    - Fluid bolus consists of 250 mL crystalloid/colloid boluses
    - Boluses are titrated to restore the hemodynamic goals
    - Volume non-responders are treated with vasoconstrictors and inotropes
  - Goals used:
    - CVP 8–12 cm H_2O
    - Mean arterial pressure > 60 mm Hg
    - Mixed venous oxygen saturation > 70%
    - Mixed venous oxygen saturation > 65%
    - Hematocrit > 30%
    - Respirophasic variations < 10% including:
      - Pulse pressure variation
      - Stroke volume variation
      - Systolic pressure variation

- Other parameters used:
  - Cardiac index
  - Stroke volume index
- Advantages:
  - Improved clinical outcomes
  - Lower risk of mortality
  - Reduced incidence of pneumonia and AKI
  - Reduced incidence of wound infections
  - Shorter duration of hospital stay
- Current status:
  - Superior to liberal fluid strategy
  - Superiority over restrictive fluid strategy is yet to be proven
  - Preferred for:
    - All major surgeries
    - Surgeries with expected blood loss > 500 mL
    - Surgeries with major intraoperative fluid shifts
    - Patients with:
      - Myocardial dysfunction
      - COPD
      - Cor pulmonale

Validation

Cristal Trial

- ❖ Multi-center randomized clinical trial
- ❖ Enrolled 2857 critically ill patients in 57 ICUs of 4 countries
- ❖ Divided into 2 groups:
  - Group 1: Used colloids for all fluid interventions other than maintenance
  - Group 2: Used NS or RL for all fluid interventions other than maintenance
- ❖ Parameters studied:
  - Primary outcome: death within 28 days
  - Secondary outcomes:
    - 90-day mortality
    - Renal replacement therapy free days
    - Mechanical ventilation free days
    - Vasopressor free days
- ❖ Conclusions:
  - Use of colloids did not result in significant difference in 28-day mortality
  - Treatment with colloids was however associated with:
    - Lower 90-day mortality
    - Earlier weaning from mechanical ventilation
    - No evidence of increased risk of renal failure

Optimize Trial

- ❖ Multicenter, randomized, observer blinded trial
- ❖ Enrolled 734 high risk patients undergoing GIT surgery
- ❖ Divided into 2 groups:
  - Group 1: Goal directed fluid therapy with cardiac output monitoring
  - Group 2: Conventional fluid therapy
- ❖ Parameters studied:
  - Primary outcomes: Composite of:
    - 30-day moderate or major complications
    - 30-day mortality
  - Secondary outcomes:
    - Morbidity on day 7 POD
    - Infection
    - Critical-care free days
    - All cause mortality at 30 days
    - All cause mortality at 180 days
    - Length of hospital stay
- ❖ Conclusions:
  - No difference in the perioperative complication rate with GDFT
  - Failed to show any benefit of CO-guided GDFT for major GIT surgery
  - GDFT cannot be routinely recommended
  - Its use should be reserved for high-risk patients

SALT-ED Trial

- ❖ Single centre, pragmatic, multiple cross-over trial
- ❖ Compares BSS with saline
- ❖ Enrolled 13,347 non-critically ill patients admitted in emergency department
- ❖ Divided in to 2 groups:
  - Group 1: Received BSS
  - Group 2: Received normal saline
- ❖ Parameters studied:
  - Primary outcome: Hospital-free days (days alive after discharge before day 28)
  - Secondary outcomes: Composite of major adverse outcomes within 30 days:
    - All-cause mortality
    - New renal-replacement therapy
    - Persistent renal dysfunction
- ❖ Conclusions:
  - No difference in hospital-free days between treatment with BSS and NS
  - Higher incidence of renal adverse outcomes in the patients treated with NS

Goal Directed Fluid Therapy

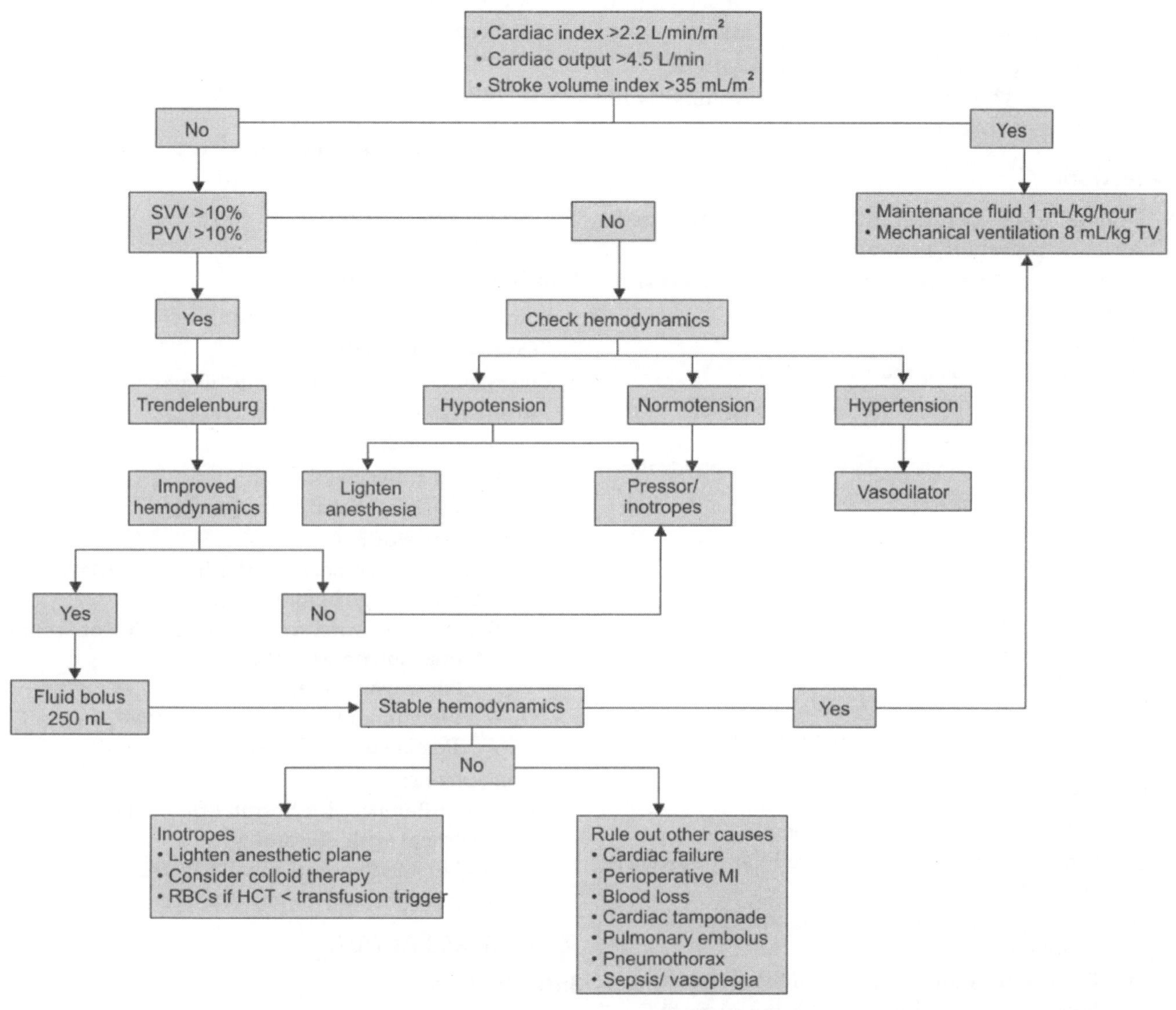

SALINE

Introduction

- Available in 2 concentrations:
  - 0.9% normal saline (isotonic)
  - 0.45% normal saline (hypotonic)
- 0.9% sodium chloride:
  - As it is isotonic, it is physiologically normal
  - Hence, this solution is called normal saline

Composition

- 0.9% normal saline:
  - Sodium 154 mmol/L
  - Chloride 154 mmol/L

Contd...

Contd...

  - Osmolarity 308 mOsm/L
  - pH 4.5–7
- 0.45% normal saline:
  - Sodium 77 mmol/L
  - Chloride 77 mmol/L
  - Osmolarity 154 mOsm/L
  - pH 4.5–7

Physiology

- NS expands intravascular volume without altering ion concentrations grossly
- Sodium ions determines distribution of fluids and other electrolytes
- Chloride ions serves as a buffering agent within the lungs and tissues

- Normal saline is iso-osmotic
- Thus, it prevents large fluid shifts between intracellular, intravascular and interstitial spaces
- NS is excreted more slowly compared with RL
- Thus, upto 40% of the administered volume is retained intravascularly

Indications

- Limited use in perioperative period except in pediatrics (to prevent hyponatremia)
- Treatment of hypochloremic metabolic alkalosis in the presence of fluid loss:
  - Vomiting
  - Continuous nasogastric aspiration
- Treatment of mild hyponatremia
- Others:
  - Extracellular fluid replacement for dehydration due to:
    - Diarrhea
    - Excessive diuresis
  - Initial fluid therapy of sepsis
  - Initial fluid therapy in diabetic ketoacidosis
  - Treatment of hypercalcemia
  - Irrigation for washing of body fluids
  - Priming solution for hemodialysis
  - Drug dilution for intravenous infusion

Contraindications

- Dehydration with severe hypokalemia:
  - In severe hypokalemia, intracellular K+ levels is also reduced
  - Administration of NS does not provide K+ supple-mentation
  - Thus, only volume deficits will be corrected
  - Associated potassium deficit is not corrected
  - This can aggravate intracellular hypokalemia
- Severe hypertension
- Preeclampsia

Adverse Effects

- Hyperchloremic metabolic acidosis:
  - Occurs with large volume resuscitation using normal saline (> 2 litres)
  - This causes iatrogenic hyperchlorhydria
  - This results in intracellular shift of HCO_3 ions to allow equilibration of pH
  - This decreases the concentration of bicarbonate available for buffering
  - This results in metabolic acidosis with hyperchloremia
- Complications of large volume resuscitation with normal saline:
  - Hyponatremia and cerebral edema seen with use of 0.45% normal saline
  - Iatrogenic fluid overload in:
    - Acute kidney injury
    - Chronic kidney injury
    - Myocardial dysfunction
- Associated with increased incidence of renal dysfunction

Validation: Salt-ED Trial

- Single centre, pragmatic, multiple cross-over trial
- Compares BSS with saline
- Enrolled 13,347 non-critically ill patients admitted in emergency department
- Divided in to 2 groups:
  - Group 1: Received BSS
  - Group 2: Received normal saline
- Parameters studied:
  - Primary outcome: Hospital-free days (days alive after discharge before day 28)
  - Secondary outcomes: Composite of major adverse outcomes within 30 days:
    - All-cause mortality
    - New renal-replacement therapy
    - Persistent renal dysfunction
- Conclusions:
  - No difference in hospital-free days between treatment with BSS and NS
  - Higher incidence of renal adverse outcomes in the patients treated with NS

RINGERS LACTATE

Introduction

- Buffered isotonic crystalloid used as a balanced salt solution for fluid replacement
- Composition of Ringers solution originally created in 1880 by Sydney Ringer
- Alexis Hartmann added lactate to modify it to Hartmanns solution or Ringer lactate

Composition

- Sodium 131 mmol/L
- Potassium 5 mmol/L
- Calcium 2 mmol/L
- Bicarbonate (as lactate or acetate) 29 mmol/L
- Chloride 111 mOsm/L
- pH 6.5
- Osmolarity 273 mOsm/L
- Calorific content 5 kcal/L

Physiology

- RL rapidly expands intravascular volume due to its sodium concentration
- It is the most physiological fluid as its electrolyte composition is similar to plasma
- Large volume resuscitation can be achieved with minimal electrolyte disturbances

Metabolism

- Volume kinetics:
  - At any given time, osmolarity is equal between:
    - Intracellular compartment
    - Extracellular compartment
  - Ringers lactate is an isotonic fluid
  - It does not alter tonicity of the plasma when administered intravenously
  - Thus, RL does not move into the intracellular compartment
  - However, it is distributed evenly across the entire extracellular compartment:
    - Interstitial compartment
    - Intravascular compartment
  - Only 30% of the administered volume is retained intravascularly
  - Redistribution to the interstitial space is completed within 25–30 minutes
  - This causes tissue edema following large volume resuscitation
- Lactate metabolism:
  - During normal anerobic metabolism:
    - Pyruvate undergoes oxidation-reduction reaction with NADH to yield:
      - NAD+ from NADH
      - Lactate via lactate dehydrogenase
      - Lactate is shuttled out of the cell to maintain NADH/NAD + ratio
  - Ringers lactate is a source of sodium lactate which acts as a buffer
  - Lactate acts as a buffer as it takes up the H+ ions formed
  - This results in the formation of lactic acid
  - Furthermore, lactate can be metabolized in liver to form bicarbonate buffer
  - Lactate acts as a buffer under ischemic conditions to prevent cell death
- Acetate metabolism:
  - Acetate is metabolised similar to lactate to yield bicarbonate
  - However, it is metabolized faster and consumes lesser oxygen for metabolism
  - Thus, O_2 consumption using acetate buffer is lesser compared to lactate buffer
  - Acetate is therefore a better buffer than lactate in the presence of shock

Indications

- Perioperative maintenance fluid therapy
- Replacement of blood loss:
  - 3:1 ratio for liberal fluid strategy
  - 1.5: 1 for restrictive fluid strategy
- Volume resuscitation in:
  - Burn injuries
  - Trauma
  - Sepsis
  - Diarrhea with hypokalemic metabolic acidosis
- Pancreatitis

Contraindications

- Cerebral edema: Isotonic and hypotonic fluids are contraindicated
- Liver dysfunction:
  - Administered lactate is predominantly metabolized in the liver
  - Thus, liver dysfunction causes accumulation of lactate levels
- Pre-existing hyperkalemia and renal failure in large volumes
- Diabetes mellitus as lactate present in RL may increase plasma glucose levels
- Severe metabolic acidosis and shock as RL may cause misinterpretation of lab results
- Hypochloremic metabolic alkalosis:
  - Bicarbonate provided by RL infusion will worsen alkalosis
  - Conditions where RL worsens alkalosis:
    - Vomiting
    - Continuous nasogastric aspiration
- Addisons disease

Adverse Effects

- Role in hyperkalemia:
  - RL was traditionally thought to worsen hyperkalemia:
  - This is because of the K^+ content in lactated ringers
  - However, the volume of distribution for K^+ in RL is large
  - Thus, administration of RL in hyperkalemic patients does not worsen hyper K^+

- Even in patients with CRF, administration of RL does not worsen hyper K+
- However, in these patients elimination of K+ is reduced
- Thus, large volumes of RL should be avoided in hyper K^+ and CRF

❖ Role in lactic acidosis:
- RL was traditionally avoided in lactic acidosis
- This was due to fear of worsening the acidosis
- However, lactate (and not lactic acid) is provided by ringer lactate
- Thus, administration of RL in these patients boosts lactate levels
- This is utilized by the body as a source of energy in anerobic conditions
- However, RL may cause elevation of measured blood lactate levels
- This may lead to erroneous interpretation of laboratory results
- Thus, alternate BSS may be preferred in patients with lactic acidosis

❖ Precipitation with blood products:
- RL has calcium ion concentration
- Coadministration with blood products causes precipitation of calcium citrate
- This may cause clotting and occlusion of IV lines
- Thus, blood products and RL should be administered in separate IV lines

❖ Complications of large volume resuscitation with RL:
- Edema:
  - Administered RL equilibrates between:
    - Intravascular compartment
    - Interstitial compartment
  - This can lead to edema with large volume resuscitation
- Hyponatremia as sodium concentration of RL is low
- Iatrogenic fluid overload in patients with:
  - Borderline myocardial function
  - Acute kidney injury
  - Chronic kidney injury

❖ Anaphylactoid reactions: urticaria, facial flushing

PLASMALYTE

Introduction

❖ Buffered isotonic crystalloid used as a balanced salt solution for fluid replacement

❖ NS and RL differ significantly from plasma with regards to electrolyte composition

❖ However, physicochemical properties of plasmalyte are similar to plasma

Composition

❖ Sodium 140 mmol/L
❖ Potassium 5 mmol/L
❖ Magnesium 1.5 mmol/L
❖ Chloride 98 mmol/L
❖ Acetate 27 mmol/L
❖ Gluconate 23 mmol/L
❖ Osmolarity 294 mOsm/L
❖ pH 7.40 (6.5–8)
❖ Caloric content 21 kcal/L

Physiology

❖ Plasmalyte has an electrolyte composition similar to plasma

❖ It causes expansion of extracellular volume including:
- Interstitial volume
- Intravascular volume

❖ However, it has a metabolic alkalinizing effect due to gluconate and acetate ions

❖ Acetate and gluconate ions act as buffering agents

❖ This is due to metabolism in muscles and peripheral tissues to H_2CO_3 using H+ ions

Indications

❖ Preferred fluid for:
- Maintenance therapy in perioperative period
- Volume resuscitation in prophylaxis and treatment of hemorrhagic shock

❖ Fluid replacement for burns patients

❖ Metabolic acidosis as RL alters laboratory values of lactate

❖ Priming of extracorporeal circuits

Contraindications

❖ Known hypersensitivity to plasmalyte A

❖ Patients with pre-existing:
- Hyperkalemia
- Renal failure

❖ Hypochloremic hypokalemic alkalosis

Adverse Effects

❖ Complications of large volume resuscitation with plasmalyte:
- Hyponatremia:
  - Especially common in patients with:
    - Cardiac failure
    - SIADH
  - Can lead to acute hyponatremic encephalopathy

- Hypernatremia: Common in patients with:
  - Primary and secondary hyperaldosteronism
  - Concomitant corticosteroid therapy
  - Renal disease
  - Preeclampsia
- Hyperkalemia: Risk may be increased in patients with:
  - Severe renal impairment
  - Extensive tissue injury
  - Burns patients
- Hypermagnesemia: Especially common in:
  - Renal failure
  - Concomitant magnesium sulphate therapy (eclampsia)
- Metabolic alkalosis and hypocalcemia
- Iatrogenic fluid overload in:
  - Acute kidney injury
  - Chronic kidney injury
  - Myocardial dysfunction

❖ Can cause false positive test results for aspergillus infections using BioRad EIA test

HYDROXYETHYL STARCH

Introduction

❖ Complex polysaccharide which is used rarely for intravenous volume expansion

❖ Amylopectin derivative structurally resembling glycogen

Chemistry

❖ Artificial colloid obtained from starch

❖ Contains amylo-pectin (highly branched and more stable component of starch)

❖ Average molecular weight 450,000 Da

❖ Available as 10%, 6%, and 3% solution

Metabolism

❖ Degraded in serum and tissues by α-amylase

❖ Smaller molecules are excreted mainly in kidneys

❖ Medium sized molecules are eliminated in the bile and feces

❖ A proportion of the infused HES is taken up in RES and eliminated gradually

❖ Long elimination $T_{1/2}$ of 5 days

❖ Complete elimination occurs in 42 days

❖ Initial volume expansion of 62% of infused volume is obtained

❖ Causes 90–100% volume expansion, similar to 5% albumin

❖ Thus, volume expansion is higher than that provided by gelatins

Strength	Plasma volume expansion period
Hestar 3%	1–2.5 hours
Hestar 6%	3–4 hours
Hestar 10%	4–8 hours

❖ Duration of volume expansion lasts around 8–12 hours

Indications

❖ As an adjunct in leukopheresis to improve harvesting

❖ Prophylaxis and treatment of hypovolemia and shock (rarely used) due to:
- Surgery
- Trauma
- Infection
- Burns

Dosage and Administration

❖ Adults:
- 500–1000 mL once
- Repeated as needed based on hemodynamics
- Maximum dose should not exceed 33–50 mL/day

❖ Pediatrics: Not recommended in pediatric patients:

❖ Recommended maximum daily dosage:
- Hestar 3%: Upto 66 mL/kg/day
- Hestar 6%: Upto 33 mL/kg/day
- Hestar 10%: Upto 20 mL/kg/day

Contraindications

❖ Severe hemorrhagic defects

❖ Severe congestive cardiac failure

❖ Renal failure with oliguria/anuria

❖ Chronic hepatic disease

❖ Patients allergic to starch

❖ Hypervolemia

❖ Early pregnancy use is contraindicated unless benefits overweigh hazards to fetus

Adverse Reactions

❖ Minor adverse effects:
- Anaphylactoid reactions are more common compared with other synthetic colloids
- Nausea and vomiting rarely
- Pruritus due to deposition of HES in skin: treated with capsaicin

- Major adverse effects:
  - Coagulopathy
  - Renal dysfunction
  - Serum macroamylasemia:
    - May occur on infusion of large volumes of HES
    - Serum amylase (for pancreatic disease) is not reliable for 3–5 days
  - Circulatory overload
  - Hyperchloremic metabolic acidosis

Advantages

- Added oncotic properties
- Increase duration of hemodynamic effects due to long elimination $T_{1/2}$
- Low antigenicity: Infrequent anaphylaxis
- Absent disease transmission
- Low cost compared with albumin
- Does not interfere with blood grouping, typing or cross matching

Disadvantages

- Coagulopathy:
  - Occurs due to:
    - Reduced circulating factor VIII and von Willebrand factor
    - Impairment of platelet function
  - This causes prolongation of PTT and aPTT
  - This may lead to increased postoperative bleeding
- Renal impairment:
  - High molecular weight causes osmotic nephrosis like lesions in renal tubules
  - HES infusion is associated with:
    - Increased creatinine levels
    - Oliguria and acute renal failure
  - These effects are augmented in patients with existing renal impairment

Current Use

- Perioperative period:
  - HES is not recommended for fluid therapy in surgical patients
  - Thus, use of HES in the perioperative period is restricted
  - This is due to risk of renal impairment and coagulopathy
- Critically ill patients:
  - Increases risk of mortality and renal replacement therapy
  - Thus, use of HES in restricted

HUMAN ALBUMIN

Introduction

- Human albumin is the most abundant circulating protein in the plasma (3.5–5 g/dL)
- It represents 50% of the total protein content in the body

Chemistry

- Small globular protein
- Molecular weight 66.5 kDa
- Contains a single chain of 585 amino acids
- These are organized into 3 domains, each of which has 2 sub-domains

Metabolism

- Approximately 10–15 grams of albumin is manufactured in the liver per day
- Synthesis of albumin is modulated by:
  - Insulin
  - Cortisol
  - Growth hormone
- Once released in circulation, 30–40% is retained intravascularly
- The remainder is distributed into the interstitium
- It is metabolised in the muscles, liver and kidney
- Intravascular circulatory $T_{1/2}$ 16–18 hours
- Total $T_{1/2}$ 12–19 *days*
- Thus, volume expansion is more long lasting with albumin

Functions

- Albumin is the main modulator of fluid distribution in the body
- It provides approximately 70–80% of the total plasma oncotic pressure
- Osmotic effect of albumin is due to:
  - Higher molecular mass
  - *Gibbs-Donnan effect*:
    - Due to negative charge of the molecule
    - This attracts positively charged cations such as sodium
    - Thus, Na^+ along with water is drawn into intravascular compartment
- Other functions:
  - Stabilizes endothelial layer and maintains normal capillary permeability
  - Transport of hydrophobic molecules:
    - Endogenous substances:
      - Thyroxine

      - Cholesterol
      - Fatty acids
      - Bilirubin
    - Exogenous substances:
      - Drugs
      - Nitric oxide
  - Donor of sulfydryl groups which is a scavenger of reactive oxygen species

Manufacture

- Source is whole blood/serum/placenta
- Contains 96% albumin and 4% other proteins
- Available in two concentrations:
  - 5% solution:
    - 50 mg albumin per mL of solution
    - Thus, 20 mL of the solution contains 1 gram of albumin
    - Iso-oncotic and osmotically equivalent to human plasma
    - Primarily used for the treatment of hypovolemia
    - Causes 90% initial volume expansion
  - 25% solution:
    - 250 mg albumin per mL of the solution
    - Thus, 4 mL of the solution contains 1 gram of abumin
    - Hyper-oncotic with colloid osmotic pressure 5 times that of plasma
    - Primarily used for the treatment of hypoproteinemia
    - Causes 400% volume expansion within 30 minutes

Indications

- Volume expansion:
  - For emergency treatment of hypovolemic shock:
    - Severe burns
    - Sepsis
    - Hemorrhagic shock
  - During exchange transfusion for neonatal hemolytic disease
  - For plasma volume expansion in ovarian hyperstimulation syndrome
- Correction of hypoalbuminemia (< 2.5 grams/dL) in critically ill patients:
  - Shock, sepsis
  - ARDS
  - Trauma, burns
  - Pulmonary edema
- Cirrhosis and ascites:
  - Type I hepatorenal syndrome
  - Refractory ascites
  - Following large volume paracentesis:
    - Prevents hepatorenal syndrome
    - Used along with diuretic therapy
    - 6–8 grams of HA given per litre of ascites fluid removed
  - Spontaneous bacterial peritonitis:
    - HA improves 3-month survival
    - Used along with broad spectrum antibiotics
    - Thus, high dose HA is recommended in patients with SBP:
      - 1.5 grams/kg at the time of diagnosis
      - 1 gram/kg on day 3 following diagnosis
- Other uncommon indications:
  - Treatment of nephrotic syndrome with refractory edema
  - Cardiothoracic surgery as pump prime in neonates
  - Postoperatively:
    - Replacement of excessive protein losses following major surgery
    - Following liver transplantation
    - Chylothorax following cardiac surgery
    - Hypoproteinemia, burns and peritonitis

Dosage

- Adults:
  - 5% albumin:
    - 12.5–25 grams/dose
    - Administered over 10–20 minutes
    - Can be repeated after 30 minutes if response is inadequate
  - 25% albumin:
    - 50–100 grams/dose
    - Administered over 4 hours
    - May be repeated at 4–12 hours intervals as required
- Pediatrics:
  - 5% albumin:
    - 0.5–1 gram/kg (10–20 mL/kg/dose)
    - Administered over 10–20 minutes
    - Rate of infusion 2–4 mL/minute
    - May increase rate of infusion in severe hypotension
    - May repeat after 30 minutes if response is inadequate

- 25% albumin:
  - 0.5–1 gram/kg/dose
  - Administered over 2–3 hours
  - Followed by diuretic therapy
  - Rate of infusion 1 mL/minute
  - May be repeated upto 3 times per day

Usage

- Requires patients consent prior to administration
- Can be used without regard to ABO type and cross match
- Administration does not require a separate blood transfusion set
- Standard IV infusion set may be used for administration
- The preparation does not contain any antimicrobial preservative
- Thus, administration should be completed within 4 hours of starting infusion

Contraindications

- Absolute contraindications:
  - Hypersensitivity to albumin
  - Severe anemia
  - Traumatic brain injury: associated with higher mortality
- Relative contraindications:
  - Renal failure
  - Low cardiac reserve

Adverse Reactions

- Mild reactions:
  - Mild hypotension
  - Flushing
  - Urticaria
  - Fever
- Severe reactions:
  - Anaphylactic reactions
  - Hypernatremia
  - Circulatory overload, especially with 20% albumin
  - Renal failure

Advantages

- Natural colloid:
  - Less incidence of anaphylactoid reactions compared with synthetic colloids
  - Lesser incidence of coagulation abnormalities
- 25% albumin results in the greatest volume expansion amongst all colloids
- Additional antioxidant, scavenging effects of albumin

Disadvantages

- Expensive compared with other colloids
- High risk of volume overload
- Associated with renal dysfunction

Validation: ALBIOS Study 2014

- Included 1818 patients with severe sepsis
- Divided in to 2 groups:
  - Group 1: 20% albumin with crystalloid solution
  - Group 2: Crystalloid solution alone
- Parameters studied:
  - Primary outcome: Death at 28 days
  - Secondary outcomes:
    - All cause mortality at 90 days
    - Organ dysfunction
    - Length of hospital and ICU stay
- Concluded that albumin administration *did not* improve survival at 28 and 90 days
- It may however be used for volume expansion to stabilize hemodynamics

HEMACCEL

Introduction

- Colloid solution of polygeline (urea-cross linked gelatin) with electrolytes
- It is iso-oncotic with similar pH and viscosity to plasma
- Used mainly for plasma volume expansion
- Not widely used due to short duration of action
- Minimal effects on coagulation and renal function

Manufacture

- Contains polygeline polypeptides of degraded bovine gelatin
- These polypeptides are cross linked via urea bridges
- Shelf life:
  - Unused bottles:
    - Up to 5 years when stored at 22–25°C
    - 2 years when stored at > 25°C
  - Once opened, the solution should be used immediately
  - Any unused solution should be immediately discarded

Chemistry

- Molecular weight 30,000 Da
- pH of solution 7–7.3
- Oncotic pressure 3.4- 3.8 kPa
- Osmolality 293 mOsm/kg

- Osmolarity 301 mOsm/L
- Pharmacologically inert

Metabolism

- Upon administration, augmentation of intravascular volume depends upon:
  - Rate of infusion
  - Existing volume deficit
- In general result in a 70–80% volume expansion
- It is broken down into smaller peptides and amino acids
- The principal mode of elimination is via the kidneys
- Elimination $T_{1/2}$ 4–8 hours
- Elimination is completed within 48 hours of infusion
- Duration of action is shorter compared to albumin and starches

Composition

- 3.5% solution (3.5 grams in 100 mL of solution)
- Sodium 145 mmol/L
- Potassium 5.1 mmol/L
- Calcium 6.25 mmol/L
- Chloride 145 mmol/L

Indications

- Prevention and treatment of hypovolemic shock:
  - Hemorrhagic shock
  - Burns
  - Peritonitis
  - Pancreatitis
  - Crush injuries
- Acute normovolemic hemodilution as a plasma substitute
- Priming of CPB circuits
- Prevention of hypotension following spinal anesthesia
- Other rare uses:
  - Isolated organ perfusion
  - For drug dilution

Dosage

- Adults:
  - Prevention of hemorrhagic shock:
    - 500–1500 mL can be administered
    - Upto 25% or 1500 mL blood loss may be replaced by hemaccel alone
  - Treatment of hemorrhagic shock:
    - Volume is determined by hemodynamic status and hematocrit
    - RBC transfusion is recommended when HCT < 8 g/dL
    - Maximum recommended volume 2000 mL
    - Rate of infusion:
      - Slowly over 30-60 minutes
      - Can be administered more rapidly in emergencies
      - Rapid administration is associated with anaphylactoid reactions
  - Burns patients:
    - 1 mL of hemaccel is infused per kg body weight
    - This is multiplied by the % BSA affected by burns
    - The volume obtained should be infused over 24 hours
    - For example: In a 70 kg adult with 10% burns:
      - 700 mL of hemaccel is the volume required
      - This is given over 24 hours
      - The remaining volume deficit is corrected with crystalloids
- Children:
  - Use is generally avoided as administration causes dilution of plasma proteins
  - Human albumin is preferred for volume resuscitation

Usage

- Can be used without regard to ABO type and cross match
- Administration does not require a separate blood transfusion set
- Standard IV infusion set may be used for administration
- Should not be coadministered with blood
- Calcium present in the hemaccel solution will cause recalcification of blood
- Preferred in hypokalemic patients as it contains potassium

Advantages

- Cost effective
- Iso-oncotic with pH and viscosity similar to plasma
- Does not interfere with blood typing
- Does not impair coagulation
- Non-immunogenic and does not induce antibody formation
- Safe in pregnant and lactating mothers
- No effect on renal function

Disadvantages

- Higher incidence of anaphylactoid reactions
- Indirect effect on coagulation due to dilutional coagulopathy
- Cause renin-aldosterone mediated circulatory disturbances in ascitic patients

Contraindications

- Absolute contraindications: hypersensitivity to any constituent of the solution
- Relative contraindications:
  - History of anaphylactoid reactions
  - Due to risk of volume overload:
    - Myocardial dysfunction
    - Pulmonary edema
    - Renal failure
  - Hemorrhagic diatheses

Adverse Effects

- Mild reactions:
  - Anaphylactoid reactions:
    - Due to histamine release
    - Skin reactions: Wheals, urticaria
    - Flushing of face and neck
  - Increased ESR
  - Fever, nausea, vomiting
- Major side effects:
  - Anaphylactic reactions
  - Volume overload
  - Mild, clinically covert hypercalcemia

GELOFUSINE

Introduction

- Most commonly used gelatin
- Colloid solution of succinylated gelatin (modified fluid gelatin) with electrolytes
- It is iso-oncotic with similar pH and viscosity to plasma
- Used mainly for plasma volume expansion
- They are frequently associated with anaphylactoid reactions
- Short duration of action (2–3 hours)
- Minimal effects on coagulation and renal function

Composition

- Succinylated gelatin 40 grams in 1000 mL
- Sodium 154 mmol/L
- Chloride 120 mmol/L

Chemistry

- Average molecular weight 30,000 Da
- Osmolarity 274 mOsm/L
- pH 7.1–7.7

Metabolism

- Leads to 70–80% volume expansion
- Eliminated primarily via renal excretion
- Volume augmentation effect lasts for approximately 3 hours
- Elimination $T_{1/2}$ 4 hours
- Duration of action is shorter compared with albumin and starches

Indications

- Prevention and treatment of hypovolemic shock:
  - Hemorrhagic shock
  - Burns
  - Peritonitis
  - Pancreatitis
  - Crush injuries
- Replacement of perioperative blood loss
- Acute normovolemic hemodilution as a plasma substitute
- Priming of CPB circuits
- Prevention of hypotension following spinal anesthesia

Dosage

- Adults:
  - Prophylaxis of hemorrhagic shock:
    - 500–1500 mL can be administered
    - First 20–30 mL infused slowly to allow early recognition of reactions
  - Treatment of hemorrhagic shock:
    - 1000–2000 mL may be given
    - First 500 mL can be given as a rapid infusion
    - Following hemodynamic stabilization, remaining volume may be given
    - Therapeutic end-point is a hematocrit < 24%
    - Maximum dosage limit is not defined for volume expansion
  - Normovolemic hemodilution:
    - Administration corresponding to blood volume removed
    - 1 mL gelofusine given per mL of blood retrieved
    - Maximum infusible dose 20 mL/kg/day

- Pediatrics:
  - Use is generally avoided as administration causes dilution of plasma proteins
  - Human albumin is preferred for volume resuscitation
  - Lack of data in children < 1 year age

Usage

- Can be used without regard to ABO type and cross match
- Administration does not require a separate blood transfusion set
- Standard IV infusion set may be used for administration
- Used with caution in hypernatremic patients

Advantages

- Low cost
- High dosage ceiling: No maximum daily dose limitation
- High safety margin
- Iso-oncotic with pH and viscosity similar to plasma
- Does not interfere with blood typing
- No adverse effect on renal function
- Does not alter coagulation system directly
- Safe in pregnant and lactating mothers

Disadvantages

- Higher incidence of anaphylactoid reactions
- Indirect effect on coagulation due to dilutional coagulopathy
- Cause renin-aldosterone mediated circulatory disturbances in ascitic patients

Contraindications

- Absolute contraindications:
  - Known hypersensitivity reactions
  - Hypervolemia
- Relative contraindications:
  - Severe myocardial dysfunction
  - Coagulopathies as administration causes dilution of coagulation factors
  - Hypernatremia due to presence of sodium in gelofusine
  - Renal insufficiency
  - Liver disease as it may cause dilutional coagulopathy

Adverse Effects

- Mild reactions:
  - Anaphylactoid reactions:
    - These are common
    - Localized erythema
    - Urticaria
    - Flushing of face and neck
  - Nausea, vomiting
  - Raised ESR
- Severe reactions:
  - Anaphylactic shock
  - Bronchospasm
  - Volume overload

MEASUREMENT OF SURGICAL BLOOD LOSS

Introduction

- Amount of blood lost during surgery can be measured by:
  - Assessing the amount of blood lost from the patient o
  - Assessing the amount remaining in the patient.

Methods

- Visual observation of degree of bleeding:
  - Measure of blood in surgical container
  - Estimating blood on surgical sponges and laparotomy pads
  - Fully soaked 4 × 4 sponge contains approximately 10 mL of blood
  - Soaked laparotomy pads contain 100–150 mL of blood
  - 1 mL blood is taken to be equal to 1 gm blood
- Clinical estimation:
  - Serial hematocrit/Hb concentration reflects ratio of blood loss to plasma
  - This does not necessarily reflect blood loss
  - Serial Hb measurement is especially useful during long procedures.
  - Clinical signs:
    - Hypotension, low CVP, tachycardia
    - Palor, diaphoresis, reduced urine output
- Gravimetric method:
  - Simplest and most commonly used method
  - Blood loss estimated by measurements of gain in weight of swabs and towels
  - This is taken together with measurements of contents of suction bottle
  - 1 mL blood assumed to weigh 1 gm
  - Disadvantages:
    - Weighing of swabs underestimates blood loss by 25%

- This is because it does not take into account:
  - Evaporation
  - Blood lost in floor, drapes and body cavities
- Overestimating of blood loss may occur if the swabs also measure urine, pus and other fluids during mopping

❖ Dilution Methods:
- Colorimetric method:
  - Swabs and towels are mixed thoroughly with known volume of fluid
  - Change in optical density of water is measured
  - This is done at the isobestic absorption wavelength of Hb
  - This is related with Hb concentration of patients blood

$$\text{Blood loss} = \frac{\text{Colorimeter reading} \times \text{volume of solution}}{200 \times \text{patients Hb (gm\%)}}$$

  - Alternatively, change in electrical resistance due to blood electrolytes in the bath can be measured
  - Uses:
    - In operations involving complex exchanges of blood
    - Extracorporeal circulation
    - Useful to wash out bladder in TURP
  - Disadvantages: Errors due to:
    - Incomplete extraction
    - Contamination with bile

❖ Use of radioactive tracer dilution methods:
- Method:
- Tracers used:
  - Patients RBCs labelled with Cr^{51} following incubation with the isotope
  - Pooled human albumin labelled with 1^{125} or I^{131}
- I^{125} is the *isotope of choice* as it emit less energy
- Tracer should remain in the compartment whose volume is being measured
- The activity of the tracer is first measured and then injected IV
- The activity remaining in the empty syringe is measured
- This is deducted from the amount of isotope injected
- After 10–15 mins, a sample of blood is withdrawn from the opposite arm
- This is to ensure that there is no contamination from isotope remaining at the injection site
- The activity of this sample is then measured and the dilution volume calculated from the result
- Repeated measurements can be made to estimate the change in blood volume
- Allowance is made for residual radioactivity from previous measurements
- Errors:
  - In a shocked patient, the time taken for mixing throughout the blood volume may be more
  - So, measurement is a better indicator of effective circulating volume than the total volume
  - Also, loss of injected isotope by vigorous hemorrhage (before mixing) may happen

American college of surgeons classes of acute hemorrhage

Factors	*Class I*	*Class II*	*Class III*	*Class IV*
Blood loss (mL)	< 750	750–1500	1500–2000	≥ 2000
Blood loss (% blood volume)	15	15–30	30–40	≥ 40%
Pulse (bpm)	100	100	120	≥ 140
Blood pressure	Normal	Normal	Reduced	Reduced
Pulse pressure	Normal or ↑	Decreased	Decreased	Decreased
Capillary refill test	Normal	Positive	Positive	Positive
Urine output (mL/hr)	30	20–30	5–10	Negligible
CNS mental status	Slightly anxious	Mildly anxious	Anxious, confused	Confused, lethargic
Respiratory rate (/min)	14–20	20–30	30–40	35
Fluid replacement (3:1 rule)	Crystalloid	Crystalloid	Crystalloid + blood	Crystalloid + blood

BLOOD COMPONENT THERAPY

Introduction

Transfusion therapy which is aimed at the need to correct deficiency of specific component of whole blood by administration of that specific fraction instead of giving whole blood.

Separation of Whole Blood

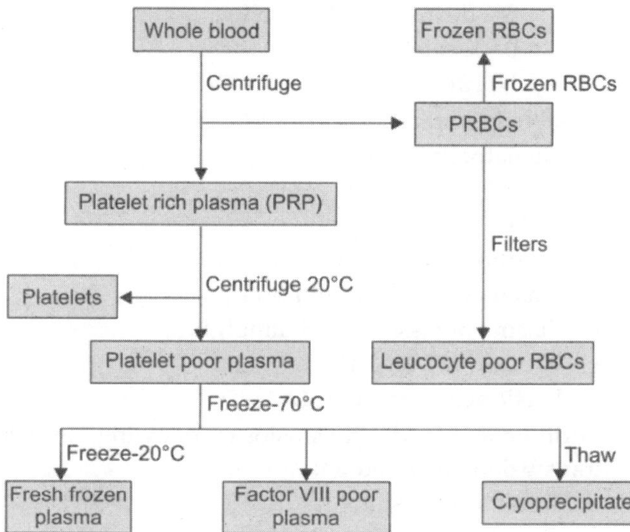

Blood Components

- Erythrocyte preparations:
  - PRBCs
  - Washed RBCs
  - Leukocyte poor RBCs
  - Frozen RBCs
- Leukocyte preparations:
  - Granulocytes
  - Mononuclear cells
- Platelets
- Plasma fractions:
  - FFP
  - Cryoprecipitate
  - Platelet rich plasma
  - Fractionated plasma:
    - Factor VIII concentrate, factor IX concentrate
    - Auto thrombin III concentrate
    - Prothrombin complex
    - Albumin
    - Intravenous immunoglobins

Hazards of Blood Component Therapy

- Immediate reactions:
  - Febrile reactions
  - Allergic reactions
  - Acute hemolytic reaction
  - Sensitivity to leukocytes and platelets
  - Non cardiogenic pulmonary edema
  - Bacterial contamination
  - Circulatory overload
  - Dilutional coagulopathy
  - Air embolism
- Delayed reactions:
  - Delayed hemolytic reaction
  - Post transfusion purpura
  - TA- GVHD
  - Transmission of hepatitis B, C, CMV, HIV, HTLV 2, WNV

ERYTHROCYTE PREPARATIONS

Packed Red Blood Cells

- Manufacture:
  - Obtained by removal of platelet-rich plasma from a unit of whole blood (WB)
  - Following centrifugation of whole blood:
    - Platelet rich plasma is removed
    - 100 mL of additive solution is added
  - Each unit contains:
    - 200 mL RBCs
    - Plasma < 50 mL
    - Additive 50–100 mL
    - Total volume of each unit is 300–350 mL
    - Each unit has a hematocrit of 55–60%
  - Thus, it has same amount of Hb as WB but most of the plasma is removed
- Storage of PRBCs:
  - Storage bags are made of PVC and di-2-ethylhexylphthalate (DEHP) plasticizer
  - Anticoagulant-preservative (A-P) solutions are used to increase the shelf life
  - First A-P solution to be used was acid-citrate dextrose (ACD)
  - This increased shelf life of PRBCs to 21 days
  - A-P solutions currently used are:
    - Citrate-phosphate dextrose (CPD)—21 days shelf life
    - CPD-adenine—35 days shelf life
    - Newer generation additive solutions—42 days shelf life
  - PRBCs are stored at 1–6°C to maintain RBC viability
  - Temperature must be maintained between 1–10°C during transport of PRBCs
  - Unit is discarded if present outside the controlled temperature for > 30 minute

- Indications:
  - Anemia:
    - Rarely required when Hb > 10 gm%
    - Almost always indicated when Hb < 6 gm%
    - The decision to transfuse between 6–10 g% depends on:
      - Cardiopulmonary risk factors
      - Ongoing blood loss
      - Clinical judgement
    - Restrictive transfusion strategy (Hb <8 g/dL) should be used
  - Acute blood loss:
    - > 1500 mL in adults
    - > 40 mL/kg in children
- Shelf life: 35–42 days depending on the additive (at 1–4°C)
- Dosage:
  - Each unit or 7.5 mL/kg increases the hematocrit by 3%
  - Effect takes upto 24 hours to manifest while intravascular volume equilibrates
  - The therapeutic effect also depends on:
    - Rapid ongoing RBC destruction
    - Splenic sequestration
- Typing and cross-matching
  - PRBC transfusion requires:
    - Matching donor and recipient RBCs according to blood type (ABO, Rh)
    - Screening recipient plasma for antibodies to minor RBC antigens
  - Screening is done with commercially available RBCs with all minor antigens
  - If the screen is positive:
    - Recipient plasma is cross matched with the specific PRBC unit
    - This unit may be used for transfusion on successful cross-matching
  - If the screen is negative cross matching may require additional blood samples
  - Type O Rh-negative blood (universal donor) may be used in emergencies
  - Type O Rh-positive blood may be used when Rh-negative blood is unavailable
  - Mismatching with Rh-positive blood is avoided in women of child bearing age
- Administration:
  - Usually transfused over 1–2 hours in the absence of hemodynamic instability
  - Initial transfusion rate should be slow to recognise transfusion reactions
  - Transfusion duration should not exceed 4 hours to prevent contamination
  - Administered after reconstitution with crystalloid/colloid which:
    - Does not contain calcium: causes clotting
    - Is not hypotonic: Causes hemolysis
  - Solutions recommended are:
    - 5% dextrose in 0.45% saline
    - 5% dextrose in 0.9% saline
    - 0.9% saline
    - Normosol R with pH of 7.4
- Metabolic characteristics of PRBCs:
  - Hematocrit 55–60%
  - pH 6.79
  - pCO_2 79 mm Hg
  - Bicarbonate 11 mmol/L
  - Plasma sodium 126 mmol/L
  - Plasma potassium 20.5 mmol/L
  - Glucose 432 mg/dL
  - Lactic acid 9.4 mmol/L
- Additional blood transfusions following initial transfusion are based on:
  - Trend of vital signs
  - Ongoing blood loss
  - Anticipated blood loss
  - Volume of intravenous fluids given
  - Assessment of hemoglobin concentration
  - Surgical concerns
- Disadvantages of storage of PRBCs:
  - Platelets present in the component are inactivated by cold storage
  - Intracellular potassium leaks into the plasma space
  - 2,3-Diphosphoglyceric acid (2,3-DPG) is depleted from RBCs
  - Other changes seen in stored PRBCs are:
    - Elevated plasma ammonia levels
    - Elevated PCO_2 levels
    - Lowered pH
    - Increased amounts of microaggregates

Leukocyte Poor Red Cells

- Leukoreduction (LR) refers to the removal of WBCs from the PRBC unit
- These cells are present in the PRBC unit due to copurification
- Each unit of PRBC contains $2–5 \times 10^9$ leukocytes
- Donor WBCs do not provide any known benefit to the recipient

- However, many adverse effects may be attributed to the presence of donor WBCs
- Thus, leukoreduction is done to reduce the risk of:
    - ***HLA alloimmunization***
    - ***Febrile non-hemolytic transfusion reactions (FNHTRs)***
    - CMV transmission
    - Leukocyte- induced immunomodulation
    - Transfusion related acute lung injury
    - Variant Creutzfeldt-Jakob disease
- LR reduces WBC content by 70–85%, from 109 WBCs/unit to 106 WBCs/unit
- Leukoreduction can also be used for platelet preparations
- Manufacture:
    - Units can be prepared during:
        - Procurement of blood (*pre-storage leukoreduction*)
        - At the time of transfusion (*bedside leukoreduction*)
    - Leukoreduction is done using specially designed leukocyte reduction filters:
        - Sedimentation
        - Inverted centrifugation
        - Filtration through nylon/cotton fibres
        - Saline batch washing
    - Leukoreduction results in reduction of WBC count by 99.9–99.99%
- Types of leukoreduction:
    - Pre-storage leukoreduction preferred as:
        - Achieves greater degree of leukocyte removal
        - Provides greater quality control and standardization
        - Avoids incorrect filter usage by unfamiliar personnel
    - Bedside leukoreduction: Associated with hypotensive reactions
- Indications:
    - Patients with recurrent febrile reactions to prevent FNHTRs
    - Frequently transfused patients to reduce HLA antigen allo-immunization
    - Patients undergoing cardiac surgery
    - All patients with solid organ/hematopoietic cell transplants
    - Acute leukemia patients and those with other malignancies
    - Prevention of transmission of CMV
- Disadvantages:
    - Does not prevent transfusion associated GVHD (irradiated blood is preferred)
    - Blood from patients with sickle cell trait may block the filter

Washed Red Cells

- Washing RBCs is done to remove plasma in those with allergic transfusion reactions
- However, it does not:
    - Affect antigens present on the cells
    - Does not remove enough RBCs to prevent GVHD or HLA alloimmunization
- Shelf life:
    - 4 hours if stored at 20–24°C
    - 24 hours if stored at 1–6°C
- Manufacture:
    - Packed red cells obtained by centrifugation are washed with 0.9% saline by:
        - Manual batch centrifugation
        - Continuous flow separation
    - Removes ≥98% plasma patients, electrolyte and antibodies
- Indications:
    - Hypersensitivity to plasma/allergy to whole blood
    - ***Patients with recurrent allergic/febrile reactions***
    - ***Patients with IgA/haptoglobin deficiency***
    - Neonatal transfusion to reduce:
        - Quantity of metabolic breakdown products
        - Extracellular potassium
        - Risk of CMV transmission
    - Patients at risk for hyperkalemia

Frozen Red Cells

- Manufacture:
    - Prepared using cryoprotective agent in the form of 40% glycerol
    - RBC may be stored continually at –80°C for up to 10 years
- Shelf life:
    - 10 years in frozen state
    - 24 hours in deglycerolized state
- Indications:
    - Maintaining an inventory of rare RBC phenotypes (Bombay phenotype)
    - Patients with multiple alloantibodies for common RBC blood group antigens
    - Patients with IgA deficiency in the absence of IgA-deficient donors

- Advantages:
  - Ready supply of rare phenotype RBCs
  - Freezing arrests biochemical changes which occur during liquid storage
  - Reduced incidence of:
    - Non-hemolytic reactions
    - Sensitization to HLA antigen
    - Transfusion hepatitis

Irradiated RBCs

- Irradiation prevents proliferation of donor T-lymphocytes in blood
- These T-lymphocytes are the immediate cause of transfusion-associated GVHD
- Viable donor T-lymphocytes attack recipient cells in immunocompromised patients
- They can attack hematopoietic cells as well as cells of other tissues
- This leads to bone marrow hypoplasia and other systemic complications
- Incidence of transfusion GVHD is rare (1 per 1,000,000 transfusions)
- However, fatality rate of transfusion GVHD is high (more than 90%)
- Thus, irradiation of cellular components is performed to prevent:
  - ***Transfusion GVHD*** from directed-donor units from blood relatives
  - Transfusion GVHD in highly immunosuppressed patients such as:
    - Leukemia
    - Lymphoma
    - Hematopoietic stem cell transplant recipients
    - Congenital cellular immunodeficiencies
    - Chemotherapy with purine analogues such as fludarabine
- Manufacture:
  - Gamma irradiation is performed with 2500 cGy to damage donor WBC DNA
  - This prevents a cellular immune proliferative response to recipients tissues
  - This in turn inhibits lymphocyte proliferation and TA-GVHD
  - Irradiation is performed in blood irradiators with:
    - Cesium-137
    - Cobalt-60
  - The blood units do not come in contact with the radioisotope
  - The units are therefore not radioactive
- Indications:
  - Fetal recipients of intrauterine transfusions
  - Infants younger than 4 months of age
  - Critically ill children
  - Children below 1 year of age on ECMO/ECLS
  - HLA matched products and transfusion from relatives
  - Severe congenital/acquired immunodeficiency:
    - Leukemia
    - Lymphoma
    - Solid organ transplant recipients
    - Hematopoietic stem cell transplant recipients
    - Congenital cellular immunodeficiencies
    - Chemotherapy with purine analogues such as fludarabine
- Disadvantages:
  - Expensive
  - Reduces shelf life of stored PRBCs (28 days):
    - Irradiation damages the RBC membrane
    - This reduces RBC viability and accelerates extracellular K^+ leakage
    - Thus, shelf life of irradiated blood is lesser

LEUKOCYTE PREPARATIONS

Granulocyte Preparations

- Collection of granulocytes requires processing between 5–10 litres of blood
- Indications:
  - Absolute granulocyte count < 500 cells/mL
  - Fever, unidentified mircro-organisms
  - No reduction in fever after 48 hrs of antibiotic therapy

Mononuclear Cells

- Manufacture:
  - Factors which stimulate stem cell release into circulation:
    - Human growth factor (best)
    - Glucocorticoids
    - Folinic acid
    - Endotoxins
  - Cell separator techniques facilitate processing large quantities of blood to collect stem cells
- Indications: Therapeutically used for bone marrow transplantation for:
  - AML
  - Hodgkins
  - Multiple myeloma
  - CA breast, ovary
  - Neuroblastomas

PLATELET PREPARATIONS

Introduction

- Platelet preparations are used when:
  - Prophylactically to prevent bleeding in thrombocytopenia
  - Therapeutically in thrombocytopenic patients with active bleeding
- Platelet preparations are *the only blood products that are stored at room temperature*

Types

- Apheresis platelets:
  - Also called Single Donor Platelets (SDP)
  - Platelets are obtained from a single donor
- Platelet concentrates:
  - Also called Random Donor Platelets (RDP)
  - These are pooled concentrates from 4-6 whole blood donations
  - Increases the risk of:
    - Disease transmission
    - Transfusion reactions
- Lymphocyte depleted platelets
- Irradiated platelets
- Cryopreserved platelets

Manufacture

- Platelet concentrates:
  - Manufactured from whole blood by centrifugation
  - Contains 5.5–7 × 1010 platelets suspended in 50 mL of plasma
  - Stored at 20–32 °C under constant agitation for 5 days
  - It is lymphocyte contaminated
  - Number of platelets per unit is inadequate to the platelet count
  - Thus, 4–6 units platelet concentrates are pooled to obtain adult dose
  - Advantages:
    - Low cost
    - Ease of collection and processing
  - Disadvantages:
    - Increased risk of infections
    - Increased risk of transfusion reactions
- Apheresis platelets:
  - From single donor in a 1–2 hour apheresis procedure
  - Platelets are selectively removed along with some WBCs and plasma
  - Most RBCs and plasma are returned back to the patient
  - Each unit contains 3–4 ×1011 platelets in 200–300 mL plasma
  - Stored at 20–22°C under constant agitation for 5 days
  - Each SDP unit is equivalent to "6 pack" platelet concentrate
- Lymphocyte depleted platelets:
  - Manufactured by passing platelets through a leukoreduction (LR) filter
  - This filter blocks the passage of 99.9-99.99% of WBCs
  - LR prevents several complications associated with WBC contamination
  - However, TA-GVHD is not prevented
- Units can be prepared during:
  - Procurement of blood (*pre-storage leukoreduction*)
  - At the time of transfusion (*bedside leukoreduction*)
- Irradiated platelets:
  - Platelet irradiation is used to prevent TA-GVHD
  - They are irradiated with 2500 cGy from a cesium-137 source
  - Platelets are enucleate and hence their function is unaffected by irradiation
  - However, platelet membrane damage may cause a reduction in shelf life
- Cryopreserved platelets:
  - Use DMSO as the preservative
  - Cryopreservation increases the shelf life of stored platelets
  - This can therefore be used:
    - As a strategy to augment blood inventories
    - Improve product availability in remote locations such as in combat
  - However, cryopreserved platelets cause a lower increment in platelet count

Storage

- Platelets are routinely stored at room temperature
- This is because cold temperature induces:
  - Clustering of von Willebrand factor receptors on platelet surface
  - Morphological changes in the platelets
- This causes enhanced clearance of platelets by hepatic macrophages
- Metabolic activity of any cell stored at room temperature is higher
- Thus, platelets are stored in bags which allow gas exchange
- Citrate is added to the unit to prevent clotting

Shelf Life

- 5 days at room temperature with constant and gentle agitation
- Can be stored up to 7 days in special FDA-approved containers
- Risk of infective complications increases after 5 days of storage especially for RDPs

Indications

- Prophylactic platelet transfusion:
  - Rarely indicated when platelet count > 1,00,000/mm^3
  - Usually indicated when platelet count < 50,000/mm^3
  - When count is between 50,000–1,00,000/mm^3 risk of bleeding is evaluated
  - Definitely when platelet count < 10, 000 cells/mm^3
- Periprocedural platelet transfusion:
  - Platelet count < 20,000 cells/mm^3 for central venous catheterization
  - Platelet count < 50,000 cells/mm^3 for:
    - Lumbar puncture
    - Neuraxial anesthesia
    - Endoscopy with biopsy
    - Liver biopsy
    - Vaginal delivery
    - Laparotomy
  - Platelet count 80,000–1,00, 000 cells/mm^3: risk of closed-cavity bleeding:
    - Ophthalmic surgery
    - Neurosurgery
- Therapeutic platelet transfusion:
  - Platelet count < 75,000 cells/mm^3 in:
    - Massive hemorrhage with ongoing loss
    - Hemorrhagic shock
  - Platelet count < 50,000 /mm^3 for:
    - DIC
    - Coagulopathies
  - Microvascular bleeds due to platelet dysfunction in:
    - Uremia
    - Liver diseases
    - Cardio pulmonary bypass
    - Massive blood transfusion

Cross Matching

- ABO compatibility:
  - Platelet transfusions are preferably ABO-type specific
  - Serological cross-matching is usually not done for platelet transfusions
  - Since platelets are stored in plasma, complications due to plasma may occur
  - Due to unavailability, non-type specific platelets may sometimes be transfused
  - Thus, *platelet concentrates need not be ABO blood group specific*
  - This may however result in:
    - Reduction in the half-life of transfused platelets
    - Rare instances of hemolytic transfusion reactions
  - Non-type specific transfusion is avoided in:
    - Children
    - Patients receiving multiple transfusions
- Rh compatibility:
  - Platelets by themselves do not express Rh antigens
  - However, platelet products may contain small volumes of RBCs
  - Rh-incompatibility may result in alloimmunization due to these RBCs
  - Thus, Rh-incompatible platelets is avoided in women of child-bearing age
  - In case of administration of Rh-incompatible platelets:
    - Risk of alloimmunization and HDFN is present
    - Thus, anti-D immunoglobulins may be co-administered
- If the volume of incompatible plasma is large as in SDP transfusion:
  - Use plasma reduced SDP
  - Replace plasma with compatible plasma
  - Replace plasma with platelet additive solutions (PAS)

Dosage: AABB 2015 Guidelines

- Children: 5–10 mL/kg
- Adults:
  - 1 unit RDP per 10 kg body weight
  - 4–6 units of RDP
  - 1 unit of SDP
- The platelet dose is usually transfused over a period of 20–30 minutes

Therapeutic Efficacy

- Therapeutic efficacy of platelet concentrates is difficult to monitor
- 1 unit of RDP increases platelet count by 7–10,000 cells/mm^3 1 hour after transfusion

- 10 units of RDPs are required to increase the count by 1,00,000 cells/mm^3
- One unit of SDP raises the platelet count by 50,000 cells/mm^3
- Factors which influence therapeutic efficacy include:
  - Sequestration due to splenomegaly
  - Previous sensitization causing platelet destruction by antibodies
  - Fever, sepsis
  - Ongoing bleeding causing active thrombosis and platelet consumption
  - Antibiotics as they may form antibiotic-platelet complexes

Contraindications

- Diseases associated with platelet activation:
  - Examples:
    - Thrombotic thrombocytopenic purpura
    - Heparin induced thrombocytopenia
  - In these disorders, platelet consumption causes thrombocytopenia
  - However, underlying platelet activation may increase risk of thrombosis
  - Thus, prophylactic administration of platelets may increase risk of thrombosis
  - However, platelet transfusion should not be withheld in the event of bleeding
- Idiopathic thrombocytopenic purpura:
  - These patients produce antiplatelet antibodies
  - These antibodies destroy:
    - Circulating platelets
    - Megakaryocytes in bone marrow
  - However, the circulating platelets in these patients are highly functional
  - Bleeding is rare in these patients even when thrombocytopenia is severe
  - Thus, platelet transfusion is avoided unless life threatening bleeding

Side Effects

- Infection:
  - As platelets are stored at room temperature, chances of infection are higher
  - Risk increases with transfusion of RDP concentrates stored for > 5 days
  - Rate of bacterial contamination is 1 per 2500 units
  - Sepsis from platelet concentrates is suspected if fever within 6 hrs of transfusion
- Febrile non-hemolytic transfusion reactions:
  - Platelet preparations contains some WBCs along with platelets
  - These WBCs may cause:
    - FNHTR
    - Alloimmunization
    - TA-GVH disease
- Plasma component of platelet preparations may cause TRALI and anaphylaxis
- Platelet refractoriness:
  - Suspected if poor increment in platelet count 20–24 hours after transfusion
  - Clinical causes:
    - Hypersplenism causing sequestration
    - Fever causing increased consumption
    - Bleeding causing increased consumption
    - Medications:
      - Aspirin
      - NSAIDs
      - Thenopyridines
      - Beta lactam antibiotics
      - Antidepressants
    - Disseminated Intravascular Coagulation
  - Immunological causes:
    - Antibodies to HLA
    - Antibodies to platelet specific antigens

PLASMA FRACTIONS

FRESH FROZEN PLASMA

Introduction

- FFP is the plasma taken from one unit of whole blood
- FFP is the most frequently used and arguably the most dangerous blood product
- FFP contains all the coagulation factors present in the original unit of blood
- These are slightly diluted by the anticoagulant solution used to collect the blood
- Levels of factor V and factor VIII fall on prolonged storage

Types

- FFP:
  - Called fresh frozen plasma
  - Can be prepared from:
    - Single units of whole blood
    - Plasma collected by apheresis techniques
  - Frozen at –18 to –30°C within 6-8 hours of collection
  - Useable for 1 year from date of collection
  - Standard units have 200–250 mL of plasma
- PF_{24}:
  - Called frozen plasma
  - Plasma is frozen within 24 hours of collection

- Useable for 1 year from date of collection
- Comparable to FFP except for:
  - 20–25% reduction in factor VIII and V levels
  - Decreased levels of protein C

❖ Thawed plasma:
- FFP which has been thawed in a water bath at 30–37 °C
- Thawed plasma may be useable for upto 5 days when refrigerated at 1–6 °C
- Has lower concentration of factor V and VIII
- Its main advantage is the availability for immediate use
- Useful in emergencies with mass trauma requiring large volumes of plasma

Manufacture

❖ Obtained by aphèresis/separation of plasma from centrifuged whole blood

❖ Plasma is frozen at –18 to –30 °C within:
- 6-8 hours of collection for FFP
- Within 24 hours for PF_{24}

❖ Each unit of FFP prepared from 1 unit of blood will have 200–250 mL

❖ Thawing of FFP prior to clinical use:
- Done in a water bath at 30–37 °C
- Time taken is approximately 20–25 minutes

❖ This process should not be hastened by artificial heating

Shelf Life

❖ Frozen plasma: Can be used within 1 year from the date of collection in frozen form

❖ Thawed plasma:
- 24 hours at room temperature
- 5 days when stored refrigerated (1–6 °C)

Contents

❖ Contains all the coagulation factors in normal concentration:
- Fibrinogen 700–800 mg/unit
- Factors II, VII, VIII, IX, X, XI, XIII
- Especially rich in factors V and VIII
- von Willebrand factor, fibronectin
- Protein C, S and albumin
- Antithrombin III

❖ Electrolytes, immunoglobulins and complement

❖ 1 unit of FFP provides coagulation factors equivalent to:
- 4–5 units of platelet concentrates
- 1 unit of apheretic platelets
- 1 unit of whole blood

❖ FFP is devoid of RBCs, WBCs and platelets

Indications

❖ Urgent reversal of warfarin therapy:
- In the presence of severe bleeding
- Prior to urgent surgery/invasive procedures

❖ Heparin resistance:
- Due to antithrombin III deficiency
- Used when antithrombin III concentrates are not available
- Helps in reducing the total heparin dose

❖ Correction of isolated factor deficiencies:
- Used when the specific concentrates are unavailable
- Conditions include:
  - Factor II, V, VII, VIII, IX, X
  - Protein C and S deficiency
  - C_1 esterase inhibitors
  - Antithrombin III deficiency

❖ Periprocedural transfusion for multifactor deficiency:
- Conditions causing multifactor deficiency include:
  - Liver dysfunction
  - DIC
  - HELLP syndrome
- Transfusion is indicated when:
  - Clinical evidence of bleeding
  - Anticipation of major surgery or invasive procedure
  - PT or aPTT > 1.5 times the control
  - INR > 2

❖ Treatment of:
- Hemolytic uremic syndrome (HUS)
- Disseminated Intravascular Coagulation (DIC)
- Plasma exchange therapy for:
  - Guillain-Barre syndrome
  - Thrombotic Thrombocytopenic Purpura (TTP)
- HELLP syndrome

❖ Massive blood transfusion when:
- Transfusion has exceeded 1 blood volume (70 mL/kg)
- When coagulation studies are not easily available

Cross Matching

❖ Plasma contains antibodies, including antibodies to RBCs

❖ All units of blood are subjected to antibody screen prior to fractionation

- The screen becomes positive when the donor has at least 1 antibody to an RBC antigen
- Plasma is not prepared from blood units which test positive on screening
- Thus, when FFP is prepared, the only alloantibodies present in it are ABO antibodies
- Rh compatibility is therefore not necessary for FFP transfusion
- ABO compatibility:
  - ABO compatibility has to be ensured for plasma transfusion
  - This is in order to avoid transfusing donor anti-A and anti-B antibodies
  - Transfusion of ABO-incompatible FFP causes hemolytic transfusion reactions
- Universal FFP donor:
  - Type O blood group is not the universal donor for FFP, as for PRBCs
  - This is because O-group plasma contains anti-A and anti-B antibodies
  - Thus, type-AB Rh-negative FFP is the universal FFP donor

Dosages

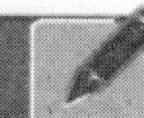

- Congenital and acquired clotting factor deficiency therapy:
  - To achieve coagulation factor concentration > 30%, dose used is:
    - 10–15 mL/kg in pediatrics
    - 4 units in adults
  - Repeat doses are guided by PT, INR and aPTT measurements
- Reversal of warfarin therapy:
  - 15–30 mL/kg of FFP in the presence of bleeding
  - Lower doses titrated to the INR for anticipated invasive procedures
- For massive blood transfusion:
  - Early administration of plasma resuscitation reduces the risk of:
    - Hemorrhagic shock
    - Mortality
  - Plasma: RBC ratio:
    - Improved outcomes are seen with FFP: RBC ratio of 2:3
    - Higher platelets: plasma: RBCs (1:1:1) ratio shows no benefit
- Rate of transfusion:
  - Healthy individuals: 2–3 mL/kg/hour (1 unit in 1.5 hours)
  - Patients with poor LV function: 1 mL/kg/hour (1 unit in 4 hours)

Therapeutic Efficacy

- 1 Unit of FFP increases most factors by approximately 3–5%
- 2 units of FFP increase most clotting factors by approximately 10%
- Thus, for clinically relevant correction of deficiency 4 FFP units are required

Side Effects

- TRALI:
  - Rare but potentially lethal complication
  - Risk is higher with plasma transfusion
  - This is because TRALI occurs due to donor antibodies in plasma against:
    - Recipient HLA antigens
    - Recipient neutrophil antigens
- TACO:
  - FFP increases risk of fluid overload and pulmonary edema
  - This may be reduced by restricting the rate of infusion to 1 mL/kg/hour
- Febrile allergic reactions:
  - FFP transfusion is commonly associated with risk of fever and chills
  - Prophylactic administration of antihistaminics and antipyretics is ineffective
- Anaphylactic reactions may occur in patients with IgA deficiency
- Infections:
  - Risk of transmitting infections is similar to that of PRBCs
  - However, since FFP is acellular, risk of CMV and HTLV transmission is lesser
- As leucocytes are absent in FFP risk is minimized for:
  - Transmission of CMV
  - TA-GVHD

Contraindications

- Role in volume replacement:
  - FFP is a reliable source of volume replacement in case of acute blood loss
  - However, other alternative therapies are equally satisfactory and safer
  - Thus, use of FFP for the sole purpose of volume replacement is avoided
- For reversal of anticoagulation by:
  - Heparin
  - Direct thrombin inhibitors
  - Direct factor Xa inhibitors
- For augmenting albumin concentration

CRYOPRECIPITATE

Introduction

- This is an insoluble material which is obtained after FFP is thawed at 4 °C
- Cryoprecipitate is rich in certain plasma proteins, especially fibrinogen
- Use of cryoprecipitate is reducing due to preference for fibrinogen concentrates

Manufacture

- Prepared as a cold insoluble precipitate by thawing FFP at 4 °C for 24 hours
- This controlled thawing enables precipitation of larger molecules
- The resultant fluid mixture has 2 components:
  - Liquid component which includes all proteins that have gone back in solution
  - Precipitated component containing cold-insoluble proteins
- The precipitant is separated from the supernatant subsequently by centrifugation
- It is then refrozen at -18 °C in a concentrated volume with 10-15 mL of plasma
- 1 unit of cryoprecipitate will have a volume of 10–20 mL only
- Cryoprecipitate can only be made from FFP which has been frozen within 8 hours
- It cannot be made from plasma frozen within 24 hours of collection (PF_{24})

Contents

- Concentration of certain clotting factors is similar to FFP:
  - Fibrinogen (factor I)
  - Factor VIII
  - Factor XIII
  - von Willebrand factor
- Concentration of individual factors:
  - Factor I fibrinogen 150–250 mg/unit
  - Factor VIII 80 IU/unit
  - Factor XIII 50–75 IU/unit
  - von Willebrand factors 100–150 IU/unit
- Trace of fibronectin and other plasma proteins
- Antibodies in cryoprecipitate is very low
- Compared to FFP, cryoprecipitate has more fibrinogen per unit volume:
  - 1500 mg/dL of fibrinogen in cryoprecipitate
  - 250 mg/dL of fibrinogen in FFP
- Thus it is used as a low-volume alternative for fibrinogen replacement

Shelf Life

- 1 year in the frozen form
- Following thawing:
  - Infusion of individual units should be completed within 6 hours of thawing
  - Pooled cryoprecipitate units should be transfused within 4 hours of thawing

Indications

- Treatment of hemophilia A:
  - Treatment with cryoprecipitate has been replaced by F VIII concentrates
  - However, cryoprecipitate may be used when factor concentrate is not available
- Treatment of congenital fibrinogen deficiency:
  - Used when specific treatment is unavailable
  - Indicated for:
    - Elective surgeries
    - Invasive procedures
    - Peri-partum period
- von Willebrand disease: Useful when specific treatment is unavailable:
  - Recombinant vWF
  - vWF concentrates
  - Desmopressin
- Factor XIII replacement when specific treatment is unavailable in:
  - Sepsis
  - Trauma
  - Burns
- Acquired hypofibrinogenemia:
  - Can occur due to:
    - Massive blood loss
    - DIC
  - Used in massive blood loss as part of massive transfusion protocols
  - Also useful in DIC patients with severe bleeding
  - Usually transfused when the fibrinogen level is low (< 150–200 mg/dL)
- Severe hepatic disease with impaired hemostasis
- Severe postpartum hemorrhage in spite of fibrinogen levels > 150 mg/dL
- Uremic bleeding:
  - Usually occurs due to platelet dysfunction
  - However, cryoprecipitate may be used when bleeding is refractory to DDAVP

Dosage

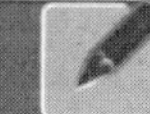

- 5–10 units of cryoprecipitate
- Typical volume for an adult dose is 50–200 mL
- For factor VIII and XIII deficiency, typical dose is 1 unit per 10 kg body weight
- Units are usually pooled in order to facilitate transfusion (5 units/pool)
- Should be administered through a filter as rapidly as possible at least 200 mL/hr

Cross Matching

- Cross matching is usually unnecessary
- ABO compatibility:
  - Concentration of antibodies in cryoprecipitate is very low
  - Thus, ABO compatible transfusion may not be essential
  - ABO compatible units are strongly recommended for:
    - Neonates
    - Small children
    - Hematopoietic cell transplant recipients
- Rh compatibility:
  - Cryoprecipitate preparations may contain RBC fragments
  - This may sensitize Rh-negative recipients to the Rh antigen
  - Thus, Rh-specific units are preferred in women of child bearing age group
  - However, Rh-specific transfusion is not mandatory in other patient types

Therapeutic Efficacy

- The fibrinogen increment with each bag is calculated as 25 mg/L plasma volume
- Each unit of cryoprecipitate raises the plasma fibrinogen levels by 7–10 mg/dL
- Thus, an adult dose of 10 U increases fibrinogen by 70–100 mg/dL

Complications

- Infections:
  - Cryoprecipitate carries similar risk of infections compared with PRBCs and FFP
  - However, incidence of infections with cryoprecipitate is higher
  - This is because more number of units are transfused
- Volume overload:
  - Less likely to cause TACO compared with FFP
  - However, transfusion of large volumes may result in TACO
- Transfusion reactions:
  - Lower risk of hemolytic transfusion reactions compared with FFP
  - This is because cryoprecipitate units have smaller volumes
  - Thus, the volume of alloantibodies is lesser than in FFP
- Risk of allergic reactions is similar to FFP

Contraindications

- Thrombocytopenic bleeding
- Reversal of warfarin therapy as it does not contain vitamin-K dependant factors
- Isolated clotting factor deficiency other than factors I, VIII, XIII and vWF

Characteristic	FFP	Cryoprecipitate
Volume	250–300 mL	10–20 mL
Time to prepare	30 minutes	30 minutes
Fibrinogen	700–800 mg	150–250 mg
Fibrinogen/unit volume	250 mg/dL	1500 mg/dL
Other clotting factors	All coagulation factors	Factors VIII, XIII, vWF

FIBRIN GLUE

- When FFP is thawed, supernatant forms cryoprecipitate
- The precipitate contains large amounts of fibrinogen
- When centrifuged, about 4 mL of concentrated precipitate results
- With added thrombin, this is locally applied as fibrin glue

ALBUMIN

Manufacture

- Source is whole blood/serum/placenta
- Contains 96% albumin and 4% other proteins
- Available in 5% and 25% solution in isotonic saline

Usage

- Can be used without regard to ABO type and cross match
- Should be administered within 4 hrs of starting infusion

Indications

- Hypoproteinemia, burns and peritonitis
- For volume expansion acutely

Side Effects

- Very costly and in short supply
- Risk of bacterial sepsis and *Creutzfeldt-Jakob disease*

ANTITHROMBIN III CONCENTRATE

Introduction

- Antithrombin III (AT III) is the primary physiological inhibitor of in-vivo coagulation
- AT III (AT III) concentrate is used in patients with hereditary antithrombin deficiency

Chemistry and Preparation

- Antithrombin III is an α_2-glycoprotein
- It has a molecular weight of 58000 DA
- There are two preparations of AT III which are available commercially:
  - Thrombate III
  - ATryn
- Thrombate III:
  - One form of AT III is Thrombate III, a sterile non-pyrogenic concentrate
  - Thrombate III is marketed in powder form for reconstitution in a sterile manner
  - It is prepared from pooled units of human plasma from normal donors
  - Viruses are removed from this pool using two methods:
    - Heat treatment
    - Nanofiltration
  - When reconstituted with sterile water, the resultant mixture constitutes:
    - pH 6–7.5
    - Sodium 110–210 mEq/L
    - Chloride 110–210 mEq/L
    - Alanine 0.075 M- 0.125 M
    - Heparin 0.1 IU per 1 unit of AT
    - 50 IU of AT III per mL of the solution
  - Once reconstituted, the solution should be administered within 3 hours
  - The solution should not be refrigerated after reconstitution
  - The reconstituted AT III should be administered slowly over 10–20 minutes
- ATryn:
  - AT III can also be manufactured using recombinant technology (rhAT)
  - This form is also known as antithrombin alfa
  - It is produced from transgenic goats expressing rhAT in their milk
  - Thus, antibodies against rhAT protein may develop
  - This can lead to immunological reactions and anaphylaxis

Mechanism of Action

- AT III is normally present in human plasma at a concentration of 12.5 mg/dL
- In the presence of thrombin, rigid covalent bond is formed between the 2 molecules
- The bond is between serine reactive site of thrombin and arginine reactive site of AT
- This results in an inactive stoichiometric complex between the two molecules
- Other coagulation factors inhibited by AT III include:
  - Factor IXa
  - Factor Xa
  - Factor XIa
  - Factor XIIa
  - Plasmin

Pharmacokinetics

- Thrombate:
  - AT III has 50% disappearance time of 17.4 + 3.9 hours
  - Elimination half life of AT III:
    - 2.5 ± 1.5 days via immunological assay of AT III
    - 3.8 ± 1.8 days vias functional assay of AT III
  - Elimination $T_{1/2}$ maybe decreased following:
    - Surgery with hemorrhage
    - Acute thrombosis
    - Following heparin administration
- ATryn:
  - Volume of distribution Vd 7.7 L
  - Elimination $T_{1/2}$ 12–18 hours

Indications

- Treatment of heparin resistance during cardiac surgery
- Treatment of thromboembolism in hereditary AT III deficiency
- Prevention of perioperative and peripartum thromboembolism in hereditaryAT III deficiency

Dosage

Type	Target At Level	Dose (Units)	Monitoring
Loading	120% of normal	Calculated loading dose	Baseline
			20 minutes post injection
			12 hrs post injection
			Pre-injection (trough)
Maintenance (Q24H)	80–120% of normal	(Calculated loading dose) × 0.6	Q24H, as needed

- Dose is individualized to achieve plasma AT III levels between 80–120% of baseline
- In cases of hereditary AT III deficiency, maintenance dose is given for 2–8 days
- For heparin resistance during cardiac surgery, 500–1000 IU is usually given:

$$\text{Calculated loading dose of AT III} = \frac{(120\%\text{–baseline }\%) \times \text{body weight in kg}}{1.4}$$

- No dosing adjustments are required in renal and hepatic impairment

Monitoring During Therapy

- Coagulation tests suitable to the anticoagulant used have to be performed regularly:
  - aPTT
  - anti-factor Xa activity
- Functional AT assays:
  - Done by two methods:
    - Amidolytic assays using chromogenic substrates
    - Clotting assays
  - Immunoassays are not used for assessing functional levels
  - This is because they do not detect all hereditary AT deficiencies

Contraindications

- Hypersensitivity reactions to thrombate III
- Recombinant antithrombin III ATryn is contra-indicated in those allergic to goat milk
- No other contraindications have been identified till date

Adverse Effects

- Dizziness, chest discomfort
- Nausea, dysgeusia, abdominal cramps
- Hypersensitivity reactions including anaphylaxis
- Transmission of infectious diseases:
  - Viruses
  - Creutzfeldt-Jakob disease and its variant
- Bleeding due to excessive anticoagulation
- Thrombosis due to inadequate Dosage
- Wound hematoma

Drug Interactions

- Anticoagulant effect of AT III is increased by 1000 times with heparin coadministration
- This interaction can be used favorably in patients with heparin resistance
- Anticoagulation may be potentiated by coad-ministration of anti-platelet agents

PROTHROMBIN CONCENTRATES

Manufacture

- Factor IX recovered from plasma by absorption with ion exchange
- These are complexes of vitamin K dependent II, VII, IX, and X
- Commercially available as ***Konyne and Proplex***

Indications

- Hemophilia B/factor IX deficiency (***Christmas disease***)
- Acquired hypoprothrombinemic bleeding disorders like warfarin overdose

Side Effects: Risk of hepatitis

INTRAVENOUS IMMUNOGLOBULIN

Manufacture: Pools of plasma fractionated to create concentrated immunoglobulin product (mainly IgG) which is virally inactivated.

Indications

- Hematological conditions:
  - Acquired hypogammaglobulinemias
  - Acquired RBC aplasia
  - HIV associated thrombocytopenia
  - Idiopathic thrombocytopenic purpura (ITP)
  - Posttransfusion pupura (PTP)
- Neurological conditions:
  - Acute disseminated encephalomyelitis
  - Dermatomyositis
  - ***Guillain-Barre syndrome***
  - ***Eaton-Lambert syndrome***
  - Myasthenia gravis

- Viral infections:
    - Cytomegalovirus
    - Pediatric HIV

Adverse Reactions

- Anaphylaxis, especially in IgA deficiency
- Headache, febrile reaction
- Renal failure

LEUCOREDUCTION

Introduction

- Involves removal of leucocytes from blood or blood components used for transfusion
- Leukoreduction (LR) is generally used for:
    - Packed red blood cell transfusions
    - Platelet transfusions

Rationale

- Leucocytes are present in the PRBC unit due to co-purification
- Each unit of PRBC contains 2–5 × 109 leukocytes
- Donor WBCs do not provide any known benefit to the recipient
- However, many adverse effects may be attributed to the presence of donor WBCs:
    - Immunologically mediated effects:
        - Allo-sensitization to HLA antigens causing:
    - Febrile non-hemolytic transfusion reactions
    - Platelet refractoriness
        - Transplant rejection
    - Infectious disease transmission:
        - CMV
        - HTLV I and II
        - Ebstein-Barr virus
    - Reperfusion injury
- Thus, leucocytes are considered as contaminants of other cellular blood components
- Leukoreduction is therefore done to reduce the risk of:
    - HLA alloimmunization
    - Febrile non-hemolytic transfusion reactions (FNHTRs)
    - CMV transmission
    - Leukocyte-induced immunomodulation
    - Transfusion related acute lung injury
    - Variant Creutzfeldt-Jakob disease

Indications

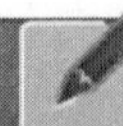

- Patients with recurrent febrile reactions to prevent FNHTRs
- Frequently transfused patients to reduce HLA antigen allo-immunization
- Patients undergoing cardiac surgery
- All patients with solid organ/hematopoietic cell transplants
- Acute leukemia patients and those with other malig-nancies
- Prevention of infection with leucocyte borne viruses in at-risk patients:
    - New variant Creutzfeldt Jakob virus (post-tonsillectomy patients)
    - Ebstein-Barr virus
    - Cytomegalo virus (CMV)
    - Human T-cell lymphotrophic virus

Advantages

- Febrile non-hemolytic transfusion reactions:
    - Seen in approximately 1% of patients who receive transfusion
    - These reactions are mediated by:
        - Donor leucocytes
        - Cytokine accumulation during storage of products
    - FNHTRs can be prevented by reducing the WBC count < 5 × 108 cells/unit
    - This can be achieved by various methods:
        - Saline washing
        - Micro-aggregate filters
        - Leukoreduction (LR)
    - LR is most effective as it produces greater reduction in WBC count
- Prevention of HLA alloimmunization:
    - HLA antigens on the surface of donor WBCs induce production of HLA Abs
    - This causes many complications in patients receiving frequent transfusions:
    - Increased risk of graft rejection for:
    - Solid organ transplants
    - Bone marrow transplants
    - Platelet refractoriness
    - Thus, LR may be an effective strategy to prevent these complications
- Prevention of bacterial contamination of RBCs:
    - Bacterial contamination of RBCs may occur due to:

- Contamination at the time of venepuncture
- Contamination during component preparation
- Subclinical infection in the donor
• Pre-storage leukoreduction results in decreased proliferation of bacteria by:
  - Removal of bacteria ingested by leukocytes
  - Filtration of bacteria
  - Prevention of release of viable bacteria from disintegrating WBCs

❖ Reperfusion injury:
  • Reperfusion injury occurs due to inflammatory responses mediated by WBCs
  • Leukoreduction prevents reperfusion injury following CPB

Methods

❖ Leukoreduced units can be prepared during:
  • Procurement of blood (*pre-storage leukoreduction*)
  • At the time of transfusion (*bedside leukoreduction*)

❖ Leukoreduction is done using specially designed leukocyte reduction filters

❖ Three generations of filters are used for:
  • Sedimentation
  • Inverted centrifugation
  • Saline batch washing

❖ Leukoreduction results in reduction of WBC count by 99.9–99.99%

❖ This results in a residual leucocyte count of 5 × 106 cells/unit

Types

❖ Pre-storage leukoreduction:
  • Done at the time of procurement of blood
  • Pre-storage leukoreduction is preferred as:
    - Achieves greater degree of leukocyte removal
    - It is immediately available
    - Decreases cytokine and histamine production
    - Has more consistent quality
    - Provides greater quality control and standardization
    - Avoids incorrect filter Usage by unfamiliar personnel

❖ Bedside leukoreduction: associated with hypo-tensive reactions

❖ Universal leukoreduction:
  • Involves leukodepletion of all leucocyte containing cellular products
  • This should ideally be performed if cost is not an issue

Disadvantages

❖ Does not prevent transfusion associated GVHD (irradiated blood is preferred)

❖ Blood from patients with sickle cell trait may block the filter

❖ Reduces hemoglobin concentration in the unit by approximately 15%

Complications

❖ *Red Eye Syndrome*:
  • Seen within 24 hours of leucoreduced RBC transfusion
  • Seen in association with use of LeukoNet cellulose acetate filters

❖ Blockade of filter by PRBCs from sickle cell trait donors:
  • This occurs due to:
    - Low oxygen content of venous blood
    - Low pH of venous blood
    - Hypertonicity of anticoagulant-preservative solutions
  • Incidence may be prevented by:
    - Storing units at 4 °C prior to filtration
    - Storage in oxygen permeable blood bags
    - Use of metered-citrate anticoagulant system

TRANSFUSION RELATED IMMUNOMODULATION

Introduction

Transfusion related immunomodulation refers to the transient depression of immune system which occurs following transfusion of blood products

Benefits: ***Allogenic survival***: Increased chances of graft survival in renal transplant if recipient is transfused with donors blood for 1 week prior to surgery

Hazards

❖ Increased postoperative infections like NVCJD, HIV

❖ Increased chances of cancer recurrence

❖ Increased transmission of non-Hodgkins lymphoma

❖ Increased chances of TRALI

❖ It is a mechanism of non-hemolytic febrile reaction

❖ Platelet refractoriness may occur

❖ Increased chances of SIRS and MODS

Mechanisms of Trim

❖ Natural killer cell activity

❖ Cytokine production

❖ Monocyte function

❖ Interleukin production

❖ CD_4/CD_8 count

- Production of anti-idiotype antibodies
- Cell mediated toxicity against certain target cells
- Response to mitogens

Types of Trim

- Antigen of specific: Occurs in renal transplant cases

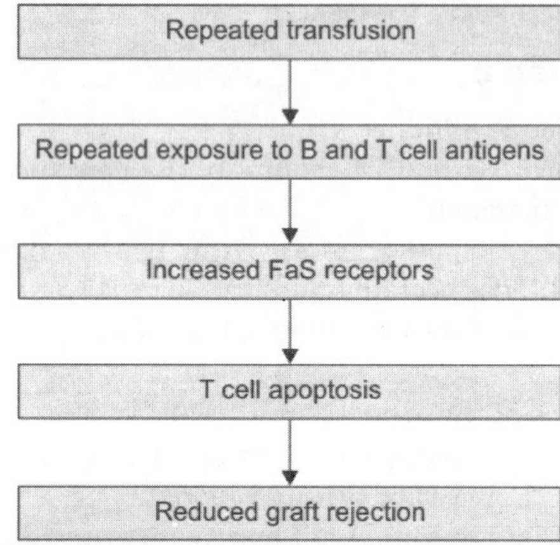

- Anti-idiotype antibodies
- Bystander suppression

Prevention of Trim

- Avoid blood products
- Use blood substitutes
- Gamma irradiation of blood
- Leucoreduction

Indications for Gamma Irradiation of Blood

Absolute Indications

- Bone marrow transplant recipients
- Intrauterine transfusion
- Congenital cell mediated immunodeficiency diseases
- Acute lymphoid leukemia, Hodgkin lymphoma
- Immunocompromised organ transplant recipient

Relative Indications

- Neonate < 1200 gm
- HIV with opportunistic infection
- Patients on immunosuppressive therapy for cancer

MASSIVE BLOOD TRANSFUSION

Introduction

Massive blood transfusion is defined as:

- Replacement of 1 circulating blood volume (around 10–12 units of PRBCS) within 24 hrs
- Loss of 50% of circulating blood volume within 3 hrs
- Loss of 10% of circulating blood volume within 10 mins
- Transfusion of 10 units of blood within 6 hrs
- Transfusion of 4 units of blood within 1 hour with continuing blood loss
- Transfusion of 1 unit of blood within 5 minutes

Preparation for Massive Blood Transfusion

- 2 large gauge venous cannula (14 G)
- Triple lumen central venous catheter via:
  - Internal jugular vein
  - Subclavian vein
  - Femoral vein
- Use of three way taps reduces the need to use needles for drug administration
- Wear gloves to prevent contamination of hands with spilled blood
- Monitors:
  - Triple lumen central venous catheter used for:
    - Rapid blood sampling
    - Measurement of CVP
  - Foleys catheter to measure urine output
  - Central and peripheral temperature should be measured
  - Pulse oximetry, arterial pressure and ECG should be monitored

Method of Administration

- Constant pressure infusion device
- Do not prime the system with fluids containing Ca^{2+} like:
  - Lactated Ringers
  - Hemaccel
- Hematomic Rapid Infuser Device with a 3 litre reservoir:
  - Cell saved or banked blood and FFP can be stored in the reservoir
  - This blood is warmed and infused at rates of 2 L/min
- For faster rates of transfusion:
  - Increase height of fluid above patient
  - Manual compression of bag
  - Using syringe and three way tap to aspirate and push volume

Warming of Stored Blood

- Double length blood warming coil
- Counter current aluminium heat exchangers
- Plastic coils/plastics cassettes in warm water bath (37–38°C)
- Warming plates which have an upper (43°C) and lower limits (33°C) is *safest*

Management of Massive Transfusion

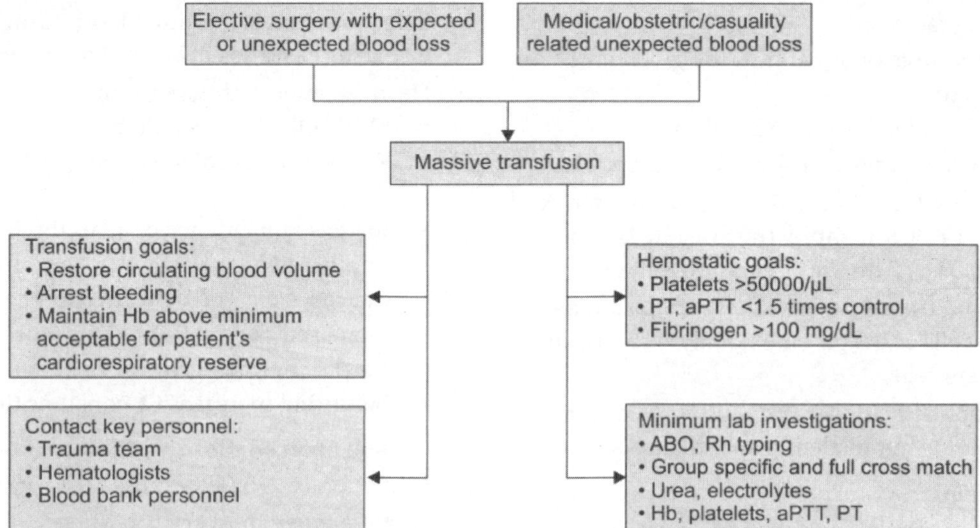

Complications of Massive Transfusion

I. Coagulopathy:

- Occurs due to the following reasons:
  - Reduced synthesis and release of clotting factors (hepatic ischemia)
  - Dilution of endogenous clotting factors with colloids/RL
  - Thrombocytopenia and DIC
  - Chelation of calcium by citrate (least important)
  - Hypothermia
- Clotting factor deficiency occurs before thrombocytopenia
- Concentration of II, V and VIII are reduced in stored blood
- *Transfusion guidelines:*
  - If platelet count < 50000/μl, platelet transfusion
  - If INR > 1.5, transfuse FFP
  - If fibrinogen < 100mg/dL, transfuse cryoprecipitate

II. Citrate Toxicity:

- Not caused by citrate ion per se, but because citrate binds to Ca^{2+}
- Each unit of blood contains 3 gm of citrate
- Increased chances of citrate toxicity possible when:
  - Pediatric patients
  - Cardiac disease and low cardiac output states
  - Hypotension and hypovolemia
  - Hepatic disease
  - Liver transplantation
  - Hyperventilation
  - Alkalosis
  - Hypothermia
  - Hyperkalemia
- Factors precipitating toxicity:
  - Rate of blood transfusion more important than total volume of blood transfused
  - Hypocalcemia occurs only when:
    - Rates of transfusion > 1 mL/kg/min
    - 1 unit blood transfused in 5 min
  - Rate of citrate metabolism reduces by 50% when body temperature reduces from 37°C to 31°C
- Clinical features:
  - Reduced myocardial function
  - Hypotension, narrow pulse press, increased diastolic pressure and CVP
  - Increased QTc, widened QRS and flattened T waves
- Treatment:
  - 1 gm calcium gluconate (10%) given IV for every 5 units blood/FPP
  - 13.4% calcium chloride contains 0.192 mmol/mL of Ca^{2+}
  - 10% calcium gluconate contains only 0.22 mmol/mL of Ca^{2+}
  - $CaCl_2$ is not used much even though it contains more Ca^{2+} as it very irritant to veins

III. Hyperkalemia:

- Serum K^+ is as high as 19–30 mEq/L in stored blood after 21 days

- This is because RBCs exchange K^+ ions to uptake H^+ ions generated by metabolism
- Precipitating factors:
  - Large amounts of blood must be given for hyper K^+ to occur
  - Rate of blood infusion ≥ 120 mL/min
  - Premature infants are especially susceptible
- Transfuse only fresh (< 8 days old) plasma reduced or washed PRBCs if rapid transfusion is required (≥ 10–15 mL/kg/2 hrs) in premature infants
- Hypokalemia occurs 24 hrs after transfusion as the transfused cells correct their electrolyte composition and K^+ enters cells.
- Thus, metabolic acidosis and hyper K^+ occur first but net result is hypokalemia and alkalosis

IV. Hypernatremia:

- Serum Na^+ of whole blood and FFP > normal blood levels due to sodium citrate
- Hypernatremia occurs when large volume of plasma is given to patients with disordered salt and water handling: Liver disease, cardiac and renal disease
- Na^+ increases to 150–160 mm/L after 3 weeks of storage of plasma

V. Acid Base Abnormalities:

- Causes of acidosis of bank blood:
  - pH of storage media like CPDA is very low (5.5). When blood is added, its pH reduces to 7.0
  - Accumulation of lactic acid and pyruvate by RBC metabolism reduces pH further to 6.9 after 21 days storage
  - PCO_2 increases to 150–220 mm Hg as the plastic container does not provide air escape mechanisms for CO_2
- On blood transfusion, the citrate present in stored blood is metabolized in liver
- This generates large amounts of bicarbonate which may neutralize metabolic acidosis initially
- Thus, prophylactic sodium bicarbonate administration is not recommended
- Thus, initially, metabolic acidosis and hyperkalemia occur while later alkalosis and hypokalemia occur.

VI. Hypothermia:

- 1 unit of PRBCs at 40 °C will reduce core temperature of 70 kg patient by 0.25 °C
- *Blood warming device must be used for any transfusion requiring > 2 U blood*
- If < 30°C ventricular irritability and cardiac arrest occurs
- Safest method is passing blood through plastic coils or plastic cassettes in warm water bath (37–38 °C)
- Harmful effects of hypothermia:
  - Shifts ODC curve to left
  - Reduces metabolism of citrate, lactate and other drugs
  - Increased incidence of arrhythmias
  - Impairs hemostasis
  - Increases oxygen consumption
  - Increased postoperative infection
  - Masks clinical signs
  - Shivering increases O_2 consumption by 400%

VII. Tissue Oxygenation:

- Depletion of 2–3 DPG shifts ODC curve to left
- Tissue oxygen delivery is reduced
- Transfusion of 2,3 DPG depleted blood while increasing Hb, results in less efficient oxygen delivery
- After transfusion, 2,3-DPG returns to normal in 12-24 hrs

VIII. Hyperbilirubinemia:

- Jaundice as significant amounts of transfused blood may not survive
- Also, liver function may be impaired, particularly in the presence of sepsis or multi organ failure, paradoxical *conjugated hyper bilirubinemia* occurs
  - Increased load of bilirubin from destroyed RBCs occurs which is conjugated
  - There may be delayed excretion which causes conjugated hyperbilirubinemia

IX. Multiorgan Dysfunction:

- Due to lysis of RBCs during storage causing free Hb release
- This causes oxidant mediated injury causing MODS

X. Microaggregates:

- Platelet aggregates form during 2–5th day
- From 10 days onwards, larger aggregates form with:
  - Fibrin
  - Degenerated WBCs
  - Platelets
  - Size of 100-200 µm which can cause:
    - Acute lung injury
    - Hypoxemia
    - DIC and tissue ischemia
    - Complement activation
- Use filter when > 1 L of blood is transfused

TRANSFUSION RELATED ACUTE LUNG INJURY

Introduction

- Non cardiogenic pulmonary edema occurring after blood product administration
- Rare and potentially fatal complication of blood transfusion
- New acute lung injury occurring within 6 hours of a completed transfusion with:
  - Ratio of $PaO_2/FiO_2 < 300$ mm Hg
  - O_2 saturation measured by pulse oximetry of < 90% on room air
  - Bilateral infiltrates on chest X-ray
  - No evidence of left atrial HTN
- Possible TRALI:
  - When criteria for TRALI are present in a patient with pre-existing ARDS
  - *Terminology is no longer used*

Incidence

- Incidence of 0.04–0.1% of transfused patients
- 1:5000 units of blood components transfused
- Incidence in critically ill patients may increase upto 5–8%
- Mortality of at least 5%

Risk Factors

- Patient related risk factors:
  - Liver transplant surgery
  - Chronic alcohol abuse
  - Current smoking
  - Transfusion in trauma patients
  - Presence of shock prior to transfusion
  - Sepsis and systemic Inflammatory Response Syndrome (SIRS)
  - High peak airway pressure on mechanical ventilation
  - Positive fluid balance prior to transfusion
- Donor related risk factors: high risk of TRALI with:
  - Female donors
  - Multiparity
  - Presence of highly-reactive anti-HLA class II antibodies
- Blood component therapy related risk factors:
  - Associated with transfusion of all blood products:
    - Whole blood
    - PRBCS
    - FFP, platelets, cryoprecipitate
    - Intravenous immunoglobulin therapy
    - Granulocytes, stem cell preparation
  - Risk is highest with high-plasma-volume components:
    - Fresh frozen plasma
    - Single donor platelets SDP/apheresis platelets)
  - Whole blood

Pathogenesis

- Anti-granulocyte antibody theory:
  - Donor blood contains antibodies against recipient WBC antigen
  - Antigen-antibody binding occurs causing cellular activation
  - The activated neutrophils lodge in pulmonary capillaries
  - Reactive oxygen metabolites are released
  - This causes pulmonary endothelial leakage, capillary leakage and TRALI
- Granulocyte priming theory:
  - Transfused products contain biologically active substances such as:
    - Bioactive lipids such as lysophosphatidyl choline
    - Cytokines
  - These substances are called Biological Response Modifiers or BRM
  - BRMs can prune the activity of granulocytes in pulmonary vasculature
  - This causes increased vascular permeability leading to TRALI
- Knudsons two-hit hypothesis:
  - Most widely accepted hypothesis
  - TRALI occurs due to two-hit mechanism
  - Neutrophil sequestration and priming:
    - This is the first event
    - Caused by the recipients underlying clinical conditions like:
      - Surgery
      - Infection
      - Inflammation
    - These conditions result in endothelial injury
    - This causes neutrophil sequestration in the lung microvasculature
    - Neutrophils are then primed to respond to weaker stimuli
  - Neutrophil activation:
    - This is the second event

- Caused by transfusion of blood components with activating factors
- Activating factors include:
  - Donor anti-leukocyte antibodies
  - Biological response modifiers such as bio-active lipids
  - This results in activation of recipient neutrophils
- Activated neutrophils degranulate and release:
  - Cytokines
  - Reactive oxygen species
  - Oxidases
  - Proteases
- This causes damage to pulmonary capillary endothelium
- This results in capillary leak phenomenon and TRALI

❖ Other possible mechanisms:
- Direct injury to pulmonary endothelium
- Immune complex formation with complement activation
- Cytokine network activation
- BRM like interleukins causing direct injury
- Monocyte activation

Classification

❖ TRALI type I:
- No pre-existing risk factors for ARDS
- New acute lung injury occurring within 6 hours of a completed transfusion
- Presence of all clinical criteria:
  - Hypoxemia with:
    - Ratio of $PaO_2/FiO_2 < 300$ mm Hg
    - SpO_2 measured by pulse oximetry of < 90% on room air
  - Bilateral infiltrates on chest X-ray
  - No evidence of left atrial HTN
- No temporal relationship to an alternative risk factor for ARDS

❖ TRALI type II:
- Presence of pre-existing risk factors for ARDS
- Presence of ARDS with stable respiratory status 12 hours prior to transfusion
- Deterioration of respiratory status within 6 hours of blood transfusion:
  - Hypoxemia with:
    - Ratio of $PaO_2/FiO_2 < 300$ mm Hg
    - SpO_2 measured by pulse oximetry of < 90% on room air
  - Bilateral infiltrates on chest X-ray
  - No evidence of left atrial HTN

Clinical Features

❖ Acute onset dyspnea
❖ Severe hypoxemia
❖ Fever, chills, rigors
❖ Non-cardiogenic pulmonary edema, hypotension/hypertension
❖ In ventilated patients:
- Increased oxygen requirements in intubated patients
- Fluid in ET tube:
  - Occurs within 1–2 hours after transfusion
  - Maximal within 6 hours of transfusion
  - PaO_2 levels usually return to normal within 48-96 hours

Investigations

❖ Chest X-ray:
- Shows bilateral chest infiltrates with normal cardiac silhouette
- Chest X-ray infiltrates may persist for 7 days post-transfusion

❖ Edema fluid analysis:
- Undiluted edema fluid obtained from ETT can be analysed
- Edema fluid protein: plasma protein ratio is calculated
- Ratio ≥ 0.6 suggests TRALI rather than TACO

❖ Complete blood count shows:
- Hemoconcentration
- Neutrophil count:
  - Initial neutropenia as pulmonary neutrophil sequestration occurs
  - This is followed by neutrophilia

❖ Sudden reduction in serum albumin

Differential Diagnosis

❖ ***Transfusion associated circulatory overload (TACO)***:
- Raised JVP
- Increased systolic BP at the time dyspnea develops
- Widened pulmonary vascular pedicle on chest X-ray
- Increased BNP shortly after transfusion

❖ ARDS
❖ Sepsis
❖ Hemolytic transfusion reaction
❖ Anaphylaxis due to transfusion of IgA containing products to a recipient with IgA deficiency

Diagnostic Criteria

- Onset of lung dysfunction within 6 hours of transfusion
- Acute lung injury as evidenced by:
  - Acute onset of signs and symptoms
  - Hypoxemia:
    - $PaO_2/FiO_2 < 300$ mm Hg
    - Room air $SpO_2 < 90\%$
    - Other clinical evidence of hypoxemia
  - Bilateral infiltrates on chest X-ray without cardiomegaly
  - No clinical evidence of left atrial HTN (PCWP) < 18 mm Hg)

Prevention

- Avoid multiparous female donors
- Avoidance of donors implicated in prior TRALI reactions
- ***Prestorage leucoreduction is useful***
- Limit preparation of high plasma volume components from donors known to be leukocyte alloimmunized
- Substitution of FFP with pooled solvent detergent plasma
- HLA antibody testing and screening

Treatment

- *Immediately stop blood transfusion*
- Mainly supportive hemodynamic& ventilatory support
- Ventilatory support:
  - Supplemental O_2 if mild manifestations
  - Non-invasive ventilation for moderate symptoms (CPAP/BiPAP)
  - Mechanical ventilation for severe TRALI: protective-lung ventilation:
    - FiO_2 titrated to maintain:
      - PaO_2 55–80 mm Hg
      - SpO_2 88–95%
    - Low tidal volume (6–7 mL/kg)
    - Optimal PEEP to prevent barotrauma (high PEEP may be required)
    - Limit plateau pressure to < 30 cm H_2O
    - Limit mean airway pressure < 40 cm H_2O
- Hemodynamic support:
  - Fluid resuscitation and vasoactive support
  - Diuretics:
    - Have no therapeutic role in TRALI
    - Can be used to differentiate TRALI from TACO
- High-dose corticosteroids:
  - Have been tried to reduce complement mediated granulocyte activation
  - Lack of evidence to support routine use
  - May cause harm when initiated > 2 weeks after syndrome onset
  - Thus, routine use is not recommended
- Additional transfusions:
  - No risk for recurrent episodes following transfusion from other donors
  - Additional products from different donors may be transfused
- Investigational therapies:
  - HMG-CoA reductase inhibitors (statins)
  - Aspirin
  - Prostaglandin E_1

JEHOVAHS WITNESS

Introduction

Christian movement with following beliefs:

- Prohibits consumption of blood
- Belief prevents them from accepting whole blood and its primary components
- Belief that blood which is removed from body is unclean and should be disposed
- Believe procedures with removal and storage of their own blood is unacceptable

Legal Issues

Consent

- Procurement of informed consent before any medical intervention
- Special consent forms with section for specific exclusion from consent
- Patient interviewed in the presence of independent witness while obtaining consent

Children

- Full and frank discussion between anesthetist, surgeon and parents
- Children under 16 yrs can give consent themselves if they understand the issues involved (***Gillicks competence***)
- If consent for transfusion is refused:
  - An application is made to high court
  - Application for specific issue order which allows transfusion without removing parental authority
- In emergencies, blood should be given.

Emergencies

- Perform blood transfusion if Jehovahs witness status unknown
- If relatives suggest patients may not accept blood transfusion, documentation of same to be done
- If refusal of transfusion consent is retracted, make a witnessed entry in patients notes

Anesthetic Considerations

- Preoperative planning, preparation essential for successful outcome
- Unlawful to administer blood to a Jehovahs Witness patient who has expressly forbidden it
- Acute Normovolemic Hemodilution often un-acceptable to JW patient as it involves removal and storage of blood before transfusion
- Intraoperative blood salvage may be acceptable to some if:
  - Blood is not stored
  - Circuitry is designed so that it remains in continuity with patients own circulation
- Patients may refuse blood component therapy too
- ***Bloodless medicine***: Team which reduces blood loss and uses best available alternatives to allogenic transfusion therapy

Preoperative Preparation

- Optimize Hb%, treat anemia
- Optimize nutritional feeding: enteral supple-mentation or TPN
- Drugs:
  - To increase RBC production: Iron, folate, Vitamin B_{12}, Erythropoietin
  - To promote clotting: Vitamin K
- Management of anticoagulant therapy and congenital/drug induced coagulopathies
- Restricted diagnostic phlebotomy
- Prophylactic embolization:
  - Pelvic tumors
  - Vascular tumor like metastasis
  - Aneurysmal bone cyst
- Prescribe for cell salvage apparatus

Intraoperative Management

- Choice of technique:
  - Prefer laparoscopic surgery
  - Prefer regional anesthetic technique
  - Invasive monitoring with IBP and CVP
  - Hypotensive anesthesia techniques
- Physiology:
  - Proper positioning: lateral position for THR
  - Maintain normothermia
  - Avoid hypoventilation and hypercarbia
  - Avoid high intrathoracic pressures
- Recent advances:
  - Intraoperative blood salvage
  - Acute normovolemic hemodilution (ANH)
  - Acute hypervolemic hemodilution (AHH)
  - Use of blood substitutes
  - Reduced transfusion trigger to 7g%
- Drugs to enhance hemostasis:
  - Factor VII a
  - Tranexemic acid: 10 mg/kg IV upto 30 mg/kg/day
  - Aprotinin
  - Ethamsylate
  - Desmopressin
- Adequate topical hemostasis:
  - Argon lazer beam cautery (diathermy)
  - Spray coagulation
  - Use of arterial tourniquet
  - Avoid large abdominal packs
  - Hemostats:
    - Collagen and cellulose pads (***Kaltostat***)
    - Fibrin glue (***Tisseal***)

Postoperative Management

- Good compressive padded dressing
- Limb elevation in TKR
- Maintain normothermia
- Adequate analgesia
- Stop bleeding sources
- Maintain hypotension/prevent normotension till bleeding stops
- Oral/parental iron therapy
- Erythropoietin therapy
- Appropriate fluid and volume management
- Reduce transfusion trigger
- Postoperative blood salvage
- Restricted diagnostic phlebotomies
- Prevent and treat coagulation disorders promptly

Hematology and Oncology

- Individualized chemotherapy regimens to reduce hematotoxicity
- Embolization of vascular tumors
- Restricted diagnostic phlebotomy
- Tolerance of anemia
- Pharmacological prophylaxis of bleeding

BLOODLESS MEDICINE

Introduction

- Bloodless medicine is defined as a team approach that reduces blood loss and uses the best available alternatives to allogenic transfusion therapy, while focusing on the provision of the best possible medical care to all patients
- Mainly started for Jehovahs Witnesses who refuse transfusion based on interpretation of Old and New testament tests

Principles of Bloodless Medicine

Preoperative Assessment and Planning

- Management of anemia, optimize preoperative Hb
- Management of anticoagulation, congenital and drug induced coagulopathies
- Prophylactic interventional radiology and embolization
- Restricted diagnostic phlebotomy
- Prescribing and scheduling of cell salvage apparatus
- Optimize nutritional status:
  - Total Parenteral Nutrition
  - Supplemental enteral feeds
- Drugs to increase RBC production:
  - Iron
  - Vitamin B_{12} and folate
  - Erythropoietin
  - Drugs to Promote Clotting: Vitamin K

Intraoperative Blood Conservation

- Argon beam diathermy
- Use of tourniquet
- Avoid large surgical packs
- Meticulous surgical hemostasis
- Pharmaceutical enhancement of hemostasis: fibrin glue
- Hypotensive anesthesia
- Regional anesthetic technique
- Reduce transfusion trigger
- Surgical positioning to minimize blood loss
- Intraoperative blood salvage
- Hypotensive anesthesia
- Recombinant factor VII, tranexemic acid, aprotinin, desmopressin

Postoperative Blood Conservation

- Adequate analgesia
- Good padded compressive dressing
- Maintenance of normothermia
- Maintain limb elevation post TKR
- Stop bleeding if active bleed present
- Avoid attempts to normalize BP until bleeding has stopped
- Oral/parenteral iron to improve iron stores.
- Exogenous erythropoietin therapy effectively increases RBC mass

Hematology and Oncology

- Aggressive exogenous erythropoietin and iron therapy for prophylaxis of anemia
- Individualized chemotherapy protocols to minimize hematologic toxicity
- Tolerance of anemia
- Pharmacological prophylaxis and treatment of bleeding
- Restricted diagnostic phlebotomy

Advantages

- Eliminates risk of transfusion reactions
- Eliminates risk of disease transmission
- Eliminates risk of alloimmunization to RBCs, WBCs
- Reduces demand on blood supply
- Eliminates risk of TA-GVHD

PERIOPERATIVE BLOOD CONSERVATION STRATEGY

Preoperative Strategies

- Preoperative autologous blood donation (PABD)
- Preoperative arterial embolization

Intraoperative Strategies

- Anesthetic modifications:
  - Regional anesthetic technique
  - Proper positioning
  - Normothermia
  - Pharmacological agents:
    - Erythropoietin
    - Blood substitutes
    - DDAVP
    - Antifibrinolytics
  - Hypotensive anesthesia
  - Acute Normovolemic Hemodilution (ANH)
  - Intraoperative blood salvage
- Surgical modification:
  - Topical hemostasis with fibrin glue
  - Tourniquet

Postoperative Strategies

- Postoperative blood salvage
- Good padded compressive dressing
- Limb elevation post-TKR

AUTOLOGOUS BLOOD TRANSFUSION

Introduction

- Refers to the transfusions in which the donor and the recipient are the same
- Aims to decrease the incidence of complications associated with allogenic transfusion

Types

- Preoperative autologous blood donation (PABD)
- Intraoperative blood salvage
- Postoperative blood salvage
- Acute normovolemic hemodilution (ANH)

Advantages

- Eliminates risk of transfusion reactions
- Eliminates risk of disease transmission:
  - HIV
  - HTLV
  - Hepatitis virus
  - Variant Creutzfeldt- Jakob disease (vCJD)
- Eliminates risk of allo-immunization to RBC, WBC, platelets
- Eliminates risk of transfusion associated-GVH disease (TA-GVHD)
- Safe transfusion in patients with:
  - Multiple allo-antibodies
  - Rare blood group
- Safe and acceptable blood cover in ***Jehovahs witness*** patients
- Readily available blood in major hemorrhage
- Reduces demand on homologous blood supply
- Hemodilution improves tissue perfusion by reducing blood viscosity
- Preoperative donation stimulates erythropoiesis prior to surgery

Disadvantages

- Expensive equipment and trained staff required: may not be cost effective
- Complex logistics required for collection, storage, and transfusion
- Bacterial contamination of collected blood bag is still possible
- Tendency to over-transfuse patient
- Patient may become grossly anemic and develop coagulation defects during collection
- Suitable for certain operative procedures only
- If surgery delayed blood becomes outdated and may cause wastage

PREOPERATIVE AUTOLOGOUS DONATION

Introduction

- Procedure in which:
  - Patients own blood is collected, through repeated phlebotomies
  - Blood is collected over a span of 4-5 weeks
  - Blood is re-transfused during the surgery
- However, use of preoperative autologous blood transfusion is declining due to:
  - Increased wastage of autologous blood
  - Improved safety of allogenic blood

Patient Selection

- Patients in whom elective surgery can be scheduled several weeks in future
- Surgical procedure for which blood is usually cross matched
- Hb $\geq$ 11 g % or HCT > 33%
- May donate upto 10.5 mL/kg excluding samples for testing
- No weight/age bar
- No medical contraindication for donation of blood

Indications

- Elective surgeries which may require > 4 units of RBC transfusion such as:
  - Cardiac surgery
  - Major vascular surgery
  - Liver transplantation
  - Prostatectomy
  - Major orthopedic surgeries: Spine, THR, TKR, etc.
- Jehovahs witness patients
- Patients with:
  - Rare blood groups
  - Multiple RBC antibodies causing difficulty in cross matching allogenic blood

Techniques

- Blood is collected at the nearest blood collection facility
- Blood collection:

- Optimal donating period begins 4–5 weeks before surgery in order to:
  - Allow sufficient number of units to be collected
  - Also to enable more complete RBC regeneration before surgery
- Blood is usually donated at weekly intervals
- Frequency of blood donation depends upon the physical status of the patient
- Approximately 450 mL of blood is collected during each phlebotomy
- Up to a maximum of 4 units of blood can be collected or 11 mL/Kg

❖ Serological testing:
- Collected blood is subjected to minimal compatibility testing
- Cross matching is recommended prior to issuing for transfusion

❖ Storage:
- Blood is collected in citrate-phosphate-dextrose bags and stored conventionally
- Volume of anticoagulant to be added depends on the collected blood volume
- Collected blood has shelf life of 35 days
- Collected blood is stored till patients are discharged/till unit become outdated

❖ Last blood donation:
- Usually done 2 weeks prior to surgery
- Not to be collected later than 72 hours before surgery
- This is to allow adequate time for restoration of intravascular volume

❖ Transfusion:
- Blood drawn last is usually given first in PABD
- Blood is usually cross matched immediately prior to transfusion
- This is to avoid clerical transfusion errors

❖ Prevention of preoperative anemia:
- Iron supplementation:
  - Administered only in previously iron-deficient patients
  - It is not helpful in patients who are iron-replete prior to PABD
  - Patient receives supplemental iron 2 mg/kg/day × 3 weeks
  - Supplementation is given in the form of:
    - Ferrous sulphate 325 mg PO TID
    - Ferrous gluconate 325 mg five times a day
  - IV supplementation is used in patients who do not tolerate PO doses
  - Iron supplementation increases RBC expansion from 14% to 19%
- Erythropoietin:
  - Useful in anemic patients undergoing PABD
  - Given in doses of 12,000–40,000 IU per week
  - Has to be accompanied by iron supplementation
  - Risk of thromboembolic events precludes routine use in all patients

Contraindications

❖ Active bacterial infection, especially with Yersinia enterocolitica

❖ History of indwelling urinary catheter/device penetrating skin Cardiac disease:
- Significant AS
- Cyanotic heart disease
- Uncontrolled HTN
- Frequent unstable angina
- High grade left-main coronary artery disease
- History of MI/CVA within 6 months of the planned donation

❖ Active seizure disorder

❖ Pre-existing anemia with Hb < 11 gm%

❖ Hemorrhagic shock

❖ Reschedulable surgical procedure to reduce the risk of wastage

Advantages

❖ Eliminates need for allogenic transfusions:
- Technique provides upto 4 units of blood prior to surgery
- This may eliminate the need for allogenic transfusion

❖ Reduces the complications associated with allogenic transfusion:
- Viral transmission
- Immunologically mediated reactions
- Febrile and allergic reactions
- Immunomodulation
- TRALI

❖ May reduce the risk of postoperative infections

❖ Metabolically superior to allogenic blood:
- Low K^+ compared to stored blood
- Relatively normal pH, normothermic
- Functionally superior cells
- High levels of 2,3 DPG

❖ Stimulates erythropoiesis:
- Repeated preoperative phlebotomies stimulates erythropoiesis
- This enables regeneration of hemoglobin at an accelerated rate postoperatively

Disadvantages

- Requires planning well ahead of surgery
- May be logistically difficult, especially if surgery is re-schedulable
- Expenses may be more than allogenic transfusions owing to:
  - Equipment used
  - Wastage of blood products
- Preoperative blood donation may not be tolerated by all patients
- Certain complications of allogenic transfusion persist:
  - Risk of bacterial infections
  - Metabolic derangements
  - Transfusion associated circulatory overload (TACO)
- Wastage:
  - Blood may have to be discarded if not transfused to the patient
  - This is because autologous blood is not subjected to testing as allogenic blood
  - Thus, it cannot be used as allogenic blood, to transfuse other patients
  - Incidence of wastage may reach up to 50% of autologous units
- Clerical error: Can administer wrong unit of blood to patients
- Preoperative anemia due to PAD:
  - Patient undergoes elective surgery with a low starting hematocrit
  - This may increase the rate of overall perioperative transfusion

Complications

- Risk of bacterial contamination during phlebotomy
- Hemolysis due to improper:
  - Collection techniques
  - Handling and storage techniques
  - Transfusion techniques
- Vasovagal attack during blood donation
- Transfusion associated circulatory overload
- Human errors in transfusing blood like transfusing wrong unit of blood
- Iatrogenic preoperative anemia, MI/cerebral hypoxia

Special Considerations

- Elderly patients above 60 years:
  - PABD is generally avoided in this age group
  - However, it may be used for rare blood phenotypes if:
    - Physiological conditions permit
    - No major underlying disease
- Pediatric patients:
  - In general, children >30 kg preferred
  - Has been done in children 8 years old also
  - Venous access and emotional tolerance of venepuncture limits collection
- Obstetric patients:
  - PABD is usually not required in obstetric patients
  - Can be considered in:
    - Patients with auto-antibodies to multiple antigens
    - Placenta previa

Cross Over Usage

- Unused autologous blood may be used for homologous transfusion to other patients
- This is called crossover ***usage***
- Advantages:
  - Increases total available blood supply
  - Reduces overall cost of blood transfusions
- No longer recommended as:
  - Autologous blood is not sufficiently tested prior to storage
  - Thus, safety for cross-over usage may be suboptimal
  - Autologous donors are not voluntary donors

INTRAOPERATIVE BLOOD SALVAGE

Introduction

- Refers to collection, processing and reinfusion of blood lost during surgery

Indications: AOA 2018 Guidelines

- Surgeries with anticipated extensive blood loss:
  - Blood loss volume:
    - More than 500 mL in adults
    - More than 8 mL/kg in children weighing >10 kg
    - More than 10% of calculated total blood volume in any age group
  - Examples:
    - Cardiac surgery, aortic reconstruction surgery
    - Orthopedic surgery:
      - Spine instrumentation
      - Joint arthroplasty
      - Liver transplant
      - Splenectomy

- Trauma patients
- Ruptured ectopic pregnancy
- May be indicated for transfusion in:
  - Patients with rare blood group phenotypes
  - Patients with multiple RBC alloantibodies
  - Jehovahs witness patients

Characteristics of Salvaged Blood

- Salvaged blood is more alkaline
- Similar oxygen carrying capacity as allogenic blood
- Better oxygen-offloading capability compared with allogenic blood
- P_{50} of salvaged blood is higher than for allogenic stored blood
- 2,3 DPG levels are normal (allogenic blood has reduced 2,3-DPG)
- Hematocrit of 50–60%
- Free Hb levels of 200–500 mg% is common
- FDP and complement activation is present
- Platelets and coagulation factors are deficient

Steps of Cell Salvage

- Suctioning of shed blood from the surgical field
- Addition of anticoagulant
- Separation and washing of RBCs
- Concentration of blood
- Re-transfusion to the patient

Technique

- Cell salvage device used to salvage blood from operative field
- Suctioning:
  - Suctioning is done from the surgical field
  - Blood can also be obtained from blood soaked surgical gauze pads
  - Recommended maximum vacuum setting for suction is < 150 mm Hg
  - Suction should be done from within the blood pool and not at blood-air interface
  - This is because suctioning at the blood-air interface causes hemolysis
- Anticoagulation:
  - Salvaged blood is anticoagulated prior to processing to prevent clotting
  - Heparin:
    - Heparin is the most commonly used anticoagulant
    - It is prepared as a solution with normal saline (30,000 IU/L)
    - This solution is slowly added to blood at a rate of 15 mL/100 mL blood
    - Thus, salvaged blood is continually washed with heparinized saline
  - Citrate based anticoagulants:
    - Used when heparin is contraindicated
    - CPD or CPD-A may be used
    - These are added in a concentration of 15 mL citrate per 100 mL blood
- RBC separation and concentration:
  - Aspirated blood is collected in a sterile, filtered reservoir
  - Processing is initiated once 350–700 mL volume has been collected
  - Salvaged blood is first pumped into a centrifugation bowl
  - Here, higher density RBCs are separated and concentrated
  - Plasma, platelets and waste components are sent to the waste bag
  - Salvaged blood is then washed with isotonic saline to separate:
    - Free hemoglobin
    - Cellular debris
  - Collected blood is not mixed with hypotonic solutions as it causes hemolysis
  - The washed blood is then pumped into a blood salvage bag for reperfusion
  - 500–70 mL collected blood produces 225–500 mL of salvaged blood
  - This salvaged PRBC unit has a HCT of 50–60%
- Re-transfusion of salvaged blood:
  - Re-transfusion is typically performed using micro-aggregate (40 μm) filters
  - LR filters should be used if available for transfusion of salvaged blood
  - Leukoreduction filters help in filtering:
    - WBCs
    - Bacteria
    - Cancer cells
    - Fat particles
    - Amniotic fluid

Shelf Life

- Storage at room temperature for recovered blood: 4 hours
- At 1–6 °C for 24 hours provided:
  - It has been collected under aseptic precautions
  - Salvaged blood has been washed
  - Storage has begun within 4 hours of completing collection

Contraindications

- Absolute contraindications:
  - Intraoperative irrigation with solutions causing intravascular toxicity:
    - Antibiotic solutions
    - Povidone-iodine solutions
    - Hydrogen peroxide
  - Intraoperative blood contamination with tissues:
    - Bowel contents
    - Amniotic fluid: risk of amniotic fluid embolism
  - Intraoperative blood contamination with hemostatic products:
    - Bone cement
    - Topical thrombin
    - Fibrin glue
- Relative contraindications:
  - Bacterial contamination of the surgical wound:
    - Minimal risk of sepsis exists
    - Reduction of risk of sepsis with salvaged blood is due to:
      - Periprocedural washing of RBCs
      - Use of leukocyte filters during transfusion
  - Active malignancy:
    - Minor risk of metastasis following cell salvage exists
    - Periprocedural washing does not reduce risk of metastasis
    - Use of leucocyte filters reduces the risk of metastasis
  - Sickle cell disease due to increased risk of hemolysis following transfusion
  - Cold agglutinin disease

Advantages

- Eliminates need for allogenic transfusions
- Reduces the complications associated with allogenic transfusion:
  - Viral transmission
  - Immunologically mediated reactions
  - Febrile and allergic reactions
  - Immunomodulation
  - TRALI
- May reduce the risk of postoperative infections
- Logistical benefits:
  - Eliminates risk of transfusing wrong unit of blood as seen with PABD
  - Avoids repeated preoperative visits as required for phlebotomy in PABD
  - Readily available as it is done in the operating room itself
- Requires no preoperative preparation of the patient
- Useful for transfusion in:
  - Patients with rare blood group phenotypes
  - Patients with multiple RBC alloantibodies
  - Jehovahs witness patients
- Eliminates side effects resulting from:
  - Antifibrinolytic agents
  - Clotting factors

Complications

- Non-immune hemolysis
- Immune hemolysis
- Renal failure due to free hemoglobin
- Bacterial contamination
- Air embolism, amniotic fluid embolism
- Reinfusion of debris from surgical field:
  - Fat, air
  - Platelets, lymphocytes, free Hb, RBC stroma
  - Heparin, bacteria
  - Debris like PMMA/bone cement
- Dilutional coagulopathy as all clotting factors and platelets are removed by washing

POSTOPERATIVE BLOOD SALVAGE

Introduction

Refers to postoperative recovery of defibrinogenated blood with immediate reinfusion of unwashed blood through 40 μm microaggregate filters.

Indications

- Cardiac surgery:
  - Entails reinfusion of blood from mediastinal tubes
  - This may affect lab tests like creatinine kinase
  - Increased CK may be present even though no peri-operative MI has occurred
  - Blood collected from heart lung machine can be transfused back after processing
  - Indications in cardiac surgery include:
    Reoperations
    When mediastinal drains exceed 100 mL/hour
- Orthopedic surgery:
  - Main setting in which postoperative blood salvage is used
  - Surgeries for which it is indicated include:
    - TKR
    - THR
    - Spinal fusion or instrumentation

- Posttraumatic salvage:
  - Following chest/abdominal trauma
  - Blood from hemothorax/hemoperitoneum

Types of Postoperative Cell Salvage

- Washed postoperative cell salvage:
  - Blood collected is subjected to centrifugation
  - Higher density RBCs are separated and concentrated
  - Salvaged RBCs are then washed with isotonic saline to separate:
    - Free hemoglobin
    - Cellular debris
  - Collected blood is not mixed with hypotonic solutions as it causes hemolysis
  - Used predominantly for cardiac surgery as recovered blood has:
    - Fat cells
    - Other contaminants due to use of bone cement
- Unwashed postoperative cell salvage:
  - Blood collected is not subjected to centrifugation
  - It is directly transfused back to the patient through microaggregate filters
  - Used predominantly for orthopedic surgery

Technique

- Blood salvaged post operatively is collected from mediastinal/chest/joint drains and transfused back without washing
- Being defibrinogenated, it does not require anti-coagulation prior to transfusion
- Upto 1400 mL of unprocessed blood can be reinfused as it has high concentration of cytokines
- If transfusion of blood has not begun within 6 hrs of initiating collection, the blood must be discarded
- Shelf life of 6 hrs

Complications

- Theoretical risk of reinfusion of:
  - Free Hb, RBC stroma
  - Marrow fat, tissue debris
  - Toxic irritants/methacrylate debris
  - FDPs and complement
- Risk of bacterial contamination if storage time > 6 hours
- Coagulopathy:
  - Postoperative blood salvage replaces only RBCs
  - Thus, mild coagulopathy develops as:
    - Platelets are deranged: prolonged bleeding time
    - No clotting factors are present: prolonged PT, aPTT
- Renal insufficiency if large amounts of free Hb present
- Air embolism:
  - The cell saver can to pump massive volumes of air into blood bag
  - This can result in air embolism during retransfusion
  - Blood bag must therefore be disconnected from cell-saver prior to transfusion
- Complement activation causing:
  - Non cardiogenic pulmonary edema
  - Upper airway edema
- Transfusion associated circulatory overload

ACUTE NORMOVOLEMIC HEMODILUTION

Introduction

- Method of intraoperative blood conservation
- Whole blood is removed from the patient while restoring intravascular volume with:
  - Crystalloids 3 mL per mL of blood removed
  - Colloids 1 mL per mL of blood removed
- For augmented hemodilution, blood is replaced with synthetic O_2 carriers
- Blood is collected on the day of surgery rather than over several weeks as in PABD
- Also in PABD, no crystalloids are given to increase the blood volume

Advantages

- Reduces amount of allogenic blood transfusion to 1–2 units/patient
- Provides fresh supply of coagulation factors and platelets
- Tissue perfusion is improved with hemodilution as blood viscosity is reduced
- Patients loses blood of low HCT intraoperatively
- Withdrawn blood is reinfused at the end of surgery: less Hb is lost in blood
- Blood component sequestration:
  - Blood is collected intraoperatively
  - It is subjected to various procedures like apheresis and centrifugation
  - Individual blood components are separated
- Acute hypervolemic hemodilution:
  - Involves rapid infusion of fluid to achieve hemodilution without prior withdrawal of blood

- Associated changes:
  - Decrease in PCV and SVRI by around 30%
  - Increase in CI and LVEDP
  - Increase in PAP and PCWP which normalize on stoppage of surgery
  - Slight increase in MAP and decrease in HR,
  - Low chance of pulmonary edema

Patient Selection Criteria

- For surgeries where likelihood of transfusion exceeds 10%
- Preoperative Hb level is at least 12 g%
- Absence of clinically significant coronary pulmonary, renal/liver disease
- Absence of severe HTN
- Absence of infection and risk of bacteremia

Contraindications

- Absolute contraindications:
  - Severe anemia with Hb < 8 gm/dL
  - Hemorrhagic shock
  - LV dysfunction with EF < 45%
  - Hemostatic disorders
  - Limited ability to increase cardiac output like AS, LV dysfunction
  - Respiratory failure
  - End Stage Renal Disease
  - Severe sepsis
- Relative contraindications:
  - Less severe anemia with Hb < 11 g/dL
  - Severe respiratory distress
  - CCF/LV dysfunction
  - History of stroke
  - CAD/carotid artery disease
  - Inadequate vascular access

Compensatory Mechanisms in ANH

- Blood:
  - Reduced blood viscosity
  - Reduced RBC aggregation
  - Shift of ODC to right
  - Reduced oxygen carrying capacity (below 30%)
- Oxygen utilization: Increased blood flow to tissues with increased O_2 extraction
- Cardiac:
  - Increased cardiac output
  - Coronary vasodilatation
- Cerebral: Increased cerebral blood flow: Hyper-ventilation avoided
- GIT:
  - Increased HbF
  - Increased O_2 extraction in liver
  - Centrilobular hepatic necrosis
- Renal: Renal vasoconstriction causing decrease in fraction of CO to kidneys
- Pregnancy: ANH done with caution as reduction in material HCT reduces placental perfusion

Technique

- Informed consent
- Timing:
  - Prior to induction of anesthesia with awake patient is better
  - Usually done after induction of anesthesia
  - Terminated when:
    - Calculated blood volume has been withdrawn
    - Surgical bleeding becomes significant
- Blood collection:
  - Site of collection:
    - Peripheral line not preferred as tube resistance and sludging occurs
    - Arterial line not used as we cannot monitor IBP during procedure
    - Central venous line is *best* and IJV/subclavian vein used
  - Calculation of volume to be collected:
    - Calculates estimated blood volume (EBV)
    - EBV = 70 mL/kg in females and 75 mL/kg in males
    - Baseline HCT noted
    - Target HCT:
      - 8 g/dL in healthy patients
      - 10 g % if CVS/RS/CNS disease

$$\text{Calculate average HCT} = \frac{\text{Baseline HCT} + \text{Target HCT}}{2}$$

$$\text{Volume of blood collectable} = \frac{\text{Baseline HCT} - \text{Target HCT}}{\text{Average HCT} \times \text{EBV}}$$

  - Anticoagulation of specimen:
    - CPD anticoagulant is added to blood collection bag
    - This is then attached to a port in the IV line
  - Sample collection:
    - 450 mL of blood is collected per bag
    - Collect whole blood and mix blood in bag with CPD
    - Typically 1–3 units of blood may be removed
    - Bag is agitated using a mechanical agitator
    - This prevents platelet aggregation and preserves platelet function

- Asanguinous fluid administration:
  - 3 mL crystalloid replaced for every 1 mL blood collected
  - 1 mL colloid replaced for every 1 mL blood collected
  - Blood collection and fluid infusion should not mix if multi-lumen CV line is used
- Storage:
  - Can be stored at room temperature (22 °C) for up to 8 hours
  - Collected blood can be refrigerated at 1-6 °C for up to 24 hours
  - Intermittent agitation done to ensure that sludging does not occur

❖ Reinfusion of whole blood:
- Given according to surgical condition
- Any remaining blood given in operating theatre or refrigerated
- Diuretic given if risk of hypervolemia
- Last collected blood infused first as when whole blood is collected with ANH, each subsequent unit becomes more dilute

❖ Monitoring during ANH:
- Heart rate, BP
- Capnography
- ECG
- Pulse oximetry
- If more advanced cases, with large volume of blood sequestered:
- CVP/PAP
- Cardiac output
- Trans-esophageal echocardiography

Complications

❖ Iatrogenic anemia may not be safe

❖ MI/cerebral hypoxia possible if severe hemodilution

❖ Bleeding diathesis during surgery due to:
- Dilutional thrombocytopenia
- Hypofibrinogenemia as coagulation factors are being sequestered

❖ Volume overload

FIBRIN GEL

❖ Blood derivatives derived from a source of fibrin and factor XIII (fibrin stabilizing factor) in which a solution of fibrinogen is mixed with a solution of thrombin and applied to surgical field

❖ Applied directly to wounds which display diffuse microvascular bleeding.

❖ Risk of anaphylaxis and HIV transmission present

❖ Also topical use of fibrin sprays, bone wax/surgical/platelet gel

DRUGS

❖ Erythropoietin:
- Indications:
  - If patient cannot undergo PABD due to anemia/limited time to donate blood
  - Now used in PABD to reduce blood transfusion in major surgeries, Jehovahs witness
  - Used for in anemic patients undergoing renal dialysis
- Efficacy:
  - Erythropoiesis is seen in 3 days
  - Equivalent of 1 unit of blood produced in 70 days
  - Always administered with iron supplementation (IV iron saccharate)
- Dosage:
  - 300 U/Kg for 15 days beginning 10 days before surgery
  - 600 U/kg weekly once starting 3 wks before surgery
  - One more 600 U/kg dose administered on the day of surgery
- HTN and seizures occur in patients with CRF and rare thrombotic events

❖ Desmopressin: Synthetic vasopressin analogue

❖ Tranexemic acid:
- Antifibrinolytic agent
- Mechanism of action:
  - Forms a reversible complex with fibrin
  - This displaces plasminogen from fibrin
- Common indications:
  - Cardiac surgery
  - Liver transplantation
  - Hip/knee arthroplasty
  - Spine surgery
  - Prostate surgery
  - Trauma surgeries
- Dose:
  - 10–30 mg/kg bolus dose at a rate < 100 mg/minute
  - This may be followed by an infusion 1–16 mg/kg/hour
  - Dose reduction is required for renal failure patients

- Pharmacokinetics:
  - Oral bioavailability: 45%
  - Volume of distribution: 9–12 litres
  - Plasma protein binding: 3%
  - Excreted > 95% unchanged in urine
  - Elimination T ½ = 2–11 hours
- Adverse effects:
  - Thrombotic events:
    - Data supporting increased risk of thrombosis is limited
    - However, risk may be patient and procedure specific
  - Seizures with high doses (> 50 mg/kg)

OTHER MEASURES

- Position of patient:
  - Bleeding during THR is less with patient in lateral position than in supine
  - Elevation of lower limb after TKR reduces postoperative blood loss
- Maintain normothermia
- Controlled hypotensive spinal/epidural/general anesthesia with additives like clonidine
- Preoperative arterial embolization for:
  - Pelvic fractures
  - Surgery on vascular tumors like:
    - Metastasis
    - Aneurysmal bone cysts
- Efficient padded compressive dressing for tamponade effect

RECOMBINANT FACTOR SEVEN

Introduction

- Recombinant factor VIIa (rf-VIIa) or novoseven manufactured by Novo Nordisk
- Produced by transfection of human factor VII gene into cultured hamster cells
- Used to promote hemostasis in patients with coagulopathies

Chemistry and Preparation

- Chemistry:
  - It is a vitamin-K dependant glycoprotein
  - Contains 406 amino acid residues with molecular weight 50 kDa
  - Is structurally similar to human plasma derived factor VIIa
- Preparation:
  - Supplied as a sterile white lyophilized powder of factor VIIa in single use vial
  - Can be stored at room temperature (up to 25 °C)
  - Diluent is a 10 mmol solution of histidine in water, for injection
- After reconstitution:
  - Each vial contains 1 mg/mL of novoseven
  - Should be administered within 4 hours of reconstitution
  - Beneficial effects are seen within 60 minutes of administration
- Pharmacokinetics:
  - Volume of distribution 103 mL/kg
  - Clearance 33 mL/kg/hour
  - $T_{1/2}$ 2 hours
- In pregnancy/lactating mothers:
  - Paucity of data for use of factor seven during pregnancy
  - *Category C drug*
  - Should be used only if potential benefits exceeds potential risks to fetus
  - Still not known if it is excreted in human milk

Mechanism of Action

- Activates *extrinsic pathway* of the coagulation cascade at physiological doses:
  - Recombinant VIIa complexes with tissue factor
  - This can activate factor X to factor Xa as well as factor IX to IXa
  - Factor Xa complexes with other factors and converts prothrombin to thrombin
  - This results in occurrence of a ***Thrombin burst***
  - This leads to the conversion of fibrinogen to fibrin
  - This results in formation of hemostatic plug and local hemostasis
- At high supra-physiological doses:
  - Binds to the surface of activated platelets
  - Promotes activation of factor X and thrombin generation
  - This accentuates platelet activation and local aggregation of platelets

Indications

- On-label indications:
  - Hemophilia A or B with inhibitors to exogenous factor VIII or IX preparations
  - Congenital factor VII deficiency
  - ***Glanzmanns thrombasthenia***

- Off-label indications:
  - Congenital hemostatic disorders:
    - Factor XI deficiency
    - von Willebrand disease
    - Inherited disorders of platelet function
  - Acquired hemostatic disorders:
    - Warfarin, LMWH, direct thrombin inhibitors
    - Antiplatelet agents
    - Selective Xa inhibitors: fondaparinux
  - Reduction of perioperative blood loss:
    - Orthotopic liver transplantation
    - Liver biopsy
    - Cardiac surgery
    - Retropubic prostatectomy
    - Jehovahs witness
  - Other causes of bleeding:
    - Liver diseases
    - Trauma
    - Gastrointestinal bleeding
    - Obstetrical hemorrhage
- Off-label indications with questionable benefit:
  - No survival benefit has been shown with use of novoseven in:
    - Trauma
    - Liver transplantation
- Off-label indications with potential harm:
  - May be associated with increased risk of thromboembolic events
  - These include:
    - Intracranial hemorrhage
    - Cardiac surgery

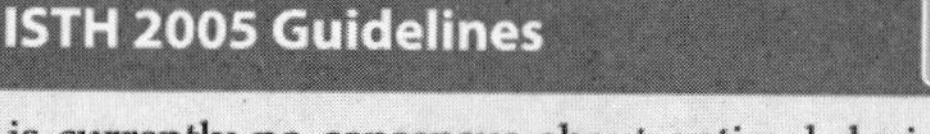

Dosage: ISTH 2005 Guidelines

- There is currently no consensus about optimal dosing of novoseven
- Hemophilia A/B with inhibitors: for bleeding episodes:
  - 90 µg/kg bolus Q2H until hemostasis is achieved
  - Posthemostatic dosing for severe bleeding: dose continued Q3-6H
- Hemophilia A/B with inhibitors: For surgery:
  - 90 µg/kg immediately before surgery
  - Dose is repeated Q2H during surgery
  - Post-surgical dosing:
    - Minor surgeries:
      - 90 µg/kg IV Q2H for first 48 hours
      - Then Q2-6H until healing is achieved
    - Major surgeries:
      - 90 µg/kg IV Q2H for first 5 days
      - Then Q4H till hemostasis is achieved

Contd...

Contd...

- Perioperative bleeding:
  - 20–80 µg/kg depending upon:
    - Type of surgery
    - Degree of bleeding
  - 120 µg/kg given for patients with massive bleeding:
    - Loss of 50% blood volume within 3 hours
    - Blood loss at > 150 mL/minute
    - Blood loss at > 1.5 mL/kg/minute for > 20 minutes
    - Transfusion of > 10 units PRBCs within 24 hours
- Trauma patients: 75–200 µg/kg
- Bleeding unresponsive to conventional therapy: 60 µg/kg
- Factor VII deficiency: 15-30 µg/kg Q4-6H until hemostasis is achieved
- Acquired hemophilia: 70-90 µg/kg Q2-3H until hemostasis is achieved

Monitoring during Therapy

- PT/INR, aPTT and factor VII levels may be useful
- Factor VII has the ability to normalize INR and shorten prolonged aPTT in hemophilia

Contraindications

- Hypersensitivity: Avoided when hypersensitivity to:
  - Novoseven
  - Mouse/hamster/bovine proteins
- Clinical states where in tissue factor is widely exposed:
  - If administered, thrombosis occurs at locations distant from site of bleeding
  - Examples:
    - DIC, crush injury, septicemia
    - Post-cardiac surgery with ECC support
    - Patients on ECMO or ventricular assist devices
- Patients with known hypercoagulability:
  - History of thrombotic complications like MI, liver disease, DIC
  - Elderly patients, post-operative immobilization
  - ***Factor-V Leiden deficiency***
  - ***Antiphospholipid antibody syndrome***
- Acidosis:
  - Acidosis decreases the efficacy of recombinant factor VIIa
  - Administration avoided when pH is less than 7.2
  - Thus pH should be maintained above 7.2 before instituting therapy
- Hypothermia (less than 33°C):
  - Hypothermia decreases the efficacy of recombinant factor VIIa
  - Hence, temperature should be maintained above 33°C

Benefits

- Anticoagulant therapy:
  - Used to reverse effect of warfarin
  - Useful when vitamin K supplementation is insufficient
  - However, fibrin burst occurs in response to factor VIIa therapy
  - This requires availability of factor X
  - Thus, in severe overdose, factor VIIa alone might be ineffective
- Cardiac surgery:
  - Has been used to control massive bleeding in cardiac surgery
  - Not associated with any survival benefit
  - Prophylactic administration is not recommended
  - Use is not recommended when on ECC support
- Orthotopic liver transplant/liver biopsy:
  - Prophylactic administration recommended in:
  - Patients with a poor MELD score
  - Patients with prolonged prothrombin
  - Reduces intra-operative bleeding
- Trauma: Owing to the high cost, use is restricted to:
  - Patients with survivable injury/medical disease
  - Patients not in terminal shock (pH less than 7, K+ more than 6 mEq/L)
  - Not in cardiac arrest
  - Not requiring vasoactive support

Side Effects

- Pyrexia, headache, pruritus
- Injection site reaction, hypertension, urticaria
- Arthralgia, hypotension, hypersensitivity
- Thrombotic events:
  - Occur at sites distant from the site of bleeding
  - Risk is increased with:
    - Septicemia
    - Crush injuries
    - Coronary artery disease
    - Cerebrovascular disease
    - History of thromboembolic events
  - Majority of these events produce arterial thrombi resulting in:
    - CVA, MI
    - Pulmonary emboli
    - Clotted devices
    - Deep veins thrombosis/superficial thrombophlebitis
- Antibody formation: should be suspected if:
  - Factor VIIa activity fails to reach expected levels
  - Prothrombin time is not corrected
  - Bleeding not controlled after treatment with recommended dose
- High cost limits its routine use in clinical situations

Drug Interactions

- Avoid simultaneous use of activated prothrombin complex/prothrombin complex concentrates
- Novoseven should not be mixed with infusion solutions

ARTIFICIAL BLOOD

Introduction

- Refers to substitutes designed to replace the oxygen carrying capacity of human RBCs
- The term oxygen therapeutics more accurately describes these substitutes
- This is because blood performs other functions besides carrying oxygen
- Also called:
  - ***Synthetic oxygen carrying substances***
  - ***Synthetic blood***

Characteristics of Ideal Blood Substitutes

- Ability to Effectively Transport Oxygen and Carbon Dioxide
- Lack of contamination
- Long shelf-life in storage
- Extended half-life in circulation
- Complete excretion from the body
- Lack of tissue accumulation
- Good safety profile:
  - Lack of toxicity
  - Non-immunogenicity
  - Non-antigenicity
  - Non-carcinogenicity
- Low cost
- Ease of access

Types

- Perfluorocarbons (PFCs) emulsion
- Modified hemoglobin solutions

Advantages of Blood Substitutes

- Unlimited source:
  - Donor blood is a limited source
  - Since oxygen therapeutics are synthetic, their supply is unlimited
- Avoids blood transfusion associated diseases:
  - HIV
  - Hepatitis B
  - *Creutzfeld-Jakob disease*
  - Mad cow disease
- Blood substitutes do not contain any antigens:
  - Can be used across all blood types without immunological reactions
  - Useful in emergencies where rapid blood transfusion would be impossible
- Long shelf life:
  - Can be stored at room temperature for much longer time
  - Most HBOCs have shelf life of 1-3 years
  - Donated blood has shelf life of 35-42 days
- Oxygen carrying capacity:
  - Blood substitutes allow for immediate full capacity oxygen transport
  - Transfused blood requires 24 hours to reach full oxygen transport capacity
  - This is due to 2-3 DPG depletion in stored blood

Parameter	Synthetic blood	Allogenic blood
Oxygen delivery	Rapid and consistent	Dependant on 2,3 DPG
Risk of disease transmission	None	Present
Storage	Room temperature	Stored refrigerated
	Stable efficacy	Loss of efficacy
Shelf life	1–3 years	42 days
Preparation	Ready to use	Cross match required
Compatibility	Universal	Type specific
Duration of action	1–3 days	60–90 days

PERFLUOROCARBONS

Chemistry

- PFCs are chemically inert synthetic molecules which consist primarily of:
  - Carbon atoms
  - Fluorine atoms
- The bond between carbon and fluoride atoms is strong
- Thus, these compounds are not metabolized
- They are colorless, inert, non-toxic liquids
- Can include both straight and cyclic hydrocarbon chains
- Straight form is a better carrier of oxygen than the cyclic form
- General chemical formula is C_nF_{2n+2}

Physical Properties

- Insoluble in water and alcohol with a low boiling point
- PFCs molecules are very small (< 0.2 µm)
- They measure about one-fourth the diameter of an RBC
- This small size enables them to traverse minute capillaries
- This can benefit damaged tissue where RBCs cannot flow through
- Also, PFCs are heat resistant and can withstand temperatures up to 300 °C
- PFCs are insoluble in water and therefore will not mix with blood
- Thus for clinical applications, they are solubilized using an emulsion agent
- This liquid is then mixed with antibiotics, vitamins, nutrients and salt

Physiology

- The main difference between oxygen transfer by hemoglobin and PFC is that:
  - Hemoglobin transports oxygen by binding to it
  - PFC transports oxygen by dissolving it
- Direct diffusion of oxygen is the mechanism by which it is delivered to the tissues
- Thus, PFCs increase dissolved O_2 content of blood without binding to O_2 molecule
- Oxygen has 100 times greater affinity for PFC solutions than in plasma
- Oxygen is dissolved in PFCs at a concentration of 40–50%
- This is twice as high as its concentration in plasma
- PFCs can also dissolve many other gases like carbon dioxide
- Thus, oxygen carrying capacity of PFC is directly related to partial pressure of O_2
- The oxygen content of PFC obeys ***Henrys laws of partial pressures:***
  - Amount of oxygen dissolved is directly related to partial pressure of oxygen
  - Thus, oxygen dissociation curve of PFC is linear
  - This fact limits use of PFCs to situations where PAO_2 are supra-normal

- Thus, alveolar O_2 tension (P_AO_2) > 400 mm Hg is required for gas exchange
- This is impossible to attain without supplemental oxygen administration
- Such high PaO_2 may be impossible at high altitudes with any maneuver

Metabolism

- After IV administration, droplets of the emulsion are taken up by cells of RES:
  - Kupffer cells
  - Macrophages
- They are slowly broken down and transported to blood
- Here, they are bound to lipids and transported to the lungs
- PFCs are mainly removed from the lungs by exhalation
- Have a plasma half-life of approximately 12 hours
- They are clinically stable for upto 2 years when refrigerated at 4 °C

Examples

- Fluosol DA:
  - Also called Pluronic F-68
  - Was the first FDA approved HBOC for use in PTCA
  - PFC based emulsion of:
    - Perfluorodecalin
    - Perfluorotripropylamine
  - Oxygen carrying capacity of only 7.2% at 37 °C
  - Approved for use in 1989
  - Withdrawn in 1994 due to:
    - Complement activation by emulsifier
    - Break down of pulmonary surfactant
    - Pulmonary side effects
    - Marginal efficacy
    - Complexity of use
    - Short effective half-life
- Oxygen
  - Contains:
    - 58% weight by volume perfluoro-octyl bromide
    - 2% weight by volume perfluoro-decyl bromide
    - Emulsified in 3.6% weight per volume egg yolk phospholipid
  - Thus, oxygen essentially consists of PFCs surrounded by lecithin surfactant
  - This differs from fluosol- DA by having:
    - Greater stability at room temperature than fluosol-DA
    - Increased oxygen carrying capacity (4–5 times higher)
  - Phase III trial were associated with increased risk of stroke
  - Clinical trials using oxygen have been stopped
- Perflubron:
  - Newer emulsion in which emulsifying agents are similar to primary compound
  - Perflubron has been developed as a stable emulsion containing:
    - Perfluoro-octyl-bromide
    - Perfluoro-decyl bromide as emulsifying agent
  - The emulsion is then buffered with egg yolk phospholipids
  - Perflubron has an O_2 carrying capacity which is 3-fold that of earlier solutions
  - Solution also has a longer half life
- Other PFC solutions that have been developed include:
  - Perftoran
  - Oxycyte: Undergoing phase II trials
  - Oxyfluor (discontinued due to safety issues)
  - PHER–O_2: Still in research phase
  - Perfluoran: Being used in Russia and Mexico

Advantages of PFCs

- Amount of oxygen dissolved in plasma is <1% of total O_2 content of arterial blood
- In contrast, PFCs can increase dissolved O_2 to 10–15% of total arterial oxygen content

Disadvantages of PFCs

- Long half-life:
  - PFC gas has a half-life of 3–4 hours in the plasma phase
  - However, they have a retention time of around 1 week in the RES
  - Thus, PFCs have a long half-life of nearly 1 week in the RES
  - This poses a problem with respect to dosage
  - Longer T ½ in RES limits additional dose of PFCs for 1–2 weeks
  - Thus, PFCs are essentially single -dose drugs
- Effective O_2 delivery occurs at supra-normal alveolar oxygen tension (400 mm Hg)

Adverse Effects

- Flu-like syndrome
- Mild thrombocytopenia

HEMOGLOBIN BASED OXYGEN CARRIERS (HBOC)

Chemistry

- Human hemoglobin derived from expired RBC bags is the main source of Hb
- Other sources include:
  - Cord blood RBCs
  - Animal blood
  - Recombinant hemoglobin
- Recombinant hemoglobin is produced from simple eschericia coli expression system

Physiology

- Outside the RBC, changes occurring to the hemoglobin include:
  - Disintegration:
    - The $\alpha_2\beta_2$ tetramers of Hb disintegrate into dimers and monomers
    - This renders the hemoglobin non-functional
    - This also results in severe renal complications as:
      - Dimers get filtered by the kidney
      - They interact with cell wall pieces in renal glomeruli
      - This results in ATN and ARF
  - Separation from 2,3-DPG:
    - Outside the RBC, hemoglobin is separated from 2,3-DPG
    - The hemoglobin becomes non-functional at physiological levels of oxygenation
    - Also, affinity to oxygen increases, shifting the ODC to left
    - The P_{50} of native *stroma free hemoglobin (SFH)* is around 17 mm Hg

Types of HBOCs

- Cellular HBOCs:
  - Hemoglobin is encapsulated into a cell-like structure
  - Since Hb is cell-encapsulated, vasoactive complications are reduced
  - Encapsulation is done using a phospholipid layer
  - This liposomal encapsulation of Hb (LEH) prolongs both:
    - Half-life in vivo
    - Shelf-life in vitro
  - These LEH are much smaller than RBCs (1:30)
  - Thus, vascular access to compromised areas are improved
- Acellular HBOCs:
  - Hemoglobin is stabilized into a stable functional tetramer by various methods
  - Thus, dissociation into monomers and dimers is prevented
  - Have been designed to:
    - Increase Hb performance
    - Decrease side effects of free hemoglobin
  - Three types of acellular HBOCs are:
    - Cross-linked HBOCs:
      - Hb chains are linked by intermolecular covalent bonds
      - These covalent bonds stabilises the Hb tetramer
      - Diaspirin has been commonly used for this purpose
    - Polymerized HBOC:
      - Hb chains are linked by intermolecular covalent bonds
      - This increases the molecular size
      - Each polymerized Hb molecule contains 4–5 Hb molecules
    - Conjugated HBOC:
      - Inert polymer is bound to the surface of Hb
      - This increases the size of the molecule
  - Limitations:
    - Most of the acellular HBOCs lack the ability to convert Fe^{3+} to Fe^{2+}
    - Thus, meth-hemoglobin with low oxygen carrying capacity results
    - This can be circumvented by attaching reducing agents to Hb surface
    - Most of these HBOCs have a shorter half-life and side effects
    - Thus, most of these have not been successful in clinical trials
- Recombinant hemoglobin:
  - Recombinant production of Hb makes it easily modifiable
  - This is done through site-directed mutagenesis
  - Hemoglobin is usually produced using E.coli expression system
  - Targeted mutations may be used to:
    - Increase oxygen affinity
    - Reduce auto-oxidation
    - Reduce nitric oxide scavenging
    - Reduce rate of heme loss
  - Recombinant hemoglobin has a P_{50} of 32 mm Hg
  - Advantages:
    - Does not require cross matching
    - Does not transmit disease
    - Maximum tolerable dose of rHb is unknown

Examples of Acellular HBOCs

- Cross-linked HBOCs:
  - HemAssist:
    - Diaspirin cross-linked hemoglobin
    - Utilizes human hemoglobin
    - Hemoglobin is cross linked with diasprin
    - Currently in phase III trials
    - Associated with increased mortality
- Polymerized HBOC:
  - Hemopure:
    - Ultrapurified bovine hemoglobin is used
    - Hemoglobin is polymerized with glutaraldehyde
    - They are then suspended in balanced salt solution
    - Contains higher amounts of free $\alpha_2\beta_2$ (31%)
    - This increases the risk of cardiovascular problems
    - Also, risk of disease transmission due to bovine hemoglobin
    - Currently in phase III trials
  - Polyheme:
    - Uses human hemoglobin
    - Polymerized using glutaraldehyde
    - Pyridoxal phosphate is used to bind 2,3-DPG to improve P50
    - Incorporated into electrolyte solution
    - Associated with cardiovascular side effects and oxidative stress
    - Rejected by the FDA
  - Oxyglobin:
    - Utilizes bovine hemoglobin
    - Contains 2% $\alpha_2\beta_2$ molecules
    - This is suspended in balanced salt solution with no RBCs
    - Risk of disease transmission due to bovine hemoglobin
    - Lower hypertensive complications compared with polyheme
    - Approved for use in veterinary animals
  - PolyHb-fibrinogen:
    - Utilizes bovine hemoglobin
    - Shows both oxygen carrying and blood coagulation properties
    - Useful in massive bleeding to augment oxygenation and coagulation
    - Risk of disease transmission due to bovine hemoglobin
- Conjugated HBOC:
  - Hemospan:
    - Utilizes human hemoglobin
    - Maleimide-polyethylene (PEG) glycol is used to reduce toxicity
    - Available in powder form which is then mixed and transfused
    - It can be stored for many years
  - MP4:
    - Utilizes human hemoglobin
    - Maleimide activated PEG modified Hb is used to reduce toxicity

Examples of Cellular HBOCS

- Neo red cell:
  - Liposome encapsulated-Hb
  - Shows higher oxygen transport efficiency compared to native RBCs
  - Readily circulated due to low viscosity
  - However, comparatively low half-life due to:
    - Removal by RES
    - Shear-induced liposomal destruction
- Hemoglobin-loaded polymeric nanoparticle (HbPNP):
  - Biodegradable nanoparticles are used to house the hemoglobin
  - Rapid clearance by phagocytes reduces the half life
- Single-protein nano-capsule:
  - Protein molecule is encapsulated with a thin polymer layer
  - The resulting nano-capsule has both mechanical and thermal resistance
  - This can be used for oxygenation along with delivery of drugs
- Other cellular HBOCs include:
  - Nanoscale hydrogel particles
  - Lipogel

Advantages of HBOCs

- Do not require supranormal oxygen tension to be effective in delivering oxygen
- Lack of iso-agglutinating antigens due to absence of RBC membrane
- This obviates the need for blood typing and screening
- Does not transmit HIV or hepatitis B/C

Disadvantages of HBOCs

- Plasma hemoglobin is not a true blood substitute:
  - Hemoglobin can replace only the oxygen transport capacity of blood
  - Lacks the coagulation/immunological aspects of blood

- Free hemoglobin avidly binds nitric oxide, causing HTN due to vasoconstriction
- Metabolism of free hemoglobin:
  - Identical to natural hemoglobin released from RBC destruction
  - This can cause increase in bilirubin levels
  - Amylase levels also increase (from pancreas)
- Consequences of HBOC metabolism may be similar to multiple blood transfusions:
  - Hemosiderosis
  - Chronic iron overload
- Risk of transmission of infections still exists (bovine spongiform encephalitis)
- Decrease in cardiac index (may be due to nitric oxide)

SICKLE CELL ANEMIA

Introduction

- Sickle cell anemia is a hemoglobinopathy in which the dominant Hb is unstable HbS instead of HbA
- Sickle cell syndrome includes:
  - Sickle cell anemia (HbSS)
  - Double heterozygote conditions like
    - Sickle cell C (HbSC)
    - Sickle thalassemia (HbSThal)

Genetics

- HbS occurs due to a mutation in chromosome 11
- Glutamic acid is replaced by valine at 6th position from N-terminus of β chain
- Sickle cell trail refers to heterozygotes who have one βA and one βS chain (HbSA)
- Sickle cell disease refers to homozygotes who have both βS genes

Incidence

- Endemic in Africa, Mediterranean, Middle east and India
- Sickle cell trait occurs in 8-10% African-Americans
- 0.2% homozygotes with sickle cell disease amongst African-Americans

Types

- Sickle cell trait: (SCT)
  - Heterozygous for sickle gene (HbSA)
  - Asymptomatic carrier state for HbS
  - RBCs have HbS concentration < 50% (38–45%)
  - Have normal blood film and Hb level
  - Are asymptomatic but have positive sickling test
  - HbAs begins to sickle only when oxygen saturation of Hb is less than 20%
  - No special treatment is required, except to avoid:
    - Hypoxia
    - Dehydration
    - Infection
    - Acidosis
    - Hypothermia
- Sickle cell disease: (SCD)
  - Homozygous for sickle gene (HbSS)
  - RBCs have HbS concentration between 70–98%
  - RBC lifespan reduced to 12–17 days in contrast to normal of 120 days
  - Characterized by chronic hemolysis, acute episodic vaso-occlusive crisis

Pathophysiology

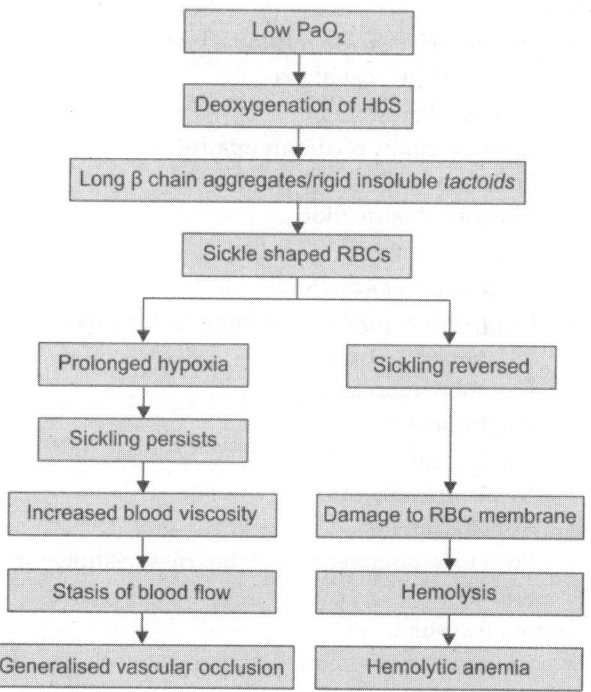

Mechanisms of Cellular Injury in SCD

- Erythrocyte and platelet adhesion to endothelium
- Endothelial dysfunction secondary to inflammation and reduction of NO
- Reduced NO due to leukocyte superoxide release
- Leucocytosis and complement system activation
- Activation of coagulation cascade with thrombosis and ischemia
- Activation of cytokine and inflammatory mediators
- Free radical injury due to leukocyte superoxide release

- Free radical injury secondary to free Hb
- Reperfusion injury
- Excessive iron stores secondary to repeated erythrocyte transfusion

Clinical Features

- Clinical features manifest at 3–4 months of age when switch from HbF to HbA occurs
- Episodic painful crisis bone and joint pains common where pain is poorly localised
- Central nervous system:
  - Stroke
  - Aneurysms
  - Meningitis
- Psychological:
  - Depression, anxiety
  - Substance abuse. narcotic dependence
- Eye:
  - ***Proliferative sickle retinopathy***
  - Hemorrhage, visual loss
- Cardiovascular system:
  - Cardiomegaly, cardiomyopathy
  - Pulmonary HTN, cor pulmonale
  - Diastolic dysfunction
- Respiratory system:
  - ***Acute chest syndrome***
  - Hypoxemia, pulmonary infarcts, fibrosis
  - Asthma, sleep apnea
  - Thromboembolism
  - Pneumonia
- Hematological:
  - ***Hemolytic anemia***
  - Aplastic anemia
  - Shift to left of oxyhemoglobin dissociation curve (ODC)
- Immune system:
  - Immunosuppression, increased infections and sepsis due to:
    - Reduced IgM levels
    - Reduced capacity for phagocytosis
    - Reduced capacity for opsonization
  - Leucocytosis
- Musculoskeletal:
  - ***Painful crisis***
  - Bone marrow hyperplasia
  - Avascular necrosis
  - Osteomyelitis
  - Bone infarcts
  - Skeletal deformities, growth retardation
  - Cutaneous ulcers
- Spleen:
  - ***Auto-infarction***
  - Hyposplenism
  - ***Splenic sequestration***
- Liver:
  - Jaundice
  - Hepatitis
  - Cirrhosis
  - Gall stones, cholestasis
- Genitourinary:
  - Priapism
  - Polyuria due to impaired concentrating ability of kidney
  - Chronic renal failure
  - Papillary necrosis, glomerular necrosis

Predictors for Increased Risk of Complications

- Age > 30 years
- Previous history of stroke/acute coronary syndrome
- Asthma, resting hypoxemia
- Frequent painful crises
- Pulmonary HTN
- Thoracic, cardiac and intracranial surgeries: High risk
- Abdominal and orthopedic surgeries: Moderate risk
- Tonsillectomy, adenoidectomy, myringotomy: Mild risk

Life Threatening Complications

- Sepsis
- Aplastic crisis
- Splenic sequestration
- Acute chest syndrome

Causes of End Organ Damage

- Sickling and adhesion of cells in blood vessels secondary to tissue ischemia
- Hemolytic crisis/aplastic crisis

Sickle Cell Crisis

- Vascular occlusion with organ infarction and pain
  - Acute chest syndrome
  - Infarctive crisis
- Hemolytic crisis with features of sudden hemolysis
- Sequestration syndrome with RBCs sequestration in liver and spleen
- Aplastic crisis with bone marrow suppression

I. Acute chest syndrome:

- Precipitated by:
  - Pulmonary infection
  - Fat embolism from bone marrow necrosis
  - Worsening of asthma
  - Perioperative respiratory dysfunction
- Clinical features:
  - Fever, cough
  - Dyspnea, tachypnea, wheezing
  - Chest pain, hypoxemia
  - Pleural effusion and pulmonary infilterates on chest X-ray
  - Progresses to ARDS, respiratory failure, pneumonia
- Treatment:
  - Bronchodilators
  - Mechanical ventilation
  - Antibiotics
  - Steroids
  - Exchange transfusion to reduce HbS concentration

II. Infarctive crises:

- Precipitated by:
  - Infection
  - Trauma
  - High temperature
- Clinical features:
  - Acute onset pain
  - Usually abdominal pain, fever, vomiting.
- Treatment:
  - Adequate hydration
  - Partial alkalinization of blood
  - Partial exchange transfusion with HbA containing RBCs
  - Antibiotics
  - Oral bicarbonate upto 20g/day to produce alkalinisation
  - Treatment of pain with opioids/epidural local anesthetics + opioids

III. Hemolytic crises:

- Drop in Hb, increase in reticulocytes and bilirubin
- Usually accompanies vaso-occlusive crisis

IV. Splenic sequestration crises:

- Occurs mainly in children
- Treatment:
  - Volume resuscitation
  - RBC transfusion
  - Splenectomy after resolution of crisis

V. Aplastic crisis:

- Temporary bone marrow shut down manifested by:
  - Precipitous fall in Hb
  - Absence of reticulocytes
- RBC transfusion given till normal marrow function is re-established

Factors Causing Increased Sickling

- HbS concentration ≥ 50%
- Low PO_2: $PaO_2 \leq 40$ mm Hg causes sickling in SCD
- $PaO_2 \leq 20$ mm Hg causes sickling in SC trait
- Reduced body temperature causes vasoconstriction causing stasis and sickling
- Increased body temperature casues increasing metabolic requirements precipitating sickling
- Dehydration
- Acidosis favours sickling which is more in veins than arteries

Investigations

- Complete blood count
  - Hb usually between 6–9 gm% in SC trait
  - Leucocytosis and thrombocytosis occur as reactive features
- Peripheral blood smear:
  - Normal in SC trait
  - Normocytic normochromic anemia
  - Increased reticulocytes, sickled cells and target cells
  - ***Howell Jolly*** bodies if atrophied spleen
- Sickling test with sodium metabisulphate
- Screening for HbS with quick solubility test Eg ***Sickledex***
- Hb electrophoresis:
  - *Definitive and confirmatory*
  - HbS level aimed at < 30% in crisis
- BUN, serum creatinine, urinalysis
- Chest X ray, ECG, ECHO
- Liver function tests, electrolytes, PT/PTT, INR
- ABG in patients with cardiac disease

Treatment

- Mainly supportive
- Early treatment of complication
- Hydroxyurea used to increase circulating levels of HbF
- Only *curative therapy is bone marrow transplant* reserved for young patients having severe presentation
- Hyperbaric O_2 therapy used in SC crises due to :
  - Reduction in rate of sickling
  - Improved tissue oxygenation by direct diffusion
- Splenic autoinfarcts require lifelong therapy with:
  - Penicillin
  - Aggressive immunization programme against pneumococcus

Preop Preparation

- Assessment of existing organ dysfunction
- Preoperative hydration aggressively is necessary
- Prophylactic antibiotic cover with correction of co-existing infection
- Preoperative alkalinisation has anti-sickling effect but shifts ODC to left
- Preoperative transfusion:
  - Hematologist advice before surgery
  - Transfusion goals:
    - To increase HbA to 40–50%
    - To decrease HbS < 30%
    - Hematocrit of 30–35%
    - Hematocrit to be kept < 35% as:
    - Increased HCT will cause increase in blood viscosity
    - This precludes stasis in circulation
    - This can cause vascular occlusion
  - If exchange transfusion needed, use only buffy coat poor, HbS free, washed RBCs
  - Compatible blood difficult to find as RBC antibodies common due to multiple transfusions
  - Sample blood for grouping and antibody screening as previous transfusion common
  - Patient selection for exchange transfusion:
    - Minor surgery: Not required unless severe SCD
    - Moderate to high risk surgery: Transfusion required

Anesthetic Goals

Maintain:
- Good oxygenation
- Good hydration
- Normothermia
- Normal acid base balance
- Avoid tourniquets/limb circulation stasis.

Intraoperative Management

Preoperative Preparation and Premedication

- NPO orders
- Informed consent
- Avoid drugs causing respiratory depression: Opioids avoided

Monitoring

- Pulse oximetry in multiple areas including ear and toe especially in pregnant patients
- NIBP
- Urine output
- ECG
- Capnography
- If pulmonary HTN or cardiac dysfunction, IBP and CVP monitoring
- Serial arterial blood gases to ensure adequate oxygenation

Induction

- Adequate pre-oxygenation with high FiO_2
- Induction with thiopentone and succinylcholine followed by tracheal intubation
- Avoid endobronchial intubation as one lung ventilation precipitates acute chest syndrome

Maintenance

- Moderate hyperventilation maintained with N_2O + O_2 + isoflurane
- Opioids + NDMR + Volatile anesthetics
- Opioids carefully titrated to prevent postoperative respiratory depression
- Guidelines for tourniquet use:
  - It should be applied as distally as possible
  - Limb should be thoroughly exsanguinated before application
  - Ischemic time should be minimized
  - Prevent respiratory and metabolic acidosis at the time of tourniquet release
- Avoid conditions which increase sickling:
  - Adequate oxygenation necessary
  - Prevent vascular stasis
  - Avoid increases in oxygen consumption: Maintain deep planes of anesthesia
  - Avoid hypothermia

Ventilation

- Titrate FiO_2 to maintain normal or increased PaO_2
- Avoid hypoventilation and hypoxia
- Prevent respiratory/metabolic acidosis

Hemodynamics

- Rapid correction of hypotension and maintenance of intravascular fluid volume
- Maintain blood viscosity at low level:
  - Limit maximum hematocrit to 35%
  - Avoid overtransfusion
- Avoid hypothermia using body warming and IV fluid warming devices
- Avoid shivering

Role of Regional Anesthesia

- Regional anesthesia is better avoided
- Administer supplemental O_2

- Compensatory vasoconstriction, stasis and reduced PaO_2 may occur in areas which are not blocked and may result in infarction

Postoperative

Complications

- Increased respiratory infections
- Acute chest syndrome in SCD patients undergoing surgery under GA
- Sequestration syndrome: Lethal in obstetric patients immediately postpartum
- CCF in patients with cardiomegaly and pulmonary HTN

Management

- Supplemental O_2
- Chest physiotherapy
- Adequate antibiotic cover to control chest infection
- Maintain intravascular volume, HCT between 30–35%
- Early mobilization
- Respiratory depression, acidosis and hypoxia, may occur with opioids
- Avoid shivering as it increases O_2 consumption

Pain

- Carefully titrated opioids for pain relief
- Tolerance to opioids possible due to frequent opioid based analgesia for sickle crises
- NSAIDs only as adjuvant therapy
- Local infilteration techniques useful-multimodal analgesia

DISSEMINATED INTRAVASCULAR COAGULATION

Introduction

- An acquired condition characterized by:
  - Intravascular activation of coagulation with loss of localization
  - Widespread intravascular coagulation
  - Consumptive coagulopathy
- Also called:
  - Consumption coagulopathy
  - Defibrination syndrome
- It should be suspected in any patient with diffuse bleeding/clotting and:
  - Altered PT/aPTT
  - Decreased platelet count

Causes

- Infections: *Most common cause of DIC*
  - Sepsis: *Most commonly associated with gram negative sepsis*
  - Gram negative toxemia
  - Rocky mountain spotted fever
  - Fungemias
  - Viremias
- Obstetric causes:
  - Amniotic fluid embolism
  - Intrauterine fetal death
  - Abruptio placentae
  - Septic abortion
  - Preeclampsia, HELLP syndrome
- Extensive tissue damage:
  - Trauma, crush injury
  - Complicated surgery
  - Burns, heat stroke
  - Rhabdomyolysis
  - Hypo/hyperthermia
  - Hemolytic transfusion reactions, multiple transfusions
- Organ damage:
  - Liver disease:
    - Fulminant hepatic failure
    - Reperfusion after liver transplantation
  - Head injury
- Malignancies:
  - Adenocarcinomas
  - Prostatic carcinoma
  - Acute promyelocytic leukemia
  - Metastatic malignancies
  - ***Trousseaus syndrome***
- Vascular anomalies:
  - Abdominal aortic aneurysm
  - Giant hemangiomas (***Kasabach-Merritt syndrome***)
  - Vasculitis
  - Multiple telangiectasias
- Fat embolism:
  - Long bone fractures
  - Sickle cell crisis
- Toxic procoagulant molecules:
  - Amphetamine overdose
  - Rattle snake venom
  - Viper venom
- Others:
  - Peritoneovenous shunts
  - Paroxysmal nocturnal hemoglobinuria
  - Acute hemolytic transfusion reactions (ABO incompatibility)
  - Purpura fulminans

Pathophysiology

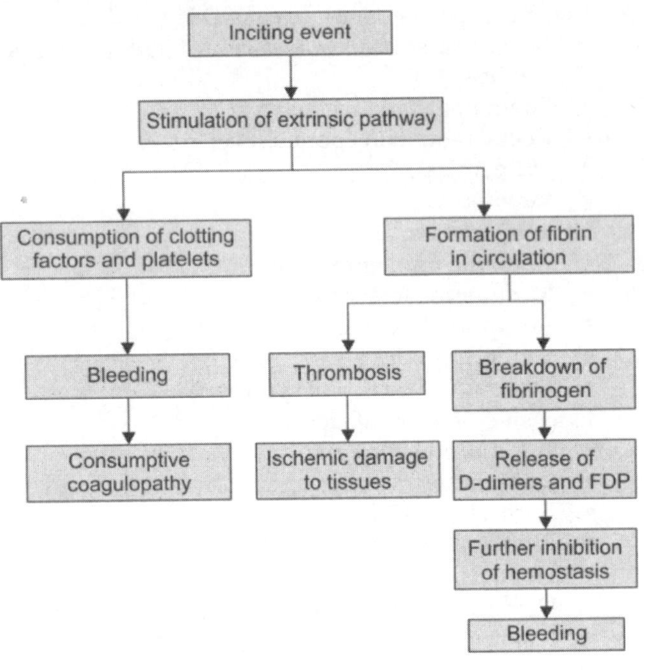

Clinical Features

- Signs of coagulopathy:
  - Bleeding:
    - Bleeding from at least 3 unrelated sites suggests DIC
    - Bleeding is more common in acute fulminant DIC
    - Signs of bleeding:
      - Petechiae, purpura, subcutaneous hematomas
      - Ecchymosis, hemorrhagic bullae, jaundice
      - Bleeding from GIT, GUT, mucosal and venepuncture sites
  - Thrombotic manifestations:
    - More commonly seen in chronic DIC
    - Only 5–10% of acute DIC present with thrombosis
    - Occur first in malignancy associated DIC
    - In other causes, hemorrhagic diathesis occurs first
    - Signs of thrombosis:
      - Acral cyanosis
      - Skin necrosis of lower limbs: purpura fulminans
      - Localized infarction and gangrene
    - Pulmonary function may be impaired due to microthrombus formation.
- Signs of multiorgan failure:
  - CNS: Altered consciousness, stupor
  - CVS: Hypotension, tachycardia, circulatory collapse
  - RS: Pleuritis, ARDS
  - GIT: Hematemesis, hematochezia
  - GUT: Renal failure, renal cortical necrosis, metrorrhagia
- Complications:
  - Purpura fulminans
  - Multiorgan failure

Differential Diagnosis

- Acute/chronic liver failure
- Hemolytic uremic syndrome
- Thrombotic thrombocytopenic purpura
- Heparin induced thrombocytopenia
- Other consumptive coagulopathies

Components of DIC

- Exposure of blood to procoagulant substances
- Fibrin deposition in microvasculature
- Impaired fibrinolysis
- Depletion of coagulation factors and platelets (***Consumptive Coagulopathy***)
- Multiple organ damage and failure

Investigations

No.	Test	Normal	DIC
Most Useful			
1.	Platelet count	2.5–4 lacs/μL	< 50 000/μL
2.	Fibrinogen level	400–650 mg/dL	< 150 mg/dL
3.	Prothrombin time	Seconds	> 100 seconds
4.	FDP and d-Dimers	<16 μg/mL	> 200 μg/mL
Helpful			
1.	aPTT	35–50 seconds	> 100 seconds
2.	Thrombin time	15–20 seconds	> 100 seconds
3.	Fragmented RBCs/ schistocytes	Absent	Present
4.	Specific factor assays:		
	II		Reduced
	V		Reduced
	VII		Reduced
	VIII		Reduced/normal/high
	IX, X		Reduced

Other Investigations

- 3P test (***plasma-protamine-paracoagulation***) test:
  - Can be used to confirm diagnosis sometimes
  - Tests for presence of soluble complexes composed of fibrin monomers (generated by excess thrombosis) and FDPS
  - The addition of protamine destabilizes these complexes forming a precipitate

- Levels of prothrombin fragments F_1+ F_2
- Levels of thrombin-antithrombin complexes
- α_2 antiplasmin levels reduced by binding to excess plasmin
- Reduced plasminogen
- Reduced protein C levels
- Thromboelastography

Diagnosis

ISTH-DIC Score

No.	Criteria	Points
1.	Platelet Count	
	> 1,00,000 cells/mm³	0
	50,000–1,00,000 cells/mm³	1
	< 50,000 cells/mm³	2
2.	Fibrin Related Markers (D-Dimer, FDP)	
	Normal	0
	Mildly elevated	2
	Markedly elevated	3
3.	Prolongation in Prothrombin Time	
	< 3 seconds	0
	3-6 seconds	1
	> 6 seconds	2
4.	Fibrinogen Level	
	> 100 milligrams/dL	0
	< 100 milligrams/dL	1

- Score > 5 points:
  - Compatible with overt/high grade DIC
  - Scoring has to be repeated daily
- Score < 5 points:
  - Suggestive (not affirmative) of non- overt/low grade DIC
  - Scoring to be repeated in 1–2 days

ISTH-DIC Score in Pregnancy

No.	Criteria	Points
1.	Platelet count	
	< 50,000 cells/mm³	0
	50,000–1,00,000 cells/mm³	2
	1,00,000–1,85,000 cells/mm³	1
	> 1,85,000 cells/mm³	0
2.	Prolongation of prothrombin time	
	< 0.5 seconds	0
	0.5–1 second	5
	1–1.5 seconds	12
	> 1.5 seconds	25
3.	Fibrinogen level	
	< 300 mg/dL	25
	300–400 dL	6
	400–450 mg/dL	1
	> 450 mg/dL	0

- Score > 26 points:
  - 88% sensitive for diagnosis of DIC
  - 96% specific for DIC

Treatment

- Treatment goals:
  - To increase fibrinogen levels to 100–150 mg/dL
  - Supportive therapy for circulatory compromise
  - Treatment of cause
- Treatment of underlying cause:
  - Antibiotics for septicemia
  - Uterine evacuation/hysterectomy for obstetric cause
  - Anti-snake venom
- Supportive therapy:
  - Correction of:
    - Hypovolemia
    - Acidosis
    - Hypothermia
  - Fluids, RBCs/inotropes to support CVS
  - Mechanical ventilation if respiratory complications
- Hemostatic therapy:
  - Platelets transfused when:
    - Platelet count < 50,000 cells/mm³ with active bleeding
    - Platelet count < 20, 000 cells/mm³ even in the absence of bleeding
  - Cryoprecipitate transfused when fibrinogen level < 50 mg/dL
  - Fresh frozen plasma transfused to replace clotting factors

Component	Dose	Lab parameter	Target lab parameter	
			No clinically significant bleeding	Clinically significant bleeding
Platelets	1 unit SDP	Platelet count	>100000/ µL	20-50000 /µL
	4-6 units RDP			
FFP	10-15 mL/ kg Usually 3-5 units	aPTT/PT		<1.5 times upper limit of normal reference range
Cryoprecipi-tate	10 units	Fibrinogen	>80-100 mg/dL	> 80–100 mg/dL

- Heparin:
  - Use restricted to conditions where thrombosis is clinically problematic
  - Also useful in chronic DIC

- 5–10 IU/kg/hour as infusion without any bolus dose
- Avoid if intracranial/GI bleed/abruption/imminent surgery
- For refractory bleeding, heparin use is controversial

❖ Antifibrinolytics:
- Used only if:
  - All other modalities are unsuccessful
  - Documented hypofibrinogenemia and fibrinolysis
- They should be avoided in the presence of widespread thrombosis
- This is because of the possibility of disseminated thromboembolism

❖ Other therapies:
- Recombinant activated protein:
  - Especially useful in patients with sepsis
  - Reduces mortality and organ failure
- Antithrombin III concentrates (ATC)
- Tumor factor inhibitors

Anesthetic Management

Preoperative Preparation

❖ Manage underlying cause:
- Antibiotics
- Correct hypovolemia
- Fluids and blood products warmed to avoid hypothermia
- Surgery to remove cause as soon as coagulopathy corrected to acceptable level

❖ Correct coagulopathy: PC and FFP, cryoprecipitate if fibrinogen < 1g/dL

❖ Heparin is best avoided before surgery

❖ Premedication avoided in critically ill

❖ IM injections are avoided

Perioperative Management

❖ Regional anesthesia contraindicated in coagulopathy

❖ Controlled ventilation and invasive monitoring preferred in critically ill patients

❖ Nasotracheal intubation avoided

❖ Insert NGT carefully to prevent trauma

❖ Large bore IV cannula with infusion of warmed IV fluids

❖ Replace blood loss promptly

❖ Measure platelet count and clotting function regularly and replace promptly

Postoperative Management

❖ May require mechanical ventilation, intensive cardiovascular monitoring and support

❖ Frequent measurement of hematological parameters

THROMBOELASTOGRAPHY

Introduction

❖ Viscoelastic technique which measures entire spectrum of clot formation including:
- Early fibrin strand formation
- Clot retraction
- Fibrinolysis

❖ Thus, this is a coagulo-viscometer which yields information about both:
- Clot formation
- Clot dissolution

❖ Developed by ***Hartert*** in 1948

❖ Provides a measure of the mechanical properties of evolving clot as a function of time

❖ Thus, it evaluates clot formation as a dynamic process

❖ Information derived includes:
- Integrity of the coagulation cascade
- Platelet function
- Platelet- fibrin interactions
- Fibrinolysis

❖ Viscoelastic tests include:
- Thromboelastography (TEG)
- Sonoclot
- Thromboelastometry (ROTEM)

Procedure

❖ 0.35 mL of whole blood is placed in a prewarmed cuvette containing:
- Calcium
- Contact activator

❖ A plastic pin is suspended into the cuvette

❖ The plastic pin is attached by a torsion wire to an electronic needle recorder

❖ The pin is lowered into the blood sample taken in the cuvette

❖ Cuvette continuously oscillates through an arc of 4°45″ at 37 °C

❖ As clot formation occurs, the pin becomes enmeshed within the clot

❖ Thus, the motion of the pin becomes coupled with the cuvette

- Rotation of the cuvette is transferred to the piston and to the electronic recorder
- Conversely, during clot lysis, bonds between the cuvette and pin are broken
- Thus, the signal progressively decreases to result in formation of thromboelastogram
- The recording paper constantly advances at a speed of 2 mm/minute
- The parameters are calculated from the tracing obtained using a software package
- The specific parameters recorded includes:
  - Reaction time (R value)
  - Coagulation time (K value)
  - α–angle
  - Maximum amplitude
  - Amplitude 60 minutes after the minimum amplitude (A60)
  - Clot lysis indices at 30 and 60 minutes after MA (LY30 and LY60)
- Interpretations:
  - A weak clot stretches and thus delays the arc movement of the piston which is expressed as a narrow TEG
  - A strong clot will move the piston simultaneously and proportionally to the cuvette movements forming a thick thromboelastogram

Advantages

- Can be used as a point of care test for coagulation
- Provides information regarding:
  - Coagulation cascade
  - Platelet function
  - Fibrinogen function
  - Fibrinolysis
- Can be used with heparinase to monitor coagulation on CPB
- More accurate predictor of postoperative bleeding

Disadvantages

- Lack of specificity associated with abnormal findings
- Qualitative assessment is not possible

Parameters Measured by TEG

- Reaction time (R-value):
  - Measurement:
    - Represents early stage of clotting cascade leading to fibrin formation
    - Period of time from initiation of test to formation of initial fibrin clot
    - Measured from the start of the test until amplitude of tracing is 2 mm

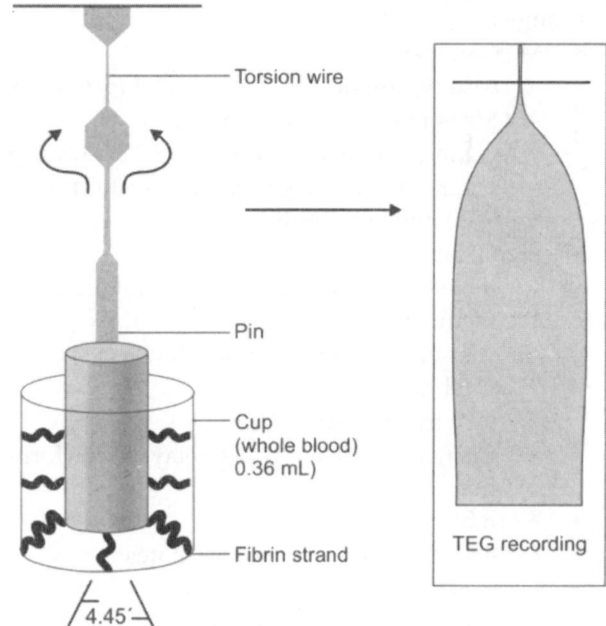

Fig. 1: TEG procedure.

  - Significance: It is a measure of:
    - Intrinsic pathway
    - Extrinsic pathway
    - Common pathway
  - Normal values vary with type of activator used:
    - 7.5–15 minutes using celite activator
    - 1–3 minutes using tissue factor activator
  - Factors causing increased R-value
    - Clotting factor deficiency
    - Liver disease
    - Anticoagulation with warfarin or heparin
    - Hypofibrinogenemia
  - Factors causing decreased R-value: hypercoagulable state
- Coagulation time (K-value):
  - Measurement:
    - It is a measure of the speed of clot formation
    - Measured from end of R-time till amplitude of the clot reaches 20 mm
    - Represents clot potentiation by activation of platelets
  - Normal values: 3-6 minutes
  - Factors causing increased K-value:
    - Clotting factor deficiency
    - Thrombocytopenia
    - Platelet dysfunction
    - Hypofibrinogenemia
  - Factors causing decreased K-value: hypercoagulable states

- α-angle:
  - Measurement:
    - Also represents the speed of clot formation
    - Measured as the angle between:
      - Line drawn in the middle of TEG tracing
      - Line drawn tangential to the clot trace at 20 mm amplitude
  - Significance:
    - Increased angle reflects rapid clot formation mediated by:
      - Thrombin-activated platelets
      - Fibrin
      - Activated factor XIII
    - Decreased angle reflects delayed clot formation
  - Normal value: 45–55°
  - Increased in: Hypercoagulable states
  - Decreased in:
    - Clotting factor deficiency
    - Hypofibrinogenemia
    - Thrombocytopenia
    - Platelet dysfunction
- Maximum amplitude:
  - Measurement:
    - Amplitude of the clot measured at peak clot strength
    - Represents peak clot strength by GPIIb/IIIa interactions between:
      - Platelets
      - Fibrin
    - Thus, it is an indicator of:
      - Platelet function
      - Interaction of platelet with fibrin
    - Percentage reduction in MA after 30 minutes represents fibrinolytic activity
  - Normal value: 50–60 mm
  - Increased in: Hypercoagulable states
  - Decreased in:
    - Clotting factor deficiency
    - Hypofibrinogenemia
    - Thrombocytopenia
    - Platelet dysfunction
- Amplitude 60 minutes after the maximum amplitude (A60):
  - Measures rate of amplitude reduction 60 minutes after MA
  - Represents stability of the clot formed
  - Decreased due to fibrinolysis
- Clot lysis indices at 30 minutes after MA (LY30):
  - Measurement:
    - Measures percentage decrease in the MA amplitude after 30 minutes
    - Represents the activation of fibrinolytic system and fibrinolysis
  - Normal value: < 7.5%
  - Increased in fibrinolytic states
- Clot viscoelasticity (G-value):
  - Calculated from maximal amplitude

$$\text{Clot viscoelasticity G} = \frac{5000 \times \text{MA}}{(96\text{-MA})}$$

  - Increased in platelet hypercoagulability

Uses of TEG

- Obstetric and postpartum bleeding:
  - Useful to predict massive transfusion in patients with mild PPH
  - Useful to identify cause of coagulopathy
  - Useful to guide blood product therapy in massive hemorrhage

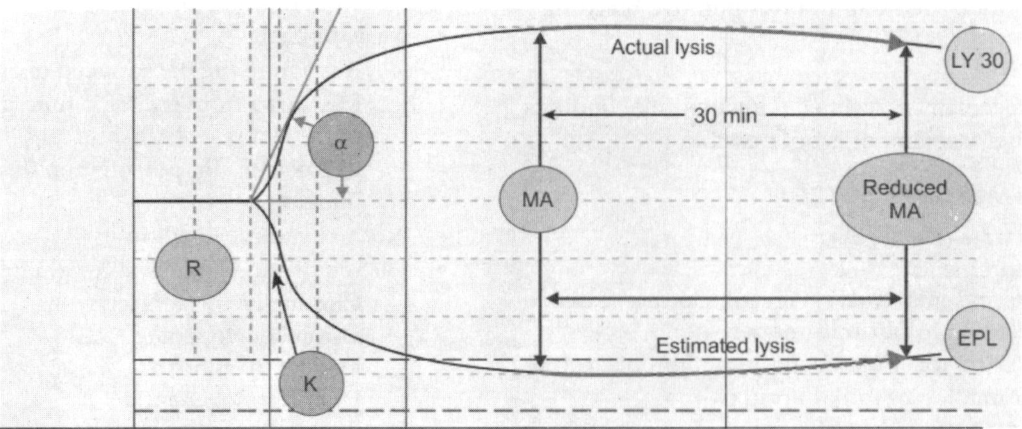

Fig. 2: Normal TEG.

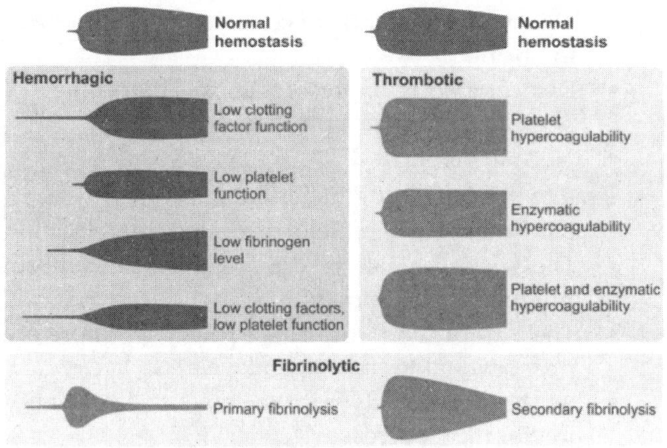

Fig. 3: Abnormalities in TEG.

- Liver disease and surgery:
  - Have a high predictive value for bleeding and coagulopathy
  - Prothrombin time does not reliably predict bleeding in these patients
  - To identify cause of coagulopathy and reduce overall transfusion
  - Standard of care for guiding blood component therapy
- Cardiac surgery:
  - *Not very effective* in predicting bleeding
  - Useful for the diagnosis of coagulopathy following cardiac surgery
  - TEG-driven protocols improve outcomes and reduce transfusions
- Trauma:
  - Insufficient data to prove that TEG is effective for prediction bleeding
  - Useful for the diagnosis of traumatic coagulopathy
  - TEG-guided protocol reduce transfusion requirement and mortality

Teg Treatment Algorithm for Bleeding

TEG finding	Interpretation	Treatment
R(plain) > R(heparinise)	Inadequate heparin reversal	Protamine
R between 11–14 mins	Reduced clotting factors	2 units FFP
R > 14 mins	Severe clotting factor deficiency	2 units FFP
40 < MA > 48	Reduced platelet number and function	1 unit platelet
MA < 40	Severe thrombocytopenia	2 units platelets
LY30 > 7.5%, EPL > 15%	Hyperfibrinolysis	Antifibrinolytics

Modifications of Thromboelastography

- Rapid TEG:
  - Utilized human recombinant tissue factor as an activator
  - This accelerates the rate of thrombin formation and thus clot formation
  - Commonly used in the trauma settings due to short test times:
  - R-value is obtained in less than 1 minute
  - MA value is obtained within 20 minutes
  - Disadvantages: Loss of sensitivity to coagulation factor component of R-value
- Functional fibrinogen test:
  - This test utilizes the MA value obtained from TEG
  - MA value reflects GPIIb/IIIa mediated interaction between platelets and fibrin
  - On addition of GPIIb/IIa antagonist, MA amplitude will be reduced
  - The resultant MA amplitude reflects the strength of fibrin alone
  - This value correlates closely with the plasma fibrinogen levels
- PlateletMapping:
  - Modification of TEG which measures platelet function by comparing:
    - Activated MA tracing with ADP receptors (MA_{pi})
    - MA achieved with no platelet activity (MA_f)
    - Maximal platelet activation (MA_{kh})
  - Test is carried out with heparinized blood
  - This is done to exclude thrombin-platelet activation
  - MA_{pi} represents the largest amplitude achieved with platelet activators (ADP)
  - MA_{kh} is the value obtained with standard kaolin-heparinase activated sample
  - MA_f represents the MA formed due to:
    - Factor XIII
    - Reptilase
  - Percentage reduction in platelet activity is then measured

  Percentage inhibition of platelet activity

$$= 100 - \left\{ \frac{(MA_{pi} - MA_f) \times 100}{(MA_{kh} - MA_f)} \right\}$$

SONOCLOT

Introduction

- Alternative viscoelastic monitor of coagulation
- Introduced by ***von Kaulla*** in 1975

Method

- In contrast to TEG, sonoclot measures changing impedance using ultrasonic probe
- The probe is immersed into a cuvette with 0.4 mL coagulating sample of blood
- The tubular probe oscillates up and down at:
  - Amplitude of 1 µm
  - Frequency of 200 Hz
- As clot formation occurs, impedance to probe movement through the blood increases
- This does not allow the ultrasonic probe to vibrate freely
- This generates an electrical signal with a characteristic ***clot signature***
- The Sonoclot Signature reflects real time coagulation including:
  - Start of fibrin formation
  - Fibrin cross linkage
  - Platelet mediated clot strengthening
  - Clot retraction
  - Fibrinolysis

Variations of Sonoclot

- kACT using kaolin activator
- SonACT using celite activator
- aiACT using celite and clay
- gbACT+ using glass beads
- H-gbACT+ using glass beads and heparinase

Parameters

- SonACT:
  - It is a measure of coagulation factor performance
  - Represents the time for initial fibrin formation
  - Time in seconds from the immersion until amplitude of 1 mm is reached
  - This is typically measured in seconds
  - Normal value: 60–130 seconds
  - Correlated with ACT derived by hemochron method
  - Shorter than R-value in TEG
  - This is because R-value is measured at a later stage of fibrin development
- Clot Rate (CR):
  - It is a measure of fibrin formation
  - CR phase includes 2 peaks on the sonoclot signature trace
  - The primary slope is called R1
  - Clot rate (CR) represents the maximal gradient of primary slope
  - This depends on rate of conversion of fibrinogen to fibrin
  - Rate of rise is expressed as the percentage of peak amplitude per unit time
  - Normal value 18–45%
- Time to peak (TP) or Platelet Function:
  - It is a measure of platelet mediated clot retraction
  - The second peak is due platelets and fibrin producing clot retraction
  - The amplitude of this peak is therefore proportional to fibrinogen levels
  - As the clot retracts from the cuvette, impedance to vibration decreases
  - The fibrinogen converts to fibrin and fibrin polymerizes
  - Speed of clot formation and platelet-fibrin interactions are represented by TP
  - Normal value of TP: 5–10 minutes
  - In the presence of more fibrinogen, the second peak has higher amplitude
  - The subsequent downward slope results from platelet mediated clot retraction

Interpretation

- Initial clot formation time: Son ACT
- Fibrin gel formation phase: T inflection
- Fibrin gel formation rate: R_1
- Clot retraction: T peak
- Rate of clot retraction: R_3
- Fibrinolysis

Advantages

- Predicts bleeding with an accuracy of 74%
- Ability to measure platelet function

Uses of Sonoclot

- Used to derive ACT
- Provides information regarding clot strength and fibrinolysis
- Helps to manage anti coagulation
- Manage blood product usage
- Identify hypercoagulable patients

ROTATIONAL THROMBOELASTOMETRY

Introduction

- Viscoelastic assay similar to TEG but with a different mode of measurement
- Has multiple advantages compared with TEG and currently preferred over TEG

Indications for ROTEM

- Coagulopathy associated with trauma and massive hemorrhage
- Liver transplant
- Cardiac surgery
- Major orthopedic surgery
- Hypothermia
- Postpartum hemorrhage
- Hypercoagulable states
- Procoagulant therapy

Uses of ROTEM

- Diagnosis of potential causes of hemorrhage
- Guide to hemostatic therapy
- Risk predictor of bleeding during surgery

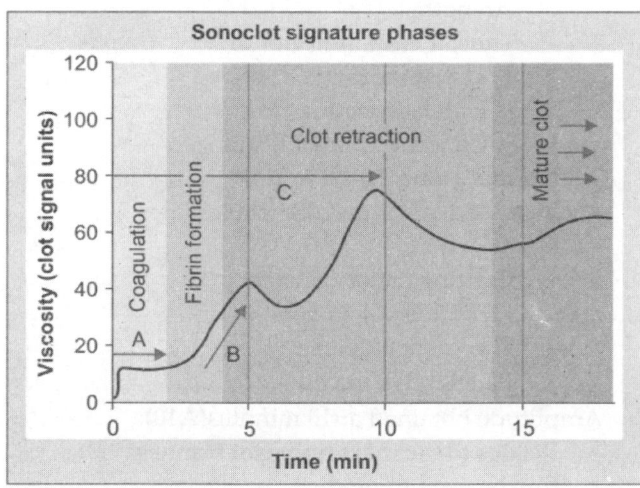

Fig. 4: Normal Sonoclot signature.

- Reducing complications due to blood products (TRALI, TACO, TRIM)
- Monitoring hypercoagulable states

Procedure

- Small amount of blood and coagulation activator is added to a disposable cuvette
- This is placed within the pre-warmed cuvette holder
- In contrast to TEG, the cuvette containing the sample is held stationary
- A rotating shaft is lowered into the blood sample within the cuvette
- The tip of the rotating shaft houses a disposable pin (sensor)
- This shaft rotates clockwise, then counter-clockwise by 4.75° repeatedly
- As the sample clots, there is a loss of elasticity in the sample
- This leads to changes in the rotation of the shaft
- This is detected by reflection of light on a small mirror attached to the shaft
- The change in the axis of the shaft is measured over time
- This is converted into a graph called the thromboelastogram, resembling TEG trace
- Typical time taken for the various test values:
  - Measurement of coagulation factor function: 10 minutes
  - Measurement of platelet and fibrinogen function: 23 minutes
  - Measurement of fibrinolysis: 40 minutes

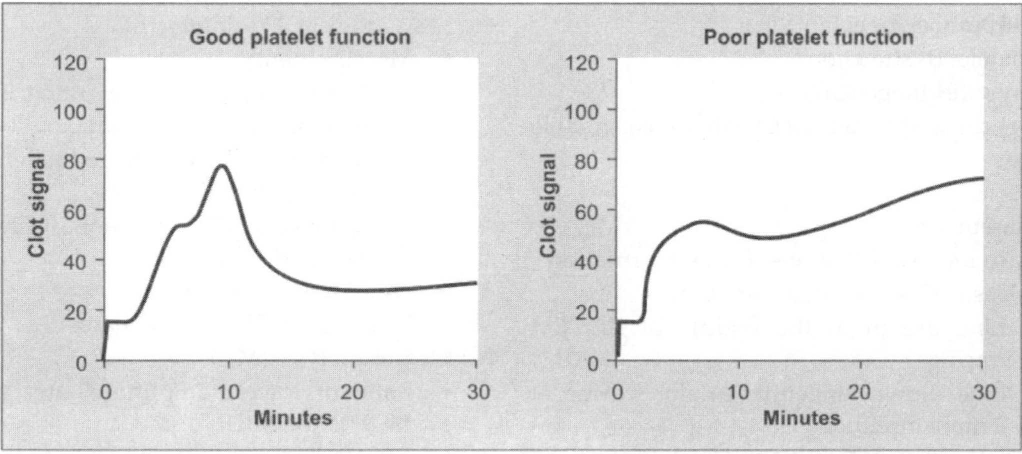

Fig. 5: Abnormal sonoclot signature.

Parameters Measured

- Clotting time (CT):
  - Measurement:
    - Represents early stage of clotting cascade comprising:
      - Initiation of clotting
      - Thrombin formation
      - Beginning of clot polymerization
    - Period of time from initiation of test to formation of initial fibrin clot
    - Measured from the start of the test until amplitude of tracing is 2 mm
    - Primarily an indication of:
      - Clotting factor concentration
      - Effect of heparin
  - Factors causing increased clotting time:
    - Clotting factor deficiency
    - Liver disease
    - Anticoagulation with warfarin or heparin
    - Hypofibrinogenemia
  - Factors causing decreased clotting time: hypercoagulable state
- Clot formation time (CFT):
  - Measurement:
    - It is a measure of the speed of clot formation
    - Primarily an indication of platelet count and function
    - Measured from end of CT till amplitude of the clot reaches 20 mm
    - Represents clot potentiation by:
      - Activation of platelets (mainly)
      - Fibrin polymerization
  - Normal values: 3–6 minutes
  - Factors causing increased CFT:
    - Clotting factor deficiency
    - Thrombocytopenia
    - Platelet dysfunction
    - Hypofibrinogenemia
  - Factors causing decreased CFT: hypercoagulable states
- α-angle:
  - Measurement:
    - Also represents the speed of clot formation
    - Measured as the angle between:
      - Line drawn in the middle of ROTEM tracing
      - Line drawn tangential to clot tracing at 2 mm amplitude
    - Primarily an indication of platelet count and function
  - Significance:
    - Increased angle reflects rapid clot formation mediated by:
      - Thrombin-activated platelets
      - Fibrin
      - Activated factor XIII
    - Decreased angle reflects shorter CFT
  - Normal value: 45–55°
  - Increased in: Hypercoagulable states
  - Decreased in:
    - Clotting factor deficiency
    - Hypofibrinogenemia
    - Thrombocytopenia
    - Platelet dysfunction
- Maximum Clot Firmness (MCF):
  - Measurement:
    - Amplitude of the clot measured at peak clot strength
    - Thus, it is an indicator of:
      - Platelet count
      - Platelet function
      - Concentration of fibrinogen
  - Normal value: 50–60 mm
  - Increased in: Hypercoagulable states
  - Decreased in:
    - Clotting factor deficiency
    - Hypofibrinogenemia
    - Thrombocytopenia
    - Platelet dysfunction
- Amplitude obtained at 10 minutes(A10):
  - Relates to the maximum clot firmness
  - Can be used to predict:
    - Maximum clot firmness
    - Platelet function
  - Represents stability of the clot formed
- Lysis index at 30 minutes (LI30):
  - Measurement:
    - It is a parameter representing fibrinolysis at a determined time point
    - Measures percentage reduction in MCF of tracing after 30 minutes
    - Represents the activation of fibrinolytic system and fibrinolysis
  - Normal value: < 7.5%
  - Increased in fibrinolytic states
- Maximum lysis (ML):
  - Ratio of lowest amplitude after reaching the MCF to the MCF
  - This parameter too represents activation of fibrinolytic system and fibrinolysis

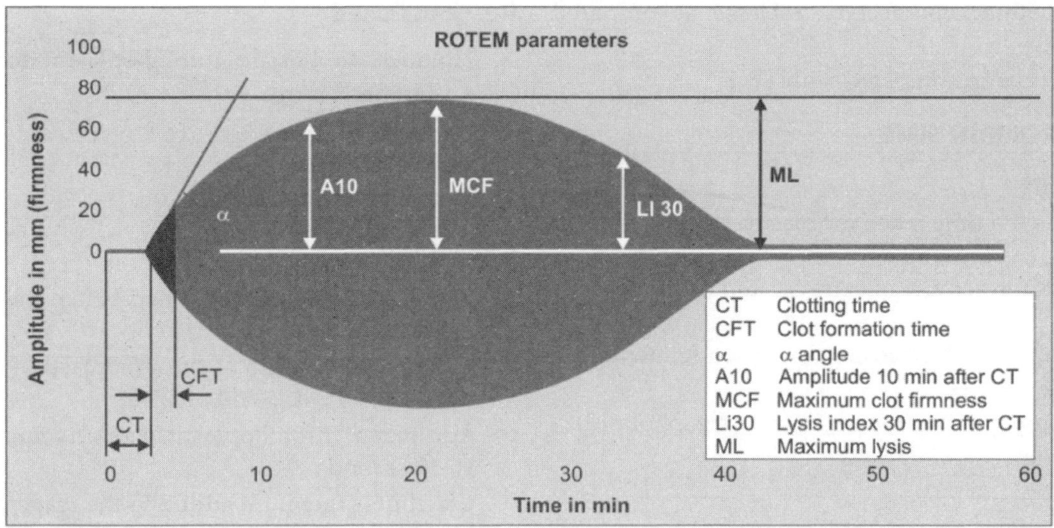

Fig. 6: ROTEM trace.

Types of ROTEM

- INTEM (intrinsic cascade)
- EXTEM (extrinsic cascade)
- HEPTEM (intrinsic cascade in the presence of heparin)
- FIBTEM (measures fibrinogen activity)
- APTEM (measures tissue factor activation and tranexamic acid)
- Platelet aggregation ROTEM:
  - ADPTEM (using ADP)
  - ARATEM (using arachidonic acid metabolites)
  - TRAPTEM (using TRAP)

Reagents Used

- INTEM: Ellagic acid
- EXTEM: Tissue factor
- HEPTEM:
  - Ellagic acid
  - Heparinase
- FIBTEM:
  - Tissue factor
  - Cytochalasin C
- APTEM:
  - Tissue factor
  - Aprotinin

Significance of ROTEM

- EXTEM:
  - Activation by thromboplastin or tissue factor (rabbit brain)
  - Used as a screening test for extrinsic pathway
  - Useful in evaluation of Factors I, II, V, VII, IX, X
  - Most sensitive to fibrinolysis
- INTEM:
  - Activation occurs in the contact phase by ellagic acid
  - Sensitive to intrinsic pathway factors
  - Useful in evaluation of Factors I, II, VIII, IX, XI, XII, von Willebrand factor
- FIBTEM:
  - Activation is similar to EXTEM
  - However, the addition of cytochalasin D inhibits platelet function
  - This allows isolated activation of fibrinogen
  - The resulting clot is dependent exclusively on fibrin polymerization
  - Thus, FIBTEM is a specific measure for fibrin concentration and function
- APTEM:
  - Activation is similar to EXTEM but with addition of aprotinin
  - Aprotinin inhibits fibrinolysis in the sample
  - Thus, APTEM is used to rule out fibrinolysis by comparing to EXTEM
- HEPTEM:
  - Activation is similar to that of INTEM
  - Refers to INTEM in the presence of heparinase
  - Useful to detect residual heparin

Advantages

- Method of recording the thromboelastogram is much more sensitive than TEG

- External vibrations affect the test lesser as compared with TEG
- Lower variance compared with TEG

PROTHROMBIN TIME

Introduction

- Measures the time taken for plasma to clot when exposed to tissue factor
- It reflects the activity of extrinsic and common pathways
- It is the reaction time to clot formation following addition of:
  - Thromboplastin (tissue factor + phospholipid)
  - Calcium

Physiology

- PT is used to evaluate adequacy of extrinsic and common pathway clotting mechanisms
- It measures the clotting ability of:
  - Factor I (fibrinogen)
  - Factor II (prothrombin)
  - Factor V
  - Factor VII
  - Factor X

Pathway Tested: Extrinsic and common coagulation pathway

Coagulation Factors Tested

- Factor I (fibrinogen)
- Factor II (prothrombin)
- Factor V
- Factor VII
- Factor X

Specimen

- Sodium-citrate (0.5 mL of 3.2%) anticoagulated *whole blood* is used
- Sodium citrate chelates the calcium and prevents premature activation of clotting
- This keeps the blood sample in stasis until ready to be tested
- 5 mL volume of blood is collected in the sample tube
- This is because low sample volume may result in falsely prolonged PT
- It is gently inverted a few times prior to storage
- The sample must be tested within:
  - 2 hours if stored at room temperature (22–24°C)
  - 4 hours if refrigerated (2–4 °C)

Reagents Used

- Homogenized tissue- thromboplastin from:
  - Human brain
  - Rabbit brain
  - Placenta
- Recombinant thromboplastin

Procedure

- Blood specimens are obtained before the daily dose of warfarin
- Calcium and excess of thromboplastin (0.2 mL) are added to 0.1 mL blood at 37°C
- Addition of thromboplastin shortens clotting time to 11–12 seconds
- Calcium is therefore added to the reagent just prior to test
- This overcomes the citrate anticoagulant and allows tissue factor to initiate coagulation
- Clot detection is usually done photo-optically
- Time taken for clot formation is the prothrombin time
- PT test result is usually given in seconds, along with a control value
- The control value varies depending upon:
  - Concentration and source of thromboplastin
  - Calcium concentration
  - Method used to detect clot formation
- The patients PT should be approximately equal to the control value
- Some laboratories may report the results as percentage of the normal activity
- Point-of-care home testing is available for those requiring long-term anticoagulation

Range

- Normal range:
  - 11–12.5 seconds
  - 85–100% of normal activity
- Healthy premature babies have normally prolonged PT which normalizes by 6 months
- If APTT is normal, prolonged prothrombin time represents F VIII deficiency
- Critical range: more than 20 seconds for non-anticoagulated specimens

Indications

- Screening for:
  - Deficiency of prothrombin
  - Dysfibrinogenemia

- Afibrinogenemia
- Liver failure
- DIC
- Vitamin K deficiency

❖ Monitoring anticoagulant therapy for:
- Valvular heart disease patients with prosthetic valves
- DVT prophylaxis
- DVT therapy
- Pulmonary embolism
- Atrial fibrillation

❖ Aid in calculation of MELD score

Causes of Prolonged Prothrombin Time

❖ Vitamin K deficiency:
- Occurs due to:
  - Malnutrition
  - Broad spectrum antibiotics
  - Fat malabsorption syndrome
- Mild deficiency causes prolongation of only prothrombin time
- However severe deficiency results in prolongation of PT and aPTT

❖ Vitamin-K antagonists:
- Warfarin interferes with post-translational modification of factors such as:
  - Factor II
  - Factor VII
  - Factor IX
  - Factor X
- Thus, it causes prolongation of prothrombin time

❖ Other anticoagulants:
- Heparin theoretically should prolong PT by inhibiting thrombin and factor Xa
- However, most PT reagents contain heparinase which block this effect
- At high doses though, heparinase gets saturated and may result in prolonged PT
- All other anticoagulants prolong PT and include:
  - Direct thrombin inhibitors
  - Direct oral anticoagulants
- However, degree of prolongation of PT is drug dependent
- Thus, PT cannot be used to titrate therapy with other anti-coagulants

❖ Liver diseases:
- Liver disease is associated with decrease in:
  - Vitamin-K dependant clotting factors (II, VII, IX, X)
  - Vitamin-K independent clotting factors (I, V)
- Mild liver disease prolongs only PT due to predominant effect on factor VII
- In severe liver disease, both PT and aPTT are prolonged

❖ DIC:
- DIC is characterized by consumptive coagulopathy of clotting factors
- Thus, both PT and aPTT may be prolonged

❖ Clotting factor deficiency of II, V, VII, IX, X

❖ Antiphospholipid antibodies:
- Lupus antibodies specific for prothrombin (factor II) may be produced
- This may cause prolongation of prothrombin time

Artefactual Prolongation

❖ Low sample volume

❖ Elevated hematocrit:
- Polycythemia
- Myelodysplastic syndromes

❖ Heparin contamination from indwelling catheters

❖ Increased plasma turbidity:
- Hyperlipidemia
- Hyperbilirubinemia
- Hemolysis

Limitations

❖ Not a very sensitive test:
- More sensitive for factors VII and X
- Less sensitive for factors I, II and V

❖ PT identifies the defect very late in course of disease:
- Factor levels as low as 40–50% may not prolong PT
- PT increases only marginally even if prothrombin reduces to as low as 10%
- PT is unaffected until fibrinogen < 100 mg/dL

❖ Does not identify the cause of hemostatic defect

❖ Results vary from lab to lab

❖ High turn-around time of 90 minutes

INTERNATIONAL NORMALIZED RATIO

Introduction

INR is a mathematical calculation developed to standardize PT values and negate differences in sensitivity between reagents in calculating PT.

Definition

❖ It is ratio of patient PT time to a control sample raised to the power of ISI value of the control sample used

❖ ISI = international sensitivity index

Formula

$$INR = \left(\frac{\text{PT of patient (seconds)} * \text{ISI}}{\text{Mean of normal range}}\right)$$

Normal Value

- INR of 1.3–1.5 (15–18 sec) recommended
- INR of 1.5–2 recommended in patients with prosthetic valves and recurrent emboli

Derivation

- Each thromboplastin reagent has an international sensitivity index (ISI) value
- ISI value shows how sensitive it is compared with the international reference thromboplastin
- ISI is usually between 1 and 1.4
- ISI of 1 ⇒ TP specimen has same sensitivity as reference TP
- ISI > 1 ⇒ TP specimen less sensitive than reference TP
- ISI < 1 ⇒ TP more sensitive than reference TP

Factors Increasing INR: Associated with Increased Risk of Bleeding

- Alcoholism with concomitant liver disease
- Drugs:
  - Amiodarone
  - Anabolic steroids
  - Cimetidine
  - Clofibrate
  - INH
  - Omeprazole
  - Piroxicam
  - Cotrimoxazole
  - Erythromycin
  - Fluconazole
  - Fluroquinolones
  - Metronidazole
  - Phenylbutazone
  - Propranolol

Factors Reducing INR: Associated with Increased Risk of Thrombosis

- Enteral feeds with high vitamin K levels
- Drugs:
  - Avocado
  - Barbiturates
  - Carbamazepine
  - Griseofulvin
  - Rifampicin
  - Sucralfate

ACTIVATED PARTIAL THROMBOPLASTIN TIME

Introduction

- Partial thromboplastin time and aPTT are identical tests used to test clotting function
- However, a contact activator is used to hasten clot formation for aPTT measurements
- Measures the activity of intrinsic and common pathways of coagulation
- Commonly used to monitor patient response to UFH infusions
- It is the reaction time to clot formation following addition of:
  - Thromboplastin with no tissue factor activity
  - Calcium
  - Contact activation factor
- Since thromboplastin with no tissue factor is used, it is termed as partial thromboplastin time

Pathway Tested: Intrinsic and Final Common Pathway

Factors Tested

- Factor I (fibrinogen)
- Factor II (prothrombin)
- Factor V
- Factor VIII
- Factor IX
- Factor X
- Factor XI
- Factor XII
- High Molecular Weight Kininogens (HMWK)
- Pre-kallikrein

Specimen

- Sodium citrate (0.5% mL of 3.2%) anticoagulated *platelet-poor plasma* is used
- Fasting sample taken as lipemia hampers photoelectric measurement of clot formation
- In patients receiving heparin, samples are taken 30–60 minutes before next dose
- In patients receiving heparin infusions, sample may be taken at any time
- 5 mL volume of blood is drawn from the patient
- The tube is inverted gently several times to enable mixing with the citrate
- After collection, the whole blood sample is centrifuged and plasma is removed
- The plasma is kept refrigerated at 4°C and transported as soon as possible
- The test has to be completed within 4 hours of collection

Additives Used

- Reaction initiated by kaolin, Ca^{2+} and phospholipids is called aPTT
- Addition of negatively charged phospholipids shortens clotting time
- Phospholipids are platelet substitutes (hence sample is platelet poor)
- Sources of phospholipids:
  - Rabbit brain
  - Cephalin (dehydrated rabbit brain)

- Bovine brain
- Soya bean

Procedure

- Calcium and contact activator (0.2 mL) are added to 0.1 mL plasma at 37 °C
- Contact activators used are:
  - Cephalin
  - Kaolin
  - Microsilicate
  - Ellagic acid
- Contact activator avoids prolonged time of natural contact activation
- Plasma sample (platelet poor plasma) added to activator
- This is incubated at 37 °C for 5 mins
- Thromboplastin preparation added, mixed with $CaCl_2$ and timer started
- Time to fibrin clot formation recorded

Mixing Studies

- Prolonged aPTT is evaluated further by mixing studies
- In this, patients plasma is mixed with normal plasma
- If the mixing corrects the prolonged aPTT, a clotting factor deficiency is suspected
- Failure to correct the aPTT within 3-4 seconds of mixing suggests:
  - Coagulation factor inhibitor (acquired factor VIII antibodies)
  - Lupus anticoagulant

Range

- Normal range:
  - aPTT: 30–40 second
  - PTT: 60–70 seconds
- Critical range causing increased risk of spontaneous bleeding:
  - aPTT more than 70 seconds
  - PTT more than 100 seconds
- Therapeutic range: aPTT is adjusted to 1 ½ to 2 times normal in heparin therapy
- Healthy premature babies have prolonged aPTT which returns to normal at 6 months

Indications

- Monitoring unfractionated heparin therapy:
  - Response to heparin therapy can be measured with aPTT
  - Heparin dose may be adjusted based on aPTT values to achieve desired effect
  - Therapeutic range usually is between 60–80 seconds
- Screening for bleeding disorders:
  - Hemophilia A and B (factor VIII, factor IX)
  - von Willebrands disease
  - Dysfibrinogenemia
  - DIC
  - Liver failure
  - Vitamin K deficiency
- Other uses:
  - For preoperative screening
  - Evaluation of unexplained bleeding
  - Evaluation for lupus anticoagulant
  - Diagnosis of activated protein C (APC) resistance

Causes of Prolonged APTT

- Heparin therapy:
  - Heparin inactivates factor II (prothrombin)
  - This prevents formation of thromboplastin and prolongs aPTT
  - Intrinsic pathway coagulation is prolonged for 4-6 hours after heparin dose
- Hemophilia A and B: Deficiency of factor VIII and factor IX
- Obstructive biliary diseases:
  - Cause a reduction in vitamin K dependant factors II, IX, X
  - This results in prolongation of aPTT
- DIC:
  - Characterized by consumptive coagulopathy of all factors
  - Thus, DIC results in prolongation of aPTT
- Normal pregnancy:
  - Associated with factor XI deficiency and anti phospholipid antibodies
  - This may result in prolonged aPTT
- Autoimmune conditions:
  - Acquired anti-factor VIII antibodies
  - Lupus anticoagulant antibodies
- Drugs:
  - Direct thrombin inhibitors
  - Direct factor Xa inhibitors
  - Antihistaminics
  - Salicylates
  - Ascorbic acid

Causes of Shortened APTT

- Early stages of DIC due to circulating procoagulants
- Extensive cancer
- Immediately following acute hemorrhage

- During acute phase response leading to high factor VIII levels

Artefactual Prolongation

- Low sample volume
- Elevated hematocrit:
  - Polycythemia
  - Myelodysplastic syndromes

Disadvantages

- Cannot be used to monitor therapy with newer low-molecular weight heparin
- Clotting factor levels must fall below 30% before aPTT is prolonged
- Thus, aPTT identifies the defect very late in course of disease
- aPTT is more sensitive to factors VIII and IX than other factors
- Thus, values may not be prolonged until levels fall below 15% for some factors
- aPTT values may be reagent specific with no reference standard
- Thus, with the lack of reference standards, aPTT values are institution specific

Interpretation

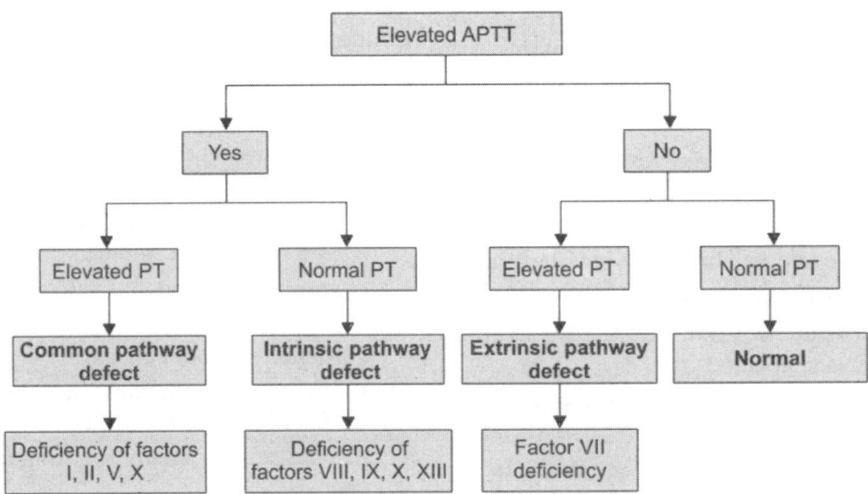

ACTIVATED CLOTTING TIME

Introduction

- First introduced by ***Hattersley*** in 1966
- It is a variation of the Lee-White whole blood clotting time
- Most widely used monitor of heparin effect during:
  - Angioplasty
  - Cardiac surgery
  - Hemodialysis
- Measures the activity of intrinsic and common pathways

Physiology

- This test measures time for whole blood to clot after addition of particulate activators
- Whole blood is added to a tube with an activator which can be:
  - Diatomaceous earth (celite)
  - Kaolin
- The presence of the activator augments contact-activation phase of coagulation
- This stimulates the intrinsic coagulation pathway by activating factor XII

Specimen: Fresh whole blood free of venepuncture derived thromboplastin

Procedure

- The required quantity of whole blood is mixed with the activator
- These tubes with freshly drawn blood are incubated at 37 °C
- Contact of blood with the activator initiates the intrinsic coagulation cascade
- Tubes are tilted at 30-second intervals until flow of blood stops
- Tilting and recording of time can be done manually or by automated machines
- Commercially available devices detect the onset of clot formation

Choice of Activator

- Heparin prolongs celite-activated ACT more than kaolin activated ACT
- Aprotinin also increases the ACT substantially with celite activator
- However, prolongation of aprotinin-ACT is only minimal with kaolin
- This is due to binding of kaolin with aprotinin, eliminating aprotinin's effect on ACT

Types

- Hemachron:
  - Manufactured by International Technidyne Corporation, Edison, New Jersey
  - Most commonly used device
  - Has a small test tube with a cylindrical magnet placed within it
  - Magnet is in contact with a proximity detection switch
  - The tube also contains the celite activator
  - 2 mL blood sample is added to test tube and incubated at 37 °C
  - The tube is then rotated gently as the test progresses
  - The cylinder rolls along the bottom of the tube continuously
  - As the fibrin clot forms, the cylinder gets enmeshed in it
  - Thus, the cylinder is pulled away from the proximity detection switch
  - This interrupts the magnetic field and activates the proximity detection switch
  - An alarm is triggered which signals the end of the clotting time
  - Hemachron ACT can also be performed using kaolin as activator
- ACT Plus (Hemotec ACT, Hepcon HMS Plus):
  - Manufactured by Medtronic Perfusion Services, Minneapolis, Minnesota
  - This consists of a cartridge with 2 chambers with kaolin activator
  - The cartridge is housed in a heat block
  - 0.4 mL blood is placed into each chamber
  - A flag-shaped plunger is raised and passively dropped into the chamber
  - The formation of a clot slows the rate of descent of the plunger
  - This decrease in velocity is detected by a photo-optical system
  - The test is signalled to an end once the plunger is enmeshed in the clot
- Comparison:
  - Hemachron ACT may over-estimate the ACT
  - This may be due to the larger volume of blood used during the test
  - This difference is even higher in the pediatric population

Range

- Normal range: 80–120 seconds
- Reflects activity of classical intrinsic pathway
- Therapeutic range: 150–600 second depending upon the therapeutic procedure

Uses

- Titrating heparin therapy during cardiac surgery:
  - Baseline ACT is determined before IV heparin
  - Sampling is repeated approximately 3 minutes after heparin administration
  - Done at 30-minute intervals thereafter
  - During CPB,
    - Accepted ACT goal > 400–480 seconds
    - ACT 180–400 seconds: Questionable effect
    - ACT < 180 seconds: Inadequate effect
- Limitation of postoperative blood transfusion:
  - ACT enables better titration of heparin therapy
  - This results in reduced blood loss and transfusion requirements post-CPB

Advantages

- ACT has several advantages over aPTT while monitoring heparin therapy
- ACT is more accurate when high doses of heparin are used
- Thus, it is more useful for monitoring heparin effect on CPB
- aPTT is not measurable at such high doses of heparin
- ACT is less expensive and can be performed more easily
- It is a point of care test which allows immediate accessibility

Limitations

- Does not correlate with plasma heparin levels
- Insensitive to low dose heparin
- Low reproducibility
- Assays overall coagulation activity
- Insensitive to factor VII deficiency (gets prolonged only if factor level < 5%)

- Prolonged values may not be exclusively due to heparin therapy
  - Hypothermia causes a dose-related increase in ACT
  - Hemodilution caused by CPB prime prolongs ACT
  - Abnormal values may also result from:
    - Thrombocytopenia below 30,000–50,000/μL prolong ACT
    - Platelet abnormality:
      - Coadministration of platelet inhibitors increase the ACT:
        - Aspirin
        - Clopidogrel
        - Prostacyclins
      - Platelet lysis causes a significant reduction in ACT values

Prolonged ACT

- Heparin therapy
- Altered heparin metabolism (liver/kidney disease)
- Heparin rebound phenomenon
- Other drugs:
  - Protamine overdose
  - Aprotinin
- Clotting factor deficiencies
- Impaired ability of blood to generate clot:
  - Warfarin administration
  - Severe thrombocytopenia
  - Platelet inhibitors:
    - Prostacyclin
    - Aspirin
    - Clopidogrel
    - Monoclonal antibodies against GP II b/IIIa
- Artefactual prolongation:
  - Aprotinin
  - Hemodilution
  - Hypothermia

Suboptimal ACT

- Heparin resistance
- Platelet lysis

Heparinase-ACT

- ACT test may be modified by the addition of heparinase
- With this, anticoagulant effect of heparin is eliminated
- Thus, coagulation status of the heparin-neutralised sample may be assessed
- The test provides a side-by-side comparison of untreated ACT with heparinase ACT
- It serves as a rapid test for assessment of:
  - Circulating heparin like substances
  - Residual heparinization after CPB

PLATELET FUNCTION TESTS

Introduction

- Platelets play a crucial role in both hemostasis and thrombosis
- Thus, measurement of platelet function is important to guide platelet therapy

Platelet Function Tests

- Bleeding time
- Platelet counting:
  - Manual platelet counting
  - Automated cell counter method
  - Optical counting method
  - Flow cytometric methods
  - Platelet count ratio
- Platelet aggregometry:
  - Turbidometric platelet aggregometry
  - Whole blood aggregometry
  - Light scattering methods
- Platelet adhesion tests:
  - Clot signature analyzer (CSA)
  - Thrombotic status analyzer (TSA)
  - Platelet function analyzer (PFA-100)
  - Cone and platelet analyzer (IMPACT)
- Measurement of platelet aggregation:
  - Hemostatus device
  - TEG and ROTEM
  - Hemodyne device
- Measurement of platelet activation:
  - VASP-P
  - Measurement of soluble activation markers
  - Flow cytometric analysis of platelet activation markers
  - Reticulated platelets
- Tests to monitor antiplatelet therapy:
  - Verify Now
  - Multiplate analyzer

Bleeding Time

- Was the first in-vivo test of platelet function developed by Duke in 1910
- Not used as a routine preoperative screening test

- Useful for identifying patients with severe hemostatic defects:
  - von Willebrands disease
  - Glanzmann's thrombasthenia
- Disadvantages:
  - Poorly reproducible
  - Invasive test
  - Insensitive assay
  - Cannot be used during surgical procedures

Platelet Counting Methods

- Manual platelet counting:
  - Platelet count continues to be the first line test of platelet function
  - Manual counting is done using phase-contrast microscopy
  - This method is inaccurate
  - Coefficients of variability (CV) is high between 15–25%
- Automated cell counter methods:
  - Uses impedance method to estimate platelet count
  - Particles within a given volume range are counted (2 fL–30 fL volume)
  - All particles within this range are counted as platelets
  - Other methods used include:
    - Optical scattering
    - Immunological methods
  - Advantages:
    - Rapid and precise
    - Easily reproducible
  - Disadvantages:
    - Over-estimate platelet count in samples with debris such as:
      - Thalassemia
      - Thrombotic thrombocytopenic purpura
      - Leukemia
    - Underestimation in patients with large platelets such as ITP
- Optical counting methods:
  - In this method, platelets are identified by their:
    - Light scattering properties
    - Fluorescence
  - These properties are studied following addition of a suitable dye
  - Advantages:
    - Both normal and large sized platelets are accurately identified
    - This method is more accurate compared to impedance methods
- Flow cytometric methods:
  - Platelets are incubated with a fluorescent monoclonal antibody
  - Antibody is directed against antigens on the surface of the platelet
  - The platelet count is derived from calculating the RBC ratio
  - RBC ratio is then multiplied by the RBC count to provide the platelet count

$$\text{RBC ratio} = \frac{\text{Number of fluorescent particles counted}}{\text{Number of red cell events}}$$

  - Advantages:
    - Method is devoid of pipetting and dilution artifacts
    - Derived platelet counts are highly accurate
    - Coefficients of variation are low (< 5%)
    - Also this method is more accurate at very low platelet counts
- Platelet count ratio:
  - Platelets within anticoagulated whole blood sample is stimulated by agonists:
    - Adenosine diphosphate (ADP)
    - Epinephrine
    - Ristocetin
  - On stimulation, aggregates are formed
  - This results in the reduction of the number of free platelets
  - The platelet count ratio is calculated using:

$$\text{Platelet count ratio} = \frac{\text{Platelet count in stimulated sample}}{\text{Platelet count in control sample}}$$

  - The platelet count ratio correlates well with platelet aggregometry
  - Test can be performed on automated cell counters using commercial agents
  - ICHOR point of care hematology counter may be used for platelet count ratio

Platelet Aggregometry

- Turbidometric platelet aggregometry:
  - Blood is centrifuged at low force to obtain platelet-rich-plasma (PRP)
  - This is stirred in a cuvette at 37 C between:
    - Light source and
    - Measuring photocell
  - Upon addition of an agonist such as ADP, platelets aggregate
  - This results in an increase in the transmission of light and reduction in turbidity

- The changes in light transmission are recorded as a function of time
- This facilitates diagnosis of platelet disorders based on pattern of aggregation
- Factors affecting the test results include:
  - Normal functioning of platelets
  - Presence of platelet inhibitors
  - Concentration of agonist

❖ Whole blood aggregometry:
- Uses electrical impedance to measure platelet aggregation
- Whole blood is stirred at 37 °C between 2 platinum wire electrodes
- These electrodes are placed at a fixed distance
- Following addition of agonists, electrodes are covered with platelet aggregates
- This changes the electrical impedance with time, which is recorded
- Results obtained are similar to the turbidometric method
- Useful for monitoring aspirin and clopidogrel therapy

❖ Light scattering methods:
- Uses laser light scattering to monitor formation of platelet aggregates
- Intensity of light scattered is proportional to the size of aggregates formed

Platelet Adhesion Tests

❖ Clot signature analyzer (CSA):
- Uses an instrument called hemostatometer
- Non-anticoagulated whole blood is taken in the test tube
- Holes are made within the tube
- This encourages hemostatic plug formation and collagen channels in the tube
- Variables measured include:
  - Time for platelets to occlude the holes punched (platelet hemostasis time or PHT)
  - Collagen induced thrombus formation time (CITF)
  - Clotting time
- Thus CSA detects abnormalities in both platelet activation and coagulation

❖ Thrombotic status analyzer (TSA):
- Measures thrombotic and thrombolytic activities in non-anticoagulated blood
- This induces platelet aggregation solely by shear forces
- It does not utilize platelet agonists
- Whole blood is taken in a capillary tube
- Platelet activation and aggregation results in capillary tube occlusion
- Subsequent thrombolysis also may be measured
- Thus, this test may be used to monitor:
  - Platelet function
  - Thrombolytic therapy
  - Anti-platelet therapy

❖ Platelet function analyzer (PFA):
- Uses citrated whole blood to measure hemostasis under high shear stress
- PFA-100 uses a test cartridge with a membrane impregnated with either:
  - Collagen and ADP (Col/ADP)
  - Collagen and epinephrine (Col/Epi)
- The blood sample is placed in a cup and aspirated through the aperture
- The sample is thus exposed to high shear within the capillary tube
- This results in platelet activation and aggregate formation
- Formation of a platelet plug results in a drop in the flow rate
- End point of the test:
  - Measured as the closure time
  - Occurs when blood flow stops due to aperture occlusion by platelets
- Normal closure time:
  - 77–133 seconds for Col/ADP membrane
  - 98–185 seconds for Col/Epi membrane
- Uses:
  - As a screening tool for hemostatic anomalies, especially in children
  - Col/ADP cartridges:
    - von Willebrand disease
    - Congenital platelet disorders
  - Col/Epi cartridges:
    - Congenital platelet function disorders
    - Aspirin ingestion
    - von Willebrand disease

❖ Cone and platelet analyzer (IMPACT):
- Immediate microscopic platelet adhesion cone and plate technology
- Tests platelet adhesion under arterial flow conditions
- Based on the adhesion of platelets to an extracellular matrix (ECM)
- Device consists of a polystyrene cone and plate system
- 130 µL blood sample is exposed to the polystyrene plate
- This is exposed to a high shear stress for 2 minutes

- Surface bound platelets are quantified using an image analyzer
- Parameters measured are:
  - Surface coverage of the plate by platelets
  - Average size of surface bound objects
- Used to diagnose:
  - Afibrinogenemia
  - von Willebrand disease
  - Glanzmann thrombasthenia
  - Bernard-Soulier syndrome

Measurement of Platelet Aggregation

❖ Hemostasus device:
- Point of care device to measure platelet function
- Analyses the effects of platelet activating factor (PAF) on kaolin-ACT
- Measures the effect of four different concentration of PAF over ACT
- Used to:
  - Monitor GP IIb/IIIa inhibitors
  - Identify Glanzmann thrombasthenia

❖ Thromboelastography and ROTEM:
- Assesses several parameters of clot formation in whole blood
- TEG monitors interaction of platelets within the fibrin mesh of the clot
- Useful as a point of care test of platelet function in surgical patients

❖ Hemodyne device:
- Measures platelet contractile force (PCF)
- It is a sensitive measure of global platelet function
- 800 μL of citrated whole blood is used
- The sample is placed within a sample cup between 2 parallel plates
- Upon addition of thrombin, platelets adhere to the plates
- Upon formation of fibrin meshwork, PCF is transmitted outwards to the plates
- Parameters measured include:
  - Platelet contractile force
  - Clot rigidity
- Uses:
  - Glanzmanns thrombasthenia
  - Dysfunction during cardiopulmonary bypass
  - Platelet dysfunction in uremia

Measurement of Platelet Activation

❖ VASP-P:
- Refers to vasodilator-stimulated phosphoprotein
- This protein triggers cell motility via its interaction with actin
- VASP-P is responsible for pseudopod formation in platelets
- Thus, it may be used as a marker for ADP-induced platelet activation

❖ Measurement of soluble activation markers:
- Sample tubes containing inhibitors of platelet activation are used
- These inhibitors include:
  - Theophylline
  - PGE_1
- This helps in the measurement of platelet release products
- Assays for platelet specific proteins include:
  - Platelet factor 4
  - Beta thromboglobulin
  - Thromboxane B_2
  - Soluble P-selectin

❖ Flow cytometric analysis of platelet activation markers:
- Activation markers commonly measured are:
  - Granule membrane markers (CD62p, CD 63, LAMP-1)
  - Ligand induced binding site (LIBS) antibodies
  - Receptor induced binding site (RIBS) antibodies
  - Thrombospondin
  - Multimerin
- Uses:
  - To optimize antiplatelet therapy
  - To predict thrombotic events after invasive procedures (angioplasty)

❖ Reticulated platelets:
- Immature platelets contain residual RNA and are called reticulated platelets
- Specific dyes may be used to measure platelets with residual RNA
- This is used to assess platelet turnover in thrombocytopenia
- Uses:
  - Bone marrow recovery following transplantation
  - Response to therapy with thrombopoietin

Tests to Monitor Antiplatelet Therapy

❖ Verify Now analyzer:
- Turbidometric based optical detection system utilizing microbeads
- Platelet induced aggregation is measured as a decrease in light transmittance

- Patients citrated whole blood is added to the assay system
- Fibrinogen-coated microbeads are used in the analyzer
- Platelets are activated using ADP which results in aggregation
- Upon platelet aggregation, the microbeads also aggregate
- The change in optical density is measured as a marker of platelet function
- Aspirin may be added to the blood sample to measure its effect
- Platelet function is reported in the form of Aspirin Reaction Units (ARU):
  - > 550 ARU: No evidence of platelet dysfunction due to aspirin
  - < 550 ARU: Platelet dysfunction is due to aspirin

❖ Multiplate analyzer:
- Based on the principle of platelet adherence following platelet activation
- Multiplate test cell contains an inlet to receive the sample
- Metal sensor wires are also present which extend into the blood sample
- Electrical resistance between the sensor wires is constantly monitored
- On activation, platelets bind to these sensor wires
- This increases the electrical resistance, which is measured by the analyzer
- Uses:
  - To titrate anti-platelet therapy
  - To predict bleeding in patients on antiplatelet therapy
  - To assess perioperative platelet function

SUGGESTED READING

1. AABB guidelines: Kaufman, R. M. et al., (2015). Platelet transfusion: A clinical practice guideline from the AABB. *Annals of Internal Medicine*, 162(3), 205–13.
2. Adcock, D. M., Kressin, D. C. and Marlar, R. A. (1998). Minimum specimen volume requirements for routine coagulation testing: dependence on citrate concentration. *American Journal of Clinical Pathology*, 109(5), 595–9.
3. Agarwal, V. K. (2014). Organo-fluorine compounds as artificial blood substitutes. *Defence Science Journal*, 30(1), 51–4.
4. ALBIOS Study Investigators: Caironi, P. et al., (2014). Albumin replacement in patients with severe sepsis or septic shock. *New England Journal of Medicine*, 370, 1412-1.
5. Barash, P. G. et al., (2017). *Clinical Anesthesia*. 8th ed. Philadelphia: Wolters Kluwer.
6. Barile, L. et al., (2017). Acute normovolemic hemodilution reduces allogenic red blood cell transfusion in cardiac surgery: A systematic review and meta-analysis of randomized trials. *Anesthesia & Analgesia*, 124(3), 743–52.
7. Benzon, H. T., Park, M., McCarthy R. J., Kendall, M. C. and Lindholm, P. F. (2018). Mixing studies in patients with prolonged activated partial thromboplastin time or prothrombin time. *Anesthesia & Analgesia*, 128(6), 1089–96.
8. Biss, T. T. and Hanley, J. P. (2007). Use of recombinant factor VIIa (rFVIIa) in the management of intractable haemorrhage: a survey of current UK practice. *British Journal of Haematology*, 138(1), 126–8.
9. Bonello, L. et al., (2013). A randomized trial of platelet reactivity monitoring-adjusted clopidogrel therapy versus prasugrel therapy to reduce high on-treatment platelet reactivity. *International Journal of Cardiology*, 168(4), 4244–8.
10. Bowles, K. M., Bloxham, D. M., Perry, D. J. and Baglin, T. P. (2006). Discrepancy between impedance and immunofluorescence platelet counting has implications for clinical decision making in patients with idiopathic thrombocytopenia purpura. *British Journal of Haematology*, 134(3), 320–2.
11. Bux, J. and Sach, U. J. H. (2007). The pathogenesis of transfusion-related acute lung injury. *British Journal of Haematology*, 136(6), 788–99.
12. Cabrales, P. and Intaglietta, M. (2013). Blood substitutes: evolution from non-carrying to oxygen and gascarrying fluids. *Journal of American Society of Artificial Internal Organs*, 59(4), 337–54.
13. Caraceni, P., Tufoni, M. and Elena Bonavita, M. (2013). Clinical use of albumin. *Blood Transfusion*, 11(Suppl 4), s18–25.
14. Carless, P. A., Henry, D. A., Moxey, A. J., O'Connell, D. L., Brown, T. and Fergusson, D. A. (2010). Cell salvage for minimizing perioperative allogeneic blood transfusion. *Cochrane Database of Systematic Reviews*, 18;(4), CD001888.
15. Chappell, D., Jacob, M., Hofman-Kiefer, K., Conzen, P. and Rehm, M. (2008). A rational approach to perioperative fluid management. *Anesthesiology*, 109(4), 723–40.
16. Cheng, D. et al., (2007). Colloids for perioperative plasma volume expansion: Systematic review with meta-analysis of controlled trials (Abstract). *Transfusion Alternatives in Transfusion Medicine*, 9, S3.
17. Cohn, C. S. and Cushing, M. M. (2009). Oxygen therapeutics: Perfluorocarbons and blood substitute safety. *Critical Care Clinics*, 25(2), 399–414.
18. CRISTAL Investigators: Annane, D. et al., (2013). Effects of fluid resuscitation with colloids vs crystalloids on mortality in critically ill patients presenting with hypovolemic shock: the CRISTAL randomized trial. *Journal of American Medical Association*, 310(17), 1809–17.
19. Crochemore, T. et al., (2017). A new era of thromboelastometry. *Einstein*, 15(3), 380–5.
20. Davis, A. L. et al., (2017). American College of Critical Care Medicine clinical practice parameters for hemodynamic support of pediatric and neonatal septic shock. *Critical Care Medicine*, 45(6), 1061–93.
21. Dellinger, R. P. et al., (2013). Surviving sepsis campaign: international guidelines for management of severe sepsis and septic shock: 2012. *Critical Care Medicine*, 41(2), 580–637.

22. Despotis, G. J. et al., (1996). Evaluation of a new point-of-care test that measures PAF-mediated acceleration of coagulation in cardiac surgical patients. *Anesthesiology*, 85(6), 1311–23.
23. Dutta, T. K. and Verma, S. P. (2014). Rational use of recombinant factor VIIa in clinical practice. *Indian Journal of Hematology & Blood Transfusion*, 30(2), 85–90.
24. Eisenhut, M. (2006). Causes and effects of hyperchloremic acidosis. *Critical Care*, 10(3), 413.
25. Esper, S. A. and Waters, J. H. (2011). Intraoperative cell salvage: A fresh look at the indications and contra-indications. *Blood Transfusion*, 9(2), 139–47.
26. Finfer, S. Myburg, J. and Bellomo, R. (2018). Intravenous fluid therapy in critically ill adults. *Nature Reviews Nephrology*, 14, 541–57.
27. Fronticelli, C. and Koehler, R. (2009). Designs of recombinant hemoglobins for use in transfusion fluids. *Critical Care Clinics*, 25(2), 357–71.
28. Funk, D. M. (2012). Coagulation assays and anticoagulant monitoring. Hematology: *American Society of Hematology Education Program*, 2012(1), 460–5.
29. Galan, A. M., Tonda, R., Altisent, C., Maragall, S., Ordinas, A. and Escolar, G. (2001). Recombinant factor VIIa (Novo-Seven®)restores deficient coagulation: experience from an ex-vivo model. *Seminars in Hematology*, 38(Suppl 12), 10–4.
30. Garcia-Martinez,R., Caraceni, P., Bernarddi, M., Gines, P., Arroyo, V. and Jalan, R. (2013). Albumin: Pathophysiological basis of its role in the treatment of cirrhosis and its complications. *Hepatology*, 58(5), 1836–46.
31. Giefer, M. J., Murray, K. F. and Colletti, R. B. (2011). Pathophysiology, diagnosis, and management of pediatric ascites. *Journal of Pediatric Gastroenterology and Nutrition*, 52(5), 503–13.
32. Gladden, L. B. (2004). Lactate metabolism: a new paradigm for the third millennium. *Journal of Physiology*, 558(Pt 1), 5–30.
33. Goldberg, A. D. and Kor, D. J. (2012). State of the art management of transfusion-related acute lung injury (TRALI). *Current Pharmacological Design*, 18(22), 3273–84.
34. Gravlee, G. P., Davis, R. F., Hammon, J. and Kussman, B. (2015). *Cardiopulmonary Bypass and Mechanical Support*. 4th ed. Philadelphia: Wolters Kluwer.
35. Guidelines, Curry, N. S. et al., (2018). The use of viscoelastic haemostatic assays in the management of major bleeding: A British Society for Haematology Guideline. *British Journal of Haematology*, 182(6), 789–806.
36. Guidelines, European Association for the Study of the Liver. (2010). EASL clinical practice guidelines on the management of ascites, spontaneous bacterial peritonitis, and hepatorenal syndrome in cirrhosis. *Journal of Hepatology*, 53(3), 397–417.
37. Guidelines, Martinowitz, U., Michaelson, M. and Israeli Multidisciplinary rFVIIa Task Force. (2005). Guidelines for the use of recombinant activated factor VII (rFVIIa) in uncontrolled bleeding: a report by the Israeli Multidisciplinary rFVIIa Task Force. *Journal of Thrombosis and Haemostasis*, 3(4), 640–8.
38. Hahn, R. G. (ed.) (2011). *Clinical Fluid Therapy in the Perioperative Setting*. New York: Cambridge Medicine.
39. Harrison, P., Robinson, M. S., Mackie, I. J. and Machin, S. J. (1997). *Reticulated platelets*. Platelets, 8(6), 379–83.
40. Harrison, P. and Lordkipanidze, M. (2013). Testing platelet function. *Hematology/Oncology Clinics of North America*, 27(3), 411–41.
41. Hayward, C. P. M., Harrison, P., Cattaneo, M., Ortel, T. L., Rao, A. K. and Platelet Physiology Subcommittee of the Scientific and Standardization Committee of the International Society on Thrombosis and Haemostasis. (2006). Platelet function analyzer (PFA)-100 closure time in the evaluation of platelet disorders and platelet function. *Journal of Thrombosis and Haemostasis*, 4(2), 312–9.
42. Hedner, U. (2000). Recombinant coagulation factor VIIa: from the concept to clinical application in hemophilia treatment in 2000. *Seminars in Thrombosis and Hemostasis*, 26(4), 363–6.
43. Hett, D. A., Walker, D., Pilkington, S. K. and Smith, D. C. (1995). Sonoclot analysis. *British Journal of Anaesthesia*, 75(6), 771–6.
44. Hines, R. (ed.) (2017). *Stoelting's Anesthesia and Co-existing Disease*. 7th ed. Philadelphia: Elsevier.
45. Holte, K., Sharrock, N. E. and Kehlet, H. (2002). Pathophysiology and clinical implications of perioperative fluid excess. *British Journal of Anaesthesia*, 89(4), 622–32.
46. Ichai, C. Orban, J. and Fontaine, E. (2014). Sodium lactate for fluid resuscitation: the preferred solution for the coming decades? *Critical Care*, 18, 163.
47. Insert, P. (2018). Gelofusine: *summary of product* characteristics.
48. Insert, P. (2018). *Piramal Healthcare*.
49. Irwin, R. S. and Rippe, J. M. (eds.) (2011). *Irwin & Rippe's Intensive Care Medicine*. 7th ed. Philadelphia: Lippincott Williams & Wilkins.
50. Jacob, E. K., Emery, R. L., Orrock, J. M., Van Buskirk, C. M. and Gandhi, M. J. (2009). Filter failures with sickling hemoglobin. *Transfusion*, 49(8), 1535–6.
51. Jacob, M., Bruegger, D., Conzen, P., Becker, B. F., Finsterer U. and Rehm, M. (2005). Development and validation of a mathematical algorithm for quantifying preoperative blood volume by means of the decrease in hematocrit resulting from acute normovolemic hemodilution. *Transfusion*, 45(4), 562–71.
52. James, M. (2008). The role of tetrastarches for volume replacement in the perioperative setting. *Current Opinion in Anesthesiology*, 21(5), 674–8.
53. Joshi, G. P. and Kehlet, H. (2016). CON: Perioperative goal-directed fluid therapy is an essential element of an enhanced recovery protocol? *Anesthesia and Analgesia*, 122(5), 1261–3.
54. Kamal, A. H., Tefferi, A. and Prithi, R. K. (2007). How to interpretand pursue an abnormal prothrombin time (PT), activated partial thromboplastin time, and bleeding time in adults. *Mayo Clinic Proceedings*, 82(7), 864–73.
55. Kaplan, J. A., Augoustides, J. G. T., Reich, D. L. and Manecke, G. R. (2017). *Kaplan's Cardiac Anesthesia*. 7th ed. Philadelphia: Elsevier.
56. Kelin, A. A. et al., (2018). Association of Anaesthetists guidelines: Cell salvage for perioperative blood conservation 2018. *Anaesthesia*, 73(9), 1141–50.
57. Kendrick, J. B. et al., (2019). Goal-directed fluid therapy in the perioperative setting. *Journal of Anaesthesiology and Clinical Pharmacology*, 35(Suppl 1), s29–34.

58. Kessler, C. M. (2000). New products for managing inhibitors to coagulation factors: A focus on recombinant factor VIIa concentrate. *Current Opinion in Hematology*, 7(6), 408–13.
59. Kleinman, S. et al., (2004). Toward an understanding of transfusion-related acute lung injury: statement of a consensus panel. *Transfusion*, 44(12), 1774–89.
60. Lecak, J., Scott, K., Young, C., Hannon, J. and Acker, J. P. (2004). Evaluation of red blood cells stored at -80 C in excess of 10 years. *Transfusion*, 44(9), 1306–13.
61. Levi, M., Toh, C. H., Thachil, J. and Watson, H. G. (2009). Guidelines for the diagnosis and management of disseminated intravascular coagulation. *British Journal of Haematology*, 145(1), 24–33.
62. Levy, J. H., Koster, A., Quinones, Q. J., Milling, T. J. and Key, N. S. (2018). Antifibrinolytic therapy and perioperative considerations. *Anesthesiology*, 128(3), 657–70.
63. Lewis, S. R. et al., (2018). Colloids versus crystalloids for fluid resuscitation in critically ill people. *Cochrane Database of Systematic Reviews*, 8(8):CD000567.
64. Li, C. K. N., Hoffmann, T. J., Hsieh, P.-Y., Malik, S. and Watson, W. C. (1998). The Xylum Clot Signature Analyzer®: a dynamic flow system that simulates vascular injury. *Thrombosis Research*, 92(6), S67–77.
65. Lier, H., Vorweg, M., Hanke, A. and Gorlinger, K. (2013). Thromboelastometry guided therapy of severe bleeding. Essener Runde algorithm. *Hamostaseologie*, 33(1), 51–61.
66. Liumbruno, G., Bennardello, F., Lattanzio, A., Piccoli, P. and Rossettias, G. as Italian Society of Transfusion Medicine and Immunohaematology (SIMTI) Working Party.(2009). Recommendations for the use of albumin and immunoglobulins. *Blood Transfusion*, 7(3), 216–34.
67. Marini, J. J. and Dries, D. J. (2019). *Critical Care Medicine: The Essentials and More*. 5th ed. Philadelphia: Wolters Kluwer.
68. Martin-Llahi, M. et al., (2008). Terlipressin and albumin vs albumin in patients with cirrhosis and hepatorenal syndrome: a randomized study. *Gastroenterology*, 134(5), 1352–9.
69. McCullough, J. (2010). Overview of platelet transfusion. *Seminars in Hematology*, 47(3), 235–42.
70. Michelson, A. D. and Furman, M. I. (1999). Laboratory markers of platelet activation and their clinical significance. *Current Opinion in Hematology*, 6(5), 342–8.
71. Miller,T. E. and Myles, P. S. (2019). Perioperative fluid therapy for major surgery. *Anesthesiology*, 130, 825–32.
72. Mitra, S. and Khandelwal, P. (2009). Are all colloids same? How to select the right colloid? *Indian Journal of Anaesthesia*, 53(5), 592–607.
73. Modi, M. P., Vora, K. S., Parikh, G. P. and Shah, V. R. (2012). A comparative study of impact of infusion of ringer's lactate solution versus normal saline on acid-base balance and serum electrolytes during live related renal transplantation. *Saudi Journal of Kidney Diseasesand Transplantation*, 23(1), 135–7.
74. Moore, E. E., Johnson, J. L., Cheng, A. M., Masuno, T. and Banerjee, A. (2005). Insights from studies of blood substitutes in trauma. *Shock*, 24(3), 197–205.
75. Moradi, S., Jahanian-Najafabadi, A. and Roudkenar, M. H. (2016). Artificial blood substitutes: first steps on the long route to clinical utility. *Clinical Medicine Insights: Blood Disorders*, 9, 33–41.
76. Myburgh, J. A. and Mythen, M. G. (2013). Resuscitation fluids. *New England Journal of Medicine*, 369, 1243–51.
77. Nakajima, S. et al., (2000). A global platelet test of thrombosis and thrombolysis detects a prothrombotic state in some patients with non-insulin dependent diabetes and in some patients with stroke. *Platelets*, 11(8), 459–66.
78. Nicholson, N. S. et al., (1998). Assessment of platelet function assays. *American Heart Journal*, 135(5), S170–8.
79. OPTIMISE Study Group: Pearse, R. M. et al., (2014). Effect of a perioperative, cardiac output-guided hemodynamic therapy algorithm on outcomes following major gastrointestinal surgery: a randomized clinical trial and systematic review. *Journal of the American Medical Association*, 311(21), 2181–90.
80. Ozaki, Y., Satoh, K., Yatomi, Y., Yamamoto, T., Shirasawa, Y. and Kume S. (1994). Detection of platelet aggregates with a particle counting method using light scattering. *Analytical Biochemistry*, 218(2), 284–94.
81. Pagana, K. D., Pagana, T. J. and Pagana, T. N. (2019). *Mosby's Diagnostic & Laboratory Test Reference*. 14th ed. Missouri: Elsevier.
82. Pandya, S. (2015). *Practical Guidelines on Fluid Therapy*. 2nd ed. Mumbai: Bhalani Medical Book House.
83. Papageorgiou, C. et al., (2018). Disseminated intravascular coagulation: an update on pathogenesis, diagnosis, and therapeutic strategies. *Clinical and Applied Thrombosis/Hemostasis*, 24(9), 76029618806424.
84. Piper, G. L. and Kaplan, L. J. (2012). Fluid and electrolyte management for the surgical patient. *Surgical Clinics of North America*, 92(2), 189–205.
85. Rana, R. et al., (2006). Transfusion-related acute lung injury and pulmonary edema in critically ill patients: a retrospective study. *Transfusion*, 46(9), 1478–83.
86. Ratko, T. A. et al., (2001). Evidence-based recommendations for the use of WBC-reduced cellular blood components. *Transfusion*, 41(10), 1310–9.
87. RGropper, M., Eriksson, L., Fleisher, L., Wiener-Kronish, J., Cohen, N. and Leslie, K. (2020). *Miller's Anesthesia*. 9th ed. Philadelphia: Elsevier Saunders.
88. Robertson, J. and Shilkofski, N.(eds.) (2005). *The Harriet Lane Handbook: A Manual for Pediatric House Officers*. 17th ed. Philadelphia: Mosby.
89. Rodgers, R. P. and Levin, J. (1990). A critical appraisal of the bleeding time. *Seminars in Thrombosis and Hemostasis*, 16(1):1–20.
90. SALT-ED Investigators: Self, W. H. et al., (2018). Balanced crystalloids versus saline in noncritically ill adults. *New England Journal of Medicine*, 378, 819–28.
91. Savion, N. and Varon, D. (2006). Impact: the cone and plate(let) analyzer: testing platelet function and anti-platelet drug response. *Pathophysiology of Haemostasis and Thrombosis*, 35(1-2), 83–88.
92. Schierhout, G. and Roberts, I. (1998). Fluid resuscitation with colloid or crystalloid solutions in critically ill patients: a systematic review of randomised trials. *British Medical Journal*, 316(7136), 961–4.
93. Schmaier, A. (1997). Contact activation: a revision. *Journal of Thrombosis and Haemostasis*, 78(1), 101–7.
94. Scott, M. G., Kucik, D. F., Goodnough, L. T. and Monk, T. G. (1997). Blood substitutes: evolution and future applications. *Clinical Chemistry*, 43(9):1724–31.

95. Sharma, A., Arora, S., Grewal, P., Dhillon, V. and Kumar, V. (2011). Recent innovations in delivery of artificial blood substitute: a review. *International Journal of Applied Pharmaceutics*, 3(2), 1–5.
96. Sirtl, C., Laubenthal, H., Zumtobel, V., Kraft, D. and Jurecka, W. (1999). Tissue deposits of hydroxyethyl starch (HES): dose-dependent and time-related. *British Journal of Anaesthesia*, 82(4), 510–3.
97. Spahn, D. R. et al., (2013). Management of bleeding and coagulopathy following major trauma: an updated European guideline. *Critical Care*, 17(2):R76.
98. Squires, J. E. (2002). Artificial blood. *Science*, 295(5557), 1002–5.
99. Stehling, L. and Zauder, H. L. (1991). Acute normovolemic hemodilution. *Transfusion*, 31(9), 857–68.
100. Tabuchi, N., de Haan, J., Gallandat Huet, R. C., Boonstra, P. W. and van Oeveren, W. (1995). Gelatin use impairs platelet adhesion during surgery. *Thrombosis and Haemostasis*, 74(6), 1447–51.
101. Tao, Z. and Ghoroghchian, P. P. (2014). Microparticle, nanoparticle, and stem cell-based oxygen carriers as advanced blood substitutes. *Trends in Biotechnology*, 32(9), 466–73.
102. Tintinalli, J., Stapczynski, J., John Ma, O., Yealy, D., Meckler, G. and Cline, D. (2016). *Tintinalli's Emergency Medicine*. 8th ed. New York: McGraw Hill.
103. Toh, C.-H., Alhamadi, Y. and Abrams, S. T. (2016). Current pathological and laboratory considerations in the diagnosis of disseminated intravascular coagulation. *Annals of Laboratory Medicine*, 306(6), 505–12.
104. Toy, P. et al., (2012). Transfusion-related acute lung injury: incidence and risk factors. Blood*, 119(7)*, 1757–67.
105. Vanderlinde, E. S., Heal, J. M. and Blumberg, N. (2002). Autologous transfusion. *British Medical Journal*, 324(7340), 772–5.
106. van Stein, D. et al., (2010). Transfusion-related acute lung injury reports in the Netherlands: an observational study. *Transfusion*, 50(1), 213–20.
107. van Werkum, J. W., Harmsze, A. M., Elsenberg, E. H. A. M., Bouman, H. J., ten Berg, J. M. and Hackeng, H. M. (2009). The use of the Verify Now system to monitor antiplatelet therapy: a review of the current evidence. *Platelets*, 19(7), 479–88.
108. Vlaar, A. P. J. et al., (2019). A consensus redefinition of transfusion-related acute lung injury. *Transfusion*, 59(7), 2465–76.
109. Walunj, A., Babb, A. and Sharper, R. (2006). Autologous blood transfusion. *Continuing Education in Anaesthesia Critical Care & Pain*, 6(5), 192–6.
110. Waters, J. H. (2013). Intraoperative blood recovery. *American Society for Artificial Internal Organs Journal*, 59(1), 11–7.
111. Wikes, N. J. et al., (2001). The effects of balanced versus saline-based hetastarch and crystalloid solutions on acid-base and electrolyte status and gastric mucosal perfusion in elderly surgical patients. *Anesthesia & Analgesia*, 93(4), 811–6.
112. Wrzosek, A. et al., (2019). Perioperative restrictive versus goal-directed fluid therapy for adults undergoing major non-cardiac surgery. *Cochrane Database of Systematic Reviews*. [Viewed 23 May 2020] Available from: https://doi.org/10.1002/14651858.CD012767.pub2.
113. Wurtz, M., Hvas, A.-M., Christensen, K. H., Rubak, P., Kristensen, S. D. and Grove, E. L. (2014). Rapid evaluation of platelet function using the Multiplate® Analyzer. *Platelets*, 25(8), 628–33.
114. Yank, V. et al., (2011). Systematic review: benefits and harms of inhospital use of recombinant factor VIIa for off-label indications. *Annals of Internal Medicine*, 154(8), 529–40.
115. Yasumura, S. et al., (2017). Evidence-based guidelines for the use of albumin products. *Japanese Journal of Transfusion and Cell Therapy*, 63(5), 641–63.

16 CHAPTER

Transplant Anesthesia

LUNG TRANSPLANT

Introduction

- Lung transplantation is an important mode of therapy for patients with end-stage liver disease (ESLD)
- Lung transplantation is the treatment of choice for ESLD patients with:
  - High risk of death (> 50%) within 2 years in the absence of lung transplant
  - High likelihood (> 80%) of survival for > 90 days following transplantation
  - High likelihood (> 80%) of 5-year post-transplant survival

Efficacy

- Median survival for all lung transplant recipients was 6.5 years
- Bilateral LT recipients have a better survival than single lung transplant (SLT) recipients (7.6 vs 4.7 years)

Indications

- Diagnostic indications:
  - COPD
  - Cystic fibrosis and bronchiectasis
  - Interstitial lung disease
  - Pulmonary vascular disease
  - Adenocarcinoma of lung
- Timing for listing on transplant for each disease:
  - COPD patients are listed for transplant when:
    - BODE index > 7
    - One episode of severe hypercapnic failure with:
      - $PaCO_2$ > 50 mm Hg
      - PaO_2 < 60 mm Hg
    - FEV_1 < 15–20% predicted
    - 6-minute walk distance < 400 metres
    - Moderate-severe PAH
  - Cystic fibrosis and bronchiectasis are listed when:
    - Chronic respiratory failure with:
      - PaO_2 < 60 mm Hg
      - $PaCO_2$ > 50 mm Hg
    - Long term non-invasive therapy
    - Moderate-severe PAH
    - Frequent hospitalization
    - Rapid decline in lung function
  - Interstitial lung disease patients are listed when:
    - Decline in FVC > 10% during last 6 months
    - Decline in DLCO > 15% during last 6 months
    - Desaturation to < 88%
    - 6-minute walk test duration < 250 metres
    - Moderate-severe PAH
    - Frequent hospitalization
    - Rapid decline in lung function
  - Pulmonary vascular disease patients are listed when:
    - NYHA class II-IV despite combination therapy including prostanoids
    - Cardiac index < 2 $L/min/m^2$
    - Mean right atrial pressure > 15 mm Hg
    - 6-minute walk test < 350 metres
    - Development of:
      - Pericardial effusion
      - Significant hemoptysis
      - Signs of progressive right heart failure
  - Minimally invasive adenocarcinoma patients are listed when:
    - Diffuse parenchymal involvement causing lung restriction
    - Significantly reduced quality of life
    - Failure of conventional medical therapy

Contraindications

- Absolute contraindications:
  - Untreatable disease of other major organ systems
  - Active malignancy within last 2 years
  - Active pulmonary tuberculosis
  - Non-curable chronic pulmonary infection

- Acute medical instability:
  - Acute sepsis
  - Myocardial infarction
  - Liver failure
- Uncorrectable bleeding diathesis
- Chest wall/spinal deformity which may cause severe RLD post-transplant
- Obesity with BMI > 35 kg/m^2
- Psychosocial conditions:
  - Untreatable psychiatric condition
  - Absence of reliable social support system
  - Severe limitation of functional status with poor rehabilitation potential
- Documented non-compliance with therapy
- Substance addiction:
  - Either active or in last 6 months
  - Non-compliance with rehabilitation therapy

❖ Relative contraindications:
- Age:
  - More than 65 years with low physiological reserve
  - More than 70 years even if physiological reserve is good
- Progressive or severe malnutrition
- Extensive prior chest surgery with lung resection
- Infection highly virulent bacteria, fungi or mycobacteria
- HIV, hepatitis B or C infections
- Obesity with BMI between 30–35 kg/m^2
- Medical conditions which have not resulted in end-organ damage:
  - Diabetes mellitus
  - Systemic HTN
  - Epilepsy
  - Central venous obstruction
  - Severe osteoporosis

Types

❖ Single lung transplant:
- Accounts for 25% of lung transplants
- Procedure can be done in lateral position
- One lung ventilation will be required during resection of the lung
- During clamping of the PA, severe RV dysfunction may occur
- This may cause RV decompensation requiring support
- Thus, CPB support or ECMO may be used during the procedure
- Thus, perfusionist team should be available and on standby during the procedure

❖ Bilateral sequential transplant:
- Performed in 75% of patients with generalized pulmonary disease
- The lungs are implanted separately and sequentially
- Usually performed via sequential technique
- Uses transverse thoracosternotomy for optimal exposure

❖ En-bloc double lung transplant: Rarely used

❖ Heart lung transplant:
- Indicated in combined ESHD with ESLD
- Usually reserved for severe PAH with concomitant severe RV failure:
  - Eisenmanger syndrome
  - Idiopathic pulmonary arterial HTN

❖ Living related lobar transplant:
- Not performed regularly
- This surgery is restricted to children and small-statured adults
- Requires lung tissue from 2 donors
- RLL from 1 donor is implanted into recipients right hemithorax
- LLL from another donor is implanted into recipients left hemithorax

Single lung transplant	Double lung transplant
Technically easier	More difficult
Not done in infections as native lung can infect new lung	Can be done
Useful for difficult recipients (prior thoracic surgery)	Not done for difficult recipients
Bad functional improvement	Good improvement
Increased VP mismatch postoperatively	No such increase
Better survival	No such increase
CPB used if severe pulmonary HTN	CPB used routinely

Surgical Considerations

❖ For single lung transplant (SLT):
- Lateral decubitus position
- Via thoracotomy
- Pelvis is angled to allow femoral cannulation for CPB
- OLV during resection and removal of lung
- Once OLV stabilized lung is dissected and PA isolated
- Progressive temporary clamping of PA done
- If temporary clamping is well tolerated, PA is clamped and stapled
- Pneumonectomy is completed
- Implant graft beginning with airway anastomosis

- Anastomosis completed with telescoping bronchial anastomoses or use of omental wrap
- PA branches attached to graft
- Cuff of left atrium anastomosed to pulmonary vein
- Partially inflate implanted lung, de-air LA cuff and pulmonary veins
- Restore circulation of organ

❖ For bilateral lung transplant (BLT):
- Supine position
- ***Clamshell incision*** and transverse thoracosternotomy
- Bilateral anterior thoracotomy with or without transverse sternotomy
- This allows complete visualization of heart and lungs
- Both the native lungs are mobilized
- En-bloc bilateral lung transplant:
  - Rarely performed
  - Uses hypothermic CPB and cardioplegia
  - OLV during dissection and removal of lung
- Sequential bilateral lung transplant:
  - Does not require CPB routinely
  - RV decompensation during PA clamping may necessitate CPB
  - It is usually done in 2 phases
  - First phase:
    - More severely compromised lung (as by V-P scan) is removed
    - Single lung ventilation of contralateral lung
    - Bronchial anastomosis is completed with new lung
  - Second phase:
    - Brief period of reperfusion of first lung allograft
    - OLV is then switched over to allograft side
    - Other lung removed during ventilation of transplanted lung

Preoperative Evaluation

❖ Same as for thoracotomy

❖ Intraoperative management may be challenging for patients with:
- High baseline oxygen requirement (>4L/minute)
- Preoperative requirement of airway secretion clearance therapy
- Elevated baseline $PaCO_2$ levels
- Pulmonary arterial HTN

Preoperative Preparation and Premedication

❖ NPO orders:
- Recipients receive surgical notification within hours of donor confirmation
- Thus, time available for fasting may be inadequate
- Rapid sequence induction may be used in these patients

❖ Blood product availability:
- Adequate availability of cross-matched blood products should be verified
- 2 units of PRBCs are sufficient for SLT without CPB
- Products required for BLT or SLT on CPB support include:
  - 4 units PRBCs
  - 4 units FFP

❖ Timing of anesthetic induction:
- Donor lung procurement and recipient induction should be carefully timed
- This is done in order to minimize cold ischemia time (CIT) of donor lung:
  - Increasing CIT adversely affects the outcome
  - CIT is preferably limited to < 6 hours
- Following resection of donor lung:
  - It is flushed with cold preservative solution
  - Partially inflated and cooled for transport
- Recipient induction is begun only after ascertaining the donor lung status

❖ Venous access:
- 2 large bore venous access is secured to enable rapid blood transfusion
- Central venous access is secured prior to anesthetic induction
- 2 CVCs may be secured at times:
  - First central venous access for PAC
  - Additional CVC access with multi-lumen catheter for inotropes

❖ Anti-aspiration prophylaxis
- Patients routine PPI is continued on the day of surgery
- Other drugs used:
  - Non-particulate antacids sodium citrate 500 mg in 15 mL
  - IV metoclopramide 0.15 mg/kg
  - H_2 receptor antagonists:
    - Cimetidine
    - Famotidine

- ❖ Preoperative sedation:
  - Generally avoided
  - ESLD patients are susceptible to respiratory depression
  - Sedation may lead to severe hypercapnea and cause RV decompensation
- ❖ Planning for postoperative analgesia:
  - Thoracic epidural catheter may be placed preoperatively
  - This has several advantages:
    - Reduced postoperative pain
    - Reduced opioid analgesic requirements
    - Reduced duration of ventilation
    - Reduced length of ICU and hospital stay
  - Disadvantages:
    - Epidural hematoma however exists due to intraoperative heparin
    - Intraoperative hypotension jeopardizing GDFT strategies
- ❖ Preoperative medications:
  - Bronchodilator therapy should be continued on the morning of surgery
  - Pulmonary vasodilator therapy also should be continued

Monitors

- ❖ Pulse oximetry
- ❖ E_TCO_2
- ❖ ECG
- ❖ Urine output
- ❖ Temperature
- ❖ Frequent arterial blood gases
- ❖ Invasive arterial BP monitoring:
  - Routinely used
  - Radial artery catheterization is usually performed for SLT
  - Femoral artery catheterization:
    - Preferred for clamshell incisions and BLT
    - Retraction of chest wall may compress subclavian artery against 1st rib
    - Thus radial pressure will be 10–20 mm Hg lower than femoral artery
  - Arterial cannula is useful for:
    - Beat-to-beat monitoring of blood pressure
    - Assessment of intravascular volume status with SVV
    - Blood sampling for ABG
- ❖ Central venous catheterization:
  - Routinely used
  - Ultrasound guided catheterization preferred
  - Ultrasound enables detection of DVT due to repeated prior cannulation
  - Subclavian vein is avoided as:
    - It may be inaccurate during retraction of chest wall
    - May cause pneumothorax which may be detrimental in ESLD
  - Central venous catheter may be used for:
    - Assessment of intravascular volume status
    - Assessment of fluid responsiveness
    - Administration of inotropes
    - Blood sampling for $ScvO_2$
- ❖ Pulmonary artery catheter:
  - Commonly used
  - Essential for patients with evidence of pulmonary HTN
  - Position of PAC tip:
    - PAC should be floated with TEE visualization
    - This is to position the tip of PAC just proximal to PA bifurcation
    - Surgeon should be notified of PAC tip position
    - This is to avoid PAC entrapment during transection of PA
  - May be used to monitor:
    - Continuous cardiac output
    - Pulmonary artery pressure
    - Changes in pulmonary vascular resistance
  - PACs with continuous MvO_2 monitoring capability may be useful
- ❖ Transesophageal echocardiography:
  - Used routinely for both SLT and BLT
  - Useful to monitor:
    - Intravascular volume status
    - Useful to diagnose etiology of hemodynamic instability
    - Monitoring of cardiovascular anatomy and function
    - Assess PAH and RV function
    - Guidance of CPB/ECMO cannula placement
- ❖ Other monitors of cardiac output:
  - Lithium-dilution based methods
  - Thermodilution based devices (PICCO)
  - Arterial-waveform based methods (Flotrac)
  - Thoracic electrical bioimpedance methods
- ❖ Neuromonitoring: NIRS may be used to monitor cerebral oxygenation

Induction

- ❖ Adequate preoxygenation
- ❖ Prolonged preoxygenation required as:
  - Patients generally have increased FRC

- Increased airway pressures
- Reduced alveolar ventilation
- Preoxygenation done for 15–20 minutes

❖ Induction in patients with no risk for aspiration:
- Small dose of midazolam (1–2 mg) may be administered just prior to induction
- This may help reduce the dose of induction agent
- In stable patients:
  - IV propofol 0.5–1 mg/kg is the preferred induction agent
  - Induction agent is administered in titrated doses slowly
  - This is due to risk of hypotension caused by loss of SVR
- In unstable patients:
  - Etomidate is agent of choice
  - IV etomidate 0.2–0.3 mg/kg may be used for induction
  - Ketamine may be used as an alternative
- Intubation is facilitated with:
  - Fentanyl 2–5 μg/kg
  - Vecuronium 0.1 mg/kg

❖ Rapid sequence induction:
- Rapid sequence induction is indicated for inadequate fasting status
- Neuromuscular blocking agent:
  - Succinylcholine (SCH):
    - May be used when serum $K^+ < 5.5$ mEq/L
    - Serum K^+ levels increase transiently by 0.5–1 mEq/L
    - Serum K^+ levels return to baseline after 10–15 minutes
  - Rocuronium:
    - Used when serum $K^+ \geq 5.5$ mEq/L
    - Provides similar intubating conditions to SCH
    - Dose used for RSI is high (0.8–1.2 mg/kg)

❖ Intubation:
- DLT is the preferred method for lung isolation
- SLT with BB may be used for difficult airway patients
- Choice of DLT:
  - Left sided DLT is preferred for BLT
  - Right sided DLT is placed for left SLT
  - Left sided DLT is placed for right SLT
- Positioning of DLT:
  - Bronchial cuff should be positioned as proximally as possible
  - Proximal positioning allows room for surgical anastomosis
- In the presence of cystic fibrosis with thick secretions:
  - Single lumen ETT is inserted first
  - This is followed by FOB guided bronchial lavage
  - This is followed by DLT insertion

❖ Nasogastric tube and Foleys catheter are secured

❖ TEE probe may be inserted following intubation

❖ Surgical antibiotic prophylaxis:
- IV ceftazidime 2 g is the most commonly used antibiotic
- Ceftazidime administration is completed 30 minutes prior to skin incision
- This is to attain adequate blood antibiotic levels prior to skin incision
- Repeat doses of 1 g IV are administered every Q8H
- Additionally, IV vancomycin 15 mg/kg (up to 2 g) is administered
- Vancomycin administration is begun 1 hour prior to surgery
- This is to enable slow infusion and prevent Redman syndrome
- IV vancomycin 15 mg/kg is repeated Q12H

❖ Hypotension at induction:
- Precipitous hypotension may occur at induction
- ESLD usually have a high preoperative sympathetic tone
- This will be lost on administration of induction agents
- Thus, precipitous hypotension on induction is possible
- Hypotension is treated with vasopressors such as:
  - Ephedrine
  - Phenylephrine
  - Norepinephrine

Position

❖ Supine if double lung transplant

❖ Lateral decubitus for single lung transplant

Maintenance

❖ TIVA preferred as:
- Frequent need for airway access during surgery for:
  - Suction
  - Bronchoscopy
- This may lighten patient if VA used

- Also VA are avoided in end stage lung disease as it inhibits HPV
- Balanced anesthesia if used, is accomplished with O_2 + air + 0.5–1 MAC isoflurane
- Alternatively, sevoflurane or desflurane may be used
- Nitrous oxide is contraindicated as it increases pulmonary arterial pressures
- Anesthesia may be supplemented with boluses of:
  - Fentanyl 1 µg/kg
  - Vecuronium 0.03 mg/kg
- Heparin:
  - IV UFH 5000 IU may be administered prior to clamping of PA
  - Dose is repeated prior to second lung transplant in BLT
- Induction dose of immunosuppression:
  - Given soon after induction:
    - IV mycophenolate mofetil 1 g infused over 2 hours
    - IV basiliximab 20 mg given over 30 minutes
  - IV methylprednisolone 500 mg–1 g is given prior to release of PA clamp

Ventilation

- Ventilatory goals:
  - Permissive hypercapnea with lung protective ventilation
  - FiO_2:
    - FiO_2 is adjusted to maintain SpO_2 88–95%
    - Usually titration of FiO_2 < 100% is not possible clinically in ESLD
    - 100% used just prior to OLV as it:
      - Minimizes desaturation during OLV
      - Promotes absorption atelectasis in non-ventilated lung
  - Tidal volume 6–7 mL/kg
  - Respiratory rate adjusted to maintain $PaCO_2$ close to baseline
  - PEEP 5–10 cm H_2O
  - Lower plateau airway pressure < 25–30 cm H_2O due to risk of bullous rupture
  - I:E ratio of 1:3 to 1:4 to reduce air trapping
- During one lung ventilation:
  - 100% FiO_2
  - Tidal volume 4–5 mL/kg
  - PEEP 7–12 cm H_2O
- Ventilation of transplanted lung:
  - Recruitment maneuvers (3–5) are performed following reperfusion of graft
  - Lung protective ventilation of transplanted lung is preferred
  - FiO_2:
    - Minimum FiO_2 to maintain SpO_2 88–95% is used
    - Hyperoxia and FiO_2 > 40% is associated with poor outcomes
  - Tidal volume < 6 mL/kg
  - Respiratory rate adjusted to maintain $PaCO_2$ close to baseline
  - PEEP < 5 cm H_2O to limit hyperinflation of native lung
  - Lower plateau airway pressure < 25–30 cm H_2O due to risk of bullous rupture
  - I:E ratio of 1:3 to 1:4 to reduce air trapping
- Watch for pulmonary tamponade during IPPV
- Prevention of auto-PEEP:
  - High I:E ratio is preferred (1:3 to 1:4)
  - Intermittent apnea is practiced with disconnection of ventilator circuit
  - This allows venting of lungs if pulmonary tamponade occurs

Hemodynamics

- Fluid therapy: Restrictive fluid strategy is used with:
  - Maintenance fluids at 1.5 mL/kg/hour of balanced salt solution
  - Replacement of evaporative losses at 1 mL/kg/hour
  - Replacement of blood loss to maintain hematocrit > 25%
  - Volume resuscitation when required is done with 5% albumin
  - Restrict fluid administration in the first 24 hours to less than 2 mL/kg/hour
  - Restrict perioperative positive fluid balance to less than 1.5 L
- Hemodynamic changes:
  - Hypotension is common during:
    - Induction of anesthesia
    - Clamping of PA
    - Side clamping of LA to complete pulmonary vein anastomosis
    - Reperfusion of lung
  - During conversion to OLV:
    - Hypoxia and hypercarbia may increase RV afterload
    - TEE is used to monitor RV dysfunction during PA clamping
  - During bronchial anastomosis watch for:
    - Low cardiac output
    - Arrhythmias
    - Systemic hypotension and pulmonary HTN

- Therapeutic options:
  - Prefer vasopressors/inotropes to treat:
    - Anesthesia induced vasodilation
    - Ongoing hypoperfusion
  - Vasopressors preferred are:
    - Vasopressin
    - Norepinephrine
  - If PA clamping is not tolerated, treat with:
    - PGE_1
    - Nitric oxide
    - Inotropes
    - CPB if RV dysfunction persists
- Increased chances of hypothermia:
  - Warm IV fluids used
  - Warm blankets
  - Forced air warmers

CPB Considerations

- Electively indicated for:
  - Severe pulmonary HTN with transpulmonary pressure gradient > 20 mm Hg
  - Pulmonary fibrosis
  - RV dysfunction with hypertrophy or fibrosis
  - Children in whom DLT may cause RUL obstruction
- Emergent indication in:
  - RV dysfunction during PA clamping
  - Early graft dysfunction during second lung transplant
  - Surgical mishaps
- ECMO is preferred over CPB as it is associated with:
  - Reduced need for tracheostomy
  - Reduced incidence of primary graft rejection
  - Better outcomes
  - Reduced hospital stay
- CPB not preferred as it:
  - Increases lung dysfunction
  - Increases bleeding and blood product use
  - Associated with increased duration of ventilation

Ischemia Time

- Cold ischemia time extends from:
  - Donor pulmonary artery cross clamp prior to harvest till
  - Removal of pulmonary artery cross clamp and reperfusion post implantation
- Minimization of cold ischemia time is vital to attain optimal graft function
- This requires close communication between donor and recipient teams
- Incision in recipient is usually begun when status of donor organ has been ascertained
- Cold ischemia time should be restricted to 6 hours

Extubation

- Generally postoperatively ventilated
- Thus, DLT is changed to SLT at the end of surgery
- FO bronchoscopy is done following SLT tube change to:
  - Examine bronchial anastomosis
  - Suction blood and secretions
- Early postoperative extubation may be planned for patients with:
  - Established thoracic epidural analgesia
  - Minimal opioid requirements intraoperatively
  - Absence of signs of fluid overload
  - Low transfusion requirement
  - No intraoperative requirement for ECMO
- Differential lung ventilation of native and transplanted lungs is also rarely done

Postoperative Care

Management

- Most patients may be weaned and extubated within 24 hours of surgery
- Early extubation is preferred to prevent:
  - Stress on bronchial anastomosis site
  - Pulmonary infections
- Nursing position:
  - Transplant side should be up for patients with:
    - Obstructive lung disease
    - Severe pulmonary HTN
  - Transplant side should be down for restrictive lung disease patients
- Immunosuppression continued for 5–10 days
- Perioperative prophylactic antibiotic therapy to be continued

Analgesia

- Pain is usually severe in patients following clamshell incision
- Adequate postoperative analgesia is essential to optimize lung function
- Analgesia offered by TEA alone may be insufficient for clamshell incision
- Thus, multimodal analgesia is preferred
- PCA with opioids may be used to supplement analgesia
- However, dose of opioids must be limited to prevent respiratory depression

- Other regional anesthetic alternatives include:
  - Paravertebral block
  - Serratus anterior plane block

Complications

- Pulmonary HTN and RV failure during PA clamping
- Systemic hypotension following transplantation as new lung has vasodilator preservatives
- Air embolism due to incomplete de-airing of LA cuff
- Anastomotic leaks at LA cuff or PA
- Early graft rejection
- Fulminant pulmonary edema
- Hypoxemia due to:
  - OLV
  - Graft rejection
  - Secretions in cystic fibrosis
- Pneumothorax
- Infections: CMV, pneumocystis carinii

Considerations in Previous Lung Transplant

- Immunocompromised status of patient
- Chemotherapy causing:
  - Tumors
  - Cardiac failure
  - Renal failure
- Cough reflex present only in native airway as transplanted lung is denervated
- Bronchiolitis obliterans common
- Capnography:
  - Differences in compliance between native and new lung present
  - This causes biphasic pattern of capnograph with two peaks
- DLT with differential lung ventilation if single lung transplant as difference in compliance and blood flow of the two lungs

RENAL TRANSPLANTATION

Introduction

- Renal transplantation is the most commonly performed organ transplant surgery
- First attempted in the 1930s and popularized in the 1950s

Types of Renal Transplantation

- Living donor renal transplant:
  - Can be performed electively and scheduled well in advance
  - Allows thorough preoperative evaluation prior to surgery
  - Better graft survival seen with living donor transplants
- Cadaveric renal transplant:
  - Usually performed as an emergency
  - This is in order to maintain viability of donor kidney
  - Donor kidneys have a cold ischemia time up to 24 hours (shelf life)

Efficacy

- Survival in patients undergoing renal transplantation has improved considerably
- Survival rate following renal transplantation is 95% at 1 year
- Survival rate at 3–5 years is almost 90%
- Life-expectancy beyond 10 years is lesser than the general population due to:
  - Associated cardiovascular comorbidities
  - Immunosuppressive therapy associated complications:
    - Malignancies
    - Infections

Indications

- Renal transplant is the preferred treatment modality for ESRD
- Compared with renal replacement therapy (RRT), transplantation is associated with:
  - Better quality of life
  - Less morbidity
  - Less mortality
- Early renal transplantation is preferred for ESRD due to:
  - Hereditary causes:
    - Polycystic kidney disease
    - Horseshoe kidney
    - Nephronophthisis
    - Hereditary nephritis
    - Tuberous sclerosis
  - Acquired causes:
    - Diabetic nephropathy
    - Hypertensive nephropathy
    - Hyperoxaluria
    - Fabrys disease
    - Analgesic nephropathy
    - Progressive systemic sclerosis
    - Acute tubular necrosis

- Delayed renal transplantation:
  - Preferred for diseases with recurrence of original disease post-transplantation
  - In these patients, RRT is preferred until the disease reaches quiescent stage
  - Indications for delayed renal transplantation:
    - Focal segmental glomerulosclerosis
    - Membranoproliferative glomerulonephritis
    - Membranous glomerulonephritis
    - IgA nephropathy
    - Anti-GBM disease

Contraindications

- Absolute contraindications:
  - Metastatic or untreated cancer
  - Active untreated infections
  - Active glomerulonephritis
  - Positive T-cell cross match
  - Severe psychiatric disease
  - Persistent substance abuse
  - Severe mental retardation
  - Refractory congestive cardiac failure
  - Active systemic disease:
    - Lupus nephritis
    - Goodpasture syndrome
    - Wegeners, granulomatosis
- Relative contraindications:
  - Treated malignancy
  - Substance abuse patients on rehabilitation therapy
  - Chronic hepatitis B or C
  - Mild-moderate cardiovascular disease
  - Morbid obesity

Pretransplant Evaluation

- Evaluation is carried out by a multidisciplinary team of:
  - Transplant surgeons
  - Nephrologists
  - Anesthesiologists
  - Nurses
  - Social workers
- Evaluation of ESRD-associated comorbidities:
  - Anemia
  - Coagulation system for hypercoagulability and platelet dysfunction
  - Gastrointestinal tract for:
    - Gastritis
    - Diverticulitis
  - Liver dysfunction due to:
    - Viral illnesses
    - Alcohol consumption
    - Toxic drugs
- Laboratory evaluation:
  - Complete blood count, coagulation profile, PTH levels
  - Chest X-ray, ECG
  - Blood grouping and typing
  - HLA typing, donor specific antibodies (DSA)
  - Urine analysis and culture
  - Abdominal ultrasound
  - CMV, EBV, hepatitis A, B, C and varicella-zoster serology
  - Rapid plasma reagin (RPR) and purified protein derivative (PPD)
  - Immunological tests:
    - C3, C4
    - Rheumatoid factor
    - Anti-nuclear antibodies
    - Anti-GBM antibodies
    - ANCA antibodies
  - In selected cases:
    - Pulmonary function tests
    - Carotid doppler, peripheral arterial doppler
    - Cardiac evaluation
    - Pap smear, mammography if any family history of malignancy
    - Upper GI endoscopy
    - Prostate specific antigen if age > 50 years
- Evaluation of cardiovascular status:
  - CV disease is the most common cause of death in renal transplant recipients
  - Thus, appropriate evaluation of CV status is important
  - Asymptomatic patients with high cardiovascular risk:
    - Non-invasive tests to evaluate myocardial perfusion
    - Resting and exercise ECG are not useful to assess myocardial perfusion
    - This is due to high prevalence of non-specific changes due to ESRD
    - Tests used include:
      - Dobutamine stress echocardiogram
      - Thallium SPECT scan
  - Coronary angiography is indicated for:
    - Symptomatic patients
    - Asymptomatic patients with impaired perfusion scan

Surgical Considerations

- Renal allograft is usually placed in the right or left extraperitoneal fossa
- Right extraperitoneal fossa is usually the preferred site
- Donor kidney receives blood supply from external iliac vessels following anastomosis
- Curvilinear incision 20–25 cm long is made from pubic symphysis to ASIS
- Abdominal musculature is divided and peritoneum is entered
- External iliac artery and vein are identified and mobilized
- Heparin may be administered prior to clamping of blood vessels
- Renal vascular anastomosis:
  - External iliac vein is clamped first
  - Thereafter, renal vein anastomosis is performed
  - This is followed by clamping of external iliac artery
  - Renal artery is then anastomosed
- Ureteral anastomosis:
  - Done following completion of vascular anastomosis
  - Donor ureter is implanted in recipient bladder
  - Bladder may be filled with antibiotic saline irrigation solution
  - This aids implantation of the donor ureter
  - Temporary ureteral stent may be inserted to aid ureteral implantation
- Recipients native kidney:
  - This is usually left in-situ and rarely removed
  - Native kidney nephrectomy may be indicated for:
    - Large, infected kidneys
    - Bleeding polycystic kidneys
    - Intractable HTN
    - Reflux nephropathy
    - Heavy proteinuria due to FSGS
- Following completion of ureteral anastomosis, abdominal wound is closed in layers

Preoperative Assessment

- Preoperative evaluation should include:
  - Complete medical and surgical history
  - Thorough physical examination
  - Assessment of all organ systems
  - Evaluation of specific history which may alter intraoperative management:
    - Cardiovascular disease
    - Neoplastic disease
    - Previous pregnancies
    - Previous blood transfusion
- Patients not on chronic dialysis:
  - Patient should be assessed for comorbidities:
    - Primary disease process causing ESRD
    - Adverse effects of ESRD
    - Adverse effects of chronic dialysis therapy
  - Maintenance dialysis may not be required for many patients of ESRD
  - Preemptive transplantation in these patients has better outcomes than those on chronic dialysis
  - However, immediate preoperative dialysis may be necessitated by:
    - Hyperkalemia:
      - Serum $K^+ > 5$ mEq/L for elective transplantation
      - Serum $K^+ > 6$ mEq/L for urgent transplantation
    - Volume overload:
      - Dialysis is indicated when diuretic therapy is ineffective
      - Ultrafiltration may be used to remove 1–2 L of fluid
- Patients on chronic dialysis therapy:
  - Patient should be assessed for comorbidities:
    - Primary disease process causing ESRD
    - Adverse effects of ESRD
    - Adverse effects of chronic dialysis therapy
  - Dialysis access site:
    - Chronic dialysis access site should be available prior to surgery
    - Patency of dialysis access site should be ascertained
    - This is to ensure availability of access site for postoperative dialysis
    - Access sites already present should be preserved carefully
  - Preoperative dialysis:
    - Usually avoided for 24 hours prior to transplantation
    - Dialysis is completed 48–72 hours prior to transplantation
    - Indications:
      - Hyperkalemia:
        - Serum $K^+ > 5$ mEq/L for elective transplantation
        - Serum $K^+ > 6$ mEq/L for urgent transplantation

- Volume overload:
  - Ultrafiltration used to treat volume overload
  - Post-dialysis weight target: 1–2 kg above dryweight
- In the event of immediate preoperative dialysis:
- Ensure heparin free dialysis
- If heparin is used during dialysis:
  - Delay surgery by 3–4 hours
  - This is to allow normalization of coagulation profile
  - Ensure aPTT < 45 seconds prior to induction

❖ Laboratory investigations:
- Complete blood count, coagulation profile, PTH levels
- Chest X-ray, ECG
- Blood grouping and typing
- HLA typing, donor specific antibodies (DSA)
- Urine analysis and culture
- Abdominal ultrasound
- CMV, EBV, hepatitis A, B, C and varicella-zoster serology
- Rapid plasma reagin (RPR) and purified protein derivative (PPD)
- Immunological tests:
  - C3, C4
  - Rheumatoid factor
  - Anti-nuclear antibodies
  - Anti-GBM antibodies
  - ANCA antibodies
- In selected cases:
  - Pulmonary function tests
  - Carotid doppler, peripheral arterial doppler
  - Cardiac evaluation
  - Pap smear, mammography if any family history of malignancy
  - Upper GI endoscopy
  - Prostate specific antigen if age > 50 years

Anesthetic Goals

❖ Provide adequate depth of anesthesia

❖ Maintain muscle relaxation to facilitate surgical exposure

❖ Maintain hemodynamic stability:
- Maintain renal blood flow to the renal graft
- Maintain optimal intravascular volume status

Preoperative Preparation and Premedication

❖ Informed consent

❖ NPO status is verified

❖ On the day of surgery, the following investigations are repeated:
- Complete blood counts especially for platelet count
- Serum electrolytes for serum K^+ levels especially
- Patients current weight for fluid overload
- Blood glucose levels

❖ Venous access:
- Two large bore venous access are secured
- Side of AV fistula is avoided for securing intravenous access
- At least 2 units of PRBCs are kept cross matched and ready for transfusion

❖ Preoperative medications on the day of surgery:
- Beta blocker therapy should be continued
- Oral hypoglycemia agents should be withheld

❖ Premedication:
- May be used in anxious patients
- Small doses of IV midazolam 0.5 mg are titrated to anxiolytic effect

❖ Gastroparetic therapy:
- Useful as ESRD patients usually have gastroparesis
- Drugs used:
  - Non-particulate antacids sodium citrate 500 mg in 15 mL
  - H_2 receptor antagonists:
    - Cimetidine
    - Famotidine
  - Metoclopramide is usually avoided

❖ Antibiotic prophylaxis:
- First generation cephalosporins:
  - These are usually preferred for surgical antibiotic prophylaxis
  - IV cefazoline 2 g is the most commonly used agent
  - Antibiotics are timed 30–60 minutes prior to surgical incision
  - This is to ensure adequate tissue levels prior to incision
  - Antibiotic dose is repeated Q4H intraoperatively
- Vancomycin:
  - Vancomycin and clindamycin should be avoided to:
    - Prevent colonization by vancomycin resistant organisms
    - Prevent postoperative diarrhea due to Clostridium difficile
  - Vancomycin may be used in patients allergic to cephalosporin

- IV vancomycin 1 g is given 60–120 minutes prior to incision
- This is to allow adequate tissue levels as it has to be infused slowly

Choice of Anesthetic Technique

- Both neuraxial and general anesthesia have been successfully used
- However, neuraxial anesthetic techniques are usually avoided due to:
  - Uremic platelet dysfunction
  - Residual heparin action post-dialysis
- General anesthesia is the preferred anesthetic technique

Monitors

- Pulse oximetry, E_TCO_2
- NIBP cuff: Limb with AV-fistula site is avoided
- ECG, temperature
- Neuromuscular monitoring
- Urine output is measured pre-grafting and post grafting
- Invasive blood pressure monitoring:
  - Routinely used
  - Site of intra-arterial monitoring:
    - Radial artery catheter is preferred
    - Catheter is placed contralateral to the side of AV fistula
    - However, this may jeopardize choice of future AV access for dialysis
    - Femoral artery catheterization is avoided on the side of transplant
    - Ipsilateral femoral artery access increases risk of:
      - Thrombosis
      - Hematoma
    - This may adversely affect the implanted graft
  - Allows monitoring of:
    - Continuous beat-to-beat blood pressure
    - Respirophasic SVV
    - Intermittent ABGs for acid-base status
- Central venous catheterization:
  - Routinely used
  - May be difficult to secure due to repeated previous cannulations for dialysis
  - Veins which have been repeatedly cannulated must be examined for DVT
  - Useful for:
    - Inotrope, vasopressor and immunosuppressant administration
    - Monitoring intravascular fluid status for GDFT (not very accurate)
  - Useful as access for:
    - Difficult venous access patients
    - Urgent postoperative dialysis in the absence of AV fistula
- Pulmonary artery catheterization and transesophageal echocardiography:
  - Indicated for:
    - Advanced coronary artery disease
    - Right or left ventricular dysfunction
    - Pulmonary HTN
  - Useful to assess:
    - Intravascular volume status
    - Cause of hemodynamic instability

Induction

- Adequate preoxygenation
- IV propofol 1–2 mg/kg is the preferred induction agent
- Induction agent is administered in titrated doses slowly
- This is due to risk of hypotension caused by arterial and venous dilatation
- Fentanyl (1 µg/kg) and atracurium (0.5 mg/kg) may be used to facilitate intubation
- Cisatracurium 0.15–0.2 mg/kg may be used as alternative
- Tachycardia at intubation is avoided with IV lidocaine 1.5 mg/kg
- Rapid sequence induction:
  - Used in patients at high risk of aspiration due to gastroparesis
  - Succinylcholine (SCH):
    - May be used when serum $K^+ < 5.5$ mEq/L
    - Serum K^+ levels increase transiently by 0.5–1 mEq/L
    - Serum K^+ levels return to baseline after 10–15 minutes
  - Rocuronium:
    - Used when serum $K^+ > 5.5$ mEq/L
    - Provides similar intubating conditions to SCH
    - Dose used for RSI is high (0.8–1.2 mg/kg)
    - At these high doses, rocuronium may cause delayed recovery
- Hypotension at induction:
  - Profound hypotension may occur on induction in:
    - Hypovolemic recipients
    - Pre-existing heart failure
    - Elderly recipients

- Hypotension may be transiently reverted due to intubation response
- Following intubation, hypotension persists till surgical incision

Position

- Careful positioning with padding of pressure points
- AV fistula is carefully protected to avoid pressure
- Pressure on the fistula site may lead to fistula thrombosis

Maintenance

- Anesthetic maintenance:
  - Balanced anesthesia technique is preferred
  - O_2 + air + isoflurane is used commonly
  - Sevoflurane and desflurane may be used as alternatives
  - Sevoflurane nephrotoxicity:
    - Nephrotoxicity may occur due to formation of sevo-olefin
    - However, incidence of sevoflurane nephrotoxicity is very low
    - Thus, sevoflurane may be used as alternative for renal transplantation
    - Fresh gas flow > 2 L/min is recommended to prevent nephrotoxicity
  - N_2O may be used to reduce the delivered volatile anesthetic volume
  - Opioids:
    - Intermittent boluses of fentanyl 1 µg/kg is preferred
    - Alternative agents which can be used include:
      - Remifentanil
      - Sufentanyl
      - Alfentanyl
    - Agents which are avoided due to active metabolites include:
      - Morphine
      - Pethidine
  - Neuromuscular blockade:
    - Adequate MR is essential up to closure of abdominal wall fascia
    - However, excessive NMBA can lead to prolonged NMB
    - This may delay recovery and necessitate postoperative ventilation
    - Thus, NMBAs should be titrated with peripheral nerve stimulator
    - This avoids both intraoperative patient movement and delayed recovery
    - Preferred neuromuscular blocking agents include:
      - Atracurium 0.1 mg/kg
      - Cisatracurium 0.01 mg/kg
    - Agents avoided due to prolonged action include:
      - Vecuronium
      - Rocuronium
      - Pancuronium
  - Intraoperative patient movement:
    - May result in disruption of venous and arterial anastomosis
    - This may require revision of anastomosis
    - This in turn leads to an increase in warm ischemia time
- Heparin 5000 IU may be administered prior to clamping of blood vessels
- Diuretic therapy:
  - Used prior to allograft reperfusion to:
    - Decrease incidence of ATN
    - Promote diuresis
  - Agents used include:
    - Mannitol:
      - Used most commonly
      - Efficacy has been proven in multiple trials
      - Advantages:
        - Prevents ATN by promoting osmotic diuresis
        - Thus, excess tissue and intravascular fluid is eliminated
        - Increases renal blood flow by releasing prostaglandins
    - Furosemide:
      - Commonly used in refractory oliguria
      - Multiple trials have shown lack of benefit with furosemide
      - Thus, its use in renal transplant surgery is not beneficial
- Immunosuppressive induction:
  - Glucocorticoids:
    - Typically administered as a bolus before reper-fusion
    - Methylprednisolone used most commonly (500 mg-1 g)
  - Anti- thymocyte globulin (ATG) preparations:
    - Administered shortly before and after reperfusion
    - Agents used:
      - IV basiliximab 20 mg (2 doses)
      - IV alemtuzumab 30 mg
      - IV rabbit ATG 1.5 mg/kg (continued for 3–14 days)
      - IV horse ATG 15 mg/kg (continued for 3–14 days)
    - Given slow IV to avoid hypotension

Ischemia Time

- Allograft viability depends on minimizing the donor ischemic kidney time
- Ischemia time begins with clamping of the donor renal blood vessels
- It ends with the release of clamp following renal vascular anastomosis in the recipient
- Warm ischemia time:
  - For living kidney donors
  - It consists of 2 phases:
    - From clamping of donor vessels to infusion of preservative solution
    - From placement of donor kidney in recipient to reperfusion following vascular anas-tomosis
  - Excessive warm ischemia time increases the risk of ATN postoperatively
- Cold ischemia time:
  - For deceased kidney donors
  - Extends from:
    - Time of preservation of donor kidney in the preservative fluid
    - To release of vascular clamp following completion of anastomosis
  - Longer cold ischemia time is associated with poor graft function
  - Cold ischemia time should be restricted to 24 hours

Hemodynamics

- Fluid therapy:
  - Goal directed liberal fluid therapy is used
  - Rate of infusion:
    - Maintenance fluid is administered at 1–3 mL/kg/hour
    - Rate of fluid infusion is increased during renal vascular anastomosis
  - Expansion of intravascular volume at this time decreases incidence of ATN
  - Fluid therapy is titrated to:
    - Increase renal blood flow
    - Improve allograft function following reperfusion
  - Targeted goals include:
    - CVP 8–12 cm H_2O
    - SVV < 10%
  - Fluids preferred:
    - Both BSS and NS should be used in equal proportions
    - This is to avoid over-administration of either solution
    - Excessive NS causes hyperchloremic metabolic acidosis
    - Excessive BSS results in hyponatremia and hyperkalemia
  - Titrated fluid boluses:
    - Indications:
      - Hemodynamic instability with SVV > 10%
      - During anastomosis of renal vessels
      - Hypotension due to release of clamp after vascular anastomosis
    - Choice of fluid for boluses:
      - BSS is usually titrated and administered
      - Amongst colloids, 5% albumin is preferred
  - Blood transfusion:
    - PRBCs are indicated when Hb < 8 g/dL
    - Washed, leucocyte depleted preparations are preferred
- Hemodynamic management:
  - Hemodynamic goals:
    - MAP 60–80 mm Hg prior to vascular anastomosis
    - Following renal reperfusion and vascular anastomosis:
      - MAP 70–90 mm Hg
      - MAP > 90 mm Hg if preoperative HTN
  - Hypotension:
    - Occurs commonly during:
      - Induction of anesthesia
      - Release of clamp following vascular anastomosis
    - Hypotension increases risk of allograft failure due to:
      - Vascular thrombosis of graft
      - Hypoperfusion of graft and renal ischemia
    - Trendelenburg position is used to identify volume responsiveness
    - Hypovolemia is treated with titrated fluid boluses
    - Euvolemic hypotension is treated with:
      - Ephedrine boluses (5–10 mg) if transient
      - Dopamine (3–5 μg/kg/min) if persistent
      - Fenoldopam is useful as an alternative agent due to:
  - Improvement in postoperative renal function
  - Dose-dependent antihypertensive effect
      - Amongst inotropes, there is no consensus on preferred agent
      - Vasopressors are avoided as they reduce allograft perfusion

- Hypertension:
  - Beta blockers:
    - IV esmolol 10–50 mg boluses
    - IV metaprolol 1 mg boluses
  - IV NTG 0.1–4 μg/kg/min used if ischemic ECG changes are present
- Urine output:
  - Urine output > 0.5 mL/kg/hour is preferred intraoperatively
  - However, fluid therapy should not be titrated based solely upon urine output
  - Most patients are anuric until ureteral anastomosis is complete
  - Intraoperative oliguria (< 0.5 mL/kg/hour) can be caused by:
    - Reduced allograft perfusion
    - Hypovolemia
    - Ureteral obstruction
    - Vascular thrombosis
- Blood sugar maintenance:
  - Intraoperative blood glucose levels maintained at 140–180 mg/dL
  - Insulin infusion may be used to treat blood sugar levels > 180 mg/dL
- Hypothermia:
  - Hypothermia < 35.5°C is avoided
  - This is achieved using:
    - Forced air warming devices
    - Insulation water mattresses
    - Fluid warmers
    - Maintenance of OR temperature
- Changes at reperfusion:
  - Allograft and lower limb perfusion is restored following vascular clamp release
  - This results in washout of:
    - Renal preservative solution
    - Stagnated blood from lower limbs
  - This can lead to sudden hyperkalemia due to:
    - Washout of K^+ containing preservative solution from allograft
    - Washout of stagnated acidotic blood from lower limbs
  - Hypotension may occur at this time due to:
    - Abrupt release of vasodilators present in stagnated blood
    - Addition of 300 mL to intravascular volume from lower limbs
  - Cardiac arrest may occur at this time due to these changes

Ventilation

- Protective lung ventilation is used
- FiO_2 titrated to maintain SpO_2 > 92%
- Tidal volume 6–7 mL/kg
- PEEP 5 cm H_2O
- Plateau pressure < 30 cm H_2O
- Mean airway pressure < 40 cm H_2O

Extubation

- Most patients can be extubated soon after surgery after ensuring:
  - Normothermia
  - Full consciousness
  - Ability to protect airway
  - Adequate neuromuscular blockade reversal with:
    - Sugammadex for RSI with rocuronium
    - Neostigmine and glycopyrrolate for all other NMBAs
- Hemodynamic response at extubation:
  - Exaggerated hemodynamic responses may occur during extubation
  - This is especially common in chronic HTN patients
  - Agents used to suppress these responses include:
    - Short acting beta-blockers
    - IV lidocaine
- Postoperative ventilation may be required for:
  - Delayed neuromuscular recovery
  - Fluid overload pulmonary edema
  - Associated coronary artery disease
  - Cerebrovascular disease
  - Delayed graft function

Postoperative Management

Management

- Euvolemia should be maintained to prevent hypoperfusion of allograft
- Postoperative dialysis may be indicated for:
  - Refractory fluid overload
  - Severe hyperkalemia with serum K^+ > 6.5 mEg/L
  - Severe metabolic acidosis with pH < 7.1
  - Uremic encephalopathy

Monitors

- Pulse oximetry
- Invasive blood pressure
- ECG
- Urine output closely monitored on hourly basis for oliguria
- Frequent ABGs for metabolic acidosis

Analgesia

- Options for multimodal analgesia are limited by ESRD:
  - Neuraxial techniques are avoided due to uremic platelet dysfunction
  - NSAIDs are avoided due to nephrotoxicity
- Opioids:
  - Opioids form the mainstay of postoperative analgesia
  - Fentanyl is most commonly used agent
  - Pethidine is contraindicated due to formation of norpethidine causing:
    - Respiratory depression
    - Seizures
  - Opioids are usually delivered with PCA pumps for the first 24–48 hours
  - Dose reduction for opioids is required due to ESRD
  - Thus, basal infusion rate is avoided in PCA infusions
- Regional anesthesia techniques which may be used include:
  - Continuous wound infiltration using OnQ pump system
  - Transversus abdominis plane block
- Paracetamol can be used following discontinuation of PCA

Complications

- Wound infection
- Hematoma
- Fluid overload and pulmonary edema
- Oliguria due to:
  - Hypovolemia
  - Ureteral obstruction
  - Vascular thrombosis
  - Delayed graft function
- Delayed graft function:
  - Refers to renal allograft dysfunction within the first week of transplantation
  - Delayed graft function is associated with:
    - Graft failure
    - Increased requirement for post-transplant dialysis
    - Increased incidence of all-cause mortality
- Graft rejection

LIVER TRANSPLANTATION

Introduction

- Liver transplant is the treatment of choice for ESLD
- First successful liver transplant was performed by Thomas Starzl in 1967
- Liver is the second most commonly transplanted organ after the kidney
- 95% of liver transplants are from deceased donors

Types of Liver Transplantation

- Living donor liver transplant (LDLT):
  - Can be performed electively and scheduled well in advance
  - Scarcity of donor organs is the limiting factor
  - Allows thorough preoperative evaluation prior to surgery
  - Better graft survival seen with living donor transplants
  - However, substantial postoperative risk exists for the donor
  - LDLT of the lateral segment of left lobe of liver is used in pediatrics
  - Right or left lobe LDLT can be performed in adults
- Cadaveric liver transplant:
  - Usually performed as an emergency
  - This is in order to maintain viability of donor liver
  - Donor livers have a cold ischemia time up to 12 hours (shelf life)

Efficacy

- Incidence of graft failure is 9.8% at 1 year for deceased-donor liver transplants
- 5-year survival rate for recipients of living donor livers is 74.6%

Indications

- Acute liver failure with complications:
  - Hepatic encephalopathy
  - INR > 1.5
- Decompensated cirrhosis:
  - Transplant can be considered for cirrhosis due to:
    - Alcoholic cirrhosis in patients with low psychosocial risk
    - Hepatitis B and C
    - Primary biliary cholangitis
    - Primary sclerosing cholangitis
    - Autoimmune hepatitis
    - Non-alcoholic steatohepatitis
  - Criteria for liver transplant in cirrhotic patients:
    - Hepatorenal syndrome
    - Encephalopathy
    - MELD score > 15
    - Child-Pugh score B/C

- Liver tumors:
  - Tumors which can be treated with transplantation include:
    - Hepatocellular carcinomas
    - Epithelioid hemangioendothelioma
    - Large hepatic adenomas
  - Tumors should meet certain criteria:
    - Single lesion < 5 cm
    - Up to 3 separate lesions all less than 3 cm with:
      - No evidence of gross vascular invasion
      - No regional lymph node metastasis
      - No distant metastasis
- Metabolic disorders:
  - Familial amyloid polyneuropathy
  - Alpha-1 antitrypsin deficiency
  - Type I and IV glycogen storage disease
  - Hemochromatosis
  - Wilson's disease
  - Acute intermittent porphyria

Contraindications

- Absolute contraindications:
  - Severe cardiac or pulmonary disease
  - Severe PAH with mean PA pressure > 45 mm Hg
  - Ongoing alcohol addiction with rehabilitation non-compliance
  - Hepatocellular carcinoma with extracellular metastasis
  - Current extrahepatic malignancies
  - Sepsis
- Relative contraindications:
  - Untreated alcohol abuse
  - Cholangiocellular carcinoma
  - Hepatic metastatic neuroendocrine tumors
  - Metastatic hemangioendothelioma
  - Morbid obesity

Surgical Considerations

- Usually described in 3 distinct stages
- Phases of liver transplantation:
  - Dissection phase:
    - Skin incision to entry into peritoneal cavity
    - Entry into peritoneal cavity is associated with loss of ascitic fluid
    - Mobilization of the liver and vascular structures
    - Identification of vascular structures:
      - Suprahepatic and infrahepatic vena cava
      - Portal vein
      - Hepatic artery
    - Isolation of bile duct
  - Anhepatic phase:
    - Clamping of hepatic artery and portal vein
    - Removal of diseased liver
    - Anastomosis of IVC and portal vein of donor liver
    - Implantation of the graft
    - Involves clamping of the IVC
    - This may reduce RV preload by up to 50–60%
    - Veno-venous bypass may be used to maintain RV preload
  - Neohepatic (reperfusion) phase:
    - Reperfusion occurs through the portal vein
    - Completion of anastomosis of hepatic artery and biliary system
    - Reperfusion of transplanted liver
    - Hemostasis
    - Evaluation of graft function
    - Ultrasound for vascular patency
    - Abdominal closure

Anesthetic Considerations

- Risk of aspiration requiring RSI due to:
  - Emergent surgery
  - Preoperative administration of immunosuppressants
  - Bowel decontamination antibiotics
  - Ascites increasing intra-abdominal pressure
- Hypoxemia due to hepatopulmonary syndrome
- RV dysfunction due to pulmonary HTN
- Hyperdynamic circulation due to vasodilatation with high cardiac output state
- Preoperative anemia due to:
  - Impaired hematopoiesis
  - Gastrointestinal bleeding
  - Hypersplenism
  - Malnutrition
- Massive surgical bleeding due to:
  - Coagulopathy from reduction in all liver derived procoagulant factors:
    - Factor II
    - Factor V
    - Factor VII
    - Factor IX
    - Factor X
    - Factor XI
    - Thrombin
  - Thrombocytopenia due to:
    - Decreased hepatic production of thrombopoietin
    - Splenic sequestration of platelets in patients with portal HTN

- ❖ Impaired renal excretion of drugs in hepatorenal syndrome
- ❖ Osteoporosis causing fracture susceptibility during positioning

Preanesthetic Assessment

- ❖ Hepatic evaluation:
  - Identification of etiology of liver disease
  - Definition of severity of liver disease and prognosis:
    - MELD score
    - Child Pugh score

MELD score = 10 × [(0.957 × in (creatinine))] + [(0.378 × in (bilirubin))] + [(1.120 × in (INR))]

- ❖ Laboratory investigations:
  - Liver function tests
  - Synthetic function of liver:
    - Albumin
    - PT, INR
  - Renal function
  - Tests of lipid and iron metabolism
  - Thyroid function tests
  - Viral hepatitis A-E
  - Ceruloplasmin
  - Alpha-1-antitrypsin genotyping
  - Autoimmune parameters:
    - Antinuclear antibodies (ANA)
    - Antimitochondrial antibodies (AMA)
    - Smooth muscle antibodies (SMA)
    - Liver kidney microsomal antibodies (LKMA)
  - Hepatic imaging:
    - Ultrasonography with doppler
    - Multi-slice CT
  - Cardiopulmonary evaluation:
    - Spirometry
    - Arterial blood gases
    - Stress echocardiography
  - Psychosocial evaluation: Alcohol and other addictions
  - Extrahepatic malignancies:
    - Gastroscopy
    - Colonoscopy
  - Evaluation for infections:
    - Cytomegalovirus
    - Ebstein Barr virus
    - Interferon gamma release assay

Preoperative Preparation and Premedication

- ❖ Blood product availability:
  - Adequate availability of cross-matched blood products should be verified
  - Products required include:
    - 10 units PRBCs
    - 10 units FFP
    - 6 units platelets
- ❖ Timing of anesthetic induction:
  - Donor liver procurement and recipient induction should be carefully timed
  - This is done in order to:
    - Minimize cold ischemia time (CIT) of donor liver:
      - Increasing CIT adversely affects the outcome
      - CIT is preferably limited to < 12 hours
    - Minimize risk of precipitating acute liver failure in recipient:
      - Anesthesia causes clinical deterioration in severe liver disease
      - Thus, delay in transplantation following anesthetic induction should be minimized
- ❖ NPO orders:
  - Recipients receive surgical notification within hours of donor confirmation
  - Thus, time available for fasting may be inadequate
- ❖ Venous access:
  - 2 large bore venous access is secured to enable rapid blood transfusion
  - Central venous access is secured prior to anesthetic induction
- ❖ Correction of coagulation abnormalities:
  - Routine preoperative correction is no longer recommended
  - Indications for preoperative correction include:
    - Active bleeding
    - Clinical signs of impaired clotting (prolonged bleeding from needle prick)
- ❖ Anti-aspiration prophylaxis
  - Patients routine PPI is continued on the day of surgery
  - Other drugs used:
    - Non-particulate antacids sodium citrate 500 mg in 15 mL
    - H_2 receptor antagonists:
      - Cimetidine
      - Famotidine

Monitors

- ❖ Pulse oximetry, E_TCO_2
- ❖ ECG
- ❖ Temperature
- ❖ Urine output

- Frequent arterial blood gases
- Invasive arterial BP monitoring:
  - Routinely used
  - No consensus exists on the ideal site of monitoring IBP
  - Femoral artery catheterization is commonly preferred
  - This is because radial artery may underestimate arterial pressure due to:
    - Vasodilatation associated with ESLD
    - Intraoperative use of high dose vasopressors
    - Compression against first rib during retraction
  - Thus radial artery pressures will be 10–20 mm Hg lower than femoral artery
  - Arterial cannula is useful for:
    - Beat-to-beat monitoring of blood pressure
    - Assessment of intravascular volume status with SVV
    - Blood sampling for ABG
- Central venous catheterization:
  - Routinely used
  - Ultrasound guided catheterization preferred
  - This is to prevent hematoma in patients with coagulopathy
  - Ultrasound also enables detection of DVT in hypercoagulable patients
  - Femoral vein is avoided as IVC is clamped during the procedure
  - Central venous catheter may be used for:
    - Assessment of intravascular volume status
    - Assessment of fluid responsiveness
    - Administration of inotropes
    - Blood sampling for $ScvO_2$ and thromboelastogram
- Pulmonary artery catheter:
  - Commonly used
  - Essential for patients with evidence of pulmonary HTN
  - May be used to monitor:
    - Continuous cardiac output
    - Pulmonary artery pressure
    - Changes in pulmonary vascular resistance
  - PACs with continuous MvO_2 monitoring capability may be useful
- Transesophageal echocardiography:
  - Should be used with caution in patients with esophageal varices
  - Useful to monitor:
    - Intravascular volume status
    - Complications due to surgery:
      - Hypovolemia due to IVC compression
      - Volume overload due to cirrhotic cardiomyopathy
      - Dynamic LVOT obstruction due to cirrhotic cardiomyopathy
      - Thromboembolic phenomenon in RV and LV
- Other monitors of cardiac output:
  - Lithium-dilution based methods
  - Thermodilution based devices (PICCO)
  - Arterial-waveform based methods (Flotrac)
  - Thoracic electrical bioimpedance methods
- Neuromonitoring:
  - Used in patients with raised ICP or hepatic encephalopathy
  - NIRS and ICP monitoring is commonly used
- Tests of coagulation:
  - Laboratory based tests:
    - PT, aPTT, INR, fibrinogen and platelet count
    - Limited utility as they do not evaluate:
      - Clot strength
      - Platelet function
      - Fibrinolysis
  - Point of care viscoelastic monitors:
    - TEG and ROTEM most commonly used
    - Provides information about the entire clotting process
    - Thus, it detects the specific abnormality leading to coagulopathy
    - This helps in reducing blood transfusion requirement perioperatively
    - However, platelet dysfunction is not detected

Induction

- Adequate preoxygenation
- Rapid sequence induction:
  - Rapid sequence induction is indicated for:
    - Inadequate fasting status
    - Moderate-severe ascites due to increased intra-abdominal pressure
  - IV propofol 1–2 mg/kg is the preferred induction agent
  - Induction agent is administered in titrated doses slowly
  - This is due to risk of hypotension caused by loss of SVR
  - Fentanyl 1 μg/kg may be used to facilitate intubation

- Neuromuscular blocking agent:
  - Succinylcholine (SCH):
    - May be used when serum $K^+ < 5.5$ mEq/L
    - Serum K^+ levels increase transiently by 0.5–1 mEq/L
    - Serum K^+ levels return to baseline after 10–15 minutes
  - Rocuronium:
    - Used when serum $K^+ > 5.5$ mEq/L
    - Provides similar intubating conditions to SCH
    - Dose used for RSI is high (0.8–1.2 mg/kg)
    - This may cause delayed recovery
    - The time of delay can be used to test the graft function
    - Extreme delay suggests poor graft function

❖ Nasogastric tube and Foleys catheter are secured

❖ Surgical antibiotic prophylaxis:
- IV cefazolin 2 g is the most commonly used antibiotic
- Alternative agents include:
  - Ceftriaxone
  - Cefotetan

❖ Hypotension at induction:
- Precipitous hypotension may occur at induction
- This is due to:
  - Pre-existing low SVR in liver failure patients
  - Loss of sympathetic tone on induction
- Hypotension is treated with high doses of vasopressors

Maintenance

❖ Balanced anesthesia with O_2 + N_2O + 0.5–1 MAC isoflurane

❖ Isoflurane is the preferred volatile agent due to:
- Splanchnic vasodilatory effect
- This optimizes hepatic circulation and oxygen supply to the graft

❖ Alternatively, sevoflurane and desflurane can be used

❖ Frequent alteration of MAC may be required to maintain hemodynamic stability

❖ Midazolam may be used to maintain amnesia during these periods

❖ Volatile agents are avoided in patients with:
- Raised ICP
- Fulminant hepatic failure

❖ Anesthesia may be supplemented with fentanyl 1 µg/kg boluses

❖ Preferred neuromuscular blocking agents include:
- Atracurium 0.1 mg/kg
- Cisatracurium 0.01 mg/kg

❖ IV magnesium sulphate 2 g may be administered during anhepatic phase

❖ Immunosuppressive induction
- Steroids are administered during anhepatic phase
- This is to ensure maximal plasma concentration during reperfusion of graft
- IV methylprednisolone 100 mg is used
- Dosage of steroids is reduced as liver is immunotolerant

Hemodynamics

❖ Fluid therapy:
- Choice of fluids:
  - Plasmalyte is preferred as the maintenance fluid intraoperatively
  - Plasmalyte contains acetate and gluconate buffers
  - These molecules do not require metabolism to be active as buffers
  - NS is avoided due to risk of hyperchloremic metabolic acidosis
  - Ringer's lactate is avoided due to:
    - Lactate:
      - RL contains lactate as buffering agent
      - However, lactate must be metabolized in liver to act as a buffer
      - Thus, in ESLD, administration of RL causes hyperlactatemia
    - Calcium:
      - RL contains calcium in solution
      - This can precipitate citrate present in transfused blood
  - Albumin:
    - 5% albumin is the preferred colloid
    - It is useful to replace albumin loss intraoperatively
    - This occurs on drainage of ascitic fluid on entering peritoneum
    - It is also indicated for patients with:
      - Hepatorenal syndrome
      - Spontaneous bacterial peritonitis

❖ Hemodynamic changes:
- Dissection phase:
  - Characterized by profound hypotension
  - Onset of hypotension occurs soon after induction
  - This is due to:
    - Vasodilatory effect associated with ESLD

- Vasodilatation associated with anesthetic agents
- Bleeding during surgical dissection especially in:
  - Portal HTN
  - Pre-existing coagulopathy
- Anhepatic phase:
  - Changes depend upon the patients cardiovascular reserve
  - Due to absence of liver, lactate metabolism is absent
  - This may lead to severe metabolic acidosis and hyperkalemia
  - This may result in:
    - Arrhythmias due to hyperkalemia
    - Hypotension due to myocardial depression
  - Thus, ABG analysis is performed Q20–30 minutes during this stage
  - Also, complete caval clamping results in decrease in RV preload
  - Preload may reduce by up to 50–60%
  - This can lead to reduced cardiac output and hypotension
- Neohepatic phase:
  - Following IVC clamp release, sudden increase in preload to RV occurs
  - This may be associated with abrupt increase in potassium levels
  - Once donor graft function is re-established, hemodynamics stabilize
  - Hypotension at this stage may occur due to:
    - Release of acid by-products of metabolism
    - Decrease in SVR
    - RV dysfunction due to volume load
    - Kink in caval anastomosis
    - Surgical bleeding

❖ Hemodynamic goals:
- Dissection phase:
  - MAP > 65–70 mm Hg
  - Low CVP 6–8 cm H_2O to minimize venous congestion and blood loss
- Anhepatic phase:
  - MAP > 65–70 mm Hg
  - CVP 8–10 cm H_2O especially if complete caval clamping
- Neohepatic phase:
  - MAP > 65–70 mm Hg
  - CVP 8–10 cm H_2O

❖ Therapeutic options:
- Dissection phase:
  - Fluid bolus with:
    - 5% albumin to replace ascitic fluid
    - BSS boluses when HB > 8 g/dL
    - PRBCs to replace blood loss when Hb < 8 g/dL
  - Vasopressors:
    - Norepinephrine 0.03–0.15 µg/kg/min
    - Vasopressin (VP):
      - 0.01–0.04 units/minute can be used as alternative
      - Benefits of vasopressin:
        - » Compensates endogenous VP deficit in ESLD
        - » Reduces portal HTN by decreasing portal venous flow
- Anhepatic phase:
  - Titrated fluid boluses:
    - CVP is maintained at 8–10 cm H_2O
    - Aggressive fluid resuscitation should be avoided
    - This may cause fluid overload following reperfusion
  - High dose vasopressor therapy to reduce fluid requirement
  - Inotropes:
    - Can be used for:
      - Impaired LV function
      - Vasopressor resistant hypotension
    - Alternatives include:
      - Dobutamine
      - Dopamine
      - Epinephrine
  - Aggressive correction of hyperkalemia in the presence of arrhythmias
- Neohepatic phase:
  - Correction of metabolic acidosis
  - Correction of hyperkalemia
  - Volume resuscitation with blood products if bleeding is present
  - Inotropes to support RV function

❖ Blood component therapy:
- PRBC transfusion:
  - Used for patients with HCT < 8 g/dL
  - Washed PRBC units are preferred
  - Rapid transfusion devices should be used
  - PRBC units > 14 days old are avoided to prevent:
    - Hyperkalemia
    - Postoperative AKI
  - Blood should be warmed prior to transfusion
  - Massive transfusion may be required to maintain Hb > 8 g/dL
  - Hyperkalemia may result from large volume transfusion

- Transfusion of other blood components may be guided by TEG/ROTEM
- Fresh frozen plasma:
  - Used during dissection phase to correct pre-existing coagulopathy
  - Risk of TRALI with large volume of FFP
- Platelets:
  - Avoided during dissection phase even in severe thrombocytopenia
  - Administration of platelets is associated with worse outcomes
  - Platelet transfusion is withheld till hepatic A anastomosis is completed
  - In the presence of precarious hepatic artery anastomosis:
    - Platelet administration may cause thrombosis
    - Thus, platelets are altogether avoided
- Cryoprecipitate:
  - Useful in the neo-hepatic phase
  - This is characterized by release of tPA from donor liver
  - This results in accelerated fibrinolysis
  - Cryoprecipitate helps in replenishing fibrinogen levels

❖ Management of blood sugar:
- Common during liver transplantation due to:
  - Catecholamine administration
  - Administration of steroids for immunosuppression
- Intraoperative blood glucose levels maintained at 140–180 mg/dL
- Blood glucose levels > 180 mg/dL is associated with surgical site infections
- Insulin infusion may be used to treat blood sugar levels > 180 mg/dL

❖ Hypothermia:
- Hypothermia < 35.5°C is avoided
- This is achieved using:
  - Forced air warming devices
  - Insulation water mattresses
  - Fluid warmers
  - Maintenance of OR temperature

❖ Hyperkalemia:
- Common during:
  - Anhepatic phase due to metabolic acidosis
  - Neohepatic phase due to washout of storage fluids
- Serum K^+ levels have to be monitored Q20–30 minutes during anhepatic phase
- Serum K^+ level < 4–4.5 mEq/L is preferred prior to reperfusion

Intraoperative Blood Conservation Techniques

❖ Intraoperative blood salvage:
- Cell saver systems are used to separate, wash and concentrate salvaged RBCs
- This minimizes allogenic blood transfusions
- Use of cell saver system has to avoided with:
  - Hepatocellular carcinoma
  - Localized infections
  - Contaminated surgical field

❖ Antifibrinolytic agents:
- Currently no consensus regarding antifibrinolytic agents
- May be used if evidence of fibrinolysis is seen on TEG
- Agents used include:
  - Tranexemic acid
  - Epsilon amino caproic acid

❖ Prothrombin complex concentrates:
- Can be used to minimize surgical bleeding
- Contains a procoagulant factor complex with:
  - Factor II
  - Factor VII
  - Factor IX
  - Factor X
- Advantages:
  - Small volume compared to FFP:
    - Reduced risk of TRALI
    - Avoids volume overload
  - Prevents transfusion reactions

❖ Recombinant activated factor VIIa:
- Use is reserved for refractory bleeding
- Its clinical benefit in liver transplant is unproven

Ventilation

❖ Protective lung ventilation is used

❖ FiO_2 titrated to maintain SpO_2 > 92%

❖ Tidal volume 6–7 mL/kg

❖ PEEP 5 cm H_2O

❖ Plateau pressure < 30 cm H_2O

❖ Mean airway pressure < 40 cm H_2O

Ischemia Time

❖ Allograft viability depends on minimizing the donor ischemic time

❖ Warm ischemia time is usually restricted to < 45 minutes

❖ Cold ischemia time is usually restricted to < 12 hours

Extubation

- Early extubation has become common and is preferred to postoperative ventilation
- Most patients can be extubated soon after surgery after ensuring:
  - Normothermia
  - Full consciousness
  - Ability to protect airway
  - Adequate neuromuscular blockade reversal with:
    - Sugammadex for RSI with rocuronium
    - Neostigmine and glycopyrrolate for all other NMBAs
- Postoperative ventilation may be required for:
  - Intraoperative complications
  - Delayed neuromuscular recovery
  - Excessive blood transfusion > 6 units of PRBCs
  - Fluid overload pulmonary edema
  - Hemodynamically unstable patients
  - Uncontrolled preoperative encephalopathy
  - Preoperative BMI > 34 kg/m^2
  - Associated severe preoperative comorbidities
  - Poor graft quality

Postoperative Management

Management

- Euvolemia should be maintained
- Postoperative nutrition:
  - May be enteral or parenteral
  - Early resumption of enteral feeds is associated with better outcomes
  - Enteral feeding is usually established within 48 hours
  - Parenteral nutrition used in:
    - Intubated patients
    - Patients unable to tolerate oral feeds
- Immunosuppression:
  - PO prednisolone 10–40 mg Q12H
  - PO tacrolimus 1–2 mg Q12H
  - Mycophenolate mofetil 1 g Q12H
- Hyperglycemia may be treated with insulin infusion
- Liver graft function should be monitored
- Liver enzyme levels usually start reducing by days 2–7 POD
- AST/ALT levels < 1500 IU/L within 72 hrs post-surgery indicates good graft function
- Grading of postoperative graft function within day 5 POD:
  - Good function:
    - AST < 1000 IU/L
    - Spontaneous PT > 50%
  - Fair function:
    - AST 1000–2500 IU/L
    - Clotting factor support < 2 days
  - Initial poor function (IPF):
    - AST > 2500 IU/L
    - Clotting support > 2 days
  - Primary graft non-function (PGNF):
    - Characterized by:
      - AST > 5000 IU/L
      - INR > 3
      - Persistent acidosis with pH < 7.3 and lactate > twice normal
    - Graft never functioned post-transplantation
    - Requires re-transplantation within 7 days for survival

Monitors

- Pulse oximetry, E_TCO_2
- ECG
- Invasive blood pressure monitoring
- Urine output
- Arterial blood gases and serum lactate levels
- Graft function:
  - Serum transaminase levels
  - Prothrombin time
  - Bilirubin levels

Analgesia

- Severe pain occurs usually due to extensive right subcostal incision
- Multimodal analgesia is useful but options available are limited
- Thoracic epidural is usually avoided due to co-existing coagulopathy
- Subcostal transversus abdominis plane (TAP) block may be used
- Opioids in the form of PCA form the mainstay of postoperative analgesia
- Opioid requirements should be reduced due to altered LFTs

Complications

- Early complications:
  - Bleeding
  - Primary allograft dysfunction
  - Primary allograft non-function
  - Post-reperfusion syndrome:
    - Decrease in MAP > 30%
    - Occurs within 5 minutes of reperfusion
    - Lasts longer than 1 minute

- Dyselectrolytemias and acid-base disturbances:
  - Metabolic acidosis
  - Hypocalcemia:
    - Occurs due to citrate toxicity from blood transfusion
    - This is because citrate is not metabolized in ESLD
  - Hyponatremia
  - Hyperkalemia
  - Thromboembolism:
    - Portal vein thrombosis
    - IVC and hepatic vein thrombosis
    - Hepatic artery thrombosis
    - Sepsis
    - Acute kidney injury
- ❖ Delayed complications:
  - Immunosuppression related side effects
  - Infection
  - Graft rejection
  - Recurrent primary disease
  - Biliary tree obstruction

HEART TRANSPLANT

Introduction

- ❖ Treatment of choice for severe ESHD patients with low 12-month survival rate
- ❖ First successful heart transplant performed by Christian Barnard in 1967

Efficacy

- ❖ Current 1-year survival rate in heart transplant recipients is 80–90%
- ❖ Current 5-year survival in recipients is approximately 70%
- ❖ Survival is better in:
  - Young age recipients (30–59 years age)
  - Non-ischemic cardiomyopathy transplant recipients
- ❖ Accelerated atherosclerosis occurs in denervated heart
- ❖ This increases the 5-year incidence of CAD in transplant recipients
- ❖ However, CAD is often dormant as angina is not appreciated in the denervated heart

Indications

- ❖ End stage heart disease (ESHD) with:
  - Refractory NYHA class IV symptoms
  - Refractory life-threatening ventricular arrhythmias
  - Ejection fraction < 20%
  - Medically refractory heart failure class D
  - Peak oxygen uptake (VO_2) during exercise < 10 mL/kg/min
- ❖ Diagnostic indications causing ESHD:
  - Common indications:
    - Ischemic cardiomyopathy
    - Idiopathic cardiomyopathy
    - Complex congenital heart defects
  - Rare indications:
    - Viral cardiomyopathy
    - Post-partum cardiomyopathy
    - Refractory valvular heart disease patients
    - Primary myocardial diseases:
      - Sarcoidosis
      - Amyloidosis
    - Drug induced myocardial disease
- ❖ Criteria for donor:
  - Age < 35 years
  - Age > 60 years with:
  - No cardiac risk factors
  - No evidence of CAD
  - Absence of HIV/hepatitis B or C

Contraindications

- ❖ Absolute contraindications:
  - Age > 70 years
  - Chronic renal failure
  - Body mass index > 35 kg/cm^2
- ❖ Relative contraindications:
  - Irreversible severe pulmonary HTN with PVR more than:
    - 6–8 wood units
    - 480–640 dynes-sec cm^{-5}
  - Presence of extensive end-organ damage or major systemic illness
  - Rehabilitation non-compliant drug abuse
  - Psychosocial issues

Surgical Considerations

- ❖ Done via median sternotomy on CPB
- ❖ Three surgical techniques exist:
  - Bicaval technique
  - Biatrial technique
  - Total technique
- ❖ Bicaval technique:
  - Used most commonly
  - Described in 1990 by Lower and Shumway
  - Technique:
    - Entire right atrium is transected

- Left atrial cuff surrounding pulmonary veins is left behind
- This is followed by:
  - End-to-end anastomosis of vena cava
  - Reconstruction of LA surrounding remaining LA cuff
- Advantages of bicaval technique:
  - Reduced incidence of sinoatrial node dysfunction
  - Lower incidence of bradycardia
  - Lower incidence of tricuspid regurgitation and RV failure
  - Reduced incidence of LA dilatation
  - Improved graft function
- Disadvantages:
  - Requires longer cross-clamp time
  - No evidence of improved survival

❖ Biatrial technique:
- Used traditionally
- Described in 1960 by Wythenshawe
- Atria are transected along AV groove
- Right and left atria of donor and recipient hearts are anastomosed
- This is followed by anastomosis of aorta and PA
- Advantages: Lesser cross clamp time
- Disadvantages:
  - Increased incidence of SA node dysfunction
  - Increased incidence of tricuspid regurgitation

❖ Total technique;
- Described in 1991 by Dreyfus and Carpentier
- Reduces recipient LA size furthermore
- Only 2 islands of LA tissue surrounding pulmonary veins are preserved

Anesthetic Considerations

❖ In all patients:
- Cardiac transplant is done usually as an emergency procedure
- Thus, insufficient time is usually available for:
  - Ensuring adequate NPO status
  - Stopping preoperative drugs with adverse perioperative outcomes:
    - ACE inhibitors
    - AT II receptor antagonists
    - Antiplatelet agents
- Post-transplant:
  - Parasympathetic tone:
    - Transplanted heart loses its parasympathetic tone
    - Thus, resting heart rate post-transplant will be faster
    - 90–110 beats/minute is required to maintain cardiac output
  - Denervation of donor heart:
    - The graft functions in isolation from recipients nervous system
    - However, direct activation of myocardial receptors is preserved
  - Intrinsic myocardial reflexes are preserved:
    - Frank- Starling mechanism
    - Anrep effect
    - Bowditch effect
  - Change in pharmacological action of drugs:
    - Loss of action of indirect acting drugs:
      - Dopamine
      - Ephedrine
      - Atropine
      - Glycopyrrolate
    - Preserved action of direct acting drugs:
      - Epinephrine
      - Isoproterenol
    - Modified action of other drugs:
      - Digoxin:
        - » Preservation of inotropic function
        - » Loss of rate-reducing action
    - Loss of rate-modifying action of co-administered drugs:
      - Fentanyl
      - Pancuronium
      - Meperidine

❖ Patients with VAD devices in situ:
- Previous sternotomy: Risk of injury to cardiac chambers during sternotomy
- Chronic anticoagulation:
  - Patients with VAD are usually on anticoagulation with warfarin
  - These patients may require reversal of anticoagulation prior to surgery
  - Anticoagulation is reversed only after confirmation of graft quality
  - Anticoagulation may be reversed with:
    - IV vitamin K
    - Fresh frozen plasma
    - Prothrombin complex concentrates
- Central line placement:
  - Right IJV is avoided for central venous access in TAH patients
  - If accessed, the catheter should be placed above innominate vein
  - This is to avoid occlusion of right sided valve by the CVC catheter
  - In the absence of CIED, left IJV or SCV are preferred

- Preoperative anemia:
  - Blood transfusion is avoided in patients listed for transplant
  - This is in order to minimize transfusion-related alloimmunization
  - Thus, transfusion trigger is usually low in these patients (< 6g/dL)
- Patients on ECMO/IABP:
  - Coagulopathy:
    - Anticoagulant agent administration leads to coagulopathy
    - This can lead to:
      - Bleeding from venous access site
      - Bleeding during TEE probe placement
  - Anemia and thrombocytopenia may be seen frequently

Preoperative Assessment

- Underlying etiology of heart failure
- Examination for:
  - Pre-existing comorbidities
  - Recent health status changes to existing comorbidities
  - New infections
  - New onset renal or liver insufficiency
  - Stroke, active malignancy
  - Tobacco/alcohol addiction
- Status as organ recipient:
  - Prior cardiac surgery
  - Echocardiography for ventricular function
  - Cardiac catheterization studies for status of pulmonary vasculature:
    - Risk of RV failure in the transplanted heart is high if:
      - PASP > 50 mm Hg
      - PVR > 3 wood units (320 dynes-sec cm^{-5})
      - Transpulmonary gradient > 12 mm Hg
    - Pulmonary vasodilators are used to reduce PVR in these patients with:
      - Milrinone
      - Sildenafil
    - Pulmonary vasodilators should be continued in the pre-bypass period
    - Heart-lung transplant is considered in patients with irreversible PAH
  - Presence of CIEDs
  - Presence of VADs
  - Blood grouping, HLA typing
- Assessment of level of requirement for:
  - Intravenous inotropes
  - Pulmonary vasodilator therapy
- Preoperative discussion and finalization of:
  - Timing of induction as:
    - Early induction prolongs anesthesia time in hemodynamically unstable patients
    - Delayed induction increases cold-ischemia time
  - Plan for immunosuppression
  - Perioperative antibiotic regimen
- Investigations:
  - Blood grouping, cross matching
  - Coagulation function tests
  - Thromboelastogram to assess baseline abnormalities
  - Ultrasound evaluation of central venous patency

Preoperative Preparation and Premedication

- Fasting status:
  - Recipients receive surgical notification within hours of donor confirmation
  - Thus, time available for fasting may be inadequate
- Reprogramming of implanted ICD or VAD:
  - Most heart transplant patients will have CIED devices
  - CIEDs should be interrogated and reprogrammed immediately prior to surgery
  - Antitachycardia function is usually turned off
  - Pacemaker is converted to asynchronous mode
  - CIED wires are usually transected during removal of native heart
  - Pulse generator and remaining leads are removed at end of surgical procedure
  - Wire remnants which cannot be removed usually have no sequelae
- Vascular access:
  - 2 large bore IV cannula are secured for volume resuscitation
  - Arterial and CVC access are secured preinduction
  - This allows aggressive resuscitation for refractory hypotension at induction
- Availability of blood products:
  - Adequate blood product availability should be verified prior to induction
  - PRBCs should be available in OT during sternotomy for redo cases

- Correction of coagulation abnormalities:
  - Patients with VAD are usually on anticoagulation with warfarin
  - These patients may require reversal of anticoagulation prior to surgery
  - Anticoagulation is reversed only after confirmation of graft quality
  - Anticoagulation may be reversed with:
    - IV vitamin K
    - Fresh frozen plasma
    - Prothrombin complex concentrates
- Preoperative sedation:
  - Usually avoided
  - This is to prevent:
    - Respiratory depression
    - Hypercarbia and increased PA pressure
    - Right ventricular decompensation
- Anti-aspiration prophylaxis
  - Patients routine PPI is continued on the day of surgery
  - Other drugs used:
    - Non-particulate antacids sodium citrate 500 mg in 15 mL
    - IV metoclopramide 0.15 mg/kg
    - H_2 receptor antagonists:
      - Cimetidine
      - Famotidine

Anesthetic Goals

- Rate: Avoid bradycardia
- Rhythm: Maintain sinus rhythm
- Contractility: Maintain contractility
- Preload: Maintain preload, avoid sudden reduction in preload
- Afterload: Avoid sudden changes in SVR (increase/decrease)
- SVR: Avoid sudden changes (increase/decrease) in SVR
- PVR: Avoid increase in PVR by avoiding:
  - Hypoxia
  - Hypercarbia
  - Acidosis
  - Hypothermia

Monitors

- Pulse oximetry
- E_TCO_2
- ECG:
  - Pre-transplant is unremarkable and similar to preoperative ECG
  - Post-transplant:
    - Residual atrial tissue of recipient heart continues to have SAN activity
    - Native P wave will have no physiological effects on the donor heart
    - However, this may result in 2 P-waves on the ECG post-CPB
- Urine output
- Temperature
- Frequent arterial blood gases
- Invasive arterial BP monitoring:
  - Routinely used
  - No consensus exists on the ideal site of monitoring IBP
  - Femoral artery catheterization is commonly preferred
  - Thus radial artery pressures will be 10–20 mm Hg lower than femoral artery
  - Arterial cannula is useful for:
    - Beat-to-beat monitoring of blood pressure
    - Assessment of intravascular volume status with SVV
    - Blood sampling for ABG
- Central venous catherization:
  - Routinely used
  - Ultrasound guided catheterization preferred
  - This is to prevent hematoma in patients with coagulopathy
  - Ultrasound also enables detection of DVT due to repeated prior cannulation
  - Central venous catheter may be used for:
    - Assessment of intravascular volume status
    - Assessment of fluid responsiveness
    - Administration of inotropes
    - Blood sampling for $ScvO_2$ and thromboelastogram
- Pulmonary artery catheter:
  - Commonly used
  - Essential for patients with evidence of pulmonary HTN
  - Floatation of PA catheter:
    - Not be routinely required pre-CPB
    - May be difficult pre-CPB due to chamber dilatation and severe TR
  - May be used post-CPB to monitor:
    - Continuous cardiac output
    - Pulmonary artery pressure
    - Changes in pulmonary vascular resistance
  - PACs with continuous MvO_2 monitoring capability may be useful

- Transesophageal echocardiography:
  - Used routinely
  - Useful to monitor:
    - Intravascular volume status
    - Useful to diagnose etiology of hemodynamic instability
    - Also useful to assess post-bypass function of donor heart
- Other monitors of cardiac output:
  - Lithium-dilution based methods
  - Thermodilution based devices (PICCO)
  - Arterial-waveform based methods (Flotrac)
  - Thoracic electrical bioimpedance methods
- Neuromonitoring:
  - NIRS may be used to monitor cerebral oxygenation
  - NIRS during cardiac transplantation has shown beneficial effects:
    - Reduced incidence of major organ dysfunction
    - Reduced length of ICU stay
    - Improved outcomes
- Tests of coagulation:
  - Laboratory based tests:
    - PT, aPTT, INR, fibrinogen and platelet count
    - Limited utility as they do not evaluate:
      - Clot strength
      - Platelet function
      - Fibrinolysis
  - Point of care viscoelastic monitors:
    - TEG and ROTEM most commonly used
    - Provides information about the entire clotting process
    - Thus, it detects the specific abnormality leading to coagulopathy
    - This helps in reducing blood transfusion requirement perioperatively
    - However, platelet dysfunction is not detected

Induction

- Adequate preoxygenation
- Defibrillator paddles are placed prior to induction
- Inotropes should be prepared and readily available during induction:
  - Dobutamine
  - Epinephrine
  - Milrinone
  - Norepinephrine
  - Vasopressin
- Induction:
  - Small dose of midazolam (1–2 mg) may be administered just prior to induction
  - This may help reduce the dose of induction agent
  - In stable patients:
    - IV propofol 0.5–1 mg/kg is the preferred induction agent
    - Induction agent is administered in titrated doses slowly
    - This is due to risk of hypotension caused by loss of SVR
  - In unstable patients:
    - Etomidate is agent of choice
    - IV etomidate 0.2–0.3 mg/kg may be used for induction
    - Ketamine may be used as an alternative
  - Intubation is facilitated with:
    - Fentanyl 2–5 µg/kg
    - Vecuronium 0.1 mg/kg
- Rapid sequence induction:
  - Rapid sequence induction is indicated for inadequate fasting status
  - Neuromuscular blocking agent:
    - Succinylcholine (SCH):
      - May be used when serum $K^+ < 5.5$ mEq/L
      - Serum K^+ levels increase transiently by 0.5–1 mEq/L
      - Serum K^+ levels return to baseline after 10–15 minutes
    - Rocuronium:
      - Used when serum $K^+ > 5.5$ mEq/L
      - Provides similar intubating conditions to SCH
      - Dose used for RSI is high (0.8–1.2 mg/kg)
- Nasogastric tube and Foleys catheter are secured
- TEE probe may be inserted following intubation
- Tranexemic acid or EACA may be used to reduce requirement of blood transfusion
- Surgical antibiotic prophylaxis:
  - IV cefazolin 2 g is the most commonly used antibiotic
  - Cefazolin administration is completed 30 minutes prior to skin incision
  - This is to attain adequate blood antibiotic levels prior to skin incision
  - Repeat doses are administered every 3 hours intraoperatively

- Additionally, IV vancomycin 15 mg/kg (up to 2 g) is administered
- Vancomycin administration is begun 1–2 hours prior to surgery
- This is to enable slow infusion and prevent Redman syndrome
- In patients who have received ATG preoperatively, fluconazole may be used

❖ Hypotension at induction:
- Precipitous hypotension may occur at induction
- This may be unresponsive to vasoactive agents such as:
  - Ephedrine
  - Phenylephrine
- This is due to chronic exposure of such patients to inotropic agents
- This is due to sudden loss of sympathetic tone on induction
- Hypotension is treated with high doses of vasopressors such as:
  - Norepinephrine
  - Vasopressin

Maintenance

❖ Balanced anesthesia with O_2 + air + 0.5–1 MAC isoflurane

❖ Alternatively, sevoflurane or desflurane may be used

❖ Nitrous oxide is contraindicated as it increases pulmonary arterial pressures

❖ Anesthesia may be supplemented with boluses of:
- Fentanyl 1 µg/kg
- Vecuronium 0.03 mg/kg

❖ Induction dose of immunosuppression:
- Given prior to CPB:
  - Mycophenolate mofetil:
    - May be started prior to induction
    - IV mycophenolate mofetil 1 g infused over 2 hours
  - Basiliximab:
    - Given soon after induction
    - IV basiliximab 20 mg given over 30 minutes
- Given on CPB:
  - Methylprednisolone 1 g bolus
  - Given just before release of aortic cross clamp

CPB Considerations

❖ IV heparin (3–5 mg/kg) is administered prior to aortic cannulation

❖ ACT is checked 3 minutes after administering heparin

❖ Transplant is conducted on CPB with aorto-bicaval cannulation

❖ Aortic cannulation site high, near the aortic arch

❖ SVC and IVC cannula are snared to completely exclude the right atrium during CPB

❖ For PA catheters floated pre-CPB:
- PA catheter is withdrawn to right heart prior to snaring of SVC
- Following CPB weaning, PA catheter may be re-floated
- Re-floating may also be done under direct vision prior to PA anastomosis

❖ Challenges during weaning from CPB:
- Transplanted hear is denervated
- Early AV nodal conduction however, is usually preserved
- Thus, chronotropic support is required in addition to inotropic support

Ventilation

❖ Protective lung ventilation is used

❖ FiO_2 titrated to maintain SpO_2 > 92%

❖ Tidal volume 6–7 mL/kg

❖ PEEP 5 cm H_2O

❖ Plateau pressure < 30 cm H_2O

❖ Mean airway pressure < 40 cm H_2O

Hemodynamics

❖ Fluid therapy:
- Goal-directed fluid therapy strategy is used to maintain euvolemia
- Maintenance fluid used is BSS at 1–3 mL/kg/hour
- Targets for GDFT are:
  - CVP 8–12 cm H_2O
  - Mean arterial pressure > 60 mm Hg
  - Mixed venous oxygen saturation > 70%
  - Central venous oxygen saturation > 65%
  - Hematocrit > 30%
  - Pulse pressure and stroke volume variations < 10%
  - Cardiac index > 2.2 L/min/m^2
  - Stroke volume index > 35 mL/m^2
- When used, blood products which are leucode-pleted and irradiated are preferred

❖ Hemodynamic challenges while coming of CPB:
- Challenges due to denervated heart:
  - Denervated heart is unresponsive to atropine
  - Combination of inotropes and chronotropes are required
  - Heart rate is maintained at 100–130 beats/minute

- Chronotropic support:
  - Epicardial atrial and ventricular pacing wires
  - Isoprenaline 0.05–0.2 µg/kg/min
  - Inotropic support:
    - Milrinone 0.5–1 µg/kg/min
    - Dobutamine 5–10 µg/kg/min
    - Adrenaline 0.05–0.2 µg/kg/min
- Challenges due to pulmonary HTN:
  - May result in RV dysfunction causing difficulty in weaning from CPB
  - This is common in patients receiving preoperative pulmonary vasodilators
  - Options to reduce PVR include:
    - IV milrinone 0.5–1 µg/kg/min
    - Inhaled nitric oxide 20 ppm dose
    - Nebulized eprostenol 0.03–0.05 µg/kg/min
- Vasoplegia:
  - Low SVR may cause vasoplegia and difficulty in weaning from CPB
  - Vasoplegia is characterized by:
    - MAP < 50 mm Hg
    - Low SVR < 800 dyne-sec-cm^{-5}
    - Normal or high cardiac index > 2.5 L/min/m^2
  - Commonly occurs in patients with:
    - Previous cardiac surgery
    - Preoperative mechanical circulatory support
    - Large body surface area
    - Thyroid disease
    - Elevated serum creatinine
    - Prolonged duration of CPB > 140 minutes
  - Therapeutic options include:
    - IV norepinephrine 0.05–0.3 µg/kg/min
    - IV vasopressin 0.01–0.04 IU/minute
    - Methylene blue:
      - 1–2 mg/kg IV bolus over 10–20 minutes
      - Followed by 0.5–1 mg/kg/hour infusion
    - IV hydroxocobalamin 5 g over 10 minutes
- Management of blood sugar:
  - Common during heart transplantation due to:
    - Catecholamine administration
    - Administration of high-dose steroids for immunosuppression
  - Intraoperative blood glucose levels maintained at 140–180 mg/dL
  - Blood glucose levels > 180 mg/dL is associated with surgical site infections
  - Insulin infusion may be used to treat blood sugar levels > 180 mg/dL

Ischemia Time

- Cold ischemia time extends from:
  - Donor aortic cross clamp prior to harvest till
  - Removal of recipient aortic cross clamp post grafting
- Minimization of cold ischemia time is vital to attain optimal graft function
- This requires close communication between donor and recipient teams
- Timing of surgery in recipient:
  - Incision is usually begun when status of donor organ has been ascertained
  - However, redo sternotomy on the recipient may require earlier start of surgery
  - Recipient heart is ideally excised as soon as donor heart arrives in hospital
- Cold ischemia time should be restricted to 6 hours

Extubation

- Patients are extubated within 24 hours after surgery after ensuring:
  - Normothermia
  - Full consciousness
  - Ability to protect airway
  - Adequate neuromuscular blockade reversal with:
    - Sugammadex for RSI with rocuronium
    - Neostigmine and glycopyrrolate for all other NMBAs
- Postoperative ventilation may be required for:
  - Hemodynamically unstable patients
  - Moderate-severe RV dysfunction
  - Intraoperative complications
  - Delayed neuromuscular recovery
  - Excessive blood transfusion > 6 units of PRBCs
  - Fluid overload pulmonary edema
  - Preoperative BMI > 34 kg/m^2
  - Associated severe preoperative comorbidities

Postoperative Management

Management

- Euvolemia should be maintained
- Postoperative nutrition:
  - Enteral nutrition is preferred
  - Early resumption of enteral feeds is associated with better outcomes
  - Enteral feeding is usually established within 48 hours

- Parenteral nutrition used in:
  - Intubated patients
  - Patients unable to tolerate oral feeds
- Immunosuppression:
  - PO prednisolone 10–40 mg Q12H
  - PO tacrolimus 1–2 mg Q12H to maintain blood levels 8–10 ng/mL
  - Mycophenolate mofetil 1 g Q12H
- Hyperglycemia may be treated with insulin infusion

Monitors

- Pulse oximetry, E_TCO_2
- ECG
- Invasive blood pressure monitoring
- Urine output
- Arterial blood gases and serum lactate levels
- Graft function with:
  - Echocardiography
  - Endomyocardial biopsy

Analgesia

- Multimodal analgesia is useful but options available are limited
- Thoracic epidural is usually avoided due to heparinization on CPB
- Erector spinae block may be useful as regional adjunct
- Opioids in the form of PCA form the mainstay of postoperative analgesia
- Opioid requirements should be reduced to avoid respiratory depression
- This may lead to:
  - Hypercarbia
  - Increased PA pressure
  - RV failure

Complications

- Early complications:
  - Bleeding
  - Acute rejection
  - Renal and hepatic dysfunction
  - Infections and sepsis
- Delayed complications:
  - Immunosuppression related side effects
  - Infection
  - Severe tricuspid regurgitation
  - RV failure
  - Accelerated atherosclerosis and CAD

ORGAN HARVEST IN BRAIN DEAD DONOR

Pathophysiology of Brain Death

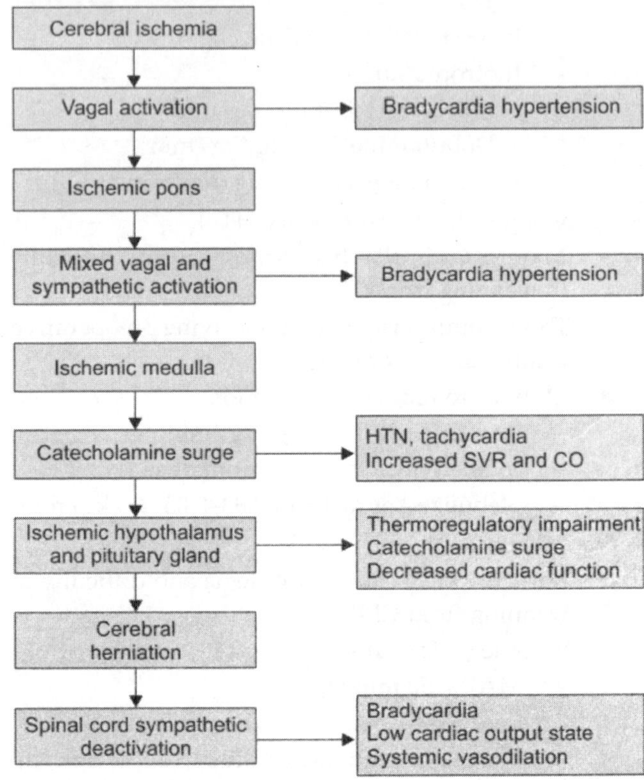

Phases of Brain Death

Hyperdynamic Phase

- Not seen in all patients
- Sympathetic overactivity
- Catecholamine surge (epinephrine and norepinephrine):
  - Increased HR, BP, cardiac output
  - Increased systemic vascular resistance
  - Altered myocardial O_2 demand supply balance

Cardiovascular Collapse Phase

- Loss of sympathetic tone
- Profound vasodilation
- Myocardial depression
- Aggravated by hypovolemia secondary to diabetes insipidus

Patient Selection

- Ideally donor < 60 years
- No end organ damage from systemic disease
- Proper intrinsic function of organ to be harvested
- Requires cessation of both cerebral and brainstem function

- Rule out reversible causes of coma:
  - Hypothermia
  - Hypotension
  - Drugs
  - Toxins

Contraindications

Absolute

- Uncontrolled sepsis
- Active viral infection
  - HIV: CMV
  - Hepatitis B and C: Herpes simplex
- Malignancies except:
  - Primary intracranial tumor
  - Non-melanotic skin cancer
  - Ca cervix in situ

Relative

- Chest trauma: Active infection
- Prolonged cardiac arrest: Major cardiac disease
- Those who have received intracardiac injections (for heart transplants)

Care of Patient Before Harvest

- Frequent turning to avoid decubitus ulcers
- Skin care and dressing changes
- Urinary and intravascular catheter care
- Nasogastric tube for gastric decompression and prevention of aspiration
- Arterial line in upper limbs as femoral line maybe inaccurate during surgery

Maintenance Therapy End Points

Hemodynamics

- SBP between 100–120 mm Hg
- MAP around 60 mm Hg
- Urine output ≥ 100–300 mL/hr
- Core temperature > 35 °C

Ventilation

- PaO_2 > 80–100 mm Hg
- SPO_2 > 95%
- pH between 7.35 –7.45
- Hematocrit around 30–35%
- Hemoglobin around 10–12 gm%

Investigations

- Hb, hematocrit, complete blood count, blood glucose
- Urine analysis, serum electrolytes, BUN, serum creatinine
- LFT, coagulation profile
- Serology for Hepatitis B, C and HIV
- Blood and urine culture if:
  - Evidence of infection
  - Duration of hospitalization > 72 hrs
- In case of multiorgan donors
  - ECHO for heart transplant
  - Bronchoscopy for lung transplant

Anesthetic Goals

General

Preservation of:

- Tissue perfusion
- Tissue oxygenation
- Mileu preservation
- Organ viability

Hemodynamics

- Maintain euvolemia
- CVP between 6–12 mm Hg
- PCWP < 12 mm Hg
- Minimize use of vasopressors (associated with renal graft failure)
- Urine output > 100 mL/hr
- Maintain hematocrit of around 30%
- Maintain INR < 1.5 using FFP
- Serum sodium < 155 mmol/L (increase associated with liver graft failure)

Ventilation

- $PaO_2/FiO_2 \geq 300$ mm Hg
- $PaCO_2$ 30–35 mm Hg
- Peak airway pressure < 30 mm Hg
- PEEP ≤ 5 cm H_2O during organ transport

Monitoring

- ECG
- BP
- Pulse oximetry
- Core temperature
- Urine output
- CVP
- PAC for PCWP and pulmonary venous oximetry for unstable donors with persistant acidosis

Hemodynamic Support

Factors Affecting Hemodynamics

- Hypovolemia secondary to ICP therapy
- Diabetes insipidus
- Hyperglycemia induced osmotic diuresis
- Coincident cardiac dysfunction
- Vasodilation secondary to brain death

Principles

- Bradycardia not treated unless symptomatic as it is seen due to *Cushings, reflex*
- Regardless of hypotension/hypertension patient is usually hypovolemic
- Maintain adequate filling pressure: CVP 6–12 mm Hg and PCW < 12 mm Hg
- Low filling pressure for lung transplant
- Higher filling pressure for renal transplant

Fluid Resuscitation

- Choice of fluids according to electrolyte status
- Maintian hematocrit around 30% and hemoglobin of 10 gm%

Drug Therapy

Vasoactive agents:

- Dopamine 1–10 μg/kg/min: Higher doses increase chances of ATN (***first choice***)
- Dobutamine 5–15 μg/kg/min (***second choice***)
- Norepinephrine 0.05–0.1 μg/kg/min Epinephrine 2–4 μg/min
- Phenylephrine 100–150 μg/min loading dose followed by 40–60 μg/min
- Vasopressin 0.01–0.04 IU/min

Chronotropic agents:

- *Atropine has no chronotropic effects after brain death*
- Isoproterenol 0.05–0.1 μg/kg/min
- Epinephrine 0.05–0.5 μg/kg/min

Hypotensive agents:

- Sodium nitroprusside 0.5–5 μg/kg/min
- Nitroglycerine 0.5 μg/kg/min
- Esmolol 0.05 mg/kg/min
- Avoid calcium channel blockers and long acting beta blockers due to negative inotropic action

Ventilatory Support

Factors Affecting Ventilation

- Aspiration
- Pulmonary contusion/effects of CPR and shock
- Pneumonia and pulmonary edema
- Atelectasis/volutrauma/barotrauma due to ventilation

Principles

- Pressure control/volume control mode depending on airway pressure
- Tidal volume 8–12 mL/kg if no lung injury
- Tidal volume 6–8 mL/kg if lung injury present
- PaO_2 between 70–100 mm Hg, $SpO_2 > 95\%$
- $FiO_2 < 60\%$
- If $FiO_2 > 40\%$ it contraindicates lung transplantation
- $PaO_2/FiO_2 > 300$
- PEEP < 5 cm H_2O
- $PaCO_2$ 35–45 mm Hg
- Plateau pressure ≤ 30 cm H_2O

Metabolic Support

Most commonly metabolic alkalosis due to mechanical hyperventilation to treat raised ICP.

Others:

- Contraction alkalosis
- Hyper hypokalemia
- Hypophosphatemia
- Hypernatremia
- Metabolic acidosis

Treatment

- Treat correctable causes
- Change ventilatory parameters
- Drugs to correct acid/base deficits

Endocrine Support

Diabetes Insipidus

- Most common endocrine disorder
- Suspect if polyuria with hypernatremia (>150 mEq/L) with hyperosmolarity (< 310 mOsm/L) with dilute urine (osmolarity < 300 mOsm/L)
- 5% Dextrose used to treat free water deficit
- Once urine output >4 mL/kg/hr desmopressin 1–4 μg IV QID
- Vasopressin 1 IU IV bolus followed by infusion 0.5–4 IU/hr alternative

Hormonal Cocktail

- Methylprednisolone 15 mg/kg Q24H
- T_3 4 μg IV followed by 3 μg/hr
- Desmopressin IU then 0.5 –4 U/hr to maintain SVR at 800–1200 dyne/s/cm^5
- Insulin infusion to maintain 120–180 mg%
- T_4 20 μg/kg bolus followed 10 μg/kg/hr infusion

Renal Support

- Maintain adequate systemic perfusion pressure and brisk urine output >1–2 mL/kg/hr
- Decreased use of vasopressor
- Volume loading to increase urine output
- Loop diuretics (furosemide)/osmotic diuretics (mannitol)

- Avoid nephrotoxic agents: Aminoglycoside and NSAIDs

Temperature Regulation

- Patient becomes poikilothermic after brain death
- Aggravating factors:
  - Systemic vasodilation
  - Administration of cold IVF and blood products
- Maintain core temperature ≥ 35°C
- Humidified and heated ventilator gases, warm IV fluids and warming blankets

Coagulation Abnormalities

Causes:

- DIC and coagulopathy
- Dilutional coagulopathy due to fluid resuscitation
- Release of thromboplastin from injured brain
- Massive blood transfusion
- Hypothermia

FFP transfusion to maintain INR < 1.5

Fibrinolytics like EACA avoided as increased microvascular thrombosis rendering organ unsuitable for transplant.

Reperfusion Injury

- Cytoprotective strategies:
  - High dose steroids
  - N-acetylcysteine
  - P-selectine inhibitors

Other Drugs

- PGE_1 to improve circulation of lung preservation solution
- Glucocorticoids
- Systemic heparinization just before exsanguination and excision
- Broad spectrum antibiotics
- Mannitol

TRANSPLANT PATIENT FOR NON-TRANSPLANT SURGERY

Pathophysiology

I. Cardiovascular Disease

- Hypertension:
  - Native kidney disease: Allograft dysfunction
  - Steroid therapy: Weight gain
  - Transplant renal artery stenosis
- Coronary artery disease
- Congestive cardiac failure—fluid overload
- Ventricular hypertrophy
- Cerebrovascular disease
- Peripheral vascular disease

II. Bone Disorders

- Persistent hyperparathyroidism:
  - Poor allograft function
  - Vitamin D deficiency
- Gout:
  - Cyclosporine
  - Impaired renal uric acid clearance
- Osteonecrosis: High dose steroids
- Osteoporosis:
  - Steroid therapy
  - Hyperparathyroidism
  - Vitamin D deficiency/resistance
  - Phosphate depletion

III. Electrolyte and Acid Base Imbalance

- Hyperkalemia:
  - Cyclosporine induced impairment of tubular potassium secretion
  - Poor graft function
  - Excessive intake
  - ACE inhibitors
- Hypophosphatemia:
  - Residual hyperparathyroidism
  - Glucocorticoids
  - Low Vitamin D state
- Hypercalcemia:
  - Persistent hyperparathyroidism
  - Coadministration of Vitamin D and calcium
- Hypomagnesemia: Cyclosporine
- Metabolic acidosis: Distal Tubular Acidosis:
  - Cyclosporine
  - Graft rejection
  - Residual hyperparathyroidism

Anesthetic Considerations

- Potential for infectious complications: Wound infections, UTI, pneumomia
- Potential for malignancies: Lymphoproliferative malignancies
- Difficult airway if lymphoproliferative disease due to tonsillar obstruction
- Drug interactions:
  - Calcium channel blockers promote cyclosporine and prednisolone toxicity
  - Cyclosporine potentiates NMBAS

- Adverse effects of immunosuppressants:
  - Cyclosporine: Nephrotoxic, hepatotoxic, neurotoxic, hyperkalemia, HTN
  - Tacrolimus: Hypertrophic obstructive cardiomyopathy, diabetes
  - Azathioprine: Bone marrow depression, hepatotoxicity, pancreatitis
  - Mycophenolate: Nephrotoxic, hepatotoxic, bone marrow depression, GI bleeds
  - Sirolimus: Bone marrow depression, buccal ulcers, diarrhea
- Transfusion of only CMV: Negative blood products
- Difficult perioperative glucose control due to steroid therapy

Preoperative Evaluation

I. Clinical Evaluation

- Evaluate complications of immune suppression:
  - CNS: Lowered seizure threshold
  - CVS: HTN, hyperlipidemia, atherosclerosis
  - Renals: Redued GFR, hyperkalemia, hypomagnesemia
  - Hematology: Increased risk of infection, increased risk of malignancy pancytopenia
  - Others: DM, osteoporosis poor wound healing
- Evaluate signs of acute graft rejection or infection—postpone surgery and optimize status
- Level of renal dysfunction to decide drugs and dose modification
- Airway evaluation especially if lymphoproliferative malignancies

II. Investigations

- Complete blood counts: Anemia, leucopenia, thrombocytopenia
- Serum electrolytes: Hyperkalemia, hypophosphatemia, hypomagnesemia
- ECG: Hyperkalemia, hypercalcemia
- ECHO
- Liver function tests:
- Coagulation studies: Hypercoagulability with cyclosporine
- Renal function tests: For graft rejection
- Pulmonary function tests
- ABG: Metabolic acidosis common
- Chest X-ray: Rule out infection
- Urine analysis: Graft function and infection

Preoperative Optimization

- Minimal disruption of antibiotics, antivirals, antifungals and immune suppression agents
- Maintain therapeutic blood levels of immunosuppressants—tacrolimus or cyclosporine 4–7 hours before surgery
- DVT prophylaxis
- Avoid drugs causing renal dysfunction:
  - Cyclosporin, tacrolimus: Amphoterecin
  - Ranitidine/cimetidine: Vancomycin/gentamicin/tobramycin
  - NSAIDs: Cotrimoxazole
- Antiaspiration prophylaxis: Avoid metaclopramide
- Antisialogogues: Glycopyrrolate has prolonged duration of action

Intraoperative Considerations

I. Monitors

- Routine:
  - ECG: NIBP
  - Pulse oximetry: Capnography
  - ABG and blood sugar monitoring
  - Neuromuscular monitoring important as:
    - Prolonged NMBA action due to cyclosporine
    - Muscle weakness due to dyselectrolytemias
- Invasive monitors:
  - Limited to minimum
  - Used only when necessary
  - Strict aseptic precautions

II. Induction

- *Rapid sequence induction* preferred: Propofol/thiopentone with reduced doses
- Ketamine best avoided
- Etomidate preferred if hemodynamic compromise
- Preoxygenation important as anemia and increased risk of CVA
- LMA and mask best avoided
- Nasal intubation avoided to reduce risk of infection
- Difficult intubation if diabetic/lymphoproliferative malignancy

III. Maintenance

- Isoflurane/desflurane preferred
- Halothane not recommended for repeat use
- Enflurane and sevoflurane avoided as nephrotoxic
- Succinylcholine avoided if hyperkalemia
- Rocuronium maybe used for RSI

- Atracurium/cisatracurium *drug of choice*
- Vecuronium may cause renal vasoconstriction and prolonged action in acidosis

IV. Hemodynamics

- Maintain euvolemic status at all times to prevent graft dysfunction
- Use potassium free fluids if hyperkalemia
- Osmotic diuretics preferred over tubular diuretics

V. Infection

- Strict aseptic technique: Gowns, gloves, handwashing
- Routine perioperative antibiotic prophylaxis: 30 minutes before skin incision
- Intravenous lines and invasive monitors only if specifically indicated, removed as soon as no longer necessary for patient care
- Use antiseptic impregnated catheters

VI. Immunosuppression

- Maintain intraoperative immunosuppressant levels
- Preoperative administration of immunosuppressants
- Postpone elective surgery if WBC count < 2000/cc^3
- Intraoperative monitoring of blood levels as hemodilution and bleeding during surgery can decrease blood levels

VII. Transfusion

- Adequate blood arranged in advance
- Cross matching might be delayed
- Transfusion reactions and transmission of infection possible
- Refractoriness to platelet transfusion common
- Leucocyte poor/irradiated blood products preferred

VIII. Renal Transplant Patients

- Maintain renal perfusion
- Adequate CVP/TEE guided volume replacement
- Avoid nephrotoxic agents

IX. Lung Transplant Patients

- Increased risk of pneumonia as cough reflex maybe reduced
- Compare preoperative CXR PFT and ABG with prior studies
- Increased risk of bronchospasm as increased airway reactivity
- Regional anesthesia techniques advantageous
- Avoid depression of intercostal muscle function
- Invasive monitors for intraoperative fluid status
- CVP inserted on side of native lung
- Tracheal cuff positioned just beyond vocal cords to avoid site of anastomoses
- Early extubation is preferred

X. Heart Transplant Patients

- Transplanted hearts usually denervated
- Do not respond to indirectly acting agents like dopamine, ephedrine and atropine
- Norepinephrine and epinephrine used for refractory cardiogenic shock
- Beta effects of epinephrine/norepinephrine exaggerated
- Isoprenaline is mainstay of chronotropic therapy
- GA preferred as denervated heart does not reflexly compensate for hemodynamic changes
- Preoperative ECG, ECHO, stress testing and myocardial biopsy as required
- ECG shows 2 P waves:
  - Native atrium not conducted
  - Implanted atriums waves

XI. Others

- Use minimally invasive techniques both for surgery and anesthesia
- Careful positioning to avoid pathological fractures
- Frequent blood gas determination for acidosis and dyselectrolytemia
- Increased risk of perioperative arrhythmias
- Impaired respiratory muscle power—Hyperkalemia, hypophosphatemia, hypomagnesemia
- Early extubation preferred

XII. Postoperative Care

Analgesia:

- NSAIDs avoided due to risk of nephrotoxicity
- Opioids may cause increased PONV due to synergism with chemotherapeutic agents
- Morphine and pethidine avoided if renal function deranged
- Epidural, regional blocks and topical infilterations useful
- Multimodal analgesia useful

Maintenance:

- Maintain hematocrit > 30% and normothermia
- Intensive physiotherapy

- Early mobilization
- Early removal of catheters and drains
- Continuation of immunosuppressive therapy
- DVT prophylaxis

Complications:

- CMV sepsis
- Infection
- Graft rejection
- B cell lymphomas
- Visceral perforation

SUGGESTED READING

1. Barash, P.G. (2017). *Clinical Anesthesia*. 8th ed. China: Wolters Kluwer.
2. Berg, C.L., et al. (2007). Improvement in survival associated with adult-to-adult living donor liver transplantation. *Gastroenterology*, 133(6), 1806–13.
3. Biancofiore, G. (2015). *Oxford Textbook of Transplant Anesthesia and Critical Care*. Oxford: Oxford University Press.
4. Bratzler, D.W., et al. (2013). Clinical practice guidelines for antimicrobial prophylaxis in surgery. *Surgical Infections*, 170(3), 73–156.
5. Briggs, J.D. (2001). Causes of death after renal transplantation. *Nephrology Dialysis and Transplantation*, 16(8), 1545–9.
6. Butterworth, J., Mackey, D., Wasnik, J. (2018). *Morgan and Mikhails Clinical Anesthesiology*. 6th ed. Lange.
7. Felten, M.L., et al. (2016). Immediate postoperative extubation in bilateral lung transplantation: predictive factors andoutcomes. *British Journal of Anesthesia*, 116(6), 847–54.
8. Flood, P. (2015). *Stoeltings Pharmacologyand Physiology in Anesthetic Practice*. 5th ed. China: Wolters Kluwer.
9. Gainsburg, D.M. (2014). *Anesthesia for Urological Surgery*. New York: Springer.
10. Graziadei, I., et al. (2016). Indications for liver transplantation in adults. *Wien Klin Wochenschr*, 128(19), 679–90.
11. Gropper, M., Eriksson, L., Fleisher, L., Wiener-Kronish, J., Cohen, N., Leslie, K. (2020). *Millers Anesthesia*. 9th ed. Philadelphia: Elsevier Saunders.
12. Hardinger, K.L., Brennan, D.C., Klein. C.L. (2013). Selection of induction therapy kidney transplantation. *Transplant International*, 662–72.
13. Hayanga, J.W., D'Cunha, J. (2014). The surgical technique of bilateral sequential lung transplantation. *Journal of Thoracic Disease*, 6(8), 1063–9.
14. Jaffe, R.A., Schmiesing, C.A., Golianu, B. (2009). *Anesthesiologists Manual of Surgical Procedures*. Baltimore: Lippincott Williams and Wilkins.
15. Kaplan, J.A. (2017). *Kaplans Cardiac Anesthesia*. 7th ed. Philadelphia: Elsevier.
16. Kashimutt, S., Kotzé, A. (2016). Anesthesia for liver transplantation. *British Journal of Anesthesia*, 17(1), 35–40.
17. Kim, W.R., et al. (2018). OPTN/ SRTR 2016 annualdata report: liver. *American Journal of Transplantation*, 18 (Suppl 1), 172–253.
18. Marschall, K., Hines, R.L. (2017). *Stoeltings Anesthesia and Coexisting Disease*. 7th ed. New York: Elsevier.
19. Martin, A.K., Renew, J.R., Jayaraman, A.L., Murray, A.W., Fritz, A.S., Ramakrishna, H. (2019). Analysis of outcomes in lung transplantation. *Journal of Cardiothoracic andVascular Anesthesia*, 33(5), 1455–66.
20. Martin, P., DiMartini, A., Feng, S., Brown, S. Jr, Fallon, M. (2014). Evaluation for liver transplantation in adults: 2013 practice guidelines by the AASLD and AST. *Hepatology*, 59(3), 1144–65.
21. Othman, M.M., Ismael, A.Z., Hammouda, G.E. (2010). The impact of timing of maximal crystalloid hydration on early graft function during kidney transplantation. *Anesthesia Analgesia*, 110(5), 1440–6.
22. Schumann, R., et al. (2013). Anesthesia for liver transplantation in United States academic centers: intraoperative practice. *Journal of Clinical Anesthesiology*, 25(7), 542–50.
23. Silberhumer, G.R., et al. (2007). Combination of extended donor criteria andchanges in the MELD score predict patient survival andprimary dysfunction in liver transplantation. *Transplantation*, 83(5), 588–92.
24. Slinger, P. (2019). *Principles and Practice Anesthesia for Thoracic Surgery*. 2nd ed. Toronto: Springer.
25. Sun, J.P., et al. (2007). Influence of different implantation techniques on long-term survival after orthotopic heart transplantation: an echocardiographi study. *Journal of Heart Lung Transplantation*, 26(12), 1243–8.
26. Tomasi, R., et al. (2018). Intraoperative anesthetic management of lung transplantation: center-specific practices andgeographic andcenters size differences. *Journal of Cardiothoracic and Vascular Anesthesia*, 32(1), 62–9.
27. Vetrugno, L., Barbariol, F., Baccarani, U., Forfori, F., Volpicelli, G., Rocca, G.D. (2017). TEE in orthotopic liver transplantation: a comprehensive intraoperative monitoring tool. *Critical Ultrasound Journal*, 9, 15.
28. Walia, A., et al. (2012). Anesthesia for liver transplantation in US academic centers: institutional structure and perioperative care. *Liver Transplantation*, 18(6), 737–43.
29. Weill, D. (2015). A consensus document for the selection of lung transplant candidates: 2014: an update from the pulmonary transplantation council of ISHLT. *The Journal of Heart and Lung Transplantation*, 34(1), 1–15.
30. Yuan, H., et al. (2013). Clinical correlates, outcomes andhealthcare costs associated with early mechanical ventilation after kidney transplantation. *American Journal of Surgery*, 206(5), 686–92.

DNB Question Papers

CARDIOVASCULAR SYSTEM

1. Air embolism during anesthesia
2. Methods, uses and complications of cannulation of internal jugular vein
3. Central venous pressure monitoring and uses
4. Cardiac arrhythmias during anesthesia
5. Discuss the etiology and management of supra-ventricular arrhythmias during surgical procedures
6. Pulmonary artery catheter
7. Prevention and treatment of intra-operative myocardial infarction
8. Preoperative preparation and evaluation of a patient with history of exertional angina for surgery under general anesthesia
9. Management of multi focal ventricular ectopics during anesthesia
10. Monitored anesthesia care in a 75 years old man with *ischemic heart disease* for cataract surgery
11. Define hypertension. How will you evaluate and prepare preoperatively a 40-year-old female patient scheduled for abdominal hysterectomy. Discuss the anesthetic and postoperative management of such a case
12. Coronary circulation, ***Goldmans*** risk index
13. Describe the basic life support (BLS) measures in an adult, who has been brought into the emergency room of the hospital in a state of cardiac arrest
14. *Myocardial protection* during cardiopulmonary bypass
15. Anesthesia in a patient with *artificial pacemaker*
16. Transesophageal echocardiography
17. Child with t*etralogy of Fallot* is posted for corrective surgery. Discuss the preoperative evaluation and anesthetic management of this case
18. Role of anesthetist in the management of a case with *thromboangiitis obliterans*
19. Factors affecting coronary circulation
20. Defibrillation
21. Cardioversion
22. Myocardial preservation
23. Pathophysiology of CAD. Discuss anesthetic management of a patient with angina
24. Cardiac evaluation for non-cardiac surgery
25. Classify congenital heart diseases. Explain with diagrams the blood flow before and after delivery in p*atent ductus arteriosus*
26. Clinical features of i*nfective endocarditis*, principle guidelines to use antibiotics as prophylaxis against, during surgery
27. Preoperative evaluation of a patient with *valvular heart disease.*
28. A patient who has undergone h*eart transplant* requires non-cardiac surgery. What precautions must be undertaken by an anesthesiologist for this surgery?
29. Define *perioperative hypertension*. Describe the causes and management
30. Discuss the anesthetic management in a patient of *myasthenia gravis* scheduled for thymectomy
31. Advantages and disadvantages of off-pump coronary artery bypass graft surgery (OPCAB)
32. Determinants of cardiac output and non-invasive methods of measurement of CO
33. Anesthetic management of *mitral stenosis and atrial fibrillation* for balloon valvotomy
34. A hypertensive man with CAD for TURP: discuss the anaesthetic management
35. Anticoagulation and cardiopulmonary bypass
36. Cardioplegia
37. Anesthetic management of mitral stenosis for closed mitral valvotomy
38. Anesthesia in a patient with *coronary stent*
39. Perioperative problems and anaesthetic management of mitral stenosis for elective LSCS
40. Anesthetic management of 3-year-old child scheduled for PDA ligation
41. Indication of mediastinoscopy, anesthetic implication
42. DVT-diagnosis, prophylaxis and management

43. Preoperative evaluation and anesthetic management of a patient with mediastinal tumor for thoracotomy
44. PCWP vs CVP
45. Anesthetic management in a patient with *abdominal aortic dissection* scheduled for aortic bypass graft
46. Describe the cardiac conduction system. How do you manage a patient with *paroxysmal supraventricular tachycardia*

ENDOCRINE SYSTEM

1. *Pheochromocytoma*-preoperative preparation, anesthetic management and complications during removal of the tumor
2. Discuss the preoperative investigations, preparation and anesthetic management of *diabetic* patient presenting for an exploratory laparotomy
3. Preoperative evaluation and preparation of a patient of *thyrotoxicosis*. Describe anesthetic and postoperative management of such a case
4. *Myasthenia gravis* - clinical features, preoperative investigations, preparation, anesthetic management and complications for an interval appendicectomy
5. Management of *diabetic ketoacidosis*
6. Role of corticosteroids in the practice of anesthesiology
7. *Thyroid crisis*
8. *Malignant hyperthermia*-clinical features, laboratory finding and anesthetic importance
9. *Myxoedematous coma*, causes of airway obstruction following thyroid surgery and its management
10. *Carcinoid tumour* for removal: anesthetic management
11. Anesthetic management of a case of diabetes scheduled for open cholecystectomy
12. Diabetic patient with *autonomic neuropathy* for abdominal hysterectomy
13. Anesthetic management of a case of pituitary adenoma who is planned for *transsphenoidal hypophysectomy*
14. A 25-year-old man presents with marked features of acromegaly and is posted for trans-sphenoidal hypophysectomy. Discuss the anesthetic management
15. A 60-year-old man presents for elective *parathyroidectomy*. Discuss the anesthetic management
16. Discuss anesthetic management of 25-year-old female with *Cushing syndrome* for bilateral adrenalectomy
17. Discuss anesthetic management of an inadequately managed diabetes mellitus patient with ketoacidosis posted for below knee amputation
18. A 50-year-old woman with *hypothyroidism* is scheduled for abdominal hysterectomy. Discuss the anesthetic management.
19. Evaluation of autonomic nervous system in diabetic autonomic neuropathy
20. Different methods used for *perioperative control of blood sugar* in diabetes with their advantages and disadvantages
21. Describe the manifestations and management of thyroid storm intraoperatively

OPHTHALMOLOGY AND ENT

1. Problems during anesthesia for *laser surgery*
2. Anesthesia for *squint surgery.*
3. Anesthesia for *perforating injury* of the eye in a 3-year-old child
4. Anesthesia for *total laryngectomy*
5. *Oculocardiac reflex*
6. Anesthesia for *intraocular surgery*
7. *Post tonsillectomy bleeding*
8. Merits and demerits of *Retro bulbar vs. Peri-bulbar block*
9. Anesthesia techniques practiced for cataract surgery and their complications
10. A 2-year-old child weighing 10 kg. is scheduled for removal of organic foreign body in right bronchus. Discuss the anesthetic management
11. Causes of hypertension in 20-years-old female patient posted for *angiofibroma* of nose
12. Anesthetic management of a child with retro-pharyngeal abscess presenting for surgical drainage
13. A 22-year-old male patient with multiple papilloma of larynx is scheduled for laser excision. Describe the anesthetic management
14. What is *monitored anesthesia care*? Describe the technique in an 80-year-old patient with ischemic heart disease scheduled for cataract surgery

GIT, LIVER AND URO

1. Anesthetic management and postoperative care in a patient with uncontrolled hypertension (B.P. 180/120 mmHg) for emergency laparotomy for *perforated duodenal ulcer*
2. *Hepato-renal syndrome* – etiology, pathophysiology prevention and management
3. Preoperative evaluation and anesthetic management of an emergency abdominal operation in a 60-year-old man who had myocardial infarction six weeks back

4. Problems of *laparoscopic surgery* and monitoring techniques used during the procedure
5. Upper intestinal obstruction for emergency laparotomy. Discuss the preoperative evaluation, preparation and anesthetic management of the case.
6. Anesthetic management of strangulated inguinal hernia in a patient with a recent myocardial infarction.
7. *TURP Syndrome*
8. Assessment, preparation and problems of anesthesia in a chronic smoker for cholecystectomy
9. Preoperative preparation and risk assessment in a patient with *cirrhosis of liver*
10. *Hepatitis B* and the anesthesiologist
11. Electrolyte disturbances and pre-anesthestic correction in small gut obstruction
12. Assessment of risk factor for patient with moderate to severe liver disease
13. *Postoperative jaundice*
14. Preoperative evaluation of a case with *chronic renal failure* posted for renal transplant
15. Describe the *countercurrent mechanism* in the kidney. Discuss the renal protection strategies during preoperative period
16. Role of kidney in acid base balance
17. Patient with permanent pacemaker posted for TURP
18. Discuss the anesthetic problems in a patient undergoing lieno-renal shunt
19. Anesthetic problems of *liver transplantation surgery*
20. Preoperative assessment and preparation for *thoraco abdominal esophagectomy*. Describe your anesthetic problem during operation
21. Preoperative preparation of diabetic patient with bleeding varices for lieno-renal shunt operation
22. Anesthetic considerations in chronic liver failure
23. What are the problems associated with anesthesia for an elective surgery in patient of chronic renal failure
24. A patient with *obstructive jaundice* is posted for Whipple's procedure. Discuss preoperative evaluation and anesthetic management of this case
25. Discuss anesthetic management of a 20-year-old male with achalasia cardia and bronchial asthma for laproscopic cardiomyotomy
26. What are the problems related to *chronic hemodialysis*
27. What are the anesthetic implications in a patient with transplanted kidney posted for incidental elective surgery
28. Physiological changes associated with pneumoperitonium for laparoscopic cholecystectomy
29. Anesthetic management of a severely jaundiced patient
30. Describe the assessment and management of a 70-year-old patient posted for transurethral resection of prostate. What are the possible complications and how will you treat them

INSTRUMENTS

1. Double lumen endotracheal tubes
2. Volutrauma
3. Application of venturi principle in anesthetic practice
4. Role of capnography during anesthesia
5. Sterlization of anesthesia equipments
6. Coaxial circuits
7. Pediatric circuit
8. Merits and demerits of laryngeal mask
9. Evolution of rotameter
10. PEEP and its application in modern ventilators
11. Check out procedure to be followed routinely before using an anaesthesia machine and other monitoring equipment
12. Pulse oximetry
13. Jugular Venous Oximetry
14. Characteristics of ideal vaporizer
15. Newer modes of ventilation
16. Physical principles of pulse oximetry
17. Operation theatre safety
18. What is minimum monitoring standard? Describe the objectives and methods
19. What is low flow anesthesia? Discuss its advantages and disadvantages
20. Discuss different methods of humidification
21. Draw a labeled diagram of a flexible fibreoptic bronchoscope and describe methods for its sterilization or high level disinfection
22. Supra glottic airway devices
23. Link 25 proportioning system in anesthesia machine
24. Laryngeal Mask Airway – various modifications
25. Functional analysis of pressure reducing valve
26. Discuss principles of monitoring $ETCO_2$
27. Classify vapourisers. Briefly mention the effects of altered barometric pressure on the performance of vapouriser
28. Compare and contrast TOF and double burst
29. Discuss in brief the sites and devices for temperature monitoring
30. Safety features in a modern day anesthesia machine.
31. I Gel airway
32. LMA
33. Evolution of Boyles anesthesia machine
34. Sterilisation of ventilators

NEUROANESTHESIA

1. Somatosensory evoked potential
2. Glasgow coma scale
3. Describe anesthetic and postoperative management of a patient undergoing intra-cranial aneurysm surgery
4. Awareness during anesthesia
5. Monitoring and control of raised intra-cranial pressure in head injury
6. Preoperative management of a neonate for meningomyelocele surgery
7. Methods of decreasing increased intracranial pressure
8. Management of a 4 years old child scheduled for computerised tomographic scanning a brain using an iodine containing solution
9. Trigeminal neuralgia, clinical features and management
10. Regulation of cerebral blood flow
11. Regulation of intracranial tension
12. Hydrocephalus and its various methods of management
13. Preoperative evaluation of autonomic function
14. Horner's syndrome
15. Minimum monitoring for post spinal fusion in scoliosis
16. Anesthetic management of a patient with suspected posterior fossa tumor
17. Methods of monitoring of neuromuscular transmission during anesthesia
18. Methods of intracranial pressure (ICP) monitoring, uses and complication of ICP monitoring
19. Medical management of head injured patient
20. Describe the criteria and neurological test for brainstem death and preparing the patient for organ donation
21. What is cerebral protection. Explain the methods adopted in clinical practice for cerebral protection
22. Discuss the peri-operative management of cerebral AVM (arteriovenous malformation)
23. Anesthesia for electro convulsive therapy
24. Discuss the causes of delayed recovery from anesthesia and the management
25. Gullian-Barre Syndrome- Discuss briefly etiology, pathogenesis, symptomatology and management including anesthetic management
26. Intra operative problems of neurosurgical procedure under anesthesia in sitting position
27. Preoperative evaluation and anaesthetic considerations of a patient with Parkinsons disease
28. Compare and contrast TOF and double burst
29. What is bispectral index monitoring. What are its clinical applications in anesthesia practice
30. How is cerebral blood flow regulated? What is the affect of various anesthetic drugs in cerebral blood flow
31. Discuss the management of intracranial hypertension
32. Hypotensive anesthesia in neurosurgery
33. What are the anesthetic problems of cranio-facial surgery. Describe an appropriate anesthetic technique
34. Central anticholinergic syndrome
35. Myasthenia gravis vs myasthenic syndrome
36. Causes of perioperative seizures

OBSTETRIC ANESTHESIA

1. HELLP syndrome
2. Discuss the pathophysiological changes in pre-eclampsia and eclampsia. Discuss your choice of anesthetic technique for such a patient for emergency caesarean section
   a. A patient of coarctation of aorta is scheduled for caesarean section. Discuss the preoperative preparation, anesthetic management and postoperative care of the patient
3. Draw a neat labeled diagram of fetal circulation and delineate the differences from adult
4. Aspiration prophylaxis in obstetrics
5. Supine hypotension syndrome
6. Describe physiologic changes occurring during pregnancy and clinical implications to the anesthesiologist
7. Modern trends in obstetrical analgesia
8. Cardiopulmonary resuscitation in pregnant women
9. Anesthetic management of emergency appendicectomy in a 16 weeks pregnant patient
10. Problems and management of pregnant patient with dilated cardiomyopathy on treatment for emergency LSCS
11. Pre-anesthetic evaluation of a patient of mitral stenosis for medical termination of pregnancy (MTP) and sterilization
12. Role of anesthesiologist in an obstetric unit
13. Regional versus GA in obstetric surgery
14. Anesthesia for a pregnant woman for non-obstetric surgery
15. Laparoscopy surgery in a pregnant patient
16. Describe innervation of female genital tract with a diagram and discuss methods of producing painless labour

17. Discuss the preoperative evaluation and anesthetic management of a 30-year-old female patient who underwent mitral valve replacement 6 months ago and is now scheduled for medical termination of pregnancy (MTP) with laparoscopic sterilization
18. Anesthetic implications of fetal surgery
19. Techniques to prevent hypotension after spinal anesthesia in caesarean section
20. Draw a labeled diagram of fetal circulation. What are the circulatory changes that occur at birth
21. Amniotic fluid embolism
22. Neonatal resuscitation in labor room

ORTHO

1. Mechanism of reflex sympathetic dystrophy
2. Management of spinal injury
3. Post traumatic fat embolism
4. The Golden Hour
5. An 80-year-old male is posted for total hip replacement. Discuss the preoperative evaluation, preparation and anesthetic management of this case
6. Discuss the preoperative assessment and the method of anesthesia in patient with TM ankylosis for the release of ankylosis
7. Minimum monitoring for post-spinal fusion in scoliosis
8. Assessment of an adult who sustained multiple trauma of few hours duration
9. Indication and contra-indication for use of arterial tourniquet. What complication may arise from the use of such tourniquet
10. Problems encountered by anesthetists during the orthopedic operative procedures
11. Anesthetic problems of total hip replacement in elderly patients
12. Anesthetic problems in scoliosis surgery
13. An 86-year-old patient is scheduled for open reduction and internal fixation of subtrochanteric fracture of femur. Discuss the preoperative evaluation and anesthetic management of patient
14. What is triage. What are the triage criteria in relation to trauma
15. Discuss the anesthetic problems, preoperative preparation and anesthetic management of a case posted for correction of kyphoscoliosis

OTHERS

1. Discuss the anesthetic techniques and postoperative problems in an obese patient for large hernia of interior abdominal wall
2. Total intravenous anesthesia
3. Peripheral nerve injury under anesthesia
4. Describe airway management of a patient of anyklosing spondylitis with severe restriction of neck movement posted for total hip replacement
5. Obesity: anesthetic problems
6. Iatrogenic complications in anesthesia
7. Anesthesia for radiotherapy
8. Attenuation of laryngoscopic reaction to intubation
9. Etiology and management of hypotension during anesthesia
10. Enumerate various positions in relation to anesthesia and discuss in detail the problems associated with them
11. Monitored anesthesia care
12. Simulator in anesthesia education
13. Computer - based patient record for anesthesia
14. APACHE score (acute physiology and chronic health evaluation)
15. Discharge criteria in outpatient anesthesia (day-stay surgery)
16. Minimum patient monitoring during anesthesia
17. Operating room pollution
18. Problems and role of anesthetists in a dental anesthesia
19. Oxygen therapy
20. Write down the physiology of sleep. How does it differ from anesthesia? What phases occur in various stages of anesthesia?
21. Informed consent
22. Infections related to anesthetic practice
23. Role of anesthetist in multiple trauma
24. MRI and anesthesia
25. Prevention of fire and explosion hazards in operation theaters
26. Jugular venous oximetry
27. Discuss the regulation of body temperature. How will you prevent hypothermia in a neonate posted for major abdominal surgery
28. Recognition and management of anaphylaxis during general anesthesia
29. Methods of monitoring of neuromuscular transmission during anesthesia
30. Possible causes of delayed recovery from general anesthesia
31. Discuss in brief the problems of adult patient with Downs syndrome for multiple teeth extraction
32. Third space loss - its importance to anesthesiologist
33. Anaphylactic reaction on the operation table
34. Pre-emptive analgesia

35. Anesthetists role in pain and palliative care
36. Acute Pain Management Service
37. Anesthetic consideration for Magnetic Resonance Imaging (MRI)
38. Myasthenic Syndrome
39. Causes and management of post anesthesia shivering.
40. Enumerate risk factors for postoperative nausea and vomiting (PONV) and discuss its management
41. A 40-year-old man weighing 140 kg has diabetes and hypertension and is scheduled for gastric banding. Discuss the anesthetic management
42. American Society of Anesthesiologists (ASA) physical status classification
43. Anesthetic management for radio-diagnostic procedures
44. Evidence based medical education
45. Principle of ultrasonography. How is ultrasound useful in anesthesia
46. Indication of mediastinoscopy, anesthetic implication
47. HIV disinfection in operating room working
48. Computers in anesthesia
49. Operating room pollution
50. Impact of cancer therapy on anesthetic management
51. Preanesthetic assessment clinic
52. Vicarious liability for negligence.
53. Preoperative evaluation, preparation and anesthetic management of a known case of bronchial asthma posted for radical mastectomy
54. Postoperative hypoxemia- its causes, prophylaxis and management

PAIN

1. Patient controlled analgesia
2. Discuss the various methods of postoperative pain relief in pediatric surgery
3. World Health Organization regimen of chronic pain management
4. Postoperative analgesia in an infant for circumcision
5. The World Health Organisation-three-step ladder pattern for pain relief in advanced cancer
6. Postoperative analgesia in children for inguinal hernia
7. What are the various routes of administration of opioids? Discuss the merits and demerits of each
8. Assessment of pain in children
9. Preemptive analgesia
10. Discuss the principles, assessment and methods of analgesia for pain relief in burns
11. Acute pain relief in opioid dependent pain
12. Caudal epidural analgesia in anesthetic practice
13. Phantom limb pain
14. Pain management options in a patient with intractable pain due to carcinoma head of pancreas
15. Patient controlled analgesia (PCA) in anesthetic practice
16. Recent views of preemptive analgesia
17. Assessment of pain
18. Commonly used techniques and drugs for postoperative pain relief
19. Pain relief in fracture ribs
20. Define and classify chronic pain. Describe the methods of treatment of complex regional pain syndrome in left upper limb in a 20-year-old male patient

PEDIATRIC ANESTHESIA

1. Anesthetic management of a 2 days neonate for primary repair of tracheo-esophageal fistula
2. Postoperative analgesia in pediatric patients
3. Heat loss during abdominal surgery in a new born child
4. Postoperative analgesia in an infant for circumcision
5. Postoperative analgesia in children for inguinal hernia
6. Discuss the problems, preoperative preparation and anesthetic management of a neonate posted for repair of gastroschisis
7. Recent advances in intraoperative pediatric fluid management
8. Neonatal resuscitation
9. Role of regional analgesia in pediatric surgery
10. Describe the anatomy and physiology of various types of Tracheo-esophageal fistula. Discuss the anesthetic management
11. Anesthetic management of a 4-year-old with foreign body in right main bronchus. Discuss the problems.
12. Temperature regulation in neonate and prevention of hypothermia in neonate during peri operative period
13. Anesthetic problems of repair of congenital diaphragmatic hernia in a neonate.
14. Preoperative considerations in pediatric patients
15. 10 months old baby for hernia repair. Discuss anesthetic and postoperative pain management
16. Anesthetic implications in neonatal anesthesia
17. Discuss the anesthetic considerations in a neonate for repair of cervical meningomyelocele
18. Perioperative fluid requirement in small pediatric patients

19. Indications, technique and complications of spinal anesthesia in pediatric patient undergoing surgery
20. Fasting guidelines for children. How does premedication in adults differ from that in children
21. New guidelines for neonatal resuscitation.
22. Preoperative assessment and anesthetic management of a 2-year-old child of hydrocephalous posted for shunt procedure
23. Preanesthetic assessment and preparation of 1 day old neonate for trachea-esophageal fistula repair
24. Anesthetic management of congenital diaphragmatic hernia
25. Indication of caudal epidural in a pediatric patient, describe its technique and complications.
26. Anesthesia for bronchoscopy in children
27. Regional analgesia in children
28. How does the pediatric airway differ from that of an adult ? What are the implications for an anesthesiologist
29. Describe anesthetic management of a 6 month old child with hydrocephalus scheduled for MRI

PHARMACOLOGY

1. Hauffman degradation
2. Midazolam
3. Remifentanyl
4. Rocuronium
5. Role of Nitric Oxide in ICU
6. Role of magnesium in anesthesia practice
7. Narcotic antagonists
8. Beta receptor blockade its relationship in anesthesia
9. What are the various routes of administration of morphine. Discuss the pharmacokinetics and pharmacokinetics of epidural morphine
10. Nephrotoxicity of halogenated anesthetics
11. Propofol
12. Enzyme induction: Describe the mechanism with routine anesthesia examples
13. Mechanism of action of local anesthetic agents
14. Manifestations and treatment of beta adrenergic agonist toxicity
15. Sevoflurane
16. Untoward effects of intravenous sodium bicarbonate
17. Hepatotoxicity of halothane
18. Compare propofol with midazolam
19. Neuro-muscular transmission
20. Propofol as compared to thiopentone
21. Elimination of atracurium from the body
22. Sevoflurane vs. Desflurane
23. Rocuronium
24. Adenosine and its clinical uses
25. Ropivacaine
26. Isoflurane Vs. Sevuflurane
27. Human Albumin
28. Transdermal opioids
29. Effect of esmolol pretreatment on cardiovascular system, neuro-muscular junction and intraocular pressure
30. Mannitol in surgery
31. Pharmacokinetics of intravenous thiopentone
32. Clinical use of alpha 2 agonists in anesthesia
33. Enumerate the problems with the muscle relaxants
34. Adrenergic agonists
35. Drug interactions
36. Compare and contrast dopamine and dobutamine as an inotropic agents
37. What are the manifestations of hyponatremia and how will you treat it
38. Perioperative β-blocker therapy
39. Concentration effect and second gas effect produced during uptake of inhalation agent
40. Mention the commonly used immunosuppressive drugs and their interaction with anesthetic drugs
41. Clonidine in anesthesia practice
42. Lipid-emulsion for the treatment of local anesthetic toxicity-mechanism and dosage.
43. Nitrous oxide – current status
44. Adverse effects of neuromuscular blocking agents
45. Compare and contrast starch and gelatin as IV fluids
46. Discuss the ECG abnormalities due to various electrolyte abnormalities
47. What are the factors affecting neuromuscular blockage. Discuss various methods to monitor neuromuscular blockage
48. Transdermal administration of drugs
49. Dexmeditomidine, clinical application and complications
50. Rationale of premedication
51. Methods of prolonging effect of local anesthetics
52. Cardiovascular effects of newer anesthetic ethers
53. Adrenergic receptor antagonists and their uses
54. Classify antihypertensive drugs. Describe the management of hypertensive emergency

POST-OP ICU, CCU AND BLOOD

1. Complications and sequel of blood transfusion
2. Weaning modes of ventilation
3. Disseminated intra-vascular coagulation

4. Pressure controlled ventilation
5. Use of muscle relaxants in intensive care unit
6. Postoperative analgesia in pediatric patients
7. Present trend of blood component therapy
8. Newer modes of ventilation
9. Autologous blood transfusion
10. Hypokalemia
11. Crystalloid and colloid
12. Anesthesia for drainage of empyema thoracis
13. Total parenteral nutrition
14. Post anesthetic vomiting
15. Long term ventilation and its complications
16. Care of organophosphorous poisoning in intensive care unit
17. Perioperative blood conservation
18. Discuss the pathophysiology, preventive and corrective measures of irreversible shock
19. Airway management in an unconscious patient
20. Oxygen therapy in postoperative period
21. Uses, advantages and disadvantages of plasma expanders
22. Define multiple organ dysfunction syndrome. How do you plan to manage such a case
23. Control of nosocomial infections in postoperative and intensive care unit
24. How is the diagnosis of dilutional hyponatremia made? What is its significance in anesthesia
25. Disinfection
26. Principles of management of diabetic ketoacidosis
27. Management of mismatched blood transfusion
28. Septic shock
29. Autologous blood transfusion
30. Plasma volume expanders
31. Causes, diagnosis and treatment of hypo and hyperkalemia
32. Describe PEEP (Positive End Expiratory Pressure) its mechanism of action, uses and complications
33. The role of sedation in intensive care unit patients
34. Recent advances in cardio-pulmonary resuscitation
35. Artificial blood (synthetic oxygen carrying substances)
36. Discuss the management of an unconscious young patient with history of drowning
37. Discuss the management of a patient with snake bite
38. What are the criteria for the diagnosis of SIRS. Discuss the principles of management in a patient of septic shock admitted in ICU
39. What is autologous blood transfusion. Describe various techniques of autologous blood transfusion
40. Anion gap
41. Recombinant Factor VII
42. Discuss the management of massive blood loss
43. What is thromboelastography. Draw a labeled diagram to show a normal tracing. What are its implications
44. Enteral feeding in critically ill patients
45. Enumerate five Hs and five Ts as possible causes of cardiac arrest. What is the management of pulseless electrical activity in an unconscious patient
46. What is Triage. What are the triage criteria in relation to trauma
47. What are the common nosocomial infections in ICU. Discuss the measures for prevention of ventilatory associated pneumonias
48. Clinical features, diagnosis and management of paracetamol poisoning
49. Anemia and anesthesia
50. Coagulation of blood and management of hemophiliac patients
51. Physiological and biochemical changes of acute blood loss
52. How would you investigate the causes of increase bleeding during surgery. Give a brief account of various techniques employed to reduce bleeding
53. Blood substitutes
54. Postoperative hypoxemia- its causes, prophylaxis and management
55. Blood transfusion related disease transmission
56. How will you diagnose mismatched blood transfusion intraoperatively? Describe its management.
57. Enumerate the indications, contraindications and complications of invasive arterial blood pressure monitoring. Describe the technique
58. What are the major buffer systems in the body? Enumerate the causes, effects and management of metabolic acidosis

REGIONAL ANESTHESIA

1. Describe the nerve innervation of the foot with diagram and discuss the local anesthetic block at the ankle for the amputation of gangrenous toes in a patient
2. Pulmonary function changes following central neuraxial blockade
3. Continuous subarachnoid block
4. Intravenous regional anesthesia
5. Postdural puncture headache
6. Management of local anesthetic toxicity
7. Regional analgesia in children
8. Epidural analgesia for postoperative pain relief

9. Peribulbar block
10. Epidural pressure and the various factors affecting the same
11. Complications of local anesthetics
12. Three in one block
13. Pulmonary edema in intra operative and immediate postoperative period
14. Effect of intrathecal neostigmine on spinal anesthesia
15. Indications and methods of stellate ganglion block
16. Combined spinal epidural block
17. Caudal block
18. Modified combined spinal and epidural analgesia
19. Spinal anesthesia in children
20. Regional anesthesia in day care surgery
21. Describe the intrathecal and epidural opioids in clinical practice and their complications
22. Describe the nerve supply of foot and the technique of ankle block for amputation of great toe
23. Various epidural narcotics for management of post-operative pain
24. Indications, technique and complications of spinal anesthesia in pediatric patient undergoing surgery
25. Anatomy of epidural space and the methods of identification
26. Discuss one method brachial plexus block through supraclavicular approach and enumerate the complications associated with it
27. Describe anatomy of paraverteberal space and describe one method of establishing paraverteberal block
28. Describe with the help of labeled diagram the anatomy of lumbar plexus and describe the technique of lumbar plexus block
29. Enumerate the guidelines for regional anesthesia in a patient on anticoagulant/antiplatelet therapy
30. Describe the anatomy of celiac plexus. Describe indications and measures to block celiac plexus
31. Regional analgesia in children
32. IVRA technique and mode of action
33. Regional anesthesia techniques for upper extremity surgery.
34. Role of anesthesiologist in managing reflex sympathetic dystrophy
35. Complications of epidural anesthesia
36. Pain relief in fracture ribs
37. Innervation of foot and technique of performing ankle block
38. What is postdural puncture headache ? What are the factors affecting it? Describe the management of such a case

RESPIRATORY

1. Minimum alveolar concentration (MAC)
2. Pressure controlled ventilation
3. Functional residual capacity
4. The factors influencing tissue oxygenation
5. Risk and management of pulmonary aspiration
6. Describe airway management of a patient of ankylosing spondylitis with severe restriction of neck movement posted for total hip replacement
7. Problems and management in one lung anesthesia
8. Management of intra-operative bronchospasm
9. Oxygen therapy
10. Relevance of pulmonary function tests
11. Inverse ratio ventilation
12. Describe the pathogenesis and management of adult respiratory distress syndrome (ARDS)
13. Discuss the current concepts in the management of a case of chronic obstructive airway disease in respiratory failure
14. Closing volume of the lungs and its measurement.
15. Discuss the patho-physiology and management of inhalational injury
16. Tracheo-bronchial tree with diagram
17. Discuss anatomy of the diaphragm with a diagram. How does it behave under different stages of anesthesia
18. Physiological changes associated with IPPV
19. Vocal cord palsies with the aid of diagrams of direct laryngoscopic view
20. Acute lung injury
21. Describe the anatomy of larynx with difference in adult and children. What is importance of recurrent laryngeal nerve in anesthesia practice
22. Pulmonary edema in intraoperative and immediate postoperative period
23. Broncho-pleural fistula
24. Evaluation of difficult airway
25. Respiratory monitoring in anesthesia
26. Difficult intubation
27. Tracheostomy techniques and complications
28. High frequency ventilation
29. Discuss the preoperative assessment and the method of anesthesia in patient with TM ankylosis for the release of ankylosis
30. Hydropneumothorax
31. Predictive factors and intubation difficulty
32. Discuss the anesthetic management of a patient posted for pneumonectomy for carcinoma of right bronchus

33. Oxygen toxicity
34. Pressure support ventilation
35. Management of an adult with smoke inhalational injury
36. Oxygen cascade, oxygen transport and oxygen dissociation curve
37. List the bed side tests available to predict the difficult intubation. Comment on their use
38. Discuss the ventilatory management of ARDS (Adult Respiratory Distress Syndrome)
39. Anesthetic management of two years old child who is scheduled for therapeutic bronchoscopy following inhalation of foreign body 2 days ago child could not exhibit any sign of airway obstruction
40. Postoperative pulmonary complications
41. What are the causes of hypercarbia during the intra-operative period. Discuss the effects and management
42. Lung compliance
43. How will you anesthetize airway of a 40-year-old man for awake intubation
44. Discuss the management of cannot intubate and cannot ventilate situation in the operation theatre
45. What is low flow anesthesia ? Discuss its advantages and disadvantages
46. Oxygen dissociation curve
47. Laryngospasm during anesthesia
48. Noninvasive ventilation: advantages, disadvantages and methods of administration
49. Discuss briefly different modes used for neonatal ventilation.
50. Criteria for weaning from prolonged ventilation
51. Percutaneous dilatational tracheostomy
52. Discuss the pathophysiology and management of a case of carbon monoxide poisoning
53. Discuss the distribution of ventilation and perfusion in a normal lung with the help of labeled diagram. What are the factors affecting ventilation perfusion ratio
54. Enumerate predictors of weaning from mechanical ventilation
55. Hypoxic pulmonary vasoconstriction
56. Describe the techniques of chest physiotherapy. What is its role in post surgical period
57. Describe with diagram the flow volume loops
58. Permissive hypercapnia.
59. Methemoglobinemia and anesthesiologist
60. Pressure Support Ventilation
61. Prolonged use of ventilators
62. High frequency jet ventilation
63. Pulse oximetry in anesthetic practice
64. Oxygen cascade and oxygen flux
65. Modes of ventilation during bronchoscopy
66. Treatment of acute pulmonary edema
67. One lung anesthesia
68. CO_2 carriage in blood and effects of hypercapnia
69. A 40-year-old male with emphysematous bulla in right lung is scheduled for thoracoscopic (VATS) excision of bulla. Describe the anesthetic management
70. Describe the metabolic functions of lung